PROFESSIONAL GUIDE TO
Diseases

Eighth Edition

PROFESSIONAL GUIDE TO
Diseases

Eighth Edition

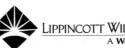

LIPPINCOTT WILLIAMS & WILKINS
A **Wolters Kluwer** Company

Philadelphia • Baltimore • New York • London
Buenos Aires • Hong Kong • Sydney • Tokyo

STAFF

Executive Publisher
Judith A. Schilling McCann, RN, MSN

Editorial Director
H. Nancy Holmes

Clinical Director
Joan M. Robinson, RN, MSN

Senior Art Director
Arlene Putterman

Editorial Project Manager
William Welsh

Editors
Scott Etkin, David P. Lenker,
Elizabeth Jacqueline Mills

Clinical Editor
Joanne M. Bartelmo, RN, MSN

Copy Editors
Kimberly Bilotta (supervisor), Scotti Cohn,
Amy Furman, Dona Perkins,
Carolyn Peterson, Irene Pontarelli,
Lisa Stockslager, Kelly Taylor,
Dorothy P. Terry, Pamela Wingrod

Designer
Linda Jovinelly Franklin (project manager)

Cover Illustration
Anatomical Chart Company

Digital Composition Services
Diane Paluba (manager), Joyce Rossi Biletz,
Donna S. Morris

Manufacturing
Patricia K. Dorshaw (director),
Beth J. Welsh

Editorial Assistants
Megan L. Aldinger, Tara L. Carter-Bell,
Karen J. Kirk, Linda K. Ruhf

Indexer
Barbara E. Hodgson

PGD8010205—020306

**Library of Congress
Cataloging-in-Publication Data**

Professional guide to diseases.— 8th ed.
    p. ; cm.
Includes bibliographical references and index.
    1. Clinical medicine—Handbooks, manuals, etc. 2. Diseases—Handbooks, manuals, etc. 3. Nursing—Handbooks, manuals, etc. I. Lippincott Williams & Wilkins.
    [DNLM: 1. Clinical Medicine—Handbooks. 2. Disease—Handbooks. WB 39 P964 2006]
    RT65.P69 2006
    616—dc22
ISBN 1-58255-370-X (alk. paper)   2004025162

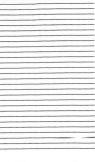

Contents

Contributors and consultants   *xi*
Foreword   *xiii*

1   **Genetic disorders**   **1**
Introduction *1*
Autosomal dominant inheritance *8*
Autosomal recessive inheritance *14*
X-linked inheritance *25*
Chromosomal abnormalities *31*
Multifactorial abnormalities *38*

2   **Malignant neoplasms**   **46**
Introduction *47*
Head, neck, and spine *56*
Thorax *72*
Abdomen and pelvis *82*
Male and female genitalia *103*
Bone, skin, and soft tissue *123*
Blood and lymph *138*

3   **Infection**   **151**
Introduction *152*
Gram-positive cocci *160*
Gram-negative cocci *176*
Gram-positive bacilli *178*
Gram-negative bacilli *187*
Spirochetes and mycobacteria *207*
Mycoses *213*
Respiratory viruses *222*
Rash-producing viruses *231*
Enteroviruses *243*
Arbovirus *246*
Miscellaneous viruses *247*
Rickettsia *257*
Protozoa *259*
Helminths *269*
Miscellaneous infections *277*

4   **Trauma**   **280**
Introduction *281*
Head *285*
Neck and spine *292*
Thorax *294*
Abdomen *299*
Extremities *301*
Whole body *308*
Miscellaneous injuries *323*

5   **Immune disorders**   **340**
Introduction *341*
Allergy *350*
Autoimmunity *364*
Immunodeficiency *389*

6   **Psychiatric disorders**   **406**
Introduction *407*
Disorders of infancy, childhood, and adolescence *414*
Substance-related disorders *426*
Psychotic disorders *439*
Mood disorders *449*
Anxiety disorders *459*
Somatoform disorders *471*
Dissociative disorders *479*
Eating disorders *490*
Sexual and gender identity disorders *495*

7   **Respiratory disorders**   **507**
Introduction *508*
Congenital and pediatric disorders *514*
Acute disorders *521*
Chronic disorders *553*
Pneumoconioses *565*

8   **Musculoskeletal disorders**   **570**
Introduction *571*
Congenital disorders *576*
Joints *583*
Bones *591*
Muscle and connective tissue *607*

9   Neurologic disorders   **616**
Introduction *617*
Congenital anomalies *626*
Paroxysmal disorders *637*
Brain and spinal cord disorders *642*
Neuromuscular disorders *668*
Cranial nerve disorders *674*
Pain disorders *680*

10   Gastrointestinal disorders   **682**
Introduction *683*
Mouth and esophagus *687*
Stomach, intestine, and pancreas *701*
Anorectum *736*

11   Hepatobiliary disorders   **747**
Introduction *747*
Liver disorders *752*
Gallbladder and duct disorders *765*

12   Renal and urologic disorders   **770**
Introduction *771*
Congenital anomalies *779*
Acute renal disorders *782*
Chronic renal disorders *795*
Lower urinary tract disorders *808*
Prostate and epididymis disorders *818*

13   Endocrine disorders   **824**
Introduction *824*
Pituitary gland *827*
Thyroid gland *834*
Parathyroid glands *844*
Adrenal glands *849*
Pancreatic and multiple disorders *863*

14   Metabolic and nutritional disorders   **869**
Introduction *870*
Nutritional imbalance *875*
Metabolic disorders *890*
Homeostatic imbalance *908*

15 Obstetric and gynecologic disorders   929
Introduction *930*
Gynecologic disorders *936*
Uterine bleeding disorders *951*
Disorders of pregnancy *956*
Abnormalities of parturition *974*
Postpartum disorders *979*
Hemolytic diseases of the neonate *984*

16 Sexual disorders   992
Introduction *992*
Sexually transmitted diseases *995*
Male reproductive disorders *1008*

17 Hematologic disorders   1015
Introduction *1015*
Anemias *1020*
Polycythemias *1035*
Hemorrhagic disorders *1040*
Miscellaneous disorders *1053*

18 Cardiovascular disorders   1057
Introduction *1058*
Congenital acyanotic defects *1064*
Congenital cyanotic defects *1072*
Acquired inflammatory heart disease *1077*
Valve disorders *1086*
Degenerative cardiovascular disorders *1091*
Cardiac complications *1115*
Vascular disorders *1134*

19 Eye disorders   1152
Introduction *1153*
Eyelid and lacrimal ducts *1157*
Conjunctival disorders *1164*
Corneal disorders *1168*
Uveal tract, retinal, and lens disorders *1172*
Miscellaneous disorders *1181*

20 Ear, nose, and throat disorders   1188
Introduction *1189*
External ear *1191*
Middle ear *1195*
Inner ear *1202*
Nose *1207*
Throat *1217*

21 **Skin disorders** **1227**
Introduction *1228*
Bacterial infections *1232*
Fungal infections *1237*
Parasitic infestations *1241*
Follicular and glandular disorders *1246*
Pigmentation disorders *1252*
Inflammatory reactions *1256*
Miscellaneous disorders *1262*

Appendices *1277*
Cultural considerations in patient care *1279*
Rare diseases *1282*
Community resources *1314*
Potential agents of bioterrorism *1318*
Acknowledgments *1320*
Index *1321*

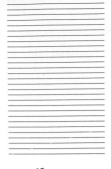

Contributors and consultants

Susan E. Antczak, RN, OCN
Clinical Instructor
Fox Chase Cancer Center
Philadelphia

Dorothy Borton, RN, BSN, CIC
Infection Control Practitioner
Albert Einstein Medical Center
Philadelphia

Cheryl L. Brady, RN, MSN
Adjunct Faculty
Mercy College of Northwest Ohio, St.
    Elizabeth Campus
Youngstown

Marissa Camanga-Reyes, RN, MN,
    CCRN, CNS
Clinical Nurse Specialist,
    Cardiopulmonary Critical Care
Harbor-University of California at Los
    Angeles Medical Center
Torrance

Shelba Durston, RN, MSN, CCRN
Nursing Instructor
San Joaquin Delta College
Stockton, Calif.
Staff Nurse
San Joaquin General Hospital
French Camp, Calif.

Carrin Dvorak, RN, MSN
Assistant Professor of Nursing
Cuyahoga Community College
Cleveland

Henry Geiter, RN, ADN, CCRN
Adjunct Instructor
St. Petersburg (Fla.) College
Critical Care Nurse
Bayfront Medical Center
St. Petersburg, Fla.
Critical Care Transport Nurse
Sunstar-AMR
Largo, Fla.

Julia Anne Isen, MS, FNP-C
Nurse Practitioner
Veterans' Administration Medical Center
San Francisco

Mary T. Kowalski, RN, BA, MSN
Professor, Nursing Educator
Cerro Coso Community College
Ridgecrest, Calif.

Carol T. Lemay, RN
Staff Nurse, Triage/Observation
University of Massachusetts
Amherst

Dawna Martich, RN, MSN
Trainer
American Healthways
Pittsburgh

Elizabeth Molle, RN, MS
Nurse Educator
Middlesex Hospital
Middletown, Conn.

E. Ann Myers, MD, FACE, FACP
Physician
Golden Gate Endocrine Associates
San Francisco

Richard O. Nenstiel, MBA, PA-C
Chairman, Department of Physician
  Assistant Studies
University of South Alabama
Mobile

Barbara L. Sauls, EdD, PA-C
Clinical Director, Physician Assistant
  Program
King's College
Wilkes-Barre, Pa.

**Janet Somlyay, Lt. Col (retired) U.S.
  Air Force,** RN, MSN, CNS, CPNP
Assistant Lecturer
University of Wyoming, Fay W. Whitney
  School of Nursing
Laramie

Dominique Alexis Thuriere, MD
Chief, Mental Health & Behavioral Sciences
Bay Pines (Fla.) Veterans' Administration
  Medical Center
Assistant Professor of Psychiatry
University of South Florida College of
  Medicine
Tampa

David Toub, MD, MBA, FACOG
Medical Director
Med Cases
Philadelphia

Daniel T. Vetrosky, MEd, PA-C, PhD(c)
Assistant Professor
University of South Alabama
Mobile

Robin Rider Wilkerson, RN, BC, PhD
Associate Professor
University of Mississippi School of Nursing
Jackson

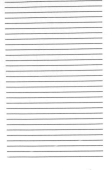

Foreword

The current state of medical economics hasn't been particularly kind to health care professionals. Budget restrictions, liability concerns, and the inflationary rise of health care costs are forcing professionals from all fields and specialties to take on more responsibility and more patients in increasingly tighter time constraints. The result is rushed, almost frenetic care that benefits no one—not you and certainly not your patients.

How can you integrate information on new innovations and research discoveries into your care when your other myriad responsibilities prevent you from learning about them? Yet, as a professional, you must ensure that your knowledge base is up-to-date. It's incumbent upon you to give your patients the best possible care—which is why it's imperative for you to have ready access to a reliable and contemporary medical guide. That guide needs to be current, easily accessible, and written in a format that has your busy schedule in mind.

Imagine how invaluable such a resource would be!

Well, imagine no more. This eighth edition of *Professional Guide to Diseases* fulfills these criteria by offering current clinical information in a format that's succinct yet entirely comprehensive. Its range of topics is impressive. The book thoroughly covers such common disorders as cancer, myocardial infarction, and Alzheimer's disease as well as such emerging diseases as West Nile encephalitis and severe acute respiratory syn-

drome. The book pays particular attention to disorders that continue to evolve, such as acquired immunodeficiency syndrome and lupus erythematosus.

The highly regarded team of clinical editors, contributors, and consultants who crafted this book made sure that each and every entry reflected the latest in disease assessment and management.

The book itself is organized into 21 chapters that each cover a specific disorder category, such as infection or trauma, and each chapter opens with an introduction that reviews pertinent disease physiology and pathophysiology. Next, each disease entry has a standardized format that quickly and efficiently provides readers with the exact information they're searching for, beginning with a concise definition and followed by a summary of etiological causes and incidence information. A description of signs and symptoms helps guide your history taking and physical examination. A section outlining the appropriate diagnostic tests and procedures shows you the path to take to reach a definitive diagnosis. A section on treatment outlines therapeutic and supportive interventions, such as medical and surgical modalities and pharmacotherapeutic regimens. A section on special considerations outlines important points to consider throughout the disease process, including supportive approaches to traditional medical interventions and patient comfort and self-care instructions.

Professional Guide to Diseases, Eighth Edition, makes excellent use of its supporting tables, graphics, algorithms, and medical illustrations. Each piece is well chosen and adds to the book's utility. Eye-catching graphic logos, such as *Alert, Confirming diagnosis, Elder tip,* and *Pediatric tip,* jump out from the text to ensure that you don't miss the valuable clinical points held within. A quick-reference guide to the management of life-threatening disorders that's found inside the front and back covers is especially useful.

Just like all the other books in the *Professional Guide* series, *Professional Guide to Diseases,* Eighth Edition, doesn't stop when the entries do. The book also features four quick-glance appendices, which include information on cultural considerations in patient care, rare diseases, community resources, and potential agents of bioterrorism. All are invaluable time-savers.

Professional Guide to Diseases, Eighth Edition, is a worthy addition to any medical library. I have no doubt that you'll benefit from its concise yet thorough approach to medical problem solving and treatment.

Howard Sachs, MD
Director, Adult Primary Care Clinic
Associate Professor of Clinical Medicine
University of Massachusetts Memorial
    Medical Center
Worcester

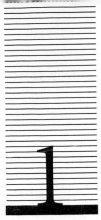

Genetic disorders

Introduction   *1*

Autosomal dominant inheritance   8
Neurofibromatosis   *8*
Osteogenesis imperfecta   *10*
Marfan syndrome   *11*
Stickler's syndrome   *13*

Autosomal recessive inheritance   14
Cystic fibrosis   *14*
Tay-Sachs disease   *17*
Phenylketonuria   *18*
Albinism   *20*
Sickle cell anemia   *21*

X-linked inheritance   25
Hemophilia   *25*
Fragile X syndrome   *29*

Chromosomal abnormalities   31
Down syndrome   *31*
Trisomy 18 syndrome   *33*
Trisomy 13 syndrome   *34*
Klinefelter's syndrome   *35*
Velocardiofacial syndrome   *37*

Multifactorial abnormalities   38
Neural tube defects   *38*
Cleft lip and cleft palate   *42*

Selected references   45

Introduction

Genetic diseases result from single-gene (Mendelian) alterations, chromosomal abnormalities, or multifactorial errors. Well over 6,000 such abnormalities have been identified in humans, ranging from mild differences (as in certain hemoglobin abnormalities) to fatal or overwhelmingly disabling conditions, such as trisomy 18 (Edwards') syndrome and trisomy 13 (Patau's) syndrome. The risk of single gene disorders is estimated at 1 in 200 births.

Although genetic disorders are determined primarily by genetic makeup, they can and do interact with environmental factors. For example, albinism (an inherited inability to generate the protective pigment melanin) greatly increases susceptibility to skin cancer after excessive exposure to sunlight.

Genetic analysis
Genetics, the study of heredity, analyzes defects in chromosomal reproduction or disease processes that can be passed from one generation to the next. It uses various tests to unravel the effects of altered genes and the patterns of inheritance. As heredity becomes better understood, genetic influences are likely to assume greater importance in health care delivery.

DNA AND HOW IT WORKS

Deoxyribonucleic acid (DNA) is a double-helix polymer (macromolecule) made up of individual units called nucleotides. Each nucleotide is composed of one sugar (deoxyribose), one phosphate, and one nitrogen-containing base—either a purine or a pyrimidine. The purine bases are adenine (A) and guanine (G). The pyrimidine bases are thymine (T) and cytosine (Q). The two polynucleotide chains of each DNA macromolecule are attached by hydrogen bonds between the bases (see illustration). The base pairing is very specific: adenine pairs only with thymine and cytosine pairs only with guanine. The DNA within the human genome (22 different autosomes and two different sex chromosomes) is made up of about 3 billion base pairs.

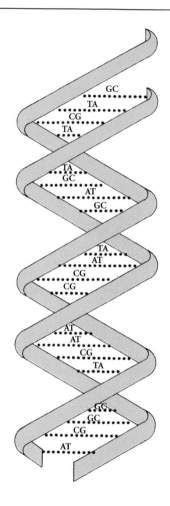

Genes make up approximately 10% of the human genome. A gene is a segment of DNA that ultimately determines the linear sequence of an amino acid chain. Through a complex process, a gene is transcribed into messenger ribonucleic acid (mRNA), which eventually is translated into an amino acid chain. A sequence of three mRNA nucleotides is called a codon. An mRNA codon can mark the beginning of translation, the end of translation, or a specific amino acid. Our genetic code is made up of 64 different codons, 61 of which actually code for amino acids. The eventual translated strand of amino acids must undergo further modification within the cell before it becomes a functional protein. The Human Genome Project is an international effort that officially began in 1990 and was completed in 2003 with the sequencing of the entire human genome. Emphasis is now on determining gene and protein function and how the environment influences these. With this information, treatment of genetic-based conditions is occurring at the molecular and cellular levels.

The essential ingredient of heredity is *deoxyribonucleic acid* (DNA), which makes up *genes,* basic units of hereditary material that are arranged into threadlike organelles called *chromosomes* in the cell nucleus. (See *DNA and how it works,* and *DNA replication.*) Together, these elements contribute to a person's genotype (gene composition) and phenotype (outward appearance). In humans, each body cell (except ova and sperm) has 46 chromosomes consisting of 22 pairs of autosomes and 1 pair of sex chromosomes. Females have a matched (homologous) pair of X sex chromosomes; males have an unmatched (heterologous) pair of sex chromosomes—an X and a Y.

Thus, the normal human chromosome complement is 46,XX in females and 46,XY in males. The 22 autosomes are all homologous. Each chromosome has a short arm (p) and a long arm (q) joined at the centromere.

The position that the gene for a given trait occupies on a chromosome is called a *locus*. Different loci exist for hair color, blood group, and so on. The number and arrangement of the loci on homologous chromosomes are the same. When the two genes are identical, the individual is homozygous at that locus. When the genes aren't identical, the individual is heterozygous at that locus. A different form of the same gene that occupies a corresponding locus on a homologous chromosome is called an *allele;* it determines alternative (and inheritable) forms of the same characteristic. Some alleles control normal trait variation such as hair color; other defective alleles may cause a congenital defect or even induce a spontaneous abortion. Both heterologous (codominant) alleles may express their own effects, or one (the dominant allele) may be expressed and the other (the recessive) suppressed.

A mutation is a permanent, inheritable change in a DNA sequence. When a mutation occurs in a gene's DNA sequence it may cause serious, even lethal defects, or it may be relatively benign. Mutations can occur spontaneously or can be caused by exposure to teratogenic agents, such as radiation, drugs, viruses, and synthetic chemicals.

Types of genetic disorders

Genetic disorders occur in several different forms. (See *Patterns of transmission in genetic disorders,* page 4.)

■ *Mendelian* or *single-gene disorders* are inherited in clearly identifiable patterns.
■ *Chromosomal aberrations or abnormalities* include structural defects within a chromosome, such as deletion and translocation, plus absence or addition of complete chromosomes.
■ *Multifactorial disorders* reflect the interaction of at least two abnormal genes and environmental factors to produce a defect.

DNA REPLICATION

The body grows and replaces all dividing cells other than germ cells (sperm and ova) by *mitosis*. In mitosis, the cell's deoxyribonucleic acid (DNA) replicates itself exactly and leads to the creation of a new daughter cell with the identical genetic makeup as the parent cell. Each new cell has a diploid number of chromosomes (in humans, 46).

Germ cells, however, form by *meiosis*. In meiosis, DNA first replicates. Then, through a complicated process, two cell divisions create four daughter cells (a sperm or ovum) from each parent cell, each of which has a haploid number of chromosomes (in humans, 23).

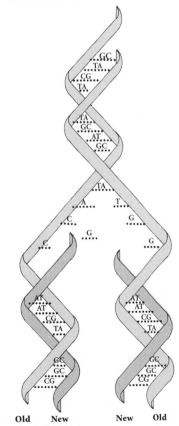

Old   New   New   Old

PATTERNS OF TRANSMISSION IN GENETIC DISORDERS

Autosomal dominant
Achondroplasia (dwarfism)
Colorectal polyposis
Hereditary hemorrhagic telangiectasia
Huntington's disease
Hyperlipidemias (some types)
Marfan syndrome
Neurofibromatosis (most cases)
Osteogenesis imperfecta (most cases)
Pituitary diabetes insipidus
Retinoblastoma
Spherocytosis

Autosomal recessive
Albinism (some cases)
Congenital adrenal hyperplasia
Cretinism
Cystic fibrosis
Cystinuria
Fabry's disease
Fanconi's anemia
Galactosemia
Niemann-Pick disease
Osteogenesis imperfecta (some cases)
Phenylketonuria
Retinitis pigmentosa (some cases)
Sickle cell anemia

Tay-Sachs disease
Thalassemia (alpha and beta)
Xeroderma pigmentosum (most cases)

X-linked
Duchenne type muscular dystrophy
Fragile X mental retardation
Glucose-6-phosphate dehydrogenase
deficiency
Hemophilia (most types)
Pseudohypoparathyroidism
Some immunodeficiencies

Chromosomal
Cri du chat syndrome
Down syndrome (trisomy 21)
Edwards' syndrome (trisomy 18)
Klinefelter's syndrome (XXY)
Patau's syndrome (trisomy 13)
Turner's syndrome (XO)

Multifactorial
Cleft lip or palate (some cases)
Congenital heart defects (some cases)
Diabetes mellitus (some cases)
Mental retardation (some cases)
Neural tube defects

Single-gene disorders

Single-gene disorders may be autosomal (resulting from a single altered gene or a pair of altered genes on one of the 22 pairs of autosomes) or X-linked (resulting from an altered gene on the X chromosome). Single-gene disorders may be further classified as dominant or recessive, depending on whether the altered gene is a dominant or a recessive allele.

Single-gene inheritance patterns

A dominant allele produces its effect in heterozygotes (people who also carry a normal gene for the same trait) because the dominant allele masks the effects of the normal paired gene *(autosomal dominant inheritance)*. Because a person with an autosomal dominant disease is usually a heterozygote and carries one dominant gene

as well as one normal gene, his children have a 50% chance of inheriting the dominant gene and the disease. This probability remains the same for each pregnancy. Unaffected people (homozygote for the normal gene) don't carry the altered gene and therefore can't transmit it, except as a new mutation. (See *Inheritance patterns.*)

Sex doesn't influence transmission of an autosomal dominant allele. However, in some autosomal dominant diseases (such as Huntington's disease) the severity of symptoms can vary in offspring, depending on which parent transmits the dominant allele. Unless the dominant allele has arisen as a new mutation or is nonpenetrant in an individual, every affected person has an affected parent. Thus, autosomal dominant traits don't skip generations. However, the severity of symptoms can range from very mild to severe among persons who inherit the allele. This variation of severity is known as *expressivity.*

Because a recessive allele can produce a disorder only when paired with another disease-causing allele *(autosomal recessive inheritance)*, offspring must receive one copy of the disease causing allele from each parent to inherit the recessive trait. A carrier has a diseased gene, but is phenotypically normal. Autosomal recessive disorders affect males and females equally. Because both parents must be heterozygous carriers, autosomal recessive disorders are more common in children of consanguineous parents (blood relatives).

In *X-linked recessive inheritance,* nearly all affected persons are males because females have two X chromosomes and males have an X and a Y chromosome. There's very little DNA sequence in common between the X and the Y chromosomes. Therefore, recessive alleles on a male's X chromosome are expressed. Females who carry a disease-causing recessive allele on only one X chromosome are usually unaffected because they have two X chromosomes—one with the disease-causing allele and one with the normal dominant allele. However, every cell in the female, except the oocytes, undergoes a normal process called X inactivation where one X chromosome is turned off. This process is random. Therefore, females who carry only one copy of a disease-causing allele may have mild symptoms if a disproportionate number of cells have the X chromosome with the disease-causing allele turned on and the X chromosome with the normal allele turned off.

In *X-linked dominant inheritance,* which is rare, females are affected to varying degrees. These disorders tend to be lethal in males. A family history of multiple male miscarriages or stillbirths is usually a clue to an X-linked dominant disorder.

Sex does influence transmission of X-linked alleles. An affected male transmit's the disease-causing allele to all of his female offspring, but to none of his male offspring. This is because males have only one X chromosome. When a sperm containing an X chromosome joins an ovum (which can only have an X chromosome), a female

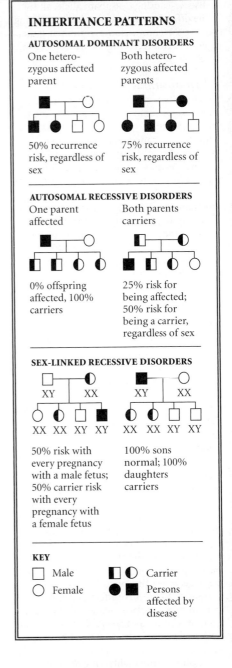

INHERITANCE PATTERNS

AUTOSOMAL DOMINANT DISORDERS

One hetero-zygous affected parent

Both hetero-zygous affected parents

50% recurrence risk, regardless of sex

75% recurrence risk, regardless of sex

AUTOSOMAL RECESSIVE DISORDERS

One parent affected

Both parents carriers

0% offspring affected, 100% carriers

25% risk for being affected; 50% risk for being a carrier, regardless of sex

SEX-LINKED RECESSIVE DISORDERS

XY	XX

| XX | XX | XY | XY |

XY	XX

| XX | XX | XY | XY |

50% risk with every pregnancy with a male fetus; 50% carrier risk with every pregnancy with a female fetus

100% sons normal; 100% daughters carriers

KEY

☐ Male   ◨ ◖ Carrier

◯ Female   ● ■ Persons affected by disease

offspring results. When the X chromosome contains a disease-causing recessive allele, female offspring are typically unaffected carriers. When the X chromosome contains a disease-causing dominant allele, all female offspring are affected. Male offspring receive a Y chromosome from their father, therefore not receiving the disease-causing allele.

Chromosomal abnormalities

During germ cell formation by meiosis, failure of chromosomes to divide *(nondisjunction)* results in a germ cell that contains fewer or more than the normal 23 pairs of chromosomes. Usually, such abnormal germ cells fail to unite at conception; if fertilization does take place, the embryo is usually miscarried early in the pregnancy. Experts believe that up to 60% of spontaneous abortions at less than 90 days' gestation result from an abnormal number of fetal chromosomes; offspring with some chromosomal abnormalities are probably never even implanted. Absence of an autosomal chromosome is incompatible with life, but absence of a sex chromosome, as in Turner's syndrome, is better tolerated. The presence of an extra chromosome *(trisomy)*, as in Down syndrome, commonly produces physical malformation, mental retardation, or both.

Chromosomal disorders may also result from structural changes within chromosomes. For instance, in *deletion,* loss of part of a chromosome during cell division produces varying effects in the offspring, depending on the type and amount of genetic material lost. An example is velocardiofacial syndrome, in which part of the long arm of chromosome 22 is missing.

In *translocation,* part of a chromosome attaches itself to another chromosome. If little or no genetic material is lost, the translocation is balanced (symmetrical) and the person displays no effects but may have reproductive problems, such as miscarriage, infertility, or children with malformations, cognitive effects, or both. The person may produce unaffected children, each of whom has a 50% chance of being a balanced translocation carrier, like the parent.

Another abnormality, *ring chromosomes,* results when a chromosome loses a section of genetic material from each end and the remaining stumps join together to form a ring. The effect varies, depending on the type of genetic material lost and on the specific chromosome that's involved.

In *mosaicism,* abnormal chromosomal division in the zygote results in two or more cell lines with different chromosomes. (One cell line may be normal and the other abnormal.) The patient's phenotype depends on the percentage of normal cells and on the varying effects of the abnormal cell line, which depend on the percentage of abnormal cells in each type of tissue.

Originally, Gregory Mendel's theories of heredity pointed to the understanding that an individual's phenotype is the same no matter which parent donates the allele. Now, it's known that this isn't always true. When a deletion on 15q11-13 is inherited from the father, the child will have Prader-Willi syndrome (obesity, short structure, hypogonadism). If the deletion is inherited from the mother, the child will have Angelman's syndrome (mental retardation, no verbal language, seizures). This indicates that different genes are active on chromosome 15 depending on which parent provided the chromosome.

Multifactorial disorders

Multifactorial disorders are abnormalities that result from the interaction of at least two inherited abnormal genes and environmental factors. They include common malformations, such as neural tube defects, cleft lip, and cleft palate, as well as disorders that may not appear until later in life such as diabetes mellitus. Such disorders don't follow the Mendelian patterns of inheritance, but the increased incidence of specific birth defects within families suggests familial transmission.

Detecting genetic disorders

Genetic testing and counseling can help prevent genetic disorders and help patients and their families deal with them when they do develop. Genetic diagnosis relies primarily on pedigree (family tree) analysis, karyotype (chromosomal) analysis, and biochemical analysis of blood, urine, or body tissues (including tissues obtained by amniocentesis or chorionic villus sampling [CVS]) to detect abnormal gene products. Neonatal screening for inherited metabolic disorders such as phenylketon uria has become standard, and prompt treatment of such disorders can prevent or minimize their effects.

Simple blood tests can detect carriers of recessive-gene disorders, such as Tay-Sachs disease and sickle cell anemia. DNA testing can detect some autosomal recessive, autosomal dominant, and X-linked recessive disorders. This gives a couple at risk the option of prenatal diagnosis (by amniocentesis or possibly CVS) for some disorders, to detect affected offspring.

A *pedigree*, a diagram of family relationships and diseases and cause of death of individual family members, helps determine a disorder's inheritance pattern, including the probability of occurrence. The pedigree chart begins with the patient (proband, or index case) and traces all living and deceased blood relatives in order of their birth, listing:
- current age or age at death
- health status of all relatives, including miscarriages and stillbirths (and the reasons for them), the site and nature of congenital anomalies, and the presence of mental and growth retardation
- relationships (if the patient is a twin, involved in a consanguineous marriage, or divorced).

This information can be obtained from the patient's memory, autopsy and pathology reports, photographs, and medical records. The pedigree chart is analyzed in relation to the clinical features of the suspected genetic disorder and appropriate laboratory tests or medical records. In one such test, the *karyotype,* white blood cells obtained from a venous blood sample are grown in a special culture until a specific stage of mitosis, when chromosomes are most easily seen with a microscope. Then the cells are broken open and stained to show specific bands on the chromosomes. Staining techniques can be varied to help identify each chromosome and the bands it contains.

Amniocentesis, needle aspiration of amniotic fluid after transabdominal puncture of the uterus under ultrasound guidance, can now detect over 600 genetic disorders before birth by:
- karyotyping cultured amniocytes

- using a special technique called fluorescent in situ hybridization on cultured amniocytes to detect submicroscopic chromosome deletions, duplications, or translocations
- measuring enzyme levels or activity on cultured amniocytes
- performing DNA mutation or linkage analysis on cultured amniocytes
- measuring proteins (for example, alpha-fetoprotein) or biochemical substrates in amniotic fluid.

Amniocentesis allows parents to make informed decisions for a pregnancy before the birth of a child with a genetic disorder. It's recommended to patients with:
- maternal age over 34 at delivery
- family history of chromosomal abnormalities
- history of previous children or a first- or second-degree relative with an open or closed neural tube defect or scoliosis with spinal dysraphism
- history of multiple reproductive losses
- parents who are known carriers of a genetic disorder that's detectable by biochemical or DNA testing.

The benefits of amniocentesis must be carefully weighed against the potential complications, which may include amniotic fluid leakage, miscarriage, and (rarely) infection. The risk of complications is estimated to be 0.5% (1 in 200) or less. Genetic counseling is done to help the patient and family weigh the risks against the benefits so they can make an informed decision about testing. For some patients, CVS, another method of collecting genetic information from the fetus, may be an alternative. Using a vaginal or abdominal approach, with ultrasound as a guide, the physician collects a small amount of chorionic tissue, which is then analyzed in much the same way as the amniocentesis. Biochemical tests that are typically done on amniotic fluid can't be done on CVS tissue.

Researchers are currently studying new methods of earlier prenatal diagnosis, such as amniocyte filtration and karyotyping of fetal cells in maternal blood.

Prenatal diagnosis may be considered even when a couple would continue an affected pregnancy because knowing the diagnosis ahead of time can help the health care team provide the optimal timing and method of delivery, thus improving the neonate's outcome. It also gives the couple more time to look into financial, educational, and psychological support services to prepare for the birth of a child with special needs.

Health care providers may recommend genetic testing for selected children and adolescents; it's indicated for prevention, decreasing the need for surveillance, and examining treatment availability.

Helping the family cope

Genetic counseling helps a family to understand its risk for a particular genetic disorder and to cope with the disorder if that risk becomes reality. Counseling sessions make it easier for the family to comprehend:
- medical facts (diagnosis, prognosis, treatment)
- how heredity works (risks to other relatives)
- options for dealing with the problem
- consequences of their decision.

Psychological support to relieve stress and improve the child's or parents' self-concept is as important as obtaining the correct information. The birth of a child with a genetic defect may provoke parental feelings of guilt, anxiety, isolation, insecurity, and helplessness and may place undue stress on all members of the family. Family members may experience a period of shock and denial, followed by grief and mourning. Following acceptance of the diagnosis, parents may continue to experience periods of denial; guilt; and chronic sorrow, a phenomenon that manifests as episodes of sadness, particularly around developmental milestones. These feelings are a normal response to having a child with a disability.

When testing confirms a genetic disorder, here's how you can provide psychological support:
- Refer the family for genetic counseling. The following organizations can be contacted to obtain a list of qualified health professionals throughout the United States who can provide genetic evaluation, diagnosis, counseling, and management services:
– American College of Medical Genetics
– International Society of Nurses in Genetics
– March of Dimes Birth Defects Foundation
– National Society of Genetic Counselors.
- Find out the services that are offered by the counseling center so you can tell the family what to expect.
- Provide the genetic professional with pertinent medical records and information about the family's special concerns, such as religious beliefs and social preferences.
- After counseling sessions, make sure family members understand the new information presented to them, and reinforce the information provided. Communicate with them in an unhurried and nontechnical manner, and make sure your facts are accurate.
- Inform the family about community resources, agencies, and available support groups to help them deal with genetic disorders. If they're interested, help them get in touch with the families of other patients with the same disorder. The Alliance of Genetic Support Groups or the National Organization for Rare Disorders are valuable resources for locating support groups and parent networking opportunities.
- Coordinate the assistance needed from other members of the health care team, such as physicians, psychologists, and social workers.
- Recognize the parents' stresses in caring for their child, and allow them to express their feelings.

AUTOSOMAL DOMINANT INHERITANCE

Neurofibromatosis

Neurofibromatosis is a group of inherited developmental disorders of the nervous system, muscles, bones, and skin that causes formation of multiple, pedunculated, soft tumors (neurofibromas), and café-au-lait spots. The most common types are

NF-1 (von Recklinghausen disease) and NF-2 (bilateral acoustic neurofibromatosis). About 80,000 Americans are known to have neurofibromatosis; in many others, the disorder is overlooked because symptoms are mild. The prognosis varies; however, spinal or intracranial tumors can shorten the patient's life span.

Causes and incidence
NF-1 is an autosomal dominant disorder of chromosome 17 that occurs in about 1 in 3,000 births. Approximately 50% of affected families have a negative family history; in many of these families, the father is older, suggesting that advanced paternal age may influence the NF-1 mutation. NF-2 is an autosomal dominant disorder of chromosome 22; however, many patients have a negative family history.

Signs and symptoms
Signs and symptoms of NF-1 vary greatly from one family to another and within members of the same family. A patient with seemingly mild symptoms initially may develop more severe problems later.

An infant with this form may present with only café-au-lait spots or may also have congenital glaucoma, plexiform neurofibromas, or pseudoarthrosis. About 90% of patients have Lisch nodules on the iris; as many as 15% develop optic pathway gliomas, which may cause a significant loss of vision.

Cutaneous and other neurofibromas may begin to develop or become more prominent at puberty; pregnancy may exacerbate tumor growth. Some tumors become malignant; approximately 8% of patients develop neurofibrosarcoma (cancer of the nerve sheath). Other less-specific features may include other types of tumors (such as meningiomas), short stature, seizures, speech and learning disabilities, mental retardation (occasionally), and abnormalities of the cerebral, GI, and renal arteries.

The first sign of NF-2 is usually a central nervous system tumor, such as a spinal or intracranial meningioma, an acoustic neuroma, and occasionally a schwannoma or spinal astrocytoma. Cutaneous neurofibromas may be less conspicuous in this form,

and café-au-lait spots may be minimal or even absent. Learning disabilities and other less-specific features characteristic of NF-1 aren't typically seen in NF-2.

Diagnosis
Diagnosis rests on typical clinical findings, especially neurofibromas and café-au-lait spots. Diagnostic criteria for NF-1 include two or more of the following:
- first-degree relative (parent, sibling, child) with known NF-1
- six or more café-au-lait spots over 5 mm in diameter in a prepubertal patient and 15 mm or more in a postpubertal patient
- freckling in the axillary or inguinal region
- optic pathway glioma
- two or more Lisch nodules on the iris
- osseous lesion, such as sphenoid dysplasia or thinning long-bone cortex.

Diagnostic criteria for NF-2 include a first-degree relative with NF-2 and two of the following:
- neurofibroma, meningioma, schwannoma, glioma, juvenile posterior subcapsular lenticular opacity
- unilateral eighth nerve mass
- bilateral eighth nerve masses seen on magnetic resonance imaging (MRI) or computed tomography (CT) scan.

X-rays, MRI, and CT scan may be indicated to determine the presence of widening internal auditory meatus and intervertebral foramen. An eye examination to look for Lisch nodules should be done on patients suspected of having NF-1. Myelography may be used to identify spinal cord tumors, and lumbar puncture with cerebrospinal fluid analysis will reveal elevated protein concentration in the presence of spinal neurofibromas and acoustic tumors. Deoxyribonucleic acid analysis and prenatal diagnosis may also be done in some families.

Treatment
Neurofibromatosis has no specific treatment. Management consists of surgical removal of intracerebral or intraspinal tumors (when possible) and correction of kyphoscoliosis. Tumors that cause pain and loss of function are removed on an individual basis.

ALERT *Tumors that grow rapidly should be removed promptly because they may become malignant.*

Cosmetic surgery for disfiguring or disabling growths may be done; however, regrowth is likely. Special schooling for individuals with learning disorders or attention deficit hyperactivity disorder may be required. Annual eye exams should be performed.

Researchers are currently investigating experimental treatments for severe tumors.

Special considerations

■ Disfigurement may cause overwhelming embarrassment and social regression. By showing acceptance, you can help the patient adjust to his condition.
■ Advise the patient to choose attractive clothing that covers unsightly nodules; suggest special cosmetics to cover skin lesions.
■ Refer the patient for genetic counseling to discuss the 50% risk of transmitting this disorder to offspring. Recommend contacting the National Neurofibromatosis Foundation.

Osteogenesis imperfecta

Osteogenesis imperfecta (brittle bones) is a hereditary disease of bones and connective tissue that may cause varying degrees of skeletal fragility, thin skin, blue sclerae, poor teeth, hypermobility of joints, and progressive deafness. This disease occurs in many forms. In the rare congenital form, fractures are present at birth. This form is usually fatal within the first few days or weeks of life. In the late-appearing form, the child appears normal at birth but develops recurring fractures (mostly of the extremities) after the first year of life.

Causes and incidence

Osteogenesis imperfecta can result from autosomal dominant inheritance of a defect in the amount of Type I collagen, an important part of the bone matrix. Clinical signs may result from defective osteoblastic activity and a defect of mesenchymal collagen (embryonic connective tissue) and its derivatives (sclerae, bones, and ligaments). The reticulum fails to differentiate into mature collagen or causes abnormal collagen development, leading to immature and coarse bone formation. Cortical bone thinning also occurs.

Type I, the most common form of osteogenesis imperfecta, occurs in about 1 in 30,000 live births. Both types I and IV are thought to be inherited as an autosomal dominant trait. Types II and III are believed to be inherited as an autosomal recessive trait.

Signs and symptoms

Clinical severity varies, depending on the type. In type I, fractures characteristically occur from minimal trauma. The sclerae are a deep blue-black color, and the teeth may be yellow or even grayish blue from opalescent dentin. Patients with dental abnormalities are shorter and have more fractures at birth, more frequent fractures, and more severe skeletal deformities than type I patients with normal teeth.

Bowing of the lower limbs is common in this type, as is kyphosis in adults. Approximately 40% of all adults with type I have severely impaired hearing, and virtually all adults have some degree of hearing impairment by age 50. The number of fractures may spontaneously decrease in adolescence.

Type II is characterized by intrauterine fractures due to extreme bone fragility, leading to intrauterine or early infant death. Death usually results from complications of bone fragility, heart failure, pulmonary hypertension, or respiratory failure. Therapeutic intervention doesn't usually increase survival.

Type III is generally nonlethal. Fractures are usually present at birth and occur frequently in childhood; they typically lead to progressive skeletal deformity and, eventually, impaired mobility. Patients have a poor growth rate; most fall below the third percentile in height for their age. Their sclerae are usually normal or light blue, and their teeth aren't usually opalescent.

Type IV is characterized by osteoporosis, which leads to increased bone fragility. The sclerae may be light blue at birth but appear normal in adolescents and adults. Bowed limbs may be present at birth, but only 25% of patients have fractures at birth. The number of fractures may decrease spontaneously at puberty, but the majority of patients are short. A few have a skull deformity.

Diagnosis

Family history and characteristic features, such as blue sclerae or deafness, establish the diagnosis. Whenever possible, collagen biochemical studies of cultured skin fibroblasts should be performed. Prenatal diagnosis may be available for certain families with an identified mutation. Prenatal ultrasound performed as early as 16 weeks may show evidence of severe osteogenesis imperfecta. X-rays showing evidence of multiple old fractures and skeletal deformities and a skull X-ray showing wide sutures with small, irregularly shaped islands of bone (wormian bones) between them support the diagnosis. These findings can help differentiate osteogenesis imperfecta from child abuse or from other disorders such as juvenile idiopathic osteoporosis.

In a family with a history of type II osteogenesis imperfecta, diagnostic serial ultrasound should be considered for future pregnancies to detect limb shortening, in utero fractures, and polyhydramnios.

Treatment

Treatment aims to prevent deformities by traction, immobilization, or both and to aid normal development and rehabilitation. Fractures must be repaired quickly to avoid deformities. Surgical procedures such as inserting metal rods through bones can help strengthen bones and prevent deformity. The use of bisphosphonates in children with osteogenesis imperfecta is being researched, as are growth hormone and gene therapies. Other medical interventions include bone marrow transplant. Supportive measures include:
- checking the patient's circulatory, motor, and sensory abilities
- encouraging the patient to walk when possible (children with osteogenesis imperfecta develop a fear of walking)
- teaching preventive measures, such as avoiding contact sports or strenuous activities or wearing knee pads, helmets, or other protective devices when engaging in sports
- assessing for and treating scoliosis, a common complication
- promoting preventive dental care and repair of dental caries.

Special considerations

- Educate the family about the disorder. Teach the parents and child how to recognize fractures and how to correctly splint them. Also teach the parents how to protect the child during diapering, dressing, and other activities of daily living.
- Advise the parents to encourage their child to develop interests that don't require strenuous physical activity and to develop his fine motor skills. These actions will promote the child's self-esteem.
- Advise the parents that physical and rehabilitation therapy is beneficial. Swimming is an excellent conditioning exercise.
- Teach the child to assume some responsibility for precautions during physical activity to help foster his independence.
- Stress the importance of good nutrition to heal bones and optimize muscle strength.
- Refer the parents and child for genetic counseling to assess the recurrence risk.
- Administer analgesics, as ordered, to relieve pain from frequent fractures, a hallmark of this disease.
- Monitor dental and hearing needs. Stress the need for regular dental care and immunizations.
- Instruct the parents to provide a medical identification bracelet for the child.

Marfan syndrome

Marfan syndrome is a rare, inherited, degenerative, generalized disease of the connective tissue that causes ocular, skeletal, and cardiovascular anomalies. It probably results from elastin and collagen abnormalities. Death is usually attributed to cardiovascular complications and may occur any time from early infancy to adulthood, depending on the severity of the symptoms. Marfan syndrome affects males and females equally.

Causes

Marfan syndrome is inherited as an autosomal dominant trait of chromosome 15. It's caused by mutations in gene fibrillin-1, producing changes in elastic tissues, especially of the aorta, eye, and skin. Mutations of fibrillin-1 also cause overgrowth of long bones. In 85% of patients with this disease, the family history confirms Marfan syndrome in one parent as well. In the remaining 15%, a negative family history suggests a fresh mutation, possibly from advanced paternal age.

Signs and symptoms

The most common signs and symptoms of this disorder are skeletal abnormalities, particularly excessively long tubular bones and an arm span that exceeds the patient's height. The patient is usually taller than average for his family (in the 95th percentile for his age), with the upper half of his body shorter than average and the lower half, longer. His fingers are long and slender (arachnodactyly). Weakness of ligaments, tendons, and joint capsules results in joints that are loose, hyperextensible, and habitually dislocated. Excessive growth of the rib bones gives rise to chest deformities such as pectus excavatum (funnel chest).

Eye problems are also common; 75% of patients have crystalline lens displacement (ectopia lentis), the ocular hallmark of Marfan syndrome. Quivering of the iris with eye movement (iridodonesis) typically suggests this disorder. Most patients are severely myopic, many have retinal detachment, and some have glaucoma.

The most serious complications occur in the cardiovascular system and include weakness of the aortic media, which leads to progressive dilation or dissecting aneurysm of the ascending aorta. Such dilation appears first in the coronary sinuses and is commonly preceded by aortic insufficiency. Less-common cardiovascular complications include mitral valve prolapse and endocarditis.

Other associated problems include sparsity of subcutaneous fat, frequent hernias, cystic lung disease, recurrent spontaneous pneumothorax, and scoliosis or kyphosis.

Diagnosis

Because no specific test confirms Marfan syndrome, diagnosis is based on typical clinical features (particularly skeletal deformities and ectopia lentis) and a history of the disease in close relatives. Useful supplementary procedures, though not definitive for diagnosis, include X-rays for skeletal abnormalities and an echocardiogram to detect aortic root dilation.

Treatment

Attempts to stop the degenerative process have met with little success. Therefore, treatment of Marfan syndrome is basically aimed at relieving symptoms — for example, surgical repair of aneurysms and ocular deformities. In young patients with early dilation of the aorta, prompt treatment with beta-adrenergic blockers may decrease ventricular ejection and protect the aorta; extreme dilation requires surgical replacement of the aorta and the aortic valve. Steroids and sex hormones have been successful (especially in girls) in inducing precocious puberty and early epiphyseal closure to prevent abnormal adult height. Genetic counseling is important, particularly because pregnancy and resultant increased cardiovascular workload can produce aortic rupture.

Special considerations

- High school and college athletes (particularly basketball players) who fit the criteria for Marfan syndrome should undergo a careful clinical and cardiac examination before being allowed to play, to avoid sudden death due to dissecting aortic aneurysm or other cardiac complications.
- Provide the patient with supportive care, as appropriate for his clinical status.
- Educate the patient and his family about the course of the disease and its potential complications.
- Stress the need for frequent checkups to detect and treat degenerative changes early.
- Emphasize the importance of taking prescribed medications as ordered and of avoiding contact sports and isometric exercise.

 PEDIATRIC TIP *To encourage normal adolescent development, advise the parents to avoid unrealistic ex-*

pectations for their child simply because he's tall and looks older than his years.

■ Refer the patient and family to the National Marfan Foundation for additional information.

Stickler's syndrome

Stickler's syndrome (arthro-ophthalmopathy) is an autosomal dominant chondrodysplasia caused by structural defects in collagen. It's characterized by ocular, skeletal, auditory, and craniofacial abnormalities. Expression of clinical features is highly variable from one individual to another.

Causes and incidence

At least 19 different types of collagen have been identified. Collagen is an essential component of connective tissues. The collagen defect in most families with Stickler's syndrome is caused by a mutation in the type II collagen gene (COL2AI) located on chromosome l2q13. Other families demonstrate linkage to the COLIIA2 gene located on chromosome 6p2l.3 and others to the COLIJAI gene located on chromosome lp2l. COL2AI and COLIJA I are expressed in the hyaline cartilage, vitreous, intervertebral disc, and inner ear. COLIIA2 isn't expressed in the vitreous. Genetic studies have identified a few families who carry the clinical diagnosis of Stickler's syndrome yet don't demonstrate linkage to any of the three aforementioned collagen genes, suggesting further genetic heterogeneity (a pattern of traits caused by genetic factors in some cases and nongenetic factors in others).

Approximately 1 in 10,000 people is affected with Stickler's syndrome. However, this incidence rate is considered conservative because persons with very mild symptoms may never be diagnosed with the syndrome.

Signs and symptoms

The clinical phenotype can consist of ocular, auditory, craniofacial, and skeletal abnormalities. The number of organ systems involved and the specific phenotypic features expressed can vary significantly between affected family members and, in particular, between unrelated affected persons.

Ocular symptoms, particularly high myopia, are common in persons with Stickler's syndrome, with the exception of those who have COLIJA2 mutations. Vitreal abnormalities are considered a hallmark of Stickler's syndrome, although the abnormalities in the vitreous differ in persons with a COL2AI mutation from those with a COLIIAI mutation. Retinal detachment resulting in blindness is the most serious ocular complication.

The vitreoretinal degeneration that leads to retinal detachment is much more common in persons with a COL2AI mutation. Persons with Stickler's syndrome can also have congenital cataracts and develop glaucoma. Ocular symptoms are typically absent in persons with linkage to COLIJA2.

Auditory symptoms include conductive hearing loss secondary to Eustachian tube dysfunction in children with cleft palate or collagen defects in the inner ear apparatus. Sensorineural hearing loss has an earlier onset and tends to be more progressive in persons with a COLIJAI mutation.

Craniofacial features may include micrognathia (small lower jaw) and a flattened midface and nasal bridge. Micrognathia may be associated with some degree of cleft palate (bifid uvula to complete cleft of the palate). Micrognathia associated with glossoptosis places neonates and infants with Stickler's syndrome at significant risk for episodic obstructive apnea during feeding and when lying flat.

Skeletal symptoms can include joint hypermobility in young children, spondyloepiphyseal dysplasia, and, later, degenerative arthropathy during early adult years. Also related to the collagen defect, scoliosis and mitral valve prolapse can develop in some persons with Stickler's syndrome.

Diagnosis

Diagnosis is based on the recognition of clinical features consistent with Stickler's syndrome. The number of genes involved in Stickler's syndrome and the complexity of sequencing large genes currently preclude the clinical utility of routine genetic testing for diagnostic purposes. Therefore, diagnosis must rely on the dysmorphology skills of the practitioner performing the physical examination.

Stickler's syndrome should be considered in neonates with the triad of micrognathia, cleft of the soft palate, and glossoptosis. This triad of features is known as *Pierre Robin syndrome.*

Severe myopia in infants and young children should be considered a possible symptom of Stickler's syndrome. The diagnosis should also be considered in persons with a family history of cleft palate and significant myopia, deafness, or spondyloepiphyseal dysplasia. A slit-lamp examination of the vitreous is necessary to determine the presence of vitreal abnormalities that are considered pathognomonic of Stickler's syndrome.

Treatment
Beginning with the first 6 months of life, annual ophthalmology evaluation must be obtained to assess for myopia, vitreal abnormalities, and retinal degeneration and detachment. Persons who experience floaters or shadows in their vision require immediate assessment.

Persons with vitreoretinal degeneration need to avoid contact sports and other physical activity that can jar and detach the retina.

An auditory brain stem–evoked response evaluation should be done during the first month of life. The schedule for regular follow-up needs to be determined based on the results of the initial evaluation, frequency of otitis media episodes, and progress in language development.

Early use of corrective lenses and hearing aids is recommended to enable developmental progression at the infant or young child's full potential.

Depending on the infant's weight and health, surgical correction of the cleft palate can occur around age 9 months. With few exceptions, surgical closure of the palate should occur before age 2 in order to maximize speech and language development.

Special considerations
■ To assess for obstructive apnea, neonates with the Pierre Robin syndrome triad need oxygen and carbon dioxide measurements while lying in different positions and while feeding.
■ Neonates and infants with cleft palate may need a specialized cleft palate nurser to obtain adequate caloric intake.
■ Screening for cardiac valvular disease should be considered in the older child and adult with Stickler's syndrome.
■ Genetic counseling by a person trained in genetics should be offered to adults with Stickler's syndrome.
■ Referral to appropriate support groups or networking groups should be offered to help with coping skills and to provide anticipatory guidance related to day-to-day needs of a person with Stickler's syndrome.

AUTOSOMAL RECESSIVE INHERITANCE

Cystic fibrosis

Cystic fibrosis is a generalized dysfunction of the exocrine glands that affects multiple organ systems. Transmitted as an autosomal recessive trait, it's the most common fatal genetic disease in white children.

Cystic fibrosis is a chronic disease. With improvements in treatment over the past decade, the average life expectancy has risen from age 16 to age 28 and more.

Causes and incidence
The gene responsible for cystic fibrosis (located on chromosome 7) encodes a protein that involves chloride transport across epithelial membranes; over 100 specific mutations of the gene are known. (See *Cystic fibrosis transmission risk.*) The immediate causes of symptoms in cystic fibrosis are increased viscosity of bronchial, pancreatic, and other mucous gland secretions and consequent obstruction of glandular ducts. Cystic fibrosis accounts for almost all cases of pancreatic enzyme deficiency in children.

CYSTIC FIBROSIS TRANSMISSION RISK

The chance that a relative of a person with cystic fibrosis or a person with no family history will carry the cystic fibrosis gene appears in the chart below.

Relative of affected person	Carrier chance
Brother or sister	2 in 3 (67%)
Niece or nephew	1 in 2 (50%)
Aunt or uncle	1 in 3 (33%)
First cousin	1 in 4 (25%)

No known family history	Carrier chance
Whites	1 in 25 (4%)
Blacks	1 in 65 (1.5%)
Asians	1 in 150 (0.67%)

In the United States, the incidence of cystic fibrosis is highest in Whites of northern European ancestry (1 in 2,000 live births) and lowest in Blacks (1 in 17,000 live births), Native Americans, and people of Asian ancestry. The disease occurs equally in both sexes.

Signs and symptoms
The clinical effects of cystic fibrosis may become apparent soon after birth or may take years to develop. They include major aberrations in sweat gland, respiratory, and GI function. Sweat gland dysfunction is the most consistent abnormality. Increased concentrations of sodium and chloride in the sweat lead to hyponatremia and hypochloremia and can eventually induce fatal shock and arrhythmias, especially in hot weather.

Respiratory symptoms reflect obstructive changes in the lungs: wheezy respirations; a dry, nonproductive paroxysmal cough; dyspnea; and tachypnea. These changes stem from thick, tenacious secretions in the bronchioles and alveoli and eventually lead to severe atelectasis and emphysema. Children with cystic fibrosis display a barrel chest, cyanosis, and clubbing of the fingers and toes. They suffer recurring bronchitis and pneumonia as well as associated nasal polyps and sinusitis.

Death typically results from pneumonia, emphysema, or atelectasis.

The GI effects of cystic fibrosis occur mainly in the intestines, pancreas, and liver. One early symptom is meconium ileus; the neonate with cystic fibrosis doesn't excrete meconium, a dark green mucilaginous material found in the intestine at birth. He develops symptoms of intestinal obstruction, such as abdominal distention, vomiting, constipation, dehydration, and electrolyte imbalance. As the child gets older, obstruction of the pancreatic ducts and resulting deficiency of trypsin, amylase, and lipase prevent the conversion and absorption of fat and protein in the GI tract. The undigested food is then excreted in frequent, bulky, foul-smelling, pale stools with a high fat content. This malabsorption induces poor weight gain, poor growth, ravenous appetite, distended abdomen, thin extremities, and sallow skin with poor turgor. The inability to absorb fats results in a deficiency of fat-soluble vitamins (A, D, E, and K), leading to clotting problems, retarded bone growth, and delayed sexual development. Males may experience azoospermia and sterility; females may experience secondary amenorrhea but can reproduce. A common complication in infants and children is rectal prolapse secondary to malnutrition and wasting of perirectal supporting tissues.

In the pancreas, fibrotic tissue, multiple cysts, thick mucus, and eventually fat replace the acini (small, saclike swellings normally found in this gland), producing symptoms of pancreatic insufficiency: insufficient insulin production, abnormal glucose tolerance, and glycosuria. About 15% of patients have adequate pancreatic exocrine function for normal digestion and, therefore, have a better prognosis. Biliary obstruction and fibrosis may prolong neonatal jaundice. In some patients, cirrhosis and portal hypertension may lead to esophageal varices, episodes of hematemesis and, occasionally, hepatomegaly.

Diagnosis

CONFIRMING DIAGNOSIS *The Cystic Fibrosis Foundation has developed certain criteria for a definitive diagnosis: Two sweat tests using a pilocarpine solution (a sweat inducer) and either obstructive pulmonary disease, confirmed pancreatic insufficiency or failure to thrive, and a family history of cystic fibrosis.*

The following test results may support the diagnosis:
- Chest X-rays indicate early signs of obstructive lung disease.
- Stool specimen analysis indicates the absence of trypsin, suggesting pancreatic insufficiency.
- Deoxyribonucleic acid testing can now locate the presence of the Delta F 508 deletion (found in about 70% of cystic fibrosis patients, although the disease can cause more than 100 other mutations). It allows prenatal diagnosis in families with a previously affected child.
- Pulmonary function tests reveal decreased vital capacity, elevated residual volume due to air entrapments, and decreased forced expiratory volume in 1 second. This test is used if pulmonary exacerbation already exists.
- Liver enzyme tests may reveal hepatic insufficiency.
- Sputum culture reveals organisms that cystic fibrosis patients typically and chronically colonize, such as *Staphylococcus* and *Pseudomonas*.
- Serum albumin measurement helps assess nutritional status.
- Electrolyte analysis assesses hydration status.

Treatment

The aim of treatment is to help the child lead as normal a life as possible. The type of treatment depends on the organ systems involved.

To combat electrolyte losses in sweat, salt foods generously and, in hot weather, administer sodium supplements.

To offset pancreatic enzyme deficiencies, give oral pancreatic enzymes with meals and snacks, as ordered. Maintain a diet that's low in fat, but high in protein and calories, and provide supplements of water-miscible, fat-soluble vitamins (A, D, E, and K).

Management of pulmonary dysfunction includes chest physiotherapy, postural drainage, and breathing exercises several times daily to aid removal of secretions from lungs. Antihistamines are contraindicated because they have a drying effect on mucous membranes, making expectoration of mucus difficult or impossible. Aerosol therapy includes intermittent nebulizer treatments before postural drainage to loosen secretions.

Dornase alfa or DNase (recombinant human deoxyribonuclease), genetically engineered pulmonary enzymes given by aerosol nebulizer, helps thin airway mucus, improving lung function and reducing the risk of pulmonary infection.

Treatment of pulmonary infection requires:
- broad-spectrum antimicrobials
- oxygen therapy as needed
- loosening and removal of mucopurulent secretions, using an intermittent nebulizer and postural drainage to relieve obstruction. Use of a mist tent is controversial because mist particles may become trapped in the esophagus and stomach and never even reach the lungs.

Lung transplantation may be considered in some cases. Genetic research is ongoing, with researchers hoping to cure cystic fibrosis by artificially inserting a "healthy" gene into a person through gene therapy. The gene would be inserted by using an intranasal form. Research on correcting the disorder before birth is promising.

Special considerations
- Throughout this illness, teach the patient and his family about the disease and its treatment. The Cystic Fibrosis Foundation can provide educational and support services.
- Although many males with cystic fibrosis are infertile, females may become pregnant (due to increased life expectancies). As a result, more cystic fibrosis patients are now facing difficult reproductive decisions. Refer such patients (or the parents of an affected child) for genetic counseling so they can discuss family planning issues or prenatal diagnosis options if they're considering having more children.
- Be aware that some patients have recently undergone lung transplants to reduce the effects of the disease. Also, aerosol gene therapy shows promise in reducing pulmonary symptoms.

Research indicates that the genetic defect responsible for cystic fibrosis has also been identified in individuals experiencing some forms of unexplained pancreatitis.

Tay-Sachs disease

The most common of the lipid storage diseases, Tay-Sachs disease results from a congenital deficiency of the enzyme hexosaminidase A. It's characterized by progressive mental and motor deterioration and is usually fatal before age 5, although some adolescents and adults with variations of hexosaminidase A deficiency have been noted.

Causes and incidence
Tay-Sachs disease (also known as GM_2 gangliosidosis) is an autosomal recessive disorder of chromosome 15 in which the enzyme hexosaminidase A is virtually absent or deficient. This enzyme is necessary for metabolism of gangliosides, water-soluble glycolipids found primarily in central nervous system (CNS) tissues. Without hexosaminidase A, accumulating lipid pigments distend and progressively destroy and demyelinate CNS cells.

Tay-Sachs disease appears in fewer than 100 neonates born each year in the United States. However, about it's 100 times more common in persons of Eastern European Jewish (Ashkenazi) ancestry than in the general population, occurring in about 1 in 3,600 live births in this ethnic group. About 1 in 30 Ashkenazi Jews, French Canadians, and American Cajuns are heterozygous carriers. If two such carriers have children, each of their offspring has a 25% chance of having Tay-Sachs disease.

Signs and symptoms
A neonate with classic Tay-Sachs disease appears normal at birth, although he may have an exaggerated Moro reflex. By age 3 to 6 months, he becomes apathetic and responds only to loud sounds. His neck, trunk, arm, and leg muscles grow weaker, and soon he can't sit up or lift his head. He has difficulty turning over, can't grasp objects, and has progressive vision loss.

By age 18 months, the infant is usually deaf and blind and has seizures, generalized paralysis, and spasticity. His pupils are dilated and don't react to light. Decerebrate rigidity and a vegetative state follow. The child suffers recurrent bronchopneumonia after age 2 and usually dies before age 5. A child who survives may develop ataxia and progressive motor retardation between ages 2 and 8.

The "juvenile" form of Tay-Sachs disease generally appears between ages 2 and 5 as a progressive deterioration of psychomotor skills and gait. Patients with this type can survive to adulthood.

Diagnosis
CONFIRMING DIAGNOSIS *Typical clinical features point to Tay-Sachs disease, but serum analysis showing deficient hexosaminidase A is the key to diagnosis. An ophthalmologic examination showing optic nerve atrophy and a distinctive cherry-red spot on the retina supports the diagnosis. (The cherry-red spot may be absent in the juvenile form.)*

Diagnostic screening is essential for all couples when at least one partner is of Ashkenazi Jewish, French Canadian, or Cajun ancestry and for others with a family history of the disease. A blood test evaluating hexosaminidase A levels can identify carriers. Amniocentesis or chorionic villus sampling can detect hexosaminidase A deficiency in the fetus.

Treatment

Tay-Sachs disease has no known cure. Supportive treatment includes tube feedings of nutritional supplements, suctioning and postural drainage to remove pharyngeal secretions, skin care to prevent pressure ulcers in bedridden children, and mild laxatives to relieve neurogenic constipation. Anticonvulsants usually fail to prevent seizures. Because these children need constant physical care, many parents have full-time skilled home nursing care or place them in long-term special care facilities.

Special considerations

Your most important job is to help the family deal with inevitably progressive illness and death.

■ Offer carrier testing to all couples from high-risk ethnic groups.
■ Refer the parents for genetic counseling, and stress the importance of considering an amniocentesis in future pregnancies. Refer siblings for screening to determine if they're carriers. If they're carriers and are adults, refer them for genetic counseling, but stress that there's no danger of transmitting the disease to offspring if they don't marry another carrier.
■ Some in-vitro fertilization centers have recently started offering preimplantation genetics. Refer the couple to an appropriate center if they express interest in assisted reproductive technology.
■ Because the parents of an affected child may feel excessive stress or guilt because of the child's illness and the emotional and financial burden it places on them, refer them for counseling if indicated.
■ If the parents care for their child at home, teach them how to do suctioning, postural drainage, and tube feeding. Also teach them how to provide good skin care to prevent pressure ulcers.

For more information on this disease, refer parents to the National Tay-Sachs and Allied Diseases Association.

Phenylketonuria

Phenylketonuria (PKU) is an inborn error in phenylalanine metabolism that results in the accumulation of high serum levels of the enzyme phenylalanine in the blood. When left untreated, it results in cerebral damage and mental retardation.

Causes and incidence

PKU is transmitted by an autosomal recessive gene on chromosome 12. Patients with this disorder have insufficient hepatic phenylalanine hydroxylase, an enzyme that acts as a catalyst in the conversion of phenylalanine to tyrosine. As a result, phenylalanine and its metabolites accumulate in the blood, eventually causing mental retardation if left untreated. The exact biochemical mechanism that causes this retardation is unclear.

In the United States, this disorder occurs in 1 in approximately 14,000 births. (About 1 person in 60 is an asymptomatic carrier.) The gene is most common in Ireland, Scotland, Belgium, and West Germany and rare in Blacks, Asians, Native Americans, Finns, and Ashkenazi Jews.

Signs and symptoms

An infant with undiagnosed and untreated PKU appears normal at birth but by 4 months begins to show signs of arrested brain development, including mental retardation and, later, personality disturbances (schizoid and antisocial personality patterns and uncontrollable temper). Such a child may have a lighter complexion than unaffected siblings and typically has blue eyes. He may also have microcephaly; eczematous skin lesions or dry, rough skin; and a musty (mousy) odor due to skin and urinary excretion of phenylacetic acid. Approximately 80% of these children have abnormal EEG patterns, and about one-third have seizures, usually beginning between ages 6 and 12 months.

Children with PKU show a precipitous decrease in IQ in their first year, are usually hyperactive and irritable, and exhibit purposeless, repetitive motions. They have increased muscle tone and an awkward gait.

Although blood phenylalanine levels are near normal at birth, they begin to rise within a few days. By the time they reach significant levels (approximately 30 mg/dl), cerebral damage has begun. Such irreversible damage probably is complete by age 2 or 3. However, early detection and treatment can minimize cerebral damage, and children under strict dietary control can lead normal lives.

Diagnosis

All states require screening for PKU at birth; the Guthrie screening test on a capillary blood sample (bacterial inhibition assay) reliably detects PKU. However, because phenylalanine levels may be normal at birth, the neonate should be reevaluated after he has received dietary protein for 24 to 48 hours. The common practice of discharging new mothers from the hospital within 24 hours of delivery has resulted in failure to detect some neonates with PKU. For this reason, some states now require a minimum hospital stay of 48 hours after a vaginal delivery.

Adding a few drops of 10% ferric chloride solution to a wet diaper is another method of detecting PKU. If the area turns a deep, bluish green, phenylpyruvic acid is present in the urine.

CONFIRMING DIAGNOSIS *Detection of elevated blood levels of phenylalanine and the presence of phenylpyruvic acid in the infant's urine confirm the diagnosis. (Urine should also be tested 4 to 6 weeks after birth because urinary levels of phenylpyruvic acid vary with the amount of protein ingested.)*

Chorionic villi sampling can be used to detect fetal PKU as a prenatal diagnosis. Enzyme assay can be used to detect the carrier state in parents.

Treatment

Treatment consists of restricting dietary intake of the amino acid phenylalanine to keep phenylalanine blood levels between 3 and 9 mg/dl. Because most natural proteins contain 5% phenylalanine, they must be limited in the child's diet. An enzymatic hydrolysate of casein, such as Lofenalac powder or Pregestimil powder, is substituted for milk in the diets of affected infants. This milk substitute contains a minimal amount of phenylalanine, normal amounts

of other amino acids, and added amounts of carbohydrate and fat. Dietary restrictions usually continue throughout life.

The special diet for PKU calls for careful monitoring. Because the body doesn't make phenylalanine, overzealous dietary restriction can induce phenylalanine deficiency, producing lethargy, anorexia, anemia, rashes, and diarrhea.

Special considerations

In caring for a child with PKU, it's especially important to teach both the parents and child about this disease and to provide emotional support and counseling. (Psychological and emotional problems may result from the difficult dietary restrictions.)

■ Emphasize to the child and his parents the critical importance of adhering to the special diet. The child must avoid breads, cheese, eggs, flour, meat, poultry, fish, nuts, milk, legumes, and phenylalanine sugar substitutes.

■ Inform the parents that the child will need frequent tests for urine phenylpyruvic acid and blood phenylalanine levels to evaluate the diet's effectiveness.

■ As the child grows older and is supervised less closely, his parents will have less control over what he eats. As a result, deviation from the restricted diet becomes more likely, as does the risk of brain damage. Encourage the parents to allow the child some choices in the kinds of low-protein foods he wants to eat; this will help make him feel trusted and more responsible.

■ Teach the parents about normal physical and mental growth and development so that they can recognize any developmental delay that may point to excessive phenylalanine intake.

 PEDIATRIC TIP *Infants should be routinely screened for PKU because detection of the disorder and control of phenylalanine intake soon after birth can prevent severe mental retardation.*

■ Refer females with PKU who reach reproductive age for genetic counseling because recent research indicates that their offspring may have a higher-than-normal incidence of brain damage, mental retardation, microcephaly, and major congenital malformations, especially of the heart and central nervous system. Such damage may be minimized with a low-phenylalanine diet before conception and during pregnancy, but even patients under good control remain at increased risk for offspring with this defect.

Albinism

Albinism is a rare inherited defect in melanin metabolism of the skin and eyes (oculocutaneous albinism) or just the eyes (ocular albinism). Ocular albinism impairs visual acuity. Oculocutaneous albinism also causes severe intolerance to sunlight and increases susceptibility to skin cancer. Other forms are associated with deafness.

Causes and incidence
Oculocutaneous albinism results from autosomal recessive inheritance; ocular albinism, from an X-linked recessive trait that causes hypopigmentation only in the iris and the ocular fundus.

Normally, melanocytes synthesize melanin. Melanosomes, melanin-containing granules within melanocytes, diffuse and absorb the sun's ultraviolet light, thus protecting the skin and eyes from its dangerous effects. In *tyrosinase-negative albinism* (the most common type), melanosomes don't contain melanin because they lack tyrosinase, the enzyme that stimulates melanin production. In *tyrosinase-positive albinism*, melanosomes contain tyrosine, a tyrosinase substrate, but a defect in the tyrosine transport system impairs melanin production.

In *tyrosinase-variable albinism* (rare), an unidentified enzyme defect probably impairs synthesis of a melanin precursor. Other rare forms of albinism are *Chédiak-Higashi syndrome* (tyrosine-negative albinism with hematologic and neurologic manifestations); *Hermansky-Pudlak syndrome* (tyrosinase-positive albinism with platelet dysfunction, bleeding abnormalities, and ceroidlike inclusions in many organs); and *Cross-McKusick-Breen syndrome* (tyrosinase-positive albinism with neurologic involvement).

In the United States, both types of albinism are more common in Blacks than in Whites. Native Americans have a high incidence of the tyrosine-positive form.

Signs and symptoms
Light-skinned Whites with tyrosinase-negative albinism have pale skin and hair color ranging from white to yellow; their pupils appear red because of translucent irides. Blacks with the same disorder have hair that may be white, faintly tinged with yellow, or yellow-brown. Both Whites and Blacks with tyrosinase-positive albinism grow darker as they age. For instance, their hair may become straw-colored or light brown and their skin cream-colored or pink. People with tyrosinase-positive albinism may also have freckles and pigmented nevi that may require excision.

In tyrosinase-variable albinism, at birth the child's hair is white, his skin is pink, and his eyes are gray. As he grows older, though, his hair becomes yellow, his irides may become darker, and his skin may even tan slightly.

The skin of a person with albinism is easily damaged by the sun. It may look weather-beaten and is highly susceptible to precancerous and cancerous growths. The patient may also have photophobia, myopia, strabismus, and congenital horizontal nystagmus.

Diagnosis
Diagnosis is based on clinical observation and the patient's family history. Microscopic examination of the skin and of hair follicles determines the amount of pigment present. Testing plucked hair roots for pigmentation when incubated in tyrosine distinguishes tyrosinase-negative albinism from tyrosinase-positive albinism. Tyrosinase-positive hair bulbs will develop color.

Treatment
No specific treatment for albinism exists.

Special considerations
■ To help the parents work through any feelings of guilt or depression, encourage early infant-parent bonding. Also inform the parents about cosmetic measures (glasses with tinted lenses, makeup) that

can lessen the child's disfigurement when he's older.

■ Teach the child and his parents what measures best protect him from solar radiation, and inform them of its danger signals (excessive drying of skin, crusty lesions on exposed skin, changes in skin color).

■ Advise the patient to wear full-spectrum sunblocks, dark glasses, and appropriate protective clothing.

■ If the patient's appearance causes him social and emotional problems, he may need psychological counseling. Such counseling may also be in order for his family, if they too find it difficult to accept his disorder.

■ Stress the need for frequent refractions and eye examinations to correct visual defects.

■ Refer the adult patient or the parents of an affected child for genetic counseling to learn about the probability of recurrence in future offspring.

Sickle cell anemia

A congenital hemolytic anemia that occurs primarily but not exclusively in blacks, sickle cell anemia results from a defective hemoglobin (Hb) molecule (HbS) that causes red blood cells (RBCs) to roughen and become sickle-shaped. Such cells impair circulation, resulting in chronic ill health (fatigue, dyspnea on exertion, swollen joints), periodic crises, long-term complications, and premature death.

Penicillin prophylaxis can decrease morbidity and mortality from bacterial infections. Half of patients with sickle cell anemia die by their early twenties; few live to middle age.

Causes and incidence

Sickle cell anemia results from homozygous inheritance of the gene that produces HbS (chromosome 11). It's inherited as an autosomal recessive trait. Heterozygous inheritance of this gene results in sickle cell trait, a condition that usually produces no symptoms. (See *Sickle cell trait*.) Sickle cell anemia is most common in tropical Africans and in people of African descent;

> **SICKLE CELL TRAIT**
>
> Sickle cell trait is a relatively benign condition that results from heterozygous inheritance of the abnormal hemoglobin (Hb) S-producing gene. Like sickle cell anemia, this condition is most common in blacks. Sickle cell trait *never* progresses to sickle cell anemia.
>
> In persons with sickle cell trait (known as *carriers*), 20% to 40% of their total Hb is HbS; the rest is normal.
>
> Such persons usually have no symptoms. They have normal Hb and hematocrit values and can expect a normal life span. Nevertheless, they must avoid situations that provoke hypoxia, which can occasionally cause a sickling crisis similar to that in sickle cell anemia.
>
> Genetic counseling is essential for sickle cell carriers. If two sickle cell carriers produce offspring, each of their children has a 25% chance of inheriting sickle cell anemia.

---

about 1 in 10 American blacks carries the abnormal gene. However, sickle cell anemia also appears in other ethnic populations, including people of Mediterranean or East Indian ancestry.

If two parents who are both carriers of sickle cell trait (or another hemoglobinopathy) have offspring, each child has a 25% chance of developing sickle cell anemia. (See *Inheritance patterns in sickle cell anemia*, page 22.) Overall, 1 in every 400 to 600 black children has sickle cell anemia. The defective HbS-producing gene may have persisted because, in areas where malaria is endemic, the heterozygous sickle cell trait provides resistance to malaria and is actually beneficial.

The abnormal HbS found in such patients' RBCs become insoluble whenever hypoxia occurs. As a result, these RBCs become rigid, rough, and elongated, forming a crescent or sickle shape. (See *Comparing*

INHERITANCE PATTERNS IN SICKLE CELL ANEMIA

When both parents are carriers of sickle cell trait, each child has a 25% chance of developing sickle cell anemia, a 25% chance of being a normal (unaffected) noncarrier, and a 50% chance of being a carrier of sickle cell trait.

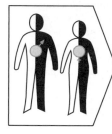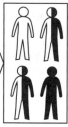

When one parent has sickle cell anemia and one is normal, all offspring will be carriers of sickle cell trait.

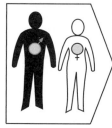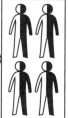

KEY

☐ Normal, noncarrier

◨ Normal, carrier of sickle cell trait

■ Sickle cell anemia (affected with sickle cell disease)

normal and sickled red blood cells.) Such sickling can produce hemolysis (cell destruction). In addition, these altered cells tend to pile up in capillaries and smaller blood vessels, making blood more viscous. Normal circulation is impaired, causing

pain, tissue infarctions, and swelling. Such blockage causes anoxic changes that lead to further sickling and obstruction.

Signs and symptoms

Characteristically, sickle cell anemia produces tachycardia, cardiomegaly, systolic and diastolic murmurs, pulmonary infarctions (which may result in cor pulmonale), chronic fatigue, unexplained dyspnea or dyspnea on exertion, hepatomegaly, jaundice, pallor, joint swelling, aching bones, chest pains, ischemic leg ulcers (especially around the ankles), and increased susceptibility to infection. Such symptoms usually don't develop until after age 6 months because large amounts of fetal Hb protect infants for the first few months after birth. Low socioeconomic status and related problems, such as poor nutrition and education, may delay diagnosis and supportive treatment.

Infection, stress, dehydration, and conditions that provoke hypoxia — strenuous exercise, high altitude, unpressurized aircraft, cold, and vasoconstrictive drugs — may all provoke periodic crises. A painful crisis (vasoocclusive crisis, infarctive crisis), the most common crisis and the hallmark of the disease, usually appears periodically after age 5. It results from blood vessel obstruction by rigid, tangled sickle cells, which causes tissue anoxia and possible necrosis. This type of crisis is characterized by severe abdominal, thoracic, muscular, or bone pain and possibly worsening jaundice, dark urine, and a low-grade fever.

Autosplenectomy, in which splenic damage and scarring is so extensive that the spleen shrinks and becomes impalpable, occurs in patients with long-term disease. This can lead to increased susceptibility to Streptococcus pneumoniae sepsis, which can be fatal without prompt treatment. Infection may develop after the crisis subsides (in 4 days to several weeks), so watch for lethargy, sleepiness, fever, or apathy.

An aplastic crisis (megaloblastic crisis) results from bone marrow depression and is associated with infection, usually viral. It's characterized by pallor, lethargy, sleepiness, dyspnea, possible coma, markedly decreased bone marrow activity, and RBC hemolysis.

In infants between ages 8 months and 2 years, an acute sequestration crisis may cause sudden massive entrapment of RBCs in the spleen and liver. This rare crisis causes lethargy and pallor and, if untreated, commonly progresses to hypovolemic shock and death.

A hemolytic crisis is quite rare and usually occurs in patients who also have glucose-6-phosphate dehydrogenase deficiency. It probably results from complications of sickle cell anemia, such as infection, rather than from the disorder itself. Hemolytic crisis causes liver congestion and hepatomegaly as a result of degenerative changes. It worsens chronic jaundice, although increased jaundice doesn't always point to a hemolytic crisis.

Suspect any of these crises in a sickle cell anemia patient with pale lips, tongue, palms, or nail beds; lethargy; listlessness; sleepiness with difficulty awakening; irritability; severe pain; a fever over 104° F (40° C); or a fever of 100° F (37.8° C) that persists for 2 days.

Sickle cell anemia also causes long-term complications. Typically, the child is small for his age and has delayed puberty. (However, fertility isn't impaired.) If he reaches adulthood, his body build tends to be spiderlike — narrow shoulders and hips, long extremities, curved spine, barrel chest, and elongated skull. An adult usually has complications from organ infarction, such as retinopathy and nephropathy. Premature death commonly results from infection or from repeated occlusion of small blood vessels and consequent infarction or necrosis of major organs (such as cerebral blood vessel occlusion causing stroke).

Diagnosis

A positive family history and typical clinical features suggest sickle cell anemia. Hb electrophoresis showing HbS or other hemoglobinopathies can also confirm it. Electrophoresis should be done on umbilical cord blood samples at birth to provide sickle cell disease screening for all neonates at risk.

COMPARING NORMAL AND SICKLED RED BLOOD CELLS

When a person with sickle cell anemia develops hypoxia, the abnormal hemoglobin S found in his red blood cells (RBCs) becomes insoluble. This causes the RBCs to become rigid, rough, and elongated, forming the characteristic sickle shape.

NORMAL RBCS

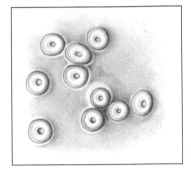

SICKLE CELLS

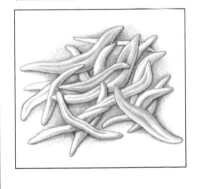

Additional laboratory studies may show a low RBC count, elevated white blood cell and platelet counts, decreased erythrocyte sedimentation rate, increased serum iron, decreased RBC survival, and reticulocytosis. Hb levels may be low or normal. During early childhood, palpation may reveal splenomegaly, but, as the child grows older, the spleen shrinks.

Treatment

Treatment begins before age 4 months with prophylactic penicillin. If the patient's Hb drops suddenly or if his condition deteriorates rapidly, he'll need to be hospitalized for a transfusion of packed RBCs. In a sequestration crisis, treatment may include sedation, administration of analgesics, a blood transfusion, oxygen administration, and large amounts of oral or I.V. fluids.

Daily folic acid supplementation is recommended to prevent megaloblastic crisis. Hydroxyurea, which causes an increase in the synthesis of fetal Hb and a significant reduction in crises, is being used for some patients with sickle cell anemia. Researchers have found it helpful for some patients because it reduces the frequency of painful crises and episodes of acute chest syndrome and decreases the need for blood transfusions.

Newer drugs are being developed to manage sickle cell anemia. Some of these agents try to induce the body to produce more fetal Hb, which helps decrease the amount of sickling. Others work by increasing the binding of oxygen to sickle cells. Currently, bone marrow transplantation offers the only cure for sickle cell anemia. Gene therapy (replacing HbS with normal HbA) may be the ideal treatment, but it's difficult to perform.

Special considerations

Supportive measures during crises and precautions to avoid them are important. Here are some actions you can take during a painful crisis:

- Apply warm compresses to painful areas, and cover the child with a blanket. (Never use cold compresses because they aggravate the condition.)
- Administer an analgesic-antipyretic, such as aspirin or acetaminophen. (Additional pain relief may be required during an acute crisis.)
- Encourage fluids and bed rest, and place the patient in a sitting position. If dehydration or severe pain occurs, hospitalization may be necessary.
- When cultures indicate, give antibiotics as ordered.

During remissions:

- Advise the patient to avoid tight clothing that restricts circulation.
- Warn against strenuous exercise, vaso-constricting medications, cold temperatures (including drinking large amounts of ice water and swimming), unpressurized aircraft, high altitude, and other conditions that provoke hypoxia.

 PEDIATRIC TIP *Stress the importance of normal childhood immunizations, meticulous wound care, good oral hygiene, regular dental checkups, and a balanced diet as safeguards against infection.*

- Emphasize the need for prompt treatment of infection.
- Inform the patient of the need to increase fluid intake to prevent dehydration due to impaired ability to concentrate urine properly. Tell parents to encourage the child to drink more fluids, especially in the summer, by offering fluids such as milkshakes and ice pops.

During pregnancy or surgery:

- Warn women with sickle cell anemia that they may have increased obstetrical risks. However, use of hormonal contraceptives may also be risky; refer them for birth control counseling to a qualified obstetric or gynecologic health care provider.
- If such women *do* become pregnant, they should maintain a balanced diet and may benefit from a folic acid supplement.
- During general anesthesia, a patient who has sickle cell anemia requires optimal ventilation to prevent hypoxic crisis. Make sure the surgeon and the anesthesiologist know that the patient has sickle cell anemia. Provide a preoperative transfusion of packed RBCs, as needed.

General tips:

- To encourage normal mental and social development, warn parents against being overprotective. Although the child must avoid strenuous exercise, he can enjoy most everyday activities.
- Refer parents of children with sickle cell anemia for genetic counseling to answer their questions about the risk to future offspring. Recommend screening of other family members to determine if they're heterozygote carriers. These parents may also need psychological counseling to cope with guilt feelings. In addition, suggest they

join an appropriate community support group.

■ Adolescents or adult males with sickle cell anemia may develop sudden, painful episodes of priapism. Such episodes are common and, if prolonged, can have serious reproductive consequences. Advise the patient to contact the physician when these episodes occur.

X-LINKED INHERITANCE

Hemophilia

Hemophilia is a hereditary bleeding disorder resulting from a deficiency of specific clotting factors. After a person with hemophilia forms a platelet plug at a bleeding site, the clotting factor deficiency impairs the blood's capacity to form a stable fibrin clot. Bleeding occurs primarily into large joints, especially after trauma or surgery. Spontaneous intracranial bleeding can occur and may be fatal.

Advances in treatment have greatly improved the prognosis for patients with hemophilia, many of whom live normal life spans. Surgical procedures can be done safely at special treatment centers under the guidance of a hematologist.

Causes and incidence

Both hemophilia A and B are inherited as X-linked recessive traits. This means that female carriers have a 50% chance of transmitting the gene to each daughter, who would then be a carrier, and a 50% chance of transmitting the gene to each son, who would be born with hemophilia. Hemophilia A (classic hemophilia), which affects more than 80% of patients with hemophilia, results from a deficiency of factor VIII-C; hemophilia B (Christmas disease), which affects approximately 15% of patients with hemophilia, results from a deficiency of factor IX-C.

The factor VIII gene is located within the Xq28 region, and the factor IX gene is located within Xq27. Females with one defective factor VIII gene are carriers of hemophilia. A large number of disease-causing mutations have been identified in both genes. A specific inversion mutation in the noncoding region of the factor VIII gene is present in approximately 45% of families with severe hemophilia A. Hemophilia A is the most common X-linked genetic disease, occurring in approximately 1 in 10,000 live male births. It is five times more common than hemophilia B.

Signs and symptoms

Hemophilia produces abnormal bleeding, which may be mild, moderate, or severe, depending on the degree of factor deficiency.

Mild hemophilia commonly goes undiagnosed until adulthood because the patient doesn't bleed spontaneously or after minor trauma but has prolonged bleeding if challenged by major trauma or surgery. Postoperative bleeding continues as a slow ooze or ceases and starts again, up to 8 days after surgery.

Severe hemophilia causes spontaneous bleeding. In many cases, the first sign of severe hemophilia is excessive bleeding after circumcision. Later, spontaneous bleeding or severe bleeding after minor trauma may produce large subcutaneous and deep intramuscular hematomas. Bleeding into joints (hemarthrosis) and muscles causes pain, swelling, extreme tenderness and, possibly, permanent deformity.

Moderate hemophilia causes symptoms similar to severe hemophilia but produces only occasional spontaneous bleeding episodes.

Bleeding near peripheral nerves may cause peripheral neuropathy, pain, paresthesia, and muscle atrophy. If bleeding impairs blood flow through a major vessel, it can cause ischemia and gangrene. Pharyngeal, lingual, intracardial, intracerebral, and intracranial bleeding may all lead to shock and death.

Diagnosis

Development of a large cephalohematoma or intracranial hemorrhage after prolonged labor or delivery by forceps or vacuum extraction may be the first indication of a bleeding problem. After the neonatal period, a history of prolonged bleeding after

FACTOR REPLACEMENT PRODUCTS

Cryoprecipitate
- Contains factor VIII (70 to 100 units/bag). Doesn't contain factor IX
- Can be stored frozen up to 12 months but must be used within 6 hours after it thaws
- Given through a blood filter; compatible with normal saline solution only
- No longer treatment of choice because of the risk of human immunodeficiency virus and hepatitis infection; can still contain viruses despite greatly improved screening and purification procedures for viral inactivation in blood products

Lyophilized factor VIII or IX
- Freeze-dried
- Can be stored up to 2 years at about 36° to 46° F (2° to 8° C), up to 6 months at room temperature not exceeding 88° F (31.1° C)
- Labeled with exact units of factor VIII or IX contained in vial
- 200 to 1,500 units of factor VIII or IX per vial; 20 to 40 ml after reconstitution with diluent
- No blood filter needed; usually given by slow I.V. push through a butterfly infusion set

Fresh frozen plasma
- Contains approximately 0.75 unit/ml of factor VII and approximately 1 unit/ml of factor IX; not practical for most people with hemophilia because a large volume is needed to raise factors to hemostatic levels
- Can be stored frozen up to 12 months but must be used within 2 hours after it thaws
- Given through a blood filter; compatible with normal saline solution only

surgery (including dental extractions) or trauma or of episodes of spontaneous bleeding into muscles or joints usually indicates some defect in the hemostatic mechanism. Hemophilia A and B may be clinically indistinguishable, but specific coagulation factor assays can diagnose the type and severity of the disease. A positive family history, prenatal diagnosis, and carrier testing can also help diagnose hemophilia, but nearly one-third of all patients have no family history.

Characteristic findings in hemophilia A include:
- factor VIII-C assay, 0% to 30% of normal
- prolonged partial thromboplastin time (PTT)
- normal platelet count and function, bleeding time, and prothrombin time.

Characteristics of hemophilia B include:
- deficient factor IX-C
- baseline coagulation results similar to hemophilia A, with normal factor VIII.

In both types of hemophilia, the degree of factor deficiency determines severity:
- mild hemophilia — factor levels 5% to 40% of normal
- moderate hemophilia — factor levels 1% to 5% of normal
- severe hemophilia — factor levels less than 1% of normal.

Treatment
Hemophilia isn't curable, but treatment can prevent crippling deformities and prolong life expectancy. Correct treatment quickly stops bleeding by increasing plasma levels of deficient clotting factors to help prevent disabling deformities that result from repeated bleeding into muscles and joints. (See *Factor replacement products*.)

Desmopressin (DDAVP — 1-deamino-8-D-arginine vasopressin) administered I.V. or intranasally is usually sufficient to manage bleeding episodes of children and adolescents with mild hemophilia A. Persons with moderate to severe hemophilia A require commercially prepared factor VIII concentrates to treat bleeding episodes. Concentrates derived from human plasma are virally attenuated by one or more available methods significantly minimizing the risk for human immunodeficiency virus (HIV)-1, HIV-2, hepatitis B, and hepatitis C contamination. However, no currently available method has been successful in eradicating parvovirus B 19 from blood products. Factor VIII concentrate derived from recombinant technology (rFVIII) has been shown in multiple clinical trials to be as effective as virally attenuated plasma-derived concentrate. Risk for viral contamination is essentially nonexistent in preparations of rFVIII that avoid human serum albumin as a stabilizer.

In hemophilia B, administration of factor IX concentrate during bleeding episodes increases factor IX levels.

The U.S. National Hemophilia Foundation first recommended prophylaxis with factor concentrates in 1994 after investigators in Sweden demonstrated repeated success with this approach. The ultimate goal is to prevent irreversible destructive arthritis that results from repeated hemarthrosis and synovial hypertrophy. Prophylaxis of persons with hemophilia A or B may begin as early as age 1 or 2.

A person with hemophilia who undergoes surgery needs careful management by a hematologist with expertise in hemophilia care. The patient will require replacement of the deficient factor before and after surgery, possibly even for minor surgery such as a dental extraction. (DDAVP may be given before dental extractions and surgery to prevent bleeding.) In addition, epsilon-aminocaproic acid is commonly used for oral bleeding to inhibit the active fibrinolytic system present in the oral mucosa.

Development of factor VIH or factor XI inhibitors occurs in up to 3.5% of children with severe hemophilia A and up to 3% of those with hemophilia B. Studies indicate that certain gene mutations predispose to an increased risk for inhibitor development. Patients with hemophilia who can't achieve hemostasis after use of previously effective factor concentrate doses should be evaluated for factor inhibitors.

Preventive measures include teaching the patient how to avoid trauma, manage minor bleeding, and recognize bleeding that requires immediate medical intervention. Genetic counseling helps carriers understand how this disease is transmitted. (See *Managing hemophilia,* page 28.)

Special considerations
During bleeding episodes:
- Give clotting agents as ordered. The body uses up factor VIII in 48 to 72 hours, so repeat infusions, as ordered, until bleeding stops.
- Apply cold compresses or ice bags and raise the injured part.
- To prevent recurrence of bleeding, restrict activity for 48 hours after bleeding is under control.
- Control pain with an analgesic, such as acetaminophen, propoxyphene, codeine, or meperidine, as ordered. Avoid I.M. injections because of possible hematoma formation at the injection site. Aspirin and aspirin-containing medications are contraindicated because they decrease platelet adherence and may increase the bleeding. Caution should be used when trying other nonsteroidal anti-inflammatory drugs, for example, ibuprofen or ketoprofen.

If the patient has bled into a joint:
- Immediately elevate the joint.
- To restore joint mobility, begin range-of-motion exercises, if ordered, at least 48 hours after the bleeding is controlled. Tell the patient to avoid weight bearing until bleeding stops and swelling subsides.

After bleeding episodes and surgery:
- Watch closely for signs of further bleeding, such as increased pain and swelling, fever, or symptoms of shock.
- Closely monitor PTT.
- Teach parents special precautions to prevent bleeding episodes.
- Refer new patients to a hemophilia treatment center for evaluation. The center will devise a treatment plan for such patients' primary physicians and is a resource for other medical and school personnel, dentists, and others involved in their care.
- Persons who have been exposed to HIV through contaminated blood products need special support.
- Refer patients and carriers for genetic counseling.

MANAGING HEMOPHILIA

The following guidelines can help parents care for their child with hemophilia.

- Instruct parents to notify the physician immediately after even a minor injury, but especially after an injury to the head, neck, or abdomen. Such injuries may require special blood factor replacement. Also, tell them to check with the physician before allowing dental extractions or any other surgery.
- Educate the patient and his parents on the early signs and symptoms of hemarthrosis: stiffness, tingling, or ache in joint, followed by decreased range of motion. If signs and symptoms are recognized early, treatment can begin earlier, potentially decreasing the possibility of long-term disability.
- Stress the importance of regular, careful toothbrushing with a soft-bristled toothbrush to prevent the need for dental surgery.
- Teach parents to be alert for signs of severe internal bleeding, such as severe pain or swelling in a joint or muscle, stiffness, decreased joint movement, severe abdominal pain, blood in urine, black tarry stools, and severe headache.
- Advise parents that the child is at risk for hepatitis from blood components. Early signs — headache, fever, decreased appetite, nausea, vomiting, abdominal tenderness, and pain over the liver — may appear 3 weeks to 6 months after treatment with blood components. Tell them to discuss with their physician the possibility of hepatitis vaccination.
- Discuss the increased risk of human immunodeficiency virus (HIV) infection if the child received a blood product before routine screening of blood products for HIV began. Tell parents to ask the physician about periodic testing for HIV.
- Urge parents to make sure their child wears a medical identification bracelet at all times.

- *Teach parents never to give their child aspirin,* which can aggravate the tendency to bleed. Advise them to give acetaminophen instead.
- Instruct parents to protect their child from injury, but to avoid unnecessary restrictions that impair his normal development. For example, they can sew padded patches into the knees and elbows of a toddler's clothing to protect these joints during falls. They should forbid an older child to participate in contact sports such as football but can encourage him to swim or to play golf.
- Teach parents to elevate and apply cold compresses or ice bags to an injured area and to apply light pressure to a bleeding site. To prevent recurrence of bleeding, advise parents to restrict the child's activity for 48 hours after bleeding is under control.
- If parents have been trained to administer blood factor components at home to avoid frequent hospitalization, make sure they know proper venipuncture and infusion techniques and don't delay treatment during bleeding episodes.
- Instruct parents to keep blood factor concentrate and infusion equipment on hand at all times, even on vacation.
- Emphasize the importance of having the child keep routine medical appointments at the local hemophilia center.
- Daughters of individuals with hemophilia should undergo genetic screening to determine if they're hemophilia carriers. Affected males should undergo counseling as well. If they produce offspring with a noncarrier, all of their daughters will be carriers; if they produce offspring with a carrier, each child has a 25% chance of being affected.
- For more information, refer parents to the National Hemophilia Foundation.

Fragile X syndrome

Fragile X is the most common inherited cause of mental retardation. The condition is typically caused by a well-defined mutation at a specific locus of the fragile X mental retardation 1 (FMR1) gene on the X chromosome. Approximately 85% of males and 50% of females who inherit the FMR1 mutation will demonstrate clinical features of the syndrome. Post-pubescent males with fragile X syndrome usually have distinct physical features, behavioral difficulties, and cognitive impairment. Females with fragile X syndrome tend to have more subtle symptoms.

Causes and incidence

Fragile X syndrome is an X-linked condition that doesn't follow a simple X-linked inheritance pattern. The normal sequence of the FMR1 gene was identified at Xq27.3 in 1991. The unique mutation that results in fragile X syndrome consists of an expanding region of a specific triplet of nitrogenous bases: cytosine, guanine, guanine (CGG) within the gene's deoxyribonucleic acid (DNA) sequence. Normally, FMR1 contains 6 to 50 sequential copies of the CGG triplet. When the number of CGG triplets expands to the range of 50 to 200 repeats, the region of DNA becomes unstable and is referred to as a premutation. A full mutation consists of over 200 CGG triplet repeats.

The full mutation typically causes abnormal methylation (methyl groups attach to components of the gene) of FMR1. Methylation inhibits gene transcription and thus protein production. The reduced or absent protein product (FNIRP) is responsible for the clinical features of fragile X syndrome. Approximately 15% to 20% of males with a full mutation don't have fragile X. This may be explained by either the ability of unmethylated portions (of their mutated FMR1) to be transcribed for eventual protein production, or that these males are mosaic for the FMR1 premutation. In asymptomatic mosaic males it's believed that the cells with a premutation can produce enough protein to compensate for the cells that contain a full mutation and consequently produce no protein.

Approximately 50% of females who inherit a full mutation from their mother have clinical features of fragile X syndrome. This is primarily due to the normal process of random X inactivation. At the time of meiosis, both X chromosomes must be activated. However, shortly after the zygote stage, an X chromosome is inactivated in every cell. Clinically measurable effects of the full FMR1 mutation will be more likely in relevant tissues or organs that have a disproportionate number of cells in which the normal X chromosome has been inactivated.

Males with a premutation don't have fragile X. They're considered unaffected or normal-transmitting males. Because males have only one X chromosome, all daughters of a transmitting male will inherit their father's X chromosome with the premutation. None of the male's sons will inherit the premutation because they inherit their father's Y chromosome rather than the X chromosome.

Females with the premutation don't have fragile X syndrome. However, the premutation can expand into the full mutation range (>200 CGG triplets) when it's transmitted from a premutation carrier mother to her offspring. This expansion can occur during or after maternal meiosis. Therefore, the following possibilities exist for every pregnancy of a mother with a premutation.

- A female conceptus receives the mother's X chromosome with the nonmutated FMR1 gene. She won't be affected with fragile X. None of her future offspring will be at risk for inheriting the syndrome from her.
- A male conceptus receives the mother's X with the nonmutated FMR1 gene. He won't be affected with fragile X. None of his future offspring will be at risk for inheriting the syndrome from him.
- A female conceptus receives the mother's X chromosome with the FMR1 premutation. She'll be a carrier like her mother but won't have fragile X syndrome. Her future offspring will be at risk for inheriting a full mutation from her.
- A male conceptus receives the mother's X with the FMR1 premutation. He won't be affected with fragile X. All of his future

daughters but none of his future sons will inherit the premutation from him.

■ A female conceptus receives the mother's X chromosome with the FMR1 gene whose premutation expanded into a full mutation during or after maternal meiosis. Depending on the outcome of random X inactivation, the daughter may have clinically definable fragile X syndrome. Her future offspring will be at risk for inheriting the full mutation and, thus, the syndrome from her.

■ A male conceptus receives the mother's X chromosome with the FMR1 gene whose premutation has expanded into a full mutation during or after maternal meiosis. In 85% of cases, the son in this situation will have fragile X syndrome. Evidence indicates, however, that the FMR1 gene in the son's gametes will have the CGG triplet repeat within the premutation range, not the full mutation range like his somatic cells. Therefore, his future daughters wouldn't be expected to have fragile X syndrome.

It should be noted that most commonly the FMR1 status of a mother is subsequently determined after her son is clinically and later molecularly diagnosed with fragile X syndrome. Health care professionals need to be sensitive to the fact that the mother could either find out she's a carrier of a premutation or she has a full mutation. Consequently, not only will she learn her son's diagnosis but she, herself, could be diagnosed with fragile X if she has a full mutation and clinical symptoms.

Fragile X syndrome is estimated to occur in about 1 in 1,500 males and 1 in 2,500 females. It has been reported in almost all races and ethnic populations.

Signs and symptoms

Small children may have relatively few identifiable physical characteristics; behavioral or learning difficulties may be the initial presenting features.

Many adult male patients display a prominent jaw and forehead and a head circumference exceeding the 90th percentile. A long, narrow face with long or large ears that may be posteriorly rotated can be a helpful finding at all ages. Connective tissue abnormalities — including hyperextension of the fingers, a floppy

mitral valve (in 80% of adults), and mild to severe pectus excavatum — have also been reported. Unusually large testes, found in most affected males after puberty, are an important identifying factor of the disorder.

The average IQ of a person with fragile X syndrome is comparable to that of a person with Down syndrome; however, the behavioral characteristics are quite different. Hyperactivity, speech difficulties, language delay, and autistic-like behaviors may be attributed to other disorders, such as attention deficit hyperactivity disorder, and thus delay the diagnosis.

Approximately 50% of females with the FMR1 full mutation will have clinical symptoms, although the degree of severity and number of symptoms vary widely among females with fragile X syndrome. Those who are symptomatic typically have a much milder clinical presentation than males due to having an unaffected X chromosome in addition to the one with an FMR1 full mutation. Some degree of cognitive impairment is usually present in symptomatic females. Learning disabilities — math difficulties, language deficits, and attentional problems — are most common. Some females can have IQ scores in the mental retardation range. Although affected females can have autistic-like features, excessive shyness or social anxiety are the more common behavioral symptoms. Prominent ears and the connective tissue manifestations may be as significant as in males. Although males with the FMR1 premutation are asymptomatic, some female carriers of an FMR1 premutation can have associated symptoms. These symptoms include significantly earlier menopause and a low normal performance IQ.

Diagnosis

CONFIRMING DIAGNOSIS *Diagnosis of fragile X syndrome requires identification of clinical symptoms and a positive genetic test. DNA analysis of blood or buccal samples is used to detect the size of the CGG repeat and the methylation status of FMR1.*

A specific genetic test (polymerase chain reaction) can also be performed to diagnose this disease. This test looks for an expanded mutation (called a triplet repeat*) in the FRAXA gene.*

Before identification of the FMR1 mutation, a special cytogenetic (chromosome) blood test was used to microscopically detect the fragile site on the long arm of the affected X chromosome. It's now common knowledge that a full FMR1 mutation doesn't always result in a cytogenetically detectable fragile site. Therefore, chromosome analysis alone can provide false-negative results. Chromosome analysis still has utility together with FMR1 mutation analysis when performing a genetic evaluation on a male with mental retardation of unknown etiology.

In addition to diagnosing fragile X syndrome, genetic testing can determine whether the mother of a diagnosed individual is a carrier of the FMR1 premutation or has a full mutation. This information can be used for preconceptional genetic counseling by a trained professional and prenatal testing if the woman so chooses. FMR1 mutation analysis can also be subsequently performed on at-risk family members. It should be noted, however, that communication of genetic test results to at-risk family members constitutes a breech of patient confidentiality and privacy unless prior written permission to communicate results has been obtained from the previously tested patients.

Treatment
Fragile X syndrome has no known cure. Treatment is aimed at controlling individual symptoms. Surgery may be needed to repair a defective mitral valve.

Special considerations
■ Individuals who have been identified as carriers may experience guilt and grief; provide support to help the carrier and family members accept the diagnosis.
■ Parents of an affected child may need help to deal with their grief over unmet expectations for the child; refer them for appropriate counseling if necessary.
■ Refer the family (and possibly the extended family) to a professional trained in genetics to discuss the diagnosis, testing, and the risk of recurrence in future offspring.

■ Recurrent otitis media is common. To maximize the affected child's potential for language development, early diagnosis and aggressive treatment of otitis media are essential.
■ Throughout childhood, assess and refer the patient and his family for history of seizure activity.

 PEDIATRIC TIP *Encourage parents to enroll infants and toddlers in early intervention programs. Advocate for special education services and individualized speech, language, and occupational therapy services for this child during school years.*
■ Assess and refer for hyperactivity, attention deficit, or both.
■ The patient and his family can contact the National Fragile X Foundation for additional information and support.

CHROMOSOMAL ABNORMALITIES

Down syndrome

The first disorder attributed to a chromosome aberration, Down syndrome (trisomy 21) characteristically produces mental retardation, dysmorphic facial features, and other distinctive physical abnormalities. It's commonly associated with congenital heart defects (in approximately 60% of patients) and other abnormalities.

Life expectancy for patients with Down syndrome has increased significantly because of improved treatment for related complications (heart defects, respiratory and other infections, acute leukemia). Nevertheless, up to 44% of such patients who have congenital heart defects die before age 1 year.

Causes and incidence
Down syndrome usually results from trisomy 21, a spontaneous chromosomal abnormality in which chromosome 21 has three copies instead of the normal two because of faulty meiosis (nondisjunction) of the ovum or, sometimes, the sperm. This results in a karyotype of 47 chromosomes

instead of the normal 46. In about 4% of patients, Down syndrome results from an unbalanced translocation in which the long arm of chromosome 21 breaks and attaches to another chromosome. Most commonly, this is a robertsonian translocation and results in an increased risk of having multiple children with Down syndrome. The disorder may also be due to chromosomal mosaicism with two cell lines — one with a normal number of chromosomes (46) and one with 47 (an extra chromosome 21).

Down syndrome occurs in 1 in 660 live births, but the incidence increases with advanced parental age, especially when the mother is age 34 or older at delivery or the father is older than age 42. At age 20, a woman has about one chance in 2,000 of having a child with Down syndrome; by age 49, she has one chance in 12. However, if a woman has had one child with Down syndrome, the risk of recurrence is 1% to 2% unless the trisomy results from translocation.

Signs and symptoms

The physical signs of Down syndrome (especially hypotonia) as well as some dysmorphic facial features and heart defects may be apparent at birth. The degree of mental retardation may not become apparent until the infant grows older. People with Down syndrome typically have craniofacial anomalies, such as slanting, almond-shaped eyes with epicanthic folds; a flat face; a protruding tongue; a small mouth and chin; a single transverse palmar crease (simian crease); small white spots (Brushfield's spots) on the iris; strabismus; a small skull; a flat bridge across the nose; slow dental development, with abnormal or absent teeth; small ears; a short neck; and cataracts.

Other physical effects may include dry, sensitive skin with decreased elasticity; umbilical hernia; short stature; short extremities, with broad, flat, and squarish hands and feet; clinodactyly (small little finger that curves inward); a wide space between the first and second toe; and abnormal fingerprints and footprints. Hypotonic limb muscles impair reflex development, posture, coordination, and balance.

Congenital heart disease (septal defects or pulmonary or aortic stenosis), duodenal atresia, megacolon, and pelvic bone abnormalities are common. The incidence of leukemia and thyroid disorders (particularly hypothyroidism) may be increased. Frequent upper respiratory infections can be a serious problem. Genitalia may be poorly developed and puberty delayed. Females may menstruate and be fertile. Males are infertile with low serum testosterone levels; many have undescended testicles.

Patients with Down syndrome may have an IQ between 30 and 70; however, social performance is usually beyond that expected for mental age. The level of intellectual function depends greatly on the environment and the amount of early stimulation received in addition to the IQ.

Diagnosis

Physical findings at birth, especially hypotonia, may suggest this diagnosis, but no physical feature is diagnostic in itself.

CONFIRMING DIAGNOSIS *A karyotype showing the specific chromosomal abnormality provides a definitive diagnosis. Amniocentesis allows prenatal diagnosis and is recommended for pregnant women older than age 34 even if the family history is negative. Amniocentesis is also recommended for a pregnant woman of any age when either she or the father carries a translocated chromosome.*

Treatment

Down syndrome has no known cure. Surgery to correct heart defects and other related congenital abnormalities and antibiotic therapy for recurrent infections have improved life expectancy considerably. Plastic surgery is occasionally done to correct the characteristic facial traits, especially the protruding tongue. Benefits beyond improved appearance may include improved speech, reduced susceptibility to dental caries, and fewer orthodontic problems later. Most patients with Down syndrome are now cared for at home and attend special education classes. As adults, some may work in a sheltered workshop or live in a group home facility.

Special considerations

Support for the parents of a child with Down syndrome is vital. By following the guidelines listed below, you can help them meet their child's physical and emotional needs.

- Establish a trusting relationship with the parents, and encourage communication during the difficult period soon after diagnosis. Recognize signs of grieving.
- Teach parents the importance of a balanced diet for the child. Stress the need for patience while feeding the child, who may have difficulty sucking and may be less demanding and seem less eager to eat than normal babies.
- Encourage the parents to hold and nurture their child.
- Emphasize the importance of adequate exercise and maximum environmental stimulation; refer the parents for early intervention as soon as the diagnosis of Down syndrome is made.

 PEDIATRIC TIP *Balanced nutrition and exercise gain increased importance as the child ages. Obesity commonly becomes problematic.*

 PEDIATRIC TIP *All children with Down syndrome need to be checked for atlantoaxial instability before they engage in exercise or sports.*

- Refer the parents and older siblings for genetic and psychological counseling, as appropriate, to help them evaluate future reproductive risks. Discuss options for prenatal testing.
- Encourage the parents to remember the emotional needs of other children in the family.
- Refer the parents to national or local Down syndrome organizations and support groups such as the National Down Syndrome Congress.

Trisomy 18 syndrome

Trisomy 18 syndrome (also known as *Edwards' syndrome*) is the second most common multiple malformation syndrome. Most affected infants have *full trisomy 18*, involving an extra (third) copy of chromosome 18 in each cell, but *partial trisomy 18* (with varying phenotypes) and *transloca-*

tion types have also been reported. Most infants with this disorder present with intrauterine growth retardation, congenital heart defects, microcephaly, and other malformations.

Full trisomy 18 syndrome is generally fatal or has an extremely poor prognosis; 30% to 50% of infants with full trisomy 18 syndrome die within the first 2 months of life; 90% die within the first year. Most patients who survive exhibit profound mental retardation.

Causes and incidence

Most cases of trisomy 18 syndrome are caused by spontaneous meiotic nondisjunction. The risk of chromosomal abnormalities typically increases with maternal age; however, the mean maternal age for this disorder is 32½. Incidence is 1 in 3,000 neonates, with females three times more likely to be affected than males.

Signs and symptoms

Growth retardation begins in utero and remains significant after birth. Initial hypotonia may soon give way to hypertonia. Common findings include microcephaly and dolichocephaly, micrognathia, genital and perineal abnormalities (including imperforate anus), diaphragmatic hernia, and various renal defects. Congenital heart defects, such as ventricular septal defect, tetralogy of Fallot, transposition of the great vessels, and coarctation of the aorta, occur in 80% to 90% of patients and may be the cause of death in many infants.

Other findings may include a short and narrow nose with upturned nares; unilateral or bilateral cleft lip and palate; low-set, slightly pointed ears; a short neck; a conspicuous clenched hand with overlapping fingers (usually seen on ultrasound as well); neural tube defects; omphalocele; cystic hygroma; choroid plexus cysts (also seen in some healthy infants); and oligohydramnios.

Diagnosis

Multiple marker maternal serum screening tests involving different combinations of alpha-fetoprotein, human chorionic gonadotropin, and unconjugated estriol may be abnormal in many pregnant women with an affected fetus; however; these tests aren't diagnostic. Fetal ultrasound may reveal varying degrees of abnormalities, but many fetuses have few detectable defects. Diagnosis should be based on karyotype, done either prenatally or using peripheral blood of skin fibroblasts after birth.

Treatment
Treatment is aimed at providing comfort for the infant and emotional support for the parents. Because the infant's sucking reflex is poor, nutrition is maintained using gavage feedings. Teach parents about home care and feeding techniques.

Special considerations
■ Allow adequate time for the parents to bond with and hold their child.
■ Refer the parents to early intervention if the infant is medically stable.
■ Refer the parents of an affected child for genetic counseling to explore the cause of the disorder and discuss the risk of recurrence in a future pregnancy.
■ Refer the parents to a social worker or grief counselor for additional support if needed.
■ Refer the parents to the Support Organization for Trisomy 18, 13 and Related Disorders (S.O.F.T.) national support group to allow them interaction with other parents of infants with trisomy 18 and trisomy 13.

Trisomy 13 syndrome

Trisomy 13 syndrome (also known as *Patau's syndrome*) is the third most common multiple malformation syndrome. Most affected infants have *full trisomy 13* at birth; a few have the rare *mosaic partial trisomy 13* syndrome (with varying phenotypes) or *translocation types*. Infants with this disorder typically have brain and facial abnormalities as well as major cardiac, GI, and limb malformations. Full trisomy 13 syndrome is fatal. Many trisomic zygotes are spontaneously aborted; 50% to 70% of infants with full trisomy 13 syndrome die within 1 month after birth and 75% by the first year. Only isolated cases of survival beyond 5 years have been reported in full

trisomy 13 patients. All survivors have profound mental retardation.

Causes and incidence
Approximately 75% of all cases of trisomy 13 syndrome are caused by chromosomal nondisjunction. About 20% are due to chromosomal translocation involving a rearrangement of chromosomes 13 and 14. About 5% are estimated to be mosaics; the clinical effects in these cases may be less severe.

Incidence is estimated to be 1 in every 5,000 neonates. The risk of chromosomal abnormalities typically increases with advanced maternal age; however, the mean maternal age for this abnormality is about 31 years.

Signs and symptoms
Infants with trisomy 13 syndrome may present with microcephaly, varying degrees of holoprosencephaly, sloping forehead with wide sutures and fontanel, and a scalp defect at the vertex. Micro-ophthalmia, cataracts, and other eye abnormalities are seen in most patients with full trisomy 13. Bilateral cleft lip with associated cleft palate is seen in at least 45% of patients. Most are born with a congenital heart defect, especially hypoplastic left heart, ventricular septal defect, patent ductus arteriosus, or dextroposition, which may significantly contribute significantly to the cause of death.

Other possible findings include a flat and broad nose, low-set ears and inner ear abnormalities, polydactyly of the hands and feet, club feet, omphaloceles, neural tube defects, cystic hygroma, genital abnormalities, cystic kidneys, hydronephrosis, and musculoskeletal abnormalities. Affected infants may also experience failure to thrive, seizures, apnea, and feeding difficulties.

Diagnosis
Multiple marker maternal serum screening tests, involving different combinations of alpha-fetoprotein, human chorionic gonadotropin (HCG) or free beta-HCG in some labs, and unconjugated estriol, may be abnormal in some pregnant women with an affected fetus; however, these tests aren't diagnostic.

Ultrasound commonly reveals multiple abnormalities in the fetus; however, because many multiple malformation syndromes have similar features, the diagnosis should be based on karyotype, done either prenatally or on peripheral blood lymphocytes or skin fibroblasts in a neonate or an aborted fetus. The neonate may have a single umbilical artery at birth. Magnetic resonance imaging or a computed tomography scan of the head may reveal a structural abnormality of the brain (holoprosencephaly) where the two cerebral hemispheres are fused.

Treatment
Supportive care is the only treatment for the infant with trisomy 13 syndrome.

Special considerations
- Maintain the infant's fluid balance, and position him for comfort.
- Refer the parents to early intervention if the infant is medically stable.
- Provide the family with emotional support.
- Allow adequate time for the parents to bond with and hold their child.
- Refer the parents of an affected infant for genetic counseling to explore the cause of the disorder and to discuss the risk of recurrence in future pregnancies.
- Refer the parents to a social worker or grief counselor for additional support if needed.
- Refer the parents to the Support Organization for Trisomy 18, 13 and Related Disorders (S.O.F.T.) national support group to allow them interaction with other parents of infants with trisomy 18 and trisomy 13.

Klinefelter's syndrome

Klinefelter's syndrome is a relatively common genetic abnormality that results from an extra X chromosome. It affects only males and usually becomes apparent at puberty, when the secondary sex characteristics develop; the testicles fail to mature, and degenerative testicular changes begin that eventually result in irreversible infertility. It commonly causes gynecomastia and is also associated with a tendency toward learning disabilities.

Klinefelter's syndrome is unlike Turner's syndrome, which results from the loss of an X chromosome. (See *Turner's syndrome*, page 36.)

Causes and incidence
Klinefelter's syndrome, probably the most common cause of hypogonadism, appears in approximately 1 in every 500 males. This disorder usually results from one extra X chromosome, giving such patients a 47,XXY complement instead of the normal 46,XY. (See *Fertilization in Klinefelter's syndrome*, page 36.) In the rare mosaic form of this syndrome, some cells contain the extra X chromosomes, whereas others contain the normal XY complement.

The extra chromosome responsible for Klinefelter's syndrome probably results from either meiotic nondisjunction during parental gametogenesis or from meiotic nondisjunction in the zygote. The incidence of meiotic nondisjunction increases with maternal age.

Signs and symptoms
Klinefelter's syndrome may not be apparent until puberty or later in mild cases. Because many of these patients aren't mentally retarded, behavioral problems in adolescence or infertility may be the only presenting features initially.

The syndrome's characteristic features include a small penis and prostate gland, small testicles, sparse facial and abdominal hair, feminine distribution of pubic hair (triangular shape), sexual dysfunction (impotence, lack of libido) and, in fewer than 50% of patients, gynecomastia. Aspermatogenesis and infertility result from progressive sclerosis and hyalinization of the seminiferous tubules in the testicles and from testicular fibrosis during and after puberty. In the mosaic form of Klinefelter's syndrome, such pathologic changes and resulting infertility may be delayed.

Klinefelter's syndrome may also be associated with osteoporosis, abnormal body build (long legs with short, obese trunk), tall stature, learning disabilities characterized by poor verbal skills and, in some individuals, behavioral problems beginning

TURNER'S SYNDROME

In Turner's syndrome, one of the X chromosomes (or part of the second X chromosome) may be lost from the ovum or sperm through nondisjunction or chromosome lag. Mixed aneuploidy may result from mitotic nondisjunction.

This disorder occurs in 1 in 3,000 births; up to 95% of affected fetuses are spontaneously aborted.

Signs and symptoms

In utero, the fetus may have a cystic hygroma, seen on ultrasound; however, these may also be seen in fetuses that don't have Turner's syndrome. The mother may have elevated or low levels of serum alpha-fetoprotein.

At birth, 50% of neonates with this syndrome measure below the third percentile in length. Many have swollen hands and feet, a wide chest with laterally displaced nipples, and a low hairline that becomes more obvious as they grow. They may have webbing of the neck and coarse, enlarged, prominent ears. Gonadal dysgenesis is seen at birth and typically causes sterility in adult females (unless they have the mosaic form).

Cardiovascular defects, such as a bicuspid aortic valve and coarctation of the aorta, occur in 10% to 40% of patients. Short stature (usually under 59" [150 cm]) is the most common adult sign.

Most patients have average or slightly below-average intelligence; they commonly exhibit spatial defects, right-left disorientation for extrapersonal space, and defective figure drawing.

Diagnosis and treatment

Turner's syndrome can be diagnosed by chromosome analysis. Differential diagnosis should rule out mixed gonadal dysgenesis, Noonan's syndrome, and other similar disorders.

Treatment should begin in early childhood and may include hormonal therapy (androgens, human growth hormone and, possibly, small doses of estrogen). Later, progesterone and estrogen can induce sexual maturation, but most patients remain sterile.

FERTILIZATION IN KLINEFELTER'S SYNDROME

Fertilization by a sperm with X and Y chromosomes produces an XXY zygote.

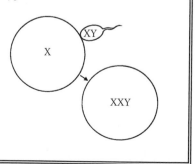

in adolescence. It's also associated with an increased incidence of pulmonary disease and varicose veins and a significantly increased rate of breast cancer because of the extra X chromosome.

Diagnosis

CONFIRMING DIAGNOSIS *Typical clinical features suggest Klinefelter's syndrome, but only a karyotype (chromosome analysis) determined by culturing lymphocytes from the patient's peripheral blood can unequivocally confirm the disorder.*

Characteristically, Klinefelter's syndrome decreases urinary 17-ketosteroid levels, increases the excretion of follicle-stimulating hormone, and decreases the levels of plasma testosterone after puberty.

Treatment

Depending on the severity of symptoms, treatment may include mastectomy in patients with persistent gynecomastia and supplemental testosterone to induce secondary sexual characteristics of puberty.

Special considerations

■ Psychological counseling may be indicated for body image problems or emotional maladjustment due to sexual dysfunction.

■ Genetic counseling is essential for patients with the mosaic form of the syndrome who are fertile; they may transmit this chromosomal abnormality as well as others.

■ Encourage patients to discuss feelings of confusion and rejection that may arise, and try to reinforce their male identity.

■ Improve compliance with hormone replacement therapy by making sure patients understand the potential benefits and adverse effects of testosterone administration.

Velocardiofacial syndrome

Velocardiofacial syndrome (VCFS) is considered a chromosomal microdeletion syndrome. Most persons with VCFS have a de novo submicroscopic deletion. However, the deletion is dominantly inherited from an affected parent in up to one-third of reported cases. The phenotype demonstrates interfamilial variability consisting of over 150 possible clinical features.

Causes and incidence

VCFS occurs in at least 1 in 5,000 live births. The syndrome is caused by a submicroscopic deletion of chromosome 22q1 1.2. In most persons with VCFS, the chromosome deletion is too small to be detected by routine chromosome analysis. Although small, the deleted region, containing 1.5 to 3 megabases, is thought to contain several genes. Neonates or infants clinically diagnosed with DiGeorge syndrome (a similar disorder) commonly test positive for a 22q1 1.2 deletion. Therefore, in most cases, persons with DiGeorge syndrome represent the severe end of the VCFS clinical spectrum.

Signs and symptoms

Clinical features of VCFS vary greatly among affected persons. Neonates with complex heart malformations, dysmorphic features, hypocalcemia, missing thymus, and renal anomalies represent the severe end of the VCFS clinical presentation. On the other hand, the clinical features can be so mild that an affected parent isn't identified until an offspring is diagnosed and genetic testing is subsequently done on the parents. Symptoms have been reported in the cardiac, craniofacial, neuropsychological, renal, ocular, neurologic, skeletal, endocrine, immune, and hematologic systems. The most common symptoms can be classified as cardiac, craniofacial, and neuropsychological.

Clinical studies indicate that 70% to 85% of persons with VCFS have cardiac anomalies, of which conotruncal defects (for example, tetralogy of Fallot, interrupted aortic arch, truncus arteriosis) are the most common. This incidence may decrease over time as persons with only mild symptoms, such as learning difficulties in school or subtle dysmorphic features, are tested and found to be deletion positive.

Craniofacial features include palatal abnormalities, dysmorphic facial features, and dysphagia usually due to velopharyngeal incompetence with or without pharyngoesophageal dysmotility. Therefore, feeding problems during infancy are common. The palate may be hypotonic and hypoplastic or have a midline cleft (ranging from bifid uvula to complete clefts of the palate). Related to palate problems are speech delays and abnormalities—particularly hypernasal speech and dyspraxia. Typical dysmorphic features include malformed ears, narrow palpebral fissures, hooded upper eyelids, ptosis, a broad square nasal root, a bulbous nasal tip (typically with a midline vertical crease), and micrognathia.

Neuropsychological symptoms are present to some degree in most persons with VCFS. Hypotonia during the neonatal stage through early childhood period has been reported in more than 75% of cases.

Even as hypotonia resolves with maturation, coordination and balance remain problematic. Cognitive symptoms, which can range from learning difficulties to varying levels of mental retardation, have been reported in over 80% of persons with VCFS. Children with VCFS typically have difficulties in visual-spatial activities, planning, attention, and concentration. Their strengths tend to be in rote verbal memory skills. Reading skills usually exceed math skills; however, reading comprehension tends to be problematic. The behavior of children with VCFS can be either shy and withdrawn or disinhibited and impulsive. Thought problems can be recognized during childhood and adolescence. Adults with VCFS are at risk for psychiatric disorders, particularly schizophrenia.

Diagnosis

Fluorescence in situ hybridization (FISH) using 22q 11.2 specific and chromosome 22 control probes is the preferred diagnostic test for VCFS and DiGeorge syndrome. Chromosome analysis with high-resolution banding detects only about one-third of affected persons. However, high-resolution chromosome analysis may be ordered in conjunction with FISH analysis for patients whose clinical presentation suggests a chromosome abnormality and 22ql 1.2 deletion is only one of several possible diagnoses in the differential.

Prenatal diagnosis is possible by performing a 22ql 1.2 FISH analysis on chorionic villi or cultured amniocytes. Prenatal diagnosis may be considered when a biologic parent is known to have a 22ql 1.2 deletion or when a level 2 prenatal ultrasound reveals anomalies that can be present in persons with VCFS. A 22ql 1.2 FISH analysis is recommended in neonates with cardiac anomalies and any one or more of the other clinical features of VCFS.

Treatment

Treatment is aimed at preventing, ameliorating, or managing symptoms.

Special considerations

- Infants with palatal abnormalities and suck and swallow coordination difficulties will likely require feeding interventions,

such as the use of cleft palate nursers and, in some cases, nasogastric or gastric tube feedings.
- Infants with heart malformations may require increased caloric intake.
- Management of heart malformations ranges from careful monitoring to multiple surgical interventions.
- Repair of cleft or abnormally functioning palate may improve hypernasal speech.
- Referral of the patient to speech pathology for evaluation of language delays or speech problems can be helpful.
- Infants may require occupational and physical therapy to minimize the developmental effects of hypotonia.

 PEDIATRIC TIP *Encourage the parents to have the child participate in early intervention programs and educational services to optimize learning abilities.*

- Designate a case manager to optimize care given by professionals from multiple disciplines and specialty areas.
- Refer the parents of an infant diagnosed with VCFS for genetic testing and counseling services.
- When providing patient and family teaching, assess for parental cognitive impairments and adjust teaching interventions accordingly.
- Anticipate, assess, and provide support for shock, denial, anger, and guilt reactions by parents discovered to have VCFS after their child's diagnosis.
- Help parents to identify and use effective coping strategies, and make referrals to mental health professionals as needed.
- Refer parents to appropriate support groups.
- Provide anticipatory guidance related to the physical, emotional, and neuropsychological effects of VCFS.

MULTIFACTORIAL ABNORMALITIES

Neural tube defects

Neural tube defects (NTDs) are serious birth defects that involve the spine or brain; they result from failure of the neural tube to close at approximately 28 days after conception. The most common forms of NTDs are spina bifida (50% of cases), anencephaly (40%), and encephalocele (10%).

Spina bifida occulta is the most common and least severe spinal cord defect. It's characterized by incomplete closure of one or more vertebrae without protrusion of the spinal cord or meninges.

However, in more severe forms of spina bifida, incomplete closure of one or more vertebrae causes protrusion of the spinal contents in an external sac or cystic lesion (spina bifida cystica). Spina bifida cystica has two classifications: myelomeningocele (meningomyelocele) and meningocele. In myelomeningocele, the external sac contains meninges, cerebrospinal fluid (CSF), and a portion of the spinal cord or nerve roots distal to the conus medullaris. When the spinal nerve roots end at the sac, motor and sensory functions below the sac are terminated. In meningocele, less severe than myelomeningocele, the sac contains only meninges and CSF. Meningocele may produce no neurologic symptoms.

In encephalocele, a saclike portion of the meninges and brain protrudes through a defective opening in the skull. Usually, it's in the occipital area, but it may occur in the parietal, nasopharyngeal, or frontal area.

In anencephaly, the most severe form of NTD, the closure defect occurs at the cranial end of the neuroaxis and, as a result, part or the entire top of the skull is missing, severely damaging the brain. Portions of the brain stem and spinal cord may be missing. No diagnostic or therapeutic efforts are helpful; this condition is invariably fatal.

Causes and incidence

NTDs may be isolated birth defects, may result from exposure to a teratogen, or may be part of a multiple malformation syndrome (for example, chromosomal abnormalities such as trisomy 18 or 13 syndrome). Isolated NTDs (those not due to a specific teratogen or associated with other malformations) are believed to be caused by a combination of genetic and environmental factors. Although most of the specific environmental triggers are unknown, recent research has identified a lack of folic acid in the mother's diet as one of the risk factors.

The incidence of NTDs varies greatly among countries and by region in the United States. For example, the incidence is significantly higher in the British Isles and low in southern China and Japan. In the United States, North and South Carolina have at least twice the incidence of NTDs as most other parts of the country. These birth defects are also less common in blacks than in whites.

Signs and symptoms

Spina bifida occulta is usually accompanied by a depression or dimple, tuft of hair, soft fatty deposits, port wine nevi, or a combination of these abnormalities on the skin over the spinal defect; however, such signs may be absent. Spina bifida occulta doesn't usually cause neurologic dysfunction but occasionally is associated with foot weakness or bowel and bladder disturbances. Such disturbances are especially likely during rapid growth phases, when the spinal cord's ascent within the vertebral column may be impaired by its abnormal adherence to other tissues.

In both myelomeningocele and meningocele, a saclike structure protrudes over the spine. Like spina bifida occulta, meningocele seldom causes neurologic deficit. But myelomeningocele, depending on the level of the defect, causes permanent neurologic dysfunction, such as flaccid or spastic paralysis and bowel and bladder incontinence. Associated disorders include trophic skin disturbances (ulcerations, cyanosis), clubfoot, knee contractures, hydrocephalus (in about 90% of patients), and possibly mental retardation, Arnold-Chiari syndrome (in which part of the brain protrudes into the spinal canal), and curvature of the spine.

Clinical effects of encephalocele vary with the degree of tissue involvement and location of the defect. Paralysis and hydrocephalus are common. Infants with this defect have a better chance of survival than anencephalic infants and usually suffer less paralysis; however, surviving infants are usually severely mentally retarded.

Diagnosis

CONFIRMING DIAGNOSIS *Amniocentesis can detect elevated alpha fetoprotein (AFP) levels in amniotic fluid, which indicates the presence of an open NTD. Measuring acetylcholinesterase levels can confirm the diagnosis. (Biochemical testing will usually miss closed NTDs.) Because 5% to 7% of NTDs are associated with chromosomal abnormalities, a fetal karyotype should be done in addition to the biochemical tests.*

Maternal serum AFP screening in combination with other serum markers, such as human chorionic gonadotropin (HCG), free beta-HCG, or unconjugated estriol, may be offered to some patients who aren't scheduled for amniocentesis, such as those with a lower risk of NTDs and those who will be younger than age 34½ at the time of delivery. Although this screening test can't diagnose either an open NTD or a chromosomal abnormality, it can estimate a fetus's risk of such a defect. Most patients with abnormal maternal serum AFP levels *won't* have an affected child; however, they may be at increased risk for perinatal complications, such as premature rupture of the membranes, abruptio placentae, or fetal death.

Ultrasound may be used when the fetus has an increased risk of an open NTD based on either the family history or abnormal serum screening results; however, this test alone can't identify all open NTDs or ventral wall defects.

If the NTD isn't diagnosed before birth, other tests are used to make the diagnosis. For example, spina bifida occulta is commonly overlooked, although it's occasionally palpable and spinal X-ray can show the bone defect. Myelography can differentiate it from other spinal abnormalities, especially spinal cord tumors.

Myelomeningocele and meningocele are obvious on examination; transillumination of the protruding sac can sometimes distinguish between them. (In meningocele, it typically transilluminates; in myelomeningocele, it doesn't.) In myelomeningocele, a pinprick examination of the legs and trunk shows the level of sensory and motor involvement; skull X-rays, cephalic measurements, and computed tomography

(CT) scan demonstrate associated hydrocephalus. Other appropriate laboratory tests in patients with myelomeningocele include urinalysis, urine cultures, and tests for renal function starting in the neonatal period and continuing at regular intervals.

In encephalocele, X-rays show a basilar bony skull defect. CT scan and ultrasonography further define the defect.

Treatment

Prompt neurosurgical repair and aggressive management may improve the condition of children with some NTDs, but serious and permanent disability is likely.

Spina bifida occulta usually requires no treatment. Treatment of meningocele consists of surgical closure of the protruding sac and continual assessment of growth and development. Treatment of myelomeningocele requires repair of the sac and supportive measures to promote independence and prevent further complications. Surgery doesn't reverse neurologic deficits. A shunt may be needed to relieve associated hydrocephalus.

Treatment of encephalocele includes surgery during infancy to place protruding tissues back in the skull, excise the sac, and correct associated craniofacial abnormalities.

Special considerations

■ When an NTD has been diagnosed prenatally, refer the prospective parents to a genetic counselor, who can provide information and support the couple's decisions on how to manage the pregnancy.

■ Recent research sponsored by the March of Dimes and others has indicated that the risk of an open NTD may be reduced 50% to 70% in pregnant women who take a daily multivitamin with folic acid. Urge all women of childbearing age to take such a vitamin supplement until menopause or the end of childbearing potential. (See *Folic acid supplement recommendations.*)

 PEDIATRIC TIP *The parents of a child with an NTD will need assistance from physicians, nurses, surgeons, rehabilitation providers, and social workers. Help to coordinate such assistance as needed. Obviously, care is most complex when the neurologic deficit is severe. Imme-*

diate goals include psychological support to help parents accept the diagnosis and preoperative and postoperative care. Long-term goals include patient and family teaching, and measures to prevent contractures, pressure ulcers, urinary tract infections (UTIs), and other complications.

Before surgery:
- Prevent local infection by cleaning the defect gently with sterile saline solution or other solutions, as ordered. Inspect the defect often for signs of infection, and cover it with sterile dressings moistened with sterile saline solution. Prevent skin breakdown by placing sheepskin or a foam pad under the infant. Keep skin clean, and apply lotion to knees, elbows, chin, and other pressure areas. Give antibiotics as ordered.
- Handle the infant carefully, and don't apply pressure to the defect. Usually, the infant can't wear a diaper or a shirt until after surgical correction because it will irritate the sac, so keep him warm in an infant Isolette. Hold and cuddle the infant; on your lap, position him on his abdomen; teach parents to do the same.
- Provide adequate time for parent-child bonding if possible.
- Measure head circumference daily, and watch for signs of hydrocephalus and meningeal irritation, such as fever or nuchal rigidity. Be sure to mark the spot so you get accurate readings.
- Contractures can be minimized by passive range-of-motion exercises and casting. To prevent hip dislocation, moderately abduct hips with a pad between the knees or with sandbags and ankle rolls.
- Monitor intake and output. Watch for decreased skin turgor, dryness, or other signs of dehydration. Provide meticulous skin care to genitals and buttocks to prevent infection.
- Ensure adequate nutrition.

After surgery:
- Watch for hydrocephalus, which commonly follows surgery. Measure the infant's head circumference as ordered.
- Monitor vital signs often. Watch for signs of shock, infection, and increased intracranial pressure (ICP) such as projectile vomiting. Frequently assess the infant's fontanels. Remember that, before age 2, infants don't show typical signs of increased

---

FOLIC ACID SUPPLEMENT RECOMMENDATIONS

The following recommendations for folic acid supplement dosages have been endorsed by the Centers for Disease Control and Prevention, the American Academy of Pediatrics, and the Spina Bifida Association of America, among other groups.

All women of childbearing age
All women who can become pregnant should consume 0.4 mg of folic acid daily to reduce their risk of having a child with spina bifida or another neural tube defect (NTD).

Women at high risk
Women with a previous pregnancy affected by an NTD should:
- receive genetic counseling before their next pregnancy
- consume 0.4 mg of folic acid daily
- when actively trying to become pregnant (at least 1 month before conception), increase their intake of folic acid to 4 mg daily and continue to take 4 mg of folic acid daily through the first 3 months of pregnancy.

ICP because suture lines aren't fully closed. In infants, the most telling sign is bulging fontanels.
- Change the dressing regularly as ordered, and check and report any signs of drainage, wound rupture, and infection.
- Place the infant in the prone position to protect and assess the site.
- If leg casts have been applied to treat deformities, watch for signs that the child is outgrowing the cast. Regularly check distal pulses to ensure adequate circulation.

To help parents cope with their infant's physical problems and successfully meet long-term treatment goals:
- Teach them to recognize early signs of complications, such as hydrocephalus, pressure ulcers, and UTIs.

- Provide psychological support and encourage a positive attitude. Help parents work through their feelings of guilt, anger, and helplessness.
- Encourage parents to begin training their child in a bladder routine by age 3. Emphasize the need for increased fluid intake to prevent UTIs. Teach intermittent catheterization and conduit hygiene, as ordered.
- To prevent constipation and bowel obstruction, stress the need for increased fluid intake, a high-bulk diet, exercise, and a stool softener, as ordered. If possible, teach parents to help empty their child's bowel by telling him to bear down, and giving a glycerin suppository as needed.
- Urge early recognition of developmental lags (a possible result of hydrocephalus). The child may need to attend a school with special facilities. Also, stress the need for stimulation to ensure maximum mental development. Help parents plan activities appropriate to their child's age and abilities. Refer to early intervention.
- Refer parents for genetic counseling, and suggest that parents consider an amniocentesis in future pregnancies. Also refer parents to the Spina Bifida Association of America.

Cleft lip and cleft palate

Cleft lip and cleft palate — an opening in the lip or palate — may occur separately or in combination. These deformities originate in the second month of pregnancy, when the front and sides of the face and the palatine shelves fuse imperfectly. Cleft deformities usually occur unilaterally or bilaterally, rarely midline. Only the lip may be involved, or the defect may extend into the upper jaw or nasal cavity.

Cleft lip and cleft palate occur in twice as many males as females; isolated cleft palate is more common in females.

Causes and incidence
Cleft lip or palate most commonly occurs as an isolated birth defect. Isolated cleft lip with or without cleft palate and cleft palate only are the result of a disruption in the normal development of the orofacial structures. This disruption in development is thought to be the result of a combination of genetic and environmental factors. Cleft lip or cleft palate may also occur as part of a chromosomal or Mendelian syndrome (cleft defects are associated with over 300 syndromes). Exposures to specific teratogens during fetal development may also produce these defects.

Cleft lip with or without cleft palate occurs in approximately 1 in 1,000 births among Whites; the incidence is higher in Asians (1.7 in 1,000) and Native Americans (over 3.6 in 1,000) but lower in Blacks (1 in 2,500).

A family history of cleft defects increases the risk of a couple having a child with a cleft defect. Likewise, an individual with a cleft defect is at an increased risk for having a child with a cleft defect. Children with cleft defects and their parents or adult individuals should be referred for genetic counseling for accurate diagnosis of cleft type and recurrence risk counseling. Recurrence risk information is based on family history, the presence or absence of other physical or cognitive traits within a family, and prenatal exposure information.

Signs and symptoms
Orofacial cleft defects are divided into two major groups: cleft lip with or without cleft palate or cleft palate only. Cleft of the lip may involve the alveolus (premaxilla) and may extend through the palate (hard and soft). Congenital clefts of the face occur most commonly in the upper lip. They can range from a simple notch to a complete cleft from the lip edge, through the floor of the nostril and through the alveolus. Cleft lip can occur on either or both sides of the midline but rarely along the midline itself. A cleft lip involving only one side is a *unilateral* cleft lip, and a cleft on both sides of the midline is a *bilateral* cleft lip. When a bilateral cleft lip involves clefting of the alveolus on both sides of the premaxilla, the premaxilla is separated from the maxilla into a freely moving segment.

A cleft of the palate only may be partial or complete, involving only the soft palate or extending from the soft palate complete-

VARIATIONS OF CLEFT LIP AND CLEFT PALATE

The illustration below shows the four variations of cleft lip and cleft palate.

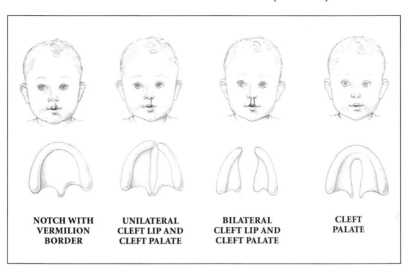

| NOTCH WITH VERMILION BORDER | UNILATERAL CLEFT LIP AND CLEFT PALATE | BILATERAL CLEFT LIP AND CLEFT PALATE | CLEFT PALATE |

ly through the hard palate. A cleft palate can occur alone or with a cleft lip. Isolated cleft palate is more commonly associated with congenital defects other than isolated cleft lip with or without cleft palate. (See *Variations of cleft lip and cleft palate.*) The constellation of U-shaped cleft palate, mandibular hypoplasia, and glossoptosis is known as Pierre Robin syndrome, or Robin syndrome. Robin syndrome can occur as an isolated defect or one feature of many different syndromes; therefore, a comprehensive genetic evaluation is suggested for infants with Robin syndrome. Because of the mandibular hypoplasia and glossoptosis, careful evaluation and management of the airway are mandatory for infants with Robin syndrome.

Diagnosis

A typical clinical picture confirms the diagnosis. Cleft lip with or without cleft palate is obvious at birth; occasionally, more severe defects may be seen with diagnostic prenatal ultrasonography. Cleft palate without cleft lip may not be detected until a mouth examination is done or until feeding difficulties develop.

Treatment

Treatment consists of surgical correction, but the timing of surgery varies. Some plastic surgeons repair cleft lips within the first few days of life to make feeding the baby easier. However, many surgeons delay lip repairs for 8 to 10 weeks (sometimes as long as 6 to 8 months) to allow the infant to grow and mature, thereby minimizing surgical and anesthesia risks, ruling out associated congenital anomalies, and allowing time for parental bonding. Cleft palate repair is usually completed by the 12th to 18th month. Still other surgeons repair cleft palates in two steps, repairing the soft palate between ages 6 and 18 months and the hard palate as late as age 5 years. In any case, surgery is performed only after the infant is gaining weight and infection-free.

Surgery must be coupled with speech therapy. Because the palate is essential to speech formation, structural changes, even in a repaired cleft, can permanently affect speech patterns. To compound the problem, children with cleft palates commonly have hearing difficulties because of middle ear damage or infections.

Special considerations

■ Recent research has indicated that ingestion of 0.4 mg of folic acid twice daily before conception *may* decrease the risk of isolated cleft defects.

 ALERT *Never place a child with Robin syndrome on his back because his tongue could fall back and obstruct his airway. Place these infants on their side for sleeping. Most other infants with a cleft palate can sleep on their backs without difficulty.*

■ Maintain adequate nutrition to ensure normal growth and development. Experiment with feeding devices. A baby with a cleft palate has an excellent appetite but often has trouble feeding because of air leaks around the cleft and nasal regurgitation. He usually feeds better from a bottle and nipple designed specifically for feeding infants with cleft defects. These bottles come with special nipples or regular nipples with enlarged holes and may be used with cleft palate bottles.

Teach the parents how best to feed the infant. Advise them to hold the infant in a near-sitting position, with the flow directed to the side or back of the baby's tongue. Tell them to burp the baby frequently because he tends to swallow a lot of air. If the underside of the nasal septum becomes ulcerated and the child refuses to suck because of the pain, instruct the parents to direct the nipple to the side of his mouth to give the mucosa time to heal. Tell them to gently clean the palatal cleft with a cotton-tipped applicator dipped in half-strength hydrogen peroxide or water after each feeding.

■ Encourage the mother of a baby with cleft lip to breast-feed if the cleft doesn't prevent effective sucking. Breast-feeding an infant with a cleft palate or one who has just had corrective surgery usually isn't possible. (Postoperatively, the infant can't suck for 6 to 10 weeks.) However, if the mother desires, suggest that she use a breast pump to express breast milk and then feed it to her baby from a bottle.

■ Following surgery, record intake and output and maintain good nutrition. To prevent atelectasis and pneumonia, the physician may gently suction the nasopharynx (this may be necessary before surgery, too). Restrain the infant to prevent him from hurting himself. Elbow restraints allow the baby to move his hands while keeping them away from his mouth. When necessary, use an infant seat to keep the child in a comfortable sitting position. Hang toys within reach of restrained hands.

■ Surgeons sometimes place a curved metal bow over a repaired cleft lip to minimize tension on the suture line. Remove the gauze before feedings, and replace it often. Moisten it with normal saline solution until the sutures are removed. Check your hospital policy to confirm this procedure.

■ Help the parents deal with their feelings about the child's disability. Start by telling them about it and showing them their baby as soon as possible. Because society places undue importance on physical appearance, many parents feel shock, disappointment, and guilt when they see the child. Help them by being calm and providing positive information.

Direct the parents' attention to their child's assets. Stress the fact that surgical repairs can be made. Include the parents in the care and feeding of the child right from the start to encourage normal bonding. Provide the instructions, emotional support, and reassurance that the parents will need to take proper care of the child at home.

■ Refer the parents to a social worker who can guide them to community resources, if needed, and to a genetic counselor to determine the recurrence risk. Refer the family to the American Cleft Palate-Craniofacial Association for information and support.

Selected references

Allen, P.J., et al., eds. *Primary Care of the Child with a Chronic Condition,* 4th ed. St. Louis: Mosby–Year Book, Inc., 2003.

De Santis, M., et al. "Hemangiomas and Other Congenital Malformations in Infants Exposed to Antiretroviral Therapy In Utero," *JAMA* 291(3):305, January 2004.

Elles, R., and Mountford, R., eds. *Molecular Diagnosis of Genetic Diseases,* 2nd ed. Totowa, N.J.: Humana Press, 2004.

Hamptom, T. "Physicians Apply Genome Research To Treat Critical Illness and Injury," *JAMA* 291(3):287-88, January 2004.

Hatfield, N. *Broadribb's Introductory Pediatric Nursing,* 6th ed. Philadelphia: Lippincott Williams & Wilkins, 2003.

Haws, P.S. *Care of the Sick Neonate: Quick Reference for Health Care Providers.* Philadelphia: Lippincott Williams & Wilkins, 2004.

Jorde, L.B., et al. *Medical Genetics,* 3rd ed. St. Louis: Mosby–Year Book, Inc., 2003.

Milunsky, A., ed. *Genetic Disorders and the Fetus: Diagnosis, Prevention, and Treatment,* 5th ed. Baltimore: Johns Hopkins University Press, 2004.

Minkovitz, C.S., et al. "A Practice-based Intervention To Enhance Quality of Care in the First 3 Years of Life: The Healthy Steps for Young Children Program," *JAMA* 290(23): 3081-91, December 2003.

White, L. *Essentials of Maternal and Pediatric Nursing.* Albany, N.Y.: Delmar Pubs., 2002.

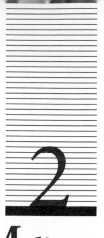

Malignant neoplasms

Introduction *47*

Head, neck, and spine *56*
Malignant brain tumors *56*
Pituitary tumors *62*
Laryngeal cancer *64*
Thyroid cancer *67*
Malignant spinal neoplasms *70*

Thorax *72*
Lung cancer *72*
Breast cancer *76*

Abdomen and pelvis *82*
Gastric cancer *82*
Esophageal cancer *85*
Pancreatic cancer *87*
Colorectal cancer *91*
Kidney cancer *94*
Liver cancer *96*
Bladder cancer *98*
Gallbladder and bile duct cancer *101*

Male and female genitalia *103*
Prostatic cancer *103*
Testicular cancer *105*
Penile cancer *107*
Cervical cancer *108*
Uterine cancer *112*
Vaginal cancer *115*

Ovarian cancer *117*
Cancer of the vulva *120*
Fallopian tube cancer *122*

Bone, skin, and soft tissue *123*
Primary malignant bone tumors *123*
Multiple myeloma *127*
Basal cell epithelioma *129*
Squamous cell carcinoma *130*
Malignant melanoma *132*
Kaposi's sarcoma *136*

Blood and lymph *138*
Hodgkin's disease *138*
Non-Hodgkin's lymphoma *141*
Mycosis fungoides *143*
Acute leukemia *144*
Chronic granulocytic leukemia *147*
Chronic lymphocytic leukemia *149*

Selected references *150*

COMPARING BENIGN AND MALIGNANT TUMORS

Factor	Benign	Malignant
Differentiation	Well differentiated	Variable
Effect on body	Cachexia rare; usually not fatal but may obstruct vital organs, exert pressure, produce excess hormones; can become malignant	Cachexia typical, with such symptoms as anemia, loss of weight, and weakness; fatal if untreated
Growth	Slow expansion; push aside surrounding tissue but don't infiltrate	Usually infiltrate surrounding tissues rapidly, expanding in all directions
Limitation	Commonly encapsulated	Seldom encapsulated; in many cases poorly delineated
Mitotic activity	Variable	Extensive
Morphology	Cells closely resemble cells of tissue of origin	Cells may differ considerably from those of tissue of origin
Recurrence	Rare after surgical removal	When removed only by surgery, commonly recur due to infiltration into surrounding tissues
Spread	No metastasis	Spread via blood and lymph systems; establish secondary tumors
Tissue destruction	Usually slight	Extensive due to infiltration and metastatic lesion

Introduction

Primarily a disease of older adults, cancer is second only to cardiovascular disease as the leading cause of death in the United States (more than 560,000 deaths annually). More than 67% of patients who die of cancer are older than age 65. The most common cancers in the United States are prostate, breast, lung, and colorectal.

Cancer results from a malignant transformation (carcinogenesis) of normal cells. A characteristic feature of cancer cells is their ability to proliferate uncontrollably, thus establishing themselves at other tissues to form secondary foci (metastasis). Additionally, cancer cells serve no useful purpose. (See *Comparing benign and malignant tumors.*) Cancer cells metastasize via the circulation through the blood or lymphatics, by unintentional transplantation from one site to another during surgery, and by local extension. (See *How cancer metastasizes,* pages 48 and 49.)

Classified by their histologic origin, tumors derived from epithelial tissues are called carcinomas; from epithelial and glandular tissues, adenocarcinomas; from connective, muscle, and bone tissues, sarcomas; from glial cells, gliomas; from pigmented cells, melanomas; and from plasma cells, myelomas. Cancer cells derived from erythrocytes are known as *erythroleukemia;* from lymphocytes, *leukemia;* and from lymphatic tissue, *lymphoma.*

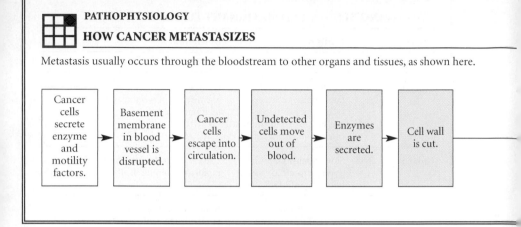

Metastasis usually occurs through the bloodstream to other organs and tissues, as shown here.

| Cancer cells secrete enzyme and motility factors. | → | Basement membrane in blood vessel is disrupted. | → | Cancer cells escape into circulation. | → | Undetected cells move out of blood. | → | Enzymes are secreted. | → | Cell wall is cut. |

What causes cancer?

Researchers have found that cancer develops from mutations within the genes of cells. Thus, cancer is a genetic disease. Cancer susceptibility genes are of two types. Some are *oncogenes,* which activate cell division and influence embryonic development, and some are *tumor suppressor genes,* which halt cell division.

These genes are typically found in normal human cells, but certain kinds of mutations may transform the normal cells. Inherited defects may cause a *genetic mutation,* whereas exposure to a carcinogen may cause an *acquired mutation.* Current evidence indicates that carcinogenesis results from a complex interaction of carcinogens and accumulated mutations in several genes.

In animal studies of the ability of viruses to transform cells, some human viruses exhibit carcinogenic potential. For example, the Epstein-Barr virus, the cause of infectious mononucleosis, has been linked to Burkitt's lymphoma and nasopharyngeal cancer.

High-frequency radiation, such as ultraviolet and ionizing radiation, damages the genetic material known as *deoxyribonucleic acid (DNA),* possibly inducing genetically transferable abnormalities. Other factors, such as a person's tissue type and hormonal status, interact to potentiate radiation's carcinogenic effect. Examples of substances

that may damage DNA and induce carcinogenesis include:
- alkylating agents — leukemia
- aromatic hydrocarbons and benzopyrene (from polluted air) — lung cancer
- asbestos — mesothelioma of the lung
- tobacco — cancer of the lung, oral cavity and upper airways, esophagus, pancreas, kidneys, and bladder
- vinyl chloride — angiosarcoma of the liver.

Diet has also been implicated, especially in the development of GI cancer as a result of a high animal fat diet. Additives composed of nitrates and certain methods of food preparation — particularly charbroiling — are also recognized factors.

The role of hormones in carcinogenesis is still controversial, but it seems that excessive use of some hormones, especially estrogen, produces cancer in animals. Also, the synthetic estrogen diethylstilbestrol causes vaginal cancer in some daughters of women who were treated with it. It's unclear, however, whether changes in human hormonal balance retard or stimulate cancer development.

Some forms of cancer and precancerous lesions result from genetic predisposition either directly (as in Wilms' tumor and retinoblastoma) or indirectly (in association with inherited conditions such as Down syndrome or immunodeficiency diseases). Expressed as autosomal recessive,

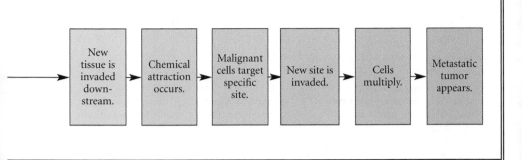

| New tissue is invaded downstream. | Chemical attraction occurs. | Malignant cells target specific site. | New site is invaded. | Cells multiply. | Metastatic tumor appears. |

X-linked, or autosomal dominant disorders, their common characteristics include:
- early onset of malignant disease
- increased incidence of bilateral cancer in paired organs (breasts, adrenal glands, kidneys, and eighth cranial nerve [acoustic neuroma])
- increased incidence of multiple primary malignancies in nonpaired organs
- abnormal chromosome complement in tumor cells.

Immune response

Other factors that interact to increase susceptibility to carcinogenesis are immunologic competence, age, nutritional status, hormonal balance, and response to stress. Theoretically, the body develops cancer cells continuously, but the immune system recognizes them as foreign cells and destroys them. This defense mechanism, known as *immunosurveillance*, has two major components: humoral immune response and cell-mediated immune response. Their interaction promotes antibody production, cellular immunity, and immunologic memory. Presumably, the intact human immune system is responsible for spontaneous regression of tumors.

Theoretically, the *cell-mediated immune response* begins when T lymphocytes become sensitized by contact with a specific antigen. After repeated contacts, sensitized T cells release chemical factors called *lymphokines,* some of which begin to destroy the antigen. This reaction triggers the transformation of an additional population of T lymphocytes into "killers" of antigen-specific cells — in this case, cancer cells.

Similarly, the *humoral immune response* reacts to an antigen by triggering the release of antibodies from plasma cells and activating the serum-complement system, which destroys the antigen-bearing cell. However, an opposing immune factor, a "blocking antibody," enhances tumor growth by protecting malignant cells from immune destruction.

Theoretically, cancer arises when any one of several factors disrupts the immune system:
- Aging cells, when copying their genetic material, may begin to err, giving rise to mutations. The aging immune system may not recognize these mutations as foreign and thus may allow them to proliferate and form a malignant tumor.
- Cytotoxic drugs decrease antibody production and destroy circulating lymphocytes.
- Extreme stress or certain viral infections can depress the immune system.
- Increased susceptibility to infection commonly results from radiation, cytotoxic drug therapy, and lymphoproliferative and myeloproliferative diseases, such as lymphatic and myelocytic leukemia. These cause bone marrow depression, which can impair leukocyte function.
- Acquired immunodeficiency syndrome weakens cell-mediated immunity.

- Cancer itself is immunosuppressive; advanced cancer exhausts the immune response. (The absence of immune reactivity is known as *anergy*.)

Diagnostic methods

A thorough medical history and physical examination should precede sophisticated diagnostic procedures. Useful tests for the early detection and staging of tumors include X-ray, endoscopy, isotope scan, computed tomography scan, and magnetic resonance imaging, but the single most important diagnostic tool is a biopsy for direct histologic study of tumor tissue. Biopsy tissue samples can be taken by curettage, fluid aspiration (pleural effusion), fine-needle aspiration biopsy (breast), dermal punch (skin or mouth), endoscopy (rectal polyps), and surgical excision (visceral tumors and nodes).

An important tumor marker, carcinoembryonic antigen (CEA), although not diagnostic by itself, can signal malignancies of the large bowel, stomach, pancreas, lungs, and breasts. CEA titers range from normal (less than 5 ng) to suspicious (5 to 10 ng) to suspect (over 10 ng). CEA serves many valuable purposes:
- as a baseline during chemotherapy to evaluate the extent of tumor spread
- to regulate drug dosage
- to prognosticate after surgery or radiation
- to detect tumor recurrence.

Although no more specific than CEA, alpha-fetoprotein — a fetal antigen uncommon in adults — can suggest testicular, ovarian, gastric, and hepatocellular cancers. Beta human chorionic gonadotropin may point to testicular cancer or choriocarcinoma. Other commonly used tumor markers include prostate-specific antigen to detect and monitor prostatic cancer, and CA-125, useful for monitoring ovarian, colorectal, and gastric cancers.

Staging and grading

Choosing effective therapeutic options depends on correct *staging* of malignant disease, commonly with the internationally known TNM staging system (*t*umor size, *n*odal involvement, *m*etastatic progress). This classification system provides an accu-

rate tumor description that's adjustable as the disease progresses. TNM staging allows reliable comparison of treatments and survival rates among large population groups; it also identifies nodal involvement and metastasis to other areas.

Grading, another way to define a tumor, classifies the lesion according to corresponding normal cells, such as lymphoid or mucinous lesions; it compares tumor tissue to normal cells (differentiation); and it estimates the tumor's growth rate. For example, a low-grade tumor typically has cells more closely resembling normal cells, whereas a high-grade tumor has poorly differentiated cells.

Five major therapies

Cancer treatments include surgery, radiation, chemotherapy, biotherapy (also called *immunotherapy*), and hormonal therapy. Therapies may be used alone or in combination, depending on the type, stage, localization, and responsiveness of the tumor and on limitations imposed by the patient's clinical status.

Surgery, once the mainstay of cancer treatment, is usually combined with other therapies. Surgery may be performed as a biopsy to obtain tissue for study; as continued surgery to remove the bulk of the tumor; or before chemotherapy or radiation to debulk the tumor in hope of a better outcome. Surgery can be curative as well.

Later, other therapies may be used to discourage proliferation of residual cells. Surgery can also relieve pain, correct obstruction, and alleviate pressure. Today's less radical surgical procedures (such as lumpectomy instead of radical mastectomy) are more acceptable to patients.

Radiation therapy aims to destroy the dividing cancer cells while damaging nonmalignant cells as little as possible. Therapeutic radiation is either particulate or electromagnetic. Both types ionize matter and have cellular DNA as their target.

Radiation treatment approaches include external beam radiation and intracavitary and interstitial implants. The latter therapy requires personal radiation protection for all staff members who come in contact with the patient.

Normal and malignant cells respond to radiation differently, depending on blood supply, oxygen saturation, previous irradiation, and immune status. Generally, normal cells recover from radiation faster than malignant cells. The success of the treatment and damage to normal tissue also vary with the intensity of the radiation. Although a large single dose of radiation has greater cellular effects than fractions of the same amount delivered sequentially, a protracted schedule allows time for normal tissue to recover in the intervals between individual sublethal doses.

Radiation may be used palliatively to relieve pain, obstruction, malignant effusions, cough, dyspnea, ulcerations, and hemorrhage; it can also promote the repair of pathologic fractures after surgical stabilization and delay tumor spread.

Combining radiation and surgery can minimize radical surgery, prolong survival, and preserve anatomic function. For example, preoperative doses of radiation shrink a tumor, making it operable, while preventing further spread of the disease during surgery. After the wound heals, postoperative doses prevent residual cancer cells from multiplying or metastasizing.

Systemic adverse effects, such as weakness, fatigue, anorexia, nausea, vomiting, and anemia, may subside with antiemetics, steroids, frequent small meals, fluid maintenance, and rest. They are seldom severe enough to require discontinuing radiation but may require a dosage adjustment. (For localized adverse effects, see *Radiation's adverse effects,* page 52.)

Radiation therapy involves frequent blood counts (particularly of white blood cells and platelets), especially if the target site involves areas of bone marrow production. Radiation also requires special skin care, such as covering the irradiated area with loose cotton clothing and avoiding deodorants, colognes, and other topical agents during treatment. (See *How to prepare the patient for external radiation therapy,* page 53.)

Chemotherapy includes a wide array of drugs, which may induce regression of a tumor and its metastasis. It's particularly useful in controlling residual disease and, as an adjunct to surgery or radiation thera-

py, it can induce long remissions and sometimes effect cures, especially in patients with childhood leukemia, Hodgkin's disease, choriocarcinoma, or testicular cancer. As a palliative treatment, chemotherapy aims to improve the patient's quality of life by temporarily relieving pain and other symptoms.

Some major chemotherapeutic agents include:

■ alkylating agents and nitrosoureas, which inhibit cell growth and division by reacting with DNA

■ antimetabolites, which prevent cell growth by competing with metabolites in the production of nucleic acid

■ antitumor antibiotics, which block cell growth by binding with DNA and interfering with DNA-dependent ribonucleic acid synthesis

■ plant alkaloids, which prevent cellular reproduction by disrupting cell mitosis

■ steroid hormones, which inhibit the growth of hormone-susceptible tumors by changing their chemical environment.

The adverse effects of chemotherapy vary. Antineoplastic agents, toxic to cancer cells, can also cause transient changes in normal tissues, especially among proliferating body cells. For example, antineoplastic agents typically suppress bone marrow, causing anemia, leukopenia, and thrombocytopenia; irritate GI epithelial cells, causing nausea and vomiting; and destroy the cells of the hair follicles and skin, causing alopecia and dermatitis. Some chemotherapy drugs can also have permanent effects such as peripheral neuropathy.

Some I.V. chemotherapy drugs are irritants; others are vesicants. Irritants can cause pain at the injection site and along the vein but usually don't cause tissue necrosis. However, vesicants, extravasated, may cause deep cutaneous necrosis requiring debridement and skin grafting. (*Note:* Most drugs with the potential for direct tissue injury are now given through a central venous catheter.)

Therefore, all patients undergoing chemotherapy need special care:

■ Watch for any signs of infection, especially if the patient is receiving simultaneous radiation treatment. Be alert for even a low-grade fever when the granulocyte

RADIATION'S ADVERSE EFFECTS

Area radiated	Effect	Management
Abdomen and pelvis	Cramps, diarrhea, nausea	Administer loperamide and diphenoxylate with atropine. Provide a low-residue diet. Maintain fluid and electrolyte balance. Administer antiemetics as ordered.
Chest	Esophagitis	Give pain medication. Provide total parenteral nutrition or tube feedings. Maintain fluid balance.
	Lung tissue irritation, persistent nonproductive cough	Tell the patient to stop smoking and to avoid people with upper respiratory infections. Provide steroid therapy as ordered. Provide humidifier if necessary. Administer cough suppressants as ordered.
	Pericarditis, myocarditis	Control arrhythmias with appropriate agents, such as procainamide, disopyramide, and phosphate. Monitor for heart failure.
Head and neck	Alopecia	Gently comb and groom scalp. Use a soft head covering.
	Dental caries	Apply fluoride to teeth prophylactically, and provide gingival care.
	Mucositis	Provide a non-alcohol-based mouthwash with viscous lidocaine; cool carbonated drinks; ice pops; and a soft, nonirritating diet. Use soft toothbrushes or swabs. Avoid spicy food and alcohol.
	Xerostomia (dry mouth)	Encourage good oral hygiene. Consider prescribing an oral saliva replacement. Moist foods are better tolerated than dry foods.
Kidneys	Nephritis, lassitude, headache, edema, dyspnea, hypertensive nephropathy, azotemia, anemia	Maintain fluid and electrolyte balance, and watch for signs of renal failure. Consider prescribing erythropoietin.

count falls below 500/µl; take the patient's temperature often.
- Increase the patient's fluid intake before and throughout chemotherapy.
- Inform the patient of possible temporary hair loss, and reassure him that his hair should grow back after therapy ends. Suggest a wig or other head covering, and

encourage the patient to purchase it before the hair loss.
- Check skin for petechiae, ecchymoses, chemical cellulitis, and secondary infection during treatment.
- Minimize tissue irritation and damage by checking needle placement before and during infusion if you administer the drug by a peripheral vein. Tell the patient to re-

port any discomfort during infusion. If a vesicant extravasates, stop the infusion, aspirate the drug from the needle, and give the appropriate antidote if available.

Chemotherapeutic drugs can be given orally, subcutaneously, I.M., I.V., intracavitarily, intrathecally, intraperitoneally, topically, intralesionally, and by arterial infusion, depending on the drug and its pharmacologic action; usually, administration is intermittent to allow for bone marrow recovery between doses. Dosages are calculated according to the patient's body surface area, with adjustments for general condition, degree of myelosuppression, and weight changes. When calculating dosage, make sure your information is current because dosages change periodically.

Because many patients approach chemotherapy with apprehension, allow them to express their concerns, and provide simple and truthful information. Explain that not all patients who undergo chemotherapy experience nausea and vomiting and, for those who do, antiemetic drugs, relaxation therapy, and diet can minimize these problems.

Biotherapy (also known as *immunotherapy*) relies on treatment agents known as biological response modifiers. Biological agents are usually combined with chemotherapeutic drugs or radiation therapy. Much of the work done in biotherapy is still experimental. However, the Food and Drug Administration has approved several new drugs, which are providing promising results. For example, rituximab — a monoclonal antibody — is effective for treatment of relapsed or refractory B-cell non-Hodgkin's lymphoma.

The main biotherapy agent classifications include *interferons, interleukins, hematopoietic growth factors,* and *monoclonal antibodies.* Interferons have antiviral, antiproliferative, and immunomodulary effects. The interleukins exert their effects on the T lymphocytes. Monoclonal antibodies such as rituximab provide the most tumor-specific therapy for cancer by selectively binding to tumor cell surfaces.

Although not used to treat cancer directly, hematopoietic growth factors are used to increase the patient's blood counts when

> ## HOW TO PREPARE THE PATIENT FOR EXTERNAL RADIATION THERAPY
>
> ■ Show the patient where radiation therapy takes place, and introduce him to the radiation therapist.
> ■ Tell him to remove all metal objects (pens, buttons, jewelry) that may interfere with therapy. Explain that the areas to be treated will be marked with indelible ink and that *he must not scrub these areas* because it's important to radiate the same areas each time.
> ■ Reinforce the physician's explanation of the procedure, and answer any questions as honestly as you can. If you don't know the answer to a question, refer the patient to the physician.
> ■ Teach the patient to watch for and report any adverse effects. Because radiation therapy may increase susceptibility to infection, warn him to avoid people with colds or other infections during therapy. However, emphasize the benefits (such as outpatient treatment) instead of the adverse effects.
> ■ Reassure the patient that treatment is painless and won't make him radioactive. Stress that he'll be under constant surveillance during radiation administration and should call out if he needs anything.

chemotherapy or radiation causes a decrease.

The adverse effects of biotherapeutic agents mimic the body's normal immune response with flulike symptoms being the most common.

Hormonal therapy is based on studies showing that certain hormones affect the growth of certain cancer types. For example, the gonadotropin-releasing hormone analogue leuprolide is used to treat prostate cancer. With long-term use, this hormone inhibits testosterone release and tumor growth, and tamoxifen, an anti-estrogen hormonal agent, blocks estrogen receptors in breast tumor cells that require estrogen to thrive. Additionally, tamoxifen can be given prophylactically to women at high risk for breast cancer.

Hormone-receptive tumors may be treated with aromatase inhibitors (anastro-zole, exemestane, letrozole, testolactone), which inhibit the conversion of adrenal androgens to estrogens, thereby inhibiting the growth of hormone-dependent tumors.

Some adverse effects of these hormonal agents include hot flashes, sweating, impotence, decreased libido, nausea and vomiting, and blood dyscrasias (with tamoxifen).

Maintaining nutrition and fluid balance

Tumors grow at the expense of normal tissue by competing for nutrients; consequently, the cancer patient commonly suffers protein deficiency. Cancer treatments themselves produce fluid and electrolyte disturbances, such as vomiting and anorexia. Maintaining adequate nutrition, fluid intake, and electrolyte balance should be a major focus in cancer care.
- Obtain a comprehensive dietary history to pinpoint nutritional problems and their past causes such as diabetes; help plan the diet accordingly.
- Ask the dietitian to provide a liquid diet high in proteins, carbohydrates, and calories if the patient can't tolerate solid foods. If the patient has stomatitis, provide soft, bland, nonirritating foods.
- Encourage the patient's family to bring foods from home, if he requests.
- Make mealtime as relaxed and pleasant as possible. Encourage the patient to dine with visitors or other patients. Allow choices from a varied menu.
- With the physician's approval, you may suggest that the patient drink a glass of wine before dinner to stimulate the appetite and aid relaxation.
- Encourage the patient to drink eight 8-oz (236.6 ml) glasses of noncaffeinated liquids per day. Urge him to drink juice or other caloric beverages instead of water.
- Suggest small, frequent meals if he can't tolerate normal ones.
- Avoid strong-smelling foods.

If the patient can't eat

The patient who has had recent head, neck, or GI surgery or who has pain when swallowing can receive nourishment through a nasogastric (NG) tube. If the patient still needs to use the tube after he's discharged, teach him how to insert it, how to test its position in his stomach by aspirating stomach contents, and how to use it to feed himself.

If an NG tube isn't appropriate, other alternatives are gastrostomy, jejunostomy and, occasionally, esophagostomy. These procedures make it possible for you to feed the patient prescribed protein formulas and semiliquids, such as cream soups and eggnog; they also make it easier for the patient to feed himself.

Remember to forewarn the patient that if spilled gastric or intestinal juices come in contact with the abdominal skin, they'll cause excoriation if they aren't washed off immediately. Always flush the tube well with water following each feeding.

Also, to provide adequate hydration, instill about 4 to 6 oz (118 to 177.5 ml) of water or another clear liquid between meals.

After jejunostomy, begin with small feedings, slowly and carefully increasing the amounts. Provide additional fluids and calories during these days of limited food intake by supplementing jejunostomy feedings with I.V. fat emulsions.

Total parenteral nutrition

Commonly considered an important component of cancer care if the patient can't tolerate enteral nutrition, total parenteral nutrition (TPN) can improve a severely debilitated patient's protein balance. In doing so, TPN characteristically strengthens and conditions the patient, allowing him to better tolerate treatment.

TPN can produce a slight weight gain in the patient receiving radiation therapy, provide optimum nutrition for wound healing, and help the patient combat infection after radical surgery.

Pain control critical

Typically, cancer patients have a great fear of overwhelming pain. Therefore, controlling pain is a major consideration at every

PATIENT-CONTROLLED ANALGESIA SYSTEM

The patient-controlled analgesia (PCA) system is an option for pain treatment in cancer care. It's typically used in the postoperative clinical setting, where I.V. pain management is needed for acute intervention. This system permits the patient to self-administer a premeasured dose of analgesic by pressing a button at the bedside that activates a pump fitted with a prefilled syringe containing the analgesic. Small, intermittent doses of the analgesic administered I.V. maintain blood levels that ensure comfort and minimize the risk of oversedation. The physician or the nursing staff presets doses and time intervals (usually 8 to 10 minutes) that allow the patient to determine his comfort level. The syringe is locked inside the pump as a safety feature, and the system will only dispense the analgesic until the correct (preset) time interval has elapsed.

Clinical studies report that patients on PCA tend to titrate analgesic drugs effectively and maintain comfort without oversedation. They also tend to use less of the drug than the amount normally given by I.M. injection.

PCA provides other significant advantages:
- Patients are alert and active during the day.
- Patients no longer need to suffer pain while awaiting their injections.
- Patients are free from pain caused by injections.
- The nursing staff is free for other clinical duties.

stage of managing cancer — from localized cancer to advanced metastasis. In cancer patients, pain may result from inflammation of or pressure on pain-sensitive structures, tumor infiltration of nerves or blood vessels, or metastatic extension to bone. Such chronic and unrelenting pain can wear down the patient's tolerance to treatment, interfere with eating and sleeping, and color his life with anger, despair, and anxiety.

Opioid analgesics — either alone or in combination with nonopioid analgesics, antianxiety agents, or tricyclic antidepressants — are the mainstay of pain relief in patients with advanced cancer. In terminal stages of cancer, effective opioid dosages may be quite high because drug tolerance invariably develops. Provide such analgesics generously. Anticipate the need for pain relief, and provide it on a schedule that doesn't allow pain to break through. Don't wait to relieve pain until it becomes severe. Reassure the patient that you'll provide pain medication whenever he needs it. (See *Patient-controlled analgesia system.*)

Nonpharmacologic pain-relief techniques can be used alone or, more commonly, in combination with drug therapy. Popular techniques include cutaneous stimulation, relaxation, biofeedback, distraction, and guided imagery.

Surgical excision of the tumor can relieve pressure on sensitive tissues and pain caused by inflamed necrotic tissue; treatment with antibiotics can combat inflammation; radiation therapy can shrink metastatic tissue and control bone pain. When a tumor invades nerve tissue, effective pain control requires anesthetics, destructive nerve blocks, electronic nerve stimulation with a dorsal column or transcutaneous electrical nerve stimulator, rhizotomy, or chordotomy.

The hospice approach

A holistic approach to patient care modeled after St. Christopher's Hospice in London, hospice care provides comprehensive physical, psychological, social, and spiritual care for terminally ill patients. Although some hospices are located in inpatient settings, most hospice programs serve terminally ill patients amid the more familiar and relaxed surroundings of their own home.

The goal of the hospice care team is to help the patient achieve as full a life as possible, with minimal pain, discomfort, and restriction. Of the many medications provided for pain control, morphine is considered the drug of choice.

Hospice care also emphasizes a coordinated team effort to help the patient and family members overcome the severe anxiety, fear, and depression that occur with terminal illness. As a means to this end, hospice staffs encourage family members to help with the patient's care, thereby providing the patient with warmth and security and helping the family caregivers begin the grieving process before the patient dies.

Everyone involved in this method of care must be committed to high-quality patient care, unafraid of emotional involvement, and comfortable with personal feelings about death and dying. Good hospice care also requires open communication among team members, not just for evaluating patient care but also for helping the staff cope with their own feelings.

Psychological aspects

No illness evokes as profound an emotional response as the diagnosis of cancer. Patients express this response in several ways. A few face this difficult reality from the outset of diagnosis and treatment. Many use denial as a coping mechanism and simply refuse to accept the truth, but this stance is increasingly difficult for them to maintain. As evidence of the tumor becomes inescapable, the patient may experience clinical depression. Family members may express denial in attempts to cope by encouraging unproven methods of cancer treatment, which can delay effective care. Some patients cope by intellectualizing about their disease, enabling them to obscure the reality of the cancer and regard it as unrelated to themselves. Generally, intellectualization is a more productive coping behavior than denial because the patient is receiving treatment. Be aware of the possible behavioral responses so you can identify them and then interact supportively with the patient and his family. For many malignancies, you can offer realistic hope for long-term survival or remission; even in advanced disease, you can offer short-term achievable goals. To help a patient cope with cancer, make sure you understand your own feelings about it. Then listen sensitively to the patient so you can offer genuine understanding and support. When caring for a patient with terminal cancer, increase your effectiveness by seeking out someone to help you through your own grieving.

HEAD, NECK, AND SPINE

Malignant brain tumors

Primary malignant brain tumors account for about 10% to 30% of adult cancers. These tumors may occur at any age. The most common tumor types in adults are gliomas and meningiomas, which usually occur supratentorially (above the covering of the cerebellum). In children, incidence is generally highest before age 12, affecting 3 out of every 100,000 children; more than 1,200 new cases occur each year. The most common types in children are astrocytomas, medulloblastomas, ependymomas, and brain stem gliomas. In children, brain tumors of the central nervous system (CNS) account for 20% of all childhood cancers; they're similar in incidence to leukemias.

Causes and incidence

The cause of most brain tumors is unknown, but exposure to ionizing radiation is a known environmental risk. Additionally, most malignant tumors of the brain are of metastatic origin; 20% to 40% of patients with cancer develop brain metastasis.

Signs and symptoms

Brain tumors cause CNS changes by invading and destroying tissues and by secondary effect — mainly compression of the brain, cranial nerves, and cerebral vessels; cerebral edema; and increased intracranial pressure (ICP). (See *Comparing malignant brain tumors*.) Generally, clinical features result from increased ICP; these features vary with the type of tumor, its location,

COMPARING MALIGNANT BRAIN TUMORS

Tumor	Clinical features
Astrocytoma ■ Second most common malignant glioma (approximately 30% of all gliomas) ■ Occurs at any age; incidence higher in males ■ Usually occurs in white matter of cerebral hemispheres; may originate in any part of the central nervous system ■ Cerebellar astrocytomas usually confined to one hemisphere	*General* ■ Headache; mental activity changes ■ Decreased motor strength and coordination ■ Seizures; scanning speech ■ Altered vital signs *Localizing* ■ Third ventricle: changes in mental activity and level of consciousness, nausea, pupillary dilation and sluggish light reflex; later — paresis or ataxia ■ Brain stem and pons: early — ipsilateral trigeminal, abducens, and facial nerve palsies; later — cerebellar ataxia, tremors, other cranial nerve deficits ■ Third or fourth ventricle or aqueduct of Sylvius: secondary hydrocephalus ■ Thalamus or hypothalamus: various endocrine, metabolic, autonomic, and behavioral changes
Ependymoma ■ Rare glioma ■ Most common in children and young adults ■ Usually locates in fourth and lateral ventricles	*General* ■ Similar to oligodendroglioma ■ Increased intracranial pressure (ICP) and obstructive hydrocephalus, depending on tumor size
Glioblastoma multiforme *(spongioblastoma multiforme)* ■ Peak incidence at 50 to 60 years; twice as common in males; most common glioma ■ Unencapsulated, highly malignant; grows rapidly and infiltrates the brain extensively; may become enormous before diagnosed ■ Usually occurs in cerebral hemispheres, especially frontal and temporal lobes (rarely in brain stem and cerebellum) ■ Occupies more than one lobe of affected hemisphere; may spread to opposite hemisphere by corpus callosum; may metastasize into cerebrospinal fluid (CSF), producing tumors in distant parts of the nervous system	*General* ■ Increased ICP, nausea, vomiting, headache, papilledema ■ Mental and behavioral changes ■ Altered vital signs (increased systolic pressure; widened pulse pressure, respiratory changes) ■ Speech and sensory disturbances ■ In children, irritability, projectile vomiting *Localizing* ■ Midline: headache (bifrontal or bioccipital); worse in the morning; intensified by coughing, straining, or sudden head movements ■ Temporal lobe: psychomotor seizures ■ Central region: focal seizures ■ Optic and oculomotor nerves: visual defects ■ Frontal lobe: abnormal reflexes, motor responses

(continued)

COMPARING MALIGNANT BRAIN TUMORS *(continued)*

Tumor	Clinical features
Medulloblastoma • Rare glioma • Incidence highest in children ages 4 to 6 • Affects males more commonly than females • Commonly metastasizes via CSF	*General* • Increased ICP *Localizing* • Brain stem and cerebrum: papilledema, nystagmus, hearing loss, flashing lights, dizziness, ataxia, paresthesia of face, cranial nerve palsies (V, VI, VII, IX, X, primarily sensory), hemiparesis, suboccipital tenderness; compression of supratentorial area produces other general and focal signs and symptoms
Meningioma • Most common nongliomatous brain tumor (15% of primary brain tumors) • Peak incidence among 50-year-olds; rare in children; more common in females (ratio 3:2) • Arises from the meninges • Common locations include parasagittal area, sphenoidal ridge, anterior part of the base of the skull, cerebellopontile angle, spinal canal • Benign, well-circumscribed, highly vascular tumors that compress underlying brain tissue by invading overlying skull	*General* • Headache • Seizures (in two-thirds of patients) • Vomiting • Changes in mental activity • Similar to schwannomas *Localizing* • Skull changes (bony bulge) over tumor • Sphenoidal ridge, indenting optic nerve: unilateral visual changes and papilledema • Prefrontal parasagittal: personality and behavioral changes • Motor cortex: contralateral motor changes • Anterior fossa compressing both optic nerves and frontal lobes: headaches and bilateral vision loss • Pressure on cranial nerves causing varying symptoms
Oligodendroglioma • Third most common glioma • Occurs in middle adult years; more common in women • Slow-growing	*General* • Mental and behavioral changes • Decreased visual acuity and other vision disturbances • Increased ICP *Localizing* • Temporal lobe: hallucinations, psychomotor seizures • Central region: seizures (confined to one muscle group or unilateral) • Midbrain or third ventricle: pyramidal tract symptoms (dizziness, ataxia, paresthesia of the face) • Brain stem and cerebrum: nystagmus, hearing loss, dizziness, ataxia, paresthesias of the face, cranial nerve palsies, hemiparesis, suboccipital tenderness, loss of balance

COMPARING MALIGNANT BRAIN TUMORS *(continued)*

Tumor	Clinical features

Schwannoma
(acoustic neurinoma, neurilemoma, cerebellopontile angle tumor)

- Accounts for approximately 10% of all intracranial tumors
- Higher incidence in women
- Onset of symptoms between ages 30 and 60
- Affects the craniospinal nerve sheath, usually cranial nerve (CN) VIII; also, V and VII and, to a lesser extent, VI and X on the same side as the tumor
- Benign, but commonly classified as malignant because of its growth patterns; slow-growing — may be present for years before symptoms occur

General
- Unilateral hearing loss with or without tinnitus
- Stiff neck and suboccipital discomfort
- Secondary hydrocephalus
- Ataxia and uncoordinated movements of one or both arms due to pressure on brain stem and cerebellum

Localizing
- CN V: early — facial hypoesthesia or paresthesia on side of hearing loss; unilateral loss of corneal reflex
- CN VI: diplopia or double vision
- CN VII: paresis progressing to paralysis (Bell's palsy)
- CN X: weakness of palate, tongue, and nerve muscles on same side as tumor

---

and the degree of invasion. (See *What happens in increased ICP*, page 60.) Onset of symptoms is usually insidious, and brain tumors are commonly misdiagnosed.

Diagnosis

 CONFIRMING DIAGNOSIS *In many cases, a definitive diagnosis follows a tissue biopsy performed by stereotactic surgery. In this procedure, a head ring is affixed to the skull, and an excisional device is guided to the lesion by a computed tomography (CT) scan or magnetic resonance imaging (MRI).*

Other diagnostic tools include a patient history, a neurologic assessment, skull X-rays, a brain scan, a CT scan, MRI, and cerebral angiography. An EEG may reveal focal abnormalities. Lumbar puncture shows increased pressure and protein levels, decreased glucose levels and, occasionally, tumor cells in cerebrospinal fluid (CSF).

Treatment

Treatment includes removing a resectable tumor; reducing a nonresectable tumor; relieving cerebral edema, increased ICP, and other symptoms; and preventing further neurologic damage.

The mode of therapy depends on the tumor's histologic type, radiosensitivity, and location and may include surgery, radiation, chemotherapy, or decompression of increased ICP with diuretics, corticosteroids, or possibly ventriculoatrial or ventriculoperitoneal shunting of CSF.

A glioma usually requires resection by craniotomy, followed by radiation therapy and chemotherapy. The combination of nitrosoureas (carmustine [BCNU], lomustine [CCNU], or procarbazine) and postoperative radiation is more effective than radiation alone.

Surgical resection of low-grade cystic cerebellar astrocytomas brings long-term survival. Treatment of other astrocytomas includes repeated surgery, radiation therapy, and shunting of fluid from obstructed CSF pathways. Some astrocytomas are highly radiosensitive, but others are radioresistant.

Treatment of oligodendrogliomas and ependymomas includes resection and radiation therapy; for medulloblastomas, resection and possibly intrathecal infusion of methotrexate or another antineoplastic drug. Meningiomas require resection, including dura mater and bone (operative

PATHOPHYSIOLOGY
WHAT HAPPENS IN INCREASED ICP

Increased intracranial pressure (ICP) is the force exerted within the intact skull by intracranial volume: about 10% blood, 10% cerebrospinal fluid (CSF), and 80% brain tissue and water. The rigid skull allows little space for expansion of these substances. When ICP increases dramatically, brain damage can result.

The brain compensates for increases by regulating the volume of the three substances by limiting blood flow to the head, displacing CSF into the spinal canal, and increasing absorption or decreasing production of CSF. When compensatory mechanisms become overworked, small changes in volume lead to large changes in pressure.

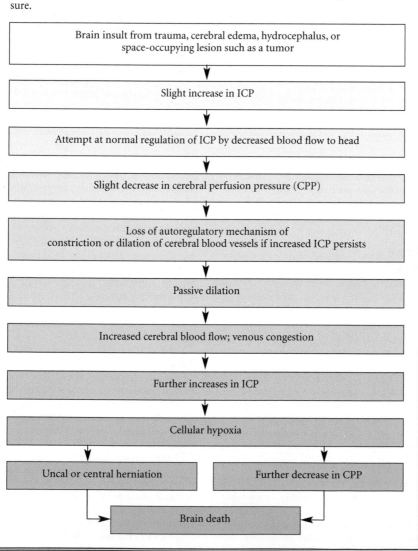

mortality may reach 10% because of large tumor size).

For schwannomas, microsurgical technique allows complete resection of the tumor and preservation of facial nerves. Although schwannomas are moderately radioresistant, postoperative radiation therapy is necessary.

Chemotherapy for malignant brain tumors includes the nitrosoureas that help break down the blood-brain barrier and allow other chemotherapeutic drugs to go through as well. Intrathecal and intraarterial administration of drugs maximizes drug actions.

Palliative measures for gliomas, astrocytomas, oligodendrogliomas, and ependymomas include dexamethasone for cerebral edema; osmotic diuretics, such as urea and mannitol, to reduce brain swelling; analgesics to control pain; and antacids and histamine receptor antagonists for stress ulcers. These tumors and schwannomas may also require anticonvulsants such as phenytoin to reduce seizures.

Special considerations
A patient with a brain tumor requires comprehensive neurologic assessment, teaching, and supportive care. During your first contact with the patient, perform a comprehensive assessment (including a complete neurologic evaluation) to provide baseline data and to help develop your care plan. Obtain a thorough health history concerning onset of symptoms. Help the patient and his family cope with the treatment, potential disabilities, and changes in lifestyle resulting from his tumor.

Throughout hospitalization:
- Carefully document seizure activity (occurrence, nature, and duration).
- Maintain airway patency.
- Monitor patient safety.
- Administer anticonvulsive drugs as ordered.
- Check continuously for changes in neurologic status, and watch for an increase in ICP.

ALERT *Watch for and immediately report sudden unilateral pupillary dilation with loss of light reflex; this is an ominous change that indicates imminent transtentorial herniation.*

- Monitor respiratory changes carefully (abnormal respiratory rate and depth may point to rising ICP or herniation of the cerebellar tonsils from expanding infratentorial mass).
- Monitor temperature carefully. Fever commonly follows hypothalamic anoxia but might also indicate meningitis. Use hypothermia blankets preoperatively and postoperatively to keep the patient's temperature down and minimize cerebral metabolic demands.
- Administer steroids and osmotic diuretics such as mannitol as ordered to reduce cerebral edema. Fluids may be restricted to 1,500 ml/24 hours. Monitor fluid and electrolyte balance to avoid dehydration.
- Observe and report signs and symptoms of stress ulcers: abdominal distention, pain, vomiting, and tarry stools. Administer antacids as ordered.

Surgery requires additional nursing care. After craniotomy, continue to monitor general neurologic status and watch for signs of increased ICP, such as an elevated bone flap and typical neurologic changes. To reduce the risk of increased ICP, restrict fluids to 1,500 ml/24 hours. To promote venous drainage and reduce cerebral edema after supratentorial craniotomy, elevate the head of the patient's bed about 30 degrees. Position him on his side to allow drainage of secretions and prevent aspiration. As appropriate, instruct the patient to avoid Valsalva's maneuver or isometric muscle contractions when moving or sitting up in bed; these can increase intrathoracic pressure and thereby increase ICP. Withhold oral fluids, which may provoke vomiting and consequently raise ICP.

After infratentorial craniotomy, keep the patient flat for 48 hours, but logroll him every 2 hours to minimize complications of immobilization. Prevent other complications by paying careful attention to ventilatory status and to cardiovascular, GI, and musculoskeletal functions.

- Radiation therapy is usually delayed until after the surgical wound heals, but it can induce wound breakdown even then, so observe the wound carefully for infection and sinus formation. Because radiation may cause brain inflammation, watch for signs of rising ICP.

■ Because the nitrosoureas — BCNU, CCNU, and procarbazine — used as adjuncts to radiotherapy and surgery can cause delayed bone marrow depression, tell the patient to watch for and immediately report any signs of infection or bleeding that appear within 4 weeks after the start of chemotherapy. Before chemotherapy, give prochlorperazine or another antiemetic, as ordered, to minimize nausea and vomiting.

■ Teach the patient and his family signs of recurrence; urge compliance with treatment regimen.

■ Because brain tumors may cause residual neurologic deficits that disable the patient physically or mentally, begin rehabilitation early. Consult with occupational and physical therapists to encourage independence in daily activities and improve the quality of life. As necessary, provide aids for self-care and mobilization, such as bathroom rails for the wheelchair patient. If the patient is aphasic, arrange for consultation with a speech pathologist.

■ Legal advice is helpful in forming advance directives such as power of attorney in cases where continued physical or intellectual decline is likely.

■ Refer the patient for counseling and to national and local support groups to help him cope with this disorder.

Pituitary tumors

Pituitary tumors, which constitute 10% of intracranial malignant neoplasms, usually originate in the anterior pituitary (adenohypophysis). They occur in adults of both sexes, usually during the 3rd and 4th decades of life. The three tissue types of pituitary tumors are chromophobe adenoma (90%), basophil adenoma, and eosinophil adenoma.

The prognosis for patients with this type of tumor is fair to good, depending on the extent to which the tumor spreads beyond the sella turcica.

Causes and incidence

Although the exact cause is unknown, a predisposition to pituitary tumors may be inherited through an autosomal dominant trait. Pituitary tumors aren't malignant in the strict sense but, because their growth is invasive, they're considered a neoplastic disease.

Chromophobe adenoma may be associated with production of corticotropin, melanocyte-stimulating hormone, growth hormone (GH), and prolactin; basophil adenoma, with evidence of excess corticotropin production and, consequently, with signs of Cushing's syndrome; eosinophil adenoma, with excessive GH.

Pituitary tumors develop in 1 in 10,000 people. About 15% of tumors located within the skull are pituitary tumors.

Signs and symptoms

As pituitary adenomas grow, they replace normal glandular tissue and enlarge the sella turcica, which houses the pituitary gland. The resulting pressure on adjacent intracranial structures produces these typical clinical manifestations:

Neurologic:

■ frontal headache

■ visual symptoms, beginning with blurring and progressing to field cuts (hemianopias) and then unilateral blindness

■ cranial nerve involvement (III, IV, VI) from lateral extension of the tumor, resulting in strabismus; double vision, with compensating head tilting and dizziness; conjugate deviation of gaze; nystagmus; lid ptosis; and limited eye movements

■ increased intracranial pressure (ICP) (secondary hydrocephalus)

■ personality changes or dementia, if the tumor breaks through to the frontal lobes

■ seizures

■ rhinorrhea, if the tumor erodes the base of the skull

■ pituitary apoplexy secondary to hemorrhagic infarction of the adenoma. Such hemorrhage may lead to both cardiovascular and adrenocortical collapse.

Endocrine:

■ hypopituitarism, to some degree, in all patients with adenoma, becoming more obvious as the tumor replaces normal gland tissue (signs and symptoms include amenorrhea, decreased libido and impotence in men, skin changes [waxy appearance, decreased wrinkles, and pigmenta-

tion], loss of axillary and pubic hair, lethargy, weakness, increased fatigability, intolerance to cold, and constipation [because of decreased corticotropin and thyroid-stimulating hormone production])
- addisonian crisis, precipitated by stress and resulting in nausea, vomiting, hypoglycemia, hypotension, and circulatory collapse
- diabetes insipidus, resulting from extension to the hypothalamus
- prolactin-secreting adenomas (in 70% to 75%), with amenorrhea and galactorrhea
- GH-secreting adenomas, with acromegaly
- corticotropin-secreting adenomas, with Cushing's syndrome.

Diagnosis
- Skull X-rays with tomography show enlargement of the sella turcica or erosion of its floor; if GH secretion predominates, X-rays show enlarged paranasal sinuses and mandible, thickened cranial bones, and separated teeth.
- Carotid angiogram shows displacement of the anterior cerebral and internal carotid arteries if the tumor mass is enlarging; it also rules out intracerebral aneurysm.
- Computed tomography scan may confirm the existence of the adenoma and accurately depict its size.
- Cerebrospinal fluid (CSF) analysis may show increased protein levels.
- Endocrine function tests may contribute helpful information, but results are commonly ambiguous and inconclusive.
- Magnetic resonance imaging differentiates healthy, benign, and malignant tissues as well as arteries and veins.

Treatment
Surgical options include transfrontal removal of large tumors impinging on the optic apparatus and transsphenoidal resection for smaller tumors confined to the pituitary fossa. (See *Transsphenoidal pituitary surgery.*)

Radiation is the primary treatment for small, nonsecretory tumors that don't extend beyond the sella turcica or for patients who may be poor postoperative risks; otherwise, it's an adjunct to surgery.

TRANSSPHENOIDAL PITUITARY SURGERY

This illustration shows the placement of the bivalve speculum and rongeur for pituitary gland removal.

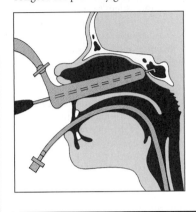

Postoperative treatment includes hormone replacement with cortisone, thyroid, and sex hormones; correction of electrolyte imbalance; and, as necessary, insulin therapy.

Drug therapy may include bromocriptine, an ergot derivative that shrinks prolactin- and GH-secreting tumors. Cyproheptadine, an antiserotonin drug, can reduce increased corticosteroid levels in the patient with Cushing's syndrome.

Adjuvant radiation therapy is used when only partial removal of the tumor is possible. Cryohypophysectomy (freezing the area with a probe inserted by transsphenoidal route) is a promising alternative to surgical dissection of the tumor.

Special considerations
- Conduct a comprehensive health history and physical assessment to establish the onset of neurologic and endocrine dysfunction and provide baseline data for later comparison.
- Establish a supportive, trusting relationship with the patient and his family to assist them in coping with the diagnosis, treatment, and potential long-term changes. Make sure they understand that

POSTCRANIOTOMY CARE

- Monitor vital signs (especially level of consciousness), and perform a baseline neurologic assessment from which to plan further care and assess the patient's progress.
- Maintain the patient's airway; suction as necessary.
- Monitor intake and output carefully.
- Give the patient nothing by mouth for 24 to 48 hours to prevent aspiration and vomiting, which increases intracranial pressure.
- Observe for cerebral edema, bleeding, and leakage of cerebrospinal fluid.
- Provide a restful, quiet environment.

the patient needs lifelong evaluations and, possibly, hormone replacement.
- Reassure the patient that some of the distressing physical and behavioral signs and symptoms caused by pituitary dysfunction (for example, altered sexual drive, impotence, infertility, loss of hair, and emotional instability) will disappear with treatment.
- Maintain a safe, clutter-free environment for the visually impaired or acromegalic patient. Reassure him that he'll probably recover his sight.
- Position patients who have undergone supratentorial or transsphenoidal hypophysectomy with the head of the bed elevated about 30 degrees to promote venous drainage from the head and reduce cerebral edema. Place the patient on his side to allow drainage of secretions and prevent aspiration.
- Withhold oral fluids, which can cause vomiting and subsequent increased ICP. Don't allow a patient who has had transsphenoidal surgery to blow his nose. Watch for CSF drainage from the nose. Monitor for signs of infection from the contaminated upper respiratory tract. Make sure the patient understands that he'll lose his sense of smell.

- Regularly compare the patient's postoperative neurologic status with your baseline assessment. (See *Postcraniotomy care.*)
- Monitor intake and output to detect fluid and electrolyte imbalances.
- Before discharge, encourage the patient to purchase and wear a medical identification bracelet or necklace that identifies his hormone deficiencies and their proper treatment.

Laryngeal cancer

The most common form of laryngeal cancer is squamous cell cancer (95%); rare forms include adenocarcinoma, sarcoma, and others. Such cancer may be intrinsic or extrinsic. An *intrinsic* tumor is on the true vocal cord and doesn't tend to spread because underlying connective tissues lack lymph nodes. An *extrinsic* tumor is on some other part of the larynx and tends to spread early.

Causes and incidence
In laryngeal cancer, major predisposing factors include smoking and alcoholism; minor factors include chronic inhalation of noxious fumes and familial tendency. Cancer of the larynx rarely occurs in nonsmokers.

Laryngeal cancer is classified according to its location:
- supraglottis (false vocal cords)
- glottis (true vocal cords)
- subglottis (downward extension from vocal cords [rare]).

The ratio of male to female incidence is 3.8:1. Most victims are between ages 50 and 65.

Signs and symptoms
In intrinsic laryngeal cancer, the dominant and earliest symptom is hoarseness that persists longer than 3 weeks; in extrinsic cancer, it's a lump in the throat or pain or burning in the throat when drinking citrus juice or hot liquid. Later clinical effects of metastasis include dysphagia, dyspnea, cough, enlarged cervical lymph nodes, and pain radiating to the ear.

Diagnosis

Any hoarseness that lasts longer than 2 weeks requires visualization of the larynx by laryngoscopy. (See *Staging laryngeal cancer,* pages 66 and 67.)

CONFIRMING DIAGNOSIS *Firm diagnosis also requires xeroradiography, biopsy, laryngeal tomography, computed tomography scan, or laryngography to define the borders of the lesion and chest X-ray to detect metastasis.*

Treatment

Early lesions are treated with surgery or radiation; advanced lesions with surgery, radiation, and chemotherapy. In early stages, laser surgery can excise precancerous lesions; in advanced stages it can help relieve obstruction caused by tumor growth. Surgical procedures vary with tumor size and can include cordectomy, partial or total laryngectomy, supraglottic laryngectomy, or total laryngectomy with laryngoplasty. The treatment goal is to eliminate the cancer and preserve speech. If speech preservation isn't possible, speech rehabilitation may include esophageal speech or prosthetic devices; surgical techniques to construct a new voice box are still experimental.

Special considerations

Provide psychological support and good preoperative and postoperative care to minimize complications and speed recovery.

Before partial or total laryngectomy:
- Instruct the patient to maintain good oral hygiene. If appropriate, instruct a male patient to shave off his beard.
- Encourage the patient to express his concerns before surgery. Help him choose a temporary nonspeaking communication method (such as writing).
- If appropriate, arrange for a laryngectomee to visit him. Explain postoperative procedures (suctioning, nasogastric [NG] feeding, laryngectomy tube care) and their results (breathing through neck, speech alteration). Also prepare him for other functional losses: He won't be able to smell, blow his nose, whistle, gargle, sip, or suck on a straw.

After partial laryngectomy:
- Give I.V. fluids and, usually, tube feedings in the initial postoperative period; then resume oral fluids. Keep the tracheostomy tube (inserted during surgery) in place until edema subsides.
- Keep the patient from using his voice until he has medical permission (usually 2 to 3 days postoperatively). Then caution him to whisper until healing is complete.

After total laryngectomy:
- As soon as the patient returns to his bed, place him on his side and elevate his head 30 to 45 degrees. When you move him, remember to support his neck.
- The patient will probably have a laryngectomy tube in place until his stoma heals (about 7 to 10 days). This tube is shorter and thicker than a tracheostomy tube but requires the same care. Watch for crusting and secretions around the stoma, which can cause skin breakdown. To prevent crust formation, provide adequate room humidification. Remove crusting with petroleum jelly, antimicrobial ointment, and moist gauze.
- Teach stoma care.
- Watch for and report complications: fistula formation (redness, swelling, secretions on suture line), carotid artery rupture (bleeding), and tracheostomy stenosis (constant shortness of breath). A fistula may form between the reconstructed hypopharynx and the skin. This eventually heals spontaneously but may take weeks or months. Carotid artery rupture usually occurs in patients who have had preoperative radiation, particularly those with a fistula that constantly bathes the carotid artery with oral secretions. If carotid rupture occurs, apply pressure to the site; call for help immediately and take the patient to the operating room for carotid ligation. Tracheostomy stenosis occurs weeks to months after laryngectomy; treatment includes fitting the patient with successively larger tracheostomy tubes until he can tolerate insertion of a large one. If the patient has a fistula, feed him through an NG tube; otherwise, food will leak through the fistula and delay healing. Monitor vital signs (be especially alert for fever, which indicates infection). Record fluid intake and output, and watch for dehydration.
- Give frequent mouth care.

STAGING LARYNGEAL CANCER

The TNM (tumor, node, metastasis) classification system developed by the American Joint Committee on Cancer describes laryngeal cancer stages and guides treatment. The T stages cover supraglottic, glottic, and subglottic tumors.

Primary tumor
TX — primary tumor unassessible
T0 — no evidence of primary tumor
Tis — carcinoma in situ

Supraglottic tumor stages
T1 — tumor confined to one subsite in supraglottis; vocal cords retain motion
T2 — tumor extends to other sites in supraglottis or to glottis; vocal cords retain motion
T3 — tumor confined to larynx, but vocal cords lose motion; or tumor extends to the postcricoid area, the pyriform sinus, or the pre-epiglottic space, and vocal cords lose motion; or both
T4 — tumor extends through thyroid cartilage or extends to tissues beyond the larynx (such as the oropharynx or soft tissues of the neck) or both
T4a — tumor invades through the thyroid cartilage or invades tissues beyond the larynx (trachea, soft tissues of neck including deep extrinsic muscle of the tongue, strap muscles, thyroid, or esophagus)
T4b — tumor invades prevertebral space, encases carotid artery, or invades mediastinal structures

Glottic tumor stages
T1 — tumor confined to vocal cords, which retain normal motion; may involve anterior or posterior commissures

T2 — tumor extends to supraglottis or subglottis or both; vocal cords may lose motion
T3 — tumor confined to larynx, but vocal cords lose motion
T4 — tumor extends through thyroid cartilage or extends to tissues beyond the larynx (such as the oropharynx or soft tissues of the neck) or both
T4a — tumor invades through the thyroid cartilage or invades tissues beyond the larynx (trachea, soft tissues of neck including deep extrinsic muscle of the tongue, strap muscles, thyroid, or esophagus) or both
T4b — tumor invades prevertebral space, encases carotid artery, or invades mediastinal structures.

Subglottic tumor stages
T1 — tumor confined to subglottis
T2 — tumor extends to vocal cords; vocal cords may lose motion
T3 — tumor confined to larynx with vocal cord fixation
T4 — tumor extends through cricoid or thyroid cartilage or extends to tissues beyond the larynx, or both
T4a — tumor invades through the thyroid cartilage or invades tissues beyond the larynx (trachea, soft tissues of neck including deep extrinsic muscle of the tongue, strap muscles, thyroid, or esophagus) or both
T4b — tumor invades prevertebral space, encases carotid artery, or invades mediastinal structures

---

■ Suction gently; unless ordered otherwise. Don't attempt deep suctioning, which could penetrate the suture line. Suction through both the tube and the patient's nose because the patient can no longer blow air through his nose; suction his mouth gently.

■ After insertion of a drainage catheter (usually connected to a wound-drainage system or a GI drainage system), don't stop suction without the physician's consent. After catheter removal, check dressings for drainage.
■ Give analgesics as ordered.

tion of Laryngectomees and other sources of support.
- Support the patient through the grieving process. If the depression seems severe, consider a psychiatric referral.

Regional lymph nodes
NX — regional lymph nodes can't be assessed
N0 — no evidence of regional lymph node metastasis
N1 — metastasis in a single ipsilateral lymph node, 3 cm or less in greatest dimension
N2 — metastasis in one or more ipsilateral lymph nodes, or in bilateral or contralateral nodes, larger than 3 cm but less than 6 cm in greatest dimension
N3 — metastasis in a node larger than 6 cm in greatest dimension

Distant metastasis
MX — distant metastasis unassessible
M0 — no evidence of distant metastasis
M1 — distant metastasis

Staging categories
Laryngeal cancer progresses from mild to severe as follows:
STAGE 0 — Tis, N0, M0
STAGE I — T1, N0, M0
STAGE II — T2, N0, M0
STAGE III — T3, N0, M0; T1, N1, M0; T2, N1, M0; T3, N1, M0
STAGE IVA — T4, N0, M0; T4, N1, M0; Any T, N2, M0
STAGE IVB — any T, N3, M0
STAGE IVC — any T, any M, MI

- If the patient has an NG feeding tube, check tube placement and elevate the patient's head to prevent aspiration.
- Reassure the patient that speech rehabilitation may help him speak again. Encourage contact with the International Associa-

Thyroid cancer

Papillary and follicular carcinomas are the most common types of thyroid cancer and are usually associated with a longer survival. Papillary carcinoma accounts for half of all thyroid cancers in adults; it's most common in young adult females and metastasizes slowly. It's the least virulent form of thyroid cancer. Follicular carcinoma is less common but more likely to recur and metastasize to the regional nodes and through blood vessels into the bones, liver, and lungs. Medullary carcinoma originates in the parafollicular cells derived from the last branchial pouch and contains amyloid and calcium deposits. It can produce calcitonin, histaminase, corticotropin (producing Cushing's syndrome), and prostaglandin E_2 and F_3 (producing diarrhea). This rare form of thyroid cancer is familial, associated with pheochromocytoma, and completely curable when detected before it causes symptoms. Untreated, it progresses rapidly. Seldom curable by resection, anaplastic tumors resist radiation and metastasize rapidly.

Causes and incidence
Predisposing factors to thyroid cancer include radiation exposure (especially childhood radiation therapy), prolonged thyroid-stimulating hormone (TSH) stimulation (through radiation or heredity), familial predisposition, or chronic goiter.
Thyroid cancer occurs in all age-groups, especially in people who have had radiation treatment of the neck area. It affects 1 in 1,000 people.

Signs and symptoms
The primary signs of thyroid cancer are a painless nodule, a hard nodule in an enlarged thyroid gland, or palpable lymph nodes with thyroid enlargement. Eventual-

STAGING THYROID CANCER

The classification and staging systems adopted by the American Joint Committee on Cancer describe thyroid cancer according to the tumor's (T) size and extent at its origin, its invasion of regional (cervical and upper mediastinal) lymph nodes (N), and the disease's metastasis (M) to other structures.

Primary tumor

TX — primary tumor can't be assessed

T0 — no evidence of primary tumor

T1 — tumor 2 cm or less in greatest dimension and limited to the thyroid

T2 — tumor more than 2 cm but less than 4 cm in greatest dimension and limited to the thyroid

T3 — tumor more than 4 cm in greatest dimension and limited to the thyroid or any tumor with minimal extrathyroid extension, such as extension to the sternothyroid muscle or perithyroid soft tissues

T4a — tumor of any size extending beyond the thyroid capsule to invade subcutaneous soft tissues, larynx, trachea, esophagus, or recurrent laryngeal nerve

T4b — tumor invades prevertebral facia or encases carotid artery or mediastinal vessels (All anaplastic carcinomas are considered T4 tumors.)

Regional lymph nodes

NX — regional lymph nodes can't be assessed

N0 — no evidence of regional lymph node metastasis

N1 — regional lymph node metastasis

N1a — metastasis to level IV (pretracheal, paratracheal, prelaryngeal, and Delphian lymph nodes)

N1b — metastasis to unilateral, bilateral, or contralateral cervical or superior mediastinal lymph nodes

Distant metastasis

MX — distant metastasis can't be assessed

M0 — no evidence of distant metastasis

M1 — distant metastasis

Staging categories for papillary or follicular cancer

Papillary or follicular cancer progresses from mild to severe as follows:

STAGE I — any T, any N, M0 (patient younger than age 45); T1, N0, M0 (patient age 45 or older)

STAGE II — any T, any N, M1 (patient younger than age 45); T2, N0, M0 (patient age 45 or older)

STAGE III — T3, N0, M0; T1, N1a, M0; T2, N1a, M0; T3, N1a, M0 (patient age 45 or older)

STAGE IVa — T4a, N0, M0; T4a, N1a, M0; T1, N1b, M0; T2, N1b, M0; T3, N1b, M0; T4a, N1b, M0 (patient age 45 or older)

STAGE IVb — T4b, any N, M0 (patient age 45 or older)

STAGE IVc — any T, any N, MI (patient age 45 or older)

Staging categories for medullary cancer

Medullary cancer progresses from mild to severe as follows:

STAGE I — T1, N0, M0

STAGE II — T2, N0, M0; T3, N0, M0

STAGE III — T3, N0, M0; T1, N1a, M0; T2, N1a, M0; T3, N1a, M0

STAGE IVa — T4a, N0, M0; T4a, N1a, M0; T1, N1b, M0; T2, N1b, M0; T3, N1b, M0; T4a, N1b, M0

STAGE IVb — T4b, any N, M0

STAGE IVc — any T, any N, M1

Staging categories for anaplastic cancer

All cases are stage IV:

STAGE IVa — T4a, any N, M0

STAGE IVb — T4b, any N, M0

STAGE IVc — any T, any N, M1

ly, the pressure of such a nodule or enlargement causes hoarseness, dysphagia, dyspnea, and pain on palpation. If the tumor is large enough to destroy the gland, hypothyroidism follows, with its typical symptoms of low metabolism (mental apathy and sensitivity to cold). However, if the tumor stimulates excess thyroid hormone production, it induces symptoms of hyperthyroidism (sensitivity to heat, restlessness, and hyperactivity). Other clinical features include diarrhea, anorexia, irritability, vocal cord paralysis, and symptoms of distant metastasis.

Diagnosis

The first clue to thyroid cancer is usually an enlarged, palpable node in the thyroid gland, neck, lymph nodes of the neck, or vocal cords. A patient history of radiation therapy or a family history of thyroid cancer supports the diagnosis. However, tests must rule out nonmalignant thyroid enlargements, which are much more common. Thyroid scan differentiates between functional nodes (rarely malignant) and hypofunctional nodes (commonly malignant) by measuring how readily nodules trap isotopes compared with the rest of the thyroid gland. In thyroid cancer, the scintiscan shows a "cold," nonfunctioning nodule. Other tests include needle biopsy, computed tomography scan, ultrasonic scan, chest X-ray, serum alkaline phosphatase, and serum calcitonin assay to diagnose medullary cancer. Calcitonin assay is a reliable clue to silent medullary carcinoma. (See *Staging thyroid cancer*.)

Treatment

- Total or subtotal thyroidectomy, with modified node dissection (bilateral or unilateral) on the side of the primary cancer (papillary or follicular cancer)
- Total thyroidectomy and radical neck excision (for medullary, giant, or spindle cell cancer)
- Radiation (^{131}I) with external radiation (for inoperable cancer and sometimes postoperatively in lieu of radical neck excision) or alone (for metastasis)

- Adjunctive thyroid suppression, with exogenous thyroid hormones suppressing TSH production, and simultaneous administration of an adrenergic blocking agent such as propranolol, increasing tolerance to surgery and radiation
- Chemotherapy for symptom-producing, widespread metastasis is limited, but doxorubicin is sometimes beneficial.

Special considerations

Before surgery, tell the patient to expect temporary voice loss or hoarseness lasting several days after surgery.

Plan meticulous postoperative care:
- When the patient regains consciousness, keep him in semi-Fowler's position, with his head neither hyperextended nor flexed, to avoid pressure on the suture line. Support his head and neck with sandbags and pillows; when you move him, continue this support with your hands.
- After monitoring vital signs, check the patient's dressing, neck, and back for bleeding. If he complains that the dressing feels tight, loosen it and call the physician immediately. Check serum calcium levels daily; hypocalcemia may develop if parathyroid glands are removed. Watch for and report other complications: hemorrhage and shock (elevated pulse rate and hypotension), tetany (carpopedal spasm, twitching, and seizures), thyroid storm (high fever, severe tachycardia, delirium, dehydration, and extreme irritability), and respiratory obstruction (dyspnea, crowing respirations, retraction of neck tissues). (See *What happens in thyroid storm*, page 70.)
- Keep a tracheotomy set and oxygen equipment handy in case of respiratory obstruction. Use continuous steam inhalation in the patient's room until his chest is clear.
- The patient may need I.V. fluids or a soft diet, but many patients can tolerate a regular diet within 24 hours of surgery.

Care of the patient after extensive tumor and node excision is identical to other radical neck postoperative care. Referral to a local or national support group can help relieve the patient's stress.

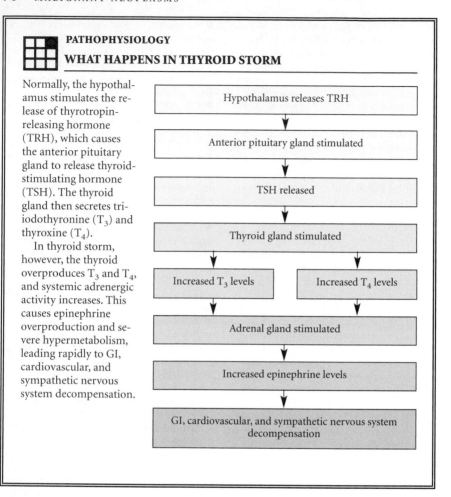

PATHOPHYSIOLOGY
WHAT HAPPENS IN THYROID STORM

Normally, the hypothalamus stimulates the release of thyrotropin-releasing hormone (TRH), which causes the anterior pituitary gland to release thyroid-stimulating hormone (TSH). The thyroid gland then secretes triiodothyronine (T_3) and thyroxine (T_4).

In thyroid storm, however, the thyroid overproduces T_3 and T_4, and systemic adrenergic activity increases. This causes epinephrine overproduction and severe hypermetabolism, leading rapidly to GI, cardiovascular, and sympathetic nervous system decompensation.

Hypothalamus releases TRH

Anterior pituitary gland stimulated

TSH released

Thyroid gland stimulated

Increased T_3 levels

Increased T_4 levels

Adrenal gland stimulated

Increased epinephrine levels

GI, cardiovascular, and sympathetic nervous system decompensation

Malignant spinal neoplasms

Malignant spinal neoplasms may be any one of many tumor types similar to intracranial tumors; they involve the cord or its roots and, if untreated, can eventually cause paralysis. As primary tumors, they originate in the meningeal coverings, the parenchyma of the cord or its roots, the intraspinal vasculature, or the vertebrae. They can also occur as metastatic foci from primary tumors.

Causes and incidence
Primary tumors of the spinal cord may be extramedullary (occurring outside the spinal cord) or intramedullary (occurring within the cord itself). Extramedullary tumors may be intradural (meningiomas and schwannomas), which account for 60% of all primary malignant spinal cord neoplasms, or extradural (metastatic tumors from breasts, lungs, prostate, leukemia, or lymphomas), which account for 25% of these malignant neoplasms.

Intramedullary tumors, or gliomas (astrocytomas or ependymomas), are comparatively rare, accounting for only about 10%. In children, they're low-grade astrocytomas.

Spinal cord tumors are rare compared with intracranial tumors (ratio of 1:4). They occur equally in men and women, with the exception of meningiomas, which occur mostly in women. Spinal cord tumors can occur anywhere along the length of the cord or its roots.

Signs and symptoms

Extramedullary tumors produce symptoms by pressing on nerve roots, the spinal cord, and spinal vessels; intramedullary tumors, by destroying the parenchyma and compressing adjacent areas. Because intramedullary tumors may extend over several spinal cord segments, their symptoms are more variable than those of extramedullary tumors.

The following clinical effects are likely with all malignant spinal cord neoplasms:
- Pain — Most severe directly over the tumor, radiates around the trunk or down the limb on the affected side and is unrelieved by bed rest. It may worsen when lying down or with straining, coughing, or sneezing. Pain can be diffuse, occurring over all extremities. Generally, it progressively worsens and isn't relieved by medication.
- Motor symptoms — Asymmetric spastic muscle weakness, decreased muscle tone, exaggerated reflexes, and a positive Babinski's sign. If the tumor is at the level of the cauda equina, muscle flaccidity, muscle wasting, weakness, and progressive diminution in tendon reflexes are characteristic.
- Sensory deficits — Contralateral loss of pain, temperature, and touch sensation (Brown-Séquard's syndrome). These losses are less obvious to the patient than functional motor changes. Caudal lesions invariably produce paresthesias in the nerve distribution pathway of the involved roots.
- Bowel and bladder symptoms — Urine retention is an inevitable late sign with cord compression. Early signs include incomplete emptying or difficulty with the urine stream, which is usually unnoticed or ignored. Cauda equina tumors cause bladder and bowel incontinence due to flaccid paralysis.

Diagnosis
- Spinal and lumbosacral magnetic resonance imaging confirm spinal tumor.
- X-rays show distortions of the intervertebral foramina; changes in the vertebrae

or collapsed areas in the vertebral body; and localized enlargement of the spinal canal, indicating an adjacent block.
- Myelography identifies the level of the lesion by outlining it if the tumor is causing partial obstruction; it shows anatomic relationship to the cord and the dura. If obstruction is complete, the injected dye can't flow past the tumor. (This study is dangerous if cord compression is nearly complete because withdrawal or escape of cerebrospinal fluid (CSF) will allow the tumor to exert greater pressure against the cord.)
- Radioisotope bone scan demonstrates metastatic invasion of the vertebrae by showing a characteristic increase in osteoblastic activity.
- Computed tomography scan shows cord compression and tumor location.
- Frozen section biopsy at surgery identifies the tissue type.
- Lumbar puncture may be normal, abnormal, or nonspecific. It may show clear yellow CSF as a result of increased protein levels if the flow is completely blocked. If the flow is partially blocked, protein levels rise, but the fluid is only slightly yellow in proportion to the CSF protein level. Cytology of the CSF may show malignant cells of metastatic carcinoma.

Treatment

Treatment of spinal cord tumors generally includes decompression or radiation. Laminectomy is indicated for primary tumors that produce spinal cord or cauda equina compression; it *isn't* usually indicated for metastatic tumors. If the tumor is slowly progressive or if it's treated before the cord degenerates from compression, symptoms are likely to disappear, and complete restoration of function is possible. In a patient with metastatic carcinoma or lymphoma who suddenly experiences complete transverse myelitis with spinal shock, functional improvement is unlikely, even with treatment, and his outlook is ominous. If the patient has incomplete paraplegia of rapid onset, emergency surgical decompression may save cord function. Steroid therapy with dexamethasone minimizes cord edema and temporarily relieves symptoms until surgery can be performed.

Partial removal of intramedullary gliomas, followed by radiation, may alleviate symptoms for a short time. Metastatic extradural tumors can be controlled with radiation, analgesics and, in the case of hormone-mediated tumors (breast and prostate), appropriate hormone therapy. Transcutaneous electrical nerve stimulation (TENS) may control radicular pain from spinal cord tumors and is a useful alternative to opioid analgesics. In TENS, an electrical charge is applied to the skin to stimulate large-diameter nerve fibers and thereby inhibit transmission of pain impulses through small-diameter nerve fibers. Chemotherapy generally hasn't proven effective against most spinal tumors, but may be recommended in some cases.

Special considerations
The care plan for patients with spinal cord tumors should emphasize emotional support and skilled intervention during acute and chronic phases, early recognition of recurrence, prevention and treatment of complications, and maintenance of quality of life.

■ On your first contact with the patient, perform a complete neurologic evaluation to obtain baseline data for planning future care and evaluating changes in his clinical status.

■ Care of the patient with a spinal cord tumor is basically the same as that for the patient with spinal cord injury and requires psychologic support, rehabilitation (including bowel and bladder retraining), and prevention of infection and skin breakdown. After laminectomy, care includes checking neurologic status frequently, changing position by logrolling, administering analgesics, monitoring frequently for infection, and aiding in early walking. Physical therapy may be needed to improve muscle strength and to improve the ability to function independently when permanent neurologic losses occur.

■ Help the patient and his family to understand and cope with the diagnosis, treatment, potential disabilities, and necessary changes in lifestyle.

■ Take safety precautions for the patient with impaired sensation and motor deficits. Use side rails if the patient is bedridden; if he isn't, encourage him to wear flat shoes, and remove scatter rugs and clutter to prevent falls.

■ Encourage the patient to be independent in performing daily activities. Avoid aggravating pain by moving the patient slowly and by making sure his body is well aligned when giving personal care. Advise him to use TENS to block radicular pain.

■ Administer steroids and antacids, as ordered, for cord edema after radiation therapy. Monitor for sensory or motor dysfunction, which indicates the need for more steroids.

■ Enforce bed rest for the patient with vertebral body involvement until the physician says he can safely walk because body weight alone can cause cord collapse and cord laceration from bone fragments.

■ Logroll and position the patient on his side every 2 hours to prevent pressure ulcers and other complications of immobility.

■ If the patient is to wear a back brace, make sure he wears it whenever he gets out of bed.

THORAX

Lung cancer

Even though it's largely preventable, lung cancer has long been the most common cause of cancer death in men and is an increasing cause of cancer death in women. Lung cancer usually develops within the wall or epithelium of the bronchial tree. Its most common types are epidermoid (squamous cell) carcinoma, small cell (oat cell) carcinoma, adenocarcinoma, and large cell (anaplastic) carcinoma. Although the prognosis is usually poor, it varies with the extent of metastasis at the time of diagnosis and the cell type growth rate. Only about 14% of patients with lung cancer survive 5 years after diagnosis.

Causes and incidence
Most experts agree that lung cancer is attributable to inhalation of carcinogenic pollutants by a susceptible host. Who's most susceptible? Any smoker older than

age 40, especially if he began to smoke before age 15, has smoked a whole pack or more per day for 20 years, or works with or near asbestos.

Pollutants in tobacco smoke cause progressive lung cell degeneration. Lung cancer is 10 times more common in smokers than in nonsmokers; 80% of patients with lung cancer are smokers. Cancer risk is determined by the number of cigarettes smoked daily, the depth of inhalation, how early in life smoking began, and the nicotine content of cigarettes. Two other factors also increase susceptibility: exposure to carcinogenic industrial and air pollutants (asbestos, uranium, arsenic, nickel, iron oxides, chromium, radioactive dust, and coal dust) and familial susceptibility.

Signs and symptoms
Because early-stage lung cancer usually produces no symptoms, this disease is usually in an advanced state at diagnosis. These late-stage symptoms commonly lead to diagnosis:
- Epidermoid and small cell carcinomas — smoker's cough, hoarseness, wheezing, dyspnea, hemoptysis, and chest pain
- Adenocarcinoma and large cell carcinoma — fever, weakness, weight loss, anorexia, and shoulder pain.

In addition to their obvious interference with respiratory function, lung tumors may also alter the production of hormones that regulate body function or homeostasis. Clinical conditions that result from such changes are known as *hormonal paraneoplastic syndromes:*
- Gynecomastia may result from large cell carcinoma.
- Hypertrophic pulmonary osteoarthropathy (bone and joint pain from cartilage erosion due to abnormal production of growth hormone) may result from large cell carcinoma and adenocarcinoma.
- Cushing's and carcinoid syndromes may result from small cell carcinoma.
- Hypercalcemia may result from epidermoid tumors.

Metastatic signs and symptoms vary greatly, depending on the effect of tumors on intrathoracic and distant structures:
- bronchial obstruction: hemoptysis, atelectasis, pneumonitis, dyspnea

- cervical thoracic sympathetic nerve involvement: miosis, ptosis, exophthalmos, reduced sweating
- chest wall invasion: piercing chest pain, increasing dyspnea, severe shoulder pain, radiating down arm
- esophageal compression: dysphagia
- local lymphatic spread: cough, hemoptysis, stridor, pleural effusion
- pericardial involvement: pericardial effusion, tamponade, arrhythmias
- phrenic nerve involvement: dyspnea, shoulder pain, unilateral paralyzed diaphragm, with paradoxical motion
- recurrent nerve invasion: hoarseness, vocal cord paralysis
- vena caval obstruction: venous distention and edema of face, neck, chest, and back.

Distant metastasis may involve any part of the body, most commonly the central nervous system, liver, and bone.

Diagnosis
Typical clinical findings may strongly suggest lung cancer, but firm diagnosis requires further evidence.
- Chest X-ray usually shows an advanced lesion, but it can detect a lesion up to 2 years before symptoms appear. It also indicates tumor size and location.
- Sputum cytology, which is 75% reliable, requires a specimen coughed up from the lungs and tracheobronchial tree, *not* postnasal secretions or saliva.
- Computed tomography (CT) scan of the chest may help to delineate the tumor's size and its relationship to surrounding structures.
- Bronchoscopy can locate the tumor site. Bronchoscopic washings provide material for cytologic and histologic examination. The flexible fiber-optic bronchoscope increases the test's effectiveness.
- Needle biopsy of the lungs uses biplane fluoroscopic visual control to detect peripherally located tumors. This allows firm diagnosis in 80% of patients.
- Tissue biopsy of accessible metastatic sites includes supraclavicular and mediastinal node and pleural biopsy. Directed needle biopsy may be performed in conjunction with CT scan.

STAGING LUNG CANCER

Using the TNM (tumor, node, metastasis) classification system, the American Joint Committee on Cancer stages lung cancer as follows.

Primary tumor

TX — primary tumor can't be assessed or malignant tumor cells detected in sputum or bronchial washings but undetected by X-ray or bronchoscopy

T0 — no evidence of primary tumor

Tis — carcinoma in situ

T1 — tumor 3 cm or less in greatest dimension, surrounded by normal lung or visceral pleura; no bronchoscopic evidence of cancer closer to the center of the body than the lobar bronchus

T2 — tumor larger than 3 cm; one that involves the main bronchus and is 2 cm or more from the carina; one that invades the visceral pleura; or one that's accompanied by atelectasis or obstructive pneumonitis that extends to the hilar region but doesn't involve the entire lung

T3 — tumor of any size that extends into neighboring structures, such as the chest wall, diaphragm, or mediastinal pleura; tumor in the main bronchus that doesn't involve but is less than 2 cm from the carina; or tumor that's accompanied by atelectasis or obstructive pneumonitis of the entire lung

T4 — tumor of any size that invades the mediastinum, heart, great vessels, trachea, esophagus, vertebral body, or carina; or tumor with malignant pleural effusion

Regional lymph nodes

NX — regional lymph nodes can't be assessed

N0 — no detectable metastasis to lymph nodes

N1 — metastasis to the ipsilateral peribronchial or hilar lymph nodes or both

N2 — metastasis to the ipsilateral mediastinal or subcarinal lymph nodes or both

N3 — metastasis to the contralateral mediastinal or hilar lymph nodes, the ipsilateral or contralateral scalene lymph nodes, or the supraclavicular lymph nodes

Distant metastasis

MX — distant metastasis can't be assessed

M0 — no evidence of distant metastasis

M1 — distant metastasis

Staging categories

Lung cancer progresses from mild to severe as follows:

Occult carcinoma — TX, N0, M0

Stage 0 — Tis, N0, M0

Stage I — T1, N0, M0; T2, N0, M0

Stage II — T1, N1, M0; T2, N1, M0

Stage IIIa — T1, N2, M0; T2, N2, M0; T3, N0, M0; T3, N1, M0; T3, N2, M0

Stage IIIb — any T, N3, M0; T4, any N, M0

Stage IV — any T, any N, M1

■ Thoracentesis allows chemical and cytologic examination of pleural fluid.

Additional studies include preoperative mediastinoscopy or mediastinotomy to rule out involvement of mediastinal lymph nodes (which would preclude curative pulmonary resection).

Other tests to detect metastasis include bone scan, bone marrow biopsy (recommended in small cell carcinoma), CT scan of the brain or abdomen, and positron emission tomography.

After histologic confirmation, staging determines the extent of the disease and helps in planning the treatment and predicting the prognosis. (See *Staging lung cancer.*)

Treatment

Recent treatment, which consists of combinations of surgery, radiation, and chemotherapy, may improve the prognosis and prolong survival. Nevertheless, because treatment usually begins at an advanced stage, it's largely palliative.

Surgery is the primary treatment for stage I, stage II, or selected stage III squamous cell cancer; adenocarcinoma; and large cell carcinoma, unless the tumor is nonresectable or other conditions rule out surgery.

Surgery may include partial removal of a lung (wedge resection, segmental resection, lobectomy, or radical lobectomy) or total removal (pneumonectomy or radical pneumonectomy).

Preoperative radiation therapy may reduce tumor bulk to allow for surgical resection. Preradiation chemotherapy helps improve response rates. Radiation therapy is ordinarily recommended for stage I and stage II lesions, if surgery is contraindicated, and for stage III lesions when the disease is confined to the involved hemithorax and the ipsilateral supraclavicular lymph nodes.

Generally, radiation therapy is delayed until one month after surgery, to allow the wound to heal, and is then directed to the part of the chest most likely to develop metastasis. High-dose radiation therapy or radiation implants may also be used.

Research has shown that chemotherapy combinations of paclitaxel, gemcitabine, docetaxel, irinotecan, and vinorelbine are more active and better tolerated when combined with cisplatin or carboplatin. Many of these drugs are also being utilized as single agents for the treatment of small-cell and non–small-cell lung cancers.

In laser therapy, laser energy is directed through a bronchoscope to destroy local tumors.

Special considerations

Comprehensive supportive care and patient teaching can minimize complications and speed recovery from surgery, radiation, and chemotherapy.

Before surgery:
■ Supplement and reinforce the information given to the patient by the health care team about the disease and the surgical procedure.
■ Explain expected postoperative procedures, such as insertion of an indwelling catheter, use of an endotracheal tube or chest tube (or both), dressing changes, and I.V. therapy.
■ Teach the patient how to perform coughing, deep diaphragmatic breathing, and range-of-motion (ROM) exercises.
■ Reassure the patient that analgesics will be provided and proper positioning will be implemented to control postoperative pain.
■ Inform the patient that he may take nothing by mouth beginning after midnight the night before surgery, that he'll shower with a soaplike antibacterial agent the night or morning before surgery, and that he'll be given preoperative medications, such as a sedative and an anticholinergic to dry secretions.

After thoracic surgery:
■ Maintain a patent airway, and monitor chest tubes to reestablish normal intrathoracic pressure and prevent postoperative and pulmonary complications.
■ Check vital signs every 15 minutes during the 1st hour after surgery, every 30 minutes during the next 4 hours, and then every 2 hours. Watch for and report abnormal respiration and other changes.
■ Suction the patient as needed, and encourage him to begin deep breathing and coughing as soon as possible. Check secretions often. Initially, sputum will be thick and dark with blood, but it should become thinner and grayish yellow within a day.
■ Monitor and record closed chest drainage. Keep chest tubes patent and draining effectively. Fluctuation in the water-seal chamber on inspiration and expiration indicates that the chest tube is patent. Watch for air leaks, and report them immediately. Position the patient on the surgical side to promote drainage and lung reexpansion.
■ Watch for and report foul-smelling discharge and excessive drainage on dressing. Usually, the dressing is removed after 24 hours, unless the wound appears infected.
■ Monitor intake and output. Maintain adequate hydration.

■ Watch for and treat infection, shock, hemorrhage, atelectasis, dyspnea, mediastinal shift, and pulmonary embolus.

■ To prevent pulmonary embolus, apply antiembolism stockings and encourage ROM exercises.

If the patient is receiving chemotherapy and radiation:

■ Explain possible adverse effects of radiation and chemotherapy. Watch for, treat and, when possible, try to prevent them.

■ Ask the dietary department to provide soft, nonirritating foods that are high in protein, and encourage the patient to eat high-calorie between-meal snacks.

■ Give antiemetics and antidiarrheals, as needed.

■ Schedule patient care activities in a way that helps the patient conserve his energy.

■ During radiation therapy, administer skin care to minimize skin breakdown. If the patient receives radiation therapy in an outpatient setting, warn him to avoid tight clothing, exposure to the sun, and harsh ointments on his chest. Teach him exercises to help prevent shoulder stiffness.

Educate high-risk patients in ways to reduce their chances of developing lung cancer:

■ Present the benefits of quitting to smokers and encourage them to consider this lifestyle change.

■ Refer smokers who want to quit to local branches of the American Cancer Society or smoking-cessation programs or suggest group therapy, individual counseling, or support the patient's use of smoking-cessation products.

■ Encourage patients with recurring or chronic respiratory infections and those with chronic lung disease who detect any change in the character of a cough to see their physician promptly for evaluation.

Breast cancer

Breast cancer occurs more commonly in the left breast than the right and more commonly in the outer upper quadrant. Growth rates vary. Theoretically, slow-growing breast cancer may take up to 8 years to become palpable at 1 cm. It spreads by way of the lymphatic system

and the bloodstream, through the right side of the heart to the lungs, and eventually to the other breast, the chest wall, liver, bone, and brain.

The estimated growth rate of breast cancer is referred to as "doubling time," or the time it takes the malignant cells to double in number. Survival time for breast cancer is based on tumor size and spread; the number of involved nodes is the single most important factor in predicting survival time.

Breast cancer is classified by histologic appearance and location of the lesion, as follows:

■ adenocarcinoma — arising from the epithelium

■ intraductal — developing within the ducts (includes Paget's disease)

■ infiltrating — occurring in parenchyma of the breast

■ inflammatory (rare) — reflecting rapid tumor growth, in which the overlying skin becomes edematous, inflamed, and indurated

■ lobular carcinoma in situ — reflecting tumor growth involving lobes of glandular tissue

■ medullary or circumscribed — large tumor with rapid growth rate.

These histologic classifications should be coupled with a staging or nodal status classification system for a clearer understanding of the extent of the cancer. The most commonly used system for staging cancer, both before and after surgery, is the TNM staging (tumor size, nodal involvement, metastatic progress) system. (See *Staging breast cancer*.)

Causes and incidence

The cause of breast cancer isn't known, but its high incidence in women implicates estrogen.

Certain predisposing factors are clear; women at *high risk* include those who have a family history of breast cancer, particularly first-degree relatives (mother, sister, and maternal aunt).

Other women at high risk include those who:

■ have long menstrual cycles or began menses early (before age 12) or menopause late (after age 55)

STAGING BREAST CANCER

Cancer staging helps form a prognosis and a plan of treatment. For breast cancer, most clinicians use the TNM (tumor, node, metastasis) system developed by the American Joint Committee on Cancer.

Primary tumor

TX — primary tumor can't be assessed
T0 — no evidence of primary tumor
Tis — carcinoma in situ: intraductal carcinoma, lobular carcinoma in situ, or Paget's disease of the nipple with no tumor
T1 — tumor 2 cm or less in greatest dimension
T1a — tumor 0.5 cm or less in greatest dimension
T1b — tumor more than 0.5 cm but not more than 1 cm in greatest dimension
T1c — tumor more than 1 cm but not more than 2 cm in greatest dimension
T2 — tumor more than 2 cm but not more than 5 cm in greatest dimension
T3 — tumor more than 5 cm in greatest dimension
T4 — tumor of any size that extends to the chest wall or skin
T4a — tumor extends to the chest wall
T4b — tumor accompanied by edema, ulcerated breast skin, or satellite skin nodules on the same breast
T4c — both T4a and T4b
T4d — inflammatory carcinoma

Regional lymph nodes

NX — regional lymph nodes can't be assessed
N0 — no evidence of nodal involvement
N1 — movable ipsilateral axillary nodal involvement
N2 — metastasis in ipsilateral axillary lymph nodes fixed or matted, or in clinically apparent ipsilateral internal mammary nodes in the absence of clinically evident axillary lymph-node metastasis
N2a — metastasis in ipsilateral axillary lymph nodes fixed to one another (matted) or to other structures
N2b — metastasis only in clinically apparent ipsilateral internal mammary nodes in the absence of clinically evident axillary lymph-node metastasis
N3 — metastasis in ipsilateral infraclavicular lymph nodes, with or without axillary lymph node involvement; or in clinically apparent ipsilateral internal mammary lymph nodes in the presence of clinically evident axillary lymph-node metastasis; or metastasis in ipsilateral supraclavicular lymph nodes, with or without axillary or internal mammary lymph node involvement
N3a — metastasis in ipsilateral infraclavicular lymph nodes
N3b — metastasis in ipsilateral internal mammary lymph nodes and axillary lymph nodes
N3c — metastasis in ipsilateral supraclavicular lymph nodes

Pathologic staging

pN0 — no lymph node metastasis histologically, no additional examination for isolated tumor cells
pN0(i!) — no regional lymph node metastasis histologically, negative isolated tumor cells (ITC)
pN0(i+) — no regional lymph node metastasis histologically, positive ITC, no ITC cluster greater than 0.2 mm
pN0(mol!) — no regional lymph node metastasis histologically, negative molecular findings reverse transcriptase and polymerase chain reaction
pN1 — metastasis in 1 to 3 axillary lymph nodes and in internal mammary nodes with microscopic disease detected by sentinel lymph node dissection, but not clinically apparent
pN1mi — micrometastasis (greater than 0.2 mm, none greater than 2 mm)
pN1a — metastasis in 1 to 3 axillary lymph nodes

(continued)

STAGING BREAST CANCER *(continued)*

pN1b — metastasis in internal mammary nodes with microscopic disease detected by sentinel lymph node dissection, but not clinically apparent.

pN1c — metastasis in 1 to 3 axillary lymph nodes and in internal mammary nodes with microscopic disease detected by sentinel lymph node dissection, but not clinically apparent (If associated with more than 3 positive axillary lymph nodes, the internal mammary nodes are classified as pN3b to reflect increased tumor burden.)

pN2 — metastasis in 4 to 9 axillary lymph nodes or in clinically apparent internal mammary lymph nodes in the absence of axillary lymph-node metastasis

pN2a — metastasis in 4 to 9 axillary lymph nodes with at least 1 tumor deposit greater than 2 mm

pN2b — metastasis in clinically apparent internal mammary lymph nodes in the absence of axillary lymph-node metastasis.

pN3 — metastasis in 10 or more axillary lymph nodes, or in infraclavicular lymph nodes, or in clinically apparent ipsilateral internal mammary lymph nodes in the presence of 1 or more positive axillary lymph nodes, or in more than 3 axillary lymph nodes with clinically negative microscopic metastasis in internal mammary lymph nodes, or in ipsilateral supraclavicular lymph nodes

pN3a — metastasis in 10 or more axillary lymph nodes with at least 1 tumor deposit greater than 2 mm, or metastasis to the infraclavicular lymph nodes

pN3b — metastasis in clinically apparent ipsilateral internal mammary lymph nodes in the presence of 1 or more positive axillary lymph nodes, or in more than 3 axillary lymph nodes and in internal mammary lymph nodes with microscopic disease detected by sentinel lymph-node dissection, but not clinically apparent

pN3c — metastasis in ipsilateral supraclavicular lymph nodes

Distant metastasis

M1 — distant metastasis

Staging categories

Breast cancer progresses from mild to severe as follows:

STAGE 0 — Tis, N0, M0

STAGE I — T1, N0, M0

STAGE IIA — T0, N1, M0; T1, N1, M0; T2, N0, M0

STAGE IIB — T2, N1, M0; T3, N0, M0

STAGE IIIA — T0, N2, M0; T1, N2, M0; T2, N2, M0; T3, N1 or N2, M0; T3, N2, M0

STAGE IIIB — T4, N0, M0; T4, N1, M0; T4, N2, M0

STAGE IIIC — any T, N3, M0

STAGE IV — any T, any N, M1

Note: Clinically apparent is defined as detected by imaging studies (excluding lymphoscintigraphy) or by clinical examination or grossly visible pathologically.

- have taken hormonal contraceptives
- used hormone replacement therapy for more than 5 years
- who took diethylstilbestrol to prevent miscarriage
- have never been pregnant
- were first pregnant after age 30
- have had unilateral breast cancer
- have had ovarian cancer — particularly at a young age

- were exposed to low-level ionizing radiation.

Recently, scientists have discovered the BRCA1 and BRCA2 genes. Mutations in these genes are thought to be responsible for less than 10% of breast cancers. However, these discoveries have made genetic predisposition testing an option for women at high risk for breast cancer.

Women at *lower risk* include those who:

- were pregnant before age 20

- have had multiple pregnancies
- are Native American or Asian.

Most breast cancer deaths occur in women age 50 and older (84% of cases), and 77% of new breast cancer cases occur in this age-group. However, it may develop any time after puberty. It occurs in men, but rarely; male cases of breast cancer account for less than 1% of all cases.

The 5-year survival rate for localized breast cancer has improved because of earlier diagnosis and the variety of treatments now available. According to the most recent data, mortality rates continue to decline in White women and, for the first time, are also declining in younger Black women. Lymph node involvement is the most valuable prognostic predictor. With adjuvant therapy, 70% to 75% of women with negative nodes will survive 10 years or more compared with 20% to 25% of women with positive nodes.

Signs and symptoms
Warning signals of possible breast cancer include:
- a lump or mass in the breast (a hard, stony mass is usually malignant)
- change in symmetry or size of the breast
- change in skin, thickening, scaly skin around the nipple, dimpling, edema (peau d'orange), or ulceration
- change in skin temperature (a warm, hot, or pink area; suspect cancer in a non-lactating woman older than childbearing age until proven otherwise)
- unusual drainage or discharge (a spontaneous discharge of any kind in a non-breast-feeding, nonlactating woman warrants thorough investigation; so does any discharge produced by breast manipulation (greenish black, white, creamy, serous, or bloody.) (If a breast-fed infant rejects one breast, this may suggest possible breast cancer.)
- change in the nipple, such as itching, burning, erosion, or retraction
- pain (not usually a symptom of breast cancer unless the tumor is advanced, but it should be investigated)
- bone metastasis, pathologic bone fractures, and hypercalcemia
- edema of the arm.

Diagnosis
The most reliable method of detecting breast cancer is the clinical breast examination, followed by immediate evaluation of any abnormality. Other diagnostic measures include mammography, ultrasound, needle biopsy, and surgical biopsy. Mammography is indicated for any woman whose physical examination suggests breast cancer. It should be done as a baseline on women between ages 35 and 39 and annually on all women older than age 40, on those who have a family history of breast cancer, and on those who have had unilateral breast cancer (to check for new disease).

 ELDER TIP *Unfortunately, many older women don't receive regular mammograms, even when recommended by health care professionals, either because they fear radiation, discovering cancer, or discomfort during the procedure or because they're embarrassed about exposing their breasts.*

The value of mammography is questionable for women under age 35 (because of the density of the breasts), except for those women who are strongly suspected of having breast cancer. False-negative results can occur in as many as 30% of all tests. Consequently, with a suspicious mass, a negative mammogram should be disregarded, and a fine-needle aspiration or surgical biopsy should be done. Ultrasonography, which can distinguish a fluid-filled cyst from a tumor, can also be used instead of an invasive surgical biopsy.

Bone scan, brain scan, computed tomography scan, measurement of alkaline phosphatase levels, liver function studies, and liver biopsy can detect distant metastases. A hormonal receptor assay done on the tumor can determine if the tumor is estrogen or progesterone dependent. (This test guides decisions to use therapy that blocks the action of the estrogen hormone that supports tumor growth.)

Treatment
Much controversy exists over breast cancer treatments. In choosing therapy, the patient and physician should take into consideration the stage of the disease, the woman's age and menopausal status, and

the disfiguring effects of the surgery. Treatment of breast cancer may include one or any combination of the following:
■ Surgery involves either mastectomy or lumpectomy. A lumpectomy may be done on an outpatient basis and may be the only surgery needed, especially if the tumor is small and there's no evidence of axillary node involvement. In many cases, radiation therapy is combined with this surgery.

A two-stage procedure, in which the surgeon removes the lump and confirms that it's malignant and then discusses treatment options with the patient, is desirable because it allows the patient to participate in her plan of treatment. Sometimes, if the tumor is diagnosed as clinically malignant, such planning can be done before surgery. In lumpectomy and dissection of the axillary lymph nodes, the tumor and the axillary lymph nodes are removed, leaving the breast intact. A simple mastectomy removes the breast but not the lymph nodes or pectoral muscles. Modified radical mastectomy removes the breast and the axillary lymph nodes. Radical mastectomy, the performance of which has declined, removes the breast, pectoralis major and minor, and the axillary lymph nodes.

The spread of breast cancer to regional lymph nodes is considered a vital prognostic indicator. Sentinel lymph-node biopsy, a reliable and minimally invasive procedure, is used to identify and sample the sentinel lymph node closest to the breast tumor. During the patient's surgery, the axillary node is injected with dye to help with identification and then sent to the pathologist to assess for cancer spread. If the node is negative, the patient can be spared an axillary node dissection, which carries its own risks and the potential for long-term complications.

Reconstructive breast surgery can be performed at the same time as mastectomy or it can be planned for a later date. Several options are available for breast reconstruction, including the insertion of breast implants or a transverse rectus abdominis musculocutaneous flap.
■ Chemotherapy, involving various cytotoxic drug combinations, is used as either adjuvant or primary therapy, depending on several factors, including the TNM staging

and estrogen receptor status. The most commonly used antineoplastic drugs are cyclophosphamide, fluorouracil, methotrexate, doxorubicin, vincristine, and paclitaxel. A common drug combination used in both premenopausal and postmenopausal women is cyclophosphamide, doxorubicin, and paclitaxel.

Tamoxifen, an estrogen antagonist, is the adjuvant treatment of choice for postmenopausal patients with positive estrogen receptor status. It's also been found to reduce the risk of breast cancer in women at high risk.
■ Peripheral stem cell therapy is an option, but it's rarely used for advanced breast cancer.
■ Primary radiation therapy before or after tumor removal is effective for small tumors in early stages with no evidence of distant metastasis; it's also used to prevent or treat local recurrence. Presurgical radiation to the breast in inflammatory breast cancer helps make tumors more surgically manageable.
■ Estrogen, progesterone, androgen, or antiandrogen aminoglutethimide therapy may also be given to breast cancer patients. The success of these drug therapies — along with growing evidence that breast cancer is a systemic, not local, disease — has led to a decline in ablative surgery.

Special considerations
To provide good care for a patient with breast cancer, begin with a history, assess the patient's feelings about her illness, and determine what she knows about it and what she expects. Preoperatively, make sure you know what kind of surgery is scheduled, so you can prepare her properly. If a mastectomy is scheduled, in addition to the usual preoperative preparation (for example, skin preparations and not allowing the patient anything by mouth), provide the following information:
■ Teach her how to deep-breathe and cough to prevent pulmonary complications and how to rotate her ankles to help prevent thromboembolism.
■ Tell her she can ease her pain by lying on the affected side or by placing a hand or pillow on the incision. Preoperatively, show her where the incision will be. Inform her

that she'll receive pain medication and that she need not fear addiction. Remember, adequate pain relief encourages coughing and turning and promotes general well-being. Positioning a small pillow anteriorly under the patient's arm provides comfort.

■ Encourage her to get out of bed as soon as possible (even as soon as the anesthesia wears off or the first evening after surgery).

■ Explain that, after mastectomy, an incisional drain or suction device will be used to remove accumulated serous or sanguineous fluid, thereby promoting healing.

Postoperative care:

■ Inspect the dressing anteriorly and posteriorly, reporting bleeding promptly.

■ Measure and record the amount of drainage; also note the color. Expect drainage to be bloody during the first 4 hours and afterward to become serous.

■ Check circulatory status (blood pressure, pulse, respirations, and bleeding).

■ Monitor intake and output for at least 48 hours after general anesthesia.

■ Prevent lymphedema of the arm, which may be an eventual complication of any breast cancer treatment that involves lymph node manipulation. Help the patient prevent lymphedema by instructing her to exercise her hand and arm regularly and to avoid activities that might cause infection or impairment in this hand or arm, which increases the chance of developing lymphedema. (See *Postoperative arm and hand care.*)

■ Inform the patient to not let anyone draw blood, start an I.V., give an injection, or take a blood pressure on the affected side because these activities will also increase the chances of developing lymphedema.

■ Inspect the incision. Encourage the patient and her partner to look at her incision as soon as possible, perhaps when the first dressing is removed.

■ Advise the patient to ask her physician about reconstructive surgery or to call the local or state medical society for the names of plastic reconstructive surgeons who regularly perform surgery to create breast mounds. In many cases, reconstructive surgery may be planned before the mastectomy.

POSTOPERATIVE ARM AND HAND CARE

Hand exercises for the patient who's prone to lymphedema can begin on the day of surgery. Plan arm exercises with the physician because he can anticipate potential problems with the suture line.

■ Have the patient open her hand and close it tightly six to eight times every 3 hours while she's awake.

■ Elevate the arm on the affected side on a pillow above the heart level.

■ Encourage the patient to wash her face and comb her hair — an effective exercise.

■ Measure and record the circumference of the patient's arm 2¼" (5.7 cm) from her elbow. Indicate the exact place you measured. By re-measuring a month after surgery, and at intervals during and following radiation therapy, you can determine whether lymphedema is present. The patient may complain that her arm is heavy — an early symptom of lymphedema.

■ When the patient is home, she can elevate her arm and hand by supporting it on the back of a chair or a couch.

■ Instruct the patient about breast prostheses. The American Cancer Society's Reach to Recovery group can provide instruction, emotional support and counseling, and a list of area stores that sell prostheses.

■ Give psychological and emotional support. Most patients fear cancer and possible disfigurement and worry about loss of sexual function. Explain that breast surgery doesn't interfere with sexual function and that the patient may resume sexual activity as soon as she desires after surgery.

■ Also explain to the patient that she may experience "phantom breast syndrome" (a phenomenon in which a tingling or a pins-

and-needles sensation is felt in the area of the amputated breast tissue) or depression following mastectomy. Listen to the patient's concerns, offer support, and refer her to an appropriate organization such as the American Cancer Society's Reach to Recovery, which offers caring and sharing groups to help breast cancer patients in the hospital and at home.

ABDOMEN AND PELVIS

Gastric cancer

Gastric cancer can be classified as polypoid, ulcerating, ulcerating and infiltrating, or diffuse, according to gross appearance. The parts of the stomach affected by gastric cancer, listed in order of decreasing frequency, are the pylorus and antrum, the lesser curvature, the cardia, the body of the stomach, and the greater curvature. (See *Sites of gastric cancer.*)

Gastric cancer infiltrates rapidly to regional lymph nodes, omentum, liver, and lungs by the following routes: walls of the stomach, duodenum, and esophagus; lymphatic system; adjacent organs; bloodstream; and peritoneal cavity.

Causes and incidence

The cause of gastric cancer is unknown. It's commonly associated with gastritis with gastric atrophy, which may result from gastric cancer and may not be a precursor state. Predisposing factors include environmental influences, such as smoking and high alcohol intake. Genetic factors have also been implicated because this disease occurs more commonly among people with type A blood than among those with type O; similarly, it's more common in people with a family history of gastric cancer. Dietary factors also seem related, including types of food preparation, physical properties of some foods, and certain methods of food preservation (especially smoking, pickling, or salting). There's a strong correlation between infection with *Helicobacter pylori* and distal gastric cancer.

Gastric cancer is common throughout the world and affects all races; however, unexplained geographic and cultural differences in incidence occur — for example, a higher mortality in Japan, Iceland, Chile, and Austria. In the United States, during the past 25 years, incidence has decreased by 50% and the resulting death rate is one-third what it was 30 years ago. Incidence is higher in males older than 40. Hispanic, Native, and African Americans are twice as likely to develop gastric cancer than Whites. The prognosis depends on the stage of the disease at the time of diagnosis; however, the overall 5-year survival rate is approximately 19%.

The decrease in gastric cancer in the United States has been attributed, without proof, to the balanced American diet and to refrigeration, which reduces nitrate-producing bacteria in food.

Signs and symptoms

Early clues to gastric cancer are chronic dyspepsia and epigastric discomfort, followed in later stages by weight loss, anorexia, feeling of fullness after eating, anemia, and fatigue. If the cancer is in the cardia, the first sign or symptom may be dysphagia and, later, vomiting (commonly coffee-ground vomitus). Affected patients may also have blood in their stools.

The course of gastric cancer may be insidious or fulminating. Unfortunately, the patient typically treats himself with antacids or histamine blockers until the symptoms of advanced stages appear.

Diagnosis

Diagnosis depends primarily on reinvestigations of any persistent or recurring GI changes and complaints. To rule out other conditions producing similar symptoms, diagnostic evaluation must include the testing of blood, stools, and stomach fluid samples.

Diagnosis of gastric cancer generally requires these studies:
- Barium X-rays of the GI tract with fluoroscopy show changes (tumor or filling defect in the outline of the stomach, loss of flexibility and distensibility, and abnormal gastric mucosa with or without ulceration).

SITES OF GASTRIC CANCER

The most common site of gastric cancer is the pyloric area, accounting for about 50% of cases. The next most common area is the lesser curvature of the stomach, accounting for about 25% of cases.

Cardia — 10%

10%

Lesser curvature —

25%

Pyloric area —

Body and fundus

3% to 5%

50%

Greater curvature

■ Gastroscopy with fiber-optic endoscopy helps rule out other diffuse gastric mucosal abnormalities by allowing direct visualization and gastroscopic biopsy to evaluate gastric mucosal lesions.

■ Photography with fiber-optic endoscope provides a permanent record of gastric lesions that can later be used to determine disease progression and effect of treatment.

Certain other studies may rule out specific organ metastasis: computed tomography scans, chest X-rays, liver and bone scans, and liver biopsy. (See *Staging gastric cancer,* page 84.)

Treatment

In many cases, surgery is the treatment of choice. Excision of the lesion with appropriate margins is possible in over one-third of patients. Even in patients whose disease isn't considered surgically curable, resection offers palliation and improves poten-

tial benefits from chemotherapy and radiation.

The nature and extent of the lesion determine what kind of surgery is most appropriate. Common surgical procedures include subtotal gastric resection (subtotal gastrectomy) and total gastric resection (total gastrectomy). When carcinoma involves the pylorus and antrum, gastric resection removes the lower stomach and duodenum (gastrojejunostomy or Billroth II). If metastasis has occurred, the omentum and spleen may also have to be removed.

If gastric cancer has spread to the liver, peritoneum, or lymph glands, palliative surgery may include gastrostomy, jejunostomy, or a gastric or partial gastric resection. Such surgery may temporarily relieve vomiting, nausea, pain, and dysphagia, while allowing enteral nutrition to continue.

STAGING GASTRIC CANCER

The prognosis and treatment of gastric cancer depend on its type and stage. Using the TNM (tumor, node, metastasis) system, the American Joint Committee on Cancer describes the following stages of gastric cancer.

Primary tumor

TX — primary tumor can't be assessed

T0 — no evidence of primary tumor

Tis — carcinoma in situ: intraepithelial tumor doesn't penetrate the lamina propria

T1 — tumor penetrates the lamina propria or submucosa

T2a — tumor penetrates the muscularis propria

T2b — tumor invades the subserosa

T3 — tumor penetrates the serosa (visceral peritoneum) without invading adjacent structures

T4 — tumor invades adjacent structures

Regional lymph nodes

NX — regional lymph nodes can't be assessed

N0 — no evidence of regional lymph node metastasis

N1 — involvement of perigastric lymph nodes within 3 cm of the edge of the primary tumor

N2 — involvement of the perigastric lymph nodes more than 3 cm from the edge of the primary tumor or in lymph nodes along the left gastric, common hepatic, splenic, or celiac arteries

Distant metastasis

MX — distant metastasis can't be assessed

M0 — no evidence of distant metastasis

M1 — distant metastasis

Staging categories

Gastric cancer stages progress from mild to severe as follows:

STAGE 0 — Tis, N0, M0

STAGE IA — T1, N0, M0

STAGE IB — T1, N1, M0; T2a/b, N0, M0

STAGE II — T1, N2, M0; T2a/b, N1, M0; T3, N0, M0

STAGE IIIA — T2a/b, N2, M0; T3, N1, M0; T4, N0, M0

STAGE IIIB — T3, N2, M0

STAGE IV — T4, N1-3, M0; T1-3, N3, M0; any T, any N, M1

Chemotherapy for GI cancers may help to control symptoms and prolong survival. Adenocarcinoma of the stomach has responded to several agents, including fluorouracil, paclitaxel, doxorubicin, cisplatin, methotrexate, and mitomycin. Antiemetics can control nausea, which increases as the cancer advances. In the more advanced stages, sedatives and tranquilizers may be necessary to control overwhelming anxiety. Opioids are commonly necessary to relieve severe and unremitting pain.

Radiation has been particularly useful when combined with chemotherapy in patients who have unresectable or partially resectable disease. It should be given on an empty stomach and shouldn't be used preoperatively because it may damage viscera and impede healing.

Treatment with antispasmodics and antacids may help relieve GI distress.

Special considerations

■ Before surgery, prepare the patient for its effects and for postsurgical procedures such as insertion of a nasogastric (NG) tube for drainage and I.V. lines.

■ Reassure the patient who's having a partial gastric resection that he may eventually be able to eat normally. Prepare the patient who's having a total gastrectomy for slow recovery and only partial return to a normal diet.

■ Include the family in all phases of the patient's care.

- Emphasize the importance of changing position every 2 hours and of deep breathing.
- After surgery, give meticulous supportive care to promote recovery and prevent complications.
- After any type of gastrectomy, pulmonary complications may result, and oxygen may be needed. Regularly assist the patient with turning, coughing, and deep breathing. Turning the patient hourly and administering analgesic opioids, as ordered, may prevent pulmonary problems. Incentive spirometry may also be needed for complete lung expansion. Proper positioning is important as well; semi-Fowler's position facilitates breathing and drainage.
- After gastrectomy, little (if any) drainage comes from the NG tube because no secretions form after stomach removal. Without a stomach for storage, many patients experience dumping syndrome. Intrinsic factor is absent from gastric secretions, leading to malabsorption of vitamin B_{12}. To prevent vitamin B_{12} deficiency, the patient must take a replacement vitamin for the rest of his life as well as an iron supplement.
- During radiation treatment, encourage the patient to eat high-calorie, well-balanced meals. Offer fluids such as ginger ale to minimize such radiation adverse effects as nausea and vomiting.

Watch for the following complications of surgery:

- Patients who experience poor digestion and absorption after gastrectomy need a special diet: frequent feedings of small amounts of clear liquids, increasing to small, frequent feedings of bland food. After total gastrectomy, patients must eat small meals for the rest of their lives. (Some patients need pancreatin and sodium bicarbonate after meals to prevent or control steatorrhea and dyspepsia.)
- Wound dehiscence and delayed healing, stemming from decreased protein, anemia, and avitaminosis, may occur. Preoperative vitamin and protein replacement can prevent such complications. Observe the wound regularly for redness, swelling, failure to heal, or warmth. Parenteral administration of vitamin C may improve wound healing.

- Vitamin deficiency may result from obstruction, diarrhea, or an inadequate diet. Ascorbic acid, thiamine, riboflavin, nicotinic acid, and vitamin K supplements may be beneficial. Good nutrition promotes weight gain, strength, independence, a positive outlook, and tolerance for surgery, radiation therapy, or chemotherapy. Aside from meeting caloric needs, nutrition must provide adequate protein, fluid, and potassium intake to facilitate glycogen and protein synthesis. Anabolic agents such as methandrostenolone may induce nitrogen retention. Steroids, antidepressants, wine, or brandy may boost the appetite.
- When all treatments have failed, concentrate on keeping the patient comfortable and free from pain, and provide as much psychological support as possible. If the patient is going home, discuss continuing care needs with the caregiver or refer the patient to an appropriate home health care agency or hospice. Encourage the patient and the caregivers to express their feelings and concerns. Answer their questions honestly with tact and sensitivity.

Esophageal cancer

Esophageal cancer is a malignant tumor that occurs in the esophagus, the muscular tube that propels food from the mouth to the stomach. It's difficult to treat, but can be cured if the cancer is confined to the esophagus. For patients whose cancer has spread beyond the esophagus, cure generally isn't possible; treatment is directed toward symptom relief.

Causes and incidence

The cause of esophageal cancer is unknown, but among predisposing factors are chronic irritation caused by heavy smoking and excessive use of alcohol, stasis-induced inflammation, nutritional deficiency, and diets high in nitrosamines. A genetic link has been proposed concerning an overexpression and mutation of the p53 tumor suppressor gene. Esophageal tumors are usually fungating and infiltrating. Most arise in squamous cell epithelium. However, the number of adenocarcinomas is

---

STAGING ESOPHAGEAL CANCER

The TNM (tumor, node, metastasis) staging system accepted by the American Joint Committee on Cancer classifies esophageal cancer as follows.

Primary tumor
TX — primary tumor can't be assessed
T0 — no evidence of primary tumor
Tis — carcinoma in situ
T1 — tumor invades lamina propria or submucosa
T2 — tumor invades muscularis propria
T3 — tumor invades adventitia
T4 — tumor invades adjacent structures

Regional lymph nodes
NX — regional lymph nodes can't be assessed
N0 — no regional lymph node metastasis
N1 — regional lymph node metastasis

Distant metastasis
MX — distant metastasis can't be assessed
M0 — no known distant metastasis
M1 — distant metastasis

Staging categories
Esophageal cancer progresses from mild to severe as follows:
STAGE 0 — Tis, N0, M0
STAGE I — T1, N0, M0
STAGE IIA — T2, N0, M0; T3, N0, M0
STAGE IIB — T1, N1, M0; T2, N1, M0
STAGE III — T3, N1, M0; T4, any N, M0
STAGE IV — any T, any N, M1

---

greatly rising in the United States. Melanomas and sarcomas are few.

Regardless of type, esophageal cancer is usually fatal, with a 5-year survival rate of approximately 10% and regional metastasis occurring early via submucosal lymphatics. Metastasis produces such serious complications as tracheoesophageal fistulas, mediastinitis, and aortic perforation. Common sites of distant metastasis include the liver and lungs. (See *Staging esophageal cancer.*)

Esophageal cancer most commonly develops in men older than age 60 and is nearly always fatal. This disease occurs worldwide, but incidence varies geographically. It's most common in Japan, China, the Middle East, and parts of South Africa.

Signs and symptoms

Dysphagia and weight loss are the most common presenting symptoms. Dysphagia is mild and intermittent at first, but it soon becomes constant. Pain, hoarseness, coughing, and esophageal obstruction follow. Cachexia usually develops.

Diagnosis

X-rays of the esophagus, with barium swallow and motility studies, reveal structural and filling defects and reduced peristalsis.

CONFIRMING DIAGNOSIS *Endoscopic examination of the esophagus (esophagogastroduodenoscopy), punch and brush biopsies, and exfoliative cytologic tests confirm esophageal tumors. Usually, magnetic resonance imagining of the chest and thoracic computed tomography are helpful in determining disease staging. Positron emission tomography is useful in determining disease staging and whether surgery is possible.*

Treatment

Multimodal therapy is usually indicated. Whenever possible, treatment includes resection to maintain a passageway for food. This may require such radical surgery as esophagogastrectomy with jejunal or colonic bypass grafts. Palliative surgery may include a feeding gastrostomy. Chemotherapy with 5-fluorouracil or cisplatin may be used. Insertion of prosthetic tubes to bridge the tumor alleviates dysphagia. Other treatments to improve the patient's ability to swallow include endoscopic dilation of the esophagus (sometimes with placement of a stent) and photodynamic therapy.

Treatment complications may be severe. Surgery may precipitate an anastomotic leak, a fistula, pneumonia, and empyema. Rarely, radiation may cause esophageal perforation, pneumonitis and pulmonary fibrosis, or myelitis of the spinal cord. Prosthetic tubes may dislodge and perforate the mediastinum or erode the tumor.

Special considerations

■ Before surgery, answer the patient's questions and let him know what to expect after surgery, such as gastrostomy tubes, closed chest drainage, and nasogastric suctioning.

■ If surgery included an esophageal anastomosis, keep the patient flat on his back to avoid tension on the suture line.

■ Promote adequate nutrition and assess the patient's nutritional and hydration status to determine the need for supplementary parenteral feedings.

■ Prevent aspiration of food by placing the patient in Fowler's position for meals and allowing plenty of time to eat. Provide high-calorie, high-protein, "blenderized" food, as needed. Because the patient will probably regurgitate some food, clean his mouth carefully after each meal. Keep mouthwash handy.

■ If the patient has a gastrostomy tube, give food slowly — by gravity — in prescribed amounts (usually 200 to 500 ml). Offer something to chew before each feeding to promote gastric secretions and a semblance of normal eating.

■ Instruct the family in gastrostomy tube care (checking tube patency before each feeding, adequate flushing after feedings and medications, providing skin care around the tube, keeping the patient upright during and after feedings).

■ Provide emotional support for the patient and his family; refer them to appropriate organizations such as the American Cancer Society.

■ When all treatments have failed, concentrate on keeping the patient comfortable and free from pain, providing as much psychological support as possible. If the patient is going home, discuss continuing care needs with the caregiver or refer the patient to an appropriate home health care agency or hospice. Encourage the patient and caregiver to express their feelings and concerns. Answer their questions honestly, with tact and sensitivity.

Pancreatic cancer

A deadly GI cancer, pancreatic cancer progresses rapidly. Most pancreatic tumors are adenocarcinomas and arise in the head of the pancreas. Rarer tumors are those of the body and tail of the pancreas and islet cell tumors. The two main tissue types are cylinder cell and large, fatty, granular cell.

Causes and incidence

Evidence suggests that pancreatic cancer is linked to inhalation or absorption of the following carcinogens, which are then excreted by the pancreas:

■ cigarettes

■ food additives

■ industrial chemicals, such as beta-naphthalene, benzidine, and urea.

Possible predisposing factors are chronic pancreatitis, diabetes mellitus, and chronic alcohol abuse (both pancreatitis and diabetes mellitus may be early manifestations of the disease as well).

Pancreatic cancer incidence increases with age, peaking between ages 60 and 70. Geographically, the incidence is highest in Israel, the United States, Sweden, and Canada.

Signs and symptoms

The most common features of pancreatic cancer are weight loss, abdominal or low back pain, jaundice, and diarrhea. Other generalized effects include fever, skin lesions (usually on the legs), and fatigue. (See *Types of pancreatic cancer,* page 88.)

Diagnosis

Definitive diagnosis requires a laparotomy with a biopsy.

Other tests used to detect pancreatic cancer include:

■ ultrasound of the abdomen — can identify a mass but not its histology

TYPES OF PANCREATIC CANCER

Type and pathology	Clinical features
Head of pancreas ■ Commonly obstructs ampulla of Vater and common bile duct ■ Directly metastasizes to duodenum ■ Adhesions anchor tumor to spine, stomach, and intestines.	■ Jaundice (predominant sign)—slowly progressive, unremitting; may cause skin, especially of the face and genitals, to turn olive green or black ■ Pruritus—in many cases severe ■ Weight loss—rapid and severe, possibly as great as 30 lb [13.6 kg]); may lead to emaciation, weakness, and muscle atrophy ■ Slowed digestion, gastric distention, nausea, diarrhea, and steatorrhea with clay-colored stools ■ Liver and gallbladder enlargement from lymph node metastasis to biliary tract and duct wall resulting in compression and obstruction; gallbladder may be palpable (Courvoisier's sign) ■ Dull, nondescript, continuous abdominal pain radiating to right upper quadrant; relieved by bending forward ■ GI hemorrhage and biliary infection common
Body and tail of pancreas ■ Large nodular masses become fixed to retropancreatic tissues and spine ■ Direct invasion of spleen, left kidney, suprarenal gland, diaphragm ■ Involvement of celiac plexus results in thrombosis of splenic vein and spleen infarction.	**Body** ■ Pain (predominant symptom)—usually epigastric, develops slowly and radiates to back; relieved by bending forward or sitting up; intensified by lying supine; most intense 3 to 4 hours after eating; when celiac plexus is involved, pain is more intense and lasts longer ■ Venous thrombosis and thrombophlebitis common; may precede other symptoms by months ■ Splenomegaly (from infarction), hepatomegaly (occasionally), and jaundice (rarely) **Tail** Symptoms result from metastasis: ■ Abdominal tumor (most common finding) producing a palpable abdominal mass and abdominal pain radiating to left hypochondrium and left side of the chest ■ Anorexia leading to weight loss, emaciation, and weakness ■ Splenomegaly and upper GI bleeding

■ computed tomography scan of the abdomen—similar to ultrasound but shows greater detail

■ angiography—shows vascular supply of tumor

■ endoscopic retrograde cholangiopancreatography—allows visualization, instillation of contrast medium, and specimen biopsy

■ magnetic resonance imaging of the abdomen—shows tumor size and location in great detail.

Laboratory tests supporting this diagnosis include serum bilirubin (increased); serum amylase and serum lipase (sometimes elevated); prothrombin time (prolonged); aspartate aminotransferase and alanine aminotransferase (elevations indicate necrosis of liver cells); alkaline phosphatase (marked elevation occurs with biliary obstruction); plasma insulin immunoassay (shows measurable serum insulin in the presence of islet cell tumors) (see *Islet cell tumors*); hemoglobin (Hb) and hematocrit (HCT) (may show mild anemia); fasting blood glucose (may indicate hypoglycemia or hyperglycemia); and stools (occult blood may signal ulceration in GI tract or ampulla of Vater).

Treatment
Treatment of pancreatic cancer is rarely successful because this disease has usually metastasized widely at diagnosis. Therapy consists of surgery and, possibly, radiation and chemotherapy. Standard chemotherapy for patients with locally unresectable cancer includes gemcitabine. Gemcitabine has been demonstrated to improve the quality of life through better pain control, adequate performance status, decreased analgesic consumption, shrinkage of tumor, and prolonged survival. (See *Staging pancreatic cancer,* page 90.)

Other medications used in pancreatic cancer include:
- antacids (by mouth or by nasogastric [NG] tube) — to decrease secretion of pancreatic enzymes and to suppress peptic activity, thereby reducing stress-induced damage to gastric mucosa
- antibiotics (oral, I.V., or I.M.) — to prevent infection and relieve symptoms
- anticholinergics (particularly propantheline) — to decrease GI tract spasm and motility and reduce pain and secretions
- diuretics — to mobilize extracellular fluid from ascites
- insulin — to provide adequate exogenous insulin after pancreatic resection
- opioids — to relieve pain, but only after analgesics fail because morphine, meperidine, and codeine can lead to biliary tract spasm and increase common bile duct pressure
- pancreatic enzymes (average dose 0.5 to 1 mg with meals) — to assist in digestion of proteins, carbohydrates, and fats when pancreatic juices are insufficient because of surgery or obstruction.

Small advances have been made in the survival rate with surgery:

ISLET CELL TUMORS
Relatively uncommon, islet cell tumors (insulinomas) may be benign or malignant and produce signs and symptoms in three stages:

1. Slight hypoglycemia — fatigue, restlessness, malaise, and excessive weight gain
2. Compensatory secretion of epinephrine — pallor, clamminess, perspiration, palpitations, finger tremors, hunger, decreased temperature, and increased pulse and blood pressure
3. Severe hypoglycemia — ataxia, clouded sensorium, diplopia, episodes of violence, and hysteria.

Usually, insulinomas metastasize to the liver alone but may metastasize to bone, brain, and lungs. Death results from a combination of hypoglycemic reactions and widespread metastasis. Treatment consists of enucleation of tumor (if benign) and chemotherapy with streptozocin or resection to include pancreatic tissue (if malignant).

- Total pancreatectomy may increase survival time by resecting a localized tumor or by controlling postoperative gastric ulceration.
- Cholecystojejunostomy, choledochoduodenostomy, and choledochojejunostomy have partially replaced radical resection to bypass obstructing common bile duct extensions, thus decreasing the incidence of jaundice and pruritus.
- Whipple's operation, or pancreatoduodenectomy, has high mortality but can produce wide lymphatic clearance, except with tumors located near the portal vein, superior mesenteric vein and artery, and celiac axis. This rarely used procedure removes the head of the pancreas, the duodenum, and portions of the body and tail of the pancreas, stomach, jejunum, pancreatic duct, and distal portion of the bile duct.

STAGING PANCREATIC CANCER

Using the TNM (tumor, node, metastasis) system, the American Joint Committee on Cancer has established the following stages for pancreatic cancer.

Primary tumor
TX—primary tumor can't be assessed
T0—no evidence of primary tumor
T1—tumor limited to the pancreas
T1a—tumor 2 cm or less in greatest dimension
T1b—tumor more than 2 cm in greatest dimension
T2—tumor penetrates the duodenum, bile duct, or peripancreatic tissues
T3—tumor extends beyond the pancreas, but without involvement of the celiac axis or the superior mesenteric artery
T4—tumor involves the celiac axis or the superior mesenteric artery (unresectable primary tumor)

Regional lymph nodes
NX—regional lymph nodes can't be assessed

N0—no evidence of regional lymph node metastasis
N1—regional lymph node metastasis

Distant metastasis
MX—distant metastasis can't be assessed
M0—no known distant metastasis
M1—distant metastasis

Staging categories
Pancreatic cancer progresses from mild to severe as follows:
Stage 0—Tis, N0, M0
Stage IA—T1, N0, M0
Stage IB—T2, N0, M0
Stage IIA—T3, N0, M0
Stage IIB—T1, N1, M0; T2, N1, M0; T3, N1, M0
Stage III—T4, any N, M0
Stage IV—any T, any N, M1

■ Gastrojejunostomy is performed if radical resection isn't indicated and duodenal obstruction is expected to develop later.

Radiation therapy is usually ineffective except as an adjunct to chemotherapy or as a palliative measure.

Special considerations

Before surgery:
■ Ensure that the patient is medically stable, particularly regarding nutrition (this may take 4 to 5 days). If the patient can't tolerate oral feedings, provide total parenteral nutrition and I.V. fat emulsions to correct deficiencies and maintain positive nitrogen balance.
■ Give blood transfusions (to combat anemia), vitamin K (to overcome prothrombin deficiency), antibiotics (to prevent postoperative complications), and gastric lavage (to maintain gastric decompression), as ordered.

■ Tell the patient about expected postoperative procedures and expected adverse effects of radiation and chemotherapy.

After surgery:
■ Watch for and report complications, such as fistula, pancreatitis, fluid and electrolyte imbalance, infection, hemorrhage, skin breakdown, nutritional deficiency, hepatic failure, renal insufficiency, and diabetes.
■ If the patient is receiving chemotherapy, treat adverse effects symptomatically.

Throughout this illness, provide meticulous supportive care:
■ Monitor fluid balance, abdominal girth, metabolic state, and weight daily. In weight loss, replace nutrients I.V., by mouth, or by NG tube; in weight gain (due to ascites), impose dietary restrictions, such as a low-sodium or fluid-retention diet, as ordered. Maintain a 2,500-calorie diet.

■ Serve small, frequent, nutritious meals by enlisting the dietitian's services. Administer an oral pancreatic enzyme at mealtimes if needed. Give an antacid to prevent stress ulcers as ordered.

■ To prevent constipation, administer laxatives, stool softeners, and cathartics, as ordered; modify diet; and increase fluid intake. To increase GI motility, position the patient properly at mealtime, and help him walk when he can.

■ Ensure adequate rest and sleep. Assist with range-of-motion (ROM) and isometric exercises, as appropriate.

■ Administer pain medication, antibiotics, and antipyretics, as ordered. Note time, site (if injected), and response.

■ Watch for signs of hypoglycemia or hyperglycemia; administer glucose or an antidiabetic agent, as ordered. Monitor blood glucose levels and response to treatment.

■ Document progression of jaundice.

■ Provide meticulous skin care to avoid pruritus and necrosis. Prevent excoriation in a pruritic patient by clipping his nails and having him wear cotton gloves.

■ Watch for signs of upper GI bleeding, test stools and vomitus for occult blood, and keep a flow sheet of Hb levels and HCT. To control active bleeding, promote gastric vasoconstriction with prescribed medication. Replace any fluid loss. Ease discomfort from pyloric obstruction with an NG tube.

■ To prevent thrombosis, apply antiembolism stockings and assist in ROM exercises. If thrombosis occurs, elevate the patient's legs, and give an anticoagulant or aspirin, as ordered.

■ When all treatments have failed, concentrate on keeping the patient comfortable and free from pain, and provide as much psychological support as possible. If the patient is going home, discuss continuing care needs with the caregiver or refer the patient to an appropriate home health care agency or hospice. Encourage the patient and caregiver to express their feelings and concerns. Answer their questions honestly, with tact and sensitivity.

Colorectal cancer

Colorectal cancer is the second most common visceral malignant neoplasm in the United States and Europe. Incidence is equally distributed between men and women. Colorectal malignant tumors are almost always adenocarcinomas. About one-half of these are sessile lesions of the rectosigmoid area; the rest are polypoid lesions.

Colorectal cancer tends to progress slowly and remains localized for a long time. Consequently, it's potentially curable in about 90% of patients if early diagnosis allows resection before nodal involvement. With improved diagnosis, the overall 5-year survival rate is about 60% for adjacent organ or nodal spread, and greater than 90% for early localized disease. (See *Staging colorectal cancer,* page 92.)

Causes and incidence

The exact cause of colorectal cancer is unknown, but studies showing concentration in areas of higher economic development suggest a relationship to diet (excess saturated animal fat). Other factors that magnify the risk of developing colorectal cancer include:

■ other diseases of the digestive tract

■ age (older than age 40)

■ history of ulcerative colitis (average interval before onset of cancer is 11 to 17 years)

■ familial polyposis (cancer almost always develops by age 50).

There are more than 130,000 cases of colorectal cancer diagnosed in the United States each year. It's the second-leading cause of cancer-related death, accounting for more than 50,000 per year. However, in almost all cases, it's treatable if caught early by colonoscopy.

Signs and symptoms

Signs and symptoms of colorectal cancer result from local obstruction and, in later stages, from direct extension to adjacent organs (bladder, prostate, ureters, vagina, sacrum) and distant metastasis (usually liver). In the early stages, signs and symptoms are typically vague and depend on the anatomic location and function of the

STAGING COLORECTAL CANCER

Named for pathologist Cuthbert Dukes, the Dukes cancer classification system assigns tumors to four stages. These stages (with substages) reflect the extent of bowel-mucosa and bowel-wall infiltration, lymph node involvement, and metastasis.

Stage A
Malignant cells are confined to the bowel mucosa, and the lymph nodes contain no cancer cells. Treated promptly, about 90% of these patients remain disease-free 5 years later.

Stage B
Malignant cells extend through the bowel mucosa but remain within the bowel wall. The lymph nodes are normal. In substage B2, all bowel wall layers and immediately adjacent structures contain malignant cells, but the lymph nodes remain normal. About 63% of patients with substage B2 survive for 5 or more years. Duke's B is a composite of better (T3, N0, M0) and worse (T4, N0, M0) prognostic groups.

Stage C
Malignant cells extend into the bowel wall and the lymph nodes. In substage C2 malignant cells extend through the entire thickness of the bowel wall and into the lymph nodes. The 5-year survival rate for patients with stage C disease is about 25%. Duke's C is a composite of any T, N1, M0; and any T, N2, M0. MAC is the modified Astler-Coller Classification.

 ELDER TIP *Older patients may ignore bowel symptoms, believing that they result from constipation, poor diet, or hemorrhoids. Evaluate your older patient's responses to your questions carefully.*

On the right side of the colon (which absorbs water and electrolytes), early tumor growth causes no signs of obstruction because the tumor tends to grow along the bowel rather than surround the lumen, and the fecal content in this area is normally liquid. It may, however, cause black, tarry stools; anemia; and abdominal aching, pressure, or dull cramps. As the disease progresses, the patient develops weakness, fatigue, exertional dyspnea, vertigo and, eventually, diarrhea, obstipation, anorexia, weight loss, vomiting, and other signs or symptoms of intestinal obstruction. In addition, a tumor on the right side may be palpable.

On the left side, a tumor causes signs of an obstruction even in early stages because in this area stools are of a formed consistency. It commonly causes rectal bleeding (in many cases ascribed to hemorrhoids), intermittent abdominal fullness or cramping, and rectal pressure. As the disease progresses, the patient develops obstipation, diarrhea, or "ribbon" or pencil-shaped stools. Typically, he notices that passage of stools or flatus relieves the pain. At this stage, bleeding from the colon becomes obvious, with dark or bright red blood in the feces and mucus in or on the stools.

With a rectal tumor, the first symptom is a change in bowel habits, in many cases beginning with an urgent need to defecate on arising (morning diarrhea) or obstipation alternating with diarrhea. Other signs are blood or mucus in stools and a sense of incomplete evacuation. Late in the disease, pain begins as a feeling of rectal fullness that later becomes a dull, and sometimes constant, ache confined to the rectum or sacral region.

Diagnosis
Only a tumor biopsy can verify colorectal cancer, but other tests help detect it:
- Digital rectal examination can detect almost 15% of colorectal cancers.

bowel segment containing the tumor. Later signs or symptoms usually include pallor, cachexia, ascites, hepatomegaly, or lymphangiectasis.

■ Fecal occult blood test can detect blood in stools. However, it's commonly negative in patients with colon cancer.

■ Proctoscopy or sigmoidoscopy can detect up to 66% of colorectal cancers.

■ Colonoscopy permits visual inspection (and photographs) of the colon up to the ileocecal valve, and gives access for polypectomies and biopsies of suspected lesions.

■ Computed tomography scan helps to detect areas affected by metastasis.

■ Barium X-ray, using a dual contrast with air, can locate lesions that are undetectable manually or visually. Barium examination should *follow* endoscopy or excretory urography because the barium sulfate interferes with these tests.

■ Carcinoembryonic antigen, though not specific or sensitive enough for early diagnosis, is helpful in monitoring patients before and after treatment to detect metastasis or recurrence.

Treatment

The most effective treatment of colorectal cancer is surgery to remove the malignant tumor and adjacent tissues and any lymph nodes that may contain cancer cells. The type of surgery depends on the location of the tumor:

■ Cecum and ascending colon — right hemicolectomy (for advanced disease) may include resection of the terminal segment of the ileum, cecum, ascending colon, and right half of the transverse colon with corresponding mesentery

■ Proximal and middle transverse colon — right colectomy to include transverse colon and mesentery corresponding to midcolic vessels, or segmental resection of transverse colon and associated midcolic vessels

■ Sigmoid colon — surgery is usually limited to sigmoid colon and mesentery

■ Upper rectum — anterior or low anterior resection (newer method, using a stapler, allows for resections much lower than were previously possible)

■ Lower rectum — abdominoperineal resection and permanent sigmoid colostomy.

Chemotherapy is indicated for patients with metastasis, residual disease, or a recurrent inoperable tumor. Drugs used in such treatment commonly include fluorouracil with leucovorin, irinotecan, and oxaliplatin.

Radiation therapy induces tumor regression and may be used before or after surgery or combined with chemotherapy, especially fluorouracil.

Special considerations

Before surgery:

■ Monitor the patient's diet modifications, laxatives, enemas, and antibiotics — all used to clean the bowel and to decrease abdominal and perineal cavity contamination during surgery. If the patient is having a colostomy, teach him and his family about the procedure:

■ Emphasize that the stoma will be red, moist, and swollen and that postoperative swelling will eventually subside.

■ Show them a diagram of the intestine before and after surgery, stressing how much of the bowel will remain intact. Supplement your teaching with instructional aids. The patient can benefit from a consultation with an enterostomal therapist or wound and ostomy care nurse. Also arrange a postsurgical visit from a recovered ostomate.

■ Prepare the patient for postoperative I.V. infusions, nasogastric tube, and indwelling urinary catheter.

■ Discuss the importance of performing deep-breathing and coughing exercises.

After surgery:

■ Explain to the patient's family the importance of their positive reactions to the patient's adjustment. Consult with an enterostomal therapist, if available, to help set up a regimen for the patient.

■ Encourage the patient to look at the stoma and participate in its care as soon as possible. Teach good hygiene and skin care. Allow him to shower or bathe as soon as the incision heals. If appropriate, instruct the patient with a sigmoid colostomy to do his own irrigation as soon as he can after surgery. Advise him to schedule irrigation for the time of day when he normally evacuated before surgery. Many patients find that irrigating every 1 to 3 days is necessary for regularity. If flatus, diarrhea, or constipation occurs, eliminate suspected causative foods from the patient's diet. He may reintroduce them later.

■ After several months, many patients with sigmoid colostomies establish control with irrigation and no longer need to wear a pouch. A stoma cap or gauze sponge placed over the stoma protects it and absorbs mucoid secretions.

■ Before achieving such control, the patient can resume physical activities, including sports, provided that there's no threat of injury to the stoma or surrounding abdominal muscles. However, he should avoid heavy lifting because herniation or prolapse may occur through weakened muscles in the abdominal wall. A structured, gradually progressive exercise program to strengthen abdominal muscles may be instituted under medical supervision.

■ If appropriate, refer the patient to a home health agency for follow-up care and counseling. Suggest sexual counseling for male patients; most are impotent after an abdominoperineal resection.

■ Anyone who has had colorectal cancer is at increased risk for recurrence and should have yearly screening and testing.

Kidney cancer

Kidney cancer (also known as *nephrocarcinoma, renal cell carcinoma, hypernephroma,* and *Grawitz's tumor*) usually occurs in older adults. Renal pelvic tumors and Wilms' tumor occur primarily in children. Kidney tumors, which usually are large, firm, nodular, encapsulated, unilateral, and solitary, can be separated histologically into clear cell, granular, and spindle cell types. (See *Staging kidney cancer.*) The prognosis ranges from 66% for Stage I to 11% for Stage IV.

Causes and incidence
The causes of kidney cancer aren't known, although smokers develop more renal cell tumors than nonsmokers. However, the incidence of this malignancy is rising, possibly as a result of exposure to environmental carcinogens as well as increased longevity. Even so, this cancer accounts for only about 2% of all adult cancers. Kidney cancer is more common in men than women and peaks in incidence between ages 50 and 70.

Signs and symptoms
Kidney cancer produces a classic clinical triad (hematuria, pain, and a palpable mass), but any one may be the first sign of cancer. Microscopic or gross hematuria (which may be intermittent) suggests that the cancer has spread to the renal pelvis. Constant abdominal or flank pain may be dull or, if the cancer causes bleeding or blood clots, acute and colicky. The mass is generally smooth, firm, and nontender. All three signs coexist in only about 10% of patients.

Other signs include fever (perhaps from hemorrhage or necrosis), hypertension (from compression of the renal artery with renal parenchymal ischemia), rapidly progressing hypercalcemia (possibly from ectopic parathyroid hormone production by the tumor), and urine retention. Weight loss, edema in the legs, nausea, and vomiting signal advanced disease.

Diagnosis
Studies to identify kidney cancer usually include computed tomography scans, excretory urography, retrograde pyelography, ultrasound, cystoscopy (to rule out associated bladder cancer), and nephrotomography or renal angiography to distinguish a kidney cyst from a tumor.

Related tests include liver function studies showing increased levels of alkaline phosphatase, bilirubin, alanine aminotransferase and aspartate aminotransferase, and prolonged prothrombin time. Such results may point to liver metastasis, but if metastasis hasn't occurred, these abnormalities reverse after tumor resection.

Routine laboratory findings of hematuria, anemia (unrelated to blood loss), polycythemia, hypercalcemia, and increased erythrocyte sedimentation rate call for more testing to rule out kidney cancer.

Treatment
Radical nephrectomy, with or without regional lymph node dissection, offers the only chance of cure. Because the disease is radiation resistant, radiation is used only if the cancer spreads to the perinephric re-

STAGING KIDNEY CANCER

Using the TNM (tumor, node, metastasis) system, the American Joint Committee on Cancer has established the following stages for kidney cancer.

Primary tumor

TX — primary tumor can't be assessed

T0 — no evidence of primary tumor

T1a — tumor 4 cm or less in greatest dimension and limited to the kidney

T1b — tumor greater than 4 cm, but not more than 7 cm, in greatest dimension and limited to the kidney

T2 — tumor greater than 2.5 cm in greatest dimension and limited to the kidney

T3 — tumor extends into major veins or invades adrenal gland or perinephric tissues but not beyond Gerota's fascia

T3a — tumor extends into adrenal gland or perinephric tissues but not beyond Gerota's fascia

T3b — tumor grossly extends into renal veins or vena cava

T4 — tumor extends beyond Gerota's fascia

Regional lymph nodes

NX — regional lymph nodes can't be assessed

N0 — no evidence of regional lymph node metastasis

N1 — metastasis in a single lymph node, 2 cm or less in greatest dimension

N2 — metastasis in a single lymph node, between 2 and 5 cm in greatest dimension, or metastasis to several lymph nodes, none more than 5 cm in greatest dimension

N3 — metastasis in a lymph node, more than 5 cm in greatest dimension

Distant metastasis

MX — distant metastasis can't be assessed

M0 — no known distant metastasis

M1 — distant metastasis

Staging categories

Kidney cancer progresses from mild to severe as follows:

STAGE I — T1, N0, M0

STAGE II — T2, N0, M0

STAGE III — T1, N1, M0; T2, N1, M0; T3a, N0, M0; T3a, N1, M0; T3b, N0, M0; T3b, N1, M0

STAGE IV — T4, any N, M0; any T, N2, M0; any T, N3, M0; any T, any N, M1

gion or the lymph nodes or if the primary tumor or metastatic sites can't be fully excised. In these cases, high radiation doses are used.

Chemotherapy has been only erratically effective against kidney cancer. Fluorouracil, cyclophosphamide, vinblastine, vincristine, cisplatin, tamoxifen, teniposide, interferons, and hormones such as medroxyprogesterone and testosterone have been used, usually with poor results. Biotherapy (interferon and interleukins), commonly used in advanced disease, has produced few durable remissions.

Special considerations

Meticulous postoperative care, supportive treatment during other therapy, and psychological support can hasten recovery and minimize complications.

■ Before surgery, assure the patient that his body will adapt to the loss of a kidney.

■ Teach the patient about such expected postoperative procedures as diaphragmatic breathing, coughing properly, splinting his incision, and others.

■ After surgery, encourage diaphragmatic breathing and coughing.

■ Assist the patient with leg exercises, and turn him every 2 hours.

■ Check dressings often for excessive bleeding. Watch for signs of internal bleeding, such as restlessness, sweating, and increased pulse rate.

■ Place the patient on the operative side to allow the pressure of adjacent organs to fill

the dead space at the operative site, improving dependent drainage. If possible, help the patient walk within 24 hours after surgery.
- Maintain adequate fluid intake, and monitor intake and output. Monitor laboratory results for anemia, polycythemia, or abnormal blood values that may point to bone or liver involvement or may result from radiation or chemotherapy.
- Treat drug adverse effects.
- Stress compliance with the prescribed outpatient treatment regimen.

Liver cancer

Liver cancer, also known as *primary* and *metastatic hepatic carcinoma,* is a rare form of cancer in the United States, with a high mortality. Most primary liver tumors (90%) originate in the parenchymal cells and are hepatomas (hepatocellular carcinoma, primary lower-cell carcinoma). Some primary tumors originate in the intrahepatic bile ducts and are known as *cholangiomas* (cholangiocarcinoma, cholangiocellular carcinoma). Rarer tumors include a mixed-cell type, Kupffer cell sarcoma, and hepatoblastomas (which occur almost exclusively in children and are usually resectable and curable). The liver is one of the most common sites of metastasis from other primary cancers, particularly colon, rectum, stomach, pancreas, esophagus, lung, breast, or melanoma. In the United States, metastatic carcinoma is over 20 times more common than primary carcinoma and, after cirrhosis, is the leading cause of liver-related death. At times, liver metastasis may appear as a solitary lesion, the first sign of recurrence after a remission.

Causes and incidence

The immediate cause of liver cancer is unknown, but it may be a congenital disease in children. Adult liver cancer may result from environmental exposure to carcinogens, such as the chemical compound aflatoxin (a mold that grows on rice and peanuts), thorium dioxide (a contrast medium formerly used in liver radiography), *Senecio* alkaloids, and possibly androgens and oral estrogens.

Roughly 30% to 70% of patients with hepatomas also have cirrhosis. (Hepatomas are 40 times more likely to develop in a cirrhotic liver than in a normal one.)

Whether cirrhosis is a premalignant state or alcohol and malnutrition predispose the liver to develop hepatomas is still unclear. Other risk factors are exposure to the hepatitis C virus and the hepatitis B virus.

Liver cancer accounts for roughly 1% of all cancers in the United States and for 10% to 50% in Africa and parts of Asia. Liver cancer is most prevalent in men (particularly men older than age 60), and incidence increases with age. It's rapidly fatal, usually within 6 months, from GI hemorrhage, progressive cachexia, hepatic failure, or metastasis.

Signs and symptoms

Clinical effects of liver cancer include:
- a mass in the right upper quadrant
- tender, nodular liver on palpation
- severe pain in the epigastrium or the right upper quadrant
- bruit, hum, or rubbing sound if tumor involves a large part of the liver
- weight loss, weakness, anorexia, fever
- occasional jaundice or ascites
- occasional evidence of metastasis through venous system to lungs, from lymphatics to regional lymph nodes, or by direct invasion of portal veins
- dependent edema.

Diagnosis

 CONFIRMING DIAGNOSIS *The confirming test for liver cancer is liver biopsy by needle or open biopsy.*

Liver cancer is difficult to diagnose in the presence of cirrhosis, but several tests can help identify it:
- Serum glutamic-oxaloacetic transaminase, serum glutamic-pyruvic transaminase, alkaline phosphatase, lactic dehydrogenase, and bilirubin all show abnormal liver function.
- Alpha-fetoprotein rises to a level above 500 mcg/ml.
- Chest X-ray may rule out metastasis.
- Liver scan may show filling defects.

- Arteriography may define large tumors.
- Electrolyte studies may indicate an increased retention of sodium (resulting in functional renal failure) and hypoglycemia, leukocytosis, hypercalcemia, or hypocholesterolemia.

Treatment

Because liver cancer is commonly in an advanced stage at diagnosis, few hepatic tumors are resectable. A resectable tumor must be a single tumor in one lobe, without cirrhosis, jaundice, or ascites. Resection is done by lobectomy or partial hepatectomy.

Radiation therapy for unresectable tumors is usually palliative. Because of the liver's low tolerance for radiation, external beam radiation hasn't increased survival. However, radiolabeled antibodies have been used to selectively target cancer tissue; when used concurrently with chemotherapy, patients can convert from nonresectable to resectable.

Another method of treatment is chemotherapy with I.V. fluorouracil, mitomycin, or doxorubicin, or with regional infusion of fluorouracil or floxuridine (catheters are placed directly into the hepatic artery or left brachial artery for continuous infusion for 7 to 21 days, or permanent implantable pumps are used on an outpatient basis for long-term infusion).

Appropriate treatment for liver metastasis may include resection by lobectomy or chemotherapy with mitomycin or fludarabine (results similar to those in hepatoma). Liver transplantation is now an alternative for a small subset of patients.

Special considerations

The patient care plan should emphasize comprehensive supportive care and emotional support.

- Control edema and ascites. Monitor the patient's diet throughout. Most patients need a special diet that restricts sodium, fluids (no alcohol allowed), and protein. Weigh the patient daily, and note intake and output accurately. Watch for signs of ascites (peripheral edema, orthopnea, or dyspnea on exertion). If ascites is present, measure and record abdominal girth daily. To increase venous return and prevent edema, elevate the patient's legs whenever possible.
- Monitor respiratory function. Note any increase in respiratory rate or shortness of breath. Bilateral pleural effusion (noted on chest X-ray) is common, as is metastasis to the lungs. Watch carefully for signs of hypoxemia from intrapulmonary arteriovenous shunting.
- Relieve fever. Administer sponge baths and aspirin suppositories if there are no signs of GI bleeding. Avoid acetaminophen, because the diseased liver can't metabolize it. High fever indicates infection and requires antibiotics.
- Give meticulous skin care. Turn the patient frequently and keep his skin clean to prevent pressure ulcers. Apply lotion to prevent chafing, and administer an antipruritic such as diphenhydramine for severe itching.
- Watch for encephalopathy. Many patients develop end-stage signs or symptoms of ammonia intoxication, including confusion, restlessness, irritability, agitation, delirium, asterixis, lethargy and, finally, coma. Monitor the patient's serum ammonia level, vital signs, and neurologic status. Be prepared to control ammonia accumulation with sorbitol (to induce osmotic diarrhea), neomycin (to reduce bacterial flora in the GI tract), lactulose (to control bacterial elaboration of ammonia), and sodium polystyrene sulfonate (to lower potassium level).
- If a transhepatic catheter is used to relieve obstructive jaundice, irrigate it frequently with prescribed solution (normal saline or, sometimes, 5,000 units of heparin in 500 ml dextrose 5% in water). Monitor vital signs frequently for any indication of bleeding or infection.
- After surgery, give standard postoperative care. Watch for intraperitoneal bleeding and sepsis, which may precipitate coma. Monitor for renal failure by checking urine output, blood urea nitrogen, and creatinine levels hourly. Remember that, throughout the course of this intractable illness, your primary concern is to keep the patient as comfortable as possible.
- When all treatments have failed, concentrate on keeping the patient comfortable and free from pain, and provide as much

psychological support as possible. If the patient is going home, discuss continuing care needs with the caregiver or refer the patient to an appropriate home health care agency or hospice. Encourage the patient and caregiver to express their feelings and concerns. Answer their questions honestly, with tact and sensitivity.

Bladder cancer

Bladder tumors can develop on the surface of the bladder wall (benign or malignant papillomas) or grow within the bladder wall (generally more virulent) and quickly invade underlying muscles. Ninety percent of bladder tumors are transitional cell carcinomas, arising from the transitional epithelium of mucous membranes. Less common are adenocarcinomas, epidermoid carcinomas, squamous cell cancers, sarcomas, tumors in bladder diverticula, and carcinoma in situ. Cancer of the bladder is the most common cancer of the urinary tract.

Causes and incidence

Certain environmental carcinogens, such as 2-naphthylamine, benzidine, tobacco, and nitrates, predispose people to transitional cell tumors. Thus, workers in certain industries (rubber workers, weavers and leather finishers, aniline dye workers, hairdressers, petroleum workers, and spray painters) are at high risk for such tumors. The period between exposure to the carcinogen and development of symptoms is about 18 years.

Squamous cell cancer of the bladder is most common in geographic areas where schistosomiasis is endemic. It's also associated with chronic bladder irritation and infection (for example, from renal calculi, indwelling urinary catheters, and cystitis caused by cyclophosphamide).

Bladder tumors are most prevalent in men older than age 50 and are more common in densely populated industrial areas.

Signs and symptoms

In early stages, approximately 25% of patients with bladder tumors have no symptoms. Commonly, the first sign is gross, painless, intermittent hematuria (in many cases with clots in the urine). Many patients with invasive lesions have suprapubic pain after voiding. Other signs and symptoms include bladder irritability, urinary frequency, nocturia, and dribbling.

Diagnosis

 CONFIRMING DIAGNOSIS *Only cystoscopy and biopsy confirm bladder cancer. Cystoscopy should be performed when hematuria first appears. When it's performed under anesthesia, a bimanual examination is usually done to determine if the bladder is fixed to the pelvic wall. A thorough history and physical examination may help determine whether the tumor has invaded the prostate or the lymph nodes. (See* Comparing staging systems for bladder cancer.*)*

The following tests can provide essential information about the tumor:
- Urinalysis can detect blood in the urine and malignant cytology.
- Excretory urography can identify a large, early stage tumor or an infiltrating tumor, delineate functional problems in the upper urinary tract, assess hydronephrosis, and detect rigid deformity of the bladder wall.
- Retrograde cystography evaluates bladder structure and integrity. Test results help to confirm the diagnosis.
- Pelvic arteriography can reveal tumor invasion into the bladder wall.
- Computed tomography scan reveals the thickness of the involved bladder wall and detects enlarged retroperitoneal lymph nodes.
- Ultrasonography can detect metastasis beyond the bladder and can distinguish a bladder cyst from a tumor.
- Excretory urography evaluates the upper urinary tract for tumors or blockage.

Treatment

Superficial bladder tumors are removed by transurethral (cystoscopic) resection and fulguration (electrical destruction). This

COMPARING STAGING SYSTEMS FOR BLADDER CANCER

Staging helps determine the most appropriate treatment for bladder cancer. One or two staging systems may be used: the TNM (tumor, node, metastasis) system or the JSM (Jewett-Strong-Marshall) system. The JSM system grades cancers 0 and A through D. Both systems distinguish superficial bladder cancers from invasive bladder cancers, which penetrate bladder muscle and may spread to other sites.

TNM	STAGE	JSM
Superficial tumor		
TX	Primary tumor can't be assessed	—
T0	No tumor	0
Tis	Carcinoma in situ	0
Ta	Noninvasive papillary tumor	0
Invasive tumor		
T1	Tumor invades subepithelial connective tissue	—
T2	Tumor invades superficial muscle (inner half)	B_1
T3a	Tumor invades deep muscle	B_2
T3b	Tumor invades perivesical fat	C
T4	Tumor invades prostate, uterus, vagina, pelvic wall, or abdominal wall	D_1
NX	Regional lymph nodes can't be assessed	—
N0	No evidence of lymph node involvement	—
N1	Metastasis in a single lymph node, 2 cm or less in greatest dimension	D_1
N2	Metastasis in a single lymph node, between 2 and 5 cm in greatest dimension, or metastasis to several lymph nodes, none greater than 5 cm in greatest dimension	—
N3	Metastasis in a lymph node more than 5 cm in greatest dimension	—
MX	Distant metastasis can't be assessed	—
M0	No evidence of distant metastasis	—
M	Distant metastasis	D_2

procedure is adequate when the tumor hasn't invaded the muscle.

Intravesicular chemotherapy is also used for superficial tumors (especially those that occur in many sites) and to prevent tumor recurrence. This treatment involves washing the bladder directly with antineoplastic drugs — most commonly, thiotepa, doxorubicin, mitomycin, or Bacillus Calmette-Guérin immunotherapy.

If additional tumors develop, fulguration may have to be repeated every 3 months for years. However, if the tumors penetrate the muscle layer or recur frequently, cystoscopy with fulguration is no longer appropriate.

Tumors too large to be treated through a cystoscope require segmental bladder resection to remove a full-thickness section of the bladder. This procedure is feasible only if the tumor isn't near the bladder neck or ureteral orifices. Bladder instillation of thiotepa, mitomycin-C, or doxorubicin after transurethral resection may also help control such tumors.

For infiltrating bladder tumors, radical cystectomy is the treatment of choice. The week before cystectomy, treatment may include external beam therapy to the bladder. Surgery involves removal of the bladder with perivesical fat, lymph nodes, urethra, the prostate and seminal vesicles (in males), and the uterus and adnexa (in females). The surgeon forms a urinary diversion, usually an ileal conduit. The patient must then wear an external pouch continuously. Other diversions include ureterostomy, nephrostomy, vesicostomy, ileal bladder, ileal loop, and sigmoid conduit.

Males are impotent following radical cystectomy and urethrectomy because these procedures damage the sympathetic and parasympathetic nerves that control erection and ejaculation. At a later date, the patient may desire a penile implant to make sexual intercourse (without ejaculation) possible.

Treatment of patients with advanced bladder cancer includes cystectomy to remove the tumor, radiation therapy, and systemic chemotherapy with such drugs as doxorubicin, methotrexate, vinblastine, and cisplatin. This combination sometimes is successful in arresting bladder cancer. Cisplatin is the most effective single agent. Investigational treatments include photodynamic therapy and intravesicular administration of interferon-alfa and tumor necrosis factor. Photodynamic therapy involves I.V. injection of a photosensitizing agent such as hematoporphyrin ether, which malignant cells readily absorb. Then a cystoscopic laser device introduces laser energy into the bladder, exposing the malignant cells to laser light, which kills them. Because this treatment also produces photosensitivity in normal cells, the patient must totally avoid sunlight for about 30 days.

Special considerations

■ Before surgery, assist in selecting a stoma site that the patient can see (usually in the rectus muscle to minimize the risk of herniation). Do so by assessing the abdomen in various positions.

■ After surgery, encourage the patient to look at the stoma. Provide a mirror to make viewing easier.

■ To obtain a specimen for culture and sensitivity testing, catheterize the patient using sterile technique. Insert the lubricated tip of the catheter into the stoma about 2″ (5.1 cm). In many facilities, a double telescope-type catheter is available for ileal conduit catheterization.

■ Advise the patient with a urinary stoma that he may participate in most activities, except for heavy lifting and contact sports.

■ When a patient with a urinary diversion is discharged, arrange for follow-up home health care or refer him to an enterostomal therapist, who will help coordinate the patient's care.

■ Teach the patient about his urinary stoma. Encourage his spouse, a friend, or a relative to attend the teaching session. Advise this person beforehand that a negative reaction to the stoma can impede the patient's adjustment.

■ First, show the patient how to prepare and apply the pouch, which may be reusable or disposable. If he chooses the reusable type, he'll need at least two.

■ To select the right pouch size, measure the stoma and order a pouch with an opening that clears the stoma with a ⅛″

(3 mm) margin. Instruct the patient to re-measure the stoma after he goes home, in case the size changes. The pouch should have a drainage valve at the bottom. Tell the patient to empty the pouch when it's one-third full or every 2 to 3 hours.

■ To ensure a good skin seal, select a skin barrier that contains synthetics and little or no karaya (which urine tends to destroy). Check the pouch frequently to make sure that the skin seal remains intact. A good skin seal with a skin barrier may last for 3 to 6 days, so change the pouch only that often. Tell the patient that he can wear a loose-fitting elastic belt to help secure the pouch.

■ The ileal conduit stoma reaches its permanent size 2 to 4 months after surgery. Because the intestine normally produces mucus, mucus will appear in the draining urine.

■ Keep the skin around the stoma clean and free from irritation. After removing the pouch, wash the skin with water and mild soap. Rinse well with clear water to remove soap residue, and then gently pat the skin dry; don't rub. Place a gauze sponge soaked with vinegar-water (1 part to 3 parts) over the stoma for a few minutes to prevent uric acid crystal buildup. While preparing the skin, place a rolled-up dry sponge over the stoma to collect draining urine. Coat the skin with skin protectant, and cover with the collection pouch. If skin irritation or breakdown occurs, apply a layer of antacid precipitate to the clean, dry skin before coating with the skin protector.

■ The patient can level uneven surfaces on his abdomen, such as gullies, scars, or wedges, with various specially prepared products or skin barriers.

■ All high-risk people — for example, chemical workers and people with a history of benign bladder tumors or persistent cystitis — should have periodic cytologic examinations and learn about the danger of disease-causing agents.

■ Refer patients with ostomies to such support organizations as the American Cancer Society and the United Ostomy Association.

Gallbladder and bile duct cancer

Gallbladder cancer is rare, accounting for fewer than 1% of all cancers. It's normally found by accident in patients with chole-cystitis; 1 in 400 cholecystectomies reveals a malignant tumor. The disease is most prevalent in females older than age 60. It's rapidly progressive and usually fatal; patients seldom live a year after diagnosis. The poor prognosis is due to late diagnosis; gallbladder cancer isn't usually diagnosed until after cholecystectomy, when in many cases it's in an advanced, metastatic stage.

Causes and incidence

Gallbladder cancer may result from a complication of gallstones. However, this inference rests on circumstantial evidence from postmortem examinations: 60% to 90% of gallbladder cancer patients also have gallstones, but postmortem data from patients with gallstones show gallbladder cancer in only 0.5%.

The predominant tissue type in gallbladder cancer is adenocarcinoma, 85% to 95%; squamous cell, 5% to 15%. Mixed-tissue types are rare.

Lymph node metastasis is present in 25% to 70% of patients at diagnosis. Direct extension to the liver is common (in 46% to 89%); direct extension to both the cystic and the common bile ducts, stomach, colon, duodenum, and jejunum also occurs and produces obstructions. Metastasis also spreads by portal or hepatic veins to the peritoneum, ovaries, and lower lung lobes.

The cause of extrahepatic bile duct cancer isn't known; however, statistics report an unexplained increased incidence of this cancer in patients with ulcerative colitis. This association may be due to a common cause — perhaps an immune mechanism, or chronic use of certain drugs by the colitis patient.

Extrahepatic bile duct cancer is the cause of approximately 3% of all cancer deaths in the United States. It occurs in both males and females (incidence is slightly higher in males) between ages 60 and 70. The usual site is at the bifurcation in the common duct. Cancer at the distal end of the common duct is commonly confused with cancer of the pancreas. Characteristically, metastatic spread occurs to local lymph nodes, the liver, lungs, and the peritoneum.

Signs and symptoms

Clinically, gallbladder cancer is almost indistinguishable from cholecystitis — pain in the epigastrium or right upper quadrant, weight loss, anorexia, nausea, vomiting, and jaundice. However, chronic, progressively severe pain in an afebrile patient suggests malignancy. In patients with simple gallstones, pain is sporadic. Another telling clue to malignancy is palpable gallbladder (right upper quadrant), with obstructive jaundice. Some patients may also have hepatosplenomegaly.

Progressive profound jaundice is commonly the first sign of obstruction due to extrahepatic bile duct cancer. The jaundice is usually accompanied by chronic pain in the epigastrium or the right upper quadrant, radiating to the back. Other common signs or symptoms, if associated with active cholecystitis, include pruritus, skin excoriations, anorexia, weight loss, chills, and fever.

Diagnosis

No test or procedure, by itself, can diagnose gallbladder cancer. However, the following laboratory tests support the diagnosis when they suggest hepatic dysfunction and extrahepatic biliary obstruction:
■ baseline studies — complete blood count, routine urinalysis, electrolyte studies, enzymes
■ liver function tests — typically reveal elevated serum bilirubin, urine bile and bilirubin, and urobilinogen levels in more than 50% of patients as well as consistently elevated serum alkaline phosphatase levels
■ occult blood in stools — linked to the associated anemia
■ cholecystography — may show calculi or calcification
■ cholangiography — may locate the site of common duct obstruction
■ magnetic resonance imaging — detects tumors.

The following tests help compile data that confirm extrahepatic bile duct cancer:
■ liver function studies — indicate biliary obstruction: elevated levels of bilirubin

[5 to 30 mg/dl], alkaline phosphatase, and blood cholesterol as well as prolonged prothrombin time
■ endoscopic retrograde cannulization of the pancreas — identifies the tumor site and allows access for obtaining a biopsy specimen.

Treatment

Surgical treatment of gallbladder cancer is essentially palliative and includes various procedures, such as cholecystectomy, common bile duct exploration, T-tube drainage, and wedge excision of hepatic tissue.

If the cancer invades gallbladder musculature, the survival rate is less than 5%, even with massive resection. Although some cases of long-term survival (4 to 5 years) have been reported, few patients survive longer than 6 months after surgery for gallbladder cancer.

Surgery is normally indicated to relieve obstruction and jaundice that result from extrahepatic bile duct cancer. The procedure used to relieve obstruction depends on the cancer site. Such procedures may include cholecystoduodenostomy or T-tube drainage of the common duct.

Other palliative measures for both kinds of cancer include radiation, radiation implants (mostly used for local and incisional recurrences), and chemotherapy (with combinations of fluorouracil, irinotecan, and gemcitabine). All of these treatment measures have limited effects.

Special considerations

After biliary resection:
■ Monitor vital signs.
■ Use strict sterile technique when caring for the incision and the surrounding area.
■ Place the patient in low Fowler's position.
■ Prevent respiratory problems by encouraging deep breathing and coughing. The high incision makes the patient want to take shallow breaths; using analgesics and splinting his abdomen with a pillow or an abdominal binder may aid in greater respiratory efforts.
■ Monitor bowel sounds and bowel movements. Observe the patient's tolerance to diet.
■ Provide pain control.

ELDER TIP *Check intake and output carefully. Watch for electrolyte imbalance; monitor I.V. solutions to avoid overloading the cardiovascular system, especially in older patients.*
■ Monitor the nasogastric tube, which will be in place for 24 to 72 hours postoperatively to relieve distention, and the T tube. Record amount and color of drainage each shift. Secure the T tube to minimize tension on it and prevent its being pulled out.
■ Help the patient and his family cope with their initial fears and reactions to the diagnosis by offering information and support.
■ Before discharge, teach the patient how to manage the biliary catheter.
■ Advise the patient of the adverse effects of both chemotherapy and radiation therapy, and monitor him for these effects.
■ When all treatments have failed, concentrate on keeping the patient comfortable and free from pain and provide as much psychological support as possible. If the patient is going home, discuss continuing care needs with the caregiver or refer the patient to an appropriate home health care or hospice agency. Encourage the patient and caregiver to express their feelings and concerns. Answer their questions honestly, with tact and sensitivity.

MALE AND FEMALE GENITALIA

Prostatic cancer

Prostatic cancer is the most common cancer in men older than age 50. Adenocarcinoma is its most common form; sarcoma occurs only rarely. Most prostatic cancers originate in the posterior prostate gland; the rest originate near the urethra. Malignant prostatic tumors seldom result from the benign hyperplastic enlargement that commonly develops around the prostatic urethra in elderly men. Prostatic cancer seldom produces symptoms until it's advanced.

Causes and incidence

Four factors have been suspected in the development of prostatic cancer: family or racial predisposition, exposure to environmental elements, co-existing sexually transmitted diseases, and endogenous hormonal influence. Eating fat-containing animal products has also been implicated. Although androgens regulate prostate growth and function and may also speed tumor growth, no definite link between increased androgen levels and prostatic cancer has been found. When primary prostatic lesions metastasize, they typically invade the prostatic capsule and spread along the ejaculatory ducts in the space between the seminal vesicles or perivesicular fascia.

Incidence is highest in Blacks and lowest in Asians. In fact, Black Americans have the highest prostate cancer incidence in the world and are considered at high risk for the disease. Incidence also increases with age more rapidly than any other cancer.

Signs and symptoms

Signs and symptoms of prostatic cancer appear only in the advanced stages and include difficulty initiating a urine stream, dribbling, urine retention, unexplained cystitis and, rarely, hematuria. Pain may be present with urination, ejaculation, and bowel movement. (See *Staging prostatic cancer*, page 104.)

Diagnosis

A digital rectal examination that reveals a small, hard nodule may help diagnose prostatic cancer. The American Cancer Society advises a yearly digital examination for men older than age 40, a yearly blood test to detect prostate-specific antigen (PSA) in men older than age 50, and ultrasound if abnormal results are found.

CONFIRMING DIAGNOSIS *A biopsy confirms the diagnosis of prostatic cancer. PSA levels will be elevated in all men with metastatic prostatic cancer. Serum acid phosphatase levels will be elevated in two-thirds of men with metastatic prostatic cancer.*

Therapy aims to return the serum acid phosphatase level to normal; a subsequent rise points to recurrence. Magnetic resonance imaging, computed tomography

STAGING PROSTATIC CANCER

The American Joint Committee on Cancer recognizes the TNM (tumor, node, metastasis) cancer staging system for assessing prostatic cancer.

Primary tumor
TX — primary tumor can't be assessed
T0 — no evidence of primary tumor
T1 — tumor an incidental histologic finding
T1a — three or fewer microscopic foci of cancer
T1b — more than three microscopic foci of cancer
T2 — tumor limited to the prostate gland
T2a — tumor involves one-half of 1 lobe or less
T2b — tumor involves more than one-half of 1 lobe but not both lobes
T2c — tumor involves both lobes
T3 — unfixed tumor extends into the prostatic apex or into or beyond the prostatic capsule, bladder neck, or seminal vesicle
T4 — tumor fixed or invades adjacent structures not listed in T3

Regional lymph nodes
NX — regional lymph nodes can't be assessed
N0 — no evidence of regional lymph-node metastasis

N1 — metastasis in a single lymph node, 2 cm or less in greatest dimension
N2 — metastasis in a single lymph node, between 2 and 5 cm in greatest dimension, or metastasis to several lymph nodes, none more than 5 cm in greatest dimension
N3 — metastasis in a lymph node more than 5 cm in greatest dimension

Distant metastasis
MX — distant metastasis can't be assessed
M0 — no known distant metastasis
M1 — distant metastasis

Staging categories
Prostatic cancer progresses from mild to severe as follows:
STAGE 0 or STAGE I — T1a, N0, M0; T2a, N0, M0
STAGE II — T1b, N0, M0; T2b, N0, M0
STAGE III — T3, N0, M0
STAGE IV — T4, N0, M0; any T, N1, M0; any T, N2, M0; any T, N3, M0; any T, any N, M1

---

scan, and excretory urography may also aid diagnosis.

Elevated alkaline phosphatase levels and a positive bone scan point to bone metastasis.

Treatment

Management of prostatic cancer depends on clinical assessment, tolerance of therapy, expected life span, and the stage of the disease. Treatment must be chosen carefully, because prostatic cancer usually affects older men, who commonly have coexisting disorders, such as hypertension, diabetes, or cardiac disease.

Therapy varies with each stage of the disease and generally includes radiation, prostatectomy, orchiectomy to reduce androgen production, and hormone therapy with synthetic estrogen (diethylstilbestrol [DES]) and antiandrogens, such as cyproterone, megestrol, and flutamide. Radical prostatectomy is usually effective for localized lesions.

Radiation therapy is used to cure some locally invasive lesions and to relieve pain from metastatic bone involvement. A single injection of the radionuclide strontium 89 is also used to treat pain caused by bone metastasis.

If hormone therapy, surgery, and radiation therapy aren't feasible or successful, chemotherapy (using combinations of mitoxantrone with prednisone, estramustine,

of miracles. May, the month Jesus sat with her on the grass in Golden Gate Park, spoke her name tenderly, and sent her home. She hadn't known she carried a child then, but God had. "That sounds perfect, Mitch." She placed her hand on his chest and felt his warmth, his strength, the steady beat of his heart. God had given her a man she could trust. Even so, it took courage to say the words. "I love you."

"I know." His mouth tipped in a teasing smile. "But I've loved you longer."

"You're getting the raw end of the deal, Mitch."

"No, I'm not. And don't ever say that again." He touched her as though she were the most precious thing in the world to him. "I'm getting the woman I want. I feel as though I've loved you forever."

She knew he meant it.

❄ ❄ ❄

Their wedding day turned out to be a perfect, sunny day. Carolyn's father gave her away while Mom and May Flower Dawn sat in the front row of folding chairs. Dawn didn't want to be her flower girl, so Carolyn didn't have one. Mitch's pastor performed the wedding ceremony before a gathering of Mitch's close friends and Carolyn's relatives. She was surprised they all came, including Aunt Rikka, who flew in from New York. Boots drove up from Topanga Canyon. Mitch had arranged for a professional photographer who took candid shots as well as formal poses. He'd also hired a catering service to put on a wedding luncheon.

Oma patted Carolyn's cheek before she and Mom and Dad headed home. "You've done well for yourself. I'm proud of you." Mitch bent down to receive her kiss of blessing. "Take good care of my girl." He promised he would. He had a honeymoon planned, but wouldn't tell Carolyn anything about it. May Flower Dawn was "going home with Granny and Papa." Mitch reminded Dawn home was now Alexander Valley, and he and her mother would be picking her up in ten days. Dawn looked less defiant after that.

Mitch saw the last guests out while the caterers cleared everything away. Within a few hours, the folding chairs and tables, the linens, trays, and china had been loaded into vans, leaving the gardens and house spotless and silent.

Mitch took Carolyn's hand and led her to the master suite. She felt a bubbling fear in her belly as all the old memories rose up. Mitch sensed something was wrong. He didn't push. He took his time. Even so, he knew she hadn't experienced the pleasure he had. He didn't ask questions, just held her close. Emotionally exhausted, she fell asleep in his arms. He awakened her with kisses and coffee at three thirty in the morning. "Time to get dressed."

"Where are we going?"

"Hawaii. A limo is picking us up."

"What? I haven't packed!"

"Your mom took care of that. Anything you don't have, we'll buy when we get there."

Dear Rosie,

Carolyn and Mitch are married. I am so happy for them. The wedding was lovely and held in the backyard of Mitch's rather palatial home in Alexander Valley. The place looks like a Tuscan villa, with cypress trees lining his driveway and a vineyard on the hills behind the house with all its grand landscaping, pool, and gazebo. Bernhard was all praises about it. I was equally impressed. I remember Mitch when he was a skinny, freckled redhead on a bicycle, riding off with Charlie to do some mischief and, later, a gangly young man with eyes for Carolyn, though she never seemed aware of his adoration. He has grown handsome, competent, confident—a man who always did know what he wanted: Carolyn. My prayers for her are answered. Mitch sees her as a gift from God and will treat her accordingly.

Carolyn asked May Flower Dawn to be her flower girl, but the child refused. She sat in the front row and sulked. Hildemara made no effort to correct her rude misbehavior. I wanted to turn both of them over my knee. Dawn will stay with Hildemara and Trip until Carolyn and Mitch return from a Hawaiian honeymoon.

Hildemara understands she must relinquish May Flower Dawn. Or says she does. I wonder.

I tried to talk with Hildemara about our past, but she cut the conversation short. All I can do is keep holding out the olive branch and hope one day she will accept it.

Oh, Rosie, I look back and wish I had handled things differently. . . .

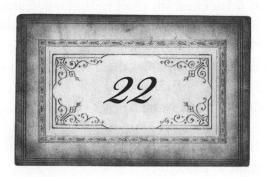

22

Mom and Dad greeted them on their return from a glorious week in Hawaii. While Dad took Mitch into the living room, Mom took Carolyn into the kitchen. She looked worried. "What's wrong, Mom? Where's Dawn?"

"In her room. We explained everything to her, but she doesn't fully understand." She offered Carolyn a cup of tea or coffee. "This is the only real home she's ever known."

What about the house on Vineyard Avenue? Carolyn wanted to say. *Didn't that count?* "She doesn't want to go with me. Is that what you're trying to tell me?"

"She's only seven, Carolyn."

"She's my daughter."

"I know that. It's just going to be very hard for her to adjust to all these changes."

Mom's red-rimmed eyes told Carolyn her daughter wasn't the only one having a hard time.

"I'm sorry about that, but I think the sooner we go, the better."

"You won't even stay for dinner?"

"Is she packed?"

May Flower Dawn clung to her grandfather. Pried loose and strapped into the backseat, she cried for an hour. Carolyn and Mitch tried to reassure her. It didn't help. When she finally fell asleep in the backseat, Mitch took Carolyn's hand. "Give her time."

Mitch carried their things into the house. Carolyn unpacked Dawn's clothes, hanging her dresses in the closet and putting the rest into the dresser. She left the Barbies and doll clothes in the box for Dawn to unpack the next morning. When she told Dawn to get ready for bed, she did. As she tucked her in, Dawn started to cry again. "I want to go home!"

"This is your home."

"I want *Granny*!"

Pierced through the heart, Carolyn bent down and kissed her daughter's head. "Sorry, May Flower Dawn. You're stuck with your *mother*."

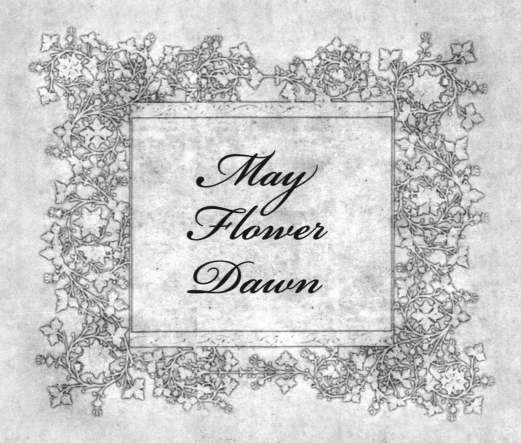

May
Flower
Dawn

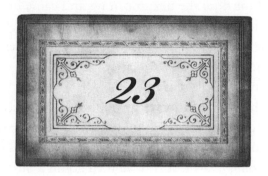

WIDE-AWAKE AND MISERABLE, Dawn lay curled in a ball in the middle of her fancy new bed. Her mother had turned off the light and closed the door, leaving only a tiny night-light in the bathroom to contend against total darkness. Even though she was seven and a half, Dawn was a little nervous in this big, dark, silent room. Unlike her mother's bungalow on Vineyard Avenue, Mitch's house stood at the end of a long driveway lined with cypress trees, too far from the road to hear cars or see headlights.

Dawn didn't want to live in this house so far away from Granny and Papa. Her mother wouldn't have time for her. She'd never see her school friends again. Granny said she and Papa would come to visit soon, but what did "soon" mean? Tomorrow? Next week?

Dawn wiped away angry tears. She had initially liked Mitch, but now that he'd married Mom, she wasn't so sure.

A soft wind and moonlight cast frightening shadows outside her window. Dawn huddled deep under the blankets, covered her head, and cried herself to sleep.

❄ ❄ ❄

Mom opened the door the next morning and came in, all smiles and cheer. "Breakfast will be ready soon."

Dawn hated that her mother looked so happy when she was so miserable. "I'm not hungry."

"I'm making bacon and waffles."

Dawn set her jaw, refusing to be tempted by her favorite breakfast. "I'm not going to eat anything until you take me home." She felt triumphant when the joy dimmed in her mother's face.

"You *are* home, Dawn. If you want to go on a hunger strike, that's fine. If you want to come out and sit with us, even better. Either way, I won't force you." Her mother quietly closed the door behind her.

Dawn stared, furious. When fifteen minutes passed and Mom didn't come back, Dawn shoved her covers off and went into the pink, green, and white bathroom. Her hair looked like a blonde mop on her head. Granny used to brush it for her every morning. Her clothes lay in a mess on the floor where she'd dropped them. Granny would have picked them up and folded them for her. Her mother always expected her to do everything herself! She'd probably force her to do dishes, too!

As Dawn approached the kitchen archway, she heard Mom talking. "A private Christian school is too expensive, Mitch. She's my daughter. I wouldn't feel right having you pay tuition—"

"Whoa. What's mine is yours now. Remember? You need to get that into your head, Carolyn. We're partners."

"She's been going to a public school. I'm not sure I want her in a Christian school."

"Why not?"

Her mother spoke too quietly for Dawn to hear. Dawn walked around the corner and through the archway into the kitchen.

Mitch grinned. "Well, good morning, sleepyhead." Dawn glared at him. His brows rose. "Oops. I guess you're not a morning person."

Her mother studied her coolly. "I thought you weren't hungry."

"I won't eat if you don't want me to. I can go back to my room and stay there and starve, if that's what you want!"

Mitch breathed out a laugh. "Trying hard to be a pita, aren't you?"

"Pita?"

"Pain in the . . . Never mind." He stood, pulled out a chair, and bowed. "It would please us humble folk to have Your Majesty grace us with your presence at our table." He waved his arm for her to sit.

Dawn stayed where she was, trying not to cry. Mitch had always been nice to her. She wanted him to like her, not think she was a spoiled brat.

His face softened. "Relax, Dawn. Sit with us." Mitch scooted her chair in comfortably when she did. He squeezed her shoulders before he took his seat again. Mom put two strips of crisp bacon and a golden brown waffle on her plate, but Dawn had lost her appetite. She kept her head down, blinking back tears. Mitch and Mom had already finished breakfast. They hadn't even waited for her.

Mitch sighed. "Think I'll leave you two alone." He cleared his dishes while Mom loaded the dishwasher. "Are you going to be okay?" Mitch spoke tenderly. Dawn glanced up and then realized he wasn't talking to her. He had his arm around Mom's waist. Mom shrugged. He kissed her. Grimacing, Dawn looked away. Mitch came over to the table and leaned down to plant a kiss on top of her head. "See you later, alligator. . . ."

She used to laugh and say, "After a while, crocodile." That was before he married her mother.

Mom poured another cup of coffee and returned to the table. "Something wrong with the waffle?"

Granny's waffles were darker and crisper. "It's okay, I guess." She nibbled the edges.

Her mother sighed. "If you're done, you can put your plate on the counter." Her mother put her hands around her coffee cup. "I was going to wait a few days to put you in school. Now, I think the sooner, the better. The sooner you make new friends, the sooner you'll settle in."

"I want to go to my old school with all my friends!"

"You'll make new friends at your new school. Go get cleaned up, and we'll head over there. They'll probably even let you start today."

Fear coursed through Dawn. "It'll be just like when Susan came." The girls had whispered about her and made her cry. It had been a game at first, one that made Dawn uncomfortable, but she hadn't wanted to go against the crowd. "Nobody wanted to be her friend."

Her mother stood and looked at her. "Well, let's hope the people you meet in Healdsburg will be nicer than the 'friends' you had in Paxtown."

Dawn felt as though her mother had slapped her.

Mom's expression softened. "I know life isn't easy, May Flower Dawn. Believe me, I do. I could fix your hair in a French braid and help you pick out a skirt and—"

"I don't want to look like you!" She fled to the doorway. "And don't call me May Flower Dawn. It's a stupid, hippy name! I'm *Dawn*."

❄   ❄   ❄

Granny called that night. Dawn poured out her loneliness and anger over having to live so far away. Granny said she was sorry about that, too, and then asked if she liked second grade. "Did you make any friends today?" Several girls had come up to her and wanted to be friends. Dawn had been surprised at how nice they were.

Granny called again the next night—and the night after that.

After a few weeks, Dawn realized she enjoyed riding the bus to school with her friends. Getting off the bus after school proved harder. Granny wouldn't be waiting at the house. She had always given Dawn a snack, then played board games or let Dawn watch TV. Mom told her to play outside or with her Barbies. "You've been sitting in a classroom all day. I don't want you sitting in front of a television all afternoon."

Every evening, Granny called right about the time Mom started clearing dishes. After a while, Mom stopped answering the telephone and let Dawn run to her room and catch it. At least she had her very own phone. That was one nice thing about living in Mitch's house.

❄ ❄ ❄

Dawn knew something was wrong the moment she heard Granny's voice. "What is it, Granny?" Her heart began to pound. "Is Papa sick?"

"No. Papa is fine." Granny sniffled. "Everything is fine."

"No, it's not. I can tell." Something had made her grandmother cry.

"I'm going to stop calling you every evening, honey. I'll call you once a week instead."

"Why? Are you mad at me?"

"No! Of course not. It's just that . . . your mother says— "

"She's so mean!" Dawn was crying now too. "I want to come home! Please come and get me!"

"Honey, I can't. I love you so much, but she's your mother." Granny sniffled again. "She and Mitch love you very much, Dawn. I have to go now." Her voice broke. "I'll talk to you in a week."

Dawn marched down the hall to the kitchen, where her mother was putting the last plate into the dishwasher. "You made Granny cry!"

Mom turned and looked at her. "I'm sorry about that, but—"

"You're not sorry! You're not sorry at all! You said she couldn't call me anymore!" Hands in fists, she screamed. "And I hate you! I wish you were dead so I could go home and live with Granny!"

All the color drained from her mother's face, leaving her skin the color of ashes. She opened her mouth, but no sound came out. Her blue eyes filled with tears, and she turned away.

Feeling sick rather than triumphant, Dawn fled to her room.

❄ ❄ ❄

Someone tapped on the door. Limp from crying, Dawn sat up, expecting her mother to retaliate. She tensed when the door opened. Mitch stood in the doorway, looking grim and unhappy. "May I come in?"

She shrugged, trying to pretend she didn't care. Her palms felt moist. Had her mother told him what she'd said?

Mitch crossed the room, took her desk chair, and turned it around, straddling it and resting his arms on the back. "So, Pita. Feeling any better now that you got things off your chest?"

He'd called her Pita. Dawn heard the disappointment in his tone and felt the heat of guilt pouring into her face. She decided to lie. "I don't know what you mean."

"I was home, in my office. I heard every word you said. Not *said*—screamed, like a spoiled two-year-old having a tantrum."

"She told Granny not to talk to me anymore!"

"That's the second lie you've told me, unless your grandmother lied to you."

"Granny never lies!"

"Then how about the truth this time?" He spoke gently.

Dawn plucked at her skirt, eyes smarting with tears. "I want to go home."

"Granny isn't the only one who loves you. She's not the only one who cries. Your mother loves you, too."

She covered her face and sobbed. Mitch sat for a while, silent. He got up, put the chair back, and came over to her. She felt too ashamed to lift her head. "Your mother loves you, Dawn, and so do I." She felt him kiss the crown of her head. "Maybe you could give us a chance."

❋ ❋ ❋

Dawn didn't sleep well. Gathering her courage the next morning, she headed for the kitchen to say she was sorry. Her mother was at the sink.

Dawn stood in the doorway, chewing her lower lip, not sure what to do. "Where's Mitch?"

Her mother's head lifted slightly. "He went to work." She turned mechanically, removed the lid from a frying pan, and scooped a portion of scrambled eggs onto a plate. She brought it to the table, poured a glass of orange juice, and moved away.

Dawn poked at her breakfast. The hollow feeling in her stomach had nothing to do with hunger. She didn't know what to say to break the silence. Her mother went back to the sink and stood there, staring out the window, arms wrapped around herself. Did she have a stomachache, too? After a few minutes, she went into the laundry room off the kitchen and began sorting clothes.

Dawn scraped her uneaten eggs into the garbage disposal. Rinsing her plate and silverware, she put them in the dishwasher. Trembling inside, she went to the laundry room door. She gulped. "Can I talk to you for a minute?" Her voice came out tight.

Her mother went still. She didn't look up. "If you want to talk, call Granny when you get home from school."

It didn't matter that she'd won. Dawn felt awful. She wanted to say she was sorry; she didn't hate her; she'd just been so mad. She wished she could take the words back, but they still hung in the air like a foul stench. *Mommy,* she wanted to cry out. *Mommy, I'm sorry.* "I . . . I . . ." She couldn't get the words past the hard, hot lump in her throat.

24

Dawn called Granny as soon as she got home from school. "Mommy said I can call you—"

"I know, sweetie. Your mother called me. She didn't tell me what made her change her mind. Do you know?"

Dawn knew, but didn't want to say. "She said she knows I love you." That was true, at least.

"Oh. Good. I was afraid . . . Oh, never mind. Why don't you tell me all about your day, honey? I'm eager to hear everything. Who did you play with?"

Dawn didn't want to tell Granny it was the worst day of her life. Her teacher asked a question twice before Dawn realized she was supposed to answer. Everyone laughed. She spent recess crying in the back stall of the girls' bathroom. On the way home, she sat in the back of the bus, worrying about how things would be when she got home, but Mom acted normal, even asked how Dawn's day had gone. Dawn could muster only one word: "Fine." Her mother sighed and said she could go call Granny.

"You're a little quiet tonight, sweetie."

Dawn couldn't think of anything to say. "I have homework, Granny." It was true.

"I suppose I should get Papa's dinner going. I'll call you tomorrow. I love you, honey."

"I love you, too." Dawn hung up and put her head in her arms.

When Mitch came home, he stuck his head in her room to say hello. "Apologize yet?"

She shrugged. "I tried."

Later, Mitch called her to the dinner table. He talked easily about his day. Mom paid close attention to everything he said. She glanced in Dawn's direction several times, passed serving dishes, asked if Dawn wanted more milk, more mashed potatoes. But whenever Dawn looked at her, Mom turned away without meeting her eyes. When Mom started to clear dishes, Dawn picked up her own. Mom held her hand out for them. "I can do that."

Mom carried the dishes to the sink. Dawn looked at Mitch, hoping he could do something to make things better. He gave her a sad smile. Pushing his chair back, he went to her mother. He draped his arm around her shoulders and whispered something in her ear.

Feeling left out, Dawn wandered away from the table.

❊　❊　❊

Without consulting her, Mom registered Dawn for soccer. "Your friends play, don't they? Mitch is going to be your coach."

"Assistant coach," Mitch clarified. "Football is my game. Joaquin Perez is coach. He knows everything there is to know about soccer." He grinned at Dawn. "We'll both be learning from scratch."

On the first day of practice, she spotted four classmates: Torie Keyes, Tiffany Myers, Leanne Stoddard, and Susan Mackay. They had all played soccer since kindergarten. "Swarm ball," Torie laughed.

After several practices, Coach made Dawn a forward. "You're a natural." Mom encouraged Dawn to invite her friends over to play. Soon they were practicing soccer on the big lawn behind the house.

Dawn's days filled with activity. She went to church with Mitch, though her mother never attended, staying home alone. Mitch said Mom liked being alone with God, and she had fellowship when she went to AA twice a week in Santa Rosa.

❋ ❋ ❋

1979

Dawn dumped her backpack in her bedroom, changed for soccer practice, and went searching for Mitch, eager to leave. "Mitch! Where are you? It's time to go!"

"We're in here!"

She found Mom and Mitch sitting close together in the family room. Mitch had a grin on his face. Her mother looked oddly uncomfortable. "What's going on? We're going to be late for practice."

"Sit down, Dawn. We have some good news to share." He kissed Mom's temple. "Go ahead. Tell her."

"She'll take it better from you."

Mitch laughed, his eyes alight. "We're going to have a baby! You're going to have a little brother or sister about six months from now. What do you think of that?"

Dawn didn't know what to say. "That's great." But was it?

"I think she's in shock." Mitch kissed Mom again and stood. He clapped his hands on Dawn's shoulders. "You'll get used to the idea." He turned her around. "Let's go."

"Go where?" Her mind had gone blank.

"Soccer practice!"

Mitch told Coach Joaquin, and a few players overheard. Soon everyone knew Dawn's mother was pregnant. Dawn swung between embarrassment and worry. Where would she fit into the family after a baby came?

"Oh, wow, do I pity you," Torie said. "It's bad enough when

you have a brother or sister close to your own age, but eight years apart . . . The baby will be the star, and you'll be the babysitter."

Soon after soccer season ended, Granny called and asked to speak with Mom. Dawn knew something was wrong. She handed the telephone over to Mom and stayed around to watch and listen.

"What? When? Why didn't you call us sooner?" Mom sounded shaken. "We'll come right down. . . . Why? . . . Does he have to be so stubborn? This weekend then." She listened again, her expression growing more troubled. "I don't know, Mom." She glanced at Dawn and then turned away. "The weekend. A couple of days." She hung up.

She held up calming hands at Dawn's flurry of questions. "Papa had a mild heart attack, but he's okay. He's spending another two nights in the hospital just to be sure."

Dawn started to cry. Didn't people die of heart attacks? When her mother put her arms around her, Dawn stiffened at the unexpected show of affection. Mom let go and stepped back.

"He'll be home for a while," Mom added. "On bed rest. We'll go see him this weekend. Granny wants you to stay at the house."

Papa looked more disgruntled than sick when Dawn came flying into the house. He was in plaid pajamas and a robe, wearing old, worn leather slippers and sitting in his recliner in the living room. When he started to get up, Granny told him she'd march him straight back to bed if he did. He grinned at Dawn. "Granny's got her nursing cap on. Heaven help me. Climb on up here and give me a hug!"

Mom had noticed Oma's car was missing. Granny said she was gone again. "She came home to see Trip—I mean Dad—and then decided to spend a week with Uncle Bernie and Aunt Elizabeth."

Mom and Mitch asked Papa questions, but Granny answered. Papa glowered. "I'm still alive. I can speak for myself. It's not as bad as she makes it sound."

Granny scowled back at him. "It was bad enough."

Granny's lips trembled. Papa took her hand and kissed it and suggested she start dinner.

Mom offered to help. Granny said she could manage, then asked Dawn to set the table. Papa kissed Dawn's cheek before she got off his lap. Mitch and Papa talked in low voices. Mom didn't say anything. In the kitchen, Granny ran her hand over Dawn's hair. "Papa looks better now that you're home."

Papa was too tired to sit at the dinner table. Dawn went along while Granny walked with him back to the master bedroom and settled him into the hospital bed they'd rented. She prepared a dinner tray for him. "Why don't I make up a tray for you too, honey? You're better medicine for Papa than anything the doctor prescribed." Granny stayed at the dining room table with Mom and Mitch.

While they ate dinner together, Papa asked Dawn how she liked living in Alexander Valley. She had grown to like it a lot, and she told him about her new friends, about Mitch acting as assistant soccer coach. She loved soccer. Did he want to know how many goals she'd kicked? Twenty-six! Mitch was teaching her to swim now, and she practiced every day in the backyard pool. Papa's eyelids drooped, and he fell asleep while she was talking. She kissed his cheek, then left the bedroom. She heard Granny talking in the kitchen.

"Well, you could ask her, couldn't you? The school year is almost over. She wouldn't miss anything."

"We didn't plan on leaving Dawn behind, Hildie."

"Well, I told Carolyn—"

"We were talking about this weekend, Mom. Two days, not the whole summer."

Dawn walked into the kitchen just as Mom got up and left the table. Mitch gave Granny a grim look and pushed his chair back, following Mom into the living room. Mom picked up her sweater and pulled it on, then picked up her shoulder bag. They spoke in low voices. Dawn asked Granny what was wrong. Granny said nothing, nothing at all; it was just a little misunderstanding and nothing to worry about. Mom stood in the entryway. "We'll be at the Paxtown Hotel. We'll be back in the morning, Dawn."

Granny looked furious. "You're leaving now? What about dessert? I made a chocolate cake. It's your favorite!"

"It's Dawn's favorite." Mom turned to Dawn. "We'll be back tomorrow." She went out the door.

Mitch said he'd be right with her. He leaned down and whispered in Dawn's ear. "Be wise. Don't take sides."

"It's just like your mother to run away!" Granny stacked dinner dishes and headed into the kitchen. She asked if Dawn wanted to play a board game. Dawn hadn't played games since moving to Alexander Valley. There were too many other things to do now. When she didn't say anything right away, Granny added, "Or we could watch TV."

Granny checked on Papa and joined her in the living room. She talked more than she watched. She and Papa sure missed Dawn. Wouldn't it be nice if she could stay longer than the weekend? How long before school ended? Two weeks? She didn't have any plans for summer, did she? Remember how much she loved the county fair? And with the baby coming, her mother would have all kinds of things to do: doctors' appointments, getting the nursery ready, shopping, that sort of thing. She wouldn't have time for Dawn, not like Granny and Papa. They would have all the time in the world for her.

Dawn knew what Granny wanted. Maybe she *should* spend the summer. Granny seemed so certain Papa would get better fast if she did.

She loved Granny and Papa, but this wasn't her home anymore. She wanted to be in Alexander Valley with Mom and Mitch. She wanted to be there when her baby brother or sister was born. But how could she say that to Granny without hurting her feelings?

Mom and Mitch came back in the morning. Granny said she would have breakfast ready shortly, but Mitch said they'd eaten at the hotel. Granny seemed hurt. She said she thought Dawn wanted to spend the summer. Mom said that didn't surprise her. Mitch asked, "Is that what you want, Dawn?"

"Granny said Papa will get well faster if I'm here."

He frowned at Granny. "No one can argue with that without sounding like a heartless wretch."

Granny's face turned beet red. "I wasn't pressuring—"

"It's probably true, Mitch," Mom said quietly. "Dad will do better if Dawn is here. But she has two more weeks of school. I'm not leaving her now."

"That'll be fine." Granny smiled, relieved. She hugged Dawn against her side. "We'll have all summer together."

"One month, Mom. Not the whole summer."

"What about the county fair?"

Mom turned to Dawn. She held her gaze for the first time in months. "One month or the whole summer, Dawn?"

Mitch interrupted. "Your little brother or sister is expected the middle of July. Remember?"

"I . . ." Dawn looked from Mom to Granny and then at Mitch. "Um . . ." She felt pulled and torn. "I . . ." She wanted to cry. No matter what she decided, someone would be hurt and upset.

"One month," Mitch decided. He smiled at Granny. "I'll miss her too much. She can come home the end of June and stay until the baby comes. Then she can make up her mind about the rest of the summer. Is that agreeable to everyone?" He looked to Mom to answer. She nodded.

Granny harrumphed. "I guess I don't have anything to say about it."

Papa spoke from the doorway. "I think you've had too much say already."

❄ ❄ ❄

Dawn enjoyed her time with Granny and Papa, but was ready to go home by the end of June. Mitch drove down to get her. Her friends had been calling. When she asked how Mom was doing, he said, "Bursting at the seams."

She settled in again and spent hours on the telephone with Torie and Tiffany. She swam every day. She rode double on Torie's horse. Mom vetoed any idea of having one of her own. "I just can't imagine you mucking out a stable. . . ."

"Dawn!" Mitch awakened her in the middle of the night. "Baby's coming. Up and at it, sugar. I've already called Tiff's folks. They're expecting us." He dropped her off on the way to the hospital, Mom huffing and puffing and saying they'd better hurry.

Two days later, Tiffany's mom brought her home. Dawn charged into the house, dumped her duffel bag. "I'm home! Where are you?"

Mitch appeared at the master room door, finger to his lips. Mom sat in a new rocking chair by the windows, holding the most adorable creature Dawn had ever seen.

"May Flower Dawn, meet your brother, Christopher Charles Hastings." Dawn had never seen that look on her mother's face. She was enraptured, in love, her lips curved in a soft smile. She held the baby so close, as though he were the most precious human on the planet.

Mitch put his hands on Dawn's shoulders. "So? What do you think of your baby brother?"

She looked at the baby again, her mouth wobbling. "He's so cute." She stepped forward. "Can I hold him?"

Mom seemed slightly alarmed at the idea. "Not yet. In a few days. We'll see." She studied Dawn's face and looked relieved. Gazing down again, she ran a tender finger along the baby's smooth cheek. "I think your sister likes you." His tiny mouth worked.

"Uh-oh." Mitch laughed. "He's hungry again." He ushered Dawn out of the room so her mother could nurse the baby.

❊ ❊ ❊

Dawn decided not to go back to Paxtown. She wanted to stay in Alexander Valley with Mom, Mitch, and her new baby brother. Christopher fascinated her. He had the cutest little ears, and he was so soft. She loved when he grasped her finger, holding on tight.

Mitch let her hold him once, but Mom took him back after a few minutes.

Once, she snuck into the master bedroom to watch him sleeping in his crib. She touched his hand and watched him start, his fingers opening wide, then closing on her thumb. Leaning down, she kissed his forehead. He even smelled good.

Granny and Papa came at the end of August. Mom didn't hand Christopher over to Granny, not even for a minute. She did let Papa hold him once. When Mom placed Christopher in his arms, Dawn watched his face soften.

Mom smiled. "I need to step out for a few minutes. Are you going to be okay alone with him?" He nodded, gaze fixed on his grandson.

Tears ran down his face as he cupped Christopher's head and leaned down to kiss him. "You look just like Charlie. . . ."

❄ ❄ ❄

Granny and Papa came up for Thanksgiving and stayed four days. Mom didn't relax until they left. Mitch invited them back for Christmas. Mom invited Oma, too, but she said Aunt Cloe had already insisted she come to Hollywood. Dawn overheard Mom talking to Mitch in the kitchen. "Something's wrong, but she won't say what."

Over Christmas Eve dinner, Papa announced he'd put in for retirement. He figured it was about time. He didn't want to have another heart attack. Besides, the law was now working against police officers. Arrest a criminal and the courts would let him loose.

"We've been thinking about moving," Granny said.

"Moving?" Dawn gaped. "But you love Paxtown!"

"Well, of course we do, but we love our family more. We only get to see you a couple of times a year."

That wasn't true. They came to visit for every holiday, and Dawn spent time with them every time she had a school break.

Mom set her knife and fork down. "What about Oma?"

"We invited her to come with us." Granny sawed at a tender slice of turkey like it was shoe leather. "She said no."

Papa put his hand on Granny's wrist. "I told you not to bring it up, Hildie." He faced Mom. "We haven't made a final decision yet. We wanted to ask if it would be all right with you if we moved closer."

Dawn couldn't bear the look on Granny's face. "That'd be great, Mom! Wouldn't it?" *Say something!* Mom opened her mouth, but no words came.

Mitch spoke. "It'd be great to have you two closer. You're the last set of parents I have."

"Thanks, Mitch," Papa said. Granny relaxed a little. Papa glanced at her, his face softening. Then he looked at Mom. "We've missed you more than you know, Carolyn."

Mom winced. Dawn jumped in again to break the tension. "You could live right next door!"

Papa laughed. "Sorry, honey. We can't afford this neighborhood."

Granny's shoulders relaxed. "Healdsburg seems like a nice little town."

Christopher started to fuss in his high chair. Mom got up quickly and released him, lifting him in her arms and holding him closer while Papa talked.

"I was thinking of something a little farther out. We don't want to park ourselves on your front doorstep."

Mitch poured more sparkling cider. "Stay with us while you're looking. We have plenty of room."

When Dawn came into the kitchen the next morning, she found her mother sitting at the table, rubbing her forehead while she talked on the telephone. "I'd feel better if you were coming, too." When she saw Dawn, she got up and took the portable phone into the family room. "We have plenty of room. You could live with us. Mitch would . . . Why not? Why would she care?"

Dawn knew Mom was talking to Oma. Pouring herself a bowl of cereal, she lingered and listened.

"Just think about it, Oma. Please?" Mom pleaded.

Dawn knew her mother loved Oma, but she didn't know why. Granny stayed away from her, so Dawn did too.

Dear Rosie,

My daughter doesn't know how to let go. She has decided to sell the big house and property (including my cottage) and move to Sonoma County. She would like it if she could live right next door to May Flower Dawn, though I think Trip will put his foot down over that. I'm not sure what I will do. I had hoped to live here for the rest of my life. I should have seen this coming when Trip put in for retirement.

I'm not sure where I will live now. Hildemara said I can come with them, but doing so might make it look like I approve. She doesn't consider how this will affect Carolyn's budding relationship with Dawn. In truth, I think Hildemara is a little jealous, though she would never admit it.

Bernhard and Elizabeth think I should move in with them. Clotilde offered a condo in North Hollywood. Rikka invited me to stay part of the year in her Soho apartment. She has many artistic friends, all like tropical birds chattering about their flights of fancy. Two weeks and I'm ready to migrate back to California.

As much as I love my children, I can be on my own.

Why do they think I need a keeper? I may have gray hair, wear glasses, have certain limitations, but I am not in my dotage. I still have dreams. They say I'm being stubborn. So be it.

I miss the Central Valley. I miss the heat, the scent of sand, orchards, and vineyards. I miss putting flowers on Niclas's grave. Merced is centrally located. I can afford a bungalow there. I could drive to Yosemite in an hour and enjoy the mountains for a day. Who knows? Maybe, after all these years, I could finally go to college. . . .

25

1980

Granny and Papa's Paxtown property sold quickly. A moving company stored everything while they stayed in Alexander Valley and looked for another home. They stayed in the second suite at the other end of the house from Mom and Mitch. Dawn was in-between. Granny made afternoon and evening appointments with their Realtor. That way, Dawn could go with them to see houses. Granny wanted to live at the north end of Healdsburg. Papa wanted to look at Cloverdale. Granny said that was too far away. So were Windsor and Santa Rosa. Granny said maybe they'd find something on Dry Creek Road.

Finally Granny decided on a house in Healdsburg. She talked about the nice guest bedroom with private bath, the neat houses along the street, the small, easily maintained backyard. And it was so close to Dawn's school. "You could have lunch with us!"

Papa looked at Dawn in the rearview mirror and didn't say a word until they got back to Alexander Valley. "Go on in the house, Dawn. Granny and I are going to have a little talk before we come in."

They sat in the car for almost an hour. When Granny came inside, she headed straight for the guest suite. Papa went into the family room and sank into an easy chair. Mitch raised his brows. "Is everything okay?"

"We're going to take a long drive tomorrow, by ourselves, and see a little more of the area." Mom came into the family room, Christopher in her arms. Papa looked at her with a sad smile. "Healdsburg is a nice little town, but I'd like to be forty-five minutes to an hour away. Somewhere on the coast, if we could afford it."

Papa found just the house he wanted at the end of the Russian River in Jenner by the Sea. The house was tucked into a hillside, almost hidden by a row of overgrown, shaggy cypress trees. He said the place needed some work, but he claimed it would have a "million-dollar view" when the trees were topped and the dead-wood cut out and hauled away. Granny argued vehemently against buying it, but Papa won in the end.

❄ ❄ ❄

Just before Christopher's first birthday, Mitch flabbergasted Dawn by asking if he could adopt her.

Her stepdad was the coolest guy she knew, and she loved him, but she was torn. She asked for some time to think about it. Her mother didn't like that, but Dawn didn't want to make a rash decision and hurt anyone's feelings. She went out to Jenner by the Sea for the weekend and talked it over with her grandparents. She hoped they'd give their blessing.

Papa didn't say much about it other than, "It's up to you, honey." Granny remained silent on the subject until the next morning, when she insisted she and Dawn go to the beach for a walk. They hadn't gone to the beach in months, so Dawn knew Granny had something to say. Granny let loose in the car on the drive over. She reminded Dawn that Mitch wasn't her father; that Papa had paid all the bills for the first five years of her life; Papa had rocked her to sleep. Papa had read stories to her; Papa had played with her. Of course, he'd been hurt when Dawn told him about Mitch's offer. How could he not be? Of course, he'd hide his feelings and say it was up to Dawn! Granny parked and wiped tears away. Besides all that, Dawn was the last Arundel in the family. Yes, of course, she'd get married someday and take her husband's name, but until then, it meant a lot to them.

Dawn couldn't bear to hurt her grandparents, and she knew Mitch would understand.

When she came home, she told Mitch she was honored, but thought she'd like to leave things as they were. Mitch looked disappointed, but accepted her decision with grace. He even kissed her cheek. "Don't worry about it."

Her mother stood silent, eyes glacier blue. She opened her mouth to say something, then pressed her lips together and left the room without speaking. Mitch followed her, closing the door of the master suite behind them. Her mother talked then, loud enough for Dawn to hear the tone, but not the words.

Dawn tried to talk to her the next morning. She wanted to explain it had nothing to do with Mitch. She loved Mitch. "I'm sorry if you're upset, Mom. I just don't want to hurt anyone's feelings."

"You don't want to hurt Granny's feelings. You don't care who else you hurt."

"Mitch seemed okay with it."

"They're your *grand*parents, Dawn! Isn't that enough?"

"*They've* always been there for me."

Her mother blinked. "So you hurt Mitch to get back at me?"

"No!"

Mom turned her back and continued making Dawn's bag lunch. She didn't have to say she didn't believe Dawn; her posture said it all.

"Can we talk about it, Mom?"

"Why? You made your decision. Everything will be the way Granny wants it, and it'll stay that way. It always does." She shoved the sandwich into a Baggie and put it in the paper bag. "You'd better get your stuff together, or you'll be late for the bus."

❇ ❇ ❇

1985

Dawn struggled with feelings of ecstasy, anger, and misery. She had kicked the winning goal in the final junior high team championship soccer game, and Mom wasn't even in the stands. Mitch had come. Her stepfather always made an effort to support her. Just once, couldn't Mom make the effort, too—especially since this was the last and most important game of Dawn's life? Of course, Mom would have an excuse. Chris always had something going on somewhere else. Mom hadn't even bothered to show up at Mary's Pizza Shack for the season-ending party. When Dawn and Mitch came into the kitchen, there they were, sitting at the table, Mom smiling over something Chris had said. She glanced up. "How'd it go?"

"Dawn kicked the winning goal. I got it all on film."

"That's great. Congratulations, Dawn. Chris's game started late. We just got home. He wanted to stop at Burger King."

Mitch ruffled Christopher's curly red hair. "How'd you do, Tiger?"

"We lost." Her little brother—still adorable at almost six—never got upset about anything. "Can we watch Dawn's game?"

"Whenever you're ready."

Christopher was on his feet, hamburger forgotten. He and Mitch trooped into the family room while Mom gathered up the remains of their take-out meal. "You seem upset."

"No, Mom. Why would I be?"

"Where are you going?"

"To my bedroom."

"Aren't you going to watch the game video?"

"I *played* the game, remember? Seeing it on video isn't the same as being there, is it?"

Her mother stood at the trash compactor. "You had a cheering section. Mitch went. And Granny and Papa were there."

"Why should it matter whether Granny and Papa are there? It'd be nice to have you and Chris at one of my games."

"Well, Chris couldn't come. His team needed him."

"He's in peewees! They play swarm ball! Just once, just for a couple of hours, couldn't *I* be first in your life?"

"You came first for a long time, Dawn. Not that it ever mattered to anyone, especially you."

Dawn gave up. Storming out of the kitchen, she went down the hall and slammed her bedroom door. She sat on the end of her bed and cried. Someone tapped on the door. Dawn shouted, "Go away!"

Sometimes she wished her mother would yell back instead of walking away—or responding in that cool, calm tone. Dawn wondered sometimes: How could she miss her mother so much when she'd never had her love in the first place?

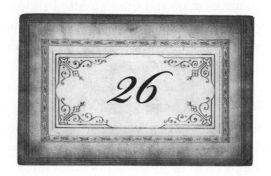

1986

Dawn still felt adrift after nine months as a freshman. High school had turned out to be a complete bust. She'd gone from junior high Sky Hawks star soccer player to outcast and dweeb. The girls who had been her friends since second grade left her behind by mid-September, charging like forwards into new groups. Torie Keyes now ran with the Mexican gangbangers. Dawn saw her every day in the corridor, draped around Juan Alvarez like a bun around a hot dog. Susan Mackay hacked her hair into a butch, donned button-down shirts and black pants, and "came out of the closet" as a lesbian. Two other buddies from the Sky Hawks soccer team, Tiffany Myers and Leanne Stoddard, still hung out together. They smoked pot behind the modular buildings lining the football field. If Dawn wanted to go to a big party where booze and drugs and sex would be in abundance, all she had to do was ask Tiff and Lee. They'd know where to find one.

She scribbled more loops on her notepaper. Summer break loomed a week away with the promise of endless boredom.

She'd be stuck at home for three months without even Christopher's company. Her little brother had an army of little buddies; hence, places to go and things to do. In addition to friends, Mom signed him up for swimming lessons and, not one, but four different vacation Bible schools. Why? Because he had four "best friends," all in different churches, and he didn't want to play favorites. *Must be nice to be so popular, not to mention the blessing of being the first and only son.*

Even more annoying, Mom, who never went to church, would volunteer at every VBS. She'd take snacks, help with art projects, do whatever she could to be involved in Chris's life. She acted like a mother bear sometimes, as though someone might snatch Christopher away and molest him.

Tossing the pen aside, Dawn rubbed her forehead. Thinking about her mother always brought on a stress headache—ironically, the one thing they had in common. After they argued, Mom always retreated into the master suite and put cold compresses on her head or went to an AA meeting.

But their arguments were infrequent. You had to have feelings for someone to fight with them. Her mother didn't seem to care one way or the other about Dawn. She didn't hover over her; she just stepped back and watched from a distance, if she watched at all.

Mitch made time for her. Every month, they went on a "date." The last time, they couldn't find a movie worth watching and ended up eating dinner at the Western Boot. He talked about Uncle Charlie all evening. She loved hearing about Uncle Charlie. He sounded so cool. He and Mitch had gotten away with major mischief that left her laughing and in awe.

"And what about Mom? Did she get into any trouble?"

"She was a good girl."

"Yeah, right. She never did anything wrong."

"Nope."

"She waited until she got to Haight-Ashbury."

Mitch didn't say anything to that.

"Does she ever talk to you about those years?"

He shook his head.

"And you don't ask?" When he just looked at her, she pressed a little harder. "Shouldn't you know?"

"Your mother laid her life bare in less than a minute the first time I managed to corner her for lunch. She tore the skin off old wounds, and no, I am not going to betray her trust and tell you anything."

"Did she say anything about my father? Does she even know who he is?"

Mitch put his napkin on the table and signaled the waiter.

Dawn hung her head. "I'm sorry." She looked up at her stepfather through her tears. "I don't want to go yet, Mitch. Please. I'll behave."

Mitch told the waiter they'd like to see the dessert selection. Dawn looked at the menu, but she wasn't hungry. Was it so wrong for her to want to know? "I must remind her of things she'd rather forget."

Mitch put the menu aside. "You should sit down with *her* and ask your questions, Dawn."

"She'd never tell me anything. Every time I even hint, she changes the subject or says she has to go to a meeting. Maybe just talking to me makes her want a drink."

"I'm not going to get in the middle."

"Mom and I don't even speak the same language."

Dawn tried to put herself in her mother's shoes. How would she feel if she had a kid out of wedlock, living proof of how she'd messed up her life and needed her parents to pick up the pieces and put her back together? As painful as it might be to go over the past, Dawn wanted to know something about her biological father. Not that Mitch wasn't a great dad; he was the best. But she didn't come from his gene pool.

Rubbing her temples, Dawn stared at the wall clock, noting another fifteen minutes before study hall ended. Maybe she'd ask her mother if she could sign up for summer school; at least it would be something to do. She'd already checked at McDonald's about a job, but she had to be sixteen. If she didn't find something to do, Granny and Papa would expect her to spend the summer at Jenner by the Sea again, just like last summer and the summer before that and every summer since they'd moved from Paxtown. She loved them dearly, but three months around their house with nothing to do wore her down.

They had books, of course, lots of them, most about building a house from foundation to roof, how to remodel, how to make repairs, plumbing and wiring, etc. Granny collected cookbooks. Dawn wouldn't have minded learning to cook, but they had a "one-butt kitchen," as Papa called it, and Granny liked being the only "butt" at the sink and stove. Last summer, Dawn found herself so desperate, she weeded every inch of Granny's garden below the house.

The class bell rang, jolting Dawn from her reverie. She stuffed her notebook into her backpack, slung it over her shoulder, and headed for the door.

If she wanted to stay home this summer, she was just going to have to spell it out. She'd beg if needed. If Mom said no, she'd enlist Mitch and Christopher's help. They always had better luck with Mom than she did.

❄ ❄ ❄

Dinner was almost over before Dawn gathered enough courage to say she wanted to spend summer at home. Mom glanced up, surprised. "But you always spend the summer at Jenner."

"I know, but I'd rather stay home this year."

"What's Granny said about this?"

"I haven't told her yet." Avoiding her mother's look, Dawn smiled at Christopher. "Maybe I can help keep an eye on Little Dweeb when you have an open house."

"I only do open houses on the weekends, and Mitch is here."

So much for trust.

"What do you plan to do for three months?" Mitch cut a piece of roast beef and forked it into his mouth.

She batted her eyelashes at him. "You could teach me to drive."

He laughed in mock horror. "No way! Besides, you're not old enough."

"I could learn to drive one of your tractors."

"And risk my vineyard? I don't think so."

"I can help with laundry and cooking."

Mom spooned a second helping of mashed potatoes onto Christopher's plate. "Your grandparents will be disappointed. They expect you to spend time with them."

"I could go out one weekend a month. It's not like I'm saying I don't want to spend any time with them."

Mitch gave her mother a look. "It might be nice having Pita here for a summer. She's not going to be around that much longer, you know. Three more years and she'll be off to college."

"I'm not looking for a fight, Mitch. You know how things are."

Mitch put his napkin on the table. "I'm going to be late for the elders' meeting." He leaned down and kissed Dawn on the cheek. "It'll be good to have you around this summer, Pita." He came around the table and kissed her mother full on the mouth. "Won't it?" He kissed her again. He ruffled Christopher's thatch of curling reddish brown hair. "No dragging your feet about going to bed tonight, buster. You still have a couple of days of school left."

Her mother sent Christopher to take a bath and gathered the dinner dishes. She glanced at Dawn's plate. "You didn't eat much."

"Wasn't hungry. I can help around the house, Mom. Do the dishes. Do the laundry."

"That'd be nice." Mom stood at the sink. "Okay." She turned and looked at Dawn. "On one condition."

"Anything."

"*You* have to tell your grandparents."

Dawn gave her a half-pleading smile. "I was hoping you would help me with that."

"No way." Her mother turned to rinse the plates before putting them in the dishwasher. "They wouldn't believe me if I told them you'd rather be here than out there with them."

❄ ❄ ❄

Dawn worried and rehearsed the call for two days.

"Was it your mother's idea to make you stay home all summer?"

"No." *Just say it, Dawn!* She let her breath out slowly. "I've never been home for an entire summer, Granny."

Silence.

"You'll still come out on weekends, won't you?"

Dawn chewed her lip. "Not every weekend, Granny."

Another silence.

"We were thinking about taking you on a trip to Yellowstone. Papa isn't getting any younger. This will probably be the last year for doing this kind of thing."

Granny knew how to apply the screws. "I know you and Papa will have a great time." She plucked at her bedspread. "I love you, Granny. I'll call you soon." She hung up before Granny could add anything else to make her feel even more guilty.

"Everything all right?" Mom stood in the doorway, expression guarded, hands tucked into her apron pockets.

"Everything's fine."

"Good." Her mother took her hands out of her pockets and smiled. "Come on in the kitchen. You can go through my cookbooks and decide what you want to fix for dinner tomorrow night."

"Tomorrow night? But I don't know how to cook."

"Cooking is easy. All you have to do is follow directions."

Panic set in.

Her mother walked ahead of her down the hall, pulled several cookbooks off a shelf, took a pad of paper and a pen from a drawer, and dropped them on the kitchen table. "Figure out what you'd like to cook, make a list of ingredients, and I'll pick up whatever you need tomorrow morning." Her mother slung her purse onto her shoulder.

"Aren't you going to help me?"

"I can't. Chris's class is having an end-of-year party." She opened the refrigerator and took out a bowl of potato salad.

"Mom?"

Her mother paused in the doorway and looked back at her. Dawn wanted to say she hadn't stayed home to be alone, but to spend time with her mother. The silence stretched, the words sticking in her throat.

Her mother's expression softened. "Don't look so worried, Dawn. You'll do fine without me."

Dawn listened to the garage door open and close. She flipped open the *Joy of Cooking* and turned the pages. Shoving the book aside, she put her head in her arms and cried.

Two weeks at home felt like a year. Christopher had a packed social calendar, Mom as chauffeur, while Dawn got to hang around the house, do laundry, plan and fix meals. At least she had company today. Christopher had a rare day at home, and Mom trusted her enough to act as lifeguard while he swam in the backyard pool.

Dawn rubbed sunscreen on her legs while keeping an eye on her little brother. Christopher stopped and sputtered, wiping hair back from his face and treading water in the deep end. Tossing the tube of Coppertone aside, she stood. "Need me to fish you out?"

"No!" He set off again.

Dawn walked to the end of the pool and waited for him. When he grabbed hold of the edge, she tapped him on the head. "Enough already, Chris." He cleared his eyes and looked at her. She held his wrist. "You're doing great. Just take a rest, would you please? You've done four laps. If you do another, I'm going to have to drag you out and give you mouth-to-mouth resuscitation."

"Gross!" He let her haul him out of the water. Christopher's wet feet slapped along the smooth concrete. He threw his towel around his shoulders, but still looked like a half-drowned mouse.

She grabbed her towel off the chaise longue and rubbed his hair dry. "I couldn't even do one lap when I was six."

"If I can do six laps without stopping, I can be a dolphin. And then I can learn to dive." Her little brother flipped out his towel and sprawled on his stomach. "Dawn, will you go to VBS with me tomorrow?"

"I'm too old for VBS, buddy."

"You could be a helper."

"Doing what? Handing out graham crackers and apple juice? Taking kids to the potty?"

"Come on. Please." He put his hands together and gave her his practiced puppy-dog look. "Pretty please. I'm supposed to invite someone."

"Someone from kindergarten to fifth grade, Chris. I'm telling you they don't sign up sophomores for VBS."

"High school kids come. They have a band! They help in the classes; they play outdoor games with us."

"Sounds like VBS has more than enough help already."

"I told the band kids I have a sister. I said you were pretty."

"Thanks."

"I said I'd bring you tomorrow."

When she glared at him, he stuck out his lip. He could be cute. "Do you get extra points or something?"

"No. But if you go to VBS, you can't do the wash and Daddy won't have to wear pink T-shirts." He grinned broadly.

"Okay. That's it!" Dawn jumped up, grabbed him by an arm and a leg, and headed for edge of the pool. "Time for a few more laps!" He squealed with laughter as she swung him back and forth and launched him into the deep end of the pool. He popped up quickly, grinning from ear to ear and hollering for her to do it again.

❄ ❄ ❄

Cornerstone Covenant Church turned out to be a large warehouse with metal roll-up doors in the Windsor Industrial Park. Volunteers had pitched two huge tents in the empty back lot. It looked more like a circus than a church.

Christopher grabbed Dawn's hand. "We have to go to chapel first!" He hauled her into a huge concrete-floored room with basketball hoops on either end. No pews, just folding chairs. Bright colored banners hung on the walls. *Faith. Hope. Joy. Love One Another.* The largest was purple with gold names appliquéd: *Mighty God, Everlasting Father, Wonderful Counselor, Prince of Peace, Jesus, King of Kings.*

Mom laughed. "It's not exactly what I expected either." She carried a tray of iced cupcakes and nodded toward a door. "The kitchen is that way."

"No, Mom. Dawn has to come with me." Christopher pulled her into the throng of kids. "Come on! They're going to start in a minute. My class is down front."

Her heart jumped when she spotted Jason Steward, one of the best-looking guys at school, on the raised platform with four other teens. They wore black Levis and canary yellow T-shirts with *Christ is Lord* emblazoned in red letters. Kim Archer, a pretty brunette who was a cheerleader at Healdsburg High, and another girl, Sharon something-or-other, had been in Dawn's PE class. Both had seemed nice. One of the guys plugged a guitar into an amplifier while the other did a drumroll and hit the cymbals. Jason caught a hand microphone tossed by a man near the stage. Raising one hand, he held the mike to his mouth. "Good morning, everybody!"

The children shouted back. "Good morning!"

He laughed. "Is that the best you can do?" He put his hand to his ear. "I can barely hear you!" The guitar player made a loud, warbling chord that had everyone shouting good morning again. Jason called out, "This is a day the Lord has made!" Another loud chord, more cheering. "Let's rejoice and be glad in it! Let's hear you! *Good morning!*"

Dawn wanted to cover her ears.

"That's better! Come on, everybody! Let's worship the Lord!"

The drummer went wild, his head bobbing up and down, while Jason and Sharon sang and Kim played keyboard. It seemed more like a rock concert than vacation Bible school.

A hundred children, plus teachers and volunteers, clapped their hands and sang the words projected on an overhead screen. Christopher kept pulling her forward, waving wildly. "Hey, Jason! I brought my big sister!"

Dawn wanted to duck down among the throng and hide. She pulled Christopher's arm down. Too late. Jason Steward looked straight at her and smiled broadly as he sang.

"What do you think you're doing?"

"That's Jason Steward! He told me to bring you! Isn't he the coolest?"

"I'm going to kill you."

"Don't go!" Christopher grabbed her hand again. Dawn pried loose and looked for escape. Boxed in with children all around her, there was no path out of this mob. Christopher joined in the clapping and singing. Dawn locked her attention on the overhead screen and lip-synched the words.

She'd spotted Jason her first day of high school. Who wouldn't? He was drop-dead gorgeous with black hair, hazel eyes, and olive skin. He looked a mix of Caucasian, Hispanic, and Asian. He'd been standing in the corridor of lockers, talking with a couple of guys. He had a contagious laugh. Later, she had seen him sitting at a picnic table under the redwoods, having lunch with a group of kids. She caught a glimpse of him every day on her way to English class. He'd caught her staring at him once and smiled. Mortified, she'd been careful not to stare after that.

Instead, she'd sit where he wouldn't notice her, watching him toss a football back and forth with the jocks during lunch break. Jason Steward was nice to everyone—geeks; pretty, popular cheerleaders; and even gangster types. She'd see him standing under the redwood trees near the student parking lot, talking with people. She'd seen him alone only a couple of times during the whole year, and she had never had the courage to utter hello.

Was her face still as red as it felt?

After three more songs, Jason handed the microphone over to Pastor Daniel Archer, who prayed, made some announcements, and then dismissed the children by groups.

"I'm going to go help Mom."

"No, you're not!" Christopher grabbed her hand again. "You have to come to my class."

"What am I? your show-and-tell?"

"I told Jason you'd help."

She let her brother lead her out of the chapel into the blinding morning sunlight and through the gate in the cyclone fence. "Come on!" He pulled her along. Glancing back, he let go, and his face broke into a broad smile. "Hey, Jason!"

Dawn gulped, but didn't turn around. She prodded Christopher. "You have to get to your class. Where is it?"

"Wait for Jason."

She wanted to throttle him. "We've gotta go."

Jason caught up with them. "Hi." He smiled at her, and she felt the heat rising into her cheeks again.

"Hi." She cast a quick smile in his general direction. "Bye." She ducked inside the tent after her brother. Heart knocking, she stayed in back as Christopher grabbed a square of carpet and ran forward to sit among a gaggle of other leggy boys and girls his age. His teacher, Mrs. Preston, had a felt board. *Oh, boy. Oh, boy.*

Jason came inside the tent and stood beside her. "Christopher said he'd bring his sister today. You go to Healdsburg High, don't you? I've seen you around."

"Yeah." Gawking at him, most likely. She glanced up briefly and then fixed her gaze on the back of Christopher's head.

"Chris didn't tell me your name."

"May Flower Dawn Arundel." Her face went hot again. What possessed her to say her whole name? "People call me Dawn."

"People call me Jason." He stepped in front of her and held his hand out. "Nice to meet you, Dawn. Thanks for agreeing to help." When his fingers closed around her hand, she tingled all over. His expression turned curious. "Arundel? Not Hastings."

Once he released her hand, she breathed easier. "Christopher is my half brother."

"He's a great kid."

"He has his moments." She swallowed hard. "Now that I'm here, I'm just not sure what I'm supposed to do."

"Help me set up the art project." He smiled and gestured toward two long tables covered with butcher paper on the left side of the tent. "They're making burning bushes today." While Mrs. Preston gave a dramatic reading of Moses fleeing into the wilderness, Jason laid out the trays of supplies. "They're going to glue down twigs to make a bush, drop paint, and use a straw to blow it around like flames."

"Clever."

His dark eyes shone with amusement. "Yeah, well, tomorrow's lesson is on the plagues of Egypt. They're making green paper-plate frogs. You are coming back to help, aren't you?"

"Let's see how today goes." She'd be back. She just didn't want to sound too eager. She laid a piece of paper and a small pile of twigs by each folding chair.

Jason put out paint, brushes, and straws. "Christopher told me he wants to be in a rock band."

"Last week, he wanted to be an astronaut; yesterday he wanted to be a dolphin in swim class so he can learn to dive."

Jason laughed. "Reminds me of myself at his age." It took them less than five minutes to put everything needed on the table. "Our work's done for the moment." He pulled out a folding chair for her, turned another around, and straddled it. Crossing his arms on the back, he looked her straight in the eyes and smiled warmly. "What about you?"

She was close enough to see the flecks of gold in the green, the rim of brown around his pupil. "What about me?"

"Do you know what you want to do with your life?"

"I haven't got a clue. Have fun, I guess." Could she have said anything more inane and shallow? "You'll be a senior, right? You probably have your future all planned out."

"I have a couple of ideas. My mom would like me to be an engineer. Pastor Daniel thinks I should go into the ministry. Maybe I can figure out a way to do both."

"How?" They seemed diametrically opposed.

"There's a lot more to ministry than just working at a church. God needs workers in all kinds of businesses, too. I've been asking Him to show me which direction to go, and I know He will."

She'd never heard anyone talk so naturally about God, though she didn't see what God would have to do with Jason's decision. Wasn't it all about free will? "Why would God care what you do? I mean, doesn't He want us to decide for ourselves? That's what I've been told. It's up to us to find out what makes us happy."

He tilted his head to one side. "Well, yes, God wants us to be happy. But there's a whole lot more to it than that."

"Really? What do you mean?" Jason Steward sure wasn't what she had expected.

"God gave each of us specific talents and abilities. He has plans for us. He has a purpose for your life."

"My life? I'm not so sure about that."

"You can be. It starts with being in an intimate relationship with Him. Then, just like any other relationship, it will influence what you want, what you do, what you believe."

The conversation was starting to make her uncomfortable. "*Intimate* isn't exactly a word I'd use about God."

Jason stood. "Hey, just think about it. If you open the door and let Him in, everything in your life is going to change. I promise."

Maybe that's why he'd told Christopher to bring her. To evangelize her. She didn't care one way or another about God. She just wanted to keep Jason talking. "Is that what happened to you?"

His eyes glowed. "Yeah." He looked behind her. "Ready or not, here they come." He swung his chair back into place as Christopher and his friends surrounded the table and found seats. Dawn helped her brother get started on his project, then helped a couple of the other kids. Jason introduced her to Mrs. Preston, who said Christopher was a terrific kid and a pleasure to have in class. As if Dawn hadn't heard that a thousand times before.

It didn't take long to finish the burning bushes. Mrs. Preston called the children together and took them outside, where she handed them over to other volunteers who gave them a choice of games to play.

Jason stood beside Dawn. "Do you go to church?"

She said, "Of course," and told him where. When he asked about their youth group, she shrugged and said with a congregation of less than a hundred and comprised mostly of people older than her stepdad, who was in his forties, there weren't enough teenagers to have one.

"Come to ours then. We meet here tonight at seven thirty. We hang out, play basketball, eat junk food, and have a Bible study. Give it a try. See what you think."

"I'd have to ask my mother." Mom might disapprove, but she wouldn't have grounds for argument. She was bringing Christopher to VBS here, after all.

"Do you need a ride?"

Her heart fluttered. Would he offer to pick her up if she said yes? "We live in Alexander Valley."

"I can introduce you to someone who lives up that way."

"Never mind."

A piercing whistle came from the parking lot. Jason gave a wave. "I have to get back to the sanctuary and set up for the closing. Thanks for helping today, Dawn. Hope I see you tonight . . . and tomorrow."

She looked for Jason when she accompanied Christopher's class back into the warehouse. He stood on the platform, talking and laughing with the two girls who had been onstage with him while the classes settled into their designated seats. Pastor Daniel had the microphone again and encouraged everyone to get settled quickly. He explained how the children's offerings would buy books for an orphanage in Mexico. He asked if anyone had a guest. Dawn held Christopher's hand down. Pastor Daniel went on. "Keep giving out those invitations! We have plenty of room for more."

He tossed the microphone to Jason, who had everyone up and singing again. After several songs, Jason gave a short closing prayer and called out, "See you all tomorrow!"

Dawn grabbed Christopher's hand and headed for Mom standing against the wall with several other women. She came toward them and smiled at Dawn. "I see you survived."

"It was okay, I guess." She didn't want to sound overly enthusiastic and have Mom wonder why. "I said I'd help again tomorrow. One of the guys invited me to youth group tonight."

"Invited?" Her mother gave her a quick glance. "As in asking you for a date?"

"No. He just said to come. He thought I might enjoy it."

"I'd rather you didn't go."

Dawn bristled. "Why not?" Christopher could do anything he wanted, but she asked for something and the answer was no?

"You have a church."

"So does Christopher, but that didn't stop you from signing him up for VBS at Cornerstone."

"Because Mitch's church doesn't have one."

"It doesn't have a youth group either."

"VBS only lasts three more days, Dawn."

"I'm not asking if I can join the church, Mom. I just want to see what youth group is like. I'd like to hang out with kids my own age, Christian kids."

"Let me think about it."

THE CCC YOUTH group consisted of fewer than twenty kids, mostly girls grouped together and talking while five guys played basketball. Another guest invited by Jason, Tom Barrett, had come to stick his toes carefully in religious waters. As soon as he was introduced, Jason took him to join in the basketball game. Kim Archer, the pastor's daughter, took charge of Dawn, inviting her to grab a folding chair from those stacked against a wall and join the gaggle of girls. Dawn knew some of them already, their names at least. She'd seen Sharon Bright, Pam Preston, Linda Doile, and Amy King at school, not that they would recognize her.

"Hey," Sharon said. "You were in my PE class. Dawn ran right past everyone during track."

Dawn added her chair to the circle. "I played soccer for six years. Coach Perez made us run a mile before every practice."

Pam twisted her hair up and put a clip in it. "Why didn't you try out for the team? We could use you."

"Thought I'd take a break. Try something else."

"Such as?"

"Studying."

"That's where I've seen you." Linda crossed her ankles. "In study hall. You sat in the back row by the windows."

"Yep."

The girls talked about school and how their summers were shaping up. Dawn took quick, surreptitious glances at Jason playing basketball with the guys. Sharon said her family was heading for Tahoe next week for a family gathering. Linda had a job in a pizza parlor near the downtown mall. Amy wished she had a job at the mall. She was working as a nanny for three children. She almost hadn't come this evening. Bed had looked pretty good, and she had to be back at the Johnsons' by six thirty in the morning. Kim answered the church telephone. She was filling in for the church secretary, Mrs. Carson, who was in Los Angeles helping move her mother into a residential care facility.

"What about you, Dawn?" Kim asked. "What are you doing this summer?"

Dawn pulled her gaze away from Jason. "Not much. I don't have a driver's license, and we live out in Alexander Valley." She shrugged. "I'm doing laundry and cooking for the family. So far, no one has died."

Pam laughed. "My mother says you were a big help in her VBS class this morning."

"All I did was put out some art supplies."

"I'll say thank you anyway. You saved me from being drafted into duty." She shuddered expressively.

The basketball bounced their way. "Hey, ladies!" Jason called. "Save us some steps?" Dawn got up, caught it, and gave it a light kick so that it landed right in his hands. "Good kick!" He grinned and dribbled the ball halfway down the court, passing it to Tom Barrett, who took two steps, jumped, and shot it smoothly over the heads of three others. It dropped perfectly into the basket. Jason and Tom gave each other high fives.

Sharon laughed as Dawn sat down. "Well, we all know why you came tonight."

"What?" Dawn pretended not to know.

"Jason Steward." Sharon stretched out her long, jean-clad legs. "Join the club. We've all had a crush on him at one time or another."

When she glanced over, Jason was looking at her. He quickly looked away. Raising his hand, he called out to Tom, who passed him the ball.

❅ ❅ ❅

When Pastor Daniel came in, everyone made a circle of chairs. Everyone but Dawn had brought a Bible, even Tom Barrett. Kim said not to worry about it and shared hers. The pastor called on the regulars to read portions of the book of Daniel, then pointed out how a few teenagers made an impact on a godless society. He challenged them to make a difference wherever they were: high school, mall, babysitting.

When the study portion ended, everyone hung around, nibbling chips, eating leftover VBS cupcakes, drinking sodas, and talking. Jason had picked up Tom Barrett. They walked out and stood talking to a couple of the guys in the parking lot. Dawn spotted her mom's tan Suburban and headed for it. Pam Preston caught up with her. "I'm glad you came tonight. Can I meet your mom?"

"Sure. I guess." Dawn opened the car door. "Mom, this is Pam Preston; Pam, my mom, Mrs. Hastings."

Pam leaned in to shake her hand. "It's nice to meet you, Mrs. Hastings. We live on the north side of Healdsburg. I could pick up Dawn next week."

Mom looked dubious. "It's nice of you, but—"

"I've had my license for two years and haven't gotten a ticket. My mom says I drive like an old lady. You can ask her when you bring Christopher to VBS tomorrow."

Mom smiled politely. "I'll take your word for it, Pam." Dawn got into the car and closed the door. "She seems nice enough. How well do you know her?"

"She's on the high school soccer team." Dawn watched Pam talking to Kim and Pastor Daniel.

"So what was it like?"

"We read about Daniel." Dawn leaned back as her mother drove out of the parking lot. "There's a lot more to him than surviving a night in a lion's den. I felt like such an idiot. Everyone had a Bible. I don't even know where mine is."

"I'm sorry they made you feel inferior."

"No, Mom." Dawn didn't want her getting the wrong idea. "It wasn't like that at all. It's just that I've been going to church with Mitch since second grade, but I don't know a fraction of what those kids know."

"Granny and Papa read you Bible stories when you were little, didn't they?"

"Yeah. Simplified versions with pictures. Pastor Daniel made something written thousands of years ago sound like current events. Rev. Jackson doesn't exactly light my fire when he preaches."

"Boots gave me a Bible when I lived with her."

"Wasn't she Granny's friend? the one who died of cancer a few years ago?"

"Yes. She was my friend, too. She's the one who encouraged my interest in Scripture."

"I didn't know you even had a Bible, let alone read one."

"I didn't mean to shock you."

"Well, it's not like I've ever seen you reading it."

"I have a quiet time every morning. In the privacy of my room, so I can think about what I'm reading."

"But you never go to church."

Mom kept her eyes straight ahead.

"Why don't you?"

Her mother lifted one shoulder and shifted her hands on the steering wheel. "I'm not comfortable in church."

"Did Boots go?"

"Christmas and Easter. Like me, she felt more at home in AA meetings. We both have the same Higher Power: Jesus."

"AA isn't the same as church, Mom."

"How would you know?"

Dawn hadn't meant to sound critical. This was the first time her mom had talked to her about anything remotely personal. Dawn didn't want to ruin it. "Is it?"

"For me, it's better." She gave Dawn a bleak smile. "We all know we're sinners in AA. No one wears a mask."

❄ ❄ ❄

Every Wednesday, Dawn hitched a ride to Cornerstone youth group with Pam Preston. After meetings, they hung out until Pastor Daniel locked up and headed home with Kim. Then Dawn piled into Pam's Honda with Sharon, Linda, and Amy; and they all went to Taco Bell to have sodas and nachos and talk about boys, movies, movie stars, clothes, makeup, and the latest diet craze. Tom Barrett called Dawn for a date. So did Steven Dial. Dawn made excuses, hoping Jason would call. He didn't. She saw him at youth group, but he didn't talk to her much.

Pastor Daniel started a new summer study on chastity and talked at length about running from sin and avoiding youthful passions and how rebellion against God led to a ruined life. "Joseph had to run from Potiphar's wife when she tried to seduce him. Learn from Joseph. God wants you to be pure, and that's not going to be easy in a world that encourages promiscuity."

Jason glanced at her once, but she didn't look back at him. Discussion moved to advertising, movies, music, attitudes at school, the media, new provocative styles of dress.

Jason didn't come to the next meeting.

"He can't come for the rest of the summer," Kim told Dawn. "My dad knows someone at Raley's, and they helped Jason get a job there. He's working nights stocking shelves and cleaning floors."

"Oh. That's great." Dawn tried to sound enthusiastic. "So he's not coming back?"

"Not until school starts. Maybe not then either. He has to save money for college."

She felt niggling jealousy. She liked Kim. She liked her a lot, but she seemed to know quite a bit about Jason's private life. "Well, say hi when you see him."

"I don't see him. He comes by and talks with my dad." She gave Dawn a knowing smile. "If you want to see him, you'll have to come to church."

"I can't."

Kim's brows went up. "Why not?"

"I promised my mother I'd keep going to Mitch's church if she let me come to youth group."

"Oh." Kim looked sympathetic. "Then I guess you're going to have to wait five weeks until school starts." She gave Dawn a curious look. "You said 'Mitch's church.' Doesn't your mom go with you?"

Dawn shook her head. "No."

"Why not?"

"I have no idea. My grandmother said she used to go all the time, and then she just quit."

She couldn't get Jason out of her mind for the rest of the week. The thought of going through the rest of the summer without so much as a glimpse of him depressed her.

"Why so glum, Pita?" Mitch asked over dinner. "The spaghetti and salad are great. You're becoming a fine cook."

Dawn lifted one shoulder and poked at her food. "Doesn't take a lot of talent to boil noodles, dump Ragu on them, and tear up a head of lettuce."

He chuckled. "Maybe you need to challenge yourself more. Try some fancy French cuisine tomorrow night."

She sighed heavily. "Getting through the rest of summer is going to be challenge enough."

Mom frowned as she lifted her glass of ice water. "Since

Christopher won't go to camp for two weeks, I thought this might be a good time to go down to Merced and see Oma." She sipped and set her glass down without looking at Dawn. "We'll be back in plenty of time for camp."

Christopher's exuberant mood collapsed. He groaned and launched into excuses. He wanted to play with his friends. He wanted to swim and Oma only had sprinklers. He wanted . . .

Mom glowered at him. "Be quiet, Christopher."

Mitch leaned back in his chair. "Why don't you take Dawn this year?"

"She wants to stay home for the summer."

"Granny called." Christopher jumped in again. "She and Papa are coming in to pick Dawn up and take her out to Jenner by the Sea for the weekend."

Dawn's heart sank. She'd forgotten all about it. "You could go instead of me. Granny and Papa would love to have you spend a weekend with them. Or a week, for that matter."

"The beach! Cool!" Christopher turned a bright smile on Mom. "Could I, Mom?"

"No." Her tone came out flat and hard enough to keep Christopher from asking again. Dawn wondered why it was fine for her to spend an entire summer, but her mother wouldn't even allow Christopher to spend a night. What sense did that make? They were his grandparents, too, for heaven's sake.

Mitch spoke up. "Christopher can stay home with me. Take Dawn. You two haven't had a trip alone together in a long time." Dawn wanted to snort. They had never been on a trip together. Mitch looked at Christopher. "What do you say we make it men only for a week?" He winked. "Pizza delivery, steak at the Western Boot, rent a dozen movies. We could play some golf. What do you say, buddy? Wanna stick around the hacienda with dear old Dad?"

"Yeah!" Christopher turned to Mom and made prayer hands. He stuck out his lower lip and made it quiver pathetically. "Please, Mom." Not waiting to see if his playacting worked, he jumped up and wrapped his arms around her neck and kissed her cheek three or four times.

Mitch laughed. "How can you turn the boy down?"

Mom, mouth twitching, rolled her eyes at Mitch. "Okay, Christopher, okay. . . ." She laughed.

Sometimes Dawn felt like an outsider watching the three of them. She was a cuckoo left in a warbler's nest.

"Only promise me one thing, Mitch."

His eyes grew warm as he looked at Mom. "Anything."

"Please don't take him out on your Harley."

"Aw, Mom!" Christopher groaned.

Dawn chewed her lower lip. Her mother was going to Merced for a week. Just because she'd agreed to leave Christopher home with Mitch didn't mean she wanted to take her daughter with her. Dawn remembered how Mom and Oma would have afternoon tea on the wisteria-covered patio in Paxtown. Granny never sat with them, and when Dawn had, the conversation felt stilted. Mom and Oma always seemed to have things to talk about. And Mom was one of the most reticent people Dawn knew; she hardly talked to anyone, except Mitch, and then mostly in quiet voices or behind closed doors.

While Christopher came up with a dozen more ideas on how he wanted to be entertained for a week, making Mom and Mitch laugh, Dawn spoke up. "Can I go with you to Merced, Mom?" She held her breath as her mother considered it.

"I think it's time you did."

29

MOM WANTED TO leave early. Dawn packed shorts and tops, sandals and toiletries in a duffel bag and set her alarm for five. She didn't want Mom leaving without her. She lay in bed wide-awake thinking about Jason. He'd be working right now, stacking cans on shelves or sweeping and polishing the floors of the grocery store. He'd probably met some pretty checker a couple of years older and wiser, some fast girl who'd promise him a good time and know how to keep herself out of trouble. Rolling over, Dawn punched her pillow. She hoped Jason had been listening to Pastor Daniel. She hoped he'd run like Joseph did when Potiphar's wife tried to seduce him. *Run, Jason! Run!*

Bleary-eyed in the morning, Dawn dressed and took her duffel bag into the kitchen. Mom sat with a cup of coffee, a pensive look on her face. She glanced up in surprise. "I thought I'd have to wake you."

"I set my alarm. I didn't want you sneaking off without me."

Her mother gave a soft, humorless laugh. "I wouldn't do that. Would you like breakfast before we leave?"

"I'd rather eat along the way. Could we?"

Mitch came out in sweatpants and a T-shirt, his red hair sticking up all over his head like a little boy's. Mom's eyes softened and glowed.

"Didn't want you going without a kiss."

Dawn rolled her eyes. "I'll be in the car." She grabbed her duffel bag. One thing hadn't changed in the eight years Dawn had known Mitch. He still couldn't keep his hands off her mother.

It would be nice if Jason felt that way about her. Just thinking about him made Dawn's blood warm.

Mom followed her out. "I thought we'd take our time and use country roads. Do you know how to read a map?"

"Not really."

Mom opened a California map and refolded it. "We're here. Just follow the yellow highlighted roads. We're going to follow this little black line to Calistoga and meet up with Highway 29 through Yountville and Napa." She traced the route with her finger. "We connect here with Highway 12 and then head east through Rio Vista."

"Great." Dawn tried to make sense of the map. "Have you gone this way before?"

"Yes, but you haven't."

"We could end up in Sacramento with me as guide."

"You'll be fine."

Christopher probably talked Mom's ear off when they went on their excursions. Dawn didn't feel much like talking. She kept thinking about Jason, trying to figure out a way to see him before school started. She looked out the window at the hedgerows of blooming roses. Mitch had rosebushes all around his vineyard too. He told her they drew bees for pollination, but were sensitive to disease and gave vintners early warning so they could take preventive measures if necessary to save their vines.

The road went through Napa and took them south of town onto Highway 12. Dawn watched for signs. "There's the turnoff to

Interstate 80." The road snaked through the hills and curved onto the interstate. Dawn warned of the exit to Rio Vista.

Mom smiled as she took the off-ramp. "Good job."

Dawn felt inordinately pleased. "Thanks." She gave her mother a bright smile. "I can relax now, right? We're on the road to Lodi."

"Oh, Lord, stuck in Lodi again."

Dawn looked at her, wondering what on earth her mother meant.

"It was a Creedence Clearwater song." Mom shrugged. "Way back when."

The road narrowed and took them over undulating hills covered with dry grass. A C-130 military transport took off from Travis Air Force Base and flew overhead. Dawn leaned forward, watching it make a wide circle. "Practice landings, probably," Mom told her, eyes straight ahead.

"Didn't you and Mitch take Christopher to an air show at Travis while I was at Jenner last summer?"

"We didn't think you'd be interested."

Dawn hadn't been asked, but then bringing that up would only build a thicker wall between them. They crossed over a delta slough and drove on to Lodi, where they found a small diner. Dawn ordered waffles and scrambled eggs with bacon.

"You must have Oma's metabolism." Mom ordered a small bowl of fruit and a cup of coffee. The waitress went off to place the order.

Dawn toyed with the menu and tucked it back into the stand that held the sugar dispenser, salt and pepper shakers, and a bottle of ketchup. "Did Papa teach you how to read a map?"

"No. I learned on my own." Mom put her hands in her lap like a schoolgirl. "I once drove from San Francisco to Bethel, New York, and back again."

Dawn stared at her, amazed. "By yourself?" That sort of an adventure didn't fit her mother.

"I was with a friend."

"What was in Bethel, New York?"

"Woodstock."

Bemused, Dawn pictured the little yellow bird in a Charlie Brown cartoon. "Woodstock."

Her mother looked amused. "Ancient history, I guess. It was a rock concert."

Dawn laughed in disbelief. "You drove thousands of miles across country to go to a rock concert?"

She tucked a strand of blonde hair behind her ear. "Me, Chel, and lots of other people from around the country. It wasn't just a rock concert. It was a happening."

Chel seemed an odd name. "Was Chel a guy?" Her father, perhaps?

"Rachel Altman. She was my best friend."

"Oh." Then why didn't her mother ever talk about her? Why hadn't she ever heard the name? Dawn played with the silverware. "How was it?" She glanced up. "Woodstock, I mean."

"Great. The music, at least."

Talking to her mother was like trying to scrape burned spaghetti out of a pot. "What wasn't great about it?"

"Well, it rained. The field turned to mud. There wasn't any shelter. The few outhouses overflowed. The food ran out." She shrugged. "The organizers didn't think any more than two hundred thousand would come. Five hundred thousand showed up."

"Five hundred thousand?" Dawn tried to imagine that many people in an open field and couldn't.

"Everyone came to celebrate the music." Mom's expression became distant. "We all talked of peace and love, though it was already too late. We were so naive."

Naiveté had never been one of the faults Granny laid at Mom's feet.

The waitress brought their breakfasts. Mom thanked her and unrolled her silverware from the paper napkin. She might as well have put up a sign: *Silence, please!* Dawn ignored it. "I've never heard you talk about Rachel Altman, Mom." Not that it was all that surprising. She'd never heard her mother talk about anyone!

Now that Dawn had a name from her mother's past, she wanted to know more.

"Haven't you?" Mom didn't raise her eyes. "I thought Granny might have mentioned her."

"Nope." If Granny had, Dawn couldn't remember. "Are you still in touch with her? I mean, if you were best friends and all . . ."

"No." The word came out firm and flat. End of conversation. Her mother poked at the fruit and speared a piece of melon. "What classes are you taking this year?"

"English, geometry, social studies, PE, biology." She'd be studying human anatomy and physiology this year, too.

"What about Spanish? You'll need a foreign language if you want to go to a university."

"Spanish, too. I forgot. Not that I'm all that excited about going to college."

Mom glanced up. "What do you want to do?"

"I want to get married. I want to have children. I want to be a housewife." Dawn laughed at herself. "Hardly considered a worthy goal, is it? I'm supposed to want a career." Dawn forked eggs into her mouth, pleased to have shocked her mother. At least she was getting some reaction out of her.

When they headed off again, Dawn yawned. "I'm so tired." She looked at the map. "I hardly slept last night."

"I wouldn't have left you behind."

Dawn had hoped they'd talk all the way down, but the silences grew longer. She might as well take a nap so the time would go more quickly. As she dozed off, she thought she felt her mother's fingers lightly brush the hair back from her face.

❄ ❄ ❄

Dawn awakened when the car stopped. "We're here!" Mom sounded light and happy. They were parked in front of a small house with a single-car garage. Dawn got out and went around the back for her duffel bag. She stood on the sidewalk looking down a long, straight street lined with old elm trees and small houses that all looked alike except for the color and landscaping. Oma's house was yellow with white trim and a bright red door. Red, yellow, and white roses bloomed profusely below a front window. A cement walk led to the front steps and postage-stamp porch.

The front door was opened by a wizened old lady with permed white hair and wire-rimmed glasses. She was wearing a blue dress with white polka dots and collar. "It's going to be a scorcher."

Mom hurried up the steps and hugged Oma. Dawn felt shy. Oma's hands looked like bird claws on Mom's back. "It's good to see you, *Liebling*. And I noticed you brought someone special with you."

Mom straightened and turned, eyes glistening with tears. "Dawn asked to come along."

"Did she?" Oma smiled at Dawn. "Well, come on in where it's cool."

An oscillating fan whirred on a stool set up in the kitchen doorway, stirring the heavy air across the tiny, simply furnished living room. A gilt-framed print of snow-covered mountains and green meadows hung on the wall. A recliner sat near the windows with a white crocheted afghan tossed over one arm. A reading lamp stood on one side and a side table stacked with books on the other.

Oma waved toward the short hall. "Carolyn, you can take the front bedroom." Mom disappeared around the corner with her suitcase. "Dawn, the family room is through the kitchen and down the steps on your right. You can use the hide-a-bed."

Dawn stepped around the stool with the oscillating fan and went into the kitchen. She liked the glossy yellow walls with white trim and colorful chicken-print curtains. An ancient gas stove and a small, round-fronted refrigerator were on her right. Three red vinyl, chrome-leg chairs and a table covered with a blue- and white-checkered oilcloth sat against the back wall. A big window looked out onto a large backyard with a stretch of green lawn and a tree loaded with lemons, oranges, and limes.

Dawn went through the side doorway at the back of the

kitchen and stepped down into the family room. It looked more like a library. Shelves laden with books covered the back wall. Dawn dumped her duffel bag beside the green hide-a-bed with needlepoint pillows and took a closer look at Oma's collection. Each shelf held books on a different topic: the ancient history of Egypt; Babylonian, Assyrian, Chinese, European, and British history; American history; biographies. Several shelves held books on farming and business management. One shelf held novels, all classics, all on Dawn's college preparatory reading list.

The backyard beckoned. Stepping outside, she inhaled the sweet scent of wisteria, roses, and sweet alyssum mingling with freshly mown lawn. Bees buzzed in the Joseph's Coat roses climbing posts supporting the white lattice patio cover. Two white wicker chairs with green- and white-striped cushions and a yellow and white couch swing looked inviting. Red, purple, and pink fuchsias spilled from hanging pots.

The kitchen window slid open. "May Flower Dawn!" Oma called out to her. "Iced tea or lemonade?"

How long since anyone had called her May Flower Dawn? Only Mom ever did it, and not very often.

"Lemonade, please." She came back inside and found Mom sitting at the kitchen table with a glass of iced tea. She looked so relaxed and pretty, her blue eyes shining. "It's so good to be here, Oma." She clearly meant it.

Oma's hand shook, spilling some lemonade, as she set a glass in front of Dawn.

"Drat it all. Lucky I didn't spill it all over you. I'm shaking worse than ever."

"What did the doctor say?" Mom wanted to know.

"He said I'm getting old." She snorted. "As if I didn't know. I see myself in the mirror every morning when I put in my dentures." She scowled. "But let's get serious. Angel food cake now or after supper?"

Mom laughed. "How about now *and* after supper?"

"That's my girl." Oma winked at Dawn. "Still has her sweet tooth. How about you, Miss May Flower Dawn?"

Just Dawn, she wanted to say, but stopped herself. She'd never seen her mother in such a lighthearted mood and didn't want to spoil it. "Any time is a good time for dessert."

"Good answer."

Mom told Oma to sit; she'd take care of serving. Oma eased herself into a chair. While Mom cut the cake, Oma asked about Christopher and Mitch. One question from Oma and words spilled from Mom's mouth. Dawn had never heard her mother talk so much or so easily. Nor had Dawn ever tasted anything as good as Oma's angel food cake. Granny's didn't come close.

"And what about you?" Oma asked Dawn. "What's going on in your life?"

"Not much." Dawn shrugged. "Other than I have a massive crush on a gorgeous guy I met at a youth group." She couldn't believe she had blurted out that bit of news. Oma was practically a stranger.

"And you left him all alone to come down here and visit an old lady? I'm flattered."

"Unfortunately, Jason barely knows I exist."

Dawn collected the empty plates and put them in the sink. "Would you mind if I sat outside on your patio? It's so pretty out there, and I love your swing."

Oma waved her hand. "Make yourself to home."

Dawn stretched out on the swing, one foot on the patio to push off. She gazed dreamily through the red, orange, and golden blossoms of the Joseph's Coat above her. She hadn't known what to expect, but she liked it here. Granny said Oma could be unapproachable and rather cold, a woman who expected perfection, but so far, Dawn hadn't gotten that feeling. Maybe age had mellowed Oma. If her great-grandmother had always expected perfection, why would she and Mom be such bosom buddies? Mom had broken moral laws and Granny's heart right along with them.

With the kitchen window cracked open, Dawn could hear

Mom and Oma talking inside the house. Though words were indistinct, the constant babble and frequent laughter told her clearly how well they got along, how much they loved each other.

It had always been that way. Granny said they had a private club with only two members and it was no use trying to break in. But Oma had welcomed Dawn today. She had seemed genuinely glad to have her come down for the week. Dawn hadn't really expected that.

The back door opened and Oma came outside. "Mind if we join you?"

Dawn grinned at her. "As long as I don't have to give up the swing."

"You stay put. I have to move the sprinkler." She went out and pulled on the hose.

Mom came outside, carrying two frosty glasses of lemonade. She set one on the side table near the swing. "I thought you might like a refill." She sat in one of the white wicker chairs. "It's hot out here, isn't it? Like a sauna."

Oma dragged the hose, the sprinkler flipping over and over. "So what do you think, Dawn?" She snapped the hose and the sprinkler righted itself. She headed back for the covered patio.

"About what?"

Oma settled into the other wicker chair. "Being down here with your mom."

"I'm glad I came."

"Good." Oma put her head back and let out her breath. Her mouth curved into a Mona Lisa smile.

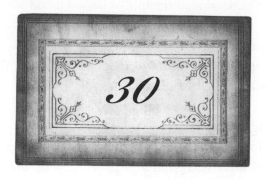

30

THE THREE OF them sat in the family room that evening and watched *Jeopardy!* Oma knew every question in every category before the contestants. Amazed, Dawn asked if she'd ever tried to go on the show. "You'd make a fortune, Oma!"

"Might have made sense thirty years ago when I needed the money, but I have more than I need now. What would I do with a fortune other than leave it to my kids and ruin their lives? And don't give me that cheeky grin. It'd be even worse giving it to grandchildren or great-grandchildren. Take away all your incentive to make something of your life. It's the hard days of scrambling for enough that you'll look back on with fondness when you're a dinosaur like me."

"Granny says every parent wants to make things easier on their children."

Oma turned the volume down with the remote while a commercial played. "Making things easier on your children is sometimes the worst thing you can do. Of course, sometimes it's easier for you. But what does it do in the long term?" She put the remote aside. "Take your granny as an example. She was a sickly baby. If I'd kept on coddling her, she'd have grown up weak. But she's strong. She developed dreams of her own and went after them."

Dawn winced. "I forgot. She said to say hi to you."

Oma grunted. "Next time you talk to her, tell her I'd rather have a call from her than a relayed message."

Mom patted Oma's hand and kissed her cheek before getting up. "I'm going to bed."

"Sleep as long as you want, Carolyn. You're on vacation."

Mom wished Dawn a good night and went up the steps into the kitchen. Oma moved to give Dawn more room on the sofa. "Since this is your bedroom, you let me know when you want it all to yourself."

"How late do you usually stay up?"

"Depends on what's on television. Not much these days. I usually end up reading in the living room, but I'm between books right now."

Glancing toward the back wall, Dawn gave a quiet laugh. "You must love reading."

"Did you find anything to interest you?"

"I have to read *Ivanhoe* next year in English."

"Have to?" Oma got up and pulled the book from the shelf. "It wouldn't be a classic if it hadn't won the respect and hearts of generations." She dropped it on Dawn's lap. "Read fifty pages. If you're not hooked, put it back. If you enjoy it, take it home as my gift."

They watched a mystery in companionable silence. When it ended at ten, Oma flipped through channels, giving terse critiques. "Rerun. Stupid. Copy of a better show. Trash. More trash. I give up!" She shut off the television and put the remote on the cabinet. At home, if nothing caught Dawn's interest, she could always load a favorite video. Oma didn't have a VCR, let alone a library of movies.

Oma struggled to her feet and headed for the kitchen steps.

"How about some hot chocolate? Now that it's cooled off, we can sit outside and enjoy the stars."

Dawn sat in a wicker chair, fascinated as her great-grandmother pointed out stars and constellations and told the mythological stories that went with them.

"How do you know all this, Oma?"

"I'm interested. I have *Bulfinch's Mythology* in my library if *Ivanhoe* doesn't catch your attention." She waved her hand. "There's a whole universe of things to learn." Crickets chirped love songs while Dawn sipped cocoa and listened to Oma until she wound down and sighed.

"You made your mother very happy by coming down here."

"I had to beg her to bring me," Dawn admitted. "She prefers Christopher's company."

"Christopher never said, 'I hate you. I wish you were dead so I could go home and live with Granny.'"

"What?" Dawn spoke weakly.

"Oh, it was a long time ago. You'd just moved to Alexander Valley. Your mother said she understood. After all, you'd spent more time with your grandmother than you had with her. And your grandmother had built her life around you."

Dawn didn't hear any condemnation in Oma's voice, but felt close to tears anyway. She hadn't thought about that in a long, long time. She remembered feeling ashamed. She remembered wanting to apologize. She remembered her mother telling her if she wanted to talk, she could call Granny. She hadn't told Granny what she had said. She'd been too ashamed to admit it. "Sometimes people say things they don't really mean."

"You meant it at the time." Oma reached out and patted her hand. "I've said things I regret, too, my dear. We all do."

"Granny's always loved me."

"So has your mother."

Dawn wanted to believe it. "Not like Granny does."

"And why would that be, do you suppose?"

Why not be frank? Maybe she'd get the truth from Oma. No

one else wanted to talk about the past. "Because I wasn't planned, I guess. I was a mistake in a long line of mistakes she made."

"When has she ever said that to you?"

"She never says much of anything to me."

"Your mother doesn't say much of anything to anyone, other than Mitch."

"She talked with you all afternoon." Dawn hadn't meant to sound resentful or jealous. "I've never heard her talk that much to anyone, not even Mitch."

"She's safe with me."

Dawn looked at her, waiting for more. She could see the sheen in Oma's eyes as she looked at the sky.

"Your mother has never had to guard words with me. She can speak her mind without fear I'll love her less." Oma gazed at the stars in silence for a few minutes, then spoke again. "We all make mistakes. It's how we learn. I'm quite certain your mother would admit to making her share of mistakes. Though I'm also certain she does not consider *you* to be one of them."

"She'd probably still be in Haight-Ashbury if she hadn't gotten pregnant with me."

Oma scowled. "Well, now, I don't know how you can believe that when she didn't even know you were on the way until a month *after* she came home."

"Granny said she came home pregnant."

"Yes. She did. But being pregnant isn't the same thing as knowing you're pregnant. Your mother found out the same day your granny did."

Dawn tried to think back on things Granny had said to her. "Maybe I got it wrong."

Oma relaxed again. "You wouldn't be the first."

Dawn chewed her lip for a moment. "Do you know who my father is?"

"I never asked. Have you?"

"Yes," Dawn said in frustration, "but she always changes the subject."

"Then you might ask yourself when and how you asked."

"I just want to know the truth, Oma. Don't I have a right to know?"

"That's all well and good, but what would you do with the truth if it was given to you?"

Oma talked in riddles! "I don't know what you mean."

Oma pushed herself up from the wicker chair. "Then you have something to ponder, haven't you?" She picked up her empty cup, said good night, and went back inside the house.

❄ ❄ ❄

Over a breakfast of scrambled eggs, sausage, and biscuits the next morning, Oma talked about what her other "kids" were doing. Dawn couldn't help but laugh at the idea of Granny, in her sixties, still being considered a kid. Uncle Bernhard had received a long-deserved prestigious award for grafting lime, lemon, and orange trees. Business boomed and their son, Ed, now managed vendor and customer accounts as well as advertising so Bernie could concentrate on his horticulture experiments.

Rumors circulated in Hollywood that Aunt Clotilde would be up for an Oscar. "Apparently the costumes she designed for some science fiction movie were out of this world," Oma joked.

Aunt Rikka still lived in her apartment in Soho. "She says she has good light for her painting and plenty of subjects. She's doing portraits now. She just finished one of a hoodlum from the Bronx with a tattooed neck and arms. She's calling it *Simon the Zealot*. She's talked an IRS officer into posing as Matthew the tax collector. I don't know who will buy these portraits, but she doesn't care. She says she's saved enough to paint whatever she wants for a while. If she runs short on money, she can always weld some more scrap metal together, give it a fancy name, and put it in that art gallery that loves her work. She told me she has a friend who mounted a urinal on a slab of wood and sold it for two hundred thousand dollars!" Oma shook her head. "People will make complete fools of themselves trying to keep up with whatever the latest art craze is."

Mom took Oma's grocery list and headed off to the store, leaving Dawn alone with Oma. Oma smirked at Dawn as Mom went out the door. "Am I babysitting you or are you babysitting me?" She got up from her recliner. "I have some watering to do. Would you like to go out in the backyard with me? We can keep an eye on each other."

Dawn lounged on the swing. "You had four children, Oma, and they're all so different."

"More similar than you might imagine." Oma tipped a watering can over a box overflowing with blue and red petunias. "All four were bright and good-looking. They all found their God-given talents. Clotilde and Rikka are both artists. Bernhard and Hildemara took to science."

Dawn put her arm behind her head. "I don't think I have any talent."

Oma straightened and glowered at her. "How would you know? You haven't tried anything yet. Other than soccer, which your mother said you play very well."

"Yeah, well, I don't think they have any professional women's soccer leagues."

Oma set the watering can down and eased herself into a chair. "You probably have a good idea already what you want to do with your life."

Get married. Have children. She didn't want to say all that after Mom's nonresponse. "I'm only fifteen. How would I know?"

"Your granny was reading books on Florence Nightingale at fifteen. I left home at fifteen. I knew what I wanted, or thought I did, and made steps to go after it."

Dawn couldn't imagine leaving home right now, let alone leaving her country. How had Oma done that? "What did you want, Oma?" Had she run away like Mom? Maybe that was part of the bond between them.

"I wanted a chance to make something of my life, and my

father thought educating a girl was a waste of time and money. He made me quit school at twelve and sent me to work at whatever menial job he could find. He didn't think I'd amount to anything. He sent me to housekeeping school in Bern to learn how to be a servant. It wasn't what I wanted, but I found ways to make good use of the training. I was going to own something as grand as the *Hotel Edelweiss* someday."

"*Hotel Edelweiss?*"

"My friend Rosie's family had a hotel. It's still in the family as far as I know."

"So you had to give up that dream?"

"Not completely. I owned a boardinghouse in Montreal and helped build a forty-acre ranch specializing in almonds and grapes. If my father had pampered and petted me, I might have ended up staying in Steffisburg and waiting on him for the rest of my life." She snorted and shook her head.

All Dawn wanted to do was get married and have children. It didn't seem like much when compared to Oma or Granny or even her mother, who had become a successful Realtor. In less than three years, Dawn would be eighteen. She'd need some kind of workable plan for her future until her dreams came true, if they did. "The idea of going out on my own scares me." The thought was daunting.

"Probably because you're too comfortable." Oma chortled. "Nice big room in a big fancy house with a swimming pool, everything taken care of for you. Why would you want to leave? The people I loved most told me to go. My mother told me to fly. Rosie couldn't wait for me to have adventures. Even my employers, Solange and then Lady Daisy, both said I had to go. They loved me, but put their needs aside for my good. People either weigh you down or give you wings. I had to shove your granny out of the nest. If I hadn't, she'd still be single and living on the farm, thinking she had to take care of me." She looked annoyed at the memory. "I love every one of my children, and I did the best I knew how in raising them. I just wasn't always the mother they wanted." She let out a soft breath. "I tried to mend the rift with your granny, but . . ." She shook her head. "It's easier to put up a wall than build a bridge."

"Are you sorry you never got your dream, Oma?"

"I can't complain. Sometimes we realize our dreams in ways we never imagined. I never thought I'd ever marry, let alone have children. I wanted an education more than anything. I don't have a high school diploma, but I can speak three languages, and I've read more great books than most college graduates. It's a good thing God isn't limited by what we have in mind for ourselves. His plan is so much bigger. When you're as old as I am, you have time to sit still and take a long, thoughtful look back over your life and see how God's plan was also a whole lot better."

"Jason talks about God the way you do."

Oma raised her brows. "And how's that?"

"Like God cares."

"And you don't think He does?"

"Well, I suppose so, but . . ."

"It's too hot out here for a philosophical conversation." Oma fanned herself. "Let's go inside."

Dawn followed Oma back inside the house. They sat at the kitchen table, the oscillating fan turned on high. "As I get older, I miss the Alps more. Then again, maybe it's just the heat."

"Have you ever gone back?"

"Once, when I was eighty-four. Rikka went with me and made drawings of the old Lutheran church, the schoolhouse where I went, Thun Castle. I was offered a job there once."

"In a castle?" Dawn was impressed.

Oma snorted derisively. "As a maid who'd've been paid a pittance for the honor of working there." She snorted again. "I said no."

"I never knew any of this. You should write all this down."

Oma pushed herself to her feet, took an old leather journal from a kitchen drawer, and tossed it on the table in front of Dawn. "Rosie gave that to me as a going-away present before I left for Bern. She told me to fill it with adventures." Oma chuckled. "I didn't expect to have any. So I filled it with bits and pieces of useful information, things I thought would get me where I wanted to go. And eventually, I suppose some of my 'adventures' made it into the pages too."

Dawn opened the journal. Oma's German script was as small and perfect as the Declaration of Independence, and she had made the most of every page. "Can you read some of it to me?"

Oma put her hands on her hips. "*Ivanhoe* will be a lot more interesting, especially for a girl with romantic inclinations. Jason, is it? He's the one you want to marry?"

Dawn blushed. "I can hope." Covering her embarrassment, she gave Oma a smug smile. "I finished *Ivanhoe* last night."

"Did you now? Well, aren't you the smart little cookie?" Oma looked pleased. "Go ahead and read my journal. It's only the first section that's in German. I started practicing my English as soon as I could. If nothing else, it'll help put you to sleep."

Dawn flipped through pages. "Any recipes for love potions or advice on how to win a boy's heart?"

Oma laughed. "You're on your own there, my girl. I only went out with one man and ended up marrying him. But there's advice on how to mend fences and build bridges. Not that I've ever been good at either."

THAT NIGHT, AFTER Mom and Oma had gone to bed, Dawn stayed up reading the worn journal. The first pages, in German, looked like lists and maybe recipes. The journal switched to English beginning with a heading, "Tea Service for Lady Daisy." A recipe for spicy chicken sandwiches was followed by advice on how to wash linens, polish silver, and clean wood floors. Sometimes a line would be written that wouldn't fit in among the rest.

Another year and I will forget why I came to England. Do I want to be as hopeless as Miss Millicent?

She'd filled one page with information on crop rotation and how to prune almond trees and grapevines.

I bought a car today. Niclas is not happy. I am!

More menus followed, along with a list of "Summer Bedlam Activities." Oma had filled the last two pages with Scripture.

Trust in the Lord with all thine heart; and lean not unto thine own understanding. In all thy ways acknowledge him, and he shall direct thy paths. Proverbs 3:5-6

Oma had made a vine and grape border around this Scripture. The second stood alone with more space around it than anything she had written on the other pages.

When I was a child, I spake as a child, I understood as a child, I thought as a child: but when I became a (wo)man, I put away childish things. For now we see through a glass, darkly; but then face to face: now I know in part; but then shall I know even as also I am known. And now abideth faith, hope, love, these three; but the greatest of these is love. 1 Corinthians 13:11-13

Dawn turned the last page.

I have lived out my mother's hope and pray I have given wings to my daughters' dreams.

Leaving space, she wrote again.

A coddled child grows up crippled.

The last entry put an ending to the journal.

I lived and loved the best way I knew how, trusting God to keep His promise never to lose one of His own. I hold fast to what Mama taught me. In Him, we live and breathe. In Him, we will one day find one another again. In Him, we are one. In this life, we will not love perfectly. In the next, God promises we will. I hold to that hope. I cling to that dream.

❄ ❄ ❄

On the way home to Alexander Valley, Mom fell into her habitual silence. It didn't bother Dawn as much this time, not after a week with Oma. "Can I go back with you next summer?"

Mom smiled, eyes straight ahead. "So you enjoyed yourself."

"Very much." She didn't want to be left out or left behind again. "Christopher and I could camp outside on Oma's lawn."

"He'd like that."

Well, her mother hadn't said she couldn't come. "Oma knows more than anyone I've ever met." She gave her mother a teasing smile. "Even Mitch."

Mom let out a soft laugh. "She's lived decades longer."

Dawn enjoyed the new rapport between them. "Could we go to a stationer's on the way home? I'd like to get a thank-you gift for Oma."

"What do you have in mind?"

"A diploma."

They stopped on the way through Santa Rosa. "I want something that looks like a real diploma. It has to look authentic. This one." She pointed. "'This certifies that Marta Waltert has graduated magna cum laude from the University of Hard Knocks.'"

Mom laughed. "She's going to love it!"

When they picked up the framed diploma, Dawn wrote a

note and put it in the box before sending it by Federal Express to Merced.

> *Dear Oma,*
>
> *I learned more from you in one week than I've learned in ten years of school. I hope to visit again soon.*
>
> *Love, Dawn*

Ten days later, a package arrived Priority Mail from Oma. Dawn opened it at the kitchen table with Mom watching. "A leather journal! Just like the one her friend Rosie gave her." Dawn ran her hand over the beautifully etched tan cover. When she opened it, a note fluttered to the floor. Mom picked it up and handed it to her.

> *If you learned more from me in one week than you learned in ten years of school, you weren't paying attention! Open those lovely blue eyes and look at the world around you! Open those cute shell-shaped ears and listen! Get busy on going after your dream. Thank you for my diploma. I have it hanging on my bedroom wall where I can admire it every night and pray for the blessed child who sent it.*
>
> *Love, Oma*

Dear Rosie,

Carolyn brought May Flower Dawn with her this
year. I had given up hope of ever getting to know my great-
granddaughter. She was such an obnoxious child, so
full of herself, so spoiled by Hildemara and critical of
Carolyn—not that it was entirely her fault. Christopher
usually comes with Carolyn, but Dawn asked to come this
time. I see that as a miracle. I didn't think she liked me.

Dawn has a "crush" on a young man who barely knows
she exists. I doubt that. The girl is a beauty—long blonde
hair, blue eyes, nicely proportioned. I was taken aback.
She is the mirror image of Elise. Thankfully, she is
very different in temperament. May Flower Dawn and
I had several very nice, long conversations. I was surprised
to discover she has a teachable spirit. I am quite taken
with her. She may very well turn out to have the best of
Hildemara Rose and Carolyn in her, and perhaps a little
of me as well. Not too much, I hope.

Dawn sent a gift. According to the diploma she had
made, I graduated magna cum laude from the University
of Hard Knocks. I laughed and wept when I saw it, and I
wept more when I read her sweet note. May Flower Dawn

wants to come again. I am filled with joy! Dare I hope she might be the one to bring my daughter home to me? Oh, how I would love to sit and serve Hildemara, Carolyn, and May Flower Dawn tea on my patio. Think of it, Rosie! Four generations of women together at last. We could drink in the scent of summer roses and talk. Oh, how I would love that. . . .

THREE WEEKS LATER, Granny called. When Oma didn't answer her telephone, her neighbor had gone over to check on her. She found Oma sitting in her recliner. She'd died peacefully, Alexis de Tocqueville's *Democracy in America* open on her lap.

The memorial service took place in a Methodist church in Merced, the front two rows packed with relatives and the rest packed with friends. No air-conditioning and late August heat made the sanctuary almost unbearable. Uncle Bernie and Aunt Elizabeth; Ed; Granny and Papa; Aunt Cloe and her producer husband, Ted; and Aunt Rikki and an old friend and widower named Melvin were all there. Dawn sat beside Mom in the pew behind Granny and Papa. Mitch sat on the other side of Mom, his arm wrapped around her as though holding her together. Christopher sat on the other side of Mitch, leaning against him.

Dawn had never lost anyone, and she felt more regret than grief. She'd liked Oma immensely and wished she'd spent more time with her. But the depth of her mother's grief frightened her. Mom had cried for three days after Granny called with the news.

She hadn't eaten in a week. Now, she sat ashen-faced, tears streaming down her cheeks as the minister spoke of heaven and the hope
God gave everyone who believed in the crucifixion and resurrection of Jesus Christ our Savior and Lord.

Granny glanced back at Mom, her expression pained, almost
angry. Dawn had overheard her speaking to Mom in the pastor's
office before the service. "Are you going to be all right, Carolyn?"
She had sounded impatient.

"She'll be fine, Hildie." Papa put his arm around Granny's waist.
"Come on. We need to go in and sit down."

"No." Granny stepped away from him and kept staring
at Mom. "If you can't hold yourself together better than this,
Carolyn, maybe you should stay in here and cry your heart out."

Mom gasped as though struck.

Mitch's face darkened. Dawn had never seen him so angry.
"There's no shame in grieving over someone she loves!"

"No shame at all." Papa took Granny firmly by the arm.
Granny's face crumpled before she turned away.

Mitch looked chagrined and muttered the first foul word Dawn
had ever heard him say. He folded Mom in his arms and whispered
to her. Christopher looked confused and distressed. Dawn put her
arm around him and told him everything would be okay, though
she wondered if it would.

Now, as the service wore on, she studied her mother's worn face
and wanted to weep. She took her hand and found it cold. While
the minister droned on, Dawn remembered things Granny had
said. "Your mother was always going off by herself, even as a little
girl. She liked being on her own in her dream world. She'd play
outside with the dog for hours."

Dawn thought that meant her mother hadn't cared deeply
about anyone but herself, that she didn't need anyone. Clearly,
she cared deeply about Oma.

Mitch decided they would leave Merced shortly after the reception started. "She's taken all she can take," he told Papa.

"We have to stay," Papa said. "The lawyer will be going over the will tomorrow morning. Apparently, Oma managed to make some good investments."

Mom stared out the front passenger window on the drive home. Tears streamed down her white cheeks. Mitch looked worried. Christopher put his head in Dawn's lap and slept most of the way. Dawn didn't know what else to do but pray. *God . . . God . . .* Even then, words wouldn't come.

※　※　※

During the last two weeks before school started, Mom went about her daily chores like an automaton. Even Christopher couldn't lift her spirits with his cheerful inane chatter and repertoire of new puns and knock-knock jokes. When Granny called, Dawn escaped to Jenner by the Sea. Papa asked how her mom was doing, and Granny jumped in.

"You know very well how she's doing, Trip. I told you I called a few days ago and Mitch said she wasn't up to talking to me."

"Maybe she's feeling better now."

"She won't even speak to me!"

"She isn't talking to anyone, Granny." Fighting tears, Dawn went into the blue bedroom off the kitchen and closed the wooden folding doors. She could hear her grandparents talking in low voices at the table. Papa raised his voice.

"You're madder at Carolyn for grieving than you're sad over your mother dying."

Dawn heard Granny crying and then quick footsteps retreating to the back bedroom. Opening the door slowly, Dawn peered out and saw Papa still sitting at the kitchen table, staring out at the Russian River. When she sat with him, he gave her a pained smile and quipped, "Women. You can't live with them, and you can't live without them." He let out his breath. "Things wouldn't be nearly so bad if everything had been sorted out between your granny and Oma years ago."

"What wasn't?"

He scratched his balding head. "Nothing that's ever going to get fixed now."

❋ ❋ ❋

Home again, Dawn left Mom alone and went out to wander through the garden and vineyard alone. Mitch had started building a new tasting room last spring, and now he pitched in with the carpenters. Maybe he just wanted to be out of the house so Mom could grieve in private.

Hot and tired, Dawn came back inside and found her mother sitting at the kitchen table with a cup of steaming hot tea. Dawn sat with her. "Is there anything I can do for you, Mom?" She'd already finished the laundry and folding. She wouldn't need to start dinner for another three hours.

"It'll just take time." Mom put her hands around the cup. "I wish you'd known her better."

"So do I. It's my fault I didn't." Dawn hurt for her mother. She hurt for Granny, too. They should be comforting one another. Instead, they didn't even speak. "Do you want to talk about Oma? Would that help?"

Mom raised her head and offered a sad, rueful smile. "Maybe you should think about being a shrink."

Dawn gave a soft laugh and started to cry. Angry with herself, she covered her face. "I'm sorry. I just wish I could make things easier on you and Granny. She cried all weekend."

"Did she?"

Dawn wiped the tears from her cheeks. "She'd smile and pretend everything was fine, and then she'd disappear into the garage and cry."

Mom rubbed her temples. "You'll be a great comfort to her."

"What about you, Mom?" Dawn could see the effort it took for her to sit at the table. Her mother leaned forward, heels of her hands pressed hard against her eyes. Was she trying to stop another onslaught of tears?

"I won't run away to Haight-Ashbury," she half whispered hoarsely. "I won't run . . ."

It seemed such an odd thing to say, but Dawn didn't want to make things worse by asking what she meant. "Christopher needs you, Mom." Maybe that would be enough to shake her out of despair.

Her mother raised her head with an effort, eyes bleak. "And you don't."

Dawn felt impelled to admit what she never had before. "Yes, I do." She slid her hand across the table, lifting her fingers in invitation, hoping her mother would understand. Silent, pale, her mother stared. Dawn waited, counting the seconds. Just when she'd almost given up hope, her mother slid her hand across the table and wove her fingers into Dawn's. The first spark of life came back into her mother's eyes as they held tight to each other.

33

"You have mail." Mom came into Dawn's room and handed her two envelopes. Dawn set Jane Austen's *Pride and Prejudice* aside and tore open the large envelope first. Members of the CCC youth group had sent a condolence card with wishes she would return to meetings soon. Even Pastor Daniel had signed it. The second envelope held a note from Jason Steward.

Dear Dawn,

Kim told me about your great-grandmother passing on. I'm sorry for your family's loss and hope you take comfort in the Lord Jesus. I hope to see you when school starts again. If you'd like to talk, I'd listen.

Sincerely yours,
Jason Steward

She spent the rest of the afternoon obsessing about Jason's note. Did he want her to call? Was he inviting her into a relationship? If so, what sort? friendship only or something more?

It took all night and most of the next day to gather enough courage to look up his telephone number. Her heart pounded in her ears as she pushed the numbers. Losing her nerve, she hung up after two rings. She picked up her portable phone half a dozen times before she finally had the nerve to try again.

A woman answered. Stammering, Dawn asked if she could please speak to Jason Steward. The woman's voice became cold. "Who's calling?"

"Dawn Arundel."

"Just a moment." Dawn could hear muffled voices. Time stretched and with it Dawn's nerves. Had she made a mistake calling Jason? Maybe he'd sent the note only to be polite.

"Dawn?" His voice made her pulse skyrocket. She hadn't talked to him in weeks.

"Hi." She winced at the high-pitched tension she heard in that one word. She let out her breath and tried to calm down. "I just called to thank you for your note." When he didn't say anything, she wondered if they'd been cut off. "Jason?"

"I'm here. Hang on a second." Again, the muffled receiver, the indistinct voices. Then he came back on. "How are you doing?"

"So-so, I guess. Better than my mother. Oma's death has hit her hard. They were extremely close."

"Was it expected? Her death, I mean. Your grandmother's. I mean your great-grandmother." He let out a tense breath.

He sounded more nervous than she was. That pleased her, for some odd reason. "She was in her nineties. It wasn't exactly unexpected."

"Oh. Yeah. Dumb question."

"I didn't mean that. My mom and I spent a week with Oma this summer. She was really, really cool." Dawn rolled her eyes, thinking she sounded really, really dumb.

Jason's mother said something. He told Dawn to hang on a second again.

"Dawn?"

"Yes?"

"I have to go. I have something I have to do before I go to work tonight."

"Okay." Dawn felt heat flood her entire body. "Bye." She clicked the phone off and tossed it on the bed. She shouldn't have called. How would she face him when school started?

Kim called later that evening. "Did Jason call you?"

"No," Dawn drawled cautiously. "Why would he?"

"Well, I don't know, but he called me an hour ago and asked for your number."

"He did?"

Kim giggled. "Dad thought Jason wanted to ask me out. I didn't dare tell him he wanted your number."

"I guess your dad doesn't like me very much."

"Oh, it's not that," Kim said quickly. "It's just that Jason is exactly the sort of guy my father wants me to marry. Are you coming back to youth group? Jason said he had Wednesday night off this week."

When Jason didn't show up, Kim shrugged. "I guess he had something else he had to do."

❉ ❉ ❉

Dawn took special care getting ready for the first day of school. She wanted to catch Jason's attention and make a lasting impression. When she came out for breakfast, Mitch leaned back in his chair and gave her a wry grin. "Who's your prey?"

She blushed. Angry, she pulled her chair out and sat down. "I don't know what you mean."

"Ah, Pita. I see trouble ahead." Mitch tossed his napkin on the table and stood. He kissed Mom on the cheek. "I'll buy a shotgun on the way home." Laughing, he headed out of the kitchen.

Mom raised her brows at Dawn.

Dawn stared back at her. "What?" She had chosen jeans that fit her like a second skin and a pink scoop-neck T-shirt that showed off her tan. She'd left her hair down and put on touches of eye shadow and glossy pink lipstick. It wasn't that big a deal, was it?

"You look very nice. That's all I was going to say."

As the bus turned off Prince Street into the school driveway, Dawn caught a glimpse of Jason in the student parking lot with Tom Barrett and Kim Archer. Slinging her backpack over her shoulder, Dawn got off the bus.

"Dawn! Wait up!" Kim caught up with her. Jason held back with Tom, talking while looking at Dawn. Did he like how she looked? His expression showed nothing. He didn't even wave at her. "He bought a car!"

Dawn pulled her gaze from Jason. "Who?"

"Jason! Who else? He gave me and Tom a ride to school." She kept talking as they went inside together to their lockers. Dawn wished she lived in Windsor instead of Alexander Valley. Then, maybe, he would offer her a ride.

Jason and Tom came in the door after them. She stood with her back to them as she opened her locker. Every nerve quivered when Jason came closer. "Hi, Dawn." He spoke quietly. She gave a quick glance over her shoulder without meeting his eyes and gave what she hoped was an equally nonchalant greeting.

After that, she didn't see Jason until the lunch hour. He was with Kim and Tom again, sitting at a table in the cafeteria. Matt Cavanaugh came over and blocked her view. "I don't think I've seen you around school. My name's Matt. And you're . . . ?" He left the question hanging.

"Dawn Arundel. I was here last year."

He grinned at her. "How did I miss you?"

"Maybe you were too busy getting dents in your football helmet."

He laughed easily. "Where are you sitting for lunch?"

She peered around and saw the seats at Jason's table had already filled up. Sharon glanced toward her in question. "Outside, I guess." She headed for the door, not expecting Matt to follow.

He got to the door ahead of her and opened it. "You can sit with me in the senior court."

Joe Hernandez and two other seniors joined them. They flirted outrageously, each trying to outdo the other, which gave her a feeling of power and made her laugh. She finished her lunch quickly and excused herself, going back inside the cafeteria. Sharon, Steven Dial, Pam Preston, Linda Doile, and Amy King still sat at the table. Kim, Tom, and Jason had left.

"Where have you been?" Sharon asked.

"Sitting with Matt in the senior court."

"If you're looking for Jason, he and Kim and Tom went to do a Bible study in one of the courts. I'm not sure which one."

Dawn spotted Jason in the hallway as she headed for her Spanish class. He barely looked at her as he passed by.

The next few days were no different, other than she managed to avoid Matt and his friends. Jason hung out with Tom and Steven Dial, and sometimes Kim. He made no effort to single Dawn out or even speak to her. When she sat down, he got up and left the lunch table. She wasn't the only one who noticed.

"What's with you and Jason?" Sharon kept pace on the way to class. Dawn had just spent another miserable lunch hour of wondering why Jason seemed so determined to avoid her.

She shrugged off Sharon's question. "I've got to get my books."

Spanish passed slowly, Dawn struggling to concentrate on conjugating verbs. She kept glancing at the clock. She wouldn't see Jason until tomorrow, and he'd probably ignore her again. When the bell rang, she headed for biology and then realized she'd forgotten her textbook. She hurried to her locker and grabbed the book she needed. Turning, she bumped into Jason. Her heart jumped and she stepped back, embarrassed. "Sorry. I didn't see you."

"My fault. Can we talk?"

Now he wanted to talk? After almost a month of acting as though she didn't even exist? "I'm going to be late." She stepped around him, but he moved to block her.

"I tried calling you."

"When?"

"This summer. After you called me."

"Thanks for reminding me."

"Once I stayed on the line long enough to hear your voice on the answering machine. I didn't leave a message."

She looked at him. "Why not?"

"I chickened out." A muscle tensed in his jaw.

"Your note said if I wanted to talk, you'd listen. I guess I know now that was bull." She stepped around him and raced to class, slipping into the room just as the bell rang.

She didn't expect to see Jason waiting for her when she came out.

"Would you like to go for a soda after school? We could talk then. I have a car. I could drive you home."

After so many weeks of nothing from him, she couldn't quite take in his sudden warmth. False hope and wrong conclusions would just add to the hurt. "I know you have a car. Kim told me you've been picking her up every day."

His eyes flickered, and then he smiled, looking relieved. "I've been picking up Tom Barrett, too. But she and Tom decided to ride the bus together instead. It takes longer to get home."

She blinked, not sure what he meant. "Are you saying they like each other?"

"Yeah. Is that so surprising? Tom's a great guy."

"I know he is, but Kim is Pastor Daniel's daughter, and Tom is barely a Christian."

"The three of us have been doing a Bible study every lunch hour. Tom is talking to Pastor Daniel about getting baptized."

A Bible study every lunch hour? Was that why Jason had been leaving the table? Maybe his departure had nothing to do with her.

The warning bell rang. Jason took her books. "I'll walk you to class."

Bemused, she fell into step beside him. "You don't know where I'm going."

"You're going to algebra, which is just down the hall from my trigonometry class." He saw her to the door. "Do you want to go have a Coke after school?"

"Yes."

His eyes warmed. "Wait for me after class. We'll get your stuff and go." He headed back in the other direction.

Dawn couldn't wait for class to end. Every minute felt like torture. When the bell finally rang, she slapped her book closed, gathered her things, and headed for the door. A few minutes later, she spotted Jason weaving his way through the throng of students. When he smiled at her, Dawn went hot all over.

"How was algebra?"

"Agony."

On the way to student parking, Dawn spotted Kim and Tom walking hand in hand. "How did I miss that?"

Jason laughed as he opened the car door for Dawn. "I guess you had other things on your mind."

Jason. That's what she had on her mind. Every day, all day, and nighttime, too. She slid into the white Honda, admiring the pristine, beige interior. Jason tossed his backpack into the trunk and slid into the driver's seat. She smiled. "It's so neat and clean."

"I bought it from a lady in the trailer park. She's in her eighties and can't drive anymore." He started the engine. "She only put seven thousand miles on it and had records on oil changes and services." He put his arm on the seat behind her, backed out of the parking space, and pulled into line behind others waiting to exit the cyclone-fenced lot. "My mother is less than happy about it."

"Why?"

"I dipped into my college savings." He pulled out onto Prince Street. "She was pretty ticked off. But I'm still working five to nine as a bagger five days a week. It's good pay."

"What about a Doyle Scholarship and Santa Rosa Junior College? That would give you two extra years to save." She didn't want to think about him leaving the area in less than a year.

"My mother has her heart set on me going to the University of California."

"Which UC campus? Berkeley? Davis?" Both were close enough that Jason could come home on weekends.

"Berkeley. The hotbed of radicals." He pulled into McDonald's and asked if she wanted something to eat. She was hungry, but said no. She didn't want him spending what little money he had buying her junk food. He bought two sodas and a large order of French fries.

Jason drove to Memorial Beach. They walked across the grass and sat on the beach above the Russian River. He insisted she share the fries. They talked about their classes and teachers' expectations. He asked about her summer, and she talked about Oma.

"You're blessed." He looked at the river, expression wistful. "I've never met my grandparents."

"Do they live far away?"

He wadded up his empty bag and pitched it into a garbage can. "San Diego." He rested his forearms on his raised knees. "They don't speak to my mother."

"Why not?"

Jason turned his head and looked at her solemnly. "She had me." When her mouth fell open in surprise, he stood abruptly and walked down to the water's edge. Dawn got up, dusted off her jeans, and followed him. Jason shoved his hands in his pockets. "I thought you ought to know."

Dawn moved closer, her hand brushing his arm. "My mother came home from Haight-Ashbury and found out a month later she'd brought an unexpected package with her. Arundel is Mom's maiden name."

Jason stared at her. "I wouldn't have guessed."

"It's not something to advertise, is it? Have you met your father?"

"Once, when I was five or six. We ran into him at a park. He kept staring at me, and I asked why. Mom told me he was my father. I ran over to him and asked. His friends laughed." He gave a bleak laugh. "He told me to get lost. We moved a few weeks later. I haven't heard of or seen him since." He tilted his head. "What about you?"

She shook her head. "I have no idea who my father is."

"Have you asked?"

"Once or twice. My mother won't tell me anything."

"Maybe the memories are too painful."

"Or she doesn't know who he is."

He winced. "Ouch."

"Well, she was a hippy. Free love and all that. . . ." She lifted her shoulders. She wondered why she was telling Jason. It wasn't something she'd ever wanted to discuss with anyone.

Jason turned to her and gripped her arms. "Dawn, I've been wanting—" At the sound of a car crossing the bridge, he let go of her and stepped back. Looking grim, he glanced at his watch. "I'd better drive you home. I need to get to work." They walked slowly up the sandy hill and under the shade of the redwood trees, neither in a hurry to leave.

"When are you going to do homework, Jason?"

"Study hall, and I get up early." He opened the car door for her. When he slid into the driver's seat again, he turned to her. "I'm not going to have a lot of free time, but what I have I'd like to spend with you. How do you feel about that?" He searched her face.

Everything bloomed inside her. "I'd like that very much."

34

JASON MET DAWN at the bus stop every morning and walked her
to her locker and first class. They ate lunch together with other
members of the CCC youth group, then met every afternoon,
after their last class. Filling their backpacks with textbooks and
homework assignments, they'd head for the parking lot and drive
to the library. They'd find a small, empty table and sit opposite
one another. When she had trouble with math assignments, Jason
moved his chair beside hers, leaning close and whispering help. The
brush of his shoulder against hers and warmth of his body made
her blood race. She savored the exquisite torture of being so close
to him. When he looked at her, she studied the gold flecks in his
eyes, the black depths of his widening pupils.

Dawn was disappointed, but not surprised, when Jason said
they couldn't study at the library anymore. "I'm not getting my
work done, and I've got to keep my grades up."

They hung out at school every day, and he called her every
night on his work breaks. Sometimes he called when he got home,
but his mother never allowed him to talk long. Dawn could hear

her. "You need your sleep, Jason." "You have to get up at four thirty tomorrow morning to finish that report." "You'll see her in school. Get off the phone!"

Sometimes he called her back. "Mom's asleep. We can talk now." And they did, for two hours sometimes.

Pastor Daniel came by. Jason fumed over the telephone. "Mom must have called him. He said rebellion against God leads to a ruined life."

"You haven't rebelled against God."

"I told him that, but he's right, too. I'm not exactly where I was a year ago. I can't go to youth group because of work, and I'm not reading my Bible every day like I was. I'm not praying like I did either. Other than getting my homework done, all I think about is you."

"Maybe we both have a problem." Dawn rolled over and tucked her arm beneath her pillow. "We'll bring our Bibles to school and find a nice quiet place where we can be alone and study. Do you think that will help?"

He gave a hoarse laugh. "When I'm with you, the last thing on my mind is studying."

The sound of his voice stroked her senses, and she knew hers did the same to him. Stirring him up stirred her as well. She liked the rush of blood in her veins, the warmth in her belly. "I wish you were here, Jason."

"Imagine I am."

"Dawn?"

Dawn jumped a foot off the bed. "Christopher!" She hissed in annoyance. "You scared me!"

Her little brother stood in the doorway in his pajamas. "I had a bad dream."

She wanted to tell him to go back to bed, to leave her alone, but he looked so distressed, she stretched out her arm. "Speaking of dreams, I think my little brother just had a bad one." She made room for him. "He likes to curl up in bed with me when that happens." Christopher climbed in and snuggled close.

"Lucky Christopher." He wished her a good night and hung up. She tucked the telephone back in its cradle on her bedside table.

"You love Jason, don't you?" Christopher pressed tight against her.

"More than anyone."

"More than Granny and Papa? More than Mom and Dad and me?"

"It's a different kind of love, Chris. It doesn't take love away from anyone else." She pushed down the palm tree of hair tickling her nose and kissed his head. "Now, go to sleep."

❄ ❄ ❄

On Thanksgiving Day, Granny and Papa arrived for the annual gathering. Mom and Granny acted like polite strangers. No one mentioned Oma. Before the table had even been set, Granny said she wanted to have the family come out to Jenner by the Sea for Christmas. Mom said she'd think about it. Granny said she had all the rooms ready and decorated. Mom and Mitch could have the downstairs apartment with Christopher in the small sitting room.

"I'll put a nice little tree downstairs with ornaments and lights." Dawn would have the blue bedroom upstairs, of course, just as she always did. Mom kept laying out silverware, not saying anything.

"Well, Carolyn?"

"I said I'd think about it."

"I know what that means." Granny stood by the table, fiddling with the silverware Mom had carefully laid out. "Why don't you ask Dawn what she wants to do?"

Dawn hated to be pulled into the middle of the argument. When Mom glanced at her, she winced. She didn't want to tell her grandmother she'd rather stay home. She knew Jason would be working extra hours over Christmas break, but she still wanted to be at home in case he had time to see her.

"It's not up to Dawn." Mom laid out the last set of silverware and left the dining room. Dawn heard her telephone. She'd turned the volume up on the ring so she wouldn't miss it. Excusing herself quickly, she ran down the hall, swinging her door shut before she grabbed the phone.

"Hello."

"You sound like you've been running," Jason said.

"It's crazy around here. Granny and Mom are circling one another with me right in the middle."

"We're going over to the Archers' for dinner."

Uh-oh. "Pastor Daniel probably wants a private talk with you."

"Why do you say that?"

"Because he talked to me last night after the meeting." Pastor Daniel had done a lot of talking about relationships over the last few youth group meetings. He said if anyone thought they were standing strong, they'd better be careful not to fall. Sometimes he'd look right at her when he talked. Last night, Pastor Daniel called her aside after the kids dispersed. Sharon cast a worried glance and said she'd wait in the car.

Pastor Daniel got right to the point. "Georgia tells me you and Jason are seeing a lot of each other."

Dawn felt her cheeks heating up. She had met Jason's mother only once. She'd sensed Georgia Steward didn't like her very much. "We see each other at school. That's about it." Pastor Daniel didn't say anything, but Dawn could tell he was waiting for more of a confession than that. "And we talk on the telephone." Clearly, he already knew that.

"My intention wasn't to upset you, Dawn."

"I'm not upset." What did he want her to say? "We haven't done anything wrong."

"I didn't say you had. You're members of our youth group, and I care about you both. I'll see you next week?"

She forced a smile. "Sure." She watched him walk away. His words had seemed bland enough, but she felt a stab of guilt. Hadn't he read last week that Jesus said thinking about sinning was tantamount to committing the sin? Well, then she sinned all the time! Not a day passed that she didn't wonder what it would be like to make love with Jason.

"What'd Pastor Daniel say?"

"He said he heard we were seeing each other. I got the impression he thinks I'm some kind of Delilah tempting Samson."

Jason didn't laugh. "Mom must have talked to him. She told me the other day she thinks I'm losing my focus."

"And that's my fault?"

"She didn't say that. She just reminded me that I have to keep my focus on where I want to be in five years. We've had this same conversation a hundred times before you and I started hanging out."

She could hear Jason's mother speaking in the background. "You need to get off the phone, Jason. We have to go. You can talk to her at school. . . ." *Yada, yada.*

"I've got to go, Dawn. Can I call you tomorrow?"

"I don't know." Her voice choked up. "*Can* you?" She hung up.

❄ ❄ ❄

Mom fixed turkey with all the trimmings, but Dawn didn't feel like eating. As soon as everyone finished, Mom started clearing platters. Mitch, Papa, and Christopher went into the family room to watch football. Granny stayed to help clear the table. "You've been quiet all evening."

"I just have a lot on my mind." Dawn stacked Villeroy & Boch dinner dishes and headed for the kitchen. She didn't feel like talking about Jason or his mother. She wondered if he was having a good time with Kim. His mother probably would have no problem with Jason going out with Pastor Daniel's daughter. Mom positioned herself at the sink so Granny couldn't step in and wash anything. The dishwasher door yawned, wide-open, from the wall on the other side.

Granny asked what she could do to help. Mom suggested she go relax with Papa and Mitch and Christopher; everything would be done in a few minutes.

"What about the pies? I could cut the pies," Granny insisted.

Dawn wanted to scream at both of them. Why couldn't Mom give in and Granny shut up?

The doorbell rang. Relieved, Dawn said she'd go, then fled the kitchen.

"Don't just open the door," Granny called after her. "Check the peephole first."

Jason stood on the front door stoop. He looked like a *GQ* model in his navy blue sports jacket and gray slacks. He'd loosened his tie and unbuttoned his shirt collar. Her insides knotted. He was clearly upset. "Jason." Her voice came out breathy. "I thought you were going to the Archers'."

"I did. I left." He stepped closer. "Dawn, I—"

"Ask him in." Mitch spoke from behind her. "Jason." He extended his hand in welcome. "Come on into the family room. Dawn's grandparents are visiting."

Jason winced. "I'm sorry. I didn't mean to interrupt your Thanksgiving. I should've called first."

"I'm glad you came," Dawn said quickly.

"We've already finished eating or we would've invited you to join us." Mitch put his hand on Jason's shoulder and half pushed him toward the family room. "Dawn? Are you coming? You can make the introductions."

Jason's arrival distracted Granny from trying to help Mom. Papa shook hands with him. Mitch told Jason to sit and relax. Dawn sat beside him, every nerve stretched tight while Papa asked questions like a police detective. Granny told him to stop interrogating the boy. Mitch seemed to be enjoying the scene. Mom came out of the kitchen and sat. She listened and watched, but didn't say anything.

Dawn gave Mitch a pleading look. How long did they have to sit and make small talk before they could escape and Jason could tell her why he had come?

Christopher provided the way when he insisted Jason had to see his latest LEGO creation. Thankful, Dawn followed and sat on Christopher's bed while Jason hunkered down and admired Christopher's castle and knights. Her little brother chattered on and on about King Arthur and Sir Lancelot, Galahad, Gawain, and Perceval. When Jason glanced at her, Dawn rolled her eyes. "Mom's reading him a book on the knights of the Round Table."

"You want to see it?" Christopher jumped up.

Jason straightened. "Maybe another time, Chris. I came to talk to your sister."

Dawn preceded him down the hall. "We can use the library." The double pocket doors were open. As Jason moved into the center of the room, she closed them quietly. He stood on the yellow and blue Aubusson rug. He glanced around at the mahogany bookcases with colorful amphoras and expensive American Indian pottery tucked in here and there. When he turned, his expression was pained. "I keep forgetting . . ."

She came toward him, drinking in the sight of him. He had left the Archers and his mother and driven all the way to Alexander Valley on Thanksgiving to see her. That had to mean something, didn't it? "Forgetting what?"

He shook his head. "It shouldn't matter, but it does." His gaze swept the room again, pointedly, and she understood.

"It *doesn't* matter." Dawn stood right in front of him. "I'm sorry I hung up on you." She lowered her voice. "I was upset."

"I know."

"Do you want to sit down?"

"No." He reached out, his hand sliding down her arm and taking hold of her hand. He toyed with her fingers. When she looked at him, he let go and stepped away. Sitting on the couch, he rested his forearms on his knees.

Dawn sat beside him. "What happened?" She put her hand on his arm.

"We weren't there five minutes before Pastor Daniel invited me into his office. When he closed the door, I knew something was up. He picked up right where Mom left off on our drive over, and I saw red. I asked if Mom had asked him to talk to me. He said she had concerns. He started talking about how he met his wife. I know all that. He didn't even date until he was a senior in college.

He met her in class and didn't ask her out until he'd asked around about her and knew she loved the Lord as much as he did. They didn't kiss until they were engaged. I didn't want to hear the whole story again." He raked his hands into his hair and held his head. "I lost it."

"What did you say?"

He looked at her bleakly. "I asked him whatever happened to trusting in the Lord, and then I left."

"What about your mother?"

"She's still there." He grimaced. "I can imagine what she's going to say." He came to his feet as though he couldn't bear to sit still any longer. "I've never done anything like that before. I don't know what's the matter with me. I'm going to have to go back and apologize." He stood at the window, looking out. "And if they find out I came here to see you, it's going to make things a hundred times worse."

His words hit like a punch to her stomach. "Oh." She closed her eyes tightly, fighting tears. "I guess they don't like me very much."

Jason turned around to face her again. "They're just trying to protect us."

"Not *us*, Jason." She blinked away tears. "*You*. They don't think I'm good enough."

Someone tapped on the door and slid one side open. Mitch held out the phone. "Your mother wants to speak with you, Jason."

Jason's face darkened as he took the telephone and walked over to the window again, facing out. Mitch pushed the pocket doors into the walls and motioned Dawn over. "Leave the doors open."

Dawn glared at him. "We're not doing anything!"

His gaze narrowed. "Maybe not, but emotions are running a little too high in here."

Jason came back and handed the telephone to Mitch. "Thanks, Mr. Hastings."

"Everything okay?"

"Just some things that need sorting out." Tense, angry, Jason said he had to leave. He apologized to Mitch for the interruption and went into the family room to say good-bye to Mom and tell Granny and Papa it was a pleasure meeting them. Frustrated and worried about whatever his mom had said, Dawn walked with him to the front door. "Will I see you at all this weekend?"

He took her hand. Out of sight of the others, he didn't pretend he wasn't upset. "I doubt it. I'll probably be grounded."

"And it's my fault."

"No, it isn't. This has been brewing for a long time. It's got nothing to do with you, Dawn." He leaned down and whispered, "Can I kiss you?" She said please. His mouth was firm and warm, moving tentatively over hers. When he straightened, she drew in a shaky breath. They stared at one another, and then he stepped closer and kissed her again. His arms slid around her, and she felt his heart pounding against hers. At the sound of footsteps, they broke apart, panting softly, shocked that their feelings could skyrocket so fast. He stared at her, eyes dark, face flushed. "I'll call you." He went quickly out the door, closing it behind him.

Dawn turned and found her mother standing in the archway. "Is everything all right?"

Heart pounding, body swimming with sensation, Dawn shrugged. "No. Not really." Not yet, anyway, but things were going to change. She felt ecstatic and triumphant. When Jason kissed her the second time, she knew his mother and Pastor Daniel wouldn't be able to keep them apart.

35

JASON DIDN'T CALL. She didn't see him until Monday morning at school. He'd gone back to the Archers' and apologized to everyone. When he and his mother got home, she exploded. Yes, he was grounded. For two weeks. No telephone privileges, no going anywhere with friends. *Friends*, Dawn knew, meant her.

Every morning when Dawn got off the bus, Jason stood waiting for her. They hung out under the maple trees along Prince Avenue before going to their lockers and on to class. They met as often as their schedules allowed. They sat alone together on the field during lunch hour, rather than eat with their friends. He never kissed her, but sometimes he held her hand when they walked around campus.

Dawn still attended youth group with Sharon on Wednesday evenings, but she barely paid attention to what Pastor Daniel had to say. She came to be with her friends, not listen to him lecture. Kim and Tom sat together, but didn't touch, and Kim still rode home with her father after the meetings while the rest of the kids, including Tom, met up at Taco Bell or McDonald's to talk for another hour or two. "Does Pastor Daniel know you and Kim are going out yet?" Steven Dial asked, stirring up trouble.

"Yeah, he knows." Tom shrugged. "He was pretty cool about it."

"Cool? How so?"

"He invited me to a baseball game. We spent most of the time talking."

Steven laughed. "You mean *he* talked."

"Not all the time. He asked me if I loved Kim. I said I did. He told me love between a man and woman can be a beautiful thing, but it's fragile, too. It only takes one mistake to turn life into a tangled mess." Everyone knew what he meant, though few believed him.

Two weeks felt like two years, but finally Jason's mother paroled him. Jason called Dawn that night. He called on breaks at work. He called when he got home, when he finished his homework. They often talked until after midnight. She worried about him. He seemed so tired all the time. She'd tell him not to call, to go to bed; she'd see him at school first thing in the morning. He said he liked hearing the sound of her voice just before he went to sleep, although sometimes they talked about things that kept them both awake long into the night.

Christmas break approached, and Dawn went shopping with Sharon, Amy, and Kim. Kim bought Tom a Bible and a silver chain and a cross made of nails. Dawn bought a gold identity bracelet with *Forever* engraved on it for Jason.

The day school let out for winter break, Jason drove her out on Dry Creek Road and parked in the empty visitors' center lot at the base of Warm Springs Dam. The skies opened up, rain pounding the roof of his Honda and sheets of water pouring over the windshield. He kept the car running and the heater on, though it wasn't necessary. The knowledge they were alone and the desire swimming in their bellies kept them warm. Eager to see if he liked his gift, she insisted he open hers first. As soon as he opened it, she took it from the box and attached it around his wrist. "So everyone will know you're mine."

Jason gave her a small white box tied with a red ribbon. He seemed nervous. "I hope you like it." She told him she'd love anything he gave her, but drew in a soft breath of pleasure when she saw a delicate gold bracelet coiled on the cotton. She touched the small heart and glistening white pearl. She asked him to put it on her wrist. As he did, she kept her gaze fixed upon his face. "I love it, Jason. I'll never take it off." When he raised his head, she leaned toward him, lips parted.

The windows steamed up. The rain pounded harder and faster, as though trying to keep pace with their hearts. Murmuring his name, she clutched his shirt. He pressed her back against the seat. She wanted him closer. Pushing his jacket open, she slipped one hand beneath his sweater. She felt the smooth skin of his back, the hard muscle from lifting boxes of canned goods. His hand went under her thigh, gripping, sliding her down on the seat. She gave a soft cry as her head bumped hard against the armrest. Jason pulled back abruptly. "Are you okay?"

"Yes." Her voice came out raspy. She rubbed her head as he pulled her back up.

"I'm sorry."

"Don't be." When she leaned toward him again, he drew back.

"We've got to stop." He shifted over and shut his eyes tightly, then opened them again, face taut. "We'd better go."

"We were only kissing, Jason. There's nothing wrong with that, is there?"

"No, but I wanted more."

Swallowing hard, pulse pounding, she looked straight into his eyes. "I wouldn't have stopped you."

"That's why we have to leave." He released the emergency brake and put the car into reverse.

She pressed the heels of her hands against her eyes and gulped a sob.

Jason stopped, rammed on the emergency brake, and put his arms around her. "Don't cry. It's my fault. I shouldn't have brought you out here. It's my fault things got out of hand." He tipped her chin and kissed her softly. "I'm sorry, Dawn. I won't let it happen again."

She believed him, which only hurt and frustrated her more. "You're good all the time, Jason. All the time you're good. And all I want is you."

Jason touched her arm gently. "It isn't what God wants for us, Dawn."

God again. "Sometimes you talk as though He's in the backseat."

"He's closer than that. He's inside us."

Us. Maybe that was the real problem. The Holy Spirit did live inside Jason. She had no doubt about that.

But she wondered . . . what about her?

❋ ❋ ❋

Granny called, trying to wear Mom down about having the family Christmas dinner at Jenner by the Sea. Failing, Granny called Mitch at his office. Dawn arrived in time to overhear the end of the conversation. "I'll talk to her, Hildie. Sure, I understand, but . . ." He rubbed his forehead. Dawn slipped into the chair in front of his desk, mouthed *no*, and shook her head. "What's wrong with Trip? If it's serious, Carolyn is going to insist you two come in." He gave Dawn a pained look. Dawn leaned forward. Mitch shook his head and mouthed, *He's okay.* She put her head back against the red leather wing chair. Just Granny applying the emotional screws again. "Let me talk to her. If she agrees, she'll call you. Okay? That's the most I can promise. I love you, too."

Hanging up, Mitch gave her a wry grin. "And how was your day?"

"Are we going to Jenner for Christmas?"

"You heard what I said. Maybe. We'll see. It's up to your mother."

"Then we'll be going. I'm surprised she's held out this long."

"You don't look pleased about it."

"What's wrong with Papa?"

"He doesn't feel up to driving in and spending a few days in Alexander Valley. He wants to stay home."

Dawn went into her bedroom and dumped her backpack. Flinging herself onto her bed, she stared at the ceiling. Jason had hoped to take her out over break, but it all depended on his work schedule and what plans his mother made.

Mitch had probably told Mom about Granny's call by now. She decided to go to the kitchen, hoping to encourage her mother to hold her ground and insist Granny and Papa come in this year.

"Well, at least, let me bring something. . . ." Mom was on the phone, perched on a kitchen table, knees together, feet up like a little girl.

So much for that idea. Dawn returned to her room and threw herself across the bed again.

Mom announced at dinner that they'd be going to Jenner by the Sea for Christmas Eve dinner. "She wants to serve dinner at six instead of four."

"Then we'll stay over," Mitch decided. "It'll be after ten before we finish unwrapping presents. No point in driving back in the dark on a windy road with the weather such as it is."

"With the weather such as it is, they should come in," Dawn said. "You know how Jenner gets this time of year. If there's a real storm, we could end up stuck out there."

"Too late, Pita." Mitch gave her a cajoling smile. "Your mom agreed, and rightfully so. Granny said this is probably the last year she'll have the family gathering, and she has her heart set on it." He looked across at Mom. "She'll pass you the baton."

"Did she say that?" Mom sounded hopeful.

"Not exactly, but it's only a matter of time."

"It's not about time, Mitch." Mom looked defeated. She glanced at Dawn. "You'd better pack extra clothes. They'll want you to stay through New Year's."

Dawn's heart sank. "Maybe Christopher could stay this time."

"No, Christopher can't. Besides, you haven't spent a weekend out there in over two months."

Before Dawn could protest, Mitch spoke up. "If Jason wants to see you badly enough, he'll drive out."

※ ※ ※

Christmas went exactly as Dawn expected. When Mom tried to help, Granny acted like a pit bull guarding her territory. Only Dawn was allowed into the kitchen "so she'll know what to do when she has a home of her own." Sometimes Dawn wondered if Granny just wanted Mom out of the way and things back to the way they used to be when she was a little girl and Granny was her nanny.

After hours of labor, dinner disappeared in less than thirty minutes. Mom insisted on doing the dishes. "You cooked; I clean." It started to turn into an argument before Papa and Mitch stepped in. Mitch said he'd help, and they'd open gifts when the dishes were washed and put away.

Papa took Granny by the arm and escorted her into the living room, where she sat nervous as a cat, staring at the closed door to the kitchen. She couldn't stand to be idle. Papa told her to put on one of her old Christmas movies. "How about *Ben-Hur*?" Dawn suggested, knowing it was one of her favorites.

"There's no time for *Ben-Hur*," Papa grumbled.

"How about *How the Grinch Stole Christmas*?" Christopher piped up.

"We don't have that one," Granny said.

"How about *A Christmas Story*?" Christopher tried again. "The one where the boy wants a rifle."

"A BB gun," Dawn corrected him.

"We don't have that one either," Granny said.

"How about *Hatari*?" Papa said. "We have *Hatari*."

"It's not a Christmas story."

When Papa put his head back and let out a heavy sigh, Granny got up. "We can have some nice Christmas music."

Things eased up after Mom and Mitch came into the living

room. Mom looked more relaxed. Mitch held her hand. When they sat on the couch, he put his arm around her and pulled her in tight against him. Christopher played elf and passed out the presents. Papa put out a big box so they could wad up wrapping paper and "shoot baskets." Christopher pleaded to camp out in the living room so he could enjoy the colorful Christmas lights on the tree and the fire burning low in the fireplace. Mitch thought that was a grand idea and whispered something in Mom's ear that made her blush.

"How's Santa going to come if you're here in the living room?" Papa teased Christopher.

"He's not coming. We already opened all the presents." Christopher grinned. "Besides, Papa, how'd he get down your chimney with a fire burning?"

They all laughed, even Granny, who sat with the robin's-egg blue velvet robe with embroidered trim Mom had given her. She kept stroking it.

Mitch stood, drawing Mom up with him, and bid everyone good night. Granny smiled and nodded and told them to feel free to sleep in the following morning, then watched Mom leave the room, a pained and wistful look on her face.

Long after Granny and Papa had gone to bed and Christopher had settled down in a sleeping bag on the living room floor, Dawn lay awake.

Jason didn't call.

❄ ❄ ❄

Mom, Mitch, and Christopher piled everything into the Suburban and headed home after breakfast the next morning, leaving Dawn at Jenner with Granny and Papa. "We're going to have such a good time together," Granny promised, and Dawn didn't want to disappoint her. While Papa dozed in front of the television, Granny made an angel food cake. Dawn sat at the kitchen table and talked about Jason. She showed off the bracelet he'd given her, though she left out personal details of what had happened during their gift exchange.

"Your first love." Granny smiled. "It's a milestone."

"He's my last love, too, Granny."

"That's the way it was for me and Papa. He was the first man I dated and the only one I've ever loved." She slid the angel food cake into the oven. "I think it was that way with Oma, too. Fidelity must run in the family, just skipped one generation."

Dawn recognized the reference to Mom's hippy years and ignored it. "What was Opa like?"

Granny sat across from her. "He was grand. Tall, blond, handsome. He was at least a head taller than Mama. And strong as Atlas. I remember him lifting me as though I didn't weigh more than a feather. He worked hard. So did Mama, of course, but my father enjoyed life more. He didn't allow things to worry him the way Mama did. He sang in the orchard. My mother never sang, except in church. And he had the patience of Job, especially with Mama. She'd get so het up about things, had to have her way."

Dawn held back a smile, thinking Granny could fit that description, not that she'd like hearing it. "Do you have any pictures of him?"

"Just a couple. There's one in the bedroom on my dresser. They had it taken before Bernie went away to college. Bernie had copies made later on. Photographs were expensive in those days, and they never had a lot of money to spare. Rikka drew pictures of Papa and Mama and had them framed. They're probably in one of the storage boxes out in the garage."

Dawn followed Granny into the bedroom later while she put some towels away. She picked up the portrait and sat on her grandparents' old king bed to study it. Oma, with dark hair cut short and pushed back from her plain face, stood straight, shoulders back, chin up, eyes straight ahead, lips curved into a taut smile. She stared straight into the camera lens, expression grim, as though having her picture taken was the last thing she wanted to do. Opa, on the other hand, looked at ease, a relaxed smile on his lips.

Strikingly handsome in a dark suit, white shirt, and tie, he stood with one shoulder behind Oma, his head tilted toward her. Dawn imagined he had his arm around her waist, holding her in place. "Opa was sure handsome."

"Blond hair and blue eyes." Granny tucked away the towels and came out of the pink- and black-tiled bathroom. She took the picture and studied it with a smile. "Bernie got his looks. All the girls at school fell in love with him. Cloe and Rikka got his coloring, too." She set the picture firmly on her dresser. "I took after Mama."

36

JASON CALLED TWO days after Christmas. "We just got back from LA." When she asked if he'd gone to Hollywood or down to Disneyland, he said no. His mom wanted him to walk the campuses at UCLA and USC and Pepperdine.

"I thought she wanted you to go to Berkeley."

"We're not talking about Berkeley anymore." He changed the subject before she could ask why. "When are you coming home?"

"New Year's Day." She turned her back on Granny when she came into the kitchen. She lowered her voice. "I miss you, Jason."

"Would your grandparents mind if I came out to see you?"

Heart singing, she told Granny and Papa her boyfriend was coming for a visit. She was so excited she couldn't sit still. She changed from sweats to fitted jeans and a pink sweater. She put on a touch of makeup. Maybe they could visit with Granny and Papa for a little while and then go over to the beach.

How long before he got there? It only took forty minutes and it had been forty-five. She sat at the kitchen table watching cars come around the bend before crossing to tiny Bridgehaven with its trailer park—flooded now—two-room motel, and restaurant overlooking the river.

The rain started again. So much for taking a walk on the beach.

An hour passed, and then another. "Road might be closed," Papa told her while eating a sandwich at the kitchen table. "Aren't many places to stop and call."

Finally, she spotted his car zinging along Highway 1. When the car slowed through Jenner and turned right onto Willig, she darted out the back door to unlatch the gate. Swinging it open, she stayed under the wooden cover and watched him park. Heart knocking, she smiled as he got out of the car. "I was worried you got stuck somewhere!"

"I didn't want to come empty-handed." He leaned back into the car, sweater stretching taut over his shoulders, jeans snug, and lifted out a cellophane-wrapped potted poinsettia and box of Russell Stover chocolates. When she reached for the chocolates, he drew them back and grinned at her. "For your grandparents, not for you." She laughed. He looked toward the house and then leaned down to brush a kiss against her cheek. "Not sure I can stay long. There were a lot of fallen limbs on the road, and water just after Guerneville."

"If the road closes, you can always stay over."

"I don't think my mom would go for that idea."

The sky opened up, rain pounding the roof and streaking down over the living room windows. Papa said he'd better go down and get some presto logs out from under the garage in case the power went off. Jason insisted he'd take care of it. "Nice young man," Papa said.

"And handsome, too," Granny added. Dawn felt smug. At least she had her family's approval.

Granny suggested an early afternoon dinner "so Jason can eat before he heads home." Jason became so engrossed in Papa's World War II stories that Dawn went into the kitchen to help Granny make a tossed green salad and a casserole of turkey, dressing, and gravy. They all sat to eat at three. By four, the sky had darkened.

The rain hadn't let up. Jason gave Dawn an apologetic look and said he'd better go. Papa said he'd better call highway patrol first and see if the road was open through Guerneville.

It wasn't. Papa said Jason would have to take the road south through Bodega and go back through Sebastopol in order to get the highway north to Windsor.

Granny protested. "It's dark. And that's too far to go in driving rain, especially if you aren't familiar with the coast highway. Jason should stay here with us." She suggested he call his mom so she wouldn't worry. Dawn suggested Granny go on into the living room with Papa and let her take care of washing the dishes. For once, Granny didn't quibble. Maybe she understood how desperately Dawn wanted to be alone with Jason, even if only for a few minutes, before his mother insisted he get back in his car and come home no matter how bad the weather.

Jason sighed. "She'll be ticked off."

"It's not like you started the storm, Jason."

"No, but she told me it was a bad idea coming out here."

Dawn wondered if she'd been talking about the weather or seeing her. Jason punched in the numbers. His mother must have been sitting by the telephone because it barely had time to ring before Jason said, "Hi, Mom."

Dawn squirted dish soap into the old porcelain sink, turned on the hot water, and pretended not to listen.

"The road's closed. I'm going to have to stay out here." He listened briefly. "It'd take two hours to go that way, and I only have half a tank of gas. . . ." Jason turned away. Elbows on knees, shoulders tense, he hunched over the receiver and growled. "Jeez louise, Mom, would you rather I ended up over a cliff in the ocean—"

Apparently his mother cut him off. Dawn added some cold to the hot and grabbed one of the glasses.

"Nice to know how much you trust me." Jason grew more angry. "We're not alone out here, Mom. *Both* of Dawn's grandparents are with us, and it's a small house. Two chaperones. Is that good enough?" He listened for another few seconds. "Okay. I'm

sorry, but—" He sat up and let out a steamed breath. "Yeah, I hear
you. First thing in the morning. Okay, okay. Yes! I'll drive south if
the roads are still closed. I promise." He hung up. His expression
looked faintly triumphant. "Need some help with those dishes?"

"Sure." She smiled. He'd be here all night! "The towels are in
that drawer." When he stepped close beside her, she looked up,
melting inside. He told her how much he liked her grandfather
as he dried glasses and then silverware, asking where things went.
Dawn daydreamed. Someday, when they got married, they'd stand
like this every night and do dishes together.

They'd just finished putting everything away when Granny
came into the kitchen with a pile of burgundy sheets, a pillowcase,
and flannel pajamas. "Here's an extra pair of Papa's pajamas for
you, Jason, and Dawn can make up the bed downstairs."

Jason looked blank. "Downstairs?"

"The apartment. There's an electric blanket on the bed, but
we'll keep the heat on so you don't get too cold. You'll be snug as
a bug down there."

"Please don't go to any trouble. I can sleep on the couch."

"Nonsense." Granny dumped the pile into Dawn's waiting
arms. "We like our guests to be comfortable." She went back into
the living room.

Dawn headed for the back door. "Come on. I'll show you where
you'll be." He opened the door for her as she called out to her
grandparents that they would be back in a few minutes.

The frosty air of the downstairs apartment struck Dawn as she
stepped inside. Jason followed her. Mom had folded up the hide-a-
bed—Chris hadn't slept in it anyway—and put the coffee table back.
Granny's small writing desk sat in the corner. A Victorian lounge
chair sat in the back room facing the stripped queen-size bed. Mom
had left the thermal and electric blankets and blue chenille spread
folded neatly across the end. Jason straddled the flowery lounge and
watched Dawn shake out the bottom flannel sheet. She worked
quickly. "You look like you know how to make a bed."

She laughed, excited to have him here, even more excited at

the thought of him sleeping just down the stairs from her room. "Granny taught me how to do square corners. She was a nurse." Shaking out the top sheet, she glanced at him and saw something in his expression that made her breath catch.

She unfolded the electric blanket, making sure it was plugged in properly, before spreading it over the burgundy sheets. Dawn didn't notice any cold air now, and no warm air blasted yet from the heating vent. Jason got up and helped spread the thermal blanket over the top. They didn't speak. Pillowcase fitted, she plumped the pillow, pulled the bedspread up, and tucked it neatly under.

They stood on opposite sides of the bed, staring at one another.

Jason came around the side of the bed and took her hand. "Can I kiss you again?"

Trembling, she looked at him. "I wish you would."

Tilting his head toward her, he whispered, "I was afraid your grandparents might get the wrong idea. . . ." When his mouth covered hers, she stepped closer, putting her arms around his neck and pressing her body fully and firmly against him. His soft groan lit a fire inside her. His hands moved down her back to her waist and hips and then up again, encircling her tightly. He dragged his mouth away. "I don't think I'm going to get much sleep down here. I'll be lying awake, staring at the ceiling, knowing you're right above me." When he kissed her again, she fitted her body to his and heard his sharp intake of breath. They were both shaking when Jason finally set her away from him. "We'd better go upstairs before your grandparents wonder what's going on down here."

❄ ❄ ❄

Granny and Papa stayed up later than usual. When Papa pushed himself out of his recliner and said it was time to hit the sack, Jason stood and said he'd better go to bed, too, and thank you for everything. Dawn said good night to him from the couch and watched him go out the back door. He glanced back at her through the glass before heading for the wooden steps to the downstairs. Granny paused in the bedroom doorway and looked at her. "Are you staying up, Dawn?"

"I'm not sleepy yet. I thought I'd watch television for a while."

"Turn down the thermostat when you go to bed." Granny wished her a good night and closed the French glass doors with their sheer privacy curtains. Dawn pulled a crocheted afghan around her shoulders. She lowered the volume and changed the channel. She heard Papa's loud snores. He always fell asleep the moment his head hit the pillow. It wasn't long before Granny made it a duet. Dawn waited another fifteen minutes before turning off the television and resetting the thermostat. She took a quick shower and slipped on her nightgown. Pulling the covers back, she rumpled them and stuffed two pillows underneath in the off chance Granny awakened and felt the need to look in on her.

She closed the accordion doors before carefully opening the back door. She made sure it was unlocked before quietly closing it behind her. Then she hurried tiptoe down the wooden steps, feeling the icy drops of rain soaking through her cotton gown. A soft light shone above the apartment door. She hesitated. Then, shivering with cold, she pushed the door open. Her heart lurched as it creaked. As she stepped inside the door, Jason turned on the bedside light. "What are you doing?" Throwing the covers off, he got out of bed.

Jason looked so comical in Grandpa's pajamas, Dawn giggled nervously. "I couldn't sleep."

"Shhh. . . . You'd better go before they—"

"Listen!" she whispered, pointing up. Papa snored so loudly, they could hear him downstairs. She grinned at him. "They both sleep like logs. They won't know a thing."

"You're shivering." He put his arms around her. "You're wet!"

"It's raining." She inhaled his scent. It went right to her head. "I'm freezing." She shivered, loving the feel of his arms around her. His heart pounded harder. "I'd be warmer in bed."

"Not a good idea."

"We won't do anything." She slipped her arms around him. "We'll just talk."

Beneath the covers, Jason held her close and asked if she was warm enough. She said no and snuggled closer, pressing her body against the length of his. She heard his breath quicken. They did talk, for a little while. Then they kissed. Heating up fast, they had to push the covers off. Niggling doubts flitted into Dawn's mind as passion grew.

Fear gripped her at the last. Too late. She sucked in her breath at the unexpected pain. Jason stopped, rasping an apology. She said, "It's okay; it's okay." They both knew it wasn't. Worse, they couldn't go back.

This wasn't how she imagined it would be.

When it was all over, Jason sat on the edge of the bed, head in his hands. Dawn pulled the blankets up to her chin. Silent, rigid, eyes welling, she felt sick with regret. What had she done?

Jason was silent so long, she felt driven to speak. "I love you." That's why she'd done it. "I love you, Jason." She sounded like a frightened child afraid of being chastised.

"I love you, too." Jason's voice was thick with tears. And regret.

Ashamed, Dawn shoved the covers off and fled to the door. Jason caught up with her and wrapped his arms around her. Pulling her firmly against him, he whispered against her hair, "It's my fault." He drew in a ragged breath. "I should've gone home."

Hurt by his remorse, ashamed of her own behavior, she spoke tersely, voice breaking. "I wish you had."

❄ ❄ ❄

Of course, Granny insisted Jason have breakfast before he left. Jason glanced at her once when she came out of her bedroom. He had dark shadows under his eyes, as though he hadn't slept any better than she had. Dawn could tell it took concentrated effort for Jason to smile and act normal, to talk with her grandparents as though nothing had happened last night.

Sitting there at the table, Granny and Papa chattering away, Jason giving distracted answers, she kept thinking, *I had sex with Jason downstairs last night in the bed Mom and Mitch slept in a few days ago. Granny and Papa were right upstairs. They all trust me. They respect Jason. What would they think of us now if they knew?* She felt cold prickles along her arms. What if Jason confessed what they'd done to Pastor Daniel? What if he told Tom Barrett and Tom told Kim?

She hadn't expected to feel sick with guilt and shame. She knew Jason felt even worse than she did. He didn't hurry, but he didn't linger over breakfast the way he might have if she'd stayed in her own bedroom last night.

"I'd better get going." Jason said his good-byes and thank-yous. Dawn followed him out to his car. She stood under the overhang, arms wrapped around herself, afraid of what he might say. Jason gave her the same chaste peck on the cheek that he had when he arrived yesterday. Only his eyes looked different. "The sheets are . . ." He winced. "They're going to know."

Dawn's face went hot. "I'll strip the bed and wash them." Thank goodness Granny had given her burgundy sheets rather than white ones, or she'd never be able to wash away their sin.

Sin!

Shocked, Dawn felt the word stab her heart like a spear, leaving her wounded. *We sinned. I sinned.*

"I'm sorry, Jason." She pressed her lips together, tears spilling from her eyes.

He stepped close, his hand at her waist as he whispered into her ear. "I love you. Nothing's going to change that."

But something already had.

37

1987

Dawn didn't hear from or see Jason until school started again. He stood waiting when the bus pulled in and fell into step beside her as she headed inside to her locker. "We have to talk."

"You could've called." Hurt, angry, she walked on.

"I couldn't. Mom and I had a big fight when I got home."

The blood drained from her head, and she felt faint with fear. "Did you tell her?"

"*No.*" Glancing around, he leaned closer while she worked the combination and opened her locker. "How long before we know if you're . . . ?" She could feel his embarrassment. She looked at him and let him see her fear and hurt, and he frowned. "Things will work out." When Jason took her hand, she wove her fingers through his and held tight, afraid he'd fall out of love with her as quickly as she had fallen in love with him.

Every day, he gave her that questioning look, and she shook her head. After three weeks had passed, he said he'd try to get a home pregnancy test. "I might not be able to buy one this week. Bill is working the same shift I am, and if he sees, he'll say something to Mom." Agitated, he raked a hand through his hair.

Mom awakened Dawn Saturday morning. "Your grandparents are going to be here in an hour."

Dawn sat up and rubbed her eyes.

"Are you all right?"

Fear shot through her. Did her mother know? Had she some extrasensory perception that she could guess? "I'm fine."

She showered, dressed, and threw her hair into a ponytail. A car honked loudly, and she drew back the sheer curtains. Granny and Papa had arrived in separate cars, Papa in a white Buick and Granny in their shiny black Sable. When Dawn opened the front door, Granny dangled the keys. "The Sable is all yours."

Papa grinned. "Happy sixteenth birthday!"

"What?" Dawn stared. "You're kidding, aren't you?"

"Of course not." Granny took her limp hand and dropped the keys into it, closing Dawn's fingers around them. "We wouldn't kid about something like that."

Dawn shrieked and threw her arms around Granny and then Papa. "Thank you, thank you!"

Mitch, Christopher, and Mom appeared and asked what was going on. Dawn darted out the door and ran her hands over the freshly polished Sable. "They said it's mine!" she called back, happy for the first time in weeks. "I have wheels!"

Mom's eyes widened. "You should've talked to me about it first."

Granny scowled. "We're doing it as much for you as for Dawn, Carolyn. You have Christopher in sports and music lessons and church group. Dawn can't take a bus everywhere, you know. She needs a car. Now she has one."

Mom's face reddened. "It's not for you to make that decision." She turned to Mitch, who stood beside her. He looked grim.

Dawn came back, wanting the freedom the car offered. "You won't have to drive me to Jenner, Mom. I can drive out all by myself."

Granny beamed. Papa patted Dawn's shoulder. "Everything's been checked out. It's a good car, Carolyn."

"I know, Dad. That's not—"

"That little baby won't need any repairs for a long time to come. All the paperwork is in the glove compartment, Dawn. This car will run for another hundred thousand miles easily. You won't find a better used car anywhere, and it gets good gas mileage."

"It's beautiful, Papa." She kissed his cheek and embraced her grandmother. "I love it."

Mom headed for the house. Granny's expression soured. "Oh, for heaven's sake, Carolyn . . ." She stepped around Dawn and went after her.

Papa looked worried now. "Maybe we did get a little ahead of ourselves."

"Yeah," Mitch said solemnly. "You did. But it's too late now to take it back, isn't it?"

Dreading the argument she knew was brewing, Dawn went to the kitchen. Granny stood with her hands gripping the back of a kitchen chair, making her case, while Mom stood, back to her, at the sink peeling potatoes. "I'm sorry if I've done something wrong." Granny sounded exasperated, not sorry.

"Can I say something?" Dawn pleaded. The swelling fear of the last three weeks made her feel even more vulnerable when Granny and Mom were at odds. "I really, really want the car, Mom, but I won't even ask to drive it until after I have my license and you and Mitch are both satisfied that I'm a safe driver."

Mom turned slowly and studied her. "What about insurance and gas?"

"We'll pay for her insurance and give her an allowance, since it seems you won't."

Spots of pink bloomed in Mom's cheeks. "No, we won't, and you won't either." She blinked as she said it, as though surprising herself. Granny's lips parted.

Things were going from bad to worse, and Dawn knew she was in the middle of the battlefield. "I have some savings, Granny, and

I can get a part-time job after school at Java Joe's." At Granny's blank expression, she added, "It's a coffee shop near the square." She looked between them. "It'd be fun. It'd be good for me."

"We'll talk about it later, Dawn." Mom turned her back to both of them and resumed peeling potatoes.

Granny pulled the chair out and wilted into it. "I should've asked first. I'm sorry, Dawn, but maybe . . ."

Mom put her hands on the sink. "Dawn can keep the car." She sounded tired and defeated.

Dawn stood between the two women she loved most in the world and wanted to weep. Oma suddenly popped into her mind like a specter. "Wouldn't it be nice if we all had tea?" Oma had said the same thing every day when she and Mom visited her in Merced. Mom turned toward her. Face crumpling, she muttered a soft excuse and left the kitchen.

"She hasn't gotten over Oma yet." Dawn spoke into the silence.

Granny's shoulders drooped. "I don't think she ever will."

Mitch and Papa and Christopher carried the conversation through dinner. When Mom got up to clear the table, Mitch suggested they all go into the family room. Papa kept glancing at Granny, who sat silent and distracted. Mom called everyone into the kitchen. She had set out a sheet cake decorated with pink flowers and *Happy 16th Birthday, May Flower Dawn* written in white across the icing. "Chocolate!" Dawn forced a brightness into her voice that she didn't feel. "My favorite." She smiled at her mother and thanked her. She felt Mitch squeeze her shoulder.

Leaning down, he kissed her cheek the way Jason had the morning before Dawn changed everything between them. "You're growing up, Dawn."

Maybe more than he could even imagine.

She opened Christopher's gift first and raised her brows at him. "A soccer ball? Are you sure this is for me?"

"You played really, really well." He grinned impishly. "You can teach me."

"Thanks, sport." She ruffled his hair and gave him a hard hug.

Mom and Mitch gave her a pearl necklace and pearl stud earrings. "Pearls for innocence." Dawn felt Mitch's hand on her shoulder.

Her mother spoke from across the table. "They're also a rite of passage into womanhood."

Dawn couldn't raise her head for fear of what they might see in her face. She wasn't innocent anymore, and she didn't feel like a woman either. She touched the luminous pearls and swallowed the tears gathering and almost choking her. "They're beautiful. Thank you."

She lay in bed that night crying softly, silently confessing her sin and pleading with God that no baby had been made. Startled, she heard a tap on the door, and Mom came in. She sat on the end of Dawn's bed. "What's wrong, Dawn? Are you upset because Jason didn't remember your birthday?"

"I didn't tell him." She'd forgotten all about it. Her mind had been too filled with worries and fears to think about anything else.

"Do you want to talk about what's bothering you? You haven't been yourself for the last few weeks."

"I'm okay." *One lie.* "I just feel so stirred up all the time." *True.* "I don't know what's wrong with me." *Another lie.* They didn't come as easily after she'd just been begging God for mercy.

"I'm just worrying about the future." That was true, at least. She wanted to bury her head in the pillow again and sob, but she couldn't do that with her mother sitting so close. Dawn felt her mother's hand through the blanket.

"You won't turn eighteen for another two years. You have plenty of time to make decisions."

Dawn gave a hoarse laugh. "I know." She'd already made one. A bad one.

Her mother squeezed her foot. "You can talk to me, you know." She waited a moment. "About anything." She waited again. Minutes passed. She let out a soft sigh and got up. "Good night, May Flower Dawn." She stood at the open doorway. "If you can't talk to me, you know you can always go to Granny." She closed the door quietly behind her.

After two more days of feverish prayers of repentance and promises of chastity and obedience, God answered her prayers.

Jason met her at the bus stop the next morning. His mouth curved in an uncertain smile. "Everything okay?"

"Everything is perfect!"

For the first time, Jason kissed her there in front of everyone. He took her hand as they walked into school together, both forgetting the door they had opened and the untamed beast that now prowled loose.

❊ ❊ ❊

Mitch and Mom thought it would be a good idea if she got a part-time job. Java Joe's manager, Dennis Bingley, didn't even ask her to fill out an application, but hired her on the spot. "The boys will be lining up for coffee when they see you." She worked Monday through Friday afternoons from three to five. Jason drove her downtown, bought one coffee, and stationed himself at one of the small tables tucked in a back corner, where he did homework until four thirty. Boys did line up, but she didn't pay any attention. Whenever she cleared and cleaned a table, she'd stop by Jason's. Mitch picked Dawn up on his way home.

After six weeks, and hours of practice driving with Mitch, Dawn felt ready to face the DMV test. She passed with flying colors and drove the Sable home. Mom told her over dinner that night she could drive the car to school. Dawn said she'd take turns with Sharon driving to youth group, but she wanted to continue riding the bus to school. That way, she'd save money for the next insurance premium as well as gas.

"And Jason will still give you a ride to work." Mitch gave her a smirk that said she wasn't fooling anyone. She conceded that was part of her reasoning.

The first Saturday after she gained driving privileges, she drove to the Windsor Trailer Park. The double-wide looked old, but well-tended, with potted flowers on a small deck with green- and white-striped awning and a pebble driveway, where Jason's Honda was parked. Jason, dressed in sweatpants and a sleeveless T-shirt, opened the door before she even knocked. He came out barefoot and admired her car. An elderly lady opened her screen door just across the way. "A friend of yours, Jason?"

"Study partner," he called back. "How are you doing this morning, Mrs. Edwards?"

"Can't complain." She sat in a rocker on her little porch.

Jason opened the front door, and Dawn entered a carpeted living room with a worn green plaid couch, two matching chairs, and a coffee table facing a small television on an old cabinet. Beige drapes and sheers let a shaft of light through the front window.

"It must feel claustrophobic to you," Jason said grimly.

"It's cozy. Comfortable."

A small Early American table with two chairs was cluttered with books, an open binder, and papers. "You're studying."

"Every spare minute." He drew her into his arms. "I needed a break." He kissed her. One gentle, tentative kiss led to another and another.

Breathless, she began to worry. "Where's your mom?"

"Working. Until noon."

"Maybe I should go." When he didn't let go, she wondered if she had said the words aloud or just thought them. He asked if she wanted to see his room. Of course, she did. Things quickly got out of hand, not that either tried to stop, not until someone rapped on the door. Jason pulled away and got off the bed. "It's probably Mrs. Edwards." Another rap sounded, louder this time. "If I don't answer, she's going to think something's going on."

Think something is going on? Dawn wanted to laugh hysterically. "Wait!" She ducked into the bathroom and leaned against the door. Adjusting her clothing, she raked fingers through her hair. She could hear Mrs. Edwards.

"I don't think your mother would want a girl here when she's not."

Jason said they were just talking. "Then where is she? I don't see her sitting on the sofa."

Dawn flushed the toilet and ran the water noisily before stepping out of the bathroom. She pretended surprise. "Oh, hi." Mrs. Edwards muttered something to Jason and went down the steps. "What'd she say?"

He gave a brief laugh. "She told me I'd better behave myself."

Blushing, Dawn shrugged her purse onto her shoulder. Neither one of them had been doing a good job of that lately. "I'd better go."

Jason walked her to her car. He said he wished she wouldn't go. They stood and talked awhile. Mrs. Edwards sat in her rocker watching them. Jason asked if Dawn was planning to go on the mission trip to Mexico. She said she was and had already gotten the financial backing she needed from Mom and Mitch and her grandparents. "Plus I'm putting in some of my own money," she added, proud of herself. "What about you?" He said he wasn't sure yet, but he hoped so. Before Dawn got into her car, she waved at Mrs. Edwards and said it was nice meeting her.

The following Saturday, Dawn brought her backpack full of books, and they did study, for a little while. She left an hour before Georgia Steward was due home. The Saturday after that, they didn't even bother to open a book.

THE NEXT SATURDAY, Georgia Steward's white van with *Georgia's Housekeeping Services* painted in red on the side was parked behind Jason's white Honda. Disappointed, Dawn figured she and Jason would just have to study today. At least they'd be together. Grabbing her book bag, Dawn slid out of her Sable. Mrs. Edwards wasn't sitting on the porch this morning, but movement in the front curtains told Dawn the old lady was still watching. Annoyed, Dawn went up the steps and tapped at the door, expecting Jason to answer. His mother opened the door. "Hello, Dawn."

"Hi." Dawn plastered a smile on her face despite the cool look on Georgia's. "I'm here to study with Jason."

"Come in." Georgia opened the door all the way. The drapes had been pulled back, allowing sunlight to stream in. Jason's bedroom door was wide-open. She had seen his car in the drive-way. Where was he? "Have a seat." Georgia closed the front door.

Dawn felt her body tense. She put her book bag down and took a seat at the table. "Where's Jason?"

Georgia sat across from her and folded her hands. "He's gone for the day."

"Gone?" Dawn's heart pounded in alarm. Why hadn't he called her? She felt increasingly uncomfortable under his mother's scrutiny.

"He and Pastor Daniel took a little fishing trip. He didn't know he was going until early this morning."

Dawn felt the urge to take flight. "I should go then." She reached for her book bag.

"Not yet." Georgia's tone was firmer this time, colder.

Leaving the book bag on the floor, Dawn eased back into the seat, knees trembling beneath the table. "Is something wrong?"

Georgia's expression turned to one of disdain. "You could say that, couldn't you?" Her knuckles whitened. "I knew what was going on between the two of you when Jason came home from Jenner. He couldn't look me in the eye. I watched him sweat for a month and thought maybe the two of you had learned your lesson. And then Mrs. Edwards told me yesterday that you've been coming over every Saturday . . . to study."

"We do study."

Georgia reached into her pocket and put a crumpled, empty condom wrapper on the table between them.

Dawn felt all the blood draining from her face. She met Georgia's glare. "I love him. And he loves me."

Georgia's face flushed. Her brown eyes grew hotter. "You don't know anything about love! You're a spoiled, self-centered little girl who wants what she wants and wants it *now*." She leaned forward. "Your *love* has single-handedly ruined most of Jason's chances to escape this trailer park. His grades have dropped. He no longer has the qualifications to get into UC Berkeley—or get a full scholarship to Stanford. He spent most of his savings buying that car so he could take you out. He hardly reads his Bible anymore, and his relationship with God used to be *the most important thing in his life!*"

Dawn flinched as Georgia stood abruptly and stepped away from the table. After a moment, she continued in a taut, restrained tone. "If you get pregnant, Jason will do the right thing. But I'd like to give you a picture of what your lives will be like if that should happen." She sat again, more in control, eyes like black ice.

"Jason will have to give up all his dreams of college. He'll have to find a job to support you and your baby. And what sort of job will he find with only a high school diploma? Minimum wage. Of course, he won't make enough working nine to five to pay rent on a place as grand as this." Her eyes swept the room derisively. "So Jason, being Jason, will want to do better. He'll get a second job, which won't please you because you'll never see him. He'll be working all the time just to keep a roof over your head and food on the table for the three of you. And then there are the utilities and medical expenses. Of course, you'll be lonely. You'll carry the full responsibility of taking care of your baby: changing diapers, nursing, getting up at all hours of the night. You'll be exhausted. You'll feel overwhelmed. The baby will be your only company. After a while, you'll get bored sitting around the trailer. When Jason finally does make it home, you'll complain he's never around. He's no fun anymore. He doesn't make you happy."

Dawn started to cry.

"Tears don't work with me, honey."

"Why do you hate me so much?" Wrapping her arms around herself, Dawn fought for control.

"I don't hate you. I just don't like you. Why should I? *You're ruining my son's life!*" Georgia sounded distraught, close to tears. She released her breath slowly. "He's in love with you. Anyone can see that. He's so in love he can't think straight. He won't listen to a word of caution. You've stripped him of his dreams, taken his innocence, and now you're on the road to destroying his potential." She let out her breath in frustration.

Dawn couldn't raise her head.

"Look at me, Dawn." When she managed to raise her head, Georgia stared at her. "What I see in front of me is a very pretty sixteen-year-old girl with no character and no substance. You have nothing at all to offer Jason, and you're too willfully stupid and selfish to see or even care about the damage you're doing to him. That's not love. Not by any stretch of the imagination. You think you can live with your romantic daydreams. Fairy tales always end with 'happily ever after,' don't they? You don't know how wrong you are."

When Georgia didn't say anything more, Dawn spoke in a small voice. "Can I go now?"

"Please do. And don't you dare come into this house again, not unless *I* invite you."

Dawn got up quickly and headed for the door.

"One last thing." Georgia still sat at the table, face turned away. "You'll probably run straight to Jason and tell him everything I've said to you . . . or those parts that serve your purpose." She looked at Dawn then, eyes glistening with unshed tears. "But remember this: Someday, Jason will grow up. And when he does, he'll see the truth for himself."

❄ ❄ ❄

Dawn's first instinct was to go to Granny and sob out her woe, but she quickly dismissed that idea. Dawn knew she could do no wrong in Granny's eyes. Granny always took her side. If Granny knew she'd seduced Jason in the downstairs apartment, she'd be deeply hurt. She might start thinking Dawn was the kind of person who could live the wild life in Haight-Ashbury like her mother had.

What was Pastor Daniel saying to Jason right now? Was he hearing the same things Georgia Steward believed? *That girl isn't good enough for you. She has nothing at all to offer. She's selfish, spoiled, carnal, and probably not even a Christian. What are you thinking, Jason? Why would you want to be with her?*

She drove aimlessly for an hour, then went home. Her mother had an open house. Mitch and Christopher had gone bowling. Dawn went straight to her bedroom. Stripping off her clothes, she took a long, hot shower. She scrubbed and still felt unclean. Hunkered in the corner of the shower, she sobbed as the water pounded her. The air thickened with steam. She felt no better when she stepped out and dried off. Pulling on sweats, she got into bed. She lay there for the rest of the day, going over and over what Jason's mother had said.

"Dawn?" Mom tapped at the door. "Dinner's almost ready."

"I'm not hungry." When Mom opened the door, Dawn covered her head with a pillow.

"Are you sick?"

Lovesick. Heartsick. Sick with shame. "Just go away, Mom. Please." She half hoped her mother would press harder this time, but she left quietly, closing the door behind her.

❄ ❄ ❄

Hours later, the door opened again, a spear of light from the hallway intruding. Mom came in this time. She didn't turn on a light. She sat on the end of the bed, but didn't say a word.

After fifteen minutes, Dawn couldn't bear the silence. She whispered, "Would you hate me if I told you Jason and I have been having sex?"

"No." No questions, just a firm response, then silence again.

Dawn sat up slowly, bunching the pillow tight against her chest, thankful for the darkness. She wouldn't be able to see her mother's disappointment. "I went to see him this morning. He wasn't there. His mother talked to me."

When Mom still didn't ask anything, Dawn went on talking, slowly, painfully, until everything spilled out in a flood of tears. When Dawn finished, she pressed her face into the pillow already damp from an afternoon of weeping. She felt her mother's hand on her head.

"Words can be a sword to the heart, Dawn." Mom ran her fingers gently through Dawn's hair. "Sometimes there's truth in them. Sometimes there isn't. Go over what Jason's mother said to you. If there's any truth in it, you'll have to decide what to do with it. As to the rest, try to let it go." Her hand lifted.

Dawn curled into a fetal position. Her mother stood and pulled the covers up, tucking them in around her as though she were a little girl again. Leaning down, she kissed Dawn and whispered, "And try to forgive."

❄ ❄ ❄

Jason called Sunday night. He said his mom told him she'd come by. He apologized for not being there. "Pastor Daniel took me out to the coast. I didn't know he was coming until he showed up."

She said it was okay. She and his mother talked. He wanted to know what about. She said nothing much. Just small talk. *No character. No substance. Nothing to offer . . .*

"Dawn . . ." She knew by his tone what was coming. "I think maybe we should stop hanging out for a while."

She couldn't have prepared for the pain his words brought. She tried to press her lips together to keep from crying out. She hunched over, mouth open in agony. Shutting her eyes, she wanted to beg. She wanted to remind him they said they loved each other. Instead, she heard the echo of Georgia's voice. *Someday, Jason will grow up. And when he does, he'll see the truth . . .*

"Are you okay with that?" Jason sounded uncertain. Did he want her to say no? Did he want her to talk him out of it? And if she did, what then?

You'll ruin his life. . . .

Dawn had spent all of Saturday night and all of Sunday thinking about what Jason's mother had said, seeing the awful truth in it. Only one thing was false. She did love Jason.

She'd dreamed about Oma last night. She'd come like a vision, speaking words of wisdom. *"When you know what you want in life, May Flower Dawn, go after it. Sometimes it doesn't end up the way you planned. Trust God and it'll turn out better."*

Dawn knew what she wanted. She wanted to be Jason's wife. She wanted to have his children. She wanted to spend her life with him. And now she'd ruined it all. What had she brought into his life? Sin. Regret. Fear. Shame.

"Dawn? Are you there?"

Her breath caught softly, throat thick with pain and tears. "I think you're right."

She went into the kitchen and told Mom and Mitch she and Jason had broken up. She asked if she could transfer to the independent study program. She didn't have to explain why. Mom said she'd call the school Monday morning and do everything she could to make that happen.

❄ ❄ ❄

Dawn didn't return to youth group until Kim and Sharon told her Jason wouldn't be coming back because of his job. "About the only time I see Jason is at church on Sunday," Kim told her. "He comes with his mom. He doesn't come by the house and talk with Dad anymore."

A month after Jason broke up with her, Dawn came home from independent study and found a message on her answering machine. "I love you, Dawn." His voice roused all the pain and longing she had tried so hard to push down. He cleared his throat as though having trouble speaking. "I'll love you forever." *Click.* She sat on the bed and replayed it, letting herself wallow in regrets.

She didn't know what to do about the Mexico mission trip over spring break. She'd received pledges of financial backing from Mitch and her grandparents. She had a certified copy of her birth certificate. But if Jason was going, she knew she shouldn't. It would be too hard to be together. Sharon asked her why she hadn't said yes or no, and Dawn admitted her dilemma. Sharon called the next day. "I talked to Jason. He's not going to Mexico. He has to work. He said you ought to feel free to go now that you know he isn't."

Pastor Daniel might not share that opinion. She had no doubt Georgia Steward had talked with him about Dawn's relationship with Jason. He might not want someone like her to be part of his team. Dawn needed to know one way or the other, but it took days to gather the courage to call him.

Pastor Daniel seemed surprised by her question. "Of course, I want you on our team."

Maybe he didn't know everything. Maybe Georgia Steward hadn't wanted to share that information. "I didn't want to take anything for granted, Pastor Daniel."

"God loves a broken and contrite spirit, Dawn." His quiet words dispelled any illusions about whether Jason's mother had spoken to him. They also reassured her that Pastor Daniel wasn't going to throw stones.

❄ ❄ ❄

After all the talk of how a mission trip could change a person's outlook on life, Dawn didn't know what to expect. Hearing about poverty or seeing it on television ads wasn't the same as being in the middle of it, smelling it, tasting it in the air. They drove down streets with houses tucked tight together, garbage dumped and rotting in the streets. Some people lived in shelters that couldn't even be called shanties. What surprised Dawn most was the people: They smiled and shouted greetings as the Amor ministry team arrived. Children ran alongside the van, waving and calling out in Spanish.

After a night's sleep, she and the others rose early and went to work building a twelve-by-fourteen-foot house for the Guttierez family. Dawn's hands blistered, her back ached, and she smelled of sweat like any common laborer. When Pastor Daniel told her to take a break, she sat in the shade and watched some children kicking an old soccer ball back and forth. She wasn't a great hod carrier or carpenter, but she knew how to play soccer. Dawn joined the children and showed off a few tricks she'd learned while playing for the Sky Hawks. Soon, children swarmed around her whenever she wasn't working on the house.

On the last night, house complete, Senor and Senora Guttierez insisted on hosting dinner for the entire team. Leftover boards propped up on sawhorses acted as a dining table. Senora Guttierez and her teenage daughter, Maria, made a big pot of beans and chicken enchiladas with cheese. Senor Guttierez stood at the head of the table, tears running down his rugged cheeks, as he told them in broken English what it meant to him to have a house for his family. Senora Guttierez added her shy thanks, as did their five children.

Dawn went outside, sat hunched against the wall, and wept. Pastor Daniel came out and sat beside her. "What's on your mind?"

"My bedroom is bigger than their entire house." She covered her face. Had she ever once said thank you for the blessings she had received? Not that she could remember. And the Guttierez family hadn't stopped thanking all of them since the day the team arrived.

"From those to whom much is given, much is required."

And there it was again, that piercing stab of conscience. "I think they spent everything they have to put on this dinner." What had she ever given to anyone?

"Probably, and they're proud and pleased to do it. They count the ability to give as a blessing, too." He got up and smiled at her. "Come back inside when you're ready."

Dawn sat for a while longer. These people worked hard and barely managed to get by. They wanted the opportunity for a better life for their children. Georgia Steward popped into her mind. *"Your* love *has single-handedly ruined most of Jason's chances to escape this trailer park."* Dawn leaned her head against the wall she'd helped build. Was that true? Not entirely, but enough so that it stung. Jason still had opportunities. So did she.

Before leaving the next morning, the CCC crew left the remaining food supplies, bottled water, building materials, and some tools. As soon as they crossed the border and started the long drive north to Anaheim, where they would stop and spend a day at Disneyland as reward for their labors, everyone fell asleep except Pastor Daniel, Mr. Jackson in the passenger seat, and Dawn in the back. While they talked, she sat in the back row, staring out the window and praying.

Who am I, God? Who do You want me to be? Oma said the plans

You have are better for us than the ones we make for ourselves. My plans led me into sin and pain and regret and fear. God, I want to become a woman of character and faith. I don't want to be a selfish, spoiled little girl with nothing to offer. Change me, Lord. Please change me.

Weary, head aching, Dawn leaned her head back against the seat. Pastor Daniel looked at her in the rearview mirror. His eyes crinkled the way they did when he smiled.

❄ ❄ ❄

Back in Windsor, everyone piled out of the church van and started unloading. Some met up with waiting parents. Dawn had left the Sable in the church parking lot. Running a finger over the dusty trunk, she imagined what Papa would say and decided to go through a car wash on the way home. She stowed her duffel bag. Closing the trunk, she found Pastor Daniel standing by the car. "Thanks for going with us, Dawn."

"My pleasure."

"You worked harder than anyone on the team." He gave her a teasing smile. "I didn't know you had it in you."

She gave him a sad smile. "Neither did I."

Maybe it was a start.

When she pulled into the last space in Mitch's four-car garage, Christopher bounded out to greet her. Mitch took her duffel bag. He said Mom was manning an open house. "You look worn-out, Pita."

"I'm exhausted." Dawn hugged him around the waist. "Thank you for my big, beautiful bedroom and the beautiful home and yard and pool and good food on the table and for loving me even when I'm a pain in the—"

"Wow!" Mitch laughed. "What happened to you?" He put his arm around her shoulders and steered her toward the door into the house. "It's been my pleasure, Dawn. You look dead on your feet. They must've worked you hard in old Mexico. Why don't you take a nap?" She thanked him and headed down the hall to her room. Mitch called after her, "Forgot to mention it, but you'll never guess who stopped by my office for a visit."

"Who?"

"Jason. He stayed more than an hour."

Just the mention of his name was enough to make Dawn's heart race. "Did he ask about me?"

"Briefly. He had some questions. He has to make decisions about his future. He's weighing all his options. He said to say hi."

✳ ✳ ✳

Independent study helped keep Dawn's mind occupied. She didn't have to worry about facing Jason. She didn't have friends or class disturbances to distract her. She could fix her mind on the work ahead. Rather than coast by, Dawn dove into her studies. She only had to go to Healdsburg High once a week to check in with the independent studies supervisor, turn in work assignments, and take exams.

All Sharon, Amy, and Pam talked about at youth group was the upcoming prom. Kim and Tom were going together. Steven Dial had asked Pam. Sharon held out hope hunk-of-the-month football fullback Tomás Perez would ask her. Amy worried that if anyone did ask, she wouldn't be able to afford a dress. Dawn wondered if Jason was going and with whom, but didn't ask.

Prom came and went, and conversations at youth group turned to finals and graduation, summer jobs and college plans. Half the members were finishing high school. Sharon and Kim were graduating and going to college. Amy's father had been offered a better job in Dallas. With so many of her friends leaving, Dawn wondered if she'd even attend the CCC youth group next year. She felt out of it, on the edge again, not really part of anything anymore. She didn't know what was happening on the Healdsburg High campus, nor did she care. What did all that matter, especially now that Jason was going away to college? "Somewhere in

Southern California," Sharon told her. "I just can't remember which college. And he's working construction over the summer. Down in San Jose, I think, with a friend of a friend of Pastor Daniel."

Dawn had the feeling Jason Steward had walked out of her life. Whatever plans God might have for her now clearly did not include him.

She didn't think her grief could go any deeper until Granny called on a hot August morning and said Papa was dead.

39

THE APPALLING CALL about Papa's death sent Mom into panic mode. They needed to get out to Jenner *now*. Dawn insisted on going with them. Mitch called the Eckhards and asked if they would keep Christopher. They dropped him off on the way out. Dawn sat in the backseat in a state of shock. When they arrived, they found Granny sitting in the corner chair in the living room. Face white, eyes red, she pointed to the closed French doors to the bedroom. Mom stepped back and bumped into Mitch. He grasped her shoulders and whispered something.

Trembling, Dawn went into the bedroom first. She refused to believe Papa was dead. He apeared to be asleep. She went closer and laid her hand on his forehead. He felt so cold. He wasn't breathing. She drew in a sharp breath as though to do it for him. She felt warmth behind her. Mitch, standing ready. "He looks peaceful, doesn't he, honey? He's with the Lord." Sobbing, she turned and fell into his arms.

Granny spoke in the living room. "He said he was tired. He gave me a kiss good night. He was snoring when I went to bed.

And then when I woke up this morning, it was so quiet." She cried. "It was too quiet. I knew."

Mitch ushered Dawn back into the living room. Mom's face twitched. Her fingers pleated her tiered skirt. Face ashen, wide-eyed, she turned toward the bedroom, but didn't move. Dawn sat next to her on the couch. They didn't look at one another. They didn't touch. Mitch seemed the only one in the room capable of thought. "Have you called anyone, Hildie?"

"I called you." Granny blew her nose.

Mitch went down on one knee beside her and put his hand over hers. "I mean about his body."

She jerked. "No. I'm not ready to send him away yet."

"You'll be able to say good-bye at his memorial. . . ."

"There's not going to be a memorial service!" Granny sounded broken, but adamant. Her hand fluttered like a wounded bird. "We don't know anyone up here." It had been too far to drive in from Jenner to church on Sundays. She and Papa only made it to Easter cantatas— and one Christmas pageant when Christopher had played a little shepherd boy.

Mom shook, hands clenching her skirt. "You can have the service in Paxtown, Mom." She spoke in a dull voice. "Mitch can call Rev. Elias." Her face was shuttered. "Dad was one of his elders. He would want to officiate."

Granny dabbed her eyes. "Rev. Elias retired five years ago. He and Janice moved up to Silverton, Oregon. I think. I don't remember. We haven't even exchanged Christmas cards with them in the last few years."

"You have friends in Paxtown. The MacPhersons, Dr. Griffith, Doc and Thelma Martin." Mom's voice came out flat as she listed names.

Granny glared at her. "As if any of them remember us."

Mom raised her head, clearly distressed. "Is that my fault?" She sounded as though she thought it might be.

"No! Did I say it was? Did I? Thelma Martin was never my friend."

"Hildie." Mitch spoke gently.

Granny cried again. "We *had* friends, Carolyn. We've been gone eight years. Life goes on. People move away. People *die*." She started to sob.

Mom stared at Mitch with huge eyes. She was like a frightened little girl, frozen in her seat, afraid to move. Dawn couldn't bear seeing her like that or Granny crying her heart out. Someone had to do something! She fled into the kitchen, pulled out the telephone directory, and flipped frantically through pages. Scrubbing away tears, she read the number for Cornerstone Covenant Church and punched it into Granny's ancient phone.

Kim answered. She must be standing in for the church secretary again. Dawn started talking and knew she was making no sense. She started to cry. Pastor Daniel came on the line. "What's wrong, Dawn?" Fighting down the tears and rising hysteria, she told him her grandfather had died and his body was still in his bed and Granny didn't want a service and Mitch was going to call the mortuary and have his body taken away and she couldn't bear the thought of that being the end of him and—

"I'm on my way," Pastor Daniel interrupted her.

Mitch called the mortuary as soon as she hung up the telephone. Dawn went outside and paced on the deck, watching the road. When she saw Pastor Daniel's blue Chevy coming, she stood outside the gate. He got out of the car and held her close. "Did he know Christ, Dawn?" She nodded against his shirt, soaking it with her tears. "Then you know where he is right now."

"It doesn't help."

"It will."

She led him into the house and introduced him to Granny. He sat on her hassock and talked to her. Mom went outside and stood on the deck. Mitch went out and wrapped his arms around her, holding her tight against him. Dawn sat on the couch, hands pressed between her knees, not knowing what to do. *Jesus. Jesus.* That's all she could think to pray. Just His name over and over again.

"Why don't you get your mother and stepfather, Dawn?" When they came inside, Pastor Daniel led them all into the bedroom, where they gathered around Papa. Pastor Daniel held Granny's hand and talked about Jesus' life and death and resurrection and the promise He made, a promise that would never be broken. Mom kept looking at him. Granny grew calmer as he spoke.

Pastor Daniel stayed until after Papa's body had been taken away. He had been the one to remember to ask for Papa's wedding ring. He said he'd come and talk with Granny again if she liked. Would she be staying with the Hastings?

Granny shook her head.

Mitch leaned forward on the couch, one hand still holding Mom's, the other resting on the arm of the sofa closest to Granny. "Why don't you come home with us, Hildie?"

"No." Granny gripped the arms of her corner chair, letting everyone know she wouldn't be pried from her home. "I'm staying right here."

"You shouldn't be alone, Hildie."

Granny glared at Mitch, a stubborn tilt to her chin. "It's my home. I'm going to have to get used to being alone, aren't I?"

Dawn could tell Mitch was exasperated and torn. She knew he would take good care of Mom, who seemed as undone as she had been when Oma died. But Granny shouldn't be alone. When Pastor Daniel stood, Dawn took his place on the hassock. "I'll stay."

❄ ❄ ❄

Dennis Bingley gave her time off. Over the next week, Dawn cried almost as much as Granny. Instead of sleeping in the blue room, she slept with Granny. Once, while Granny slept in the easy chair, Dawn went downstairs and sat on the bed where she had given herself to Jason. She then cried for other reasons. If she'd followed Jesus instead of her own desires, she wouldn't be spending the rest of her life living in regret.

On the sixth morning, she awakened when Granny brushed

hair back from her face. Granny smiled faintly, head on her own pillow. "You're a very sweet girl. Do you know that?"

"Are you going to be all right, Granny?"

"Yes. I'll have to be because you have to go home today."

Dawn took her hand and held it against the mattress. "I'll call you every night and come out next weekend."

"I know you will." Granny's hazel eyes filled with tears. "All this is just part of life. Still it feels unexpected. You'll have to call home for a ride. Maybe your mother will come out and pick you up." She sounded hopeful.

Mitch came for Dawn. On the way home, he asked how things went. She told him Granny was going to have a hard time, but was too stubborn to talk about moving into town. "How's Mom doing?"

"She's bottled up inside again. It's going to take time. One good thing came out of all this."

How could anything good come from losing Papa? "What's that?"

"She asked me to take her to your church this morning."

❄ ❄ ❄

1988

Senior year proved grueling as Dawn combined afternoon college courses with her remaining high school requirements. The previous year she had taken one class at Santa Rosa Junior College, and she enjoyed it so much she decided to take two this year. She didn't have a spare minute for R & R, as Mitch put it, not between commuting to Santa Rosa, attending classes, studying, writing papers, and working twenty hours a week at Java Joe's. When she did get a weekend off, she often drove out to Jenner and stayed with Granny until Sunday morning, when she'd drive back to attend CCC with Mom, Mitch, and Christopher.

With dismay, but no protest, Mitch had given up his old church. Dawn knew he was glad Mom had finally found a church where she felt comfortable. Christopher couldn't have been happier now that he could spend even more time with his friend Tim Eckhard. People had welcomed the family with open arms, even Georgia Steward, who came and shook Mitch's hand and gave Mom a quick hug. She greeted Dawn with cool courtesy.

Kim always made a point of telling Dawn when Jason planned to come home. Dawn didn't attend services on those Sundays. It wasn't until Thanksgiving and Dawn's suggestion that she and Granny go back to Jenner Saturday afternoon that Mom spoke up about it.

"You can't avoid Jason forever, Dawn."

When Christmas came around, Mom, Mitch, and Granny ganged up on her and insisted she attend church with the family. She said she would if she could drive her own car.

Jason sat in the third row with his mother. Dawn and her family sat in the middle on the same side. She tried to concentrate on what Pastor Daniel said, but her eyes kept drifting to Jason. He'd cut his hair, had grown a little taller, broader. As soon as the service ended, Dawn stood and made her way toward the exit. Kim stopped her, a perplexed expression on her face when Dawn made a quick excuse, gave her a quick hug, and headed for the door, where Pastor Daniel stood shaking hands.

"Great sermon, Pastor Daniel." When he offered his hand, she took it. He gripped her hand firmly and asked why she seemed in such a hurry to get out the door. She didn't dissemble. "You know why. Jason's here." He gave her a sad smile and let go.

She didn't stop until she was safely inside her car, key in the ignition. Jason stood at the door with his mother. When he looked toward her, she started her car, backed out, and put it quickly into gear. She glanced in her rearview mirror one last time before she pulled out onto the street and headed home. Jason stood with all their old friends, home from college.

Her telephone was ringing when she walked into the house. She put her purse on her desk and sat on the bed as her answering machine picked up with her recorded message. "This is Dawn.

Sorry I missed your call. Please leave a message at the sound of the beep." No one spoke. Her heart pounded harder the longer the silence stretched. The answering machine clicked. She breathed again. The phone rang again. The machine picked up. Again, the long silence.

You have nothing to offer Jason.

She hadn't forgotten what Georgia Steward said or the truth of most of it. She *didn't* have anything to offer Jason.

The phone rang again. Sobbing, she put her hands over her ears.

A few days later, Dawn drove Granny home to Jenner by the Sea. "That young man you used to date, Jason what's-his-name . . . ?"

"Steward."

"He was at church on Christmas."

Dawn focused on the road.

Granny studied her. "When you got up and headed out, he never took his eyes off you. I think he was trying to catch up with you, but people kept getting in the way."

"He has a lot of friends." Her voice came out with a soft catch in it. She adjusted her sunglasses.

"So do you, Dawn." Granny spoke quietly and didn't ask about Jason again.

❋ ❋ ❋

1989

Mom and Mitch gave her the gift of another mission trip to Mexico. Since she had the equivalent of four years of Spanish classes under her belt, Pastor Daniel lined her up with another church that planned to put on a vacation Bible school in Tijuana. He also thought the preparatory meetings held on Thursday evenings rather than five in the morning on Wednesdays would be an added benefit to her. "Your parents said you're burning your candle at both ends."

The work in Mexico felt like a vacation after her grueling school and work schedule at home. And though she loved the children, she knew by the end of Easter week she was not meant to be a teacher. When she shared that conviction, Granny talked about her nursing days.

❄ ❄ ❄

Fall enrollment at Santa Rosa Junior College rolled around, and Dawn signed up for human anatomy. By midterm, she decided to work toward a bachelor of science degree in nursing. Mom didn't seem surprised by the idea, saying Granny would be pleased to know Dawn intended to follow in her footsteps. Mitch said Dawn could always do real estate later if nursing didn't pan out, to which Dawn replied she hoped to finish at the junior college and transfer to a four-year college by the end of the following year. Mom seemed a little taken aback by that announcement. "You'll be going off to college."

Mitch leaned down and kissed her. "You'll still have Christopher around. And me." He straightened. "With your grades, Dawn, you can go anywhere you want. Why not consider UC Berkeley? It's not too far from home."

UCB was a great school, but Dawn knew the competition would devour her. She'd considered UC Santa Cruz, but it had the reputation as a party school. UC Davis was too close, UC San Diego too far away. Her counselor had graduated from Cal Poly, and she spoke highly of it. Dawn researched a dozen colleges, all good, some too expensive. Something had nudged her toward Cal Poly. Maybe it was the location—half a day from home, close to the coast. When people asked why there, her inclination was to ask, "Why not?" She couldn't really explain.

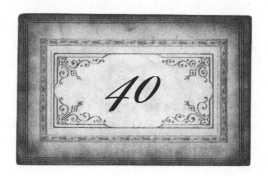

40

1990

All Dawn's old friends came home from college that summer, except Sharon, who had found a job in Santa Rosa and moved into an apartment near the Coddingtown Mall. Dawn caught up with their news after Sunday services. Most had lined up summer jobs at the downtown mall or various businesses in Healdsburg or Windsor. Kim called a few days after coming home from Pepperdine. "We're going to get together every Wednesday evening. It'll be better than old times."

"Who all is coming?"

"Everyone but Jason. He's off doing some kind of training this summer."

"I'll come when I can." Rather than drive back and forth twice a day to Healdsburg, she had quit the job at Java Joe's and worked at a coffee shop near the junior college, saving time and gas money.

All the old gang turned up at the Archer house the next Wednesday evening, eager to hang out with old friends. Kim and

Tom had become engaged. Amy King had lost twenty-five pounds and added blonde streaks to her brown hair. Steven Dial had shot up six inches and now towered over Dawn.

Kim's mom stood in the front doorway and announced she was going to have a ladies' night out with friends from church. "Coffee's ready, and there's hot water for any who prefer tea. Lots of cookies. Popcorn for those of you who are worried about your weight, which seems to be just about everyone these days." She waggled her fingers at Kim. "You're in charge. If it turns into a wild party, it'll be your head on the block, not mine. Good night, children." She closed the door behind her.

Everyone lounged around the living room talking about old times. Two hours passed before they got around to talking about what Bible book to study over summer. Tom Barrett suggested Song of Solomon and earned a round of guffaws and teasing remarks, while Kim reminded him, in hushed tones, they would be going through premarital counseling and could discuss *all that* some other time.

"Oh, yeah." Tom groaned loudly. "Like I'm going to feel so at ease talking about sex with your father."

Kim blushed crimson. "I hadn't thought about that."

The unattached of the bunch voted Song of Solomon down and suggested Proverbs. "It's practical." Pam grinned. "And God knows, we need practical advice on how to live the Christian life in the midst of a pagan culture."

"As long as we skip chapter 31." Kim smirked at Tom, and she added in an aside to Dawn and Pam, "Last thing I need right now is hearing what *I* have to do to be the perfect wife."

Grinning, Tom slung an arm around her shoulders and hugged her close. "Come on now, babe. Aren't you the one who's been telling me all Scripture is inspired by God and profitable for teaching, for reproof, for correction, for training . . ." He let out a yelp. "She pinched me!"

While the others laughed, Steven paged through his Bible. "We don't have time to finish all this."

Amy reached into a bowl of popcorn. "How about Philippians? Only four chapters and lots of encouraging words." They put it to a quick vote and settled it.

Lying in bed that night, Dawn thought about all the steps she had taken over the past three years to grow closer to the Lord. Even though she knew she didn't have a future with Jason, she still harbored a dream of being a wife and mother, God willing. She hadn't considered God would have a definition for the perfect wife. Pushing the covers aside, she turned on the desk light and opened her Bible. She felt depressed after reading Proverbs 31. How could any woman be all those things? Of course, it had taken the woman time. Her children were old enough to call their mother blessed, and her husband had gained enough standing in the community to be respected as a leader, and she managed servants.

Dawn covered her face. *Lord, I've worked so hard to become better, to become someone who could be a proper helpmate to a godly man. I know I was all wrong in the way I pursued Jason. Is it too much to hope that even so, You might have a husband and children in store for me someday?*

I love you. The answer came from the depths of her. Nothing was ever wasted, not even the damage she had done. Hadn't shame and guilt sent her down a new path?

I'll never be perfect, Lord. I'll never be good enough for someone like Jason.

My grace is sufficient for you, for power is perfected in weakness. Bible?

Slipping the leather journal Oma had given her from the top drawer, Dawn wrote: *How to Be a Good Wife.* But as she wrote, she searched for traits that would please God rather than a man.

❄ ❄ ❄

Pam called and asked Dawn if she'd like to get together. "We could do a little shopping and then go to Bakers Square for pie." Dawn knew something was up. Pam hated to shop. She suggested possible days and times, and they set a date to meet at the entrance of Ross Dress for Less.

Spotting her friend coming across the parking lot, Dawn laughed. Pam looked like she had an appointment for a root canal rather than an afternoon of shopping. "What are we looking for, Pam?"

"I don't know. You're the one who always loved to shop." Pam shrugged and stood outside the store. "I need your help. You always look like a fashion model, so put-together. I sort of agreed to a date with Steven."

"What sort of date?" Dawn knew they'd gone to their high school prom together as friends, but she hadn't noticed anything more between them.

"Dinner."

"Sounds serious."

"Oh, shut up. I wish I'd never . . ."

Dawn took her by the arm and pulled her through the front doors. "Did he say where you're going?"

"How would I know? I mean, he could've meant he was taking me to Taco Bell. Something casual, I guess." She looked around, her expression one of panic.

"You could've asked him where he plans to take you."

"I did! All he'd say is it would take us an hour to get there."

"Well, then it's not Taco Bell. Someplace nice, probably. No jeans. No T-shirt."

Pam rolled her eyes. "Just shoot me now."

Dawn laughed. "Relax. This is going to be fun!" She started pulling things off racks. "Start with these. The dressing room is back there." She pointed. "I'm going to keep looking. I'll be there before you have the first outfit on."

Holding half a dozen garments on hangers, Pam looked baffled. "What outfit?"

"This skirt, this top. Now go!"

After a few changes, Pam grumbled. One hand behind her head and the other on her hip, she struck a pose. "How about this one?"

"Not bad, but not all that great either. Take it off. Try these." She hung more garment possibilities on the hook and took the discards. After an hour, Pam had had enough of being a model and pleaded for an end to the torture. Dawn pointed. "The black skirt and tunic with the red belt. It looks great on you. What about shoes?"

"Shoes?" Pam sounded horrified.

Ignoring further protest, Dawn thrust the favored garments into her friend's arms, grabbed the others, and handed them over to the attendant on the way out of the dressing rooms. Dawn ushered Pam to the racks of shoes. She pointed out several pairs that would look nice. Pam found reasons not to try them on—too high, too red, too fancy, "You have got to be kidding me. No way!" When Pam picked up a pair of purple sneakers, Dawn grabbed them and shoved them back on the shelf. Pam reached for them again, and Dawn slapped her hand. They both laughed like little girls and finally settled on a pair of black slip-ons with two-inch heels.

"Boring, but serviceable." Dawn shook her head in dismay. "Do you have new nylons?"

Pam seemed to shrink. "I'll get them on the way home. I promise!"

They went to Bakers Square and sat in a booth by the front windows. Pam ordered apple pie à la mode, Dawn, caramel pecan silk supreme. They lingered and talked about college. Pam attended Arizona State and had declared a physical education major.

"How many applications have you sent out?"

Dawn debated whether to say anything. "One."

"One? You know what they say about putting all your eggs in one basket. Which college?"

"Cal Poly."

"Why there? I thought it was an engineering college."

"High rep for technology and sciences. I'll be in the nursing program."

"Is that where Jason went?"

"Jason?" Dawn's heart turned over.

"Jason Steward." Pam gave her a wry smile. "Don't pretend you've forgotten him."

"No, but I thought he went to UCLA."

"He applied, but didn't qualify for a scholarship."

"Oh." Pinched by guilt, Dawn winced.

Pam frowned. "I can't remember where he went. He doesn't come home very often." She shrugged. "San Diego, maybe." She moved on to other subjects.

Jason Steward. Dawn's mind drifted into a vortex of bittersweet memories. Sending up a quick prayer, she asked God's blessing on him and let him go.

❄ ❄ ❄

Mom and Mitch sat Dawn down and told her they intended to pay for her last two years of college. The first two years hadn't cost them anything, and they'd set aside money that would enable her to concentrate on school instead of having to work a part-time job. When she argued, Mitch turned adamant. "You've done nothing but study and work the last three years, Dawn. You have no life."

"I go to church. I go to the college group."

"Two hours a week."

"Everyone works. You work; Mom works."

"You're nineteen. You should have a little time to enjoy life."

Mitch handed her a checkbook and told her how much would be deposited each month—enough for tuition, books, and a studio apartment. He also handed over a credit card and gave her a limit, plenty for living expenses like food and gas. She'd even have enough to pay for car insurance.

Stunned, Dawn felt the tears coming. "You don't have to do this, Mitch."

Mitch's mouth tipped. "I'm not, Pita. It's all your mother's doing."

Mom shook her head. "Don't, Mitch."

He ignored her. "She's been banking her commissions since we married just so she could give you this gift. If you say no, I swear I'll turn you over my knee."

"Mom . . . I . . ."

Mom shrugged. "I didn't get to give you a car."

Dawn's smile trembled. "This is a whole lot more than a car."

"It hurts to see you work so hard to . . ." Mom stood abruptly and went to the kitchen counter, where she picked up some papers. "You'll need to find a place soon. I have a list of apartment complexes that offer furnished studios." She put them on the table. "The ones closest to campus are highlighted. You'll have to stay in a hotel while you're looking. I have a list of those as well." She stood, hands gripping the back of a chair. "You're going to be on your own." Her eyes filled.

"She'll be coming home for vacations." Mitch put his arm around Dawn's shoulders. "Won't you?"

It sounded more a command than a question. "Yes." She looked at her mother. "And you'll come down, too, I hope."

Dawn drove to San Luis Obispo the beginning of August. She listened to the radio on the drive, music interspersed with news reports of the Iraqi invasion of Kuwait, and the first U.S. troops being deployed to Saudi Arabia. Mitch had told her many high-ranking U.S. military officers were veterans of Vietnam. This war would be swift and decisive. Dawn thought of the uncle she had never met who died in Vietnam, and she turned off the radio.

The skies were clear that afternoon and cloudy the next morning when she arose. She left her things at Motel 6 and headed out to find a furnished studio apartment close to campus for a price she was willing to pay. She didn't want to blow through her mother's gift like found money, but use it wisely.

After three days, she signed a rental agreement with Bishop Peak Apartments. Her studio had a kitchenette with a small table and two chairs. The living room and bedroom were divided by an accordion partition. On one side was a sofa, one chair, a coffee table, and a hanging lamp, and on the other a full-size bed with two simple side tables and two cheap lamps. After her designer-decorated bedroom in Alexander Valley, it seemed drab, but she reminded herself of Mexico and felt thankful.

As soon as the phone service had been turned on, she called Mom with the new number. Then she called Granny and talked about the trip down, the hunt for an apartment, what she had seen of the town. "I'm going to try one of the churches tomorrow."

"You sound lonely, honey."

"A little, I guess. I'll get used to being on my own."

Over the next few days, Dawn took long walks around campus, familiarizing herself with its main buildings, the library, the dining complex. Hills dotted with oaks rose around campus with Bishop Peak in the distance. Sitting on a bench, Dawn watched others pass by. Was she really hearing God's voice about Cal Poly? Or had she come three hundred miles from home on some sort of delusion?

Once Dawn knew her way around the campus, she took drives to the Pacific beaches, coastal dunes, ridges, forests, and nearby lakes. She spent an afternoon at the mission, wandering through the garden with its fountain and statue of Father Junípero Serra and sitting in the chapel praying God would lead her in the days ahead.

She met with Mrs. Townsend, a college counselor, who helped her plan out schedules to earn her degree as quickly as possible. Mrs. Townsend looked dubious. "If you find what we've laid out too ambitious, you can drop a course."

Classes started, and the first weeks felt like a grueling marathon of lectures, reading, studying. A throng of students moved from building to building. Dawn felt overwhelmed by the numbers. SRJC had nearly as many students, but somehow it had felt smaller to her, less intense.

She hated studying in her drab apartment and started going to the Robert Kennedy Library instead. She preferred the smell of books, the soft sound of footsteps and hushed voices, to the silence in her studio or someone partying nearby. She felt more at home in the stacks than in her flat.

Around lunchtime one day in the library, her stomach growled, reminding her she hadn't eaten since breakfast. Glancing at her wristwatch, she saw she had less than an hour before chemistry class. She didn't have time to run to the dining complex and stand in line for a full meal. The eggs and toast she'd eaten for breakfast wouldn't carry her through the whole day.

Gathering her notes, textbook, and purse, she headed for the library café. Better a cup of coffee and pastry than nothing.

She'd just finished a blueberry scone and half her coffee when Jason Steward walked in. Dawn's heart dropped into the pit of her stomach.

She stared, trying to calm the tumble of emotions. Jason was even more handsome than she remembered. Short hair suited him. He looked tan and fit, taller and broader through the shoulders. He was with two other young men and a pretty girl with shoulder-length dark hair and a bright, sunny smile. Was she his girlfriend? A sharp stab of pain went through her heart. She thought she'd gotten over him.

As the four made their selections, paid, got their coffee, and sat across the room, Dawn drank in the sight of him. He talked easily, laughing at something one of the boys said. He pulled out the chair for the girl. He sat with his back to Dawn, but one of his friends noticed her and smiled. She'd seen that same smile on a dozen other male faces in the last few weeks. It usually predicated an attempt to start a conversation or ask her out. Dawn averted her eyes so he wouldn't be encouraged.

A few seconds later, she glanced over again and found Jason half turned in his chair, staring at her. Surprise didn't begin to describe the expression on his face. A flood of feelings swept over Dawn. Her smile felt stiff, her insides like Jell-O. When Jason scraped his chair back, she went hot and cold all over. He said something to the others and rose. The girl looked past him to Dawn.

Breathing in slowly, trying to slow her rapid-fire heartbeat, Dawn watched Jason cross the room. She offered a tremulous smile. He didn't seem happy to see her. He stood at her table, hands gripping the back of the chair. "What are you doing here?"

Why did he sound angry? He'd been the one to initiate their breakup. "I'm having coffee."

"I don't mean that. I mean here, on campus."

"I'm a student."

"A student?" He frowned.

"I'm in the nursing program."

Emotion flickered, and then his mouth flattened. "You could've gone anywhere." His hazel eyes cooled.

His last telephone message came back to her so clearly. She remembered pressing the button and hearing his voice. *"I love you, Dawn. I'll love you forever."* Pain lanced through her. She'd listened to that message over and over, for days, weeks, before she finally surrendered to God and erased it. *Jesus, where is Your purpose in this?* If she'd known Jason was attending Cal Poly, she never would have applied. She didn't know what to say to him now, so she resorted to the mundane. "It's good to see you again, Jason." She spoke as though they had been mere acquaintances, not lovers.

"Really." He sounded doubtful.

She blinked, wishing her heart would slow down. "How are you?"

"Fine." He mocked her. "I'm doing great." He nodded toward his friends at the other table, the girl watching their exchange. He didn't ask Dawn if she wanted to be introduced. The dark-haired girl gave her a curious smile. Jason moved enough to block her from view. Dawn could feel his animosity.

"It took me a long time to get over you, Dawn. I don't even know why I'm talking to you."

What could she say to that? She'd never gotten over him, never would. She hadn't realized that fully until now. *Oh, Lord, why?* Lowering her eyes, she put her hands around the cooling cup of coffee. She didn't know what to say.

"You're wearing the bracelet I gave you."

She glanced at the gold chain with the delicate heart and glistening pearl. "I've never taken it off."

He looked as though she'd punched him in the stomach. "I don't get it."

"Get what?"

"I called, Dawn. You never called back. I left you a message. I never heard a word from you. Not one. You want to explain?"

"You know why, Jason."

"Yeah, right." He sneered. "Why don't you enlighten me?"

She hadn't planned on a public confession, but she didn't feel like being a silent martyr. "We went too far, Jason. It was always going to be all or nothing with us. And it was all sin three years ago." Her eyes burned. "I . . ." She had to swallow before she could confess more. "I wanted to get right with God."

Jason studied her face and then turned his back and walked away. Suffocating with pain, Dawn watched him sit with his friends. Was he telling them who she was, what they had once been to each other, what he thought of her now? The dark-haired girl leaned back and looked at her again. One of the guys looked, too, scraped his chair back, and got up until Jason said something that made him sit down again.

Why was she still sitting here, torturing herself with regret and shame? She couldn't change the past. She couldn't undo what she had done. She had no control over what Jason thought about her now.

Gathering her things, Dawn threw away the cup and crumpled napkin and left the café. Her throat burned with tears as she hurried down the steps and along the walkway away from the library.

Oh, God, I must've misunderstood. Why did I come here? This is the last place I should be. Oh, Lord, the look on his face . . . I thought I was over him. She brushed tears away and kept walking. *You are my first love, Jesus, my forever love. But it hurts, Lord. I wish You had arms to hold me.*

She headed for her chemistry class.

DAWN CONTINUED STUDYING in the library every afternoon, but didn't go back to the café. She got up early every morning and sat at her nook window, with the sun coming in, and read her Bible. Sometimes she felt she was walking in the valley of the shadow of death, her heart trembling and broken. She feared running into Jason. She couldn't bear to see the coldness in his eyes.

Studying held off the pain. She'd pushed herself through class after class for three years. She would do it again. Surely God had a purpose in all this. She prayed constantly. Sometimes she talked aloud to Him when she sat alone in her apartment. *What do You want me to do with the rest of my life?* She could never be the Proverbs 31 wife. Maybe God intended her for the mission field. There must be dozens of organizations who needed nurses. Maybe she'd serve on an Indian reservation or in Africa or the Far East. *Someplace far away, Lord, at the ends of the earth.*

Every night, she dreamed of Jason. Every morning, she woke up and cried. She begged God to stop the dreams.

Day after day, she set her mind on attending classes, taking notes, completing assignments to the best of her ability. God had a plan for her. She would trust God to work it all out.

She thought of Oma and how she had said she had made plans of her own and then found God had made better ones for her. She searched for God's promises and wrote them in the leather-bound journal Oma had given her.

I have loved you, my people, with an everlasting love. With unfailing love I have drawn you to myself. . . . I know the plans I have for you . . . plans for good and not for disaster, to give you a future and a hope.

I want to believe You, Lord. Help me believe.

Eventually, she found a church similar to CCC and finally felt at home, comforted among the flock of believers, less vulnerable than when she was by herself battling loneliness and loss. The second week she attended, she spotted Jason in the third row. She would have left if the service hadn't already started.

God, why are You doing this to me?

When the pastor called for prayer, Jason didn't just bow his head; he hunched over. Dawn felt grateful. She'd stolen his innocence, but at least she hadn't destroyed his faith. When the congregation rose to sing, Jason stood taller than the others around him. He looked like a soldier, shoulders back, head up. Throat tight, Dawn mouthed the praise songs, unable to make a sound.

The service ended. She thought about heading quickly for the door, but Jason rose and started down the aisle. Afraid he'd see her, she kept her head turned away as he made his way toward the doors. Departing parishioners greeted him, drawing him into conversation. She leaned down as though to get her purse as he passed by and then sat up and watched him go out the door.

The sanctuary emptied. The praise band stowed their instruments. Dawn rose. She'd try another church next Sunday. Or maybe she'd just stay home and read her Bible.

Monday, Dawn dragged herself out of bed and did her morning Bible reading. She barely made it to her anatomy class and had to struggle to keep her eyes open. She downed a cup of coffee before she went to her nursing history course, then went to the dining complex for a slice of pizza at BackStage. She had two hours before her next class, enough time to study in the library.

After an hour, she felt drained. She massaged her forehead, wishing the coffee had helped the headache. She'd lived in San Luis Obispo two whole months; it felt like ten years. She didn't know if she could stay here. Maybe she should transfer. Maybe it had been a mistake coming here, even though she had felt certain God had been directing her. She hadn't expected more pain, more sleepless nights, more confusion. If she transferred, she wouldn't face the risk of seeing Jason every day. She might have a chance to see what God wanted her to do.

Someone pulled out a chair and sat opposite her. She didn't feel like sharing her space. Gathering her notes, she tucked them quickly into a folder. She leaned over for her backpack.

"I've been trying to find you."

Her heart lurched to a stop and then raced.

Jason folded his arms on the table. "How are you doing?"

Why now, Lord? I don't know what You want from me anymore. She gave Jason a bleak smile. "I'm managing." All the old attraction swam through her blood as he looked her over.

Standing, she lifted her backpack onto the table and began putting her books away.

"You look tired, Dawn."

"I haven't been sleeping very well."

"Neither have I." He leaned forward, keeping his voice low. "Do you want to go somewhere? talk?"

She recognized the glint in his eyes and went hot all over. She remembered all too well how it had been between them. Reason enough to withdraw. *Now.* "I have a chemistry class."

"I joined the Army."

"Very funny, Jason."

Jason caught hold of her arm and pulled her to a stop. "I joined the Army, Dawn." When she pulled back, his hand slid away. "They're paying for my education. When I finish, I'll be on active service for six years."

Dawn went cold with guilt. "And it's my fault." She thought of Iraq and Kuwait and the young men being deployed. Mitch had told her things would heat up before it was over. What would that mean for Jason? Would he finish college and end up shipped off to a war? All because she'd distracted him from his studies and he couldn't get a scholarship? Georgia Steward had every right to hate her. "I'm sorry, Jason." An apology would never be enough. Her eyes blurred with tears. "I'm so sorry." She stepped back. "I *was* the worst thing that ever happened to you." She turned away.

Jason caught hold of her again. "Will you just wait a minute?"

She wrenched free. "You had everything planned out before I messed things up. You'd be at Berkeley on scholarship right now if we hadn't . . ." Unable to say more, she spun from him and wove quickly into the throng of students, half-running.

❄ ❄ ❄

Chemistry class passed in a blur. She took notes, trying to make sense of things, but she kept thinking about Jason's announcement. The Army! He'd wanted to be an engineer or a Christian business-man—or maybe even a pastor. Now he'd be a soldier building bridges or roads into some godforsaken battle zone. What a mess she'd made!

Dawn emerged from class and saw Jason leaning against the wall. Pushing away, he caught up with her. "We need to talk."

"I think your first instincts three years ago were right on, Jason. We need to let things go."

"Please, Dawn." He took her hand and pressed it flat against his chest. She felt his heart pounding hard and fast. He leaned closer. "I could barely catch my breath when I saw you sitting in the café. It's not over, Dawn. It's never going to be over between us."

Her body filled with sensations. Unthinking, she stepped forward and slid her arms around his waist. As she pressed herself against him, she heard him suck in his breath. He put his arms around her and let it out again, slowly. "I love you, Dawn. I'll love you forever." Dawn felt the heat of his hand press against the small of her back. His breath was ragged. "Are you finished with classes for the day?"

"Yes."

"Let's find someplace to be alone and talk. I have a couple of roommates. What about you?" When he stepped back, she watched his eyes go dark the same way they had every time she came to the trailer while his mother had been away working. That look had intoxicated her then. It still sent curling heat into the pit of her stomach and down her legs.

"I live alone." She could feel the heat coming off him at that, or was it her?

"It's been too long, Dawn." Jason took her hand. "Let's go."

The Spirit within Dawn warned her. Alert to Him after three years of walking close, she listened and obeyed. "No." She pulled her hand free and didn't move from where they stood. "We can't be alone, not with our history." And not with the way she was feeling right then. If they were alone and he touched her, she'd forget all about what God wanted of her. Three years had obviously changed Jason. She had to find out how much.

He didn't pretend not to understand. Running his hands down her arms, he gave her a slow smile that melted her insides. "Okay. We'll set rules. Kissing, but no petting, no—"

Dawn shook her head. "I'm not strong enough, Jason, and I'm not willing to go down that road again."

Jason let out a shuddering breath. "Okay." He took her hand and wove his fingers through hers. "Make a suggestion."

"Someplace public, so we'll have to behave ourselves."

He laughed. "Then I guess it's going to be the Dexter Lawn." When he smiled at her this time, he looked like the Jason she remembered.

EVERY MORNING, DAWN and Jason met on the Dexter Lawn after he finished ROTC classes. They met on the walkways between classes and at the dining complex for lunch. They talked on the telephone every night until they couldn't keep their eyes open.

Jason introduced her to his friends: Dod Henson, Jack Kohl, and Alice Jeffries, the pretty, dark-haired girl who turned out to be Dod's girl. None were Christians and they seemed surprised to find out Jason was. "When did that happen?" Dod wanted to know, and Jason said a long time ago, but he just hadn't been walking with the Lord lately. He'd been ticked at God and hadn't felt like talking to Him. He laughed when he said it, grimacing in self-mockery. They all went into town and talked over Chinese food or hamburgers. On Saturdays, Dawn and Jason studied in the library. On Sunday mornings, they went to church together.

A month passed like a Santana wind, and Jason wanted to do something special to celebrate their "anniversary." Dawn suggested a Sunday afternoon picnic on the beach and brought homemade fried chicken, potato salad, and fresh-baked cookies. They ate at a table, with the wind blowing cold off the ocean, and stowed the leftovers in the backseat of his white Honda. Throwing a blanket over his shoulder, Jason took her hand and said he wanted to walk awhile. He found a cove shielded from the wind and spread the blanket so they could sit and watch the waves.

Dawn talked about the sermon they'd heard that morning and raised questions. Jason's answers seemed more seasoned with life than they had when he was seventeen. Shivering, Dawn wrapped her arms around her raised knees and told Jason about the day she'd seen him sitting near the front of the church. "You came in late. I watched you pray."

Jason stretched on his back, arms behind his head. "That was the first time I'd been to church since moving down here."

Dawn stared at him in surprise. "Kim said you were in church every time you came home."

"Yeah," he drawled. "Because Mom insisted." He frowned. "Is that why you weren't there? Because I was?"

She looked out at the ocean. Seagulls dipped and floated on the wind. "It hurt to see you."

Jason's hand curved around her hip. "I didn't feel much like seeing Pastor Daniel after that surprise fishing trip he and Mom pulled on me."

"What'd Pastor Daniel say to you that weekend?"

Jason grimaced. "That a man protects those he loves, and I was putting you at risk. I won't go into the gory details, but Daniel told me what *I* thought of as protection wasn't what God had in mind. I knew he was right, which was the problem, of course. I just didn't want to hear it. I figured you'd be upset when I wasn't there, but—"

"Your mom was there."

"Well, I know, but I'm sure you and she didn't have much to talk about. "

"Oh, your mom had a few things to say."

"What?" He exploded to his feet and raked his hands through his hair. "I asked you what the two of you talked about, and you said nothing! Now you're telling me she said something to you? Did she say something that made you build such a wall between us?"

Dawn had had three years to think over what Georgia Steward had said that day. "She told me the truth."

"I'll bet she did." His eyes darkened. "Her version of it." He swore.

"Sit down, Jason. Please."

He did, body tense, jaw clenching, fists against the sand. "Like my mother has any right to cast stones. She had me out of wedlock, remember?"

"Yes, so who better to recognize the danger we were putting ourselves in? Your mom spoke God's truth, Jason. And the Lord used her words to open my eyes to what *He* wanted. I see that as a great kindness. We both owe Pastor Daniel and your mother a debt of gratitude."

"You think so? What about the pain they caused?"

"Pain builds character, and *they* didn't cause it. *We* did that to ourselves. I knew what I was doing that night at Jenner. I wanted you. That's all I cared about. Not how I went about getting you or what the price might be. Sin always has consequences. When I look back now, I see God's mercy in the way it all turned out."

Jason's eyes softened. "You're not the girl you were, Dawn."

"I hope not."

"God got hold of you." Jason pulled her down on top of him. "But I want to hold you, too." He dug his fingers into her hair and kissed her the way he used to when they were alone in his bedroom. "You still taste like heaven." Rolling her onto her back, he kissed her again. "Will you marry me?"

Dawn smiled and brushed some sand off his sweater. "I think you already know the answer. Of course I will."

Joy and then determination filled his face. "We'll get married during Christmas break."

She laughed. "Thanksgiving is only ten days away."

"I know, and I wasn't planning to go home until now."

"You mean it!"

"Yes. I mean it." He stood, pulling her up with him. "Now we'll go home together, in my car. I'm calling my mother tonight, so she'll have fair warning. And then I'm calling Pastor Daniel and finding out what day he has open for a wedding." He shook out the blanket. "You'd better call your folks before they hear from someone else."

Dawn tried to catch her breath. "They'll probably suggest we wait until we graduate."

"That's not for another two years—or maybe even three. I don't think either one of us can wait that long." Jason stopped folding the blanket. "Say something." He frowned. "You don't want to wait, do you?"

"No." Joy bubbled up inside her. God had given her the desire of her heart. She laughed. "No, Jason, I don't want to wait." She threw herself into his arms.

❄ ❄ ❄

Jason said his mother didn't have a lot to say about them getting married. Pastor Daniel said he'd check his calendar and they could talk when Jason and Dawn came home for Thanksgiving. Expecting resistance, Jason rehearsed arguments on the long drive north. Despite her fears, Dawn counseled him to listen and not storm in the front door of the trailer half-cocked for a gunfight. "Your mom and Pastor Daniel love you, Jason. They want the best for you."

He glanced at her. "This is about *us*, Dawn, not *me*." He frowned. "You haven't said much about your folks' reaction. If Mitch and your mom say wait, are you going to listen?"

"I'm going to hear them out without interrupting." She shoved her hands under her thighs. "This isn't about what makes *us* happy, Jason. It's about God. Let's try to focus on what will make *Him* happy. Okay? You told me a long time ago the Lord knows better than any of us."

Jason cast an apologetic smile. "I guess I needed the reminder."

When he dropped her off, Mitch and Mom came out to welcome them. Eleven-year-old Christopher darted out and hugged Dawn, telling her how much he'd missed her and she was getting married and did that mean Jason would move in with them for the summer and why didn't Jason come in and see the city he'd built with his LEGOs. They all laughed. Jason was clearly relieved by the warm greeting.

Mom threw cold water on both of them with an announcement. "Jason, you and your mom are having Thanksgiving dinner with us." She looked at Dawn. "And Granny's coming, too, of course. She called me right after you called her about your engagement."

Dawn winced inwardly. No wonder her mother had been so quiet when Dawn called with the news she and Jason wanted to get married.

❋ ❋ ❋

Dawn answered the door when Jason and his mom arrived. Georgia Steward's smile was tense as Dawn ushered them into the house. As his mother walked ahead, Jason stole a kiss from Dawn. Mitch and Mom greeted them in the family room, offering sparkling cider and appetizers. Mitch made a toast. Granny chattered happily, eager to help plan the nuptials. "We'll have to work fast if we're going to pull everything together before Christmas. Dawn will need a wedding gown. We'll have to find a photographer, order flowers and engraved invitations."

Pensive and silent, Mom went into the kitchen. Georgia followed, asking if she could help.

Jason took Dawn's hand. "Can we take a walk in the garden?"

Out of view of the windows, Jason took her in his arms and kissed her. "You look like a deer in the headlights."

"A gown, wedding invitations, photographer, flowers . . ."

"I didn't stop to ask what kind of wedding you want. Something big and white, I guess."

"I think Granny is dreaming about all that because she and Papa didn't have it. And she didn't get to put on a big wedding for my mom, either."

"What do you want?"

"You!"

"You've got me." He kissed her again, pressing her to him. He raised his mouth, then whispered against her ear. "Maybe we should save everyone the trouble and elope."

Conversation didn't lull around the dinner table. Even Georgia seemed loquacious when Mitch asked about her business. Booming, she said. She'd hired two more maids over the past two months and was on the lookout for another. Christopher barely spoke, too busy stuffing himself with turkey and dressing. Mom said she and Georgia would work out some of the details regarding the wedding. "We just have to know what you two have in mind."

"Something simple." Dawn's smile wobbled. "Close friends and family."

"What about flowers?" Georgia lifted her glass of sparkling cider to sip and peered at her over the rim.

"Poinsettias." They could be left in the church to decorate through Christmas.

Georgia set her glass down carefully. "What about your bouquet?"

"Gardenias smell wonderful," Granny volunteered. "And roses . . . or white orchids . . ."

"I want to carry five long-stemmed white roses."

Granny looked surprised and then disheartened. "That's not a bridal bouquet, Dawn."

"Maybe not." Dawn leaned over and kissed Granny's cheek to take away any sting of disappointment. "But it's what I want."

❄ ❄ ❄

Pastor Daniel sat behind his desk when Jason ushered Dawn into the office Friday morning. They held hands as they sat on the couch in front of him. "You two act like you're facing a firing squad instead of coming in to talk about a wedding."

Jason sat straight and tall, poised for a fight. "Don't try to shoot us down. We want to get married as soon as possible."

It occurred to Dawn what Pastor Daniel might think about hasty wedding plans. "I'm not pregnant, Pastor Daniel."

Jason shot her a glance. His hand tightened around hers as he faced their pastor again. "And we're not sleeping together either, nor will we until we're married."

Pastor Daniel blushed. "Wow! Last time we talked, Jason, I must've come across as judge and jury. I hope you'll both forgive me."

Dawn smiled. "We do. You were right. I'm thankful that God gave us enough time to realize that for ourselves. Not to mention a second chance." She turned her smile on Jason.

Jason's hand loosened. "You said something about a premarital Bible study." He had said on the way home he thought Pastor Daniel or his mother might come up with some sort of delaying tactic.

Pastor Daniel lifted two workbooks and put them on the front of his desk. "These are for you two to take back to Cal Poly." Leaning forward, he folded his hands on the desk. "There's lots of Scripture to read and things to ponder together. The intent is for you to be forewarned so you'll be able to work through problems that will come up in the course of your marriage, not just in the first year, but in the years to come."

Pastor Daniel smiled warmly at Dawn. "I've watched your relationship with Jesus grow over the last three years." His expression turned grim when he shifted his focus to Jason. "I'm not so sure about you. Still wandering in the wilderness?"

"Not anymore. I'm back in church and I plan to stay." Jason let go of Dawn's hand and leaned forward to take the workbooks. "Thanks, Daniel." Smiling, he relaxed on the sofa.

"I hoped it would all work out this way."

"Did you?" Jason sounded dubious.

"What do you say we take a bike ride tomorrow? Talk a little more."

Jason agreed.

Leaning back in his chair, Pastor Daniel gave them a smug smile. "You'll be the first couple to meet and marry in our church. December is a nice month for a wedding."

Dawn laughed. "What about Kim and Tom?"

Pastor Daniel chuckled. "Ah, but they're not getting married until June. We'll tie your knot on December 21."

❄ ❄ ❄

When Dawn got home, a light blinked on her answering machine. She pressed the button, thinking it might be Kim or Pam or one of her other friends. Instead, she heard Georgia Steward's invitation to the trailer for coffee Saturday afternoon at three. "We have a few things to settle between us, Dawn." Her voice sounded cool and detached. "If three isn't convenient, please call so we can set another time."

Dawn sank onto her bed. What would Jason's mother say to her this time? Was she afraid this marriage would ruin his chances of getting through college? that Dawn might get in the way again? that she might be pregnant?

Dawn wanted to call and make some excuse not to go. How could she face Georgia again, after all that had been said the last time? *God, help me. What do I do?*

Reason took hold. Georgia Steward would be her mother-in-law in a few weeks. She deserved respect and consideration. Georgia might not like her, but for Jason's sake they needed to make some kind of peace. Dawn didn't want to become a stumbling block between mother and son. She prayed about it all afternoon.

Jason called that night. When he didn't mention his mother's invitation, Dawn knew Georgia hadn't told him. That did not bode well.

Jason said he had a great idea for their honeymoon. They'd

have only a few days before they needed to come back for a family Christmas. "It won't be the Ritz, but I think you'll like it." He wanted it to be a surprise.

"I'll love it, wherever it is."

Unable to sleep, Dawn sat at her desk, reading her Bible until well after midnight.

She covered her face and prayed for Georgia's heart to soften toward her. When she finally went to bed, she dreamed she wore a scarlet wedding dress, and Georgia, dressed in black, wept in the front row.

43

Dawn's insides quivered as she parked her Sable behind Georgia's van. Mrs. Edwards peered through her living room curtains. Georgia opened the door, leaned out to wave to her neighbor, and then beckoned Dawn inside. Blushing, Dawn went up the steps onto the small porch. One glance over her shoulder confirmed Mrs. Edwards still waited with bated breath to witness the outcome of this meeting between Georgia and the girl who had seduced Jason.

A small potted plant sat on the table where Dawn and Jason used to spread their books out before going into his bedroom. Georgia moved tensely about the kitchen. Dawn pressed her damp palms on her dark skirt.

"Do you like coffee, Dawn, or would you prefer tea?"

"Whatever you're having will be fine, ma'am."

Georgia gave a sharp laugh. "*Ma'am* makes me feel like a nasty old woman. Call me Georgia. I'm a coffee drinker. Do you like cream or sugar?"

"Nothing, thank you."

Georgia carried a wooden tray with saucers and cups of coffee and a plate of homemade chocolate chip cookies into the living room and set it on the low table. "Sit down. You're making me nervous." She waved her hand toward the sofa. "We both know we have to have this conversation. We might as well get it over with, don't you think?"

Dawn took her coffee. The cup rattled in the saucer. Mortified, she set them on the table before she could spill coffee all over the beige rug.

Georgia cleared her throat softly. "This is difficult for both of us, Dawn. I wanted to talk with you alone and try to clear up a few things." Georgia closed her eyes for a moment and released a slow breath before she looked at Dawn again. "I said awful things to you the last time you were here." She turned her face away. "Afterward, I knew I'd jeopardized my relationship with my son. You had the power to make Jason hate me."

"I didn't tell him anything about that day."

"Oh, honey, I know you didn't. He asked me after the two of you broke up if I'd ever spoken to you. I asked if you'd said I had—implying, of course, I hadn't. He said you'd pulled out of school and wouldn't return his calls."

Georgia gripped her saucer and stared into the cup for a moment. "When Jason said you two should stop seeing each other for a while, he meant a few weeks. But you backed out of his life entirely. I watched him suffer. I heard him sobbing one night. A few days later, he put his fist through the wall. And I watched you suffer, too."

"I couldn't . . ." Dawn pressed her trembling lips together and tried again. "I knew if we saw each other, we'd go right back—"

Georgia held up her hand. "I'm not finished, Dawn. Please, let me finish." She drew in a breath, her mouth working. When she regained control, she spoke quietly. "I watched you. I listened to everything people said about you. For three years. You sat in church and soaked in every word Daniel said. I heard how well you were doing in independent study—high grades, taking college courses while you finished high school. You went on mission trips. Daniel said he'd never seen God work in a person's life the way the Lord worked in yours. You fixed your eyes on Jesus and never looked away. But while I watched your faith grow, I saw Jason struggling. When I heard you'd transferred to Cal Poly, I prayed harder than I ever had in my life."

Dawn hung her head. She could imagine how hard Georgia Steward had prayed. She must have assumed the girl who'd caused her son so much grief had gone after him again.

Georgia's eyes glistened. "Jason thanked me the other day. When I asked him what for, he said you told him I'd been kind to you." She smiled bleakly. "He apologized for assuming I'd said the same things to you that I'd been saying *about* you for weeks before that last fiasco." She shook her head. "And I know everything you've done, even forgiving me, has been out of love for my son." Her voice broke.

Dawn realized she wasn't the only one consumed by guilt. "You weren't wrong about me."

"Oh, I was very wrong. I couldn't have been more wrong. When I looked at you, I saw myself at fifteen—arrogant, selfish, defiant. I wanted what I wanted when I wanted it. I didn't care what anyone thought. *You* listened. *You* repented. When I got pregnant, my world fell apart. My boyfriend dumped me and moved on to a new girl. My parents kicked me out. I was living on the streets when Jason was born. It took five years to crawl up out of the gutter life I'd made for myself. I don't even want to remember the things I did to put bread on our table. And then, feeling holier-than-thou, I had the audacity to ambush you. I dug a hole and tried to bury you under my hurt and bitterness. Everything I said to you was all about the girl I'd been. I didn't even see you."

Dawn let out a shuddering breath. She'd prayed so hard about this meeting and now felt the warmth of God's answer filling her. "But don't you see? I *was* all the things you said, Georgia."

When Georgia opened her mouth, Dawn raised her hand. "Let *me* finish. If you'd been gentle, I might not have listened. It took you speaking the truth the way you did to get through to me. I'm grateful that you did. God used your words to draw me to Himself, and that's when the Lord started working. Maybe if someone had spoken to you the way you spoke to me, things would have turned out differently for you too." She'd been afraid she wouldn't be able to say a word when she walked through the front door, but words flowed naturally and with a love she hadn't known she possessed for Jason's mother.

Georgia let out a long breath. "Just to be clear: I couldn't be more pleased you're marrying my son."

"Me, too."

They laughed together.

"Well. All that being said . . ." Georgia leaned forward and lifted the plate. "Have a cookie. And then let's talk about how I can help put on a beautiful wedding."

❄   ❄   ❄

From the day Dawn told her family she and Jason were getting married, Granny had pressured Dawn to go shopping for a white wedding dress. Dawn didn't feel entitled to wear a white gown, but she didn't want to hurt Granny by explaining why not. She didn't know what to do until her mother offered the pale pink gown and veil she'd worn when she married Mitch. "I think it'll fit you." Her mother seemed shy about it. "If you want it."

"I do." She'd felt her mother stiffen slightly when she hugged her. Sometimes Dawn wondered why her mother seemed so uncomfortable with physical affection, unless it came from Christopher or Mitch.

On the morning of the wedding, deaconesses were on hand to decorate the church with the poinsettias Georgia had delivered, and by eleven, the place was packed with well-wishers. Dawn saw Jason's gaze fixed on her as Mitch walked her down the aisle. She gave white roses to Granny and Mom. When Pastor Daniel pronounced them man and wife, the congregants erupted in applause and cheers. On the way back up the aisle, Dawn paused and gave Georgia a white rose and kissed her cheek. She had two left, one to throw and one to keep.

While pictures were being taken, deacons rearranged chairs and set up tables. Caterers covered everything with linens and spread platters with enough fancy sandwiches and salads to feed an army. A three-tiered wedding cake stood on a central table. The stack of beautifully wrapped packages grew on two back tables. After the receiving line, Jason and Dawn sat at the head table and nibbled at lunch. They cut the cake, carefully feeding each other small bites, and then danced to the music of the professional band Mitch had hired.

Jason held Dawn close as they waltzed, his warm breath sending shivers down her spine. "Can we go now?" he whispered against her ear. His hand spread on the small of her back. "We've cut the cake and had our dance."

She laughed softly. "The reception is supposed to last another hour."

Mitch cut in. "Dad's turn." Grinning broadly at Jason, he took Dawn in his arms. "You look like you can't wait to get her out of here, but you won't want to drive your Honda anywhere until you run it through a car wash."

Jason grimaced. "I'm going to—"

"Do nothing." Mitch chuckled. "Carolyn will give you the keys to my Bonneville."

"Thanks, Mitch." Jason stepped forward. "Can I have my wife back now?"

"Not so fast. You have duties to perform. Dance with your mother and mother-in-law first. And I've been informed Dawn still has to throw her rose to a gaggle of single girls. And you have to toss her garter to that pack of wolves you call friends. Then Pita's all yours for the rest of your life, buddy boy."

Laughing, Dawn punched him.

It was a long, dark drive and well after ten before they reached Fort Bragg and signed into the Harbor Lite Lodge as Mr. and Mrs. Jason Steward. The suite was larger than Dawn's studio apartment.

Someone had already lit the fire in the small Franklin stove. She opened the sliding-glass door and went out on the small balcony overlooking the Noyo River. A light rain sprinkled, and fog curled around the security lights on the docks below.

Jason slid his hands around her waist and drew her back against him. "Finally. We're alone." He kissed the curve of her neck, sending warm tendrils through her body. "And married."

❄ ❄ ❄

After spending two nights and two days in their suite, with only brief outings for meals, Dawn and Jason returned to Alexander Valley for the family Christmas celebration. "Wait until you see!" Christopher bounded ahead of them to her bedroom and threw the door open. All the wedding presents had been stacked, waiting to be unwrapped. Dawn gaped.

Jason dumped their two small suitcases inside the door and stared. "Holy cow!"

Mom peered in. "Welcome home, you two." Her eyes shone. "It seems you both have a lot of friends who wanted to help you set up housekeeping."

Mitch, standing right behind her, nudged her into the room. "Don't panic. Once everything is opened, pick what you need and leave the rest here for later."

Granny asked Dawn and Jason to come out to Jenner for a few days after Christmas, but Jason said they needed to go home to San Luis Obispo. He had to move his stuff into Dawn's apartment, and they needed to get settled in before classes started.

Dawn knew another reason Jason didn't want to go to Jenner. She waited until they were alone that night to ask his forgiveness for what she brought about in the downstairs apartment.

"You weren't alone, you know." Jason touched her cheek. "I stayed overnight *hoping* you'd come downstairs. I could have stopped things if I'd wanted, Dawn. It wasn't all your idea." He drew her close and kissed her.

❊ ❊ ❊

1991

It didn't take long for Jason and Dawn to decide they had to study
somewhere other than in the apartment. With two small desks and
the nook table, they didn't have room to spread their books and
reports. They made other adjustments as well. Dawn liked to do
her Bible study before the sun came up pink-yellow over the hills.
Jason, a night owl, studied Scripture at night.

They walked to campus together. They ate lunch together, and
they spent every spare minute studying at the library. Dawn cooked
and did laundry on Saturdays. Sunday, they went to the early
service and then took long walks, went to the beach, talked over
Chinese food, and hung out with Dod Henson and Alice Jeffries,
their closest friends on campus. Sometimes Jack Kohl joined them,
if he had a new girlfriend.

They talked of nothing but the war in Iraq, the need to protect
the oil fields and Persian Gulf, the hope for success with the air
campaign and bombing of leadership targets in Baghdad. Coalition
ground forces drove on Iraqi forces in Kuwait. After four days,
Iraqi forces agreed to a cease-fire and retreated from Kuwait. The
push to reach Baghdad halted. Jason and Dod sneered over U.N.
objectives being met. Even when Iraq agreed to a permanent cease-
fire, they saw trouble ahead. "Saddam Hussein fancies himself the
second Nebuchadnezzar. He's not done. They've just given him
time to coil for another strike."

LIFE FELT REGIMENTED, but comfortable and with frequent moments of delight. The only dark cloud was approaching summer break. Jason would be leaving for two months, undergoing military training at Fort Lewis, Washington. Dawn knew she had to keep busy or be miserable while he was gone. Still intent upon finishing college as quickly as possible, she registered for a summer session psychology class.

The week before finals, Dawn had difficulty sleeping. One morning she rose while it was still dark and quietly slid the partition between the living room and bedroom closed. Turning on the swag lamp over the kitchen nook table, she opened her Bible and workbook. She and Jason had been married five months, and she still hadn't finished all the sections. She'd been taking her time, praying over the questions, and examining herself, asking God to reveal areas of her life that needed change.

As the warmth of the sun spilled in the window, she heard a soft click. Startled, she glanced toward the bedroom. Jason stood there holding a camera. "Perfect." Grinning, he set it on the coffee table.

"You took a picture?" She was still in her robe and slippers, her hair loose and wild.

Leaning down, he hemmed her in with his hands planted on the table. He nuzzled her neck. "I love the way the sun lights up your hair in the morning. You look like an angel studying God's directives for the day." Straightening, he put his hands on her shoulders. "And I wanted something more natural than a wedding picture to keep me company while I'm at Fort Lewis."

❄ ❄ ❄

The first thing Dawn saw when she walked into the apartment after her last final exam was Jason's physical training uniform hooked on the closet trim, ready to be worn. She burst into tears. They'd been married only five months, and he'd be gone tomorrow morning. He'd spend a month in cadet troop leadership training and then be off to airborne school right after that. "Two months," she muttered. "Two months!"

He said the camp was designed to develop leadership skills, teamwork, water safety, land navigation, fire support, weapons use, and tactical and physical training. Portions of it sounded ominous and dangerous to her, but he dismissed her worries. Thankfully, the war in Iraq had ended in March. Lord willing, Jason would not see actual combat during his military service. Dawn didn't know how she would cope with that.

Jason had told her he first started thinking about ROTC after her grandfather had regaled him with World War II stories. After their breakup, Jason started thinking more about the military. He'd sought out Mitch and asked questions about the Vietnam War and his military experience. Mitch had told him the military had a lot to offer and the country always needed good men trained and ready. His school counselor told him to talk to the ROTC recruiting officer at Cal Poly. When he learned the Army would give him the financial aid he needed to get through college in exchange for six years of his life, Jason decided it was a generous offer. Without discussing it with his mother or Pastor Daniel, he entered the program freshman year.

Dawn dumped her backpack on the bed. Jason admitted he hadn't consulted God about that decision, but whether he had or had not wasn't an issue now. God was sovereign. Man might plan, but God would prevail. She believed that with all her heart. She just hadn't realized how much military life might suit Jason—or how much it might demand of her.

Jason took her in his arms. "I'm not gone yet."

"You'll be jumping out of airplanes, Jason."

"Yeah."

He sounded excited about it. She pushed away and looked at him. He looked excited, too. "You can't wait, can you?"

"I'm not going to lie to you."

"I know." She'd overheard him talking with Dod and Jack. In truth, all three were looking forward to the training, like it was some kind of grand adventure!

Letting out her breath, she withdrew. "I'm just being ridiculous." Would she rather he was miserable and wishing he didn't have to follow through on his obligations to the military? When she reached for the duffel bag, he grabbed it and slung it onto the bed. She started packing for him. "I'll be all right. I'll keep busy."

"I'll call you every chance I get."

❄ ❄ ❄

Jason called to let her know he'd arrived safely at Fort Lewis. After less than a minute, she heard another man asking to use the phone. After that, she waited in vain to hear from him. His second call came before he headed into airborne training, though Dawn still couldn't understand why an engineer needed to know how to jump out of an airplane. She didn't waste time asking. They talked for fifteen minutes before he had to hang up so someone else could make a call.

To keep from being depressed, Dawn poured herself into her psychology class. While going through lecture notes on symptoms of abuse, she thought about her mother for some odd reason. Dawn realized she knew very little about her mother's past, other than what Granny had told her.

What had kept Mom away from church for so many years? Why did she withdraw from any show of affection, unless it came from Mitch or Christopher? Granny took a step toward her, and Mom retreated. What caused the tension between them? When Dawn thought more about it, she realized her mother had always had difficulty with relationships, especially if they were casual. She served, but didn't mingle; she watched from a distance, but didn't attempt to participate. Dawn had this mental picture of her mother peering over a protective wall while keeping the gate to the outside world locked.

What might have caused that? Could it have something to do with the Haight-Ashbury years? Dawn didn't know much about that time in her mother's life. Granny said the past was best forgotten, and Mom never talked about it. Anytime anyone mentioned the turbulent sixties, Mom became very quiet.

Maybe she should ask. . . .

Dawn tried to during one of her weekly calls home. As usual, Mom stayed on the phone less than five minutes, leaving it to Christopher to report the family's news. Dawn didn't even get close to broaching the subject with her.

Dawn asked Granny what Mom had been like as a little girl. "Beautiful." Granny sounded wistful. "Quiet. There weren't any other little girls her age on our road, but she always seemed content playing by herself."

"Did she ever seem nervous or exhibit any odd behavior?"

Granny chuckled. "The trouble with studying psychology is you begin to imagine symptoms of all kinds of neuroses in everyone you know. Your mother was a perfectly normal child, just a little quieter than most."

"So Mom never had nightmares or sucked her thumb . . . ?"

"Oh, there was a while when she used to sneak into Charlie's room and sleep with him or on the floor beside his bed. It didn't last long. I put a stop to it as soon as I knew."

"And she was fine with that, no crying or arguments?"

Silence for a moment. "She started sleeping in her closet. But really, Dawn, you're making way too much of it."

"I know, Granny. I'm just curious. That's all."

"We started leaving a night-light on in the bathroom. She seemed fine after that. Or maybe it was Oma."

"Oma?"

"She came to live with us about that time." Her tone turned brisk. "Either way, your mom stayed in her own bed after that."

On impulse, Dawn called her mother that evening and asked if she remembered having nightmares as a child.

"Why do you ask?"

"I'm taking psychology."

"Oh. Well. I suppose all children have bad dreams. Don't they?"

"Granny said you used to sneak in and sleep with Uncle Charlie."

"Did she?"

"And when she put a stop to it, you slept in your closet."

Silence.

"Mom?"

"What started this line of questioning?"

Dawn winced. Mom might as well have said *interrogation*. "I'm taking psychology, and the lectures have been on child abuse."

"I was never beaten, May Flo—" She stopped. "Dawn." She spoke the correction quietly.

"We'll have to talk about my name someday." Dawn tried to keep her tone light. When her mother didn't respond, she apologized for asking such personal questions. "I was just curious."

Her mother's reticence only served to make *her* more so.

❄ ❄ ❄

Dawn sat at the nook table, flipping through her class notes. Slapping her binder closed, she stared out the window. She'd studied enough. She didn't want to think about psychology or come up with any more theories on why her mother was the way she was. She'd never know anything more about her than she did now. It wasn't her business anyway.

She knew what the problem was: she had too much time on her hands. She needed something to do other than go to class, study, and hang around the apartment, waiting for Jason to call. She had to stop counting the days until he'd come home. She looked at the bare white walls, the worn beige couch, the drab chipboard coffee table sitting on the beige rug. Life without Jason was as colorless as the apartment.

The place needed cheering up. It needed *color*!

Grabbing her keys and purse, Dawn left the apartment. She drove downtown and bought half a dozen women's magazines. She spotted notices on the coffee shop bulletin board: garage sales popped up like weeds every Friday afternoon. She'd always thought it might be fun to visit a few, see what treasures she might find among the piles of junk. On the way back to the apartment, Dawn stopped by a hardware store and picked out paint color strips.

"Walls have to be back to white before you leave," Mr. Cooper, the apartment manager told her when she explained what she'd like to do. "Otherwise, you forfeit your security deposit."

After psychology class, Dawn went to the library and looked for books on interior design. She jotted down ideas, then went back to the apartment to take measurements and map out furnishings. She tore pages from magazines.

Early Saturday morning, Dawn drove south to Santa Maria, hoping to be the first arrival at the *Huge Neighborhood Garage Sale: furnishings, fine linens, china . . .* She wasn't. Already a crowd wandered the cul-de-sac, picking through racks of cloth-ing, looking over electronic gadgets, tools, toys, and totally useless knickknacks. Dawn bargained for two matching crested chairs with burgundy upholstery and got them for twenty dollars. She fitted them carefully into the backseat of the Sable and continued her search. She bought two Talavera plates for five dollars; an old, worn, imitation Persian rug in jewel tones for twenty-five; and a glass bowl full of seashells for a buck.

Still on the hunt, Dawn wandered, looking for anything that caught her eye. She became engrossed with a shoe box full of maps and another of postcards. She bought three framed posters of rock groups. On her way back to the car, she bargained for two large sky-blue blankets and a somewhat-faded yellow and blue French provincial tablecloth with deep pink peonies and daisies.

Mr. Cooper saw her pull up and laughed. "When the dog's away, the cat will play. Need some help unloading all that junk?"

She laughed, excited about getting to work on decorating. "Yes, please." She started pulling the rolled carpet through the back window. "And I'll have you know these are *treasures*."

Over the next week, Dawn painted the living room wall butter yellow, folded and pinned one blue blanket around the body of the sofa and the other around the two large cushions, unrolled the Persian rug, tucking it beneath the sofa, and set the oval-backed chairs in opposite corners, the coffee table in the middle. Making do without a sewing machine, Dawn folded and pinned colorful cloth covers over cheap pillows and arranged them on the sofa.

Removing the rock concert pictures, she used two of the frames to mount maps of Monterey and Washington, D.C. As the center-piece of wall art, she created a colorful collage of old postcards from national parks across the country. She hung the two Talavera plates in the kitchen, put a yellow valance over the nook window, and spread the Provence tablecloth. Last touches included the glass bowl of seashells on the coffee table, the new issue of *VIA* from the California Automobile Association, and a bouquet of yellow roses in a lime green Fiesta water pitcher.

Arms akimbo, she admired the room. Eclectic, she decided, already imagining other things she could do to make the room more interesting. A potted palm in the corner would be nice, and some nice coverings for the ugly end tables. Changing the lamp shades . . .

She stopped the train of thoughts running through her head. The living room looked warm and cozy. Now she needed to read another chapter in her psychology text and review her notes. She still had five more days for decorating before Jason came home.

Flipping through her notes, she became distracted. She had a great idea for adding a little wow factor to the bedroom.

❄ ❄ ❄

Dawn spotted Jason in his uniform coming down the steps of the small jet disgorging its twenty passengers. She wanted to hurtle herself into his arms, but had already been warned the military frowned on public displays of affection. Apparently, Jason forgot. When she got her breath back, she noticed Dod Henson and Jack Kohl approaching and called out a greeting as Jason took her hand.

They all waited at the conveyor belt that would deposit passenger luggage.

Jason brushed his other hand against her cheek. "What've you been doing while I've been away?"

"Keeping busy."

"How's your psychology class going?"

"Fascinating, but I've discovered another passion."

"What's that?"

She gave him an impish smile. "Wait and see."

When he stepped through the door of the apartment, he stared. "Wow! Did you call in a decorator?"

"Nope. I did it all by myself. I spent less than two hundred dollars on the whole place. What do you think?"

"Classy." He looked closer at the maps on the wall. "Where did you come up with all these ideas?"

"Women's magazines, garage sales . . ."

He stepped around the partition. "I'm impressed." He stared at the ceiling medallion where she'd tucked and hot-glued mosquito netting that draped the top half of the bed. He turned to grin at her. "Reminds me of a pasha's tent. Do you have harem girls in the closet?"

"There's only room for one girl in this apartment, Jason." She stepped close and unfastened the top button on his camouflage shirt. She looked up at him as she unbuttoned the next and the next. "And don't even think about adding another to your life."

Jason swept her up in his arms and tossed her into the middle of the bed. "Not unless we have a daughter."

1992

When she finally started student nursing, Dawn was distressed
to discover that working in a hospital wasn't anything like taking
nursing classes. She could make beds and cheer the patients. She
could do sponge baths and plump pillows. She could take vitals
and fill out charts. But she felt queasy every time she watched a
procedure. When called to help change dressings, she sucked in her
breath every time the patient did. The sight of more than a table-
spoon of blood made yellow and black spots dance before her eyes.

It wasn't her calling. That was the problem. She watched the
other nursing students and knew they loved what they were doing,
while she dreaded every minute. She felt tense and uncomfortable
the moment she stepped into the hospital, afraid she wouldn't be
up to whatever emergency she'd face.

Jason tried to cheer her up. "You should've majored in art and
interior design."

Too late now. Mom and Mitch, Christopher, and Granny came
down together for Dawn's graduation. Georgia arrived a day ahead,

thought the apartment "stunning," and accepted the invitation to sleep on the sofa rather than pay for a motel room.

The rest agreed with Georgia. "I think you missed your calling, Pita."

Great. Just what she needed to hear.

Jason sat proudly in the audience as Dawn received honors for her academic work. He needed another year to finish his engineering degree, especially now that he'd decided to add on a master's.

Christopher begged Dawn and Jason to come home for the summer. Everyone else joined in. Georgia said Kim and Tom were coming home. "She's pregnant."

Dawn couldn't wait for the day when she and Jason could start a family.

Granny patted Jason's arm. "You haven't been out to Jenner since before Papa died." Dawn felt heat flood her face and lowered her head, hoping no one noticed. Granny rushed on. "You two can stay in the downstairs apartment as long as you like, take drives along the coast, walk on the beach. Spend a week . . . or a month."

Mom looked at Dawn. "It'd be nice if you'd spend a few weeks with us, too."

"Don't forget you have a mother, Jason."

Under the table, Jason's hand slid to Dawn's thigh. "Nice to be in such demand." He gave her a teasing smile. "We wouldn't have to pay rent for two months."

❄ ❄ ❄

Dawn and Jason spent the first two weeks with Georgia. Dawn felt odd the first night, sleeping in Jason's old bed with Georgia just across the narrow hall. Both tense, they spoke in whispers and barely touched.

After their stay with Georgia, they moved to Alexander Valley to spend time with Mom, Mitch, and Christopher. Christoper jabbered all through the first dinner and left shortly afterward for an overnight at a friend's house. Dawn insisted on doing the dishes.

When the phone rang, Mom answered. Dawn could tell by her shuttered expression Granny was on the other end of the line.

"They just got here. . . . I don't know. They haven't said anything. They were over at Georgia's for two weeks." She listened for a moment, shoulders drooping. "They have friends to see and things to do. . . . Yes. I know." She looked at Dawn and mouthed, *Granny wants to talk to you.*

Dawn dried her hands and took the phone. Mom went into the family room, where Mitch and Jason were watching a golf tournament. Mitch said something, and Mom sat next to him. He draped an arm around her and she leaned into his side.

Granny wanted to know how soon Dawn and Jason were coming to Jenner. Feeling guilty, Dawn said they wouldn't come for three weeks, at least. So long? Granny didn't try to cover her disappointment. "I'd like to spend as much time with Mom and Mitch and Christopher as I can, Granny."

"Oh. Well. Of course, I understand." Her tone hinted the opposite. "There are three of them to visit with and only one of me."

Dawn winced with guilt. "We could come out for a visit on Saturday."

"I'll fix a nice lunch."

When Dawn told Jason, Mitch gave her an odd look. Mom kept her focus on the television.

Later that night, Jason slipped his arm around her as they lay in bed. "What's with your mom and grandmother?"

"I'm not sure, but I think I'm the bone of contention."

"How so?"

"Mom came home from Haight-Ashbury pregnant. Granny had to give up her nursing career to take care of me."

"Somehow I don't think she minded." He ran a finger over her brow. "Where was your mom while your grandmother was taking care of you?"

"Going to school, working. I think she was trying to piece her life back together."

"She picked a good man to help her."

"Mitch picked *her*. As far as I know, my mother never even went on a date until he rode into town on his motorcycle. He was Uncle Charlie's best friend. He told me once he's been in love with Mom since high school."

"Sounds like someone else I know." Jason leaned down and kissed her.

When he raised his head, she ran her fingers through his short hair. "Mitch is the only person Mom allows close." She sighed. "Mothers and daughters should be close, too. I know Mom and Granny love each other, but they can't talk. I'm not sure who put up the wall first or why. I just wish I knew how to tear it down."

They curled together like two spoons in a drawer. Jason wrapped his arm around her. "Ask God to do it for you."

❄ ❄ ❄

1993

Everyone came for Jason's graduation. Jason wore a black cap and gown to receive his bachelor's and master's diplomas. Later that same day, he wore his Army uniform with red trim and socks to designate he was an engineer. Dawn had never seen him more handsome.

The past year had been difficult, but she knew harder days were to come.

While Dawn sat silent, Jason told everyone what was coming. He had orders to Fort Sill, Oklahoma, where he'd go through three months of basic infantry training. After that, he'd train with the corps of engineers at Fort Leonard Wood in Missouri. Then he could apply for Airborne, Ranger, or Special Forces training.

Granny jumped in and pressed Dawn with advice to quit her nursing job at the clinic and stay at Jenner until Jason had a duty station.

Mom spoke quietly. "That could be months away."

Granny looked annoyed. "It's not easy chasing all over the country. I've done it." She turned to Dawn. "You move into a room somewhere and wait until he has a weekend off. You'll be lonely and depressed."

Jason frowned as though that side of things hadn't even occurred to him until Granny brought it up.

Mom interrupted. "Dawn should decide."

"I wasn't saying she shouldn't. I just think Dawn would be better off spending time with family *now*."

Dawn jumped in before things could get worse. "I've already decided what I'm going to do."

Jason looked at her in surprise. "You have?"

"Yes." She smiled at him, trying to project more confidence than she felt. "Where you go, I go." She glanced around the table, at Mitch, Mom, Christopher, Granny, and Georgia. "I love all of you very much, but Jason is my husband."

"But . . . ," Granny stammered.

"If I have to live in a tent, Granny, it's all right by me. I belong with Jason."

A few seconds of silence could feel like an eternity.

"Okay then." Jason's eyes shone. He took her hand and kissed it.

Granny's shoulders slumped. "Thank God there's no war."

"What, Hildie?" Mitch grinned down the table. "Dawn might strap on a rifle and follow him into battle?"

Everyone laughed, even Granny, though not as brightly. "I shouldn't be surprised. Dawn is my granddaughter." She told the gathering she'd almost enlisted in the nursing corps during World War II, but Trip made her ineligible.

"How'd he do that?" Christopher wanted to know.

"He got me pregnant!"

More laughter resounded around the table. Georgia winked at Dawn. "Now, there's a welcome idea."

❄ ❄ ❄

Dawn put in her two-week notice at the clinic. They offered a bonus if she would stay until they could find a replacement. After discussing it with Jason, Dawn agreed to stay on staff for a month. Jason had his Honda serviced, packed, and headed for Oklahoma, leaving Dawn to decide what to take, sell, or give away before following him to Fort Sill.

Until Jason walked out the door, Dawn had no qualms about the decisions they had made. After he left, she lay awake at night, filled with anxiety. What had ever given her the idea she could drive cross-country alone? What if the car overheated or broke down? What if she ran out of gas on some long stretch across Arizona or New Mexico? Where would she stay when she arrived in Lawton, Oklahoma?

Burying her face in her hands, Dawn prayed. Her mind wandered to Abraham and Sarah. God had told Abraham to go forth from his country, his relatives, and his father's house to the land God would show him. And he'd gone without question, just like Jason. Maybe she should have been like Sarah and gone with him rather than stay behind and follow later.

Lord, help me not to be afraid.

Oma came to mind. She'd never been afraid of anything, had left home at fifteen and gone out alone into the world to make her own way. Oma had lived in Montreaux and then moved to France and on to England. She boarded a ship, crossed the Atlantic, and started all over again in Montreal, Canada. When she married, her husband went off to the wheat fields to work, leaving her behind to run a boardinghouse and then travel by herself with a babe in arms to join her husband. Then she gave birth to Granny in a cabin out in the middle of nowhere—no hospital, no doctor, not even a midwife to help her. Later, with three children, she packed and came with her husband to California, where they lived in a tent before finally having a place of their own.

Fear lost its grip when Dawn thought about her great-grandmother. Granny had always said Oma was hard, but Dawn hadn't found her that way during that week in Merced. Crusty on the outside, perhaps, but she'd revealed a softness inside that had made Dawn wish she'd spent more time with her, gotten to know her better. Still, she had assurance Oma's blood ran in her veins.

God didn't give His children a heart of timidity, but of power and love and discipline. She would get maps, lay out her route, and take the journey one day at a time. What sense did it make to worry about tomorrow?

❄ ❄ ❄

Dawn talked with her mother before setting off. She half hoped Mom would volunteer to come with her. Instead, she talked about Oma. "She loved to take long drives and explore. She would've loved the kind of trip you're going on."

Doodling on a notepad, Dawn tossed out another hint. "It's a little daunting driving so far without any company."

"I know. I did it once."

"You had a friend with you."

"Half-comatose from drugs and alcohol."

"Oh."

"You don't have to go alone, Dawn. You could ask Granny."

Dawn's heart sank, and she rubbed her forehead. "I think I should go alone. I might as well grow up now and not put it off."

"You're growing up quite nicely, May Flower Dawn."

The softly spoken compliment brought tears to Dawn's eyes. "Do you really think so, Mom?" She felt like a baby, wanting to wail.

"Yes. I do. I'm proud of you."

Dawn almost blurted out that she wanted her mother to come with her. She wanted time alone with her so they could talk. She wanted to get to know her mother before they were separated by half a continent. "I'm a little nervous about the trip."

"Understandable, but you won't be alone, Dawn. You're never alone. God is with you. He goes ahead and He watches your back. He walks with you and dwells inside you. Just keep listening to Him."

"I'm glad you finally started believing in God."

"I've believed in Jesus for twenty-four years, Dawn. It's people I never learned to trust. I'll be praying for you. So will Georgia and a host of others. Granny, too. You know that. If you wouldn't mind, I'd like you to call me, let me know how far you make it each day. You don't have to talk long."

"Jason insisted I check in with someone every day."

"Good for Jason."

When they hung up, Dawn finished packing the last few things and went to bed, hoping for a good night's sleep before she set off the next morning. But her mind wouldn't shut down.

Twenty-four years. Isn't that what her mother had said? That would make it right around the time she had gotten pregnant. Maybe it had been the hardship and accidental pregnancy that had driven her mother to her knees. A desperate surrender.

Dawn yearned for the open affection Mom gave Christopher. But at least now her mother felt pride in her. They could talk more. Their best days as mother and daughter had been during the worst time in Dawn's life. Mom had known she grieved over Jason. When she came to Dawn's bedroom that dark night of despair, and Dawn confessed, Mom never spoke a word of condemnation or disappointment. What Mom said helped Dawn change course: *Examine yourself; take what is true and do what's right. And when others hurt you, forgive.*

Maybe someday they'd be able to sit down and really talk. Maybe someday they could go back to the beginning and go deep and rise up out of the pain of the past, together.

DAWN SET OUT early Saturday morning, a disposable camera close at hand. She drove north to Atascadero, cut across to Shandon, and then took the road southeast toward the Central Valley. Orchards covered the area around Blackwells Corner. She pulled in at James Dean's Last Stop and browsed shelves of candy, dried fruit, jars of preserves and salsas, Indian art, and fifties memorabilia. After buying trail mix and a few souvenir postcards, she got back on the road. She passed rows of pink, red, and white rosebushes near Wasco before joining Highway 99 south.

She stopped at a roadside café on the other side of Bakersfield for lunch and studied the map while she ate. Later in the after-noon, she stretched her legs by walking through a Route 66 museum. Heat kept her in the car after that. Finally, as night approached, she could see a dome of light on the horizon. Las Vegas. She drove the Strip and found the hotel where she'd made a reservation.

Tossing her duffel bag on the green paisley spread, she picked up the telephone and punched the number for an open line.

Mom answered on the second ring and sounded relieved when she heard it was Dawn. "Everything go okay today?"

Dawn summarized what she'd seen in less than a minute.

"Are you in a decent place?"

"Clean, good lock, close to the Tropicana. I'm going to walk over there for dinner."

"I'm sorry. I didn't mean to delay you."

Dawn realized how abrupt she must sound. "I didn't mean to . . ." Why was it so much easier to talk to Granny than her mother?

"You go have a nice dinner, Dawn. I'll talk to you in a few days. Call me collect."

After a very reasonably priced buffet dinner, she returned to the hotel and wrote to Jason.

I wish I could sketch like Aunt Rikki. . . . I bought a copy of On the Road by Jack Kerouac. Maybe it will boost my enthusiasm for this trip. . . .

She spent half the next day at Hoover Dam and then drove nonstop to Hurricane, Utah, checked into a hotel, and ate at a small diner next door before calling Granny. She hadn't talked more than five minutes when Granny started worrying about long-distance charges. When she mentioned it again a minute later, Dawn surrendered.

She left early the next morning to see Zion National Park. Mom wanted to hear all about it, but Dawn was too tired to talk long and wanted to get a letter off to Jason before she went to bed.

This will be a short letter, my love. I miss you so much! I wish you were making this trip with me. I'm trying not to rush. I know if I do, I'll just end up sitting alone in an apartment and crying all day. . . .

The farther she drove, the lonelier she felt. She tried not to think how many more days it would take to reach Lawton, Oklahoma. Jason would be living in the barracks for three months. They'd see each other only on weekends.

She thought about her mother trying to keep her on the telephone and Granny trying to hurry her off. It seemed such a turnaround, now that she thought more about it. That night she checked in with Granny first and then called Mom.

"Jason called this afternoon. He gave me the names of two apartment complexes he wants you to check out when you get to Lawton. Both are near the base."

Dawn jotted down the information.

"Did you make it to the Grand Canyon?"

Dawn flopped back on the bed. "I'm about ten minutes away from the south rim. Japanese tourists got there ahead of me." She laughed. "They all had cameras. I had to wait an hour to get close to the rail." Mom kept asking questions and Dawn kept answering.

"Are you planning to stay over tomorrow, see a little more?"

"I don't think so. I want to keep going. I hope to make it to Monument Valley." Dawn heard Mitch talking in the background. "Does he need the phone?" She hadn't talked to her mother this long on a telephone ever.

"No. He just wants to know if you're checking oil and tire pressure and making sure you have plenty of gas before you make those long hauls across the desert."

"Tell him yes. I'm being very conscientious."

The next day seemed to last forever. Monument Valley was an endless expanse. Worried she might overheat the car, she turned off her air-conditioning and opened the window.

Granny let her talk for five minutes that night, then told Dawn she should get a good night's sleep. Dawn hung up and wrote another long letter to Jason.

❄ ❄ ❄

Dawn saw the sign for the turnoff to Mesa Verde National Park and calculated how long it would take to go in, see the ruins and museum, and drive out. *Forget it!* She headed for Durango. She'd had enough of traveling alone. Even if she and Jason couldn't live together, she still wanted to be as close to him as possible. It might cheer him up to know she was ready and waiting when he did get liberty.

Canceling reservations in Pagosa Springs and Albuquerque, Dawn headed for Amarillo, Texas. Other than stopping now and then to use a restroom, check her oil and tire pressure, fill the tank with gas, and have a fast meal, she didn't see anything that held as much interest for her as Jason Steward in Lawton, Oklahoma.

The following afternoon, exhausted, Dawn arrived, checked into a Best Western, and called her mother. "I made it."

"I wondered how long you'd last before you decided to make a run for Lawton. Will you be able to see Jason?"

"Probably not, but at least I'm close to him. When he calls you, give him this number."

Dawn let a hot shower massage her aching muscles. She put on sweatpants and one of Jason's T-shirts and fell asleep on top of the bedspread. Bleary-eyed, she looked at the time and realized she had slept five hours. The sun was going down.

Her motel room phone rang.

"You're *here?*" Jason lowered his voice. "How close?"

"Five minutes from the gate."

He laughed softly. "Didn't see Mesa Verde?"

"Waved as I drove on by."

"Durango?"

"Drove through."

"What happened to seeing some of the country?"

"I'm only interested in one natural wonder. You."

❄ ❄ ❄

Jason's old Honda was parked in the hotel lot when Dawn returned from moving their things into the apartment she'd found. He came out of the office, looking annoyed. She rolled down her window and called out to him. "Hey, handsome!" Grinning broadly, he headed straight for her like an airplane landing on a carrier. He opened her car door. She got out and threw herself into his arms. "I found us an apartment. I moved our stuff in this afternoon. All white and beige . . ."

"Don't waste time or money fixing the place up. Okay? I'm only going to be here two more months and then Missouri."

She closed her eyes. Another long, lonely drive lay ahead of her, but she wouldn't allow herself to think of that now. This was the path Jason had chosen. God had brought them back together so she could walk it with him. When her stomach growled loudly, she grimaced. "I'm so hungry, my stomach is about to digest my lungs."

"We'd better feed you then."

Dawn packed and checked out the next morning. Jason followed in his old Honda and pulled into the space beside her. "Nice complex." He liked the apartment, though after a barracks, he said even the hotel room had been Shangri-la. While Dawn pulled sheets and pillowcases from a box and made up the queen bed, Jason talked about his training, the guys he'd met in the barracks, his instructors. Dawn stowed pots and pans while Jason set up their computer on the nook table.

"We're all moved in." Jason thunked his booted feet on the coffee table and draped his arms over the back of the couch.

Dawn looked at the nook table covered with computer components and printer and wires snaking everywhere. "Not very homey."

"Functional. And we can use the coffee table for dining." He smirked at her when she stared pointedly at his boots. "Or go out."

She sat beside him, tucking herself under his arm. "We need groceries." She looked through the glass doors to the naked patio.

Their home needed color and spots of interest. Two patio chairs and a little table with a potted plant would perk up the outside. A couple of pillows, a simple cabinet to cover all the computer wires, a framed picture, and . . .

Jason gripped her head like a basketball. "I can hear your wheels turning."

❄ ❄ ❄

Monday morning, Dawn awakened alone, puffy-eyed from crying herself to sleep the night before. Jason had stayed as long as he could before heading back to base, but watching him walk out the door left an empty, aching feeling inside her. It would be five days before she saw him again. She remembered what Granny had said about sitting around all day, waiting and feeling lonely and wondering when she'd see her husband.

Standing at the kitchen counter, Dawn ate her eggs and glared at the nook. She had no place to write notes and study her Bible, and the computer was an eyesore. The apartment felt like a beige tomb. She shoved her Bible, journal, and spiral notebook into a backpack and headed out to Cameron University, only a few blocks away.

The college library felt more like home. She found a quiet table where she could read. She felt less lonely with others nearby, comfortable with the studious silence. After an hour, she looked through books on interior design. She made quick sketches and jotted down ideas. The *Lawton Constitution* and *Anadarko Daily News* had a list of upcoming garage sales.

Dawn drove to the base to fill out the paperwork for her ID, then went on a self-guided base tour of grave sites of famous Indians warriors—Geronimo and Kiowa Chief Satanta and Comanche Chief Quanah Parker.

She stopped at a large home improvement center on the way back to the apartment and bought a computer table kit, screwdriver, and small hammer. The store put on workshops for basic carpentry and home repairs. Unfortunately, most were on Saturdays. She asked if they had anything during the week; the clerk said no, but showed her a wall display of how-to books.

Jason called that night. "What did you do today?"

"Explored Lawton and the base. The wind sure blows here." She told him about the Indian Wars, the Chiricahua Apaches. "Did you know Geronimo is buried on Fort Sill?"

Lying alone in bed that night, Dawn stared at the ceiling. During the day, she could keep busy and not feel so alone. When the night rolled in around her, the wind whistling outside, the loneliness blew in and stayed. She imagined Jason lying on his bunk in a barracks full of other soldiers. Bunching up Jason's pillow, she hugged it close.

Seven weeks later, she packed up and followed Jason again.

❄ ❄ ❄

Dear Granny,

Jason and I are now settled in on-base housing at "Fort Lost in the Woods," Missouri. Jason has been told he'll be here for "a while," though that can mean anything from a few weeks to a few years in the Army. Wherever Jason is needed, we'll go.

Driving on snowy roads is an experience. I wouldn't want to drive cross-country this time of year! There'd have to be a good reason! We are looking forward to a white Christmas, though we will miss you and the rest of our family.

We looked for apartments in Devil's Elbow, Hooker,

Gospel Ridge (don't you just love those names!) but decided to choose on-base housing. A two-bedroom, one-bathroom unit opened up. Our little house shares a wall with Ricardo and Alicia Martinez and little Lalo, their adorable two-year-old. Alicia had him outside making snow angels.

Jason sold his old Honda, and we used the money to buy a secondhand bedroom set, an "antique" round oak table with claw feet, and two chairs. We also bought a new sofa and television, which we will pay off quickly now that I have a part-time job at the FLW hospital. . . .

1994

Dawn checked the calendar again, trying not to get her hopes up. When they moved into this little house a year ago, Jason had taken her birth control pills out of the medicine cabinet, looked her square in the eye, and with a grin, tossed them into the bathroom wastebasket. She'd been ecstatic, and she'd expected to get pregnant right away. After six months, she tried not to obsess. They'd thought she might be pregnant once, but the test had come up negative. But each day for the past two weeks, her hopes had been slowly building again. It was time to tell Jason.

Jason came home for lunch, as he did every day. Dawn never got over how handsome he was in his Army combat uniform. He left his hat on the hall table, kissed her, and frowned. "You look awfully pale."

"I'm fine. Just . . . have something on my mind, that's all." She smoothed mayonnaise onto one slice of bread and mustard on another, laid on two thick slices of bologna, tomato, purple onion, lettuce.

Jason sat waiting. "Well?"

"I wondered if you could run an errand for me on your way home tonight." She put Jason's sandwich on a plate and put it in the refrigerator.

Laughing, he got up and retrieved it. "I guess I'd better, because you're obviously not thinking straight. What is it?"

"Well, I thought we might want to take another pregnancy test."

"Really? Okay. Will do. We'll know tonight." He set his plate on the table and made another sandwich for her. "Wait until my mother hears."

"Don't say anything to anyone, Jason." Both sides of the family would be ecstatic. Georgia and Granny had been campaigning for a grandchild since Jason graduated and received his commission. Dawn thought they should wait until Jason received orders for his duty station.

Jason turned her around and kissed her. When she relaxed in his arms, he held her closer, his hands moving up and down her back, then resting on her hips. When he drew back, he gave her a purely male smile. "Doesn't change how we feel."

"Did you think it would?"

"It occurred to me." He put his arm around her. "Maybe you should quit working."

"Let's talk about that when we have a firm answer."

Jason came home with a small plastic bag from the pharmacy. She took it into the bathroom. When she came out, Jason sat on the edge of the bed, head bowed, hands clasped between his knees. She waited until he raised his head.

"Well?" He stared at her intently.

"Which way do you want it to go, Jason?"

He frowned. "Whichever way God wants it." He tucked her hair back. "We can always keep trying."

"You make it sound like work." She ran her hands over his chest. "I guess it is time you took a vacation."

It took him a few seconds to catch her meaning. Then he laughed, lifted her in his arms, and swung her around.

❊ ❊ ❊

Mom didn't shriek like Granny. "I'm happy if you're happy, May Flower Dawn." Dawn knew when her mother used her full name, she felt more deeply than she let on.

"I am happy, Mom. I'm so happy I could burst!"

"We've been thinking about flying out to see you. Would that be all right?"

"Of course!"

"We'll fly into Branson as soon as Christopher is out of school. Second week of June. We'd love to have you and Jason meet us there. We'll put you up in a nice hotel, eat out, and see some shows. You wouldn't have to do a thing."

Dawn chuckled. "Oh. I get it. You don't want to stay in guest housing."

"Oh, we'll come up to Fort Leonard Wood for a few days. You've written about all you've done with the house. I'd like to see it. If that's all right."

"Mom! Of course! Any chance you could bring Granny with you? She's been wanting to come, but she's never been on an airplane before." Nearing eighty, she was afraid to come alone. "We could help pay for her plane ticket."

A momentary silence. "No, that's fine, Dawn. We can take care of her ticket. I'm sure Granny would love to come along. Do you want to call and tell her? Or shall I?"

Dawn heard the subtle change in her mother's voice, then realized she had hurt her feelings. "I'll leave it up to you, Mom. I'm sorry. I shouldn't have asked."

"No. I should have thought of it first." Voices in the background. "Christopher wants to talk to you." Mom was gone, and Dawn's little brother took her place. Although Dawn had to remind herself that he wasn't "little" anymore; he'd just turned fifteen. And he'd been taller than she was the last time she'd seen him.

He talked nonstop for five minutes, excited about soccer, excited about summer, excited about coming to see her and Jason.

"I want to see the Indian caves. . . ." Dawn heard Mom say something to him. "Mom said to tell you she'll call Granny as soon as we're off the phone."

Granny called an hour later, excited but nervous about flying, eager to see Dawn and Jason. "I hope we'll have a little one-on-one time together, honey. I've missed you so much."

One-on-one time meant cutting Mom out.

"I always end up hurting one of them," Dawn told Jason over dinner.

"You probably won't get any time alone with your mother."

"No." Dawn cleared dishes. "I won't." She had only herself to blame for that.

❄ ❄ ❄

Granny, Mom, Mitch, and Christopher visited for only four days. It was nerve-racking trying to make sure she had time with Granny *and* Mom. She never had to worry about how to entertain Mitch and Christopher. They took off to see the Indian caves or talked Jason into going bowling "so the girls can talk."

Granny talked. Mom didn't get the chance to say much of anything.

Mom went out for long walks every afternoon. She always retreated when she felt uncomfortable. Dawn wondered if she did it so Granny could have more time with Dawn. If so, Granny didn't return the favor. Even when the three of them sat together, the men off somewhere, Granny dominated the conversation, asking questions or reminiscing about Dawn as a baby, a toddler, a child.

Dawn was certain that they loved each other. They just didn't know how to talk to each other. There was a lot of unfinished business between them. And she was a big part of it.

She hadn't realized how stressful it would be having Mom and Granny together for four days. Not that anything untoward had been said. Jason had to get up early, and he found it hard to keep his eyes open after nine o'clock. Mitch would suggest it was time to head back to the Ramada Inn. Mom would then ask Granny if she was ready to go. It became a ritual, leaving it up to Granny to decide.

If there had been an extra bed in the second room instead of the new crib, Dawn would have asked Mom to spend the night. With Granny, Mitch, and Christopher back at the Ramada Inn, maybe she and Mom could've talked more.

Her mother never said much, but what she said counted.

❄ ❄ ❄

Over the next few days, Dawn couldn't shake the feeling something was wrong. Granny called to thank her for the wonderful time. Now that Granny had been on an airplane, she might make the next trip on her own. "Your mom can drive me to the airport."

Mom called, but didn't talk long. Christopher talked for half an hour. He hadn't cared all that much about the bright lights and entertainment in Branson, but he'd loved hanging out with Jason and hiking with Dad. They'd explored the bluffs above the Big Piney.

Dawn went to bed shortly after dinner. Jason followed. "Are you okay, honey?"

"Just tired." Lying on her side, she went over her prayer list. She didn't make it halfway through before sleep pulled her down.

She stood knee-deep in murky swamp water, surrounded by cypress trees with low-hanging Spanish moss. Something moved close by, rippling the water and making her heart quicken with fear. She moved carefully forward toward a savanna with solid ground and grassland undulating like a golden sea. The thick mud pulled at her feet. She managed another step. Gasping, she went deeper, the dark water around her rib cage. Her body felt like a heavy weight. Something slick slithered between her legs. Grasping hold of a cypress root, she kicked free. A broad, diamond-shaped head appeared, black eyes staring at her. The huge snake coiled around her middle. She groaned as the pain grew worse. She couldn't get her breath.

A hand moved across her face. "Dawn." Jason caressed her cheek. "Wake up, honey. You're having a bad dream."

She stared into the darkness; her heart still pounded. "Hold me, Jason."

Jason tucked her into him. Wide-awake now, she felt it again. No dream this time. Her abdomen cramped. Searing pain spread downward. "Jason . . ."

Jason turned on the light. When she pushed the covers off, he sucked in his breath. "Don't move! I'm calling 911."

❄   ❄   ❄

Dawn awakened in a hospital room, white ceiling overhead, white curtain blocking her view, an IV drip hanging beside the bed. A monitor beeped. Somewhere close by, Jason talked in a low voice, tone questioning. A stranger answered. ". . . lost a lot of blood. . . . couple more hours in recovery. . . . taking precautions. . . . Try not to worry. . . ."

Jason stepped around the curtain. He looked haggard and pale, but his expression filled with relief when he met her eyes. "You're awake. Are you in pain?"

"No." But she felt so tired she didn't think she could move.

He took her hand and kissed it. "You're going to be all right."

She knew what that meant. She couldn't see him through her tears. "Our baby, Jason," she sobbed. "I lost our baby."

Jason slipped his arms around her, and he held her close, his voice raspy. "I almost lost you."

The nurse came in and added something to the IV. "She'll sleep now."

Dawn fought to keep her eyes open. "You should go home, Jason."

"I'm staying."

She awakened on the gurney as they moved through the

hospital corridor to another room. Two orderlies lifted her gently onto a bed. Jason stepped around one of them and took her hand again. A nurse tucked warm covers around her, checked her vitals and the IV.

Rousing again later, she saw Jason in a chair beside her bed. He slept with his head on his crossed arms. Running her hand over the short-cropped hair, she thanked God she had a husband who loved her enough to stay so long at her side. He woke and leaned over her. "Do you need anything?"

"No." Just him.

He sat down again and took her hand, rubbing it against his cheek. He needed a shave.

"You must be AWOL."

"I called Cap." Jason put his hand on her forehead. "Good. No fever." He let out a deep breath. He looked older than his twenty-six years. "Try to go back to sleep. Everything's going to be okay."

Okay? Without their baby?

Once, at fifteen, she had feared she might be pregnant. Now, Dawn wondered if she and Jason would ever have children. God willing, someday. She would hold on to that hope.

❄ ❄ ❄

Alicia came over to visit. Watching Lalo play made Dawn feel her loss more acutely. She grieved even more when she went to the commissary and saw young mothers with babies. Unwilling to burden Jason with her emotional state, she called Granny, who told her it wasn't unusual to have a miscarriage and not to let it get her down. Then she talked about how wonderful it would be when Dawn had babies, how she'd forget all about the pain of losing this one.

On the phone, Mom listened while Dawn talked. Dawn had to ask her to say something. "I turned away from the Lord, Dawn, and I learned my lesson. I turned back because He was the only One who understood. He became my comfort."

Dawn hadn't opened her Bible in a week. "Why did you turn away?"

"I was afraid of Him."

Dawn had learned to wait until Mom was ready to speak. Mom wasn't uncomfortable with silence the way Granny was.

"I didn't think God loved me. I thought everything that happened to me was punishment because I couldn't measure up."

"But now you know that's not true. Don't you?"

"Do you?"

Dawn cried then. She'd been asking herself for weeks what she had done wrong. "Oh, Mom . . ." Shoulders heaving, she sobbed into the telephone.

"I learned God loves me. Even when I felt down for the count, May Flower Dawn. He loves you that way, too. He'll lift you up. Just hold out your hands and give your sorrow to Him."

48

1996

Jason got orders for Fort Bragg, North Carolina. Dawn admonished herself for being surprised. After three years at Fort Leonard Wood, she forgot Jason could be transferred anytime and anywhere the Army wanted. She'd just put in roses. She wouldn't be around when they bloomed.

The inspecting officer came through. All the walls would have to be repainted white. She had known the rules, but the thought of her hard work being undone depressed her.

Jason hired two privates to paint the interior walls on their off-duty hours. They needed the extra money. Dawn needed their help. The Army movers arrived. Dawn supervised. She had all the boxes labeled and kept an inventory list in her purse. As soon as the moving van left, Jason and Dawn threw two suitcases into the trunk of the Sable and headed out.

Jason had leave before reporting in at Fort Bragg. So they took the scenic route, wanting to see more of the country on the way. They spent nights in St. Louis, Nashville, and Chattanooga. After

the flatlands and wind of Fort Sill and the low hills and bluffs
of Fort Leonard Wood, Dawn drank in the beauty of the Great
Smoky Mountains. They took their time driving the Blue Ridge
Parkway, stopping at overlooks, snapping pictures of one another,
and staying two nights in a bed-and-breakfast. Fall had come with
a burst of reds, oranges, and yellows among the myriad evergreens.

❆ ❆ ❆

Fort Bragg wasn't like little Fort Lost in the Woods. It had over
170,000 inhabitants, schools, churches, hospitals, golf courses,
bowling alleys, and theaters. It even had a mall! While Jason
worked, Dawn drove around, getting acclimated to her new
surroundings. When the Sable broke down, Jason decided it was
time to sell it and buy another car. Dawn spotted a van and said it
would come in handy when she started going to garage and estate
sales. Jason took it for a test drive, had a mechanic look it over, and
made an offer. After a few months, with things so spread out, Jason
decided they both needed transportation and bought a used GMC
Jimmy. Dawn teased him about his "cheap jeep."

Their new house was twice the size of the last.

Uninspired, she made a replica of their last master bedroom,
turned another into an office, and left the door of the last bedroom
closed. The living room looked bare and uninteresting. She needed
to find one piece of *something* to inspire her, so she drove eighty
miles up to Raleigh to see an art sale. Within the first hour, she
found what she needed to fire her imagination: an oil-painted
reproduction of John William Waterhouse's *Knight.* The handsome
young man in full armor sat on a stone wall, his sword set aside, a
beautiful red-haired lady kneeling at his feet with her hand over his
and an expression of adoration.

"You like that, huh?" The vendor, an old man with thinning
gray hair and one arm missing, said he had worked twenty years for
a museum in New York, painting reproductions of various masters.

"It's gorgeous." She could see the whole living room coming together around it.

He wanted three hundred dollars for the painting. Dawn's heart sank. He might as well have asked for a million. Dawn smiled with regret, told him it was worth that and more. Unfortunately a knight's wife couldn't afford it.

She searched for two more hours and came up empty-handed. She had to get home so she'd be in time to fix dinner.

"Milady," the old vendor called to her as she came abreast of his booth. "I still have it."

Surprised, she walked over. "No offers at all?"

"Oh, I had offers, but none that made me want to hand it over. I took a lot of time on this one. It's special." The old man propped it up so she had to look at it again. "Is your husband as handsome as the knight?"

Dawn studied the painting and smiled. "As handsome as that knight is, mine is more so. Thanks for letting me look at it again. I know you'll find the right buyer." She started to walk away.

He called after her. "Where would you hang it if you could afford it?"

She turned and looked at him. "In the living room, of course, where everyone would see it first thing when they walked in. And I'd tell everyone who did the reproduction, if he gave me his card."

"Well, that's a whole lot better than having it hang in a guest room." He wagged his fingers at her. "Give me whatever you've got before I change my mind. Okay, okay. Calm down. You're welcome. I'll even wrap it for you."

Dawn drove home, singing praise songs. She couldn't wait to get started!

Jason noticed the painting when he walked in the door. He stood in the living room staring at it. Dawn slipped her arm through his. "Romantic, isn't it?"

He grinned at her. "I can hardly wait to see what you do with the rest of the place."

A laugh bubbled out of her. "A man's home should be his castle. Don't you think?"

He pulled her close. "It's good to hear you laugh again, Dawn."

They both knew why she hadn't.

❊ ❊ ❊

1997

They'd been stationed at Fort Bragg six months when Dawn took a home pregnancy test. She hadn't mentioned the morning sickness. She didn't want to get Jason's hopes up or worry him. When she checked the test results, joy flooded her. Fear quickly followed. She saw it in Jason's eyes, too, when she told him the news.

He pulled her close. "If you are pregnant, you're quitting work. We're not taking any chances."

She'd already decided that. Two ladies from her Wednesday Bible study had offered to pay her to help decorate their houses, so they could easily do without her part-time nursing income.

Jason held her hand tightly in the examining room as the nurse practitioner moved the monitor over Dawn's abdomen. They both heard the baby's heartbeat at the same time. Jason frowned. "It's so fast." The nurse and Dawn smiled and assured him it should be.

Jason wanted to call their families that night, but Dawn asked him to wait. He asked why. "I don't know, Jason. I just . . . I don't know." She couldn't dispel the feeling something might go wrong.

At five months, Jason insisted. "You're fine. You haven't been sick for two months. The baby is growing. So are you!"

Dawn gave in.

Georgia and Granny were ecstatic. So were Christopher and Mitch. When Mom came on the phone, Dawn poured out her fears. Mom didn't dismiss them. "I'll pray for you, May Flower Dawn." Dawn knew it wasn't a platitude.

Granny called every few days to check on her. Dawn called Mom and did most of the talking.

At six months, Dawn sensed something wrong. The flutters had stopped. Rather than wait for her scheduled checkup, she called the doctor. Jason went with her. The stethoscope felt ice-cold on her abdomen. The doctor moved it several times, listening intently. His expression became increasingly grim. Jason stroked her shoulders. "It's going to be okay," he said again and again, like a litany of prayer.

When the doctor straightened, Dawn held her breath. "I'm sorry." He looked at Jason first, then Dawn. "There's no heartbeat."

Jason stood silent, his hands gripping her shoulders. He looked down at her, love and tears spilling from his eyes. "It's going to be okay, Dawn."

She sobbed. They both knew nothing was okay.

The doctor admitted Dawn to the hospital and induced labor. Dawn gave birth to a perfectly formed little boy who weighed just under two pounds.

It would take longer to get over the loss this time.

❄ ❄ ❄

Jason took Dawn home to California for Christmas. They spent the first few nights with Georgia, Christmas Eve and Day with Mom, Mitch, and Christopher, home on break from his first year at Stanford.

Granny came in from Jenner, but kept pressing them to come out and stay with her on the coast. Approaching her eighty-first birthday, she had aged. Her hair was almost completely gray now, and she bore signs of osteoporosis. Mom, who had turned fifty last spring, still wore long, colorful tiered skirts and tunics with leather belts. Her hair had streaks of silver. Mom still didn't ask for Granny's help, and Granny no longer offered. Dawn could see the rift had widened. Granny talked to Dawn and spared some attention for Jason, Mitch, and Christopher. Mom listened from the kitchen.

No one talked about the baby, though Dawn knew her stillborn son was on everyone's mind. Christopher sat beside her on the couch and took her hand. He had grown six inches since she last saw him. He called her his little-big sister now. He had Mitch's dark red hair and their mother's blue eyes. "You're turning into a hunk, Chris."

Mitch laughed. "He's got girls calling him all the time. The phone hasn't stopped ringing since he got home last week."

Christopher blushed to the roots of his hair.

"Good for you. You've always been good at making friends." Dawn tried to keep things light. It was Christmas, after all. Had all gone well, she would have had a newborn in her arms.

And a child shall be born to you . . .

Jason agreed to go to Jenner. They spent the last four days with Granny. Dawn and Jason walked on the beach every afternoon. They sat on the sand and watched the waves. On the last night, he went to bed before she did. Granny broached the subject everyone else had avoided. "You'll have a baby, Dawn. I know it. I feel it!"

Dawn cried and blew her nose. She felt like Hannah in the Old Testament, begging God for a child. "It's up to God, Granny. I have to accept that it may not be His will for me."

"Nonsense. You have time, honey. You're young. Keep trying."

Dawn knew trying wasn't the answer. God was. And she was going to trust Him with her future, no matter how difficult it might be right now.

On the long flight home, Dawn dreamed she sat on the beach north of Goat Rock. The wind blew warmer than usual, sun sparkling off turquoise and green waves. Dawn felt the wind in her hair, the sun on her face. Granny and Mom sat nearby, talking together as they never had before. A little girl with long blonde hair pranced along the edge of the waves. Water splashed up like white flashing lights around the child's knees. She flapped her arms like a bird learning to fly. Now and then, she stooped and picked up a sea-washed rock, a bit of driftwood, a seagull feather, then raced up the beach to show off her treasures. Dawn got up and went down to join the child. She danced with her in the frothy, foaming waves. She felt happy. She felt free.

Dawn awakened in the darkness, the hum of jet engines

soothing. Jason slept, his knees wedged against the seat in front of him. She saw the moon outside the airplane window and city lights below. She felt at peace for the first time since losing the baby, hope rising inside her like a sunrise.

Jason awakened and took her hand. "Are you okay?"

"Yes." More than okay. "I had a wonderful dream, Jason." She told him all about it.

"Sounds like a promise."

"It was."

❄ ❄ ❄

1998

Dawn painted the spare bedroom a pale pink. She added furnishings: a crib; a white dresser; a gliding rocker; a plush, pale blue area rug. She hung an embroidered alphabet sampler she found at a garage sale.

As each month passed, Jason seemed less certain. He brought up adoption. She said, yes, that was something they might consider. Eventually. His suggestion didn't diminish her faith. The dream would come to pass. In God's perfect timing—not hers, not Jason's.

"You know I can get transferred at any time, Dawn."

"I know."

"You're putting a lot of time in that bedroom." The house didn't belong to them. "We may have to move. What then?"

"We'll take the furniture. I'll start over."

Jason's six-year commitment to the Army was coming to an end, too. By next year he would need to make a decision about his future. They talked about what Jason could do as a civilian. The opportunities seemed endless.

"If I stay in the Army, I'd only have fourteen more years before I could retire. I'd still be young enough to start another career." She asked if that's what he wanted, if he believed that was what God wanted him to do. Jason said yes.

"We may still get transferred, Dawn. There's no guarantee we're going to stay here."

Dawn knew what really worried Jason, what worried him all the time. He feared she might be crushed if she didn't become pregnant again soon. She told him God was sovereign. God was trustworthy. Whatever happened, they could trust God with the outcome. Even so, she kept the door to the baby's room closed, so he wouldn't have the constant reminder. She held God's promise close to her heart.

Even after a year, Dawn didn't lose hope.

When two passed, then three, the ache grew, but her faith didn't diminish.

49

2001

Dolores, one of Dawn's Bible study ladies, called. She sounded on the verge of hysteria. "Are you watching your television?"

"No. Why?"

"Two airliners just crashed into the twin towers of the World Trade Center!"

Dawn sat frozen in front of the television for the rest of the day. She watched the World Trade Center buildings crumble in a cloud of dust and debris over and over. She listened to minute-by-minute reports on how terrorists had hijacked two airliners out of Boston, another hijacked jetliner crashed into the Pentagon, and a fourth went down in a Pennsylvania field after passengers on board the aircraft called family members on cell phones and learned how the other airliners had been used. They fought back, or the fourth plane might have gone into the White House. No one knew yet how many had died. Fifty thousand people worked in and around the World Trade Center.

The front door opened. Dawn jumped up. "Jason!" She flew into his arms.

He held her close for a minute, rubbing his chin on the top of her head. "How long have you been watching the news?"

"All day. Jason, what does this mean for us?"

"We're at war. That's what it means."

"Will you have to go?"

"We'll have to find out who we're fighting and where, first."

Airports shut down. President George Bush flew into New York and stood at ground zero speaking to the rescue workers. He assured them the nation was on bended knee in prayer. When some cried out because they couldn't hear, Bush said *he* could hear *them*, everyone could hear them, and those who had knocked down the buildings "will hear all of us soon!"

People chanted, "USA, USA . . ."

President Bush called out, "God bless America," a hope all would cling to in the coming days.

Dawn spent her days reading newspaper stories about heroes: a man who stayed behind to help another man in a wheelchair— both died when the buildings crumbled; firefighters and police officers who worked tirelessly searching for survivors; cadaver dogs and their handlers searching the rubble. The Salvation Army responded to the tragedy. New Yorkers pulled together.

War loomed, but against what country?

Jason was deployed to New York to work with civil engineers. The mammoth job of clearing a city block began. Jason would be gone for months, maybe more if terrorists found other ways to blow up more Americans. Every newscaster speculated on what terrorists might do next—poison water systems, unleash deadly viruses, tote backpack-size atomic bombs.

People flooded into the churches for the first few weeks. Crowds dwindled after three months.

Jason came home to Fort Bragg on weekend leave, burning with anger against Osama bin Laden, who had denied responsibility for the attacks, though the U.S. government still considered him the prime suspect.

Exhausted, he slept twenty-four hours straight, leaving only half a day before he had to go back. "Why didn't you wake me up?" Dawn said she'd come to him next time. Jason ordered her to stay home. He didn't want her in New York. He wasn't sure he wanted her at Fort Bragg. What better target for another attack than one of the biggest military bases in the world? He wanted her to go home. She said no. They argued. She cried after he left.

Jason returned to Fort Bragg after three months away. He and Dawn flew home for Christmas again. CCC was packed with new people. "You should have seen it after 9/11," Mitch told them. Chris asked a dozen questions. Jason made it clear he didn't want to talk about what he'd seen at ground zero. Granny worried about war and what part Jason would have to play in it. Dawn still prayed diplomacy would work. Mitch and Jason talked behind closed doors. Mom and Dawn had tea and didn't talk at all.

❄ ❄ ❄

2002

When Dawn and Jason returned to Fort Bragg, Jason bought a new laptop computer and a Rosetta Stone program on Arabic. "If I get sent anywhere, it'll be the Middle East."

Everyone knew it was only a matter of time before the Army started deploying troops. America couldn't ignore the murder of three thousand citizens. It was a miracle there hadn't been tens of thousands. But three thousand was more than the number of lives lost at Pearl Harbor, and the country couldn't let it go.

Dawn knew the waiting had come to an end when Jason came home and said he had orders to Fort Dix, New Jersey. Dawn packed and followed. She rented a two-bedroom, one-bathroom bungalow off base. She didn't paint the walls. Every hour with Jason was too precious to waste.

❄ ❄ ❄

2003

The first U.S. troops were deployed to the Persian Gulf region on January 1. On March 17, President Bush issued an ultimatum to Saddam Hussein, giving him forty-eight hours to leave the country or face war. On March 19, the deadline passed, and Operation Iraqi Freedom began. By April, they took Baghdad and toppled Saddam Hussein's statue to Iraqi and American cheers.

The hunt for weapons of mass destruction intensified. Hussein had used chemical weapons on the Kurds. Had he buried bombs in the desert the same way he had buried airplanes? Had they been sold and scattered to neighboring countries? Or had it all been an empty boast by a mad dictator?

May rolled around, and Jason received orders for deployment to Iraq. Dawn wept. They made love the way they had when they were first married—hungry, with abandon. They said everything they wanted to say to one another, knowing they might never have another opportunity.

"It's up to God." He held her close. "There's a time for peace, and there's a time for war. Remember Nehemiah. He ordered the people to keep their weapons close at hand while they worked. The biggest job we're going to face in Iraq is rebuilding the country, giving the Iraqi people the protection and resources they need to hold on to the freedom they've never had before. I'll have my weapon strapped to me, Dawn. We're trained to watch each other's back."

Jason wanted no public displays of affection when she saw him off. She had to be brave and tearless for his sake. He kissed her. "Write to me." He spoke roughly, his hands gripping her head. He kissed her again. "I'll e-mail you when I can."

She took his hand in both of hers before he walked away. "May the Lord bless you and keep you, Jason. He goes ahead of you. He stands at your side. He dwells within you. He is your rear guard." And though she saw tears in his hazel eyes, she smiled at him and said the rest. "This isn't our home, Jason. Heaven is. And there, nothing can ever part us."

❄ ❄ ❄

Two months later, at the end of July, Dawn sent her sixtieth e-mail, knowing it might be days before Jason could read it.

> God is good, Jason. He always keeps His promises. Our baby is due on Valentine's Day. The doctor won't know the baby's gender for a few more months, but I told him God already promised us a little girl. She's going to have blonde hair, and she's going to run on the beach, collect rocks and seashells and bird feathers, and dance at the edge of the sea. . . .

Jason e-mailed whenever he could.

> Hey, Mama, I miss you so much I ache. I started a Bible study with three men in my unit. We're rebuilding a hospital. We're reading Nehemiah. Thought it appropriate. We do a lot of praying as we work.
> . . . went into one of Saddam Hussein's palaces. Marble floors, mosaics, pillars, fountains—the guy had it. Figured he was the next Nebuchadnezzar. Must have forgotten the end of the story—the king on his hands and knees eating grass like an animal. God said pride comes before a fall.
> I wish I could see you getting as round as a pumpkin, big as a house, weighing in at 185 with my baby inside you. . . .

Dawn wrote letters every day. She wanted Jason to have something at mail call, not just on his computer.

> *Hello, my love.*
> *I went for my checkup this morning and heard our daughter's heartbeat. I may not weigh 185 pounds yet, but*

everything is fine. I walk two miles every evening (yes, dear, before it gets dark). Since everyone works, this is the best time to meet people.

Only Maura Kerwin and LaShaye Abbot have come for tea. Neither is ready to commit to a Bible study. Maura's husband (Mick) just got shipped over. LaShaye is pregnant for the third time in four years. They're still paying hospital bills for the last baby. Rory told her to get an abortion. I got weepy and told them about our lost babies. LaShaye left.

I keep remembering the prayer Mom gave me when you and I weren't seeing each other. "God, grant me the serenity to accept the things I can't change, the courage to change the things I can, and the wisdom to know the difference. Thy will, not mine, be done." I've been saying it a lot lately. . . .

❄ ❄ ❄

A suicide bomber blew himself up in the middle of a market this morning. He took innocent women and children with him. All in the name of his god! These people need to hear the gospel, and we're forbidden to evangelize. I'll probably get busted, but I'm not going to be silent when given an opportunity to talk about the difference between Allah and Jesus. Only Christ can make men free! The enemy of our souls wants to keep these people captive. . . .

LaShaye didn't come for tea. So I dropped by. She
couldn't even look at me. I told her I love her and I'm praying for her. If she ever wants to talk, my door is open. She
closed hers, and I haven't seen her since. Maura came.
She and LaShaye were friends long before I came on the
scene. Maura took her to the clinic.

I pray. I still take my walks.

Picture attached. Notice the nice little bulge under my
new sweater!

Thanks for the photo! You look beautiful. But so thin!
You look like you're losing weight instead of gaining. Are
you eating enough? Maybe you shouldn't be walking so
much. . . .

I don't have to look like a pumpkin or a house to be
healthy, Jason. I'm eating constantly. I don't know why I'm
not gaining a lot of weight. Must be my metabolism. The
doctor said walking is good for me. Don't worry—I'm not
overdoing it.

Good news! LaShaye came over. We talked for hours!
She and Rory are struggling. I found a crisis pregnancy
center in the area. They have a postabortion class. I said
I'd take her and sit with her if that would help. I'm praying
LaShaye and Rory can work things out. They have enough
grief between them without discarding their marriage.

I have another checkup tomorrow. I know everything
is fine, Jason. I've been feeling our little girl move for a
couple weeks now. Only four months to go before I meet
her face-to-face.

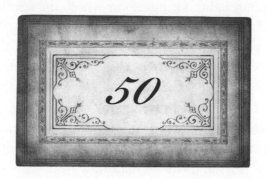

50

Dawn gulped down sobs as she headed home from her prenatal appointment. The doctor had put her through a battery of tests over the last two weeks and insisted that she see a specialist besides. He gave her the results this morning. "We have a problem. . . ." She had sat stunned and silent as he talked in quiet, grim tones, hands folded on his desk. "I advise you not to wait, Dawn. I know it's going to be difficult for you, especially with your history, but the alternative is—"

"You don't need to say any more!" Dawn had stood abruptly, slinging her bag over her shoulder with shaking hands.

"Please sit down, Mrs. Steward. We need to discuss this. The longer you wait, the more—"

"I understand everything you've said, Doctor. I was a nurse." And she wouldn't do it! She'd rather die than do it.

She yanked the door open and walked out.

Two other pregnant mothers sat in the waiting room. Dawn managed to get out the door before the tears came. She sat in her car until she thought she had regained enough control to drive home. Now she couldn't even see the road. Swiping tears away, she pulled onto the shoulder, jammed on her parking brake, and put on her emergency lights. Gripping the wheel, she screamed. "Why, Lord? Why? *I don't understand!*"

Cars flew past. Sobbing, Dawn ran her hands over the slight bulge in her belly. A police officer tapped on her window. She hadn't even noticed the cruiser pull in behind her. She let her window down and fumbled through her shoulder bag for her license. She found the car registration in the glove compartment. He glanced at them and handed them back. Leaning down, he looked at her. "Anything wrong, ma'am?"

"I've just had some very bad news." She gulped down sobs. "I'm sorry. I just thought it'd be safer for everyone if I sat here for a little while. Is that okay?" She wiped her cheeks.

"I noticed the Fort Dix base sticker on your car."

"My husband's in Iraq."

"Sit until you're ready, ma'am." The officer walked back to his cruiser. She glanced in the rearview mirror. He talked into his radio. She thought he'd drive away, but he didn't. Regaining some control over her emotions, Dawn took the brake off, put on her blinker, and pulled out onto the highway again. The police cruiser pulled out right behind her. He stayed with her all the way to off-base housing, gave her a salute, and kept going.

Dawn raised her hand in thanks. *God puts angels all around us. Some in uniform.*

Dumping her keys on the coffee table, Dawn sank onto the couch. She felt her baby move and ran her hand over her abdomen. "What am I going to tell your daddy, sweetie?" She hadn't mentioned the tests to Jason. Why worry him? He needed to keep his mind on what was happening around him, not on her and the baby. Now, she didn't dare tell him.

Lord, help me. Please help me.

Someone knocked on the door. Dawn didn't answer. They knocked again. She waited before going to the front door. Peering through the peephole, she watched LaShaye walk down the path to the sidewalk where Maura stood waiting. They both talked for a few minutes, then went their separate ways.

Dawn went into the bathroom, turned on the shower, and undressed while she waited for the water to get warm. Stepping in, she closed the glass door and let the water rain down on her.

Lord, You breathed out the universe. You made the stars in the heavens, the earth, everything. Nothing is too difficult for You! You made me Your vessel. Your Holy Spirit lives within me. You opened my womb so I could carry this child. You showed her to me. I saw my daughter on the beach, dancing, flapping her arms like a little bird. She is strong. She is full of the life You gave her. Oh, God, You are merciful! Please. Be merciful.

She didn't stop praying or get out of the shower until the warm water gave out.

❄ ❄ ❄

Dawn fixed a square meal and sat alone in the dining room. She needed to eat, whether she felt like it or not. She and the baby needed nourishment. The telephone rang.

I'm not ready to talk, Lord, not to anyone but You.

The answering machine picked up. "It's Granny, sweetheart. Just thinking about you and wanted to talk. You said something about joining the choir. You're probably at church. Call back when you have a minute. I love you."

Church. She'd forgotten about the choir. Those sweet old ladies would take one look at her and want to know what was wrong. They'd have all kinds of wisdom to share.

She'd already made her decision. No matter what the doctor said, she would have this baby. She'd face everything else later.

She had to e-mail Jason. If a day passed and she didn't, he would wonder why. He always checked dates. Did he look at the times, too? It was getting late. She put her dish and utensils in the dishwasher, then went to the computer.

What was she going to say to him? She didn't like keeping

secrets from her husband, but she couldn't write about what she'd been told today.

Hands resting on the keyboard, she tried to think. She double-clicked the e-mail icon; nothing from Jason today, but several others, including one from her brother. Christopher wrote like he talked. He was taking classes part-time toward a master's degree. He had a job at a trendy, expensive restaurant.

> Hardest part of the job is warding off advances from cougars. Even when I turn them down, they leave nice tips. I'll have enough saved to go to London this summer.

Leaning on her elbows, Dawn rubbed her temples.

I will trust in You, Lord, no matter what happens. I believe the dream You gave me on the airplane about our little girl. I believe, Father! Oh, God, help my unbelief.

Dawn clicked *New Mail* and typed *Ja* and Jason's address filled the send-to line. Subject? *How do I love thee? Let me count the ways.* Words flowed out of her as she recounted the first time she'd seen Jason in the high school corridor, then being dragged by Christopher to CCC VBS and working with Jason. His faith and dedication to God had awed her. She had felt blessed every time he told her he loved her. When they broke up, she set her heart and mind upon becoming like the wife in Proverbs 31, a woman of character, substance, faith, and purpose—for God and for whomever He might have in store for her, never dreaming He would give the two of them a second chance. She reminisced about their wedding day and the intense joy he'd given her on their wedding night and every time he'd made love to her since.

> I just miss you so much, Jason. I wish I could curl up with your arms around me. I wish . . .

Weeping, Dawn got up without sending the message. She puttered, fluffing pillows, wandering through the house, trying to step back, trying to think more clearly and not allow her emotions to rule. After an hour, she went back and reread what she had written. He would know something was wrong. She deleted everything and started again.

> I saw the doctor again today. Our daughter is strong and healthy. I can feel her moving inside me right now as I write this note. Maybe she's waving hello to her daddy. Your wife and daughter have both had a big day today. I'm exhausted. I'm going to make this short and head for bed.
>
> I love you so much, Jason. I pray constantly that God will command angels to guard you. Remember Elisha and how he opened Gehazi's eyes so he could see the fiery chariots all around? The Lord is with you. He hears our prayers. I'll love you forever, Jason.
>
> Always yours,
> Dawn

❄ ❄ ❄

Dawn dreamed about Granny and Mom. They argued over something, but Dawn couldn't hear what. They turned their backs to one another, both weeping. Dawn wanted to call out to them, but she'd lost her voice.

She awakened as the sun came in the window. It had snowed the night before, and everything lay beneath a cover of white. She sat at the dining room table, where she could see everything, and opened her Bible. She couldn't get Granny and Mom out of her mind. She felt an intense longing for both of them. She wasn't Moses, but wouldn't it be nice to have her mother holding up one arm and Granny holding up the other as Dawn beseeched God for victory in the battle she now faced? But another picture came to mind. Granny pulling one way and Mom the other.

❄ ❄ ❄

2004

Dawn had made excuses not to fly home for the holidays. Just before Thanksgiving, she'd passed the six-month mark in her pregnancy and breathed easier. The baby had an excellent chance of survival now, even if she should come early. But Dawn still prayed every day for a full-term, healthy delivery for their daughter.

Mom had said she'd fly to Newark when Dawn got closer to delivery. And then, just as she always did, Dawn had said it would be nice to have Granny come, too.

Why did she have to choose between them?

As Christmas came and went, she found herself wishing she were at home. Now, January rolled around. She'd have a birthday soon. *What do I do, Lord?* Dawn covered her face. *Lord, I want to go home!*

She couldn't fly now. It was too risky to fly at seven and a half months. She could drive. Four thousand miles alone, in winter? Jason would have a fit!

Jason didn't have to know.

Dawn shrugged into her heavy parka and went out for a walk. It was midmorning. Blank spaces on the street showed where cars had been during the snowfall last night. Everyone had gone to work by now. Maura worked at a co-op preschool. LaShaye never stepped outside her door. *Okay, Lord, if I'm supposed to drive home to California, Maura and LaShaye will be home and both will want to talk with me.*

She'd just passed LaShaye's when the front door opened. "Dawn! Wait a minute!" LaShaye hurried down the path to the sidewalk. "You look awful. Is Jason all right?"

"He's fine."

She took Dawn by the arm. "Come inside out of the cold. I'll fix some tea. Tell me what's going on." The phone was ringing when they walked in. Maura wanted to come over.

An hour later, they all sat crying in LaShaye's kitchen. LaShaye gripped Dawn's arm. "What are you going to do?"

"I'm going home to California. I want to be with my family. I'm going to need Mom and Granny's help. The hard part is going to be getting them to work things out between them so they can."

Maura held out her hands. "What can we do?"

Dawn took hold. "I have to call the landlord, then call the base to store our furniture. Or sell some of it. I don't know which."

"If you're driving across the country, you should have your car serviced," LaShaye said. "Rory can do that for you."

Between the three of them, they worked out the details. Dawn held out her hands. Maura and LaShaye each took one. "It's been a pleasure, ladies." She blinked back tears. "I didn't have as long as I wanted with you."

LaShaye squeezed tight. "Maybe we ought to pray."

Dawn thanked God for these friends. "Yes. Please." She felt a quiver of apprehension at the journey ahead of her. "And don't stop."

Dawn made all her calls the next morning. She didn't think the landlord would return the security deposit, but when he heard the reasons, he brought the check over that afternoon. She bought a new laptop so she could continue e-mailing Jason every day on the long drive home. She studied routes on MapQuest. She decided against the straight route across the country. She didn't want to go through Colorado and deal with heavy snows. Better to go south.

Maura came over when the movers arrived. Everything would be stored until Jason returned from Iraq. Suitcases packed, Dawn spent the night with Maura.

"How long do you think it'll take, Dawn?"

"I don't know. I'll have to take it one day at a time." She would need to get out and walk around every hour or risk thrombo-phlebitis and edema. Main highways had rest stops. She planned to use them. "I'll drive until I need rest."

"The weather's bad all across the country. You couldn't have picked a worse time to travel."

"I don't have a lot of choice. I can't wait."

"You should have someone with you."

"I will. I'll have Jesus. He'll get me home."

She got up early the next morning, showered, dressed, and left a note on the kitchen counter beside the coffeepot.

Dear Maura,

Thanks for everything. I'll be in touch. May the Lord bless you and yours.

Love, Dawn

For the first time in days, it didn't snow.

51

Dawn knew, even before she had driven the short distance to
Baltimore, the trip would test her physical and emotional endur-
ance. She took one hour at a time, trying not to think how many
miles she had to go. Each afternoon, after checking into a hotel
and having dinner, she hooked up the laptop.

She wrote regular e-mails to Jason, as though still in New
Jersey. She wrote about the baby, tidbits of good news she found in
whatever newspapers she picked up in hotel lobbies, anything that
might keep his spirits bolstered, and not hint she was driving cross-
country alone, nearly eight months pregnant, in January. Once the
e-mail was sent and the others answered, she unhooked and packed
away the computer, watched television weather reports, and went
to bed. After a week on the road, she awakened with night sweats
and back pain. She lay in the darkness praying God would give her
strength and peace of mind. She had a long, long way to go.

Christian music stations kept her spirits up throughout the day.
When she made it to Oklahoma City, she felt more at home. She
thought of the friends she and Jason had made, all scattered now

like seeds in the wind. Some had settled in other U.S. bases, others in Germany; many had gone to Iraq. A few hadn't made it home.

After a good night's rest, she pushed on to Amarillo, Texas.

The baby moved vigorously, reminding her of why she was on this trip. Dawn draped her arm over her expanding abdomen. She wanted desperately to call home, but knew if she did, Mom and Mitch would be frantic. They worried enough already. "Be good, little one. Hang in there! You need to grow a little more. You need to be strong for Mommy."

It took three days to drive from Amarillo to Flagstaff, Arizona. Pushing harder, Dawn made it all the way to Barstow the next day, but got no farther than Buttonwillow the day after. *One more day,* she told herself. *God, help me.* One more day and she could rest.

Dawn dreamed she stood on a stone arch over a black chasm. Granny stood on solid ground on one side and Mom on the other. The bridge began crumbling beneath Dawn's feet. Granny and Mom both reached out and caught hold. Both called for the other to let go. Dawn begged them to stop! Please stop! Gripped by pain, she cried out. Her child broke free of her body and dropped into the darkness below.

❄ ❄ ❄

Exhausted, Dawn pulled in next to Georgia Steward's trailer and parked. Rain pounded on the roof of the car and slicked over the windshield. Mrs. Edwards peered through her living room curtains. Dawn barely had strength to get out of the car. She hadn't walked often enough today, and her legs felt swollen and stiff. The baby had turned and now pressed down heavily inside her. Gripping the rail, Dawn climbed the few steps and knocked on the door.

"Dawn!" After a split second of shock, Georgia stepped outside and hugged her. "You've been on my mind for days. I called, but couldn't get through. Your mom said she talked to you the other day and everything was fine."

Dawn leaned on Georgia as they went inside. She had kept to

her schedule of calling Granny and Mom. She apologized for not calling Georgia. "I'm sorry. I've been driving for days. . . ."

"You *drove*?"

"I couldn't fly. I was past seven months." Dawn sank gratefully onto the sofa and let out a deep sigh of relief.

"Honey, you look pale as a ghost." Georgia lifted Dawn's feet onto the couch. "Your ankles are swollen. Lie back." She tucked a pillow under Dawn's feet and put a blanket over her. "Are you hungry? thirsty?"

Dawn smiled weakly. "Both." She hadn't stopped for dinner, too eager to finish the long journey and rest. "But don't go to a lot of trouble, please."

Georgia opened the refrigerator. "Now I know why God had me praying for you."

Covered with the blue fleece, Dawn listened to the rain pounding the metal roof of Georgia's trailer. She could barely keep her eyes open. Georgia brushed her forehead. "You're perspiring." Her mother-in-law leaned over her, brow furrowed with worry.

"Night sweats."

"And fever, too. I'll find some Tylenol. Can you sit up and eat?"

Struggling into a sitting position, Dawn gave a weary laugh. "My center of gravity is off." The baby moved strongly. "Our little Steward is protesting." Dawn took Georgia's hand and held it against the side of her abdomen. "I think that's her foot."

Georgia sat beside her. Heads together, they waited for the baby to stretch again. They didn't have to wait long, and this time the baby kicked. Georgia laughed. "A soccer player like her mama." She patted Dawn's swollen abdomen. "We should call your mom. Let her know you got here."

"No one knew I was coming."

"No one?"

"I didn't want everyone fretting the entire time I drove."

"What about Jason?"

Dawn shook her head, but the question served to remind her.

"I need to get the laptop out of the car and e-mail him, or he'll wonder what happened to me."

Georgia looked troubled. "What's going on?"

Dawn fought tears. She shook her head and looked away, struggling with her rising emotions. She had done nothing but ponder her circumstances and plead with God for days. She didn't have the strength to talk about what was wrong. Now now. Not tonight. Swallowing her tears, Dawn met Georgia's worried gaze. "Don't call anyone. I'll explain everything in the morning."

❄ ❄ ❄

Pushing the covers off, Dawn was thankful the swelling in her ankles had gone down. Her stomach growled. Georgia had left a blue velour robe on the end of the bed. Pulling it on, Dawn opened the door. The rain had stopped. Daylight streamed in the living room window. Georgia set aside her book and got up from her easy chair. "You look better. How do you feel?"

"Rested. Can I take a shower?"

"After dinner."

"Dinner?" She noticed the table had already been set.

"You've slept eighteen hours." Slipping on mitts, Georgia opened the oven and took out a casserole dish. "I hope you like lasagna."

"Love it." She pushed her fingers back through her hair.

Georgia set it on a trivet in the center of the table. She opened the refrigerator and took out a tossed green salad and small carafe of dressing. "Milk or water?"

"Milk." The baby needed protein.

Georgia said the blessing and filled Dawn's salad bowl. She scooped lasagna onto Dawn's plate. "We should call your family doctor and get you in for an appointment. You're still awfully pale. And so thin."

"I need to work things out with Granny and Mom first."

"They're both in for a shock when they find out you're here."

Georgia served herself a smaller portion. "Are you ready to tell me what's going on?"

Dawn had had days to plan her words, but found them stilted and tremulous now. Georgia didn't utter a word or eat a bite. Dawn didn't have much appetite either by the time she finished. But she had a good reason to eat at least half of what Georgia had served her, and she intended to do so, even if it took an hour.

"I don't believe it, Dawn." Georgia's mouth wobbled. "God wouldn't do that to you." She pressed her lips together. "Jason should have some say about this. You can't leave him in the dark."

"Jason needs to know when to duck. He doesn't need to be worrying about us."

"You and the baby are not distractions. You're his family!"

Georgia's fierceness frightened Dawn. "Georgia. I'm begging you. Don't tell him! He worries about me and the baby enough already." Her eyes filled. There was a time to be gentle and a time to be blunt, even if it bordered on cruelty. "I don't want Jason coming home in a body bag."

Georgia closed her eyes in anguish.

"Pray. That's what I need you to do, Georgia. That's why I came to you first. I have to get Granny and Mom to work together and help me through this. I have to get them in one place. And they've never been able to talk. I have to be the bridge this time, not the wall between them."

❉ ❉ ❉

Dawn called Mitch at his office. She told him everything and what she wanted to do. "I have to spend time with them both, alone. Can you help that to happen?"

He cleared his throat before speaking. "You sure you don't want to have your grandmother come to our place?"

"Granny will do better in her own territory. I'm going to call her and have her call Mom to invite her out there. Don't tell Mom anything yet, okay?"

"I'm not sure how your mom will do. I don't think either one of them realizes how they've pitted themselves against each other."

"God got me home, Mitch. He'll get us through all the rest."

"What about Chris?"

"You can tell him after Mom leaves for Jenner." She wiped tears from her cheeks. "Tell him I'll see him in a few days and we can talk then. And . . ." She had to swallow and draw a slow breath before she could go on. "Pray. Pray hard."

"I am. Right now and every minute from here on out." He made a hoarse sound. "Pita?" He spoke gruffly. "I've always loved you like you were my own flesh and blood."

"I know. Dad."

❄ ❄ ❄

Dawn called Granny. "I want to spend a few days with you and Mom at Jenner."

"When do you plan to come home? spring? The baby will be—"

"I'm here, Granny."

"Here? Where? Alexander Valley?"

"I'm staying with Georgia right now. Mom doesn't know I'm home yet."

"Why didn't you come out and stay with me?"

"I wanted to see my mother-in-law, too. And I was pretty tired when I got here."

"Well, come now. We can visit for a few days and then call your mom."

She needed to make things clear. "I'm not coming out until Mom's there. I don't want her feelings hurt."

"I would never hurt your mother's feelings."

"You'd never hurt her intentionally, Granny, and neither would I; but we both do it all the time, and it has to stop."

"What's happened, Dawn? Something's wrong. Tell me."

"When the three of us are together, Granny, we're all going to talk."

"I'll call your mother as soon as we're off the phone."

"Let me know when she gets to Jenner. Then I'll come."

Georgia sat on the sofa, waiting. When Dawn sat down, Georgia took her hand. "So?"

"I don't know where to start, Georgia. I'm not a psychologist. I don't know what's going to happen at Jenner."

Georgia enfolded her in her arms and leaned back into the sofa so Dawn's head rested against her shoulder. "God didn't bring you home to let you down, honey. And I'm going to pray for a miracle."

Dawn closed her eyes. "We need one."

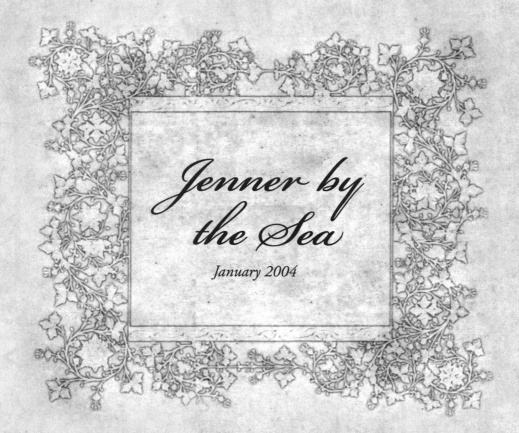

Jenner by
the Sea

January 2004

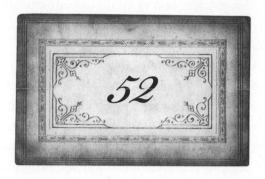

52

HILDEMARA PICKED UP the phone and punched in Carolyn's number. Her son-in-law answered. "Mitch, I don't know if you've heard, but Dawn's home. She's staying with Georgia Steward."

"I know. She called me at the office a little while ago. I'll get Carolyn." He put her on hold. His abruptness surprised her.

Hildie chewed her lip. She pulled out a chair at the kitchen nook table and sat staring out at the Russian River. It was running high, as it often did this time of year. Hildie hunched deeper into her terry-cloth bathrobe.

Winters had always been too long out here on the coast, but bearable as long as Trip had been with her. Then, even if the roads closed and phone and power lines went down, Hildie hadn't been alone. She and Trip joked about "roughing it" without lights, heat, television, or stove, like it was a grand adventure.

The sense of adventure died with Trip. While Hildie was still reeling from Trip's death, Carolyn suggested Hildie sell the house and move into town. It had seemed utterly insensitive. Give up the Jenner house? after all the work Trip had put into it? He'd spent five years—and more money than they'd paid for the place—improving it and bringing it up to his standards. Throwing it all away seemed disloyal. She said as much to Carolyn, and her daughter didn't mention moving again until a few months ago, after Hildie had taken a fall.

This year, winter had become a black hole sucking Hildie down into a vortex of despair. The last time Carolyn came out "for a visit," she broached the subject of moving again. Hildie told her *no*. When Carolyn tried to keep talking about it, Hildie ignored her and turned on the television. Carolyn didn't say anything for a long time. Hildie felt guilty and uncomfortable with the silence, but she didn't know any other way to get her point across. Sure, she was almost eighty-seven, but so what? She still had all her faculties. She didn't need to be put away. "All right, Mom," Carolyn said after fifteen minutes. "Have it your way." She left two residential care facility brochures sitting like cemetery contracts on the coffee table.

Unease filled Hildemara. Had Carolyn called Dawn and enlisted her help in getting old Granny to give up her home and move? Why else would her granddaughter fly to California when she was eight months pregnant and then insist the three of them get together at Jenner and talk? Hildemara felt her anger boiling.

"Mom?" Carolyn sounded breathless. "Are you all right?"

"Why wouldn't I be all right?"

"You never call unless something's wrong."

Was that true? When had she last called Carolyn? two weeks? a month? "Nothing is wrong. Not unless you said something to Dawn about trying to move me into an old folks' home. She's *here*."

"At Jenner?" Carolyn sounded shocked.

"No. Not Jenner. In town. She's staying with Georgia. She called a few minutes ago. She wants you to come to Jenner so the three of us can talk."

"I don't understand. Is it the baby?"

"She said she's fine."

"This isn't about Jason, is it? If she's with Georgia—"

"She sounded fine. She wouldn't be fine if anything had

happened to Jason. Just pack and get out here. Dawn said she wouldn't come to Jenner until you arrive. I don't know what that's all about." Hildie could hear Mitch saying something in the background.

"The roads are terrible, Mom. Mitch can come out and bring you back here. I could pick up Dawn."

"Didn't you hear what I said? We need to meet *here*, at *Jenner*." Hildie knew she sounded angry and impatient, but she didn't want Carolyn wasting any more time.

"It can't always be the way you want it."

Hildie hated that phrase. Mama used to say it. "It's not my way. It's Dawn's way."

Carolyn sighed. "I'll be on the road in half an hour."

"I'll call Dawn and let her know." Hildie hung up, flipped through her address book, and punched in Jason's old number. Georgia answered and said Dawn was sleeping and could she take a message. "Tell Dawn her mom is on her way out here. Jason is all right, isn't he?"

"Jason's fine. He e-mailed Dawn yesterday."

"Thank God." Hildie felt some relief, but then had to ask, "And the baby?"

"Dawn is as big as a house. Hang on a second. She's awake." Hildie heard muffled voices, then Georgia again. "Dawn will head out to Jenner in an hour."

"Tell her to be careful. The weather is mean."

As soon as Hildie got off the telephone, she opened the wooden accordion doors into the small bedroom off the kitchen. She had bought a pretty blue and white Laura Ashley comforter and curtains in the hope Carolyn might come out and spend a weekend now and then. No such luck. Dawn could sleep in here and use the nice, new, plush pink towels and pretty seashell soaps. Carolyn could sleep downstairs. Hildie switched on the lamp before leaving the room. The glow could be seen outside through the lacy sheer curtains. She liked the house to look like a Thomas Kinkade painting.

She debated turning on the downstairs thermostat, then

decided to wait until after Carolyn arrived. Propane was expensive, and the delivery truck had gotten stuck on a nearby ranch, delaying the refilling of her tank.

How could she be so tired after doing so little? She sat in her recliner and put her feet up. Oh, for heaven's sake! She was still wearing her fuzzy slippers and bathrobe! Maybe she *was* entering her dotage.

Slamming the recliner, she headed for the bathroom and turned on the electric wall heater. She put on her shower cap and washed, rinsed, and stepped out of the tub in under five minutes. Toweling dry before the heater, she pulled on her white silk Cuddl Duds leggings, a long-sleeved T-shirt, and the red velour pantsuit Carolyn had given her for Christmas. She brushed tangles from her gray hair. Carolyn had treated her to a perm three months ago. Wash-and-wear hair, her friend Marsha called it. They'd been neighbors until Marsha's daughter flew out, packed her up, and took her back to Colorado Springs. No old folks' home for Marsha. Her daughter *insisted* she move in with her family. Hildie tossed the brush in the drawer and banged it shut.

Standing in the living room, Hildie looked at the Russian River flowing wide and muddy, swollen and treacherous, from heavy rains. Rain hit the window like pebbles tossed against the glass. Surf pounded in the distance. She hadn't been to the beach since Trip's heart condition worsened. "My wings are clipped," he'd said. So were hers. She hadn't wanted to leave him alone, and he'd been irritated by his limitations. No more fishing in the surf. No more volunteer work at the visitors' center. No long walks up the hill for the panoramic view of the coastline.

Now, the closest Hildie came to the beach was the wide spot on the curve of Highway 1 where she parked her Buick Regal and used Trip's binoculars to watch the sea lions on the other side of the river. Her big outing these days was walking down the hill to the post office in a trailer next door to the Jenner Gift Shop. And going to the Guerneville Safeway store every two weeks for groceries.

How long could she manage that steep walk? She didn't like to go when the road was wet and slick. How long before she would have to give up driving?

It galled her that Carolyn was right. She *was* getting too old to live alone.

The last time she had seen Dr. Kirk, he'd told her she had a strong heart and she'd probably live to be a hundred. Considering how difficult it was for her to get around now, the prospect had been annoying.

She picked up the information Carolyn had left and looked at the glossy photos. If she moved into one of those facilities, would she see more or less of Carolyn? Since Trip had died, Carolyn had called once a week. Duty calls, right up there with the groceries Carolyn brought every two weeks, not that Hildie needed them. With professional attendants keeping watch, her daughter wouldn't need to check on her.

What Hildie needed and wanted was a relationship with her daughter. After so many years, it was just wishing for the moon. She'd never known how to bridge the gap to Carolyn any more than she'd ever been able to make a bridge to Mama.

Depressed, Hildie tossed the brochures on the coffee table. *So be it, Lord. If Carolyn wants to put me away, I'll let her.* Maybe it'd be the one thing she did that finally made her daughter happy.

❄ ❄ ❄

Carolyn hung up the telephone and turned to Mitch. His gaze slid away from hers. He poured himself a cup of coffee. "I can take care of everything here, Carolyn. You don't have to worry about anything."

"Have you talked to Dawn?"

"Briefly."

"What's going on, Mitch?"

"She wants you to meet her out at Jenner."

"Why?"

He set his cup down and took her in his arms. "She's been away from home a long time, Carolyn. She wants time alone with the two women she loves most in the world."

"Why now? Why out there?" Pushing away from him, she headed for the master bedroom. He said her name, dumped his coffee, and followed. She felt him watching her as she took her small duffel bag from the closet and threw it on the bed. When had Dawn arrived? today? yesterday? Why had she gone to Georgia instead of coming home? Was something wrong? Carolyn packed two tunic sweaters and two pairs of leggings that coordinated with her tiered skirt. Jenner would be cold. She added socks, cashmere scarves, and a flannel nightgown. What else did she need? She went into the bathroom for her toothbrush, toothpaste, brush, and deodorant, stuffing them into a cosmetics bag.

Mitch stood in the doorway, watching her. "You'd better take a raincoat and umbrella. It's pouring." He didn't say anything else, and she worried even more. He looked grim, hands shoved in his pockets.

He took her duffel bag and walked her to the garage. "Take the Suburban." She didn't argue. She took the keys from the hook and tossed her coat and umbrella onto the passenger seat. Before she could slip in and get away, Mitch turned her around. "She loves you, you know."

"I know, Mitch, but given a choice, she always goes to someone else."

Mitch held her shoulders firmly, not letting her turn away. "Don't make her choose, Carolyn. Love the two of them the way Jesus loves you."

"I do."

"Maybe you should stop stuffing your feelings. Talk to them."

"What would that do, other than make things worse?"

"You won't know unless you try." Mitch gave her a tender, lopsided smile. "No kiss?" She went into his arms and held on tight. She burrowed her face against his chest until she had control of her emotions. "I love you, Carolyn. I wouldn't let you go out there if I didn't think it was important. Call me."

"The phones might go out. You know how it is."

"Stay put when you get to Jenner. Don't come back until it's over." Mitch shut the door as she settled into the driver's seat. He raised his hand as though in blessing.

Carolyn had been watching the news and knew not to take East Side Road. Wohler Bridge was underwater. She took the freeway south and headed west on River Road. Wind-whipped eucalyptus trees cast debris on the road, filling the air with their pungent scent. She slowed, driving cautiously through flooded areas. She drove between hills covered with oak and pine, wound through groves of towering redwoods, root-locked against wind and rising water. Madrones dressed in red bark and green leaves hugged steep hillsides draped with fern boas.

Carolyn pulled into the Safeway parking lot in Guerneville, threw on her raincoat, and ran for the front door. Mom probably hadn't been able to get to the grocery store since the storm hit, and now she would have company for who knew how long. She quickly filled a cart with milk, vegetables, meat, and cookies. Shelves were emptying fast. "Everyone's picking up supplies for the next storm." The checker weighed broccoli and slid it across to the bagger. "Good thing, too. I hear another one is coming in this afternoon."

On the road again, Carolyn slowed through low areas where runoff had collected. Mitch was right. The Jag never would have made it. The river raged to her left, swollen and boiling with debris. The houses along the bank were flooded. How long before the road was closed?

As she headed up Willig Drive, she had to stop and drag part of an old apple tree off the road. Drenched, she climbed back into the Suburban and drove the last hundred yards. The old redwood on the corner of Mom's property had dropped piles of small branches. Carolyn pulled around its massive trunk and parked parallel to the house.

The gate was locked. Carolyn dumped her duffel bag and rang the bell, then returned to the car to unload the groceries. She set down the first three plastic bags and went back for the rest.

Shivering, she rang the bell again. Maybe Georgia had dropped Dawn off already, and she and Mom were too busy talking to hear the bell.

The door slammed. "All right! I'm coming!" The latch clicked and the heavy gate swung open. Mom held an umbrella. She looked at the bags of groceries. "I didn't tell you to bring anything."

"I just picked up a few things on the way through Guerneville."

"It looks like you shopped for a week!"

"Could we discuss this inside? I'm soaked and freezing."

Her mother took two bags and headed for the back door, leaving Carolyn to bring everything else after she closed the gate and latched it. "Is Dawn here yet?"

"No." Mom shook off the umbrella at the back door. "I don't know what I'm going to do with all these groceries, Carolyn. I don't have a big Deepfreeze like you do, you know."

Carolyn's frustration rose like a tide. She let it crest and recede as she put the laden bags on the counter. When would she learn her mother wanted nothing from her? "I'll take care of it." She wondered if her mother ate the home-cooked, packaged meals she brought out every two weeks. Probably not.

"Dawn will be in the blue room. Take your things downstairs."

Carolyn hadn't even been in the house two minutes and already felt unwelcome. "Okay." She went back into the cold rain. It was warmer than the kitchen.

The apartment was as chilly as a meat locker. Carolyn's breath puffed steam as she dumped her bag on the end of the queen-size bed with its chintz spread. At least it had an electric blanket. She could hear Mom tromping around upstairs in the kitchen, probably unloading the bags. Carolyn hurried upstairs. Mom looked annoyed. "Potatoes, carrots, turnips, rutabagas, celery, onions, canned tomatoes . . . Let me guess. You want to make stone soup."

Carolyn nudged her aside and took out round steak. "It's good for a cold, rainy day like this, don't you think?"

"And a lot of work, but you go right ahead if that's what you want. What does it matter that it's *my* house and I might have other plans."

"Did you?"

"That's not the point. I was getting around to it." Her mother sat at the kitchen nook table. "Go ahead." She waved her hand and looked out the window. "I'm just a little out of sorts today."

"What time did Dawn say she was coming?"

"She'll be here any minute."

Carolyn put the milk, eggs, bacon, and cheese into the refrigerator. "What's this all about, Mom?" She rummaged in a drawer for a potato peeler and paring knife.

"I thought you knew."

"Me?" Carolyn felt confused. "You called me."

Her mother looked disgruntled. "Are you sure you haven't said anything to her about pressuring me to move?"

"I'm not pressuring you. And no, I haven't discussed it with Dawn."

Carolyn let the silence settle as she rinsed potatoes and carrots. How long before her mother realized she couldn't stay out here alone, miles from a grocery store and medical care? She'd lost power for five days last winter! Mitch had to fight with the Coastal Commission to put in a generator. Not that she'd ever thanked him.

Carolyn dumped peels into the coffee can under the sink. The meat browned in an iron skillet while she diced vegetables. Her mother hadn't said a word in thirty minutes. Carolyn wanted to suggest her mother think about moving in with her and Mitch. They had plenty of room. Mom could have the never-used maid's quarters. The apartment had a nice bedroom, private bathroom, sitting room, and kitchenette. Her mother wouldn't even have to eat at the same table with them if she didn't want to. But Carolyn knew better. Her mother would make some lame excuse about not wanting to be a burden. If May Flower Dawn wasn't there, Mom had no interest in being there either.

Still, she needed to make amends. Carolyn sat at the nook table. "I never meant to hurt your feelings, Mom. I worry about you out here all by yourself." She didn't want to remind her of the fall that had left her limping for weeks.

Her mother looked like a little girl lost. "Do you?"

"Yes. Especially this time of the year. If this rain keeps up, the roads will close. What if something happened?"

"I haven't fallen again." Hildie looked toward the back door. "I hope Dawn gets here soon."

Dawn. Mom's only concern.

Carolyn let the hurt slide like water off a gull's back and admonished herself for wishing Mom could make a little space in her heart for her. Life didn't always work out the way you wished. At least she had Mitch and Christopher. "I forgot to call Mitch. My cell phone won't work out here. Do you mind if I use your phone?"

"Go ahead."

Carolyn lifted the receiver. Nothing. She checked the cord, just to be sure it hadn't been unplugged accidentally. "Too late. The phone lines are down."

"Here comes a car. Do you think it could be Dawn?" Mom headed for the door, flipping on the porch light before going out with her umbrella.

Carolyn shoved the chair back and followed. Mom had left her standing in the rain for five minutes, but now opened the gate and stood waiting with the umbrella as May Flower Dawn drove up the hill. Carolyn stood under the gate overhang as her daughter parked.

Mom didn't wait for Dawn to get out of the car before going out and making sure she was protected from the rain. Carolyn could barely catch a glimpse of her daughter as she maneuvered herself out of the front seat. "Well, look at you!" Mom laughed. They hugged. They chattered.

Carolyn shivered, rain dripping down the back of her neck. Wrapping her arms around herself to ward off the chill, she waited for them to remember her.

Not surprisingly, it was Dawn who did. She stepped out of her grandmother's embrace and came to Carolyn. "I'm so glad you came."

"Why wouldn't I?" Carolyn smiled, feeling teary at the sight of her daughter. "You're looking in full bloom." Dawn and Jason had waited a long time for this baby. It was a time for joy. When Dawn threw her arms around her, she gave a soft gasp.

Dawn held tight. "I've been dreaming about this for days."

Carolyn lifted a tentative hand to her daughter's back, disturbed by the embrace. It wasn't their usual way. "Of coming home to Jenner?"

Dawn drew back and gave a wobbly smile. "Of having a few days alone with you and Granny. I . . ." She wiped rain from her face—or was she crying? "I'm just so *happy!*"

"Well, that's good, honey, but you're getting wet." Carolyn's mother looped her arm around Dawn and herded her through the gate. "Let's get you inside where it's warm." She glanced over her shoulder. "Are you coming?"

Carolyn supposed that was as warm an invitation as she would get.

❄ ❄ ❄

Dawn smelled something wonderful when she walked in the back door. "Stone soup!" She hadn't had it in over a year.

Granny chuckled, hazel eyes bright with joy. "You'd better be hungry. Your mother made enough to feed an army." She took Dawn's bag. "You're sleeping in the blue room, honey. I don't want you having to go out in the rain, and those stairs can be awfully slick. We can't have any accidents." She set the bag inside the bedroom, then drew Dawn into the living room. "Why did you rent a car? Someone could have met you at the airport." Granny sat in her recliner.

Dawn eased her body onto the faded blue sofa. "It's not a rental. It's my car."

Mom sat in one of the swivel chairs near the fireplace. "You drove?"

"Yep." Dawn tried to make light of it.

"All the way across country in winter?" Granny stared at her. "In your condition?"

Dawn felt the tears coming. "I wanted to come home." She bowed her head and ran her hand over her swollen belly. "Don't ask me why. I know it was crazy. I just packed and came." She raised her head and smiled at her mom first, then Granny. "I want to have my baby here."

Granny frowned. "In Jenner?"

Dawn giggled. "No, Granny. In California, in Healdsburg or Santa Rosa. I want to be close to family and friends." She wasn't ready to talk about everything, not five minutes after she'd arrived, maybe not tonight or tomorrow morning either. "I didn't want to be alone."

"Well, that makes perfect sense." Granny leaned back, making herself comfortable. "When the baby is born, you can come out here and stay until Jason comes home. Then you can fly back to New Jersey to meet him." Granny, taking over again. Mom didn't argue. Dawn sensed the hurt she tried to hide and gave her an apologetic smile. "I hope you can get your money back for the airline tickets, Mom. It was important I be with both of you."

"Well, of course, it is." Granny nodded. "Your mom understands. This is where you belong."

Granny meant with her, at Jenner. Dawn saw that's the way her mother understood it, too, and spoke quietly. "I don't want to be in between anymore."

Granny frowned. "What do you mean 'in between'?"

"Between you and Mom." Dawn glanced from one to the other. "We three have a lot to talk about."

Granny's expression soured. "I should've known. Dawn drives all the way across country in the winter, and you say you don't know a thing about it." Granny glared at Mom. "I suppose you want me to believe you didn't tell her you've been after me to sell and move."

"I didn't."

"I don't believe you!"

Mom hunched her shoulders and looked away, fixing her gaze somewhere outside the window. How many times had Dawn seen this happen before? Anytime an argument arose between her and Granny, Mom pulled inside herself like a turtle in its shell. The only one who had ever been able to coax her out was Mitch, and he kept Mom's confidences.

"Mom didn't say anything to me, Granny. This is the first I've heard of any discussion of you leaving Jenner."

"You don't have to pretend, Dawn." Rain blasted the window, even as the storm in Granny's eyes grew.

"Are you going to accuse me of lying, too?"

"It's all right, Dawn. Don't put yourself in the middle. I think I'll see about dinner." Mom got up slowly and went into the kitchen, closing the door behind herself.

Dawn hurt inside. This wasn't the beginning she wanted. She looked at Granny sadly. "I wouldn't lie to you and neither would Mom." She held out her hand. Granny took it. "But now that you've brought it up, it might be time to think about moving." She squeezed Granny's hand before she let go and pushed herself up. She didn't want Mom hiding in the kitchen.

"Just leave her alone." Granny gave a weary sigh. "She'll come back when she's ready."

"I need to use the bathroom." Dawn rubbed the small of her back. "I hope you'll apologize when she comes back." *God, You got me all the way across the country. Please get me through this, too!*

When she came out of the bathroom, Mom sat at the kitchen nook table, face in her hands. Granny still sat in the corner recliner in the living room. Dawn felt the tears rise again; she hadn't been here fifteen minutes and she was right back in the middle. Granny's head lifted as Dawn stepped toward the living room. "Come on in and sit down, Dawn."

"Why don't you come in here, Granny? I'll fix some tea."

Granny glowered at both of them. "I don't want to talk about moving."

"Why not?"

"Look around." Granny's shoulders slumped. "And I'm not talking about the million-dollar view. I'm talking about—" she waved her hand like a white flag—"everything."

Dawn understood. "I have to pare down every time Jason and I move, Granny. I pick what means the most and sell or give away the rest."

"Well, it all means something to me, honey. There's a story behind everything in this house. You know how much Papa loved this place. It was his last big project." Granny's eyes grew moist as she looked at Mom. "It might not mean anything to you, Carolyn, but Dawn understands."

Mom didn't even try to defend herself.

"I understand, Granny, but Papa wouldn't want you living here alone." She didn't let Granny's look of hurt silence her. "If you wait too long, someone else will have to make all the decisions—what to keep, what to throw away."

Granny got up. "Well, that would be fine with me. When I'm dead, I won't care anymore." She dumped her tea in the sink. "Have it your way, Carolyn. If you're that set on getting me out of this house, go on down to the garage and get started sorting." She slammed her mug on the counter. "I'm going to turn on the TV and see how bad this storm is going to be." Granny went into the living room.

Dawn sighed. "I'm sorry, Mom. I was trying to help."

Mom shrugged. "It's not your fault. It is overwhelming."

Dawn smiled at her. "What was that you used to say? First things first."

"One day at a time."

"Granny loves you, Mom."

Mom made a soft sound of doubt, got up, and put her mug carefully on the counter. "I think I'll take advantage of the moment." She took her jacket by the door and went out.

Dawn went into the living room. Granny tipped her recliner up and peered around her. "Your mother isn't leaving, is she?"

"Would you care if she did?"

"Of course, I'd care." She started to push herself up from the chair.

"It's all right, Granny. She's going to the garage."

"Why?"

"You told her to get started, didn't you?"

Granny sank back in her chair. "I didn't mean *now*." She frowned. "It's freezing out there. It'll be dark soon."

"She's not going anywhere, Granny. I think she just needs to be alone for a while."

"She's always preferred her own company."

Dawn sat on the couch. Sonoma County was on the national news. "Another storm coming in tonight . . ." Aerial film crews showed the Russian River at flood level. The vineyards around Wohler Bridge were underwater. So were the ones near the Korbel Winery. The roads had closed. The river had risen high enough to close the Safeway in Guerneville.

53

SHIVERING, CAROLYN STOOD in the garage, surveying the massive project ahead of her. Dad's white Buick Regal still took up half the garage. Mom had forgotten to take the keys out of the ignition. Carolyn backed the car out of the garage and parked it behind Dawn's car.

Shelves lined the walls. One section displayed canned vegetables and soups; jars of peanut butter, jelly, and jam; cans of tuna; and boxes of macaroni and cheese. Another rack of shelves held small appliances in their original boxes and enough Costco plastic-wrapped boxes of Kleenex, toilet paper, and paper towels to last a year. Carolyn set a kerosene lamp near the door. They might need it. Cabinets lined the back wall: one held shelves of vases in all shapes and sizes; another Korbel champagne, Johnnie Walker Scotch, bottles of Mondavi cabernet sauvignon, Wente Brothers zinfandel and chardonnay, all dusty. *The devil prowls like a lion.* After more than thirty years of sobriety, Carolyn felt the sharp urge to drown her sorrows.

She still attended AA meetings, but Cornerstone Christian

Church filled another gap in her life. It had started with Pastor Daniel's compassion the day Dad died. Then Georgia openly shared her life on the streets before God got ahold of her. Others with less-than-pristine pasts rejoiced over restored lives and made others, still struggling, welcome. Carolyn made friends, though she never let anyone as close as Chel, with whom she had shared all her secrets, even the one she had never told Mitch.

Why was she thinking about all that now?

Carolyn looked over Dad's tools, mounted neatly above his worktable, all rusting in the sea air. She counted five boxes tucked in the rafters. She set up the ladder, pulled her tiered skirt up between her legs and tucked it into her leather belt, and climbed. Brushing away cobwebs, she brought them down one by one. She was warm by the time she lined the boxes on the cement floor. Mom had labeled each: *Family Pictures*, *Clothing*, *Trip*, *China/ FRAGILE*, and *Mama*.

Carolyn pulled open the top flaps of the box marked *Mama* and drew out a hand-crocheted granny-square afghan. It reeked of damp and mold, holes eaten away by mice or rats. She folded it into the garbage can, annoyed that Oma's labor of love had been stuffed in a box to rot. Next was a shoe box. Carolyn uttered a soft gasp when she found Oma's leather journal on top of bundles of thin, folded airmail letters with Swiss stamps. She took out the journal and carefully opened it. A picture slipped out and fell on the floor: Oma sitting on a chair holding a baby, a little boy beside her, and a tall, blond, very handsome man in a dark suit standing behind them. He was holding a little brown-haired girl and had his other hand on Oma's shoulder. Carolyn picked up the picture and turned it over. *Winnipeg, 1919.*

"Mom?" Dawn stood in the doorway, bundled in a down coat. "Please come back inside."

"I was just going through a few boxes." She tucked the picture back into Oma's journal and glanced around. "It is going to be a big job."

"Not one you can finish tonight. Granny fixed corn bread. The table is set for dinner. We can bring in a few boxes and go through them later, if you'd like." She examined one of them. "Might be kind of fun."

Carolyn put Oma's journal on top of the shoe box and stacked them on the box labeled *Family Pictures*. May Flower Dawn lifted the box marked *Trip*. They carried the two boxes into the house and put them in the living room. "It'll just take me a minute to get the others." When she'd stacked the other boxes in the middle of the living room, she washed her hands in the kitchen sink before sitting down with May Flower Dawn and her mother, who gave the blessing.

Carolyn put her napkin on her lap. "I found Oma's journal."

"My inheritance." Her mother snorted, scooping stone soup into bowls. "She gave Rikka a few pieces of jewelry. She'd already given Bernie her car. Cloe earns a stipend for handling the college trust Mama set up. I got her recipe book and a box of letters, written in German." She set a bowl in front of Dawn and filled another for Carolyn.

Dawn took a spoonful of soup and smiled. "Yummy." She glanced across at Carolyn. "It's not just a collection of recipes, Granny. When we visited her, Oma gave it to me to read one night. She told me she only wrote important things that made a difference in her life: tips on how to keep a house, yes, and some recipes, but also quotes from people she met, important dates like when you were born and the circumstances, ranch schedules, a funny poem a boy wrote about Summer Bedlam, her thoughts on life. It's wonderful. It defines her. I'd love to read it again." She looked at Carolyn. "She sent me a journal after that visit. Remember?"

"You sent her a diploma." Carolyn smiled, pleased to know that week had meant something to May Flower Dawn, that those few days in Merced had left her daughter with fond memories of Oma.

"The journal she sent me is leather and has my name engraved in gold. *May Flower Dawn*. I have it with me. I think of Oma every time I open it. I followed Oma's lead. I didn't write a lot of teenage nonsense in it. I wrote goals, favorite Scriptures, meaningful dates, places Jason and I have lived, dreams . . ." She smiled wistfully. "I wish I'd known Oma better. Oma's journal meant more to her than jewelry, a car, or money, Granny. She gave you the best of herself."

Carolyn's mother looked surprised—and a little perplexed.

The lights flickered and went out, enclosing them in complete darkness. "Wow." Dawn's voice sounded louder in the inky wrapping. "I can't see my hand in front of my face."

Carolyn hated the darkness. "I forgot the kerosene lantern in the garage. Where's a flashlight?"

"In one of the kitchen drawers, under the dish cabinets—middle I think—but the batteries are probably dead."

Carolyn fumbled around in the darkness, opening drawers and feeling through contents.

"Just wait a minute, Carolyn. Or did you forget you and Mitch put in a generator? There it goes." A distant whir sounded, and then noise.

Dawn laughed. "No muffler on that baby."

The lights came on. Relieved, Carolyn returned to her seat. Her mother sat calmly, hands folded on the table. "I don't think I ever thanked you, did I?"

"No. You didn't. But then we didn't ask your permission either." If they couldn't get her to move, they'd make sure she had heat and power. Four thousand dollars, not to mention the money spent on a lawyer who took over the fight with the Coastal Commission, and not one word of thanks until now.

❄ ❄ ❄

After clearing and washing the dishes, Carolyn joined her daughter and mother in the living room. She hesitated on the threshold when she saw them on the couch, May Flower Dawn holding her granny's hand on her abdomen. They spoke in whispers. Biting her lip, Carolyn stepped back. She felt like an intruder. Mom glanced up and frowned. "Why are you standing there? Come feel the baby moving."

Carolyn treaded carefully around the stacked boxes and knelt in front of them. Dawn took her hand and placed it on her abdomen. Carolyn didn't feel anything. Dawn sighed. "Little Miss must have fallen asleep again." Carolyn rose and sat in the yellow swivel rocker.

Her mother pushed herself up and settled into her recliner. "This is nice, having the two of you here, together."

Dawn grinned. "Three girls on a sleepover." She winced in pain and shifted on the couch until she looked more comfortable. Carolyn remembered the final month of pregnancy when her babies had pressed against her rib cage and bore down on her pelvis. The last month was the hardest.

Dawn yawned. She looked so tired.

"Why don't you go to bed, May Flower Dawn?"

"It's only eight, Carolyn."

"She looks exhausted, Mom."

"I'm not ready for bed yet." Dawn gave them both a tired smile. "I want to sit and visit."

"You can lie down and visit." Carolyn got up and lifted Dawn's legs onto the couch. "Your ankles are swollen." Dawn murmured a weary thank-you and said not to worry. Carolyn tucked a needle-point pillow under her head and draped a soft, white knitted blanket over her. She brushed a wayward strand of blonde hair back from her daughter's face. She was perspiring. "Do you have a fever?"

Dawn took her hand. "Relax, Mom. It's a lot of work carrying around an extra thirty pounds."

Carolyn took her seat and watched Dawn fall asleep. She snored softly. "I guess she is tired." After a few minutes, she fidgeted in her chair. She felt night fold tight around them, the glass their only barrier against it. "I guess we could go through the boxes."

"I don't want to go through those boxes." Her mother shook her head. "Not tonight. Besides, Dawn would probably get a kick out of it." She rubbed her leg as though it ached. "You stood in the doorway just now. Why do you do that?"

"Do what?"

"Stand outside a door, peer around corners, listen in."

Carolyn felt the words like a slap. "Like a sneaky little mouse, you mean. Like I'm planning to steal a bit of cheese?"

Mom looked shocked. "No." She shook her head. "Like you don't belong. Like you're waiting for an invitation."

"I was told to stay out."

"Who told you that?"

Why not tell the truth? Mom never spared her feelings. "You did. You said you never wanted me anywhere near you."

"That's a lie!" Her eyes darkened in anger.

Carolyn pressed her lips together. She should have known better than to say anything.

"I suppose Oma told you that!"

Heat flooded Carolyn. "You always blame Oma for everything, but I remember you yelling right into my face, 'Get out of here. . . . Get away from me.' Not Oma."

"When did I ever do such a thing?"

"It's the earliest memory I have."

Mom's expression changed, as though remembering. "When you brought me a bouquet of flowers . . ."

"Wildflowers. You didn't want them."

"You dropped them. They scattered all over the floor. I picked them up. Oma brought me a vase."

Picked them up? Put them in a vase? "I never went into your room after that."

Mom looked stricken. "I was sick, Carolyn. Don't you remember how sick I was?"

Carolyn didn't want to go back and visit that time. She wanted to close the trapdoor that had sprung open. She didn't want to look down into the darkness and see what lay hidden there.

"I had tuberculosis. No one but Dad and Oma were allowed in my room, and they had to take precautions. Do you remember any of that?"

"It doesn't matter."

"It does matter."

"It was a long time ago."

"I *loved* you, Carolyn."

Loved. Past tense. Why talk about the past? Why bring it up at all? Chel told her once that just because you were family didn't mean you got along. Her father hadn't liked her. "You just live with it and move on," Chel said. "Don't waste energy trying to make them love you."

Chel. Why was she thinking about Rachel Altman now? Why were her words ringing in Carolyn's head after all these years? Twice in the last few hours.

Carolyn tried to close that door on the past, but memories kept flooding in. She remembered sitting in the tall grass, plucking petals from a daisy. *She loves me; she loves me not; she loves me; she loves me not . . .*

Oma loved her.

Mom and Dad loved Charlie.

Charlie. Oh, Charlie. The pain came up quick, squeezing her heart.

"What are you thinking about, Carolyn?"

"Charlie." She spoke without thinking. Did the mention of her brother still bring Mom pain? "Sorry."

Mom appeared calm, pensive. "What about Charlie?"

"He told me you got sick after I was born."

"Not right away. I let myself get run-down. I knew better. I'd had TB before."

"When?"

"Your father and I were courting. I thought you knew all this."

"I guess I don't know anything."

"I spent months in Arroyo del Valle Sanatorium. I got better, but the disease is always there, hiding, waiting. When I got sick again after you were born, I thought I was going to die. Oma came so I could come home. Die at home, I thought. I didn't want to leave your dad in debt. So Oma moved in and . . . took over everything." She smiled sadly. "That may be what gave me the incentive to get well—watching Oma take over my family."

The rain pounded harder, like fists on the roof. "Oma loved me, Mom."

"Yes. And you loved her. Exclusively. You never came to me. You always went to Oma. That's why I told her to go home."

"So I wouldn't have anyone?"

Mom looked crushed. "You were *my* little girl, not Oma's."

Carolyn's fingers curled around the seat cushion. She remembered Dad shaking her and telling her to stop crying or else. "I felt so alone."

"You had *me*."

When had that ever been true? "No. I didn't."

"Yes, you did!"

Carolyn refused to let it pass this time. "We moved out to the new property! You and Dad worked all the time on the house and gardens."

"Not all the time."

"You told me to stay out from underfoot, to go off somewhere and play. I'd wait for Charlie, but when he got home from school, he always grabbed his bicycle and took off."

"You were right there with me. You picked flowers. You made mud cookies. You flattened down a little private place in the mustard flowers where you played with your rag doll."

That wasn't the way Carolyn remembered it. She didn't want to tell Mom what she did remember. "I think I'll go to bed." She got up.

"Carolyn. Please. Can't we talk about this a little more? I didn't know you—"

"I'll see you in the morning."

"It'll be cold downstairs." Mom tried to push herself out of the chair. "I haven't opened the heating vent to the downstairs yet. It'll take half an hour to warm up the apartment."

"Save the energy. I'll be under the covers anyway."

Carolyn struggled into her jacket at the back door. She had to get out of the house, away from her mother, away from the past that shoved its way up like a demon coming from Hades.

The cold hit Carolyn in the face. Rain pelted her. She held the rail as she hurried downstairs. The screen door stuck. She yanked twice before it creaked open. She flicked the light switch and stood in the sitting room, heart pounding. A whoosh of cold air hit her. It warmed quickly. Mom had opened the vent. Wrapping her arms around herself, Carolyn turned her face into it.

She heard muted voices. Dawn must have awakened. Carolyn thought about going upstairs again, but that might put a damper on their conversation. Mom and Dawn had always been able to talk. Carolyn knew there was more to Dawn's cross-country trip than she'd said. She didn't look well at all. Maybe she'd tell her grandmother what she couldn't tell her mother.

Carolyn turned on the electric blanket before going into the bathroom. She brushed her teeth, then sat on the side of the bed, brushed and braided her hair. Changing quickly into her pajamas, she pulled on a pair of Mitch's athletic socks and slipped quickly between the warming sheets. Shivering violently, she snuggled down deep into the covers, waiting for the warmth to soak in, while above her, Mom and Dawn went on talking.

Carolyn felt her throat close. Hadn't it always been this way? How could it be any other way when her daughter had spent the first six years of her life completely dependent on Mom? Carolyn didn't want to be bitter. She owed Mom gratitude for taking care of Dawn. If not her mother, it would have been some indifferent babysitter earning minimum wage in an overcrowded day care center.

Footsteps crossed the room above her—two pairs this time, one toward the master bedroom, the other toward the refurbished front bedroom. After that, she listened to the storm rattle the windows.

Closing her eyes, Carolyn listened to the surf and wind and rain. She dreamed she was a child again, walking in a forest of mustard flowers. Bees hummed around her, but she wasn't frightened of them. She came to a barbed-wire fence and climbed through. Her dress caught and tore. She stood behind a white house watching a man in overalls walk among two rows of white boxes on wooden pedestals. He removed a lid, setting it aside, and then carefully and slowly lifted out a wooden frame filled in with honeycomb. Breaking off a piece, he turned and smiled at her. "Come on over, honeybee. I won't hurt you."

Carolyn awakened abruptly, heart pounding. It took a few minutes for the dream to recede. Shivering, she turned the electric blanket to ten and pulled the covers over her head.

54

D AWN AWAKENED WHEN the Black Forest cuckoo clock struck three. She curled onto her side, listening to the rain coming down like the cadence of a marching band. She and Granny had talked after Mom went to bed. Granny wanted to know about Jason, and she wondered what Dawn had done with her latest house. Dawn wanted to talk about Granny's future. After some resistance, Granny gave in.

"You know your mother wanted me to move right after Papa died. It was just too soon to make any changes. And I've been fine here by myself." She let out her breath. "At least until this past year."

"What happened?"

"Last winter the power went out for five days. If your mom could've gotten out here, I would've started packing. As soon as the weather improved, your mom and Mitch went to all the trouble of putting in that generator. They had to hire a lawyer. Heaven knows how much they spent on the whole project. It wouldn't have been much of a thank-you if I'd said 'Oh, by the way, I'm ready to move now.' And besides, it can be very nice out here most of the year."

Dawn grinned. "And you always said Oma was stubborn."

Granny put her head back. "I didn't think I was being stubborn. But I guess that's how it looked. Then after my fall a few months back, your mother brought up the idea again."

"But you're ready to move now. Aren't you?"

"As ready as I'm ever going to be." Granny glowered. "But I want a place of my own, not a room in some senior care facility."

"You don't want to live with anyone, Granny?"

"I don't want to live with *strangers.*"

Dawn caught something in Granny's tone that gave her hope. "What about moving in with Mom and Mitch?"

Granny gave a derisive laugh. "That's not going to happen."

"Why not?"

"It just won't, that's all. And don't go asking your mother about it. You'll just put her in an awkward position." Granny had changed the subject after that.

Sleepless, Dawn pulled the covers over her shoulders and snuggled down into the flannel sheets. *Lord, they never really talk to each other, do they? They love each other, but they don't see love is shared.*

Dawn ran her hand over her belly. Her daughter would be arriving soon. She wanted it to be a time of joy, a chance to come together and celebrate. Dawn didn't want them at odds with one another, seeing one another through past hurts. The stakes were too high for that now.

Love one another, You said, Lord. Help me show them how.

❄ ❄ ❄

Hildie awakened early. The house creaked like a ship adrift in rough seas; the rain still pounded. She had a flashlight on her side table and pointed it at her clock. Six fifteen. Trip had always been first up and started the coffee. Oh, how she missed that man! Trip had been the only man she ever loved.

If she wasn't careful, she could sink into despair over her losses. She still missed her son, Charlie. She missed Carolyn, too, aching for what might have been. It was too late now. And she would never stop missing Mama—or wishing they had somehow made peace before the end. Dawn had been the light that pulled her up out of the darkness after Charlie was killed and Carolyn came home like a starving waif. Feeling needed, Hildie stepped in, wanting to help. Dawn had been God's blessing.

Hildie pushed the covers off, tucked her feet into her fuzzy slippers, pulled on her robe, and went into the bathroom. When she finished her morning ablutions, she turned on the lamp in the living room and went into the kitchen to set up the coffeemaker, decaf.

A few minutes later, the back door opened. "I heard you get up." Carolyn came in, hair in a French braid, and wearing another sweater over her long hippy skirt and leggings, blue this time, the exact shade of her eyes. Trip's eyes.

Hildie apologized. She hadn't meant to awaken anyone. In truth, she was glad of the company. "Did you sleep all right?"

"Okay." She poured herself a cup of coffee.

"Do you realize how long it's been since you stayed overnight out here?"

"Christmas, before Dad died." Carolyn sat at the table.

"I want a house, Carolyn, not an apartment or a room."

Carolyn raised her brows in surprise. "Like the one you and Dad built for Oma?"

Wouldn't it be nice to have a little house on Carolyn and Mitch's property? Close enough to be a part of their lives, but not so close she'd be in their way. A dream for her, probably a nightmare for Carolyn. She'd better set her daughter's mind at ease. "There's a nice trailer park in Windsor, seniors only, right around the corner from the church." Why was Carolyn frowning like that?

"Well, we can look there if you like."

"What's wrong with that idea?"

"I just can't see you in a trailer park, Mom."

No doubt, she'd like it better if her mother were under lock and key with guardians to keep an eye on her. "We had wonderful trips in our trailer."

"Yes. I guess we did."

"You guess?"

"It was a travel trailer. Not something to live in."

"Well, I'm not talking about moving into a travel trailer. I'm talking about one of those double-wides."

"Okay. Don't get upset." Carolyn sipped her coffee. "Did Dawn tell you why she drove out here?"

"She told both of us."

"Did she give you any other reason why she wanted to do something as foolish as drive cross-country in winter when she's about to have a baby?"

"Being with family isn't foolish, Carolyn. It's a good enough reason, if you ask me." She had thanked God countless times Carolyn came home when she did. They might never have known what happened to her otherwise, though at times she wondered if she knew much of anything about her daughter.

"I hope so."

"I wouldn't worry too much." Carolyn had always been overly sensitive. "A girl usually wants her husband or mother around when her time comes." A shadow flickered across her daughter's face, and Hildie felt a twinge of remorse. She had sent Carolyn to Boots. Hildie had cried buckets over that decision, but she and Trip knew it was the only way to protect Carolyn from all the gossip. They'd both been depressed for ages after she left. They'd lost Charlie in Vietnam. They'd no sooner gotten their daughter back than they had to send her away. It had hurt even more believing she would give up their only grandchild for adoption.

When Boots told them Carolyn wanted to keep the baby, Hildie had been overjoyed. Boots said she'd love to have Carolyn live with her, but Hildie wanted her daughter back. She wanted to hold her grandchild. She told Trip she wanted to quit nursing and stay home. They didn't need the money, and Carolyn would need help. They sat down and laid out a plan to help their daughter recover from the lost years in Haight-Ashbury. They wouldn't ask questions. They'd leave the past behind them. And Carolyn had done so well. She'd finished college and excelled in the real estate office.

Hildie thought they'd go on as they were. It had been a shock when Carolyn said she wanted to move out. Hildie had seen something in her eyes. Her daughter couldn't wait to get away from them. And, oh, the pain, when she had to give up Dawn.

"The sun's coming up," Carolyn said. "Not that we can see much of it through the clouds."

"More rain through today and tomorrow." Hildie sipped her lukewarm coffee. "I'm a little worried we'll run out of propane. The truck is supposed to try again on Monday."

Carolyn got up. "'Through waves and clouds and storms, He *Bible* gently clears the way.' Let's hope the roads are open on Monday." She took the carafe from the coffeemaker. "Would you like your coffee warmed up?"

"One cup is about all I can handle these days."

Carolyn replenished her own. "Didn't Dad buy presto logs?"

"They're under the garage."

"I'll bring some up, just in case." She sat again. "I should take a look at what's under there anyway."

"Why don't you wear a pair of my pants so you don't ruin your nice skirt? Take a look in my closet." While Carolyn went to see about the pants, Hildie took out eggs and bacon. Carolyn came into the kitchen wearing a pair of red polyester slacks that hit midcalf. What a difference four inches in height could make. Hildie laughed. "High-water pants."

"Clam-diggers." Carolyn laughed with her.

Dawn opened the accordion door. Hair mussed, bleary-eyed, and pale, she wore a pair of white athletic socks and Trip's old navy blue terry-cloth bathrobe. Her blue eyes still looked shadowed with exhaustion. Carolyn greeted her before getting her jacket and going out the door.

"Where are you going, Mom? Aren't you having breakfast with us?"

"I'm going to check under the garage, bring up some presto logs for a fire."

Hildie turned bacon in the frying pan. "Forget the presto logs for now, Carolyn. Just open the safe downstairs and bring up whatever's inside." She told her the combination. "If I'm going to be downsizing, a good place to start is some of the jewelry I've been keeping locked up and never wear."

Carolyn went out into the rain. Dawn eased into a chair, rested her elbow on the window, and looked out at the glutted Russian River.

Hildie studied her granddaughter. It was such a pleasure having Dawn under her roof again. "It is a beautiful view, even in flood season, isn't it, honey?"

Silent, Dawn rubbed her back in an abstracted manner.

"You okay, honey?" In the morning light, Hildie noticed even more clearly the signs that something was wrong. Other than her swollen abdomen, the girl was skin and bones. Was she just worried, anxious about Jason and the baby they'd both hoped and prayed for, for so long?

"Hmmm? Oh." Dawn smiled, still distracted. "Just tired."

"Thinking about Jason?"

"I think about Jason all the time, Granny. I miss him so much, especially now. But God is using him where he is. Two guys in his unit have become Christians."

"You picked a good man, Dawn."

"I won't be able to e-mail him until I get back to town. He'll be worried. I should've thought of that."

"Georgia will let him know you're fine."

"Jason didn't know I was coming home."

Hildie found that information disturbing. "I should've come into town instead of having you drive all the way out here. We could have been warm as toast in Alexander Valley. And you could've kept in touch with your husband."

"I wanted to be out here."

"At least someone besides me loves the place."

"I didn't want any interruptions."

Troubled, Hildie looked at her, but before she could ask what was going on, Carolyn came back in the door with a stack of papers and a box covered with flowery contact paper. "Set it over there on the counter, Carolyn. We'll go through everything after breakfast."

❄ ❄ ❄

Carolyn watched May Flower Dawn pick at her food. Her blue eyes didn't have any sparkle, and her cheeks were pale. "Didn't you sleep at all last night, Dawn?"

"I couldn't shut off my mind."

Her mother offered more toast. "She's been thinking about Jason."

"Not surprising." Carolyn took a piece and buttered it. "The whole church is praying for him. So are we." Carolyn noticed Dawn grimace. "Are you having contractions?"

Dawn rubbed her sides. "She's running out of room in there."

Carolyn folded her hands and watched her daughter closely. "You're sure the baby is a girl?"

"She would've had a sonogram, Carolyn. Of course, she knows."

"I knew long before that, Granny. I had a dream about her. She was running and playing along the edge of the surf at Goat Rock Beach." She smiled at Carolyn. "And you and Granny were sitting together on the sand, talking like good friends."

A nice dream. Carolyn cleared dishes. She scraped Dawn's cold scrambled eggs into the garbage while imagining talking with her mother like that. When had there ever been a time when she hadn't needed to be careful about every word she said?

Her mother set the pile of papers and box on the table. "Let's see what we've got here." While Carolyn washed dishes, her mother and Dawn sat at the table, going through papers. "Deed to the house, car and life insurance policies, Social Security cards, wedding and death certificates, living trust, burial arrangements, list of bank accounts . . ." She fanned the papers, pausing over one. "Oma's naturalization papers. I forgot I had them. She was so proud when she passed the test."

Mom set the certificate aside. "Oma said we were the *real* American citizens. Those born to it didn't appreciate it. She made us all study as if we had to take the test too, to earn the right to call ourselves Americans. She thought that until Trip went to war and then Charlie . . ." She picked up an envelope yellowed by age. "The letter from Charlie's commanding officer . . ." She held it for a moment and set it aside unopened.

Carolyn dried her hands and picked it up. While her mom opened the box filled with smaller boxes, Carolyn opened the letter and read.

> . . . offer my heartfelt condolences on the death
> of your son. . . . excellent young man . . . well-
> respected by everyone who served with him. . . .
> could always count on him . . . brave . . . a
> pleasure to know him. . . . will never forget . . .

Mom lifted out a black velvet box and snapped it open. "Papa gave me these pearls on our twenty-fifth wedding anniversary." She took them out and handed them to Dawn.

"They're beautiful."

"You keep them."

"I can't, Granny. They should go to Mom."

Carolyn folded the letter back into the yellowed envelope and put it on the table. "Granny wants you to have the pearls."

"You and Mitch gave me pearls for my sixteenth birthday. Remember?"

Carolyn's mother looked hurt. "I'm not slighting your mother, Dawn. Mitch gave her better pearls than these for Christmas two years ago and a bracelet and earrings to go with them."

Dawn fingered the necklace. "They're lovely." Her eyes grew moist. "Save them for my daughter."

Her mother closed the box and opened another. Unfolding a lace-trimmed embroidered handkerchief, she showed off a gold, pearl, and jade brooch. "I gave this to Oma on her eightieth birthday. You . . ." Her voice faltered. "You were gone. Anyway, Oma would want you to have it."

Touched, Carolyn accepted the box. "I don't remember ever seeing Oma wear this."

"She didn't. Not once. I doubt she ever took it out of the box." Mom pointed. "That's real, not cheap costume jewelry. I wanted to give her something special, something she would never buy for herself."

Carolyn understood all too well. "Like the cashmere shawl I gave you for Christmas a few years ago? or the pendant I gave you for Mother's Day?"

Mom's eyes widened. "They're too special to use for every day."

Carolyn searched her face. "I thought you didn't like them."

"Of course I like them. They're the nicest gifts I've ever received."

Dawn interrupted. "Maybe Oma felt the same way about the brooch, Granny."

Mom shook her head. "I thought she'd love it, but she said I'd wasted my money."

Seeing the sheen of tears in her mother's eyes, Carolyn took the brooch out of the box. "This is exquisite, Mom. Maybe she was afraid to wear it." She pinned the brooch to her sweater. "It's beautiful. I'll cherish it. Thank you."

Eyes glistening, Mom gave her a wobbly smile. "You're welcome."

Dawn's blue eyes shone. "Perfect." She propped her chin in the heels of her hands. "This is exactly what I prayed for all across the country."

"What?" Carolyn's mother looked blank.

"That we three could just sit and talk about things that shaped our lives and our relationships."

Carolyn had spent years sidestepping questions, pushing memories back, training herself to live in the present. Dredging up the past wasn't her idea of an answer to prayer. She felt her mom's glance and didn't meet it.

Dawn rose. "Why don't we go through the boxes from the garage?" She went into the living room, not waiting for them to follow. "They should be full of memorabilia."

Carolyn's mother studied her. "You don't seem particularly enthused."

Carolyn hadn't moved from her seat. "Are you?"

Her mom pushed her chair back, but didn't get up. "Maybe we *should* talk about the past, Carolyn. God knows, you've been weighed down by it for years. And so have I."

Was that how she saw it? "There are some things I don't want Dawn to know."

"Do you think anything could change how much Dawn loves you?"

"What about you?"

"Me?" Her mom searched her face, comprehension seeping into her eyes. "I'm your mother." She shook her head. "I wonder if we know one another at all."

"Are you two coming?" Dawn called from the living room.

Dawn had already opened a box and pulled out a navy blue dress with white cuffs, faded red buttons, and a red belt. "Wow! This looks like old Hollywood, Granny."

"Your great-aunt Cloe designed and made that for me when I went away to nursing school."

"You'd get a small fortune for it on eBay now. Clotilde Waltert Renny first design . . ."

"Hardly the first."

Carolyn opened the *Pictures* box and found all the pictures that had once hung inside the front door of the Paxtown home: Charlie in his football uniform, in his cap and gown, with his Army buddies; his Army portrait with the ribbons mounted below. A dozen pictures of Charlie, all framed beautifully. Not one of her. Carolyn rocked back on her heels.

"What's wrong?" Carolyn's mother looked from her to the box. "What did you find?"

"Pictures of Charlie."

Dawn lowered an ashes-of-roses dressing gown. "Are you okay, Mom?"

The hurt rose, squeezing tight around her heart. "I'd better get the presto logs. Just in case the generator goes out."

❄ ❄ ❄

Dawn put the dressing gown aside and pulled over the box her mother had opened. "Pictures of Uncle Charlie." She took out a high school graduation picture. "I remember these. They were on the wall in the Paxtown house." Every picture was of Charlie, a few of Granny and Papa with him.

"Our memorial wall."

Granny used to tell her stories about her uncle: how well he played football, baseball, basketball; how popular he had been, how handsome. Mitch had added to her uncle's legend by telling stories about their teenage angst and antics, things Granny and Papa wouldn't have known. "Did he and my mom get along?"

"More than got along, honey. She idolized him. They were polar opposites. He always watched out for her. Charlie was outgoing. Your mom was shy. He had lots of friends. She was a loner. Charlie was like my brother, Bernie. Everyone was so taken with him they never noticed his little sister."

"Mitch told me he had a crush on Mom in high school. He wanted to ask her out, but never got up the nerve. That's why he came back to Paxtown—to look her up." Dawn set Uncle Charlie's picture on the coffee table. "Did you ever meet Mom's friend, Rachel Altman?"

Granny tilted her head. "So she told you about her."

"A little."

"Carolyn brought her home once, just before Charlie went to Vietnam. They were both still attending Berkeley at the time. Rachel came from wealth. She rented a house. That's when things started to go downhill. They dropped out and disappeared. We didn't hear from your mother for two years, and then one day, I came home and there she was sitting by the front door."

Dawn sat on the couch and curled her legs up under her. "Were you angry with her?"

"Angry?"

"She was gone so long. It must have been awful for you and Papa."

"You can't even imagine how awful." Granny sounded distressed. "Don't ask her about those days. She was worrying just now in the kitchen, thinking it would make a difference in how you feel about her. She doesn't want to talk about it. We tried a few times to open the subject, but learned to leave well enough alone."

Dawn wasn't convinced. "Maybe if she talks about it, it won't haunt her so much."

"She put it all behind her and moved on with her life."

"I'd like to know who my father was."

Dismayed, Granny shook her head. "Did you ever think she might not know? And asking would just make her feel worse about it."

"I love her, Granny. No matter what she tells me, that's not going to change."

"So do I. That's why I don't ask." Granny's mouth worked, as though she fought tears. "Just leave things alone. I lost her once; I don't want—"

The back door clicked open. Mom came in with a box of presto logs and set them beside the fireplace. She gave Dawn a questioning glance. "Is something wrong?"

Dawn shook her head and couldn't think of what to say.

Mom looked at both of them and headed for the back door again.

Dawn struggled to her feet. Pain stabbed into her side. Sucking in her breath, she went outside and leaned over the rail above the stairs. "Mom, wait."

Mom glanced at her, expression bleak.

"You don't have to leave."

Her mouth curved in disbelief. "You should go back inside and stay warm. You don't want to catch cold. " She went down the steps and disappeared around the corner.

55

CAROLYN STEPPED INSIDE the storage area under the garage and pulled the string attached to a swaying overhead light. She hefted another box of presto logs and set it near the door. She'd take it up in a little while. She wasn't in any hurry to go back upstairs and walk into another private conversation.

She could use an AA meeting right now. She felt at home among others who had struggled with life. She felt Jesus' presence there. He'd come to redeem sinners, hadn't He? He'd raised her up from out of the mire and planted her feet on His sacred ground. Sometimes, she forgot the past entirely, until something or someone reminded her again.

Carolyn breathed in slowly and exhaled. She had other things to think about . . . and no time to feel sorry for herself.

Most of the stuff under the house would have to be hauled away, like the red vinyl and chrome kitchen stools from the Paxtown house. Why had Mom and Dad hung on to them all these years? The metal frames had rusted and the seats cracked. Dad's fishing poles, net, creel, and box of flies hung on one wall, along with his brown chest-waders, two pairs of hiking boots, and an old backpack. An old AM/FM radio sat between stacks of *National Geographic*s bound in bundles of twelve. Dad said they'd be worth something, someday. Water-damaged and worthless now, the whole collection would have to be lugged up to the road and taken to the dump. She wondered what Dad would say if he knew the entire collection was now available on CD-ROM.

Removing a canvas cover, Carolyn found a fertilizer spreader and push mower. The Jenner house didn't have a lawn. She opened a coffinlike chest and stepped back from the stench of molding blankets and towels. Not even a rat or mouse would make a nest in there. She found Charlie's old Lionel train, complete with engine, cars, caboose, tracks and railroad signs, station house and town buildings. Christopher would have enjoyed setting this up when he was a little boy. Had Dad forgotten about it or left it in storage because it hurt too much to be reminded of Charlie?

Another box held Charlie's high school yearbooks. She sat in the red Adirondack chair she'd given Dad for his sixtieth birthday and opened the 1962 *Amadon* yearbook. Leafing through the pages, she found his senior picture, hair neat and short. She found Mitch's picture. She loved his smile. She found other pictures of Charlie and Mitch: kneeling in the front row of the varsity football team, helmets on their knees; standing with other members of the basketball team; Charlie, head back as he laughed while hanging out on the senior lawn with friends. Friends had scrawled notes everywhere.

"I still miss you, Charlie," Carolyn whispered and closed the book. Her brother had always had a contagious laugh. Had he lived, he'd be married with grown children and grandchildren by now.

She put her head back against the chair and closed her eyes. Her heart still ached. Being cooped up and feeling like a third wheel didn't help. Mom and May Flower Dawn were close. That was good.

God, grant me the serenity to accept the things I cannot change.

She couldn't undo the past. She couldn't reclaim what had never belonged to her.

God, grant me the courage to change the things I can.

Maybe it was time to talk about the past . . . if she could do so with love. As much as she wanted to say it didn't matter, it still had the power to torment her. She'd come out to the beach a hundred times and written her sins in the sand, watching them wash away. But the guilt and shame always came back to haunt her.

"God won't take you where His love won't protect you," Boots had told her. "You lived through it. You're a survivor. The past doesn't have any power over you anymore."

Only the power she gave it.

Boots knew about the circumstances of her pregnancy. Carolyn had told her about her life in Haight-Ashbury and Rachel Altman. She'd even confessed her relationship with Ash—sordid, abusive, heart- and soul-crushing. But she'd never told her about the bee-keeper who lived next door and what she'd done with him.

God, grant me the wisdom . . . Your will, not mine be done.

Your will, Lord. Not Mom's or mine or even May Flower Dawn's.

Calm again, she stacked the yearbooks on top of the box of presto logs and headed back upstairs.

Mom sat in her recliner, reading a magazine. She glanced up as Carolyn came in the back door. "It must be freezing down there."

"Cold and damp, but not too bad." Dawn was asleep on the couch, the white afghan tucked around her. Carolyn set the box of presto logs on top of the other one and put the yearbooks on the coffee table. "She's awfully pale."

Mom put the magazine away. "She is, isn't she? And so thin."

"Did she tell you what made her drive across the country?"

"Just what she told us already. Pregnant women get strange urges. Maybe we're like salmon. We want to return to the stream where we were born."

"Then she should've headed for LA." Carolyn saw Mom wince and wished she hadn't said it. "I found Charlie's high school yearbooks."

Pain flickered across Mom's face. "I haven't looked at them in years. I won't have any room for them when I move."

When she moved, not *if.* "I'd like to keep them, if it's all right with you."

"Of course. You probably want some of the pictures in that box, too. I have my favorites hanging in the bedroom. I'll take those with me."

The lights flickered. Carolyn opened a box of presto logs. "I need to break a couple of these so we have kindling, and I'd better do it now before we lose power." Mom told her where to find Dad's hatchet and suggested taking one of the grocery bags under the sink to carry the pieces.

Carolyn chopped two logs into thick, pancake-size chunks; tucked a few old newspapers in the bag; and went back inside. Just as she closed the door behind herself, the lights went out and the heater shut down.

"Well, there it goes." Mom sighed. "At least we still have some daylight, but the house is going to get cold. There won't be heat downstairs. Why don't you bring your things up? Dawn can sleep with me in my bed and you can have that room. We'll keep the fire going and leave the bedroom doors ajar."

Carolyn rearranged several boxes. "First things first, Mom. We've got fuel; now we need to figure out how to cook."

"There's a Coleman stove under Dad's workbench."

Carolyn went out to find it.

❄ ❄ ❄

Dawn awakened to rain splattering the windows and a crackling fire. Granny sat quietly reading Oma's journal. "Where's Mom?" Dawn pushed herself up slowly, rubbing at her side.

"Out in the garage." Granny put the journal aside.

It was growing darker by the minute. "How long have I been asleep?"

"A couple of hours. You must have needed it." Granny studied her. "How do you feel now?"

"Groggy. Hungry."

"Your mom is trying to find the Coleman stove. We'll need it if we're going to cook. The generator went off. I'm out of propane. No light, no heat, no stove."

Dawn heard her mother come in the back door and move around in the kitchen before entering the living room. She sank wearily into the chair closest to the fire. "Finally found it under the garage. It was with Dad's fishing poles."

"Logical place for it." Granny nodded. "Did you see a down sleeping bag?"

"Yep, but it's mildewed."

"More stuff for the dump," Granny muttered.

"I'll use Dawn's bedding, Mom."

Granny took the flashlight and went into the master bedroom. She came back with a pile of clothes. She dropped a dark green sweatshirt and pants onto Mom's lap and a navy blue set beside Dawn. "Dad's. I meant to offer these things to Mitch and Christopher, but I kept forgetting. Take off those dirty pants, Carolyn, and put on the sweats. You must be frozen through."

Mom laughed. "After all the trips in and out of the garage and up and down those stairs, I'm nice and toasty."

"Well, you won't be for long."

Mom went to change. Dawn pulled on the extra layer. Papa's sweatpants pooled around her feet. She laughed. At least they fit her waistline. "Don't I look fetching?"

Granny chuckled. She went back into the bedroom and returned with thick pairs of Papa's socks. She insisted on warming the stone soup. "It's my house. I'm supposed to be the hostess." They ate in the living room, Mom sitting cross-legged on the rug in front of the fireplace, Dawn and Granny in the two yellow swivel chairs on either side of her.

Dawn relished the closeness. This was a first—the three of them sitting and talking, like three buddies at a sleepover. "I'm glad the roads are closed and the power is off."

Granny shook her head. "Being cut off from the world is the last thing a lady in your condition should want."

"This is fun, don't you think? The three of us sitting around the fire, enjoying one another's company." Deeper conversations could happen under these circumstances. She wouldn't push yet. *God, You do it. Strip away their resistance. Open their hearts. Get them talking.*

Granny tucked her hands inside Papa's old sweatshirt. "It's why Papa and I moved out here. We hoped this would become a gathering place for the whole family. Maybe I should keep the place, for you and Jason and your children to enjoy."

Mom looked at her with dismay. She set her empty bowl aside and pulled her legs up against her chest, gazing into the fire. Dawn didn't have to guess what she was thinking, and she decided it was time to make a few things clear. "Jason intends to stay in the military, Granny. He could be transferred anywhere anytime."

"Just a thought." Granny sighed. "Things don't always turn out the way we hope."

"I noticed you were reading Oma's journal again. Did she ever come up here, Granny?"

"She drove up once to see the place, stayed for two days, and went back to Merced. We invited her to live with us, but Mama said there wasn't anything in Jenner that mattered to her." She pinched lint off the sweatpants.

Dawn felt her hurt, but saw no reason for it. "I doubt she meant you and Papa didn't matter, Granny."

"Well, what else could she mean?"

Mom glanced at her. "Oma liked meeting people."

"There are people here."

"She liked exploring in her car."

"She had to give it up soon after that."

"And she wasn't happy about it. She started taking walks around the neighborhood, then started riding the city bus. She said it took a while to feel comfortable riding around town with strangers, but she got to know the drivers and some of the regular passengers. She rode the bus to the community college and took classes there. She was enrolled in another American history course when she passed away."

Granny leaned back, taking in that news. "I didn't know that." She sat quietly, contemplating what Mom had told her. "Oma always valued education. College for Bernie, trade school for Chloe, art classes for Rikka. She was disappointed when I chose nurses' training."

"Why?" Dawn curled her legs into the chair and pulled Papa's sweatshirt over her knees.

"She thought I was training to be a servant. Oma wanted me to go to the University of California."

Mom glanced up. "Her father made her quit school. Oma told me she would have loved to have gone to a university and I should take advantage of the opportunity."

Granny gave a soft laugh. "She said she'd pay my way if I'd go to the school she had picked out for me. I enrolled in nurses' training anyway. It was the first time I bucked her about anything." Her smile turned sardonic. "It makes sense she set up that fund for girls wanting to go to college. And it never occurred to me that might be the reason Mama didn't want to live up here."

"Did Oma ever earn a degree?"

Granny shrugged. "I don't know. She would've told you, Carolyn."

Mom smiled. "Dawn gave her the only diploma she ever received. I think Oma just liked learning new things. She took art history once so she and Aunt Rikki would have things to talk about."

"Did she ever take biology?" Granny asked.

"She took anatomy, physiology, and biology by correspondence course while living at the cottage. When she moved to Merced, she took chemistry. She said she could've used your help with that one."

Granny frowned. "Why didn't she ever tell me?"

"She tried. She invited you over for tea every day. You always had other things to do."

Granny sat with her lips parted, a deep frown furrowing her brow. Dawn remembered that when Oma died, Granny had grieved deeply. Was it because things had been left unsettled between them?

Granny crossed her arms, hugging herself. "I've been reading her journal. I'd hoped it might share some of her feelings. But it's just recipes, housekeeping information, boardinghouse rules, farm schedules—"

"You haven't read all of it yet, Granny."

"I'm sure it's unrealistic to think she'd have written anything about me, when she could never be bothered to talk to me. Or to say she loved me. She never said that to me, not once in my entire life."

Mom turned to her. "Maybe we have something in common."

"Don't you dare sit there and say Oma never told you she loved you. I heard her say it to you all the time! Every day when I was sick in bed, I'd hear her say it. 'I love you, Carolyn. I love you. I love you.'" Granny's voice broke.

"I didn't mean Oma." Mom turned her face toward the warmth of the fire.

Granny looked as though Mom had slapped her. Her eyes shone with tears as she stared at Mom.

Dawn wanted to weep for both of them. "Oma loved you, Granny."

Granny hadn't taken her eyes off Mom. "I'd like to believe she did, but she never said it. Not to me."

"Not everyone knows how to say it, Granny. They show it. Did Oma tell anyone she loved them? Uncle Bernie? Aunt Chloe?"

"She never said it to anyone, not even my father."

Mom frowned. "She loved him, didn't she?"

"So much so, I worried she'd grieve herself to death after he died. She'd go out into the orchard and scream and pound the earth. . . ." Her eyes filled. "I never understood her."

"Oma wrote about love in her journal, Granny." Dawn got up and retrieved the worn leather book from the side table. She turned pages. "Here. From 1 Corinthians 13. 'Love is patient, love is kind and is not jealous; love does not brag and is not arrogant. . . .'"

She turned more pages until she found what she was looking for near the end. "'We try to do a little better than the previous generation and find out in the end we've made the same mistakes without intending. Instead of striving to love as God first loved us, we let past hurts and grievances rule. Ignorance is no excuse.'" She looked up. "It's right here in her handwriting."

Dawn sat down. "Oma told me she only wrote important thoughts in her journal, things that helped her in life." She turned more pages. "Here's more about love. 'I know how Abraham felt when he placed Isaac on the altar. I know that pain. But what did Isaac feel lying there, bound, his father holding the knife? afraid? abandoned? expendable? Or did he, too, understand God would rescue him? God tested Abraham, and He showed Isaac what it meant to trust God. Will my Isaac ever understand that what I do, I do for love?'"

Dawn looked pointedly at Granny. "Who do you suppose Oma's Isaac was?"

"Bernie or Papa. Perhaps. How would I know?"

Mom's face filled with compassion. She met Dawn's eyes, but spoke to Granny. "I think it was you, Mom."

Granny closed her eyes and shook her head, as though the idea was too painful to consider. "We'll never really know, will we?"

56

CAROLYN LAY AWAKE on the couch after Mom and Dawn went to bed. She imagined them curled up together, sharing warmth under the covers. Why couldn't she get warm? She got up and dragged the blankets with her as she sat closer to the fire. She kept thinking about what Oma had written about Abraham and Isaac. That kind of love seemed a mystery. She understood Jacob better. Like Jacob, she had worked to earn the one she loved—May Flower Dawn—and felt cheated in the end. She also identified with Leah, the least loved, always second best.

God caused all things to work together for the good for those who love Him, and she did. Would she have learned to center her life on Jesus if she'd gotten everything she wanted? She might have poured all of her love and hope onto her daughter. God had seen that that wouldn't happen. Even Mitch, the love of her life, came in second to Jesus.

Why this sudden, deep, inexplicable desire to understand her mother, and have her understand as well? After all these years . . . Carolyn had learned, slowly, to let other people in. She opened the door of her heart to Mitch first, then allowed him free access to all her rooms. Christopher had never had to struggle with that.

She wondered if her mother had been knocking all these years, and she'd been too afraid to look through the peephole, let alone open the door. Oma once told her not to waste time on regrets, but to grasp opportunities. She remembered something else Oma had said, something that had made no sense to her at the time. "Your mother will take good care of May Flower Dawn. She never really had the chance to take care of you."

Carolyn looked up when she saw a movement in the shadows. Mom came out in her thick bathrobe and fuzzy pink slippers. "Are you cold?"

Carolyn forced a smile. "I shouldn't be. You should go back to bed. Keep warm."

"Maybe you caught cold working out in the garage. I can get you another blanket out of the closet."

"I'm fine, Mom. Really."

Her mother eased herself into the yellow swivel chair. "I've been thinking . . ." She folded her hands in her lap. "It's easier to talk about lesser sorrows, but we're silent about the ones that break our hearts and change everything."

Carolyn wanted to apologize. "Charlie." Maybe she should've left that box of pictures in the garage. She should've left the year-books under the house.

"I wasn't thinking about Charlie. I've been thinking about you, Carolyn." She looked uncertain. "It was hard for me to turn you over to Oma. I don't think you have any idea how much I love you. I do, you know. I always have."

Carolyn couldn't catch her breath. When she did, she put her head against her knees and cried.

❄ ❄ ❄

Dawn awakened when Granny got out of bed. She didn't move or speak as Granny quietly left the room. Dawn heard Granny speaking softly. Then Mom started to cry. Easing out from under the covers, Dawn wrapped Papa's old robe around herself and approached the door.

Finally, Lord.

She pressed her fingers against her trembling lips.

Mom didn't say anything.

God, please, help her speak. I don't mean to be selfish, but I need them to work things out.

"Carolyn?" Granny spoke softly, tentatively. "Why are you crying?"

Dawn covered her face and prayed.

❄ ❄ ❄

Carolyn turned her head and gave her mother a watery smile. "I didn't think you even liked me."

"Can you tell me why you thought that?"

Her mother looked so bleak, so concerned, Carolyn decided it was time to unlock the door and open it a little. "A lot of reasons."

"You said I yelled at you to get out of my bedroom. Is that why?"

"Yes, but I understand that now." It wasn't what her mother had done as much as what she hadn't. "You never allowed me to sit close to you. You never held me on your lap or kissed me."

"I couldn't, Carolyn. The TB."

"You couldn't wait to get your hands on May Flower Dawn, Mom. You held and kissed her all the time."

"I wasn't sick anymore then."

Carolyn smiled sadly. "You weren't sick when we moved to the property."

Mom bowed her head. "Maybe it became a habit with us." She raised her head. "I wanted to hold you, Carolyn, but by then you didn't want anyone but Oma to hold you. I sent her home so I could win you back, but instead, you withdrew. You didn't seem to want me; you didn't seem to want friends. You never showed interest until you met Rachel Altman."

Carolyn's heart started to pound the way it did in AA meetings when she knew God was nudging her to share. She looked into the fire. She could remain silent and let Mom believe what she did, or she could risk everything and tell the truth. The tension inside her built until she thought her heart would explode if she didn't say something. "I had one friend."

"Who?"

She could say Suzie, the girl who moved away. Mom might remember her. "Dock." His name came out before she thought better of it.

"Dock?"

Her mother didn't even remember him. It seemed so strange she wouldn't when Dock had dominated so much of Carolyn's childhood. "Hickory, dickory, dock." He didn't chase mice up a clock. He offered cheese and crackers to a little girl, then drew her slowly into his lair.

❄ ❄ ❄

It was a moment before Hildie remembered him, but when she did, she went cold. "You don't mean Lee Dockery, do you?" She could picture the beekeeper next door, his disturbing smile, the way he never looked her in the eye. He'd been polite, but something about him had made Hildie's skin crawl. They'd told the children to steer clear of him.

She studied her daughter. Carolyn sat hunched, arms locked around her knees, face turned away. Was she trembling? "How did you meet him?"

"Charlie took me over to his house. Before you and Dad told us to stay away."

Hildie pressed a hand against her stomach, trying to ignore the uneasy feelings stirring inside her. The man had mysteriously vanished around the same time Carolyn started having nightmares. Hildie had worried that there might be a connection, but Trip had assured her there couldn't be. *No. Please, God, no.* "Did you go back to see him?

"Yes."

"Often?"

"Yes." Carolyn pulled her knees in tighter to her chest and kept her head down. "At first, I sat by the fence and just watched him take honeycombs from the hives. He'd talk to me. He told me all about his bees. He gave me pieces of honeycomb. It dripped all over me once, and I started crying because I thought Daddy would be mad and he'd give me another spanking. Dock said I could come inside his house and wash off. He let me take a bath while he washed my clothes. He told me how lonely he was all by himself."

Hildie closed her eyes tightly. *Oh, God, oh, God! Why couldn't my little girl come to me?*

"I went back the next day and the next. He'd give me crackers and honey . . ."

Hildie clenched her hands. Her daughter had always loved baths. Hildie remembered being so tired by the end of the day; she'd wash Carolyn quickly, efficiently, like a nurse with a patient. Just get the job done. "Don't dawdle, Carolyn," she'd say. "It's time for bed." Hildie had been so tired, afraid she would get sick again. She needed to get some rest.

"Dock put the lid down on the toilet and talked to me while I was in the tub. He'd tell me stories." She closed her eyes tightly. "Later . . ."

The fire cracked. The rain drummed on the roof. A pulse beat in Hildie's head.

"What happened later?"

"He washed me."

Hildie fought rage and sorrow. What had she been doing that had been so important she hadn't noticed her daughter missing? Was she tending the vegetable garden? planting walnut trees? hanging up laundry? Busy, always busy with something! There had always been something to do. Charlie had been off on his bike visiting friends. She'd assumed her quiet, timid little girl was close by, picking flowers, making mud pies, watching butterflies. How could she have been so blind?

"We played games."

Hildie bit her lip. She and Trip had moved to the country so their children would be safe, so they'd have plenty of fresh air and sunshine. She felt sick with premonition, but had to know. "What sort of games, Carolyn?"

"Secret games, he called them. Touching games." Carolyn spoke so softly.

Hildie gave a soft sob and pressed her hands over her mouth. Carolyn glanced up sharply, eyes wide. She looked down quickly, putting her arms over her head. "I'm sorry. I shouldn't have told you. I'm sorry. I'm sorry." Her body shook.

When Carolyn tried to get up, Hildie reached out and pulled her back against her legs, pinning her there, arms wrapped around her. Sobbing, she rested her head on Carolyn's until she could speak. "It's not your fault, honey. It's mine." She felt a shudder go through Carolyn and held on tighter. "It's my fault, sweetheart. I'm so sorry."

Carolyn started to cry again, body relaxing, giving in. Hildie didn't let go of her. She stroked her hair and kissed the top of her head. She hadn't been there when her little girl needed her, and she might never be able to forgive herself for that. But she could try to comfort the woman in her arms now.

Carolyn wiped her face with her sleeve. "I knew I wasn't supposed to go there, Mom, but he was nice to me. He held me and kissed me and said he loved me." She gulped down a sob. "I was stupid. I was so stupid!"

"You weren't stupid. You were a *child*."

"He didn't hurt me until the last time. And then there was blood, a lot of blood, and he cried. I was so scared. And he wouldn't let me go until I promised . . . He said we'd both be in big trouble if I told anyone what we'd been playing. At first, he told me not to come back. Then he came to my window that night and said he loved me. He wanted me to be his little girl. He said he was going to look for a safe place for us. I'd know when he found it because he'd leave some honey at the front door. I don't think I dreamed it all. It was so real."

Horror filled Hildie. That man would have kidnapped Carolyn. She and Trip never would've found her. *Oh, God, thank You.* She hadn't been looking out for her daughter. But God had.

"That's why you crept into Charlie's room and slept with him."

"Yes, and when you told me to stop, I'd hide in my closet." She shuddered and moved away slightly so they could face one another. "I heard you and Dad talking about Dock. I was afraid you'd figured out what I'd done and I would be in trouble. But you never did."

Hildie wanted to reach out again and pull her daughter close. She wanted to brush her hair the way she had when Carolyn was a toddler. She ached for the time lost, hating the disease that had made her push her daughter away in the first place. She couldn't bear the thought of her precious little girl living in fear, having nightmares about the monster next door, allowing only Oma inside the walls she built to protect herself. Had Mama known? Surely she would have said something!

Hildie's arms ached to simply hold her. But it was important to keep talking, to get it all out in the open. "Lee Dockery was killed in an accident, Carolyn."

"When?" Carolyn looked up at her, face pale and strained.

"A few weeks after your nightmares started. No one disappears without a reason. Dad knew something had happened to him. He went over to see if he'd had a heart attack or something. He went into the house and found everything in order."

Hildie leaned forward, clasping her hands tensely, uncertain how her daughter would take what she had to tell her. "Lee Dockery's place stood vacant until the bank repossessed the property and sold it at auction. A year after the new family moved in, a couple of boys found Lee Dockery's truck in a ravine down in Niles Canyon. Apparently, he'd swerved off the road and gone over the edge where it wouldn't have been seen from the road."

"Was Dock in the car?"

What was left of him, after the animals had gotten to his body and time had stripped his flesh. "Yes, he was. So were his bees." They'd built a hive inside the cab of his truck.

Carolyn let out a long breath and closed her eyes. Her face looked serene. "All those years, I thought he'd come and take me away."

"He would have, Carolyn. God protected you."

"I know."

"Did Charlie know about Dock?"

"No."

It hurt to ask, but she had to know. "Did you tell Oma?"

"No. The only person I ever told about Dock was Chel. And I was drunk at the time."

❋ ❋ ❋

Dawn winced at the growing pain. Gripping the edge of the dresser, she pulled herself up. It eased a little. She sat on the edge of the bed. She felt warm, but the chill made her breath visible. Her daughter kicked twice. Smiling, Dawn ran her hand over her belly. "Sorry I woke you up." She took a pillow and put it at the end of the bed, then stretched out on her side so she could listen to Mom and Granny talk. She stroked her belly slowly, rhythmically. "They're going to love you, sweetie."

The sound of their voices filled her with hope for the future. "No tug-of-war this time."

57

"Can we talk about what happened in Berkeley, Carolyn? Please."

Carolyn braced her back against the other chair. Her mother hadn't blamed her for what happened. She'd blamed Dock. Maybe it was time to get everything out in the open. Haight-Ashbury and all the rest.

"I wanted to end the war, Mom. I wanted to save Charlie. I didn't care about school. It seemed pointless to attend classes when my brother was risking his life every minute of the day. So I quit and went on protest marches. When I wasn't doing that, I drank to forget. All I could think about was trying to get Charlie out of Vietnam. And I failed. When Charlie died, I just lost it."

"You were gone before you knew about Charlie."

"No, I wasn't."

"Yes. You were. We called the day after the officers came to the house, and your phone was disconnected. We drove to Berkeley. Your neighbors said they hadn't seen either of you in a while. The landlord was there. He said the place was trashed."

"Oma called the day the soldiers came to the house. I knew

what that meant. I remember screaming and Chel giving me something. The next thing I remember is Chel driving me across the
Bay Bridge, Janis Joplin screaming on the radio, Chel screaming
along with her." She closed her eyes so she wouldn't have to see
Mom's face when she said the rest. "I woke up in a strange house,
in a strange bed, with a guy I'd never seen before. It got worse
after that."

Carolyn pressed the heels of her hands against her eyes. "I used
to dream about Charlie all the time." She gulped down tears. "I'd
see him in a rice paddy. I'd see him burning in napalm. I'd see
him—" She stopped, appalled, realizing what her words must be
doing to her mother. She took her hands away. "I'm sorry."

"Don't stop, honey." Her mother spoke in a soft, choked voice.
"Tell me the rest."

"I stayed stoned and drunk, trying to deal with his death."

"You looked so frail when you came home."

Carolyn remembered all too well. She'd been starving slowly,
living on garbage. And then a young vet gave her a chocolate bar
and kept her warm. A young woman gave her hope and a ticket
home. "I lived in Golden Gate Park for a while. I don't remember
how long. I had to get out of that house and away from Ash."

"What house? And who is Ash?"

"We lived in a big house on Clement Street. He moved in
while Chel and I were in New York, celebrating rock and roll at
Woodstock." She spoke wryly, then went on. "She was messed
up on drugs. I didn't know if she'd come out of it. Her mind
cleared in Wyoming. When we got back, we found this beautiful
stranger sitting in the living room. He used to wear white robes
like Jesus and spoke in poetry. A fake guru, speaking bull, seduc-
ing everyone. Everyone was stoned all the time and sleeping with
whoever. Chel was the one with the money. Ash took her over the
minute she walked in the door, or he thought he did. Chel always
knew what was what. She knew Ash for what he was long before
I did. When she got tired of him, he turned to me. All I saw was
the beautiful mask, not the devil behind it. I thought I loved

him. Lee Dockery was a lot kinder." She saw the anguish in her mother's face. "I'm sorry, Mom. Maybe you don't want to hear about this."

"I need to know what happened to my daughter. Don't you think it's time?"

"I guess." Carolyn rubbed her face.

"I always wondered, but I was afraid to ask. Did Chel live in the park with you?"

"No. She overdosed on heroin. A few weeks before, we went out for a long walk in the park. She gave me her father's telephone number and said if anything happened to her, I was to call him. It scared me. I watched over her for days. The one day I didn't . . ." Her voice broke.

"I'm so sorry, honey."

"I found her sprawled across her bed. Ash was furious. He told me to lie if the paramedics asked for her name."

"Why?"

"Why do you suppose? The money would keep being deposited as long as her father thought she was alive. When the ambulance came, I waited outside. Before they took her body away, I gave them her full name. I called her father. And then I just walked away. I didn't look back. I didn't care where I went or what happened to me after that."

Carolyn raked her fingers into her hair and held her head. "I begged, Mom. I slept on benches and under bushes. I ate out of trash bins and slept in a few. I wanted to die, but I didn't have the courage to drown myself in the ocean." She gave a mocking laugh. "It was cold." Sighing, she leaned back against the front of the swivel rocker. "One night I was sitting on the beach and thinking about how nice it would be to have it all over. And then I heard a guitar playing. I saw a young man wearing an Army jacket. I thought it was Charlie, at first." Her eyes swam with tears. "Of course, it couldn't be, but I followed him anyway. He'd made a camp in the park. He had a fire and an old sleeping bag. I was so hungry. He gave me a chocolate bar. He was a veteran. He hadn't just bought the jacket from a surplus store; he'd served in Vietnam. I told him about Charlie. He told me about friends he'd lost in the war."

She drew her knees up against her chest again, hugging them close. "He shared his sleeping bag. He kept me warm. I got up and wandered off. When I couldn't find my way back, I slept on the grass. I woke up at dawn." Tears came and spilled down her cheeks. "It was May, and little white flowers grew in the grass like stars had dropped from heaven. I felt someone touch me. He sat right there on the grass with me."

"The young veteran?"

"No." She shook her head, chewing her lip a moment before she had the courage to say it aloud. She never had before. "I know you won't believe me. You'll think I was drunk or stoned. But I hadn't had anything since leaving Ash." She couldn't see Mom through her tears.

"I'll believe anything you tell me, Carolyn."

Carolyn drew a shuddering breath and prayed she would. "I saw Jesus." She let the memory fill her. "He said it was time to go home. I thought He meant I was going to die. I wasn't afraid. When I sat up, He was gone." She had sat for hours, praying He would come back and take her with Him. "A young woman came and set up a picnic for her two children. She called her little boy Charlie." Her voice wavered.

Her mother put a hand over her mouth.

Carolyn kept going. "It was like watching me and Charlie play together. She invited me to sit with her; she offered me a sandwich. I was so hungry. We talked. I told her about Charlie; she told me about her husband. He was MIA in Vietnam. She called her kids and loaded all of us in a van and took me to the bus station. She bought my ticket home. Her name was Mary."

Carolyn felt the weight lifting as she talked. "She gave me her telephone number and said if you didn't want me, she'd come and get me. I lost the slip of paper on the way home. I've thanked God a thousand times for her over the years, Mom. When the planes landed at Travis Air Force Base in 1973, and all those POWs came off, I cried and prayed Mary's husband stood among them. But I'll never know for sure if he did."

Mom wiped tears from her cheeks, but didn't say anything. She didn't seem shocked or disgusted. Carolyn wondered if she could keep going and decided it was worth the risk. "You asked me why I didn't believe you loved me. When I came home, you and Dad were ashamed of me. I could see it in your faces. When you found out I was pregnant, that was the last straw."

"No, Carolyn. It was a shock, that's all."

"You and Dad asked Rev. Elias to talk to me. He told me not to come back to church."

"What?" Mom spoke weakly, eyes wide.

"He didn't believe I was truly repentant. He said enough to convince me I wasn't good enough to set foot inside any church. When I came home, Dad made a point of asking me if I'd taken everything Rev. Elias said to heart. I did. Then you and Dad told me you were sending me to Los Angeles to live with Boots. You couldn't wait to be rid of me."

"No. *No!*" Mom looked furious, tears streaming down her white cheeks. "We asked Rev. Elias to talk to you because we thought he'd give you wise counsel. For heaven's sake, if we'd known what he said to you, we would've left the church! Why didn't Oma tell me about this?"

"Oma didn't know, Mom. I never told anyone."

"Then she must have guessed, because she left the church right after you did."

"I assumed you and Dad felt the same way he did."

"Of course not! If your father had known, he would've raised holy hell. We sent you away to protect you, not get rid of you." She took a handkerchief from her pocket and blew her nose. "I sent you to Boots. She was my best friend! I knew she'd love you and take good care of you." Her mouth wobbled, tears still streaming. "I wouldn't have entrusted you to anyone else."

Carolyn wanted to believe her, but evidence stood in the way.

"The day I walked into the house, I saw a wall of pictures, all of Charlie."

"We wanted to honor his memory."

"I looked around the house when you and Dad went to work. There wasn't a single picture of me anywhere. Not one."

Her mother clenched the crumpled, damp handkerchief in her lap and looked straight into her eyes. "I put them away a few months after you disappeared. We loved you, Carolyn. We agonized over you. The truth is we grieved more over you than Charlie. We knew what happened to him. He was killed in the line of duty. Don't forget your father was a police officer. He worked in forensics. He dealt with homicides. He had nightmares when he came home from the war. He had worse ones when you disappeared. I put your pictures away because he died a little more inside every time he looked at one. I couldn't bear to lose everyone I loved."

Carolyn's heart hurt. She pressed her hands against her chest, wanting to make it go away. She had spent so many years hiding the pain, not asking why things had been the way they were, afraid the answers might hurt even more.

Mom's eyes warmed, and she gestured toward her bedroom. "I cherish your pictures. Your wedding portrait is on my dresser, your senior picture on my wall, where I can see both of them every night before I go to sleep. All the rest are in an album over there in the cabinet." Her mouth trembled. "I love you. How could I not? You're my own flesh and blood."

Carolyn searched her mother's face and saw raw pain. "How would I know? I haven't stepped foot in your bedroom since I was three years old." She never opened any cabinets except those in the kitchen. She gave a broken laugh. "Oh, Mom . . . we've both been so good at hiding what we feel."

"I just told you I love you, Carolyn. Do you believe me?"

Carolyn looked into her eyes, eyes the same color as Oma's. "Yes." She felt all the tension drain from her body. She smiled. "And in case you don't know it, I love you, too."

❄ ❄ ❄

Dawn was thankful Mom and Granny weren't arguing anymore. She shifted her body, trying to get more comfortable. She could feel the pressure of tiny arms and legs stretching inside her. Taking two pillows and the comforter from the bed, she sat near the door. She covered herself with the comforter, scooted down, and tucked the pillows under her knees. The solid carpeted floor felt better than the soft bed.

Let the words keep flowing, Lord. Dawn knew others were praying for them, too. Georgia and the women of CCC, Pastor Daniel, Mitch, all the people who loved Mom and Granny. Her eyes grew heavy, but she forced herself to stay awake. It gave her joy and hope to hear them talking openly with one another. She probably shouldn't be eavesdropping, but she had been praying for this for so long that she felt she had to hear it to believe it.

Her mom was talking again. "I used to be afraid to love anyone. Charlie died. Then Chel. Oma. Dad. I don't even want to think about losing Mitch."

"Your dad and I rooted for him."

"Mitch told me he was going to marry me that first time he came over for dinner."

"And not for your cooking, I'll bet," Granny teased.

Dawn's mother laughed. "Thanks a lot."

"We knew he had a crush on you when he was a boy. It was hard to miss when he came over all the time."

"To see Charlie."

"And you. It is frightening to lose someone you love. I loved your dad every bit as much as you love Mitch . . . and the way Mama must have loved Papa. We all die sometime. Someday you'll lose me, too, you know."

"Yes, but I'd rather not think about that."

"At least we'll be speaking to one another."

Dawn put her hands over her face and tried not to cry. Some

things might never be worked out. Granny might never believe Oma had loved her.

Granny spoke. "I'm sorry about Rev. Elias, Carolyn. God forgive him. And I'm sorry you didn't understand why we sent you to Boots."

"It was the best thing you could have done for me. She recognized a dry drunk when she saw one and took me to my first AA meeting. She had a band of friends who were full of hope and experience and didn't mind sharing. They all thought I should give up my baby. Boots wanted me to keep May Flower Dawn and stay with her."

"You'll never know how happy Dad and I were when you decided to come home."

"I didn't know I could until you sent that car seat. And then Dad laid down all the rules, and you quit your job so you could take care of May Flower Dawn. . . ."

"We wanted to help you get back on your feet."

"I know."

"I didn't want you staying with Boots."

Dawn heard the tension building in Granny's voice, as though quick words could ward off something she didn't want to hear. But Mom wasn't going to let her get away with it this time. She spoke gently. "I loved Boots, but I didn't want to depend on her. I'd lived off Chel for too long."

"I wanted to help, Carolyn."

"I know."

"You wouldn't have made it on your own." Granny sounded defensive.

"Georgia did."

"Because she didn't have any choice. Her parents kicked her out. We wanted to help."

"Yes. You helped yourself to May Flower Dawn."

Dawn sat up and held her breath. She'd known for years she was the cause of much of their contention. She'd grown up in the middle. Granny had stepped in when needed, then held on. For a long time, Dawn had helped Granny win the tug-of-war. It wasn't until she had sex downstairs with Jason that she understood how guilt and shame could imprison a person, keep her silent, keep her distant. Like Mom.

When Georgia held up the mirror before Dawn's face, and Jason suggested they stop seeing one another, it had been her mother who came in and sat silently on the end of Dawn's bed, empathizing with her pain. It had been Mom's careful words that planted the seeds to let go and let God work, to follow the Lord and not her own deceitful heart and flesh. Mom had understood what Granny couldn't.

And now, Dawn had come home to create a bridge between them, one built on truth and love. She needed them to mend their relationship. She prayed fervently they wouldn't allow Satan to rebuild his stronghold. *Please, God, not now. Not ever again.*

"I'll take the blame for everything else, Carolyn, but don't you dare accuse me of stealing your daughter. That's not fair!"

"You didn't steal her." Mom spoke tenderly. "I placed her in your arms."

"I was helping!"

"Yes, but you didn't leave room for me."

"Of course I did!"

Dawn wept at Granny's pain and defensive tone. *God, help her see the truth!*

"When? I came home aching to nurse her, and you'd already given her a bottle. You wouldn't even let me hold her. You'd tell me she'd been fussy and you'd just put her down and I shouldn't wake her. I worked on Saturdays. You took her to church every Sunday. I never had time with her."

Granny cried, but insisted, "It wasn't my fault Dawn bonded to me. I was the one with her all the time."

"But I wanted to be. You even changed her name."

"Because people thought she was named after the Pilgrims' ship."

"Because you and Dad thought it was a hippy name. Dawn told me. It wasn't a suitable name for an Arundel."

Granny blew her nose. "I suppose I did cut you out."

"I saw how much you loved her, Mom. I was jealous, but I was grateful, too. You and Dad didn't give me a handout. You gave me a hand up. When I finally got on my feet, I tried to win Dawn back. When I married Mitch and we moved to Alexander Valley, I thought I might have a chance."

"And we followed you." Granny sniffled. "I would've lived next door if Trip would've allowed it."

"Dawn told me she hated me for making you cry, and I gave up. Dad reminded me you wanted to help. Looking back now, I think he saw how much we were both hurting."

"My mother 'helped,' too," Granny said bleakly, "and I never really forgave her. It still hurts. Can you forgive me?"

Dawn heard movement and turned so she could see into the living room. Mom knelt in front of Granny. "I forgave you a long time ago."

Granny laid a hand against Mom's cheek. "But it still hurts."

"Yes, but maybe we'll heal now. I saw as a child, but now I see through a woman's eyes. I'm glad it was you and not some stranger in a day care center."

Granny cupped Mom's face and kissed her. "I'm glad it was Oma and not Mrs. Haversal."

Dawn got up carefully. She braced herself against the dresser until the pain eased. Stooping cautiously, she gathered the pillows and comforter and put them back on the bed. She slipped beneath the covers and thanked God for answering her prayers.

She knew her biological father, though nameless, had been a kind, young vet suffering post-traumatic stress like her mother. She knew why Mom named her May Flower Dawn. And Mom and Granny were finally talking. Love would win this time.

CAROLYN GOT UP first, stoked the fire and added two presto logs, then went into the kitchen to start the Coleman and get some water boiling for coffee. She heard a loud, ominous crack from somewhere outside. The house shuddered. Another loud boom, and the house jumped on its foundations. The kitchen picture window cracked. Carolyn clambered away.

"What happened?" Her mother came rushing in, gray hair sticking out in all directions, her robe half-on. "What crashed?" She tied the sash around her waist and opened the back door.

"Wait! Mom, don't go out there." Carolyn pulled her back.

The redwood tree had fallen on the garage. Two-by-fours protruded in all directions. The deck tilted.

"My car!"

"I parked it on the road yesterday so I could sort things in the garage. It should be okay."

"Oh. Good." Her mother started to giggle. "We're going to have a lot less to sort through now."

Carolyn took her by the arm. "Let's go sit in the living room."

"Why? Because the kitchen seems to be tilting?"

"It's not. Is it?" Carolyn's insides quivered as her gaze darted around the room.

As they headed for the living room, her mother glanced out the door again. "At least we won't have to worry about firewood. We have a mountain of it."

Carolyn sat near the fire. "I can't believe Dawn slept through that!"

Mom sat across from her. "Thank goodness that's the only tree in front of the house."

"As long as the house doesn't slide down the hill."

"Well, aren't you the optimist." Mom gave her a humorless smile. "Dad said this house is built on rock."

"Did he mean granite . . . or Jesus?"

"Let's hope he meant both." They sat in companionable silence. "I wonder what all that redwood is worth," Mom mused. "Maybe enough to pay for a new garage." She shook her head. "I'll tell you one thing. I'm more than ready to get out of here now."

Carolyn chortled. "I would hope so."

Dawn came out of the bedroom, bleary-eyed. "What's all the noise?"

They told her while she made herself comfortable on the couch, the white afghan around her shoulders again. "Can we get out?"

"I don't know." Carolyn studied her. "Do we need to?"

Dawn smiled. "No."

Carolyn brushed aside a niggling worry. "I'm going to take a look around, anyway."

The gate was stuck, but she managed to shove it open after several tries. The unearthed roots of the redwood tree stood seven to eight feet high, and they had pulled up most of the road. A steady flow of rainwater raced down the hill, undercutting the cracked macadam. She went back inside. "I have four-wheel drive. We can drive up the hill and around."

"No, we can't," her mother informed her. "That road has been closed for the last week. There's a big crack down the middle of it."

"We're nice and cozy and all together," Dawn said, perfectly calm. "Let's not worry about it. Let's just talk."

"Granny and I talked most of the night."

"I know. I'm afraid I was eavesdropping. I heard everything."

Heat spilled into Carolyn's cheeks. What "everything" did she mean?

Dawn hugged the blanket closer. "The young veteran who played the guitar was my father, wasn't he?"

So her daughter had heard everything. Carolyn desperately wanted Dawn to understand. "Biologically. But I never thought of him as your father. To me, you were always a gift from God."

Dawn smiled. "I know, Mom. That's why you named me May Flower Dawn."

"Oh!" Carolyn's mother spoke with sudden comprehension. "You said it was May and the flowers were blooming in the grass, and the Lord appeared to you at dawn." Mom's eyes grew moist. "No wonder you were so hurt when I changed it." Her mouth softened. "You couldn't have chosen a better name, Carolyn."

Dawn grinned. "You could've called me Epiphany."

Carolyn laughed as the tension dissolved. "I almost did."

Mom spoke slowly, in wonder, eyes glowing. "May . . . Flower . . . Dawn."

❄ ❄ ❄

After a breakfast of cereal, they went through the other boxes. Dawn felt odd and edgy. She wanted things settled. Now. She didn't have time to wait anymore.

"Now that you don't have a garage, Granny, are you going to park your car in front of an American bungalow in Santa Rosa or a pretty Tuscany villa in Windsor?" She had something else in mind, but her mom would have to bring it up.

"Windsor's closer to Alexander Valley."

Dawn looked pointedly at her mother and raised her brows.

Dawn's mother frowned slightly and sat back on her heels. Then she turned to Granny. "Do you want to live with me and Mitch?"

Granny gaped. "Well, I didn't think you'd want me too close."

"We have maid's quarters we've never used. There's a living room, bedroom with full bath, and a little kitchen."

Granny just stared at her.

"You don't have to live with us. I just thought maybe you'd think about it. I wanted to ask you after Dad died, but you wouldn't even discuss it. You insisted you wanted your independence."

"Then it's your own fault for believing every stupid thing I say!" Granny burst into tears. But she was smiling. "And I thought Marsha had all the luck!"

Mom said they could remove the furnishings, and Granny could bring whatever she wanted, within reason. "Not that old faded couch, please. Let's get a new one."

Dawn felt everything recede in a gray cloud of pain and pressure. Then silence.

"Dawn?" Mom spoke. She and Granny were both staring at her. "What's wrong?"

"I wanted to wait—" Something popped inside her, like a balloon. She gasped as she felt a pool of warm slickness spreading beneath her. "Oh!" Drawing in her breath sharply, she struggled to lift herself off the couch. The moisture went down her legs, soaking through Papa's old sweats and spilling onto his thick socks. "Oh, *no!*"

❄   ❄   ❄

Carolyn tried not to panic while she helped Dawn lie down in the bedroom.

Her mother stood close, speaking with authority. There was an eighty-six-year-old nurse in the house, and she'd just gone on duty. "Raise up, honey. Okay. Carolyn? Get the wastebasket." She peeled off Dawn's sodden sweats and panties and dumped them into the can.

Dawn wept. "I'm so sorry, Granny. I ruined your couch."

"Didn't you just hear your mother say it was ready for the junk-yard? She wasn't going to let me keep it."

"Your nice sheets . . ."

"Oh, hush!"

Carolyn wanted to scream. A couch? Sheets? They had other things to worry about! The baby was coming *early*. The telephone didn't work. The roads were closed. A giant redwood had just upchucked its massive root system all over the road and turned the garage into a pile of giant splinters!

"Another contraction?" Carolyn's mother picked up her wrist-watch and checked Dawn's pulse.

Dawn groaned low and spoke through clenched teeth. "I thought first babies took a long time. . . ."

"Not always. Take a big breath and blow it out. Rest as much as you can, honey."

In less than a minute, another contraction came. Dawn looked at Carolyn. "Mom. You brought the Suburban."

"Yes, but Granny said we can't drive out of here."

"No." Dawn panted. "But you have GPS and OnStar, don't you?"

"Yes!" Carolyn rushed out. Rummaging through her purse, she found her keys and ran for the door.

❄ ❄ ❄

Hildie wiped Dawn's forehead. The poor girl was burning up. Though it had been decades since Hildie had assisted at a child-birth, she could still recognize a serious situation when she saw it. "Is there anything else I should know about your condition, sweet-heart? You haven't looked well ever since you arrived. Do you want to tell me what's going on?"

Dawn met her eyes briefly, then glanced away. "Hodgkin's lymphoma. It's why I came home. Well, partly why." Dawn grabbed her hand. "Don't you dare cry. Not now. And don't say anything to Mom. Please, Granny. I was going to talk to both of you at the same time, but I wanted you two to work things out first." Another contraction came, harder than the last. "God won't take this baby. He won't."

Hildie stroked Dawn's hair back and told her to ride on top of the pain, like a surfer on a wave. "When did you find out?"

Dawn panted, beads of perspiration on her face. "October. The doctor wanted me to start chemo." Tears streamed from her eyes into her hair. "They told me they could limit the dose to protect the baby, but I just couldn't take that chance. Not after waiting so long for her."

"Why didn't you tell us? Your mom and Mitch would have flown out to be with you—or to bring you back here. We could have helped you."

The back door opened. "Don't tell her! Please. Not yet. Let me—"

"Shhh." Hildie wiped her cheeks quickly. "Don't worry. Concentrate on having your daughter."

Carolyn came back into the bedroom. "I got through. They're calling it in." She came around the bed and took Dawn's hand. "How're you doing?"

Dawn gave her a tremulous smile. "Fine, Mom."

"There's a rescue helicopter at Santa Rosa Memorial, but it's going to take a while." Carolyn squeezed Dawn's hand. "It stopped raining a few minutes ago. God's clearing the way. They'll have to land on the road down by the Jenner Inn and hike up."

Another contraction had Dawn crying out and pushing down. Hildie put her hand on Dawn's abdomen again, timing the contraction. "What about the tree? Can they get by it?"

"I wish I had a chain saw!" Carolyn didn't take her eyes off Dawn.

Trip had bought one, but Hildie wasn't about to tell Carolyn where to find it. She didn't even want to think about the damage her daughter could do to herself with one of those things. "Bring the Coleman stove into the bathroom. Get a big pot, fill it with water, and get it boiling. There should be string in one of the kitchen drawers, and bring my sharp paring knife. And tongs."

Dawn giggled. "Granny sounds like my nursing instructor at San Luis Obispo. Bossy!"

"Thank God!" Smiling, Carolyn rushed out again. She set everything up. "I put some of your new towels on a kitchen chair in front of the fire. They'll be warm enough for the baby."

"Not too close, I hope," Granny muttered. "The last thing we need right now is a fire."

They all laughed a little wildly.

Five minutes later, they knew the baby wasn't going to wait for the helicopter.

"Wash your hands carefully, Carolyn, but hurry up about it." Hildie knew she didn't have the physical strength to finish the job. Dawn's body shook through transition. Her granddaughter had no break now, one contraction rolling right over into another, crushing her with pain.

Now that she knew it wasn't just childbirth racking Dawn's frail body, Hildie had to will herself not to weep. All her knowledge and training kicked into overdrive, but her legs had begun to ache so much she could barely stand. "I need that vanity chair, Carolyn."

Carolyn set it where she pointed.

"Stand there. You're going to deliver your granddaughter."

"What?"

"I'm going to tell you what to do. Don't argue or say you can't. You can."

Carolyn obeyed. Hildie put her hand on Dawn's arm and talked them both through it. She told Dawn to let nature take its course. "Don't hold back. Push!" She gave Carolyn instructions and watched her do exactly as told. Dawn's daughter broke into the world, red-faced and screaming.

Carolyn laughed joyously. "She's beautiful, Dawn. She's perfect, just like you were."

"Put the baby on Dawn's abdomen. Tie the cord, Carolyn. That's it. You can cut it now. I'll get the towels."

The *womp-womp* of a helicopter went over the house.

Hildie took the warm towels draped over the chair in front of the fireplace and brought them back to her girls. "Early bird or not, her lungs are in great condition." Dawn and Carolyn laughed in relief. Carolyn wrapped the baby and placed her in Dawn's arms.

Dawn drew the soft toweling down and gazed into her daughter's face. Smiling, she kissed her. "Your name is Faith." She looked up at her mother and sorrow mingled with joy. "Sit here close to me, Mom. You, too, Granny. I have to tell you something."

Hildie already knew. When Dawn finished, Carolyn was white. "No." Hildie reached for her hand and held it tightly, her own heart breaking.

"I didn't want it to be true either, Mom. But we can't hide from the truth. You and Granny will need to work together. Jason's life isn't his own. You'll be Faith's guardian, Mom. Granny, you're going to help her. So will Georgia. God is going to give back all the years the locusts ate, Mom."

"May Flower Dawn." Carolyn crumbled, head against Dawn's side.

Dawn put her hand on her mother's head as though offering a blessing. "You're stronger than anyone I know. Keep Faith, Mom." She smiled at Hildie. "Promise me you'll share."

❄ ❄ ❄

When the paramedics arrived, they worked quickly, efficiently. They said they had room for only one more in the helicopter. Hildie almost said she'd go, but stopped herself. "You go." She cupped Carolyn's face. "You're her mother."

"Mitch and I will come out and get you as soon as we can."

Hildie kissed Dawn and the baby. "I'll see you both soon." She tucked a strand of golden hair away from Dawn's cheek. "You hold on to faith, honey. Don't you dare give up."

When they left, Hildie went back inside. She sat in her recliner and cried. Then she prayed. She kept praying until dusk came. She forgot to stoke the fire, and it went out. She took the blanket off the couch and bundled up in it. She had weathered other winters without fire or light. She could weather this one. The darkness fit her despair.

She awakened to someone calling her name. She saw a flash of light. The back door opened, and the beam caught and blinded her. "Who . . . ?"

"Sorry it took so long to get out here, Hildie." *Mitch.* "I had to come around through Sebastopol and Bodega. The river's gone down enough to come across from Bridgehaven."

Her son-in-law had come to her rescue. God had already sent him to rescue her daughter years ago.

"You want to pack a few things?"

"I think I should, don't you?" She was still in her pajamas.

Mitch helped her around the tree roots and buckled road. He'd driven the Jaguar. It roared to life. He told her Dawn and the baby were both doing well. The baby weighed almost six pounds. Hildie asked him if he knew the reason May Flower Dawn had driven across country in the dead of winter.

"Yes. I know. The only one who doesn't know yet is Jason, and I've got a few friends in high places moving heaven and earth to get him home."

Hildie didn't learn until later how many had been praying for the restorative miracle that had taken place at Jenner—and went on praying Dawn wouldn't be called home. Not yet.

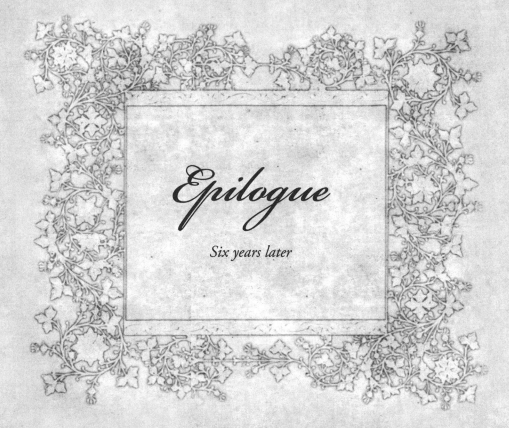

Epilogue

Six years later

CAROLYN PUT HER shoulder bag and two tote bags into the compartment beside her seat in the mammoth Lufthansa 747 aircraft. Mitch had made the arrangements and, as usual, spared no expense to make sure she was comfortable. Her husband had put her, Faith, and Georgia in business class for the long flight to Frankfurt. Faith, blonde hair in pigtails, sat on the big leather seat, jean-clad legs straight out, feet dangling, Puppy Brown hugged in a protective embrace. She looked so much like May Flower Dawn at six years of age, it pierced Carolyn's heart. She buckled Faith's seat belt before her own and brushed her knuckles down her grand-daughter's satiny cheek. "Excited to see Daddy, sweetheart?"

Faith nodded. Carolyn leaned forward and looked across the aisle. "How's GeeGee doing over there?"

Georgia sat across the aisle, face pale and strained. She gave a nervous smile. "I'm fine." She looked anything but fine, but Carolyn understood all too well. Learning Jason had been seriously wounded in Afghanistan and flown to Landstuhl had them all on their knees.

They'd gotten the news two weeks ago that Jason had been

wounded, but didn't know until a few days later the extent of his
injuries and where he had been transferred. Eventually, Jason would
end up in the States, but how long before that happened? weeks? a
month? two? Just as he'd done in the days following Faith's birth,
Mitch had moved mountains to get family members together during
this time of crisis. He had gotten Jason home from Iraq within five
days of Faith's birth at Jenner. May Flower Dawn had spent a week
in the hospital after Faith was born. Tests confirmed what she already
knew: she didn't have much time. The doctor ordered palliative radiation to control the pain. Dawn came home, and hospice was called
in. Christopher withdrew from classes at Stanford and came home to
spend as much time with his big sister as possible.

Everyone had worried about Jason. He'd been strong through
Dawn's last weeks, but grieved hard when she died. He lost weight,
couldn't sleep, wouldn't talk. Pastor Daniel took him away for a
few days, and Jason seemed better when they returned, less lost and
broken. He held Faith close. When called back to duty, he went
with God before him and as his rear guard.

Carolyn looked at the beautiful little girl sitting in the big,
cushy leather seat next to her. If not for this adorable little munchkin, they all would have fallen to pieces.

"Champagne, madame?" A pretty, dark-haired flight attendant carried a tray of tulip glasses filled with juice or champagne.
Georgia took orange juice.

Faith looked eagerly at Carolyn. "Can I have some juice,
Grammy?" Carolyn said yes and declined anything for herself.
She felt a little queasy with nerves. The last time she'd traveled
any distance on her own was driving Chel across country after
Woodstock, and that didn't offer the best of memories. Dawn
would have told her not to worry. God would be flying with them.
She smiled as she imagined Jesus in uniform, sitting in the cockpit.

Faith squealed in delight and spread her arms. "GeeGee, we're
flying!" Georgia closed her eyes and gripped the arms of her seat.
After what seemed a surprisingly short amount of time, the bell
pinged and the captain announced the 747 had reached its cruising

altitude and everyone was free to move around the cabin. Dinner was served. Carolyn took Faith to the bathroom, then strapped her back into her seat, covered her with a blanket, and read her favorite book to her, *Horton Hears a Who!* Faith fell asleep halfway through the third reading. Georgia had lowered her seat and finally looked peaceful.

Carolyn took out her wireless laptop. While she waited for it to boot up, she thought of how many times she'd used the computer over the past few years to connect with Jason on the other side of the world, Faith perched in her lap. When he came on the screen, she'd point. "There's your daddy. Say hello, sweetheart."

Jason would grin. "How's my little girl?" Carolyn hadn't wanted Jason to miss anything. She'd posted movies of Faith rolling over, sitting up, crawling. Faith had been walking by the time he came home from Iraq. Jason made the most of what little time he had with his daughter. Eighteen months after returning from Iraq, he was deployed again.

Georgia went to pieces when Jason was called up for a third tour of duty, this time in Afghanistan. "They'll keep sending him," Mitch told Carolyn. With so few men, the military had no choice but to reuse the ones they had. "As long as there's war in the Middle East, he'll be going in and coming back." It didn't look like it would end anytime soon.

Every night, Faith said the same prayer. "God, please bless Daddy and bring him home safe and soon. Help GeeGee not to worry so much. God bless Grammy Caro, Bumpa Mitch, Granny H, and Uncle Chris. In Jesus' name, amen."

Then word came that Jason had been wounded and was being airlifted to a hospital in Germany. He wouldn't be sent back into a war zone again. His war-won disabilities would bring him a Purple Heart and commendation, but also very likely an early out from the military. Jason had hoped to serve his full twenty years before returning to civilian life.

Mitch came on the screen. "Hey, darlin'. I miss you two already."

"Thank you for putting us in business class, Mitch. It's luxurious." They talked for a few minutes, and then he let Carolyn's mother take his seat. Even Mom had grown accustomed to sitting in front of a computer and carrying on a conversation via webcam.

"How's our munchkin, honey? Behaving?"

"Momentarily. She's asleep. So is Georgia. They both conked out right after dinner, which was served on white tablecloths with china and silver. Can you believe it?"

"We had pizza on paper plates." Mom winked, so Carolyn knew she was needling Mitch again. Carolyn could hear Mitch laughing and speaking in the background. "Oh, shut up." Mom sighed. "He wants me to tell you I almost lost my dentures. Not to worry though. Your man is taking good care of me."

"Don't forget to use your walker, Mom."

"Now don't you start!"

Mitch leaned down so Carolyn could see both their faces. "Don't worry about us. We get along just fine. If your mother misbehaves, I'll send her to her room." He gave Mom's cheek a brisk kiss. "My turn." Mitch helped Mom off the chair, then sat in front of the monitor. "Someone will be waiting for you at the airport. I arranged a ride to the train station."

Mom leaned down. "I put something in your suitcase, honey. If you have time . . . well, you'll understand. Give Jason a big hug from his granny-in-law."

"The whole church is praying, Carolyn."

Carolyn slept easily after that.

❄ ❄ ❄

As the train flew down the tracks toward Landstuhl, Carolyn felt Faith pressed close beside her, Puppy Brown still tucked under her arm. He'd fallen from Faith's seat while she slept on the plane. They'd been so busy gathering their things, they had forgotten him. Fortunately, one of the flight attendants spotted the well-worn, well-loved stuffed animal tangled in the blue blanket and caught up with them in the Jetway. Faith had held him at arm's length and told him not to get lost again.

Carolyn kissed Faith on the top of her head. "Your great-great-grandfather came from this country, Faith. He grew up somewhere near Hamburg." Carolyn imagined Oma making her way through Europe to England and eventually boarding a ship to cross the Atlantic, then marrying a German boarder who rented a room in her house. Under other circumstances, they could have been on a heritage trip with Mom and May Flower Dawn.

She and Mitch had talked about Mom's coming, but she refused. "No, no. You need to get to Jason as soon as you can, and I'd hold you back. If I were younger, maybe, but not now. I'm not up to it."

In truth, Carolyn had been relieved. Even with a wheelchair, the trip would have been too grueling for Mom, who had just turned ninety-three. She had a hard enough time getting from her rooms to the dining room table these days. Carolyn and Faith often served tea in Granny's "parlor" rather than have Granny make the long walk to the kitchen.

Carolyn dreaded the time when she wouldn't have Mom with her. The last six years had been precious, a time of finally getting to know each other. God had given them back the years the locusts had eaten, just as Dawn had prayed He would.

When they reached the *Schloss Hotel*, they checked in, went upstairs, dumped their luggage, and then took a cab to the hospital. Georgia had to provide Jason's full name, serial number, and doctor's name at the reception desk. The nurse gave them directions to intensive care. Only one person could go into the room at a time.

Carolyn sat in the waiting room with Faith. "Am I going to see Daddy, Grammy?"

"I hope so, sweetheart. That's why we've come so far."

When Georgia came out, Carolyn knew things weren't good. Her smile wobbled as she took Faith on her lap and said Daddy was sleeping and it might be a while before he'd wake up.

Carolyn went in next. Jason looked like death, with tubes and IVs and everywhere machines beeping and blinking, his head swathed in white. His left leg had been amputated above the knee, his right set in a cast. His left arm was bandaged from wrist to shoulder. Carolyn took Jason's right hand and leaned down. "It's Carolyn, Jason. Faith is here with us. Everyone sends their love. They're all praying. You hold on, soldier. You come back to us." She kissed his brow. "You have Faith, Jason. She needs her daddy."

When Carolyn came out, Georgia stood, holding Faith's hand. The nurse had said she could stay as long as she wanted, and it would be good if she talked to her son. She leaned down and kissed Faith. "Don't wait around here, Carolyn. She needs to go to bed. I'll be fine."

After dinner in the hospital cafeteria and looking in on Jason once more, Carolyn took Faith back to the hotel. She tucked her granddaughter into bed and read *Horton Hears a Who!* again.

"Grammy? Is Daddy going to die?"

Carolyn didn't want to lie. "I don't know, sweetheart."

"Does he still want to be with Mommy?"

Children never missed anything. "Mommy would want him to stay here until you're all grown-up." She held her granddaughter close, and they prayed Daddy would wake up soon and get better.

Georgia didn't come back to the hotel that night.

Getting ready the next morning, Carolyn found the bundle of letters from Oma's friend Rosie Brechtwald tucked under her clothes.

When Carolyn and Faith arrived at the hospital, Georgia was just coming out of Jason's room in intensive care. Tears streamed down her cheeks.

❄ ❄ ❄

"He's going to be okay!" Carolyn cried as she shared the news with Mitch and her mother. Mom leaned down behind Mitch and asked for medical details. "He came out of the coma

last night. They're moving him into another room tomorrow morning. That's all I know."

"How's Georgia holding up?"

"She's exhausted, but a lot better than she was." Carolyn ran her hand over her granddaughter's head. Faith grinned around her straw and then went back to drinking her milk. People milled around the hospital cafeteria. "Faith got to see Jason this morning. He's pretty weak right now, but he smiled." She winked at Faith. "A big smile when he saw his little girl."

Mitch asked questions, and Carolyn told him as much as she knew. "He'll be sent back to the States for rehabilitation. Texas, I think." Carolyn spotted Georgia entering the cafeteria and waved her over. "Georgia just came in. She's smiling. There must be more good news."

Georgia leaned in to say hi to Mitch and Hildie, then asked Faith if she wanted to talk with Daddy. He was asking for her. Georgia took Faith by the hand, and Carolyn said she'd follow in a minute.

"Mitch, I've been thinking about going to Switzerland in a few days, as soon as we know everything is fine with Jason. I'd like to see Oma's hometown. Would that be all right with you?"

Mitch nodded. "Mom told me about the letters. Maybe you can even find someone from your grandmother's friend's family to give them to."

"I don't know if *Hotel Edelweiss* is still there, but I'll see what I can find. Georgia will keep Faith here. We bought a few games and crayons and a coloring book to keep her occupied. She's been good as gold. Jason told her she's going to grow up to be as beautiful as her mommy. He's been carrying a picture of May Flower Dawn he took when they were first married and living in San Luis Obispo. Faith thought she was an angel with a halo of light. Jason told Faith her mommy always read her Bible in the morning as the sun was coming up. I told Jason I want a copy of that picture. It would make a wonderful portrait."

Mom leaned closer so Carolyn could see her on the screen. "Take lots of pictures, honey. I'd love to see where Oma grew up."

❄ ❄ ❄

Carolyn searched the Internet and booked one night at the *Hotel Schweizerhof* in Zurich. The grand old hotel was expensive, but it was right across the street from the train station. Now that her plans were falling into place, she felt like a child facing the first day of school. She laughed silently at herself. Oma had gone around the world by the age of twenty-three! It seemed ludicrous to hesitate in the face of any challenge with Oma's blood running through her veins. "You have to take life by the horns," Oma said once.

Oma had certainly done that. Oma had told her about the fake Count and Countess Saintonge who ran the housekeeping school in Bern, about Herr Derry Weib and Chef Warner Brennholtz at the *Hotel Germania* in Interlaken. She had talked about Lady Daisy Stockhard and her spinster daughter, Miss Millicent, always on the hunt for a suitable husband. It had surprised Carolyn to find out Mom hadn't heard any of those stories.

She got up early, packed, and kissed Faith on the forehead. Georgia walked her to the door. "I don't know how to thank you and Mitch for flying me over here, Carolyn."

Carolyn hugged her. "Jason's our son, too. I'll call tonight so you can tell me how our boy is doing."

She caught the early train to Zurich. The scenery was glorious, the passengers friendly. *Hotel Schweizerhof* couldn't have been more convenient. She checked in and asked where she might do some shopping. Her winter coat kept her warm in Sonoma County, California, but she knew after walking from the train station that it wouldn't suffice in the Alpine country of Switzerland. And she'd need boots instead of walking shoes.

She hunted from store to store until she found a coat and boots at reasonable prices. After a late lunch in Old Town, she headed back toward *Hotel Schweizerhof.* She spotted the ornately beautiful

Swiss National Museum, but it was too late in the day to visit. She
went inside the Central Station and had dinner in a café where she
could watch travelers come and go.

She called Georgia that evening.

"Jason was in a lot of pain today. Faith and I went out for a long
walk." Georgia laughed. "I needed to wear her out before we went
back to the hospital." Faith had crawled up into bed with Jason
while Georgia was in the bathroom. "The nurse found her asleep
next to her father, with Puppy Brown tucked under her chin.
When she started to move her, Jason told her to leave her there."

Before calling it a night, Carolyn e-mailed Mitch.

> Hotel Schweizerhof is a grand, glorious old hotel right
> across from the train station where I dined this evening. I'm
> having dessert now—a bar of Lindt white chocolate with
> almonds, which was delivered, free of charge, to my room.
> Tell Mom I'll bring her some. Off to Steffisburg tomorrow.

❄ ❄ ❄

Carolyn caught the morning train to Thun. Resting her chin in her
hand, she gazed out the window at one picture-perfect Christmas
scene after another passing by. Small bursts of color, painted or
natural, splashed against the white. The Alps rose like mighty senti-
nels on guard.

The two-hour train ride passed quickly, and she found herself
standing once again in the crisp Swiss air, her breath steaming like
a dragon's. The station manager spoke English. Yes, *Hotel Edelweiss*
was still in business, though it didn't take in as many guests as it
once had. He knew the family very well. "Ilse Bieler and I went to
school together." He made two calls. A room was available. A taxi
was on its way.

While she waited, snow fell like goose down after a pillow fight.
The driver took her along a small river, across a bridge, and along
the main street of what had been Oma's childhood hometown. A

white church with a thick bell tower stood at the end before the road curved right. He drove up the hill overlooking Steffisburg and parked in front of a two-story Bernese-style house. A small sign with *Hotel Edelweiss* painted in red had been bolted to the dark wood of the house.

As Carolyn walked up the steps, a woman wearing ski pants and a heavy blue and red sweater opened the door. She had dark hair and brown eyes and looked to be in her late thirties, around the same age May Flower Dawn would be, had she lived. Carolyn felt a sudden welling sense of loss. She introduced herself. "Ludwig Gasel called earlier. He said you have a room."

"Come in, please. I'm Ilse Bieler. My family owns the hotel." The woman stepped back, leaving the doorway open.

Carolyn liked the cozy feel of the stained wood walls, red sofa and chairs, multicolored woven carpet, and fire ablaze and crackling. Ilse Bieler showed her to a room upstairs with a view of the church steeple among the trees. "We have coffee and cookies downstairs," Ilse told her, then closed the door as she went out. Carolyn quickly unpacked and went downstairs. She hadn't come all this way to hide in her room. Ilse Bieler offered coffee. "What brings you to Steffisburg?"

"My grandmother grew up here. I was curious to see if any family members might still be here. She had a special friend who lived here at the *Hotel Edelweiss*."

"Really? What was your grandmother's name?"

"Schneider."

"A common name. Do you know anything about them?"

"Oma said her father was a tailor and her mother a dressmaker. She had an older brother, Hermann. I don't know what happened to him. Her mother died young. And she had a younger sister, too. Her name was Elise."

"Elise." Ilse lifted her shoulders. "Also a common name."

The telephone rang and Ilse excused herself. She spoke German for several minutes and hung up. "The church may have information on your grandmother's family." Ilse suggested Carolyn check the public records as well, and she told her how to find the building where they were stored. "And you'll meet my grandmother later. She's napping right now. But she knows everyone in town."

The church records gave the date of her great-grandparents' wedding as well as her grandmother's baptism. The town records office yielded drawers of family information that went back to the seventeen hundreds! Overwhelmed, Carolyn said thank you and left. Maybe she would just take lots of pictures around town and then return to Landstuhl. She headed up the hill to *Hotel Edelweiss*.

Ilse introduced her to her grandmother, Etta, a lovely, gray-haired lady around the age of Carolyn's own mother. She switched from German to English and back again with enviable ease, while Ilse served cabbage soup, sausages and vegetables, fried potatoes and onion salad.

Ilse asked Carolyn if she'd found any information about her family at the church or records office.

"A few important dates at the church, and I practically ran out of the records office when I saw how much they had. I could spend the rest of my life going through all of it." She shrugged. "My mother wanted me to take lots of pictures. I think that's what I'll do."

Etta passed the plate of sausages around again. Carolyn told her they were delicious.

"An old family recipe," Etta said with a smile. She cocked her head and studied Carolyn. "You mentioned that your grandmother had a friend here at *Hotel Edelweiss*. Do you know her name?"

"Yes. Rosie Brechtwald. Have you heard of her?"

Etta gasped. "Rosie Brechtwald was my mother! My granddaughter is named after her—Ilse Rose. My mother wrote letters to a friend who ended up in America, but her name was Waltert. Is that your grandmother?"

"Yes! Marta Schneider Waltert. I have your mother's letters with me." Carolyn went to her room, retrieved the bundle, and returned downstairs.

Etta looked delighted. "I grew up on stories of your *oma*. My mother used to read her letters aloud to us. They wrote back and forth for over fifty years! When Mama died, I wrote to Marta, but the letter came back. I would like to hear the end of the story."

"I'd like to hear the beginning and the middle." Carolyn smiled. "I have a hundred questions."

"Do you still have Marta's letters, Mama?" Ilse glanced at Carolyn. "She never throws anything away."

"I'll look in the family trunk after dinner is finished."

❄ ❄ ❄

Etta Bieler brought a box into the living room and set it on the coffee table in front of the fireplace. She took out bundles of letters, tied with faded ribbons. "My mother learned about organization from her father. When he died, she took over this little hotel. She kept perfect files." The letters had been kept in chronological order.

When Carolyn started looking through Oma's letters, her heart sank. "They're written in German." Why hadn't she thought of that? All of Rosie's letters to Oma had been in German.

"Ah, but look in the bottom of the box." Carolyn removed the rest of the letters and found a thick sheaf of papers under them. Etta's eyes twinkled. "My children found the story of their grandmother's friend so fascinating, I encouraged them to translate the letters when they were studying English in school. They enjoyed the practice, and we all enjoyed reading through them again. I remember them very well. Marta's father made her leave school. He sent her to Bern to become a servant." She chuckled. "But your *oma* had bigger dreams than being someone's maid. She wanted to learn French and English so she could have a hotel like this one. Mama said what Marta set out to do, Marta *did*."

"She never had a hotel."

"No, but she owned a boardinghouse in Montreal. That's where she met her husband. They moved to the Canadian wheat fields and, later, to California. It's all in the letters. I think the only thing she didn't plan was meeting your *opa*. We all loved that romantic story. Marta didn't think she would ever marry; then she met handsome Niclas, graduate of Berlin University, also an immigrant. Marta taught him to speak English."

Ilse yawned and said she needed to get to bed. She had to get up early and have breakfast ready for some guests who wanted to go out cross-country skiing. Carolyn apologized for keeping them up so late. "Would you mind if I took these upstairs to read?"

Etta had already begun opening Rosie's letters. "They're yours to keep. Our family enjoyed them, but you must have them. They're part of your family history."

"I can't wait to read them. There is so much I'd like to know about my grandparents. Maybe she wrote about her sister, Elise, too. She sometimes mentioned her to me—even used to tell me I looked like her. But she'd never tell me anything more than that."

Etta looked troubled. "My mother told me the story. It's in the early letters—references to it, not details. You may not want to know."

"I think it's important I do."

"Mama said Elise was very beautiful. I'm sure you do look like her. She was very quiet and painfully shy. She stayed in the shop with her mother while Marta was sent out to work. Mama didn't say much about what went on in your grandmother's family, just that Marta did not have an easy life. Her father sent her to Bern."

"To housekeeping school."

"*Ja*, but Mama said Marta wanted more than that. She went to Interlaken."

"And worked at the *Hotel Germania*."

"That's when her father sent Elise to work for a wealthy family in Thun. It turned out very badly."

Carolyn saw how Etta hesitated. "How badly?"

"The master of the house and his son abused her." She lowered her eyes and Carolyn understood. "Marta took her sister out of that house and brought her home, but Elise was already pregnant. No one knew yet, but the girl never went out after she was brought home. She stayed inside the house. Everyone assumed she was taking care of her mother, who was very ill with consumption. Marta confided in my mother that she feared for Elise. Apparently the girl was very dependent on her mother, whom Marta felt coddled her all too much. Then when her mother died, Elise disappeared. Everyone went searching for her. It was my mother who found Marta's sister by the river. She had frozen to death. And she was heavy with child."

Carolyn closed her eyes. Oma had kept secrets, too. Her sister's rape, an unwed pregnancy, suicide.

Etta went on with the rest of what her mother had told her about a plain girl wounded by a father who didn't love her, but used her as a source of income for the family while her mother languished with consumption and her exquisitely beautiful and delicate sister remained hidden away like Rapunzel inside a tower. When Marta went away to work, her father had demanded a portion of her wages, and Marta capitulated until Rosie Brechtwald had written the truth. "Mama knew Marta would never come back after her mother and sister died."

Carolyn ached for Oma.

"I'm sorry. Perhaps I should not have told you."

"I'm glad you did. It explains so much." No wonder Oma had been so determined to make sure her own children could stand on their own two feet. Cloistered by fear, weakened by a needy mother's coddling, Elise had been unprepared for the world. In the end, she gave up her life without a fight.

How many times had Carolyn considered doing the same thing? Once she had almost walked into the sea. God had used a man wounded by war to draw her back. He'd used an unexpected pregnancy to give her reason to keep on living, to work hard, to accept consequences and blessings along the way. But she had kept silent, too, keeping the pain locked in and pressed down.

"You look like Elise. She was my little sister, and she was very, very pretty, just like you," Oma once said, but wouldn't explain. Yet, Oma hadn't treated Carolyn the same way she had treated Mom. Oma had held her close, told her repeatedly she loved her,

encouraged her to step out in faith. Oma had learned that with-holding love might make a daughter strong, but also left deep wounds. On both sides.

❆ ❆ ❆

Carolyn read the letters translated by Etta's children and tucked them into the corresponding originals written by Oma in German. She read until her eyes blurred.

> I am in England. Papa sent a wire telling me to come home. He said nothing about either Elise or Mama, and I knew he would expect me to spend the rest of my life in the shop. . . .
>
> Cousin Felda said it was you who found Elise. I dream of her every night. . . .

Later, Oma moved away from London to "better air" and lived and worked in the "fine Tudor home" of Lady Daisy Stockhard, who loved high tea every afternoon at four o'clock. When one of the other servants left to get married, Oma replaced her as Lady Daisy's companion.

> She is a most unusual lady. I have never known anyone to discuss so many interesting topics. She doesn't treat her servants like slaves, but is genuinely interested in our lives. She had me sit with her in church last Sunday.
>
> Her daughter is never happy with anything, not even her mother. She is off on another hunt for a husband, and when she's gone, everyone in the house breathes easier, even Lady Stockhard.

Oma wrote of the long voyage to Canada:

I had days when I would have jumped overboard to end my misery if I could have climbed the stairs to reach the deck. They have packed us like cattle in a barn. The woman in the bunk next to me moans day and night. I know how she feels, but sometimes think about putting a pillow over her head, if I had a pillow. I can laugh about it now that I am on terra firma again.

And in Canada, she found so much more than she was looking for.

Dear Rosie,
I am married!
I never thought anyone would want me, and certainly never a man like Niclas Bernhard Waltert. . . . I thought I was happy when I bought my boardinghouse, but I have never been as truly happy as this. It makes me afraid sometimes. . . .

Carolyn understood the feeling of unworthiness all too well. She continued reading. Oma's letters changed. Disappointment set in when Niclas lost his job at the railroad and decided to become a farmer. Oma couldn't understand how a man of learning would want to work the land.

Dearest Rosie,
Niclas has left me and gone off to work on a wheat farm in Manitoba. He went away three weeks ago and I

have not heard from him since. I begin to understand how Elise felt when she walked out into the snow. . . .

I would have given anything for an education, but Papa said schooling was wasted on a girl. And Niclas, who has the knowledge to be a professor, wants to throw it all away and live out in the middle of nowhere tilling soil and planting wheat. He wants me to sell the boardinghouse. He wants me to go on this "adventure" with him. I would kill him if I didn't love him so much. . . .

Opa had gone alone, and Oma's letters showed how much she suffered for her decision.

Why must I give up everything I have worked so hard to gain to follow a man whose dream will impoverish us? But how can I not? Life is barren without Niclas. I will have his child soon. . . .

Carolyn read of life on a wheat farm miles from the nearest town, winters when the temperature dropped well below zero, a landlord who cared nothing about their plight and cheated them out of their share of the profits. She wrote lovingly of Bernhard, and she worried about the new baby coming.

Several months passed before Oma wrote another letter, and it held the first mention of Hildemara Rose.

I fear for this little one. I understand now how Mama's heart broke every time she held Elise. She was small and frail, too. . . .

Pray for your namesake, Rosie. One breath from heaven could blow her away, but God forbid I go too far in protecting her and bring her up to be weak like Elise.

Opa and Oma left the farm and went to Winnipeg. Opa went back to work for the railroad. Another child came.

Our third child, Clotilde Anna, arrived a month after Niclas went back to work. She is as robust as Bernhard, and every bit as loud in her demands.

Soon, Opa began to talk about farming again. This time he was dreaming of California.

The man will not be happy until he has his way. And I am tired of fighting with him.

Life in California was difficult. First the family lived in a tent by an irrigation ditch, then in a structure not much better on a farm owned by . . .

. . . Mrs. Miller, who orders us around like serfs while she and her daughter, Miss Charlotte, sit on their behinds and listen to radio programs in the big house. The wind and rain blow through ours, and she expects us to pay for "improvements." The children have constant colds. I fear most for Hildemara Rose. She has Mama's constitution. . . .

Oma reported on the achievements of Bernhard and Clotilde and Rikka in a matter-of-fact way, but her eldest daughter perplexed her and seemed a constant worry.

What must I do to make my girl strong? Niclas tells me to be gentle with her, to love her for the child she is. But he doesn't understand what happens to a child who cannot stand up for herself. I can't give in and become like Mama, coddling and protecting her. . . . I would rather she hate me than end up like Elise.

And then the day came when Hildemara got the courage to speak up. Carolyn could hardly imagine the scene as Oma's letter described it.

After all this time, my girl speaks up to me and what do I do? I slap her across the face. I did it without even thinking. I had said something hurtful to Niclas, and he left the table, and Hildemara Rose exposed my shame. . . .

I could see the hurt in her eyes. I wanted to shake her. I wanted to tell her she had every right to scream at me. She doesn't have to sit there and take it! She would have turned the other cheek if I'd raised my hand to her again.

I have not cried so much in years, Rosie. Not since Mama and Elise died.

Carolyn lay back and closed her eyes. She'd never seen Oma cry, never guessed the depth of pain she carried. Oma had gone to her grave in silence, still wounded. Carolyn realized how alike they were, and Mom, too. *How many other unhealthy coping tools have we passed down, Lord? Show us, so we can turn swords into plowshares.* Wiping tears away, she thanked God again for May Flower Dawn. God had used her and other prayer warriors to bring the walls between generations tumbling down. *I miss her, Lord. I had so little time with her.*

And she felt His answer. *You have time and eternity.*

Then Hildemara further asserted herself by choosing to go to nursing school, against Oma's wishes. But when she graduated at the head of her class, Oma's pride was evident.

She is not a timid child anymore. My girl knows her place in the world. I am so proud of her, Rosie.

Opa got cancer.

I had no choice but to ask Hildemara to give up her life and come home. He needs a nurse. He worsens by the day and I can't bear to see him in such pain. She is a great comfort to us both.

Oma grieved over Opa's passing, then began to worry about Hildemara Rose again. She didn't return to Merritt Hospital, where she had been working before Oma asked her to come home and take care of Papa. Carolyn knew a crisis was on the horizon, and in the next letter, it had happened.

A young man came to Niclas's funeral. I had never seen him before, and Hildemara had never mentioned him. But I knew when I saw them together, they love each other. She had it in her head that she had to stay and take care of me. As if I cannot take care of myself! I said enough yesterday to make her pack and leave. I appreciate all she's done, but enough is enough.

I offered to drive her to the bus station this morning, hoping for a chance to explain myself a little better. But she had already asked her brother to take her.

She was hurt and angry, once again misunderstanding my intentions. When will she understand how much I love her? How easy it would have been to let her stay and be my comfort! But at what cost to her? Elise was Mama's comfort and suffered for it. So did Mama in the end, though she didn't live with the fullness of it. No matter how much it hurts, I must be strong for Hildemara Rose's sake.

When Hildemara became sick with tuberculosis, Oma lived in fear of her dying.

I went to Arroyo del Valle to see Hildemara Rose. She had Mama's pallor and the deep shadows under her eyes. I could see no life in them when I first arrived. It terrified me. . . . I called her a coward. Though it broke my heart, I mocked and belittled her. Thank God she got good and mad. Her eyes spit fire at me and I wanted to laugh with joy.

Better she hate me for a while than give up on life and be put in an early grave. She was trying to get up when I walked away. . . .

Carolyn blinked back tears as she read Oma's description of Charlie's birth. *Oh, Charlie. I still miss you so much it hurts.* Oma was concerned even then about the breach between herself and Mom.

Hildemara Rose and I get along, but there is a wall between us. I know I built it. I doubt she's forgiven me for my harsh words at the sanatorium, and I will not apologize for them. I may have to prod her again. I'll do whatever I must to keep her spirits up. Oh, but it hurts me so to do it. I wonder if she will ever understand me.

No, Oma, I don't think she ever did. At least not yet.

Years later, Oma wrote about the gold, jade, and pearl brooch. Carolyn fingered it as she read.

I was so stunned and touched by Hildemara's gift, I said something stupid. I could see the hurt in her eyes. It's become a bad habit, saying hurtful things to her. I reached out, but she'd already turned away, and I had no voice to call her back. I take out the brooch every day and look at it. My girl has a fine, generous heart. . . .

Oma had tried to reach out to Mom in those later years, and Mom shrank back. Mom and Oma never had someone who pulled them together the way May Flower Dawn had done for Carolyn and Mom. She had built a bridge so the same mistake wouldn't be carried into the next generation.

Sometimes seeds fell on rock, but they still found a way to grow, to press up toward the sun, to cling to life no matter what. Oma had done that. She had left a legacy. *Endure whatever life dishes out.*

Learn all you can. Count your blessings. Never give up. Keep growing in the Lord.

One week with Oma had changed May Flower Dawn. Oma said once her great-granddaughter had a teachable spirit.

Dawn had been the best of all the women in their family. She had Oma's drive and ambition, not for possessions, but to become the woman God intended her to be. She had become a nurse like her grandmother, caring for others. Carolyn often wondered what qualities she might have passed along to Dawn, and she realized her daughter had been broken, too, and humbled. But God had not crushed the tender reed.

❄ ❄ ❄

Carolyn came down for breakfast and found the other guests already on their way out. Etta set a basket of fresh rolls on the sideboard as Carolyn poured herself a cup of coffee. "I was up most of the night reading the letters. I've certainly learned a lot about my grandparents . . . and my mother. Thank you so much for giving them to me."

Etta smiled. "I grew up on stories of Marta's adventures. Your *oma* was a remarkable woman. I would love to have met her."

The telephone rang. Etta held it out. "It's for you."

Georgia. "Jason is being transferred to Brooke Army Medical Center in San Antonio. He'll be flown to the States in a few days. We're ready to go home anytime you are."

Carolyn Skyped Mitch and gave him the good news, then asked, "Is Mom already in bed?"

"No, she fell asleep on the couch while we were watching the news." He chuckled. "I'm in my office and I can hear her snoring."

"Can you get her? I have something important to tell her."

It took several minutes before Mom appeared in front of the monitor. "Mitch said you wanted to talk to me."

"I'm at *Hotel Edelweiss* with Rosie Brechtwald's daughter. Oma loved you, Mom. She was proud of you."

"I know."

"No, Mom, you don't know. But I have proof, lots of it, and it's all in Oma's handwriting. Rosie Brechtwald saved all of Oma's letters. Her daughter gave them to me. You'll be able to read them when I get home."

"Did you take lots of pictures?" Mom's voice had a tremor.

"Yes, Mom. At least a hundred."

"When you and Faith get home, we'll have tea and cookies and make an album together."

"Sounds wonderful."

They would talk about things they had kept hidden, shine light on the shadows, cast out any remaining doubts.

"I love you, Mom. I'll see you soon."

"I love you, too, honey. I always have."

❄ ❄ ❄

Love one another, Jesus said. Sometimes it took a lifetime to learn how. Sometimes it took hitting rock bottom to make someone reach up and grasp hold and be lifted from the mire to stand on a firm foundation.

Sometimes a child had to show them how to love, and another child, left behind, had to remind them to take one step at a time.

Faith. How appropriately Dawn had named her child. Every time Carolyn said it, she remembered what May Flower Dawn had dreamed. So did Mom. So did Jason. So did every member of the family. *Keep faith. Nurture it. Let it grow. Watch what can happen when you do.*

God would light the way. Faith would keep them on the right path.

A Note from the Author

Dear Reader,

Since I became a Christian, my stories have begun with struggles I'm having in my own faith walk, or issues that I haven't worked out. That's how this two-book series started. I wanted to explore what caused the rift between my grandma and my mom during the last years of my grandmother's life. Was it a simple misunderstanding that they never had time to work out? or something deeper that had grown over the years?

Many of the events of this story were inspired by family history that I researched and events I read about in my mother's journals or experienced in my own life. You may have guessed that Carolyn is my alter ego. But only some of my life is interwoven through hers. Mom did have tuberculosis when I was a little girl, and Grandma did move in to help while Mom recuperated at home. When Mom was well enough, we moved to a piece of property where they built their own home from the founda-tion up. I still love the scent of sawdust. But unlike the Arundels, our family was close.

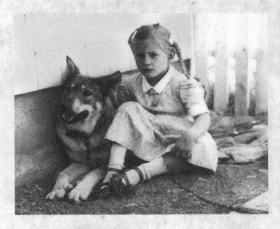

Francine as a little girl with her dog Dusty

We had sit-down dinners and lingered around the table, talking. In many ways, growing up in the fifties and early sixties in California was like living in Camelot. I had an idyllic childhood, despite the serious things happening—the "Red Scare," the Cuban Missile Crisis, and Kennedy's assassination. My dad, along with other neighbors, built a bomb shelter. (Last I heard, people have converted them into wine cellars.)

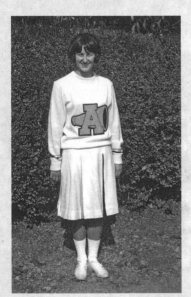

Francine as a high school student

Like Carolyn, I've known my husband, Rick, since we were children. My brother, Everett King, served in the armed forces like Trip, Charlie, and Jason. He was in Army intelligence and was wounded and captured during the Tet Offensive of '68. By the grace of God, he escaped. It was his story in the hometown paper that brought Rick back into my life. Rick was serving in the Marine Corps and stationed in Vietnam at the same time my brother was. Rick's mom sent him a newspaper clipping about my brother being MIA and, later, one about his escape. Rick wrote to me and said I was lucky to have my brother back alive. We started a correspondence, dated when he returned, and married a year after he came home.

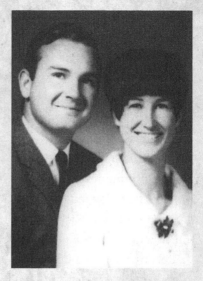

Rick got an early out for Vietnam service and went back to college, first to Chabot junior college and then to UC Berkeley, where he graduated with a degree in American history. However, aviation was in his blood, and he started his own business— Rivers Aviation Services. We had three small children by then, and all of us spent time together at the office. Our children played in the

Francine and Rick's engagement photo

packing materials, hiding in the Styrofoam peanuts, thinking we didn't know where they were. They grew up helping out and learning what it means to work hard and build something together.

Like Carolyn, I lost faith in God for a time and then (much later than she) cried out to Him. Carolyn suffered more insecurities and hardships, but many of us have to "hit bottom" before we acknowledge our need for Jesus as Savior *and* Lord. Rescue is never enough. We still have to walk through the rest of our lives. Trusting God has a plan and purpose for each of us frees us to move forward, knowing— in Christ—we have great potential.

Though this saga often focuses on mother-daughter relationships, the men in both books play important roles, too. I never knew my grandfather, though I like to imagine he was like Niclas. He died of liver cancer before I was born. He was Mom's first private patient. Mom once told me he sang German hymns in the orchard when he was working. Trip reminds me of my father, who served as a captain in the U.S. Army during World War II and was a medic during the second wave on D-day. He had dreamed of being a doctor, but gave it up to be a police officer and, eventually, coroner and public administrator of Alameda County. He never shared details of the war. (Neither did Rick's father, who spent three and a half years in Los Baños, an infamous Japanese prison camp in the Philippines.)

Mitch is very much like my husband, Rick. He loves me despite my faults. We've grown up together and encourage one another in our faith. He's given me the freedom to do what God has called me to and is my biggest encourager and supporter (literally—for years while I didn't make a cent off my writing). And Jason has similari-

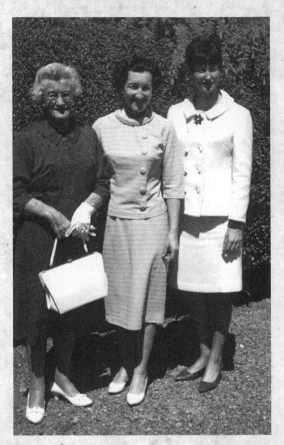

Francine (far right) with her mother and grandmother

ties to our son-in-law, Rich, a hardworking young man of faith who joined the military to offer our daughter, Shannon, a better life. After four years on the other side of the country, he left the Air Force and entered the private sector. We are blessed to have them living in the same town (blessed also that our sons and their spouses and children are all close by). Rich is my "tech support," and Shannon manages my Web site.

During the past three years of working on Marta's Legacy, I have come away with a heart full of wonderful memories and valuable lessons hard-won by Grandma and Mom, but passed down lovingly to me. I am grateful. Neither ever felt she measured up, but that did not stop them from encouraging me. May Flower Dawn begins as a self-centered child and grows into a grace-filled, wise woman. Her journey is one every woman hopes to witness in her daughter, as I am witnessing in mine.

Our experiences may be different. The times in which we have grown up may be poles apart. Yet I know I share the same longings of my grandmother, mother, and daughter. I want to be loved and accepted as I am. I want purpose. As I grow older and look back over my life, I want to leave a legacy of faith in Jesus Christ. Like Marta, I want my children and grandchildren to stand firm in faith no matter what the world throws at them. I want them to know that while they wait for heaven, God has a good purpose for them right here in this chaotic world filled with lost souls longing for the kind of love, acceptance, and purpose they will find only in Christ Jesus.

And, like Marta, I dream we will all one day be together with our Lord, having cast off the imperfection of human nature, transformed into Christlike children of the King of kings.

Proverbs 3:5-6
Francine Rivers

Discussion Guide

1. Both Hildie and Trip miss some obvious signs that something traumatic has happened to Carolyn. What are they? Later, in chapter 4, when Hildie and Trip argue about Hildie's going back to work, Trip says, "A little girl shouldn't be alone so much. Things could happen." Discuss the irony in that statement. What is it about their family dynamics that makes Carolyn vulnerable to a predator like Dock?

2. Do you think Hildie's character changes from book 1 to book 2? If so, how does she change and why? Did you like her more or less in this book?

3. Carolyn runs away—literally and figuratively—after getting the news of her brother's tragic death. Is that a realistic response? Why or why not? Have you ever wished you could run away from a painful reality? How did you deal with it? Have you ever been in the place of Carolyn's parents and grandmother—not knowing the whereabouts of someone you love? What was that like? What advice would you give someone who is facing such a situation?

4. When Carolyn meets Mary in Golden Gate Park, Mary says she felt an impulse to make extra sandwiches that morning, even though she had no idea why. Have you ever felt God nudging you to do something you didn't understand? Did you follow through on that impulse? Why or why not?

5. After Carolyn comes home following her two-year disappearance, neither Hildie nor Trip presses her for details about what happened. Do you think that is wise? How does this both help and hurt Carolyn? In your own life, how can you balance being nosy with being concerned for those you love?

6. When Carolyn graduates from college and pays off her debt to her parents, Trip and Hildie give the money back to her. Were you surprised by Trip and Hildie's action? Why or why not? Why is it hard for Carolyn to accept their gift? Have you ever given or received an unexpected, extravagant gift? What was the motivation behind it? What was the response?

7. For many years, Carolyn finds more appealing fellowship and support in AA than she does in the church. Why is that? What does that say about AA? about the church? What finally changes Carolyn's view of Christians? Do you know anyone who has a negative view of the church? What could you say or do to encourage that person to give the church another chance? What other influences does God bring into Carolyn's life to show her the truth of His love for her?

8. Near the end of the story, Hildie reflects that God sent Mitch to rescue her, just as he had rescued Carolyn years earlier. In what ways does Mitch "rescue" Carolyn? How might her life have been different if she had never married? if she had married someone less understanding and supportive?

9. Marta's choice not to move to Jenner by the Sea with Hildie and Trip seems to finally make the gap between mother and daughter so wide it can't be crossed. Why does Hildie think

Marta doesn't want to move in with them? What does Marta really want? Why are they unable to discuss it rationally?

10. In chapter 30, when Dawn and Carolyn go to visit Marta for a week, Marta says that "making things easier on your children is sometimes the worst thing you can do." Do you agree or disagree? How do you see this illustrated in the story? in your own life?

11. How does Marta change over the course of the two books? What changes her the most? In what ways is she still the same?

12. When Dawn confesses to her mother that she slept with Jason, Carolyn's response is gracious and nonjudgmental. How do Carolyn's own experiences play into her response to Dawn? How would you respond to such a confession from your son or daughter? How would you like to respond?

13. How does Dawn's experience of the church after she sleeps with Jason differ from Carolyn's experience after returning from Haight-Ashbury? Why is it different? How does Paster Daniel's gracious response affect Dawn's future and her walk with Christ? Have you ever been in a position to counsel someone who has made a mistake they think cannot be forgiven? What did (or would) you say?

14. Near the end of the story, Dawn makes an important decision that affects the life of her unborn child. How might her struggle with miscarriage and infertility have affected her decision? What would you have done in Dawn's place? Discuss her choice not to talk about it with either her husband or her family. Was that the right way to handle it? Why or why not? How do you think Jason felt when he learned what had happened?

15. In chapter 55, Dawn reads this excerpt from Marta's journal: "We try to do a little better than the previous generation and find out in the end we've made the same mistakes without intending." How do you see this illustrated in the story? How

have you seen negative behaviors easily turn into a habit in your own life, as Hildie mentions in chapter 56?

16. When the three generations (Hildemara, Carolyn, and May Flower Dawn) finally sit down to talk, they discuss many of their "family secrets." Discuss the revelations and the effect of finally getting them out into the open. Are you satisfied with what they talk about and how it goes? In what way do you wish it had been handled differently? Are the responses realistic and/or what you expected?

17. At one point, Marta tells Dawn that people either weigh you down or give you wings. How do some of the characters in this saga give people wings? What can you do in your own relationships to give those you love wings instead of weighing them down?

18. While Scripture makes it clear that children are not held responsible for their parents' sins (see Ezekiel 18:20), it's also true that destructive patterns tend to continue in families and have a negative impact on successive generations (see Exodus 20:5). Over the span of these two novels, what relationship patterns are repeated between mothers and daughters? between grandmothers and granddaughters? In what ways are the patterns finally broken? Is the resolution realistic? What relationship patterns—either negative or positive—have occurred in your family? If the patterns are negative, what have you done or what could you do to break them?

19. Are there secrets in your family—either from generations past or from the present? To whom would you like to talk about these secrets? What kind of response do you think you would get? What response would you hope for?

20. This novel contains many relationships, conversations, rifts, and moments of reconciliation. Take a few minutes to list some of your favorite scenes and tell why you were especially touched or challenged by them.

About the Author

New York Times best-selling author Francine Rivers began her literary career at the University of Nevada, Reno, where she graduated with a bachelor of arts degree in English and journalism. From 1976 to 1985, she had a successful writing career in the general market, and her books were highly acclaimed by readers and reviewers. Although raised in a religious home, Francine did not truly encounter Christ until later in life, when she was already a wife, a mother of three, and an established romance novelist.

Shortly after becoming a born-again Christian in 1986, Francine wrote *Redeeming Love* as her statement of faith. First published by Bantam Books, and then rereleased by Multnomah Publishers in the mid-1990s, this retelling of the biblical story of Gomer and Hosea, set during the time of the California Gold Rush, is now considered by many to be a classic work of Christian fiction. *Redeeming Love* continues to be one of CBA's top-selling titles, and it has held a spot on the Christian best-seller list for nearly a decade.

Since *Redeeming Love*, Francine has published numerous novels with Christian themes—all best sellers—and she has continued to win both industry acclaim and reader loyalty around the globe. Her Christian novels have been awarded or nominated for numerous honors, including the RITA Award, the Christy Award, the ECPA Gold Medallion, and the Holt Medallion in Honor of Outstanding Literary Talent. In 1997, after winning her third RITA Award for inspirational fiction, Francine was inducted into the Romance Writers of America Hall of Fame. Francine's novels have been translated into more than twenty different languages, and she enjoys best-seller status in many foreign countries, including Germany, the Netherlands, and South Africa.

Francine and her husband, Rick, live in northern California and enjoy time spent with their three grown children and taking every opportunity to spoil their grandchildren. Francine uses her writing to draw closer to the Lord, and she desires that through her work she might worship and praise Jesus for all He has done and is doing in her life.

Visit her Web site at www.francinerivers.com.

BOOKS BY BELOVED AUTHOR
FRANCINE RIVERS

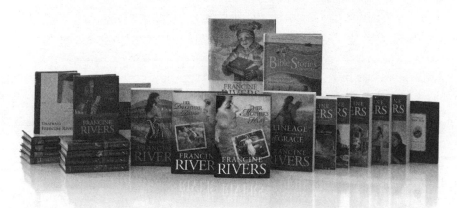

The Mark of the Lion series
(available individually or as a boxed set)
  A Voice in the Wind
  An Echo in the Darkness
  As Sure as the Dawn

A Lineage of Grace series
(available individually or in an anthology)
  Unveiled
  Unashamed
  Unshaken
  Unspoken
  Unafraid

Sons of Encouragement series
  The Priest
  The Warrior
  The Prince
  The Prophet
  The Scribe

Marta's Legacy series
  Her Mother's Hope
  Her Daughter's Dream

Children's Titles
  The Shoe Box
  Bible Stories for Growing Kids
    (coauthored with Shannon
    Rivers Coibion)

Stand-alone Titles
  Redeeming Love
  The Atonement Child
  The Scarlet Thread
  The Last Sin Eater
  Leota's Garden
  And the Shofar Blew
  The Shoe Box (a Christmas novella)

www.francinerivers.com

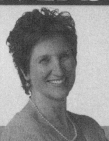

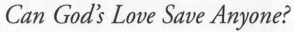
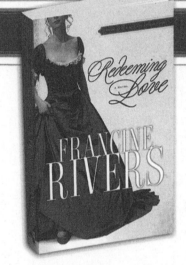

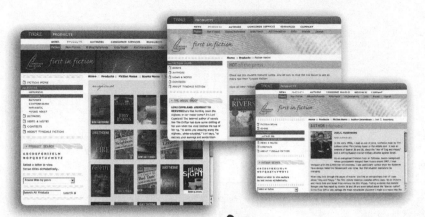

3 1333 03915 2424

docetaxel, and paclitaxel) may be tried. However, current drug therapy offers limited benefit. Combining several treatment methods may be most effective.

Special considerations

The care plan for the patient with prostatic cancer should emphasize psychological support, postoperative care, and treatment of radiation adverse effects.

Before prostatectomy:
- Explain the expected aftereffects of surgery (such as impotence and incontinence) and radiation. Discuss tube placement and dressing changes.
- Teach the patient to do perineal exercises 1 to 10 times an hour. Have him squeeze his buttocks together, hold this position for a few seconds, then relax.

After prostatectomy or suprapubic prostatectomy:
- Regularly check the dressing, incision, and drainage systems for excessive bleeding; watch the patient for signs of bleeding (pallor, falling blood pressure, rising pulse rate) and infection.
- Maintain adequate fluid intake.
- Give antispasmodics, as ordered, to control postoperative bladder spasms. Give analgesics as needed.
- Urinary incontinence is common after surgery; keep the patient's skin clean, dry, and free from drainage and urine.
- Encourage perineal exercises within 24 to 48 hours after surgery.
- Provide meticulous catheter care — especially if a three-way catheter with a continuous irrigation system is in place. Check the tubing for kinks and blockages, especially if the patient reports pain. Warn him not to pull on the catheter.

After transurethral prostatic resection:
- Watch for signs of urethral stricture (dysuria, decreased force and caliber of urine stream, and straining to urinate) and for abdominal distention (from urethral stricture or catheter blockage). Irrigate the catheter as ordered.

After perineal prostatectomy:
- Avoid taking a rectal temperature or inserting any kind of rectal tube. Provide pads to absorb urine leakage, a rubber ring for the patient to sit on, and sitz baths for pain and inflammation.

After perineal and retropubic prostatectomy:
- Explain that urine leakage after catheter removal is normal and will subside.
- When a patient receives hormonal therapy, watch for adverse effects. Gynecomastia, fluid retention, nausea, and vomiting are common with DES. Thrombophlebitis may also occur, especially with DES.

After radiation therapy:
- Watch for common adverse effects: proctitis, diarrhea, bladder spasms, and urinary frequency. Internal radiation usually results in cystitis in the first 2 to 3 weeks. Urge the patient to drink at least 67½ oz (2,000 ml) of fluid daily. Provide analgesics and antispasmodics, as ordered.

Testicular cancer

Malignant testicular tumors primarily affect young to middle-aged men and are the most common solid tumor in this group. (In children, testicular tumors are rare.) Most testicular tumors originate in gonadal cells. About 40% are seminomas — uniform, undifferentiated cells resembling primitive gonadal cells. The remainder are nonseminomas — tumor cells showing various degrees of differentiation. The prognosis varies with the cell type and disease stage, but testicular cancer is considered curable. When treated with surgery and radiation, almost all patients with localized disease survive beyond 5 years.

Causes and incidence

The cause of testicular cancer isn't known, but incidence (which peaks between ages 20 and 40) is higher in men with cryptorchidism (even when surgically corrected) and in men whose mothers used diethylstilbestrol during pregnancy. Testicular cancer is rare in nonwhite males and accounts for fewer than 1% of male cancer deaths. Testicular cancer spreads through the lymphatic system to the iliac, paraaortic, and mediastinal lymph nodes and may metastasize to the lungs, liver, viscera, and bone.

STAGING TESTICULAR CANCER

The TNM (tumor, node, metastasis) staging system adopted by the American Joint Committee on Cancer has established the following stages for testicular cancer.

Primary tumor
TX — primary tumor can't be assessed (this stage is used in the absence of radical orchiectomy)

T0 — histologic scar or no evidence of primary tumor

Tis — intratubular tumor: preinvasive cancer

T1 — tumor limited to testicles, including the rete testis

T2 — tumor extends beyond tunica albuginea or into epididymis

T3 — tumor extends into spermatic cord

T4 — tumor invades scrotum

Regional lymph nodes
NX — regional lymph nodes can't be assessed

N0 — no evidence of regional lymph-node metastasis

N1 — metastasis in a single lymph node, 2 cm or less in greatest dimension

N2 — metastasis in a single lymph node, between 2 and 5 cm in greatest dimension, or metastasis to several lymph nodes, none more than 5 cm in greatest dimension

N3 — metastasis in a lymph node more than 5 cm in greatest dimension

Distant metastasis
MX — distant metastasis unassessable

M0 — no known distant metastasis

M1 — distant metastasis

Staging categories
Testicular cancer progresses as follows:
STAGE 0 — Tis, N0, M0
STAGE I — T1, N0, M0; T2, N0, M0
STAGE II — T3, N0, M0; T4, N0, M0
STAGE III — any T, N1, M0
STAGE IV — any T, N2, M0; any T, N3, M0; any T, any N, M1

Signs and symptoms
The first sign is usually a firm, painless, and smooth testicular mass, varying in size and sometimes producing a sense of testicular heaviness. When such a tumor causes chorionic gonadotropin or estrogen production, gynecomastia and nipple tenderness may result. In advanced stages, signs and symptoms include ureteral obstruction, abdominal mass, cough, hemoptysis, shortness of breath, weight loss, fatigue, pallor, and lethargy.

Diagnosis
Two effective means of detecting a testicular tumor are regular self-examinations and testicular palpation during a routine physical examination. Transillumination can distinguish between a tumor (which doesn't transilluminate) and a hydrocele or spermatocele (which does). Follow-up measures should include an examination for gynecomastia and abdominal masses.

Diagnostic tests include excretory urography to detect ureteral deviation resulting from para-aortic node involvement, urinary or serum luteinizing hormone levels, blood tests, lymphangiography, ultrasound, and abdominal computed tomography scan. Serum alpha-fetoprotein and beta-human chorionic gonadotropin levels — indicators of testicular tumor activity — provide a baseline for measuring response to therapy and determining the prognosis.

Surgical excision and biopsy of the tumor and testis permits histologic verification of the tumor cell type — essential for effective treatment. Inguinal exploration determines the extent of nodal involvement. (See *Staging testicular cancer*.)

Treatment
The extent of surgery, radiation, and chemotherapy varies with tumor cell type and stage. Surgery includes orchiectomy

and retroperitoneal node dissection. Most surgeons remove the testis, not the scrotum (to allow for a prosthetic implant). Hormone replacement therapy may be needed after bilateral orchiectomy.

Radiation of the retroperitoneal and homolateral iliac nodes follows removal of a seminoma. All positive nodes receive radiation after removal of a nonseminoma. Patients with retroperitoneal extension receive prophylactic radiation to the mediastinal and supraclavicular nodes.

Essential for tumors beyond stage 0, chemotherapy combinations include bleomycin, etoposide, and cisplatin; etoposide and cisplatin; and cisplatin. Chemotherapy and radiation followed by autologous bone marrow transplantation may help unresponsive patients.

Special considerations

Develop a care plan that addresses both the patient's psychological and physical needs.

Before orchiectomy:

■ Reassure the patient that sterility and impotence need not follow unilateral orchiectomy, that synthetic hormones can restore hormonal balance, and that most surgeons don't remove the scrotum. In many cases, a testicular prosthesis can correct anatomic disfigurement.

After orchiectomy:

■ For the first day after surgery, apply an ice pack to the scrotum and provide analgesics, as ordered.

■ Check for excessive bleeding, swelling, and signs of infection.

■ Provide a scrotal athletic supporter to minimize pain during ambulation.

During chemotherapy:

■ Give antiemetics, as needed, for nausea and vomiting. Encourage small, frequent meals to maintain oral intake despite anorexia. Establish a mouth care regimen and check for stomatitis. Watch for signs of myelosuppression. If the patient receives vinblastine, assess for neurotoxicity (peripheral paresthesia, jaw pain, and muscle cramps). If he receives cisplatin, check for ototoxicity. To prevent renal damage, encourage increased fluid intake and provide I.V. fluids, a potassium supplement, and diuretics, as ordered.

Penile cancer

The most common form of penile cancer, epidermoid squamous cell cancer, is usually found in the glans but may also occur on the corona glandis and, rarely, in the preputial cavity. This malignancy produces ulcerative or papillary (wartlike, nodular) lesions, which may become quite large before spreading beyond the penis; such lesions may destroy the glans prepuce and invade the corpora.

The prognosis varies according to staging at time of diagnosis. If begun early enough, radiation therapy increases the 5-year survival rate to over 60%; surgery only, to over 55%. Unfortunately, many men delay treatment of penile cancer because they fear disfigurement and loss of sexual function.

Causes and incidence

The exact cause of penile cancer is unknown; however, it's generally associated with poor personal hygiene and with phimosis in uncircumcised men. This may account for the low incidence among Jews, Muslims, and people of other cultures that practice circumcision at birth or shortly thereafter. (Incidence isn't decreased in cultures that practice circumcision at a later date.) Early circumcision seems to prevent penile cancer by allowing for better personal hygiene and minimizing inflammatory (and commonly premalignant) lesions of the glans and prepuce. Such lesions include:

■ leukoplakia — inflammation, with thickened patches that may fissure

■ balanitis — inflammation of the penis associated with phimosis

■ erythroplasia of Queyrat — squamous cell cancer in situ; velvety, erythematous lesion that becomes scaly and ulcerative

■ penile horn — scaly, horn-shaped growth.

Penile cancer rarely affects circumcised men in modern cultures; when it does occur, it's usually in men who are older than age 50.

Signs and symptoms

In a circumcised man, early signs of penile cancer include a small circumscribed lesion, a pimple, or a sore on the penis. In an uncircumcised man, however, such early symptoms may go unnoticed, so penile cancer first becomes apparent when it causes late-stage signs or symptoms, such as pain, hemorrhage, dysuria, purulent discharge, and obstruction of the urinary meatus. Rarely is metastasis the first sign of penile cancer.

Diagnosis

Diagnosis of penile cancer requires a tissue biopsy.

CONFIRMING DIAGNOSIS *Preoperative baseline studies include complete blood count, urinalysis, an electrocardiogram, and a chest X-ray. Enlarged inguinal lymph nodes due to infection (caused by primary lesion) make detection of nodal metastasis by preoperative computed tomography scan difficult.*

Treatment

Depending on the stage of progression, treatment includes surgical resection of the primary tumor and, possibly, chemotherapy and radiation. Local tumors of the prepuce only require circumcision. Invasive tumors, however, require partial penectomy if there's at least a 2-cm, tumor-free margin; tumors of the base of the penile shaft require total penectomy and inguinal node dissection (procedure is less common in the United States than in other countries where incidence is higher). Radiation therapy may improve treatment effectiveness after resection of localized lesions without metastasis; it may also reduce the size of lymph nodes before nodal resection. It's not adequate primary treatment for groin metastasis, however. Topical 5-fluorouracil is used for precancerous lesions. A combination of bleomycin, methotrexate, and vincristine with or without cisplatin is used for metastasis.

Special considerations

Penile cancer calls for good patient teaching, psychological support, and comprehensive postoperative care. The patient with penile cancer fears disfigurement, pain, and loss of sexual function.

Before penile surgery:

- Spend time with the patient, and encourage him to talk about his fears.
- Supplement and reinforce what the physician has told the patient about the surgery and other treatment measures, and explain expected postoperative procedures, such as dressing changes and catheterization. Show him diagrams of the surgical procedure and pictures of the results of similar surgery to help him adapt to an altered body image.
- If the patient needs urinary diversion, refer him to the enterostomal therapist.

Although postpenectomy care varies with the procedure used and the physician's protocol, certain procedures are always applicable:

- Constantly monitor the patient's vital signs and record his intake and output accurately.
- Provide comprehensive skin care to prevent skin breakdown from urinary diversion or suprapubic catheterization. Keep the skin dry and free from urine. If the patient has a suprapubic catheter, make sure the catheter is patent at all times.
- Administer analgesics as ordered. Elevate the penile stump with a small towel or pillow to minimize edema.
- Check the surgical site often for signs of infection, such as foul odor or excessive drainage on dressing.
- If the patient has had inguinal node dissection, watch for and immediately report signs of lymphedema, such as decreased circulation or disproportionate swelling of a leg.
- After partial penectomy, reassure the patient that the penile stump should be sufficient for urination and sexual function. Refer him for psychological or sexual counseling if necessary.

Cervical cancer

One of the most common cancers of the female reproductive system, cervical cancer is classified as either preinvasive or invasive.

Preinvasive cancer ranges from minimal cervical dysplasia, in which the lower third of the epithelium contains abnormal cells, to carcinoma in situ, in which the full thickness of epithelium contains abnormally proliferating cells (also known as *cervical intraepithelial neoplasia*). Preinvasive cancer is curable 75% to 90% of the time with early detection and proper treatment. If untreated (and depending on the form in which it appears), it may progress to invasive cervical cancer.

In invasive cancer, cancer cells penetrate the basement membrane and can spread directly to contiguous pelvic structures or disseminate to distant sites by lymphatic routes.

Causes and incidence

Although the cause is unknown, several predisposing factors have been related to the development of cervical cancer: frequent intercourse at a young age (younger than age 16), multiple sexual partners, multiple pregnancies, exposure to sexually transmitted diseases (particularly genital human papillomavirus), and smoking.

In almost all cases of cervical cancer (95%), the histologic type is squamous cell cancer, which varies from well-differentiated cells to highly anaplastic spindle cells. Only 5% are adenocarcinomas. Usually, invasive cancer occurs between ages 30 and 50; rarely, in patients younger than age 20.

In 2000, 12,800 women were diagnosed with cervical cancer and there were 4,600 deaths from this disease.

Signs and symptoms

Preinvasive cervical cancer produces no symptoms or other clinically apparent changes. Early invasive cervical cancer causes abnormal vaginal bleeding, persistent vaginal discharge, and postcoital pain and bleeding. In advanced stages, it causes pelvic pain, vaginal leakage of urine and feces from a fistula, anorexia, weight loss, and anemia.

Diagnosis

A cytologic examination (Papanicolaou [Pap] smear) can detect cervical cancer before clinical evidence appears. (Systems of Pap smear classification may vary from facility to facility.) Abnormal cervical cytology routinely calls for colposcopy, which can detect the presence and extent of preclinical lesions requiring biopsy and histo-

logic examination. Staining may identify areas for biopsy when the smear shows abnormal cells but there's no obvious lesion. Although the tests are nonspecific, they do distinguish between normal and abnormal tissues. Normal tissues absorb the iodine and turn brown; abnormal tissues are devoid of glycogen and won't change color. Additional studies, such as lymphangiography, cystography, and scans, can detect metastasis. (See *Staging cervical cancer,* page 110.)

Treatment

Appropriate treatment depends on accurate clinical staging. Preinvasive lesions may be treated with total excisional biopsy, cryosurgery, laser destruction, conization (and frequent Pap smear follow-up) or, rarely, hysterectomy. Therapy for invasive squamous cell cancer may include radical hysterectomy and radiation therapy (internal, external, or both). Chemotherapy may be used alone or in combination with radiation therapy in treating cervical cancer. Cisplatin and fluorouracil are the agents used.

Special considerations

Management of cervical cancer requires skilled preoperative and postoperative care, comprehensive patient teaching, and emotional and psychological support.

■ If you assist with a biopsy, drape and prepare the patient as for routine Pap smear and pelvic examination. Have a container of formaldehyde ready to preserve the specimen during transfer to the pathology laboratory. Explain to the patient that she may feel pressure, minor abdominal cramps, or a pinch from the punch forceps. Reassure her that pain will be minimal because the cervix has few nerve endings.

■ If you assist with cryosurgery, drape and prepare the patient as if for a routine Pap smear and pelvic examination. Explain that the procedure takes approximately 15 minutes, during which time the physician will use refrigerant to freeze the cervix. Warn the patient that she may experience abdominal cramps, headache, and sweating, but reassure her that she'll feel little, if any, pain.

STAGING CERVICAL CANCER

Cervical cancer treatment decisions depend on accurate staging. The International Federation of Gynecology and Obstetrics defines cervical cancer stages as follows.

Stage 0
Carcinoma in situ, intraepithelial carcinoma

Stage I
Cancer confined to the cervix (extension to the corpus should be disregarded); T1, N0, M0
STAGE IA — preclinical malignant lesions of the cervix (diagnosed only microscopically); T1, N0, M0
STAGE IA1 — minimal microscopically evident stromal invasion
STAGE IA2 — lesions detected microscopically, measuring 5 mm or less from the base of the epithelium, either surface or glandular, from which it originates; lesion width shouldn't exceed 7 mm
STAGE IB — lesions measuring more than 5 mm deep and 7 mm wide, whether seen clinically or not (preformed space involvement shouldn't alter the staging but should be recorded for future treatment decisions); T1b, N0, M0

Stage II
Extension beyond the cervix but not to the pelvic wall; the cancer involves the vagina but hasn't spread to the lower third; T2, N0, M0
STAGE IIA — no obvious parametrial involvement
STAGE IIB — obvious parametrial involvement

Stage III
Extension to the pelvic wall; on rectal examination, no cancer-free space exists between the tumor and the pelvic wall; the tumor involves the lower third of the vagina; this includes all cases with hydronephrosis or nonfunctioning kidney; T3, N0, M0
STAGE IIIA — no extension to the pelvic wall
STAGE IIIB — extension to the pelvic wall and hydronephrosis, nonfunctioning kidney, or both

Stage IV
Extension beyond the true pelvis or involvement of the bladder or the rectal mucosa
STAGE IVA — spread to adjacent organs
STAGE IVB — spread to distant organs

■ If you assist with laser therapy, drape and prepare the patient as if for a routine Pap smear and pelvic examination. Explain that the procedure takes approximately 30 minutes and may cause abdominal cramps.
■ After excisional biopsy, cryosurgery, and laser therapy, tell the patient to expect a discharge or spotting for about 1 week after these procedures, and advise her not to douche, use tampons, or engage in sexual intercourse during this time. Tell her to watch for and report signs of infection. Stress the need for a follow-up Pap smear and a pelvic examination within 3 to 4 months after these procedures and periodically thereafter.

■ Tell the patient what to expect postoperatively if she'll have a hysterectomy.
■ After surgery, monitor vital signs every 4 hours.
■ Watch for and immediately report signs or symptoms of complications, such as bleeding, abdominal distention, severe pain, and breathing difficulties.
■ Administer analgesics, prophylactic antibiotics, and subcutaneous heparin, as ordered.
■ Encourage deep-breathing and coughing exercises.
For radiation therapy:

INTERNAL RADIATION SAFETY PRECAUTIONS

There are three cardinal safety rules in internal radiation therapy:

■ *Time.* Wear a radiosensitive badge. Remember, your exposure increases with time, and the effects are cumulative. Therefore, carefully plan your time with the patient to prevent overexposure. (However, don't rush procedures, ignore the patient's psychological needs, or give the impression you can't get out of the room fast enough.)

■ *Distance.* Radiation loses its intensity with distance. Avoid standing at the foot of the patient's bed, where you're in line with the radiation.

■ *Shield.* Lead shields reduce radiation exposure. Use them whenever possible.

In internal radiation therapy, remember that the patient is radioactive while the radiation source is in place, usually 48 to 72 hours.

■ Pregnant women shouldn't be assigned to care for these patients.

■ Check the position of the source applicator every 4 hours. If it appears dislodged, notify the physician immediately. If it's completely dislodged, remove the patient from the bed; pick up the applicator with long forceps, place it on a lead-shielded transport cart, and notify the physician immediately.

■ *Never* pick up the source with your bare hands. Notify the physician and radiation safety officer whenever there's an accident, and keep a lead-shielded transport cart on the unit as long as the patient has a source in place.

POSITIONING OF INTERNAL RADIATION APPLICATOR FOR UTERINE CANCER

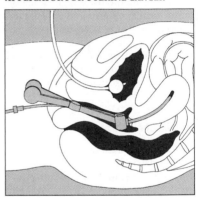

■ Find out if the patient is to have internal or external therapy, or both. Usually, internal radiation therapy is the first procedure.

■ Explain the internal radiation procedure, and answer the patient's questions. Internal radiation requires a 2- to 3-day hospital stay, bowel preparation, a povidone-iodine vaginal douche, a clear liquid diet, insertion of an indwelling urinary catheter, and nothing by mouth the night before the implantation.

■ Explain to the patient that she'll have less contact with staff and visitors while the implant is in place.

■ Tell the patient that the internal radiation applicator will be inserted in the operating room under general anesthesia and that the radioactive material (such as radium or cesium) will be loaded into it when she's back in her room.

■ Remember that safety precautions — time, distance, and shielding — begin as soon as the radioactive source is in place. Inform the patient that she'll require a private room. (See *Internal radiation safety precautions.*)

■ Encourage the patient to lie flat and limit movement while the implant is in place. If she prefers, elevate the head of the bed slightly.

■ Check vital signs every 4 hours; watch for skin reaction, vaginal bleeding, abdominal discomfort, or evidence of dehydration. Make sure the patient can reach everything she needs without stretching or straining. Assist her in range-of-motion *arm* exercises (leg exercises and other body movements could dislodge the implant). If ordered, administer a tranquilizer to help the patient relax and remain still. Organize the time you spend with the patient to minimize your exposure to radiation.

- Inform visitors of safety precautions, and hang a sign listing these precautions on the patient's door.
- Explain that external outpatient radiation therapy, when necessary, continues for 4 to 6 weeks.
- Teach the patient to watch for and report uncomfortable adverse effects. Because radiation therapy may increase susceptibility to infection by lowering the white blood cell count, warn the patient to avoid persons with obvious infections during therapy.
- Teach the patient to use a vaginal dilator to prevent vaginal stenosis and to facilitate vaginal examinations and sexual intercourse.
- Reassure the patient that this disease and its treatment shouldn't radically alter her lifestyle or prohibit sexual intimacy.

Uterine cancer

Uterine cancer involves cancerous growth of the endometrial lining. The five-year survival rate is 75% to 95% for stage I cancers; as the stages progress, the survival rate diminishes. For stage II, there's a 50% survival rate; stage III, 30%; and there's less than a 5% survival rate for stage IV.

Causes and incidence
Uterine cancer seems linked to several predisposing factors:
- abnormal uterine bleeding
- diabetes
- familial tendency
- history of uterine polyps or endometrial hyperplasia
- hypertension
- low fertility index and anovulation
- nulliparity
- obesity
- uninterrupted estrogen stimulation.

In most cases, uterine cancer is an adenocarcinoma that metastasizes late, usually from the endometrium to the cervix, ovaries, fallopian tubes, and other peritoneal structures. It may spread to distant organs, such as the lungs and the brain,

through the blood or the lymphatic system. Lymph node involvement can also occur. Less common are adenoacanthoma, endometrial stromal sarcoma, lymphosarcoma, mixed mesodermal tumors (including carcinosarcoma), and leiomyosarcoma.

Uterine cancer usually affects postmenopausal women between ages 50 and 60; it's uncommon between ages 30 and 40 and extremely rare before age 30. Most premenopausal women who develop uterine cancer have a history of anovulatory menstrual cycles or other hormonal imbalance. About 37,000 new cases of uterine cancer are reported annually, with approximately 6,400 deaths predicted for 1999.

Signs and symptoms
Uterine enlargement, and persistent and unusual premenopausal bleeding, or any postmenopausal bleeding, are the most common indications of uterine cancer. The discharge may at first be watery and blood-streaked, but it gradually becomes more bloody. Other signs or symptoms, such as pain and weight loss, don't appear until the cancer is well advanced.

Diagnosis
Unfortunately, a Papanicolaou test, so useful for detecting cervical cancer, doesn't dependably predict early-stage uterine cancer. Diagnosis of uterine cancer requires endometrial, cervical, and endocervical biopsies. (See Staging uterine cancer.) Negative biopsies call for a fractional dilatation and curettage to determine the diagnosis. Positive diagnosis requires the following tests for baseline data and staging:
- multiple cervical biopsies and endocervical curettage to pinpoint cervical involvement
- Schiller's test, staining the cervix and vagina with an iodine solution that turns healthy tissues brown; cancerous tissues resist the stain
- complete physical examination
- chest X-ray or computed tomography scan
- excretory urography and, possibly, cystoscopy
- complete blood studies
- electrocardiogram

■ proctoscopy or barium enema studies, if bladder and rectal involvement are suspected.

Treatment
Treatment varies, depending on the extent of the disease:
■ Surgery — Rarely curative, surgery generally involves total abdominal hysterectomy, bilateral salpingo-oophorectomy, or possibly omentectomy with or without pelvic or para-aortic lymphadenectomy. Total exenteration involves removal of all pelvic organs, including the vagina, and is done only when the disease is sufficiently contained to allow surgical removal of diseased parts. (See *Managing pelvic exenteration*, page 114.)
■ Radiation therapy — When the tumor isn't well differentiated, intracavitary or external radiation (or both), given 6 weeks before surgery, may inhibit recurrence and lengthen survival time.
■ Hormonal therapy — Synthetic progesterones, such as medroxyprogesterone or megestrol, may be administered for systemic disease. Tamoxifen (which produces a 20% to 40% response rate) may be given as a second-line treatment.
■ Chemotherapy — Varying combinations of cisplatin, doxorubicin, carboplatin, topotecan, paclitaxel, and gemcitabine are usually tried when other treatments have failed.

Special considerations
Patients with uterine cancer require patient teaching to help them cope with surgery, radiation, and chemotherapy. Also provide good postoperative care and psychological support.
Before surgery:
■ Reinforce what the physician told the patient about the surgery, and explain the routine tests (for example, repeated blood tests the morning after surgery) and postoperative care. If the patient is to have a lymphadenectomy *and* a total hysterectomy, explain that she'll probably have a wound drainage system for about 5 days after surgery. Also explain indwelling urinary catheter care. Fit the patient with antiembolism stockings for use during and

---

STAGING UTERINE CANCER

The International Federation of Gynecology and Obstetrics defines uterine (endometrial) cancer stages as follows.

Stage 0
Carcinoma in situ

Stage I
Carcinoma confined to the corpus
STAGE IA — length of the uterine cavity 8 cm or less
STAGE IB — length of the uterine cavity more than 8 cm
   Stage I disease is subgrouped by the following histologic grades of the adenocarcinoma:
■ G1 — highly differentiated adenomatous carcinoma
■ G2 — moderately differentiated adenomatous carcinoma with partly solid areas
■ G3 — predominantly solid or entirely undifferentiated carcinoma

Stage II
Carcinoma has involved the corpus and the cervix but hasn't extended outside the uterus

Stage III
Carcinoma has extended outside the uterus but not outside the true pelvis

Stage IV
Carcinoma has extended outside the true pelvis or has obviously involved the mucosa of the bladder or rectum
STAGE IVA — spread of the growth to adjacent organs
STAGE IVB — spread of the growth to distant organs

---

after surgery. Make sure the patient's blood has been typed and cross-matched. If the patient is premenopausal, inform her that

MANAGING PELVIC EXENTERATION

Before pelvic exenteration
- Teach the patient about ileal conduit and possible colostomy, and make sure she understands that her vagina will be removed.
- To minimize the risk of infection, supervise a rigorous bowel and skin preparation procedure. Decrease the residue in the patient's diet for 48 to 72 hours, and then maintain a diet ranging from clear liquids to nothing by mouth. Administer oral or I.V. antibiotics, as ordered, and prep skin daily with antibacterial soap.
- Instruct the patient about postoperative procedures: I.V. therapy, central venous pressure catheter, blood drainage system, and an unsutured perineal wound with gauze packing.

After pelvic exenteration
- Check the stoma, incision, and perineal wound for drainage. Be especially careful to check the perineal wound for bleeding after the packing is removed. Expect red or serosanguineous drainage, but notify the physician immediately if drainage is excessive, continuously bright red, foul-smelling, or purulent or if there's bleeding from the conduit.
- Provide excellent skin care because of draining urine and feces. Use warm water and saline solution to clean the skin, because soap may be too drying and may increase skin breakdown.

- If the patient has received subcutaneous heparin, continue administration, as ordered, until the patient is fully ambulatory again. Give prophylactic antibiotics as ordered, and provide good indwelling urinary catheter care.
- Check vital signs every 4 hours. Watch for and immediately report any sign of complications, such as bleeding, abdominal distention, severe pain, wheezing, or other breathing difficulties. Provide analgesics as ordered.
- Regularly encourage the patient to breathe deeply and cough to help prevent complications. Promote the use of an incentive spirometer several times every waking hour to help keep lungs expanded.

  For radiation therapy:
- Find out if the patient is to have internal or external radiation or both. Usually, internal radiation therapy is done first.
- Explain the internal radiation procedure, answer the patient's questions, and encourage her to express her fears and concerns.
- Explain that internal radiation usually requires a 2- to 3-day hospital stay, bowel preparation, a povidone-iodine vaginal douche, a clear liquid diet, and nothing taken by mouth the night before the implantation.
- Mention that internal radiation also requires an indwelling urinary catheter.
- Tell the patient that, if the procedure is performed in the operating room, she'll receive a general anesthetic. She'll be placed in a dorsal position, with her knees and hips flexed and her heels resting in footrests.
- Inform her that the radioactive source may be implanted in the vagina by the physician, or it may be implanted by a member of the radiation team while the patient is in her room.
- Remember that safety precautions, including time, distance, and shielding, must be imposed immediately after the patient's radioactive source has been implanted.
- Tell the patient that she'll require a private room.
- Encourage the patient to limit movement while the source is in place. If she prefers, elevate the head of the bed slightly. Make sure the patient can reach everything

removal of her ovaries will induce menopause.

  After surgery:
- Measure fluid contents of the wound drainage system every shift. Notify the physician immediately if drainage exceeds 400 ml.

she needs (call bell, telephone, water) without stretching or straining. Assist her in range-of-motion *arm* exercises (leg exercises and other body movements could dislodge the source). If ordered, administer a tranquilizer to help the patient relax and remain still. Organize the time you spend with the patient to minimize your exposure to radiation.

■ Check the patient's vital signs every 4 hours; watch for skin reaction, vaginal bleeding, abdominal discomfort, or evidence of dehydration.

■ Inform visitors of safety precautions and hang a sign listing these precautions on the patient's door.

If the patient receives external radiation:

■ Teach the patient and her family about the therapy before it begins. Tell the patient that treatment is usually given 5 days a week for 6 weeks. Warn her not to scrub body areas marked with indelible ink for treatment because it's important to direct treatment to exactly the same area each time.

■ Instruct the patient to maintain a high-protein, high-carbohydrate, low-residue diet to reduce bulk and yet maintain calories. Administer diphenoxylate with atropine, as ordered, to minimize diarrhea, a possible adverse effect of pelvic radiation.

■ To minimize skin breakdown and reduce the risk of skin infection, tell the patient to keep the treatment area dry, to avoid wearing clothes that rub against the area, and to avoid using heating pads, alcohol rubs, or any skin creams.

■ Teach the patient how to use a vaginal dilator to prevent vaginal stenosis and to facilitate vaginal examinations and sexual intercourse.

Remember, a patient with uterine cancer needs special counseling and psychological support to help her cope with this disease and the necessary treatments. Fearful about her survival, she may also be concerned that treatment will alter her lifestyle and prevent sexual intimacy. Explain that except in total pelvic exenteration, the vagina remains intact and that after she recovers, sexual intercourse is possible. Your presence and interest will help the patient, even if you can't answer every question she may ask.

Vaginal cancer

Vaginal cancer accounts for approximately 2% of all gynecologic cancers. It usually appears as squamous cell cancer, but occasionally as melanoma, sarcoma, or adenocarcinoma.

Causes and incidence

The exact cause of vaginal cancer remains unknown. This cancer generally occurs in women in their early to mid-50s, but some of the rarer types occur in younger women, and rhabdomyosarcoma appears in children. (Clear cell adenocarcinoma has an increased incidence in young women whose mothers took diethylstilbestrol).

Vaginal cancer varies in severity according to its location and effect on lymphatic drainage. (The vagina is a thin-walled structure with a rich lymphatic drainage.) Vaginal cancer is similar to cervical cancer in that it may progress from an intraepithelial tumor to an invasive cancer. However, it spreads more slowly than cervical cancer.

A lesion in the upper third of the vagina (the most common site) usually metastasizes to the groin nodes; a lesion in the lower third (the second most common site) usually metastasizes to the hypogastric and iliac nodes; but a lesion in the middle third metastasizes erratically. A posterior lesion displaces and distends the vaginal posterior wall before spreading to deep layers. By contrast, an anterior lesion spreads more rapidly into other structures and deep layers because, unlike the posterior wall, the anterior vaginal wall isn't flexible.

Signs and symptoms

Commonly, the patient with vaginal cancer has experienced abnormal bleeding and discharge. Also, she may have a small or large, in many cases firm, ulcerated lesion in any part of the vagina. As the cancer progresses, it commonly spreads to the bladder (producing frequent voiding and bladder pain), the rectum (bleeding), vulva (lesion), pubic bone (pain), or other surrounding tissues.

STAGING VAGINAL CANCER

The International Federation of Gynecology and Obstetrics uses the following staging system as a prognostic and treatment guide to vaginal cancer.

STAGE 0 — carcinoma in situ, intraepithelial carcinoma
STAGE I — the carcinoma is limited to the vaginal wall
STAGE II — the carcinoma has involved the subvaginal tissue but hasn't extended to the pelvic wall
STAGE III — the carcinoma has extended to the pelvic wall
STAGE IV — the carcinoma has extended beyond the true pelvis or has involved the mucosa of the bladder or rectum

Diagnosis

The diagnosis of vaginal cancer is based on the presence of abnormal cells on a vaginal Papanicolaou smear. Careful examination and a biopsy rule out the cervix and vulva as the primary sites of the lesion. In many cases, however, the cervix contains the primary lesion that has metastasized to the vagina. Then, any visible lesion is biopsied and evaluated histologically. It's sometimes difficult to visualize the entire vagina because the speculum blades may hide a lesion, or the patient may be uncooperative because of discomfort. When lesions aren't visible, colposcopy is used to search out abnormalities. Painting the suspected vaginal area with Lugol's solution also helps identify malignant areas by staining glycogen-containing normal tissue, while leaving abnormal tissue unstained. (See *Staging vaginal cancer.*)

Treatment

In early stages, treatment aims to preserve the normal parts of the vagina. Topical chemotherapy with 5-fluorouracil and laser surgery can be used for stages 0 and I. Radiation or surgery varies with the size, depth, and location of the lesion and the patient's desire to maintain a functional vagina. Preservation of a functional vagina is generally possible only in the early stages. Survival rates are the same for patients treated with radiation as for those treated with surgery.

Surgery is usually recommended only when the tumor is so extensive that exenteration is needed because close proximity to the bladder and rectum permits only minimal tissue margins around resected vaginal tissue.

Radiation therapy is the preferred treatment of advanced vaginal cancer. Most patients need preliminary external radiation treatment to shrink the tumor before internal radiation can begin. Then, if the tumor is localized to the vault and the cervix is present, radiation (using radium or cesium) can be given with an intrauterine tandem or ovoids; if the cervix is absent, a specially designed vaginal applicator is used instead.

To minimize complications, radioactive sources and filters are carefully placed away from radiosensitive tissues, such as the bladder and rectum. Internal radiation lasts 48 to 72 hours, depending on the dosage. (See *Safe time for radiation implant.*)

Special considerations

For internal radiation:
■ Explain the internal radiation procedure, answer the patient's questions, and encourage her to express her fears and concerns.
■ Because the effects of radiation are cumulative, wear a radiosensitive badge and a lead shield (if available) when you enter the patient's room, and adhere to internal radiation safety precautions.
■ Check with the radiation therapist concerning the maximum recommended time that you can safely spend with the patient when giving direct care.
■ While the radiation source is in place, the patient must lie flat on her back. Insert an indwelling urinary catheter (usually done in the operating room), and don't change the patient's linens unless they're soiled. Give only partial bed baths, and make sure the patient has a call bell, phone,

SAFE TIME FOR RADIATION IMPLANT

Internal radiation with cesium or radium can be administered if the cancer is localized to the vault. Distance defines safe exposure to the radioactive implant, in this case, cesium.

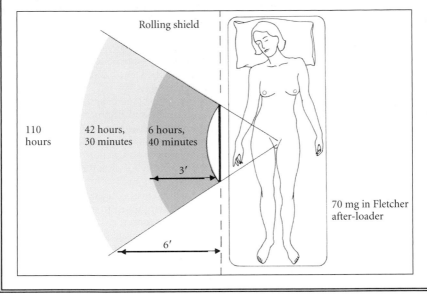

Rolling shield

110 hours

42 hours, 30 minutes

6 hours, 40 minutes

3′

6′

70 mg in Fletcher after-loader

---

water, or anything else she needs within easy reach. The physician will order a clear liquid or low-residue diet and an antidiarrheal drug to prevent bowel movements.

■ To compensate for immobility, encourage the patient to do active range-of-motion exercises with both arms.

■ Before radiation treatment, explain the necessity of immobilization, and tell the patient what it entails (such as no linen changes and the use of an indwelling urinary catheter). Throughout therapy, encourage her to express her anxieties.

■ Instruct the patient to use a stent or do prescribed exercises to prevent vaginal stenosis. Coitus is also helpful in preventing stenosis.

Ovarian cancer

Ovarian cancer is one of the leading causes of gynecological deaths in the United States. In women with previously treated breast cancer, metastatic ovarian cancer is more common than cancer at any other site and may be linked to mutations in the BRCA1 or BRCA2 gene.

The prognosis varies with the histologic type and stage of the disease but is generally poor because ovarian tumors produce few early signs and are usually advanced at diagnosis. Although about 46% of women with ovarian cancer survive for 5 years, the overall survival rate hasn't improved significantly.

Three main types of ovarian cancer exist:

■ Primary epithelial tumors account for 90% of all ovarian cancers and include serous cystadenocarcinoma, mucinous cystadenocarcinoma, and endometrioid and mesonephric malignancies. Serous cystadenocarcinoma is the most common type and accounts for 50% of all cases.

■ Germ cell tumors include endodermal sinus malignancies, embryonal carcinoma (a rare ovarian cancer that appears in children), immature teratomas, and dysgermi-noma.

■ Sex cord (stromal) tumors include granulosa cell tumors (which produce estrogen and may have feminizing effects), granulosa-theca cell tumors, and the rare arrhenoblastomas (which produce androgen and have virilizing effects).

Causes and incidence

Exactly what causes ovarian cancer isn't known, but the greatest number of cases occurs in the fifth decade of life. However, it can occur during childhood. Other contributing factors include infertility; nulliparity; familial tendency; ovarian dysfunction; irregular menses; and possible exposure to asbestos, talc, and industrial pollutants.

Primary epithelial tumors arise in the ovarian surface epithelium; germ cell tumors, in the ovum itself; and sex cord tumors, in the ovarian stroma. Ovarian tumors spread rapidly intraperitoneally by local extension or surface seeding and, occasionally, through the lymphatics and the bloodstream. Generally, extraperitoneal spread is through the diaphragm into the chest cavity, which may cause pleural effusions. Other metastasis is rare.

Signs and symptoms

Typically, symptoms vary with the size of the tumor. An ovary may grow to considerable size before it produces overt symptoms. Occasionally, in the early stages, ovarian cancer causes vague abdominal discomfort, dyspepsia, and other mild GI disturbances. As it progresses, it causes urinary frequency, constipation, pelvic discomfort, distention, and weight loss. Tumor rupture, torsion, or infection may cause pain, which, in young patients, may mimic appendicitis. Granulosa cell tumors have feminizing effects (such as bleeding between periods in premenopausal women); conversely, arrhenoblastomas have virilizing effects. Advanced ovarian cancer causes ascites, rarely postmenopausal bleeding and pain, and symptoms relating to metastatic sites (most commonly pleural effusions).

Diagnosis

Diagnosis of ovarian cancer requires clinical evaluation, complete patient history, surgical exploration, and histologic studies. Preoperative evaluation includes a complete physical examination, including pelvic examination with Papanicolaou smear (positive in only a small number of women with ovarian cancer) and the following special tests:

■ abdominal ultrasonography, computed tomography scan, or X-ray (may delineate tumor size)

■ complete blood count, blood chemistries, and electrocardiogram

■ excretory urography for information on renal function and possible urinary tract anomalies or obstruction

■ chest X-ray for distant metastasis and pleural effusions

■ barium enema (especially in patients with GI symptoms) to reveal obstruction and size of tumor

■ lymphangiography to show lymph node involvement

■ mammography to rule out primary breast cancer

■ liver function studies or a liver scan in patients with ascites

■ ascites fluid aspiration for identification of typical cells by cytology

■ laboratory tumor marker studies, such as Ca-125, carcinoembryonic antigen, and human chorionic gonadotropin.

Despite extensive testing, accurate diagnosis and staging are impossible without exploratory laparotomy, including lymph node evaluation and tumor resection. (See *Staging ovarian cancer.*)

Treatment

According to the staging of the disease and the patient's age, treatment of ovarian cancer requires varying combinations of surgery, chemotherapy and, in some cases, radiation.

Occasionally, in girls or young women with a unilateral encapsulated tumor who wish to maintain fertility, the following conservative approach may be appropriate:

■ resection of the involved ovary

■ biopsies of the omentum and the uninvolved ovary

STAGING OVARIAN CANCER

The International Federation of Gynecology and Obstetrics uses the staging system below for ovarian cancer.

Stage I
Growth limited to the ovaries; T1, N0, M0
STAGE IA — growth limited to one ovary; no ascites; no tumor on the external surface; capsule intact
STAGE IB — growth limited to both ovaries; no ascites; no tumor on the external surfaces; capsules intact
STAGE IC — tumor either stage IA or IB but on surface of one or both ovaries; or with capsule ruptured; or with ascites containing malignant cells or with positive peritoneal washings

Stage II
Growth involving one or both ovaries with pelvic extension; T2, N0, M0
STAGE IIA — extension or metastasis, or both, to the uterus or tubes (or both)
STAGE IIB — tension to pelvic tissues
STAGE IIC — tumor either stage IIA or IIB, but with tumor on surface of one or both ovaries; with capsule (or capsules) ruptured; or with ascites present containing malignant cells or with positive peritoneal washings

Stage III
Tumor involving one or both ovaries with peritoneal implants outside the pelvis or positive retroperitoneal or inguinal nodes; superficial liver metastasis equals stage III; tumor limited to the true pelvis but with confirmed extension to small bowel or omentum; T3, N0, M0
STAGE IIIA — tumor grossly limited to the true pelvis with negative nodes but with confirmed microscopic seeding of abdominal peritoneal surfaces
STAGE IIIB — tumor of one or both ovaries with confirmed implants of abdominal peritoneal surfaces none exceeding 2 cm in dimension; nodes are negative
STAGE IIIC — abdominal implants greater than 2 cm or positive retroperitoneal or inguinal nodes or both

Stage IV
Growth involving one or both ovaries with distant metastasis (such as pleural effusion and abnormal cells or parenchymal liver metastasis)

■ peritoneal washings for cytologic examination of pelvic fluid
■ careful follow-up, including periodic chest X-rays to rule out lung metastasis.

Ovarian cancer usually requires more aggressive treatment, including total abdominal hysterectomy and bilateral salpingo-oophorectomy with tumor resection, omentectomy, appendectomy, lymph node biopsies with lymphadenectomy, tissue biopsies, and peritoneal washings. Complete tumor resection is impossible if the tumor has matted around other organs or if it involves organs that can't be resected. Bilateral salpingo-oophorectomy in a prepubertal girl necessitates hormone replacement therapy, beginning at puberty,

to induce the development of secondary sex characteristics.

Chemotherapy extends survival time in most ovarian cancer patients, but it's largely palliative in advanced disease. However, prolonged remissions are being achieved in some patients.

Chemotherapeutic drugs useful in ovarian cancer include carboplatin, docetaxel, cyclophosphamide, doxorubicin, paclitaxel, cisplatin, and topotecan. These drugs are usually given in combination and they may be administered intraperitoneally.

Radiation therapy generally isn't used for ovarian cancer because the resulting myelosuppression would limit the effectiveness of chemotherapy.

Radioisotopes have been used as adjuvant therapy, but they cause small-bowel obstructions and stenosis.

Special considerations

Because the treatment of ovarian cancer varies widely, so must the patient care plan.

Before surgery:

■ Thoroughly explain all preoperative tests, the expected course of treatment, and surgical and postoperative procedures.

■ Reinforce what the surgeon has told the patient about the surgical procedures listed in the surgical consent form. Explain that this form lists multiple procedures because the extent of the surgery can only be determined after the surgery itself has begun.

■ In premenopausal women, explain that bilateral salpingo-oophorectomy artificially induces early menopause, so they may experience hot flashes, headaches, palpitations, insomnia, depression, and excessive perspiration.

After surgery:

■ Monitor vital signs frequently, and check I.V. fluids often. Monitor intake and output, while maintaining good catheter care. Check the dressing regularly for excessive drainage or bleeding, and watch for signs of infection.

■ Provide abdominal support, and watch for abdominal distention. Encourage coughing and deep breathing. Reposition the patient often, and encourage her to walk shortly after surgery.

■ Monitor and treat adverse effects of radiation and chemotherapy.

■ Provide psychological support for the patient and her family. Encourage open communication, while discouraging overcompensation or "smothering" of the patient by her family. If the patient is a young woman who grieves for her lost ability to bear children, help her (and her family) overcome feelings that "there's nothing else to live for."

 PEDIATRIC TIP *If the patient is a child, find out whether her parents have told her she has cancer, and deal with her questions accordingly. Also, enlist the help of a social worker, chaplain, and other members of the health care team for additional supportive care.*

Cancer of the vulva

Cancer of the vulva most commonly affects the skin folds around the vagina, called the *labia*. It isn't very common, but is considered serious because it makes sexual intercourse painful and difficult. If found early, it has a high cure rate.

Causes and incidence

Although the cause of cancer of the vulva is unknown, several factors seem to predispose women to this disease:

■ chronic pruritus of the vulva, with friction, swelling, and dryness

■ chronic vulvar granulomatous disease

■ diabetes

■ hypertension

■ irradiation of the skin such as nonspecific treatment for pelvic cancer

■ leukoplakia (white epithelial hyperplasia) — in about 25% of patients

■ obesity

■ pigmented moles that are constantly irritated by clothing or perineal pads

■ sexually transmitted diseases (herpes simplex, condyloma acuminatum caused by human papilloma virus).

Cancer of the vulva accounts for approximately 4% of all gynecologic malignancies. It can occur at any age, even in infants, but its peak incidence is in the mid-60s. The most common vulval cancer is squamous cell cancer. Early diagnosis increases the chance of effective treatment and survival. Lymph node dissection allows 5-year survival in 85% of patients if it reveals no positive nodes; otherwise, the survival rate falls to less than 75%.

Signs and symptoms

In 50% of patients, cancer of the vulva begins with vulval pruritus, bleeding, or a small vulval mass (which may start as a small ulcer on the surface; eventually, it becomes infected and painful), so such symptoms call for immediate diagnostic evaluation. Less common indications include a mass in the groin or abnormal urination or defecation.

Diagnosis

A Papanicolaou smear that reveals abnormal cells, pruritus, bleeding, or a small vulvar mass strongly suggests vulvar cancer.

Firm diagnosis requires histologic examination. Abnormal tissues for biopsy are identified by colposcopic examination to pinpoint vulvar lesions or abnormal skin changes and by staining with toluidine blue dye, which, after rinsing with dilute acetic acid, is retained by diseased tissues.

Other diagnostic measures include complete blood count, X-ray, electrocardiogram, and thorough physical (including pelvic) examination. Occasionally, a computed tomography scan may pinpoint lymph node involvement. (See *Staging vulvar cancer*.)

Treatment

Depending on the stage of the disease, cancer of the vulva usually calls for radical or simple vulvectomy (or laser therapy, for some small lesions). Radical vulvectomy requires bilateral dissection of superficial and deep inguinal lymph nodes. Depending on the extent of metastasis, resection may include the urethra, vagina, and bowel, leaving an open perineal wound until healing—about 2 to 3 months. Plastic surgery, including mucocutaneous graft to reconstruct pelvic structures, may be done later.

Small, confined lesions with no lymph node involvement may require a simple vulvectomy or hemivulvectomy (without pelvic node dissection). Personal considerations (young age of patient, active sexual life) may also mandate such conservative management. However, a simple vulvectomy requires careful postoperative surveillance because it leaves the patient at higher risk for developing a new lesion.

Chemotherapy alone or in combination with radiation therapy can be used in advanced cases of vulvar cancer. Cisplatin, fluorouracil, bleomycin, and doxorubicin have shown some effectiveness as a palliative treatment option.

If extensive metastasis, advanced age, or fragile health rules out surgery, irradiation of the primary lesion can offer palliative treatment.

Special considerations

Patient teaching, preoperative and postoperative care, and psychological support can help prevent complications and speed recovery.

STAGING VULVAR CANCER

The International Federation of Gynecology and Obstetrics uses the following staging system as a prognostic and treatment guide to vulvar cancer.

STAGE 0 — carcinoma in situ
STAGE I — tumor confined to skin surface of vulva — 2 cm or less in diameter; nodes are not palpable or are palpable in either groin, not enlarged, mobile (not clinically suspicious of neoplasm); T1, N0, M0
STAGE II — tumor confined to the vulva or the perineum, or both — more than 2 cm in diameter; nodes aren't palpable or are palpable in either groin, not enlarged, mobile (not clinically suspicious of neoplasm)
STAGE III — tumor of any size with (1) adjacent spread to the urethra and any or all of the vagina, the perineum, and the anus or (2) nodes palpable in either or both groins (enlarged, firm, and mobile but clinically suspicious of neoplasm)
STAGE IV — tumor of any size (1) infiltrating the bladder mucosa or the rectal mucosa or both, including the upper part of the urethral mucosa or (2) fixed to the bone or other distant metastases; fixed or ulcerated nodes in either or both groins

---

Before surgery:
■ Supplement and reinforce what the physician has told the patient about the surgery and postoperative procedures, such as the use of an indwelling urinary catheter, preventive respiratory care, and exercises to prevent venous stasis.
■ Encourage the patient to ask questions, and answer them honestly.

After surgery:
■ Provide scrupulous routine gynecologic care and special care to reduce pressure at the operative site, reduce tension on suture lines, and promote healing through better air circulation.

- Place the patient on an air mattress or convoluted foam mattress, and use a cradle to support the top covers.
- Periodically reposition the patient with pillows. Make sure her bed has a half-frame trapeze bar to help her move.
- For several days after surgery, the patient will be maintained on I.V. fluids or a clear liquid diet. As ordered, give her an anti-diarrheal drug three times daily to reduce the discomfort and possible infection caused by defecation. Later, as ordered, give stool softeners and a low-residue diet to combat constipation.
- Teach the patient how to clean the surgical tube thoroughly.
- Check the operative site regularly for bleeding, foul-smelling discharge, or other signs of infection. The wound area will look lumpy, bruised, and battered, making it difficult to detect occult bleeding. This situation calls for a physician or a primary nurse, who can more easily detect subtle changes in appearance.
- Within 5 to 10 days after surgery, as ordered, help the patient to walk. Encourage and assist her in coughing and range-of-motion exercises.
- To prevent urine contamination, the patient will have an indwelling urinary catheter in place for about 2 weeks. Record fluid intake and output, and provide standard catheter care.
- Counsel the patient and her partner about resumption of sexual activity. Explain that sensation in the vulva will eventually return after the nerve endings heal and that they'll probably be able to have sexual intercourse 6 to 8 weeks following surgery. Explain that they may want to try different sexual techniques, especially if surgery has removed the clitoris. Help the patient adjust to the drastic change in her body image.

Fallopian tube cancer

Primary fallopian tube cancer is extremely rare and accounts for fewer than 0.5% of all gynecologic malignancies. Because this disease is generally well advanced before diagnosis (up to 30% of such cancers are bilateral with extratubal spread), prognosis is poor.

Causes and incidence

The causes of fallopian tube cancer aren't clear, but this disease appears to be linked with nulliparity. In fact, over one-half of the women with this disease have never had children.

Fallopian tube cancer usually occurs in postmenopausal women in their 50s and 60s but occasionally is found in younger women.

Signs and symptoms

Generally, early stage fallopian tube cancer produces no symptoms. Late-stage disease is characterized by an enlarged abdomen with a palpable mass, amber-colored vaginal discharge, excessive bleeding during menstruation or, at other times, abdominal cramps, frequent urination, bladder pressure, persistent constipation, weight loss, and unilateral colicky pain produced by hydrops tubae profluens. (This last symptom occurs when the abdominal end of the fallopian tube closes, causing the tube to become greatly distended until its accumulated secretions suddenly overflow into the uterus.) Metastasis develops by local extension or by lymphatic spread to the abdominal organs or to the pelvic, aortic, and inguinal lymph nodes. Extra-abdominal metastasis is rare.

Diagnosis

CONFIRMING DIAGNOSIS *Unexplained postmenopausal bleeding and an abnormal Papanicolaou smear (suspicious or positive in up to 50% of all cases) suggest fallopian tube cancer, but laparotomy is usually necessary to confirm this diagnosis.*

When fallopian tube cancer involves both the ovary and fallopian tube, the primary site is difficult to identify. The preoperative workup includes:
- ultrasound or plain film of the abdomen to help delineate tumor mass
- excretory urography to assess renal function and show urinary tract anomalies and ureteral obstruction
- chest X-ray to rule out metastasis
- barium enema to rule out intestinal obstruction
- computed tomography of the abdomen and pelvis
- routine blood studies

■ electrocardiogram.

Treatment

Treatment of fallopian tube cancer consists of total abdominal hysterectomy, bilateral salpingo-oophorectomy, and omentectomy; chemotherapy with progestogens, cyclophosphamide, and cisplatin; and external radiation for 5 to 6 weeks. All patients should receive some form of adjunctive therapy (radiation or chemotherapy), even when surgery has removed all evidence of the disease.

Special considerations

Good preoperative patient preparation and postoperative care, patient instruction, psychologic support, and symptomatic measures to relieve radiation and chemotherapy adverse effects can promote a successful recovery and minimize complications.

For example, reinforce the physician's explanation of the diagnostic and treatment procedures. Explain the need for preoperative studies, and tell the patient what to expect: fasting from the evening before surgery, an enema to clear the bowel, insertion of an indwelling urinary catheter attached to a drainage bag, placement of an I.V. line and, possibly, sedative medication. Describe the tubes and dressings the patient can expect to have in place when she returns from surgery. Teach the patient deep-breathing and coughing techniques to prepare her for postoperative exercises.

After surgery:
■ Check vital signs every 4 hours. Report fever, tachycardia, and hypotension to the physician.
■ Monitor I.V. fluids.
■ Change dressings regularly, and check for excessive drainage and bleeding and signs of infection.
■ Provide antiembolism stockings as ordered.
■ Encourage regular deep breathing and coughing.
■ If necessary, institute incentive spirometry.
■ Turn the patient often, and help her reposition herself, using pillows for support.
■ Auscultate for bowel sounds. When the patient's bowel function returns, ask the

dietitian to provide a clear liquid diet; then, when tolerated, a regular diet.
■ Encourage the patient to walk within 24 hours after surgery. Reassure her that she won't harm herself or cause wound dehiscence by sitting up or walking.
■ Provide psychological support. Encourage the patient to express anxieties and fears. If she seems worried about the effect of surgery on her sexual activity, reassure her that this surgery will not inhibit sexual intimacy.
■ Before radiation therapy begins, explain that the area to be irradiated will be marked with ink to precisely locate the treatment field. Explain that radiation may cause a skin reaction, bladder irritation, myelosuppression, and other systemic reactions.
■ During and after treatment, watch for and treat adverse effects of radiation and chemotherapy.
■ Before discharge, to minimize adverse effects during outpatient radiation and chemotherapy, advise the patient to maintain a high-carbohydrate, high-protein, low-fat, low-bulk diet to maintain caloric intake but reduce bulk. Suggest that she eat several small meals per day instead of three large ones.
■ Include the patient's husband or other close relatives in patient care and teaching as much as possible.

Stress the importance of a regular pelvic examination to patients, and tell them to contact a physician promptly about any gynecologic symptom.

BONE, SKIN, AND SOFT TISSUE

Primary malignant bone tumors

Primary malignant bone tumors (also called *sarcomas of the bone* and *bone cancer*) are rare, constituting less than 1% of all malignant tumors. Most bone tumors are secondary, caused by seeding from a primary site. Primary malignant bone tumors are more common in males, especially in children and adolescents, although some types do occur in people between ages 35 and 60. They may originate in osseous or nonosseous tissue. Osseous bone tumors arise from the bony structure itself and include osteogenic sarcoma (the most common), parosteal osteogenic sarcoma, chondrosarcoma, and malignant giant cell tumor. Together they make up 60% of all malignant bone tumors. Nonosseous tumors arise from hematopoietic, vascular, and neural tissues and include Ewing's sarcoma, fibrosarcoma, and chordoma. Osteogenic and Ewing's sarcomas are the most common bone tumors in childhood. (See *Comparing primary malignant bone tumors.*)

Causes and incidence

Causes of primary malignant bone tumors are unknown. Some researchers suggest that primary malignant bone tumors arise in areas of rapid growth because children and young adults with such tumors seem to be much taller than average. Additional theories point to heredity, trauma, and excessive radiotherapy.

For incidence information, see *Comparing primary malignant bone tumors.*

Signs and symptoms

Bone pain is the most common indication of primary malignant bone tumors. It's generally more intense at night and isn't usually associated with mobility. The pain is dull and is usually localized, although it may be referred from the hip or spine and result in weakness or a limp. Another common sign is the presence of a mass or tumor. The tumor site may be tender and may swell; the tumor itself is in many cases palpable. Pathologic fractures are common. In late stages, the patient may be cachectic, with fever and impaired mobility.

Diagnosis

 CONFIRMING DIAGNOSIS *A biopsy (by incision or by aspiration) is essential to confirm primary malignant bone tumors. Bone X-rays and radioisotope bone and computed tomography scans show tumor size. Serum alkaline phosphatase level is usually elevated in patients with sarcoma.*

Treatment

Excision of the tumor with a 3″ (7.6 cm) margin is the treatment of choice. It may be combined with preoperative chemotherapy.

In some patients, radical surgery (such as hemipelvectomy or amputation) is necessary; however, surgical resection of the tumor (commonly with preoperative *and* postoperative chemotherapy) has saved limbs from amputation.

Intensive chemotherapy includes administration of doxorubicin, vincristine, cyclophosphamide, cisplatin, dacarbazine, and etoposide in various combinations. Chemotherapy may be infused intraarterially into the long bones of the legs.

Special considerations

■ Be sensitive to the emotional strain caused by the threat of amputation. Encourage communication and help the patient set realistic goals. If the surgery will affect the patient's lower extremities, have a physical therapist teach him how to use assistive devices (such as a walker) preoperatively.
■ Teach the patient how to readjust his body weight so that he can get in and out of the bed and wheelchair.
■ Before surgery, start I.V. infusions to maintain fluid and electrolyte balance and to have an open vein available if blood or plasma is needed during surgery.
■ After surgery, check vital signs every hour for the first 4 hours, every 2 hours for the next 4 hours, and then every 4 hours if the patient is stable. Check the dressing periodically for oozing. Elevate the foot of the bed or place the stump on a pillow for the first 24 hours. (Be careful not to leave the stump elevated for more than 48 hours because this may lead to contractures.)
■ To ease the patient's anxiety, administer analgesics for pain before morning care. If necessary, brace the patient with pillows, keeping the affected part at rest.
■ Urge the patient to eat foods high in protein, vitamins, and folic acid and to get plenty of rest and sleep to promote recovery. Encourage some exercise. Administer laxatives, if necessary, to maintain proper elimination.

COMPARING PRIMARY MALIGNANT BONE TUMORS

Type	Clinical features	Treatment
Osseous origin		
Chondrosarcoma	▪ Develops from cartilage ▪ Painless; grows slowly, but is locally recurrent and invasive ▪ Occurs most commonly in pelvis, proximal femur, ribs, and shoulder girdle ▪ Usually in males ages 30 to 50	▪ Chemotherapy ▪ Hemipelvectomy, surgical resection (ribs) ▪ Radiation (palliative)
Malignant giant cell tumor	▪ Arises from benign giant cell tumor ▪ Found most commonly in long bones, especially in knee area ▪ Usually in females ages 18 to 50	▪ Curettage ▪ Radiation (recurrent disease) ▪ Total excision
Osteogenic sarcoma	▪ Osteoid tumor present in specimen ▪ Tumor arises from bone-forming osteoblast and bone-digesting osteoclast ▪ Occurs most commonly in femur, but also tibia and humerus; occasionally, in fibula, ileum, vertebra, or mandible ▪ Usually in males ages 10 to 30	▪ Chemotherapy ▪ Surgery (tumor resection, high thigh amputation, hemipelvectomy)
Parosteal osteogenic sarcoma	▪ Develops on surface of bone instead of interior ▪ Progresses slowly ▪ Occurs most commonly in distal femur, but also in tibia, humerus, and ulna ▪ Usually in females ages 30 to 40	▪ Chemotherapy ▪ Surgery (tumor resection, possible amputation, hemipelvectomy) ▪ Combination of above
Nonosseous origin		
Chordoma	▪ Derived from embryonic remnants of notochord ▪ Progresses slowly ▪ Usually found at end of spinal column and in spheno-occipital, sacrococcygeal, and vertebral areas ▪ Characterized by constipation and vision disturbances ▪ Usually in males ages 50 to 60	▪ Radiation (palliative, or when surgery not applicable, as in occipital area) ▪ Surgical resection (commonly resulting in neural defects)
Ewing's sarcoma	▪ Originates in bone marrow and invades shafts of long and flat bones ▪ Usually affects lower extremities, most commonly femur, innominate bones, ribs, tibia, humerus, vertebra, and fibula; may metastasize to lungs ▪ Pain increasingly severe and persistent ▪ Usually in males ages 10 to 20	▪ Amputation (only if there's no evidence of metastasis) ▪ Chemotherapy (to slow growth) ▪ High-voltage radiation (if tumor is radiosensitive)

(continued)

COMPARING PRIMARY MALIGNANT BONE TUMORS *(continued)*

Type	Clinical features	Treatment
Nonosseous origin (continued)		
Fibrosarcoma	<ul><li>Relatively rare</li><li>Originates in fibrous tissue of bone</li><li>Invades long or flat bones (femur, tibia, mandible) but also involves periosteum and overlying muscle</li><li>Usually in males ages 30 to 40</li></ul>	<ul><li>Amputation</li><li>Bone grafts (with low-grade fibrosarcoma)</li><li>Chemotherapy</li><li>Radiation</li></ul>

■ Encourage fluids to prevent dehydration. Record intake and output accurately. After a hemipelvectomy, insert a nasogastric tube to prevent abdominal distention. Continue low gastric suction for 2 days after surgery or until the patient can tolerate a liquid diet. Administer antibiotics to prevent infection. Give transfusions, if necessary, and administer medication to control pain. Keep drains in place to facilitate wound drainage and prevent infection. Use an indwelling urinary catheter until the patient can void voluntarily.

■ Keep in mind that rehabilitation programs after limb salvage surgery will vary, depending on the patient, the body part affected, and the type of surgery performed. For example, one patient may have a surgically implanted prosthesis (for example, after joint surgery), whereas another may have reconstructive surgery requiring an allograft (such as bone from a bone bank) or an autograft (bone from the patient's own body).

Encourage early rehabilitation for patients with amputated limbs as follows:

■ Start physical therapy 24 hours postoperatively. Pain is usually not severe after amputation. If it is, watch for a wound complication, such as hematoma, excessive stump edema, or infection.

■ Be aware of the "phantom limb" syndrome, in which the patient "feels" an itch or tingling in an amputated extremity. This can last for several hours or persist for years. Explain that this sensation is normal and usually subsides.

■ To avoid contractures and ensure the best conditions for wound healing, warn the patient not to hang the stump over the edge of the bed; sit in a wheelchair with the stump flexed; place a pillow under his hip, knee, or back or between his thighs; lie with knees flexed; or rest an above-the-knee stump on the crutch handle or abduct it.

■ Wash the stump, massage it gently, and keep it dry until it heals. Make sure the bandage is firm and is worn day and night. Know how to reapply the bandage to shape the stump for a prosthesis.

■ To help the patient select a prosthesis, consider his needs and the types of prostheses available. The rehabilitation staff will help him make the final decision, but because most patients are uninformed about choosing a prosthesis, give some guidelines. Keep in mind the patient's age and possible vision problems.

 PEDIATRIC TIP *Generally, children need relatively simple devices. Children also outgrow prostheses, so advise parents to plan accordingly.*

 ELDER TIP *Elderly patients may need prostheses that provide more stability. Consider finances, too.*

■ The same points are applicable for a patient with an arm amputation, but losing an arm causes a greater cosmetic problem. Consult an occupational therapist, who can teach the patient how to perform daily activities with one arm.

■ Try to instill a positive attitude toward recovery. Urge the patient to resume an independent lifestyle. Refer elderly patients to community health services if necessary. Suggest tutoring for children to help them keep up with schoolwork.

Multiple myeloma

Multiple myeloma, also known as *malignant plasmacytoma, plasma cell myeloma,* and *myelomatosis,* is a disseminated malignant neoplasm of marrow plasma cells that infiltrates bone to produce osteolytic lesions throughout the skeleton (flat bones, vertebrae, skull, pelvis, ribs). In late stages, it infiltrates the body organs (liver, spleen, lymph nodes, lungs, adrenal glands, kidneys, skin, and GI tract). Prognosis is usually poor because diagnosis is commonly made after the disease has already infiltrated the vertebrae, pelvis, skull, ribs, clavicles, and sternum. By then, skeletal destruction is widespread and, without treatment, leads to vertebral collapse; 52% of patients die within 3 months of diagnosis, 90% within 2 years. Early diagnosis and treatment prolong the lives of many patients by 3 to 5 years. Death usually follows complications, such as infection, renal failure, hematologic imbalance, fractures, hypercalcemia, hyperuricemia, or dehydration.

Causes and incidence
Multiple myeloma mainly affects older adults, but its causes and other risk factors are unknown. It's rare, with a yearly incidence of 3 new cases in 100,000 people.

Signs and symptoms
The earliest indication of multiple myeloma is severe, constant back and rib pain that increases with exercise and may be worse at night. Arthritic symptoms may also occur: achiness, joint swelling, and tenderness, possibly from vertebral compression. Other effects include fever, malaise, slight evidence of peripheral neuropathy (such as peripheral paresthesia), and pathologic fractures. As multiple myeloma progresses, symptoms of vertebral compression may become acute, accompanied by anemia, weight loss, thoracic deformities (ballooning), and loss of body height (5″ [12.7 cm] or more) due to verte-

---

BENCE JONES PROTEIN

The hallmark of multiple myeloma, the Bence Jones protein (a light chain of gamma globulin) was named for Henry Bence Jones, an English physician who in 1848 noticed that patients with a curious bone disease excreted a unique protein — unique in that it coagulated at 113° to 131° F (45° to 55° C) and then redissolved when heated to boiling.

It remained for Otto Kahler, an Austrian, to demonstrate in 1889 that Bence Jones protein was related to myeloma. Bence Jones protein isn't found in the urine of *all* multiple myeloma patients, but it's almost never found in the urine of patients without this disease.

---

bral collapse. Renal complications such as pyelonephritis (caused by tubular damage from large amounts of Bence Jones protein, hypercalcemia, and hyperuricemia) may occur. Severe, recurrent infection such as pneumonia may follow damage to nerves associated with respiratory function.

Diagnosis
CONFIRMING DIAGNOSIS *After a physical examination and a careful medical history, the following diagnostic tests and nonspecific laboratory abnormalities confirm the presence of multiple myeloma:*

■ *Bone marrow aspiration and biopsy detects myelomatosis cells (abnormal number of immature plasma cells).*
■ *Urine studies may show Bence Jones protein and hypercalciuria. Absence of Bence Jones protein doesn't rule out multiple myeloma; however, its presence almost invariably confirms the disease. (See Bence Jones protein.)*
■ Complete blood count shows moderate or severe anemia. The differential may show 40% to 50% lymphocytes but seldom

more than 3% plasma cells. Rouleau formation (usually the first clue) seen on differential smear results from elevation of the red cell sedimentation rate.

- Serum electrophoresis shows elevated globulin spike that's electrophoretically and immunologically abnormal.
- X-rays during early stages may show only diffuse osteoporosis. Eventually, they show multiple, sharply circumscribed osteolytic (punched out) lesions, particularly on the skull, pelvis, and spine — the characteristic lesions of multiple myeloma.
- Excretory urography can assess renal involvement. To avoid precipitation of Bence Jones protein, iothalamate or diatrizoate is used instead of the usual contrast medium and, although oral fluid restriction is usually the standard procedure before excretory urography, patients with multiple myeloma receive large quantities of fluid, generally orally but sometimes I.V., before excretory urography is done.

Treatment

Long-term treatment of multiple myeloma consists mainly of chemotherapy to suppress plasma cell growth and control pain. Commonly used combinations include cyclophosphamide, doxorubicin, and prednisone as well as carmustine, doxorubicin, and prednisone. Adjuvant local radiation reduces acute lesions, such as collapsed vertebrae, and relieves localized pain. Other treatments usually include a melphalan-prednisone combination in high intermittent doses or low continuous daily doses and analgesics for pain. Oral thalidomide (with or without steroids) has shown promise in relapsed multiple myeloma, and velcade, a proteasome inhibitor, is a newer agent that has shown promise in myeloma treatment. For spinal cord compression, the patient may require a laminectomy; for renal complications, dialysis.

Clinical trials are currently under way to evaluate the role of biological response modifiers (interferon) in the management of multiple myeloma. In addition, high-dose chemotherapy and radiotherapy with peripheral stem cell rescue have been helpful in select cases.

Because the patient may have bone demineralization and may lose large amounts of calcium into blood and urine, he's a prime candidate for renal calculi, nephrocalcinosis and, eventually, renal failure due to hypercalcemia. Hypercalcemia is managed with hydration, diuretics, corticosteroids, oral phosphate, mithramycin I.V., or bisphosphonates I.V. (such as pamidronate or zoledronic acid) to decrease serum calcium levels.

Special considerations

- Push fluids; encourage the patient to drink 101.5 to 135 oz (3,000 to 4,000 ml) of fluids daily, particularly before his excretory urography. Monitor fluid intake and output (daily output shouldn't be less than 1,500 ml).
- Encourage the patient to walk (immobilization increases bone demineralization and vulnerability to pneumonia), and give analgesics, as ordered, to lessen pain. Never allow the patient to walk unaccompanied; make sure that he uses a walker or other supportive aid to prevent falls. Because the patient is particularly vulnerable to pathologic fractures, he may be fearful. Give reassurance, and allow him to move at his own pace.
- Prevent complications by watching for fever or malaise, which may signal the onset of infection, and for signs of other problems, such as severe anemia and fractures. If the patient is bedridden, change his position every 2 hours. Give passive range-of-motion and deep-breathing exercises. When he can tolerate them, promote active exercises.
- If the patient is taking melphalan (a phenylalanine derivative of nitrogen mustard that depresses bone marrow), make sure his blood count (platelet and white blood cell) is taken before each treatment. If he's taking prednisone, watch closely for infection because this drug commonly masks it.
- Whenever possible, get the patient out of bed within 24 hours after laminectomy. Check for hemorrhage, motor or sensory deficits, and loss of bowel or bladder function. Position the patient as ordered, maintain alignment, and logroll when turning.
- Provide much-needed emotional support for the patient and his family, as they're likely to be anxious. Help relieve

their anxiety by truthfully informing them about diagnostic tests (including painful procedures, such as bone marrow aspiration and biopsy), treatment, and prognosis. If needed, refer them to an appropriate community resource for additional support.

Basal cell epithelioma

Basal cell epithelioma, also known as *basal cell carcinoma,* is a slow-growing, destructive skin tumor. It's the most common form of cancer in the United States, accounting for 75% of all skin cancers. If caught and treated early, it has a cure rate of 95%. Regular follow-up is required because new sites of basal cell epithelioma can occur.

Causes and incidence
Prolonged sun exposure is the most common cause of basal cell epithelioma, but arsenic ingestion, radiation exposure, burns, and immunosuppression are other possible causes.

Although the pathogenesis of basal cell epithelioma is uncertain, some experts now hypothesize that it originates when, under certain conditions, undifferentiated basal cells become carcinomatous instead of differentiating into sweat glands, sebum, and hair.

This cancer usually occurs in people older than age 40; it's more prevalent in blond, fair-skinned males and is the most common malignant tumor affecting whites.

Signs and symptoms
Three types of basal cell epithelioma occur:
■ Noduloulcerative lesions usually occur on the face, particularly the forehead, eyelid margins, and nasolabial folds. In early stages, these lesions are small, smooth, pinkish, and translucent papules. Telangiectatic vessels cross the surface, and the lesions are occasionally pigmented. As the lesions enlarge, their centers become depressed and their borders become firm and elevated. Ulceration and local invasion eventually occur. These ulcerated tumors, known as *rodent ulcers,* rarely metastasize; however, if untreated, they can spread to

vital areas and become infected or cause massive hemorrhage if they invade large blood vessels.
■ Superficial basal cell epitheliomas are multiple in many cases and commonly occur on the chest and back. They're oval or irregularly shaped, lightly pigmented plaques, with sharply defined, slightly elevated threadlike borders. Due to superficial erosion, these lesions appear scaly and have small, atrophic areas in the center that resemble psoriasis or eczema. They're usually chronic and don't tend to invade other areas. Superficial basal cell epitheliomas are related to ingestion of or exposure to arsenic-containing compounds.
■ Sclerosing basal cell epitheliomas (morphea-like epitheliomas) are waxy, sclerotic, yellow to white plaques without distinct borders. Occurring on the head and neck, sclerosing basal cell epitheliomas commonly look like small patches of scleroderma.

Diagnosis
All types of basal cell epitheliomas are diagnosed by clinical appearance, incisional or excisional biopsy, and histologic study.

Treatment
Depending on the size, location, and depth of the lesion, treatment may include curettage and electrodesiccation, chemotherapy, surgical excision, irradiation, or chemosurgery.
■ Curettage and electrodesiccation offer good cosmetic results for small lesions.
■ Topical 5-fluorouracil is commonly used for superficial lesions. This medication produces marked local irritation or inflammation in the involved tissue but no systemic effects.
■ Microscopically controlled surgical excision carefully removes recurrent lesions until a tumor-free plane is achieved. After removal of large lesions, skin grafting may be required.
■ Irradiation is used for tumor locations that require it and for elderly or debilitated patients who might not withstand surgery.
■ Cryosurgery with liquid nitrogen freezes and kills the cells.
■ Chemosurgery generally is necessary for persistent or recurrent lesions. Chemo-

surgery consists of periodic applications of a fixative paste (such as zinc chloride) and subsequent removal of fixed pathologic tissue. Treatment continues until tumor removal is complete.

Special considerations

■ Instruct the patient to eat frequent small meals that are high in protein. Suggest "blenderized" foods or liquid protein supplements if the lesion has invaded the oral cavity and caused eating problems.

■ Tell the patient that, to prevent disease recurrence, he needs to avoid excessive sun exposure and use a strong sunscreen or sunshade to protect his skin from damage by ultraviolet rays.

■ Advise the patient to relieve local inflammation from topical fluorouracil with cool compresses or corticosteroid ointment.

■ Instruct the patient with noduloulcerative basal cell epithelioma to wash his face gently when ulcerations and crusting occur; scrubbing too vigorously may cause bleeding.

Squamous cell carcinoma

Squamous cell carcinoma of the skin is an invasive tumor with metastatic potential that arises from the keratinizing epidermal cells. Any change in an existing skin lesion, such as a wart or mole, or the development of a new lesion that ulcerates and doesn't heal may indicate skin cancer. If caught and treated early, there's a high cure rate. However, if squamous cell carcinoma is allowed to spread, it can result in disability or death.

Causes and incidence

Predisposing factors associated with squamous cell carcinoma include overexposure to the sun's ultraviolet rays, the presence of premalignant lesions (such as actinic keratosis or Bowen's disease), X-ray therapy, ingestion of herbicides containing arsenic, chronic skin irritation and inflammation, exposure to local carcinogens (such as tar and oil), and hereditary diseases (such as xeroderma pigmentosum and albinism). (See *Premalignant skin lesions.*) Rarely, squamous cell carcinoma may develop on the site of smallpox vaccination, psoriasis, or chronic discoid lupus erythematosus.

Squamous cell carcinoma usually occurs in fair-skinned white males older than age 60. Outdoor employment and residence in a sunny, warm climate (southwestern United States and Australia, for example) greatly increase the risk of developing squamous cell carcinoma.

Signs and symptoms

Squamous cell carcinoma commonly develops on the skin of the face, the ears, the dorsa of the hands and forearms, and other sun-damaged areas. Lesions on sun-damaged skin tend to be less invasive and less likely to metastasize than lesions on unexposed skin. Notable exceptions to this tendency are squamous cell lesions on the lower lip and the ears. These are almost invariably markedly invasive metastatic lesions with a generally poor prognosis.

Transformation from a premalignant lesion to squamous cell carcinoma may begin with induration and inflammation of the preexisting lesion. When squamous cell carcinoma arises from normal skin, the nodule grows slowly on a firm, indurated base. If untreated, this nodule eventually ulcerates and invades underlying tissues. (See *Staging squamous cell carcinoma,* page 132.) Metastasis can occur to the regional lymph nodes, producing characteristic systemic symptoms of pain, malaise, fatigue, weakness, and anorexia.

Diagnosis

An excisional biopsy provides definitive diagnosis of squamous cell carcinoma. Other appropriate laboratory tests depend on systemic symptoms.

Treatment

The size, shape, location, and invasiveness of a squamous cell tumor and the condition of the underlying tissue determine the treatment method used; a deeply invasive tumor may require a combination of techniques. All the major treatment methods have excellent cure rates; generally, the prognosis is better with a well-differentiated lesion than with a poorly differentiated one in an unusual location. Depending on the lesion, treatment may consist of:

PREMALIGNANT SKIN LESIONS

Disease	Cause	Patient	Lesion	Treatment
Actinic keratosis	Solar radiation	White men with fair skin (middle-aged to elderly)	Reddish brown lesions 1 mm to 1 cm in size (may enlarge if untreated) on face, ears, lower lip, bald scalp, dorsa of hands and forearms	Topical 5-fluorouracil, cryosurgery using liquid nitrogen, or curettage by electrodesiccation
Bowen's disease	Unknown	White men with fair skin (middle-aged to elderly)	Brown to reddish-brown lesions, with scaly surface on exposed and unexposed areas	Surgical excision, topical 5-fluorouracil
Erythroplasia of Queyrat	Bowen's disease of the mucous membranes	Men (middle-aged to elderly)	Red lesions with a glistening or granular appearance on mucous membranes, particularly the glans penis in uncircumcised males	Surgical excision
Leukoplakia	Smoking, alcohol use, chronic cheek-biting, ill-fitting dentures, misaligned teeth	Men (middle-aged to elderly)	Lesions on oral, anal, and genital mucous membranes vary in appearance from smooth and white to rough and gray	Elimination of irritating factors, surgical excision, or curettage by electrodesiccation (if lesion is still premalignant)

■ wide surgical excision
■ electrodesiccation and curettage (offer good cosmetic results for small lesions)
■ radiation therapy (generally for older or debilitated patients)
■ chemosurgery (reserved for resistant or recurrent lesions).

Special considerations

The care plan for patients with squamous cell carcinoma should emphasize meticulous wound care, emotional support, and thorough patient instruction.

■ Coordinate a consistent care plan for changing the patient's dressings. Establishing a standard routine helps the patient

STAGING SQUAMOUS CELL CARCINOMA

The American Joint Committee on Cancer uses the following TNM (tumor, node, metastasis) system for staging squamous cell carcinoma.

Primary tumor
TX — primary tumor can't be assessed
T0 — no evidence of primary tumor
Tis — carcinoma in situ
T1 — tumor 2 cm or less in greatest dimension
T2 — tumor between 2 and 5 cm in greatest dimension
T3 — tumor more than 5 cm in greatest dimension
T4 — tumor invades deep extradermal structures (such as cartilage, skeletal muscle, or bone)

Regional lymph nodes
NX — regional lymph nodes can't be assessed
N0 — no evidence of regional lymph node involvement
N1 — regional lymph node involvement

Distant metastasis
MX — distant metastasis can't be assessed
M0 — no known distant metastasis
M1 — distant metastasis

Staging categories
Squamous cell carcinoma progresses from mild to severe as follows:
STAGE 0 — Tis, N0, M0
STAGE I — T1, N0, M0
STAGE II — T2, N0, M0; T3, N0, M0
STAGE III — T4, N0, M0; any T, N1, M0
STAGE IV — Any T, any N, M1

and family learn how to care for the wound.
- Keep the wound dry and clean.

- Try to control odor with balsam of Peru, yogurt flakes, oil of cloves, or other odor-masking substances, even though they're typically ineffective for long-term use. Topical or systemic antibiotics also temporarily control odor and eventually alter the lesion's bacterial flora.
- Be prepared for other problems that accompany a metastatic disease (pain, fatigue, weakness, anorexia).
- Help the patient and his family set realistic goals and expectations.
- Disfiguring lesions are distressing to the patient and you. Try to accept the patient as he is and to increase his self-esteem and strengthen a caring relationship.

To prevent basal and squamous cell carcinoma, tell patients to:
- avoid excessive sun exposure
- wear protective clothing (hats, long sleeves)
- periodically examine the skin for precancerous lesions; have any removed promptly
- use strong sunscreening agents containing para-aminobenzoic acid, benzophenone, and zinc oxide. Apply these agents 30 to 60 minutes before sun exposure
- use lip screens to protect the lips from sun damage.

Malignant melanoma

A malignant neoplasm that arises from melanocytes, malignant melanoma is relatively rare and accounts for only 1% to 2% of all malignancies. However, the incidence is greatly increasing with a noted 300% increase in the past 40 years. The four types of melanomas are superficial spreading melanoma, nodular malignant melanoma, lentigo maligna, and acral lentiginous melanoma.

Melanoma spreads through the lymphatic and vascular systems and metastasizes to the regional lymph nodes, skin, liver, lungs, and central nervous system (CNS). Its course is unpredictable, however, and recurrence and metastasis may not appear for more than 5 years after resection of the primary lesion. The prognosis varies with tumor thickness. Generally, superficial lesions are curable, whereas deeper lesions tend to metastasize. The Breslow level method measures tumor depth from the granular level of the epidermis to the deepest melanoma cell. Melanoma lesions less than 0.76 mm deep have an excellent prognosis, whereas deeper lesions (more than 0.76 mm) are at risk for metastasis. The prognosis is better for a tumor on an extremity (which is drained by one lymphatic network) than for one on the head, neck, or trunk (drained by several networks).

Causes and incidence
Several factors seem to influence the development of melanoma:
- Excessive exposure to sunlight — Melanoma is most common in sunny, warm areas and usually develops on parts of the body that are exposed to the sun.
- Skin type — Most persons who develop melanoma have blond or red hair, fair skin, and blue eyes; are prone to sunburn; and are of Celtic or Scandinavian ancestry. Melanoma is rare among Blacks; when it does develop, it usually arises in lightly pigmented areas (the palms, plantar surface of the feet, or mucous membranes).
- Hormonal factors — Pregnancy may increase risk and exacerbate growth.
- Family history — Melanoma is slightly more common within families.
- Past history of melanoma — A person who has had one melanoma is at greater risk of developing a second.

Melanoma is slightly more common in women than in men and is rare in children. Peak incidence occurs between ages 50 and 70, although the incidence in younger age-groups is increasing.

Signs and symptoms
Common sites for melanoma are on the head and neck in men, on the legs in women, and on the backs of persons exposed to excessive sunlight. Up to 70% arise from a preexisting nevus. It rarely appears in the conjunctiva, choroid, pharynx, mouth, vagina, or anus.

Suspect melanoma when any skin lesion or nevus enlarges, changes color, becomes inflamed or sore, itches, ulcerates, bleeds, undergoes textural changes, or shows signs of surrounding pigment regression (halo nevus or vitiligo). (See *Recognizing potentially malignant nevi*, page 134.)

Each type of melanoma has special characteristics:
- Superficial spreading melanoma, the most common, usually develops between ages 40 and 50. Such a lesion arises on an area of chronic irritation. In women, it's most common between the knees and ankles; in Blacks and Asians, on the toe webs and soles (lightly pigmented areas subject to trauma). Characteristically, this melanoma has a red, white, and blue color over a brown or black background and an irregular, notched margin. Its surface is irregular, with small, elevated tumor nodules that may ulcerate and bleed. Horizontal growth may continue for many years; when vertical growth begins, prognosis worsens.
- Nodular melanoma usually develops between ages 40 and 50, grows vertically, invades the dermis, and metastasizes early. Such a lesion is usually a polypoidal nodule, with uniformly dark discoloration (it may be grayish), and looks like a blackberry. Occasionally, this melanoma is flesh-colored, with flecks of pigment around its base (possibly inflamed).
- Lentigo maligna melanoma is relatively rare. It arises from a lentigo maligna on an exposed skin surface and usually occurs between ages 60 and 70. This lesion looks like a large (3- to 6-cm) flat freckle of tan, brown, black, whitish, or slate color and has irregularly scattered black nodules on the surface. It develops slowly, usually over many years, and eventually may ulcerate. This melanoma commonly develops under the fingernails, on the face, and on the back of the hands.

Diagnosis
A skin biopsy with histologic examination can distinguish malignant melanoma from a benign nevus, seborrheic keratosis, and pigmented basal cell epithelioma; it can also determine tumor thickness. Physical examination, paying particular attention to lymph nodes, can point to metastatic involvement. (See *Staging malignant melanoma*, page 135.)

Baseline laboratory studies include complete blood count with differential, erythrocyte sedimentation rate, platelet count,

RECOGNIZING POTENTIALLY MALIGNANT NEVI

Nevi (moles) are skin lesions that are usually pigmented and may be hereditary. They begin to grow in childhood (occasionally they're congenital) and become more numerous in young adults. Up to 70% of patients with melanoma have a history of a preexisting nevus at the tumor site. Of these, approximately one-third are reported to be congenital; the remainder develop later in life.

Changes in nevi (color, size, shape, texture, ulceration, bleeding, or itching) suggest possible malignant transformation. The presence or absence of hair within a nevus has no significance.

Types of nevi

- *Junctional nevi* are flat or slightly raised and light to dark brown, with melanocytes confined to the epidermis. Usually, they appear before age 40. These nevi may change into compound nevi if junctional nevus cells proliferate and penetrate into the dermis.
- *Compound nevi* are usually tan to dark brown and slightly raised, although size and color vary. They contain melanocytes in both the dermis and epidermis, and they rarely undergo malignant transformation. Excision is necessary only to rule out malignant transformation or for cosmetic reasons.
- *Dermal nevi* are elevated lesions from 2 to 10 mm in diameter, and vary in color from flesh to brown. They usually develop in older adults and generally arise on the upper part of the body. Excision is necessary only to rule out malignant transformation.
- *Blue nevi* are flat or slightly elevated lesions from 0.5 to 1 cm in diameter. They appear on the head, neck, arms, and dorsa of the hands and are twice as common in women as in men. Their blue color results from pigment and collagen in the dermis, which reflect blue light but absorb other wavelengths. Excision is necessary to rule out pigmented basal cell epithelioma or melanoma or for cosmetic reasons.

- *Dysplastic nevi* are generally greater than 5 mm in diameter, with irregularly notched or indistinct borders. Coloration is usually a variable mixture of tan and brown, sometimes with red, pink, and black pigmentation. No two lesions are exactly alike. They occur in great numbers (typically over 100 at a time), never singly, usually appearing on the back, scalp, chest, and buttocks. Dysplastic nevi are potentially malignant, especially in patients with a personal or familial history of melanoma. Skin biopsy confirms diagnosis; treatment is by surgical excision, followed by regular physical examinations (every 6 months) to detect any new lesions or changes in existing lesions.
- *Lentigo maligna* (melanotic freckles, Hutchinson freckles) are a precursor to malignant melanoma. (In fact, about one-third of them eventually give rise to malignant melanoma.) Usually, they occur in people older than age 40, especially on exposed skin areas such as the face. At first, these lesions are flat, tan spots, but they gradually enlarge and darken and develop black speckled areas against their tan or brown background. Each lesion may simultaneously enlarge in one area and regress in another. Histologic examination shows typical and atypical melanocytes along the epidermal basement membrane. Removal by simple excision (not electrodesiccation and curettage) is recommended.

---

liver function studies, and urinalysis. Depending on the depth of tumor invasion and metastatic spread, baseline diagnostic studies may also include chest X-ray and a computed tomography (CT) scan of the chest and abdomen. Signs of bone metastasis may call for a bone scan; CNS metastasis necessitates a CT scan of the brain.

STAGING MALIGNANT MELANOMA

Several systems exist for staging malignant melanoma, including the TNM (tumor, node, metastasis) system, developed by the American Joint Committee on Cancer, and Clark's system, which classifies tumor progression according to skin layer penetration.

Primary tumor

TX — primary tumor can't be assessed

T0 — no evidence of primary tumor

Tis — melanoma in situ (atypical melanotic hyperplasia, severe melanotic dysplasia), not an invasive lesion (Clark's level I)

T1 — tumor 0.75 mm thick or less that invades the papillary dermis (Clark's level II)

T2 — tumor between 0.75 and 1.5 mm thick, tumor invades the interface between the papillary and reticular dermis (Clark's level III), or both

T3 — tumor between 1.5 and 4 mm thick, tumor invades the reticular dermis (Clark's level IV), or both

T3a — tumor between 1.5 and 3 mm thick

T3b — tumor between 3 and 4 mm thick

T4 — tumor more than 4 mm thick, tumor invades subcutaneous tissue (Clark's level V), or tumor has one or more satellites within 2 cm of the primary tumor

T4a — tumor more than 4 mm thick, tumor invades subcutaneous tissue, or both

T4b — one or more satellites exist within 2 cm of the primary tumor

Regional lymph nodes

NX — regional lymph nodes can't be assessed

N0 — no evidence of regional lymph node involvement

N1 — metastasis 3 cm or less in greatest dimension in any regional lymph node

N2 — metastasis greater than 3 cm in greatest dimension in any regional lymph node, in-transit metastasis, or both

Distant metastasis

MX — distant metastasis can't be assessed

M0 — no evidence of distant metastasis

M1 — distant metastasis

M1a — metastasis in skin, subcutaneous tissue, or lymph nodes beyond the regional nodes

M1b — visceral metastasis

Staging categories

Malignant melanoma progresses from mild to severe as follows:

STAGE I — T1, N0, M0; T2, N0, M0

STAGE II — T3, N0, M0

STAGE III — T4, N0, M0; any T, N1, M0; any T, N2, M0

STAGE IV — any T, any N, M1

CLARK'S LEVELS

Epidermis —
    Level I

Papillary dermis —
    Level II
    Level III

Reticular dermis —
    Level IV

Subcutaneous tissue —
    Level V

Treatment

A patient with malignant melanoma requires surgical resection to remove the tumor. The extent of resection depends on the size and location of the primary lesion. Closure of a wide resection may require a skin graft. Surgical treatment may also include regional lymphadenectomy.

Deep primary lesions may merit adjuvant chemotherapy and biotherapy to eliminate or reduce the number of tumor cells. Clinical trials are currently under way to evaluate the effectiveness of isolated limb perfusion as chemotherapy for the management of malignant melanomas of extremities. Radiation therapy is usually reserved for metastatic disease. It doesn't prolong survival but may reduce tumor size and relieve pain.

Regardless of the treatment method, melanomas require close long-term follow-up to detect metastasis and recurrences. Statistics show that 13% of recurrences develop more than 5 years after primary surgery.

Special considerations

Management of the melanoma patient requires careful physical, psychological, and social assessment. Preoperative teaching, meticulous postoperative care, and psychological support can make the patient more comfortable, speed recovery, and prevent complications.

After diagnosis, review the physician's explanation of treatment options. Tell the patient what to expect before and after surgery, what the wound will look like, and what type of dressing he'll have. Warn him that the donor site for a skin graft may be as painful as the tumor excision site, if not more so. Honestly answer any questions he may have about surgery, chemotherapy, and radiation.

■ After surgery, be careful to prevent infection. Check dressings often for excessive drainage, foul odor, redness, or swelling. If surgery included lymphadenectomy, minimize lymphedema by applying a compression stocking and instructing the patient to keep the extremity elevated.

■ During chemotherapy, know what adverse effects to expect and take measures to minimize them. For instance, give an antiemetic, as ordered, to reduce nausea and vomiting.

To prepare the patient for discharge:

■ Emphasize the need for close follow-up to detect recurrences early. Explain that recurrences and metastasis, if they occur, are commonly delayed, so follow-up must continue for years. Tell the patient how to recognize signs of recurrence.

■ Provide psychological support. Encourage the patient to verbalize his fears.

In advanced metastatic disease:

■ Control and prevent pain with consistent, regularly scheduled administration of analgesics. *Don't* wait to relieve pain until after it occurs.

■ Make referrals for home care, social services, and spiritual and financial assistance, as needed.

■ If the patient is dying, identify the needs of the patient, his family, and friends, and provide appropriate support and care.

To help prevent malignant melanoma, stress the detrimental effects of overexposure to solar radiation, especially to fair-skinned, blue-eyed patients. Recommend that they use a sunblock or sunscreen. In all physical examinations, especially in fair-skinned persons, look for unusual nevi or other skin lesions.

Kaposi's sarcoma

Initially, this cancer of the lymphatic cell wall was described as a rare blood vessel sarcoma, occurring mostly in elderly Italian and Jewish men. In recent years, the incidence of Kaposi's sarcoma has risen dramatically along with the incidence of acquired immunodeficiency syndrome (AIDS). Currently, it's the most common AIDS-related cancer.

Kaposi's sarcoma causes structural and functional damage. When associated with AIDS, it progresses aggressively, involving the lymph nodes, the viscera, and possibly GI structures.

Causes and incidence

The exact cause of Kaposi's sarcoma is unknown, but the disease may be related to immunosuppression. Genetic or hereditary predisposition is also suspected. In people with AIDS, Kaposi's sarcoma is caused by an interaction between the human immunodeficiency virus (HIV), immune system suppression, and human herpesvirus-8 (HHV-8). Occurrence has been linked with sexual transmission of HIV and HHV-8. Approximately 3 out of every 100,000 people develop Kaposi's sarcoma each year.

Signs and symptoms

The initial sign of Kaposi's sarcoma is one or more obvious lesions in various shapes, sizes, and colors (ranging from red-brown to dark purple) appearing most commonly on the skin, buccal mucosa, hard and soft palates, lips, gums, tongue, tonsils, conjunctiva, and sclera.

In advanced disease, the lesions may join, becoming one large plaque. Untreated lesions may appear as large, ulcerative masses.

Other signs and symptoms include:

- health history of AIDS
- pain (if the sarcoma advances beyond the early stages or if a lesion breaks down or impinges on nerves or organs)
- edema from lymphatic obstruction
- dyspnea (in cases of pulmonary involvement), wheezing, hypoventilation, and respiratory distress from bronchial blockage.

The most common extracutaneous sites are the lungs and GI tract (esophagus, oropharynx, and epiglottis).

Signs and symptoms of disease progression and metastasis include severe pulmonary involvement and GI involvement leading to digestive problems.

Diagnosis

CONFIRMING DIAGNOSIS *Diagnosis is made following a tissue biopsy that identifies the lesion's type and stage. Then, a computed tomography scan may be performed to detect and evaluate possible metastasis. Endoscopy shows Kaposi's lesions. (See* Laubenstein's stages in Kaposi's sarcoma.*)*

Treatment

Treatment isn't indicated for all patients. Indications include cosmetically offensive, painful, or obstructive lesions of rapidly progressing disease.

LAUBENSTEIN'S STAGES IN KAPOSI'S SARCOMA

The following staging system was proposed by L.J. Laubenstein for use in evaluating and treating patients who have acquired immunodeficiency syndrome and Kaposi's sarcoma.

STAGE I—locally indolent cutaneous lesions
STAGE II—locally aggressive cutaneous lesions
STAGE III—mucocutaneous and lymph node involvement
STAGE IV—visceral involvement
 Within each stage, a patient may have different symptoms classified as a stage subtype—A or B—as follows:

- Subtype A—no systemic signs or symptoms
- Subtype B—one or more systemic signs and symptoms, including 10% weight loss, fever of unknown origin that exceeds 100° F (37.8° C) for more than 2 weeks, chills, lethargy, night sweats, anorexia, and diarrhea.

Radiation therapy, chemotherapy, cryotherapy, and biotherapy with biological response modifiers are treatment options. Radiation therapy alleviates symptoms, including pain from obstructing lesions in the oral cavity or extremities and edema caused by lymphatic blockage. It may also be used for cosmetic improvement.

Chemotherapy includes combinations of doxorubicin, vincristine, etoposide, paclitaxel, bleomycin, and dacarbazine. Biotherapy with interferon alfa-2b may be prescribed for AIDS-related Kaposi's sarcoma. The treatment reduces the number of skin lesions but is ineffective in advanced disease.

Special considerations

■ Listen to the patient's fears and concerns and answer his questions honestly. Stay with him during periods of severe stress and anxiety.

■ The patient who's coping poorly may need a referral for psychological counseling. His family members may also need help in coping with the patient's disease and with any associated demands that the disorder places upon them.

■ As appropriate, allow the patient to participate in care decisions whenever possible, and encourage him to participate in self-care measures as much as he can.

■ Inspect the patient's skin every shift. Look for new lesions and skin breakdown. If the patient has painful lesions, help him into a more comfortable position.

■ Follow standard precautions when caring for the patient.

■ Administer pain medications as prescribed. Suggest distractions, and help the patient with relaxation techniques.

■ To help the patient adjust to changes in his appearance, urge him to share his feelings, and provide encouragement.

■ Monitor the patient's weight daily.

■ Supply the patient with high-calorie, high-protein meals. If he can't tolerate regular meals, provide him with frequent smaller meals. Consult with the dietitian, and plan meals around the patient's treatment.

■ If the patient can't take food by mouth, administer I.V. fluids. Also provide antiemetics and sedatives, as ordered.

■ Be alert for adverse effects of radiation therapy or chemotherapy — such as anorexia, nausea, vomiting, and diarrhea — and take steps to prevent or alleviate them.

■ Reinforce the physician's explanation of treatments. Make sure the patient understands which adverse reactions to expect and how to manage them. For example, during radiation therapy, instruct the patient to keep irradiated skin dry to avoid possible breakdown and subsequent infection.

■ Explain all prescribed medications, including any possible adverse effects and drug interactions.

■ Explain infection-prevention techniques and, if necessary, demonstrate basic hygiene measures to prevent infection. Advise the patient not to share his toothbrush, razor, or other items that may be contaminated with blood. These measures are especially important if the patient also has AIDS.

■ Help the patient plan daily periods of alternating activity and rest to help him cope with fatigue. Teach energy-conservation techniques. Encourage him to set priorities, accept the help of others, and delegate nonessential tasks.

■ Explain the proper use of assistive devices, when appropriate, to ease ambulation and promote independence.

■ Stress the need for ongoing treatment and care.

■ As appropriate, refer the patient to support groups offered by the social services department.

■ If the patient's prognosis is poor (less than 6 months to live), suggest immediate hospice care.

■ Explain the benefits of initiating and executing advance directives and a durable power of attorney.

BLOOD AND LYMPH

Hodgkin's disease

Hodgkin's disease is a neoplastic disease characterized by painless, progressive enlargement of lymph nodes, spleen, and other lymphoid tissue resulting from proliferation of lymphocytes, histiocytes, eosinophils, and Reed-Sternberg giant cells. The latter cells are its special histologic feature. Untreated, Hodgkin's disease follows a variable but relentlessly progressive and ultimately fatal course. However, recent advances in therapy make Hodgkin's disease potentially curable, even in advanced stages; appropriate treatment yields a 5-year survival rate in approximately 80% of patients.

Causes and incidence

Although the cause of Hodgkin's disease is unknown, a viral etiology is suspected, with the Epstein-Barr virus as a leading candidate. The disease is most common in young adults, with a higher incidence in males than in females. It occurs in all races but is slightly more common in whites. Its incidence peaks in two age-groups: 15 to 38 and after age 50 — except in Japan, where it occurs exclusively among people older than 50.

Signs and symptoms

The first sign of Hodgkin's disease is usually a painless swelling of one of the cervical lymph nodes (but sometimes the axillary, mediastinal, or inguinal lymph nodes), occasionally in a patient who gives a history of recent upper respiratory infection. In older patients, the first signs and symptoms may be nonspecific — persistent fever, night sweats, fatigue, weight loss, and malaise. Rarely, if the mediastinum is initially involved, Hodgkin's may produce respiratory symptoms.

Another early and characteristic indication of Hodgkin's disease is pruritus, which, although mild at first, becomes acute as the disease progresses. Other symptoms depend on the degree and location of systemic involvement.

Lymph nodes may enlarge rapidly, producing pain and obstruction, or enlarge slowly and painlessly for months or years. It isn't unusual to see the lymph nodes "wax and wane," but they usually don't return to normal. Sooner or later, most patients develop systemic manifestations, including enlargement of retroperitoneal nodes and nodular infiltrations of the spleen, the liver, and bones. At this late stage other symptoms include edema of the face and neck, progressive anemia, possible jaundice, nerve pain, and increased susceptibility to infection.

Diagnosis

Diagnostic measures for confirming Hodgkin's disease include a thorough medical history and a complete physical examination, followed by a lymph node biopsy checking for Reed-Sternberg's abnormal histiocyte proliferation and nodular fibrosis and necrosis. (See *Reed-Sternberg cells.*)

Other appropriate diagnostic tests include bone marrow, liver, mediastinal, lymph node, and spleen biopsies and routine chest X-ray, abdominal computed to-

---

REED-STERNBERG CELLS

These enlarged, abnormal histiocytes (Reed-Sternberg cells) from an excised lymph node suggest Hodgkin's disease. Note the large, distinct nucleoli. Reed-Sternberg cells indicate Hodgkin's disease when they coexist with one of these four histologic patterns: lymphocyte predominance, mixed cellularity, lymphocyte depletion, or nodular sclerosis.

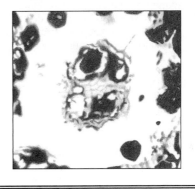

---

mography scan, positron emission tomography, lung scan, bone scan, and lymphangiography to detect lymph node or organ involvement. Laparoscopy and lymph node biopsy are performed to complete staging.

Hematologic tests show mild to severe normocytic anemia; normochromic anemia (in 50%); elevated, normal, or reduced white blood cell count and differential showing any combination of neutrophilia, lymphocytopenia, monocytosis, and eosinophilia. Elevated serum alkaline phosphatase indicates liver or bone involvement.

The same diagnostic tests are also used for staging. A staging laparotomy is necessary for patients younger than age 55 or without obvious stage III or stage IV disease, lymphocyte predominance subtype histology, or medical contraindications. Diagnosis must rule out other disorders that also enlarge the lymph nodes.

STAGING HODGKIN'S DISEASE

Treatment of Hodgkin's disease depends on the stage it has reached — that is, the number, location, and degree of involved lymph nodes. The Ann Arbor classification system, adopted in 1971, divides Hodgkin's disease into four stages. Physicians subdivide each stage into categories. Category A includes patients without defined signs and symptoms, and category B includes patients who experience such defined signs as recent unexplained weight loss, fever, and night sweats.

Stage I
Hodgkin's disease appears in a single lymph node region (I) or a single extralymphatic organ (IE).

Stage II
The disease appears in two or more nodes on the same side of the diaphragm (II) and in an extralymphatic organ (IIE).

Stage III
Hodgkin's disease spreads to both sides of the diaphragm (III) and perhaps to an extralymphatic organ (IIIE), the spleen (IIIS), or both (IIIES).

Stage IV
The disease disseminates, involving one or more extralymphatic organs or tissues, with or without associated lymph node involvement.

Treatment

Appropriate therapy (chemotherapy or radiation, or both, varying with the stage of the disease) depends on careful physical examination with accurate histologic interpretation and proper clinical staging. (See *Staging Hodgkin's disease.*) Correct and timely treatment allows longer survival and even induces an apparent cure in many patients. Radiation therapy is used alone for stages I and II and in combination with chemotherapy for stage III. Chemotherapy is used for stage IV, sometimes inducing a complete remission. The well-known MOPP protocol (mechlorethamine, vincristine [Oncovin], procarbazine, and prednisone) was the first to provide significant cures to patients with generalized Hodgkin's; another useful combination is ABVD (doxorubicin [Adriamycin], bleomycin, vinblastine, and dacarbazine). Another chemotherapy regimen — bleomycin, etoposide, cyclophosphamide, vincristine, procarbazine, and prednisone — has also shown promise in advanced Hodgkin's disease. Treatment with these drugs may require concomitant antiemetics, sedatives, or antidiarrheals to combat GI adverse effects.

New treatments include high-dose chemotherapeutic agents with autologous bone marrow transplantation or autologous peripheral blood stem cell transfusions. Biotherapy alone hasn't proven effective.

Special considerations

Because many patients with Hodgkin's disease receive radiation or chemotherapy as outpatients, tell the patient to observe the following precautions:
- Watch for and promptly report adverse effects of radiation and chemotherapy (particularly anorexia, nausea, vomiting, diarrhea, fever, and bleeding).
- Minimize adverse effects of radiation therapy by maintaining good nutrition (aided by eating small, frequent meals of his favorite foods), drinking plenty of fluids, pacing his activities to counteract therapy-induced fatigue, and keeping the skin in irradiated areas dry.
- Control pain and bleeding of stomatitis by using a soft toothbrush, cotton swab, or anesthetic mouthwash such as viscous lidocaine (as prescribed), by applying petroleum jelly to his lips, and by avoiding astringent mouthwashes.
- If a female patient is of childbearing age, advise her to delay pregnancy until prolonged remission because radiation and

chemotherapy can cause genetic mutations and spontaneous abortions.

■ Because the patient with Hodgkin's disease has usually been healthy up until this point, he's likely to be especially distressed. Provide emotional support and offer appropriate reassurance. Ease the patient's anxiety by sharing your optimism about his prognosis.

■ Make sure both the patient and his family know that the local chapter of the American Cancer Society is available for information, financial assistance, and supportive counseling.

■ The development of further malignancies, such as acute myeloid leukemia and myelodysplastic syndrome, in patients successfully treated for Hodgkin's disease is a concern. Patients must be educated as to the importance of long-term follow-up care following completion of treatment.

Non-Hodgkin's lymphoma

Non-Hodgkin's lymphomas, also known as *malignant lymphomas* and *lymphosarcomas,* are a heterogeneous group of malignant diseases originating in lymph glands and other lymphoid tissue. Nodular lymphomas have a better prognosis than the diffuse form of the disease, but in both, the prognosis is worse than in Hodgkin's disease.

Causes and incidence

The cause of non-Hodgkin's lymphoma is unknown, although some theories suggest a viral source. Since the early 1970s, the incidence of these lymphomas has increased more than 80%, with about 53,000 new cases appearing annually in the United States. The reason for the increase is unknown, although it has been partly attributed to acquired immunodeficiency syndrome. Non-Hodgkin's lymphomas are two to three times more common in males than in females and occur in all age-groups. Compared to Hodgkin's disease, they occur about one to three times more often and cause twice as many deaths in children younger than age 15. Incidence rises with age (median age is 50). These lymphomas seem linked to certain races and ethnic groups, with increased incidence in whites and people of Jewish ancestry.

Signs and symptoms

Usually, the first indication of non-Hodgkin's lymphoma is swelling of the lymph glands, enlarged tonsils and adenoids, and painless, rubbery nodes in the cervical supraclavicular areas. In children, these nodes are usually in the cervical region, and the disease causes dyspnea and coughing. As the lymphoma progresses, the patient develops symptoms specific to the area involved and systemic complaints of fatigue, malaise, weight loss, fever, and night sweats.

Diagnosis

Diagnosis requires histologic evaluation of biopsied lymph nodes; of tonsils, bone marrow, liver, bowel, or skin; or of tissue removed during exploratory laparotomy. (Biopsy differentiates non-Hodgkin's lymphoma from Hodgkin's disease.) (See *Classifying non-Hodgkin's lymphomas,* page 142.)

Other tests include bone and chest X-rays, lymphangiography, liver and spleen scan, computed tomography scan of the abdomen and chest, positron emission tomography, and excretory urography. Laboratory tests include complete blood count (may show anemia), uric acid (elevated or normal), serum calcium (elevated if bone lesions are present), serum protein (normal), and liver function studies.

Treatment

Radiation therapy is used mainly in the early localized stage of the disease. Total nodal irradiation is generally effective for both nodular and diffuse histologies.

Chemotherapy is most effective with multiple combinations of antineoplastic agents. For example, cyclophosphamide, vincristine, Adriamycin, and prednisone can induce a complete remission in 70% to 80% of patients with nodular histology and in 20% to 55% of patients with diffuse histology. Other combinations — such as methotrexate, bleomycin, Adriamycin, Cytoxan, Oncovin, and prednisone

CLASSIFYING NON-HODGKIN'S LYMPHOMAS

Staging and classifying systems for non-Hodgkin's lymphomas include the National Cancer Institute's (NCI) system, the Rappaport histologic classification, and Lukes classification. (*Note:* The NCI also cites a "miscellaneous" category, which includes these lymphomas: composite, mycosis fungoides, histiocytic, extramedullary plasmacytoma, and unclassifiable.

NCI	Rappaport	Lukes
Low grade ▪ Small lymphocytic ▪ Follicular, predominantly small cleaved cell ▪ Follicular mixed, small and large cell	▪ Diffuse well-differentiated lymphocytic ▪ Nodular poorly differentiated lymphocytic ▪ Nodular mixed lymphoma	▪ Small lymphocytic and plasmacytoid lymphocytic ▪ Small cleaved follicular center cell, follicular only, or follicular and diffuse ▪ Small cleaved follicular center cell, follicular; large cleaved follicular center cell, follicular
Intermediate grade ▪ Follicular, predominantly large cell ▪ Diffuse, small cleaved cell ▪ Diffuse mixed, small and large cell ▪ Diffuse large cell, cleaved or noncleaved	▪ Nodular histiocytic lymphoma ▪ Diffuse poorly differentiated lymphoma ▪ Diffuse mixed lymphocytic-histiocytic ▪ Diffuse histiocytic lymphoma	▪ Large cleaved or noncleaved follicular center cell, or both, follicular ▪ Small cleaved follicular center cell, diffuse ▪ Small cleaved, large cleaved, or large noncleaved follicular center cell, diffuse ▪ Large cleaved or noncleaved follicular center cell, diffuse
High grade ▪ Diffuse large cell immunoblastic ▪ Large cell, lymphoblastic ▪ Small noncleaved cell	▪ Diffuse histiocytic lymphoma ▪ Lymphoblastic, convoluted or nonconvoluted ▪ Undifferentiated, Burkitt's and non-Burkitt's diffuse undifferentiated lymphoma	▪ Immunoblastic sarcoma, T-cell or B-cell type ▪ Convoluted T cell ▪ Small noncleaved follicular center cell

(M-BACOP)—induce prolonged remission and sometimes cure the diffuse form.

In recent years, the development of monoclonal antibodies, specifically rituximab, has provided additional options for the treatment of non-Hodgkin's lymphomas either alone or in combination with traditional chemotherapy regimens. Additionally, radioimmunotherapy for the treatment of these lymphomas has shown promise. Monoclonal antibodies are labeled with beta-emitting isotopes. Currently, ibritumomab tiuxetan is being used alone and in combination with rituximab.

Special considerations
▪ Observe the patient who's receiving radiation or chemotherapy for anorexia, nausea, vomiting, or diarrhea. Plan small, frequent meals scheduled around treatment.
▪ If the patient can't tolerate oral feedings, administer I.V. fluids and, as ordered, give antiemetics and sedatives.

■ Instruct the patient to keep irradiated skin dry.

■ Provide emotional support by informing the patient and family about the diagnosis and prognosis and by listening to their concerns. If needed, refer them to the local chapter of the American Cancer Society for information and counseling. Stress the need for continued treatment and follow-up care.

Mycosis fungoides

Mycosis fungoides (MF), also known as *malignant cutaneous reticulosis* and *granuloma fungoides,* is a rare, chronic malignant T-cell lymphoma of unknown cause that originates in the reticuloendothelial system of the skin, eventually affecting lymph nodes and internal organs. Unlike other lymphomas, MF allows an average life expectancy of 7 to 10 years after diagnosis. If correctly treated, particularly before it has spread beyond the skin, MF may go into remission for many years. However, after MF has reached the tumor stage, progression to severe disability or death is rapid.

Causes and incidence
The cause of MF is unknown. Most persons with MF have it for years and it can lead to death, but this is unusual.

In the United States, MF strikes more than 1,000 people of all races annually; most are between ages 40 and 60.

Signs and symptoms
The first sign of MF may be generalized erythroderma, possibly associated with itching. Eventually, MF evolves into varied combinations of infiltrated, thickened, or scaly patches, tumors, or ulcerations.

Diagnosis
CONFIRMING DIAGNOSIS *Clear diagnosis of MF depends on a history of multiple, varied, and progressively severe skin lesions associated with characteristic histologic evidence of lymphoma cell infiltration of the skin, with or without involvement of lymph nodes or visceral organs. Consequently, this diagnosis is commonly missed during the early stages until lymphoma cells are sufficiently numerous in the skin to show up in biopsy.*

Other diagnostic tests help confirm MF: complete blood count and differential; a finger-stick smear for Sézary cells (abnormal circulating lymphocytes), which may be present in the erythrodermic variants of MF (Sézary syndrome); blood chemistry studies to screen for visceral dysfunction; chest X-ray; liver-spleen isotopic scanning; lymphangiography; and lymph node biopsy to assess lymph node involvement. These tests also help to stage the disease— a necessary prerequisite to treatment.

Treatment
Depending on the stage of the disease and its rate of progression, past treatment and results, the patient's age and overall clinical status, treatment facilities available, and other factors, treatment of MF may include topical, intralesional, or systemic corticosteroid therapy; phototherapy; methoxsalen photochemotherapy; radiation; topical, intralesional, or systemic treatment with mechlorethamine (nitrogen mustard); and other systemic chemotherapy.

Application of topical nitrogen mustard is the preferred treatment for inducing remission in pretumorous stages. Plaques may also be treated with sunlight and topical steroids.

Total body electron beam radiation, which is less toxic to internal organs than standard photon beam radiation, has induced remission in some patients with early stage MF.

Chemotherapy is employed primarily for patients with advanced MF; systemic treatment with chemotherapeutic agents (cyclophosphamide, methotrexate, doxorubicin, bleomycin, etoposide, and steroids) and interferon-alfa produces transient regression.

Special considerations
■ If the patient has difficulty applying nitrogen mustard to all involved skin surfaces, provide assistance. However, wear gloves to prevent contact sensitization and to protect yourself from exposure to chemotherapeutic agents.

- If the patient is receiving drug treatment, report adverse effects and infection at once.
- The patient who's receiving radiation therapy will probably develop alopecia and erythema. Suggest that he wear a wig to improve his self-image and protect his scalp until hair regrowth begins, and suggest or give medicated oil baths to ease erythema.
- Because pruritus is generally worse at night, the patient may need larger bedtime doses of antipruritics or sedatives, as ordered, to ensure adequate sleep. When the patient's symptoms have interrupted sleep, postpone early morning care to allow him more sleep.
- The patient with intense pruritus has an overwhelming need to scratch — in many cases to the point of removing epidermis and replacing pruritus with pain, which some patients find easier to endure. Realize that you can't keep such a patient from scratching; the best you can do is help minimize the damage. Advise the patient to keep fingernails short and clean and to wear a pair of soft, white cotton gloves when itching is unbearable.
- The malignant skin lesions are likely to make the patient depressed, fearful, and self-conscious. Fully explain the disease and its stages to help the patient and family understand and accept the disease. Provide reassurance and support by demonstrating a positive but realistic attitude. Reinforce your verbal support by touching the patient without any hint of anxiety or distaste.

Acute leukemia

Acute leukemia is a malignant proliferation of white blood cell (WBC) precursors (blasts) in bone marrow or lymph tissue and their accumulation in peripheral blood, bone marrow, and body tissues. Its most common forms are acute lymphoblastic (lymphocytic) leukemia (ALL), an abnormal growth of lymphocyte precursors (lymphoblasts); acute myeloblastic (myelogenous) leukemia (AML), the rapid accumulation of myeloid precursors (myeloblasts); and acute monoblastic (mono-

cytic) leukemia, or *Schilling's type,* a marked increase in monocyte precursors (monoblasts). Other variants include acute myelomonocytic leukemia and acute erythroleukemia.

Untreated, acute leukemia is invariably fatal, usually because of complications that result from leukemic cell infiltration of bone marrow or vital organs. With treatment, prognosis varies. In ALL, treatment induces remissions in 90% of children (average survival time: 5 years) and in 65% of adults (average survival time: 1 to 2 years). Children between ages 2 and 8 have the best survival rate — about 50% — with intensive therapy. In AML, the average survival time is only 1 year after diagnosis, even with aggressive treatment. In acute monoblastic leukemia, treatment induces remissions lasting 2 to 10 months in 50% of children; adults survive only about 1 year after diagnosis, even with treatment.

Causes and incidence

Research on predisposing factors isn't conclusive but points to some combination of viruses (viral remnants have been found in leukemic cells), genetic and immunologic factors, and exposure to radiation and certain chemicals. (See *Predisposing factors to acute leukemia.*)

Pathogenesis isn't clearly understood, but immature, nonfunctioning WBCs appear to accumulate first in the tissue where they originate (lymphocytes in lymph tissue, granulocytes in bone marrow). These immature WBCs then spill into the bloodstream and from there infiltrate other tissues, eventually causing organ malfunction because of encroachment or hemorrhage.

Acute leukemia is more common in males than in females, in whites (especially people of Jewish descent), in children (between ages 2 and 5; 80% of all leukemias in this age-group are ALL), and in people who live in urban and industrialized areas. Acute leukemia accounts for 20% of all adult leukemias. Among children, however, it's the most common form of cancer. Incidence is 6 out of every 100,000 people.

Signs and symptoms

Signs of acute leukemia are sudden onset of high fever accompanied by thrombocy-

topenia and abnormal bleeding, such as
nosebleeds, gingival bleeding, purpura,
ecchymoses, petechiae, easy bruising after
minor trauma, and prolonged menses.
Nonspecific signs and symptoms, such as
low-grade fever, weakness, and lassitude,
may persist for days or months before visible symptoms appear. Other insidious
signs and symptoms include pallor, chills,
and recurrent infections. In addition, ALL,
AML, and acute monoblastic leukemia may
cause dyspnea, anemia, fatigue, malaise,
tachycardia, palpitations, systolic ejection
murmur, and abdominal or bone pain.
When leukemic cells cross the blood-brain
barrier and thereby escape the effects of
systemic chemotherapy, the patient may
develop meningeal leukemia (confusion,
lethargy, headache).

Diagnosis

 CONFIRMING DIAGNOSIS *Typical
clinical findings and bone marrow
aspirate showing a proliferation of
immature WBCs confirm acute leukemia.*
A bone marrow biopsy, usually of the
posterior superior iliac spine, is part of the
diagnostic workup. Blood counts show
thrombocytopenia and neutropenia. Differential leukocyte count determines cell
type. Lumbar puncture detects meningeal
involvement.

Treatment

Systemic chemotherapy aims to eradicate
leukemic cells and induce remission (less
than 5% of blast cells in the marrow and
peripheral blood are normal). Chemotherapy varies:

■ Meningeal leukemia — intrathecal instillation of methotrexate or cytarabine with
cranial radiation.

■ ALL — vincristine, prednisone, high-
dose cytarabine, L-asparaginase, AMSA,
and daunorubicin. Because there's a 40%
risk of meningeal leukemia in ALL, intrathecal methotrexate or cytarabine is giv-
en. Radiation therapy is given for testicular
infiltration.

■ AML — a combination of I.V. daunorubicin and cytarabine or, if these fail to induce remission, a combination of cyclophosphamide, vincristine, prednisone, or
methotrexate; high-dose cytarabine alone

PREDISPOSING FACTORS TO ACUTE LEUKEMIA

Although the exact causes of most
leukemias remain unknown, increasing evidence suggests a combination of contributing factors:

Acute lymphoblastic leukemia
■ Congenital disorders, such as
Down syndrome, Bloom syndrome,
Fanconi's anemia, ataxia-telangiec-
tasia, and congenital agammaglobu-
linemia
■ Familial tendency
■ Monozygotic twins
■ Viruses

Acute myeloblastic leukemia
■ Congenital disorders, such as
Down syndrome, Bloom syndrome,
Fanconi's anemia, ataxia-telangiec-
tasia, and congenital agammaglobu-
linemia
■ Exposure to the chemical benzene
and cytotoxins such as alkylating
agents
■ Familial tendency
■ Ionizing radiation
■ Monozygotic twins
■ Viruses

Acute monoblastic leukemia
■ Unknown (irradiation, exposure
to chemicals, heredity, and infections show little correlation to this
disease)

or with other drugs; amsacrine; etoposide;
and 5-azacytidine and mitoxantrone. A
subtype of AML called acute promyelocytic
leukemia (APL) is treated with all-
transretinoic acid (ATRA), which causes
leukemic cells to mature into normal
WBCs. ATRA has increased the cure rate of
this type of AML. Arsenic trioxide has been
approved for patients with APL who have
failed ATRA as the usual chemotherapy.

- Acute monoblastic leukemia — cytarabine and thioguanine with daunorubicin or doxorubicin.

Bone marrow transplant or a stem-cell transplant may be possible. Treatment also may include antibiotic, antifungal, and antiviral drugs and granulocyte injections to control infection and transfusions of platelets to prevent bleeding and of red blood cells to prevent anemia.

Special considerations

The care plan for the leukemic patient should emphasize comfort, minimize the adverse effects of chemotherapy, promote preservation of veins, manage complications, and provide teaching and psychological support.

 PEDIATRIC TIP *Because many of these patients are children, be especially sensitive to their emotional needs and those of their families.*

Before treatment:
- Explain the disease course, treatment, and adverse effects.
- Teach the patient and his family how to recognize infection (fever, chills, cough, sore throat) and abnormal bleeding (bruising, petechiae) and how to stop such bleeding (pressure, ice to area).
- Promote good nutrition. Explain that chemotherapy may cause weight loss and anorexia, so encourage the patient to eat and drink high-calorie, high-protein foods and beverages. However, chemotherapy and adjunctive prednisone may cause weight gain, so dietary counseling and teaching are helpful.
- Help establish an appropriate rehabilitation program for the patient during remission.

Plan meticulous supportive care:
- Watch for symptoms of meningeal leukemia (confusion, lethargy, headache). If these occur, know how to manage care after intrathecal chemotherapy. After such instillation, place the patient in Trendelenburg's position for 30 minutes. Force fluids, and keep the patient in the supine position for 4 to 6 hours. Check the lumbar puncture site often for bleeding. If the patient receives cranial radiation, teach him about potential adverse effects, and do what you can to minimize them.

- Prevent hyperuricemia, a possible result of rapid chemotherapy-induced leukemic cell lysis. Encourage fluids to about 67½ oz (2,000 ml) daily, and give acetazolamide, sodium bicarbonate tablets, and allopurinol. Check urine pH often — it should be above 7.5. Watch for rash or other hypersensitivity reaction to allopurinol.
- Watch for early signs of cardiotoxicity such as arrhythmias and signs of heart failure if the patient receives daunorubicin or doxorubicin.
- Control infection by placing the patient in a private room and instituting neutropenic precautions. Coordinate patient care so the leukemic patient doesn't come in contact with staff who also care for patients with infections or infectious diseases. Avoid using indwelling urinary catheters and giving I.M. injections because they provide an avenue for infection. Screen staff and visitors for contagious diseases, and watch for and report any signs of infection.
- Provide thorough skin care by keeping the patient's skin and perianal area clean, applying mild lotions or creams to keep skin from drying and cracking, and thoroughly cleaning skin before all invasive skin procedures. Change I.V. tubing according to your facility's policy. Use strict sterile technique and a metal scalp vein needle (metal butterfly needle) when starting I.V. therapy. If the patient receives total parenteral nutrition, give scrupulous subclavian catheter care.
- Monitor temperature every 4 hours; patients with fever over 101° F (38.3° C) and decreased WBC counts should receive prompt antibiotic therapy.
- Watch for bleeding; if it occurs, apply ice compresses and pressure, and elevate the extremity. Avoid giving I.M. injections, aspirin, and aspirin-containing drugs. Also avoid taking rectal temperatures, giving rectal suppositories, and doing digital examinations.
- Prevent constipation by providing adequate hydration, a high-residue diet, stool softeners, and mild laxatives and by encouraging walking.
- Control mouth ulceration by checking often for obvious ulcers and gum swelling and by providing frequent mouth care and

saline rinses. Tell the patient to use a soft toothbrush and to avoid hot, spicy foods and overuse of commercial mouthwashes.
■ Check the rectal area daily for induration, swelling, erythema, skin discoloration, or drainage.
■ Provide psychological support by establishing a trusting relationship to promote communication. Allow the patient and his family to verbalize their anger and depression. Let the family participate in his care as much as possible.
■ Minimize stress by providing a calm, quiet atmosphere that's conducive to rest and relaxation.

 PEDIATRIC TIP *For children, be flexible with patient care and visiting hours to promote maximum interaction with family and friends and to allow time for schoolwork and play.*

■ For those patients who are refractory to chemotherapy and in the terminal phase of the disease, supportive nursing care is directed to comfort; management of pain, fever, and bleeding; and patient and family support. Provide the opportunity for religious counseling. Discuss the option of home or hospice care.

Chronic granulocytic leukemia

Chronic granulocytic leukemia (CGL), also known as *chronic myelogenous leukemia* and *chronic myelocytic leukemia,* is characterized by the abnormal overgrowth of granulocytic precursors (myeloblasts, promyelocytes, metamyelocytes, and myelocytes) in bone marrow, peripheral blood, and body tissues.

CGL's clinical course proceeds in two distinct phases: the *insidious chronic phase,* with anemia and bleeding abnormalities and, eventually, the *acute phase (blastic crisis),* in which myeloblasts, the most primitive granulocytic precursors, proliferate rapidly. This disease is invariably fatal. Average survival time is 3 to 4 years after onset of the chronic phase and 3 to 6 months after onset of the acute phase.

Causes and incidence
About 95% of patients with CGL have the Philadelphia, or Ph[1], chromosome, an abnormality discovered in 1960 in which the long arm of chromosome 22 is translocated, usually to chromosome 9. Radiation and carcinogenic chemicals may induce this chromosome abnormality. Myeloproliferative diseases also seem to increase the incidence of CGL, and some clinicians suspect that an unidentified virus causes this disease.

CGL is most common in young and middle-aged adults and is slightly more common in men than in women; it's rare in children. In the United States, approximately 4,300 cases of CGL develop annually, accounting for roughly 20% of all leukemias.

Signs and symptoms
Typically, CGL induces the following clinical effects:
■ anemia (fatigue, weakness, decreased exercise tolerance, pallor, dyspnea, tachycardia, and headache)
■ thrombocytopenia, with resulting bleeding and clotting disorders (retinal hemorrhage, ecchymoses, hematuria, melena, bleeding gums, nosebleeds, and easy bruising)
■ hepatosplenomegaly, with abdominal discomfort and pain in splenic infarction from leukemic cell infiltration.

Other signs and symptoms include sternal and rib tenderness from leukemic infiltrations of the periosteum; low-grade fever; weight loss; anorexia; renal calculi or gouty arthritis from increased uric acid excretion; occasionally, prolonged infection and ankle edema; and, rarely, priapism and vascular insufficiency.

Diagnosis
CONFIRMING DIAGNOSIS *In patients with typical clinical changes, chromosomal analysis of peripheral blood or bone marrow showing the Philadelphia chromosome and low leukocyte alkaline phosphatase levels confirms CGL.*

Other relevant laboratory results show:
■ white blood cell abnormalities — leukocytosis (leukocytes more than 50,000/μl, ranging as high as 250,000/μl), occasional

leukopenia (leukocytes less than 5,000/µl), neutropenia (neutrophils less than 1,500/µl) despite high leukocyte count, and increased circulating myeloblasts
- hemoglobin—commonly below 10 g/dl
- hematocrit—low (less than 30%)
- platelets—thrombocytosis (more than 1 million/µl) is common
- serum uric acid—possibly more than 8 mg/dl
- bone marrow aspirate or biopsy—hypercellular; characteristically shows bone marrow infiltration by significantly increased number of myeloid elements (biopsy is done only if aspirate is dry); in the acute phase, myeloblasts predominate
- computed tomography scan—may identify the organs affected by leukemia.

Treatment
Aggressive chemotherapy has so far failed to produce remission in CGL. Consequently, the goal of treatment in the chronic phase is to control leukocytosis and thrombocytosis. The most commonly used oral agents are busulfan and hydroxyurea. Interferon-alfa–based therapy has been used as well. However, the development and introduction of imatinib mesylate, a tyrosine kinase inhibitor that has shown significant long-term effectiveness, has remarkably changed CGL treatment.

Aspirin is commonly given to prevent stroke if the patient's platelet count is more than 1 million/µl.

Ancillary CGL treatments include:
- local splenic radiation or splenectomy to increase platelet count and decrease adverse effects related to splenomegaly
- leukapheresis (selective leukocyte removal) to reduce leukocyte count
- allopurinol to prevent secondary hyperuricemia or colchicine to relieve gout caused by elevated serum uric acid levels
- prompt treatment of infections that may result from chemotherapy-induced bone marrow suppression.

During the acute phase of CGL, lymphoblastic or myeloblastic leukemia may develop. Treatment is similar to that for acute lymphoblastic leukemia. Remission, if achieved, is commonly short lived. Bone marrow transplant may produce long asymptomatic periods in the early phase of illness but has been less successful in the accelerated phase. Despite vigorous treatment, CGL can progress after onset of the acute phase.

Special considerations
In patients with CGL, meticulous supportive care, psychological support, and careful patient teaching help make the most of remissions and minimize complications. When the disease is diagnosed, be prepared to repeat and reinforce the physician's explanation of the disease and its treatment to the patient and his family.

Throughout the chronic phase of CGL when the patient is hospitalized:
- If the patient has persistent anemia, plan your care to help avoid exhausting the patient. Schedule laboratory tests and physical care with frequent rest periods in between, and assist the patient with walking, if necessary. Regularly check the patient's skin and mucous membranes for pallor, petechiae, and bruising.
- To minimize bleeding, suggest a soft-bristle toothbrush, an electric razor, and other safety precautions.
- To minimize the abdominal discomfort of splenomegaly, provide small, frequent meals. For the same reason, prevent constipation with a stool softener or laxative, as needed. Ask the dietary department to provide a high-bulk diet, and maintain adequate fluid intake.
- To prevent atelectasis, stress the need for coughing and deep-breathing exercises.

Because many patients with CGL receive outpatient chemotherapy throughout the chronic phase, sound patient teaching is essential:
- Explain expected adverse effects of chemotherapy: pay particular attention to dangerous adverse effects such as bone marrow suppression.
- Tell the patient to watch for and immediately report signs and symptoms of infection: any fever over 100° F (37.8° C), chills, redness or swelling, sore throat, and cough.
- Instruct the patient to watch for signs of thrombocytopenia, to immediately apply ice and pressure to any external bleeding site, and to avoid aspirin and aspirin-

containing compounds because of the risk of increased bleeding.

■ Emphasize the importance of adequate rest to minimize the fatigue of anemia. To minimize the toxic effects of chemotherapy, stress the importance of a high-calorie, high-protein diet.

For more information on treatment during the acute phase, see "Acute leukemia" on page 144.

Chronic lymphocytic leukemia

A generalized, progressive disease that's common in the elderly, chronic lymphocytic leukemia (CLL) is marked by an uncontrollable spread of abnormal, small lymphocytes in lymphoid tissue, blood, and bone marrow. Nearly all patients with CLL are men older than age 50. According to the American Cancer Society, this disease accounts for about 25% of all new leukemia cases annually.

Causes and incidence

Although the cause of CLL is unknown, researchers suspect hereditary factors (higher incidence has been recorded within families), still-undefined chromosome abnormalities, and certain immunologic defects (such as ataxia-telangiectasia or acquired agammaglobulinemia). The disease doesn't seem to be associated with radiation exposure, carcinogenic chemicals, or viruses.

Approximately 2 out of every 100,000 people develop CLL annually, with 90% of cases found in people who are older than age 50. Many cases go undetected by routine blood tests in people who are asymptomatic. The disease is common in Jewish people of Russian or Eastern European descent, and is uncommon in Asia.

Signs and symptoms

CLL is the most benign and the most slowly progressive form of leukemia. Clinical signs derive from the infiltration of leukemic cells in bone marrow, lymphoid tissue, and organ systems.

In early stages, patients usually complain of fatigue, malaise, fever, and nodal en-largement. They're particularly susceptible to infection.

In advanced stages, patients may experience severe fatigue and weight loss, with liver or spleen enlargement, bone tenderness, and edema from lymph node obstruction. Pulmonary infiltrates may appear when lung parenchyma is involved. Skin infiltrations, manifested by macular to nodular eruptions, occur in about one-half of the cases of CLL.

As the disease progresses, bone marrow involvement may lead to anemia, pallor, weakness, dyspnea, tachycardia, palpitations, bleeding, and infection. Opportunistic fungal, viral, and bacterial infections commonly occur in late stages.

Diagnosis

Typically, CLL is an incidental finding during a routine blood test that reveals numerous abnormal lymphocytes. In early stages, white blood cell (WBC) count is mildly but persistently elevated. Granulocytopenia is the rule, but the WBC count climbs as the disease progresses. Blood studies also show hemoglobin levels under 11 g, hypogammaglobulinemia, and depressed serum globulins. Other common developments include neutropenia (neutrophils less than 1,500/µl), lymphocytosis (lymphocytes more than 10,000/µl), and thrombocytopenia (platelets less than 150,000/µl). Bone marrow aspiration and biopsy show lymphocytic invasion.

Treatment

Systemic chemotherapy includes alkylating agents — usually chlorambucil, cyclophosphamide, vincristine, or fludarabine (singly or in combination) — and steroids (prednisone) when autoimmune hemolytic anemia or thrombocytopenia occurs.

An advance in the treatment of CLL has been the emergence of the humanized monoclonal antibodies rituximab and alemtuzumab. Alemtuzumab acts as an antibody against the surface of CLL cells and is used when fludarabine fails. Rituximab, a monoclonal antibody, acts similiarly to alemtuzumab; studies are ongoing.

When chronic lymphocytic leukemia causes obstruction or organ impairment or enlargement, local radiation treatment can be used to reduce organ size. Allopurinol can be given to prevent hyperuricemia, a relatively uncommon finding.

Prognosis is poor if anemia, thrombocytopenia, neutropenia, bulky lymphadenopathy, and severe lymphocytosis are present.

Special considerations
■ Plan patient care to relieve symptoms and prevent infection. Clean the patient's skin daily with mild soap and water. Frequent soaks may be ordered. Watch for signs or symptoms of infection: temperature over 100° F (37.8° C), chills, redness, or swelling of any body part.

■ Watch for signs and symptoms of thrombocytopenia (black tarry stools, easy bruising, nosebleeds, bleeding gums) and anemia (pale skin, weakness, fatigue, dizziness, palpitations). Advise the patient to avoid aspirin and products containing aspirin. Explain that many medications contain aspirin, even though their names don't make this clear. Teach him how to recognize aspirin variants on medication labels.

■ Explain chemotherapy and its possible adverse effects. If the patient is to be discharged, tell him to avoid coming in contact with obviously ill people, especially children with common contagious childhood diseases. Urge him to eat high-protein foods and drink high-calorie beverages.

■ Stress the importance of follow-up care, frequent blood tests, and taking all medications exactly as prescribed. Teach the patient the signs and symptoms of recurrence (swollen lymph nodes in the neck, axilla, and groin; increased abdominal size or discomfort), and tell him to notify his physician immediately if he detects any of these signs.

ELDER TIP *Most patients with CLL are elderly; many are frightened. Provide emotional support and be a good listener. Try to keep their spirits up by concentrating on little things, such as improving their personal appearance, providing a pleasant environment, and asking questions about their families. If possible, provide opportunities for their favorite activities.*

Selected references

American Joint Committee on Cancer. *AJCC Comparison Guide: Cancer Staging Manual, Fifth Versus Sixth Edition.* New York: Springer-Verlag, 2003. Available at www. cancerstaging.net.

Antoch, G., et al. "Whole Body Dual-Modality PET/CT and Whole Body MRI for Tumor Staging in Oncology," *JAMA* 290(24):3199-206, December 2003.

Craven, R.F., and Hirnle, C.J., eds. *Fundamentals of Nursing: Human Health and Function,* 4th ed. Philadelphia: Lippincott Williams & Wilkins, 2003.

Curiel, D.T., and Douglas, J., eds. *Cancer Gene Therapy.* Totowa, N.J.: Humana Press, 2004.

Forastiere, A.A., et al. "Concurrent Chemotherapy and Radiotherapy for Organ Preservation in Advanced Laryngeal Cancer," *The New England Journal of Medicine* 349(22): 2091-98, November 2003.

Giaccone, G., et al., eds. *Cancer Chemotherapy and Biological Response Modifiers Annual 21.* Philadelphia: Elsevier Science, 2003.

Le Marchand, L., et al. "Association of the Cyclin D1 A870G Polymorphism with Advanced Colorectal Cancer," *JAMA* 290(21):2843-48, December 2003.

Prabhudesai, A.G., and Kumar, D. "Adjuvant Therapy of Colorectal Cancer: The Next Step Forward," *Current Medical Research and Opinion* 18(5):249-57, 2002.

Remington, P.L., and Trentham-Dietz, A. "Measuring Progress in Cancer Control: A Bird's Eye View," *Oncologist* 8(6):539-40, December 2003.

Singletary, S.E., et al. "Revision of the American Joint Committee on Cancer Staging System for Breast Cancer," *Journal of Clinical Oncology* (20)17:3628-36, September 2002.

Vogel, W.H., et al. *Advanced Practice Oncology and Palliative Care Guidelines.* Philadelphia: Lippincott Williams & Wilkins, 2003.

Weber, J.R. *Nurse's Handbook of Health Assessment,* 5th ed. Philadelphia: Lippincott Williams & Wilkins, 2005.

Weir, H.K., et al. "Annual Report to the Nation on the Status of Cancer, 1975-2000, Featuring the Uses of Surveillance Data for Cancer Prevention and Control," *The Journal of the National Cancer Institute* 95(17):1276-99, September 2003.

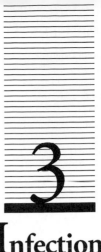

3

Infection

Introduction *152*

Gram-positive cocci *160*
Staphylococcal infections *160*
Methicillin-resistant *Staphylococcus aureus* infection *161*
Streptococcal infections *167*
Necrotizing fasciitis *167*
Vancomycin-resistant enterococcus infection *175*

Gram-negative cocci *176*
Meningococcal infections *176*

Gram-positive bacilli *178*
Diphtheria *178*
Listeriosis *179*
Tetanus *180*
Botulism *182*
Gas gangrene *183*
Actinomycosis *185*
Nocardiosis *186*

Gram-negative bacilli *187*
Salmonellosis *187*
Shigellosis *190*
Escherichia coli and other Enterobacteriaceae infections *191*
Pseudomonas infections *193*
Cholera *194*
Septic shock *196*

Haemophilus influenzae infection *198*
Whooping cough *199*
Plague *200*
Brucellosis *202*
Anthrax *204*
Campylobacteriosis *205*
Tularemia *205*
Ehrlichiosis *206*

Spirochetes and mycobacteria *207*
Lyme disease *207*
Relapsing fever *209*
Leprosy *210*

Mycoses *213*
Candidiasis *213*
Cryptococcosis *215*
Aspergillosis *216*
Histoplasmosis *217*
Blastomycosis *218*
Coccidioidomycosis *220*
Sporotrichosis *221*

Respiratory viruses *222*
Common cold *222*
Respiratory syncytial virus infection *224*
Parainfluenza *225*
Adenovirus infection *226*
Influenza *227*
Hantavirus pulmonary syndrome *229*

Rash-producing viruses   *231*
Varicella   *231*
Herpes simplex   *233*
Herpes zoster   *234*
Rubella   *236*
Rubeola   *238*
Variola   *240*
Monkeypox   *241*
Roseola infantum   *242*

Enteroviruses   *243*
Herpangina   *243*
Poliomyelitis   *244*

Arbovirus   *246*
Colorado tick fever   *246*

Miscellaneous viruses   *247*
Mumps   *247*
Infectious mononucleosis   *248*
Rabies   *250*
Cytomegalovirus infection   *251*
Lassa fever   *253*
Ebola virus infection   *253*
West Nile encephalitis   *255*

Rickettsia   *257*
Rocky Mountain spotted fever   *257*

Protozoa   *259*
Pneumocystis carinii pneumonia   *259*
Malaria   *261*
Amebiasis   *265*
Giardiasis   *266*
Toxoplasmosis   *267*

Helminths   *269*
Trichinosis   *269*
Hookworm disease   *270*
Ascariasis   *271*
Taeniasis   *272*
Enterobiasis   *273*
Schistosomiasis   *274*
Strongyloidiasis   *276*

Miscellaneous infections   *277*
Ornithosis   *277*
Toxic shock syndrome   *278*

Selected references   *279*

Introduction

Despite improved methods of treatment and prevention — potent antibiotics, complex immunizations, and modern sanitation — infection still accounts for much serious illness, even in highly industrialized countries. In developing countries, infection is one of the most critical health problems.

What is infection?

Infection is the invasion and multiplication of microorganisms in or on body tissue that produce signs and symptoms as well as an immune response. Such reproduction injures the host by causing cellular damage from microorganism-produced toxins or intracellular multiplication or by competing with host metabolism. The host's own immune response may compound the tissue damage, which may be localized (as in infected pressure ulcers) or systemic. The severity of the infection varies with the pathogenicity and number of the invading microorganisms and the strength of host defenses. The very young and the very old are especially susceptible to infections.

Why are the microorganisms that cause infectious diseases so difficult to overcome? There are many complex reasons:
- Some bacteria develop a resistance to antibiotics.
- Some microorganisms — such as human immunodeficiency virus — include so many different strains that a single vaccine can't provide protection against them all.
- Most viruses resist antiviral drugs.
- Some microorganisms localize in areas that make treatment difficult, such as the central nervous system and bone.

Moreover, certain factors that contribute to improved health — such as the affluence that allows good nutrition and living conditions and advances in medical science — can increase the risk of infection. For example, travel can expose people to diseases for which they have little natural immunity. The expanded use of immunosuppressants, surgery, and other invasive procedures also increases the risk of infection.

Kinds of infections

A laboratory-verified infection that causes no signs and symptoms is called a *subclinical, silent,* or *asymptomatic infection.* A multiplication of microbes that produces no signs, symptoms, or immune response is called a *colonization.* A person with a subclinical infection or colonization may be a carrier and transmit the infection to others. A *latent infection* occurs after a microorganism has been dormant in the host, sometimes for years. An *exogenous infection* results from environmental pathogens or sources other than the host; an *endogenous infection,* from the host's normal flora (for instance, *Escherichia coli* displaced from the colon, which causes urinary tract infection).

The varied forms of microorganisms responsible for infectious diseases include bacteria, viruses, rickettsiae, chlamydiae, fungi (yeasts and molds), and protozoa; larger organisms such as helminths (parasitic worms) may also cause infectious disease.

Bacteria are single-cell microorganisms with well-defined cell walls that can grow independently on artificial media without the need for other cells. Bacteria inhabit the intestines of humans and other animals as normal flora used in the digestion of food. Also found in soil, bacteria are vital to soil fertility. These microorganisms break down dead tissue, which allows it to then be used by other organisms.

Despite the numerous types of known bacteria, only a small percentage are harmful to man. (See *How bacteria damage tissue,* page 154.) In developing countries, where poor sanitation increases the risk of infection, bacterial diseases commonly result in death and disability. In industrialized countries, bacterial infections are the most common fatal infectious diseases.

Bacteria can be classified according to shape. Spherical bacterial cells are called *cocci;* rod-shaped bacteria, *bacilli;* and spiral-shaped bacteria, *spirilla.* Bacteria can also be classified according to their response to staining (gram-positive, gram-negative, or acid-fast bacteria); their motility (motile or nonmotile bacteria); their tendency toward encapsulation (encapsulated or nonencapsulated bacteria); and

their capacity to form spores (sporulating or nonsporulating bacteria).

Spirochetes are bacteria with flexible, slender, undulating spiral rods that have cell walls. Most are anaerobic. The three forms pathogenic in humans include *Treponema, Leptospira,* and *Borrelia.*

Viruses are subcellular organisms made up only of a ribonucleic acid or a deoxyribonucleic acid nucleus covered with proteins. They're the smallest known organisms (so tiny they're visible only through an electron microscope). Independent of host cells, viruses can't replicate. Rather, they invade a host cell and stimulate it to participate in the formation of additional virus particles. The estimated 400 viruses that infect humans are classified according to their size; shape (spherical, rod shaped, or cubic); or means of transmission (respiratory, fecal, oral, or sexual).

Rickettsiae are relatively uncommon in the United States. They're small, gram-negative organisms classified as bacteria that commonly induce life-threatening infections. Like viruses, they require a host cell for replication. Three genera of rickettsiae include *Rickettsia, Coxiella,* and *Rochalimaea.*

Chlamydiae are smaller than rickettsiae and bacteria but larger than viruses. They too depend on host cells for replication but, unlike viruses, they're susceptible to antibiotics.

Fungi are single-cell organisms, with nuclei enveloped by nuclear membranes. They have rigid cell walls like plant cells but lack chlorophyll, the green matter necessary for photosynthesis; they also show relatively little cellular specialization. Fungi occur as yeasts (single-cell, oval-shaped organisms) or molds (organisms with hyphae, or branching filaments). Depending on the environment, some fungi may occur in both forms. Fungal diseases in humans are called *mycoses.*

Protozoa are the simplest single-cell organisms of the animal kingdom. However, they show a high level of cellular specialization. Like other animal cells, they have cell membranes rather than cell walls, and their nuclei are surrounded by nuclear membranes.

PATHOPHYSIOLOGY

HOW BACTERIA DAMAGE TISSUE

The human body is constantly infected by bacteria and other infectious organisms. Some are beneficial such as the intestinal bacteria that produce vitamins. Others are harmful, causing illnesses ranging from the common cold to life-threatening septic shock.

To infect a host, bacteria must first enter it. They do this either by adhering to the mucosal surface and directly invading the host cell, or by attaching to epithelial cells and producing toxins that eventually invade the host cells. To survive and multiply within a host, bacteria or their toxins adversely affect biochemical reactions in cells. The result is a disruption of normal cell function or cell death (see illustration below). For example, the diphtheria toxin damages heart muscle by inhibiting protein synthesis. Also, as some organisms multiply, they extend into deeper tissues and eventually gain access to the bloodstream.

Some toxins cause blood to clot in the smaller blood vessels. As a result, the tissues supplied by these vessels may become deprived of blood and subsequently damaged (see illustration below).

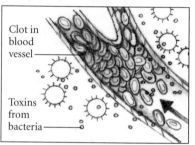

Clot in blood vessel

Toxins from bacteria

Other toxins can damage the cell walls of the smaller blood vessels, causing leakage. This fluid loss can result in decreased blood pressure, which in turn impairs the heart's ability to pump enough blood to the vital organs (see illustration below).

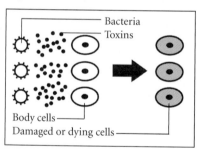

Bacteria
Toxins

Body cells
Damaged or dying cells

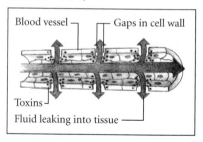

Blood vessel
Gaps in cell wall

Toxins
Fluid leaking into tissue

In addition to these microorganisms, infectious diseases may also result from larger parasites, such as roundworms or flatworms.

Modes of transmission

Most infectious diseases are transmitted in one of four ways (see *Standard precautions;* also see *CDC isolation precautions,* page 157):

■ In *contact transmission,* the susceptible host comes into direct contact (as in contact with blood or body fluids) or indirect contact (contaminated inanimate objects or the close-range spread of respiratory droplets) with the source. The most common method of contact transmission is contaminated hands.

■ *Airborne transmission* results from the inhalation of contaminated aerosolized droplet nuclei (as in pulmonary tuberculosis).

■ In *enteric (oral-fecal) transmission,* the infecting organisms are found in feces and

STANDARD PRECAUTIONS

The Centers for Disease Control and Prevention recommends that the following standard blood and body-fluid precautions be used for *all* patients. This is especially important in emergency care settings, where the risk of blood exposure is high and the patient's infection status is usually unknown.

It's important to remember that implementing standard precautions doesn't eliminate the need for maintaining other transmission-based precautions designed for specific airborne, droplet, and contact infectious diseases.

Sources of potential exposure
Standard precautions apply to blood, semen, vaginal secretions, and cerebrospinal, synovial, pleural, peritoneal, pericardial, and amniotic fluids. Standard precautions also apply to other body substances, such as feces, urine, nasal secretions, saliva, sputum, tears, vomitus, and breast milk.

Barrier precautions
■ Wear gloves when touching blood and body fluids, mucous membranes, or the broken skin of patients; when handling items or touching surfaces soiled with blood or body fluids; and when performing venipuncture and other vascular access procedures.
■ Change gloves and wash hands after contact with each patient.
■ Wear a mask and protective eyewear, or a face shield, to protect the mucous membranes of the mouth, nose, and eyes during procedures that may generate the splatter of blood or other body fluids.
■ In addition to the mask and protective eyewear or face shield, wear a gown or an apron during procedures that are likely to cause splashing of blood or other body fluids.
■ After removing gloves and other protective equipment, thoroughly wash hands and other skin surfaces that may be contaminated with blood or other body fluids.

Precautions for invasive procedures
■ During all invasive procedures, wear gloves and a surgical mask and goggles or a face shield as appropriate.

■ During procedures that commonly cause droplets or splashes of blood or other body fluids, or for those that generate bone chips, wear protective eyewear and a surgical mask or a face shield.
■ During invasive procedures that are likely to cause splashing or a splattering of blood or other body fluids, wear a gown or an impervious apron.
■ If performing or assisting in a vaginal or cesarean delivery, wear gloves and a gown when handling the placenta or the infant and during umbilical cord care.

Work practice precautions
■ To prevent needle-stick injuries, don't recap used needles, bend or break needles, remove needles from their disposable syringes or phlebotomy blood tube holders, or manipulate them.
■ Use sharps safety devices. Activate safety mechanisms as directed.
■ Place disposable syringes and needles, scalpel blades, and other sharps items in puncture-resistant containers for disposal. Make sure these containers are always located near the area of use.
■ Place large-bore reusable needles in a puncture-resistant container for transport to the reprocessing area immediately after a procedure.
■ If a glove tears or a needle-stick or other injury occurs, remove the gloves, wash your hands and the site of the needle-stick thoroughly, and put on new gloves as quickly as patient safety permits. Remove the needle or instrument involved in the incident from the sterile field. Promptly report injuries and

(continued)

STANDARD PRECAUTIONS *(continued)*

---

mucous-membrane exposure to the appropriate infection control practitioner per facility protocol.

Hand-hygiene, either by washing with soap and water or by sanitizing with an alcohol-based sanitizer, is recognized as the most effective method of interrupting the transmission of infection. Plain soap is adequate for removing visible soil. Antimicrobial soap is encouraged for washing after contamination with blood or body fluids. Alcohol-based hand sanitizers, which reduce the number of viable microorganisms on the hands, are designed for waterless use. In the United States, these products usually contain 60% to 95% ethanol or isopropanol.

Indications for washing with either ordinary or antimicrobial soap include:
- when hands are visibly dirty or contaminated with proteinaceous material or visibly soiled with blood or other body fluids (even if gloves were worn)
- before eating and after using the restroom

- exposure to suspected or proven *Bacillus anthracis* (alcohol, chlorhexidine, iodophors, and other antiseptic agents have a poor potency against its spores)
- after caring for a patient with *Clostridium difficile* (alcohol, chlorhexidine, iodophors, and other antiseptic agents are largely ineffective against its spores).

Alcohol-based hand sanitizers may be used in all other clinical situations if the hands aren't visibly soiled.

Additional precautions
- Make sure mouthpieces, one-way valve masks, resuscitation bags, and other ventilation devices are available in areas where the need for resuscitation is likely. *Note:* Saliva has not been implicated in human immunodeficiency virus transmission.
- If you have any exudative lesions or weeping dermatitis, refrain from direct patient care and from handling patient care equipment until the condition resolves.

---

are ingested by susceptible victims, in many cases through fecally contaminated food or water (as in salmonella infections).
- *Vector-borne transmission* occurs when an intermediate carrier (vector), such as a flea, mosquito, or other animal, transfers an organism.

Much can be done to prevent the transmission of infectious diseases:
- comprehensive immunization (including the required immunization of travelers to, or emigrants from, endemic areas)
- drug prophylaxis
- improved nutrition, living conditions, and sanitation
- correction of environmental factors
- widespread disease tracking.

Immunization can now control many diseases, including diphtheria, tetanus, pertussis, measles, rubella, some forms of meningitis, poliovirus, hepatitis B, pneumococcal pneumonia, influenza, rabies, and tetanus. Smallpox (variola) — which

killed and disfigured millions — was believed to have been successfully eradicated by a comprehensive World Health Organization program of surveillance and immunization. However, in light of recent concerns regarding bioterrorism, smallpox is considered a potential agent. Health care personnel must recognize potential cases of smallpox and initiate appropriate precautions as well as notify health department officials. Smallpox vaccination may be appropriate for certain emergency and first-response health care providers.

Vaccines — which contain live but attenuated (weakened) or killed microorganisms — and toxoids — which contain modified bacterial exotoxins — induce active immunity against bacterial and viral diseases by stimulating antibody formation. Natural active immunity is produced as a patient who has the disease forms antibodies against it, thus preventing the recurrence of the disease. Immune globulins

CDC ISOLATION PRECAUTIONS

To help health care facilities maintain up-to-date isolation practices, the Centers for Disease Control and Prevention (CDC) and the Hospital Infection Control Practices Advisory Committee have developed the CDC's *Guideline for Isolation Precautions in Hospitals.*

Standard precautions

The revised guidelines contain two tiers of precautions. The first tier—called *standard precautions*—is designated for the care of all hospital patients regardless of their diagnosis or presumed infection. Standard precautions are the primary strategy for preventing nosocomial infection and take the place of universal precautions. These precautions apply to:

- blood
- all body fluids, secretions, and excretions—except sweat—regardless of whether or not they contain visible blood
- skin that isn't intact
- mucous membranes.

Transmission-based precautions

The second tier of precautions is known as *transmission-based precautions.* These precautions are instituted for patients who are known to be, or suspected of being, infected with a highly transmissible infection—one that requires precautions beyond those set forth in the standard precautions. There are three types of transmission-based precautions: airborne; droplet; and contact precautions.

Airborne precautions

Airborne precautions are designed to reduce the risk of the airborne transmission of infectious agents. Microorganisms carried through the air can be widely dispersed by air currents, making them available for inhalation or deposit on a susceptible host in the same room or at a longer distance from the infected patient if ventilation creates shared air space.

Airborne precautions include special air handling and ventilation procedures to prevent the spread of infection. They also require the use of respiratory protection such as a respirator (the N95 or higher disposable respirator or a powered air-purifying respirator)—in addition to standard precautions—when entering an infected patient's room.

Droplet precautions

Droplet precautions are designed to reduce the risk of transmitting infectious agents through large-particle (exceeding 5 micrometers) droplets. Such transmission involves the contact of infectious agents to the conjunctivae or to the nasal or oral mucous membranes of a susceptible person. Large-particle droplets don't remain in the air and generally travel short distances of 3′ (1 m) or less. They require the use of a surgical mask—in addition to standard precautions—to protect the mucous membranes.

Contact precautions

Contact precautions are designed to reduce the risk of transmitting infectious agents by direct or indirect contact. Direct-contact transmission can occur through patient care activities that require physical contact. Indirect-contact transmission involves a susceptible host coming in contact with a contaminated object, usually inanimate, in the patient's environment or with items contaminated with the patient's secretions, excretions, or blood outside of the patient's environment that may have been removed from the environment without appropriate cleaning and disinfection.

Contact precautions require the use of gloves and a gown—in addition to standard precautions—to avoid contact with the infectious agent. A mask is only required if there's a chance of splash or splatter of body fluids to the face. Stringent hand-hygiene is also necessary after removal of the protective items.

contain previously formed antibodies from hyperimmunized donors or pooled plasma and provide temporary passive immunity. Generally, passive immunization is used when active immunization is perilous or impossible or when complete protection requires both active and passive immunization. It may also be appropriate in situations requiring immediate protection such as postexposure in which active immunity from immunizations takes too long to provide the necessary — and immediate — protection. Maternal passive immunity crosses the placental barrier from mother to fetus and is also provided to the infant by antibodies present in breast milk.

Although prophylactic antibiotic therapy may prevent certain diseases, the risk of superinfection and the emergence of drug-resistant strains may outweigh the benefits. Therefore, prophylactic antibiotics are usually reserved for patients at high risk for exposure to dangerous infections. Antibiotic-resistant bacteria are on the rise mainly because antibiotics have been misused and overused. Some bacteria, such as enterococci, have developed mutant strains that don't respond to antibiotic therapy.

Health care-associated infections

A *health care-associated infection* is an infection that develops as a result of health care. Health care-associated infections were previously known as *nosocomial infections,* but the name was updated because these infections may be acquired from, or associated with, any portion of the health care-delivery system, including such areas as outpatient care, ambulatory care, home care, or long-term care.

Health care-associated infections are usually transmitted by direct contact. Less commonly, transmission occurs by inhalation or by contact with contaminated equipment and solutions. Contamination of solutions during the manufacturing process is rare.

Despite facility programs of infection control that include surveillance, prevention, and education, about 5% of patients who enter health care facilities contract a health care-associated infection. Staphylococcal infections, which had been declining since the 1960s, are currently a common

cause of infection. In contrast, gram-negative bacilli, resistant enterococci, and fungal infections are also on the rise.

Health care-associated infections continue to be a difficult problem, because today's hospital patients are older and more debilitated with chronic underlying diseases than in the past. Moreover, the increased use of invasive and surgical procedures, immunosuppressants, and antibiotics predisposes patients to infection and superinfection. At the same time, the growing number of personnel who can come in contact with each patient makes the risk of exposure greater.

The following measures can help prevent health care-associated infections:
- Follow strict infection-control procedures. (See *Standard precautions,* pages 155 and 156, and *CDC isolation precautions,* page 157.)
- Document hospital infections as they occur.
- Identify outbreaks early, and take steps to prevent their spread.
- Eliminate unnecessary procedures that contribute to infection.
- Strictly follow necessary isolation techniques.
- Observe *all* patients for signs of infection, especially those patients at high risk.
- Always follow proper hand-hygiene technique and encourage other staff members to follow these guidelines as well.
- Keep staff members and visitors with obvious infection and well-known carriers away from susceptible, high-risk patients.
- Take special precautions with vulnerable patients — those with indwelling urinary catheters, mechanical ventilators, or I.V. lines and those recuperating from surgery.

Accurate assessment vital

Accurate assessment helps identify infectious diseases and prevents avoidable complications. Complete assessment consists of patient history, physical examination, and laboratory data. The history should include the patient's sex, age, address, occupation, and place of work; known exposure to illness and recent medications, including antibiotics; and date of disease onset. Signs and symptoms, including their duration and whether they occurred suddenly or

IMMUNIZATION SCHEDULE

Before an immunization, obtain the child's medication, illness, and allergy history. Instruct the parents to report a severe reaction to the vaccine to the physician. Childhood immunizations are usually given on a fixed schedule, as follows:

Age	Immunization
Birth to 2 months	First dose: Hepatitis B vaccine (HBV)
1 to 4 months	Second dose: HBV[1]
2 months	First dose: diphtheria-tetanus acellular-pertussis (DTaP) vaccine, polio vaccine (IPV), *Haemophilus influenzae* type b conjugate (Hib) vaccine, pneumococcal vaccine (PCV)
4 months	Second dose: DTaP, IPV, Hib, PCV
6 months	Third dose: DTaP, Hib, PCV
6 to 18 months	Third dose: HBV and IPV
12 to 15 months	First dose: Measles-mumps-rubella (MMR) vaccine; fourth dose: Hib; final dose: PCV
12 to 18 months	Fourth dose: DTaP[2]; first dose: varicella zoster virus vaccine
4 to 6 years	Fifth dose: DTaP; fourth dose: IPV; second dose: MMR
11 to 12 years	MMR (if not given at age 4 to 6); varicella zoster (catch-up vaccination[3])
11 to 16 years	Tetanus (booster every 10 years)

[1] The second dose of HBV is given at least 1 month after the first dose. The first dose is given at birth but may be given 2 months after the mother's hepatitis B surface antigen returns negative. The third dose is given at least 6 months after the second dose.

[2] A fourth dose of DTaP may be given as early as age 12 months through 18 months, provided that 6 months have elapsed since the third dose. The acellular form of the vaccine can now be used for all doses in the series, even for children who started the series with standard whole-cell D vaccine.

[3] Unvaccinated children with no history of chickenpox should be vaccinated at ages 11 to 12 years.

gradually, should be included in the history as well as precipitating factors, relief measures, and weight loss or gain. Detail information about recent hospitalization; blood transfusions; blood donation denial by the Red Cross or other agencies; recent travel or camping trips; exposure to animals; and vaccinations. (See *Immunization schedule.*) If applicable, ask about possible exposure to sexually transmitted diseases or about drug abuse. Also, try to determine the patient's resistance to infectious disease. Ask about usual dietary patterns, unusual fatigue, and any conditions, such as neoplastic disease or alcoholism, that may predispose him to infection. Notice if the patient is listless or uneasy, lacks concentration, or has any obvious abnormality of mood or affect.

In suspected infection, a physical examination must assess the skin, mucous membranes, liver, spleen, and lymph nodes.

Check for and make note of the location and type of drainage from any skin lesions. Record skin color, temperature, and turgor; ask if the patient has pruritus. Take his temperature, using the same route consistently, and watch for a fever, which is the best indicator of many infections. (Keep in mind that some patients, such as those who are immunocompromised, are unable to spike a fever.) Note and record the pattern of temperature change and the effect of antipyretics. Be aware that certain analgesics may contain antipyretics. With a high fever, especially in children, watch for seizures.

Check the pulse rate. Infection commonly increases the pulse rate, but some infections, notably typhoid fever and psittacosis, may decrease it. Also observe for increased respiratory rate or a change in mental status. In severe infection or when complications are possible, watch for hypotension, hematuria, oliguria, hepatomegaly, jaundice, bleeding from gums or into joints, and an altered level of consciousness. Obtain laboratory studies and appropriate cultures as ordered.

GRAM-POSITIVE COCCI

Staphylococcal infections

Staphylococci are gram-positive bacteria, either coagulase-negative (*Staphylococcus*

COMPARING STAPHYLOCOCCAL INFECTIONS

Predisposing factors	Signs and symptoms	Diagnosis
Bacteremia ■ Infected surgical wounds ■ Abscesses ■ Infected I.V. or intra-arterial catheter sites or catheter tips ■ Infected vascular grafts or prostheses ■ Infected pressure ulcers ■ Osteomyelitis ■ Parenteral drug abuse ■ Source unknown (primary bacteremia) ■ Cellulitis ■ Burns ■ Immunosuppression ■ Debilitating diseases, such as chronic renal insufficiency or diabetes ■ Infective endocarditis (coagulase-positive staphylococci) and subacute bacterial endocarditis (coagulase-negative staphylococci) ■ Cancer (leukemia) or neutrophil nadir after chemotherapy or radiation	■ Fever (high fever with no obvious source in children younger than age 1), shaking chills, tachycardia ■ Cyanosis or pallor ■ Confusion, agitation, stupor ■ Skin microabscesses ■ Joint pain ■ Complications: shock; acute bacterial endocarditis (in prolonged infection; indicated by new or changing systolic murmur); retinal hemorrhages; splinter hemorrhages under nails and small, tender red nodes on pads of fingers and toes (Osler's nodes); abscess formation in skin, bones, lungs, brain, and kidneys; pulmonary emboli if tricuspid valve is infected ■ Prognosis poor in patients older than age 60 or with chronic illness	■ Blood cultures (two to four samples from different sites at different times): growing staphylococci and leukocytosis (usually 12,000 white blood cells [WBCs]/µl), with a shift to the left of polymorphonuclear leukocytes (70% to 90% neutrophils) ■ Urinalysis may show microscopic hematuria ■ Erythrocyte sedimentation rate (ESR) elevated, especially in chronic or subacute bacterial endocarditis ■ Severe anemia or thrombocytopenia (possible) ■ Prolonged partial thromboplastic time and prothrombin time; low fibrinogen and platelet counts, and low factor assays; possible disseminated intravascular coagulation ■ Cultures of urine, sputum, and skin lesions with discharge may identify primary infection site; chest X-rays and scans of lungs, liver, abdomen, and brain may assist with identification ■ Echocardiogram may show heart valve vegetation

epidermidis) or coagulase-positive (*Staphylococcus aureus*). Coagulase-negative staphylococci grow abundantly as normal flora on skin, but they can also cause boils, abscesses, and carbuncles. In the upper respiratory tract, they're usually nonpathogenic but can cause serious infections in some individual such as those who are immunocompromised. Pathogenic strains of staphylococci are found in many adult carriers — usually on the nasal mucosa, axilla, or groin. Sometimes, carriers shed staphylococci, infecting themselves or other susceptible people. Coagulase-positive staphylococci tend to form pus and cause many different types of infections. (See *Comparing staphylococcal infections.*)

Methicillin-resistant *Staphylococcus aureus* infection

Methicillin-resistant *Staphylococcus aureus* (MRSA) is a mutation of very common bacterium spread easily by direct person-to-person contact. Once limited to large teaching hospitals and tertiary care centers, MRSA infection is now endemic in nursing homes, long-term care facilities, and community hospitals. It's also seen in patients who haven't been hospitalized, as community-acquired MRSA infections are increasing.

Patients most at risk for MRSA infection include immunosuppressed patients, burn

(*Text continues on page 164.*)

Treatment	Special considerations
■ Semisynthetic penicillins (oxacillin, nafcillin) or cephalosporins (cefazolin) given I.V. ■ Vancomycin I.V. for patients with penicillin allergy or suspected methicillin-resistant organisms ■ Possibly, probenecid given to partially prevent urinary excretion of penicillin and to prolong blood levels ■ I.V. fluids to reverse shock ■ Removal of infected catheter or foreign body ■ Surgery	■ Report infection to authorities as required. ■ *S. aureus* bacteremia can be fatal within 12 hours. Be especially alert for it in debilitated patients with I.V. catheters or in those with a history of drug abuse. ■ Administer antibiotics on time to maintain adequate blood levels, but give them slowly, using the prescribed amount of diluent, to prevent thrombophlebitis. ■ Watch for signs of penicillin allergy, especially pruritic rash (anaphylaxis) and breathing difficulties. Keep epinephrine 1:1,000 and resuscitation equipment handy. Monitor the patient's vital signs, urine output, and mental state for signs of shock. ■ Obtain cultures carefully, and observe for clues to the primary site of infection. Never refrigerate blood cultures; it delays identification of organisms by slowing their growth. ■ Impose contact precautions if the primary site of infection is draining. Special blood precautions are not necessary because the number of organisms present, even in fulminant bacteremia, is minimal. Some facilities continue isolation if the patient has methicillin-resistant *Staphylococcus aureus* (MRSA) regardless of site. ■ Obtain peak and trough levels of vancomycin to determine the adequacy of treatment. ■ Administer vancomycin I.V. slowly over 1 hour to avoid any adverse reactions.

(*continued*)

COMPARING STAPHYLOCOCCAL INFECTIONS *(continued)*

Predisposing factors	Signs and symptoms	Diagnosis
Pneumonia ■ Immune deficiencies, especially in elderly and in children younger than age 2 ■ Chronic lung diseases and cystic fibrosis ■ Malignant tumors ■ Antibiotics that kill normal respiratory flora but spare *S. aureus* ■ Viral respiratory infections, especially influenza ■ Hematogenous (bloodborne) bacteria spread to the lungs from primary sites of infection (such as heart valves, abscesses, and pulmonary emboli) ■ Recent bronchial or endotracheal suctioning or intubation	■ High temperature: adults, 103° to 105° F (39.4° to 40.6° C); children, 101° F (38.3° C) or above ■ Cough, with purulent, yellow, or bloody sputum ■ Dyspnea, crackles, and decreased breath sounds ■ Pleuritic pain ■ In infants: mild respiratory infection that suddenly worsens: irritability, anxiety, dyspnea, anorexia, vomiting, diarrhea, spasms of dry coughing, marked tachypnea, expiratory grunting, sternal retractions, and cyanosis ■ Complications: necrosis, lung abscess, pyopneumothorax, empyema, pneumatocele, shock, hypotension, oliguria or anuria, cyanosis, loss of consciousness	■ WBC count may be elevated (15,000 to 40,000/µl in adults; 15,000 to 20,000/µl in children), with predominance of polymorphonuclear leukocytes ■ Sputum Gram stain: mostly gram-positive cocci in clusters, with many polymorphonuclear leukocytes ■ Sputum culture: mostly coagulase-positive staphylococci ■ Chest X-rays: usually patchy infiltrates ■ Arterial blood gas analysis: hypoxia and respiratory acidosis
Enterocolitis ■ Broad-spectrum antibiotics (tetracycline, chloramphenicol, or neomycin) or aminoglycosides (tobramycin, streptomycin, or kanamycin) as prophylaxis for bowel surgery or treatment of hepatic coma ■ Usually occurs in elderly patients, but also in neonates (associated with staphylococcal skin lesions)	■ Sudden onset of profuse, watery diarrhea usually 2 days to several weeks after start of antibiotic therapy, I.V. or by mouth (P.O.) ■ Nausea, vomiting, abdominal pain and distention ■ Hypovolemia and dehydration (decreased skin turgor, hypotension, fever)	■ Stool Gram stain: many gram-positive cocci and polymorphonuclear leukocytes, with few gram-negative rods ■ Stool culture: *S. aureus* ■ Sigmoidoscopy: mucosal ulcerations ■ Blood studies: leukocytosis, moderately increased blood urea nitrogen level, and decreased serum albumin level

Treatment	Special considerations
■ Semisynthetic penicillins (oxacillin, nafcillin) or cephalosporins (cefazolin) given I.V. ■ Vancomycin I.V. for patients with penicillin allergy or suspected methicillin-resistant organisms ■ Isolation until sputum shows minimal numbers of *S. aureus* (about 24 to 72 hours after starting antibiotics)	■ The Centers for Disease Control and Prevention's isolation guidelines require standard precautions unless MRSA, which requires contact precautions, is present. ■ Keep the door to the patient's room closed. Don't store extra supplies in his room. Empty suction bottles carefully. Disposable suction containers are preferred. ■ When obtaining sputum specimens, make sure you're collecting thick sputum, not saliva. The presence of epithelial cells (found in the mouth, not lungs) indicates a poor specimen. ■ Administer antibiotics strictly on time, but slowly. Watch for signs of penicillin allergy and for signs of infection at the I.V. sites. Change the I.V. site every third day. ■ Perform frequent chest physical therapy. Do chest percussion and postural drainage after intermittent positive pressure breathing treatments. Concentrate on consolidated areas (revealed by X-rays or auscultation).
■ Broad-spectrum antibiotics discontinued ■ Possibly, antistaphylococcal agents such as vancomycin P.O. ■ Normal flora replenished with yogurt that contains live cultures	■ Monitor vital signs frequently to detect early signs of shock. ■ Force fluids to correct dehydration. ■ Know serum electrolyte levels. Measure and record bowel movements when possible. Check serum chloride level for alkalosis (hypochloremia). Watch for dehydration and electrolyte imbalance. ■ Collect serial stool specimens for Gram stain and culture to confirm diagnosis. (The effectiveness of therapy is usually measured by clinical response.) ■ Observe standard precautions. ■ Follow reporting requirements, especially in a group situation such as a nursing home. They may vary per facility protocol.

(continued)

COMPARING STAPHYLOCOCCAL INFECTIONS *(continued)*

Predisposing factors	Signs and symptoms	Diagnosis
Osteomyelitis ■ Hematogenous organisms ■ Skin trauma ■ Infection spreading from adjacent joint or other infected tissues ■ *S. aureus* bacteremia ■ Orthopedic surgery or trauma ■ Cardiothoracic surgery ■ Usually occurs in growing bones, especially femur and tibia, of children younger than age 12 ■ More common in males	■ Abrupt onset of fever — usually 101° F (38.3° C) or above; shaking chills; pain and swelling over infected area; restlessness; headache ■ About 20% of children develop a chronic infection if not properly treated	■ Possible history of prior trauma to involved area ■ Positive bone and pus cultures (and blood cultures in about 50% of patients) ■ X-ray changes apparent after second or third week ■ ESR elevated with leukocyte shift to the left
Food poisoning ■ Enterotoxin produced by toxigenic strains of *S. aureus* in contaminated food (second most common cause of food poisoning in United States)	■ Anorexia, nausea, vomiting, diarrhea, and abdominal cramps 1 to 6 hours after ingestion of contaminated food ■ Symptoms usually subside within 18 hours, with complete recovery occurring in 1 to 3 days	■ Clinical findings sufficient ■ Stool cultures: usually negative for *S. aureus* ■ Epidemiologic history: if others are ill and food history is a commonality; health department may be contacted for an outbreak
Skin infections ■ Decreased resistance ■ Burns or pressure ulcers ■ Decreased blood flow ■ Possible skin contamination from nasal discharge ■ Foreign bodies ■ Underlying skin diseases, such as eczema and acne ■ Common in people with poor hygiene living in crowded quarters ■ Insulin-dependent diabetes mellitus ■ Hemodialysis ■ I.V. drug injection	■ Cellulitis — diffuse, acute inflammation of soft tissue (no discharge) ■ Pus-producing lesions in and around hair follicles (folliculitis) ■ Boil-like lesions (furuncles and carbuncles) extend from hair follicles to subcutaneous tissues; these painful, red, indurated lesions are 1 to 2 cm and have a purulent yellow discharge. ■ Small macules or skin blebs that may develop into vesicles containing pus (bullous impetigo); common in school-age children ■ Mild or spiking fever ■ Malaise	■ Clinical findings and analysis of pus cultures if sites are draining ■ Cultures of nondraining cellulitis taken from the margin of the reddened area by infiltration with 1 ml sterile saline solution (nonbacteriostatic saline) and immediate fluid aspiration

patients, intubated patients, and those with central venous catheters, surgical wounds, or dermatitis. Others at risk include those with prosthetic devices, heart valves, and postoperative wound infections. Other risk factors include prolonged hospital stays; extended therapy with multiple or broad-spectrum antibiotics; and close proximity

Treatment	Special considerations
■ Surgical debridement ■ Prolonged antibiotic therapy (4 to 8 weeks) ■ Vancomycin I.V. for patients with penicillin allergy or methicillin-resistant organisms ■ Possibly, removal of prosthesis or hardware	■ Identify the infected area, and mark it on the care plan. ■ Check the penetration wound from which the organism originated for evidence of present infection. ■ Severe pain may render the patient immobile. If so, perform passive range-of-motion exercises. Apply heat as needed, and elevate the affected part. (Extensive involvement may require casting until the infection subsides.) ■ Before procedures such as surgical debridement, warn the patient to expect some pain. Explain that drainage is essential for healing, and that he will continue to receive analgesics and antibiotics after surgery. ■ Obtain a complete history of symptoms, recent meals, and other known cases of food poisoning.
■ No treatment necessary unless dehydration becomes a problem (usually in infants and elderly); oral rehydrating solution or I.V. therapy may be necessary to replace fluids	■ Monitor vital signs, fluid balance, and serum electrolyte levels. ■ Check for dehydration if vomiting is severe or prolonged and for decreased blood pressure. ■ Observe and report the number and color of stools. ■ Report infection to authorities as required.
■ Topical ointments; gentamicin or bacitracin-neomycin-polymyxin ■ P.O. cloxacillin, dicloxacillin, or erythromycin; I.V. oxacillin or nafcillin for severe infection; I.V. vancomycin for methicillin-resistant organisms ■ Application of heat to reduce pain ■ Surgical drainage ■ Identification and treatment of sources of reinfection (nostrils, perineum) ■ Cleaning and covering the area with moist, sterile dressings	■ Identify the site and extent of infection. ■ Keep lesions clean with saline solution and peroxide irrigations, as ordered. Cover infections near wounds or the genitourinary tract with gauze pads. Keep pressure off the site to facilitate healing. ■ Be alert for the extension of skin infections. ■ Severe infection or abscess may require surgical drainage. Explain the procedure to the patient. Determine if cultures will be taken, and be prepared to collect a specimen. ■ Impetigo is contagious. Isolate the patient and alert his family. Use contact precautions for all draining lesions.

to those colonized or infected with MRSA. Also at risk are patients with acute endocarditis, bacteremia, cervicitis, meningitis, pericarditis, and pneumonia.

Causes

MRSA enters health care facilities through an infected or colonized patient or a colonized health care worker. Although MRSA

VANCOMYCIN-RESISTANT INFECTIONS

Some *Staphylococcus aureus* organisms have developed resistance to vancomycin. In some cases, the resistance is considered intermediate-strength resistance and is known as vancomycin-intermediate *S. aureus* (VISA). Another mutation, vancomycin-resistant *S. aureus* (VRSA), is fully resistant to vancomycin.

Researchers believe VISA and VRSA enter health care facilities through an infected or colonized patient or a colonized health care worker. They spread through direct contact between the patient and caregiver or between patients. They may also be spread through patient contact with contaminated surfaces.

Patients with laboratory-confirmed VISA or VRSA must be placed in a single room on contact precautions, and the number of health care workers involved in patient care should be limited. Other patients who shared the patient's room should be checked for VISA or VRSA colonization using an anterior nares culture. (Notify the laboratory to look specifically for *S. aureus* and to check sensitivity).

People involved in direct care of the patient before the initiation of contact precautions should be interviewed regarding the extent of their interactions. Those with extensive interaction should have an anterior nares culture. The local health department should be notified immediately. Antimicrobial treatment may include an increased dosage of vancomycin (for VISA only) and linezolid, quinupristin and dalfopristin, or a combination of other antimicrobials according to the sensitivity pattern of the organism.

has been recovered from environmental surfaces, it's transmitted mainly by health care workers' hands. Many colonized individuals become silent carriers. The most frequent site of colonization is the anterior nares (40% of adults and most children become transient nasal carriers). Other, less common sites are the groin, axilla, and the gut. Typically, MRSA colonization is diagnosed by isolating bacteria from nasal secretions.

In individuals where the natural defense system breaks down, such as after an invasive procedure, trauma, or chemotherapy, the normally benign bacteria can invade tissue, proliferate, and cause infection. Today, up to 90% of *S. aureus* isolates or strains are penicillin resistant, and about 50% of all *S. aureus* isolates are resistant to methicillin, a penicillin derivative, as well as to nafcillin and oxacillin. These strains may also resist cephalosporins, aminoglycosides, erythromycin, tetracycline, and clindamycin.

MRSA infection has become prevalent with the overuse of antibiotics. Over the years, this has given once-susceptible bacteria the chance to develop defenses against antibiotics. This new capability allows resistant strains to flourish when antibiotics kill their more-sensitive cousins.

Signs and symptoms
There are no signs and symptoms specifically for MRSA infection. It's often found incidently during culture.

Diagnosis
MRSA can be cultured from the suspected site with the appropriate method. For example, a wound can be swabbed for culture. Cultures of blood, urine, and sputum specimens will reveal sources of MRSA. Many laboratories use oxacillin disks to check for staphylococcus sensitivity when testing culture specimens; resistance to oxacillin indicates MRSA.

Treatment
To eradicate MRSA colonization in the nares, the physician may order topical mupirocin to be applied inside the nostrils. Other protocols involve combining a topical agent and an oral antibiotic. Most facil-

ities keep patients in isolation until surveillance cultures are negative.

To attack MRSA infection, vancomycin is the drug of choice (see *Vancomycin-resistant infections*). A serious adverse effect (mostly caused by histamine release) is itching, which can progress to anaphylaxis. Some physicians also add rifampin, but whether rifampin acts synergistically or antagonistically when given with vancomycin is controversial.

Special considerations
■ People in contact with the patient should perform hand-hygiene before and after patient care.
■ Good hand-hygiene is the most effective way to prevent MRSA infection from spreading.
■ Use an antiseptic soap such as chlorhexidine. Bacteria have been cultured from worker's hands washed with milder soap. One study showed that, without proper hand-hygiene, MRSA could survive on health care workers' hands for up to 3 hours. Chlorhexidine has a residual antimicrobial effect on the skin.
■ Contact isolation precautions should be used when in contact with the patient. A disinfected private room should be made available with dedicated equipment.
■ Change gloves when contaminated or when moving from a "dirty" area of the body to a clean one.
■ Instruct the patient's family and friends to wear protective clothing when they visit him, and show them how to dispose of it.
■ Provide teaching and emotional support to the patient and his family members.
■ Consider grouping infected patients together and having the same nursing staff care for them.
■ Don't lay equipment used on the patient on the bed or bed stand. Be sure to wipe it with appropriate disinfectant before leaving the room.
■ Ensure judicious and careful use of antibiotics. Encourage physicians to limit their use.
■ Instruct the patient to take antibiotics for the full period prescribed, even if he begins to feel better.

Streptococcal infections

Streptococci are small gram-positive bacteria, spherical to ovoid in shape, and linked together in pairs or chains. Several species occur as part of normal human flora in the respiratory, GI, and genitourinary tracts. Although researchers have identified 21 species of streptococci, three classes—groups A, B, and D—cause most of the infections. (See *Comparing streptococcal infections*, pages 168 to 173.) Organisms belonging to groups A and B beta-hemolytic streptococci are associated with a characteristic pattern of human infections. Most disorders due to group D streptococcus are caused by *Enterococcus faecalis*, formerly called *Streptococcus faecalis*, or *S. bovis*. Group C and group G streptococci have been identified as the etiologic agent in such infections as bacteremia, meningitis, pharyngitis, osteomyelitis, and neonatal sepsis.

Clinically, there are three states of streptococcal infection: carrier, acute, and delayed nonsuppurative complications. In the carrier state, the patient is infected with a disease-causing species of streptococci without evidence of infection. In the acute form, streptococci invade the tissues and cause physical symptoms. In the delayed nonsuppurative complications state, specific signs and symptoms associated with streptococcal infection occur. These include those associated with the inflammatory state of acute rheumatic fever, chorea, and glomerulonephritis. If further complications occur, they usually appear about 2 weeks after the acute illness, but they may be evident after a nonsymptomatic illness.

Necrotizing fasciitis

Most commonly referred to as *flesh-eating bacteria,* necrotizing fasciitis is a progressive, rapidly spreading inflammatory infection located in the deep fascia that destroys fascia and fat with secondary necrosis of subcutaneous tissue. Also referred to as *hemolytic streptococcal gangrene, acute dermal gangrene, suppurative fasciitis,* and *synergistic necrotizing cellulites,* necrotizing fasciitis is most commonly caused by the patho-

(Text continues on page 172.)

COMPARING STREPTOCOCCAL INFECTIONS

Causes and incidence	Signs and symptoms

Streptococcus pyogenes (Group A streptococcus)

Streptococcal pharyngitis (strep throat)

■ Accounts for 95% of all cases of bacterial pharyngitis ■ Most common in children ages 5 to 10, from October to April ■ Spread by direct person-to-person contact via droplets of saliva or nasal secretions ■ Organism usually colonizes throats of persons with no symptoms ■ Up to 20% of school children may be carriers ■ Pets may also be carriers	■ After 1- to 5-day incubation period: temperature of 101° to 104° F (38.3° to 40° C), sore throat with severe pain on swallowing, beefy red pharynx, tonsillar exudate, edematous tonsils and uvula, swollen glands along the jaw line, generalized malaise and weakness, anorexia, occasional abdominal discomfort ■ Up to 40% of small children have symptoms too mild for diagnosis ■ Fever abates in 3 to 5 days; nearly all symptoms subside within a week

Scarlet fever (scarlatina)

■ Usually follows streptococcal pharyngitis; may follow wound infections or puerperal sepsis ■ Caused by streptococcal strain that releases an erythrogenic toxin ■ Most common in children ages 2 to 10 ■ Spread by large respiratory droplets or direct contact with items soiled with respiratory secretions	■ Streptococcal sore throat, fever, strawberry tongue, fine erythematous rash that blanches on pressure and resembles sunburn with goosebumps ■ Rash usually appearing first on upper chest, then spreading to neck, abdomen, legs, and arms, sparing soles and palms; flushed cheeks, pallor around mouth ■ Skin sheds during convalescence

Erysipelas

■ Occurs primarily in infants and adults older than age 30 ■ Usually follows streptococcal pharyngitis ■ Exact mode of spread to skin unknown	■ Sudden onset, with reddened, swollen, raised lesions (skin looks like an orange peel), usually on face and scalp, bordered by areas that often contain easily ruptured blebs filled with yellow-tinged fluid; lesions sting and itch; lesions on the trunk, arms, or legs usually affect incision or wound sites ■ Other symptoms: vomiting, fever, headache, cervical lymphadenopathy, sore throat

Impetigo (streptococcal pyoderma)

■ Common in children ages 2 to 5 in hot, humid weather; high rate of familial spread ■ Predisposing factors: close contact in schools, overcrowded living quarters, poor skin hygiene, minor skin trauma ■ May spread by direct contact, environmental contamination, or arthropod vector	■ Small macules rapidly develop into vesicles, then become pustular and encrusted, causing pain, surrounding erythema, regional adenitis, cellulitis, and itching; scratching spreads infection ■ Lesions commonly affect the face, heal slowly, and leave depigmented areas

Diagnosis	Complications	Treatment and special considerations
■ Clinically indistinguishable from viral pharyngitis ■ Throat culture showing group A beta-hemolytic streptococci (carriers have positive throat culture) ■ Elevated white blood cell (WBC) count ■ Serology showing a fourfold rise in streptozyme titers during convalescence	■ Acute otitis media or acute sinusitis occurs most frequently ■ Rarely, bacteremic spread may cause arthritis, endocarditis, meningitis, osteomyelitis, or liver abscess ■ Poststreptococcal sequelae: acute rheumatic fever or acute glomerulonephritis ■ Reye's syndrome	■ Penicillin or erythromycin, analgesics, and antipyretics may be ordered. ■ Stress the need for bed rest and isolation from other children for 24 hours after antibiotic therapy begins; the patient should finish his prescription, even if symptoms subside; abscess, glomerulonephritis, and rheumatic fever can occur. ■ Tell the patient not to skip doses and to properly dispose of soiled tissues.
■ Characteristic rash and strawberry tongue ■ Culture and Gram stain showing *S. pyogenes* from nasopharynx ■ Granulocytosis	■ Although rare, complications may include high fever, arthritis, jaundice, pneumonia, pericarditis, and peritonsillar abscess	■ Penicillin or erythromycin may be ordered. ■ Keep the patient in isolation for the first 24 hours. ■ Carefully dispose of purulent discharge. ■ Stress the need for prompt and complete antibiotic treatment.
■ Typical reddened lesions ■ Culture taken from edge of lesions showing group A beta-hemolytic streptococci ■ Throat culture almost always positive for group A beta-hemolytic streptococci	■ Untreated lesions on trunk, arms, or legs may involve large body areas and lead to death.	■ Penicillin or erythromycin I.V. or by mouth (P.O.) may be ordered. ■ Cold packs, analgesics (aspirin and codeine for local discomfort), and topical anesthetics may be used to increase comfort. ■ Prevention includes prompt treatment of streptococcal infections and drainage and secretion precautions.
■ Characteristic lesions with honey-colored crust ■ Culture and Gram stain of swabbed lesions showing *S. pyogenes*	■ Septicemia (rare) ■ Ecthyma, a form of impetigo with deep ulcers	■ Penicillin I.V. or P.O., erythromycin, or antibiotic ointments may be ordered. ■ Perform frequent washing of lesions with antiseptics, such as povidone-iodine or antibacterial soap, followed by thorough drying. ■ Isolate a patient with draining wounds. ■ Prevention includes good hygiene and proper wound care.

(continued)

COMPARING STREPTOCOCCAL INFECTIONS *(continued)*

Causes and incidence	Signs and symptoms

Streptococcus agalactiae (Group B streptococcus)

Neonatal streptococcal infections

▪ Incidence of early-onset infection (age 6 days or younger): 2/1,000 live births ▪ Incidence of late-onset infection (age 7 days to 3 months): 1/1,000 live births ▪ Spread by vaginal delivery or hands of nursery staff ▪ Predisposing factors: maternal genital tract colonization, membrane rupture over 24 hours before delivery, crowded nursery	▪ Early onset: bacteremia, pneumonia, and meningitis; mortality from 14% for infants weighing more than 1,500 g at birth to 61% for infants weighing less than 1,500 g at birth ▪ Late onset: bacteremia with meningitis, fever, and bone and joint involvement; mortality 15% to 20% ▪ Other signs and symptoms, such as skin lesions, depend on the site affected

Adult group B streptococcal infection

▪ Most adult infections occur in postpartum women, usually in the form of endometritis or wound infection following cesarean section ▪ Incidence of group B streptococcal endometritis: 1.3/1,000 live births ▪ Group B streptococcal bacteremia and pneumonia: occur in the elderly and frequently in patients with diabetes ▪ Invasive group B streptococcal infection: occurs in patients with human immunodeficiency virus	▪ Fever, malaise, and uterine tenderness ▪ Change in lochia ▪ Bacteremia and pneumonia patients: can exhibit neurologic symptoms such as a change in mental status

Streptococcus pneumoniae

Pneumococcal pneumonia

▪ Accounts for 70% of all cases of bacterial pneumonia ▪ More common in men, elderly, Blacks, and Native Americans, in winter and early spring ▪ Spread by droplets and contact with infective secretions ▪ Predisposing factors: trauma, viral infection, underlying pulmonary disease, overcrowded living quarters, chronic diseases, asplenia, and immunodeficiency ▪ Among the 10 leading causes of death in the United States	▪ Sudden onset with severe shaking chills, temperature of 102° to 105° F (38.9° to 40.6° C), bacteremia, cough (with thick, scanty, blood-tinged sputum) accompanied by pleuritic pain ▪ Malaise, weakness, and prostration common ▪ Tachypnea, anorexia, nausea, and vomiting less common ▪ Severity of pneumonia usually due to host's cellular defenses, not bacterial virulence

Diagnosis	Complications	Treatment and special considerations
▪ Isolation of group B streptococcus from blood, cerebrospinal fluid (CSF), or skin ▪ Chest X-ray showing massive infiltrate similar to that of respiratory distress syndrome or pneumonia	▪ Overwhelming pneumonia, sepsis, and death	▪ Penicillin or ampicillin and an aminoglycoside I.V. may be ordered. ▪ Patient isolation is unnecessary unless an open draining lesion is present, but proper hand-hygiene is essential; for a draining lesion, take drainage and secretion precautions. ▪ Group B streptococcus prophylaxis may be ordered for women who are pregnant if vaginal or rectal cultures are positive at 35 to 37 weeks gestation or if the patient meets other criteria, such as delivery earlier or later than 3 weeks of term, amniotic fluid rupture for 18 hours or more; or an intrapartum temperature greater than or equal to 100.4° F [38.0° C]).
▪ Isolation of group B streptococcus from blood or infection site	▪ Bacteremia followed by meningitis or endocarditis	▪ Ampicillin or penicillin I.V. may be ordered. ▪ Perform careful observation for symptoms of infection following delivery. ▪ Follow drainage and secretion precautions.
▪ Gram stain of sputum showing gram-positive diplococci; culture showing *S. pneumoniae* ▪ Chest X-ray showing lobular consolidation in adults; bronchopneumonia in children and elderly patient ▪ Elevated WBC count ▪ Blood cultures usually positive for *S. pneumoniae*	▪ Pleural effusion (occurs in 25% of patients) ▪ Pericarditis (rare) ▪ Lung abscess (rare) ▪ Bacteremia ▪ Disseminated intravascular coagulation ▪ Death possible if bacteremia is present	▪ Penicillin or erythromycin I.V. or I.M. may be ordered. ▪ Monitor and support respirations, as needed. ▪ Record sputum color and amount. ▪ Prevent dehydration. ▪ Avoid sedatives and opioids to preserve cough reflex. ▪ Carefully dispose of all purulent drainage (standard precautions); advise high-risk patients to receive a vaccine and to avoid infected people. *(continued)*

COMPARING STREPTOCOCCAL INFECTIONS *(continued)*

Causes and incidence	Signs and symptoms

Streptococcus pneumoniae (continued)

Otitis media
- High incidence, with about 76% to 95% of all children having otitis media at least once (*S. pneumoniae* causes half of these cases.)

- Ear pain, ear drainage, hearing loss, fever, lethargy, and irritability
- Other possible symptoms: vertigo, nystagmus, and tinnitus

Meningitis
- Can follow bacteremic pneumonia, mastoiditis, sinusitis, skull fracture, or endocarditis
- Mortality (30% to 60%) highest in infants and elderly people

- Fever, headache, nuchal rigidity, vomiting, photophobia, lethargy, coma, wide pulse pressure, and bradycardia

Group D streptococcus

Endocarditis
- Group D streptococcus (enterococcus): causes 10% to 20% of all bacterial endocarditis
- Most common in elderly people and in those who abuse I.V. substances
- Typically follows bacteremia from an obvious source, such as a wound infection, urinary tract infection, or I.V. insertion site infection
- Most cases are subacute
- Also causes urinary tract infection

- Weakness, fatigability, weight loss, fever, night sweats, anorexia, arthralgia, splenomegaly, and new systolic murmur

---

genic bacteria *Streptococcus pyogenes*, also known as group A *Streptococcus* (GAS), although other aerobic and anaerobic pathogens may be present.

This severe and potentially fatal infection may begin at the site of a small insignificant wound or surgical incision. It's characterized by invasive and progressive necrosis of the soft tissue and underlying blood supply. The high mortality rates associated with it have been attributed to the emergence of more virulent strains of streptococci caused by changes in the bacteria's deoxyribonucleic acid.

This would account for an increase in the frequency and severity of the cases re-ported since 1985, following a 50- to 60-year span of clinical insignificance. Noted for decades and described in medical literature since the Civil War, necrotizing fasciitis accounts for 8% of reported cases of invasive GAS infections today. The mortality rate is very high, at 70% to 80%. Mortality drops significantly and prognosis improves with early intervention and treatment. Cases treated aggressively with surgery, antibiotics, and hyperbaric oxygen (HBO) therapy have seen mortality rates reduced to as low as 9% to 20%.

Diagnosis	Complications	Treatment and special considerations
▪ Fluid in middle ear ▪ Isolation of *S. pneumoniae* from aspirated fluid if necessary	▪ Recurrent attacks (may cause hearing loss)	▪ Amoxicillin or ampicillin and analgesics may be ordered. ▪ Tell the patient to report a lack of response to therapy after 72 hours.
▪ Isolation of *S. pneumoniae* from CSF or blood culture ▪ Increased CSF cell count and protein level; decreased CSF glucose level ▪ Computed tomography scan of head ▪ EEG	▪ Persistent hearing deficits, seizures, hemiparesis, or other nerve deficits ▪ Encephalitis	▪ Penicillin I.V. or chloramphenicol may be ordered. ▪ Monitor the patient closely for neurologic changes. ▪ Watch for symptoms of septic shock, such as acidosis and tissue hypoxia.
▪ Anemia, increased erythrocyte sedimentation rate and serum immunoglobulin level, and positive blood culture for group D streptococcus ▪ Echocardiogram showing vegetation on valves	▪ Embolization ▪ Pulmonary infarction ▪ Osteomyelitis	▪ Penicillin for *Streptococcus bovis* (non-enterococcal group D streptococcus) may be ordered. ▪ Penicillin or ampicillin *and* an aminoglycoside for enterococcal group D streptococcus may be ordered.

Causes and incidence

More than 80 types of the causative bacteria *S. pyrogenes* are in existence, making the epidemiology of GAS infections most complex. Wounds as minor as pinpricks, needle punctures, bruises, blisters, and abrasions or as serious as a traumatic injury or surgical incision can provide an opportunity for bacteria to enter the body.

In necrotizing fasciitis, group A beta-hemolytic *Streptococcus* and *Staphylococcus aureus*, working alone or together, are most commonly the primary infecting bacteria. They can enter the host via local tissue injury or through a breach in the integrity of a mucous membrane barrier. Other aerobic and anaerobic pathogens, including *Bacteroides, Clostridium, Peptostreptococcus,* Enterobacteriaceae, coliforms, *Proteus, Pseudomonas,* and *Klebsiella,* may be present. They can proliferate in an environment of tissue hypoxia caused by trauma, recent surgery, or medical compromise. The end product of this invasion is necrosis of the surrounding tissue, which accelerates the disease process by creating an even more favorable environment for the organisms.

Men are three times more likely to develop this rare condition than women, and the disease rarely occurs in children except in countries with poor hygienic practices.

The mean age of the population contracting the disease is 38 to 44 years.

Signs and symptoms

Pain, out of proportion to the size of the wound or injury it's associated with, is usually the first symptom of necrotizing fasciitis. It generally presents before all other physical findings.

The infective process will usually begin with a mild area of erythema at the site of insult, which will quickly progress within the first 24 hours. During the first 24- to 48-hour period, the erythema changes from red to purple in color and then to blue, with the formation of fluid-filled blisters and bullae that indicate the rapid progression of the necrotizing process. By days 4 and 5, multiple patches of this erythema form, producing large areas of gangrenous skin. By days 7 to 10, dead skin begins to separate at the margins of the erythema, revealing extensive necrosis of the subcutaneous tissue. At this stage, fascial necrosis is typically more advanced than appearance would suggest.

Other clinical symptoms include fever and hypovolemia. In later stages, hypotension and respiratory insufficiency, which are signs of overwhelming sepsis requiring supportive care, occur. In the most severe cases, necrosis advances rapidly until several large areas of the body are involved. This may cause the patient to become mentally cloudy, delirious, or even unresponsive secondary to the intoxication rendered.

Other complications include renal failure, septic shock with cardiovascular collapse, and scarring with cosmetic deformities. Without treatment, involvement of deeper muscle layers may occur, resulting in myositis or myonecrosis.

Diagnosis

Tissue biopsy is the best method of diagnosing necrotizing fasciitis. Cultures of microorganisms can be obtained locally from the periphery of the spreading infection or from deeper tissues during surgical debridement. Gram's staining and culturing of biopsied tissue are useful in establishing the type of invasive organisms and the effective treatment against them.

Radiographic studies can pinpoint the presence of subcutaneous gases, and computed tomography scans can locate the anatomic site of involvement by locating the necrosis. In combination with clinical assessment, magnetic resonance imaging determines areas of necrosis and the need for surgical debridement.

Other supportive studies include laboratory values such as complete blood count with differential, electrolytes, glucose, blood urea nitrogen and creatinine, urinalysis, and arterial blood gas levels.

Other conditions to consider in the differential diagnosis include cellulitis, testicular torsion, epididymitis and orchitis (as related to Fournier's gangrene), gas gangrene, hernias, and toxic shock syndrome (TSS).

Treatment

Prompt and aggressive exploration and debridement of suspected necrotizing fasciitis is mandatory for early, definitive diagnosis and to improve prognosis. Ninety percent of patients that present with clinical signs and symptoms will need immediate surgical debridement, fasciotomy, or amputation.

Penicillin, clindamycin, metronidazole, ceftriaxone, gentamicin, chloramphenicol, and ampicillin are among the medications given orally, I.V., or I.M. to treat the organisms involved with necrotizing fasciitis. The specific drug is determined by the sensitivity of the cultured organisms. When the infection is polymicrobial, medications must be used in combination. Recommendations for specific drugs continue to change as new antibiotics are developed and new resistance emerges.

Reports suggest that the use of HBO therapy decreases the mortality rate, significantly improves the tissues defense against infection, and prevents the necrosis from spreading by increasing the normal oxygen saturations of infected wounds by a thousandfold, causing a bactericidal effect. Typical treatment involves aggressively starting HBO therapy after the first surgical debridement and continuing for a total of 10 to 15 sessions.

Special considerations

■ Antibiotic therapy should be initiated immediately.

■ Accurate and frequent assessment of the patient's pain level, mental status, wound status, and vital signs is essential in order to recognize the progression of the wound changes or the development of new signs and symptoms. Changes must be reported and documented immediately.

■ The need for supportive care, such as endotracheal intubation, cardiac monitoring, fluid replacement, and supplemental oxygen should be assessed and provided as warranted.

■ Care of postoperative patients and patients with trauma wounds requires strict sterile technique, good hand hygiene, and barriers between health care providers and patients to prevent contamination.

■ Health care workers with sore throats should see their physician to determine if they have a streptococcal infection. If they are diagnosed positive, they shouldn't return to work until 24 hours after the initiation of antibiotic therapy.

■ Risk factors for contracting necrotizing fasciitis include patients with advanced age, human immunodeficiency infection, history of alcohol abuse, and varicellar infection. Patients with chronic illnesses, such as cancer, diabetes, cardiopulmonary disease, and kidney disease requiring hemodialysis, and those using steroids are more susceptible to GAS infection due to their debilitated immune response.

 ALERT *Be alert for signs and symptoms of TSS, which is associated with any streptococcal soft tissue infection, and the development of shock, acute respiratory distress syndrome, renal impairment, or bacteremia, any of which can lead to sudden death.*

Vancomycin-resistant enterococcus infection

Vancomycin-resistant enterococcus (VRE) is a mutation of a common bacterium normally found in the GI tract that's spread easily by direct person-to-person contact. Facilities in more than 40 states have reported VRE infection, with 30% of enterococcus infections in intensive care units (ICUs) and 25% of enterococcus infections in non-ICU areas reporting as vancomycin-resistant.

Patients most at risk for VRE infection include:

■ immunosuppressed patients or those with severe underlying disease

■ patients with a history of taking vancomycin, third-generation cephalosporins, antibiotics targeted at anaerobic bacteria (such as *Clostridium difficile*), or multiple courses of antibiotics

■ patients with indwelling urinary or central venous catheters

■ elderly patients, especially those with prolonged or repeated hospital admissions

■ patients with cancer or chronic renal failure

■ patients undergoing cardiothoracic or intra-abdominal surgery or organ transplant

■ patients with wounds opening into the pelvic or intra-abdominal area, including surgical wounds, burns, and pressure ulcers

■ patients with enterococcal bacteremia, typically associated with endocarditis

■ patients exposed to contaminated equipment or to another VRE-positive patient.

Causes

VRE enters health care facilities through an infected or colonized patient or a colonized health care worker. It can also develop following treatment with vancomycin. VRE spreads through direct contact between the patient and caregiver or between patients. It can also spread through patient contact with contaminated surfaces such as an overbed table where it's capable of living for weeks. VRE has also been detected on patient gowns, bed linens, and handrails.

Signs and symptoms

There are no specific signs and symptoms related to VRE infection. The causative agent may be found incidentally with culture results.

Diagnosis

Persons with no signs or symptoms of infection are considered colonized if VRE can be isolated from stool or a rectal swab.

Once colonized, a patient is more than 10 times as likely to become infected with VRE, for example, through a breach in the immune system.

Treatment

New antimicrobials, such as linezolid and quinupristin and dalfopristin, are available for treatment of VRE infection. Patients who are already colonized with VRE usually aren't treated with antimicrobials. Instead, the physician may stop all antibiotics and simply wait for normal bacteria to repopulate and replace the VRE strain. Combinations of various drugs may also be used, depending on the source of the infection.

To prevent the spread of VRE, some facilities perform weekly surveillance cultures on at-risk patients in the intensive care or oncology units and on patients who have been transferred from a long-term care facility. Any colonized patient is then placed in contact isolation until culture-negative or until discharged. Colonization can last indefinitely; no protocol has been established for the length of time a patient should remain in isolation.

Special considerations

■ Hand hygiene before and after care of the patient is crucial. Good hand hygiene is the most effective way to prevent VRE from spreading.
■ Use an antiseptic soap such as chlorhexidine. Bacteria have been cultured from workers' hands after they've washed with milder soap. Alcohol-based hand sanitizers are effective as well.
■ Use contact precautions when in contact with the patient or his support equipment. Provide the patient with a private room and dedicated equipment. Disinfect the environment and the equipment frequently.
■ Change gloves when contaminated or when moving from a "dirty" area of the body to a clean one.
■ Don't touch potentially contaminated surfaces such as an overbed table after removing your gown and gloves.
■ Be particularly prudent in caring for a patient with an ileostomy, colostomy, or draining wound that isn't contained by a dressing.

■ Instruct the patient's family and friends to wear protective garb when they visit him, and teach them how to dispose of it. Instruct them on proper hand hygiene.
■ Provide teaching and emotional support to the patient and his family members.
■ Consider grouping ("cohorting") infected or colonized patients together and assigning the same nursing staff to them.
■ Don't lay equipment used on the patient on the bed or on the overbed table. Wipe the equipment with the appropriate disinfectant before leaving the room.
■ Ensure judicious and careful use of antibiotics. Encourage physicians to limit their use.
■ Instruct patients to take antibiotics for the full period prescribed, even if they begin to feel better.

GRAM-NEGATIVE COCCI

Meningococcal infections

Two major meningococcal infections (meningitis and meningococcemia) are caused by the gram-negative bacteria *Neisseria meningitidis*, which also causes primary pneumonia, purulent conjunctivitis, endocarditis, sinusitis, and genital infection. Meningococcemia occurs as simple bacteremia, fulminating meningococcemia and, rarely, chronic meningococcemia. It commonly accompanies meningitis. (See "Meningitis," page 172.) Meningococcal infections may occur sporadically or in epidemics; particularly virulent infections may be fatal within a matter of hours.

Causes and incidence

Meningococcal infections usually occur among children (ages 6 months to 1 year) and men, usually military recruits or those enrolled at institutions, such as colleges, because of overcrowding.

N. meningitidis has seven serogroups (A, B, C, D, X, Y, and Z); group A causes most epidemics. Transmission takes place through inhalation of an infected droplet from a carrier (an estimated 2% to 38% of the population). The bacteria localize in the nasopharynx. After incubating approximately 3 to 4 days, they spread through the bloodstream to joints, skin, adrenal glands, lungs, and the central nervous system. The tissue damage that results (possibly due to the effects of bacterial endotoxins) produces symptoms and, in fulminating meningococcemia and meningococcal bacteremia, hemorrhage, thrombosis, and necrosis.

Signs and symptoms

Features of *meningococcal bacteremia* include sudden spiking fever, headache, sore throat, cough, chills, myalgia (in back and legs), arthralgia, tachycardia, tachypnea, mild hypotension, and a petechial, nodular, or maculopapular rash. Headache and stiff neck can also occur as the infection extends to the meninges.

In about 10% to 20% of patients, the disease progresses to *fulminating meningococcemia*, with extreme prostration, enlargement of skin lesions, disseminated intravascular coagulation (DIC), and shock. Without prompt treatment, death from respiratory or heart failure occurs in 6 to 24 hours.

Characteristics of the rare *chronic meningococcemia* include intermittent fever, rash, joint pain, and an enlarged spleen.

Diagnosis

CONFIRMING DIAGNOSIS *Gram-negative diplococci, on blood or cerebrospinal fluid (CSF) Gram stain, are highly suspicious for* N. meningitidis. *Isolation of* N. meningitidis *through a positive blood culture, CSF culture, or lesion scraping confirms the diagnosis, except in nasopharyngeal infections because* N. meningitidis *is part of the normal nasopharyngeal flora.*

Tests that support the diagnosis include counterimmunoelectrophoresis of CSF or blood, low white blood cell count and, in patients with skin or adrenal hemorrhages, decreased platelet and clotting levels. Diagnostic evaluation must rule out Rocky Mountain spotted fever and vascular purpuras.

Treatment

As soon as meningococcal infection is suspected, treatment begins with high doses of aqueous penicillin G, ampicillin, or cephalosporins such as ceftriaxone; or, for the patient who is allergic to penicillin, I.V. chloramphenicol. Therapy may also include mannitol for cerebral edema, I.V. heparin for DIC, dopamine for shock, and digoxin and a diuretic if heart failure develops. Supportive measures include fluid and electrolyte maintenance, ventilation (maintenance of a patent airway and oxygen, if necessary), insertion of an arterial or central venous pressure (CVP) line to monitor cardiovascular status, and bed rest.

Prophylaxis with ciprofloxacin or rifampin aids health care personnel who work in close contact with the patient, such as those administering cardiopulmonary resuscitation or assisting with intubation or suctioning without wearing a surgical mask.

Special considerations

- Give I.V. antibiotics, as ordered, to maintain blood and CSF drug levels.
- Enforce bed rest in early stages. Provide a dark, quiet, restful environment.
- Maintain adequate ventilation with oxygen or a ventilator, if necessary. Suction and turn the patient frequently.
- Keep accurate intake and output records to maintain proper fluid and electrolyte levels. Monitor blood pressure, pulse, arterial blood gas levels, and CVP.
- Watch for complications, such as DIC, arthritis, endocarditis, and pneumonia.
- If the patient is receiving chloramphenicol, monitor complete blood count.
- Check the patient's drug history for allergies before giving antibiotics.

To prevent the infection's spread:

- Impose droplet precautions until the patient has had antibiotic therapy for 24 hours.
- Label all meningococcal specimens. Deliver them to the laboratory quickly because meningococci are very sensitive to changes in humidity and temperature.
- Report all meningococcal infections to public health department officials.

■ The meningococcal vaccine can be administered to first-year college students living in dormitories as a preventative measure.

GRAM-POSITIVE BACILLI

Diphtheria

Diphtheria is an acute, highly contagious toxin-mediated infection caused by *Corynebacterium diphtheriae,* a gram-positive rod that usually infects the respiratory tract, primarily the tonsils, nasopharynx, and larynx. The GI and urinary tracts, conjunctivae, and ears are rarely involved.

Causes and incidence
Transmission usually occurs through intimate contact or by airborne respiratory droplets from asymptomatic carriers or convalescing patients. Many more people carry this disease than contract active infection. Diphtheria is more prevalent during the colder months because of closer person-to-person indoor contact, however it may be contracted at any time during the year.

Thanks to effective immunization, diphtheria is rare in many parts of the world, including the United States. Since 1972, the incidence of cutaneous diphtheria has been increasing, especially in the Pacific Northwest and the Southwest, in areas where crowding and poor hygienic conditions prevail. Most victims are children younger than age 15; about 10% of patients die.

Signs and symptoms
Most infections go unrecognized, especially in partially immunized individuals. After an incubation period of less than a week, clinical cases of diphtheria characteristically show a thick, patchy, grayish green membrane over the mucous membranes of the pharynx, larynx, tonsils, soft palate, and nose; fever; sore throat; and a rasping cough, hoarseness, and other symptoms similar to croup. Attempts to remove the membrane usually cause bleeding, which is highly characteristic of diphtheria. If this membrane causes airway obstruction (particularly likely in laryngeal diphtheria), symptoms include tachypnea, stridor, possibly cyanosis, suprasternal retractions, and suffocation, if untreated. Adenopathy and cervical swelling can occur. In cutaneous diphtheria, skin lesions resemble impetigo.

Complications include thrombocytopenia, myocarditis, neurologic involvement (primarily affecting motor fibers but possibly also sensory neurons), renal involvement, and pulmonary involvement (bronchopneumonia) due to *C. diphtheriae* or other superinfecting organisms.

Diagnosis
CONFIRMING DIAGNOSIS *Examination showing the characteristic membrane and a throat culture, or culture of other suspect lesions growing C. diphtheriae, confirm this diagnosis.*

Treatment
Treatment must not wait for confirmation by culture. Standard treatment includes diphtheria antitoxin administered I.M. or I.V.; antibiotics, such as penicillin or erythromycin, to eliminate the organisms from the upper respiratory tract and other sites and terminate the carrier state; measures to prevent complications; and possible tracheotomy if airway obstruction occurs.

Special considerations
Diphtheria requires comprehensive supportive care with psychological support.
■ To prevent the spread of this disease, stress the need for droplet precautions. Teach proper disposal of nasopharyngeal secretions. Maintain infection precautions until after two consecutive negative nasopharyngeal cultures — at least 1 week after discontinuing drug therapy. Treatment of exposed individuals with antitoxin remains controversial. Suggest that the patient's family receive diphtheria toxoid if they haven't been immunized.
■ Give drugs as ordered. Although time-consuming and risky, desensitization should be attempted if tests are positive, because diphtheria antitoxin is the only *specific* treatment available. If sensitivity

tests are negative, the antitoxin is given before laboratory confirmation, because mortality increases directly with any delay in antitoxin administration. Before giving diphtheria antitoxin, which is made from horse serum, obtain eye and skin tests to determine sensitivity. After giving antitoxin or penicillin, be alert for anaphylaxis; keep epinephrine 1:1,000 and resuscitation equipment handy. In patients who receive erythromycin, watch for thrombophlebitis.

■ Monitor respirations carefully, especially in laryngeal diphtheria (usually, such patients are in a high-humidity environment). Watch for signs of airway obstruction, and be ready to give immediate life support, including intubation and tracheotomy.

■ Watch for signs of shock, which can develop suddenly.

■ Obtain cultures as ordered.

■ If neuritis develops, tell the patient it's usually transient. Be aware that peripheral neuritis may not develop until 2 to 3 months after the onset of illness.

ALERT *Be alert for signs of myocarditis, such as the development of heart murmurs or electrocardiogram changes. Ventricular fibrillation is a common cause of sudden death in patients with diphtheria.*

■ Stress the need for childhood immunizations to all parents. Protective immunity doesn't last longer than 10 years after the last vaccination, so it's important to get tetanus-diphtheria boosters every 10 years.

■ Report all cases to local public health authorities.

Listeriosis

Listeriosis is an infection caused by the weakly hemolytic, gram-positive bacillus *Listeria monocytogenes*. It occurs most commonly in fetuses, in neonates (during the first 3 weeks of life), and in older or immunosuppressed adults. The infected fetus is usually stillborn or is born prematurely, almost always with lethal listeriosis. This infection produces milder illness in pregnant women and varying degrees of illness in older and immunosuppressed pa-

tients; their prognoses depend on the severity of underlying illness.

Causes

The primary method of person-to-person transmission is neonatal infection in utero (through the placenta) or during passage through an infected birth canal. Other modes of transmission may include inhaling contaminated dust; drinking contaminated, unpasteurized milk; eating unprocessed soft cheese or deli meats; coming in contact with infected animals, contaminated sewage or mud, or soil contaminated with feces containing *L. monocytogenes*; and, possibly, person-to-person transmission.

Signs and symptoms

Contact with *L. monocytogenes* commonly causes a transient asymptomatic carrier state. But sometimes it produces bacteremia and a febrile, generalized illness. In a pregnant woman, especially during the third trimester, listeriosis causes a mild illness with malaise, chills, fever, and back pain. However, her fetus may suffer severe uterine infection, abortion, premature delivery, or stillbirth. Transplacental infection may also cause early neonatal death or granulomatosis infantiseptica, which produces organ abscesses in infants.

Infection with *L. monocytogenes* commonly causes meningitis (especially in immunocompromised patients), resulting in tense fontanels, irritability, lethargy, seizures, and coma in neonates and low-grade fever and personality changes in adults. Fulminant manifestations with coma are rare.

Diagnosis

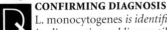 **CONFIRMING DIAGNOSIS** *L. monocytogenes is identified by its diagnostic tumbling motility on a wet mount of the culture.*

Other supportive diagnostic results include positive blood culture, spinal fluid, drainage from cervical or vaginal lesions, or lochia from a mother with an infected infant, but isolation of the organism from these specimens is generally difficult. Listeriosis also causes monocytosis.

Treatment

The treatment of choice is ampicillin or penicillin I.V. infusion for 3 to 6 weeks, possibly with gentamicin to increase its effectiveness. Alternate treatments include erythromycin, chloramphenicol, tetracycline, or co-trimoxazole.

Ampicillin or penicillin G is best for treating meningitis due to *L. monocytogenes*, because they can easily cross the blood-brain barrier. Pregnant women require prompt, vigorous treatment to combat fetal infection.

Special considerations

■ Deliver specimens to the laboratory promptly. Because few organisms may be present, take at least 10 ml of spinal fluid for culture.

■ Use standard precautions until a series of cultures are negative. Be especially careful when handling lochia from an infected mother and secretions from her infant's eyes, nose, mouth, and rectum, including meconium.

■ Evaluate neurologic status at least every 2 hours. In an infant, check fontanels for bulging. Maintain adequate I.V. fluid intake; measure intake and output accurately.

■ If the patient has central nervous system depression and becomes apneic, provide respiratory assistance, monitor respirations, and obtain frequent arterial blood gas measurements.

■ Provide adequate nutrition by total parenteral nutrition, nasogastric tube feedings, or a soft diet, as ordered.

■ Allow the patient's parents to see and, if possible, hold their infant in the neonatal intensive care unit. Be flexible about visiting privileges. Keep the parents informed of the infant's status and prognosis at all times.

■ Reassure the parents of an infected neonate who may feel guilty about the infant's illness.

■ Educate pregnant women to avoid infective materials on farms where listeriosis is endemic among livestock.

■ To avoid infection, instruct the patient and his family to avoid soft cheeses and to cook such foods as hot dogs thoroughly. Immunocompromised patients should avoid soft cheeses and deli meats.

Tetanus

Tetanus, also known as *lockjaw,* is an acute exotoxin-mediated infection caused by the anaerobic, spore-forming, gram-positive bacillus *Clostridium tetani.* This infection is usually systemic; less commonly, localized. Tetanus is fatal in up to 60% of unimmunized people, usually within 10 days of onset. When symptoms develop within 3 days after exposure, the prognosis is poor.

Causes and incidence

Normally, transmission occurs through a puncture wound that's contaminated by soil, dust, or animal excreta containing *C. tetani* or by way of burns and minor wounds. After *C. tetani* enters the body, it causes local infection and tissue necrosis. It also produces toxins that then enter the bloodstream and lymphatics and eventually spread to central nervous system tissue.

Tetanus occurs worldwide, but is more prevalent in agricultural regions and developing countries that lack mass immunization programs. It's one of the most common causes of neonatal deaths in developing countries, where infants of unimmunized mothers are delivered under unsterile conditions. In such infants, the unhealed umbilical cord is the portal of entry.

In the United States, about 75% of all cases occur between April and September.

Signs and symptoms

The incubation period varies from 3 to 4 weeks in mild tetanus to under 2 days in severe tetanus. When symptoms occur within 3 days after injury, death is more likely. If tetanus remains localized, signs of onset are spasm and increased muscle tone near the wound.

If tetanus is generalized (systemic), indications include marked muscle hypertonicity, hyperactive deep tendon reflexes, tachycardia, profuse sweating, low-grade fever, and painful, involuntary muscle contractions:

■ neck and facial muscles, especially cheek muscles — locked jaw (trismus), painful spasms of masticatory muscles, difficulty opening the mouth, and *risus sardonicus,* a

grotesque, grinning expression produced by spasm of facial muscles
- somatic muscles — arched-back rigidity (opisthotonos); boardlike abdominal rigidity
- intermittent tonic seizures lasting several minutes, which may result in cyanosis and sudden death by asphyxiation.

Despite such pronounced neuromuscular symptoms, cerebral and sensory functions remain normal. Complications can include atelectasis, pneumonia, pulmonary emboli, acute gastric ulcers, flexion contractures, and cardiac arrhythmias.

Neonatal tetanus is always generalized. The first clinical sign is difficulty in sucking, which usually appears 3 to 10 days after birth. It progresses to total inability to suck with excessive crying, irritability, and nuchal rigidity.

Diagnosis

In many cases, diagnosis must rest on clinical features, a history of trauma, and no previous tetanus immunization. Blood cultures and tetanus antibody tests are often negative; only a third of patients have a positive wound culture. Cerebrospinal fluid pressure may rise above normal. Diagnosis must also rule out meningitis, rabies, phenothiazine or strychnine toxicity, and other conditions that mimic tetanus.

Treatment

Within 72 hours after a puncture wound, a patient with no previous history of tetanus immunization first requires tetanus immune globulin (TIG) or tetanus antitoxin to neutralize the toxins and to confer temporary protection. Next, he needs active immunization with tetanus toxoid. If he hasn't received tetanus immunization within 10 years, a booster injection of tetanus toxoid is necessary. If tetanus develops despite immediate postinjury treatment, the patient will require airway maintenance and a muscle relaxant, such as diazepam, to decrease muscle rigidity and spasm. If muscle contractions aren't relieved by muscle relaxants, a neuromuscular blocker, such as metocurine iodide, may be prescribed. The patient with tetanus needs high-dose antibiotics (penicillin administered I.V. if he isn't allergic to it or such alternatives as clindamycin, erythromycin, and metronidazole.) The source of the toxin needs to be removed and destroyed through surgical exploration and wound debridement.

Special considerations

- Thoroughly debride and clean the injury site with 3% hydrogen peroxide, and check the patient's immunization history. Record the cause of injury. If it's an animal bite, report the case to local public health authorities.
- Before giving penicillin and TIG, antitoxin, or toxoid, obtain an accurate history of allergies to immunizations or penicillin. If the patient has a history of allergies, keep epinephrine 1:1,000 and resuscitation equipment available.
- Stress the importance of maintaining active immunization with a booster dose of tetanus toxoid every 10 years.

After tetanus develops:
- Maintain an adequate airway and ventilation to prevent pneumonia and atelectasis. Suction often and watch for signs of respiratory distress. Keep emergency airway equipment on hand because the patient may require artificial ventilation or oxygen administration.
- Maintain an I.V. line for medications and emergency care, if necessary.
- Monitor the electrocardiogram frequently for arrhythmias. Record intake and output accurately, and check vital signs often.
- Turn the patient frequently to prevent pressure ulcers and pulmonary stasis.
- Because even minimal external stimulation provokes muscle spasms, keep the patient's room quiet and only dimly lighted. Warn visitors not to upset or overly stimulate the patient.
- If urine retention develops, insert an indwelling urinary catheter.
- Give muscle relaxants and sedatives, as ordered, and schedule patient care — such as passive range-of-motion exercises — to coincide with periods of heaviest sedation.
- Insert an artificial airway, if necessary, to prevent tongue injury and maintain airway during spasms.

■ Provide adequate nutrition to meet the patient's increased metabolic needs. The patient may need nasogastric feedings or total parenteral nutrition.

Botulism

Botulism, a life-threatening paralytic illness, results from an exotoxin produced by the gram-positive, anaerobic bacillus *Clostridium botulinum.* It occurs with botulism food poisoning, wound botulism, and infant botulism. The mortality from botulism is about 25%; death is usually caused by respiratory failure during the first week of illness.

Causes and incidence

Botulism is usually the result of ingesting inadequately cooked contaminated foods, especially those with low acid content, such as home-canned fruits and vegetables, sausages, and smoked or preserved fish or meat. Rarely, it's a result of wound infection with *C. botulinum.*

Botulism occurs worldwide and affects more adults than children. Recently, findings have shown that an infant's GI tract can become colonized with *C. botulinum* from some unknown source, and then the exotoxin is produced within the infant's intestine. Infant botulism is usually attributed to the ingestion of honey or corn syrup. Incidence had been declining, but the current trend toward home canning has resulted in an upswing (approximately 250 cases per year in the United States) in recent years.

Signs and symptoms

Symptoms usually appear within 12 to 36 hours (range is 6 hours to 8 days) after the ingestion of contaminated food. Severity varies with the amount of toxin ingested and the patient's degree of immunocompetence. Generally, early onset (within 24 hours) signals critical and potentially fatal illness. Initial signs and symptoms include dry mouth, sore throat, weakness, dizziness, vomiting, and diarrhea. The cardinal sign of botulism, though, is acute symmetrical cranial nerve impairment (ptosis, diplopia, and dysarthria), followed by descending weakness or paralysis of muscles in the extremities or trunk, and dyspnea from respiratory muscle paralysis. Such impairment doesn't affect mental or sensory processes and isn't associated with fever.

Infant botulism usually afflicts infants between 3 and 20 weeks of age and can produce hypotonic (floppy) infant syndrome. Signs and symptoms are constipation, feeble cry, depressed gag reflex, and inability to suck. Cranial nerve deficits also occur in infants and are manifested by a flaccid facial expression, ptosis, and ophthalmoplegia. Infants also develop generalized muscle weakness, hypotonia, and areflexia. Loss of head control may be striking. Respiratory arrest is likely.

Diagnosis

CONFIRMING DIAGNOSIS *Identification of the offending toxin in the patient's serum, stool, gastric content, or the suspected food, confirms the diagnosis. An electromyogram showing diminished muscle action potential after a single supramaximal nerve stimulus is also diagnostic.*

Diagnosis also must rule out other diseases commonly confused with botulism, such as Guillain-Barré syndrome, myasthenia gravis, stroke, staphylococcal food poisoning, tick paralysis, chemical intoxications, carbon monoxide poisoning, fish poisoning, trichinosis, and diphtheria.

Treatment

Treatment consists of I.V. or I.M. administration of botulinus antitoxin (available through the Centers for Disease Control and Prevention).

If breathing difficulty develops, intubation and mechanical ventilation may be required. I.V. fluids can be given if there are swallowing problems, and a nasogastric tube can also be ordered.

Special considerations

If you suspect ingestion of contaminated food:

■ Obtain a careful history of the patient's food intake for the past several days. See if other family members exhibit similar symptoms and share a common food history.

- Observe carefully for abnormal neurologic signs. Tell the patient's family to watch for signs of weakness, blurred vision, and slurred speech after he has returned home. If such signs appear, the patient must return to the hospital immediately.
- If ingestion has occurred within several hours, induce vomiting, begin gastric lavage, and give a high enema to purge any unabsorbed toxin from the bowel.

If clinical signs of botulism appear:
- Admit the patient to the intensive care unit, and monitor cardiac and respiratory functions carefully.
- Administer botulinus antitoxin, as ordered, to neutralize any circulating toxin. Before giving the antitoxin, be sure to obtain an accurate patient history of allergies, especially to horses, and perform a skin test. Afterward, watch for anaphylaxis or other hypersensitivity and serum sickness. Keep epinephrine 1:1,000 (for subcutaneous administration) and emergency airway equipment available.
- Assess respiratory function every 4 hours. Report decreased vital capacity on inspiratory effort and any signs of respiratory distress.
- Closely assess and accurately record neurologic function, including bilateral motor status (reflexes, ability to move arms and legs).
- Give I.V. fluids as ordered. Turn the patient often, and encourage deep-breathing exercises. Isolation isn't required.
- As botulism is sometimes fatal, keep the patient and his family informed regarding the course of the disease.
- Immediately report all cases of botulism to local public health authorities.
- To help prevent botulism, encourage patients to observe proper techniques in processing and preserving foods. Warn them to avoid even *tasting* food from a bulging can or one with a peculiar odor and to sterilize by boiling any utensil that comes in contact with suspected food. Ingestion of even a small amount of food contaminated with botulism toxin can prove fatal.

Gas gangrene

Gas gangrene results from local infection with the anaerobic, spore-forming, gram-positive rod *Clostridium perfringens* (or another clostridial species). It occurs in devitalized tissues and results from compromised arterial circulation after trauma, surgery, compound fractures, or lacerations. This rare infection carries a high mortality unless therapy begins immediately; however, with prompt treatment, 80% of patients with gas gangrene of the extremities survive. The prognosis is poorer for gas gangrene in other sites, such as the abdominal wall or the bowel. The usual incubation period is 1 to 4 days but can vary from 3 hours to 6 weeks or longer.

Causes and incidence
C. perfringens is a normal inhabitant of the GI and female genital tracts; it's also prevalent in soil. Transmission occurs by entry of organisms during trauma or surgery. Because *C. perfringens* is anaerobic and spore forming, gas gangrene is usually found in deep wounds, especially those in which tissue necrosis further reduces oxygen supply. Clostridium bacteria produce four different toxins (alpha, beta, epsilon, iota) that can cause potentially fatal symptoms. When *C. perfringens* invades soft tissues, it produces thrombosis of regional blood vessels, tissue necrosis, localized edema, and damage to the myocardium, liver, and kidneys. (See *Growth cycle of* Clostridium perfringens, page 184.) Such necrosis releases both carbon dioxide and hydrogen subcutaneously, producing interstitial gas bubbles. Gas gangrene usually occurs in the extremities and in abdominal wounds; it's less common in the uterus.

Gas gangrene is rare, with only 1,000 to 3,000 cases occurring in the United States annually.

Signs and symptoms
True gas gangrene produces myositis and another form of this disease, involving only soft tissue, called *anaerobic cellulitis*. Most signs of infection develop within 72 hours of trauma or surgery. The hallmark of gas gangrene is crepitation (a crackling sensation when the skin is touched), a result of

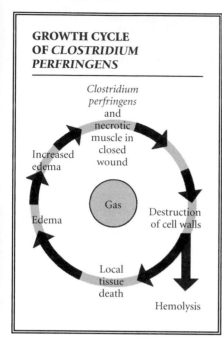

GROWTH CYCLE OF CLOSTRIDIUM PERFRINGENS

Clostridium perfringens and necrotic muscle in closed wound

Increased edema

Edema

Gas

Destruction of cell walls

Local tissue death

Hemolysis

carbon dioxide and hydrogen accumulation as a metabolic by-product in necrotic tissues. Other typical indications are severe localized pain, swelling, and discoloration (usually dusky brown or reddish), with formation of bullae and necrosis within 36 hours from onset of symptoms. The skin over the wound may rupture, revealing dark red or black necrotic muscle, a foul-smelling watery or frothy discharge, intravascular hemolysis, thrombosis of blood vessels, and evidence of infection spread.

In addition to these local symptoms, gas gangrene produces early signs of toxemia and hypovolemia (tachycardia, tachypnea, and hypotension), with moderate fever usually not above 101° F (38.3° C). Although pale, prostrate, and motionless, patients with gas gangrene may exhibit toxic delirium and are extremely apprehensive. Possible sudden death is preceded by delirium and coma and is sometimes accompanied by vomiting, profuse diarrhea, and circulatory collapse.

 ELDER TIP *Absence of a fever doesn't necessarily mean absence of infection in an elderly person. Many* older adults develop a subnormal temperature in response to infection.

Diagnosis

CONFIRMING DIAGNOSIS *A history of recent surgery or a deep puncture wound and the rapid onset of pain and crepitation around the wound suggest gas gangrene.*

Gas gangrene is confirmed by anaerobic cultures of wound drainage showing *C. perfringens;* a Gram stain of wound drainage showing large, gram-positive, rod-shaped bacteria; X-rays showing gas in tissues; and blood studies showing leukocytosis and, later, hemolysis.

Diagnosis must rule out synergistic gangrene and necrotizing fasciitis; unlike gas gangrene, both these disorders anesthetize the skin around the wound.

Treatment

Treatment includes careful observation for signs of myositis and cellulitis and *immediate treatment* if these signs appear; *immediate* wide surgical excision of all affected tissues and necrotic muscle in myositis (*delayed or inadequate surgical excision is a fatal mistake*); I.V. administration of high-dose penicillin; and, after adequate debridement, hyperbaric oxygenation, if available. For 1 to 3 hours every 6 to 8 hours, the patient is placed in a hyperbaric chamber, exposing him to pressures designed to increase oxygen tension and prevent multiplication of the anaerobic clostridia. Surgery may be performed within the hyperbaric chamber if the chamber is large enough.

Special considerations

Careful observation may result in early diagnosis. Look for signs and symptoms of ischemia (cool skin; pallor or cyanosis; sudden, severe pain; sudden edema; and loss of pulses in involved limb).

After the diagnosis:
■ Throughout this illness, provide adequate fluid replacement, and assess pulmonary and cardiac functions often. Maintain airway and ventilation.
■ To prevent skin breakdown and further infection, give good skin care. After surgery, provide meticulous wound care.

■ Before penicillin administration, obtain a patient history of allergies; afterward, watch closely for signs of hypersensitivity.

■ Psychological support is critical, because these patients can remain alert until death, knowing that death is imminent and unavoidable.

■ Deodorize the room to control foul odor from the wound. Prepare the patient emotionally for a large wound after surgical excision, and refer him for physical rehabilitation, as necessary.

■ Institute standard precautions. Dispose of drainage material properly, and wear sterile gloves when changing dressings. Spore-forming bacteria aren't destroyed by ordinary disinfecting methods. Contaminated items should be cleaned and disinfected or sterilized, as appropriate.

To prevent gas gangrene:

■ Routinely take precautions to render all wound sites unsuitable for growth of clostridia by attempting to keep granulation tissue viable; adequate debridement is imperative to reduce anaerobic growth conditions. The surgeon may delay closure of wounds.

■ Be alert for devitalized tissues, and notify the surgeon promptly.

■ Position the patient to facilitate drainage, and eliminate all dead spaces in closed wounds.

Actinomycosis

Actinomycosis is a rare infection primarily caused by the gram-positive anaerobic bacillus *Actinomyces israelii*, which produces granulomatous, suppurative lesions with abscesses. Common infection sites are the head, neck, thorax, and abdomen, but it can spread to contiguous tissues, causing multiple draining sinuses.

Causes and incidence

A. israelii occurs as part of the normal flora of the throat, tonsillar crypts, and mouth (particularly around carious teeth); infection results from its traumatic introduction into body tissues.

Actinomycosis affects twice as many males — especially those ages 15 to 35 — as females. People with dental disease or human immunodeficiency virus infection are at increased risk.

Signs and symptoms

Symptoms appear from days to months after injury and may vary, depending on the site of infection.

In *cervicofacial actinomycosis* (lumpy jaw), painful, indurated swellings appear in the mouth or neck up to several weeks after dental extraction or trauma. They gradually enlarge and form fistulas that open onto the skin. Sulfur granules (yellowish gray masses that are actually colonies of *A. israelii*) appear in the exudate.

In *pulmonary actinomycosis*, aspiration of bacteria from the mouth into areas of the lungs already anaerobic from infection or atelectasis produces a fever and a cough that becomes productive and occasionally causes hemoptysis. Eventually, empyema follows, a sinus forms through the chest wall, and septicemia may occur.

In *GI actinomycosis*, ileocecal lesions are caused by swallowed bacteria, which produce abdominal discomfort, fever, sometimes a palpable mass, and an external sinus. This follows intestinal mucosa disruption, usually by surgery or an inflammatory bowel condition such as appendicitis.

Rare sites of actinomycotic infection are the bones, brain, liver, kidneys, and female reproductive organs. Symptoms reflect the organ involved.

Diagnosis

CONFIRMING DIAGNOSIS *Isolation of* A. israelii *in exudate or tissue confirms actinomycosis. Other tests that help identify this condition are:*

■ *microscopic examination of sulfur granules*

■ *Gram staining of excised tissue or exudate to reveal branching gram-positive rods*

■ *chest X-ray to show lesions in unusual locations such as the shaft of a rib.*

Treatment

Treatment is long term, with 1 to 2 months of penicillin I.V. followed by 6 to 12 months of penicillin taken by mouth. Doxycycline usually isn't prescribed for children until after permanent teeth have erupted. In some cases, surgical drainage of the lesion may be required.

Special considerations
- Dispose of all dressings in a sealed plastic bag.
- After surgery, provide proper sterile wound management.
- Administer antibiotics as ordered. Before giving the first dose, obtain an accurate patient history of allergies. Watch for hypersensitivity reactions, such as rash, fever, itching, and signs of anaphylaxis. If the patient has a history of any allergies, keep epinephrine 1:1,000 and resuscitation equipment available.
- Stress the importance of good oral hygiene and proper dental care.

Nocardiosis

Nocardiosis is an acute, subacute, or chronic bacterial infection caused by a weakly gram-positive species of the genus *Nocardia* — usually *Nocardia asteroides*. It's most common in men, especially those with a compromised immune system. In patients with brain infection, mortality exceeds 80%; in other forms, mortality is 50%, even with appropriate therapy.

Causes
Nocardia are aerobic gram-positive bacteria with branching filaments resembling fungi. Normally found in soil, these organisms cause occasional sporadic disease in humans and animals throughout the world. Their incubation period is unknown but is probably several weeks. The usual mode of transmission is inhalation of organisms suspended in dust. Transmission by direct inoculation through puncture wounds or abrasions is less common.

Signs and symptoms
Nocardiosis originates as a pulmonary infection with a cough that produces thick, tenacious, purulent, mucopurulent, and possibly blood-tinged sputum. It may also cause a fever as high as 105° F (40.6° C), chills, night sweats, anorexia, malaise, and weight loss. This infection may lead to pleurisy, intrapleural effusions, and empye-

ma. Other potential complications include tracheitis, bronchitis, pericarditis, endocarditis, peritonitis, mediastinitis, septic arthritis, and keratoconjunctivitis.

If the infection spreads through the blood to the brain, abscesses form, causing confusion, disorientation, dizziness, headache, nausea, and seizures. Rupture of a brain abscess can cause purulent meningitis. Extrapulmonary, hematogenous spread may cause endocarditis or lesions in the kidneys, liver, subcutaneous tissue, and bone.

Diagnosis
Identifying *Nocardia* by culture of sputum or discharge is difficult. In many cases, special staining techniques must be used to make the diagnosis, in conjunction with a typical clinical picture (usually progressive pneumonia, despite antibiotic therapy). Occasionally, diagnosis requires biopsy of lung or other tissue. Chest X-rays vary and may show fluffy or interstitial infiltrates, nodules, or abscesses. Unfortunately, up to 40% of nocardial infections elude diagnosis until postmortem examination.

In brain infection with meningitis, lumbar puncture shows nonspecific changes such as increased opening pressure. Cerebrospinal fluid shows increased white blood cell and protein levels and decreased glucose levels compared with serum glucose.

Treatment
Nocardiosis requires at least 6 months of treatment, preferably with co-trimoxazole or high doses of sulfonamides. In patients who don't respond to sulfonamide treatment, other drugs, such as ampicillin, erythromycin, or minocycline, may be added. Treatment also includes surgical drainage of abscesses and excision of necrotic tissue. The acute phase requires complete bed rest; as the patient improves, activity can increase.

Special considerations
Because it isn't transmitted from person to person, nocardiosis requires no isolation.
- Provide adequate nourishment through total parenteral nutrition, nasogastric tube feedings, or a balanced diet.

■ Give the patient tepid sponge baths and antipyretics, as ordered, to reduce his fever.

■ Monitor for allergic reactions to antibiotics.

■ High-dose sulfonamide therapy (especially sulfadiazine) predisposes the patient to crystalluria and oliguria; so assess him frequently, force fluids, and alkalinize the urine with sodium bicarbonate, as ordered, to prevent these complications.

■ In patients with pulmonary infection, administer chest physiotherapy. Auscultate the lungs daily, checking for increased crackles or consolidation. Note and record the amount, color, and thickness of sputum.

■ In brain infection, regularly assess neurologic function. Watch for signs of increased intracranial pressure, such as a decreased level of consciousness and respiratory abnormalities.

■ In long-term hospitalization, turn the patient often, and assist with range-of-motion exercises.

■ Before the patient is discharged, stress the need to follow a regular medication schedule to maintain therapeutic blood levels and to continue drugs even after symptoms subside. Explain the importance of frequent follow-up examinations.

■ Provide support and encouragement to help the patient and his family cope with this long-term illness.

GRAM-NEGATIVE BACILLI

Salmonellosis

A common infection in the United States, salmonellosis is caused by gram-negative bacilli of the genus *Salmonella*, a member of the Enterobacteriaceae family. It occurs as enterocolitis, bacteremia, localized infection, typhoid, or paratyphoid fever. Nontyphoidal forms usually produce mild to moderate illness with low mortality. (See *Types of salmonellosis*, page 188.)

Typhoid, the most severe form of salmonellosis, usually lasts from 1 to 4 weeks. Mortality is about 3% in patients who are treated. In those who are untreated, 10% of cases result in fatality, usually as a result of intestinal perforation or hemorrhage, cerebral thrombosis, toxemia, pneumonia, or acute circulatory failure. An attack of typhoid confers lifelong immunity, although the patient may become a carrier. Salmonellosis is 20 times more common in patients with acquired immunodeficiency syndrome. Features are increased incidence of bacteremia, inability to identify the infection source, and tendency of infection to recur after therapy is stopped.

Causes and incidence

Of an estimated 1,700 serotypes of *Salmonella*, 10 cause the diseases most common in the United States; all 10 can survive for weeks in water, ice, sewage, or food. Nontyphoidal salmonellosis generally follows the ingestion of contaminated or inadequately processed foods, especially eggs, chicken, turkey, and duck. Proper cooking reduces the risk of contracting salmonellosis. Other causes include contact with infected people or animals or ingestion of contaminated dry milk, chocolate bars, or drugs of animal origin. Salmonellosis may occur in children younger than age 5 from fecal-oral spread. Enterocolitis and bacteremia are common (and more virulent) among infants, elderly persons, and people already weakened by other infections; paratyphoid fever is rare in the United States.

Typhoid usually results from drinking water contaminated by excretions of a carrier or from ingesting contaminated shellfish. (Contamination of shellfish occurs by leakage of sewage from offshore disposal depots.) Most typhoid patients are younger than age 30; most carriers are women older than age 50. Incidence of typhoid in the United States is increasing as a result of travelers returning from endemic areas.

Signs and symptoms

Clinical manifestations of salmonellosis vary but usually include fever, abdominal pain, and severe diarrhea with enterocolitis. Headache, increasing fever, and constipation are more common in typhoidal infection.

TYPES OF SALMONELLOSIS

Type	Cause	Clinical features
Bacteremia	Any *Salmonella* species, but most commonly *S. choleraesuis.* Incubation period: variable	Fever, chills, anorexia, weight loss (without GI symptoms), and joint pain
Enterocolitis	Any species of nontyphoidal *Salmonella,* but usually *S. enteritidis.* Incubation period: 6 to 48 hours	Mild to severe abdominal pain, diarrhea, sudden fever of up to 102° F (38.9° C), nausea, and vomiting; usually self-limiting, but may progress to enteric fever (resembling typhoid), local abscesses (usually abdominal), dehydration, and septicemia
Localized infections	Usually follows bacteremia caused by *Salmonella* species	Site of localization determines symptoms; localized abscesses may cause osteomyelitis, endocarditis, bronchopneumonia, pyelonephritis, and arthritis
Paratyphoid	*S. paratyphi* and *S. schottmuelleri* (formerly *S. paratyphi B*). Incubation period: 3 weeks or more	Fever and transient diarrhea; generally resembles typhoid but less severe
Typhoid fever	*S. typhi* enters the GI tract and invades the bloodstream via the lymphatics, setting up intracellular sites. During this phase, infection of the biliary tract leads to intestinal seeding with millions of bacilli. Involved lymphoid tissues (especially Peyer's patches in the ilium) enlarge, ulcerate, and necrose, resulting in hemorrhage. Incubation period: usually 1 to 2 weeks	Symptoms of enterocolitis may develop within hours of ingestion of *S. typhi;* they usually subside before onset of typhoid fever symptoms *First week:* gradually increasing fever, anorexia, myalgia, malaise, headache, and slow pulse *Second week:* remittent fever up to 104° F (40° C) usually in the evening, chills, diaphoresis, weakness, delirium, increasing abdominal pain and distention, diarrhea or constipation, cough, moist crackles, tender abdomen with enlarged spleen, and maculopapular rash (especially on abdomen) *Third week:* persistent fever, increasing fatigue and weakness; usually subsides by end of third week, although relapses may occur *Complications:* intestinal perforation or hemorrhage, abscesses, thrombophlebitis, cerebral thrombosis, pneumonia, osteomyelitis, myocarditis, acute circulatory failure, and chronic carrier state

Diagnosis

Generally, diagnosis depends on isolation of the organism in a culture, particularly blood (in typhoid, paratyphoid, and bacteremia) or feces (in enterocolitis, paratyphoid, and typhoid). Other appropriate culture specimens include urine, bone marrow, pus, and vomitus. In endemic areas, clinical symptoms of enterocolitis allow a working diagnosis before the cultures are positive. The presence of *Salmonella typhi* in stool 1 or more years after treatment indicates that the patient is a carrier, which is true of 3% of patients.

Widal's test, an agglutination reaction against somatic and flagellar antigens, may suggest typhoid with a fourfold rise in titer. However, drug use or hepatic disease can also increase these titers and invalidate test results. Other supportive laboratory values may include transient leukocytosis during the 1st week of typhoidal salmonellosis, leukopenia during the 3rd week, and leukocytosis in local infection.

Treatment

Antimicrobial therapy for typhoid, paratyphoid, and bacteremia depends on organism sensitivity. It may include amoxicillin, chloramphenicol and, in severely toxic patients, co-trimoxazole, ciprofloxacin, or ceftriaxone. Localized abscesses may also need surgical drainage. Enterocolitis requires a short course of antibiotics only if it causes septicemia or prolonged fever. Other treatments include bed rest and fluid and electrolyte replacement. The administration of camphorated opium tincture, kaolin with pectin, diphenoxylate, codeine, or small doses of morphine may be necessary to relieve diarrhea and control cramps in patients who must remain active.

Special considerations

■ All infections caused by *Salmonella* must be reported to the state health department.
■ Follow contact precautions if the patient is incontinent or diapered; otherwise, standard precautions are appropriate. Always wash your hands thoroughly before and after any contact with the patient, and advise other facility personnel to do the same. Teach the patient to use proper hand hygiene, especially after defecating and before eating or handling food. Wear gloves and a gown when disposing of feces or fecally contaminated objects. Continue precautions until three consecutive stool cultures are negative — the first one taken 48 hours after antibiotic treatment ends, followed by two more at 24-hour intervals.
■ Observe the patient closely for signs and symptoms of bowel perforation from erosion of intestinal ulcers: sudden pain in the lower right side of the abdomen and abdominal rigidity, possibly after one or more rectal bleeding episodes; sudden fall in temperature or blood pressure; and rising pulse rate (indicating shock).
■ During acute infection, plan care and activities to allow the patient as much rest as possible. Raise the side rails and use other safety measures, because the patient may become delirious. Assign him a room close to the nurses' station so he can be checked often. Use a room deodorizer (preferably electric) to minimize odor from diarrhea and to provide a comfortable atmosphere for rest.
■ Accurately record intake and output. Maintain adequate I.V. hydration. When the patient can tolerate oral feedings, encourage high-calorie fluids such as milkshakes. Watch for constipation.
■ Provide good skin and mouth care. Turn the patient frequently, and perform mild passive exercises, as indicated. Apply mild heat to the abdomen to relieve cramps.
■ *Don't* administer antipyretics. These mask fever and lead to possible hypothermia. Instead, to promote heat loss through the skin without causing shivering (which keeps fever high by vasoconstriction), apply tepid, wet towels (don't use alcohol or ice) to the patient's groin and axillae. To promote heat loss by vasodilation of peripheral blood vessels, use additional wet towels on the arms and legs, wiping with long, vigorous strokes.
■ After draining the abscesses of a joint, provide heat, elevation, and passive range-of-motion exercises to decrease swelling and maintain mobility.
■ If the patient has positive stool cultures on discharge, tell him to be sure to wash his hands after using the bathroom and to avoid preparing uncooked foods, such as salads, for family members. He also shouldn't work as a food handler until cultures are negative.
■ To prevent salmonellosis, advise the patient to refrigerate meat and cooked foods promptly and to avoid raw eggs or beverages mixed with raw eggs. Also teach the importance of proper hand hygiene. Advise those at high risk for contracting typhoid (laboratory workers or travelers) to seek vaccination.

Shigellosis

Shigellosis, also known as *bacillary dysentery*, is an acute intestinal infection caused by the bacteria *Shigella*, a short, nonmotile, gram-negative rod. *Shigella* can be classified into four groups, all of which may cause shigellosis: group A (*S. dysenteriae*), which is most common in Central America and causes particularly severe infection and septicemia; group B (*S. flexneri*); group C (*S. boydii*); and group D (*S. sonnei*). Typically, shigellosis causes a high fever (especially in children), acute self-limiting diarrhea with tenesmus (ineffectual straining at stool) and, possibly, electrolyte imbalance and dehydration. It's most common in children ages 1 to 4; however, many adults acquire the illness from children.

The prognosis is good. Mild infections usually subside within 10 days; severe infections may persist for 2 to 6 weeks. With prompt treatment, shigellosis is fatal in only 1% of cases, although in severe *S. dysenteriae* epidemic mortality may reach 8%.

Causes and incidence

Transmission occurs through the fecal-oral route; by direct contact with contaminated objects; or through ingestion of contaminated food or water. Occasionally, the housefly is a vector.

Shigellosis is endemic in North America, Europe, and the tropics. In the United States, about 18,000 cases appear annually, usually in children or in elderly, debilitated, or malnourished people. Shigellosis commonly occurs among confined populations, such as those in mental institutions or day-care centers.

Signs and symptoms

After an incubation period of 1 to 7 days (3 days is the average), *Shigella* organisms invade the intestinal mucosa and cause inflammation. In children, shigellosis usually produces high fever, diarrhea with tenesmus, nausea, vomiting, irritability, drowsiness, and abdominal pain and distention. Within a few days, the child's stool may contain pus, mucus, and—from the superficial intestinal ulceration typical of this infection—blood. Without treatment, dehydration and weight loss are rapid and overwhelming.

In adults, shigellosis produces sporadic, intense abdominal pain, which may be relieved at first by passing formed stools. Eventually, however, it causes rectal irritability, tenesmus and, in severe infection, headache and prostration. Stools may contain pus, mucus, and blood. Fever may be present.

Complications of shigellosis, such as electrolyte imbalance (especially hypokalemia), metabolic acidosis, and shock, aren't common but may be fatal in children and patients who are debilitated. Less common complications include conjunctivitis, iritis, arthritis, rectal prolapse, secondary bacterial infection, acute blood loss from mucosal ulcers, and toxic neuritis.

Diagnosis

CONFIRMING DIAGNOSIS *Fever (in children) and diarrhea with stools containing blood, pus, and mucus point to this diagnosis; microscopic bacteriologic studies and culture help confirm it.*

Microscopic examination of a fresh stool may reveal mucus, red blood cells, and polymorphonuclear leukocytes; direct immunofluorescence with specific antisera will demonstrate *Shigella*. Severe infection increases hemagglutinating antibodies. Sigmoidoscopy or proctoscopy may reveal typical superficial ulcerations.

Diagnosis must rule out other causes of diarrhea, such as enteropathogenic *Escherichia coli* infection, malabsorption diseases, and amebic or viral diseases.

Treatment

Treatment of shigellosis includes enteric precautions, low-residue diet and, most important, replacement of fluids and electrolytes with I.V. infusions of normal saline solution (with electrolytes) in sufficient quantities to maintain a urine output of 40 to 50 ml/hour. Antibiotics are of questionable value but may be used in an attempt to eliminate the pathogen and thereby prevent further spread. Ampicillin, tetracycline, or co-trimoxazole may be useful in severe cases, especially in children with overwhelming fluid and electrolyte loss.

Sulfamethoxazole-trimethoprim and ciprofloxacin are also used.

Antidiarrheals that slow intestinal motility are contraindicated in shigellosis because they delay fecal excretion of *Shigella* and prolong fever and diarrhea. An investigational vaccine containing attenuated strains of *Shigella* appears promising in preventing shigellosis.

Special considerations

Supportive care can minimize complications and increase patient comfort.

■ To prevent dehydration, administer I.V. fluids as ordered. Measure intake and output (including stools) carefully.

■ Correct identification of *Shigella* requires examination and culture of fresh stool specimens. Therefore, hand carry specimens directly to the laboratory. Because shigellosis is suspected, include this information on the laboratory slip.

■ Use a disposable hot-water bottle to relieve abdominal discomfort, and schedule care to conserve patient strength.

■ To help prevent spread of this disease, maintain enteric precautions until microscopic bacteriologic studies confirm that the stool specimen is negative. If a risk of exposure to the patient's stool exists, put on a gown and gloves before entering the room. Keep the patient's (and your own) nails short to avoid harboring organisms. Change soiled linen promptly and store in an isolation container.

■ During shigellosis outbreaks, obtain stool specimens from all potentially infected staff, and instruct those infected to remain away from work until two stool specimens are negative.

■ Report cases to the local health department.

Escherichia coli and other Enterobacteriaceae infections

The Enterobacteriaceae — a group of mostly aerobic, gram-negative bacilli — cause local and systemic infections, including an invasive diarrhea resembling shigella

ENTEROBACTERIAL INFECTIONS

The Enterobacteriaceae include *Escherichia coli, Arizona, Citrobacter, Enterobacter, Erwinia, Hafnia, Klebsiella, Morganella, Proteus, Providencia, Salmonella, Serratia, Shigella,* and *Yersinia.*

Enterobacterial infections are exogenous (from other people or the environment), endogenous (from one part of the body to another), or a combination of both. Enterobacteriaceae infections may cause any of a long list of bacterial diseases: bacterial (gram-negative) pneumonia, empyema, endocarditis, osteomyelitis, septic arthritis, urethritis, cystitis, bacterial prostatitis, urinary tract infection, pyelonephritis, perinephric abscess, abdominal abscesses, cellulitis, skin ulcers, appendicitis, gastroenterocolitis, diverticulitis, eyelid and periorbital cellulitis, corneal conjunctivitis, meningitis, bacteremia, and intracranial abscesses.

Appropriate antibiotic therapy depends on the results of culture and sensitivity tests. Generally, the aminoglycosides, cephalosporins, and penicillins — such as ampicillin, mezlocillin, and piperacillin — are most effective. Cefepime and quinones are also effective for some infections.

and, more commonly, a noninvasive toxin-mediated diarrhea resembling cholera. With other Enterobacteriaceae, *Escherichia coli* causes most nosocomial infections. Noninvasive, enterotoxin-producing *E. coli* infections may be a major cause of diarrheal illness in children in the United States. (See *Enterobacterial infections.*)

The prognosis in mild to moderate infection is good. Severe infection requires immediate fluid and electrolyte replacement to avoid fatal dehydration, especially among children, in whom mortality may be quite high.

Causes and incidence

Although some strains of *E. coli* exist as part of the normal GI flora, infection usually results from certain nonindigenous strains. For example, noninvasive diarrhea results from two toxins produced by strains called enterotoxic or enteropathogenic *E. coli*. Enteropathogenic *E. coli* serotype 0157:H7 is the most well-known strain in the United States. These toxins interact with intestinal juices and promote excessive loss of chloride and water. In the invasive form, *E. coli* directly invades the intestinal mucosa without producing enterotoxins, thereby causing local irritation, inflammation, and diarrhea. Normal strains can cause infection in immunocompromised patients.

Transmission can occur directly from an infected person or indirectly by ingestion of contaminated food or water or contact with contaminated utensils. Incubation takes 12 to 72 hours.

Incidence of *E. coli* infection is highest among travelers returning from other countries, particularly Mexico, Southeast Asia, and South America. *E. coli* infection also induces other diseases, especially in people whose resistance is low. The strain *E. coli* 0157:H7 has been associated with undercooked hamburger and with animals and petting zoos.

Signs and symptoms

Effects of noninvasive diarrhea depend on the causative toxin but may include the abrupt onset of watery diarrhea with cramping abdominal pain and, in severe illness, acidosis. Invasive infection produces chills, abdominal cramps, and diarrheal stools containing blood and pus.

Infantile diarrhea from an *E. coli* infection is usually noninvasive; it begins with loose, watery stools that change from yellow to green and contain little mucus or blood. Vomiting, listlessness, irritability, and anorexia commonly precede diarrhea. This condition can progress to fever, severe dehydration, acidosis, and shock. Bloody diarrhea may occur from infection with *E. coli* 0157:H7, which has also been associated with hemolytic uremic syndrome in children.

Diagnosis

Because certain strains of *E. coli* normally reside in the GI tract, culturing is of little value; a working diagnosis depends on clinical observation. However, if *E. coli* 0157:H7 is suspected, notify the laboratory so that appropriate testing of stool specimens can be performed.

A firm diagnosis requires sophisticated identification procedures, such as bioassays, that are expensive, time-consuming and, consequently, not widely available. Diagnosis must rule out salmonellosis and shigellosis, other common infections that produce similar signs and symptoms.

Treatment

Treatment consists of correction of fluid and electrolyte imbalances; for an infant or immunocompromised patient, I.V. antibiotics based on the organism's drug sensitivity; and salicylates or opium tincture for cramping and diarrhea.

Special considerations

■ Keep accurate intake and output records. Measure stool volume and note the presence of blood or pus. Replace fluids and electrolytes as needed, monitoring for decreased serum sodium and chloride levels and signs of gram-negative shock. Watch for signs of dehydration, such as poor skin turgor and dry mouth.

■ For infants, use contact precautions, give nothing by mouth, administer antibiotics as ordered, and maintain body warmth.

To prevent spread of this infection:

■ Prevent direct patient contact during epidemics. Report cases to local public health authorities. *E. coli* 0157:H7 is a reportable disease.

■ Use proper hand-hygiene technique. Teach health care personnel, patients, and their families to do the same.

■ Follow standard precautions. Provide the patient with a private room, wear protective clothing as necessary, such as when handling feces or soiled linens, and perform scrupulous hand hygiene before entering and after leaving the patient's room.

■ Advise travelers to foreign countries to avoid unbottled water and uncooked fruits and vegetables.

Pseudomonas infections

Pseudomonas is a small gram-negative bacillus that produces nosocomial infections, superinfections of various parts of the body, and a rare disease called melioidosis. This bacillus is also associated with bacteremia, endocarditis, and osteomyelitis in drug addicts. In local *Pseudomonas* infections, treatment is usually successful and complications rare; however, in patients with any type of lowered immunologic resistance— premature neonates; elderly patients; patients with debilitating disease, burns, or wounds; or patients receiving chemotherapy or radiation therapy— septicemic *Pseudomonas* infections are serious and commonly fatal.

Causes
The most common species of *Pseudomonas* is *P. aeruginosa*. Other species that typically cause disease in humans include *Xanthomonas maltophilia* (formerly known as *P. maltophilia*), *Burkholderia cepacia* (formerly known as *P. cepacia*), *P. fluorescens*, *P. testosteroni*, *P. acidovorans*, *P. alcaligenes*, *P. stutzeri*, *P. putrefaciens*, and *P. putida*. These organisms are commonly found in liquids that have been allowed to stand for a long time, such as benzalkonium chloride, saline solution, penicillin, water in flower vases, and fluids in incubators, humidifiers, and inhalation therapy equipment. *P. aeruginosa* is associated with chronic obstructive pulmonary disease. *B. cepacia* is the organism most closely associated with cystic fibrosis, although *P. aeruginosa* is also associated with it. In elderly patients, *Pseudomonas* infection usually enters through the genitourinary tract; in neonates and infants, through the umbilical cord, skin, and GI tract.

Signs and symptoms
The most common infections associated with *Pseudomonas* include skin infections (such as burns and pressure ulcers), urinary tract infections, infant epidemic diar-

MELIOIDOSIS

Melioidosis results from wound penetration, inhalation, or ingestion of the gram-negative bacteria *Pseudomonas pseudomallei*. Although it was once confined to Southeast Asia, Central America, South America, Madagascar, and Guam, incidence in the United States has risen as a result of the influx of Southeast Asians.

Melioidosis occurs in two forms: chronic melioidosis, which causes osteomyelitis and lung abscesses, and the rare acute melioidosis, which causes pneumonia, bacteremia, and prostration. Acute melioidosis is commonly fatal; however, most melioidosis infections are chronic and asymptomatic, producing clinical symptoms only with accompanying malnutrition, major surgery, or severe burns.

Diagnostic measures consist of isolation of *P. pseudomallei* in a culture of exudate, blood, or sputum; serology tests (complement fixation, passive hemagglutination); and chest X-ray (findings resemble tuberculosis). Treatment includes oral tetracycline and co-trimoxazole, abscess drainage and, in severe cases, chloramphenicol until X-rays show resolution of primary abscesses.

The prognosis is good because most patients have a mild infection and acquire permanent immunity; aggressive use of antibiotics and sulfonamides has improved the prognosis in acute melioidosis.

rhea and other diarrheal illnesses, bronchitis, pneumonia, bronchiectasis, meningitis, corneal ulcers, mastoiditis, otitis externa, otitis media, endocarditis, and bacteremia.

Drainage in *Pseudomonas* infections has a distinct, sickly sweet odor and a greenish blue pus that forms a crust on wounds. Other symptoms depend on the site of infection. (See *Melioidosis.*) For example, when it invades the lungs, *Pseudomonas* causes pneumonia with fever, chills, and a productive cough.

Diagnosis

 CONFIRMING DIAGNOSIS *Diagnosis requires isolation of the* Pseudomonas *organism in blood, spinal fluid, urine, exudate, or sputum culture.*

Treatment

In the debilitated or otherwise vulnerable patient with clinical evidence of *Pseudomonas* infection, treatment should begin immediately, without waiting for results of laboratory tests. Antibiotic treatment includes aminoglycosides, such as gentamicin or tobramycin, combined with an antipseudomonal penicillin, such as ticarcillin or piperacillin. An alternative combination is amikacin and a similar penicillin or imipenem and cilastatin. Such combination therapy is necessary because *Pseudomonas* quickly becomes resistant to ticarcillin alone.

Local *Pseudomonas* infections or septicemia secondary to wound infection requires 1% acetic acid irrigations; topical applications of colistimethate, polymyxin B, and silver sulfadiazine cream; and debridement or drainage of the infected wound.

Special considerations

- Observe and record the character of wound exudate and sputum.
- Before administering antibiotics, ask the patient about a history of drug allergies, especially to penicillin. If combinations of piperacillin or ticarcillin and an aminoglycoside are ordered, schedule the doses 1 hour apart (ticarcillin may decrease the antibiotic effect of the aminoglycoside). *Don't* give both antibiotics through the same administration set.
- Monitor the patient's renal function (output, blood urea nitrogen level, specific gravity, urinalysis, and creatinine level) during treatment with aminoglycosides. Obtain drug levels to ensure effectiveness.
- Protect immunocompromised patients from exposure to this infection. Proper hand hygiene and sterile techniques prevent further spread.

- To prevent *Pseudomonas* infection, maintain proper endotracheal and tracheostomy suctioning technique. Use strict sterile technique when caring for I.V. lines, catheters, and other tubes. Discard suction bottles, irrigating fluid, and open bottles of saline solution every 24 hours. Be sure to change I.V. tubing according to hospital policy and to empty ventilator water reservoirs before refilling them with sterile water. Remember to use suction catheters only once.

Cholera

Cholera (also known as *Asiatic cholera* or *epidemic cholera*) is an acute enterotoxin-mediated GI infection caused by the gram-negative bacillus *Vibrio cholerae*. It produces profuse diarrhea, vomiting, massive fluid and electrolyte loss and, possibly, hypovolemic shock, metabolic acidosis, and death. A similar bacterium, *Vibrio parahaemolyticus,* causes food poisoning. (See Vibrio parahaemolyticus *food poisoning.*)

Even with prompt diagnosis and treatment, cholera is fatal in up to 2% of children; in adults, it's fatal in less than 1%. However, untreated cholera may be fatal in as many as 50% of patients. Cholera infection confers only transient immunity.

Causes and incidence

Humans are the only hosts and victims of *V. cholerae*, a motile, aerobic organism. It's transmitted through food and water contaminated with fecal material from carriers or people with active infections. Cholera is most common in Africa, southern and Southeast Asia, and the Middle East, although outbreaks have occurred in Japan, Australia, and Europe. Infection also occurs after eating shellfish from recognized environmental reservoirs of cholera, including one that's along the United States' Gulf of Mexico coast.

Cholera occurs during the warmer months and is most prevalent among lower socioeconomic groups. In India, it's common among children ages 1 to 5, but in other endemic areas, it's equally distributed among all age-groups. Susceptibility to cholera may be increased by a deficiency or an absence of hydrochloric acid.

Signs and symptoms

After an incubation period ranging from several hours to 5 days, cholera produces acute, painless, profuse, watery diarrhea and effortless vomiting (without preceding nausea). As diarrhea worsens, the stools contain white flecks of mucus (rice-water stools). Because of massive fluid and electrolyte losses from diarrhea and vomiting (fluid loss in adults may reach 1 L/hour), cholera causes intense thirst, weakness, loss of skin turgor, wrinkled skin, sunken eyes, pinched facial expression, muscle cramps (especially in the extremities), cyanosis, oliguria, tachycardia, tachypnea, thready or absent peripheral pulses, falling blood pressure, fever, and inaudible, hypoactive bowel sounds.

Patients usually remain oriented but apathetic, although small children may become stuporous or develop seizures. If complications don't occur, the symptoms subside and the patient recovers within a week. However, if treatment is delayed or inadequate, cholera may lead to metabolic acidosis, uremia and, possibly, coma and death. About 3% of patients who recover continue to carry *V. cholerae* in the gallbladder; however, most patients are free from the infection after about 2 weeks.

Diagnosis

In endemic areas or during epidemics, characteristic clinical features strongly suggest cholera.

 CONFIRMING DIAGNOSIS *A culture of* V. cholerae *from feces or vomitus indicates cholera; however, definitive diagnosis requires agglutination and other clear reactions to group- and type-specific antisera.*

A dark-field microscopic examination of fresh feces showing rapidly moving bacilli (like shooting stars) allows for a quick, tentative diagnosis. Immunofluorescence also allows rapid diagnosis. Diagnosis must rule out *Escherichia coli* infection, salmonellosis, and shigellosis.

VIBRIO PARAHAEMOLYTICUS FOOD POISONING

Vibrio parahaemolyticus is a common cause of gastroenteritis in Japan. Outbreaks also occur on American cruise ships and in the eastern and southeastern coastal areas of the United States, especially during the summer.

V. parahaemolyticus, which thrives in a salty environment, is transmitted by ingesting uncooked or undercooked contaminated shellfish, particularly crab and shrimp. After an incubation period of 2 to 48 hours, *V. parahaemolyticus* causes watery diarrhea, moderately severe cramps, nausea, vomiting, headache, weakness, chills, and fever. Food poisoning is usually self-limiting and subsides spontaneously within 2 days. Occasionally, however, it's more severe, and may even be fatal in debilitated or elderly persons.

Diagnosis requires bacteriologic examination of vomitus, blood, stool smears, or fecal specimens collected by rectal swab. Diagnosis must rule out not only other causes of food poisoning but also other acute GI disorders.

Treatment is supportive, consisting primarily of bed rest and oral fluid replacement. I.V. replacement therapy is seldom necessary, but oral tetracycline may be prescribed. Thorough cooking of seafood prevents this infection.

Treatment

Improved sanitation and the administration of cholera vaccine to travelers in endemic areas can control this disease. Unfortunately, the vaccine now available confers only 60% to 80% immunity and is effective for only 3 to 6 months. Consequently, vaccination is impractical for residents of endemic areas.

Treatment requires rapid I.V. infusion of large amounts (50 to 100 ml/minute) of isotonic saline solution, alternating with isotonic sodium bicarbonate or sodium lactate. Potassium replacement may be added to the I.V. solution. Antibiotic therapy using such drugs as tetracycline, bactrim, erythromycin, and ciprofloxacin can shorten the course of infection and reduce the rehydration requirement.

When I.V. infusions have corrected hypovolemia, fluid infusion decreases to quantities sufficient to maintain normal pulse and skin turgor or to replace fluid loss through diarrhea. An oral glucose-electrolyte solution can substitute for I.V. infusions. In mild cholera, oral fluid replacement is adequate. If symptoms persist despite fluid and electrolyte replacement, treatment includes tetracycline.

Special considerations

A cholera patient requires contact precautions, supportive care, and close observation during the acute phase.

■ Wear a gown and gloves when handling feces-contaminated articles or when a danger of contaminating clothing exists, and wash your hands after leaving the patient's room.

■ Monitor output (including stool volume) and I.V. infusion accurately. To detect overhydration, carefully observe neck veins, take serial patient weights, and auscultate the lungs (fluid loss in cholera is massive, and improper replacement may cause potentially fatal renal insufficiency).

■ Protect the patient's family by administering oral tetracycline or doxycycline, if ordered.

■ Advise anyone traveling to an endemic area to boil all drinking water and avoid uncooked vegetables and unpeeled fruits.

Septic shock

Second only to cardiogenic shock as the leading cause of shock-related death, septic shock causes inadequate tissue perfusion, abnormalities of oxygen supply and demand, metabolic changes, and circulatory collapse. It typically occurs among hospitalized patients, usually as a result of bacterial infection. About 25% of patients who develop gram-negative bacteremia go into shock. Unless vigorous treatment begins promptly, preferably before symptoms fully develop, septic shock rapidly progresses to death (in many cases within a few hours) in up to 80% of these patients. Septic shock is the most common cause of death in acute care units in the United States.

Causes

In two-thirds of patients, septic shock results from infection with the gram-negative bacteria *Escherichia coli, Klebsiella, Enterobacter, Proteus, Pseudomonas,* or *Bacteroides*; in a few, from the gram-positive bacteria *Streptococcus pneumoniae, Streptococcus pyogenes, Staphylococcus aureus,* or *Actinomyces.* Infections with viruses, rickettsiae, chlamydiae, and protozoa may be complicated by shock.

These organisms produce septicemia in people whose resistance is already compromised by an existing condition; infection also results from translocation of bacteria from other areas of the body through surgery, I.V. therapy, and catheters. Septic shock commonly occurs in patients hospitalized for primary infection of the genitourinary, biliary, GI, or gynecologic tract. Other predisposing factors include immunodeficiency, advanced age, trauma, burns, diabetes mellitus, cirrhosis, and disseminated cancer.

Signs and symptoms

Signs and symptoms of septic shock vary according to the stage of shock, the organism causing it, and the patient's immune response and age:

■ *early stage*— oliguria, sudden fever (over 101° F [38.3° C]), and chills; tachypnea, tachycardia, full bounding pulse, hyperglycemia, nausea, vomiting, diarrhea, and prostration

■ *late stage*— restlessness, apprehension, irritability, thirst from decreased cerebral tissue perfusion, hypoglycemia, hypothermia, and anuria. Hypotension, altered level of consciousness, and hyperventilation may be the *only* signs among infants and the elderly.

Complications of septic shock include disseminated intravascular coagulation

(DIC), renal failure, heart failure, GI ulcers, and hepatic dysfunction.

Diagnosis

One or more typical symptoms (fever, confusion, nausea, vomiting, and hyperventilation) in a patient suspected of having an infection suggests septic shock and necessitates immediate treatment.

In early stages, arterial blood gas (ABG) levels indicate respiratory alkalosis (low partial pressure of carbon dioxide [$PaCO_2$], low or normal bicarbonate [HCO_3^-], and high pH). As shock progresses, metabolic acidosis develops with hypoxemia, indicated by decreasing $PaCO_2$ (may increase as respiratory failure ensues); partial pressure of oxygen; HCO_3^-, and pH.

The following tests support the diagnosis and determine the treatment:

- blood cultures to isolate the organism
- decreased platelet count and leukocytosis (15,000 to 30,000/µl)
- increased blood urea nitrogen and creatinine levels, decreased creatinine clearance
- abnormal prothrombin consumption and partial thromboplastin time
- simultaneous measurement of urine and plasma osmolalities for renal failure (urine osmolality below 400 mOsm, with a ratio of urine to plasma below 1.5)
- decreased central venous pressure (CVP), pulmonary artery pressure, and pulmonary artery wedge pressure (PAWP); decreased cardiac output (in early septic shock, cardiac output increases); low systemic vascular resistance
- on electrocardiogram, ST-segment depression, inverted T waves, and arrhythmias resembling myocardial infarction.

Treatment

The first goal of treatment is to monitor for and then reverse shock through volume expansion with I.V. fluids and insertion of a pulmonary artery catheter to check PAWP. Administration of whole blood or plasma can then raise the PAWP to a high normal to slightly elevated level of 14 to 18 mm Hg. A ventilator may be necessary to overcome hypoxia. Urinary catheterization allows accurate measurement of hourly urine output.

Treatment also requires immediate administration of I.V. antibiotics to control the infection. Depending on the organism, the antibiotic combination usually includes an aminoglycoside (such as amikacin, gentamicin, or tobramycin) for gram-negative bacteria combined with a penicillin (such as ticarcillin or piperacillin). Sometimes treatment includes a cephalosporin or vancomycin for suspected staphylococcal infection. Therapy may include chloramphenicol for nonsporulating anaerobes (*Bacteroides*), which may cause bone marrow depression, and clindamycin, which may produce pseudomembranous enterocolitis. Metronidazole can also be used for anaerobic infection. Appropriate antibiotics for other causes of septic shock depend on the suspected organism. Other measures to combat infection include surgery to drain and excise abscesses and debridement.

If shock persists after fluid infusion, treatment with vasopressors, such as dopamine, maintains adequate blood perfusion in the brain, liver, GI tract, kidneys, and skin. In adults with severe sepsis who have a high risk of death, drotrecogin alfa may be used to interrupt the sepsis cascade. Other treatment includes I.V. bicarbonate to correct acidosis and corticosteroids (especially in patients with gram-negative septic shock). Other experimental treatments include opioid antagonists, prostaglandin inhibitors, and calcium channel blockers, which are used to block the rapid inflammatory process.

Special considerations

Determine which of your patients are at high risk for developing septic shock. Know the signs of impending septic shock, but don't rely solely on technical aids to judge the patient's status. Consider any change in mental status and urine output as significant as a change in CVP. Report such changes promptly.

- Carefully maintain the pulmonary artery catheter. Check ABG levels for adequate oxygenation or gas exchange, and report any changes immediately.
- Record intake and output and daily weight. Maintain adequate urine output

(0.5 to 1 ml/kg/hour) and systolic pressure. Avoid fluid overload.

- Monitor serum antibiotic levels, and administer drugs as ordered.

 ALERT *Watch closely for signs of DIC (abnormal bleeding), renal failure (oliguria, increased specific gravity), heart failure (dyspnea, edema, tachycardia, distended neck veins), GI ulcers (hematemesis and melena), and hepatic abnormality (jaundice, hypoprothrombinemia, and hypoalbuminemia).*

Haemophilus influenzae infection

Haemophilus influenzae causes diseases in many organ systems but usually attacks the respiratory system. It's a common cause of epiglottitis, laryngotracheobronchitis, pneumonia, bronchiolitis, otitis media, and meningitis. Less commonly, it causes bacterial endocarditis, conjunctivitis, facial cellulitis, septic arthritis, and osteomyelitis.

Causes and incidence

H. influenzae, the cause of this infection, is a small, gram-negative, pleomorphic aerobic bacillus. Transmission occurs by direct contact with secretions or by respiratory droplets. It infects about half of all children before age 1 and virtually all children by age 3, although a haemophilus influenza b vaccine given at ages 2, 4, and 6 months has reduced this number.

Signs and symptoms

H. influenzae provokes a characteristic tissue response—acute suppurative inflammation. When *H. influenzae* infects the larynx, trachea, or bronchial tree, it leads to irritable cough, dyspnea, mucosal edema, and thick, purulent exudate. When it invades the lungs, it leads to bronchopneumonia. In the pharynx, *H. influenzae* usually produces no remarkable changes, except when it causes epiglottitis, which generally affects both the laryngeal and pharyngeal surfaces. The pharyngeal mucosa may be reddened, rarely with soft yellow exudate. Usually, though, it appears normal or shows only slight diffuse redness, even while severe pain makes swallowing diffi-

cult or impossible. *H. influenzae* infections typically cause high fever and generalized malaise. Meningitis, the most serious infection caused by *H. influenzae,* is indicated by fever and altered mental status. In young children, nuchal rigidity may be absent.

Diagnosis

 CONFIRMING DIAGNOSIS *Isolation of the organism, usually with a blood culture, confirms the diagnosis of* H. influenzae *infection.*

Other laboratory findings include:
- polymorphonuclear leukocytosis (15,000 to 30,000/μl)
- leukopenia (2,000 to 3,000/μl) in young children with severe infection
- *H. influenzae* bacteremia, found in many patients with meningitis.

Treatment

H. influenzae infections usually respond to a course of ampicillin, cefotaxime, gatifloxacin, moxifloxacin, or ceftriaxone as an initial treatment, although resistant strains are becoming more common. As an alternative, a combination of chloramphenicol and ampicillin is prescribed. If the strain proves susceptible to ampicillin, chloramphenicol is discontinued.

Special considerations

- Maintain adequate respiratory function through proper positioning, humidification (croup tent) in children, and suctioning, as needed. Monitor rate and type of respirations. Watch for signs of cyanosis and dyspnea, which require intubation or a tracheotomy. Monitor the patient's level of consciousness (LOC); decreased LOC may indicate hypoxemia. For home treatment, suggest using a room humidifier or breathing moist air from a shower or bath, as necessary.
- Check the patient's history for drug allergies before administering antibiotics. Monitor his complete blood count for signs of bone marrow depression when therapy includes ampicillin or chloramphenicol.
- Monitor the patient's intake (including I.V. infusions) and output. Watch for signs of dehydration, such as decreased skin tur-

gor, parched lips, concentrated urine, decreased urine output, and increased pulse rate.

- Organize your physical care measures beforehand, and do them quickly so as not to disrupt the patient's rest.

- Take preventive measures, such as vaccinating infants, maintaining droplet precautions, using proper hand-hygiene technique, properly disposing of respiratory secretions, placing soiled tissues in a plastic bag, and decontaminating all equipment.

Whooping cough

Whooping cough, also known as *pertussis,* is a highly contagious respiratory infection usually caused by the nonmotile, gram-negative coccobacillus *Bordetella pertussis* and, occasionally, by the related similar bacteria *B. parapertussis* and *B. bronchiseptica.* Characteristically, whooping cough produces an irritating cough that becomes paroxysmal and commonly ends in a high-pitched inspiratory whoop.

Since the 1940s, immunization and aggressive diagnosis and treatment have significantly reduced mortality from whooping cough in the United States. Mortality in children younger than age 1 is usually a result of pneumonia and other complications. The disease is also dangerous in the elderly but tends to be less severe in older children and adults.

Causes and incidence
Whooping cough is usually transmitted by the direct inhalation of contaminated droplets from a patient in the acute stage; it may also be spread indirectly through soiled linen and other articles contaminated by respiratory secretions.

Whooping cough is endemic throughout the world, usually occurring in late winter and early spring. In about 50% of cases, it strikes unimmunized children younger than age 1, because the immunization series hasn't been completed and the child has had contact with an adult harboring the organisms.

Signs and symptoms
After an incubation period of about 7 to 10 days, *B. pertussis* enters the tracheobronchial mucosa, where it produces progressively tenacious mucus. Whooping cough follows a classic 6-week course that includes three stages, each of which lasts about 2 weeks.

First, the *catarrhal stage* characteristically produces an irritating hacking, nocturnal cough, anorexia, sneezing, listlessness, infected conjunctiva and, occasionally, a low-grade fever. This stage is highly communicable.

After a period of 7 to 14 days, the *paroxysmal stage* produces spasmodic and recurrent coughing that may expel tenacious mucus. Each cough characteristically ends in a loud, crowing inspiratory whoop; excessive coughing; and choking on mucus, causing vomiting. (Patients with persistent cough should be evaluated for whooping cough, because not every patient will develop paroxysms or the distinctive whooping sound.) Paroxysmal coughing may induce such complications as nosebleed, increased venous pressure, periorbital edema, conjunctival hemorrhage, hemorrhage of the anterior chamber of the eye, detached retina (and blindness), rectal prolapse, inguinal or umbilical hernia, seizures, atelectasis, and pneumonitis. In infants, choking spells may cause apnea, anoxia, and disturbed acid-base balance. During this stage, patients are highly vulnerable to fatal secondary bacterial or viral infections. Suspect such secondary infection (usually otitis media or pneumonia) in any whooping cough patient with a fever during this stage, because whooping cough itself seldom causes fever.

During the *convalescent stage,* paroxysmal coughing and vomiting gradually subside. However, for months afterward, even a mild upper respiratory tract infection may trigger paroxysmal coughing. (Paroxysmal coughing may not be present in partially immunized individuals.)

Diagnosis
Classic clinical findings, especially during the paroxysmal stage, suggest this diagnosis; laboratory studies will confirm it. Nasopharyngeal swabs and sputum cultures

show *B. pertussis* only in the early stages of this disease; fluorescent antibody screening of nasopharyngeal smears provides quicker results than cultures but is less reliable. In addition, the white blood cell (WBC) count is usually increased, especially in children older than age 6 months and early in the paroxysmal stage. Sometimes, the WBC count may reach 175,000 to 200,000/µl, with 60% to 90% lymphocytes.

Treatment

Vigorous supportive therapy requires hospitalization of infants (commonly in the intensive care unit) and fluid and electrolyte replacement. Other measures include adequate nutrition; codeine and mild sedation to decrease coughing; oxygen therapy in apnea; and antibiotics, such as erythromycin and, possibly, ampicillin, to shorten the period of communicability and prevent secondary infections.

Because very young infants (younger than age 1) are particularly susceptible to whooping cough, immunization — most commonly with the diphtheria-tetanus acellular-pertussis vaccine — begins at ages 2, 4, and 6 months. Boosters follow at age 18 months and at ages 4 to 6. The risk of pertussis is greater than the risk of vaccine complications such as neurologic damage. However, seizures or unusual and persistent crying may be a sign of a severe neurologic reaction, and the physician may not order the other doses. The vaccine is contraindicated in children older than age 6 because it can cause a severe fever.

Special considerations

Whooping cough calls for aggressive, supportive care and droplet precautions (surgical masks only) for 5 to 7 days after initiation of antibiotic therapy.
■ Monitor acid-base, fluid, and electrolyte balances.
■ Carefully suction secretions, and monitor oxygen therapy. *Remember:* Suctioning removes oxygen as well as secretions.
■ Create a quiet environment to decrease coughing stimulation. Provide small, frequent meals, and treat constipation or nausea caused by codeine.
■ Offer emotional support to the parents of children with whooping cough.

■ To decrease exposure to organisms, empty the suction bottle and change the trash bag at least once each shift. Change soiled linens as often as needed.

Plague

Plague, also known as the *black death,* is an acute infection caused by the gram-negative, nonmotile, nonsporulating bacillus *Yersinia pestis* (formerly called *Pasteurella pestis*).

Plague occurs in several forms. *Bubonic plague,* the most common, causes the characteristic swollen, and sometimes suppurating, lymph glands (buboes) that give this infection its name. Other forms include *septicemic plague,* a severe, rapid systemic form, and *pneumonic plague,* which can be primary or secondary to the other two forms. *Primary pneumonic plague* is an acutely fulminant, highly contagious form that causes acute prostration, respiratory distress, and death — in many cases within 2 to 3 days after onset.

Without treatment, mortality is about 60% in bubonic plague and approaches 100% in both septicemic and pneumonic plagues. With treatment, mortality is approximately 18% for all forms of plague, largely due to the delay between onset and treatment and the patient's age and physical condition.

Causes and incidence

Plague is usually transmitted to humans through the bite of a flea from an infected rodent host, such as a rat, squirrel, prairie dog, or hare. (See *Carrier of bubonic plague.*) Occasionally, transmission occurs from handling infected animals or their tissues. Bubonic plague is notorious for the historic pandemics in Europe and Asia during the Middle Ages, which in some areas killed up to two-thirds of the population. This form is rarely transmitted from person to person. However, the untreated bubonic form may progress to a secondary pneumonic form, which is transmitted by contaminated respiratory droplets (coughing) and is highly contagious. In the United States, the primary pneumonic form usually occurs after inhalation of *Y. pestis* in a laboratory.

Sylvatic (wild rodent) plague remains endemic in South America, the Near East, central and Southeast Asia, north central and southern Africa, Mexico, and western United States and Canada. In the United States, its incidence has been rising, a possible reflection of different bacterial strains or environmental changes that favor rodent growth in certain areas. Plague tends to occur between May and September; between October and February it usually occurs in hunters who skin wild animals. One attack confers permanent immunity.

Signs and symptoms
The incubation period, early symptoms, severity at onset, and clinical course vary in the three forms of plague. In *bubonic plague*, the incubation period is 2 to 8 days. The milder form begins with malaise, fever, and pain or tenderness in regional lymph nodes, possibly associated with swelling. Lymph node damage (usually axillary or inguinal) eventually produces painful, inflamed, and possibly suppurative buboes. The classic sign of plague is an excruciatingly painful bubo. Hemorrhagic areas may become necrotic; in the skin, such areas appear dark—hence the name "black death."

This infection can progress extremely rapidly. A seemingly mildly ill person with only fever and adenitis may become moribund within hours. Plague may also begin dramatically, with a sudden high fever of 103° to 106° F (39.4° to 41.1° C), chills, myalgia, headache, prostration, restlessness, disorientation, delirium, toxemia, and staggering gait. Occasionally, it causes abdominal pain, nausea, vomiting, and constipation followed by diarrhea (frequently bloody), skin mottling, petechiae, and circulatory collapse.

In *primary pneumonic plague*, the incubation period is 2 to 3 days followed by a typically acute onset, with high fever, chills, severe headache, tachycardia, tachypnea, dyspnea, and a productive cough (first mucoid sputum, later frothy pink or red).

Secondary pneumonic plague, the pulmonary extension of the bubonic form, complicates about 5% of cases of untreated plague. A cough producing bloody sputum

CARRIER OF BUBONIC PLAGUE

Bubonic plague is usually transmitted to humans through the bite of a flea (*Xenopsylla cheopis*), shown here.

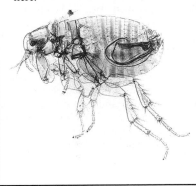

signals this complication. Both the primary and secondary forms of pneumonic plague rapidly cause severe prostration, respiratory distress and, usually, death.

Septicemic plague usually develops without overt lymph node enlargement. In this form, the patient shows toxicity, hyperpyrexia, seizures, prostration, shock, and disseminated intravascular coagulation (DIC). Septicemic plague causes widespread nonspecific tissue damage—such as peritoneal or pleural effusions, pericarditis, and meningitis. It's rapidly fatal unless promptly and correctly treated.

Diagnosis
Because plague is rare in the United States, it's commonly overlooked until after the patient dies or multiple cases develop. Characteristic buboes and a history of exposure to rodents in known endemic areas strongly suggest bubonic plague.

CONFIRMING DIAGNOSIS
Stained smears and cultures of Y. pestis *obtained from a needle aspirate of a small amount of fluid from skin lesions confirm this diagnosis.*

Postmortem examination of a guinea pig inoculated with a sample of blood or purulent drainage allows isolation of the organism. Other laboratory findings include a white blood cell count of over 20,000/μl with increased polymorphonuclear leukocytes and hemoagglutination reaction (antibody titer) studies. Diagnosis should rule out tularemia, typhus, and typhoid.

In pneumonic plague, diagnosis requires a chest X-ray to show fulminating pneumonia and stained smear and culture of sputum to identify *Y. pestis*. Other bacterial pneumonias and psittacosis must be ruled out. Stained smear and blood culture containing *Y. pestis* are diagnostic in septicemic plague. However, cultures of *Y. pestis* grow slowly; so, in suspected plague (especially pneumonic and septicemic plagues), treatment should begin without waiting for laboratory confirmation. For a presumptive diagnosis of plague, a fluorescent antibody test may be ordered.

Treatment
Antimicrobial treatment of suspected plague must begin immediately after blood specimens have been taken for culture and shouldn't be delayed for laboratory confirmation. Generally, treatment consists of large doses of streptomycin, the drug proven most effective against *Y. pestis*. Other effective drugs include gentamicin, doxycycline, tetracycline, and chloramphenicol. Penicillins are ineffective against plague.

In both septicemic and pneumonic plagues, life-saving antimicrobial treatment must begin within 18 hours of onset. Supportive management aims to control fever, shock, and seizures and to maintain fluid balance.

After antimicrobial therapy has begun, glucocorticoids can combat life-threatening toxemia and shock; diazepam relieves restlessness; and, if the patient develops DIC, treatment may include heparin.

Special considerations
■ Patients with bubonic plague require standard precautions.
■ Use an approved insecticide to rid the patient and his clothing of fleas. Carefully dispose of soiled dressings and linens, feces, and sputum. If the patient has pneumonic plague, wear a mask and follow droplet precautions. Handle all exudates, purulent discharge, and laboratory specimens with gloves. For more information, consult your infection control officer.
■ Give drugs and treat complications as ordered.
■ Treat buboes with hot, moist compresses. Never excise or drain them because this could spread the infection.
■ When septicemic plague causes peripheral tissue necrosis, prevent further injury to necrotic tissue. Avoid using restraints or armboards, and pad the bed's side rails.
■ For patients with pneumonic plague, obtain a history of patient contacts so that they can be quarantined for 7 days of observation. Administer prophylactic tetracycline or chloramphenicol, as ordered.
■ Report suspected cases of plague to local public health department officials so they can identify the source of infection.
■ To help prevent plague, discourage contact with wild animals (especially those that are sick or dead), and support programs aimed at reducing insect and rodent populations. Recommend immunization with plague vaccine to travelers to, or residents of, endemic areas, even though the effect of immunization is transient.

Brucellosis

Brucellosis (also known as *undulant fever, Malta fever,* or *Bang's disease*) is an acute febrile illness transmitted to humans from animals. It's caused by the nonmotile, nonspore-forming, gram-negative coccobacilli of the genus *Brucella*, notably *B. suis* (found in swine), *B. melitensis* (in goats and sheep), *B. abortus* (in cattle), and *B. canis* (in dogs). Brucellosis causes fever; profuse sweating; anxiety; general aching; and bone, spleen, liver, kidney, or brain abscesses.

The prognosis is good. With treatment, brucellosis is seldom fatal, although complications can cause permanent disability.

Causes and incidence
Brucellosis is transmitted through the consumption of unpasteurized dairy products and through contact with infected animals or their secretions or excretions. It's most common among farmers, stock handlers,

butchers, and veterinarians. Because of such occupational risks, brucellosis infects six times more men than women, especially those between ages 20 and 50; it's less common in children. Because hydrochloric acid in gastric juices kills *Brucella* bacteria, people with achlorhydria are particularly susceptible to this disease.

Although brucellosis occurs throughout the world, it's most prevalent in the Middle East, Africa, the former Soviet Union, India, South America, and Europe; it's seldom found in the United States. The incubation period usually lasts from 5 to 60 days, but in some cases it can last for months.

Signs and symptoms

Onset of brucellosis is usually insidious, but the disease course falls into two distinct phases. Characteristically, the acute phase causes fever, chills, profuse sweating, fatigue, headache, backache, enlarged lymph nodes, hepatosplenomegaly, weight loss, and abscess and granuloma formulation in subcutaneous tissues, lymph nodes, liver, and spleen. Despite this disease's common name — undulant fever — few patients have a truly intermittent (undulant) fever; in fact, fever is commonly insignificant. It may be observed if the patient goes without treatment for a long time.

The chronic phase produces recurrent depression, sleep disturbances, fatigue, headache, sweating, and sexual impotence; hepatosplenomegaly and enlarged lymph nodes persist. In addition, abscesses may form in the testes, ovaries, kidneys, and brain (meningitis and encephalitis). About 10% to 15% of patients with such brain abscesses develop hearing and visual disorders, hemiplegia, and ataxia. Other complications include osteomyelitis, orchitis and, rarely, subacute bacterial endocarditis, which is difficult to treat.

Diagnosis

In patients with characteristic clinical features, a history of exposure to animals, occupational exposure, or ingestion of high-risk foods suggests brucellosis. Multiple agglutination tests help to confirm the diagnosis. Approximately 90% of patients with brucellosis have agglutinin titers of 1:160 or more within 3 weeks of developing this disease. However, elevated agglutinin titers also follow vaccination against tularemia, *Yersinia* infection, or cholera; skin tests; or relapse. Agglutinin titers testing can also monitor effectiveness of treatment.

 CONFIRMING DIAGNOSIS *Three to six cultures of blood and bone marrow and biopsies of infected tissue (for example, the spleen) may provide a definite diagnosis. Culturing is best done during the acute phase.*

Hematologic studies indicate an increased erythrocyte sedimentation rate and normal or reduced white blood cell count. Diagnosis must rule out infectious diseases that produce similar symptoms, such as typhoid and malaria.

Treatment

Treatment consists of bed rest during the febrile phase. Antibiotic therapy includes a combination of doxycycline and gentamicin or doxycycline and rifampin. In severe cases, I.V. corticosteroids are given for 3 days, followed by oral corticosteroids. Standard precautions are required until lesions stop draining.

Special considerations

In suspected cases of brucellosis, take a full history. Ask the patient about his occupation and if he has recently traveled or eaten unprocessed food such as dairy products (especially unpasteurized dairy products).

■ During the acute phase, monitor and record the patient's temperature every 4 hours. Be sure to use the same route (oral or rectal) every time. Ask the dietary department to provide between-meal milk shakes and other supplemental foods to counter weight loss. Watch for heart murmurs, muscle weakness, vision loss, and joint inflammation — which may signal complications.

■ During the chronic phase, watch for depression and disturbed sleep patterns. Administer sedatives as ordered, and plan your care to allow adequate rest.

■ Keep suppurative granulomas and abscesses dry. Properly dispose of all secretions and soiled dressings. Reassure the patient that this infection *is* curable.

■ Before discharge, stress the importance of continuing medication for the prescribed duration. To prevent recurrence, advise the patient to avoid using unpasteurized milk or other dairy products. Warn meat packers and other people at risk of occupational exposure to wear gloves and goggles.

Anthrax

Anthrax is an acute bacterial infection that most commonly occurs in grazing animals, such as cattle, sheep, goats, and horses. It can also affect people who come in contact with contaminated animals or their hides, bones, fur, hair, or wool. It's also used as an agent for bioterrorism and biological warfare.

Anthrax occurs worldwide but is most common in developing countries. In humans, anthrax occurs in three forms, depending on the mode of transmission: cutaneous, inhalational, and GI.

Causes

Anthrax is caused by the bacteria *Bacillus anthracis,* which exists in the soil as spores that can live for years. Transmission to humans usually occurs through exposure to, or handling of, infected animals or animal products. Anthrax spores can enter the body through abraded or broken skin (*cutaneous anthrax*), by inhalation (*inhalational anthrax*), or through ingestion of undercooked meat from an infected animal (*GI anthrax*). Anthrax isn't known to spread from person to person.

Signs and symptoms

From the time of exposure, signs and symptoms of infection usually occur within 1 to 7 days but may take as long as 60 days to appear. The signs and symptoms of anthrax depend on the form acquired:

■ *Cutaneous anthrax:* This is the most common form of anthrax. Skin infection may begin as a small, elevated, itchy lesion that resembles an insect bite, develops into a vesicle in 1 to 2 days, and finally becomes a small, painless ulcer with a necrotic center. Enlarged lymph glands in the surrounding area are common. Without treat-

ment, mortality from cutaneous anthrax is 20%; it's less than 1% with treatment.

■ *Inhalational anthrax:* The patient may initially report flulike signs and symptoms, such as malaise, fever, headache, myalgia, and chills. These mild signs and symptoms may progress to severe respiratory difficulties, such as dyspnea, stridor, chest pain, and cyanosis, followed by the onset of shock. Even with treatment, inhalational anthrax is usually fatal.

■ *GI anthrax:* Ingestion of anthrax spores can cause acute inflammation of the intestinal tract. The patient may present with nausea, vomiting, decreased appetite, and fever, which then progress to abdominal pain, vomiting blood, and severe diarrhea. With treatment, death occurs in 25% to 60% of cases.

Diagnosis

Anthrax can be diagnosed through cultures of the blood, skin lesions, or sputum of an exposed patient. If *B. anthracis* is isolated, the diagnosis is confirmed. Additionally, specific antibodies may be detected in the blood.

Treatment

Treatment that's initiated as soon as exposure to anthrax is suspected is essential to preventing anthrax infection; early treatment may also help prevent fatality. Many antibiotics are effective against anthrax. The most widely used are penicillin, ciprofloxacin, and doxycycline.

Special considerations

■ Any case of anthrax in either livestock or a person must be reported to the appropriate public health department.

■ Supportive measures are geared toward the type of anthrax exposure.

■ An anthrax vaccine is available but, due to limited supplies, it's now administered only to United States military personnel and isn't for routine civilian use.

■ Anthrax isn't transmitted from person to person.

Campylobacteriosis

Campylobacteriosis is an intestinal infection caused by the *Campylobacter* organism, a spiral-shaped bacteria that invades and destroys the epithelial cells of the jejunum, ileum, and colon. It may spread to the bloodstream in persons with compromised immune systems, causing a life-threatening infection.

Causes and incidence

Campylobacteriosis is transmitted by the consumption of contaminated food, such as raw poultry, fresh produce, water, or unpasteurized milk; and through contact with an infected person's stool. Transmission is also possible through contact with infected pets and wild animals. Risk factors include recent family infection with *C. jejuni* and travel to an area with poor hygiene or sanitation practices.

Campylobacteriosis, which is more common in the summer months, is the most common bacterial cause of diarrheal illness in the United States.

Signs and symptoms

Signs and symptoms usually develop 2 to 4 days after exposure to *Campylobacter*. The patient's history typically reveals consumption of contaminated food or water, followed by an acute onset of mild or severe diarrhea. There may also be a history of recent close contact with a person experiencing diarrhea.

On examination, the patient may complain of cramping, abdominal pain, nausea, and vomiting. Fever may be present, and there may be traces of blood in the stool. Complications associated with campylobacteriosis include bacteremia; severe dehydration and electrolyte disturbances; Guillain-Barré syndrome; and Reiter's syndrome. Patients with campylobacteriosis who are immunocompromised are more susceptible to sepsis, endocarditis, meningitis, and thrombophlebitis because of the spread of the bacteria into the bloodstream.

Diagnosis

 CONFIRMING DIAGNOSIS *Stool culture identifying* Campylobacter *confirms the diagnosis of campylobacteriosis.*
History and physical examination help in diagnosing campylobacteriosis.

Treatment

Campylobacteriosis typically resolves on its own and isn't usually treated with antibiotics unless severe signs and symptoms are present. If severe symptoms are present, antibiotics such as ciprofloxacin and azithromycin may be ordered. Fluid and electrolyte imbalances are corrected with increased fluid intake or I.V. fluid replacement, as indicated.

Special considerations

■ Monitor the patient's intake and output and vital signs. Assess for signs of dehydration, such as tachycardia, tachypnea, and decreased urine output.
■ Monitor the patient's electrolyte levels and assess the effects of replacement electrolyte therapy and I.V. fluids.
■ Observe standard precautions.
■ Instruct the patient and his family on hand-hygiene techniques and preventive measures, including the proper handling and preparing of foods.

Tularemia

Tularemia is a highly infectious disease that can be caused by as little as 10 *Francisella tularensis* organisms, a gram-negative pleomorphic bacterium. There are six forms: ulceroglandular, glandular, oculoglandular, oropharyngeal, pneumonic, and septicemic. The disease is fatal in about 5% of patients who don't receive treatment and in less than 1% of patients who do receive treatment.

F. tularensis is considered a potential bioterrorism agent. If dispersed in aerosol form (the most likely method of dispersion), infected persons would generally develop signs and symptoms of severe respiratory illness, including pneumonia and systemic infection.

Causes and incidence

Tularemia is transmitted by the bites of infected ticks and deerflies, consuming contaminated food or water, and through contact with the blood of an infected animal (such as by skinning or handling infected carcasses), especially rabbits. The organism gains access to the host by skin or mucous membrane inoculation, inhalation, or ingestion. After inoculation, a papule and high fever develop. (The papule eventually develops into an ulcer.) The incubation period is 3 to 4 days.

In the United States, there are about 200 human cases of tularemia reported annually, with most occurring in the south-central and western areas of the country.

Signs and symptoms

Common signs and symptoms are ulcer and fever, but signs and symptoms also vary according to the form of tularemia the patient is infected with. In the ulceroglandular form, ulcers occur at the site of inoculation and are accompanied by swollen regional lymph nodes. In the glandular form, swollen regional lymph nodes are present. In the oculoglandular form, the patient exhibits a painful, red eye with purulent exudates and swollen submandibular, preauricular, or cervical lymph nodes. In the oropharyngeal form, the patient has a sore throat, abdominal pain, nausea, vomiting, diarrhea and, occasionally, GI bleeding. In the pneumonic form, the patient presents with a dry cough, dyspnea, and pleuritic chest pain. In the septicemic form, the patient has fever, chills, myalgia, malaise, and weight loss.

Complications of tularemia include pneumonia, lung abscess, respiratory failure, rhabdomyolysis, meningitis, pericarditis, and osteomyelitis.

Diagnosis

Diagnosis is based on presenting signs and symptoms, as well as the patient's history, which may include a tick bite and exposure to contaminated food or water or to contaminated blood. Other results may include a white blood cell count that is normal or elevated and blood or sputum cultures that are positive for *F. tularensis*. Chest X-ray may show pneumonia.

Treatment

General treatment involves proper skin care and increased fluid intake or supportive therapy with I.V. fluids. Medications include I.V., I.M., or oral antibiotic therapy with streptomycin or tetracycline. Antipyretics may be administered for fever.

Special considerations

■ Monitor the patient's intake and output and vital signs.

■ Assess the patient for signs of dehydration, such as tachycardia, tachypnea, and decreased urine output.

■ Monitor for complications, such as meningitis, pneumonia, pericarditis, and osteomyelitis.

Ehrlichiosis

Human ehrlichiosis, an infectious rickettsial disease that's transmitted by the bite of an infected tick, was first diagnosed in 1986. The genus Ehrlichia contains an emerging number of species that can transmit potentially life-threatening infections.

Causes and incidence

Ehrlichiosis is caused by *Ehrlichia* organisms, specifically *E. chaffeensis* and granulocytic *Ehrlichia*. Known vectors include the lone star tick (*Amblyomma americanum*), the American dog tick (*Dermacentor variabilis*), and deer ticks (*Ixodes dammini* and *Ixodes scapularis*).

In the United States, most cases of ehrlichiosis are reported in the south-central and southern Atlantic areas of the country, but it has also been reported in the upper midwest. Persons at highest risk include those who live in endemic and highly wooded areas, engage in activities in high grassy areas, and own a pet that may introduce a tick into the home.

Signs and symptoms

The incubation period for ehrlichiosis is 9 days from the time of the tick bite. Early symptoms include fever, chills, headache, muscle pain (myalgia), and nausea. A maculopapular or petechial rash appears in about half of the cases.

Most people infected with ehrlichiosis don't seek medical help, but it can be fatal.

Diagnosis

Diagnosis of ehrlichiosis is based on evaluation of signs and symptoms and supporting laboratory data. A fluorescent antibody test may return positive for *E. chaffeensis* or granulocytic *Ehrlichia*. A complete blood cell count shows decreased white blood cells (WBCs), indicative of leukopenia, and a low platelet count, indicative of thrombocytopenia. Granulocyte stain shows clumps of bacteria inside the WBCs. Liver enzymes show elevated levels of transaminase.

Treatment

Ehrlichiosis is treated with tetracycline or doxycycline, producing rapid improvement when used early in the disease's course. Death can occur if treatment is delayed.

 PEDIATRIC TIP *Oral tetracycline usually isn't prescribed for children until all permanent teeth have erupted because it can permanently discolor teeth that are still forming.*

Supportive therapy is provided to help relieve signs and symptoms.

Special considerations

■ Review with the patient measures to prevent tick bites when outdoors, such as wearing long-sleeve shirts and pants, tucking pants inside boots, and using insect repellent.

■ Advise the patient to stick to trails and avoid dense brush when hiking. Also tell him to avoid standing under overhanging foliage.

■ Tell the patient that he should examine himself for ticks after being outdoors and that he should remove any ticks found on his body; studies suggest that a tick must be attached for at least 24 hours in order to cause ehrlichiosis.

SPIROCHETES AND MYCOBACTERIA

Lyme disease

A multisystemic disorder, Lyme disease is caused by the spirochete *Borrelia burgdorferi*, which is carried by *Ixodes dammini, I. Pacificus,* and other ticks in the Ixodidae family. It commonly begins in the summer with a papule that becomes red and warm but isn't painful. This classic skin lesion is called *erythema chronicum migrans* (ECM), which may be confused with a similar rash caused by Southern tick-associated rash illness. (See *Southern tick-associated rash illness,* page 208.). Weeks or months later, cardiac or neurologic abnormalities sometimes develop, possibly followed by arthritis of the large joints.

Causes and incidence

Lyme disease occurs when a tick injects spirochete-laden saliva into the bloodstream. After incubating for 3 to 32 days, the spirochetes migrate out to the skin, causing ECM. Then they disseminate to other skin sites or organs via the bloodstream or lymph system. They may survive for years in the joints, or they may trigger an inflammatory response in the host and then die.

Initially, Lyme disease was identified in a group of children in Lyme, Connecticut. Now it's known to occur primarily in three parts of the United States: in the northeast, from Massachusetts to Maryland; in the Midwest, in Wisconsin and Minnesota; and in the west, in California and Oregon. Although it's endemic to these areas, cases have been reported in all 50 states and in 20 other countries, including Germany, Switzerland, France, and Australia.

Signs and symptoms

Typically, Lyme disease has three stages. ECM heralds stage one with a red macule or papule, commonly at the site of a tick bite. This lesion typically feels hot and itchy and may grow to over 20″ (50.8 cm) in diameter; it resembles a bull's eye or target. Within a few days, more lesions may

---

SOUTHERN TICK-ASSOCIATED RASH ILLNESS

Southern tick-associated rash illness (STARI) is a newly recognized tick-borne disease that produces a rash similar to the rash caused by Lyme disease. STARI is associated with the bite of the lone star tick, *Ambylomma americanum*, and occurs primarily in the southeastern and south-central states of the United States. Deoxyribonucleic acid analysis of the spirochetes found in the *A. americanum* tick has indicated that they are not *Borrelia burgdorferi*, the agent of Lyme disease, but are a different, newly recognized species, *Borrelia lonestari*.

Individuals living or traveling to southeastern or south-central states who develop a red, expanding rash with central clearing following a tick bite should see a physician. Mild illness, characterized by such signs and symptoms as fatigue, headache, stiff neck and, occasionally, fever, may accompany the rash.

Currently, there's no specific diagnostic test for STARI. It's suspected if diagnostic tests rule out Lyme disease, the patient's travel history is as indicated above, and a known lone star tick bite has been reported or the patient has participated in activities that may have resulted in exposure to a tick.

There are no current recommendations for treating STARI, but the rash and other accompanying signs and symptoms usually resolve with doxycycline therapy.

---

and regional lymphadenopathy. Less common effects are meningeal irritation, mild encephalopathy, migrating musculoskeletal pain, hepatitis, and splenomegaly. A persistent sore throat and dry cough may appear several days before ECM.

Weeks to months later, the second stage (disseminated infection) begins, and patients may develop additional symptoms depending on the system affected. Neurologic abnormalities — fluctuating meningoencephalitis with peripheral and cranial neuropathy — usually resolve after days or months. Facial palsy is especially noticeable. Cardiac abnormalities, such as a brief, fluctuating atrioventricular heart block, left ventricular dysfunction, or cardiomegaly may also develop. Cardiac involvement lasts only a few weeks but can be fatal.

Stage three (persistent infection) usually begins weeks or years later and is characterized by arthritis in about 80% of patients. Migrating musculoskeletal pain leads to frank arthritis with marked swelling, especially in the large joints. Recurrent attacks may precede chronic arthritis with severe cartilage and bone erosion.

Diagnosis
Because isolation of *B. burgdorferi* is difficult in humans and serologic testing isn't standardized, diagnosis is usually based on the characteristic ECM lesion and related clinical findings, especially in endemic areas. Antibodies to *B. burgdorferi* are identified by immunofluorescence or enzyme-linked immunosorbent assay (ELISA). ELISAs are confirmed with Western blot tests. Mild anemia and an elevated erythrocyte sedimentation rate, leukocyte count, serum immunoglobulin M, and aspartate aminotransferase levels support the diagnosis.

Clinicians must differentiate between Lyme disease and arthritis, encephalopathy, or polyneuropathy.

Treatment
A 28-day course of an antibiotic, such as doxycycline, is the treatment of choice for nonpregnant adults. Oral penicillin is usually prescribed for children. Alternatives include tetracycline, cefuroxime, and ceftriaxone. When given in the early stages, these

erupt, and a migratory, ringlike rash, conjunctivitis, or diffuse urticaria occurs. In 3 to 4 weeks, lesions are replaced by small red blotches, which persist for several more weeks. Malaise and fatigue are constant, but other findings are intermittent: headache, neck stiffness, fever, chills, achiness,

drugs can minimize later complications. When given during the late stages, high-dose I.V. ceftriaxone may be successful.

Special considerations

- Take a detailed patient history, asking about travel to endemic areas and exposure to ticks.
- Check for drug allergies, and administer antibiotics carefully.
- For a patient with arthritis, help with range-of-motion and strengthening exercises, but avoid overexertion. Ibuprofen helps relieve joint stiffness.
- Assess the patient's neurologic function and level of consciousness frequently. Watch for signs of increased intracranial pressure and cranial nerve involvement, such as ptosis, strabismus, and diplopia. Also check for cardiac abnormalities, such as arrhythmias and heart block.

Relapsing fever

An acute infectious disease caused by spirochetes of the genus *Borrelia*, relapsing fever (also called *tick, fowl-nest, cabin, or vagabond fever* or *bilious typhoid*) is transmitted to humans by lice or ticks and is characterized by relapses and remissions. Rodents and other wild animals serve as the primary reservoirs for the *Borrelia* spirochetes. Humans can become secondary reservoirs but cannot transmit this infection by ordinary contagion; however, congenital infection and transmission by contaminated blood are possible.

Untreated louse-borne relapsing fever normally carries a mortality of more than 10%, but during an epidemic, the mortality rate may rise to 50%. With treatment, however, the prognosis for both louse- and tick-borne relapsing fevers is excellent.

Causes and incidence

The body louse (*Pediculus humanus corporis*) carries louse-borne relapsing fever (*B. recurrentis*), which typically occurs in epidemics during wars, famines, and mass migrations. Cold weather and crowded living conditions also favor the spread of body lice.

Inoculation takes place when the victim crushes the louse, causing its infected blood or body fluid to soak into the victim's bitten or abraded skin or mucous membranes.

Louse-borne relapsing fever is most common in North and Central Africa, Europe, Asia, and South America. No cases of louse-borne relapsing fever have been reported in the United States since 1900.

Tick-borne relapsing fever, however, is found in the United States and is caused by at least 15 *Borrelia* species; the three species most commonly identified with tick carriers are *B. hermsii* (associated with *Ornithodoros hermsi*), *B. turicatae* (associated with *O. turicata*), and *B. parkeri* (associated with *O. parkeri*). This form of the disease is most prevalent in Texas and other western states, usually during the summer when ticks and their hosts (chipmunks, goats, squirrels, rabbits, mice, rats, owls, lizards, and prairie dogs) are most active. In the colder weather, outbreaks sometimes afflict people such as campers who sleep in tick-infested cabins.

Because tick bites are virtually painless and most *Ornithodoros* ticks feed at night but don't imbed themselves in the victim's skin, many people are bitten unknowingly.

Signs and symptoms

The incubation period for relapsing fever is 5 to 15 days (the average is 7 days). Clinically, tick- and louse-borne diseases are similar. Both begin suddenly, with a temperature approaching 105° F (40.6° C), prostration, headache, severe myalgia, arthralgia, diarrhea, vomiting, coughing, and eye or chest pains. Splenomegaly is common; hepatomegaly and lymphadenopathy may occur. During febrile periods, the victim's pulse and respiratory rates rise, and a transient macular rash may develop over his torso.

The first attack usually lasts from 3 to 6 days; then the patient's temperature drops quickly and is accompanied by profuse sweating. A skin rash on the trunk lasting 1 to 2 days is common after the primary febrile episode. The rash may be petechiae, macular, or papular. About 5 to 10 days later, a second febrile, symptomatic period begins. In louse-borne infection, additional relapses are unusual; but, in tick-borne cases, a second or third relapse is common. As the afebrile intervals become longer, relapses become shorter and milder because of antibody accumulation. Relapses are possibly due to antigenic changes in the *Borrelia* organism.

Complications from relapsing fever include nephritis, bronchitis, pneumonia, endocarditis, seizures, cranial nerve lesions, paralysis, and coma. Death may occur from hyperpyrexia, massive bleeding, circulatory failure, splenic rupture, or a secondary infection.

Diagnosis

 CONFIRMING DIAGNOSIS *Diagnosis requires demonstration of the spirochetes in peripheral blood smears during febrile periods, using Wright's or Giemsa stain.*

Borrelia spirochetes may be more difficult to detect in later relapses because their number declines in the blood. In such cases, injecting the patient's blood or tissue into a young rat and incubating the organism in the rat's blood for 1 to 10 days commonly allows spirochete identification.

In severe infection, spirochetes are found in the urine and cerebrospinal fluid. Other abnormal laboratory results usually include a white blood cell (WBC) count as high as 25,000/μl, with increases in lymphocytes and erythrocyte sedimentation rate; however, the WBC count may be normal. Because the *Borrelia* organism is a spirochete, relapsing fever may cause a false-positive test for syphilis in 5% to 10% of cases.

Treatment

Doxycycline or erythromycin is the treatment of choice and should continue for 4 to 5 days. In cases of drug allergy or resistance, penicillin G may be administered as an alternative. However, neither drug should be given at the height of a severe febrile attack because it may cause Jarisch-Herxheimer reaction, resulting in malaise, rigors, leukopenia, flushing, fever, tachycardia, rising respiration rate, and hypotension. This reaction, which is caused by toxic by-products from massive spirochete destruction, can mimic septic shock and

may prove fatal. Antimicrobial therapy should be postponed until the fever subsides. Until then, supportive therapy (consisting of parenteral fluids and electrolytes) should be given.

Special considerations

- During the initial evaluation period, obtain a complete history of the patient's travels and activities.
- Throughout febrile periods, monitor vital signs, level of consciousness (LOC), and temperature every 4 hours. Watch for and immediately report any signs of neurologic complications, such as decreasing LOC or seizures. To reduce fever, give tepid sponge baths and antipyretics, as ordered.
- Maintain adequate fluid intake to prevent dehydration. Provide I.V. fluids as ordered. Measure intake and output accurately, especially if the patient is vomiting or has diarrhea.
- Administer antibiotics carefully. Document and report any hypersensitive reactions (rash, fever, anaphylaxis), especially a Jarisch-Herxheimer reaction.
- Treat flushing, hypotension, or tachycardia with vasopressors or fluids, as ordered.
- Look for symptoms of relapsing fever in family members and in others who may have been exposed to ticks or lice along with the victim.
- Use proper hand-hygiene technique, and teach it to the patient. Isolation is unnecessary because the disease isn't transmitted from person to person.
- Report all cases of louse- or tick-borne relapsing fever to the local public health department, as required by law.
- To prevent relapsing fever, advise anyone traveling to tick-infested areas (Asia, North and Central Africa, and South America) to wear clothing that covers as much skin as possible and to tuck pant legs into boots or socks. Advise the use of insect repellant to reduce risk.

Leprosy

Leprosy, also known as *Hansen's disease,* is a chronic, systemic infection characterized by progressive cutaneous lesions. It's caused by *Mycobacterium leprae*, an acid-fast bacillus that attacks cutaneous tissue and peripheral nerves, producing skin lesions, anesthesia, infection, and deformities.

With timely and correct treatment, leprosy has a good prognosis and is seldom fatal. Untreated, however, it can cause severe disability. The lepromatous type may lead to blindness and deformities.

Leprosy occurs in three distinct forms:
- *Lepromatous leprosy,* the most serious type, causes damage to the upper respiratory tract, eyes, and testes as well as to the nerves and skin.
- *Tuberculoid leprosy* affects peripheral nerves and sometimes the surrounding skin, especially the face, arms, legs, and buttocks.
- *Borderline (dimorphous) leprosy* has characteristics of both lepromatous and tuberculoid leprosies. Skin lesions in this type of leprosy are diffuse and poorly defined.

Causes and incidence

Contrary to popular belief, leprosy isn't highly contagious; it actually has a low rate of infectivity. Continuous, close contact is needed to transmit it. In fact, 9 out of 10 persons have a natural immunity to it. Susceptibility appears highest during childhood and seems to decrease with age. Presumably, transmission occurs through nasal droplets containing *M. leprae* or by inoculation through skin breaks (with a contaminated hypodermic or tattoo needle, for example). The incubation period is unusually long—2 to 40 years with an average of 5 to 7 years.

Leprosy is most prevalent in the underdeveloped areas of Asia (especially India and China), Africa, South America, and the islands of the Caribbean and Pacific. About 6 million people worldwide suffer from this disease; approximately 7,000 are in the United States, mostly in California, Texas, Louisiana, Florida, New York, and Hawaii.

Signs and symptoms

M. leprae attacks the peripheral nervous system, especially the ulnar, radial, facial, anterior-tibial, and posterior-popliteal nerves. The central nervous system appears highly resistant. When the bacilli damage

the skin's fine nerves, they cause anesthesia, anhidrosis, and dryness. If they attack a large nerve trunk, motor nerve damage, weakness, and pain occur, followed by peripheral anesthesia, muscle paralysis, or atrophy. In later stages, clawhand, footdrop, and ocular complications—such as corneal insensitivity and ulceration, conjunctivitis, photophobia, and blindness—can occur. Injury, ulceration, infection, and disuse of the deformed parts cause scarring and contracture. Neurologic complications occur in both lepromatous and tuberculoid leprosy but are less extensive and develop more slowly in the lepromatous form. Lepromatous leprosy can invade tissue in virtually every organ of the body, but the organs generally remain functional.

The lepromatous and tuberculoid forms affect the skin in markedly different ways. In lepromatous disease, early lesions are multiple, symmetrical, and erythematous, sometimes appearing as macules or papules with smooth surfaces. Later, they enlarge and form plaques or nodules called *lepromas* on the earlobes, nose, eyebrows, and forehead, giving the patient a characteristic leonine appearance. In advanced stages, *M. leprae* may infiltrate the entire skin surface. Lepromatous leprosy also causes loss of eyebrows, eyelashes, and sebaceous and sweat gland function and, in advanced stages, conjunctival and scleral nodules. Upper respiratory lesions cause epistaxis, ulceration of the uvula and tonsils, septal perforation, and nasal collapse. Lepromatous leprosy can lead to hepatosplenomegaly and orchitis. Fingertips and toes deteriorate as bone resorption follows trauma and infection in these insensitive areas.

When tuberculoid leprosy affects the skin (sometimes its effect is strictly neural), it produces raised, large, erythematous plaques or macules with clearly defined borders. As they grow, they become rough, hairless, and hypopigmented and leave anesthetic scars.

In borderline leprosy, skin lesions are numerous but smaller, less anesthetic, and less sharply defined than tuberculoid lesions. Untreated, borderline leprosy may deteriorate into lepromatous disease.

Occasionally, acute episodes intensify leprosy's slowly progressing course. Whether such exacerbations are part of the disease process or a reaction to therapy remains controversial. Erythema nodosum leprosum (ENL), seen in lepromatous leprosy, produces fever, malaise, lymphadenopathy, and painful red skin nodules, usually during antimicrobial treatment, although it may occur in untreated people. In Mexico and other Central American countries, some patients with lepromatous disease develop Lucio's phenomenon. This malady produces generalized punched-out ulcers that may extend into muscle and fascia. Leprosy may also lead to secondary bacterial infection of skin ulcers and to amyloidosis.

Diagnosis

Early clinical indications of skin lesions and muscular and neurologic deficits are usually sufficiently diagnostic in patients from endemic areas. Biopsies of skin lesions are also diagnostic. Peripheral nerve biopsy or smears of the skin or of ulcerated mucous membranes help confirm the diagnosis. Blood tests show increased erythrocyte sedimentation rate; decreased albumin, calcium, and cholesterol levels; and, possibly, anemia.

Treatment

Treatment consists of antimicrobial therapy using sulfones, primarily oral dapsone, which may cause hypersensitivity reactions. Hepatitis and exfoliative dermatitis, although uncommon, are especially dangerous reactions. If they occur, sulfone therapy should be stopped immediately.

Failure to respond to sulfone or the occurrence of respiratory involvement or other complications requires the use of alternative therapy, such as rifampin in combination with clofazimine or ethionamide. Clawhand, wristdrop, or footdrop may require surgical correction.

When a patient's disease becomes inactive, as determined by the morphologic and bacterial index, treatment is discontinued according to the following schedule: tuberculoid, 3 years; borderline, depends on the severity of the disease but may be as long as 10 years; lepromatous, requires lifetime therapy.

Because ENL is commonly considered a sign that the patient is responding to treatment, antimicrobial therapy should be continued. Thalidomide and clofazimine have been used successfully to treat ENL at the National Hansen's Disease Center (NHDC); however, this treatment requires a signed consent form and strict adherence to established NHDC protocols. Corticosteroids may also be given as part of ENL therapy.

Any patient suspected of having leprosy may be referred to the Gillis W. Long Hansen's Disease Center in Carville, Louisiana, or to a regional center. At this international research and educational center, patients undergo diagnostic studies and treatment and are educated about their disease. Patients are encouraged to return home as soon as their medical condition permits. The federal government pays the full cost of their medical and nursing care.

Special considerations

Patient care is supportive and consists of measures to control acute infection, prevent complications, speed rehabilitation and recovery, and provide psychological support.

■ Give antipyretics, analgesics, and sedatives, as needed. Watch for and report ENL or Lucio's phenomenon.

■ Although leprosy isn't highly contagious, take precautions against the possible spread of infection. Tell patients to cover coughs or sneezes with a paper tissue and to dispose of it properly. Take infection precautions when handling clothing or articles that have been in contact with open skin lesions.

■ Patients with borderline or lepromatous leprosy may suffer associated eye complications, such as iridocyclitis and glaucoma. Decreased corneal sensation and lacrimation may also occur, requiring patients to use a tear substitute daily and protect their eyes to prevent corneal irritation and ulceration.

■ Stress the importance of adequate nutrition and rest. Watch for fatigue, jaundice, and other signs of anemia and hepatitis.

- Tell the patient to be careful not to injure an anesthetized leg by putting too much weight on it. Advise testing bath water carefully to prevent scalding. To prevent ulcerations, suggest the use of sturdy footwear and soaking feet in warm water after any kind of exercise, even a short walk. Advise rubbing the feet with petroleum jelly, oil, or lanolin.
- For patients with deformities, an interdisciplinary rehabilitation program employing a physiotherapist and plastic surgeon may be necessary. Teach the patient and help him with prescribed therapies.
- Provide emotional support throughout treatment. Communicating accurate information about leprosy to the general public, especially to health care professionals, is a function of primary importance for the entire staff at the NHDC.

MYCOSES
Candidiasis

Candidiasis (also called *candidosis* or *moniliasis*) is usually a mild, superficial fungal infection caused by the genus *Candida*. It usually infects the nails (onychomycosis), skin (diaper rash), or mucous membranes, especially the oropharynx (thrush), vagina (moniliasis), esophagus, and GI tract. Rarely, these fungi enter the bloodstream and invade the kidneys, lungs, endocardium, brain, or other structures, causing serious infections. Such systemic infection is most prevalent among drug abusers and patients already hospitalized, particularly diabetics, immunosuppressed patients, or patients receiving broad-spectrum antibiotics. The prognosis varies, depending on the patient's resistance.

Causes and incidence
Most cases of *Candida* infection result from *C. albicans*. Other infective strains include *C. parapsilosis, C. tropicalis, C. glabrata,* and *C. guillermondii*. These fungi are part of the normal flora of the GI tract, mouth, vagina, and skin. They cause infection when some change in the body (rising glucose levels from diabetes mellitus; low-

ered resistance from an immunosuppressive drug, radiation, aging, or a disease, such as cancer or human immunodeficiency virus [HIV] infection) permits their sudden proliferation or when they're introduced systemically by I.V. or urinary catheters, drug abuse, hyperalimentation, or surgery. However, the most common predisposing factor remains the use of broad-spectrum antibiotics, which decrease the number of normal flora and permit an increasing number of candidal organisms to proliferate. The of a mother with vaginal candidiasis can contract oral thrush while passing through the birth canal. Thrush is also found in many infants who are breastfed. The incidence of candidiasis is rising because of wider use of I.V. therapy and a greater number of immunocompromised patients, especially those with HIV infection.

Signs and symptoms
Symptoms of superficial candidiasis correspond to the site of infection:
- skin — scaly, erythematous, papular rash, sometimes covered with exudate, appearing below the breast, between fingers, and at the axillae, groin, and umbilicus; in diaper rash, papules at the edges of the rash
- nails — red, swollen, darkened nail bed; occasionally, purulent discharge and the separation of a pruritic nail from the nail bed
- oropharyngeal mucosa (thrush) — cream-colored or bluish white curdlike patches of exudate on the tongue, mouth, or pharynx that reveal bloody engorgement when scraped. They may swell, causing respiratory distress in infants, or they may be painful or cause a burning sensation in the throats and mouths of adults. (See *Recognizing candidiasis*, page 214.)
- esophageal mucosa — dysphagia, retrosternal pain, regurgitation and, occasionally, scales in the mouth and throat
- vaginal mucosa — white or yellow discharge, with pruritus and local excoriation; white or gray raised patches on vaginal walls, with local inflammation; dyspareunia.
   Systemic infection produces chills; high, spiking fever; hypotension; prostration;

RECOGNIZING CANDIDIASIS

Candidiasis of the oropharyngeal mucosa (thrush) causes cream-colored or bluish white pseudo-membranous patches on the tongue, mouth, or pharynx. Fungal invasion may extend to circumoral tissues.

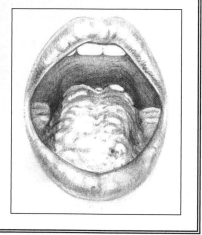

myalgias; arthralgias; and a rash. Specific signs and symptoms depend on the site of infection:

■ pulmonary—hemoptysis, cough, fever
■ renal—fever, flank pain, dysuria, hematuria, pyuria, cloudy urine
■ brain—headache, nuchal rigidity, seizures, focal neurologic deficits
■ endocardium—systolic or diastolic murmur, fever, chest pain, embolic phenomena
■ eye—endophthalmitis, blurred vision, orbital or periorbital pain, scotoma, and exudate.

Diagnosis

Diagnosis of superficial candidiasis depends on clinical signs and symptoms plus evidence of *Candida* on a Gram stain of skin, vaginal scrapings, pus, or sputum or on skin scrapings prepared in potassium hydroxide solution. Systemic infections require obtaining a specimen for blood or tissue culture.

Treatment

Treatment first aims to improve the underlying condition that predisposes the patient to candidiasis, such as controlling diabetes or discontinuing antibiotic therapy and catheterization, if possible.

Nystatin is an effective antifungal for superficial candidiasis. Clotrimazole, fluconazole, ketoconazole, and miconazole are effective in mucous-membrane and vaginal candidal infections. Ketoconazole or fluconazole is the treatment of choice for chronic candidiasis of the mucous membranes. Treatment for systemic infection consists of I.V. amphotericin B or fluconazole.

Special considerations

■ Instruct the patient using nystatin solution to swish it around in his mouth for several minutes before he swallows it.
■ Swab nystatin on the oral mucosa of an infant with thrush. Treat the infant after a feeding because feedings will wash the medication away. The infant's mother should also be treated to prevent the infection from being passed back and forth.
■ Provide the patient with a nonirritating mouthwash to loosen tenacious secretions and a soft toothbrush to avoid irritation.
■ Relieve the patient's mouth discomfort with a topical anesthetic, such as lidocaine, at least 1 hour before meals. (It may suppress the gag reflex and cause aspiration.)
■ Provide a soft diet for the patient with severe dysphagia. Tell the patient with mild dysphagia to chew food thoroughly, and make sure he doesn't choke.
■ Use dry padding in intertriginous areas of obese patients to prevent irritation.
■ Note dates of insertion of I.V. catheters, and replace them according to your hospital's policy to prevent phlebitis.
■ Assess the patient with candidiasis for underlying causes such as diabetes mellitus. If the patient is receiving amphotericin B for systemic candidiasis, he may have severe chills, fever, anorexia, nausea, and vomiting. Premedicate with acetaminophen, antihistamines, or antiemetics to help reduce adverse effects.
■ Frequently check vital signs of patients with systemic infections. Provide appropriate supportive care. In patients with renal

involvement, carefully monitor intake and output and urine blood and protein levels.

■ Check high-risk patients daily, especially those receiving antibiotics, for patchy areas, irritation, sore throat, bleeding of the mouth or gums, or other signs of superinfection. Check for vaginal discharge; record color and amount.

■ Encourage women in their third trimester of pregnancy to be examined for vaginal candidiasis to protect their neonate from infection at birth.

Cryptococcosis

Cryptococcosis, also called *torulosis* or *European blastomycosis,* is caused by the fungus *Cryptococcus neoformans.* Usually beginning as an asymptomatic pulmonary infection, it disseminates to extrapulmonary sites, usually to the central nervous system (CNS) but also to the skin, bones, prostate gland, liver, or kidneys.

With appropriate treatment, the prognosis in pulmonary cryptococcosis is good. CNS infection, however, can be fatal, but treatment dramatically reduces mortality.

Causes and incidence
Because *C. neoformans* is transmitted in particles of dust contaminated by pigeon feces that harbor this organism, cryptococcosis is primarily an urban infection. It's most prevalent in men, usually those between ages 30 and 60, and is rare in children.

Cryptococcosis is especially likely to develop in immunocompromised patients, such as those with Hodgkin's disease, sarcoidosis, leukemia, or lymphoma, and in those who are receiving immunosuppressive agents. Currently, patients with acquired immunodeficiency syndrome (AIDS) are by far the most commonly affected group.

Signs and symptoms
Typically, signs and symptoms of pulmonary cryptococcosis include fever, cough with pleuritic pain, weight loss, and CNS disturbances. CNS involvement occurs gradually (cryptococcal meningitis) and causes progressively severe frontal and temporal headache, diplopia, blurred vision, dizziness, ataxia, aphasia, vomiting, tinnitus, memory changes, inappropriate behavior, irritability, psychotic symptoms, seizures, and fever. If untreated, symptoms progress to coma and death, usually as a result of cerebral edema or hydrocephalus. Complications include optic atrophy, ataxia, hydrocephalus, deafness, paralysis, chronic brain syndrome, and personality changes.

Skin involvement produces red facial papules and other skin abscesses, with or without ulcerations; bone involvement produces painful osseous lesions of the long bones, skull, spine, and joints.

Diagnosis
Although a routine chest X-ray showing a pulmonary lesion may point to pulmonary cryptococcosis, this infection usually escapes diagnosis until it disseminates.

CONFIRMING DIAGNOSIS *Firm diagnosis requires identification of C. neoformans by culture of sputum, urine, prostatic secretions, bone marrow aspirate or biopsy, or pleural biopsy; in CNS infection, by an India ink preparation of cerebrospinal fluid (CSF) and culture. Blood cultures are positive only in severe infection.*

Supportive values include increased antigen titer in serum and CSF in disseminated infection; increased CSF pressure, protein, and white blood cell count in CNS infection; and moderately decreased CSF glucose levels in about half these patients. Diagnosis must rule out cancer and tuberculosis.

Treatment
The patient with pulmonary cryptococcosis will require close medical observation for a year after diagnosis. Treatment is unnecessary unless extrapulmonary lesions develop or pulmonary lesions progress.

Treatment of disseminated infection calls for I.V. amphotericin B, flucytosine, or fluconazole. Patients with AIDS will also need long-term therapy, usually with oral fluconazole.

Special considerations
Cryptococcosis doesn't require isolation.

- Check the patient's vital functions, and note any changes in his mental status, orientation, pupillary response, and motor function.
- Watch for headache, vomiting, and nuchal rigidity.
- Before giving I.V. amphotericin B, check for phlebitis. Infuse slowly and dilute as ordered — rapid infusion may cause circulatory collapse.
- Before therapy, draw blood for a serum electrolyte analysis to determine baseline renal status.
- During drug therapy, watch for decreased urine output, elevated blood urea nitrogen and creatinine levels, and hypokalemia.
- Monitor results of complete blood count, urinalysis, magnesium and potassium levels, and hepatic function tests. Ask the patient to report hearing loss, tinnitus, or dizziness.
- Give analgesics, antihistamines, and antiemetics, as ordered, for fever, chills, nausea, and vomiting.
- Provide psychological support to help the patient cope with long-term hospitalization.

Aspergillosis

Aspergillosis is an opportunistic infection caused by fungi of the genus *Aspergillus*, usually *A. fumigatus*, *A. flavus*, and *A. niger*. It occurs in four major forms: *aspergilloma*, which produces a fungus ball in the lungs (called a *mycetoma*); *allergic aspergillosis*, a hypersensitive asthmatic reaction to aspergillus antigens; *aspergillosis endophthalmitis*, an infection of the anterior and posterior chambers of the eye that can lead to blindness; and *disseminated aspergillosis*, an acute infection that produces septicemia, thrombosis, and infarction of virtually any organ, but especially the heart, lungs, brain, and kidneys.

Aspergillus may cause infection of the ear (otomycosis), cornea (mycotic keratitis), and prosthetic heart valves (endocarditis); pneumonia (especially in patients receiving immunosuppressants, such as antineoplastic agents or high-dose steroids); sinusitis; and brain abscesses.

The prognosis varies with each form. Occasionally, aspergilloma causes fatal hemoptysis.

Causes

Aspergillus is found worldwide, commonly in decaying vegetation, such as fermenting compost piles and damp hay. It's transmitted by inhalation of fungal spores or, in aspergillosis endophthalmitis, by the invasion of spores through a wound or other tissue injury. It's a common laboratory contaminant.

Aspergillus produces clinical infection only in people who become especially vulnerable to it. Such vulnerability can result from excessive or prolonged use of antibiotics, glucocorticoids, or other immunosuppressive agents; from radiation; from such conditions as acquired immunodeficiency syndrome, Hodgkin's disease, leukemia, azotemia, alcoholism, sarcoidosis, bronchitis, or bronchiectasis; from organ transplants; and, in aspergilloma, from tuberculosis or another cavitary lung disease.

Signs and symptoms

The incubation period in aspergillosis ranges from a few days to weeks. In aspergilloma, colonization of the bronchial tree with *Aspergillus* produces plugs and atelectasis and forms a tangled ball of hyphae (fungal filaments), fibrin, and exudate in a cavity left by a previous illness such as tuberculosis. Characteristically, aspergilloma either causes no symptoms or mimics tuberculosis, causing a productive cough and purulent or blood-tinged sputum, dyspnea, empyema, and lung abscesses.

Allergic aspergillosis causes wheezing, dyspnea, cough with some sputum production, pleural pain, and fever.

Aspergillosis endophthalmitis usually appears 2 to 3 weeks after an eye injury or surgery and accounts for half of all cases of endophthalmitis. It causes clouded vision, eye pain, and reddened conjunctiva. Eventually, *Aspergillus* infects the anterior and posterior chambers, where it produces purulent exudate.

 ALERT *In disseminated aspergillosis, Aspergillus invades blood vessels and causes thrombosis, infarctions, and the typical signs and symptoms of sep-*

ticemia (chills, fever, hypotension, delirium), with azotemia, hematuria, urinary tract obstruction, headaches, seizures, bone pain and tenderness, and soft-tissue swelling. It's rapidly fatal.

Diagnosis

In patients with aspergilloma, a chest X-ray reveals a crescent-shaped radiolucency surrounding a circular mass, but this isn't definitive for aspergillosis.

 CONFIRMING DIAGNOSIS *In aspergillosis endophthalmitis, a history of ocular trauma or surgery and a culture or exudate showing* Aspergillus *is diagnostic. In disseminated aspergillosis, culture and microscopic examination of affected tissue can confirm the diagnosis, but this form is usually diagnosed at autopsy.*

In allergic aspergillosis, sputum examination shows eosinophils. Culture of mouth scrapings or sputum showing *Aspergillus* is inconclusive because even healthy people harbor this fungus.

Treatment

Aspergillosis doesn't require isolation. Treatment requires local excision of the lesion and supportive therapy, such as chest physiotherapy and coughing, to improve pulmonary function. Endocarditis caused by *Aspergillus* is treated by surgical removal of infected heart valves and long-term amphotericin B therapy. Allergic aspergillosis requires desensitization and, possibly, steroids. Disseminated aspergillosis and aspergillosis endophthalmitis require a 2- to 3-week course of I.V. amphotericin B (as well as prompt cessation of immunosuppressive therapy). Voriconazole or itraconazole can also be used for treatment. However, the disseminated form results in an infection that's so virulent that amphotericin B therapy can't stop the systemic involvement; eventually, death ensues.

Special considerations

- Assist with chest physiotherapy and instruct the patient to cough effectively.
- Monitor the patient's vital signs, intake and output, and diagnostic test results.
- Provide emotional support for the patient and his family.

Histoplasmosis

Histoplasmosis is a fungal infection caused by *Histoplasma capsulatum*. This disease may also be called *Ohio Valley, Central Mississippi Valley, Appalachian Mountain,* or *Darling's disease.* In the United States, it occurs in three forms: primary acute histoplasmosis, progressive disseminated histoplasmosis (acute disseminated or chronic disseminated disease), and chronic pulmonary (cavitary) histoplasmosis, which produces cavitations in the lung similar to those in pulmonary tuberculosis.

A fourth form, African histoplasmosis, occurs only in Africa and is caused by the fungus *Histoplasma capsulatum duboisii.*

The prognosis varies with each form. The primary acute disease is benign; the progressive disseminated disease is fatal in approximately 90% of patients; and, without proper chemotherapy, chronic pulmonary histoplasmosis is fatal in 50% of patients within 5 years.

Causes and incidence

H. capsulatum is found in the feces of birds and bats or in soil contaminated by their feces, such as that near roosts, chicken coops, barns, caves, or underneath bridges. Transmission occurs through inhalation of *H. capsulatum* or *H. duboisii* spores or through the invasion of spores after minor skin trauma. Possibly, oral ingestion of spores may cause the disease.

The incubation period is from 5 to 18 days, although chronic pulmonary histoplasmosis may progress slowly for many years. Probably because of occupational exposure, histoplasmosis is more common in adult males. Fatal disseminated disease, however, is more common in infants and elderly men.

Histoplasmosis occurs worldwide, especially in the temperate areas of Asia, Africa, Europe, and North and South America. In the United States, it's most prevalent in the central and eastern states, especially in the Mississippi and Ohio River valleys.

Signs and symptoms

Symptoms vary with each form of this disease. Primary acute histoplasmosis may be asymptomatic or may cause symptoms of a mild respiratory illness similar to a severe cold or influenza. Typical clinical effects may include fever, malaise, headache, myalgia, anorexia, cough, chest pain, anemia, leukopenia, thrombocytopenia, and oropharyngeal ulcers.

Progressive disseminated histoplasmosis causes hepatosplenomegaly, general lymphadenopathy, anorexia, weight loss, fever and, possibly, ulceration of the tongue, palate, epiglottis, and larynx, with resulting pain, hoarseness, and dysphagia. It may also cause endocarditis, meningitis, pericarditis, and adrenal insufficiency.

Chronic pulmonary histoplasmosis mimics pulmonary tuberculosis and causes a productive cough, dyspnea, and occasional hemoptysis. Eventually, it produces weight loss, extreme weakness, breathlessness, and cyanosis.

African histoplasmosis produces cutaneous nodules, papules, and ulcers; lesions of the skull and long bones; lymphadenopathy; and visceral involvement without pulmonary lesions.

Diagnosis

A history of exposure to contaminated soil in an endemic area, miliary calcification in the lung or spleen, a positive histoplasmin skin test or urine antigen test indicate exposure to histoplasmosis. Rising complement fixation and agglutination titers (more than 1:32) strongly suggest histoplasmosis. A histoplasmosis antigen assay test can help in diagnosis.

CONFIRMING DIAGNOSIS *The diagnosis of histoplasmosis requires a morphologic examination of tissue biopsy and culture of* H. capsulatum *from sputum in acute primary and chronic pulmonary histoplasmosis and from bone marrow, lymph node, blood, and infection sites in disseminated histoplasmosis. However, cultures take several weeks to grow these organisms. Faster diagnosis is possible with stained biopsies. Also available is a deoxyribonucleic acid probe for histoplasma that can be used for difficult isolates.*

Findings must rule out tuberculosis and other diseases that produce similar symptoms. The diagnosis of histoplasmosis caused by *H. duboisii* necessitates examina-

tion of tissue biopsy and culture of the affected site.

Treatment

Treatment consists of antifungal therapy, surgery, and supportive care. Antifungal therapy is most important. Except for asymptomatic primary acute histoplasmosis (which resolves spontaneously) and the African form, histoplasmosis requires high-dose or long-term (10-week) therapy with amphotericin B, fluconazole, ketoconazole, or itraconazole. For a patient who also has acquired immunodeficiency syndrome, lifelong therapy with fluconazole is indicated.

Supportive care usually includes oxygen for respiratory distress, glucocorticoids for adrenal insufficiency, and parenteral fluids for dysphagia due to oral or laryngeal ulcerations. Histoplasmosis doesn't require isolation.

Special considerations

Patient care is primarily supportive.

■ Give medications as ordered, and teach patients about possible adverse effects. Because amphotericin B may cause chills, fever, nausea, and vomiting, give appropriate antipyretics and antiemetics, as ordered.

■ Patients with chronic pulmonary or disseminated histoplasmosis also need psychological support because of long-term hospitalization. As needed, refer the patient to a social worker or occupational therapist. Help the parents of children with this disease arrange for a visiting teacher.

■ To help prevent histoplasmosis, teach people in endemic areas to watch for early signs and seek treatment promptly. Instruct those who risk occupational exposure to contaminated soil to wear face masks.

Blastomycosis

Blastomycosis (sometimes called *North American blastomycosis* or *Gilchrist's disease*) is caused by the yeastlike fungus *Blastomyces dermatitidis*, which usually infects the lungs and produces bronchopneumonia. Less commonly, this fungus may disseminate through the blood and cause osteomyelitis and central nervous system (CNS), skin, and genital disorders. Untreated blastomycosis is slowly progressive and usually fatal; however, spontaneous remissions occasionally occur. With antifungal drug therapy and supportive treatment, the prognosis for patients with blastomycosis is good.

Causes and incidence
B. dermatitidis is probably inhaled by people who are in close contact with the soil. The incubation period may range from weeks to months. Blastomycosis is generally found in North America (where *B. dermatitidis* normally inhabits the soil), and is endemic to the southeastern United States. Sporadic cases have also been reported in Africa. Blastomycosis usually infects men ages 30 to 50, but no occupational link has been found.

Signs and symptoms
Initial signs and symptoms of pulmonary blastomycosis mimic those of a viral upper respiratory tract infection. These findings typically include a dry, hacking, or productive cough (occasionally hemoptysis), pleuritic chest pain, fever, shaking, chills, night sweats, malaise, anorexia, weight loss, and arthralgia. It can progress to pneumonia.

Cutaneous blastomycosis causes small, painless, nonpruritic, and nondistinctive macules or papules on exposed body parts. These lesions become raised and reddened and occasionally progress to draining skin abscesses or fistulas.

Dissemination to the bone causes soft-tissue swelling, tenderness, and warmth over bony lesions, which generally occur in the thoracic, lumbar, and sacral regions; long bones of the legs; and, in children, the skull.

Genital dissemination produces painful swelling of the testes, epididymis, or prostate; deep perineal pain; pyuria; and hematuria. CNS dissemination, which usually only occurs in immunocompromised hosts, causes meningitis or cerebral abscesses with resulting decreased level of consciousness (LOC), lethargy, and change in mood or affect. Other forms of dissemination may result in Addison's disease

(adrenal insufficiency), pericarditis, and arthritis.

Diagnosis
Diagnosis of blastomycosis requires:
■ culture of *B. dermatitidis* from skin lesions, pus, sputum, or pulmonary secretions
■ microscopic examination of tissue specimens from the skin or the lungs or of bronchial washings, sputum, or pus, as the physician finds appropriate
■ immunodiffusion testing, which detects antibodies for the A and B antigen of blastomycosis.

In addition, suspected pulmonary blastomycosis requires a chest X-ray, which may show pulmonary infiltrates. Other abnormal laboratory findings include increased white blood cell count and erythrocyte sedimentation rate, slightly increased serum globulin levels, mild normochromic anemia and, with bone lesions, increased alkaline phosphatase.

Treatment
All forms of blastomycosis respond to amphotericin B. Ketoconazole or fluconazole may be used as alternative agents and may be more effective with the patients who are immunocompromised. Patient care is mainly supportive.

Special considerations
■ In severe pulmonary blastomycosis, check for hemoptysis. If the patient is febrile, provide a cool room and give tepid sponge baths.
■ If blastomycosis causes joint pain or swelling, elevate the joint and apply heat. In CNS infection, watch the patient carefully for decreasing LOC and unequal pupillary response. In men with disseminated disease, watch for hematuria.
■ Infuse I.V. antifungal agents slowly (too-rapid infusion may cause circulatory collapse). During infusion, monitor vital signs (temperature may rise but should subside within 1 to 2 hours). Watch for decreased urine output and monitor laboratory results for increased blood urea nitrogen and creatinine levels. Monitor serum potassium levels for signs of amphotericin B-induced hypokalemia, which may indicate renal

toxicity. Report any hearing loss, tinnitus, or dizziness immediately. To relieve the adverse effects of amphotericin B, give antiemetics and antipyretics, as ordered.

Coccidioidomycosis

Coccidioidomycosis, also called *valley fever* or *San Joaquin Valley fever,* is caused by the fungus *Coccidioides immitis* and occurs primarily as a respiratory infection. Secondary sites include the skin, bones, joints, and meninges. Generalized dissemination is also possible. The *primary* pulmonary form is usually self-limiting and seldom fatal. The rare *secondary* (progressive, disseminated) form produces abscesses throughout the body and carries a mortality of up to 60%, even with treatment. Such dissemination is more common in dark-skinned men, pregnant women, and patients who are receiving immunosuppressants.

Causes and incidence

Coccidioidomycosis is endemic to the southwestern United States, especially between the San Joaquin Valley in California and southwestern Texas; it's also found in Mexico, Guatemala, Honduras, Venezuela, Colombia, Argentina, and Paraguay. It may result from inhalation of *C. immitis* spores found in the soil in these areas or from inhalation of spores from dressings or plaster casts of infected people. It's most prevalent during warm, dry months.

Because of population distribution and an occupational link (it's common in migrant farm laborers), coccidioidomycosis generally strikes Philippinos, Mexicans, Native Americans, and Blacks. In primary infection, the incubation period is from 1 to 4 weeks.

Signs and symptoms

Primary coccidioidomycosis usually produces acute or subacute respiratory signs and symptoms (dry cough, pleuritic chest pain, and pleural effusion), fever, sore throat, dyspnea, chills, malaise, headache, and an itchy macular rash. Chest pain, night sweats, and arthralgias can occur as well. Occasionally, the only sign is a fever

that persists for weeks. From 3 days to several weeks after onset, some patients, particularly white women, may develop tender red nodules (erythema nodosum) on their legs, especially the shins, with joint pain in the knees and ankles. Generally, primary disease heals spontaneously within a few weeks.

In rare cases, coccidioidomycosis disseminates to other organs several weeks or months after the primary infection. Disseminated coccidioidomycosis causes fever and abscesses throughout the body, especially in skeletal, central nervous system (CNS), splenic, hepatic, renal, and subcutaneous tissues. Depending on the location of these abscesses, disseminated coccidioidomycosis may cause bone pain and meningitis. Chronic pulmonary cavitation, which can occur in both the primary and the disseminated forms, causes hemoptysis with or without chest pain.

Diagnosis

CONFIRMING DIAGNOSIS *Typical clinical features and skin and serologic studies confirm this diagnosis. The primary form — and sometimes the disseminated form — produces a positive coccidioidin skin test.*

In the first week of illness, complement fixation for immunoglobulin G antibodies or, in the first month, positive serum precipitins (immunoglobulins) also establish this diagnosis. Examination or, more recently, immunodiffusion testing of sputum, pus from lesions, and a tissue biopsy may show *C. immitis* spores. The presence of antibodies in pleural and joint fluid and a rising serum or body fluid antibody titer indicate dissemination.

Other abnormal laboratory results include increased white blood cell (WBC) count, eosinophilia, increased erythrocyte sedimentation rate, and a chest X-ray showing bilateral diffuse infiltrates.

In coccidioidal meningitis, examination of cerebrospinal fluid shows WBC count increased to more than 500/μl (primarily due to mononuclear leukocytes), increased protein levels, and decreased glucose levels. Ventricular fluid obtained from the brain may contain complement fixation antibodies.

After diagnosis, the results of serial skin tests, blood cultures, and serologic testing may document the therapy's effectiveness.

Treatment
Usually, mild primary coccidioidomycosis requires only bed rest and relief of symptoms. Severe primary disease and dissemination, however, also require long-term I.V. infusion (or, in CNS dissemination, intrathecal administration) of amphotericin B, fluconazole, or itraconazole and, possibly, excision or drainage of lesions. Severe pulmonary lesions may require lobectomy. Miconazole and ketoconazole suppress *C. immitis* but don't eradicate it. Ketoconazole and itraconazole are used for oral treatment of nonmeningeal infection and for long-term therapy.

Special considerations
■ Don't wash off the circle marked on the skin for serial skin tests, because this aids in reading test results.
■ In mild primary disease, encourage bed rest and adequate fluid intake. Record the amount and color of sputum. Watch for shortness of breath that may point to pleural effusion. In patients with arthralgia, provide analgesics as ordered.
■ Coccidioidomycosis requires standard precautions, such as gloves for contact with drainage or broken skin, and good hand hygiene.
■ In CNS dissemination, monitor the patient carefully for decreased level of consciousness or change in mood or affect.
■ Before intrathecal administration of amphotericin B, explain the procedure to the patient, and reassure him that he'll receive analgesics before a lumbar puncture. If the patient is to receive I.V. amphotericin B, infuse it slowly, as ordered, because rapid infusion may cause circulatory collapse. During infusion, monitor vital signs (temperature may rise but should return to normal within 1 to 2 hours). Watch for decreased urine output, and monitor laboratory results for elevated blood urea nitrogen and creatinine levels and for hypokalemia. Tell the patient to immediately report hearing loss, tinnitus, dizziness, and all signs of toxicity. To ease adverse effects of amphotericin B, give antiemetics and antipyretics, as ordered.

Sporotrichosis

Sporotrichosis is a chronic disease caused by the fungus *Sporothrix schenckii*. It occurs in three forms: *cutaneous lymphatic*, which produces nodular erythematous primary lesions and secondary lesions along lymphatic channels; *pulmonary*, a rare form that produces a productive cough and pulmonary lesions; and *disseminated*, another rare form that may cause arthritis or osteomyelitis. The course of sporotrichosis is slow, the prognosis is good, and fatalities are rare. However, untreated skin lesions may cause secondary bacterial infection.

Causes and incidence
S. schenckii is found in soil, wood, sphagnum moss, and decaying vegetation throughout the world. Because this fungus usually enters through broken skin (the pulmonary form through inhalation), sporotrichosis is more common in horticulturists, agricultural workers, and home gardeners. Perhaps because of occupational exposure, it's more prevalent in adult men than in women and children.

Signs and symptoms
After an incubation period that lasts from 1 week to 3 months, cutaneous lymphatic sporotrichosis produces characteristic skin lesions, usually on the hands or fingers. Each lesion begins as a small, painless, movable subcutaneous nodule but grows progressively larger, discolors, and eventually ulcerates. (See *Recognizing sporotrichosis,* page 222.) Later, additional lesions form along the adjacent lymph node chain.

Pulmonary sporotrichosis causes a productive cough, lung cavities and nodules, hilar adenopathy, pleural effusion, fibrosis, and the formation of a fungus ball. It's commonly associated with sarcoidosis and tuberculosis.

Disseminated sporotrichosis produces multifocal lesions that spread from the primary lesion in the skin or lungs. The disease begins insidiously, typically causing weight loss, anorexia, synovial or bony

RECOGNIZING SPOROTRICHOSIS

Ulceration, swelling, and crusting of nodules on fingers is characteristic of cutaneous lymphatic sporotrichosis.

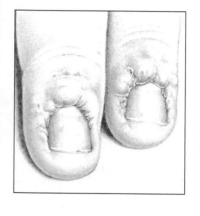

lesions and, possibly, arthritis or osteomyelitis.

Diagnosis

 CONFIRMING DIAGNOSIS *Typical clinical findings and a culture of* S. schenckii *in sputum, pus, or bone drainage confirm the diagnosis of sporotrichosis.*

Histologic identification is difficult. Diagnosis must rule out tuberculosis, sarcoidosis and, in patients with the disseminated form of sporotrichosis, bacterial osteomyelitis and neoplasm.

Treatment

Sporotrichosis doesn't require isolation. The cutaneous lymphatic form usually responds to application of a saturated solution of potassium iodide, generally continued for 1 to 2 months after lesions heal. Occasionally, cutaneous lesions must be excised or drained. The disseminated form responds to amphotericin B and itraconazole but may require several weeks of treatment. Local heat application relieves pain.

Cavitary pulmonary lesions may require surgery.

Special considerations

■ Keep lesions clean, make the patient as comfortable as possible, and carefully dispose of contaminated dressings.

■ Warn the patient about the possible adverse effects of drugs. Because amphotericin B may cause fever, chills, nausea, and vomiting, give antipyretics and antiemetics, as ordered.

■ To help prevent sporotrichosis, advise horticulturists and home gardeners to wear gloves while working.

RESPIRATORY VIRUSES

Common cold

The common cold (also known as *acute coryza*) is an acute, usually afebrile viral infection that causes inflammation of the upper respiratory tract. It's the most common infectious disease, accounting for more time lost from school or work than any other cause. Although a cold is benign and self-limiting, it can lead to secondary bacterial infections.

Causes and incidence

About 90% of colds stem from a viral infection of the upper respiratory passages and consequent mucous membrane inflammation; occasionally, colds result from a mycoplasmal infection. (See *What happens in the common cold.*)

Over a hundred viruses can cause the common cold. Major offenders include rhinoviruses, coronaviruses, myxoviruses, adenoviruses, coxsackieviruses, and echoviruses.

Transmission occurs through airborne respiratory droplets, contact with contaminated objects, and hand-to-hand transmission. Children acquire new strains from their schoolmates and pass them on to family members. Fatigue or drafts don't increase susceptibility.

PATHOPHYSIOLOGY
WHAT HAPPENS IN THE COMMON COLD

Virus-infected droplets enter the body and attack the cells lining the throat and nose. The virus particles then multiply rapidly.

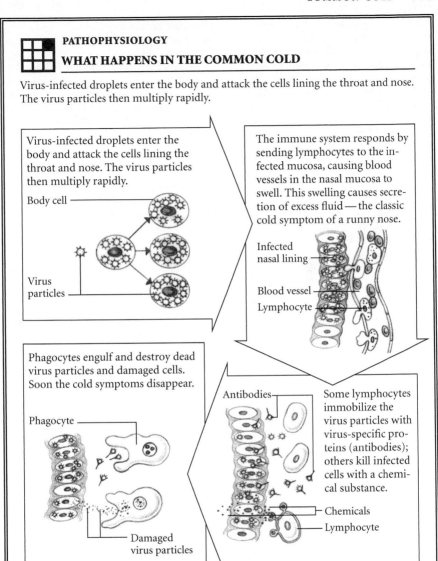

Virus-infected droplets enter the body and attack the cells lining the throat and nose. The virus particles then multiply rapidly.

Body cell

Virus particles

The immune system responds by sending lymphocytes to the infected mucosa, causing blood vessels in the nasal mucosa to swell. This swelling causes secretion of excess fluid — the classic cold symptom of a runny nose.

Infected nasal lining

Blood vessel

Lymphocyte

Phagocytes engulf and destroy dead virus particles and damaged cells. Soon the cold symptoms disappear.

Phagocyte

Damaged virus particles

Antibodies

Some lymphocytes immobilize the virus particles with virus-specific proteins (antibodies); others kill infected cells with a chemical substance.

Chemicals

Lymphocyte

The common cold is more prevalent in children than in adults; in adolescent boys than in girls; and in women than in men. In temperate zones, it's more common in the colder months; in the tropics, during the rainy season.

Signs and symptoms

After a 1- to 4-day incubation period, the common cold produces pharyngitis, nasal congestion, coryza, headache, and burning, watery eyes. Additional effects may include fever (in children), chills, myalgia, arthralgia, malaise, lethargy, and a hacking, nonproductive, or nocturnal cough.

As the cold progresses, clinical features develop more fully. After a day, symptoms include a feeling of fullness with a copious nasal discharge that commonly irritates the nose, adding to discomfort. About 3 days after onset, major signs diminish, but the "stuffed up" feeling generally persists for about a week. Reinfection (with productive cough) is common, but complications (sinusitis, otitis media, pharyngitis, and lower respiratory tract infection) are rare. A cold is communicable for 2 to 3 days after the onset of symptoms.

Diagnosis

No explicit diagnostic test exists to isolate the specific organism responsible for the common cold. Consequently, diagnosis rests on the typically mild, localized, and afebrile upper respiratory symptoms. Despite infection, white blood cell counts and differential are within normal limits. Diagnosis must rule out allergic rhinitis, measles, rubella, and other disorders that produce similar early symptoms. A temperature higher than 100° F (37.8° C), severe malaise, anorexia, tachycardia, exudate on the tonsils or throat, petechiae, and tender lymph glands may point to more serious disorders and require additional diagnostic tests.

Treatment

The primary treatments—aspirin, acetaminophen or ibuprofen, fluids, and rest—are purely symptomatic because the common cold has no cure. Aspirin eases myalgia and headache; fluids help loosen accumulated respiratory secretions and maintain hydration; and rest combats fatigue and weakness. In a child with a fever, acetaminophen is the drug of choice.

Decongestants can relieve congestion, and throat lozenges relieve soreness. Steam encourages expectoration. Nasal douching, sinus drainage, and antibiotics aren't necessary except in complications or chronic illness. Pure antitussives relieve severe coughs but are contraindicated in productive coughs, when cough suppression is harmful. The role of vitamin C remains controversial. In infants, saline nose drops and mucus aspiration with a bulb syringe may be beneficial.

Special considerations

- Emphasize that antibiotics don't cure the common cold.
- Tell the patient to maintain bed rest during the first few days, to use a lubricant on his nostrils to decrease irritation, to relieve throat irritation with hard candy or cough drops, to increase fluid intake, and to eat light meals.
- Warm baths or heating pads can reduce aches and pains but won't hasten a cure. Suggest hot- or cold-steam vaporizers. Commercial expectorants are available, but their effectiveness is questionable.
- Advise against overuse of nose drops or sprays because they may cause rebound congestion.
- To help prevent colds, warn the patient to minimize contact with people who have colds. To avoid spreading colds, teach the patient to wash his hands often and before touching his eyes, to cover coughs and sneezes, and to avoid sharing towels and drinking glasses.

Respiratory syncytial virus infection

Respiratory syncytial virus (RSV) infection results from a subgroup of the myxoviruses that resemble paramyxovirus. RSV is the leading cause of lower respiratory tract infections in infants and young children. It's the major cause of pneumonia, tracheobronchitis, and bronchiolitis in this age-group and a suspected cause of the fatal respiratory diseases of infancy.

Causes and incidence

The organism that causes RSV is transmitted from person to person by respiratory secretions and has an incubation period of 4 to 5 days. Antibody titers seem to indicate that few children younger than age 4 escape contracting some form of RSV, even if it's mild. In fact, RSV is the only viral disease that has its maximum impact during the first few months of life (incidence of RSV bronchiolitis peaks at age 2 months). School-age children, adolescents, and young adults with mild reinfections are probably the source of infection for infants and young children.

This virus occurs in annual epidemics during the late winter and early spring in temperate climates and during the rainy season in the tropics. It can also be seen in immunocompromised adults, especially patients with bone marrow transplants.

Signs and symptoms
Clinical features of RSV infection vary in severity from mild, coldlike symptoms to bronchiolitis or bronchopneumonia and, in a few patients, severe, life-threatening lower respiratory tract infections. Symptoms usually include coughing, wheezing, malaise, pharyngitis, dyspnea, and inflamed mucous membranes in the nose and throat. Reinfection is common, producing milder symptoms than the primary infection.

Otitis media is a common complication of RSV in infants. RSV has also been identified in patients with a variety of central nervous system disorders, such as meningitis and myelitis.

Diagnosis
Diagnosis is usually based on clinical findings and epidemiologic information.
- Many facilities can perform rapid tests for the virus using fluid obtained from the nose.
- Cultures of nasal and pharyngeal secretions may show RSV; however, the virus is labile, so cultures aren't always reliable.
- Chest X-rays help detect pneumonia.

Treatment
Treatment aims to support respiratory function, maintain fluid balance, and relieve symptoms. Ribavirin in aerosol form may be administered to severely ill patients or those at high risk for complications.

Special considerations
Your care plan should provide support and relief of symptoms.
- Monitor respiratory status, including rate and pattern. Watch for nasal flaring or retraction, cyanosis, pallor, and dyspnea; listen or auscultate for wheezing, rhonchi, or other signs of respiratory distress. Monitor arterial blood gas levels and oxygen saturation.

- Maintain a patent airway, and be especially watchful when the patient has periods of acute dyspnea. Perform percussion and provide drainage and suction, when necessary. Use a croup tent to provide a high-humidity atmosphere. Semi-Fowler's position may help prevent aspiration of secretions.
- Monitor intake and output carefully. Observe for signs of dehydration such as decreased skin turgor. Encourage the patient to drink plenty of high-calorie fluids. Administer I.V. fluids as needed.
- Promote bed rest. Plan your nursing care to allow uninterrupted rest.
- Hold and cuddle infants; talk to and play with toddlers. Offer diversionary activities that are appropriate for the child's condition and age. Encourage parental visits and cuddling. Restrain the child only as necessary.
- Impose droplet precautions. Enforce strict hand hygiene, because RSV may be transmitted from fomites. Avoid hand contact with nose or eyes; wear a surgical mask and eye protection.
- Make sure that staff members with respiratory illnesses don't care for infants.

Parainfluenza

Parainfluenza refers to any of a group of respiratory illnesses caused by paramyxoviruses, a subgroup of the myxoviruses. Affecting both the upper and lower respiratory tracts, these self-limiting diseases resemble influenza but are milder and seldom fatal.

Causes and incidence
Parainfluenza is transmitted by direct contact or by inhalation of contaminated airborne droplets. Paramyxoviruses occur in four forms—Para 1 to 4—that are linked to several diseases: croup (Para 1, 2, 3); acute febrile respiratory illnesses (1, 2, 3); the common cold (1, 3, 4); pharyngitis (1, 3, 4); bronchitis (1, 3); and bronchopneumonia (1, 3). Para 3 ranks second to respiratory syncytial viruses as the most common cause of lower respiratory tract infections in children. Para 4 rarely causes symptomatic infections in humans.

Parainfluenza is rare among adults but widespread among children, especially males. By age 8, most children demonstrate antibodies to Para 1 and Para 3. Most adults have antibodies to all four types as a result of childhood infections and subsequent multiple exposures. Incidence rises in the winter and spring.

Signs and symptoms

After a short incubation period (usually 3 to 6 days), signs and symptoms emerge that are similar to those of other respiratory diseases: sudden fever, nasal discharge, reddened throat (with little or no exudate), chills, and muscle pain. Bacterial complications are uncommon, but in infants and very young children, parainfluenza may lead to croup or laryngotracheobronchitis. Reinfection is usually less severe and affects only the upper respiratory tract.

Diagnosis

Parainfluenza infections are usually clinically indistinguishable from similar viral infections. A swab of nasal secretions is useful for rapid viral testing. Isolation of the virus and serum antibody titers differentiate parainfluenza from other respiratory illness but is rarely done.

Treatment

Parainfluenza may require no treatment or bed rest, antipyretics, analgesics, and antitussives, depending on the severity of the symptoms. Complications, such as croup and pneumonia, require appropriate treatment. No vaccine is effective against parainfluenza.

Special considerations

■ Throughout the illness, monitor respiratory status and temperature, and ensure adequate fluid intake and rest.

Adenovirus infection

Adenoviruses cause acute, self-limiting febrile infections, with inflammation of the respiratory or ocular mucous membranes, or both. (See *Major adenovirus infections*.)

Causes and incidence

Adenovirus has 35 known serotypes; it causes 5 major infections, all of which occur in epidemics. These organisms are common and can remain latent for years; they infect almost everyone early in life, although maternal antibodies offer some protection during the first 6 months of life.

Transmission of adenovirus can occur by direct inoculation into the eye; by the oral-fecal route (adenovirus may persist in the GI tract for years after infection); or by inhalation of an infected droplet.

Signs and symptoms

The incubation period — usually lasting less than 1 week — is followed by acute illness lasting less than 5 days. Clinical features vary, depending on the type of infection. Prolonged asymptomatic reinfection may occur.

Diagnosis

CONFIRMING DIAGNOSIS *Definitive diagnosis requires isolation of the virus from respiratory or ocular secretions or fecal smears; during epidemics, however, typical symptoms alone can confirm the diagnosis.*

Because adenoviral illnesses resolve rapidly, serum antibody titers aren't useful for diagnosis. Adenoviral diseases cause lymphocytosis in children. When they cause respiratory disease, chest X-ray may show pneumonitis.

Treatment

Supportive treatment includes bed rest, antipyretics, and analgesics. Ocular infections may require corticosteroids and direct supervision by an ophthalmologist. Hospitalization is required in cases of pneumonia (in infants) to prevent death and in epidemic keratoconjunctivitis (EKC) to prevent blindness.

Special considerations

■ During acute illness, monitor respiratory status and intake and output. Give analgesics and antipyretics, as needed. Stress the need for bed rest.
■ To help minimize the incidence of adenoviral disease, instruct all patients in prop-

MAJOR ADENOVIRUS INFECTIONS

Disease	Age-group	Clinical features
Acute febrile respiratory illness	Children	Nonspecific coldlike symptoms, similar to other viral respiratory illnesses: fever, pharyngitis, tracheitis, bronchitis, and pneumonitis
Acute respiratory disease	Adults (usually military recruits)	Malaise, fever, chills, headache, pharyngitis, hoarseness, and dry cough
Viral pneumonia	Children and adults	Sudden onset of high fever, rapid infection of upper and lower respiratory tracts, rash, diarrhea, and intestinal intussusception
Acute pharyngoconjunctival fever	Children (particularly after swimming in pools or lakes)	Spiking fever lasting several days, headache, pharyngitis, conjunctivitis, rhinitis, and cervical adenitis
Acute follicular conjunctivitis	Adults	Unilateral tearing and mucoid discharge; later, milder symptoms in other eye
Epidemic keratoconjunctivitis	Adults	Unilateral or bilateral ocular redness and edema, periorbital swelling, local discomfort, and superficial opacity of the cornea without ulceration
Hemorrhagic cystitis	Children (boys)	Adenovirus in urine, hematuria, dysuria, and urinary frequency
Diarrhea	Infants	Fever and watery diarrhea

er hand hygiene to reduce fecal-oral transmission and eye inoculation.

■ EKC can be prevented by sterilization of ophthalmic instruments, adequate chlorination in swimming pools, and avoidance of swimming pools during epidemics. Killed virus vaccine (not widely available) or a live oral virus vaccine can prevent adenoviral infection and are recommended for high-risk groups.

Influenza

Influenza (also called the *grippe* or the *flu*), an acute, highly contagious infection of the respiratory tract, results from three different types of *Myxovirus influenzae*. It occurs sporadically or in epidemics (usually during the colder months). Epidemics tend to peak within 2 to 3 weeks after initial cases and subside within a month.

Although influenza affects all agegroups, its incidence is highest in schoolchildren. However, its effects are most severe in persons who are young, elderly, or suffering from chronic disease. In these groups, influenza may even lead to death. The catastrophic pandemic of 1918 was responsible for an estimated 20 million deaths. The most recent pandemics (in 1957, 1968, and 1977) began in mainland China.

Causes and incidence

Transmission of influenza occurs through inhalation of a respiratory droplet from an infected person or by indirect contact with a contaminated object, such as a drinking glass or other items contaminated with respiratory secretions. The influenza virus then invades the epithelium of the respiratory tract, causing inflammation and desquamation.

One of the remarkable features of the influenza virus is its capacity for *antigenic variation* into numerous distinct strains, allowing it to infect new populations that have little or no immunologic resistance. Antigenic variation is characterized as *antigenic drift* (minor changes that occur yearly or every few years) and *antigenic shift* (major changes that lead to pandemics). Influenza viruses are classified into three groups:

- Type A, the most prevalent, strikes every year, with new serotypes causing epidemics every 3 years.
- Type B also strikes annually but causes epidemics only every 4 to 6 years.
- Type C is endemic and causes only sporadic cases.

Each year, tens of millions of people in the United States get the flu; about 114,000 people get sick enough to be hospitalized, and about 36,000 people die.

Signs and symptoms

After an incubation period of 24 to 48 hours, flu symptoms begin to appear: sudden onset of chills, temperature of 101° to 104° F (38.3° to 40° C), headache, malaise, myalgia (particularly in the back and limbs), a nonproductive cough and, occasionally, laryngitis, hoarseness, conjunctivitis, rhinitis, and rhinorrhea. These symptoms usually subside in 3 to 5 days, but cough and weakness may persist. Fever is usually higher in children than in adults. Also, cervical adenopathy and croup are likely to be associated with influenza in children. In some patients (especially elderly patients), lack of energy and easy fatigability may persist for several weeks.

Fever that persists longer than 3 to 5 days signals the onset of complications. The most common complication is pneumonia, which occurs as primary influenza virus pneumonia or secondary to bacterial infection. Influenza may also cause myositis, exacerbation of chronic obstructive pulmonary disease, Reye's syndrome and, rarely, myocarditis, pericarditis, transverse myelitis, and encephalitis.

Diagnosis

At the beginning of an influenza epidemic, early cases are usually mistaken for other respiratory disorders.

CONFIRMING DIAGNOSIS
Because signs and symptoms of influenza aren't pathognomonic, isolation of M. influenzae *through nose and throat cultures and increased serum antibody titers help confirm this diagnosis. Also, rapid diagnostic methods for detecting influenza are now available and help confirm this diagnosis.*

After these measures confirm an influenza epidemic, diagnosis requires only observation of clinical signs and symptoms. Uncomplicated cases show a decreased white blood cell count with an increase in lymphocytes.

Treatment

Treatment of uncomplicated influenza includes bed rest, adequate fluid intake, aspirin or acetaminophen (in children) to relieve fever and muscle pain, and dextromethorphan or another antitussive to relieve nonproductive coughing. Prophylactic antibiotics aren't recommended because they have no effect on the influenza virus.

Amantadine and rimantadine (antiviral agents) have proven to be effective in reducing the duration of signs and symptoms of influenza A infection. Oseltamivir and zanamivir are effective against influenza A and B infection. In influenza complicated by pneumonia, supportive care (fluid and electrolyte supplements, oxygen, and assisted ventilation) and treatment of bacterial superinfection with appropriate antibiotics are necessary. No specific therapy exists for cardiac, central nervous system, or other complications.

Special considerations

Unless complications occur, influenza doesn't require hospitalization; patient care focuses on relief of symptoms:

- Advise the patient to increase his fluid intake. Warm baths or heating pads may relieve myalgia. Give him nonopioid analgesics-antipyretics as ordered.
- Screen visitors to protect the patient from bacterial infection and the visitors from influenza. Use droplet precautions.
- Teach the patient proper disposal of tissues and proper hand-hygiene technique to prevent the virus from spreading.
- Watch for signs and symptoms of developing pneumonia, such as crackles, another temperature rise, or coughing accompanied by purulent or bloody sputum. Assist the patient to gradually resume his normal activities.
- Educate patients about influenza immunizations. For high-risk patients and health care personnel, suggest annual inoculations at the start of the flu season (late autumn). Remember, however, that such vaccines are made from chicken embryos and must not be given to people who are hypersensitive to eggs. (For people who are hypersensitive to eggs, amantadine is an effective alternative to the vaccine; however it must be started before the flu season and continued throughout the season.) The vaccine administered is based on the previous year's virus and is usually about 75% effective.
- Inform people receiving the vaccine of possible adverse effects (discomfort at the vaccination site, fever, malaise and, rarely, Guillain-Barré syndrome). Influenza vaccine (inactivated) is recommended for women who are pregnant and who will be in the second or third trimester during influenza season.
- Live-attenuated influenza vaccine is now available as a nasal spray. Criteria and contraindications for use vary from the inactivated, injectable vaccine. Recipients of live-attenuated influenza vaccine may shed influenza virus for up to 21 days post-immunization.

Hantavirus pulmonary syndrome

Mainly occurring in the southwestern United States, but not confined to that area, *Hantavirus* pulmonary syndrome is a viral disease first reported in May 1993. The syndrome, which rapidly progresses from flulike symptoms to respiratory failure and, possibly, death, is known for its high mortality. The hantavirus strain that causes disease in Asia and Europe — mainly hemorrhagic fever and renal disease — is distinctly different from the one currently described in North America.

Causes

A member of the Bunyaviridae family, the genus *Hantavirus* (first isolated in 1977) is responsible for *Hantavirus* pulmonary syndrome. Disease transmission is associated with exposure to aerosols (such as dust) contaminated by urine or feces from infected rodents, the primary reservoir for this virus. Data suggest that the deer mouse is the main source, but pinon mice, brush mice, and western chipmunks in close proximity to humans in rural areas are also sources. Hantavirus infections have been documented in people whose activities are associated with rodent contact, such as farming, hiking or camping in rodent-infested areas, and occupying rodent-infested dwellings.

Infected rodents manifest no apparent illness but shed the virus in feces, urine, and saliva. Human infection may occur from inhalation, ingestion (of contaminated food or water, for example), contact with rodent excrement, or rodent bites. Transmission from person to person or by mosquitoes, fleas, or other arthropods hasn't been reported.

Signs and symptoms

Noncardiogenic pulmonary edema distinguishes the syndrome. Common chief complaints include myalgia, fever, headache, nausea, vomiting, and cough. Respiratory distress typically follows the onset of a cough. Fever, hypoxia and, in some patients, serious hypotension typify its course.

SCREENING FOR *HANTAVIRUS* PULMONARY SYNDROME

The Centers for Disease Control and Prevention (CDC) has developed a screening procedure to track cases of *Hantavirus* pulmonary syndrome. The screening criteria identify potential and actual cases.

Potential cases

For a diagnosis of possible *Hantavirus* pulmonary syndrome, a patient must have one of the following:

■ febrile illness (temperature equal to or above 101° F [38.3° C]) occurring in a previously healthy person and characterized by unexplained acute respiratory distress syndrome

■ bilateral interstitial pulmonary infiltrates that develop within 1 week of hospitalization with respiratory compromise that requires supplemental oxygen

■ an unexplained respiratory illness resulting in death and autopsy findings demonstrating noncardiogenic pulmonary edema without an identifiable specific cause of death.

Exclusions

Of the patients who meet the criteria for having potential *Hantavirus* pulmonary syndrome, the CDC excludes those who have any of the following:

■ a predisposing underlying medical condition (for example, severe underlying pulmonary disease), solid tumors or hematologic cancers, congenital or acquired immunodeficiency disorders, or medical conditions or treatments — such as rheumatoid arthritis or organ transplantation — requiring immunosuppressive drug therapy (for example, steroids or cytotoxic chemotherapy)

■ an acute illness that provides a likely explanation for the respiratory illness (for example, a recent major trauma, burn, or surgery; recent seizures or history of aspiration; bacterial sepsis; another respiratory disorder such as respiratory syncytial virus in young children; influenza; or legionella pneumonia).

Confirmed cases

Cases of confirmed *Hantavirus* pulmonary syndrome must include the following:

■ at least one serum or tissue specimen available for laboratory testing for evidence of hantavirus infection

■ in a patient with a compatible clinical illness, serologic evidence (presence of hantavirus-specific immunoglobulin [Ig] M or rising titers of IgG), polymerase chain reaction for hantavirus ribonucleic acid, or positive immunohistochemistry for hantavirus antigen.

Other signs and symptoms include a rising respiratory rate (28 breaths/minute or more) and an increased heart rate (120 beats/minute or more).

Diagnosis

Despite ongoing efforts to identify clinical and laboratory features that distinguish *Hantavirus* pulmonary syndrome from other infections with similar features, diagnosis currently is based on clinical suspicion along with a process of elimination developed by the Centers for Disease Control and Prevention (CDC) with the Council of State and Territorial Epidemiologists. (See *Screening for* Hantavirus *pulmonary syndrome.*) Serologic testing for hantavirus can be performed.

Laboratory tests usually reveal an elevated white blood cell count with a predominance of neutrophils, myeloid precursors, and atypical lymphocytes; elevated hematocrit; decreased platelet count; elevated partial thromboplastin time; and a normal fibrinogen level. Usually, laboratory findings demonstrate only minimal abnormalities in renal function, with serum creatinine levels no higher than 2.5 mg/dl.

Chest X-rays eventually show bilateral diffuse infiltrates in almost all patients (findings consistent with acute respiratory distress syndrome).

Treatment
Primarily supportive, treatment consists of maintaining adequate oxygenation, monitoring vital signs, and intervening to stabilize the patient's heart rate and blood pressure.

Drug therapy includes vasopressors, such as dopamine or epinephrine, for hypotension. Fluid volume replacement may also be ordered (with precautions not to overhydrate the patient). Ribavirin in aerosol form has been used for children, but its efficacy for adults has not been proven.

Special considerations
- Assess the patient's respiratory status and arterial blood gas values often.
- Monitor serum electrolyte levels and correct imbalances as appropriate.
- Maintain a patent airway by suctioning. Ensure adequate humidification, and check ventilator settings frequently.
- In patients with hypoxemia, assess neurologic status frequently along with heart rate and blood pressure.
- Administer drug therapy, and monitor the patient's response.
- Provide I.V. fluid therapy based on results of hemodynamic monitoring.
- Provide emotional support for the patient and his family.
- Report cases of *Hantavirus* pulmonary syndrome to the appropriate state health department.
- Provide the patient with prevention guidelines. (Until more is known about *Hantavirus* pulmonary syndrome, preventive measures currently focus on rodent control.)

RASH-PRODUCING VIRUSES

Varicella

Varicella, commonly known as *chickenpox*, is a common, acute, and highly contagious infection caused by the herpesvirus varicella-zoster, the same virus that, in its latent stage, causes herpes zoster (shingles).

Causes and incidence
Chickenpox can occur at any age, but it's most common in children ages 2 to 8. Congenital varicella may affect infants whose mothers had acute infections in their first or early second trimester. Neonatal infection is rare, probably because of transient maternal immunity. However, neonates born to mothers who develop varicella 5 days before delivery or up to 2 days after delivery are at risk for developing severe generalized varicella. Second attacks are also rare. This infection is transmitted by direct contact (primarily with respiratory secretions; less commonly, with skin lesions) and indirect contact (airborne). The incubation period usually lasts 14 to 17 days but can be as short as 10 days and as long as 20 days. (See *Incubation and duration of common rash-producing infections,* page 232.) Chickenpox is probably communicable from 1 day before lesions erupt to 6 days after vesicles form (it's most contagious in the early stages of eruption of skin lesions).

Chickenpox occurs worldwide and is endemic in large cities. Outbreaks occur sporadically, usually in areas with large groups of susceptible children. It affects all races and both sexes equally. Seasonal distribution varies; in temperate areas, incidence is higher during late autumn, winter, and spring.

Most children recover completely. Potentially fatal complications may affect children on corticosteroids, antimetabolites, or other immunosuppressants and those with leukemia, other neoplasms, or immunodeficiency disorders. Congenital and adult varicella may also have severe effects.

INCUBATION AND DURATION OF COMMON RASH-PRODUCING INFECTIONS

Infection	Incubation (days)	Duration (days)
Herpes simplex	2 to 12	7 to 21
Roseola infantum	10 to 15	3 to 6
Rubella	14 to 21	3
Rubeola	8 to 14	5
Varicella	14 to 17	7 to 14

Signs and symptoms

Chickenpox produces distinctive signs and symptoms, notably a pruritic rash. During the prodromal phase, the patient has slight fever, malaise, and anorexia. Within 24 hours, the rash typically begins as crops of small, erythematous macules on the trunk or scalp. It progress to papules and then clear vesicles on an erythematous base (the so-called dewdrop on a rose petal). These become cloudy and break easily; then scabs form.

The rash spreads to the face and over the trunk of the body, then to the limbs, buccal mucosa, axillae, upper respiratory tract, conjunctivae and, occasionally, the genitalia. New vesicles continue to appear for 3 or 4 days, so the rash contains a combination of red papules, vesicles, and scabs in various stages.

Congenital varicella causes hypoplastic deformity and limb scarring; retarded growth; and central nervous system and eye manifestations. In progressive varicella, an immunocompromised patient may have lesions and a high fever for over 7 days.

Severe pruritus with this rash may provoke persistent scratching, which can lead to infection, scarring, impetigo, furuncles, and cellulitis. Rare complications include pneumonia, myocarditis, fulminating encephalitis (Reye's syndrome), bleeding disorders, arthritis, nephritis, hepatitis, and acute myositis.

Diagnosis

Diagnosis rests on the characteristic clinical signs and usually doesn't require laboratory tests. However, the virus can be isolated from vesicular fluid within the first 3 or 4 days of the rash; Giemsa stain distinguishes varicella-zoster from vaccinia and variola viruses. Serum contains antibodies 7 days after onset.

Treatment

Chickenpox calls for droplet and contact isolation until all vesicles and most of the scabs are dry (no new lesions; usually 1 week after the onset of the rash). Children with only a few remaining scabs are no longer contagious and can return to school. Congenital chickenpox requires no isolation.

In most cases, treatment consists of local or systemic antipruritics: lukewarm oatmeal baths, calamine lotion, or diphenhydramine (or another antihistamine). Antibiotics are unnecessary unless bacterial infection develops. Salicylates are contraindicated because of their link with Reye's syndrome.

Susceptible patients may need special treatment. When given up to 72 hours after exposure to varicella, varicella-zoster immunoglobulin may provide passive immunity. Acyclovir and famciclovir, antiviral agents, may slow vesicle formation, speed skin healing, and control the systemic spread of infection.

Special considerations

Care is supportive and emphasizes patient and family teaching and preventive measures.

- Teach the child and his family how to apply topical antipruritic medications correctly. Stress the importance of good hygiene.
- Tell the patient not to scratch the lesions. However, because the need to scratch may be overwhelming, parents should trim the child's fingernails or tie mittens on his hands.
- Warn parents to watch for and immediately report signs of complications. Severe skin pain and burning may indicate a serious secondary infection and require prompt medical attention.
- Varicella vaccine, part of the recommended childhood immunization schedule, effectively prevents infection. It's also effective if given 5 days post-exposure.
- To help prevent chickenpox, don't admit a child exposed to chickenpox to a unit that contains children who receive immunosuppressants or who have leukemia or immunodeficiency disorders. A vulnerable child who has been exposed to chickenpox should be evaluated for administration of varicella-zoster immunoglobulin to lessen the severity of the disease.

Herpes simplex

Herpes simplex, a recurrent viral infection, is caused by *Herpesvirus hominis* (HVH), a widespread infectious agent. Herpes type I, which is transmitted by oral and respiratory secretions, affects the skin and mucous membranes, commonly producing cold sores and fever blisters. Herpes type II primarily affects the genital area and is transmitted by sexual contact. However, cross-infection may result from orogenital sex or autoinoculation from one site to another.

Causes and incidence

About 85% of all HVH infections are subclinical; the others produce localized lesions and systemic reactions. After the first infection, a patient is a carrier susceptible to recurrent infections, which may be provoked by fever, menses, stress, heat, and cold. However, the patient usually has no constitutional signs and symptoms in recurrent infections.

Primary HVH is the leading cause of childhood gingivostomatitis in children ages 1 to 3. It causes the most common form of nonepidemic encephalitis and is the second most common viral infection in pregnant women. It can pass to the fetus transplacentally and, in early pregnancy, may cause spontaneous abortion or premature birth.

Herpes infection is equally common in males and females. Worldwide in distribution, it's most prevalent among children in lower socioeconomic groups who live in crowded environments. Saliva, stool, skin lesions, purulent eye exudate, and urine are potential sources of infection.

Signs and symptoms

In neonates, HVH symptoms usually appear 1 to 2 weeks after birth. They range from localized skin lesions to a disseminated infection of organs, such as the liver, lungs, or brain. Common complications include seizures, mental retardation, blindness, chorioretinitis, deafness, microcephaly, diabetes insipidus, and spasticity. Up to 90% of infants with disseminated disease die.

Primary infection in childhood may be localized or generalized and occurs after an incubation period of 2 to 12 days. After brief prodromal tingling and itching, localized infection causes typical primary lesions. These erupt as vesicles on an erythematous base, eventually rupture and leave a painful ulcer, followed by a yellowish crust. Vesicles may form on any part of the oral mucosa, especially the tongue, gingiva, and cheeks. Healing begins 7 to 10 days after onset and is complete in 3 weeks.

Generalized infection begins with fever, pharyngitis, erythema, and edema. Vesicles occur with submaxillary lymphadenopathy, increased salivation, halitosis, anorexia, and a fever of up to 105° F (40.6° C). Herpetic stomatitis may lead to severe dehydration in children. A generalized infection usually runs its course in 4 to 10 days. In this form, virus reactivation causes cold sores — a single or group of vesicles in and around the mouth.

Genital herpes usually affects adolescents and young adults. Typically painful, the initial attack produces fluid-filled vesicles that ulcerate and heal in 1 to 3 weeks. Fever, regional lymphadenopathy, and dysuria may also occur.

Usually, herpetic keratoconjunctivitis is unilateral and causes only local signs and symptoms: conjunctivitis, regional adenopathy, blepharitis, and vesicles on the lid. Other ocular effects may include excessive lacrimation, edema, chemosis, photophobia, and purulent exudate.

Both types of HVH can cause acute sporadic encephalitis with altered level of consciousness, personality changes, and seizures. Other effects may include smell and taste hallucinations and neurologic abnormalities such as aphasia.

Herpetic whitlow, an HVH finger infection, affects many nurses. First the finger tingles and then it becomes red, swollen, and painful. Vesicles with a red halo erupt and may ulcerate or coalesce. Other effects may include satellite vesicles, fever, chills, malaise, and a red streak up the arm.

Diagnosis

CONFIRMING DIAGNOSIS *Typical lesions may suggest HVH infection. However, confirmation requires isolation of the virus from local lesions and histologic biopsy.*

A rise in antibodies and moderate leukocytosis may support the diagnosis.

Treatment

No cure for herpes exists; however, recurrences tend to be milder and of shorter duration than the primary infection. Symptomatic and supportive therapy is essential. Generalized primary infection usually requires an analgesic-antipyretic to reduce fever and relieve pain. Anesthetic mouthwashes, such as viscous lidocaine, may reduce the pain of gingivostomatitis, enabling the patient to eat and preventing dehydration. (Avoid alcohol-based mouthwashes.) Drying agents, such as calamine lotion, ease the pain of labial or skin lesions. Avoid petroleum-based ointments, which promote viral spread and slow healing.

Refer patients with eye infections to an ophthalmologist. Topical corticosteroids are contraindicated in active infection, but idoxuridine, trifluridine, and vidarabine are effective.

Oral acyclovir may bring relief to patients with genital herpes. Frequent prophylactic use of acyclovir in immunosuppressed transplant patients prevents disseminated disease. Foscarnet can be used to treat HVH that's resistant to acyclovir. Anti-viral agents similar to acyclovir are valacyclovir and famciclovir. These agents are more active than acyclovir.

Special considerations

- Teach the patient with genital herpes to use warm compresses or take sitz baths several times per day; to use a drying agent, such as povidone-iodine solution; to increase fluid intake; and to avoid all sexual contact during the active stage.
- For pregnant women with active HVH infection at the time of delivery, a cesarean delivery is recommended to decrease the risk of infecting the neonate.
- Health care personnel should use standard precautions, such as gloves, for contact with mucous membranes to prevent acquisition of herpetic whitlow.
- Instruct patients with herpetic whitlow not to share towels or eating utensils. Educate staff members and other susceptible people about the risk of contagion. Abstain from direct patient care if you have herpetic whitlow.
- Tell patients with cold sores not to kiss infants or people with eczema. (Those with genital herpes pose no risk to infants if their hygiene is meticulous.)
- Patients with central nervous system infection alone need no isolation.

Herpes zoster

Herpes zoster (also called *shingles*) is an acute unilateral and segmental inflammation of the dorsal root ganglia caused by infection with the herpesvirus varicella-zoster, which also causes chickenpox. This infection usually occurs in adults. It produces localized vesicular skin lesions, confined to a dermatome, and severe neuralgic pain in peripheral areas innervated by the nerves arising in the inflamed root ganglia.

The prognosis is good unless the infection spreads to the brain. Eventually, most patients recover completely, except for possible scarring and, in corneal damage, visual impairment. Occasionally, neuralgia may persist for months or years.

Causes and incidence

Herpes zoster results from reactivation of varicella virus that has lain dormant in the cerebral ganglia (extramedullary ganglia of the cranial nerves) or the ganglia of posterior nerve roots since a previous episode of chickenpox. Exactly how or why this reactivation occurs isn't clear. Some believe that the virus multiplies as it's reactivated and that antibodies remaining from the initial infection neutralize it. However, if effective antibodies aren't present, the virus continues to multiply in the ganglia, destroy the host neuron, and spread down the sensory nerves to the skin.

Herpes zoster occurs primarily in adults, especially those older than age 50. It seldom recurs. It's also seen in patients with human immunodeficiency virus and other immunodeficiency disorders.

Signs and symptoms

Herpes zoster begins with fever and malaise. Within 2 to 4 days, severe deep pain, pruritus, and paresthesia or hyperesthesia develop, usually on the trunk and occasionally on the arms and legs in a dermatomal distribution. Pain may be continuous or intermittent and usually lasts from 1 to 4 weeks. Up to 2 weeks after the first symptoms, small red nodular skin lesions erupt on the painful areas. (These lesions typically spread unilaterally around the thorax or vertically over the arms or legs.) Sometimes nodules don't appear at all, but when they do, they quickly become vesicles filled with clear fluid or pus. About 10 days after they appear, the vesicles dry and form scabs. (See *Recognizing shingles.*) When ruptured, such lesions usually become infected and, in severe cases, may lead to the enlargement of regional lymph nodes; they may even become gangrenous. Intense pain may occur before the rash appears and after the scabs form.

RECOGNIZING SHINGLES

The characteristic skin lesions in herpes zoster (shingles) are fluid-filled vesicles that dry and form scabs after about 10 days.

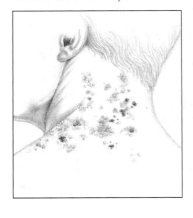

Occasionally, herpes zoster involves the cranial nerves, especially the trigeminal and geniculate ganglia or the oculomotor nerve. Geniculate zoster may cause vesicle formation in the external auditory canal, ipsilateral facial palsy, hearing loss, dizziness, and loss of taste. Trigeminal ganglion involvement causes eye pain and, possibly, corneal and scleral damage and impaired vision. Rarely, oculomotor involvement causes conjunctivitis, extraocular weakness, ptosis, and paralytic mydriasis.

In rare cases, herpes zoster leads to generalized central nervous system infection, muscle atrophy, motor paralysis (usually transient), acute transverse myelitis, and ascending myelitis. More commonly, generalized infection causes acute urine retention and unilateral diaphragm paralysis. In postherpetic neuralgia, most common in elderly persons, intractable neurologic pain may persist for years. Scars may be permanent.

Patients with immunodeficiency disorders may develop disseminated zoster. Lesions are bilateral and not limited to dermatomal distribution.

Diagnosis

Diagnosis of herpes zoster usually isn't possible until the characteristic skin lesions develop. Before then, the pain may mimic that of appendicitis, pleurisy, or other conditions. Individuals who are susceptible to varicella may develop a varicella infection following exposure to patients with zoster. Examination of vesicular fluid and infected tissue shows eosinophilic intranuclear inclusions and varicella virus. Also, a lumbar puncture shows increased pressure; examination of cerebrospinal fluid shows increased protein levels and, possibly, pleocytosis. Differentiation of herpes zoster from localized herpes simplex requires staining antibodies from vesicular fluid and identification under fluorescent light.

Treatment

Antiviral therapy is the mainstay of treatment. Acyclovir seems to stop the rash's progression and prevent visceral complications. Capsaicin, transcutaneous electrical nerve stimulation, and low-dose amitriptyline are the current treatments of choice for postherpetic neuralgia. Topical antiviral ointment is helpful if started early in the disease process.

Herpes zoster can resolve spontaneously and may only require symptomatic treatment, the goal of which is to relieve itching and neuralgic pain with calamine lotion or another antipruritic; aspirin, possibly with codeine or another analgesic; and, occasionally, collodion or compound benzoin tincture applied to unbroken lesions.

If bacteria have infected ruptured vesicles, the treatment plan usually includes an appropriate systemic antibiotic.

Trigeminal zoster with corneal involvement calls for instillation of idoxuridine ointment or another antiviral agent. To help a patient cope with the intractable pain of postherpetic neuralgia, the physician may order systemic corticosteroids — such as cortisone or possibly corticotropin — to reduce inflammation (although their use is controversial). He also may prescribe tranquilizers, sedatives, or tricyclic antidepressants with phenothiazines. In some immunocompromised patients — both children and adults — acyclovir I.V. appears to prevent disseminated, life-threatening disease. High doses of interferon (an antiviral glycoprotein) have been used in patients with cancer when the herpetic lesions are limited to the dermatome.

Special considerations

Your care plan should emphasize keeping the patient comfortable, maintaining meticulous hygiene, and preventing further infection. During the acute phase, adequate rest and supportive care can promote proper healing of lesions.

- If calamine lotion has been ordered, apply it liberally to the lesions. If lesions are severe and widespread, apply a wet dressing. Drying therapies, such as oxygen or air-loss bed, and Silvadene ointment, may also be used.
- Instruct the patient to avoid scratching the lesions.
- If vesicles rupture, apply a cold compress as ordered.
- To decrease the pain of oral lesions, tell the patient to use a soft toothbrush, eat soft foods, and use a saline or bicarbonate mouthwash.
- To minimize neuralgic pain, never withhold or delay administration of analgesics. Give them exactly on schedule because the pain of herpes zoster can be severe. In postherpetic neuralgia, consult a pain specialist to maximize pain relief without risking tolerance to the analgesic.
- Repeatedly reassure the patient that herpetic pain will eventually subside. Encourage diversionary or relaxation activity.
- Institute droplet and contact precautions. Disseminated zoster requires the same isolation precautions as primary varicella.

Rubella

Rubella, commonly called *German measles,* is an acute, mildly contagious viral disease that produces a distinctive 3-day rash and lymphadenopathy. It usually occurs among children ages 5 to 9, adolescents, and young adults. Rubella flourishes worldwide during the spring (particularly in big cities), and epidemics occur sporadically. This disease is self-limiting, with an excellent prognosis.

Causes

The rubella virus is transmitted through contact with the blood, urine, stools, or nasopharyngeal secretions of infected people and, possibly, by contact with contaminated articles of clothing. Transplacental transmission, especially in the first trimester of pregnancy, can cause serious birth defects, such as microcephaly, mental retardation, patent ductus arteriosus, glaucoma, and bone defects. (See *Congenital rubella syndrome.*) Humans are the only known hosts for the rubella virus. The disease is contagious from about 10 days before the rash appears until 5 days after it has appeared.

Signs and symptoms

In children, after an incubation period of from 14 to 21 days, an exanthematous, maculopapular rash erupts abruptly. (See *Incubation and duration of common rash-producing infections*, page 232.) In adolescents and adults, prodromal signs and symptoms — headache, malaise, anorexia, low-grade fever, coryza, lymphadenopathy and, sometimes, conjunctivitis — are the first to appear. Suboccipital, postauricular, and postcervical lymph node enlargement is a hallmark of this disease and precedes the rash.

Typically, the rubella rash begins on the face and spreads rapidly, in many cases covering the trunk and extremities within hours. Small, red, petechial macules on the soft palate (Forschheimer spots) may precede or accompany the rash but are not diagnostic of rubella. By the end of the second day, the facial rash begins to fade, but the rash on the trunk may become confluent and be mistaken for scarlet fever. The rash continues to fade in the downward order in which it appeared. It generally disappears on the third day, but it may persist for 4 or 5 days — sometimes accompanied by mild coryza and conjunctivitis. The rapid appearance and disappearance of the rubella rash distinguishes it from rubeola. In rare cases, rubella can occur without a rash. Low-grade fever may accompany the rash (99° to 101° F [37.2° to 38.3° C]), but it usually doesn't persist after the first day of the rash; rarely, temperature may reach 104° F (40° C).

CONGENITAL RUBELLA SYNDROME

Congenital rubella is by far the most serious form of the disease. Intrauterine rubella infection, especially during the first trimester, can lead to spontaneous abortion or stillbirth as well as single or multiple birth defects. (As a rule, the earlier the infection occurs during pregnancy, the greater the damage to the fetus.)

The combination of cataracts, deafness, and cardiac disease characterizes congenital rubella syndrome. Low birth weight, microcephaly, and mental retardation are other common manifestations. However, researchers now believe that congenital rubella can cause more disorders, many of which don't appear until later in life. These include dental abnormalities, thrombocytopenic purpura, hemolytic and hypoplastic anemia, encephalitis, giant-cell hepatitis, seborrheic dermatitis, and diabetes mellitus. Indeed, it now appears that congenital rubella may be a lifelong disease. This theory is supported by the fact that the rubella virus has been isolated from urine 15 years after its acquisition in the uterus.

Neonates born with congenital rubella should be isolated immediately because they excrete the virus for several months to a year after birth. Cataracts and cardiac defects may require surgery. The prognosis depends on the particular malformations that occur. The overall mortality for neonates with rubella is 6%, but it's higher for neonates born with thrombocytopenic purpura, congenital cardiac disease, or encephalitis. Parents of affected children need emotional support and guidance in finding help from community resources and organizations.

Complications seldom occur in children with rubella, but when they do, they commonly appear as hemorrhagic problems such as thrombocytopenia. Many young women, however, experience transient joint pain or arthritis, usually just as the rash is fading. Fever may then recur. These complications usually subside spontaneously within 5 to 30 days.

A significant number of cases, 20% to 50%, are asymptomatic.

Diagnosis

The rubella rash, lymphadenopathy, other characteristic signs, and a history of exposure to infected people usually permit clinical diagnosis without laboratory tests.

CONFIRMING DIAGNOSIS *The rubella rash has been confused with scarlet fever, measles (rubeola), infectious mononucleosis, roseola, erythema infectiosum, and other viral exanthems. Therefore, without exposure history, laboratory confirmation is beneficial. Cell cultures of the throat, blood, urine, and cerebrospinal fluid can confirm the virus' presence. Convalescent serum that shows a fourfold rise in antibody titers corroborates the diagnosis.*

Treatment

Because the rubella rash is self-limiting and only mildly pruritic, it doesn't require topical or systemic medication. Treatment consists of aspirin for fever and joint pain. Bed rest isn't necessary, but the patient should be isolated until the rash disappears.

Immunization with live virus vaccine RA27/3, the only rubella vaccine available in the United States, is necessary for prevention and appears to be more immunogenic than previous vaccines. The rubella vaccine should be given with measles and mumps vaccines at age 15 months to decrease the cost and number of injections.

Special considerations

■ Make the patient with active rubella as comfortable as possible. If the patient is a child, give him children's books to read or games to play to keep him occupied.
■ Explain to the patient why droplet precautions are necessary. Congenital rubella requires contact precautions until age 1. Make sure the patient understands how important it is to avoid exposing women who are pregnant to this disease.
■ Report confirmed cases of rubella to local public health officials.

Before giving the rubella vaccine:
■ Obtain a history of allergies, especially to neomycin. If the patient has this allergy or has had a reaction to immunization in the past, check with the physician before giving the vaccine.
■ Ask women of childbearing age if they're pregnant. If they are or think they may be, *don't* give the vaccine or perform a pregnancy test first. Warn women who receive rubella vaccine to use an effective means of birth control for at least 3 months after immunization.
■ Give the vaccine at least 3 months after any administration of immune globulin or blood, which could have antibodies that neutralize the vaccine.
■ Don't vaccinate patients who are immunocompromised, patients with immunodeficiency diseases, or those receiving immunosuppressive, radiation, or corticosteroid therapy. Instead, administer immune serum globulin as ordered, to prevent or reduce infection in susceptible patients.

After giving the rubella vaccine:
■ Observe the patient for signs of anaphylaxis for at least 30 minutes. Keep epinephrine 1:1,000 handy.
■ Warn the patient about possible mild fever, slight rash, transient arthralgia (in adolescents), and arthritis (in elderly patients). Suggest aspirin or acetaminophen for fever.
■ If swelling persists after the initial 24 hours, suggest a cold compress to promote vasoconstriction and prevent antigenic cyst formation.

Rubeola

Rubeola, also known as the *measles* or *morbilli*, is an acute, highly contagious paramyxovirus infection that may be one of the most common and most serious of all communicable childhood diseases. Use of the vaccine has reduced the occurrence of measles during childhood; as a result, measles is becoming more prevalent in

ADMINISTERING MEASLES VACCINE

■ Ask the patient about known allergies, especially to neomycin (each dose contains a small amount). However, a patient who's allergic to eggs may receive the vaccine because it contains only minimal amounts of albumin and yolk components.

■ Avoid giving the vaccine to a pregnant woman (ask for date of last menstrual period). Warn female patients to avoid pregnancy for at least 3 months following vaccination.

■ Don't vaccinate children with untreated tuberculosis, immunodeficiencies, leukemia, or lymphoma or those receiving immunosuppressants. If such children are exposed to the virus, recommend that they receive gamma globulin (gamma globulin won't prevent measles but will lessen its severity). Older unimmunized children who have been exposed to measles for more than 5 days may also require gamma globulin. Be sure to immunize them 3 months later.

■ Delay vaccination for 8 to 12 weeks after administration of whole blood, plasma, or gamma globulin because measles antibodies in these components may neutralize the vaccine.

■ Watch for signs of anaphylaxis for 30 minutes after vaccination. Keep epinephrine 1:1,000 handy.

■ Warn the patient or his parents that possible adverse effects are anorexia, malaise, rash, mild thrombocytopenia or leukopenia, and fever. Advise them that mild reactions may occur, usually within 7 to 10 days. If swelling occurs within 24 hours after vaccination, tell the patient to apply cold compresses to the injection site to promote vasoconstriction and to prevent antigenic cyst formation.

■ Generally, one bout of measles provides immunity (a second infection is extremely rare and may indicate a misdiagnosis); infants younger than age 4 months may be immune because of circulating maternal antibodies. Under normal conditions, measles vaccine isn't administered to children younger than age 15 months. However, during an epidemic, infants as young as 6 months may receive the vaccine and then be reimmunized at age 15 months. An alternative approach calls for administering gamma globulin to infants between ages 6 and 15 months who are likely to be exposed to measles.

---

adolescents and adults. (See *Administering measles vaccine.*) In the United States, the prognosis is usually excellent; however, measles is a major cause of death in children in underdeveloped countries.

Causes and incidence

Measles is spread by direct contact or by contaminated airborne respiratory droplets. The portal of entry is the upper respiratory tract. In temperate zones, incidence is highest in late winter and early spring. Before the availability of measles vaccine, epidemics occurred every 2 to 5 years in large urban areas.

Signs and symptoms

Incubation is from 8 to 14 days. Initial symptoms begin and greatest communicability occurs during the prodromal phase, about 11 days after exposure to the virus. This phase lasts from 4 to 5 days; signs and symptoms include fever, photophobia, malaise, anorexia, conjunctivitis, coryza, hoarseness, and hacking cough.

At the end of the prodrome, Koplik's spots, the hallmark of the disease, appear. These spots look like tiny, bluish white specks surrounded by a red halo. They appear on the oral mucosa opposite the molars and occasionally bleed. About 5 days after Koplik's spots appear, temperature rises sharply, spots slough off, and a slightly pruritic rash appears. This characteristic rash starts as faint macules behind the ears and on the neck and cheeks. The macules become papular and erythematous, rapidly spreading over the entire face, neck, eyelids, arms, chest, back, abdomen, and thighs. When the rash reaches the feet (2 to 3 days later), it begins to fade in the same sequence that it appeared, leaving a brownish discoloration that disappears in 7 to 10 days. (See *Incubation and duration of common rash-producing infections*, page 232.)

The disease climax occurs 2 to 3 days after the rash appears and is marked by a fever of 103° to 105° F (39.4° to 40.6° C), severe cough, puffy red eyes, and rhinorrhea. About 5 days after the rash appears, other symptoms disappear and communicability ends. Symptoms are usually mild in patients with partial immunity (conferred by administration of gamma globulin) or infants with transplacental antibodies. More severe symptoms and complications are more likely to develop in young infants, adolescents, adults, and patients who are immunocompromised than in young children.

Atypical measles may appear in patients who received the killed measles vaccine. These patients are acutely ill with a fever and maculopapular rash that's most obvious in the arms and legs or with pulmonary involvement and no skin lesions.

Severe infection may lead to secondary bacterial infection and to autoimmune reaction or organ invasion by the virus, resulting in otitis media, pneumonia, and encephalitis. Subacute sclerosing panencephalitis, a rare and invariably fatal complication, may develop several years after measles but it's less common in patients who have received the measles vaccine.

Diagnosis

Diagnosis rests on distinctive clinical features, especially the pathognomonic Koplik's spots. Mild measles may resemble rubella, roseola infantum, enterovirus infection, toxoplasmosis, and drug eruptions; laboratory tests are required for a differential diagnosis. If necessary, measles virus may be isolated from the blood, nasopharyngeal secretions, and urine during the febrile period. Serum antibodies appear within 3 days after onset of the rash and reach peak titers 2 to 4 weeks later.

Treatment

Treatment for measles requires bed rest, relief of symptoms, and droplet isolation throughout the communicable period. Vaporizers and a warm environment help reduce respiratory irritation, and antipyretics can reduce fever. Cough preparations and antibiotics are generally ineffective. I.V. ribavirin has reduced the severity of illness in adults. Therapy must also combat complications.

Special considerations

■ Teach the patient's parents supportive measures, and stress the need for isolation, plenty of rest, and increased fluid intake. Advise them to cope with photophobia by darkening the room or providing sunglasses and to reduce fever with antipyretics and tepid sponge baths.
■ Warn the patient's parents to watch for and report the early signs and symptoms of complications, such as encephalitis, otitis media, and pneumonia.

Variola

Variola, or *smallpox,* was an acute, highly contagious infectious disease caused by the poxvirus variola. After a global eradication program, the World Health Organization pronounced smallpox eradicated on October 26, 1979, 2 years after the last naturally occurring case was reported in Somalia. Vaccination is no longer recommended, except for certain laboratory workers. The last known case in the United States was reported in 1949. Although naturally occurring smallpox has been eradicated, variola virus preserved in laboratories remains an unlikely source of infection. In response to bioterrorism concerns, smallpox vaccination was offered to members of the military, health department officials, first responders, and key health care providers. If a bioterrorism event involving smallpox is suspected or occurs, vaccination programs can be initiated.

Smallpox developed in three major forms: *variola major* (classic smallpox), which carried a high mortality; *variola minor*, a mild form that occurred in nonvaccinated people and resulted from a less virulent strain; and *varioloid*, a mild variant of smallpox that occurred in previously vaccinated people who had only partial immunity.

Causes and incidence

Smallpox affected people of all ages. In temperate zones, incidence was highest during the winter; in the tropics, during the hot, dry months. Smallpox was transmitted directly by respiratory droplets or dried scales of virus-containing lesions or indirectly through contact with contaminated linens or other objects. Variola major was contagious from onset until after the last scab was shed.

Signs and symptoms

Characteristically, after an incubation period of 10 to 14 days, smallpox caused an abrupt onset of chills (and possible seizures in children), high fever (above 104° F [40° C]), headache, backache, severe malaise, vomiting (especially in children), marked prostration and, occasionally, violent delirium, stupor, or coma. Two days after onset, symptoms became more severe, but by the third day the patient began to feel better.

However, he soon developed a sore throat and cough as well as lesions on the mucous membranes of the mouth, throat, and respiratory tract. Within days, skin lesions also appeared, progressing from macular to papular, vesicular, and pustular (pustules were as large as 8.5 mm in diameter). All skin lesions were in the same stage of development. During the pustular stage, the patient's temperature again rose, and early symptoms returned. By day 10, the pustules began to rupture and eventually dried and formed scabs. Symptoms finally subsided about 14 days after onset. Desquamation of the scabs took another 1 to 2 weeks, caused intense pruritus, and commonly left permanently disfiguring scars.

In fatal cases, a diffuse dusky appearance came over the patient's face and upper chest. Death resulted from encephalitic manifestations, extensive bleeding from any or all orifices, or secondary bacterial infections.

Diagnosis

Before the global eradication program, smallpox was readily recognizable, especially during an epidemic or after known contact. However, most of today's health care workers aren't familiar with the disease's telltale signs and symptoms. The most conclusive laboratory test is a culture of variola virus isolated from an aspirate of vesicles and pustules. Other laboratory tests include microscopic examination of smears from lesion scrapings and complement fixation to detect virus or antibodies to the virus in the patient's blood.

Treatment

Treatment for smallpox requires hospitalization with droplet and contact precautions, antimicrobial therapy to treat bacterial complications, vigorous supportive measures, and symptomatic treatment of lesions with antipruritics, starting during the pustular stage. If the smallpox vaccination is given within 1 to 4 days of exposure to the disease, it may prevent illness or lessen symptoms. Treatment once the disease has started is limited.

Special considerations

■ Give aspirin, codeine, or (as needed) morphine to relieve pain.
■ I.V. infusions and gastric tube feedings provide fluids, electrolytes, and calories because pharyngeal lesions make swallowing difficult.
■ If smallpox is suspected, the state health department should be notified immediately.

Monkeypox

Monkeypox is a rare viral disease identified mostly in the rainforest countries of central and west Africa. The virus was originally discovered in laboratory monkeys in 1958. It was later recovered from an African squirrel, which was thought to be the natural host. It may also infect other rodents, such as rats, mice, and rabbits. The first human cases of monkeypox were reported in remote African locations in 1970. In June 2003, there was an outbreak in the United States involving people who had gotten ill following contact with infected prairie dogs.

Causes

The *monkeypox virus,* belonging to the orthopoxvirus group of viruses, causes monkeypox. It's related to variola and cowpox. People can contract monkeypox from an infected animal through a bite or direct contact with the animal's blood, body fluids, or lesions. It's spread person to person via respiratory droplets during direct and prolonged face-to face contact. It's less infectious than smallpox, but it can also be spread through direct contact with an infected person's body fluids or with virus-contaminated objects, such as bedding or clothing.

Signs and symptoms

The signs and symptoms of monkeypox are similar to smallpox, but milder. After an incubation period of about 12 days, the patient may report fever, headache, muscle aches, backache, swollen lymph nodes, and a general feeling of discomfort and exhaustion. A papular rash begins on the face or other area of the body within 1 to 3 days after onset of the fever. The lesions go through several stages before crusting and falling off. The illness' duration is 2 to 4 weeks.

In Africa, monkeypox is fatal in 10% of those who contract the disease.

Diagnosis

Diagnosis is based on history and presenting signs and symptoms. The virus may be isolated from vesicular fluid to aid in diagnosis and differentiation from other rash-producing viruses.

Treatment

There is no specific treatment for monkeypox, but the smallpox vaccine appears to reduce the risk of contracting the disease. The Centers for Disease Control and Prevention recommends that persons who are investigating monkeypox outbreaks and caring for infected individuals or animals should receive smallpox vaccination. Persons exposed to individuals or animals confirmed to have monkeypox should also receive vaccinations (up to 14 days after exposure).

Vaccinia immune globulin may be considered in some cases, such as in patients who are severely immunocompromised. There is no data available on the effectiveness of cidofovir in the treatment of human monkeypox cases.

Special considerations

- Notify the local health department immediately if you suspect monkeypox.
- A combination of standard, contact, and droplet precautions should be applied in all health care settings. Because of the risk of airborne transmission, droplet precautions should be applied whenever possible using a NIOSH-certified N95 (or comparable) filtering disposable respirator that has been fit-tested. Surgical masks may be worn if the respirator is not available. Isolation continues until all lesions are crusted over or until the local or state health department advises that isolation is no longer necessary.
- Perform scrupulous hand hygiene after contact with an infected patient or contaminated objects. Teach the patient and his family members proper hand hygiene as well.
- Eye protection should be used if splash or spray of body fluids is·possible.
- Place the patient in a private room. Use a negative pressure room if available.
- When transporting the patient, place a mask over his nose and mouth, and cover the exposed skin lesions with a sheet or gown. If the patient is to remain at home, he should maintain the same precautions.

Roseola infantum

Roseola infantum (exanthema subitum), an acute, benign, presumably viral infection, usually affects infants and young children ages 6 months to 3 years. Characteristically, it first causes a high fever and then a rash that accompanies an abrupt drop to normal temperature. It's also known as *sixth disease.*

Causes and incidence

Human herpesvirus 6 causes roseola. It affects boys and girls alike and occurs year-round. Overt roseola, the most common exanthem in children younger than age 2, affects 30% of all children; inapparent roseola (febrile illness without a rash) may affect the rest. The mode of transmission isn't known, but oral secretions are suspected. Rarely does an infected child transmit roseola to a sibling.

Signs and symptoms

After a 5- to 15-day incubation period (average, 10 days) the infant with roseola develops an abruptly rising, unexplainable fever and, sometimes, seizures. Temperature peaks at 103° to 105° F (39.4° to 40.6° C) for 3 to 5 days, then drops suddenly. In the early febrile period, the infant may be anorexic, irritable, and listless but doesn't appear particularly ill. Simultaneously, with an abrupt drop in temperature, the infant develops a maculopapular, nonpruritic rash that blanches on pressure. The rash is profuse on the trunk, arms, and neck and mild on the face and legs. It fades within 24 hours. Complications are extremely rare.

Diagnosis

Diagnosis requires observation of the characteristic rash that appears about 48 hours after fever subsides. Serologic evidence of primary infection can be determined by checking antibody levels in acute and convalescent sera.

Treatment

Because roseola is self-limiting, treatment is supportive and symptomatic: antipyretics to lower fever and, if necessary, anticonvulsants to relieve seizures.

Special considerations

■ Teach parents how to reduce their infant's fever by giving tepid baths, keeping him in lightweight clothes, and maintaining normal room temperature. Stress the need for adequate fluid intake. Strict bed rest and isolation are unnecessary. Tell parents that a short febrile seizure will not cause brain damage. Explain that seizures will cease after fever subsides and that phe-

nobarbital is likely to cause drowsiness; if it causes stupor, tell the parents to call their physician immediately.

ENTEROVIRUSES
Herpangina

Herpangina is an acute infection caused by group A coxsackieviruses (usually types 1 through 10, 16, and 22) and, less commonly, by group B coxsackieviruses and echoviruses. The disease typically produces vesicular lesions on the mucous membranes of the soft palate, tonsillar pillars, and throat.

Causes and incidence

Because fecal-oral transfer is the main mode of transmission, herpangina usually affects children younger than age 10 (except neonates because of maternal antibodies). It's also transmitted via contact with nose and throat discharges. It's slightly more common in late summer and fall and can be sporadic, endemic, or epidemic. It generally subsides in 4 to 7 days.

Signs and symptoms

After a 2- to 9-day incubation period, herpangina begins abruptly with a sore throat, pain on swallowing, and a temperature of 100° to 104° F (37.8° to 40° C) that persists for 1 to 4 days and may cause seizures, headache, anorexia, vomiting, malaise, diarrhea, and pain in the stomach, back of the neck, legs, or arms. Grayish white papulovesicles (up to 12) appear on the soft palate and, less commonly, on the tonsils, uvula, tongue, and larynx. These lesions grow from 1 to 2 mm in diameter to large, punched-out ulcers that are several millimeters in diameter and surrounded by small, inflamed margins.

Diagnosis

CONFIRMING DIAGNOSIS *Characteristic oral lesions suggest this diagnosis; isolation of the virus from mouth washings or feces and elevated specific antibody titer confirm it.*

POLIO PROTECTION

Dr. Jonas Salk's poliomyelitis vaccine, which became available in 1955, has been rightly called one of the miracle drugs of modern medicine. The vaccine contains dead (formalin-inactivated) polioviruses that stimulate production of circulating antibodies in the human body. This vaccine so effectively eliminated poliomyelitis that today it's difficult to appreciate how fearful people once were of this disease.

Oral polio vaccine is no longer used in the United States because polio had been eliminated from the Western Hemisphere and there were new cases of vaccine-associated polio. Instead, inactivated poliovirus vaccine (IPV) has been the recommended form of vaccine since January 2000. Children should receive 4 doses of IPV at ages 2, 4, and 6 to 18 months and at age 4 to 6 years. Routine poliovirus vaccination isn't generally recommended for people ages 18 or older residing in the United States.

Other routine test results are normal except for slight leukocytosis.

Diagnosis requires distinguishing the mouth lesions in herpangina from those in streptococcal tonsillitis (no ulcers; lesions confined to tonsils).

Treatment

Treatment for herpangina is entirely symptomatic, emphasizing measures to reduce fever and prevent seizures and possible dehydration. Herpangina doesn't require isolation or hospitalization but does require careful hand hygiene and sanitary disposal of excretions. Topical anesthetic agents, such as benzocaine or Xylocaine, may be applied to the mouth for discomfort.

Special considerations

■ Teach parents to provide adequate fluids and a nonirritating diet, to enforce bed rest, and to administer tepid sponge baths and antipyretics.

Poliomyelitis

Poliomyelitis, also called *polio* or *infantile paralysis*, is an acute communicable disease caused by the poliovirus. It ranges in severity from inapparent infection to fatal paralytic illness. First recognized in 1840, poliomyelitis became epidemic in Norway and Sweden in 1905. Outbreaks reached pandemic proportions in Europe, North America, Australia, and New Zealand during the first half of this century. Incidence peaked during the 1940s and early 1950s, and led to the development of the Salk vaccine. (See *Polio protection.*)

Minor polio outbreaks still occur, usually among nonimmunized groups such as the Amish of Pennsylvania. The disease usually strikes during the summer and fall. Once confined mainly to infants and children, poliomyelitis mostly occurs today in people older than age 15. Adults and girls are at greater risk for infection; boys, for paralysis.

If the central nervous system (CNS) is spared, the prognosis is excellent. However, CNS infection can cause paralysis and death. The mortality for all types of poliomyelitis is 5% to 10%.

Causes

The poliovirus has three antigenically distinct serotypes—types I, II, and III—all of which cause poliomyelitis. These viruses are found worldwide and are transmitted from person to person by direct contact with infected oropharyngeal secretions or feces. The incubation period ranges from 5 to 35 days—7 to 14 days on average.

The virus usually enters the body through the alimentary tract, multiplies in the oropharynx and lower intestinal tract, and then spreads to regional lymph nodes and the blood. Factors that increase the risk of paralysis include pregnancy; old age; localized trauma, such as a recent tonsillectomy, tooth extraction, or inoculation; and unusual physical exertion at or just before the clinical onset of poliomyelitis.

Signs and symptoms

Manifestations of poliomyelitis follow three basic patterns. Inapparent (subclinical) infections constitute 95% of all poliovirus infections. Abortive poliomyelitis (minor illness), which accounts for 4% to 8% of all cases, causes slight fever, malaise, headache, sore throat, inflamed pharynx, and vomiting. The patient usually recovers within 72 hours. Most cases of inapparent or abortive poliomyelitis go unnoticed.

Major poliomyelitis, however, involves the CNS and takes two forms: nonparalytic and paralytic. Children commonly show a biphasic course, in which the onset of major illness occurs after recovery from the minor illness stage. *Nonparalytic poliomyelitis* produces moderate fever, headache, vomiting, lethargy, irritability, and pains in the neck, back, arms, legs, and abdomen. It also causes muscle tenderness, weakness, and spasms in the extensors of the neck and back and sometimes in the hamstring and other muscles. (These spasms may be observed during maximum range-of-motion exercises.) Nonparalytic polio usually lasts about a week, with meningeal irritation persisting for about 2 weeks.

Paralytic poliomyelitis usually develops within 5 to 7 days of the onset of fever. The patient displays symptoms similar to those of nonparalytic poliomyelitis, with asymmetrical weakness of various muscles, loss of superficial and deep reflexes, paresthesia, hypersensitivity to touch, urine retention, constipation, and abdominal distention. The extent of paralysis depends on the level of the spinal cord lesions, which may be cervical, thoracic, or lumbar.

Resistance to neck flexion is characteristic in nonparalytic and paralytic poliomyelitis. The patient will "tripod" — extend his arms behind him for support — when he sits up. He'll display Hoyne's sign — his head will fall back when he's supine and his shoulders are elevated. From a supine position, he won't be able to raise his legs a full 90 degrees. Paralytic poliomyelitis also causes positive Kernig's and Brudzinski's signs.

When the disease affects the medulla of the brain, it's called *bulbar paralytic poliomyelitis*, which is the most perilous type. This form affects the respiratory muscle

---

ENTEROVIRUS FACTS

Enteroviruses (polioviruses, coxsackieviruses, and echoviruses) infect the GI tract. These viruses, among the smallest that affect humans, include 3 known polioviruses, 23 group A coxsackieviruses, 6 group B coxsackieviruses, and 34 echoviruses. They usually infect humans as a result of ingestion of fecally contaminated material, causing a wide range of diseases (hand, foot, and mouth disease; aseptic meningitis; myocarditis; pericarditis; gastroenteritis; and poliomyelitis). They can appear in the pharynx, feces, blood, cerebrospinal fluid, and central nervous system tissue. Enterovirus infections are more prevalent in the summer and fall.

---

nerves, leading to respiratory paralysis, and weakens the muscles supplied by the cranial nerves (particularly IX and X), producing symptoms of encephalitis. Other signs and symptoms include facial weakness, diplopia, dysphasia, difficulty in chewing, inability to swallow or expel saliva, regurgitation of food through the nasal passages, and dyspnea as well as abnormal respiratory rate, depth, and rhythm, which may lead to respiratory arrest. Fatal pulmonary edema and shock are possible.

Complications may result from the prolonged immobility and respiratory muscle failure. These include hypertension, urinary tract infection, urolithiasis, atelectasis, pneumonia, myocarditis, cor pulmonale, skeletal and soft-tissue deformities, and paralytic ileus.

Diagnosis

CONFIRMING DIAGNOSIS *Diagnosis requires isolation of the poliovirus from throat washings early in the disease, from stools throughout the disease, and from cerebrospinal fluid (CSF) cultures in CNS infection.*

Coxsackievirus and echovirus infections must be ruled out. (See *Enterovirus facts.*)

Convalescent serum antibody titers four times greater than acute titers support a diagnosis of poliomyelitis. Routine laboratory tests are usually within normal limits. However, CSF pressure and protein levels may be slightly increased and white blood cell count elevated initially, mostly due to polymorphonuclear leukocytes, which constitute 50% to 90% of the total count. Thereafter, mononuclear cells constitute most of the diminished number of cells.

Treatment

Treatment is supportive and includes analgesics to ease headache, back pain, and leg spasms; morphine is contraindicated because of the danger of additional respiratory suppression. Moist heat applications may also reduce muscle spasm and pain.

Bed rest is necessary only until extreme discomfort subsides; in paralytic polio, this may take a long time. Paralytic polio also requires long-term rehabilitation using physical therapy, braces, corrective shoes and, in some cases, orthopedic surgery.

Special considerations

Your care plan must be comprehensive to help prevent complications and to assist polio patients — physically and emotionally — during their prolonged convalescence.

■ Observe the patient carefully for signs of paralysis and other neurologic damage, which can occur rapidly. Maintain a patent airway, and watch for respiratory weakness and difficulty in swallowing. A tracheotomy is typically done at the first sign of respiratory distress, after which the patient is placed on a mechanical ventilator. Remember to reassure the patient that his breathing is being supported. Practice strict sterile technique during suctioning, and use only sterile solutions to nebulize medications.

■ Perform a brief neurologic assessment at least once a day, but don't demand any vigorous muscle activity. Encourage a return to mild activity as soon as the patient is able.

■ Check blood pressure frequently, especially in bulbar poliomyelitis, which can cause hypertension or shock because of its effect on the brain stem.

■ Watch for signs of fecal impaction due to dehydration and intestinal inactivity. To prevent this, give sufficient fluids to ensure an adequate daily output of low-specific-gravity urine (1.5 to 2 L/day for adults).

■ Monitor the bedridden patient's food intake for an adequate, well-balanced diet. If tube feedings are required, give liquid baby foods, juices, lactose, and vitamins.

■ Be sure to prevent pressure ulcers by providing good skin care, repositioning the patient often, and keeping the bed dry. Remember, muscle paralysis may cause bladder weakness or transient bladder paralysis.

■ Apply high-top sneakers or use a footboard to prevent footdrop. To alleviate discomfort, use foam rubber pads and sandbags, as needed, and light splints as ordered.

■ To control the spread of poliomyelitis, wash your hands thoroughly after contact with the patient, especially after contact with excretions. Instruct the ambulatory patient to do the same. (Only hospital personnel who have been vaccinated against poliomyelitis should have direct contact with the patient.)

■ Provide emotional support to the patient and his family. Reassure the nonparalytic patient that his chances for recovery are good. Long-term support and encouragement are essential for maximum rehabilitation.

■ An interdisciplinary rehabilitation program should be set up for a paralytic patient. It should include physical and occupational therapists, physicians and, if necessary, a psychiatrist to help manage the emotional problems suddenly facing severe physical disabilities.

■ Report all cases of poliomyelitis to the appropriate health department.

ARBOVIRUS

Colorado tick fever

Colorado tick fever is a benign infection caused by the Colorado tick fever arbovirus and transmitted to humans by a tick. It occurs in the Rocky Mountain region of the United States, mostly in April and May at lower altitudes and in June and July at higher altitudes. Because of occupational or recreational exposure, it's more common in men than in women. Colorado tick fever apparently confers long-lasting immunity against reinfection.

Causes and incidence
Colorado tick fever is transmitted to humans by a hard-shelled wood tick called *Dermacentor andersoni*. The adult tick acquires the virus when it bites infected rodents and remains permanently infective.

Incidence is high in Colorado, where up to 15% of people who regularly camp show past exposure. It's much less common in the rest of the United States.

Signs and symptoms
After a 3- to 6-day incubation period, Colorado tick fever begins abruptly with chills; temperature of 104° F (40° C); severe aching of back, arms, and legs; lethargy; and headache with eye movement such as extraocular movement. Photophobia, abdominal pain, nausea, and vomiting may occur. Rare effects include petechial or maculopapular rashes and central nervous system involvement. Symptoms subside after several days but return within 2 to 3 days and continue for 3 more days before slowly disappearing. Complete recovery usually follows.

Diagnosis
CONFIRMING DIAGNOSIS *A history of recent exposure to ticks along with moderate to severe leukopenia, complement fixation tests, or virus isolation confirm the diagnosis.*

Treatment
After correct removal of the tick, supportive treatment focuses on relieving symptoms, combating secondary infection, and maintaining fluid balance. Colorado tick fever needs to be differentiated from Rocky Mountain spotted fever and tularemia.

Special considerations
■ Carefully remove the tick by grasping it with forceps or gloved fingers and pulling gently. Be careful not to crush the tick's body. Keep it for identification. Thorough-

ly wash the wound with soap and water. If the tick's head remains embedded, surgical removal is necessary. Give a tetanus-diphtheria booster as ordered.
■ Be alert for secondary infection.
■ Monitor the patient's fluid and electrolyte balance, and provide replacement therapy, as indicated.
■ Reduce fever with antipyretics and tepid sponge baths.
■ To prevent tickborne infection, tell the patient to avoid tick bites by wearing long-sleeved clothing, tucking pant bottoms into the top of his boots, and carefully checking his body and scalp for ticks several times a day whenever in tick-infested areas. He should also use insect repellant.

MISCELLANEOUS VIRUSES

Mumps

Mumps, also known as *infectious* or *epidemic parotitis,* is an acute viral disease caused by a paramyxovirus. It causes painful enlargement of the salivary or parotid glands. It may also infect other organs, such as the testes, the central nervous system (CNS), and the pancreas. The prognosis for complete recovery is good, although mumps sometimes causes complications.

Causes and incidence
The mumps paramyxovirus is found in the saliva of an infected person and is transmitted by droplets or by direct contact. The virus is present in the saliva 6 days before to 9 days after onset of parotid gland swelling; the 48-hour period immediately preceding onset of swelling is probably the time of highest communicability. The incubation period ranges from 14 to 25 days (the average is 18). One attack of mumps (even if unilateral) almost always confers lifelong immunity.

Mumps is most prevalent in children between ages 6 and 8. Infants younger than age 1 seldom get this disease because of the passive immunity received from maternal antibodies. Peak incidence occurs during late winter and early spring.

Signs and symptoms

The clinical features of mumps vary widely. An estimated 30% of susceptible people have subclinical illness.

Mumps usually begins with prodromal symptoms that last for 24 hours and include myalgia, anorexia, malaise, headache, and low-grade fever followed by an earache that's aggravated by chewing; parotid gland tenderness and swelling; a temperature of 101° to 104° F (38.3° to 40° C); and pain when chewing or when drinking sour or acidic liquids. Simultaneously with the swelling of the parotid gland or several days later, one or more of the other salivary glands may become swollen.

Complications can include epididymo-orchitis and mumps meningitis. In approximately 25% of postpubertal males who contract mumps, epididymo-orchitis occurs and produces abrupt onset of testicular swelling and tenderness, scrotal erythema, lower abdominal pain, nausea, vomiting, fever, and chills. Swelling and tenderness may last for several weeks; epididymitis may precede or accompany the orchitis. In 50% of men with mumps-induced orchitis, the testicles show some atrophy, but *sterility is extremely rare.*

Mumps meningitis complicates the disease in 10% of patients and affects three to five times more males than females. Signs and symptoms include fever, meningeal irritation (nuchal rigidity, headache, and irritability), vomiting, drowsiness, and a cerebrospinal fluid lymphocyte count ranging from 500 to 2,000/µl. Recovery is usually complete. Less common effects are pancreatitis, deafness, arthritis, myocarditis, encephalitis, pericarditis, oophoritis, and nephritis.

Diagnosis

Diagnosis is usually made after the characteristic signs and symptoms develop, especially parotid gland enlargement with a history of exposure to mumps. Serologic antibody testing can verify the diagnosis when parotid or other salivary gland enlargement is absent. If comparison between a blood specimen obtained during the acute phase of illness and another specimen obtained 3 weeks later shows a fourfold rise in antibody titer, the patient most likely had mumps.

Treatment

Treatment includes analgesics for pain, antipyretics for fever, and adequate fluid intake to prevent dehydration from fever and anorexia. If the patient can't swallow, consider I.V. fluid replacement. Warm salt-water gargles, soft foods, and extra fluids may also help relieve symptoms.

Special considerations

■ Stress the need for bed rest during the febrile period. Give analgesics and apply warm or cool compresses to the neck to relieve pain. Give antipyretics and tepid sponge baths for fever. To prevent dehydration, encourage the patient to drink fluids; to minimize pain and anorexia, advise him to avoid spicy, irritating foods and those that require a lot of chewing. Offer a soft, bland diet.

■ During the acute phase, observe the patient closely for signs of CNS involvement, such as altered level of consciousness and nuchal rigidity.

■ Because the mumps virus is present in the saliva throughout the course of the disease, follow droplet precautions until symptoms subside.

■ Emphasize the importance of routine immunization with live attenuated mumps virus (paramyxovirus) at age 15 months and for susceptible patients (especially males) who are approaching or are past puberty. Remember, immunization within 24 hours of exposure may prevent or attenuate the actual disease. Immunity against mumps lasts at least 12 years.

■ Report all cases of mumps to local public health authorities.

Infectious mononucleosis

Infectious mononucleosis is an acute infectious disease caused by the Epstein-Barr virus (EBV), a member of the herpes group. It primarily affects young adults and children, although in children it's usually so mild that it's generally overlooked. This infection characteristically produces fever, sore throat, and cervical lymphadenopathy (the hallmarks of the disease) as well as hepatic dysfunction, increased lymphocyte and monocyte counts, and development and persistence of heterophil antibodies. The prognosis is excellent, and major complications are uncommon.

Causes and incidence

Apparently, the reservoir of EBV is limited to humans. Infectious mononucleosis probably spreads by the oral-pharyngeal route because about 80% of patients carry EBV in the throat during the acute infection and for an indefinite period afterward. It can also be transmitted by blood transfusions and has been reported after cardiac surgery as the post-pump perfusion syndrome. Infectious mononucleosis is probably contagious from before symptoms develop until the fever subsides and oral-pharyngeal lesions disappear.

Infectious mononucleosis is fairly common in the United States, Canada, and Europe and affects both sexes equally. Incidence varies seasonally among college students but not among the general population.

Signs and symptoms

The symptoms of mononucleosis mimic those of many other infectious diseases, including hepatitis, rubella, and toxoplasmosis. Typically, after an incubation period of about 10 days in children and from 30 to 50 days in adults, infectious mononucleosis produces prodromal symptoms, such as headache, malaise, and fatigue. After 3 to 5 days, patients typically develop a triad of symptoms: sore throat, cervical lymphadenopathy, and temperature fluctuations, with an evening peak of 101° to 102° F (38.3° to 38.9° C). Splenomegaly, hepatomegaly, stomatitis, exudative tonsillitis, or pharyngitis may also develop.

Sometimes, early in the illness, a maculopapular rash that resembles rubella develops; also, jaundice occurs in about 5% of patients. Major complications are rare but may include splenic rupture, aseptic meningitis, encephalitis, hemolytic anemia, idiopathic thrombocytopenic purpura, and Guillain-Barré syndrome. Symptoms usu-ally subside about 6 to 10 days after onset of the disease but may persist for weeks.

Diagnosis

Physical examination demonstrating the clinical triad suggests infectious mononucleosis.

 CONFIRMING DIAGNOSIS *The following abnormal laboratory results confirm the diagnosis:*

- *Monospot test is positive for infectious mononucleosis.*
- *Leukocyte count increases to 10,000 to 20,000/µl during the second and third weeks of illness. Lymphocytes and monocytes account for 50% to 70% of the total white blood cell (WBC) count; 10% of the lymphocytes are atypical.*
- *Heterophil antibodies (agglutinins for sheep red blood cells) in serum drawn during the acute illness and at 3- to 4-week intervals rise to four times the normal number.*
- *Indirect immunofluorescence shows antibodies to EBV and cellular antigens. Such testing is usually more definitive than heterophil antibodies.*
- *Liver function studies are abnormal.*

Treatment

Infectious mononucleosis resists prevention and antimicrobial treatment. Therapy is essentially supportive: relief of symptoms; bed rest during the acute febrile period; and acetaminophen or ibuprofen for headache and sore throat. Sore throat can also be helped with warm salt-water gargles. If severe throat inflammation causes airway obstruction, steroids can be used to relieve swelling and avoid tracheotomy. Splenic rupture, marked by sudden abdominal pain, requires splenectomy. About 20% of patients with infectious mononucleosis will also have streptococcal pharyngotonsillitis; these patients should receive antibiotic therapy.

Special considerations

Because uncomplicated infectious mononucleosis doesn't require hospitalization, patient teaching is essential. Convalescence may take several weeks, usually until the patient's WBC count returns to normal.

- During the acute illness, stress the need for bed rest. If the patient is a student, tell him he may continue less demanding school assignments and see his friends but should avoid long, difficult projects until after recovery.

■ To minimize throat discomfort, encourage the patient to drink milk shakes, fruit juices, and broths and to eat cool, bland foods. Suggest gargling with saline mouthwash and taking aspirin, as needed.

Rabies

Rabies, also known as *hydrophobia,* is an acute central nervous system (CNS) infection caused by a virus that's transmitted by the saliva of an infected animal (especially wild animals). If symptoms occur, rabies is almost always fatal. Treatment soon after exposure, however, may prevent fatal CNS invasion.

Causes and incidence

The rabies virus is usually transmitted to a human through the bite of an infected animal. The virus begins to replicate in the striated muscle cells at the bite site. Then it spreads up the nerve to the CNS and replicates in the brain. Finally, it moves through the nerves into other tissues, including the salivary glands. Occasionally, airborne droplets and infected tissue transplants can transmit the virus.

Rabies symptoms appear earlier if the head or face is severely bitten. If the bite is on the face, the risk of developing rabies is about 60%; on the upper extremities, 15% to 40%; and on the lower extremities, about 10%.

In the United States, dog vaccinations have reduced the incidence of rabies transmission to humans. Wild animals, such as skunks, foxes, raccoons, and bats, account for 70% of rabies cases.

Signs and symptoms

After an incubation period between 1 to 3 months, rabies typically produces local or radiating pain or burning and a sensation of cold, pruritus, and tingling at the bite site. It also produces prodromal signs and symptoms, such as a slight fever (100° to 102° F [37.8° to 38.9° C]), malaise, headache, anorexia, nausea, sore throat, and

persistent loose cough. After this, the patient begins to display nervousness, anxiety, irritability, hyperesthesia, photophobia, sensitivity to loud noises, pupillary dilation, tachycardia, shallow respirations, pain and paresthesia in the bitten area, and excessive salivation, lacrimation, and perspiration.

About 2 to 10 days after the onset of prodromal symptoms, a phase of excitation begins. It's characterized by agitation, marked restlessness, anxiety, and apprehension and cranial nerve dysfunction that causes ocular palsies, strabismus, asymmetrical pupillary dilation or constriction, absence of corneal reflexes, weakness of facial muscles, and hoarseness. Severe systemic symptoms include tachycardia or bradycardia, cyclic respirations, urine retention, and a temperature of about 103° F (39.4° C).

About 50% of affected patients exhibit hydrophobia (literally, "fear of water"). Forceful, painful pharyngeal muscle spasms expel liquids from the mouth and cause dehydration and, possibly, apnea, cyanosis, and death. Difficulty swallowing causes frothy saliva to drool from the patient's mouth. Eventually, even the sight, mention, or thought of water causes uncontrollable pharyngeal muscle spasms and excessive salivation. Between episodes of excitation and hydrophobia, the patient commonly is cooperative and lucid. After about 3 days, excitation and hydrophobia subside, and the progressively paralytic, terminal phase of this illness begins.

 ALERT *The patient experiences progressive, generalized, flaccid paralysis that ultimately leads to peripheral vascular collapse, coma, and death.*

Diagnosis

Because rabies is fatal unless treated promptly, always suspect rabies in any person who suffers an unprovoked animal bite until you can prove otherwise.

 CONFIRMING DIAGNOSIS *Virus isolation from the patient's saliva or throat and examination of his blood for fluorescent rabies antibody (FRA) are diagnostic.*

Other results typically include elevated white blood cell count, with increased polymorphonuclear and large mononuclear cells, and elevated urinary glucose, acetone, and protein levels.

Confinement of the suspected animal for 10 days of observation by a veterinarian also helps support this diagnosis. If the animal appears rabid, it should be killed and its brain tissue tested for FRA and Negri bodies (oval or round masses that conclusively confirm rabies).

Treatment
Treatment consists of wound care and immunization as soon as possible after exposure. Thoroughly wash all bite wounds and scratches with soap and water to remove any infected saliva. (See *First aid in animal bites.*) Check the patient's immunization status, and administer tetanus-diphtheria prophylaxis if needed. Take measures to control bacterial infection as ordered. If the wound requires suturing, special treatment and suturing techniques must be used to allow proper drainage.

After rabies exposure, a patient who has not been immunized before must receive passive immunization with rabies immune globulin (RIG) and active immunization with human diploid cell vaccine (HDCV). If the patient has received HDCV before and has an adequate rabies antibody titer, he doesn't need RIG immunization, just an HDCV booster.

Special considerations
■ When injecting rabies vaccine, rotate injection sites on the upper arm or thigh. Watch for and symptomatically treat redness, itching, pain, and tenderness at the injection site. Half of the RIG should be infiltrated into and around the bite wound, with the remainder given I.M.
■ Cooperate with public health authorities to determine the vaccination status of the animal. If the animal is proven rabid, help identify others at risk.

If rabies develops:
■ Monitor cardiac and pulmonary function continuously.
■ Isolate the patient. Wear a gown, gloves, and protection for the eyes and mouth when handling saliva and articles contaminated with saliva. Take precautions to avoid being bitten by the patient during the excitation phase.

FIRST AID IN ANIMAL BITES

Immediately wash the bite vigorously with soap and water for at least 10 minutes to remove the animal's saliva. As soon as possible, flush the wound with a viricidal agent, followed by a clear-water rinse. After cleaning the wound, apply a sterile dressing. If possible, don't suture the wound, and don't immediately stop the bleeding (unless it's massive) because blood flow helps to clean the wound.

Question the patient about the bite. Ask if he provoked the animal (if so, chances are it isn't rabid) and if he can identify it or its owner (because the animal may be confined for observation).

■ Keep the room dark and quiet.
■ Establish communication with the patient and his family. Provide psychological support to help them cope with the patient's symptoms and probable death.

To help prevent rabies:
■ Stress the need for vaccination of household pets that may be exposed to rabid wild animals.
■ Warn people not to try to touch wild animals, especially if they appear ill or overly docile (a possible sign of rabies)
■ Assist in the prophylactic administration of rabies vaccine to high-risk people, such as farm workers, forest rangers, spelunkers (cave explorers), and veterinarians.

Cytomegalovirus infection

Cytomegalovirus (CMV) infection is caused by the cytomegalovirus, a deoxyribonucleic acid, ether-sensitive virus belonging to the herpes family. Also known as *generalized salivary gland disease* or *cytomegalic inclusion disease*, CMV infection occurs worldwide and is transmitted by human contact.

Causes

CMV has been found in the saliva, urine, semen, breast milk, feces, blood, and vaginal and cervical secretions of infected people. The virus is usually transmitted through contact with these infected secretions, which can harbor the virus for months or even years. It may be transmitted by sexual contact and can travel across the placenta, causing a congenital infection. Immunosuppressed patients, especially those who have received transplanted organs, run a 90% chance of contracting CMV infection. Recipients of blood transfusions from donors with positive CMV antibodies are at some risk.

About four out of five people older than age 35 have been infected with CMV, usually during childhood or early adulthood. In most of these people, the disease is so mild that it's overlooked. However, CMV infection during pregnancy can be hazardous to the fetus, possibly leading to stillbirth, brain damage, and other birth defects or to severe neonatal illness. About 1% of all neonates have CMV.

Signs and symptoms

CMV probably spreads through the body in lymphocytes or mononuclear cells to the lungs, liver, GI tract, eyes, and central nervous system, where it commonly produces inflammatory reactions.

Most patients with CMV infection have mild, nonspecific complaints or none at all, even though antibody titers indicate infection. In these patients, the disease usually runs a self-limiting course. However, immunodeficient patients and those receiving immunosuppressants may develop pneumonia or other secondary infections. In patients with acquired immunodeficiency syndrome, disseminated CMV infection may cause chorioretinitis (resulting in blindness), colitis, encephalitis, abdominal pain, diarrhea, or weight loss. Infected infants ages 3 to 6 months usually appear asymptomatic but may develop hepatic dysfunction, hepatosplenomegaly, spider angiomas, pneumonitis, and lymphadenopathy.

Congenital CMV infection is seldom apparent at birth, although the neonate's urine contains the virus. CMV can cause brain damage that may not show up for months after birth. It also can produce a rapidly fatal neonatal illness characterized by jaundice, petechial rash, hepatosplenomegaly, thrombocytopenia, hemolytic anemia, microcephaly, psychomotor retardation, mental deficiency, and hearing loss. Occasionally, this form is rapidly fatal.

In some adults, CMV may cause cytomegalovirus mononucleosis, with 3 weeks or more of irregular, high fever. Other findings may include a normal or elevated white blood cell (WBC) count, lymphocytosis, and increased atypical lymphocytes.

Diagnosis

CONFIRMING DIAGNOSIS
Although virus isolation in urine is the most sensitive laboratory method, diagnosis can also be made with virus isolated from saliva, throat, cervix, WBCs, or biopsy specimens.

Other laboratory tests supporting the diagnosis include complement fixation studies, hemagglutination inhibition antibody tests and, for congenital infections, indirect immunofluorescent tests for CMV immunoglobulin M antibody.

Treatment

Treatment aims to relieve symptoms and prevent complications. In the immunosuppressed patient, CMV may be treated with acyclovir, ganciclovir, valganciclovir, cidofovir and, possibly, foscarnet. Most important, parents of children with severe congenital CMV infection need support and counseling to help them cope with the possibility of brain damage or death.

Special considerations

To help prevent CMV infection:
- Because many patients who excrete CMV are asymptomatic, standard precautions should be maintained at all times.
- Warn immunosuppressed patients and pregnant women to avoid exposure to confirmed or suspected CMV infection. (Maternal CMV infection can cause fetal abnormalities: hydrocephaly, microphthalmia, seizures, encephalitis, hepatosplenomegaly, hematologic changes, microcephaly, and blindness.)

- Urge patients with CMV infection to use good hand hygiene to prevent spreading it. Stress this particularly with young children.
- Be sure to observe standard precautions when handling body secretions.

Lassa fever

Lassa fever is an epidemic hemorrhagic fever caused by the Lassa virus, an extremely virulent arenavirus. This highly fatal disorder kills 10% to 50% of its victims, but those who survive its early stages usually recover and acquire immunity to secondary attacks.

Causes and incidence
A chronic infection in rodents, Lassa virus is transmitted to humans by contact with infected rodent urine, feces, and saliva. The virus enters the bloodstream, lymph vessels, and respiratory and digestive tracts. It then multiplies in the cells of the reticuloendothelial system. In the early stages of this illness, when the virus is in the throat, human transmission may occur through inhalation of infected droplets.

As many as 100 cases of Lassa fever occur annually in western Africa; the disease is rare in the United States.

Signs and symptoms
After a 7- to 18-day incubation period, this disease produces a fever that persists for 2 to 3 weeks, exudative pharyngitis, oral ulcers, lymphadenopathy with swelling of the face and neck, purpura, conjunctivitis, and bradycardia. Severe infection may also cause hepatitis, myocarditis, pleural infection, encephalitis, and permanent unilateral or bilateral deafness.

Virus multiplication in reticuloendothelial cells causes capillary lesions that lead to erythrocyte and platelet loss; mild to moderate thrombocytopenia (with a tendency toward bleeding); and secondary bacterial infection. These capillary lesions may also cause focal hemorrhage in the stomach, small intestine, kidneys, lungs, and brain and, possibly, hemorrhagic shock and peripheral vascular collapse.

Diagnosis
 CONFIRMING DIAGNOSIS *Isolation of the Lassa virus from throat washings, pleural fluid, or blood confirms the diagnosis.*
Recent travel to an endemic area and specific antibody titer support the diagnosis.

Treatment
Treatment of Lassa fever includes I.V. ribavirin, I.V. colloids for shock, analgesics for pain, and antipyretics for fever. Infusion of immune plasma from patients who have recovered from Lassa fever may be useful, but test results on the benefit of this type of therapy are inconclusive.

Special considerations
- Carefully monitor fluid and electrolyte status, vital signs, and intake and output. Watch for and immediately report signs of infection or shock.
- Contact precautions are necessary for at least 3 weeks, until the patient's throat washings and urine are free of the virus. To prevent the spread of this contagious disease, carefully dispose of, or disinfect, all materials contaminated with the infected patient's urine, feces, respiratory secretions, or exudates. Watch known contacts closely for at least 3 weeks for signs of the disease.
- Provide good oral care. Remember to clean the patient's mouth with a soft-bristled toothbrush to avoid irritating any oral ulcers. Ask your facility's dietary department to supply a soft, bland, nonirritating diet.
- Immediately contact the Viral Diseases Division of the Centers for Disease Control and Prevention in Atlanta to get specific guidelines for managing suspected or confirmed cases of Lassa fever.
- Report all cases of Lassa fever to the local health department.

Ebola virus infection

One of the most frightening viruses to come out of the African subcontinent, the Ebola virus first appeared in 1976. More than 400 people in Zaire (now known as Democratic Republic of Congo) and the neighboring Sudan were killed by the hemorrhagic fever that it caused. Ebola virus has been responsible for several outbreaks in the years since then, including one in Zaire in the summer of 1995.

An unclassified ribonucleic acid (RNA) virus, Ebola is morphologically similar to the Marburg virus. Both can cause headache, malaise, myalgia, and high fever, progressing to severe diarrhea, vomiting, and internal and external hemorrhage.

Four strains of the Ebola virus are known to exist: Ebola Zaire, Ebola Sudan, Ebola Tai, and Ebola Reston. All four types are structurally similar, although they have different antigenic properties. However, Ebola Reston causes illness only in monkeys, not in humans, as do the other three.

The prognosis for Ebola virus infection is extremely poor, with mortality as high as 90%. The incubation period ranges from 2 to 21 days.

Causes

Ebola virus infection is caused by an unclassified RNA virus that's passed from person to person by direct contact with infected blood, body secretions, or organs. Nosocomial and community-acquired transmission can occur. Contaminated needles can also cause the infection. Transmission through semen may occur up to 7 weeks after clinical recovery. The virus remains contagious even after the patient has died.

Signs and symptoms

The patient's health history usually reveals contact with an infected person. However, no clear line of infection may be apparent at the beginning of an Ebola virus outbreak. The patient usually complains of flulike signs and symptoms (such as headache, malaise, myalgia, fever, cough, and sore throat), which first appear within 3 days of infection.

As the virus spreads through the body, inspection reveals bruising as capillaries rupture and dead blood cells infiltrate the skin. A maculopapular eruption appears after the fifth day of infection. The patient may also display melena, hematemesis, epistaxis, and bleeding gums. As the infection progresses, severe complications, including liver and kidney dysfunction, dehydration, and hemorrhage, may develop. In pregnant women, the Ebola virus leads to abortion and massive hemorrhage.

In the final stages of the disease, the skin blisters and sloughs off, blood seeps from all body orifices, and the patient begins vomiting his liquefied internal organs. Death usually results during the second week of illness from organ failure or hemorrhage.

Diagnosis

Specialized laboratory tests reveal specific antigens or antibodies and may show the isolated virus. As with other types of hemorrhagic fever, tests also demonstrate neutrophil leukocytosis, hypofibrinogenemia, thrombocytopenia, and microangiopathic hemolytic anemia.

Treatment

No cure exists for Ebola virus infection; treatment consists mainly of intensive supportive care. Administration of I.V. fluids helps offset the effects of severe dehydration. The patient may receive replacement of plasma heparin before the onset of clinical shock.

Experimental treatments include the administration of plasma that contains Ebola virus-specific antibodies. Although this treatment has resulted in diminished levels of Ebola virus in the body, further evaluation is needed.

Throughout treatment, the patient should remain on contact precautions. If diagnostic tests indicate that the patient is free from the virus — which typically occurs 21 days after onset in those few who survive — the patient can be released.

Special considerations

■ Follow the guidelines for standard precautions formulated by the Centers for Disease Control and Prevention (CDC) when assessing a patient who may have Ebola virus.
■ Check the results of complete blood count and coagulation studies for signs of blood loss and coagulopathy.
■ Assess the patient daily for petechiae, ecchymoses, and oozing blood. Note and

document the size of ecchymoses at least every 24 hours.

- Protect all areas of petechiae and ecchymoses from further injury.
- Test stools, urine, and vomitus for occult blood.
- Watch for frank bleeding, including GI bleeding and, in women, menorrhagia. Note and document the amount of bleeding every 24 hours or more often.
- Monitor the patient's family and other close contacts for fever and other signs of infection.
- Provide emotional support for the patient and his family during the course of this devastating disease. Encourage them to ask questions and discuss any concerns they have about the disease and its treatment.
- In addition, the CDC recommends the following guidelines to help prevent the spread of this deadly disease:
  – If possible, place the patient in a negative-pressure room at the beginning of hospitalization to avoid the need for transfer as the disease progresses.
  – Restrict nonessential staff members from entering the patient's room.
  – Make sure that anyone who enters the patient's room wears gloves and a gown to prevent contact with any surface in the room that may have been contaminated.
  – Use barrier precautions to prevent skin or mucous membrane exposure to blood or other body fluids, secretions, or excretions when caring for the patient.
  – If you must come within 3′ (0.9 m) of the patient, also wear a face shield or surgical mask and goggles or eyeglasses with side shields.
  – Don't reuse gloves or gowns unless they have been completely disinfected.
- Make sure any patient who dies of the disease is promptly buried or cremated. Precautions to prevent contact with the patient's body fluids and secretions should continue even after the patient's death.

West Nile encephalitis

West Nile encephalitis is categorized as an infectious disease that primarily causes an inflammation or "encephalitis" of the brain. West Nile virus (WNV), a flavivirus commonly found in humans, birds, and other vertebrates in Africa, west Asia, and the Middle East, causes the disease, which is a part of a family of vector-borne diseases that also includes malaria, yellow fever, and Lyme disease.

The virus had not been previously documented in the Western Hemisphere until late August 1999. A virus found in numerous dead birds in New York, New Jersey, and Connecticut was definitively identified by genetic sequencing as the West Nile virus. Scientists in the United States discovered the rare strain initially in and around the Bronx Zoo and believe that infected birds may have carried the disease and that it was spread as mosquitoes fed on them.

In the temperate areas of the world, West Nile encephalitis cases occur mainly in the late summer or early fall. In the southern climates where temperatures are milder, West Nile encephalitis can occur all year round.

The risk of contracting West Nile encephalitis is greater for all residents of areas where active cases have been identified, but persons older than age 50 or those with compromised immune systems have the greatest risk. At present, there is no documented evidence that a pregnant woman's fetus is at risk due to an infection with WNV. The mortality rate of West Nile encephalitis is measured by case-fatality rates, which range from 3 % to 15 % (higher in the elderly population.)

Causes and incidence
WNV is transmitted to humans by the bite of a mosquito (primarily the *Culex* species) infected with the virus. It's considered the primary vector for WNV and the source of the August 1999 outbreak in New York, New Jersey and Connecticut. Mosquitoes become infected by feeding on birds contaminated with the West Nile virus and then transmitting it to humans and animals during a blood meal or "bite." (See *Transmission routes of West Nile virus*, page 256.)

Ticks have been found infected with WNV in Africa and Asia only. The role of ticks in the transmission and maintenance of the virus remains uncertain, and to date

TRANSMISSION ROUTES OF WEST NILE VIRUS

Birds are the reservoir of the West Nile virus. They harbor the virus but are unable to spread it. Mosquitoes serve as the vectors, spreading it from bird to bird and from birds to people. Humans are believed to be "dead-end hosts" because the virus can live and cause illness in humans, but it isn't believed that a feeding mosquito can acquire the virus from an infected person.

Brain

Mosquitoes (vector)

Human (dead-end host)

Virus

they aren't considered vectors for WNV in the United States.

The Centers for Disease Control and Prevention has reported that there is no evidence that a person can contract the virus from handling live or dead infected birds. However, avoid barehanded contact when handling dead animals, including birds, and use gloves or double plastic bags to dispose of a carcass. Report the finding to the local health department.

Signs and symptoms

Mild infections of the virus are more common and include fever, headache, and body aches, usually accompanied by a skin rash and swollen lymph glands. Severe infections can be manifested by headache, high fever, neck stiffness, stupor, disorientation, coma, tremors, occasional convulsions, paralysis and, rarely, death.

The incubation period for West Nile encephalitis is anywhere from 5 to 15 days after exposure. Most patients who are bitten by an infected mosquito won't develop symptoms. It's estimated that only 1 in 300 people who are bitten by an infected mosquito will actually get sick.

Diagnosis

The immunoglobulin (Ig) M antibody capture enzyme-linked immunosorbent assay

(MAC-ELISA) is the test of choice for rapid definitive diagnosis. The major advantage of MAC-ELISA laboratory analysis is the high probability of accurate diagnosis of WNV infection when performed with acute serum or cerebrospinal fluid specimens obtained while the patient is still hospitalized.

A new diagnostic test, the WNV MAC-ELISA, was recently approved by the Food and Drug Administration. This test detects levels of IgM antibodies in a patient's serum and is intended for use in patients with clinical symptoms consistent with viral encephalitis.

Other conditions to consider include St. Louis encephalitis, which is symptomatically similar.

Encephalitis can be caused by numerous viral and bacterial infections; all data must be examined to determine a definitive diagnosis.

Treatment

There is no specific therapy utilized to treat West Nile encephalitis and no known cure. Treatment is generally aimed at controlling the specific symptoms. Supportive care, such as I.V. fluids, fever control, and respiratory support, is rendered when necessary.

There is no vaccine present to prevent the transmission of West Nile encephalitis. Research trials are underway to determine if ribavirin, an antiviral drug, may be helpful.

Special considerations

- Obtain an extensive history of the patient's whereabouts within the past 2 to 3 weeks (especially around bodies of water, such as lakes and ponds), the presence of dead birds, and recent mosquito bites acquired.
- Perform a comprehensive physical assessment and report signs of fever, headache, lymphadenopathy, and a maculopapular rash.
- Perform a complete neurological examination and report any signs of confusion, lethargy, weakness, or slurred speech.
- Maintain adequate hydration with I.V. fluids.
- Monitor strict intake and output.

- Use fever control methods, such as cooling blankets and acetaminophen as ordered.
- Provide respiratory support measures when applicable.
- West Nile encephalitis isn't transmitted from person to person, but use standard precautions when handling body fluids and blood.
- Report any suspected cases of West Nile encephalitis to the applicable state health department.
- Teach the patient ways to reduce his risk of becoming infected with West Nile encephalitis:
  - Stay indoors at dawn, dusk, and in the early evening.
  - Wear long-sleeved shirts and long pants outdoors.
  - Apply insect repellent sparingly to exposed skin. Check the label. An effective repellent will contain 20% to 30% *N,N*-diethyl-*meta*-toluamide (DEET). DEET in high concentrations (greater than 30%) may cause adverse effects, particularly in children; avoid products containing more than 30% DEET.
  - Repellents may irritate the eyes and mouth, so avoid applying repellent to the hands of children. It's contraindicated to apply insect repellents to children younger than age 3 years.
  - Spray clothing with repellents containing DEET, as mosquitoes may bite through thin clothing.
  - Whenever you use an insecticide or insect repellent, be sure to read and follow the manufacturer's directions for use, as printed on the product.

RICKETTSIA

Rocky Mountain spotted fever

Rocky Mountain spotted fever (RMSF) is a febrile, rash-producing illness caused by *Rickettsia rickettsii*. The disease is transmitted to humans by a tick bite.

RMSF is fatal in about 5% of patients. Mortality rises when treatment is delayed and in older patients.

Causes and incidence

R. rickettsii is transmitted to a human or small animal by the prolonged bite (4 to 6 hours) of an adult tick—the wood tick (*Dermacentor andersoni*) in the west and by the dog tick (*Dermacentor variabilis*) in the east. Occasionally, it's acquired through inhalation (it can occur in laboratory settings where aerosolization of blood and specimens may occur) or through the contact of abraded skin with tick excreta or tissue juices. (This explains why people shouldn't crush ticks between their fingers when removing them from other people and animals.) In most tick-infested areas, 1% to 5% of the ticks harbor *R. rickettsii*.

Endemic throughout the continental United States, RMSF is particularly prevalent in the southeast and southwest. Because RMSF is associated with outdoor activities, such as camping and backpacking, the incidence of this illness is usually higher in the spring and summer. Epidemiologic surveillance reports for RMSF indicate that the incidence is also higher in children ages 5 to 9, men and boys, and whites.

Signs and symptoms

The incubation period is usually about 7 days, but it can range from 2 to 14 days. Generally, the shorter the incubation time, the more severe the infection. Signs and symptoms, which usually begin abruptly, include a persistent temperature of 102° to 104° F (38.9° to 40° C); a generalized, excruciating headache; nausea and vomiting; and aching in the bones, muscles, joints, and back. In addition, the tongue is covered with a thick white coating that gradually turns brown as the fever persists and rises.

Initially, the skin may simply appear flushed. Between days 2 and 5, eruptions begin around the wrists, ankles, or forehead; within 2 days, they cover the entire body, including the scalp, palms, and soles. The rash consists of erythematous macules 1 to 5 mm in diameter that blanch on pressure; if untreated, the rash may become petechial and maculopapular. By the third

week, the skin peels off and may become gangrenous over the elbows, fingers, and toes.

The pulse is strong initially, but it gradually becomes rapid (possibly reaching 150 beats/minute) and thready.

 ALERT *A rapid pulse rate and hypotension (systolic pressure less than 90 mm Hg) herald imminent death from complete vascular collapse.*

Other signs and symptoms include a bronchial cough, a rapid respiratory rate (as high as 60 breaths/minute), anorexia, constipation, abdominal pain, hepatomegaly, splenomegaly, insomnia, restlessness and, in extreme cases, delirium. Urine output falls to half of the normal level or less, is dark in color, and contains albumin. Complications, although uncommon, include lobar pneumonia, otitis media, parotitis, disseminated intravascular coagulation (DIC) and, possibly, renal failure. In rare cases, RMSF leads to death.

Diagnosis

CONFIRMING DIAGNOSIS *Diagnosis is usually based on a history of tick bite or travel to a tick-infested area and a positive complement fixation test (which shows a fourfold increase in convalescent antibody titer compared with acute titers). Blood cultures or skin biopsy at the rash site should be performed to isolate the organism and confirm the diagnosis.*

Another common but less reliable antibody test is the Weil-Felix reaction, which also shows a fourfold increase between the acute and convalescent sera titer levels. Increased titers usually develop after 10 to 14 days and persist for several months.

Additional recommended laboratory tests consist of a platelet count for thrombocytopenia (12,000 to 150,000/µl) and a white blood cell count (elevated to 11,000 to 33,000/µl) during the second week of illness.

Treatment

Treatment requires careful removal of the tick and administration of antibiotics, such as chloramphenicol or tetracycline (preferably doxycycline), until 3 days after the fever subsides. Treatment also includes symptomatic measures and, in DIC, heparin and platelet transfusion.

Special considerations
- Carefully monitor the patient's intake and output. Watch closely for decreased urine output—a possible indicator of renal failure.
- Be alert for signs of dehydration, such as poor skin turgor and dry mouth.
- Administer antipyretics as ordered, and provide tepid sponge baths to reduce fever.
- Monitor vital signs, and watch for profound hypotension and shock.
- Be prepared to administer oxygen therapy and assisted ventilation if pulmonary complications develop.
- Turn the patient frequently to prevent complications of immobility, such as pressure ulcers and pneumonia.
- Pay attention to the patient's nutritional needs; vomiting may indicate a need for parenteral nutrition or for scheduling frequent small meals.
- Instruct the patient to report any recurrent symptoms to the physician at once so that treatment measures may resume immediately.
- Advise the patient to avoid tick-infested areas (woods, meadows, streams, and canyons) in the future if possible.
- Teach the patient ways to reduce his risk of becoming infected with Rocky Mountain spotted fever:
  – Encourage him to inspect his entire body (including his scalp) every 3 to 4 hours for attached ticks.
  – Remind him to wear protective clothing, such as a long-sleeved shirt, pants securely tucked into laced boots, and a protective head covering such as a cap.
  – Advise him to apply insect repellant to exposed skin as well as to clothing.
- Offer printed and illustrated instructions, if available, to teach the patient and his family members or other caregivers how to correctly and safely remove a tick. Demonstrate how to use tweezers or forceps and apply steady traction to release the entire tick without leaving its mouth parts in the skin.
- After the patient removes the tick, caution him not to handle it or its fragments.

- Finally, instruct the patient to clean his skin with alcohol at the point of attachment.
- Report all cases to the appropriate health department.

PROTOZOA

Pneumocystis carinii pneumonia

Because of its association with human immunodeficiency virus (HIV) infection, *Pneumocystis carinii* pneumonia (PCP), an opportunistic infection, has increased in incidence since the 1980s. Before the advent of PCP prophylaxis, this disease was the first clue in about 60% of patients that HIV infection was present.

PCP was the leading cause of death in these patients. Prophylactic therapy with co-trimoxazole in HIV patients with low immune function has prevented PCP from higher mortality rates. Disseminated infection doesn't occur.

PCP is also associated with other immunocompromising conditions, including organ transplantation, leukemia, lymphoma, and steroid use.

Causes and incidence
P. carinii, the cause of PCP, usually is classified as a protozoan, although some investigators consider it more closely related to fungi. The organism exists as a saprophyte in the lungs of humans and various animals as part of the normal flora in most healthy people. It becomes an aggressive pathogen in the immunocompromised patient. Impaired cell-mediated (T-cell) immunity is thought to be more important than impaired humoral (B-cell) immunity in predisposing the patient to PCP, but the immune defects involved are poorly understood. *P. carinii* becomes activated in immunocompromised patients when the CD4$^+$ T-cell count falls below 200/μl.

P. carinii invades the lungs bilaterally and multiplies extracellularly. As the infestation grows, alveoli fill with organisms and exudate, impairing gas exchange. The alveoli hypertrophy and thicken progressively, eventually leading to extensive consolidation.

The primary transmission route seems to be air, although the organism is already present in most people. The incubation period probably lasts for 4 to 8 weeks.

Signs and symptoms

The patient typically has a history of an immunocompromising condition (such as HIV infection, leukemia, or lymphoma) or procedure (such as organ transplantation). PCP begins insidiously with increasing shortness of breath and a nonproductive cough. Anorexia, generalized fatigue, and weight loss may follow. Although the patient may have hypoxemia and hypercapnia, he may not exhibit significant symptoms. He may, however, have a low-grade, intermittent fever.

Other signs and symptoms include tachypnea, dyspnea, accessory muscle use for breathing, crackles (in about one-third of patients), marked pallor, and decreased breath sounds (in advanced pneumonia). Cyanosis may appear with acute illness; pulmonary consolidation develops later.

Diagnosis

CONFIRMING DIAGNOSIS *Histologic studies confirm P. carinii in all patients. Fiber-optic bronchoscopy remains the most commonly used study to confirm PCP. Invasive procedures, such as transbronchial biopsy and open-lung biopsy, are performed less commonly.*

In patients with HIV infection, initial examination of a first-morning sputum specimen (induced by inhaling an ultrasonically dispersed saline mist) may be sufficient; however, this technique usually is ineffective in patients without HIV infection.

Chest X-rays may show slowly progressing, fluffy infiltrates and, occasionally, nodular lesions or a spontaneous pneumothorax, but these findings must be differentiated from findings in other types of pneumonia or acute respiratory distress syndrome.

Gallium scan may show increased uptake over the lungs even when the chest X-ray appears relatively normal. Arterial blood gas (ABG) studies detect hypoxia and an increased A-a gradient.

Treatment

PCP may respond to drug therapy with co-trimoxazole. Other agents used to treat PCP include pentamidine, trimethoprim-dapsone, clindamycin, primaquine, and atovaquone. Corticosteroids are frequently used as well. However, because of immune system impairment, many patients with PCP, who also have HIV, experience severe adverse reactions to drug therapy.

Supportive measures, such as oxygen therapy, mechanical ventilation, adequate nutrition, and fluid balance, are important adjunctive therapies. Oral morphine sulfate solution may reduce the respiratory rate and anxiety, thereby enhancing oxygenation.

Special considerations

- Implement standard precautions to prevent contagion.
- Frequently assess the patient's respiratory status, and monitor ABG levels every 4 hours.
- Administer oxygen therapy as ordered. Encourage the patient to ambulate as well as to perform deep-breathing exercises and incentive spirometry to facilitate effective gas exchange.
- Administer antipyretics as ordered, to relieve fever.
- Monitor the patient's intake and output and daily weight to evaluate fluid balance. Replace fluids as ordered.
- Provide diversionary activities and coordinate health care team activities to allow adequate rest periods between procedures.
- Teach the patient energy conservation techniques.
- Supply nutritional supplements as needed. Encourage the patient to eat a high-calorie, protein-rich diet. Offer small, frequent meals if the patient cannot tolerate large amounts of food.
- Reduce anxiety by providing a relaxing environment, eliminating excessive environmental stimuli, and allowing ample time for meals.
- Give emotional support and help the patient identify and use meaningful support systems.

- Instruct the patient about the medication regimen, especially about the adverse effects.
- Emphasize the importance of continuing chemoprophylaxis for those patients at high risk of developing PCP.
- If the patient will require oxygen therapy at home, explain that an oxygen concentrator may be most effective.
- Because this infection is usually associated with acquired immunodeficiency syndrome (AIDS), provide the patient with resources and support organizations for both AIDS and HIV.

Malaria

Malaria, an acute infectious disease, is caused by protozoa of the genus *Plasmodium*: *P. falciparum*, *P. vivax*, *P. malariae*, and *P. ovale*, all of which are transmitted to humans by mosquito vectors. Falciparum malaria is the most severe form of the disease. When treated, malaria is rarely fatal; untreated, it's fatal in 10% of victims, usually as a result of complications such as disseminated intravascular coagulation (DIC).

Untreated primary attacks last from a week to a month, or longer. Relapses are common and can recur sporadically for several years. Susceptibility to the disease is universal.

Causes and incidence

Malaria literally means "bad air" and for centuries was thought to result from the inhalation of swamp vapors. It's now known that malaria is transmitted by the bite of female *Anopheles* mosquitoes, which abound in humid, swampy areas. When an infected mosquito bites, it injects *Plasmodium* sporozoites into the wound. The infective sporozoites migrate by blood circulation to parenchymal cells of the liver; there they form cystlike structures containing thousands of merozoites.

Upon release, each merozoite invades an erythrocyte and feeds on hemoglobin. Eventually, the erythrocyte ruptures, releasing heme (malaria pigment), cell debris, and more merozoites, which, unless destroyed by phagocytes, enter other erythrocytes. (See *What happens in malaria*, page 262.) At this point, the infected person becomes a reservoir of malaria who infects any mosquito that feeds on him, thus beginning a new cycle of transmission. Hepatic parasites (*P. vivax*, *P. ovale*, and *P. malariae*) may persist for years in the liver. These parasites are responsible for the chronic carrier state. Because blood transfusions and street-drug paraphernalia can also spread malaria, drug addicts have a higher incidence of the disease. Malaria is a worldwide health problem that continues to impede the development of many countries.

Malaria is a tropical and subtropical disease. It's most prevalent in Asia, Africa, and Latin America. The Centers for Disease Control and Prevention (CDC) estimates 300 to 500 million cases occur each year, with more than 1 million resulting in death. It's the greatest disease hazard for travelers in warm climates.

Signs and symptoms

After an incubation period of 12 to 30 days, malaria produces chills, fever, headache, and myalgia, interspersed with periods of well-being (the hallmark of the benign form of malaria). Acute attacks (paroxysms) occur when erythrocytes rupture. There are three stages:

- *cold stage*, lasting 1 to 2 hours, ranging from chills to extreme shaking
- *hot stage*, lasting 3 to 4 hours, characterized by a high fever (up to 107° F [41.7° C])
- *wet stage*, lasting 2 to 4 hours and characterized by profuse sweating.

Paroxysms occur every 48 to 72 hours when malaria is caused by *P. malariae* and every 42 to 50 hours when malaria is caused by *P. vivax* or *P. ovale*. All three types have low levels of parasitosis and are self-limiting as a result of early acquired immunity.

P. vivax and *P. ovale* also produce hepatosplenomegaly. Hemolytic anemia is present in all but the mildest infections.

The most severe and only life-threatening form of malaria is caused by *P. falciparum*. This species produces persistent high fever, orthostatic hypotension, and red blood cell (RBC) sludging that leads to

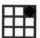

PATHOPHYSIOLOGY

WHAT HAPPENS IN MALARIA

A female Anopheles mosquito bites, injecting saliva containing sporozoites, the infective form of the malaria parasite.

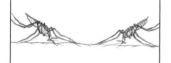

The sporozoites enter liver cells and multiply.

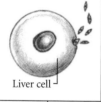

Liver cell

In the liver, the sporozoites change into merozoites, another form of the parasite.

Merozoites attack red blood cells (RBCs).

Red blood cell

Merozoites

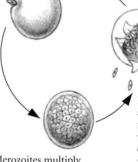

Merozoites multiply in RBCs.

RBCs burst and release the merozoites, which invade other RBCs and cause recurring chills and fever.

Merozoites are released from the liver and enter the bloodstream.

SPECIAL CONSIDERATIONS FOR ANTIMALARIAL DRUGS

Chloroquine
- Perform baseline and periodic ophthalmologic examinations, and report blurred vision, increased sensitivity to light, and muscle weakness to the physician.
- Consult with the physician about altering therapy if muscle weakness appears in a patient on long-term therapy.
- Monitor the patient for tinnitus and other signs of ototoxicity, such as nerve deafness and vertigo.
- Caution the patient to avoid excessive exposure to the sun to prevent exacerbating drug-induced dermatoses.

Primaquine
- Give with meals or antacids.
- Halt administration if you observe a sudden fall in hemoglobin concentration or in erythrocyte or leukocyte count or marked darkening of the urine, suggesting impending hemolytic reaction.

Pyrimethamine
- Administer with meals to minimize GI distress.
- Check blood counts (including platelets) twice per week. If signs of folic or folinic acid deficiency develop, reduce or discontinue dosage while the patient receives parenteral folinic acid until blood counts become normal.

Quinine
- Use with caution in patients with cardiovascular conditions. Discontinue dosage if you see any signs of idiosyncrasy or toxicity, such as headache, epigastric distress, diarrhea, rashes, and pruritus, in a mild reaction; or delirium, seizures, blindness, cardiovascular collapse, asthma, hemolytic anemia, and granulocytosis, in a severe reaction.
- Monitor blood pressure frequently while administering quinine I.V. infusion. Rapid administration causes marked hypotension.

---

capillary obstruction at various sites. Signs and symptoms of obstruction include:
- *cerebral*—hemiplegia, seizures, delirium, and coma
- *pulmonary*—coughing and hemoptysis
- *splanchnic*—vomiting, abdominal pain, diarrhea, and melena
- *renal*—oliguria, anuria, and uremia.

During blackwater fever (a complication of *P. falciparum* infection), massive intravascular hemolysis causes jaundice, hemoglobinuria, a tender and enlarged spleen, acute renal failure, and uremia. This complication is fatal in about 20% of patients.

Diagnosis

CONFIRMING DIAGNOSIS *A history showing travel to endemic areas, recent blood transfusion, or drug abuse in a person with high fever of unknown origin strongly suggests malaria. However, because symptoms of malaria mimic other diseases, unequivocal diagnosis depends on laboratory identification of the parasites in RBCs of peripheral blood smears.*

The CDC can identify donors responsible for transfusion malaria through indirect fluorescent serum antibody tests. These tests are unreliable in the acute phase because antibodies can be undetectable for 2 weeks after onset.

Supplementary laboratory values that support this diagnosis include decreased hemoglobin levels, normal to decreased leukocyte count (as low as 3,000/µl), and protein and leukocytes in urine sediment. In falciparum malaria, serum values reflect DIC: reduced number of platelets (20,000 to 50,000/µl); prolonged prothrombin time (18 to 20 seconds); prolonged partial thromboplastin time (60 to 100 seconds); and decreased plasma fibrinogen.

Treatment
Malaria is best treated with oral chloroquine in all forms except chloroquine-resistant *P. falciparum*. Symptoms and par-

HOW TO PREVENT MALARIA

- Drain, fill, and eliminate breeding areas of the *Anopheles* mosquito.
- Install screens in living and sleeping quarters in endemic areas.
- Use a residual insecticide on clothing and skin to prevent mosquito bites.
- Seek treatment for known cases.
- Question blood donors about a history of malaria or possible exposure to malaria. They *may* give blood if:
  – they haven't taken any antimalarial drugs and are asymptomatic after 6 months outside an endemic area
  – they were asymptomatic after treatment for malaria more than 3 years ago
  – they were asymptomatic after receiving malaria prophylaxis more than 3 years ago.
- Seek prophylactic drug therapy before traveling to an endemic area. Agents include mefloquine, doxycycline, chloroquine, hydroxychloroquine, or malarone (a combination of atovaquone and proguanil). They're usually started 2 weeks before visiting the endemic area and continue for 6 weeks after leaving the area.

can induce hemolytic anemia, especially in patients with glucose-6-phosphate dehydrogenase deficiency. (See *Special considerations for antimalarial drugs*, page 263.)

For travelers spending less than 3 weeks in areas where malaria exists, weekly prophylaxis includes oral chloroquine beginning 2 weeks before the trip and ending 6 weeks after it. (See *How to prevent malaria*.) Any traveler who develops an acute febrile illness should seek prompt medical attention, regardless of the prophylaxis taken.

Special considerations

- Obtain a detailed patient history, noting any recent travel, foreign residence, blood transfusion, or drug addiction. Record symptom pattern, fever, type of malaria, and any systemic signs.
- Assess the patient on admission and daily thereafter for fatigue, fever, orthostatic hypotension, disorientation, myalgia, and arthralgia. Enforce bed rest during periods of acute illness.
- Protect the patient from secondary bacterial infection by following proper hand-hygiene and sterile techniques.
- Protect yourself by wearing gloves when handling blood or body fluids.
- Activate safety devices, and use safety syringes in practice.
- Discard needles and syringes in an impervious container designated for incineration.
- Handle bed linens according to standard precautions.
- To reduce fever, administer antipyretics as ordered. Document onset, duration, and symptoms before and after episodes.
- Fluid balance is fragile, so keep a strict record of intake and output. Monitor I.V. fluids closely. Avoid fluid overload (especially in *P. falciparum*), because it can lead to pulmonary edema and aggravate cerebral symptoms. Observe blood chemistry levels for hyponatremia and increased blood urea nitrogen, creatinine, and bilirubin levels. Monitor urine output hourly, and maintain it at 40 to 60 ml/hour for an adult and at 15 to 30 ml/hour for a child. Immediately report any decrease in urine output or the onset of hematuria as a pos-

asitemia decrease within 24 hours after such therapy begins, and the patient usually recovers within 3 to 4 days. If the patient is comatose or vomiting frequently, chloroquine is given I.M.

Malaria caused by *P. falciparum*, which is resistant to chloroquine, requires treatment with oral quinine given concurrently with pyrimethamine and a sulfonamide such as sulfadiazine. Mefloquine can also be used for resistant *P. falciparum*. Relapses require the same treatment, or quinine alone, followed by tetracycline.

The only drug effective against the hepatic stage of the disease that's available in the United States is primaquine. This drug

sible sign of renal failure; be prepared to perform peritoneal dialysis for uremia caused by renal failure.

■ Slowly administer packed RBCs or whole blood while checking for crackles, tachycardia, and shortness of breath.

■ If humidified oxygen is ordered, note the patient's response, particularly any changes in rate or character of respirations, or any improvement in mucous membrane color.

■ Watch for and immediately report signs of internal bleeding, such as tachycardia, hypotension, and pallor.

■ Encourage frequent coughing and deep breathing, especially if the patient is on bed rest or has pulmonary complications. Record the amount and color of sputum.

■ Watch for adverse effects of drug therapy, and take measures to relieve them.

■ If the patient is comatose, make frequent, gentle changes in his position, and give passive range-of-motion exercises every 3 to 4 hours. If the patient is unconscious or disoriented, use restraints as needed, and keep an airway available as appropriate.

■ Provide emotional support and reassurance, especially in critical illness. Explain the procedures and treatment to the patient and his family. Suggest that other family members be tested for malaria. Emphasize the need for follow-up care to check the effectiveness of treatment and to manage residual problems.

■ Report all cases of malaria to local public health authorities.

Amebiasis

Amebiasis, also known as *amebic dysentery,* is an acute or chronic protozoal infection caused by *Entamoeba histolytica.* This infection produces varying degrees of illness, from no symptoms at all or mild diarrhea to fulminant dysentery. Extraintestinal amebiasis can induce hepatic abscess and infections of the lungs, pleural cavity, pericardium, peritoneum and, rarely, the brain.

The prognosis is generally good, although complications — such as ameboma, intestinal stricture, hemorrhage or perforation, intussusception, or abscess —

increase mortality. Brain abscess, a rare complication, is usually fatal.

Causes and incidence

E. histolytica exists in two forms: a cyst (which can survive outside the body) and a trophozoite (which can't survive outside the body). Transmission occurs through ingesting feces-contaminated food or water. The ingested cysts pass through the intestine, where digestive secretions break down the cysts and liberate the motile trophozoites within. The trophozoites multiply and either invade and ulcerate the mucosa of the large intestine or simply feed on intestinal bacteria. As the trophozoites are carried slowly toward the rectum, they are encysted and then excreted in feces. Humans are the principal reservoir of infection.

Amebiasis occurs worldwide but is most common in the tropics, subtropics, and other areas with poor sanitation and health practices. Incidence in the United States averages between 1% and 3% but may be higher among homosexuals and institutionalized people, in whom fecal-oral contamination is common.

Signs and symptoms

The clinical effects of amebiasis vary with the severity of the infestation. *Acute amebic dysentery* causes a sudden high temperature of 104° to 105° F (40° to 40.6° C) accompanied by chills and abdominal cramping; profuse, bloody, mucoid diarrhea with tenesmus; and diffuse abdominal tenderness due to extensive rectosigmoid ulcers.

Chronic amebic dysentery produces intermittent diarrhea that lasts for 1 to 4 weeks and recurs several times a year. Such diarrhea produces 4 to 8 (or, in severe diarrhea, up to 18) foul-smelling mucus- and blood-tinged stools daily in a patient with a mild fever, vague abdominal cramps, possible weight loss, tenderness over the cecum and ascending colon and, occasionally, hepatomegaly. Amebic granuloma (ameboma), commonly mistaken for cancer, can be a complication of the chronic infection. Amebic granuloma produces blood and mucus in the stool and, when granulomatous tissue covers the entire circumference of the bowel, causes partial or complete obstruction.

Parasitic and bacterial invasion of the appendix may produce typical signs of subacute appendicitis (abdominal pain and tenderness). Occasionally, *E. histolytica* perforates the intestinal wall and spreads to the liver. When it perforates the liver and diaphragm, it spreads to the lungs, pleural cavity, peritoneum and, rarely, the brain.

Diagnosis

Q **CONFIRMING DIAGNOSIS** *Isolating* E. histolytica *(cysts and trophozoites) in fresh feces or aspirates from abscesses, ulcers, or tissue confirms acute amebic dysentery.*

Diagnosis must distinguish between cancer and ameboma with X-rays, sigmoidoscopy, stool examination for amebae, and cecum palpation. In patients with amebiasis, exploratory surgery is hazardous; it can lead to peritonitis, perforation, and pericecal abscess.

Other laboratory tests that support the diagnosis of amebiasis include:
- indirect hemagglutination test — positive with current or previous infection
- complement fixation — usually positive only during active disease
- barium studies — rule out nonamebic causes of diarrhea, such as polyps and cancer
- sigmoidoscopy — detects rectosigmoid ulceration; a biopsy may be helpful.

Patients with amebiasis shouldn't have preparatory enemas because these may remove exudates and destroy the trophozoites, thus interfering with test results.

Treatment

Drugs used to treat amebic dysentery include metronidazole, an amebicide at intestinal and extraintestinal sites; emetine hydrochloride, also an amebicide at intestinal and extraintestinal sites, including the liver and lungs; iodoquinol (diiodohydroxyquin), an effective amebicide for asymptomatic carriers; chloroquine, for liver abscesses, not intestinal infections; and tetracycline (in combination with emetine hydrochloride, metronidazole, or paromomycin), which supports the antiamebic effect by destroying intestinal bacteria on which the amebae normally feed.

When nausea and vomiting are present, I.V. therapy may be necessary until medications are tolerated by mouth.

Special considerations
- Tell patients with amebiasis to avoid drinking alcohol when taking metronidazole. The combination may cause nausea, vomiting, and headache.
- Antidiarrheals aren't prescribed and can make the condition worse.
- After treatment, stools should be rechecked to make sure the infection has been cleared.

Giardiasis

Giardiasis (also called *Giardia enteritis* or *lambliasis*) is an infection of the small bowel caused by the symmetrical flagellate protozoan *Giardia lamblia*. A mild infection may not produce intestinal symptoms. In untreated giardiasis, symptoms wax and wane; with treatment, recovery is complete.

Causes and incidence

G. lamblia has two stages: the cystic stage and the trophozoite stage. Ingestion of *G. lamblia* cysts in fecally contaminated water or the fecal-oral transfer of cysts by an infected person results in giardiasis. Giardiasis may be transmitted through sexual contact (direct or indirect fecal-oral contact). When cysts enter the small bowel, they become trophozoites and attach themselves with their sucking disks to the bowel's epithelial surface. After this, the trophozoites encyst again, travel down the colon, and are excreted. Unformed feces that pass quickly through the intestine may contain trophozoites as well as cysts.

Giardiasis occurs worldwide but is most common in developing countries and other areas where sanitation and hygiene are poor. In the United States, giardiasis is most common in travelers who have recently returned from endemic areas, and in campers who drink unpurified water from contaminated streams. Probably because of frequent hand-to-mouth activity, children are more likely to become infected with *G.*

lamblia than adults. Hypogammaglobulinemia also appears to predispose people
to this disorder. Giardiasis doesn't confer
immunity, so reinfections may occur.

Signs and symptoms

Attachment of *G. lamblia* to the intestinal
lumen causes superficial mucosal invasion
and destruction, inflammation, and irritation. All of these destructive effects decrease food transit time through the small
intestine and result in malabsorption. Such
malabsorption produces chronic GI complaints—such as abdominal cramps—
and pale, loose, greasy, malodorous, and
frequent stools (from 2 to 10 daily) with
concurrent nausea. Stools may contain
mucus but not pus or blood. Chronic giardiasis may produce fatigue and weight loss
in addition to these typical signs and
symptoms.

Diagnosis

Suspect giardiasis when travelers to endemic areas or campers who may have
drunk unpurified water develop symptoms.

 CONFIRMING DIAGNOSIS *Actual
diagnosis requires laboratory examination of a fresh stool specimen for
cysts or examination of duodenal aspirate for
trophozoites. An antibody test of the stool for
giardiasis is also very effective in diagnosis. A
small bowel biopsy shows* Giardia.

A barium X-ray of the small bowel may
show mucosal edema and barium segmentation. Diagnosis must also rule out other
causes of diarrhea and malabsorption.

Treatment

Giardiasis responds readily to a 10-day
course of metronidazole or a 7-day course
of oral quinacrine and furazolidone. Severe
diarrhea may require parenteral fluid replacement to prevent dehydration if oral
fluid intake is inadequate.

Special considerations

■ Inform the patient receiving metronidazole of the possible adverse effects of this
drug: commonly, headache, anorexia, and
nausea and, less commonly, vomiting, diarrhea, and abdominal cramps. Warn against
drinking alcoholic beverages, which may
provoke a disulfiram-like reaction. If the
patient is a woman, ask if she's pregnant
because metronidazole is contraindicated
during pregnancy.
■ When talking to family members and
other suspected contacts, emphasize the
importance of stool examinations for
G. lamblia cysts.
■ If hospitalization is required, use standard precautions. A child or an incontinent
adult requires a private room. Pay strict attention to hand hygiene, particularly after
handling feces. Quickly dispose of fecal
material. (Normal sewage systems can remove and process infected feces adequately.)
■ Teach good personal hygiene, particularly proper hand-washing technique.
■ To help prevent giardiasis, warn travelers
to endemic areas not to drink water or eat
uncooked and unpeeled fruits or vegetables
(they may have been rinsed in contaminated water). Prophylactic drug therapy isn't
recommended. Advise campers to purify
all stream water before drinking it.
■ Report epidemic situations to the public
health authorities.

Toxoplasmosis

Toxoplasmosis, one of the most common
infectious diseases, is caused by the protozoa *Toxoplasma gondii*. Distributed worldwide, it's less common in cold or hot, arid
climates and at high elevations. It usually
causes localized infection but may produce
significant generalized infection, especially
in neonates and patients who are immunodeficient. Congenital toxoplasmosis, characterized by lesions in the central nervous
system, may result in stillbirth or serious
birth defects. For this reason, pregnant
women are advised to avoid cleaning cat
litter boxes because fecal-oral contamination from infected cats transmits toxoplasmosis.

Causes

T. gondii exists in trophozoite forms in the
acute stages of infection and in cystic
forms (tissue cysts and oocysts) in the latent stages. In addition to possible fecal-
oral transmission from infected cats, inges-

OCULAR TOXOPLASMOSIS

Ocular toxoplasmosis (active retinochoroiditis), characterized by focal necrotizing retinitis, accounts for about 25% of all cases of granulomatous uveitis. It's usually the result of congenital infection, but may not appear until adolescence or young adulthood, when infection is reactivated. Symptoms include blurred vision, scotoma, pain, photophobia, and impairment or loss of central vision. Vision improves as inflammation subsides but usually without recovery of lost visual acuity. Ocular toxoplasmosis may subside after treatment with prednisone.

tion of tissue cysts in raw or uncooked meat (heating, drying, or freezing destroys these cysts) can also transmit toxoplasmosis. However, toxoplasmosis also occurs in vegetarians who aren't exposed to cats, so other means of transmission may exist. Congenital toxoplasmosis follows transplacental transmission from a chronically infected mother or one who acquired toxoplasmosis shortly before or during pregnancy.

Signs and symptoms

Toxoplasmosis acquired in the first trimester of pregnancy commonly results in stillbirth. About one-third of infants who survive have congenital toxoplasmosis. The later in pregnancy that maternal infection occurs, the greater the risk of congenital infection in the infant. Obvious signs of congenital toxoplasmosis include retinochoroiditis, hydrocephalus or microcephalus, cerebral calcification, seizures, lymphadenopathy, fever, hepatosplenomegaly, jaundice, and rash. Other defects, which may become apparent months or years later, include strabismus, blindness, epilepsy, and mental retardation. (See *Ocular toxoplasmosis.*)

Acquired toxoplasmosis may cause localized (mild lymphatic) or generalized (fulminating, disseminated) infection.

Localized infection produces fever and a mononucleosis-like syndrome (malaise, myalgia, headache, fatigue, and sore throat) and lymphadenopathy. Generalized infection produces encephalitis, fever, headache, vomiting, delirium, seizures, and a diffuse maculopapular rash (except on the palms, soles, and scalp). Generalized infection may lead to myocarditis, pneumonitis, hepatitis, and polymyositis.

Diagnosis

 CONFIRMING DIAGNOSIS *Identification of* T. gondii *in an appropriate tissue specimen confirms the diagnosis of toxoplasmosis.*

Serologic tests may be useful and, in patients with toxoplasmosis encephalitis, computed tomography scans and magnetic resonance imaging disclose lesions.

Treatment

Treatment of acute disease consists of drug therapy with sulfonamides, pyrimethamine, folinic acid, clindamycin, or cotrimoxazole. In patients who also have acquired immunodeficiency syndrome, treatment continues indefinitely. No safe, effective treatment exists for chronic toxoplasmosis or toxoplasmosis occurring in the first trimester of pregnancy.

Special considerations

When caring for patients with toxoplasmosis, monitor drug therapy carefully and emphasize thorough patient teaching to prevent complications and control spread of the disease.

■ Because sulfonamides cause blood dyscrasias and pyrimethamine depresses bone marrow, closely monitor the patient's hematologic values. Also emphasize the importance of regularly scheduled follow-up care.

■ Teach all patients to wash their hands after working with soil (because it may be contaminated with cat oocysts); to cook meat thoroughly and freeze it promptly if it isn't for immediate use; to change cat litter daily (cat oocysts don't become infective until 1 to 4 days after excretion); to cover children's sandboxes; and to keep flies away from food (flies transport oocysts).

■ Advise all pregnant women to avoid cleaning and handling of cat litter boxes. If this can't be avoided, advise them to wear gloves.

■ Patients who are receiving immunosuppressants are very susceptible to toxoplasmosis. Warn them of the risks and suggest having all cats that go outdoors tested for toxoplasmosis.

■ Report all cases of toxoplasmosis to your local public health department.

HELMINTHS
Trichinosis

Trichinosis (also known as *trichiniasis* or *trichinellosis*) is an infection caused by larvae of the intestinal roundworm *Trichinella spiralis*. It occurs worldwide, especially in populations that eat pork or bear meat. Trichinosis may produce multiple symptoms; respiratory, central nervous system (CNS), and cardiovascular complications; and, rarely, death.

Causes and incidence
Transmission is through ingestion of uncooked or undercooked meat that contains *T. spiralis* cysts. Such cysts are found primarily in swine, less commonly in dogs, cats, bears, foxes, wolves, and marine animals. These cysts result from the animals' ingestion of similarly contaminated flesh. In swine, such infection results from eating table scraps or raw garbage.

After gastric juices free the worm from the cyst capsule, it reaches sexual maturity in a few days. The female roundworm burrows into the intestinal mucosa and reproduces. Larvae are then transported through the lymphatic system and the bloodstream. They become embedded as cysts in striated muscle, especially in the diaphragm, chest, arms, and legs. Human-to-human transmission doesn't take place.

Trichinosis, though common worldwide, is seldom seen in the United States because of regulations regarding animal feed and meat processing.

Signs and symptoms
In the United States, trichinosis is usually mild and seldom produces symptoms. When symptoms do occur, they vary with the stage and degree of infection:

■ *Stage 1* (invasion) occurs 1 week after ingestion. Release of larvae and reproduction of adult *T. spiralis* may cause anorexia, nausea, vomiting, diarrhea, abdominal pain, and cramps.

■ *Stage 2* (dissemination) occurs 7 to 10 days after ingestion. *T. spiralis* penetrates the intestinal mucosa and begins to migrate to striated muscle. Signs and symptoms include edema, especially of the eyelids or face; muscle pain, particularly in extremities; and, occasionally, itching and burning skin, sweating, skin lesions, a temperature of 102° to 104° F (38.9° to 40° C), and delirium. In severe respiratory, cardiovascular, or CNS infections, palpitations and lethargy can occur.

■ *Stage 3* (encystment) occurs during convalescence, generally 1 week later. *T. spiralis* larvae invade muscle fiber and become encysted.

Diagnosis
A history of ingestion of raw or improperly cooked pork or pork products, with typical clinical features, suggests trichinosis, but infection may be difficult to prove. Stools may contain mature worms and larvae during the invasion stage. Skeletal muscle biopsies can show encysted larvae 10 days after ingestion; if available, analyses of contaminated meat also show larvae.

Skin testing may show a positive histamine-like reactivity 15 minutes after intradermal injection of the antigen (within 17 to 20 days after ingestion). However, such a result may remain positive for up to 5 years after exposure. Elevated acute and convalescent antibody titers (determined by flocculation tests 3 to 4 weeks after infection) confirm this diagnosis.

Other abnormal results include elevated aspartate aminotransferase, alanine aminotransferase, creatine kinase, and lactate dehydrogenase levels during the acute stages and an elevated eosinophil count (up to 15,000/µl). A normal or increased cerebrospinal fluid lymphocyte level (to

300/µl) and increased protein levels indicate CNS involvement.

Treatment

Mebendazole effectively combats this parasite during the intestinal stage; severe infection (especially CNS invasion) may warrant glucocorticoids to combat possible inflammation. There's no treatment for trichinosis once it's in the muscles, but analgesics may be used for muscle pain.

Special considerations

■ Question the patient about recent ingestion of pork products and the methods used to store and cook them.
■ Reduce fever with alcohol rubs, tepid baths, cooling blankets, or antipyretics; relieve muscle pain with analgesics, enforced bed rest, and proper body alignment.
■ To prevent pressure ulcers, frequently reposition the patient, and gently massage bony prominences.
■ Explain the importance of bed rest. Sudden death from cardiac involvement may occur in a patient with moderate to severe infection who has resumed activity too soon. Warn the patient to continue bed rest into the convalescent stage to avoid a serious relapse and possible death.

To help prevent trichinosis:
■ Educate the public about proper cooking and storing methods not only for pork and pork products but also for meat from other carnivores. To kill trichinae, internal meat temperatures should reach 150° F (65.6° C) and meat color should change from pink to gray unless the meat has been cured or frozen for at least 10 days at low temperatures.
■ Warn travelers to foreign countries or to poor areas in the United States to avoid eating pork; swine in these areas are commonly fed raw garbage.
■ Report all cases of trichinosis to local public health authorities.

Hookworm disease

Hookworm disease, also called *uncinariasis* or *ground itch,* is an infection of the upper intestine caused by *Ancylostoma duodenale* (found in the eastern hemisphere) or *Neca-*

tor americanus (in the western hemisphere). Sandy soil, high humidity, a warm climate, and failure to wear shoes all favor its transmission. In the United States, hookworm disease is most common in the southeast. Although this disease can cause cardiopulmonary complications, it's rarely fatal, except in debilitated people and infants younger than age 1.

Causes and incidence

Both forms of hookworm disease are transmitted to humans through direct skin penetration (usually in the foot) by hookworm larvae in soil contaminated with feces containing hookworm ova. These ova develop into infectious larvae in 1 to 3 days. Larvae travel through the lymphatics to the pulmonary capillaries, where they penetrate alveoli and move up the bronchial tree to the trachea and epiglottis, where they're swallowed and enter the GI tract. When they reach the small intestine, they mature, attach to the jejunal mucosa, and suck blood, oxygen, and glucose from the intestinal wall. These mature worms then deposit ova, which are excreted in the stool, starting the cycle anew. Hookworm larvae mature in approximately 5 to 6 weeks.

Hookworm disease, affecting billions of people worldwide, is most common in moist tropical and subtropical regions. There's little risk of aquiring hookworm disease in the United States because of advances in sanitization and waste control.

Signs and symptoms

Most cases of hookworm disease produce few symptoms and may be overlooked until worms are passed in the stool. The earliest signs and symptoms include irritation, pruritus, and edema at the site of entry, which are sometimes accompanied by secondary bacterial infection with pustule formation.

When the larvae reach the lungs, they may cause pneumonitis and hemorrhage with fever, sore throat, crackles, and cough. Finally, intestinal infection may cause fatigue, nausea, weight loss, dizziness, melena, and uncontrolled diarrhea.

In severe and chronic infection, anemia from blood loss may lead to cardiomegaly (a result of increased oxygen demands), heart failure, and generalized massive edema.

Diagnosis

 CONFIRMING DIAGNOSIS *Identification of hookworm ova in the stool confirms the diagnosis. Anemia suggests severe chronic infection.*

Treatment

Treatment of hookworm infection includes administering mebendazole or albendazole, and providing an iron-rich diet or iron supplements to prevent or correct anemia.

Special considerations

■ Obtain a complete history, with special attention to travel or residency in endemic areas. Note the sequence and onset of symptoms. Interview the patient's family and other close contacts to see if they have symptoms.

■ Carefully assess the patient, noting signs of entry, lymphedema, and respiratory status.

■ Perform meticulous hand hygiene after every patient contact.

■ For severe anemia, administer oxygen, if ordered, at low to moderate flow. Be sure the oxygen is humidified because the patient may already have upper airway irritation from the parasites. Encourage coughing and deep breathing to stimulate removal of blood or secretions from involved lung areas and to prevent secondary infection. Plan your care to allow frequent rest periods because the patient may tire easily. If anemia causes immobility, reposition the patient often to prevent skin breakdown.

■ Closely monitor intake and output. Note the frequency of diarrhea and the quantity of stools. Dispose of feces promptly, and wear gloves when doing so.

■ To help assess nutritional status, weigh the patient daily. To combat malnutrition, emphasize the importance of good nutrition, with particular attention to foods high in iron and protein. If the patient receives iron supplements, explain that they will darken stools. Administer antihelmintics on an empty stomach, but without a purgative.

■ To help prevent reinfection, educate the patient in proper hand-hygiene technique and sanitary disposal of feces. Tell him to wear shoes in endemic areas.

Ascariasis

Ascariasis, also known as *roundworm infection,* is caused by *Ascaris lumbricoides.* It's the most common type of intestinal worm infection, occurring worldwide. Most patients recover without treatment, but complications can occur when adult worms move into certain organs and multiply, resulting in blockage of the intestine.

Causes and incidence

A. lumbricoides is a large roundworm resembling an earthworm. It's transmitted to humans by ingestion of soil contaminated with human feces that harbor *A. lumbricoides* ova. Such ingestion may occur directly (by eating contaminated soil) or indirectly (by eating poorly washed raw vegetables grown in contaminated soil).

Ascariasis never passes directly from person to person. After ingestion, *A. lumbricoides* ova hatch and release larvae, which penetrate the intestinal wall and reach the lungs through the bloodstream. After about 10 days in pulmonary capillaries and alveoli, the larvae migrate to the bronchioles, bronchi, trachea, and epiglottis. There they are swallowed and return to the intestine to mature into worms.

Ascariasis is most common in tropical areas with poor sanitation and in Asia, where farmers use human feces as fertilizer. In the United States, it's more prevalent in the south, particularly among people ages 4 to 12.

Signs and symptoms

Ascariasis produces two phases: early pulmonary and prolonged intestinal. Mild intestinal infection may cause only vague stomach discomfort. The first clue may be vomiting a worm or passing a worm in the stool. Severe infection, however, causes stomach pain, vomiting, restlessness, disturbed sleep and, in extreme cases, intestinal obstruction. Larvae migrating by the lymphatic and the circulatory systems cause symptoms that vary; for instance, when they invade the lungs, pneumonitis may result.

Diagnosis

 CONFIRMING DIAGNOSIS *The key to diagnosis is identifying ova in the stool or adult worms, which may be passed rectally or by mouth.*

When migrating larvae invade alveoli, other conclusive tests include X-rays that show characteristic bronchovascular markings: infiltrates, patchy areas of pneumonitis, and widening of hilar shadows. In a patient with ascariasis, these findings usually accompany a complete blood count that shows eosinophilia.

Treatment

Drug therapy, the primary treatment, consists of albendazole or mebendazole to kill intestinal parasitic worms, permitting peristalsis to expel them. No specific treatment exists for migratory infection because anthelmintics affect only mature worms.

In intestinal obstruction, nasogastric (NG) suctioning controls vomiting. If there's a blockage caused by a large number of worms, a paralyzing vermifuge (such as pyrantel pamoate or piperazine) can make the worms relax and pass through the intestine to relieve obstruction. However, ascariasis may necessitate surgery if the paralyzed worms result in intestinal blockage.

Special considerations

■ Although isolation is unnecessary, properly dispose of feces and soiled linen, and carefully wash your hands after patient contact.
■ If the patient is receiving NG suction, be sure to give him good mouth care.
■ Teach the patient to prevent reinfection with good hand hygiene, especially before eating and after defecation.

Taeniasis

Taeniasis, also called *tapeworm disease* or *cestodiasis,* is a parasitic infestation by *Taenia saginata* (beef tapeworm), *Taenia soli-* *um* (pork tapeworm), *Diphyllobothrium latum* (fish tapeworm), or *Hymenolepis nana* (dwarf tapeworm). Taeniasis is usually a chronic, benign intestinal disease; however, infestation with *T. solium* may cause dangerous systemic and central nervous system symptoms if larvae invade the brain and striated muscle of vital organs.

Causes

T. saginata, T. solium, and *D. latum* are transmitted to humans by ingestion of beef, pork, or fish that contains tapeworm cysts. Gastric acids break down these cysts in the stomach, liberating them to mature. Mature tapeworms fasten to the intestinal wall and produce ova that are passed in the feces. Transmission of *H. nana* is direct from person to person and requires no intermediate host; it completes its life cycle in the intestine. (See *Common tapeworm infestations.*)

Signs and symptoms

Taeniasis may produce mild symptoms, such as nausea, flatulence, hunger sensations, weight loss, diarrhea, and increased appetite, or no symptoms at all. Occasionally, worm segments may exit through the anus and appear on bed clothes.

Diagnosis

 CONFIRMING DIAGNOSIS *Diagnosis of tapeworm infestations requires laboratory observation of tapeworm ova or body segments in feces.*

Because ova aren't excreted continuously, confirmation may require multiple specimens. A supporting dietary or travel history aids confirmation.

Treatment

The drug of choice for tapeworm infection is niclosamide, but praziquantel and albendazole can also be used.

Laxative use or induced vomiting are contraindicated because of the danger of autoinfection and systemic disease.

After drug treatment, tapeworm infestation requires a follow-up laboratory examination of stool specimens during the next 3 to 5 weeks to check for any remaining ova or worm segments. Persistent infestation

COMMON TAPEWORM INFESTATIONS

Type and source of infection	Incidence	Clinical features
Diphyllobothrium latum (*fish tapeworm*)		
Uncooked or under-cooked infected freshwater fish, such as pike, trout, salmon, and turbot	Finland, parts of the former Soviet Union, Japan, Alaska, Australia, the Great Lakes region (United States), Switzerland, Chile, and Argentina	Anemia (hemoglobin level as low as 6 to 8 g)
Hymenolepis nana (*dwarf tapeworm*)		
No intermediate host; parasite passes directly from person to person via ova passed in stool; inadequate hand washing facilitates its spread	Most common tapeworm in humans; particularly prevalent among institutionalized mentally retarded children and in underdeveloped countries	Dependent on patient's nutritional status and number of parasites; commonly no symptoms with mild infestation; with severe infestation, anorexia, diarrhea, restlessness, dizziness, and apathy
Taenia saginata (*beef tapeworm*)		
Uncooked or under-cooked infected beef	Worldwide, but prevalent in Europe and East Africa	Crawling sensation in the perianal area caused by worm segments that have been passed rectally; intestinal obstruction and appendicitis due to long worm segments that have twisted in the intestinal lumen
Taenia solium (*pork tapeworm*)		
Uncooked or under-cooked infected pork	Highest in Mexico and Latin America; lowest among Muslims and Jews	Seizures, headaches, personality changes; commonly overlooked in adults

typically requires a second course of medication.

Special considerations

■ Obtain a complete history, including recent travel to endemic areas, dietary habits, and physical symptoms.

■ Dispose of the patient's excretions carefully. Wear gloves when giving personal care and handling fecal excretions, bedpans, and bed linens; wash your hands thoroughly, and tell the patient to do the same.

■ Use enteric precautions. Avoid procedures and drugs that may cause vomiting or gagging. If the patient is a child or is incontinent, he requires a private room. Obtain a list of contacts.

■ To prevent reinfection, teach proper hand-hygiene technique and the need to cook meat and fish thoroughly. Stress the need for follow-up evaluations to monitor the success of therapy and to detect possible reinfection.

Enterobiasis

Enterobiasis (also called *pinworm, seatworm,* or *threadworm infection,* or *oxyuriasis*) is a benign intestinal disease caused by the nematode *Enterobius vermicularis.* Found worldwide, even in temperate regions with good sanitation, it's the most prevalent helminthic infection in the United States.

Causes and incidence

Adult pinworms live in the intestine; female worms migrate to the perianal region to deposit their ova. *Direct transmission* occurs when the patient's hands transfer infective eggs from the anus to the mouth. *Indirect transmission* occurs when he comes in contact with contaminated articles, such as linens and clothing.

Enterobiasis infection and reinfection occur most commonly in children between ages 5 and 14 and in certain institutionalized groups because of poor hygiene and frequent hand-to-mouth activity. Crowded living conditions increase the likelihood of it spreading to several members of a family.

Signs and symptoms

Asymptomatic enterobiasis is commonly overlooked. However, intense perianal pruritus may occur, especially at night, when the female worm leaves the anus to deposit ova. Pruritus causes irritability, scratching, skin irritation and, sometimes, vaginitis. Rarely, complications include appendicitis, salpingitis, and pelvic granuloma.

Diagnosis

Q **CONFIRMING DIAGNOSIS** *A history of anal pruritus suggests enterobiasis; identification of Enterobius ova recovered from the perianal area with a cellophane tape swab taken before the patient bathes and defecates in the morning confirms it. A stool sample is usually ova- and worm-free because the worms deposit ova outside the intestine and die after return to the anus.*

Treatment

Drug therapy with pyrantel, mebendazole, or albendazole destroys the causative parasites. Effective eradication requires simultaneous treatment of the patient's family members and, in institutions, other patients.

Special considerations

■ If the patient receives pyrantel, tell him and his family that this drug colors the stool bright red and may cause vomiting (vomitus will also be red). The tablet form of this drug is coated with aspirin and shouldn't be given to aspirin-sensitive patients.

■ To help prevent this disease, tell parents to bathe children daily (showers are preferable to tub baths) and to change underwear and bed linens daily.

■ Tell the patient's family not to shake bed linens, to avoid aerosolization of eggs that may be on linens.

■ Educate children in proper personal hygiene, and stress the need for proper hand hygiene after defecation and before handling food. Discourage nail biting. If the child can't stop, suggest that he wear gloves until the infection clears.

■ Report *all* outbreaks of enterobiasis to school authorities.

■ Tell parents to strictly adhere to the prescribed drug dosage as directed by a physician.

Schistosomiasis

Schistosomiasis, also known as *bilharziasis,* is a slowly progressive disease caused by blood flukes of the class Trematoda. There are three major types: *Schistosoma mansoni* and *S. japonicum* infect the intestinal tract; *S. haematobium* infects the urinary tract. (See *Types of schistosomes.*) The degree of infection determines the intensity of illness. Complications — such as portal hypertension, pulmonary hypertension, heart failure, ascites, hematemesis from ruptured esophageal varices, and renal failure — can be fatal.

Causes

The mode of transmission is bathing, swimming, wading, or working in water contaminated with *Schistosoma* larvae. These larvae penetrate the skin or mucous membranes and eventually work their way to the liver's venous portal circulation. There, they mature in 1 to 3 months. The adults then migrate to other parts of the body.

The female cercariae lay spiny eggs in blood vessels surrounding the large intestine or bladder. After penetrating the mucosa of these organs, the eggs are excreted in feces or urine. If the eggs hatch in fresh water, the first-stage larvae (miracidia)

TYPES OF SCHISTOSOMES

Species and incidence	Signs and symptoms	Treatment	Adverse effects
Schistosoma mansoni Western hemisphere, particularly Puerto Rico, Lesser Antilles, Brazil, and Venezuela; also Nile delta, Sudan, and central Africa	Irregular fever, malaise, weakness, abdominal distress, weight loss, diarrhea, ascites, hepatosplenomegaly, portal hypertension, fistulas, and intestinal stricture	Praziquantel: 60 mg/kg in three equally divided doses at 4- to 6-hour intervals on the same day	Abdominal discomfort, dizziness, drowsiness, fever, headache, malaise, minimal increase in liver enzyme levels, nausea, and urticaria
Schistosoma japonicum Affects men more than women; particularly prevalent among farmers in Japan, China, and the Philippines	Irregular fever, malaise, weakness, abdominal distress, weight loss, diarrhea, ascites, hepatosplenomegaly, portal hypertension, fistulas, and intestinal stricture	Praziquantel: 60 mg/kg in three equally divided doses at 4- to 6-hour intervals on the same day	Abdominal discomfort, dizziness, drowsiness, fever, headache, malaise, minimal increase in liver enzyme levels, nausea, and urticaria
Schistosoma haematobium Africa, Cyprus, Greece, India	Terminal hematuria, dysuria, ureteral colic; with secondary infection — colicky pain, intermittent flank pain, vague GI complaints, and total renal failure	Praziquantel: 60 mg/kg in three equally divided doses at 4- to 6-hour intervals on the same day	Abdominal discomfort, dizziness, drowsiness, fever, headache, malaise, minimal increase in liver enzyme levels, nausea, and urticaria

penetrate freshwater snails, which act as passive intermediate hosts. Cercariae produced in snails escape into water and begin a new life cycle.

Signs and symptoms

Initial signs and symptoms of schistosomiasis depend on the site of infection and the stage of the disease. Initially, a transient, pruritic rash develops at the site of cercariae penetration, along with fever, myalgia,

and cough. (See *Schistosomal dermatitis,* page 276.) Later signs and symptoms may include hepatomegaly, splenomegaly, and lymphadenopathy. Worm migration and egg deposition may cause such complications as flaccid paralysis, seizures, and skin abscesses.

SCHISTOSOMAL DERMATITIS

Schistosomal dermatitis, also known as *swimmer's itch* or *clam digger's itch*, affects those who bathe in and camp along freshwater lakes in the eastern and western United States. It's caused by schistosomal cercariae, which are harbored by migratory birds and able to penetrate the skin, causing a pruritic papular rash. Initially mild, the reaction grows more severe with repeated exposure. Treatment consists of 5% copper sulfate solution as an antipruritic and 2% methylene blue as an antibacterial agent.

Diagnosis

CONFIRMING DIAGNOSIS *Typical symptoms and a history of travel to endemic areas suggest the diagnosis; ova in the urine or stool or a mucosal lesion biopsy confirms it.*

The white blood cell count shows eosinophilia.

Treatment

The treatment of choice is the anthelmintic drug praziquantel. Between 3 and 6 months after treatment, the patient will need to be examined again. If this checkup detects any living eggs, treatment may be resumed. With acute infection, corticosteroids may be ordered.

Special considerations

■ To help prevent schistosomiasis, teach people in endemic areas to work for a pure water supply and to avoid swimming or bathing in water that's known to be contaminated or potentially contaminated. If they must enter the water, tell them to wear protective clothing and to dry themselves afterward.

Strongyloidiasis

Strongyloidiasis, also called *threadworm infection*, is a parasitic intestinal infection caused by the helminth *Strongyloides stercoralis*. This worldwide infection is endemic in the tropics and subtropics. Susceptibility to strongyloidiasis is universal. Infection doesn't confer immunity, and people who are immunocompromised may suffer overwhelming disseminated infection. Because the threadworm's reproductive cycle may continue in the untreated host for up to 45 years, autoinfection is highly probable. Most patients with strongyloidiasis recover, but debilitation from protein loss may result in death.

Causes

Transmission to humans usually occurs through contact with soil that contains infective *S. stercoralis* filariform larvae; such larvae develop from noninfective rhabdoid (rod-shaped) larvae in human feces. The filariform larvae penetrate the human skin, usually at the feet. They migrate by way of the lymphatic system to the bloodstream and the lungs.

Once they enter into pulmonary circulation, the filariform larvae break through the alveoli and migrate upward to the pharynx, where they are swallowed. They then lodge in the small intestine, where they deposit eggs that mature into noninfectious rhabdoid larvae. Next, these larvae migrate into the large intestine and are excreted in feces, starting the cycle again. The threadworm life cycle, which begins with penetration of the skin and ends with excretion of rhabdoid larvae, takes 17 days.

In autoinfection, rhabdoid larvae mature within the intestine to become infective filariform larvae.

Signs and symptoms

The patient's resistance and the extent of infection determine the severity of symptoms. Some patients have no symptoms, but many develop an erythematous maculopapular rash at the site of penetration that produces swelling and pruritus and that may be confused with an insect bite. As the larvae migrate to the lungs, pulmonary signs develop, including minor hemorrhage, pneumonitis, and pneumonia; later, intestinal infection produces frequent, watery, and bloody diarrhea, accompanied by intermittent abdominal pain.

Severe infection can cause malnutrition from substantial fat and protein loss, anemia, and lesions resembling ulcerative colitis, all of which invite secondary bacterial infection. Ulcerated intestinal mucosa may lead to perforation and, possibly, potentially fatal dissemination, especially in patients with malignancy or immunodeficiency diseases or in those who receive immunosuppressants.

Diagnosis
Diagnosis requires observation of *S. stercoralis* larvae in a fresh stool specimen (2 hours after excretion, rhabdoid larvae look like hookworm larvae). Duodenal aspirations show larvae present in duodenal fluid, and an antigen test that's positive for *S. stercoralis.* During the pulmonary phase, sputum shows *S. stercoralis;* marked eosinophilia also occurs in disseminated strongyloidiasis.

Treatment
The goal of treatment is to eliminate the larvae with antithelmintics, such as ivermectin or thiabendazole. Patients may need protein replacement, blood transfusions, and I.V. fluids. Retreatment is necessary if *S. stercoralis* remains in stools after therapy.

Special considerations
■ Keep accurate intake and output records. Ask the dietary department to provide a high-protein diet. The patient may need tube feedings to increase caloric intake.
■ Use standard precautions when handling bedpans or giving perineal care, and dispose of feces promptly.
■ Because direct person-to-person transmission doesn't occur, isolation isn't required.
■ In pulmonary infection, reposition the patient frequently, encourage coughing and deep breathing, and administer oxygen as ordered.
■ To prevent reinfection, teach the patient proper hand-washing technique. Stress the importance of proper hand hygiene before eating and after defecating and of wearing shoes when in endemic areas. Check the patient's family and close contacts for signs of infection. Emphasize the need for follow-up stool examination, continuing for several weeks after treatment.

MISCELLANEOUS INFECTIONS

Ornithosis

Ornithosis (also called *psittacosis* or *parrot fever*) is caused by the gram-negative intracellular parasite *Chlamydia psittaci* and is transmitted by infected birds. This disease occurs worldwide and is mainly associated with occupational exposure to birds (such as poultry farming). With adequate antimicrobial therapy, ornithosis is fatal in fewer than 4% of patients.

Causes and incidence
Psittacine birds (parrots, parakeets, and cockatoos), pigeons, and turkeys may harbor *C. psittaci* in their blood, feathers, tissues, nasal secretions, liver, spleen, and feces. Transmission to humans occurs primarily through inhalation of dust containing *C. psittaci* from bird droppings; less commonly, through direct contact with infected secretions or body tissues, as in laboratory personnel who work with birds. Person-to-person transmission seldom occurs but usually causes severe ornithosis.

Incidence is higher in women and in people ages 20 to 50.

Signs and symptoms
After an incubation period of 4 to 15 days, onset of symptoms may be insidious or sudden. Clinical effects include chills and a low-grade fever that increases to 103° to 105° F (39.4° to 40.6° C) for 7 to 10 days then, with treatment, declines during the second or third week. Other signs and symptoms include headache, myalgia, sore throat, cough (may be dry, hacking, and nonproductive or may produce blood-tinged sputum), abdominal distention and tenderness, nausea, vomiting, photopho-

bia, decreased pulse rate, slightly increased respiratory rate, secondary purulent lung infection, and a faint macular rash. Severe infection also produces delirium, stupor and, in extensive pulmonary infiltration, cyanosis. Ornithosis may recur but is usually milder.

Diagnosis
Characteristic symptoms and a recent history of exposure to birds suggest ornithosis.

CONFIRMING DIAGNOSIS *Firm diagnosis requires recovery of C. psittaci from mice, eggs, or tissue culture that has been inoculated with the patient's blood or sputum. Culture of C. psittaci can be dangerous for laboratory personnel, making serology the preferred method of confirming diagnosis.*

Comparison of acute and convalescent serum shows a fourfold rise in *Chlamydia* antibody titers. In addition, a patchy lobar infiltrate appears on chest X-rays during the first week of illness.

Treatment
Ornithosis calls for treatment with tetracycline. If the infection is severe, tetracycline may be given via I.V. infusion until the fever subsides. Fever and other symptoms should begin to subside 48 to 72 hours after antibiotic treatment begins, but treatment must continue for 2 weeks after temperature returns to normal. Other antibiotics used to treat ornithosis include doxycycline, erythromycin, and azithromycin.

Special considerations
■ Monitor the patient's fluid and electrolyte balance. Give I.V. fluids as needed.
■ Carefully monitor the patient's vital signs. Watch for signs of overwhelming infection.
■ Reduce fever with tepid alcohol or sponge baths and a hypothermia blanket.
■ Observe standard precautions. Instruct the patient to use tissues when he coughs and to dispose of them in a closed plastic bag. Also instruct him to wash his hands afterward.
■ To prevent ornithosis, persons who raise birds for sale should feed them tetracycline-treated birdseed and follow regulations on bird importation. However, routine use of antibiotics in animal and bird feed may contribute to antimicrobial resistance. Infected or possibly infected birds should be segregated from healthy birds, and the structures that housed the infected ones should be disinfected.
■ Report all cases of ornithosis to public health authorities.

Toxic shock syndrome

Toxic shock syndrome (TSS) is an acute bacterial infection caused by toxin-producing, penicillin-resistant strains of *Staphylococcus aureus*, such as TSS toxin-1 and staphylococcal enterotoxins B and C. Initially, the disease was thought to primarily affect menstruating women younger than age 30 and was associated with continuous use of tampons during the menstrual period; however, only about 55% of cases are associated with menses. TSS is fatal in 50% of cases.

Causes
Theoretically, tampons may contribute to development of TSS by introducing *S. aureus* into the vagina during insertion (insertion with fingers instead of the supplied applicator increases the risk) or traumatizing the vaginal mucosa during insertion, thus leading to infection.

When TSS isn't related to menstruation, it appears to be linked to *S. aureus* infections, such as abscesses, osteomyelitis, and postsurgical infections. It's also associated with prior antibiotic use.

Risk factors include recent use of barrier contraceptives (diaphragms or vaginal sponges), childbirth, and surgery.

Signs and symptoms
Typically, TSS produces intense myalgias, fever over 104° F (40° C), vomiting, diarrhea, headache, decreased level of consciousness, rigors, conjunctival hyperemia, and vaginal hyperemia and discharge. Severe hypotension occurs with hypovolemic shock. Within a few hours of onset, a deep red rash develops—especially on the palms and soles—and later desquamates.

Major complications include persistent neuropsychological abnormalities, mild renal failure, rash, and cyanotic arms and legs.

Diagnosis

Diagnosis is based on several criteria: fever, hypotension, rash that peels after 1 to 2 weeks, and at least 3 organs with signs of dysfunction. In some cases, blood cultures may be positive for *S. aureus*. Organs with signs of dysfunction may include:
- GI effects, including vomiting and profuse diarrhea
- muscular effects, with severe myalgias or a fivefold or greater increase in creatine kinase levels
- mucous membrane effects such as frank hyperemia
- renal involvement with elevated blood urea nitrogen or creatinine levels (at least twice the normal levels)
- liver involvement with elevated bilirubin, aspartate aminotransferase, or alanine aminotransferase levels (at least twice the normal levels)
- blood involvement with signs of thrombocytopenia and a platelet count of less than 100,000/µl
- central nervous system effects such as disorientation without focal signs.

Negative results on blood tests for Rocky Mountain spotted fever, leptospirosis, and measles help rule out these disorders.

Treatment

Treatment involves examination and removal of foreign material, such as tampons, vaginal sponges, or nasal packing; and drainage of any identified site of infection such as surgical wounds. Antistaphylococcal antibiotics that are beta-lactamase resistant, such as oxacillin and nafcillin, are given I.V. To reverse shock, expect to replace fluids with saline solution and colloids, as ordered. Blood pressure support and dialysis may be necessary. In some cases, I.V. immunoglobulin may be required.

Special considerations

- Instruct women to change their tampons frequently and to always wash their hands before and after doing so.

- Monitor the patient's vital signs frequently.
- Administer antibiotics slowly and strictly on time. Be sure to watch for signs of penicillin allergy.
- Check the patient's fluid and electrolyte balance.
- Obtain specimens of vaginal and cervical secretions for culture of *S. aureus*, or other sites of TSS infection.
- Implement standard precautions.

Selected references

Centers for Disease Control and Prevention. "Guideline for hand hygiene in health-care settings: Recommendations of the Healthcare Infection Control Practices Advisory Committee and the HICPAC/SHEA/APIC/IDSA Hand Hygiene Task Force," *Morbidity and Mortality Weekly Report* 51(RR-16):1-45, October 2002.

Centers for Disease Control and Prevention. "Recommended Childhood and Adolescent Immunization Schedule — United States, January — June 2004," *Morbidity and Mortality Weekly Report* 53(01):Q1-4, January 2004.

Mayhall, C.G. *Hospital Epidemiology and Infection Control,* 3rd ed. Philadelphia: Lippincott Williams & Wilkins, 2004.

Scheld, W.M., et al., eds. *Infections of the Central Nervous System,* 3rd ed. Philadelphia: Lippincott Williams & Wilkins, 2004.

Tierney, L.M., et al. *Current Medical Diagnosis and Treatment,* 43rd ed. New York: McGraw-Hill Book Co., 2004.

Zuckerman, A.J., et al, eds. *Principles and Practice of Clinical Virology,* 4th ed. New York: John Wiley & Sons, 2000.

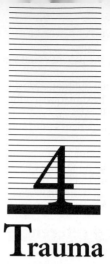

4

Trauma

Introduction *281*

Head *285*
Concussion *285*
Cerebral contusion *286*
Skull fractures *287*
Fractured nose *290*
Dislocated or fractured jaw *291*
Perforated eardrum *292*

Neck and spine *292*
Acceleration-deceleration
cervical injuries *292*
Spinal injuries *293*

Thorax *294*
Blunt chest injuries *294*
Penetrating chest wounds *298*

Abdomen *299*
Blunt and penetrating
abdominal injuries *299*

Extremities *301*
Sprains and strains *301*
Arm and leg fractures *302*
Dislocations and subluxations *306*
Traumatic amputation *307*

Whole body *308*
Burns *308*
Electric shock *312*
Cold injuries *313*
Heat syndrome *316*
Asphyxia *316*
Near drowning *318*
Decompression sickness *319*
Radiation exposure *320*

Miscellaneous injuries *323*
Poisoning *323*
Poisonous snakebites *325*
Insect bites and stings *329*
Open trauma wounds *332*
Rape trauma syndrome *335*

Selected references *339*

Introduction

Trauma is one of the leading causes of death in the United States. Emergency trauma care basics include triage; assessing and maintaining airway, breathing, and circulation (the ABCs); protecting the cervical spine; assessing the level of consciousness (LOC); and, as needed, preparing the patient for transport and possibly surgery. Common mechanisms of trauma include motor vehicle and bicycle accidents, automobile-pedestrian accidents, drowning, firearms, burns, and falls.

Triage: First things first

Triage is the setting of medical priorities for emergency care by making sound, rapid assessments. The need for triage usually arises at the scene of injury and continues in the emergency department. Following health care facility protocol, you'll decide which patient to treat first, which injury to treat first, how to best utilize other members of the medical team, and how to control patient and staff traffic.

In most cases, victims are assigned to the following categories:

- *emergent*—life-threatening or limb-threatening injury requiring treatment within a few minutes to prevent death or further injury; includes patients with moderate to severe respiratory distress, cardiopulmonary arrest, compensated or uncompensated shock, extremity injury with neurovascular compromise, alteration in neurologic status, and patients who have attempted suicide
- *urgent*—serious, but not immediately life-threatening injury that should receive treatment within 2 hours; includes patients with mild wheezing and mild or no respiratory distress, mild to moderate dehydration, and suspected forearm fracture (These patients require periodic assessment because they can deteriorate and become emergent.)
- *nonurgent*—presence of minor or stable illness or injury that doesn't require treatment within 2 hours; includes patients with ear discomfort, minor or isolated soft tissue wounds, and sore throat.

At any point during the assessment, if the patient is discovered to have a life-threatening condition, appropriate interventions should be initiated immediately. It may also be necessary to prioritize patients within the same triage category based on the severity of each patient's symptoms.

Trauma care generates a great deal of stress, and much of it falls on your shoulders. In many cases, you must deal with patients and families who are upset, angry, belligerent, intoxicated, or frightened; some may speak only a foreign language. Therefore, you must work calmly and rationally, employing crisis-intervention techniques. You can help the patient a great deal by talking to him. Be sure to tell him what you're going to do before you touch him. You must also handle difficult situations diplomatically and intelligently, recognize your limitations, and ask for help when you need it.

Begin with the ABCs

Begin your care of an injured patient with a brief primary assessment of the ABCs. Also assess for disability or neurologic status.

To assess airway patency, routinely check for respiratory distress or signs of obstruction, such as stridor, choking, or cyanosis. Be especially alert for respiratory distress in a patient who inhaled chemicals, was in a fire, or has upper body burns. If the airway is obstructed, remove vomitus, dentures, blood clots, or foreign bodies from the mouth.

In a semiconscious or unconscious patient, open the airway using a jaw-thrust maneuver. (*Don't* use the head-tilt maneuver for a trauma patient. Suspect cervical spine injury until X-rays rule it out.) Then insert an oropharyngeal or nasopharyngeal airway. A nasopharyngeal airway is contraindicated in patients with massive facial trauma and those with possible basal skull fractures. Assist with endotracheal tube insertion as necessary. If rescue personnel have inserted an esophageal obturator airway, leave it in place until the patient has been tracheally intubated. This will prevent him from vomiting and possibly aspirating.

MANAGING TETANUS PROPHYLAXIS

History of tetanus immunization (number of doses)	Tetanus-prone wounds		Non-tetanus-prone wounds	
	Td*	TIG**	Td	TIG
Uncertain	Yes	Yes	Yes	No
0 to 1	Yes	Yes	Yes	No
2	Yes	No (*yes* if 24 hours since wound was inflicted)	Yes	No
3 or more	No (*yes* if more than 10 years since last dose)	No	No (*yes* if more than 10 years since last dose)	No

*Td = Tetanus and diphtheria toxoids adsorbed (for adult use), 0.5 ml

**TIG = Tetanus immune globulin (human), 250 units

Note: When Td and TIG are given concurrently, separate syringes and separate sites should be used.

Note: For children younger than age 7, tetanus and diphtheria toxoids and pertussis vaccine, adsorbed (DPT) are preferred over tetanus toxoid alone. If pertussis vaccine is contraindicated, administer tetanus and diphtheria toxoids, adsorbed (DT).

Next, make sure the patient's breathing is adequate. Look, listen, and feel for respirations. If the patient isn't breathing, call for help immediately, begin bag-valve-mask resuscitation, and prepare for intubation. Give supplemental oxygen, then draw samples for arterial blood gas measurement and calculate the supplemental oxygen's effects to establish a baseline for oxygen and acid-base therapy. Multiple injuries always create a need for supplemental oxygen because of blood loss and overwhelming physiologic stress. A conscious multiple-injury patient should display compensatory hyperventilation. If he doesn't, expect neurologic involvement or chest injury. Needle thoracentesis may be done to decompress tension pneumothorax.

To assess circulation, check for central and peripheral pulses, as well as capillary refill (which should be less than 2 seconds).

If a carotid pulse is absent, institute cardiopulmonary resuscitation. If external hemorrhage is evident, apply direct pressure to the bleeding site and, if the wound is on an extremity, elevate it above heart level if possible. Apply a tourniquet only if the hemorrhage is life-threatening.

Monitor the patient's vital signs even if he appears stable. Because vital signs can change rapidly, taking them serially can identify subtle and overt changes. Document baseline readings, and obtain new readings every 5 to 15 minutes until the patient is stable. Assess trends in vital sign readings to detect changes. Place him on a cardiac monitor and a pulse oximeter. Remember that the patient may have up to a 25% volume loss before it's reflected in vital sign readings.

Draw blood for type and crossmatch, complete blood count, prothrombin time, partial thromboplastin time, platelet count, and routine blood studies, including amylase levels. Begin at least two I.V. lines with 14G or 16G catheters for fluid resuscitation with normal saline or lactated Ringer's solution. Administer tetanus prophylaxis as ordered. (See *Managing tetanus prophylaxis*.)

Immobilize the patient's head and neck with an immobilization device, sandbags, backboard, and tape, if this hasn't been done. Obtain cervical spine X-rays as appropriate and rule out cervical spine injury before moving the patient again. Presume spinal injury and take precautions to prevent further injury, such as logrolling and using adequate staff to move the patient, until spinal injury has been ruled out.

Proceed with assessment of the patient's disability; assess the patient's LOC and pupillary and motor response to check the patient's neurologic status. Determine and report LOC by using a stimulus-response method of reporting, rather than categorizing; don't use such words as "semiconscious" or "stuporous." Report decorticate or decerebrate responses immediately. The patient need not have a head injury to exhibit an abnormal neurologic response. Any injury that impairs ventilation or perfusion can cause cerebral edema and raise intracranial pressure.

Expose the patient

Secondary assessment includes removal of the patient's clothes for a more thorough examination. The clothing is placed in bags, which are labeled with the patient's name and the date and time he was brought to your facility. The bag will be given to the patient's family, or to the authorities if an investigation into the circumstances of the trauma is necessary. If the clothing must be given to the authorities, document having done so. Institute environmental controls by providing warming measures, such as warming blankets and units, warmed oxygen and I.V. solutions, and increased environmental temperature.

Assess the patient's vital signs, and inform the patient's family of his status. They can help to provide his history, especially his immunization status. Assess the need for comfort measures; pain medication may be given as appropriate, and other techniques may be used to make the patient comfortable.

Head-to-toe assessment

Secondary assessment also includes a thorough head-to-toe assessment of the patient. Quickly and carefully look for multiple injuries by systematically examining the patient. If you detect no spinal injury, carefully logroll the patient over to inspect his back for other wounds.

In chest trauma, assess for open wounds, tension pneumothorax, hemothorax, cardiac tamponade, bruises and hematomas, flail chest, and fractured larynx. Cover open wounds and apply direct pressure to the wound as necessary. Be ready to assist with insertion of chest tubes, pericardiocentesis, cricothyrotomy, or tracheotomy, as appropriate.

Insert an indwelling urinary catheter and a nasogastric tube, and give prophylactic antibiotics and immunizations, as indicated. Appropriate diagnostic studies — such as X-rays, computed tomography (CT) scans, peritoneal lavage, magnetic resonance imaging (MRI), and excretory urography — may be performed based on assessment findings and patient stabilization. Notify medical or surgical specialists, as appropriate.

Stabilize the patient

Because severe injuries commonly lead to shock, check skin temperature, color, and moisture. To control shock, administer I.V. fluids (lactated Ringer's or normal saline solution) followed by blood or blood products, and use a pneumatic antishock garment as ordered. Don't inflate the abdominal compartment if the patient is pregnant. Be aware that this garment's use remains controversial, and it's primarily used to stabilize pelvic fractures.

In all cases of massive external bleeding or suspected internal bleeding, watch for hypovolemia and estimate blood loss. Remember, however, that a blood loss of 500 to 1,000 ml might not change systolic blood pressure but may elevate the pulse rate. Stay alert for signs of occult bleeding, which commonly occurs in the chest, abdomen, and thigh. Repeat abdominal examinations frequently to assess the patient for abdominal distention; this could be a sign of internal injuries and bleeding.

Increased diameter of the legs or abdomen usually means that blood has leaked into these tissues (as much as 4,000 ml into the abdomen, 3,000 ml into the chest, and 2,000 ml into a thigh). Such blood loss will induce characteristic signs of hypovolemic shock (tachycardia, tachypnea, hypotension, restlessness, decreasing urine output, delayed capillary refill, and cold, clammy skin).

If the patient has renal injuries or a fractured pelvis, look for the classic sign of retroperitoneal hematoma — numbness or pain in the leg on the affected side as a result of pressure on the lateral femoral cutaneous nerve in L1 to L3. Retroperitoneal bleeding may not cause abdominal tenderness. If the patient shows clinical signs of hypovolemia, immediately begin I.V. therapy with two or more large-bore catheters, and regulate fluids according to the hypovolemia's severity. Although the initial resuscitation fluids are crystalloids, significant hypovolemia due to hemorrhage requires blood transfusion. Assist with insertion of a central venous pressure or pulmonary artery catheter to monitor circulating blood volume.

If spinal trauma is suspected, methylprednisolone may be given I.V. If head trauma is present, the patient may be given emergency medication such as mannitol and ventilation may be controlled. The patient may also require emergency surgery — either exploratory or lifesaving — to help with stabilization depending on the injury's type and extent.

Extremity fractures can be a source of blood loss. Look for limb fractures and dislocations. Check circulation and neurovascular status distal to the injury by palpating pulses distal to the injury and looking for the classic signs of arterial insufficiency: decreased or absent pulse, pallor, paresthesia, pain, and paralysis. Splint and apply traction as needed.

The patient will require X-rays, CT scan, or an MRI to determine the extent of injury to the extremity, so prepare the patient for transport. Use special care in suspected cervical spinal injury. If necessary, after splinting the injury site, also splint the areas above and below it to prevent further soft-tissue and neurovascular damage and to minimize pain. For example, if the forearm is injured, splint the wrist and elbow, too.

Types of splints include:
- *air splint* — an inflatable splint
- *hard splint* — a rigid splint with a firm surface, such as a long or short board, an aluminum ladder splint, or a cardboard splint
- *soft splint* — a nonrigid splint, such as a pillow or blanket
- *traction splint* — a splint that uses traction to decrease angulation and reduce pain.

Tips on applying a splint
- Splint most injuries "as they lie," except when the patient's neurovascular status is compromised.
- Whenever possible, have one person support the injured part while another applies padding and the splint.
- Secure the splint with straps or gauze, *not* an elastic bandage.
- To apply an air splint, slide the splint backward over your arm and grasp the distal portion of the injured limb. Then slip the splint from your arm onto the injured extremity and inflate the splint. Don't apply the splint too tightly; be sure to reassess neuromuscular integrity often while the splint is in place.

Special considerations
After the patient is stabilized, he'll need ongoing care and assessment and, possibly, rehabilitation to ensure recovery. Specialists may be consulted for certain types of trauma.
- Regularly evaluate the patient's ABCs, as well as his neurologic status.
- Keep the patient's family informed about his condition and provide support as indicated.

Depending on the type of injury, the patient may be admitted to your facility or transferred to another facility.

HEAD

Concussion

By far the most common head injury, a concussion results from a blow to the head — a blow hard enough to jostle the brain and make it strike the skull, causing temporary neural dysfunction, but not hard enough to cause a cerebral contusion. Most concussion patients recover completely within 24 to 48 hours. Repeated concussions, however, exact a cumulative toll on the brain.

Causes and incidence

The blow that causes a concussion is usually sudden and forceful. It occurs when the head strikes a stationary object (as in a fall to the ground), or when a moving object strikes the head (as in a punch to the head). Such blows may also result from automobile accidents or child abuse. Significant jarring can lead to unconsciousness. Microscopic shearing of nerve fibers is thought to occur in the brain from sudden acceleration or deceleration from the head injury.

In 2001, death resulted in 5 of every 100,000 patients with trauma related to falls.

Signs and symptoms

A concussion may produce vomiting and a short-term loss of consciousness. The patient may also suffer from anterograde and retrograde amnesia, in which the patient not only can't recall what happened immediately after the injury, but also has difficulty recalling events that led up to the traumatic incident. The presence of anterograde amnesia and the duration of retrograde amnesia reliably correlate with the injury's severity. The length of the unconsciousness may also relate to the concussion's severity.

This type of injury commonly causes adults to be irritable or lethargic, to behave out of character, and to complain of dizziness, nausea, or severe headache. Some children have no apparent ill effects, but many grow lethargic and somnolent in a few hours. Postconcussion syndrome —

characterized by headache, dizziness, vertigo, anxiety, and fatigue — may persist for several weeks after the injury.

Diagnosis

Differentiating between a concussion and more serious head injuries requires a thorough history of the injury and a neurologic examination. Such an examination must evaluate the patient's level of consciousness (LOC), mental status, cranial nerve and motor function, deep tendon reflexes, and orientation to time, place, and person. If no abnormalities are found and if a severe head injury appears unlikely, the patient should be observed for signs of more severe cerebral trauma. Observation provides a baseline for gauging any deterioration in the patient's condition. Whenever you suspect a severe head injury, obtain a computed tomography scan or magnetic resonance imaging to rule out fractures and more serious injuries. A neurosurgeon should be consulted immediately.

Treatment

Treatment for concussion varies according to the type of injury. Supportive care may include application of an ice pack to the site of injury, analgesics for mild headache, and sutures or steri-strips for lacerations.

If the neurologic examination revealed no abnormalities, observe the patient in the emergency department. Check vital signs, LOC, and pupil size every 15 minutes. The patient who remains stable after 4 or more hours of observation can be discharged in the care of a responsible adult.

Special considerations

ALERT *Before discharge, provide a head injury instruction sheet and advise the patient to be alert for vomiting, worsening of headache, and signs of an earbleed or cerebrospinal fluid leak.*

■ Instruct the family or caregiver to wake the patient every few hours at night for observation of his mental state and for medication administration. Tell them they should follow these precautions for at least 3 days. Review the head injury instruction sheet and ensure that the family or caregiver is aware of signs necessitating a return to the emergency department.

HEMORRHAGE, HEMATOMA, AND TENTORIAL HERNIATION

Among the most serious consequences of a head injury are hemorrhage, hematoma, and tentorial herniation. An epidural hematoma results from a rapid accumulation of blood between the skull and the dura mater; a subdural hematoma results from a slow accumulation of blood between the dura mater and the subarachnoid membrane. Intracerebral hemorrhage occurs within the cerebrum itself. Tentorial herniation occurs when injured brain tissue swells and squeezes through the tentorial notch, constricting the brain stem.

Epidural hemorrhage or hematoma can cause immediate loss of consciousness, followed by a lucid interval lasting minutes to hours, which eventually gives way to a rapidly progressive decrease in the level of consciousness. Other effects are contralateral hemiparesis, progressively severe headache, ipsilateral pupillary dilation, and signs of increased intracranial pressure (ICP).

With a subacute or chronic subdural hemorrhage or hematoma, blood accumulates slowly, so symptoms may not occur until days after the injury. In an acute subdural hematoma, symptoms appear within 24 hours of the injury. Loss of consciousness occurs, commonly with weakness or paralysis. Intracerebral hemorrhage usually causes nuchal rigidity, photophobia, nausea, vomiting, dizziness, seizures, decreased respiratory rate, and progressive obtundation.

Tentorial herniation causes drowsiness, confusion, dilation of one or both pupils, hyperventilation, nuchal rigidity, bradycardia, and decorticate or decerebrate posturing. Irreversible brain damage or death can occur rapidly.

Intracranial hemorrhage may require a craniotomy or burr holes to locate and control bleeding and to aspirate blood. Increased ICP may be controlled with I.V. mannitol, steroids, hyperventilation, or induced coma, but emergency surgery is usually required.

Cerebral contusion

A cerebral contusion is a bruising of brain tissue as a result of a severe blow to the head. More serious than a concussion, a contusion disrupts normal nerve function in the bruised area and may cause loss of consciousness, hemorrhage, edema, and even death.

Causes

A cerebral contusion results from coup-contrecoup or acceleration-deceleration injuries. Such injuries can occur directly beneath the site of impact when the brain rebounds against the skull from the force of a blow (such as in a beating with a blunt instrument), when the force of the blow drives the brain against the opposite side of the skull, or when the head is hurled forward and stopped abruptly (as in an automobile accident when a driver's head

strikes the windshield). The brain continues moving and slaps against the skull (acceleration) and then rebounds (deceleration). These injuries can also cause the brain to strike against bony prominences inside the skull (especially the sphenoidal ridges), causing intracranial hemorrhage or hematoma that may result in tentorial herniation. (See *Hemorrhage, hematoma, and tentorial herniation*.)

Signs and symptoms

The patient with a cerebral contusion may have severe scalp wounds and labored respirations. He may lose consciousness for a few minutes or longer. If conscious, he may be drowsy, confused, disoriented, agitated, or even violent. He may display hemiparesis, unequal pupillary response, and decorticate or decerebrate posturing. Eventually, he should return to a relatively alert state, perhaps with temporary aphasia, slight hemiparesis, or unilateral numbness. A lucid period followed by rapid deterioration suggests epidural hematoma.

Diagnosis

An accurate history of the injury and a neurologic examination are the principal diagnostic tools. A computed tomography (CT) scan or magnetic resonance imaging shows ischemic tissue, hematomas, and fractures. Intracranial hemorrhage contraindicates lumbar puncture.

Treatment

Treatment of a cerebral contusion focuses on establishing a patent airway and performing regular evaluations of the patient's level of consciousness (LOC), motor responses, and intracranial pressure. If needed, assist with a tracheotomy or endotracheal intubation. Start an I.V. fluid infusion with lactated Ringer's or normal saline solution. Mannitol I.V. may be given in consultation with a neurosurgeon to reduce cerebral edema. Dexamethasone I.V. or I.M. may be given for several days to control cerebral edema.

Special considerations

■ Verify that a head CT scan has been performed to assess for a basilar skull fracture.
■ Restrict total fluid intake to 1,200 to 1,500 ml/day to reduce volume and intracerebral swelling.
■ If spinal injury is ruled out, elevate the bed's head 30 degrees. Enforce bed rest.
■ If the patient is intubated, hyperventilate him until his partial pressure of arterial carbon dioxide reaches 25 to 35 mm Hg.
■ Type and crossmatch blood for a patient suspected of having an intracerebral hemorrhage. Such a patient may need a blood transfusion, and possibly a craniotomy, to control bleeding and to aspirate blood.
■ Insert an indwelling urinary catheter as ordered and monitor intake and output. If the patient is unconscious, insert a nasogastric tube to prevent aspiration.
■ Observe carefully for leakage of cerebrospinal fluid (CSF) from the nostrils and ear canals. If you detect blood in the canal and aren't sure whether CSF is mixed in, place a drop on a white sheet or a piece of filter paper and check for a central spot of blood surrounded by a lighter ring (halo sign). If CSF leakage develops, raise the bed's head 30 degrees. If you detect CSF leaking from the nose, place a gauze pad under the nostrils. Be sure to tell the patient not to blow his nose, but to wipe it instead. If CSF leaks from the ear, position the patient so that the ear drains naturally, and don't pack the ear or nose.
■ Monitor the patient's vital signs and respirations regularly (usually every 15 minutes). Abnormal respirations could indicate a breakdown in the respiratory center in the brain stem and, possibly, impending tentorial herniation—a critical neurologic emergency.
■ Check his neurologic status frequently. Assess for restlessness, LOC, and orientation.
■ After the patient is stabilized, clean and dress any superficial scalp wounds. (If the skin has been broken, tetanus prophylaxis may be in order.) Assist with suturing if necessary.

Skull fractures

Because of possible brain damage, a skull fracture is considered a neurosurgical condition. Skull fractures may be classified as simple (closed) or compound (open) and may displace bone fragments. Skull fractures are further described as linear, comminuted, or depressed. A linear fracture is a common hairline break, without displacement of structures; a comminuted fracture splinters or crushes the bone into several fragments; a depressed fracture pushes the bone toward the brain.

In children, the skull's thinness and elasticity allow a depression without a fracture. (A linear fracture across a suture line increases the possibility of epidural hematoma.) Skull fractures are also classified according to location, such as cranial vault fracture and basilar fractures. Because of the danger of grave cranial complications and meningitis, basilar fractures are usually far more serious than cranial vault fractures.

Causes and incidence

Skull fractures invariably result from a traumatic blow to the head. Motor vehicle accidents, bad falls, sports injuries, and physical assaults top the list of causes. The brain can be directly affected by damage to the nervous system and by bleeding. Closed head injuries occur in 200 out of every 100,000 patients. Severe head trauma carries a 30% mortality rate.

Signs and symptoms

Many skull fractures are accompanied by scalp wounds—abrasions, contusions, lacerations, or avulsions. If the scalp has been lacerated or torn away, bleeding may be profuse because the scalp contains many blood vessels. Occasionally, bleeding may be heavy enough to induce hypovolemic shock. The patient may also be in shock from other injuries or from medullary failure in severe head injuries.

Linear fractures that are associated only with concussion don't produce loss of consciousness. They require evaluation, but not definitive treatment. A fracture that results in a cerebral contusion or laceration, however, may cause the classic signs of brain injury: agitation and irritability, loss of consciousness, changes in respiratory pattern (labored respirations), abnormal deep tendon reflexes, and altered pupillary and motor responses.

If the patient with a skull fracture remains conscious, he is apt to complain of a persistent, localized headache. A skull fracture may also result in cerebral edema, which may cause compression of the reticular activating system. This cuts off the normal flow of impulses to the brain and results in possible respiratory distress. The patient may experience alterations in level of consciousness (LOC), progressing to unconsciousness or even death.

When jagged bone fragments pierce the dura mater or the cerebral cortex, skull fractures may cause subdural, epidural, or intracerebral hemorrhage or hematoma. With the resulting space-occupying lesions, clinical findings may include hemiparesis, unequal pupils, dizziness, seizures, projectile vomiting, progressive unresponsiveness, and decreased pulse and respiratory rates. Sphenoidal fractures may also dam-age the optic nerve, causing blindness, whereas temporal fractures may cause unilateral deafness or facial paralysis. Symptoms reflect the head injury's severity and extent. However, some elderly patients may have cortical brain atrophy, with more space for brain swelling under the cranium, and consequently may not show signs of increased intracranial pressure (ICP) until it's very high.

Vault fractures commonly produce soft-tissue swelling near the fracture, making it difficult to detect without a computed tomography (CT) scan.

Basilar fractures commonly produce a hemorrhage from the nose, pharynx, or ears; blood under the periorbital skin (raccoon eyes) and under the conjunctiva; and Battle's sign (supramastoid ecchymosis), sometimes with bleeding behind the eardrum (hemotympanum). This type of fracture may also cause cerebrospinal fluid (CSF) or even brain tissue to leak from the nose or ears.

Depending on the extent of brain damage, the patient with a skull fracture may suffer residual effects, such as seizures, hydrocephalus, and organic brain syndrome. Children may develop headaches, giddiness, easy fatigability, neuroses, and behavior disorders.

Diagnosis

Suspect brain injury in all patients with a skull fracture until clinical evaluation proves otherwise. Consequently, you'll need to obtain a thorough injury history and magnetic resonance imaging (MRI) or a CT scan (to locate the fracture) for every suspected skull injury. (Keep in mind that many vault fractures aren't visible or palpable.)

A fracture also requires a neurologic examination to check cerebral function (mental status and orientation to time, place, and person), LOC, pupillary response, motor function, and deep tendon reflexes.

Using reagent strips, test the draining nasal or ear fluid for CSF. The tape will turn blue in the presence of CSF but will remain the same in the presence of blood alone. However, the tape will also turn blue if the patient is hyperglycemic. Also check the patient's bedsheets for the halo sign — a blood-tinged spot surrounded by a lighter ring — from leakage of CSF.

Brain damage can be assessed by a CT scan and MRI, which reveal intracranial hemorrhage from ruptured blood vessels and swelling. Expanding lesions contraindicate a lumbar puncture.

Treatment

Although occasionally even a simple linear skull fracture can tear an underlying blood vessel or cause a CSF leak, linear fractures generally require only supportive treatment, including mild analgesics such as acetaminophen, and cleaning, debridement, and repair of any wounds after injection of a local anesthetic.

If the patient with a skull fracture hasn't lost consciousness, observe him in the emergency department for at least 4 hours. Following this observation period, if his vital signs are stable and if the neurosurgeon concurs, you can discharge him. Before discharge, give the patient an instruction sheet to follow for 24 to 48 hours of observation at home.

More severe vault fractures, especially depressed fractures, usually require a craniotomy to elevate or remove fragments that have been driven into the brain and to extract foreign bodies and necrotic tissue. This reduces the risk of infection and further brain damage. Other treatments for severe vault fractures include antibiotic therapy and, in profound hemorrhage, blood transfusions.

Basilar fractures call for immediate prophylactic antibiotics to prevent the onset of meningitis from CSF leaks as well as close observation for secondary hematomas and hemorrhages. Surgery may be necessary. In addition, both basilar and vault fractures commonly require I.V. or I.M. dexamethasone to reduce cerebral edema and minimize brain tissue damage.

Special considerations

■ Establish and maintain a patent airway; nasal airways are contraindicated in patients who may have a basilar skull fracture. Intubation may be necessary. Suction the patient through the mouth, not the nose, to prevent introducing bacteria if a CSF leak is present.

■ Be sure to obtain a complete history of the traumatic injury from the patient, family members, any eyewitnesses, and emergency medical services personnel. Ask whether the patient lost consciousness and, if so, for how long.

■ Assist with diagnostic tests, including a complete neurologic examination, CT scan, and other studies.

■ Check for abnormal reflexes such as Babinski's reflex.

■ Look for CSF draining from the patient's ears, nose, or mouth. Check pillowcases and linens for CSF leaks and look for a halo sign. If the patient's nose is draining CSF, wipe it — don't let him blow it. If an ear is draining, cover it lightly with sterile gauze — don't pack it.

■ Position the patient with a head injury so that secretions can drain properly. Elevate the bed's head 30 degrees if intracerebral injury is suspected.

■ Cover scalp wounds carefully with a sterile dressing; control any bleeding as necessary.

■ Take seizure precautions, but don't restrain the patient. Agitated behavior may be due to hypoxia or increased ICP, so check for these symptoms. Speak in a calm, reassuring voice, and touch the patient gently. Don't make any sudden, unexpected moves.

■ Don't give the patient opioids or sedatives because they may depress respirations, increase carbon dioxide levels, lead to increased ICP, and mask changes in neurologic status. Give acetaminophen or another mild analgesic for pain as ordered.

If a skull fracture requires surgery, proceed as follows:

■ Obtain consent, as needed, to shave the patient's head. Explain that you're performing this procedure to provide a clean area for surgery. Type and crossmatch blood. Obtain orders for baseline laboratory studies, such as a complete blood count, serum electrolyte studies, prothrombin time, partial thromboplastin time, and urinalysis.

■ After surgery, monitor the patient's vital signs and neurologic status frequently (usually every 5 minutes until the patient is stable and then every 15 minutes for 1 hour), and report any changes in LOC. Because skull fractures and brain injuries heal slowly, don't expect dramatic postoperative improvement.

■ Monitor intake and output frequently, and maintain the patency of the indwelling urinary catheter. Monitor fluid intake carefully. Because hypotonic fluids (such as dextrose 5% in water) can increase cerebral edema, give fluids only as ordered.

■ If the patient is unconscious, provide parenteral nutrition. (Remember, the patient may regurgitate and aspirate food if you use a nasogastric tube for feedings.)

If the fracture doesn't require surgery, proceed as follows:

■ Wear sterile gloves to examine the scalp laceration. With your finger, probe the wound for foreign bodies and a palpable fracture. Gently clean lacerations and the surrounding area; cover them with sterile gauze. Assist with suturing if necessary.

■ Provide emotional support for the patient and his family. Explain the need for procedures to reduce the risk of brain injury.

■ Before discharge, instruct the patient's family to watch closely for changes in mental status, LOC, or respirations and to give the patient acetaminophen for a headache. Tell them to return him to the hospital immediately if his LOC decreases, if his headache persists after several doses of mild analgesics, if he vomits more than once, or if he develops weakness in his arms or legs.

■ Teach the patient and his family how to care for his scalp wound. Emphasize the need to return for suture removal and follow-up evaluation.

Fractured nose

The most common facial fracture, a fractured nose usually results from blunt injury and may be associated with other facial fractures. The fracture's severity depends on the direction, force, and type of the blow. A severe, comminuted fracture may cause extreme swelling or bleeding that may partially obstruct the airway. Inadequate or delayed treatment may cause

permanent nasal displacement, septal deviation, and obstruction.

Signs and symptoms

Immediately after injury, a nosebleed may occur, and soft-tissue swelling may quickly obscure the break. After several hours, pain, periorbital ecchymoses, and nasal displacement and deformity are prominent. Possible complications include septal hematoma, which may lead to abscess formation, resulting in avascular septal necrosis and saddle nose deformity.

Diagnosis

CONFIRMING DIAGNOSIS *Palpation, X-rays, and clinical findings such as a deviated septum confirm a nasal fracture.*

Diagnosis also requires a complete patient history, including the injury's cause and the amount of nasal bleeding. Watch for clear fluid drainage, which may suggest a cerebrospinal fluid (CSF) leak and a basilar skull fracture. If the patient is pregnant, a computed tomography (CT) scan is necessary.

Treatment

Treatment restores normal facial appearance and re-establishes bilateral nasal passage after swelling subsides. Reduction of the fracture corrects alignment; immobilization (intranasal packing and an external splint shaped to the nose and taped) maintains it. Reduction is best accomplished in the operating room under local anesthesia for adults and general anesthesia for children. Severe swelling may delay treatment. CSF leakage calls for close observation, a CT scan of the basilar skull, and antibiotic therapy; septal hematoma requires incision and drainage to prevent necrosis.

Start treatment immediately. While waiting for X-rays, apply ice packs to the nose to minimize swelling. Wrap the ice packs in a light towel to prevent ice from directly contacting the skin. To control anterior bleeding, gently apply local pressure. Posterior bleeding is rare and requires an internal tamponade applied in the emergency department.

Special considerations
■ Because the patient will find breathing more difficult as swelling increases, instruct him to breathe slowly through his mouth. To warm the inhaled air during cold weather, tell him to cover his mouth with a handkerchief or scarf. To prevent subcutaneous emphysema or intracranial air penetration (and potential meningitis), warn him not to blow his nose.
■ After packing and splinting, apply ice in a plastic bag.
■ Before discharge, tell the patient that ecchymoses should fade after about 2 weeks.

Dislocated or fractured jaw

Dislocation of the jaw is a displacement of the temporomandibular joint. A jaw fracture is a break in one or both of the two maxillae (upper jawbones) or the mandible (lower jawbone). Treatment can usually restore jaw alignment and function.

Causes
Simple fractures or dislocations are usually caused by a manual blow along the jawline; more serious compound fractures commonly result from automobile accidents. Other causes include industrial accidents, recreational or sports injuries, assaults, or other trauma. Recurrence of a dislocated jaw is common.

Signs and symptoms
Malocclusion is the most obvious sign of a dislocation or fracture. Other signs include mandibular pain, swelling, ecchymosis, loss of function, and asymmetry. In addition, mandibular fractures that damage the alveolar nerve produce paresthesia or anesthesia of the chin and lower lip. Maxillary fractures produce infraorbital paresthesia and commonly accompany fractures of the nasal and orbital complex.

Diagnosis
CONFIRMING DIAGNOSIS *Abnormal maxillary or mandibular mobility during the physical examination and a history of traumatic injury suggest a fracture or dislocation; X-rays confirm it.*

Treatment
As in all traumatic injuries, check first for a patent airway, adequate ventilation, and pulses; then control hemorrhage and check for other injuries. As necessary, maintain a patent airway with an oropharyngeal airway, nasotracheal intubation, or a cricothyrotomy. Relieve pain with analgesics as needed.

After the patient stabilizes, surgical reduction and fixation by wiring restores mandibular and maxillary alignment. Maxillary fractures may also require reconstruction and repair of soft-tissue injuries. Teeth and bones are never removed during surgery unless unavoidable. If the patient has lost teeth from trauma, the surgeon will decide whether they can be reimplanted. If they can, he'll reimplant them within 6 hours, while they're still viable. Viability is increased if the tooth is placed in milk, saliva, or normal saline solution. Dislocations are usually reduced manually under anesthesia.

Special considerations
After reconstructive surgery, perform the following:
■ Position the patient on his side with his head slightly elevated. He'll usually have a nasogastric tube in place, with low suction to remove gastric contents and prevent nausea, vomiting, and aspiration of vomitus. As necessary, suction the nasopharynx through the nose or by pulling the cheek away from the teeth and inserting a small suction catheter through any natural gap between teeth.
■ If the patient isn't intubated, provide nourishment through a straw. If he has a natural gap between his teeth, insert the straw there; if not, one or two teeth may have to be extracted. After the patient can tolerate clear liquids, offer milkshakes, broth, juices, pureed foods, and nutritional supplements.
■ If the patient can't tolerate oral fluids, I.V. therapy can maintain hydration postoperatively.
■ Administer antiemetics as ordered to minimize nausea and prevent aspiration of vomitus (a real danger in a patient whose jaw is wired). Keep a pair of wire cutters at

the bedside to snip the wires should the patient vomit.

■ A dental water-pulsator may be used for mouth care while the wires are intact.

■ Because the patient will have difficulty talking while his jaw is wired, provide a Magic Slate or pencil and paper and suggest appropriate diversionary activities.

Perforated eardrum

Perforation of the eardrum is a rupture of the tympanic membrane that may cause otitis media and hearing loss.

Causes
The usual cause of perforated eardrum is trauma, such as the deliberate or accidental insertion of foreign objects (cotton swabs or bobby pins) or sudden excessive changes in pressure (explosion, a blow to the head, flying, or diving). The injury may also result from untreated otitis media and, in children, from acute otitis media.

Signs and symptoms
Sudden onset of a severe earache and bleeding from the ear are the first signs of a perforated eardrum. Other symptoms include hearing loss, tinnitus, and vertigo. Purulent otorrhea within 24 to 48 hours of injury signals infection.

Diagnosis
ALERT *A severe earache and bleeding from the ear with a history of trauma strongly suggest a perforated eardrum; direct visualization of the perforated tympanic membrane with an otoscope confirms it.*

Additional diagnostic measures include audiometric testing and a check of voluntary facial movements to rule out facial nerve damage.

Treatment
If you detect bleeding from the ear, use a sterile, cotton-tipped applicator to absorb the blood, and check for purulent drainage or evidence of cerebrospinal fluid leakage. A culture of the specimen may be ordered.

ALERT *Irrigation of the ear is absolutely contraindicated in a patient with perforation of the eardrum.*

Apply a sterile dressing over the outer ear, and refer the patient to an ear specialist. A large perforation with uncontrolled bleeding may require immediate surgery to approximate the ruptured edges. Other measures may include administration of a mild analgesic, a sedative to decrease anxiety, and an oral antibiotic.

Special considerations
■ Before discharge, tell the patient not to blow his nose or get water in his ear canal until the perforation heals.

■ Advise the patient to follow-up with an ear specialist, as appropriate.

■ Instruct the patient and his family to notify the physician if he develops signs of infection, such as fever, increasing discomfort, and continued or purulent drainage.

■ Inform the authorities if child abuse is suspected as the cause of injuries.

NECK AND SPINE

Acceleration-deceleration cervical injuries

Acceleration-deceleration cervical injuries (commonly known as whiplash) result from sharp hyperextension and flexion of the neck that damages muscles, ligaments, disks, and nerve tissue. The prognosis for this type of injury is excellent; symptoms usually subside with treatment.

Causes
Whiplash commonly results from rear-end automobile accidents. A seat belt keeps a person's body from being thrown forward, but the head may snap forward, then backward, causing a whiplash injury to the neck. Other causes include roller coasters or other amusement park rides, sports injuries, or punches or shoves.

Signs and symptoms
Although symptoms may develop immediately, they're often delayed 12 to 24 hours if the injury is mild. Whiplash produces moderate to severe anterior and posterior neck pain. Within several days, the anterior pain diminishes, but the posterior pain

persists or even intensifies, causing patients to seek medical attention if they didn't do so before. Whiplash may also cause dizziness, gait disturbances, vomiting, headache, nuchal rigidity, neck muscle asymmetry, and rigidity or numbness in the arms.

Diagnosis
Full cervical spine X-rays are required to rule out cervical fractures. If the X-rays are negative, the physical examination focuses on motor ability and sensation below the cervical spine to detect signs of nerve root compression.

Treatment
Treatment aims to control symptoms and includes:
- a mild analgesic — such as aspirin with codeine or ibuprofen — and possibly a muscle relaxant — such as diazepam, cyclobenzaprine, or chlorzoxazone with acetaminophen
- ice or cool compresses to the neck to relieve pain
- immobilization with a soft, padded cervical collar for several days or weeks
- in severe muscle spasms, short-term cervical traction.

Most whiplash patients are discharged immediately.

Special considerations
ALERT *In all suspected spinal injuries, assume that the spine is injured until proven otherwise. Until an X-ray rules out a cervical fracture, move the patient as little as possible. Before the X-ray is taken, remove any ear and neck jewelry carefully. Don't undress the patient; cut clothes away if necessary. Caution him to avoid making movements that could injure his spine.*

- Teach the patient to watch for possible adverse drug effects; to avoid alcohol if he's taking diazepam, opioids, or muscle relaxants; and to rest for a few days and avoid lifting heavy objects.
- Instruct the patient to return to the hospital immediately if he experiences persistent pain or develops numbness, tingling, or weakness on one or both sides.

Spinal injuries

Spinal injuries (without cord damage) include fractures, contusions, and compressions of the vertebral column, usually as a result of head or neck trauma. The real danger lies in possible spinal cord damage. Spinal fractures most commonly occur in the 5th, 6th, and 7th cervical, 12th thoracic, and 1st lumbar vertebrae.

Causes and incidence
Most serious spinal injuries result from motor vehicle accidents, falls, dives into shallow water, and gunshot wounds. Less serious injuries result from heavy object lifting and minor falls. Spinal dysfunction may also result from hyperparathyroidism and neoplastic lesions.

Spinal cord injuries occur in 12,000 to 15,000 people per year in the United States. About 10,000 of these injuries cause permanent paralysis; many other patients die as a result of these injuries. Most spinal cord injuries occur in males between the ages of 15 to 35 years; about 5% occur in children. Mortality is higher in pediatric spinal cord injuries.

Signs and symptoms
The most obvious symptoms of spinal injury are muscle spasm and back pain that worsen with movement. In cervical fractures, pain may produce point tenderness; in dorsal and lumbar fractures, it may radiate to other body areas such as the legs. After mild injuries, symptoms may be delayed for several days or weeks. If the injury damages the spinal cord, clinical effects range from mild paresthesia to quadriplegia and shock.

Diagnosis
The diagnosis is typically based on the patient's history, physical examination, X-rays, computed tomography (CT) scan, and magnetic resonance imaging (MRI).

The patient history may reveal a traumatic injury, a metastatic lesion, an infection that could produce a spinal abscess, or an endocrine disorder. The physical examination (including a neurologic evaluation) locates the level of injury and detects cord damage.

Spinal X-rays, the most important diagnostic measure, locate the fracture. In spinal compression, a lumbar puncture may show increased cerebrospinal fluid pressure from a lesion or trauma; a CT scan or MRI can locate a spinal mass.

Treatment

The primary treatment after a spinal injury is immediate immobilization to stabilize the spine and prevent cord damage; other measures are supportive. Cervical injuries require immobilization, using a type of cervical immobilization device (CID) on both sides of the patient's head, a hard cervical collar, or skeletal traction with skull tongs or a halo device.

Treatment of stable lumbar and dorsal fractures consists of bed rest on firm support (such as a bed board), analgesics, and muscle relaxants until the fracture stabilizes (usually in 10 to 12 weeks). Later measures include exercises to strengthen the back muscles and use of a back brace or other device to provide support while walking.

An unstable dorsal or lumbar fracture requires a plaster cast, a turning frame and, in severe fracture, a laminectomy and spinal fusion.

When the spinal injury results in compression of the spinal column, neurosurgery may relieve the pressure. If the cause of compression is a metastatic lesion, chemotherapy and radiation may relieve it. Surface wounds accompanying the spinal injury require tetanus prophylaxis unless the patient has been immunized recently.

Special considerations

In all spinal injuries, suspect cord damage until proven otherwise.

■ During the initial assessment and X-ray studies, immobilize the patient on a firm surface, with sandbags or CID on both sides of his head. Tell him not to move and avoid moving him yourself because hyperflexion can damage the cord. If you must move the patient, get at least three other members of the staff to help you logroll him to avoid disturbing body alignment.

■ Throughout assessment, offer comfort and reassurance. Remember, the fear of possible paralysis will be overwhelming.

Talk to the patient quietly and calmly. Allow a family member who isn't too distraught to accompany him.

■ If the injury requires surgery, administer prophylactic antibiotics as ordered. Catheterize the patient as ordered to avoid urine retention, and monitor bowel elimination patterns to avoid impaction.

■ Explain traction methods to the patient and his family. Reassure them that traction devices don't penetrate the brain. If the patient has a halo or skull-tong traction device, clean pin sites daily, trim hair short, and provide analgesics for persistent headaches. During traction, turn the patient often to prevent pneumonia, embolism, and skin breakdown; perform passive range-of-motion exercises to maintain muscle tone. If available, use a CircOlectric bed or Stryker frame to facilitate turning and to avoid spinal cord injury.

■ Turn the patient on his side during feedings to prevent aspiration. Create a relaxed atmosphere at mealtimes.

■ Suggest appropriate diversionary activities to fill the patient's hours of immobility.

■ Watch closely for neurologic changes. Immediately report changes in skin sensation and loss of muscle strength — either of which might indicate pressure on the spinal cord, possibly as a result of edema or shifting bone fragments.

■ Help the patient walk as soon as the physician allows; he'll probably need to wear a back brace.

■ Before discharge, instruct the patient about continuing analgesics or other medication, and stress the importance of regular follow-up examinations.

■ To help prevent a spinal injury from becoming a spinal *cord* injury, educate firemen, policemen, paramedics, and the general public about the proper way to handle such injuries.

THORAX

Blunt chest injuries

Chest injuries, including blunt chest injuries, consist of myocardial contusion as well as rib and sternal fractures that may be

FLAIL CHEST: PARADOXICAL BREATHING

A patient with a blunt chest injury may develop flail chest, in which a portion of the chest "caves in." This results in paradoxical breathing, described below.

Inhalation
- Injured chest wall collapses in.
- Uninjured chest wall moves out.

Exhalation
- Injured chest wall moves out.
- Uninjured chest wall moves in.

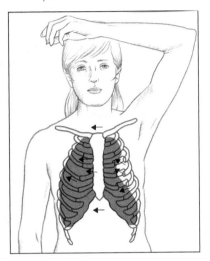 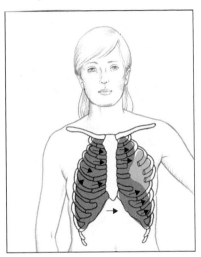

simple, multiple, displaced, or jagged. Such fractures may cause potentially fatal complications, such as hemothorax, pneumothorax, hemorrhagic shock, and diaphragmatic rupture.

Causes and incidence

Motor vehicle accidents cause two-thirds of major chest injuries in the United States. Other common causes include sports and blast injuries and cardiopulmonary resuscitation. About 50% of these injuries affect the chest wall; 80% of those with significant blunt chest trauma also have extrathoracic injuries.

Chest injuries account for 70% of all trauma-related deaths in the United States.

Signs and symptoms

Rib fractures produce tenderness, slight edema over the fracture site, and pain that worsens with deep breathing and movement; this painful breathing causes the pa-

tient to display shallow, splinted respirations that may lead to hypoventilation. Sternal fractures, which are usually transverse and located in the middle or upper sternum, produce persistent chest pains, even at rest. If a fractured rib tears the pleura and punctures a lung, it causes pneumothorax. This usually produces severe dyspnea, cyanosis, agitation, extreme pain and, when air escapes into chest tissue, subcutaneous emphysema.

Multiple rib fractures within two or more places may cause flail chest, in which a portion of the chest wall "caves in," causing a loss of chest wall integrity and preventing adequate lung inflation. (See *Flail chest: Paradoxical breathing*.)

Signs and symptoms of flail chest include bruised skin, extreme pain caused by rib fracture and disfigurement, paradoxical chest movements, tachycardia, hypotension, respiratory acidosis, cyanosis, and rapid, shallow respirations. Flail chest can also cause tension pneumothorax, a condition in which air enters the chest but can't be ejected during exhalation. This life-threatening thoracic pressure buildup causes lung collapse and subsequent mediastinal shift. The cardinal symptoms of tension pneumothorax include severe dyspnea, absent breath sounds (on the affected side), agitation, jugular vein distention, tracheal deviation (away from the affected side), cyanosis, and shock.

Hemothorax occurs when a rib lacerates lung tissue or an intercostal artery, causing blood to collect in the pleural cavity, thereby compressing the lung and limiting respiratory capacity. It can also result from rupture of large or small pulmonary vessels.

Massive hemothorax is the most common cause of shock after a chest injury. Although slight bleeding occurs even with mild pneumothorax, such bleeding resolves very quickly, usually without changing the patient's condition. Rib fractures may also cause pulmonary contusion (resulting in hemoptysis, hypoxia, dyspnea, and possible obstruction), large myocardial tears (which can be rapidly fatal), and small myocardial tears (which can cause pericardial effusion).

Myocardial contusions — actual bruising of the heart muscle — produce electrocardiographic (ECG) abnormalities. Laceration or rupture of the aorta is almost always immediately fatal. Because aortic laceration may develop 24 hours after blunt injury, patient observation is critical. Diaphragmatic rupture (usually on the left side) causes severe respiratory distress. Unless treated early, abdominal viscera may herniate through the rupture into the thorax (with resulting bowel sounds in the chest), compromising both circulation and the lungs' vital capacity.

Other complications of blunt chest trauma may include cardiac tamponade, pulmonary artery tears, ventricular rupture, and bronchial, tracheal, or esophageal tears or rupture.

Diagnosis
A history of trauma with dyspnea, chest pain, and other typical clinical features suggest a blunt chest injury. To determine its extent, a physical examination and diagnostic tests are needed.

- In hemothorax, percussion reveals dullness. In tension pneumothorax, it reveals tympany. Auscultation may reveal a change in position of the loudest heart sound.
- Chest X-rays may confirm rib and sternal fractures, pneumothorax, flail chest, pulmonary contusions, lacerated or ruptured aorta, tension pneumothorax, diaphragmatic rupture, lung compression, or atelectasis with hemothorax.
- With cardiac damage, the ECG may show abnormalities, including unexplained tachycardias, atrial fibrillation, bundle-branch block (usually right), ST-segment changes, and ventricular arrhythmias such as multiple premature ventricular contractions.
- Serial aspartate aminotransferase, alanine aminotransferase, lactate dehydrogenase, creatine kinase (CK), and CK-MB levels are elevated. However, cardiac enzymes fail to detect up to 50% of patients with myocardial damage.
- Retrograde aortography and transesophageal echocardiography reveal aortic laceration or rupture.
- Contrast studies and liver and spleen scans detect diaphragmatic rupture.
- Echocardiography, computed tomography scans, and cardiac and lung scans show the injury's extent.

Treatment
Blunt chest injuries call for immediate physical assessment, control of bleeding, patent airway maintenance, adequate ventilation, and fluid and electrolyte balance.

Special considerations
- Check all pulses and level of consciousness. Evaluate skin color and temperature, depth of respiration, use of accessory muscles, and length of inhalation compared to exhalation.
- Check pulse oximetry values for adequate oxygenation.
- Observe tracheal position. Look for distended jugular veins and paradoxical chest motion. Listen to heart and breath sounds carefully; palpate for subcutaneous emphysema (crepitation) or a lack of structural integrity of the ribs.

■ Obtain a history of the injury. Unless severe dyspnea is present, have the patient locate the pain, and ask if he's having trouble breathing. Obtain an order for laboratory studies (arterial blood gas analysis, cardiac enzyme studies, complete blood count, type, and crossmatch).

■ For simple rib fractures, have the patient cough and breathe deeply to mobilize secretions while splinting to decrease pain. Give adequate analgesics, encourage bed rest, and apply heat. Don't strap or tape the chest.

■ For more severe fractures, assist with administration of intercostal nerve blocks. (Obtain X-rays before and after the nerve blocks to rule out pneumothorax.) Intubate the patient with excessive bleeding or hemopneumothorax. Chest tubes may be inserted to treat hemothorax and to assess the need for thoracotomy. To prevent atelectasis, turn the patient frequently and encourage coughing and deep-breathing exercises.

■ For pneumothorax, assist during placement of a chest tube anterior to the midaxillary line at the fourth intercostal space to aspirate as much air as possible from the pleural cavity and to re-expand the lungs. When time permits, insert chest tubes attached to water-seal drainage and suction.

■ For flail chest, place the patient in semi-Fowler's position. Re-expanding the lung is the first definitive care measure. Administer oxygen at a high flow rate under positive pressure. Suction the patient frequently, as completely as possible. Maintain acid-base balance. Observe carefully for signs of tension pneumothorax. Start I.V. therapy, using lactated Ringer's or normal saline solution. Beware of both excessive and insufficient fluid resuscitation.

ALERT *For hemothorax, treat shock with I.V. infusions of lactated Ringer's or normal saline solution. Administer packed red blood cells for blood losses greater than 1,500 ml or circulating blood volume losses exceeding 30%. Autotransfusion is an option. Administer oxygen, and assist with insertion of chest tubes in the fourth intercostal space anterior to the midaxillary line to remove blood. Monitor and document vital signs and blood loss. Watch for and immediately report falling blood pressure, rising*

pulse rate, and hemorrhage—all require a thoracotomy to stop bleeding.

■ For a pulmonary contusion, give limited amounts of colloids (such as salt-poor albumin, whole blood, or plasma) as ordered to replace volume and maintain oncotic pressure. Give analgesics, diuretics and, if necessary, corticosteroids as ordered. Monitor blood gas levels to ensure adequate ventilation; provide oxygen therapy, mechanical ventilation, and chest tube care.

■ For suspected cardiac damage, close intensive care or telemetry may detect arrhythmias and prevent cardiogenic shock. Impose bed rest in semi-Fowler's position (unless the patient requires shock position); administer oxygen, analgesics, and supportive drugs to control heart failure or supraventricular arrhythmias as needed. Watch for cardiac tamponade, which calls for pericardiocentesis. (Provide essentially the same care as you would for a patient with a myocardial infarction.)

ALERT *For myocardial rupture, septal perforation, and other cardiac lacerations, immediate surgical repair is mandatory. Less severe ventricular wounds require use of a digital or balloon catheter; atrial wounds require a clamp or balloon catheter.*

ALERT *For patients with aortic rupture or laceration, immediate surgery is mandatory, using synthetic grafts or anastomosis to repair the damage. Give large volumes of I.V. fluids (lactated Ringer's or normal saline solution) and whole blood, along with oxygen at very high flow rates; then transport the patient promptly to the operating room.*

ALERT *For tension pneumothorax, expect to assist with insertion of a 14G to 16G angiocatheter in the second intercostal space at the midclavicular line to release pressure in the chest. After this, insert a chest tube to normalize pressure and re-expand the lung. Administer oxygen under positive pressure along with I.V. fluids.*

■ For a diaphragmatic rupture, insert a nasogastric tube to temporarily decompress the stomach, and prepare the patient for surgical repair.

Penetrating chest wounds

Depending on their size, penetrating chest wounds may cause varying degrees of damage to bones, soft tissue, blood vessels, and nerves. Mortality and morbidity from such wounds depend on the wound's size and severity. Gunshot wounds are usually more serious than stab wounds because they cause more severe wounds with rapid blood loss. Ricochet within a gunshot wound commonly damages large areas and multiple organs. Despite prompt, aggressive treatment, up to 90% of patients with penetrating chest wounds die.

Causes and incidence

Stab wounds from a knife or an ice pick are the most common penetrating chest wounds; gunshot wounds are a close second. Wartime explosions or firearms fired at close range are the usual sources of large, gaping wounds.

Penetrating chest injuries cause one in every four deaths in the United States. Many patients with this type of injury die after reaching the hospital.

Signs and symptoms

In addition to the obvious chest injuries, penetrating chest wounds can also cause:
- a sucking sound as the diaphragm contracts and air enters the chest cavity through the opening in the chest wall
- tachycardia due to anxiety and blood loss
- weak, thready pulse due to massive blood loss and hypovolemic shock
- varying levels of consciousness, depending on the injury's extent. If the patient is awake and alert, the severe pain will make him splint his respirations, thereby reducing his vital capacity.

Penetrating chest wounds may also cause lung lacerations (bleeding and substantial air leakage through the chest wall), arterial lacerations (loss of more than 100 ml blood/hour through the chest tube), exsanguination, pneumothorax (air in pleural space causes loss of negative intrathoracic pressure and lung collapse), tension pneumothorax (intrapleural air accumulation causes potentially fatal mediastinal shift), and hemothorax. Other effects may include arrhythmias, cardiac tamponade, mediastinitis, subcutaneous emphysema, esophageal perforation, bronchopleural fistula, and tracheobronchial, abdominal, or diaphragmatic injuries.

Diagnosis

 CONFIRMING DIAGNOSIS *An obvious chest wound and a sucking sound during breathing confirm the diagnosis of a penetrating chest wound. Consider any lower thoracic chest injury a thoracoabdominal injury until proven otherwise.*

Baseline tests include:
- pulse oximetry and arterial blood gas analysis to assess respiratory status
- chest X-rays before and after chest tube placement to evaluate the injury and tube placement; however, in an emergency, don't wait for chest X-ray results before inserting the chest tube
- complete blood count, including hemoglobin (Hb) level, hematocrit (HCT), and differential (low Hb level and HCT reflect severe blood loss; in early blood loss, these values may be normal)
- palpation and auscultation of the chest and abdomen to evaluate damage to adjacent organs and structures.

Treatment

Penetrating chest wounds require immediate support of respiration and circulation, prompt surgical repair, and measures to prevent complications.

Special considerations

- Immediately assess airway, breathing, and circulation. Establish a patent airway, support ventilation, and monitor pulses frequently.
- Place an occlusive dressing over the sucking wound. Monitor for signs of tension pneumothorax (respiratory distress, tachycardia, tachypnea, and diminished or absent breath sounds on the affected side [tracheal shift]); if tension pneumothorax develops, temporarily remove the occlusive dressing to create a simple pneumothorax.
- Control blood loss (remember to look *under* the patient to estimate loss), type and crossmatch blood, and replace blood and fluids as necessary.
- Assist with chest X-ray and placement of chest tubes (using water-seal drainage) to re-establish intrathoracic pressure and to

drain blood in a hemothorax. A second X-ray will evaluate the position of tubes and their function.
- Emergency surgery may be needed to repair the damage caused by the wound.
- Throughout treatment, monitor central venous pressure and blood pressure to detect hypovolemia, and assess vital signs. Provide analgesics as appropriate. Tetanus and antibiotic prophylaxis may be necessary.
- Reassure the patient, especially if he's been the victim of a violent crime. Report the incident to the police in accordance with local laws. Help contact the patient's family and offer them reassurance as well.

ABDOMEN

Blunt and penetrating abdominal injuries

Blunt and penetrating abdominal injuries may damage major blood vessels and internal organs. Their most immediate life-threatening consequences are hemorrhage and hypovolemic shock; later threats include infection. The prognosis depends on the extent of the injury and the specific organs damaged, but it's usually improved by prompt diagnosis and surgical repair.

Causes and incidence

Blunt (nonpenetrating) abdominal injuries usually result from automobile accidents, falls from heights, or sports injuries; penetrating abdominal injuries, from stab and gunshot wounds.

The most commonly injured organs associated with penetrating abdominal trauma are the small intestine (29%), liver (28%), and colon (23%). Penetrating abdominal trauma affects 35% of those admitted to urban trauma centers and 1% to 12% of those admitted to suburban and rural centers.

Signs and symptoms

Symptoms vary with the degree of injury and the organs damaged. Penetrating abdominal injuries cause obvious wounds

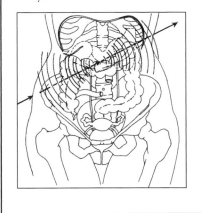

PROJECTILE PATHWAY

In a penetrating abdominal injury, you can estimate probable internal damage by determining the organs lying on the pathway between the entry and exit sites.

(gunshots commonly produce both entrance and exit wounds) with variable blood loss, pain, and tenderness. They commonly result in pallor, cyanosis, tachycardia, shortness of breath, and hypotension. (See *Projectile pathway*.) Blunt abdominal injuries cause severe pain (which may radiate beyond the abdomen to the shoulders), bruises, abrasions, contusions, or distention. They may also result in tenderness, abdominal splinting or rigidity, nausea, vomiting, pallor, cyanosis, tachycardia, and shortness of breath. Rib fractures commonly accompany blunt injuries. (See *Effects of blunt abdominal trauma*, page 300.)

In both blunt and penetrating injuries, massive blood loss may cause hypovolemic shock. Damage to solid abdominal organs (liver, spleen, pancreas, and kidneys) generally causes hemorrhage. Damage to hollow organs (stomach, intestine, gallbladder, and bladder) causes rupture and release of the organs' contents (including bacteria) into the abdomen, which in turn produces inflammation and, possibly, infection.

EFFECTS OF BLUNT ABDOMINAL TRAUMA

When a blunt object strikes a person's abdomen, it raises intra-abdominal pressure. Depending on the blow's force, the trauma can lacerate the liver and spleen, rupture the stomach, bruise the duodenum, and damage the kidneys.

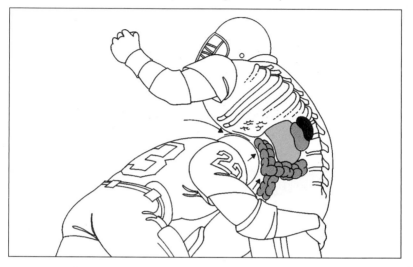

Diagnosis

CONFIRMING DIAGNOSIS *A history of abdominal trauma, clinical features, and laboratory test results confirm the diagnosis of blunt or penetrating abdominal injury and determine organ damage.*

Consider any upper abdominal injury a thoracicoabdominal injury until proven otherwise. Laboratory studies vary with the patient's condition but usually include:
- chest X-rays (preferably done with the patient upright to show free air)
- abdominal X-rays
- examination of stools and stomach aspirate for blood
- blood studies (decreased hematocrit and hemoglobin levels point to blood loss; coagulation studies evaluate hemostasis; white blood cell count is usually elevated but doesn't necessarily point to infection; type and crossmatch to prepare for a blood transfusion)
- arterial blood gas analysis to evaluate respiratory status

- serum amylase levels, which may be elevated in pancreatic injury
- aspartate aminotransferase and alanine aminotransferase levels, which increase with tissue injury and cell death
- excretory urography and cystourethrography to detect renal and urinary tract damage
- radioisotope scanning and ultrasound to detect liver, kidney, or spleen injury
- angiography to detect specific injuries, especially to the kidneys
- computed tomography scan to detect abdominal, head, or other injuries
- exploratory laparotomy to detect specific injuries when other clinical evidence is incomplete
- other laboratory studies to rule out associated injuries
- peritoneal lavage with insertion of a lavage catheter to check for blood, GI content, vegetable fibers, and bile. In blunt trauma with equivocal abdominal findings, this procedure helps establish the need for exploratory surgery.

Treatment

Emergency treatment of abdominal injuries controls hemorrhage and prevents hypovolemic shock through the infusion of I.V. fluids and blood components. After stabilization, most abdominal injuries require surgical repair; some patients, however, require immediate surgery. Analgesics and antibiotics increase patient comfort and prevent infection. Most patients require hospitalization; if they're asymptomatic, they may require observation for only 6 to 24 hours.

Special considerations

Emergency care in patients with abdominal injuries supports vital functions by maintaining airway, breathing, and circulation. At admission, immediately evaluate respiratory and circulatory status and, if possible, obtain a history. Follow these guidelines:

- To maintain airway and breathing, intubate the patient and provide mechanical ventilation as necessary; otherwise, provide supplemental oxygen.
- Using a large-bore needle, start two or more I.V. lines for rapid infusion of normal saline solution, lactated Ringer's solution, or blood. Then draw a blood sample for laboratory studies, and type and crossmatch blood. Also, insert a nasogastric tube and, if necessary, an indwelling urinary catheter. Monitor stomach aspirate and urine for blood.
- Obtain baseline vital signs, and continue to monitor them every 15 minutes.
- Apply a sterile dressing to open wounds. After assessing the patient, splint a suspected pelvic injury by tying the patient's legs together with a pillow between them. Most trousers may be used to splint pelvic fractures. Try not to move the patient.
- Give analgesics as ordered. Opioids usually aren't recommended, but if the pain is severe, give opioids in small, titrated I.V. doses.
- Give tetanus prophylaxis and prophylactic I.V. antibiotics as ordered.
- Prepare the patient for surgery. Have the patient or a responsible relative sign a consent form. Remove dentures.
- If the injury was caused by a motor vehicle accident, find out if the police were notified; if not, notify them. If the patient suffered a gunshot or stab wound, notify the police. Place the patient's clothes in a paper bag, labeled with the patient's name and the date and time he was brought to your facility; the police will require the clothing as part of their investigation into the circumstances surrounding the patient's injury. Document the number and sites of the wounds. Contact the patient's family and offer them reassurance.

EXTREMITIES

Sprains and strains

A sprain is a complete or incomplete tear in the supporting ligaments surrounding a joint that usually follows a sharp twist. A strain is an injury to a muscle or tendinous attachment. Both injuries usually heal without surgical repair.

Causes and incidence

Sprains and strains may result from accidental injury, various sports-related injuries, or from simple household or work-related tasks. More than 4 of 10 injuries resulting in time absent from work are due to sprains and strains, mostly affecting the back.

Signs and symptoms

A sprain causes local pain (especially during joint movement), swelling, loss of mobility (which may not occur until several hours after the injury), and a black-and-blue discoloration from blood extravasating into surrounding tissues. A sprained ankle is the most common joint injury. (See *Muscle-tendon ruptures*, page 302.)

A strain may be acute (an immediate result of vigorous muscle overuse or overstress) or chronic (a result of repeated overuse). An acute strain causes a sharp, transient pain (the patient may report having heard a snapping noise) and rapid swelling. When severe pain subsides, the muscle is tender; after several days, ecchymoses appear. A chronic strain causes stiffness, soreness, and generalized tenderness several hours after the injury.

MUSCLE-TENDON RUPTURES

Perhaps the most serious muscle-tendon injury is a rupture of the muscle-tendon junction. This type of rupture may occur at any such junction, but it's most common at the Achilles' tendon, extending from the posterior calf muscle to the foot. An Achilles' tendon rupture produces a sudden, sharp pain and, until swelling begins, a palpable defect. Such a rupture typically occurs in men between ages 35 and 40, especially during such physical activities as jogging and tennis.

To distinguish an Achilles' tendon rupture from other ankle injuries, the physician performs this simple test: With the patient prone and his feet hanging off the foot of the table, the physician squeezes the calf muscle. If this causes plantar flexion, the tendon is intact; if it causes ankle dorsiflexion, it's partially intact; if there's no flexion of any kind, the tendon is ruptured.

An Achilles' tendon rupture usually requires surgical repair, followed first by a long leg cast for 4 weeks, and then by a short cast for an additional 4 weeks.

Diagnosis

A history of a recent injury or chronic overuse, clinical findings, and an X-ray to rule out fractures establish the diagnosis.

Treatment

Treatment of sprains consists of controlling pain and swelling and immobilizing the injured joint to promote healing. Immediately after the injury, control swelling by elevating the joint above the level of the heart and by applying ice intermittently for 24 to 48 hours. To prevent a cold injury, place a towel between the ice pack and the skin.

Support the joint, using an elastic bandage. If the sprain is severe, immobilize the joint with a splint, and instruct the patient to stay off his feet (nonweight-bearing). Codeine or another analgesic may be necessary if the injury is severe. If the patient has a sprained ankle, he may need crutch gait training. Because patients with sprains seldom require hospitalization, provide patient teaching.

An immobilized sprain usually heals in 2 to 3 weeks, after which the patient can gradually resume normal activities. Occasionally, however, torn ligaments don't heal properly and cause recurrent dislocation, requiring surgical repair. Some athletes may request immediate surgical repair to hasten healing; to prevent sprains, they may tape their wrists and ankles before sports activities.

Acute strains require analgesics and application of ice for up to 48 hours and then application of heat. Complete muscle rupture may require surgery. Chronic strains usually don't require treatment, but heat application, nonsteroidal anti-inflammatory drugs such as ibuprofen, or an analgesic-muscle relaxant can relieve discomfort.

Special considerations

- Tell the patient to elevate the joint for 48 to 72 hours after the injury (pillows can be used while sleeping) and to apply ice intermittently for 24 to 48 hours.
- If an elastic bandage has been applied, teach the patient to reapply it by wrapping from below to above the injury, forming a figure eight. For a sprained ankle, apply the bandage from the toes to midcalf. Tell the patient to remove the bandage before going to sleep and to loosen it if it causes the leg to become pale, numb, or painful.
- Instruct the patient to call the physician if the pain worsens or persists; if so, an additional X-ray may reveal a previously undetected fracture.

Arm and leg fractures

Arm and leg fractures usually result from trauma and commonly cause substantial muscle, nerve, and other soft-tissue damage. The prognosis varies with the extent of disablement or deformity, the amount of tissue and vascular damage, the adequacy of reduction and immobilization, and the patient's age, health, and nutritional status. Children's bones usually heal rapidly and without deformity. Bones of adults in poor health and with impaired circulation may never heal properly. Severe open fractures, especially of the femoral shaft, may cause substantial blood loss and life-threatening hypovolemic shock.

Causes and incidence

Most arm and leg fractures result from major traumatic injury, such as a fall on an outstretched arm, a skiing accident, or child abuse (suggested by multiple or repeated episodes of fractures). However, in a person with a pathologic bone-weakening condition, such as osteoporosis, bone tumors, or metabolic disease, a mere cough or sneeze can also produce a fracture. Prolonged standing, walking, or running can cause stress fractures of the foot and ankle — usually in soldiers, nurses, postal workers, and joggers.

Fractures are among the most common orthopedic problems; about 6.8 million people seek medical attention for fractures in the United States each year.

ELDER TIP *Brittle bones make an older person especially vulnerable to fractures. A fall on an outstretched arm or hand or a direct blow to the arm or shoulder is likely to fracture the radius or humerus.*

Signs and symptoms

Arm and leg fractures may produce any or all of the "5 Ps": pain and point tenderness, pallor, pulse loss, paresthesia, and paralysis. (The last three occur distal to the fracture site.) Other signs include deformity, swelling, discoloration, crepitus, and loss of limb function. Numbness and tingling, mottled cyanosis, cool skin at the end of the extremity, and loss of pulses distal to the injury indicate possible arterial compromise or nerve damage. Open fractures also produce an obvious skin wound.

Complications of arm and leg fractures include:
■ permanent deformity and dysfunction if bones fail to heal (nonunion) or heal improperly (malunion)
■ aseptic necrosis of bone segments from impaired circulation

FAT EMBOLISM

A complication of long bone fracture, fat embolism may also follow severe soft-tissue bruising and fatty liver injury. Posttraumatic embolization may occur as bone marrow releases fat into the veins. The fat can lodge in the lungs, obstructing the pulmonary vascular bed, or pass into the arteries, eventually disturbing the respiratory and circulatory systems.

Fat embolism occurs 12 to 48 hours after an injury, typically producing fever, tachycardia, tachypnea, blood-tinged sputum, cyanosis, anxiety, restlessness, altered level of consciousness, seizures, coma, and a rash. Diagnostic test results reveal decreased hemoglobin level, increased serum lipase levels, leukocytosis, thrombocytopenia, hypoxemia, and fat globules in urine and sputum. A chest X-ray may show mottled lung fields and right ventricular dilation. An electrocardiogram may reveal tachycardia and large S waves in lead I, large Q waves and an inverted T wave in lead III, and right axis deviation.

Although some treatment measures are controversial, they may include steroids to reduce inflammation, heparin to prevent thrombosis, and oxygen to correct hypoxemia. Expect to immobilize fractures early. Assist with endotracheal intubation and ventilation as ordered.

■ hypovolemic shock as a result of blood vessel damage (this is especially likely to develop in patients with a fractured femur)
■ muscle contractures
■ renal calculi from decalcification (due to prolonged immobility)
■ fat embolism (See *Fat embolism*.)
■ compartment syndrome. (See *Recognizing compartment syndrome*, page 304.)

RECOGNIZING COMPARTMENT SYNDROME

Compartment syndrome occurs when pressure within the muscle compartment, resulting from edema or bleeding, increases to the point of interfering with circulation. Crush injuries, burns, bites, and fractures requiring casts or dressings may cause this syndrome. Compartment syndrome most commonly occurs in the lower arm, hand, lower leg, and foot. Symptoms include:

- increased pain
- decreased touch sensation
- increased weakness of the affected part
- increased swelling and pallor
- decreased pulses and capillary refill.

Treatment of compartment syndrome includes:

- placing the limb at heart level
- removing constricting forces
- monitoring neurovascular status
- monitoring compartment pressures
- emergency fasciotomy.

Diagnosis

A history of traumatic injury and the results of the physical examination, including gentle palpation and a cautious attempt by the patient to move parts distal to the injury, suggest an arm or leg fracture.

Note: When performing the physical examination, also check for other injuries.

CONFIRMING DIAGNOSIS *Anteroposterior and lateral X-rays of the suspected fracture as well as X-rays of the joints above and below it confirm the diagnosis. (See* Classifying fractures.*)*

Treatment

Emergency treatment consists of splinting the limb above and below the suspected fracture, applying a cold pack, and elevating the limb to reduce edema and pain.

In severe fractures that cause blood loss, apply direct pressure to control bleeding, and administer fluid replacement as soon as possible to prevent or treat hypovolemic shock.

After confirming a fracture diagnosis, begin treatment with reduction (which involves restoring displaced bone segments to their normal position).

After reduction, the fractured arm or leg must be immobilized by a splint or a cast or with traction. In closed reduction (accomplished by manual manipulation), a local anesthetic such as lidocaine and an analgesic such as I.V. morphine help relieve pain; a muscle relaxant such as I.V. diazepam or a sedative such as midazolam facilitates the muscle stretching necessary to realign the bone.

X-rays are ordered to confirm that the reduction was successful and that proper bone alignment was achieved.

When closed reduction is impossible, open reduction during surgery reduces and immobilizes the fracture by means of rods, plates, or screws. Afterward, a cast is usually applied.

When a splint or cast fails to maintain the reduction, immobilization requires skin or skeletal traction, using a series of weights and pulleys. In skin traction, elastic bandages and sheepskin coverings are used to attach traction devices to the patient's skin. In skeletal traction, a pin or wire inserted through the bone distal to the fracture and attached to a weight allows more prolonged traction.

Treatment of open fractures also requires tetanus prophylaxis, prophylactic antibiotics, surgery to repair soft-tissue damage, and thorough debridement of the wound.

Special considerations

- Watch for signs of shock in the patient with a severe open fracture of a large bone such as the femur.

 ALERT *Monitor vital signs and be especially alert for rapid pulse, decreased blood pressure, pallor, and cool, clammy skin—all of which may indicate that the patient is in shock.*

- Administer I.V. fluids as ordered.

CLASSIFYING FRACTURES

One of the best-known systems for classifying fractures uses a combination of terms, such as simple, nondisplaced, and oblique, to describe fractures. An explanation of these terms appears below.

General classification of fractures
- *Simple (closed)* — Bone fragments don't penetrate the skin.
- *Compound (open)* — Bone fragments penetrate the skin.
- *Incomplete (partial)* — Bone continuity isn't completely interrupted.
- *Complete* — Bone continuity is completely interrupted.

Below you'll find definitions of the terms used to describe fractures according to fragment positions and fracture lines.

Classification by fragment position
- *Comminuted* — The bone breaks into small pieces.
- *Impacted* — One bone fragment is forced into another.
- *Angulated* — Fragments lie at an angle to each other.
- *Displaced* — Fracture fragments separate and are deformed.
- *Nondisplaced* — The two sections of bone maintain essentially normal alignment.

- *Overriding* — Fragments overlap, shortening the total bone length.
- *Segmental* — Fractures occur in two adjacent areas with an isolated central segment.
- *Avulsed* — Fragments are pulled from normal position by muscle contractions or ligament resistance.

Classification by fracture line
- *Linear* — The fracture line runs parallel to the bone's axis.
- *Longitudinal* — The fracture line extends in a longitudinal (but not parallel) direction along the bone's axis.
- *Oblique* — The fracture line crosses the bone at roughly a 45-degree angle to the bone's axis.
- *Spiral* — The fracture line crosses the bone at an oblique angle, creating a spiral pattern.
- *Transverse* — The fracture line forms a right angle with the bone's axis.

- Offer reassurance to the patient, who's likely to be frightened and in pain.
- Ease pain with analgesics as needed.
- Help the patient set realistic goals for recovery.
- If the fracture requires long-term immobilization with traction, reposition the patient often to increase comfort and prevent pressure ulcers. Assist with active range-of-motion exercises to prevent muscle atrophy. Encourage deep breathing and coughing to avoid hypostatic pneumonia.
- Urge adequate fluid intake to prevent urinary stasis and constipation. Watch for signs of renal calculi (flank pain, nausea, and vomiting).

- Provide good cast care and support the cast with pillows. Observe for skin irritation near cast edges and check for foul odors or discharge. Tell the patient to report signs of impaired circulation (skin coldness, numbness, tingling, or discoloration) immediately. Warn him not to get the cast wet and not to insert foreign objects under the cast.
- Encourage the patient to start moving around as soon as he's able. Help him to walk. (Remember, a patient who has been bedridden for some time may be dizzy at first.) Demonstrate how to use crutches properly.
- After cast removal, refer the patient to a physical therapist to restore limb mobility.

COMMON DISLOCATION

Children commonly dislocate elbow joints as a result of an adult pulling the child by the hand, as occurs when crossing the street; the stress on the joint causes the dislocation.

NORMAL ELBOW JOINT

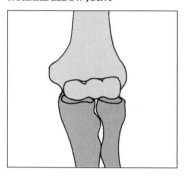

ELBOW JOINT WITH LATERAL DISLOCATION

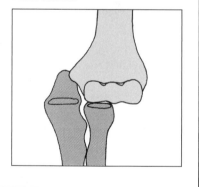

ticulating surfaces. (See *Common dislocation*.) Dislocations and subluxations occur at the joints of the shoulders, elbows, wrists, digits, hips, knees, ankles, and feet. These injuries may accompany joint fractures or result in deposition of fracture fragments between joint surfaces. Prompt reduction can limit the resulting damage to soft tissue, nerves, and blood vessels.

Causes
A dislocation or subluxation may be congenital (as in congenital hip dislocation) or it may follow trauma or disease of surrounding joint tissues.

Signs and symptoms
Dislocations and subluxations produce deformity around the joint, change the involved extremity's length, impair joint mobility, and cause point tenderness. When the injury results from trauma, it's extremely painful and commonly accompanies joint surface fractures. Even in the absence of concomitant fractures, the displaced bone may damage surrounding muscles, ligaments, nerves, and blood vessels and may cause bone necrosis, especially if reduction is delayed.

Diagnosis
Patient history, X-rays, and a physical examination rule out or confirm a fracture.

Treatment
Immediate reduction (before tissue edema and muscle spasm make reduction difficult) can prevent additional tissue damage and vascular impairment. Closed reduction consists of manual traction under general anesthesia (or local anesthesia and sedatives). During such reduction, I.V. morphine controls pain; I.V. midazolam controls muscle spasm and facilitates muscle stretching during traction. Some injuries require open reduction under regional block or general anesthesia. Such surgery may include wire fixation of the joint, skeletal traction, and ligament repair.

After reduction, a splint, a cast, or traction immobilizes the joint. In most cases, immobilizing the digits for 2 weeks, hips for 6 to 8 weeks, and other dislocated joints for 3 to 6 weeks allows surrounding liga-

■ If the patient is a child who sustained the fracture at or near the growth plate, have the family continue to follow-up with the child's pediatrician to ensure that there are no problems as the limb grows.

Dislocations and subluxations

Dislocations displace joint bones so that their articulating surfaces totally lose contact; subluxations partially displace the arments to heal. Follow-up with a physical therapist is usually required to maintain optimal joint function.

Special considerations

- Until reduction immobilizes the dislocated joint, don't attempt manipulation. Apply ice to ease pain and edema. Splint the extremity "as it lies," even if the angle is awkward. If severe vascular compromise is present or is indicated by pallor, pain, loss of pulses, paralysis, or paresthesia, an immediate orthopedic examination (and possibly immediate reduction) is necessary.
- Because a patient who receives opioids or benzodiazepines I.V. may develop respiratory depression or arrest, keep an airway and a bag-valve-mask in the room. Monitor respirations and pulse rate closely. Also have opioids and benzodiazepine reversal agents readily available.
- To avoid injury from a dressing that's too tight, instruct the patient to report numbness, pain, cyanosis, or coldness of the extremity below the cast or splint.
- To avoid skin damage, watch for signs of pressure injury (pressure, pain, or soreness) both inside and outside the dressing.
- After the cast or splint is removed, inform the patient that he may gradually return to normal joint activity.
- A dislocated hip needs immediate reduction. At discharge, stress the need for follow-up visits to detect aseptic femoral head necrosis from vascular damage.

Traumatic amputation

Traumatic amputation is the accidental loss of a body part, usually a finger, toe, arm, or leg. In a complete amputation, the member is totally severed; in a partial amputation, some soft-tissue connection remains. The prognosis for such injuries has improved as a result of earlier emergency and critical care management, new surgical techniques, early rehabilitation, prosthesis fitting, and new prosthesis design. New limb reimplantation techniques have been moderately successful, but incomplete nerve regeneration remains a major limiting factor.

Causes and incidence

Traumatic amputations usually result directly from accidents involving factory, farm, power tools, or motor vehicles. Natural disasters, wars, and terrorist attacks can also cause traumatic amputations.

Below the knee amputations account for 53% of traumatic leg amputations; with about 33% above the knee. Lower limb amputations account for 91.7% of traumatic amputations. Incidence of below the elbow amputation is 4.4%, and above the elbow amputations account for 2%.

Signs and symptoms

The obvious sign of amputation is a body part that has been cut off. Every traumatic amputee requires careful monitoring of vital signs. If amputation involves more than a finger or toe, assessment of airway, breathing, and circulation is also required. Because profuse bleeding is likely, watch for signs of hypovolemic shock, and draw blood for a hemoglobin level, hematocrit, and type and crossmatch. In partial amputation, check for pulses distal to the amputation site. After any traumatic amputation, assess for other traumatic injuries as well. The patient may exhibit crushed body tissue, in which the body part is badly mangled but still partially attached by muscle, bone, tendon, or skin.

Treatment

Because the greatest immediate threat after traumatic amputation is blood loss and hypovolemic shock, emergency treatment consists of local measures to control bleeding, fluid replacement with normal saline solution and colloids, and blood replacement as needed. Reimplantation remains controversial, but it's becoming more common and successful because of advances in microsurgery techniques. If reconstruction or reimplantation is possible, surgical intervention attempts to preserve usable joints.

When arm or leg amputations are done, the surgeon creates a stump to be fitted with a prosthesis. A rigid dressing permits early prosthesis fitting and rehabilitation.

ELDER TIP *Leg amputation can be a life-threatening procedure, especially in patients older than age 60* *with peripheral vascular disease. Such patients suffer significant morbidity with above-the-knee amputations because of associated poor health, disease, or malnutrition; complications such as sepsis; and the physiologic insult of amputation.*

Special considerations

- During emergency treatment, monitor vital signs (especially in hypovolemic shock), clean the wound, and give tetanus prophylaxis, analgesics, and antibiotics as ordered.
- After a complete amputation, wrap the amputated part in wet dressings soaked in normal saline solution. Label the part, seal it in a plastic bag, and float the bag in ice water. Flush the wound with sterile saline solution, apply a sterile pressure dressing, and elevate the limb. Notify the reimplantation team.
- After a partial amputation, position the limb in normal alignment and drape it with towels or dressings soaked in sterile normal saline solution.
- Preoperatively, irrigate and debride the wound thoroughly (using a local block). Postoperatively, perform dressing changes using sterile technique to help prevent skin infection and ensure skin graft viability.
- Help the amputee cope with his altered body image. Encourage him to perform prescribed exercises while taking care to prevent stump trauma.

WHOLE BODY

Burns

A major burn is a horrifying injury, requiring painful treatment and a long period of rehabilitation. It's commonly fatal or permanently disfiguring and incapacitating (both emotionally and physically).

Causes and incidence

Thermal burns, the most common type, are commonly the result of residential fires, automobile accidents, children playing with matches, improperly stored gasoline, space heater or electrical malfunctions, or arson. Other causes include improper handling of firecrackers, scalding accidents, and kitchen accidents (such as a child climbing on top of a stove or grabbing a hot iron). Some burns in children are traced to parental abuse.

Chemical burns result from the contact, ingestion, inhalation, or injection of acids, alkalis, or vesicants. Electrical burns usually occur after contact with faulty electrical wiring or high-voltage power lines; many children sustain them by chewing on electric cords. Friction, or abrasion, burns happen when the skin is rubbed harshly against a coarse surface. Sunburn, of course, follows excessive exposure to sunlight.

In the United States, about 2.4 million people suffer burns annually. Fire ranks fifth among accidental injuries, after motor vehicle accidents, poisoning, falls, and drowning.

Signs and symptoms

One goal of assessment is to determine the *depth* of skin and tissue damage. A partial-thickness burn damages the epidermis and part of the dermis, whereas a full-thickness burn affects the full dermis and, possibly, subcutaneous tissue. A more traditional method gauges burn depth by degrees. However, most burns are a combination of different degrees and thicknesses. (See *Gauging burn depth.*)

Burn degrees are classified as follows:
- *First degree* — Damage is limited to the epidermis, causing erythema and pain.
- *Second degree* — The epidermis and part of the dermis are damaged, producing blisters and mild to moderate edema and pain.
- *Third degree* — The epidermis and the dermis are damaged. No blisters appear, but white, brown, or black leathery tissue and thrombosed vessels are visible.
- *Fourth degree* — Damage extends through deeply charred subcutaneous tissue to muscle and bone.

Another assessment goal is to estimate the *size* of a burn, which is usually expressed as the percentage of body surface area (BSA) covered by the burn. The Rule of Nines chart usually provides this estimate, but the Lund and Browder chart is more accurate because it allows for BSA changes with age.

GAUGING BURN DEPTH

One method of assessing burns is by determining the burn's depth. A partial-thickness burn damages the epidermis and part of the dermis, whereas a full-thickness burn damages the epidermis, dermis, subcutaneous tissue, and muscle, as shown below.

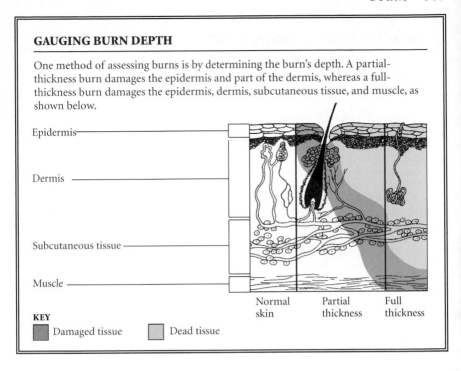

Epidermis

Dermis

Subcutaneous tissue

Muscle

Normal skin   Partial thickness   Full thickness

KEY

Damaged tissue   Dead tissue

A correlation of the burn's depth and size permits an estimate of its severity as follows:

- *major* — third-degree burns on more than 10% of BSA; second-degree burns on more than 25% of adult BSA (more than 20% in children); burns of hands, face, feet, or genitalia; burns complicated by fractures or respiratory damage; electrical burns; all burns in poor-risk patients
- *moderate* — third-degree burns on 2% to 10% of BSA; second-degree burns on 15% to 25% of adult BSA (10% to 20% in children)
- *minor* — third-degree burns on less than 2% of BSA; second-degree burns on less than 15% of adult BSA (10% in children).

Here are other important factors in assessing burns:

- Location — Burns on the face, hands, feet, and genitalia are the most serious because of possible function loss.
- Configuration — Circumferential burns can cause total occlusion of circulation in an extremity as a result of edema. Burns on the neck can produce airway obstruction, whereas burns on the chest can lead to restricted respiratory expansion.
- History of complicating medical problems — Note any disorders that impair peripheral circulation, especially diabetes, peripheral vascular disease, and chronic alcohol abuse.
- Patient age — Victims younger than age 4 or older than age 60 have a higher incidence of complications and, consequently, a higher mortality.
- Smoke inhalation — This can result in pulmonary injury. Inhalation injury should be suspected if the victim was in an enclosed space.
- Other injuries sustained at the time of the burn — Explosion and blast injuries can be caused by the person being thrown or falling from a height, resulting in other traumatic injuries.

Treatment

Immediate, aggressive burn treatment increases the patient's chances of survival. Later, supportive measures and strict sterile technique can minimize infection. Because burns require such comprehensive care,

---

MANAGING BURNS WITH SKIN GRAFTS

When a patient has a limited, well-defined burn, he may need a temporary graft to minimize fluid and protein loss from the burn surface, to prevent infection, and to reduce pain. Types of temporary grafts include:

- *allografts (homografts),* which are usually cadaver skin
- *xenografts (heterografts),* which are typically pigskin
- *biosynthetic grafts,* which are a combination of collagen and synthetics.

To treat a full-thickness burn, a patient may need an *autograft.* This method uses the patient's own skin — usually a split-thickness graft — to replace the burned skin. For areas where appearance or joint movement is important, the autograft will be transplanted intact. In flat areas where appearance is less critical, the graft may be meshed (fenestrated) to cover up to three times its original size.

When burns cover the entire body surface, epithelial cells grown in culture for autograft may provide lifesaving treatment. In this method, a small full-thickness biopsy yields epidermal cells that are cultured into sheets and then grafted onto the burns. It takes several weeks to grow confluent sheets and the process is costly. The cells are produced in a fragile sheet that's sensitive to infection.

Bilayer collagen matrices — porous, spongelike lattices are composed of bovine collagen, chondroitin-6-sulfate, and glycosaminoglycans — are another option. These matrices serve as a dermal substitute and a scaffold to support developing fibroblasts and blood vessels, which eventually replace the matrices. A silicone membrane is sealed over the surface, becoming progressively less adherent as it's incorporated into the body After 3 weeks, it's peeled off and replaced with cultured epithelial cells or thin, split-thickness grafts.

---

good nursing can make the difference between life and death. (See *Managing burns with skin grafts.*)

Moderate or major burns

- Immediately assess the patient's airway, breathing, and circulation (ABCs). Be especially alert for signs of smoke inhalation and pulmonary damage: singed nasal hairs, mucosal burns, voice changes, coughing, wheezing, soot in the mouth or nose, and darkened sputum. Assist with endotracheal intubation and administer 100% oxygen as ordered.
- When you have ensured the patient's ABCs, take a brief history of the burn. Draw blood samples for complete blood count, type and crossmatch, and electrolyte, glucose, blood urea nitrogen, creatinine, and arterial blood gas levels, including a carboxyhemoglobin level.
- Control bleeding and remove smoldering clothing (soak it first in normal saline solution if it's stuck to the patient's skin), rings, and other constricting items. Be sure to cover burns with a clean, dry, sterile bed sheet. (*Never* cover large burns with saline-soaked dressings because they can drastically lower body temperature.)
- Begin I.V. therapy immediately to prevent hypovolemic shock and maintain cardiac output. Use lactated Ringer's solution or a fluid replacement formula as ordered. (See *Fluid replacement after a burn.*) Closely monitor intake and output and frequently check vital signs. Although doing so may make you nervous, don't be afraid to take the patient's blood pressure because of burned limbs.

Minor burns

For minor burns, immerse the burned area in cool normal saline solution (55° F [12.8° C]) or apply cool compresses. Administer pain medication as ordered. Debride the devitalized tissue, taking care not to break any blisters. Cover the wound with an antimicrobial agent and a nonstick bulky dressing, and administer tetanus prophylaxis as ordered.

Electrical or chemical burns

■ Tissue damage from electrical burns is difficult to assess because internal destruction along the conduction pathway is usually greater than the surface burn would indicate. Electrical burns that ignite the patient's clothes may cause thermal burns as well. If the electric shock caused ventricular fibrillation with cardiac and respiratory arrest, begin cardiopulmonary resuscitation at once. Get a voltage estimate. (For more details, see "Electric shock," page 312.)

■ Irrigate a chemical burn with copious amounts of water or normal saline solution. Using a weak base such as sodium bicarbonate to neutralize hydrofluoric acid, hydrochloric acid, or sulfuric acid on skin or mucous membrane is contraindicated because the neutralizing agent can actually produce more heat and tissue damage.

If the chemical entered the patient's eyes, flush them with large amounts of water or normal saline solution for at least 30 minutes; in an alkali burn, irrigate until the pH of the cul-de-sacs returns to 7. Have the patient close his eyes, and cover them with a dry, sterile dressing. Note the type of chemical that caused the burn and the presence of any noxious fumes. The patient will need an emergency ophthalmologic examination.

Special considerations

■ Don't treat the burn wound itself in the emergency department if the patient is to be transferred to a specialized burn care unit within 4 hours after the burn. Instead, prepare the patient for transport by wrapping him in a sterile sheet and a blanket for warmth and elevating the burned extremity to decrease edema. Then transport him immediately.

While the patient is hospitalized:

■ A central venous pressure line and additional I.V. lines (using venous cutdown if necessary) and an indwelling urinary catheter may be inserted. To combat fluid evaporation through the burn and the re-

> **FLUID REPLACEMENT AFTER A BURN**
>
> Use the Parkland formula as a general guideline for the amount of fluid replacement. Administer 4 ml/kg of crystalloid x % total burn surface area; give half of the solution over the first 8 hours (calculated from the time of the injury) and the balance over the next 16 hours. Vary the specific infusions according to the patient's response, especially urine output.

lease of fluid into interstitial spaces (possibly resulting in hypovolemic shock), continue fluid therapy as ordered.

■ Check vital signs every 15 minutes (the physician may insert an arterial line if blood pressure is unobtainable with a cuff). Send a urine specimen to the laboratory to check for myoglobinuria and hemoglobinuria.

■ Consult nutritional therapy to provide tube feeding, total parenteral nutrition, or a high-calorie diet, as appropriate.

■ Insert a nasogastric tube to decompress the stomach and avoid aspiration of stomach contents.

Before the patient is released from the hospital:

■ Ensure that the patient's immunizations are current, particularly tetanus.

■ Arrange physical and occupational therapy consultations for the severely burned patient, as indicated.

■ Provide referral to a reconstructive surgeon for the patient disfigured by burns. Psychological counseling may also be beneficial.

■ Provide thorough teaching and complete aftercare instructions for the patient. Stress the importance of keeping the dressing dry and clean, elevating the burned extremity for the first 24 hours, taking analgesics as ordered, and returning for a wound check in 1 to 2 days.

 PEDIATRIC TIP *Consult the pediatrician if the patient is a child; consultation with a child life therapist*

may also help to ensure the child's normal growth and development.

Electric shock

When an electric current passes through the body, the damage it does depends on the current's intensity (amperes, milliamperes, or microamperes), the resistance of the tissues through which it passes, the kind of current (AC, DC, or mixed), and the frequency and duration of current flow. Electric shock may cause ventricular fibrillation, respiratory paralysis, burns, and death. The prognosis depends on the site and extent of damage, the patient's health, and the speed and adequacy of treatment.

Causes and incidence
Electric shock usually follows accidental contact with exposed parts of electrical appliances or wiring, but it may also result from lightning or the flash of electric arcs from high-voltage power lines or machines. The increased use in hospitals of electrical medical devices, many of which are connected directly to the patient, has raised serious concerns about electrical safety and has led to the development of electrical safety standards. But even well-designed equipment with reliable safety features can cause electric shock if mishandled.

Electric current can cause injury in three ways: true electrical injury as the current passes through the body, arc or flash burns from current that doesn't pass through the body, and thermal surface burns caused by associated heat and flames.

In the United States, about 1,000 people die of electric shock each year.

Signs and symptoms
Severe electric shock usually causes muscle contraction, followed by unconsciousness and loss of reflex control, sometimes with respiratory paralysis (by way of prolonged contraction of respiratory muscles or as a direct effect on the respiratory nerve center). After momentary shock, hyperventilation may follow initial muscle contraction. Passage of even the smallest electric current (if it passes through the heart) may induce ventricular fibrillation or another arrhythmia that progresses to fibrillation or myocardial infarction.

Electric shock from a high-frequency current (which generates more heat in tissues than a low-frequency current) usually causes burns, local tissue coagulation, and necrosis. Low-frequency currents can also cause serious burns if the contact with the current is concentrated in a small area (for example, when a toddler bites into an electric cord). Contusions, fractures, and other injuries can result from violent muscle contractions, falls, or being thrown during the shock; later, the patient may develop renal shutdown. Residual hearing impairment, latent rhythm effects on the heart (such as ventricular fibrillation), cataracts, and vision loss may persist after severe electric shock.

Diagnosis
In most cases, the cause of electrical injuries is either obvious or suspected. However, an accurate history can identify the voltage and the length of contact.

Treatment
Immediate emergency treatment consists of carefully separating the victim from the current source, quick assessment of vital functions, and emergency measures, such as cardiopulmonary resuscitation (CPR) and defibrillation.

To separate the victim from the current source, immediately turn it off or unplug it. If this isn't possible, pull the victim free with a nonconductive device, such as a loop of dry cloth or rubber, a dry rope, or a leather belt — with metal buckle detached. Emergency treatment then begins as follows:

■ Quickly assess vital functions. If you don't detect a pulse or breathing, start CPR at once. Continue until vital signs return or emergency help arrives with a defibrillator and other advanced life-support equipment. Then monitor the patient's cardiac rhythm continuously and obtain a 12-lead electrocardiogram.

■ Because internal tissue destruction may be much greater than indicated by skin damage, give I.V. lactated Ringer's solution as ordered to maintain urine output of 50 to 100 ml/hour. Insert an indwelling urinary catheter and send the first specimen to the laboratory. Measure intake and output hourly and watch for tea- or port wine-colored urine, which occurs when coagulation necrosis and tissue ischemia liberate myoglobin and hemoglobin. These proteins can precipitate in the renal tubules, causing tubular necrosis and renal shutdown. To prevent this, give mannitol and furosemide as ordered.

■ Administer sodium bicarbonate as directed to counteract acidosis caused by widespread tissue destruction and anaerobic metabolism.

■ Assess the patient's neurologic status frequently because central nervous system damage may result from ischemia or demyelination. Because a spinal cord injury may follow cord ischemia or a compression fracture, watch for sensorimotor deficits.

■ Check for neurovascular damage in the extremities by assessing peripheral pulses and capillary refill and by asking the patient if he feels numbness, tingling, or pain. Elevate any injured extremities.

■ Apply a temporary sterile dressing, and admit the patient for surgical debridement and observation as needed. Frequent debridement and use of topical and systemic antibiotics can help reduce the risk of infection. As ordered, prepare the patient for grafting or, if his injuries are extreme, for amputation.

Special considerations
Certain measures can be taken to prevent electric shock in patients:

■ Check for cuts, cracks, or frayed insulation on electric cords, call buttons (also check for warm call buttons), and electric devices attached to the patient's bed; keep these away from hot or wet surfaces and sharp corners. Don't set glasses of water, damp towels, or other wet items on electrical equipment. Wipe up accidental spills before they leak into electrical equipment. Avoid using extension cords because they may circumvent the ground; if they're absolutely necessary, don't place them under carpeting or in areas in which they'll be walked on.

■ Make sure ground connections on electrical equipment are intact. Line cord plugs should have three prongs, which should be straight and firmly fixed. Check that the prongs fit wall outlets properly and that outlets aren't loose or broken. Don't use adapters on plugs.

■ Report faulty equipment promptly to maintenance personnel. If a machine sparks, smokes, seems unusually hot, or gives you or your patient a slight shock, unplug it immediately if doing so won't endanger the patient's life. Check inspection labels and report equipment overdue for inspection.

■ Be especially careful when using electrical equipment near patients with pacemakers or direct cardiac lines because a cardiac catheter or pacemaker can create a direct, low-resistance path to the heart; even a small shock may cause ventricular fibrillation.

■ Remember that dry, calloused, unbroken skin offers more resistance to electric current than mucous membranes, an open wound, or thin, moist skin.

■ Make sure defibrillator paddles are free of dry, caked gel before applying fresh gel because poor electric contact can cause burns. Also, don't apply too much gel. If the gel runs over the paddle's edge and touches your hand, you'll receive some of the defibrillator shock while the patient loses some of the energy in the discharge.

■ Tell all patients how to avoid electrical hazards at home and at work. Warn them not to use electrical appliances while showering or wet. Warn them *never* to touch electrical appliances while touching faucets or cold water pipes in the kitchen because these pipes often provide the ground for all the house's circuits.

 PEDIATRIC TIP *Advise parents of small children to put safety guards on all electrical outlets and to keep children away from electrical devices.*

Cold injuries

Cold injuries result from overexposure to cold air or water and occur in two major forms: localized injuries such as frostbite and systemic injuries such as hypothermia. Untreated or improperly treated frostbite

RECOGNIZING FROSTBITE

Blackened areas in this photo show tissue necrosis and gangrene—the result of deep frostbite that extends beyond subcutaneous tissue.

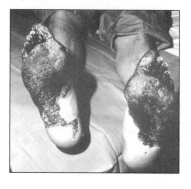

 ELDER TIP *The following risk factors put elderly people at increased risk for cold injuries: cardiovascular disease, alcohol abuse, malnutrition, diabetes, skin diseases, scarring from major burns, inadequate fluid intake, working outdoors, wearing inappropriate clothing, and living in poor environmental conditions. The use of anticholinergics, phenothiazines, diuretics, antihistamines, antidepressants, or beta-adrenergic blockers also increases the risk.*

Signs and symptoms

Frostbite may be deep or superficial. Superficial frostbite affects skin and subcutaneous tissue, especially of the face, ears, extremities, and other exposed areas. Although it may go unnoticed at first, frostbite produces burning, tingling, numbness, swelling, and a mottled, blue-gray skin color when the person returns to a warm place.

Deep frostbite extends beyond subcutaneous tissue and usually affects the hands or feet. The skin becomes white until it's thawed; then it turns purplish blue. Deep frostbite also produces pain, skin blisters, tissue necrosis, and gangrene. (See *Recognizing frostbite.*)

Indications of hypothermia (a core body temperature below 95° F [35° C]) vary with severity:

■ *mild hypothermia*—temperature of 89.6° to 95° F (32° to 35° C), severe shivering, slurred speech, and amnesia
■ *moderate hypothermia*—temperature of 86° to 89.6° F (30° to 32° C), unresponsiveness or confusion, muscle rigidity, peripheral cyanosis and, with improper rewarming, signs of shock
■ *severe hypothermia*—temperature of 77° to 86° F (25° to 30° C), loss of deep tendon reflexes, and ventricular fibrillation. The patient may appear dead (in a state of rigor mortis), with no palpable pulse or audible heart sounds. His pupils may be dilated. A temperature drop below 77° F causes cardiopulmonary arrest and death.

Diagnosis

A history of severe and prolonged exposure to cold may make this diagnosis obvious. Nevertheless, hypothermia can be over-

can lead to gangrene and may require amputation; severe hypothermia can be fatal.

Causes and incidence

Localized cold injuries occur when ice crystals form in the tissues and expand extracellular spaces. With compression of the tissue cell, the cell membrane ruptures, interrupting enzymatic and metabolic activities. Increased capillary permeability accompanies histamine release, resulting in aggregation of red blood cells and microvascular occlusion. Hypothermia effects chemical changes that slow the functions of most major organ systems, such as decreased renal blood flow and decreased glomerular filtration. Frostbite results from prolonged exposure to dry temperatures far below freezing; hypothermia, from near drowning in cold water and prolonged exposure to cold temperatures.

The risk of serious cold injuries, especially hypothermia, is increased by youth, old age, lack of insulating body fat, wet or inadequate clothing, drug abuse, cardiac disease, smoking, fatigue, hunger and depletion of caloric reserves, and excessive alcohol intake (which draws blood into capillaries and away from body organs).

looked if outdoor temperatures are above freezing or if the patient is comatose.

Treatment

In a localized cold injury, treatment consists of rewarming the injured part, supportive measures and, sometimes, a fasciotomy to increase circulation by lowering edematous tissue pressure. However, if gangrene occurs, amputation may be necessary. In hypothermia, therapy consists of immediate resuscitative measures, careful monitoring, and gradual rewarming of the body. If cold injuries in children suggest neglect or abuse, a thorough history should be performed.

Treat localized cold injuries as follows:
■ Remove constrictive clothing and jewelry and slowly rewarm the affected part in tepid water (100° to 108° F [37.8° to 42.2° C]). Give the patient warm fluids to drink. *Never* rub the injured area — this aggravates tissue damage.
■ When the affected part begins to rewarm, the patient will feel pain, so give analgesics as ordered. Check for a pulse. Be careful not to rupture any blebs. If the injury is on the foot, place cotton or gauze sponges between the toes to prevent maceration. Instruct the patient not to walk.
■ If the injury has caused an open skin wound, give antibiotics and tetanus prophylaxis as ordered.
■ If a pulse fails to return, the patient may develop compartment syndrome and need a fasciotomy to restore circulation. (See *Recognizing compartment syndrome*, page 304.) If gangrene occurs, prepare the patient for amputation.
■ Before discharge, teach the patient about possible long-term effects: increased sensitivity to cold, burning and tingling, and increased sweating. Warn him against smoking, which causes vasoconstriction and slows healing.

Systemic hypothermia is treated as follows:
■ If you detect no pulse or respiration, begin cardiopulmonary resuscitation (CPR) immediately and, if necessary, continue it for 2 to 3 hours. (Remember that hypothermia helps protect the brain from anoxia, which normally accompanies prolonged cardiopulmonary arrest. Therefore, even after the patient has been unresponsive for a long time, resuscitation may be possible, especially after cold-water near drownings.) Perform CPR until the patient is adequately rewarmed.
■ Move the patient to a warm area, remove wet clothing, and keep him dry. If he's conscious, give warm fluids with a high sugar content such as tea with sugar. If the patient's core temperature is above 89.6° F (32° C), use external warming techniques. Bathe him in water that is 104° F (40° C), cover him with a heating blanket set at 97.9° to 99.9° F (36.6° to 37.7° C), and cautiously apply hot water bottles at 104° F to the groin and axillae, guarding against burns.
■ If the patient's core temperature is below 89.6° F (32° C), use internal and external warming methods. Rewarm his body core and surface 1° to 2° F (−0.5° to −1.1° C) per hour concurrently. (If you rewarm the surface first, rewarming shock could cause potentially fatal ventricular fibrillation.) To warm inhalations, provide oxygen heated to 107.6° to 114.8° F (42° to 46° C). Infuse I.V. solutions that have been warmed to 98.6° F (37° C) and perform nasogastric lavage with normal saline solution that has been warmed to the same temperature. Assist with peritoneal lavage, using normal saline solution (full or half-strength) warmed to 104° to 113° F (40° to 45° C); in severe hypothermia, assist with heart and lung bypass at controlled temperatures and thoracotomy with direct cardiac warm saline bath.

Special considerations

■ Throughout treatment, monitor arterial blood gas levels, intake and output, central venous pressure, temperature, and cardiac and neurologic status every 30 minutes. Also monitor laboratory test results, such as complete blood count, blood urea nitrogen and electrolyte levels, prothrombin time, and partial thromboplastin time.
■ If the patient has developed a cold injury because of inadequate clothes or housing, refer him to a community social service agency, if appropriate.

Cold injuries can be prevented:
■ Tell the patient to wear mittens (not gloves); windproof, water-resistant, multi-

layered clothing; two pairs of socks (cotton next to skin, then wool); and a scarf and hat that cover the ears (to avoid substantial heat loss through the head).
- Advise the patient not to drink alcohol or smoke and to get adequate food and rest before prolonged exposure.
- Caution the patient to find shelter early or to increase physical activity if he's caught in a severe snowstorm.

Heat syndrome

Heat syndrome may result from environmental or internal conditions that increase heat production or impair heat dissipation. The three categories of heat syndrome are heat cramps, heat exhaustion, and heatstroke.

Causes
Normally, people adjust to excessive temperatures via complex cardiovascular and neurologic changes that are coordinated by the hypothalamus. Heat loss offsets heat production to regulate the body temperature. It does this by evaporation (sweating) or vasodilation, which cools the body's surface by radiation, conduction, and convection.

However, heat production increases with exercise, infection, and the use of certain drugs such as amphetamines, and heat loss decreases with high temperatures or humidity, lack of acclimatization, excess clothing, obesity, dehydration, cardiovascular disease, sweat gland dysfunction, and the use of such drugs as phenothiazines and anticholinergics. When heat loss mechanisms fail to offset heat production, the body retains heat and may develop heat syndrome.

Treatment
For specific guidelines on treating heat syndrome, see *Managing heat syndrome.*

Special considerations
Heat illnesses are easily preventable, so it's important to educate the public about the various factors that cause them. This information is especially vital for athletes, laborers, and soldiers in field training.

- Advise your patients to avoid heat syndrome by taking these precautions in hot weather: wearing loose-fitting, lightweight clothing; resting frequently; avoiding hot places; and drinking adequate fluids.

ELDER TIP *Vigorous fluid replacement in elderly people or those with underlying cardiovascular disease may cause pulmonary edema.*
- Advise patients who are obese, elderly, or taking drugs that impair heat regulation to avoid becoming overheated.
- Tell patients who have had heat cramps or heat exhaustion to exercise gradually and to increase their salt and water intake.
- Tell patients with heatstroke that residual hypersensitivity to high temperatures may persist for several months.

Asphyxia

A condition of insufficient oxygen and accumulating carbon dioxide in the blood and tissues due to interference with respiration, asphyxia results in cardiopulmonary arrest. Without prompt treatment, it's fatal.

Causes
Asphyxia results from any condition or substance that inhibits respiration such as the following:
- hypoventilation due to opioid abuse, medullary disease or hemorrhage, pneumothorax, respiratory muscle paralysis, or cardiopulmonary arrest
- intrapulmonary obstruction, as in airway obstruction, severe asthma, foreign body aspiration, pulmonary edema, pneumonia, and near drowning
- extrapulmonary obstruction, as in tracheal compression from a tumor, strangulation, trauma, or suffocation
- inhalation of toxic agents, as in carbon monoxide poisoning, smoke inhalation, and excessive oxygen inhalation.

Signs and symptoms
Depending on the asphyxia's duration and degree, common symptoms include anxiety, dyspnea, agitation and confusion leading to coma, altered respiratory rate (apnea, bradypnea, occasional tachypnea),

MANAGING HEAT SYNDROME

Management of heat syndrome depends on the injury's severity.

Type and predisposing factors	Signs and symptoms	Management
Heat cramps ■ Commonly affect young adults ■ Strenuous activity without training or acclimatization ■ Normal to high temperature or high humidity	■ Muscle twitching and spasms, weakness, severe muscle cramps ■ Nausea ■ Normal temperature or slight fever ■ Diaphoresis	■ Hospitalization is usually unnecessary. ■ Replace fluids and electrolytes. ■ Loosen the patient's clothing and have him lie down in a cool place. Massage his muscles. If muscle cramps are severe, start an I.V. infusion with normal saline solution.
Heat exhaustion ■ Commonly affects young people ■ Physical activity without acclimatization ■ Decreased heat dissipation ■ High temperature and humidity	■ Nausea and vomiting ■ Decreased blood pressure ■ Thready, rapid pulse ■ Cool, pallid skin ■ Headache, mental confusion, syncope, giddiness ■ Oliguria, thirst ■ Elevated temperature ■ Muscle cramps	■ Hospitalization is usually unnecessary. ■ *Immediately* give salt tablets and a balanced electrolyte drink. ■ Loosen the patient's clothing and put him in a shock position in a cool place. Massage his muscles. If cramps are severe, start an I.V. infusion as ordered. ■ Give oxygen if needed.
Heatstroke ■ Exertional type — commonly affects young, healthy people involved in strenuous activity ■ Classical type — commonly affects elderly, inactive people who have cardiovascular disease or who take drugs that influence temperature regulation ■ High temperature and humidity without any wind	■ Hypertension followed by hypotension ■ Atrial or ventricular tachycardia ■ Hot, dry, red skin, which later turns gray; no diaphoresis ■ Confusion, progressing to seizures and loss of consciousness ■ Temperature higher than 104° F (40° C) ■ Dilated pupils ■ Slow, deep respiration; then Cheyne-Stokes	■ Hospitalization is needed. ■ Maintain airway, breathing, and circulation. ■ To lower body temperature, cool the patient rapidly with ice packs on arterial pressure points and hypothermia blankets. ■ To replace fluids and electrolytes, start an I.V. infusion. ■ Insert a nasogastric tube to prevent aspiration. ■ Give diazepam to control seizures. ■ Monitor the patient's temperature, intake and output, and cardiac status. Give dobutamine, as ordered, to correct cardiogenic shock. (Vasoconstrictors are contraindicated.)

decreased breath sounds, central and peripheral cyanosis (cherry-red mucous membranes in late-stage carbon monoxide poisoning), seizures, and fast, slow, or absent pulse.

Diagnosis

Diagnosis is based on the patient's history and laboratory results. Arterial blood gas measurement, the most important test, indicates decreased partial pressure of oxygen (less than 60 mm Hg) and increased partial pressure of carbon dioxide (more than 50 mm Hg). Chest X-rays may show a foreign body, pulmonary edema, or atelectasis. Toxicology tests may show drugs, chemicals, or abnormal hemoglobin (carboxihemoglobin). Pulmonary function tests may indicate respiratory muscle weakness.

Treatment

Asphyxia requires immediate respiratory support—with cardiopulmonary resuscitation, endotracheal intubation, and supplemental oxygen, as needed, and elimination of the underlying cause as follows: bronchoscopy for a foreign body extraction, an opioid antagonist such as naloxone for an opioid overdose, gastric lavage for poisoning, and withholding of supplemental oxygen for carbon dioxide narcosis due to excessive oxygen therapy.

Special considerations

Respiratory distress is frightening, so reassure the patient during treatment. Give prescribed drugs. Suction carefully as needed and encourage deep breathing. Closely monitor vital signs and laboratory test results. To prevent drug-induced asphyxia, warn patients about the danger of taking alcohol with other central nervous system depressants.

Near drowning

Near drowning refers to surviving—temporarily, at least—the physiologic effects of hypoxemia and acidosis that result from submersion in fluid. Hypoxemia and acidosis are the primary problems in victims of near drowning.

Near drowning occurs in three forms: "dry," in which the victim doesn't aspirate fluid, but suffers respiratory obstruction or asphyxia (10% to 15% of patients); "wet," in which the victim aspirates fluid and suffers from asphyxia or secondary changes due to fluid aspiration (about 85% of patients); and "secondary," in which the victim suffers a recurrence of respiratory distress (usually aspiration pneumonia or pulmonary edema) within minutes or 1 to 2 days after a near-drowning incident.

Causes and incidence

Near drowning results from an inability to swim or, in swimmers, from panic, a boating accident, a heart attack or blow to the head while in the water, a fall through ice, heavy drinking prior to swimming, or a suicide attempt. Children can also suffer near drowning from swimming accidents, bathing, or falling into a container of water such as a bucket or a body of water such as a pond.

Regardless of the tonicity of the fluid aspirated, hypoxemia is the most serious consequence of near drowning, followed by metabolic acidosis. Other consequences depend on the kind of water aspirated. If the water is contaminated, such as water from a stagnant pool or contaminated stream, bacteria, fungus, or algae may be aspirated as well, causing infection or sepsis. After fresh water aspiration, changes in lung surfactant character result in exudation of protein-rich plasma into the alveoli. This, plus increased capillary permeability, leads to pulmonary edema and hypoxemia.

After saltwater aspiration, the hypertonicity of seawater exerts an osmotic force, which pulls fluid from pulmonary capillaries into the alveoli. The resulting intrapulmonary shunt causes hypoxemia. Also, the pulmonary capillary membrane may be injured and induce pulmonary edema. In both kinds of near drowning, pulmonary edema and hypoxemia occur secondary to aspiration.

In the United States, drowning claims nearly 6,500 lives annually. No statistics are available for near-drowning incidents.

Signs and symptoms

Near-drowning victims can display a host of clinical problems: apnea, shallow or gasping respirations, substernal chest pain, asystole, tachycardia, bradycardia, restlessness, irritability, lethargy, fever, confusion, unconsciousness, vomiting, abdominal distention, and a cough that produces a pink, frothy fluid.

Diagnosis

Diagnosis requires a history of near drowning, including the type of water aspirated along with characteristic features and auscultation of crackles and rhonchi if respirations are present or if the patient is being ventilated.

Arterial blood gas (ABG) analysis shows decreased oxygen content, low bicarbonate levels, and low pH. Electrolyte levels may be elevated or decreased, depending on the type of water aspirated. Leukocytosis may occur. Electrocardiogram shows arrhythmias and waveform changes.

Treatment

Emergency treatment begins with cardiopulmonary resuscitation (CPR) and administration of 100% oxygen.

■ Stabilize the patient's neck in case he has a cervical injury.

■ When the patient arrives at the hospital, assess for a patent airway. Establish one if necessary. Continue CPR, intubate the patient, and provide respiratory assistance such as mechanical ventilation with positive end-expiratory pressure, if needed.

■ Assess ABG and pulse oximetry values.

■ If the patient's abdomen is distended, insert a nasogastric tube. (Intubate the patient first if he's unconscious.)

■ Start I.V. lines and insert an indwelling urinary catheter.

■ Drug treatment for near drowning may include sodium bicarbonate for documented acidosis, corticosteroids and osmotic diuretics for cerebral edema, antibiotics to prevent infections, and bronchodilators to ease bronchospasms.

Special considerations

■ Remember that all near-drowning victims should be admitted for an observation period of 24 to 48 hours because of the possibility of developing delayed drowning symptoms.

■ Observe for pulmonary complications and signs of delayed drowning (confusion, substernal pain, adventitious breath sounds). Suction often. Pulmonary artery catheters may be useful in assessing cardiopulmonary status.

■ Monitor vital signs, intake and output, and peripheral pulses. Check for skin perfusion and watch for signs of infection.

■ To facilitate breathing, raise the bed's head slightly.

■ To prevent near drowning, advise swimmers to avoid drinking alcohol before swimming, to observe water safety rules, and to take a water safety course sponsored by the Red Cross or YMCA.

Decompression sickness

Decompression sickness (the "bends") is a painful condition that results from a too-rapid change from a high- to low-pressure environment (decompression). Most victims are scuba divers who ascend too quickly from water deeper than 30′ (9.1 m) and pilots and passengers of unpressurized aircraft who ascend too quickly to high altitudes.

Causes

Decompression sickness results from an abrupt change in air or water pressure that causes nitrogen to spill out of tissues faster than it can be diffused through respiration. It causes gas bubbles to form in blood and body tissues, which produce excruciating joint and muscle pain, neurologic and respiratory distress, and skin changes.

Signs and symptoms

Symptoms usually appear during or within 30 minutes of rapid decompression, although they may be delayed up to 24 hours. Typically, decompression sickness results in:

■ "the bends," deep and usually constant joint and muscle pain so severe that it may be incapacitating

■ transitory neurologic disturbances, such as difficult urination (from bladder paralysis), hemiplegia, deafness, visual distur-

bances, dizziness, aphasia, paresthesia and hyperesthesia of the legs, unsteady gait and, possibly, coma
- respiratory distress (known as the "chokes"), which includes chest pain, retrosternal burning, and a cough that may become paroxysmal and uncontrollable.

Such symptoms may persist for days and result in dyspnea, cyanosis, fainting and, occasionally, shock. Other symptoms include decreased temperature, pallor, itching, burning, mottled skin, fatigue and, in some patients, tachypnea.

Diagnosis

CONFIRMING DIAGNOSIS *A history of rapid decompression and a physical examination showing characteristic clinical features confirm the diagnosis.*

Treatment

Treatment consists of recompression and oxygen administration, followed by gradual decompression. In recompression, which takes place in a hyperbaric chamber (not available in all hospitals), air pressure is increased to 2.8 absolute atmospheric pressure over 1 to 2 minutes. This rapid rise in pressure reduces the size of the circulating nitrogen bubbles and relieves pain and other clinical effects. During recompression, intermittent oxygen administration, with periodic maximal exhalations, promotes gas bubble diffusion. After symptoms subside and diffusion is complete, a slow decrease of air pressure in the chamber allows for gradual, safe decompression.

Supportive measures include fluid replacement in hypovolemic shock and, sometimes, corticosteroids to reduce the risk of spinal edema. Opioids are contraindicated because they further depress impaired respiration.

Special considerations

- To avoid oxygen toxicity during recompression, tell the patient to alternate breathing oxygen for 5 minutes with breathing air for 5 minutes.
- During oxygen administration, make sure all electrical equipment is grounded. Prohibit smoking, the use of electric appliances such as razors, and the use of blankets made of wool or other materials that produce static electricity in the patient's room.
- If the patient with bladder paralysis needs catheterization, monitor intake and output.
- To prevent decompression sickness, advise divers and pilots to follow the U.S. Navy's ascent guidelines.

Radiation exposure

Expanded use of ionized radiation (X-rays, protons, neutrons, and alpha, beta, and gamma rays) has vastly increased the incidence of radiation exposure. Cancer patients receiving radiation therapy and nuclear power plant workers are the most likely victims of this modern anomaly.

The amount of radiation absorbed by a human body is measured in radiation absorbed doses (rads), not to be confused with roentgens, which are used to measure radiation emissions. A person can absorb up to 200 rads without fatal consequences. A dose of 240 to 340 rads is fatal in about 50% of cases; more than 500 rads is nearly always fatal. (See *Effects of whole body irradiation.*) However, when radiation is focused on a small area, the body can absorb and survive many thousands of rads if they're administered in carefully controlled doses over a long period of time. This basic principle is the key to safe and successful radiation therapy.

Causes

Exposure to radiation can occur by inhalation, ingestion, or direct contact. The existence and severity of tissue damage depend on the amount of body area exposed (the smaller, the better), length of exposure, dosage absorbed, distance from the source, and presence of protective shielding. Ionized radiation may cause immediate cell necrosis or disturbed deoxyribonucleic acid synthesis, which impairs cell function and division. Rapidly dividing cells — bone marrow, hair follicles, gonads, and lymph tissue — are most susceptible to radiation damage; highly differentiated cells — nerve,

EFFECTS OF WHOLE BODY IRRADIATION

Symptoms after whole body irradiation are dose-dependent. Below you'll find the effects of radiation dosages ranging from 5 to 5,000 rads.

Radiation dosage (rad)	Clinical and laboratory findings
5 to 49	Patient asymptomatic; conventional blood studies normal; chromosome aberrations detectable
50 to 74	Patient asymptomatic; minor decreases in white blood cell (WBC) and platelet counts in a few patients, especially if baseline values were established
75 to 124	Prodromal symptoms (anorexia, nausea, vomiting, fatigue) in 10% to 20% of patients within 2 days; mild decrease in WBC and platelet counts in some patients
125 to 239	Transient disability and clear hematologic changes in a majority of patients; lymphocyte count decreased by about 50% within 48 hours
240 to 499	Serious, disabling illness in most patients, with about 50% mortality if untreated; lymphocyte count decreased by 75% or more within 48 hours
500 to 4,999	Accelerated version of acute radiation syndrome with GI complications within 2 weeks; bleeding; death in most patients
5,000+	Fulminating course with cardiovascular, GI, and central nervous system complications, resulting in death within 24 to 72 hours

bone, and muscle — resist radiation more successfully.

Signs and symptoms

The effects of ionized radiation can be immediate and acute or delayed and chronic. Acute effects may be hematopoietic (after 200 to 500 rads), GI (after 400 rads or more), cerebral (after 1,000 rads or more), or cardiovascular (gross after 5,000 rads). They depend strictly on the amount of radiation absorbed.

Acute hematopoietic radiation exposure induces nausea, vomiting, diarrhea, and anorexia, which subside after 24 to 48 hours. Pancytopenia develops during the latent period that follows. Within 2 to 3 weeks, thrombocytopenia, leukopenia, lymphopenia, and anemia produce nosebleeds, hemorrhage, petechiae, pallor, weakness, oropharyngeal abscesses, and increased susceptibility to infection because of impaired immunologic response.

GI radiation exposure causes ulceration, infection, intractable nausea, vomiting, and diarrhea, resulting in severe fluid and electrolyte imbalance. Breakdown of intestinal villi later causes plasma loss, which can lead to circulatory collapse and death.

Cerebral radiation poisoning after brief exposure to large amounts of radiation causes nausea, vomiting, and diarrhea within hours. Lethargy, tremors, seizures, confusion, coma, and even death may follow within hours or days.

Repeated, prolonged exposure to small doses of radiation over a long time can seriously damage skin, causing dryness, erythema, atrophy, and malignant lesions. Such damage can also follow acute exposure. (See *Radiation dermatitis*, page 322.)

RADIATION DERMATITIS

Repeated prolonged exposure to radiation — even small doses — often induces erythematous dermatitis and atrophy of skin at the site of radiation treatment.

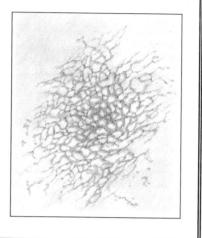

Other delayed effects include alopecia, brittle nails, hypothyroidism, amenorrhea, cataracts, decreased fertility, anemia, leukopenia, thrombocytopenia, malignant neoplasms, bone necrosis and fractures, and a shortened life span. Long-term exposure to radiation may retard fetal growth or cause genetic defects.

Diagnosis

An accurate history offers the best clues to radiation exposure. Supportive laboratory findings show decreased hematocrit; decreased white blood cell, platelet, and lymphocyte counts; and decreased hemoglobin, serum potassium, and chloride levels due to vomiting and diarrhea. Bone marrow studies show blood dyscrasia; X-rays may reveal bone necrosis. A Geiger counter may help determine the amount of radiation in open wounds.

Treatment

Treatment is essentially aimed at relieving symptoms and includes antiemetics to counter nausea and vomiting, fluid and electrolyte replacement, antibiotics, and possibly sedatives (if seizures occur). Transfusions of plasma, platelets, and red blood cells may be necessary. Bone marrow transplantation is a controversial treatment but may be the only recourse in extreme cases. When radiation exposure results from inhalation or ingestion of large amounts of radioactive iodine, potassium iodide or a strong iodine solution may be given to block thyroid uptake.

Special considerations

- To minimize radiation exposure, dispose of contaminated clothing properly. If the patient's skin is contaminated, wash his body thoroughly with mild soap and water. Debride and irrigate open wounds. If he recently ingested radioactive material, induce vomiting and start lavage.
- Monitor intake and output and maintain fluid and electrolyte balance. Give I.V. fluids and electrolytes as ordered. If the patient can take oral feedings, encourage a high-protein, high-calorie diet. Tell him to use a soft toothbrush to minimize gum bleeding. Offer lidocaine to soothe painful mouth ulcers.
- To prevent skin breakdown, make sure the patient avoids extreme temperatures, tight clothing, and drying soaps. Use rigid sterile technique.
- Prevent complications. Monitor vital signs and watch for signs of hemorrhage.
- Provide emotional support for the patient and his family, especially after severe exposure. Suggest genetic counseling and screening as needed.

Hospital personnel can avoid exposure to radiation by wearing proper shielding devices when supervising X-ray and radiation treatments. If you work in these vulnerable areas, wear radiation detection badges and turn them in periodically for readings.

MISCELLANEOUS INJURIES

Poisoning

Poisoning — inhalation, ingestion, or injection of, or skin contamination with, a harmful substance — is a common problem. The prognosis depends on the amount of poison absorbed, the poison's toxicity, and the time interval between poisoning and treatment.

Causes and incidence
In the United States, approximately 2.5 million people are poisoned annually, 1,000 of them fatally. Because of their curiosity and ignorance, children are the primary victims of poisoning. Accidental poisoning — usually from ingestion of salicylates (aspirin), acetaminophen, cleaning agents, insecticides, paints, or cosmetics — is the fourth leading cause of death in children.

In adults, poisoning is most common among chemical company employees, particularly those in companies that use chlorine, carbon dioxide, hydrogen sulfide, nitrogen dioxide, and ammonia, and in companies that ignore safety standards. Other causes of poisoning in adults include improper cooking, canning, and storage of food; ingestion of, or skin contact with, plants (see *Common poisonous plants,* page 324); and drug overdose (usually barbiturates or tricyclic antidepressants).

Signs and symptoms
Signs and symptoms vary according to the type of poison.

Diagnosis
A history of ingestion, inhalation, or injection of, or skin contact with, a poisonous substance and typical clinical features suggest the diagnosis. Suspect poisoning in any unconscious patient with no history of diabetes, seizure disorders, or trauma. Odors, such as from kerosene or cleaning fluid, may be detected on the breath or clothing of some poison victims.

CONFIRMING DIAGNOSIS *Toxicologic studies (including drug screens) of poison levels in the mouth, vomitus, urine, feces, or blood or on the victim's hands or clothing confirm the diagnosis.*

If possible, have the family or patient bring the container holding the poison to the emergency department for comparable study. In inhalation poisoning, chest X-rays may show pulmonary infiltrates or edema; in petroleum distillate inhalation, X-rays may show aspiration pneumonia.

Effects of some poisonous substances don't become apparent for hours or days.

Treatment
Treatment includes emergency resuscitation and support, prevention of further absorption of poison, continuing supportive or symptomatic care and, when possible, a specific antidote. If barbiturate, glutethimide, or tranquilizer poisoning causes hypothermia, use a hyperthermia blanket to control the patient's temperature. Dialysis may be considered in some situations.

Special considerations
- Assess cardiopulmonary and respiratory function. If necessary, begin cardiopulmonary resuscitation. Carefully monitor vital signs and level of consciousness.
- Depending on the type of poison, prevent further absorption of ingested poison by inducing vomiting using syrup of ipecac or by administering gastric lavage and cathartics. The treatment's effectiveness depends on absorption speed and the time elapsed between ingestion and removal. With syrup of ipecac, give warm water (usually less than 1 qt [1 L]) until vomiting occurs, or give another dose of ipecac as ordered.
- Never induce vomiting if you suspect corrosive acid poisoning, if the patient is unconscious or has seizures, or if the gag reflex is impaired (even in a conscious patient). Instead, neutralize the poison by instilling the appropriate antidote by nasogastric tube. Common antidotes include milk, magnesium salts (milk of magnesia), activated charcoal, or other chelating agents (deferoxamine, edetate disodium). When possible, add the antidote to water or juice.

COMMON POISONOUS PLANTS

ELEPHANT EAR PHILODENDRON

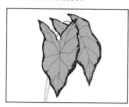

Symptoms: burning throat and GI distress
Treatment: gastric lavage or emesis; antihistamines and lime juice; symptomatic treatment

DIEFFENBACHIA

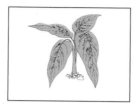

Symptoms: burning throat, edema, GI distress
Treatment: gastric lavage or emesis; antihistamines and lime juice; symptomatic treatment

POINSETTIA (MILKY JUICE)

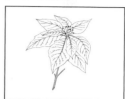

Symptoms: inflammation and blisters
Treatment: none; condition will disappear after several days

RHUBARB

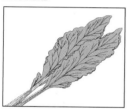

Symptoms: GI and respiratory distress, internal bleeding, coma
Treatment: gastric lavage or emesis with lime water; calcium gluconate and force fluids

MUSHROOMS

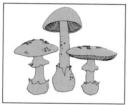

Symptoms: GI, respiratory, central nervous system, and parasympathomimetic effects
Treatment: gastric emesis with syrup of ipecac; decontamination with activated charcoal with sorbitol for catharsis; atropine

MISTLETOE

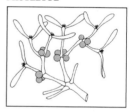

Symptoms: GI distress and slow pulse
Treatment: gastric lavage or emesis; cardiac drugs, potassium, and sodium

POISON IVY

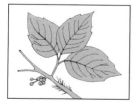

POISON OAK

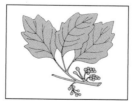

POISON SUMAC (SAP)

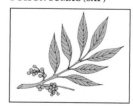

Symptoms: allergic skin reactions; if ingested, GI distress, liver and kidney damage.
Treatment: if ingested: demulcents, morphine, fluids, and high-protein, low-fat diet; for skin reactions: antihistamines and topical antipyretics.

Note: The removal of hydrocarbon poisons is controversial. For a conscious patient, gastric lavage is preferred over syrup of ipecac, especially in the emergency department. Some believe that because of poor absorption, kerosene (a hydrocarbon) doesn't require removal from the GI tract; others believe removal depends on the amount ingested.

■ To perform gastric lavage, instill 150 to 200 ml of fluid using a large-bore gastric evacuation tube; then aspirate the liquid. Repeat until aspirate is clear. Save vomitus and aspirate for analysis. (To prevent aspiration in an unconscious patient, insert an endotracheal tube before lavage.)

■ When you want to induce emesis and the patient has already taken syrup of ipecac, don't give activated charcoal to neutralize the poison until *after* emesis. Activated charcoal absorbs ipecac.

■ If several hours have passed since the patient ingested the poison, administer large quantities of I.V. fluids to induce diuresis. The kind of fluid you'll use depends on the patient's acid-base balance and cardiovascular status as well as on the flow rate.

■ Severe ingested poisoning may call for peritoneal dialysis or hemodialysis.

■ To prevent further absorption of inhaled poison, move the patient to fresh or uncontaminated air. Alert the anesthesia department and provide supplemental oxygen. Some patients may require intubation. To prevent further absorption from skin contamination, remove the clothing covering the contaminated skin and immediately flush the area with large amounts of water.

■ If the patient is in severe pain, give analgesics as ordered; frequently monitor fluid intake and output, vital signs, and level of consciousness.

■ Keep the patient warm and provide support in a quiet environment.

■ If the poison was ingested intentionally, maintain suicide precautions and refer the patient for counseling to prevent future suicide attempts.

■ For more specific treatment, contact your local poison center.

To prevent accidental poisoning:

■ Instruct patients to read the label before they take medicine. Tell them to store all medications and household chemicals properly, to keep them out of reach of children, and to discard old medications.

■ Warn patients not to take medicines prescribed for someone else, not to transfer medicines from their original bottles to other containers without labeling them properly, and never to transfer poisons to food containers.

■ Advise parents not to take medicine in front of their young children and not to call medicine "candy" to get children to take it.

■ Stress the importance of using toxic sprays only in well-ventilated areas and of following instructions carefully.

■ Tell patients to use pesticides carefully and to keep the number of their poison control center handy.

Poisonous snakebites

Poisonous snakebites are medical emergencies. With prompt, correct treatment, they need not be fatal. The only poisonous snakes in the United States are pit vipers (*Crotalidae*) and coral snakes (*Elapidae*). Pit vipers, such as rattlesnakes, water moccasins (cottonmouths), and copperheads, have a pitted depression between their eyes and nostrils and two fangs, $\frac{3}{4}''$ to $1\frac{1}{4}''$ (2 to 3 cm) long. Because fangs may break off or grow behind old ones, some snakes may have one, three, or four fangs. The fangs of coral snakes are short, but have teeth behind them. Coral snakes have distinctive red, black, and yellow bands (yellow bands always border red ones).

Causes and incidence

Of the approximately 45,000 snakebites that occur in the United States each year, 7,000 to 8,000 are from poisonous snakes, resulting in 5 to 6 deaths. Such bites are most common during summer afternoons in grassy or rocky habitats.

Pit vipers are nocturnal but active snakes that are responsible for 99% of venomous snake bites in the United States. Coral snakes are also nocturnal, but their placidity makes coral snake bites less common than pit viper bites. Coral snakes tend to bite with a chewing motion, and may leave

AFTER A SNAKEBITE

Severe edema of the affected extremity, as shown below, occurs within hours after a snakebite.

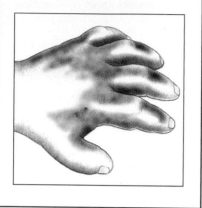

multiple fang marks, small lacerations, and extensive tissue destruction.

Signs and symptoms

Most snakebites happen on the arms and legs, below the elbow or knee. Bites to the head or trunk are most dangerous, but any bite into a blood vessel is dangerous, regardless of location.

Most pit viper bites that result in envenomation cause immediate and progressively severe pain and edema, local elevation in skin temperature, fever, skin discoloration, petechiae, ecchymoses, blebs, blisters, bloody wound discharge, and local necrosis. (See *After a snakebite.*)

Because pit viper venom is neurotoxic, pit viper bites may cause local and facial numbness and tingling, fasciculation and twitching of skeletal muscles, seizures (especially in children), extreme anxiety, difficulty speaking, fainting, weakness, dizziness, excessive sweating, occasional paralysis, mild to severe respiratory distress, headache, blurred vision, marked thirst and, in severe envenomation, coma and death. Pit viper venom may also impair coagulation and cause hematemesis, hematuria, melena, bleeding gums, and internal bleeding. Other symptoms of pit

viper bites include tachycardia, lymphadenopathy, nausea, vomiting, diarrhea, hypotension, and shock.

The reaction to coral snakebite is usually delayed — sometimes up to several hours. These snakebites cause little or no local tissue reaction (local pain, swelling, or necrosis). However, because coral snake venom is neurotoxic, a reaction can progress swiftly, producing such effects as local paresthesia, drowsiness, nausea, vomiting, difficulty swallowing, marked salivation, dysphonia, ptosis, blurred vision, miosis, respiratory distress and possible respiratory failure, loss of muscle coordination and, possibly, shock with cardiovascular collapse and death.

Diagnosis

The patient's history and account of the injury, observation of fang marks, snake identification (when possible), and progressive symptoms of envenomation all point to poisonous snakebite. Laboratory test results help identify the extent of envenomation and provide guidelines for supportive treatment.

Abnormal test results in poisonous snakebites may include:
- prolonged bleeding time and partial thromboplastin time
- decreased hemoglobin level and hematocrit
- sharply decreased platelet count (less than 200,000/mm^3)
- urinalysis disclosing hematuria
- increased white blood cell count in victims who develop an infection (a snake's mouth typically contains gram-negative bacteria)
- pulmonary edema or emboli as shown on chest X-ray
- possibly tachycardia and ectopic heartbeats on the electrocardiogram (usually necessary only in cases of severe envenomation for a patient older than age 40)
- possibly abnormal EEG findings in cases of severe envenomation.

Treatment

Prompt, appropriate first aid can reduce venom absorption and prevent severe symptoms.

- If possible, identify the snake, but don't waste time trying to find it.
- Place the victim in the supine position to slow venom metabolism and absorption.
- Don't give the victim any food, beverage, or medication orally.
- Authorities disagree about what constitutes appropriate prehospital care. Some recommend against placing a constrictive tourniquet (band) on the affected limb unless the victim is far from a medical facility.
- Whether you apply a tourniquet or not, immediately immobilize the victim's affected limb below heart level, and instruct the victim to remain as quiet as possible.
- If a tourniquet is applied, the victim or the person applying the tourniquet should check the victim's distal pulses regularly and loosen the tourniquet slightly as needed to maintain circulation. Remember that the goal of applying a tourniquet is to obstruct lymphatic drainage, not blood flow.
- When indicated, apply the tourniquet so that it's slightly constrictive, obstructing only lymphatic and superficial venous blood flow. Apply the band about 4″ (10 cm) above the fang marks or just above the first joint proximal to the bite. The tourniquet should be loose enough to allow a finger between the band and the skin. After the tourniquet is in place, don't remove it until a physician has examined the victim.

ALERT *Don't apply a tourniquet if more than 30 minutes have elapsed since the bite. Keep in mind also that total tourniquet time shouldn't exceed 2 hours and that the use of a tourniquet shouldn't delay antivenin administration. Loss of a limb is possible if a tourniquet is too tight or if tourniquet time is too long.*

- If the patient is more than a few hours away from a hospital, wash the skin over the fang marks. Within 5 to 15 minutes of a pit viper bite, make an incision through the fang marks about ½″ (1.3 cm) long and ⅛″ (3.2 mm) deep. Be especially careful if the bite is on the hand, where blood vessels and tendons are close to the skin surface.

Using a bulb syringe — or, if no other means is available, mouth suction — apply suction for up to 1 hour in the absence of antivenin administration.

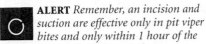

ALERT *Remember, an incision and suction are effective only in pit viper bites and only within 1 hour of the bite. Suction is also indicated if transport time to an emergency facility would exceed 30 minutes. Mouth suction is contraindicated if the rescuer has oral ulcers, if the victim is close to a medical facility, or if antivenin can be given promptly.*

ALERT *Never give the victim alcoholic drinks or stimulants because they speed venom absorption. Never apply ice to a snakebite because it will increase tissue damage.*

- Record the signs and symptoms of progressive envenomation and when they develop. Most snakebite victims are hospitalized for only 24 to 48 hours. Treatment usually consists of antivenin administration, but minor snakebites may not require antivenin. Other treatments include tetanus toxoid or tetanus immune globulin; various broad-spectrum antibiotics; and, depending on respiratory status, severity of pain, and the type of snakebite, acetaminophen, codeine, morphine, or meperidine. (Opioids are contraindicated for the treatment of coral snakebites.)

Necrotic snakebites usually need surgical debridement after 3 or 4 days. Intense, rapidly progressive edema requires fasciotomy within 2 or 3 hours of the bite; extreme envenomation may require amputation of the limb and subsequent reconstructive surgery, rehabilitation, and physical therapy.

Special considerations

When the patient arrives at the hospital, immobilize the extremity if this hasn't already been done. If a tight tourniquet has been applied within the past hour, apply a loose tourniquet proximally and remove the first tourniquet. Release the second tourniquet gradually during antivenin administration as ordered. A sudden release of venom into the bloodstream can cause cardiorespiratory collapse, so keep emergency equipment handy.

- On a flow sheet, document vital signs, level of consciousness, skin color, swelling, respiratory status, a description of the bite and surrounding area, and symptoms. Monitor vital signs every 15 minutes and check for a pulse in the affected limb.

- Start an I.V. line with a large-bore needle for antivenin administration. Severe bites that result in coagulotoxic signs and symptoms may require two I.V. lines: one for antivenin and one for blood products.
- Before antivenin administration, obtain a patient history of allergies and other medical problems. Perform hypersensitivity tests as ordered and assist with desensitization as needed. During antivenin administration, keep epinephrine, oxygen, and vasopressors available to combat anaphylaxis from horse serum.
- Give packed red blood cells, I.V. fluids and, possibly, fresh frozen plasma or platelets, as ordered, to counteract coagulotoxicity and maintain blood pressure.
- If the patient develops respiratory distress and requires endotracheal intubation or a tracheotomy, provide good tracheostomy care.

COMPARING INSECT BITES AND STINGS

In addition to maintaining airway, breathing, and circulation and assessing neurologic function, treatment varies according to the type of bite or sting.

General information

Clinical features

Tick
- Common in woods and fields throughout the United States
- Attaches to host in any of its life stages (larva, nymph, or adult); fastens to host with its teeth, then secretes a cementlike material to reinforce attachment
- Flat, brown, speckled body about ¼" (6.4 mm) long; has eight legs
- Also transmits Rocky Mountain spotted fever and Lyme disease

- Itching may be the sole symptom or, after several days, the host may develop tick paralysis (acute flaccid paralysis, starting as paresthesia and leg pain and resulting in respiratory failure from bulbar paralysis).

Brown recluse (violin) spider
- Common to south-central United States; usually found in dark areas (outdoor privy, barn, or woodshed)
- Dark brown violin on its back; three pairs of eyes; female more dangerous than male
- Most bites occur between April and October

- Venom is coagulotoxic. Reaction begins within 2 to 8 hours after bite.
- Localized vasoconstriction causes ischemic necrosis at bite site. A small, reddened puncture wound forms a bleb and becomes ischemic. In 3 to 4 days, the center becomes dark and hard. Within 2 to 3 weeks, an ulcer forms.
- Minimal initial pain increases over time.
- Other symptoms include fever, chills, malaise, weakness, nausea, vomiting, edema, seizures, joint pain, petechiae, cyanosis, and phlebitis.
- Rarely, thrombocytopenia and hemolytic anemia develop, leading to death within the first 24 to 48 hours (usually in a child or a patient with a previous history of cardiac disease). Prompt and appropriate treatment results in recovery.

■ Give analgesics as needed. *Don't* give opioids to coral snakebite victims. Clean the snakebite using sterile technique. Open, debride, and drain any blebs and blisters because they may contain venom. Change dressings daily.

■ If the patient requires hospitalization for more than 48 hours, position him carefully to avoid contractures. Perform passive exercises until the fourth day after the bite; after that, perform active exercises and give whirlpool treatments as ordered.

Insect bites and stings

Among the most common traumatic complaints are insect bites and stings, the more serious of which include those of ticks, brown recluse spiders, black widow spiders, scorpions, bees, wasps, and yellow jackets. (See *Comparing insect bites and stings.*)

(Text continues on page 332.)

Treatment	Special considerations
■ Removal of tick ■ Local antipruritics for itching papule ■ Mechanical ventilation for respiratory failure	■ To remove a tick, cover it with a tissue or gauze pad soaked in mineral, salad, or machine oil or alcohol. This blocks the tick's breathing pores and causes it to withdraw from the skin. If the tick doesn't disengage after the pad has been in place for a half hour, carefully remove it with tweezers, taking care to remove all parts. ■ To reduce the risk of being bitten, teach the patient to keep away from wooded areas, to wear protective clothes, and to carefully examine his body for ticks after being outdoors. ■ Teach patients how to safely remove ticks.
■ No known specific treatment ■ Combination therapy with corticosteroids, antibiotics, antihistamines, tranquilizers, I.V. fluids, and tetanus prophylaxis ■ Dapsone 100 mg b.i.d. to suppress the leukocyte response ■ Surgical debridement and skin grafting (large ulcerative lesions) ■ Skin grafting (large chronic ulcer)	■ Clean the lesion with a 1:20 Burow's aluminum acetate solution, and apply antibiotic ointment as ordered. ■ Take a complete patient history, including allergies and other pre-existing medical problems. ■ Monitor vital signs, general appearance, and any changes at bite site. ■ Reassure the patient with a disfiguring ulcer that skin grafting can improve his appearance. ■ To prevent brown recluse bites, tell the patient to spray areas of infestation with creosote at least every 2 months, to wear gloves and heavy clothing when working around woodpiles or sheds, to inspect outdoor work clothing for spiders before use, and to discourage children from playing near infested areas.

(continued)

COMPARING INSECT BITES AND STINGS *(continued)*

General information	Clinical features

Black widow spider
- Common throughout the United States, particularly in warmer climates; usually found in dark areas (outdoor privy, barn, or woodshed)
- Female: coal black with red or orange hourglass on ventral side; larger than male (male doesn't bite)
- Mortality less than 1% (increased risk among elderly people, infants, and those with allergies)

- Venom is neurotoxic. Age, size, and sensitivity of the patient determine the severity and progression of symptoms.
- Pinprick sensation, followed by dull, numbing pain (may go unnoticed).
- Edema and tiny, red bite marks appear.
- Rigidity of stomach muscles and severe abdominal pain occur (10 to 40 minutes after bite).
- Muscle spasms occur in the extremities.
- Ascending paralysis develops, causing difficulty swallowing and labored, grunting respirations.
- Other symptoms include extreme restlessness, vertigo, sweating, chills, pallor, seizures (especially in children), hyperactive reflexes, hypertension, tachycardia, thready pulse, circulatory collapse, nausea, vomiting, headache, ptosis, eyelid edema, urticaria, pruritus, and fever.

Scorpion
- Common throughout the United States (30 different species); two deadly species in southwestern states
- Curled tail with stinger on end; eight legs; 3″ (7.6 cm) long
- Most stings occur during warmer months
- Mortality less than 1% (increased risk among elderly people and children)

Local reaction
- Local swelling and tenderness, sharp burning sensation, skin discoloration, paresthesia, and lymphangitis with regional gland swelling occur.

Systemic reaction (neurotoxic)
- Immediate sharp pain; hyperesthesia; drowsiness; itching of the nose, throat, and mouth; impaired speech (due to sluggish tongue); generalized muscle spasms (including jaw muscle spasms, laryngospasms, incontinence, and seizures) nausea, vomiting, and drooling occur.
- Symptoms last from 24 to 78 hours; the bite site recovers last.
- Anaphylaxis is rare.
- Death may follow cardiovascular or respiratory failure.
- The prognosis is poor if symptoms progress rapidly in the first few hours.

Bee, wasp, and yellow jacket
- Honeybee (rounded abdomen) or bumblebee (over 1″ [2.5 cm] long; furry, rounded abdomen) — stinger remains in the victim; bee flies away and dies
- Wasp or yellow jacket (slender body with elongated abdomen) — retains stinger and can sting repeatedly

Local reaction
- Painful wound (protruding stinger from bees), edema, urticaria, and pruritus can occur.

Systemic reaction (anaphylaxis)
- Symptoms of hypersensitivity usually appear within 20 minutes and may include weakness, chest tightness, dizziness, nausea, vomiting, abdominal cramps, and throat constriction. The shorter the interval between the sting and systemic symptoms, the worse the prognosis. Without prompt treatment, symptoms may progress to cyanosis, coma, and death.

Treatment	Special considerations
■ Neutralization of venom using antivenin I.V., preceded by desensitization when skin or eye tests show sensitivity to horse serum ■ Calcium gluconate I.V. to control muscle spasms ■ Muscle relaxants such as diazepam for severe muscle spasms ■ Adrenaline or antihistamines ■ Oxygen by nasal cannula or mask ■ Tetanus immunization ■ Antibiotics to prevent infection	■ Take a complete patient history, including allergies and other pre-existing medical problems. ■ Have epinephrine and emergency resuscitation equipment on hand in case of anaphylactic reaction to antivenin. ■ Keep the patient quiet and warm and the affected part immobile. ■ Clean the bite site with an antiseptic; apply ice to relieve pain and swelling and to slow circulation. ■ Check vital signs frequently during the first 12 hours after the bite. Report any changes to the physician. Symptoms usually subside in 3 to 4 hours. ■ When giving analgesics, monitor respiratory status. ■ To prevent black widow spider bites, tell the patient to spray areas of infestation with creosote at least every 2 months, to wear gloves and heavy clothing when working around woodpiles or sheds, to inspect outdoor work clothing for spiders before use, and to discourage children from playing near infested areas.
■ Antivenin (made from goat serum) if available, to neutralize toxins ■ Calcium gluconate I.V. for muscle spasm ■ Phenobarbital I.M. for seizures ■ Emetine subcutaneously (S.C.) to relieve pain (opiates, such as morphine and codeine, contraindicated because they enhance the venom's effects)	■ Take a complete patient history, including allergies and other pre-existing medical conditions. ■ Immobilize the patient, and apply a tourniquet proximal to the sting. ■ Pack the area extending beyond the tourniquet in ice. After 5 minutes of ice pack, remove the tourniquet. ■ Monitor vital signs. Watch closely for signs of respiratory distress. (Keep emergency resuscitation equipment available.)
■ Antihistamines and corticosteroids (in urticaria) ■ Tetanus prophylaxis ■ In anaphylaxis, oxygen by nasal cannula or mask and epinephrine 1:1,000 S.C. or I.M. ■ In bronchospasm, albuterol and corticosteroids ■ In hypotension, epinephrine and isoproterenol	■ If the stinger is in place, scrape it off. Don't pull it; this action releases more toxin. ■ Clean the site and apply ice. ■ Watch the patient carefully for signs of anaphylaxis. Keep emergency resuscitation equipment available. ■ Tell a patient who's allergic to bee stings to wear a medical identification bracelet or carry a card and to carry an anaphylaxis kit. Teach him how to use the kit, and refer him to an allergist for hyposensitization. ■ To prevent bee stings, tell the patient to avoid wearing fragrant cosmetics during insect season, to avoid wearing bright colors and going barefoot, to avoid flowers and fruit that attract bees, and to use insect repellent.

Open trauma wounds

Open trauma wounds (abrasions, avulsions, crush wounds, lacerations, missile injuries, and punctures) are injuries that commonly result from home, work, or motor vehicle accidents and from acts of violence.

Signs and symptoms

In all open wounds, assess the extent of injury, vital signs, level of consciousness (LOC), obvious skeletal damage, local neurologic deficits, and general patient condition. Obtain an accurate history of the injury from the patient or witnesses, including such details as the mechanism and time of injury and any treatment already provided. If the injury involved a weapon, notify the police.

Also assess for peripheral nerve damage—a common complication in lacerations and other open trauma wounds—as well as for fractures and dislocations. Signs of peripheral nerve damage vary with location:

- *radial nerve*—weak forearm dorsiflexion, inability to extend thumb in a hitchhiker's sign
- *median nerve*—numbness in tip of index finger; inability to place forearm in prone position; weak forearm, thumb, and index finger flexion
- *ulnar nerve*—numbness in tip of little finger, clawing of hand
- *peroneal nerve*—footdrop, inability to extend the foot or big toe
- *sciatic and tibial nerves*—paralysis of ankles and toes, footdrop, leg weakness, numbness in sole.

Most open wounds require emergency treatment. In those with suspected nerve involvement, however, electromyography, nerve conduction, and electrical stimulation tests can provide more detailed information about possible peripheral nerve damage.

Diagnosis

A thorough physical examination of the patient will reveal traumatic wounds. They may be seen during the primary and secondary assessment of the patient.

Treatment

If hemorrhage occurs, stop bleeding by applying direct pressure on the wound and, if necessary, on arterial pressure points. If the wound is on an extremity, elevate it if possible. Don't apply a tourniquet except in a life-threatening hemorrhage. If you must do so, be aware that resulting lack of perfusion to tissue could require limb amputation. (For a description of types of wounds and specific management, see *Managing open trauma wounds.*)

Special considerations

- Frequently assess vital signs in patients with major wounds. Be alert for a 20-beat increase in pulse and 20 mm Hg drop in blood pressure (compare the patient's pulse and blood pressure taken when he's sitting with those taken when he's lying down), increased respiratory rate, decreased LOC, thirst, and cool, clammy skin — all indicate blood loss and hypovolemic shock.
- Administer oxygen as ordered.
- Send blood samples to the laboratory for type and crossmatch, complete blood count (including hematocrit and hemoglobin level), and prothrombin and partial thromboplastin times.
- Prepare the patient for surgery if needed.
- As much as possible, tell the patient about the procedures that he'll undergo (even if he's unconscious) and provide reassurance.
- Start I.V. lines, using two large-bore catheters, and infuse lactated Ringer's solution, normal saline solution, or whole blood as ordered.
- Insert a central venous pressure line and place the patient in a modified V position (with his head flat and his legs elevated). If the modified V position doesn't help, Trendelenburg's position may be an alternative.

MANAGING OPEN TRAUMA WOUNDS

After securing airway, breathing, circulatory, and neurologic status, specific treatment of the wound will depend on its severity.

Type	Clinical action
Abrasion ■ Open surface wounds (scrapes) of epidermis and possibly the dermis, resulting from friction; nerve endings exposed ■ Diagnosis based on scratches, reddish welts, bruises, pain, and history of friction injury	■ Obtain a history to distinguish injury from second-degree burn. ■ Clean the wound gently with topical germicide, and irrigate it. Too vigorous scrubbing of abrasions will increase tissue damage. ■ Remove all imbedded foreign objects. Apply a local anesthetic if cleaning is very painful. ■ Apply a light, water-soluble antibiotic cream to prevent infection. ■ If the wound is severe, apply a loose protective dressing that allows air to circulate. ■ Administer tetanus prophylaxis if necessary.
Avulsion ■ Complete tissue loss that prevents approximation of wound edges, resulting from cutting, gouging, or complete tearing of skin; frequently affects nose tip, earlobe, fingertip, and penis ■ Diagnosis based on full-thickness skin loss, hemorrhage, pain, history of trauma; X-ray required to rule out bone damage	■ Check the patient's history for bleeding tendencies and use of anticoagulants. ■ Record the time of injury to help determine if tissue is salvageable. Preserve tissue (if available) in cool normal saline solution for a possible split-thickness graft or flap. ■ Control hemorrhage with pressure, an absorbable gelatin sponge, or topical thrombin. ■ Clean the wound gently, irrigate it with normal saline solution, and debride it if necessary. Cover with a bulky dressing. ■ Tell the patient to leave the dressing in place until the return visit, to keep the area dry, and to watch for signs of infection (pain, fever, redness, and swelling). ■ Administer analgesics and tetanus prophylaxis, if necessary.
Crush wound ■ Heavy falling object splits skin, causes necrosis along split margins, and damages tissue underneath; may look like a laceration ■ Diagnosis based on history of trauma, edema, hemorrhage, massive hematomas, damage to surrounding tissues (fractures, nerve injuries, or loss of tendon function), shock, and pain; X-rays required to determine extent of injury to surrounding structures; complete blood count (CBC) and differential and electrolyte count also required	■ Check the patient's history for bleeding tendencies and use of anticoagulants. ■ Clean open areas gently with soap and water. ■ Control hemorrhage with pressure and a cold pack. ■ Apply a dry, sterile bulky dressing; wrap the entire extremity in a compression dressing. ■ Immobilize the injured extremity, and encourage the patient to rest. Monitor vital signs, and check peripheral pulses and circulation often. ■ Administer tetanus prophylaxis if necessary. ■ A severe injury may require I.V. infusion of lactated Ringer's or normal saline solution with a large-bore catheter as well as surgical exploration, debridement, and repair.

(continued)

MANAGING OPEN TRAUMA WOUNDS *(continued)*

Type	Clinical action

Laceration

- Open wound, possibly extending into deep epithelium, resulting from penetration with knife or other sharp object or from a severe blow with a blunt object
- Diagnosis based on hemorrhage, torn or destroyed tissues, pain, and history of trauma

In a laceration less than 8 hours old and in all lacerations of the face and areas of possible functional disability (such as the elbow):

- Apply pressure and elevate the injured extremity to control hemorrhage.
- Clean the wound gently with normal saline solution or water; irrigate with normal saline solution.
- As necessary, debride necrotic margins and close the wound, using strips of tape or sutures.
- A severe laceration with underlying structural damage may require surgery.

In grossly contaminated lacerations or lacerations more than 8 hours old (except lacerations of the face and areas of possible functional disability):

- Administer a broad-spectrum antibiotic for at least a 5-day course.
- *Don't* close the wound immediately.
- Instruct the patient to elevate the injured extremity for 24 hours after the injury to reduce swelling.
- Tell him to keep the dressing clean and dry and to watch for signs of infection.
- If, after 5 to 7 days, the wound appears uninfected with healthy granulated tissue, you may close it with sutures or a butterfly dressing or allow it to heal by itself.
- Apply a sterile dressing and splint.

In all lacerations:

- Check the patient's history for bleeding tendencies and anticoagulant use.
- Determine the approximate time of injury, and estimate the amount of blood lost.
- Assess for neuromuscular, tendon, and circulatory damage.
- Administer tetanus prophylaxis as needed.
- Stress the need for follow-up and suture removal.
- If sutures become infected, culture the wound and scrub with surgical soap preparation. Remove some or all sutures, and give a broad-spectrum antibiotic as ordered. Instruct the patient to soak the wound in warm, soapy water for 15 minutes, three times daily, and to return for a follow-up visit every 2 to 3 days until the wound heals.
- If the injury is the result of foul play, report it to the police department.

MANAGING OPEN TRAUMA WOUNDS (continued)

Type	Clinical action
Missile injury ■ High-velocity tissue penetration, such as a gunshot wound ■ Diagnosis based on entry and possibly exit wounds, signs of hemorrhage, shock, pain, and history of trauma; X-rays, CBC and differential, and electrolyte levels required to assess extent of injury and estimate blood loss	■ Check the patient's history for bleeding tendencies and use of anticoagulants. ■ Control hemorrhage with pressure if possible. If the injury is near vital organs, use large-bore catheters to start two I.V. lines, using lactated Ringer's or normal saline solution for volume replacement. Prepare for possible exploratory surgery. ■ Maintain a patent airway, and monitor for signs of hypovolemia, shock, and cardiac arrhythmias. Check vital signs and neurovascular response often. ■ Cover a sucking chest wound during exhalation with an occlusive dressing. ■ Clean the wound gently with normal saline solution or water; debride as necessary. ■ If damage is minor, apply a dry, sterile dressing. ■ Administer tetanus prophylaxis if necessary. ■ Obtain X-rays to detect retained fragments. ■ If possible, determine the caliber of the weapon. ■ Report the injury to the police department.
Puncture wound ■ Small-entry wounds that probably damage underlying structures, resulting from sharp, pointed objects ■ Diagnosis based on hemorrhage (rare), deep hematomas (in chest or abdominal wounds), ragged wound edges (in bites), small-entry wound (in very sharp object), pain, and history of trauma; X-rays can detect retention of injuring object	■ Check the patient's history for bleeding tendencies and use of anticoagulants. ■ Obtain a description of the injury, including force of entry. ■ Assess the extent of the injury. ■ Don't remove impaling objects until the injury has been completely evaluated. (If the eye is injured, call an ophthalmologist immediately.) ■ Thoroughly clean the injured area with soap and water. Irrigate all minor wounds with normal saline solution after removing a foreign object. ■ Unless they're on the face, very large, or gaping, leave human and animal bite wounds open. Apply a dry, sterile dressing to other minor puncture wounds. ■ Tell the patient to apply warm soaks daily. ■ Administer tetanus prophylaxis and, if necessary, a rabies vaccine. ■ Deep wounds that damage underlying tissues may require exploratory surgery; retention of the injuring object requires surgical removal.

Rape trauma syndrome

The term *rape* refers to illicit sexual intercourse without consent. It's a violent assault in which sex is used as a weapon. Rape inflicts varying degrees of physical and psychological trauma. Rape trauma syndrome occurs during the period following the rape or attempted rape; it refers to the victim's short-term and long-term reactions and to the methods the victim uses to cope with this trauma.

In most cases, the rapist is a man and the victim is a woman. However, rapes do occur between persons of the same sex, especially in prisons, schools, hospitals, and

IF THE RAPE VICTIM IS A CHILD

Carefully interview the child to assess how well she'll be able to deal with the situation after going home. Interview the child alone, away from the parents. Tell the parents that this is being done for the child's comfort, not to keep secrets from them. Ask them what words the child is comfortable with when referring to parts of the anatomy.

History and examination

A young child will place only as much importance on an experience as others do, unless there's physical pain. A good question to ask is, "Did someone touch you when you didn't want to be touched?" As with other rape victims, record information in the child's own words. A complete pelvic examination is necessary only if penetration has occurred; such an examination requires parental consent and an analgesic or a local anesthetic.

Need for counseling

The child and the parents will need counseling to minimize possible emotional disturbances. Encourage the child to talk about the experience, and try to alleviate any confusion. After a rape, a young child may regress; an older child may become fearful about being left alone. The child's behavior may change at school or at home.

Help the parents understand that it's normal for them to feel angry and guilty, but warn them against displacing or projecting these feelings onto the child. Instruct them to assure the child that they aren't angry with her; that the child is good and didn't cause the incident; that they're sorry it happened, but glad the child is all right; and that the family will work the problems out together.

other institutions. In some cases, the victim is a man and a woman is the rapist.

The prognosis is good if the rape victim receives physical and emotional support and counseling to help her deal with her feelings. Victims who articulate their feelings are able to cope with fears, interact with others, and return to normal routines faster than those who don't.

Causes and incidence

Rape isn't primarily about sex. It's a violent crime linked to feelings of rage or hatred in the assailant. Some of the cultural, sociological, and psychological factors that contribute to rape are increased exposure to sex, permissiveness, cynicism about relationships, feelings of anger, and powerlessness amid social pressures. Many rapists have feelings of violence or hatred toward women or sexual problems, such as impotence or premature ejaculation. They may feel socially isolated and be unable to form warm, loving relationships. Some rapists may be psychopaths who need violence for physical pleasure, no matter how it affects their victims; others rape to satisfy a need for power. Some were abused as children.

In the United States, a rape is reported every 6 to 7 minutes. The incidence of reported rape is highest in large cities and continues to rise. However, many rapes — possibly even most — are never reported.

Known victims of rape range in age from 2 months to 97 years. The age group most affected is 10- to 19-year-olds; the average victim's age is $13\frac{1}{2}$. About one in seven reported rapes involves a prepubertal child; most of these cases involve manual, oral, or genital contact with the child's genitals by a member of the child's family. More than 50% of rapes occur in the home; about one-third of these involve a male intruder who forces his way into a home. In about half the cases, the victim has some casual acquaintance with the attacker. Most rapists are between ages 25 and 44 and have planned the attack. Alcohol is involved in one-third of cases.

Signs and symptoms

When a rape victim arrives in the emergency department, assess her physical injuries. If she isn't seriously injured, allow her to remain clothed and take her to a private room where she can talk with you or a counselor before the necessary physical examination. (See *If the rape victim is a child.*) Remember, immediate reactions to rape differ and can include crying, laughing, hostility, confusion, withdrawal, or outward calm; anger and rage may not surface until later. During the attack, the victim may have felt demeaned, helpless, and afraid for her life; afterward, she may feel ashamed, guilty, shocked, and vulnerable and have a sense of disbelief and lowered self-esteem. Offer support and reassurance. Help her explore her feelings; listen, convey trust and respect, and remain nonjudgmental. Don't leave her alone unless she asks you to do so.

Being careful to upset the victim as little as possible, obtain an accurate history of the rape, pertinent to physical assessment. (Remember, your notes may be used as evidence if the rapist is tried.) Record the victim's statements in the first person, using quotation marks. Also, document objective information provided by others. Never speculate as to what may have happened or record subjective impressions or thoughts. Include in your notes the time the victim arrived at the facility, the date and time of the alleged rape, and the time that the victim was examined. Ask the victim if she's allergic to penicillin or other drugs, if she has had recent illnesses (especially venereal disease), and if she was pregnant before the attack. Find out the date of her last menstrual period and details of her obstetric and gynecologic history.

Thoroughly explain the examination she'll have, and tell her it's necessary to rule out internal injuries and obtain a specimen for venereal disease testing. Obtain her informed consent for treatment and for the police report. Allow her some control if possible; for instance, ask her if she's ready to be examined or if she would rather wait a bit.

Before the examination, ask the victim whether she douched, bathed, or washed before coming to the hospital. Note this on her chart. Have her change into a hospital gown, and place her clothing in paper bags. Label each bag and its contents.

 ALERT *Never use plastic bags because secretions and seminal stains will mold, destroying valuable evidence.*

Tell the victim she may urinate, but warn her not to wipe or otherwise clean the perineal area. Stay with her, or ask a counselor to stay with her, throughout the examination.

Diagnosis

Even if the victim wasn't beaten, the physical examination (including a pelvic examination by a gynecologist) will probably show signs of physical trauma, especially if the attack was prolonged. Depending on specific body areas attacked, a patient may have a sore throat, mouth irritation, difficulty swallowing, ecchymoses, or rectal pain and bleeding.

If additional physical violence accompanied the rape, the victim may have hematomas, lacerations, bleeding, severe internal injuries, and hemorrhage; if the rape occurred outdoors, she may suffer from exposure. X-rays may reveal fractures. If severe injuries require hospitalization, introduce the victim to her primary nurse if possible.

Assist throughout the examination and carefully label all possible evidence. Before the victim's pelvic area is examined, take vital signs; if she's wearing a tampon, remove it, wrap it, and label it as evidence. The pelvic examination is typically very distressing for the victim. Reassure her and allow her as much control as possible. During the examination, assist in specimen collection, including those for semen and gonorrhea. Carefully label all specimens with the patient's name, the physician's name, and the location from which the specimen was obtained. List all specimens in your notes. If the case comes to trial, specimens will be used for evidence, so accuracy is essential. (See *Legal considerations*, page 338.) Most emergency departments have "rape kits" that include containers for specimens.

Carefully collect and label fingernail scrapings and foreign material obtained by combing the victim's pubic hair; these also provide valuable evidence. Note to whom you give these specimens.

LEGAL CONSIDERATIONS

If your facility observes a protocol for emergency care of rape victims, it may include a rape evidence kit. If it does, follow the kit's instructions carefully. Include only medically relevant information in your notes.

If you're called as a witness during a trial, try to provide the judge and jury with pertinent facts while maintaining your own credibility.

Tips for the courtroom
- Go to court tastefully dressed and well-groomed.
- Keep your posture erect and look confident.
- Look the prosecuting and defense attorneys in the eye when answering their questions, but avoid long eye contact with the victim—this may cause you to appear biased.
- Don't offer speculations about the rape or volunteer information. Just answer questions that you're asked. If you don't know an answer, don't be afraid to say so.

For a male victim, be especially alert for injury to the mouth, perineum, and anus. As ordered, obtain a pharyngeal specimen for a gonorrhea culture and rectal aspirate for acid phosphatase or sperm analysis.

Assist in photographing the patient's injuries (this may be delayed for 1 day or repeated when bruises and ecchymoses are more apparent).

Most states require medical facilities to report rape. The patient may not press charges and not assist the police. If the patient doesn't go to a facility, she may not report the rape.

If the police interview the patient in the facility, be supportive and encourage her to recall details of the rape. Your kindness and empathy are invaluable.

The patient may also want you to call her family. Help her to verbalize anticipation of her family's response.

Treatment

Treatment consists of supportive measures and protection against venereal disease, human immunodeficiency virus (HIV) testing and, if the patient wishes, testing for pregnancy.

Special considerations

- Give antibiotics, as ordered, to prevent venereal disease.
- Because cultures can't detect gonorrhea or syphilis for 5 to 6 days after the rape, stress the importance of returning for follow-up venereal disease testing.
- To prevent pregnancy as a result of the rape, the patient may be given two Norgestrel and ethinyl-estradiol (Ovral) tablets orally immediately, plus two tablets 12 hours later. If so, explain the possible adverse effects of Ovral. The victim may wait 3 to 4 weeks and undergo dilatation and curettage or vacuum aspiration to abort a pregnancy.
- If the patient has vulvar lacerations, the physician will clean the area and repair the lacerations after all the evidence is obtained. Topical use of ice packs may reduce vulvar swelling.
- Offer all victims of rape testing for HIV infection as well as medical counseling and follow-up. If there's a chance that the rapist was infected with HIV, postexposure prophylaxis may be done to reduce the odds of infection by the immediate use of antiretroviral organisms.
- Refer the patient for psychological counseling, if needed, to cope with the aftereffects of the attack. Recovery from rape, which may be prolonged, consists of the acute phase (immediate reaction) and the reorganization phase. During the acute phase, physical effects include pain, loss of appetite, and wound healing; emotional reactions typically include shaking, crying, and mood swings. Feelings of grief, anger, fear, or revenge may color the victim's social interactions. Counseling helps the victim identify her coping mechanisms. She may relate more easily to a counselor of the same sex.

During the reorganization phase, which usually begins 1 to 3 weeks after the rape and may last months or years, the victim is concerned with restructuring her life. Initially, she often has nightmares in which she's powerless; later dreams show her gradually gaining more control. When she's alone, she may also suffer from "daymares" — frightening thoughts about the rape. She may have reduced sexual desire or may develop fear of intercourse or mistrust of men.

■ If the patient is engaged in legal proceedings during this time, she'll be forced to relive the trauma, leaving her feeling lonely and isolated, perhaps even temporarily halting her emotional recovery. To help her cope, encourage her to write her thoughts, feelings, and reactions in a daily diary, and refer her to organizations such as Women Organized Against Rape or a local rape crisis center for empathy and advice.

Selected references

American College of Surgeons. *Advanced Trauma Life Support for Doctors,* 7th ed. Chicago: American College of Surgeons, 2004.

Campbell, J.E. *Basic Trauma Life Support for Paramedics and Other Advanced Providers,* 5th ed. Upper Saddle River, N.J.: Prentice Hall Health, 2003.

Critical Care Nursing Made Incredibly Easy. Philadelphia: Lippincott Williams & Wilkins, 2004.

Derr, P. *Emergency and Critical Care Pocket Guide, ACLS Version,* 3rd ed. Tigard, Ore.: InforMed, 2003.

Emergency Nurses Association. *Core Curriculum for Pediatric Emergency Nursing,* 2nd ed. Sudbury, Mass.: Jones & Bartlett Pubs., Inc., 2003.

Freivalds, A. *Biomechanics of the Upper Limbs: Mechanics, Modeling, and Musculoskeletal Injuries.* New York: Taylor & Francis, 2004.

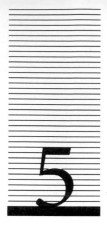

Immune disorders

Introduction *341*

Allergy *350*
Asthma *350*
Allergic rhinitis *354*
Atopic dermatitis *356*
Latex allergy *357*
Anaphylaxis *359*
Urticaria and angioedema *361*
Blood transfusion reaction *363*

Autoimmunity *364*
Rheumatoid arthritis *364*
Juvenile rheumatoid arthritis *370*
Psoriatic arthritis *372*
Ankylosing spondylitis *373*
Sjögren's syndrome *375*
Lupus erythematosus *376*
Goodpasture's syndrome *380*
Reiter's syndrome *381*
Scleroderma *382*
Vasculitis *384*
Polymyositis and dermatomyositis *388*

Immunodeficiency *389*
X-linked infantile
  hypogammaglobulinemia *389*
Common variable immunodeficiency *390*
IgA deficiency *391*
DiGeorge syndrome *392*
Acquired immunodeficiency syndrome *393*

Chronic mucocutaneous candidiasis *397*
Chronic fatigue syndrome *398*
Wiskott-Aldrich syndrome *399*
Chronic granulomatous disease *401*
Severe combined immunodeficiency
  disease *402*
Complement deficiencies *403*

Selected references *404*

Introduction

The environment contains thousands of pathogenic microorganisms — viruses, bacteria, fungi, and parasites. Ordinarily, we protect ourselves from infectious organisms and other harmful invaders through an elaborate network of safeguards — the host defense system. Understanding how this system functions provides the framework for studying various immune disorders.

Host defense system

The host defense system includes physical and chemical barriers to infection, the inflammatory response, and the immune response. Physical barriers, such as the skin and mucous membranes, prevent invasion by most organisms. Those organisms that penetrate this first line of defense simultaneously trigger the inflammatory and immune responses. Both responses involve cells derived from a hematopoietic stem cell in the bone marrow.

Chemical barriers include lysozymes (found in body secretions, such as tears, mucus, and saliva) and hydrochloric acid (found in the stomach). Lysozymes destroy bacteria by removing cell walls. Hydrochloric acid breaks down food and mucus that contains pathogens.

The inflammatory response involves polymorphonuclear leukocytes, basophils, mast cells, platelets and, to some extent, monocytes and macrophages.

The immune response primarily involves the interaction of lymphocytes (T and B), macrophages, and macrophage-like cells and their products. These cells may be circulating or may be localized in the immune system's tissues and organs, including the thymus, lymph nodes, spleen, and tonsils. The thymus participates in the maturation of T lymphocytes (cell-mediated immunity); here these cells are "educated" to differentiate "self" from "nonself." In contrast, B lymphocytes (humoral immunity) mature in the bone marrow. The key humoral effector mechanism is the production of immunoglobulin by B cells and the subsequent activation of the complement cascade. The lymph nodes, spleen, liver, and intestinal lymphoid tissue help remove and destroy circulating antigens in the blood and lymph.

Antigens

An antigen is any substance that can induce an immune response. T and B lymphocytes have specific receptors that respond to specific antigen molecular shapes (epitopes). In B cells, this receptor is an immunoglobulin (Ig) (antibody) cell: IgD or IgM, sometimes referred to as a surface immunoglobulin. The T-cell antigen receptor recognizes antigens only in association with specific cell surface molecules known as the major histocompatibility complex (MHC). (See *The major histocompatibility complex*, page 342.) MHC molecules, which differ among individuals, identify substances as self or nonself. Slightly different antigen receptors can recognize a phenomenal number of distinct antigens, which are coded by distinct, variable region genes.

Groups, or clones, of lymphocytes exist with identical receptors for a specific antigen. The clone of a lymphocyte rapidly proliferates when exposed to the specific antigen. Some lymphocytes further differentiate, and others become memory cells, which allow a more rapid response — the memory or anamnestic response — to subsequent challenge by the antigen.

Many factors influence antigenicity. Among them are the antigen's physical and chemical characteristics, its relative foreignness, and the individual's genetic makeup, particularly the MHC molecules. Most antigens are large molecules, such as proteins or polysaccharides. (Smaller molecules such as drugs that aren't antigenic by themselves are known as haptens. These haptens can bind with larger molecules, or carriers, and become antigenic or immunogenic.) The antigen's relative foreignness influences the immune response's intensity. For example, little or no immune response may follow transfusion of serum proteins between humans; however, a vigorous immune response (serum sickness) commonly follows transfusion of horse serum proteins to a human. Genetic makeup may also determine why some individuals respond to certain antigens, whereas others

THE MAJOR HISTOCOMPATIBILITY COMPLEX

The major histocompatibility complex (MHC) is a cluster of genes on human chromosome 6 that plays a pivotal role in the immune response. Also known as *human leukocyte antigen (HLA) genes,* these genes are inherited in an autosomal codominant manner. That is, each individual receives one set of MHC genes (haplotype) from each parent, and both sets of genes are expressed on the individual's cells. These genes play a role in the recognition of self versus nonself and the interaction of immunologically active cells by coding for cell-surface proteins.

HLA antigens are divided into three classes. Class I antigens appear on nearly all of the body's cells and include HLA-A, HLA-B, and HLA-C antigens. During tissue graft rejection, they're the chief antigens recognized by the host. When killer (CD8+) T cells use a virally infected antigen, they recognize it in the context of a class I antigen. Class II antigens only appear on B cells, macrophages, and activated T cells. They include the HLA-D and HLA-DR antigens. Class II antigens promote efficient collaboration between immunocompetent cells.

Helper (CD4+) T cells require that antigen be presented in the context of a class II antigen. Because these antigens also determine whether an individual responds to a particular antigen, they're also known as immune response genes. Class III antigens include certain complement proteins (C2, C4, and Factor B).

---

don't. The genes responsible for this phenomenon encode the MHC molecules.

B lymphocytes

B lymphocytes and their products, immunoglobulins, contribute to humoral immunity. The binding of soluble antigen with B-cell antigen receptors initiates the humoral immune response. The activated B cells differentiate into plasma cells that secrete immunoglobulins or antibodies. This response is regulated by T lymphocytes and their products, lymphokines. These lymphokines, which include interleukin (IL)-2, IL-4, IL-5, and interferon 8, are important in determining the class of immunoglobulins made by B cells.

The immunoglobulins secreted by plasma cells are four-chain molecules with two heavy (H) and two light (L) chains. (See *Structure of the immunoglobulin molecule.*) Each chain has a variable (V) region and one or more constant (C) regions, which are coded by separate genes. The V regions of both L and H chains participate in the binding of antigens. The C regions of the H chain provide a binding site for crystallizable fragment (Fc) receptors on cells and govern other mechanisms.

Any clone of B cells has one antigen specificity determined by the V regions of its L and H chains. However, the clone can change the class of immunoglobulin that it makes by changing the association between its V region genes and H chain C region genes (a process known as isotype switching). For example, a clone of B cells genetically preprogrammed to recognize tetanus toxoid initially will make an IgM antibody against tetanus toxoid and later an IgG or other antibody against it.

The five known classes of immunoglobulins — IgG, IgM, IgA, IgE, and IgD — are distinguished by the constant portions of their H chains. However, each class has a kappa or a lambda L chain, which gives rise to many subtypes. The almost limitless combinations of L and H chains give immunoglobulins their specificity.

■ *IgG,* the smallest immunoglobulin, appears in all body fluids because of its ability to move across membranes as a single structural unit (a monomer). It constitutes 75% of total serum immunoglobulins and

STRUCTURE OF THE IMMUNOGLOBULIN MOLECULE

The immunoglobulin molecule consists of four polypeptide chains — two heavy (H) and two light (L) chains — held together by disulfide bonds. The H chain has one variable (V) and at least three constant (C) regions. The L chain has one V and one C region. Together, the V regions of the H and L chains form a pocket known as the antigen-binding site. This site is located within the antigen-binding fragment (Fab) region of the molecule. Part of the C region of the H chains forms the crystallizable fragment (Fc) region of the molecule. This region mediates effector mechanisms such as complement activation and is the portion of the immunoglobulin molecule bound by Fc receptors on phagocytic cells, mast cells, and basophils. Each immunoglobulin molecule also has two antibody-combining sites (except for the immunoglobulin [Ig] M molecule, which has 10, and IgA, which may have 2 or more).

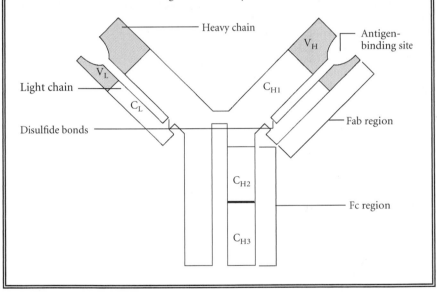

is the major antibacterial and antiviral antibody.

■ *IgM*, the largest immunoglobulin, appears as a pentamer (five monomers joined by a J-chain). Unlike IgG — which is produced mainly in the secondary, or recall, response — IgM dominates in the primary, or initial, immune response. However, like IgG, IgM is involved in classic antibody reactions, including precipitation, agglutination, neutralization, and complement fixation. Because of its size, IgM can't readily cross membrane barriers and is usually present only in the vascular system. IgM constitutes 5% to 10% of total serum immunoglobulins.

■ *IgA* exists in serum primarily as a monomer; in secretory form, IgA exists almost exclusively as a dimer (two monomer molecules joined by a J-chain and a secretory component chain). As a secretory immunoglobulin, IgA defends external body surfaces and is present in colostrum, saliva, tears, nasal fluids, and respiratory, GI, and genitourinary secretions. This antibody is considered important in preventing antigenic agents from attaching to epithelial surfaces. IgA makes up 15% to 20% of total serum immunoglobulins.

- *IgE,* present in trace amounts in serum, is involved in the release of vasoactive amines stored in basophils and tissue mast cell granules. When released, these bioamines cause the allergic effects characteristic of this type of hypersensitivity (erythema, itching, smooth-muscle contraction, secretions, and swelling).
- *IgD,* present as a monomer in serum in minute amounts, is the predominant antibody found on the surface of B lymphocytes and serves mainly as an antigen receptor. It may function in controlling lymphocyte activation or suppression.

T lymphocytes

T lymphocytes and macrophages are the chief participants in cell-mediated immunity. Immature T lymphocytes are derived from the bone marrow. Upon migration to the thymus, they undergo a maturation process that is dependent upon products of the MHC, human leukocyte antigen (HLA) genes. Thus, mature T cells can distinguish between self and nonself. T cells acquire certain surface molecules, or markers; these markers combined with the T-cell antigen receptor promote the particular activation of each type of T cell. T-cell activation requires presentation of antigens in the context of a specific HLA antigen. Helper T cells require class II HLA antigens; cytotoxic T cells require class I HLA antigens. T-cell activation also involves IL-1, produced by macrophages, and IL-2, produced by T cells.

Natural killer (NK) cells are a discrete population of large lymphocytes, some of which resemble T cells. NK cells recognize surface changes on body cells infected with a virus; they then bind to and, in many cases, kill the infected cells.

Macrophages

Important cells of the reticuloendothelial system, macrophages influence both immune and inflammatory responses. Macrophage precursors circulate in the blood. When they collect in various tissues and organs, they differentiate into macrophages with varying characteristics. Unlike B and T lymphocytes, macrophages lack surface receptors for specific antigens; instead, they have receptors for the C region of the H chain (Fc region) of immunoglobulin, for fragments of the third component of complement (C3), and for nonimmunologic factors such as carbohydrate molecules.

One of the most important functions of macrophages is the presentation of antigen to T lymphocytes. Macrophages ingest and process antigen, then deposit it on their own surfaces in association with HLA antigen. T lymphocytes become activated upon recognizing this complex. Macrophages also function in the inflammatory response by producing IL-1, which generates fever. Additionally, macrophages synthesize complement proteins and other mediators that produce phagocytic, microbicidal, and tumoricidal effects.

Cytokines

Cytokines are low-molecular-weight proteins involved in communication between cells. Their purpose is to induce or regulate a variety of immune or inflammatory responses. However, disorders may occur if cytokine production or regulation is impaired. Cytokines are categorized as follows:

- *Colony-stimulating factors* function primarily as hematopoietic growth factors, guiding the division and differentiation of bone marrow stem cells. They also influence the functioning of mature lymphocytes, monocytes, macrophages, and neutrophils.
- *Interferons* act early to limit the spread of viral infections. They also inhibit tumor growth. Mainly, they determine how well tissue cells interact with cytotoxic cells and lymphocytes.
- *Interleukins* are a large group of cytokines. (Those produced primarily by T lymphocytes are called lymphokines. Those produced by mononuclear phagocytes are called monokines.) They have a variety of effects, but most direct other cells to divide and differentiate.
- *Tumor necrosis factors* are believed to play a major role in mediating inflammation and cytotoxic reactions (along with IL-1, IL-6, and IL-8).
- *Transforming growth factor* demonstrates both inflammatory and anti-inflammatory effects. It's believed to be partially responsible for tissue fibrosis associated with many

diseases. It demonstrates immunosuppressive effects on T cells, B cells, and NK cells.

Complement system

The chief humoral effector of the inflammatory response, the complement system consists of more than 20 serum proteins. When activated, these proteins interact in a cascadelike process that has profound biological effects. Complement activation takes place through one of two pathways.

In the classical pathway, binding of IgM or IgG and antigen forms antigen-antibody complexes that activate the first complement component, C1. This, in turn, activates C4, C2, and C3. In the alternate pathway, activating surfaces such as bacterial membranes directly amplify spontaneous cleavage of C3. Once C3 is activated in either pathway, activation of the terminal components — C5 to C9 — follows.

The major biological effects of complement activation include phagocyte attraction (chemotaxis) and activation, histamine release, viral neutralization, promotion of phagocytosis by opsonization, and lysis of cells and bacteria. Other mediators of inflammation derived from the kinin and coagulation pathways interact with the complement system.

Polymorphonuclear leukocytes

Besides macrophages and complement, other key participants in the inflammatory response are the polymorphonuclear leukocytes (also known as *granulocytes*) — neutrophils, eosinophils, and basophils.

Neutrophils, the most numerous of these cells, derive from bone marrow and increase dramatically in number in response to infection and inflammation. Highly mobile cells, neutrophils are attracted to areas of inflammation (chemotaxis); in fact, they're the primary constituent of pus.

Neutrophils have surface receptors for immunoglobulin and complement fragments, and they avidly ingest opsonized particles such as bacteria. Ingested organisms are then promptly killed by toxic oxygen metabolites and enzymes such as lysozyme. Unfortunately, neutrophils not only kill invading organisms but may also damage host tissues.

Also derived from bone marrow, *eosinophils* multiply in both allergic disorders and parasitic infestations. Although their phagocytic function isn't clearly understood, evidence suggests that they participate in host defense against parasites. Their products may also diminish the inflammatory response in allergic disorders.

Two other types of cells that function in allergic disorders are basophils and mast cells. (Mast cells, however, aren't blood cells.) *Basophils* circulate in peripheral blood, whereas *mast cells* accumulate in connective tissue, particularly in the lungs, intestines, and skin. Both types of cells have surface receptors for IgE. When cross-linked by an IgE-antigen complex, they release mediators characteristic of the allergic response.

Immune disorders

Because of their complexity, the processes involved in host defense and immune response may malfunction. When the body's defenses are exaggerated, misdirected, or either absent or depressed, the result may be a hypersensitivity disorder, autoimmunity, or immunodeficiency, respectively.

Hypersensitivity disorders

An exaggerated or inappropriate immune response may lead to various hypersensitivity disorders. Such disorders are classified as type I through type IV, although some overlap exists. (See *Classification of hypersensitivity reactions*, pages 346 and 347.)

TYPE I HYPERSENSITIVITY (ALLERGIC DISORDERS)

In individuals with type I hypersensitivity, certain antigens (allergens) activate T cells. These, in turn, induce B-cell production of IgE, which binds to the Fc receptors on the surface of mast cells. When these cells are re-exposed to the same antigen, the antigen binds with the surface IgE, cross-links the Fc receptors, and causes mast cell degranulation with release of various mediators. (Degranulation may also be triggered by complement-derived anaphylatoxins — C3a and C5a — or by certain drugs such as morphine.)

CLASSIFICATION OF HYPERSENSITIVITY REACTIONS

Type	Cause	Antibody or cell involved	Pathophysiology
I - Immediate hypersensitivity (anaphylaxis, atopy)	Foreign protein (antigen)	Immunoglobulin (Ig) E	IgE attaches to the surface of the mast cell and specific antigen, triggers release of intracellular granules from mast cells
II - Cytotoxic hypersensitivity	Foreign protein (antigen)	IgG or IgM	IgG or IgM reacts with antigen, activates complement, and causes cytolysis or phagocytosis
III - Immune complex disease	Foreign protein (antigen) Endogenous antigens	IgG, IgM, IgA	Antigen-antibody complexes precipitate in tissue, activate complement, and cause inflammatory reaction
IV - Delayed cell-mediated	Foreign protein, cell, or tissue	T lymphocytes	Sensitized T-cells react with specific antigen to induce inflammatory process by direct cell action or by activity of lymphokines

Some of these mediators are preformed, whereas others are newly synthesized upon activation of mast cells. Preformed mediators include heparin, histamine, proteolytic and other enzymes, and chemotactic factors for eosinophils and neutrophils. Newly synthesized mediators include prostaglandins and leukotrienes. Mast cells also produce a variety of cytokines. The effects of these mediators include smooth-muscle contraction, vasodilation, bronchospasm, edema, increased vascular permeability, mucus secretion, and cellular infiltration by eosinophils and neutrophils. Among classic associated signs and symptoms are hypotension, wheezing, swelling, urticaria, and rhinorrhea.

Examples of type I hypersensitivity disorders are anaphylaxis, atopy (an allergic reaction related to genetic predisposition), hay fever (allergic rhinitis) and, in some cases, asthma.

TYPE II HYPERSENSITIVITY (ANTIBODY-DEPENDENT CYTOTOXICITY)
In type II hypersensitivity, antibody is directed against cell surface antigens. (Alternately, though, antibody may be directed against small molecules adsorbed to cells

or against cell surface receptors rather than against cell constituents themselves.) Type II hypersensitivity then causes tissue damage through several mechanisms. Binding of antigen and antibody activates complement, which ultimately disrupts cellular membranes.

Another mechanism is mediated by various phagocytic cells with receptors for immunoglobulin (Fc region) and complement fragments. These cells envelop and destroy (phagocytose) opsonized targets, such as red blood cells, leukocytes, and platelets. Antibody against these cells may be visualized by immunofluorescence. Cytotoxic T cells and NK cells also contribute to tissue damage in type II hypersensitivity.

Examples of type II hypersensitivity include transfusion reactions, hemolytic disease of the neonate, autoimmune hemolytic anemia, Goodpasture's syndrome, and myasthenia gravis.

TYPE III HYPERSENSITIVITY (IMMUNE COMPLEX DISEASE)
In type III hypersensitivity, excessive circulating antigen-antibody complexes (immune complexes) result in the deposition of these complexes in tissue — most com-

Clinical examples

Extrinsic asthma, allergic rhinitis, anaphylaxis, reactions to stinging insects, some food and drug reactions

Transfusion reaction, hemolytic drug reaction, Goodpasture's syndrome, hemolytic disease of the neonate

Rheumatoid arthritis, systemic lupus erythematosus, serum sickness to some drugs or viral hepatitis antigen, glomerulonephritis

Contact dermatitis, graft-versus-host disease, granulomatous diseases

monly in the kidneys, joints, skin, and blood vessels. (Normally, immune complexes are effectively cleared by the reticuloendothelial system.) These deposited immune complexes activate the complement cascade, resulting in local inflammation. They also trigger platelet release of vasoactive amines that increase vascular permeability, augmenting deposition of immune complexes in vessel walls.

Type III hypersensitivity may be associated with infections, such as hepatitis B and bacterial endocarditis; certain cancers in which a serum sickness-like syndrome may occur; and autoimmune disorders such as lupus erythematosus. This hypersensitivity reaction may also follow drug or serum therapy.

TYPE IV HYPERSENSITIVITY (DELAYED HYPERSENSITIVITY)

In type IV hypersensitivity, antigen is processed by macrophages and presented to T cells. The sensitized T cells then release lymphokines, which recruit and activate other lymphocytes, monocytes, macrophages, and polymorphonuclear leukocytes. The coagulation, kinin, and

complement pathways also contribute to tissue damage in this type of reaction.

Examples of type IV hypersensitivity include tuberculin reactions, contact hypersensitivity, and sarcoidosis.

Autoimmune disorders

Autoimmunity is characterized by a misdirected immune response in which the body's defenses become self-destructive. Autoimmune diseases aren't transmitted from one person to another, and the causes of autoimmunity aren't clearly understood. However, the process of autoimmunity is related to genes or a combination of genes, hormones, and environmental stimuli. Individuals with specific genes or gene combinations may be at a higher risk for developing autoimmune disorders, which may be triggered by outside stimuli, such as sun exposure, infection, drugs, or pregnancy.

Recognition of self through the MHC is of primary importance in an immune response. However, how an immune response against self is prevented and which cells are primarily responsible isn't well understood.

Many autoimmune disorders are characterized by B-cell hyperactivity, marked by proliferation of B cells and autoantibodies and by hypergammaglobulinemia. B-cell hyperactivity is probably related to T-cell abnormalities, but the molecular basis of autoimmunity is poorly understood. Hormonal and genetic factors strongly influence the incidence of autoimmune disorders; for example, lupus erythematosus predominantly affects females of childbearing age, and certain HLA haplotypes are associated with an increased risk of specific autoimmune disorders.

Autoimmune diseases may not follow a clear pattern of symptoms; therefore, a definitive diagnosis may be delayed. Diagnosis may rely on the patient's medical history; family history; physical examination, including signs and symptoms; and laboratory tests. Autoantibodies are usually found with such disorders as rheumatoid arthritis or systemic lupus erythematosus, but confusion may occur because individuals with these disorders may have false negative results to laboratory tests.

(Text continues on page 350.)

IATROGENIC IMMUNODEFICIENCY

Iatrogenic immunodeficiency may be a complicating adverse effect of chemotherapy or other treatments. At times, though, it's the goal of therapy—for example, to suppress immune-mediated tissue damage in autoimmune disorders or to prevent rejection of an organ transplant. As explained below, iatrogenic immunodeficiency may be induced by immunosuppressive drugs, radiation therapy, or splenectomy.

Immunosuppressive drug therapy

Immunosuppressive drugs fall into several categories:

- Cytotoxic drugs. These drugs kill immunocompetent cells while they're replicating. However, most cytotoxic drugs aren't selective and thus interfere with all rapidly proliferating cells. As a result, they reduce the number of lymphocytes as well as phagocytes. Besides depleting their number, cytotoxic drugs interfere with lymphocyte synthesis and release of immunoglobulins and lymphokines.

Cyclophosphamide, a potent and commonly used immunosuppressant, initially depletes the number of B cells, suppressing humoral immunity. However, chronic therapy also depletes T cells, suppressing cell-mediated immunity as well. Cyclophosphamide may be used in systemic lupus erythematosus, Wegener's granulomatosis, other systemic vasculitides, and in certain autoimmune disorders. Because it nonselectively destroys rapidly dividing cells, this drug can cause severe bone marrow suppression with neutropenia, anemia, and thrombocytopenia; gonadal suppression with sterility; alopecia; hemorrhagic cystitis; and nausea, vomiting, and stomatitis. It may also increase the risk of lymphoproliferative neoplasms.

Among other cytotoxic drugs used for immunosuppression are azathioprine (commonly used in kidney transplantation) and methotrexate (occasionally used in rheumatoid arthritis and other autoimmune disorders).

If the patient is receiving cytotoxic drugs, monitor his white blood cell (WBC) count. If it falls too low, the drug dosage may need to be adjusted. Also monitor urine output and watch for signs of cystitis, especially if the patient is taking cyclophosphamide. Ensure adequate fluid intake (2 qt [2 L] daily). Give mesna as ordered to help prevent hemorrhagic cystitis. Provide antiemetics to relieve nausea and vomiting as ordered. Give meticulous oral hygiene and report signs of stomatitis.

Teach the patient about the early signs and symptoms of infection. If his WBC count falls too low, granulocyte colony-stimulating factor may be used to boost the count. Suggest wearing a scarf, hat, or wig to hide temporary alopecia. Make sure the male patient understands the risk of sterility; advise sperm banking if appropriate. Young women may take hormonal contraceptives to minimize ovarian dysfunction and to prevent pregnancy during administration of these potentially teratogenic drugs.

- Corticosteroids. These adrenocortical hormones are used to treat immune-mediated disorders because of their potent anti-inflammatory and immunosuppressive effects. Corticosteroids stabilize the vascular membrane, blocking tissue infiltration by neutrophils and monocytes, thus inhibiting inflammation. They also "kidnap" T cells in the bone marrow, causing lymphopenia. Because these drugs aren't cytotoxic, lymphocyte concentration can return to normal within 24 hours after they're withdrawn. Corticosteroids also appear to inhibit immunoglobulin synthesis and to interfere with the binding of immunoglobulin to antigen or to cells with crystallizable fragment receptors. These drugs have many other effects as well.

The most commonly used oral corticosteroid is prednisone. For long-term therapy, prednisone is best given early in the morning to minimize exogenous suppression of cortisol production and with food or milk to minimize gastric irritation. After the acute phase, it's usually reduced to an alternate-day schedule and then gradually withdrawn to minimize potentially harmful adverse effects. Other corticosteroids used for immunosuppression include hydrocortisone, methylprednisolone, and dexamethasone.

Chronic corticosteroid therapy can cause numerous adverse effects, which are sometimes more harmful than the disease itself. Neurologic adverse effects include euphoria, insomnia, or psychosis; cardiovascular effects include hypertension and edema; and GI effects include gastric irritation, ulcers, and increased appetite with weight gain. Other possible effects are cataracts, hyperglycemia, glucose intolerance, muscle weakness, osteoporosis, delayed wound healing, and increased susceptibility to infection.

During corticosteroid therapy, monitor the patient's blood pressure, weight, and intake and output. Instruct the patient to eat a well-balanced, low-salt diet or to follow the specially prescribed diet to prevent excessive weight gain. Remember that even though the patient is more susceptible to infection, he'll show fewer or less dramatic signs of inflammation.

■ Cyclosporine. Cyclosporine selectively suppresses the proliferation and development of helper T cells, resulting in depressed cell-mediated immunity. This drug is used primarily to prevent rejection of kidney, liver, and heart transplants but is also being investigated for use in several other disorders. Significant toxic effects of cyclosporine primarily involve the liver and kidney, so treatment with this drug requires regular evaluation of renal and hepatic function. Some studies also link cyclosporine with increased risk of lymphoma. Adjusting the dose or the duration of therapy helps minimize certain adverse effects.

■ Antilymphocyte serum or antithymocyte globulin (ATG). This anti-T cell antibody reduces T-cell number and function, thus suppressing cell-mediated immunity. It has been used effectively to prevent cell-mediated rejection of tissue grafts or transplants. Usually, ATG is administered immediately before the transplant and continued for some time afterward. Potential adverse effects include anaphylaxis and serum sickness. Occurring 1 to 2 weeks after injection of ATG, serum sickness is characterized by fever, malaise, rash, arthralgias and, occasionally, glomerulonephritis or vasculitis. It presumably results from the deposition of immune complexes throughout the body.

Radiation therapy
Because irradiation is cytotoxic to proliferating and intermitotic cells, including most lymphocytes, radiation therapy may induce profound lymphopenia, resulting in immunosuppression. Irradiation of all major lymph node areas — a procedure known as total nodal irradiation — is used to treat certain disorders such as Hodgkin's disease. Its effectiveness in severe rheumatoid arthritis, lupus nephritis, and the prevention of kidney transplant rejection is still under investigation.

Splenectomy
After splenectomy, the patient has increased susceptibility to infection, especially with pyogenic bacteria such as *Streptococcus pneumoniae*. This risk of infection is even greater when the patient is young or has an underlying reticuloendothelial disorder. The incidence of fulminant, rapidly fatal bacteremia is especially high in splenectomized patients and often follows trauma. These patients should receive Pneumovax immunization for prophylaxis and be warned to avoid exposure to infection and trauma.

Treatment for autoimmune disorders focuses on relieving symptoms, preserving organ function, and providing medication that can target the immune system, such as cyclophosphamide and cyclosporine. Autoimmune and immunological disorders are being researched. Web sites for the National Institutes of Health *(www.nih.gov)* and other organizations offer substantial health care information relevant to both the patient and the physician.

Immunodeficiency

In immunodeficiency, the immune response is absent or depressed, resulting in increased susceptibility to infection. This disorder may be primary or secondary. Primary immunodeficiency reflects a defect involving T cells, B cells, or lymphoid tissues. The National Primary Immunodeficiency Resource Center is a source of information on primary immunodeficiency syndromes.

Secondary immunodeficiency results from an underlying disease or factor that depresses or blocks the immune response. The most common forms of immunodeficiency are caused by viral infection (as in acquired immunodeficiency syndrome). Other forms are iatrogenic. (See *Iatrogenic immunodeficiency*, pages 348 and 349.)

ALLERGY

Asthma

Asthma is a reversible lung disease characterized by obstruction or narrowing of the airways, which are typically inflamed and hyperresponsive to a variety of stimuli. It may resolve spontaneously or with treatment. Its symptoms range from mild wheezing and dyspnea to life-threatening respiratory failure. (See *Determining asthma's severity*.) Symptoms of bronchial airway obstruction may persist between acute episodes.

Causes and incidence

Asthma that results from sensitivity to specific external allergens is known as *extrinsic*. In cases in which the allergen isn't obvious, asthma is referred to as *intrinsic*. Allergens that cause extrinsic asthma include pollen, animal dander, house dust or mold, kapok or feather pillows, food additives containing sulfites, and any other sensitizing substance. Extrinsic (atopic) asthma usually begins in childhood and is accompanied by other manifestations of atopy (type I, immunoglobulin [Ig] E-mediated allergy), such as eczema and allergic rhinitis. In intrinsic (nonatopic) asthma, no extrinsic allergen can be identified. Most cases are preceded by a severe respiratory infection. Irritants, emotional stress, fatigue, exposure to noxious fumes as well as changes in endocrine, temperature, and humidity may aggravate intrinsic asthma attacks. In many asthmatics, intrinsic and extrinsic asthma coexist.

Several drugs and chemicals may provoke an asthma attack without using the IgE pathway. Apparently, they trigger release of mast-cell mediators by way of prostaglandin inhibition. Examples of these substances include aspirin, various nonsteroidal anti-inflammatory drugs (such as indomethacin and mefenamic acid), and tartrazine, a yellow food dye. Exercise may also provoke an asthma attack. In exercise-induced asthma, bronchospasm may follow heat and moisture loss in the upper airways.

The allergic response has two phases. When the patient inhales an allergenic substance, sensitized IgE antibodies trigger mast-cell degranulation in the lung interstitium, releasing histamine, cytokines, prostaglandins, thromboxanes, leukotrienes, and eosinophil chemotaxic factors. Histamine then attaches to receptor sites in the larger bronchi, causing irritation, inflammation, and edema. In the late phase, inflammatory cells flow in. The influx of eosinophils provides additional inflammatory mediators and contributes to local injury.

Although this common condition can strike at any age, half of all cases first occur in children younger than age 10; in this age-group, asthma affects twice as many males as females. Nearly 1 in 13 children have asthma, which is increasing worldwide. Emergency department visits, hospitalizations, and mortality from asthma

DETERMINING ASTHMA'S SEVERITY

Asthma is classified by severity using these features:
- frequency, severity, and duration of symptoms
- degree of airflow obstruction (spirometry measure) or peak expiratory flow (PEF)
- frequency of nighttime symptoms and the degree that the asthma interferes with daily activities.

Severity can change over time, and even milder cases can become severe in an uncontrolled attack. Long-term therapy depends on whether the patient's asthma is classified as mild intermittent, mild persistent, moderate persistent, or severe persistent. For all patients, quick relief can be obtained by using a short-acting bronchodilator (2 to 4 puffs of short-acting inhaled beta$_2$-adrenergic agonists as needed for symptoms). However, the use of a short-acting bronchodilator more than twice a week in patients with intermittent asthma or daily or increasing use in patients with persistent asthma may indicate the need to initiate or increase long-term control therapy.

Mild intermittent asthma
The signs and symptoms of mild intermittent asthma include:
- daytime symptoms no more than twice a week
- nighttime symptoms no more than twice a month
- lung function testing (either PEF or forced expiratory volume in 1 second) is 80% of predicted value or higher
- PEF varies no more than 20%.

Severe exacerbations, separated by long, symptomless periods of normal lung function, indicate mild intermittent asthma. A course of systemic corticosteroids is recommended for these exacerbations; otherwise, daily medication isn't required.

Mild persistent asthma
The signs and symptoms of mild persistent asthma include:
- daytime symptoms 3 to 6 days a week
- nighttime symptoms 3 to 4 times a month
- lung function testing is 80% of predicted value or higher
- PEF varies between 20% and 30%.

The preferred treatment for mild, persistent asthma is low-dose inhaled corticosteroids, but alternative treatments include cromolyn, leukotriene modifier, nedocromil, or sustained-release theophylline.

Moderate persistent asthma
The signs and symptoms of moderate persistent asthma include:
- daily daytime symptoms
- at least weekly nighttime symptoms
- lung function testing is 60% to 80% of predicted value
- PEF varies more than 30%.

The preferred treatment for moderate persistent asthma is low- or medium-dose inhaled corticosteroids combined with a long-acting inhaled beta$_2$-adrenergic agonist. Alternative treatments include increasing inhaled corticosteroids within the medium-dose range or low- or medium-dose inhaled corticosteroids with either leukotriene modifier or theophylline.

For recurring exacerbations, the preferred treatment is to increase inhaled corticosteroids within the medium-dose range and add a long-acting inhaled beta$_2$-adrenergic agonist. The alternative treatment is to increase inhaled corticosteroids within the medium-dose range and add either leukotriene modifier or theophylline.

Severe persistent asthma
The signs and symptoms of severe persistent asthma include:
- continual daytime symptoms

(continued)

DETERMINING ASTHMA'S SEVERITY *(continued)*

- frequent nighttime symptoms
- lung function testing is 60% of predicted value or lower
- PEF varies more than 30%.

The preferred treatment for severe, persistent asthma includes high-dose inhaled corticosteroids combined with

long-acting inhaled $beta_2$-adrenergic agonists. Long-term administration of corticosteroid tablets or syrup (2 mg/kg/day, not to exceed 60 mg/day), may be used to reduce the need for systemic corticosteroid therapy.

---

have been increasing for more than 20 years, especially among children and blacks.

Signs and symptoms

An asthma attack may begin dramatically, with simultaneous onset of many severe symptoms, or insidiously, with gradually increasing respiratory distress. It typically includes progressively worsening shortness of breath, cough, wheezing, and chest tightness or some combination of these signs or symptoms.

During an acute attack, the cough sounds tight and dry. As the attack subsides, tenacious mucoid sputum is produced (except in young children, who don't expectorate). Characteristic wheezing may be accompanied by coarse rhonchi, but fine crackles aren't heard unless associated with a related complication. Between acute attacks, breath sounds may be normal.

The intensity of breath sounds in symptomatic asthma is typically reduced. A prolonged phase of forced expiration is typical of airflow obstruction. Evidence of lung hyperinflation (use of accessory muscles, for example) is particularly common in children. Acute attacks may be accompanied by tachycardia, tachypnea, and diaphoresis. In severe attacks, the patient may be unable to speak more than a few words without pausing for breath. Cyanosis, confusion, and lethargy indicate the onset of respiratory failure.

Diagnosis

Laboratory studies in patients with asthma commonly show these abnormalities:
- Pulmonary function studies reveal signs of airway obstruction (decreased peak ex-

piratory flow rates and forced expiratory volume in 1 second), low-normal or decreased vital capacity, and increased total lung and residual capacity. However, pulmonary function studies may be normal between attacks.
- Pulse oximetry may reveal decreased arterial oxygen saturation (SaO_2).
- Arterial blood gas (ABG) analysis provides the best indications of an attack's severity. In acutely severe asthma, the partial pressure of arterial oxygen is less than 60 mm Hg, the partial pressure of arterial carbon dioxide ($PaCO_2$) is 40 mm Hg or more, and pH is usually decreased.
- Complete blood count with differential reveals increased eosinophil count.
- Chest X-rays may show hyperinflation with areas of focal atelectasis.

Before initiating tests for asthma, rule out other causes of airway obstruction and wheezing. In children, such causes include cystic fibrosis, tumors of the bronchi or mediastinum, and acute viral bronchitis; in adults, other causes include obstructive pulmonary disease, heart failure, and epiglottitis.

Treatment

Treatment of acute asthma aims to decrease bronchoconstriction, reduce bronchial airway edema, and increase pulmonary ventilation. After an acute episode, treatment focuses on avoiding or removing precipitating factors, such as environmental allergens or irritants.

If asthma is known to be caused by a particular antigen, it may be treated by desensitizing the patient through a series of injections of limited amounts of the antigen. The aim is to curb the patient's immune response to the antigen.

If asthma results from an infection, antibiotics are prescribed. Drug therapy is most effective when begun soon after the onset of signs and symptoms. For relief of symptoms in adults and children older than age 5, short-acting inhaled beta$_2$-adrenergic agonists for bronchodilation may be used, and a course of systemic corticosteroids may be needed. The goal of therapy is asthma control with minimal or no adverse effects from medication.

Acute attacks that don't respond to self-treatment may require hospital care, beta$_2$-adrenergic agonists by inhalation or subcutaneous (S.C.) injection (in three doses over 60 to 90 minutes) and, possibly, oxygen for hypoxemia. If the patient responds poorly, systemic corticosteroids and, possibly, S.C. epinephrine may help. Beta$_2$-adrenergic agonist inhalation continues hourly. I.V. aminophylline may be added to the regimen and I.V. fluid therapy is started. Patients who don't respond to this treatment, whose airways remain obstructed, and who have increasing respiratory difficulty are at risk for status asthmaticus and may require mechanical ventilation.

Treatment of status asthmaticus consists of aggressive drug therapy with a beta$_2$-adrenergic agonist by nebulizer every 30 to 60 minutes, possibly supplemented with S.C. epinephrine, I.V. corticosteroids, I.V. aminophylline, oxygen administration, I.V. fluid therapy, and intubation and mechanical ventilation for hypercapnic respiratory failure (PaCO$_2$ of 40 mm Hg or more). (See *How status asthmaticus progresses*, pages 354 and 355.)

Special considerations

During an acute attack, proceed as follows:
- First, assess the severity of asthma.
- Administer the prescribed treatments and assess the patient's response.
- Place the patient in high Fowler's position. Encourage pursed-lip and diaphragmatic breathing. Help him to relax.
- Monitor the patient's vital signs. Keep in mind that developing or increasing tachypnea may indicate worsening asthma or drug toxicity. Blood pressure readings may reveal pulsus paradoxus, indicating severe

asthma. Hypertension may indicate asthma-related hypoxemia.
- Administer prescribed humidified oxygen by nasal cannula at 2 L/minute to ease breathing and to increase SaO$_2$. Later, adjust oxygen according to the patient's vital signs and ABG levels.
- Anticipate intubation and mechanical ventilation if the patient fails to maintain adequate oxygenation.
- Monitor serum theophylline levels to ensure they're in the therapeutic range. Observe your patient for signs and symptoms of theophylline toxicity (vomiting, diarrhea, and headache), as well as for signs of subtherapeutic dosage (respiratory distress and increased wheezing).
- Observe the frequency and severity of your patient's cough, and note whether it's productive. Then auscultate his lungs, noting adventitious or absent breath sounds. If his cough isn't productive and rhonchi are present, teach him effective coughing techniques. If the patient can tolerate postural drainage and chest percussion, perform these procedures to clear secretions. Suction an intubated patient as needed.
- Treat dehydration with I.V. fluids until the patient can tolerate oral fluids, which will help loosen secretions.
- If conservative treatment fails to improve the airway obstruction, anticipate bronchoscopy or bronchial lavage when a lobe or larger area collapses.

During long-term care, proceed as follows:
- Monitor the patient's respiratory status to detect baseline changes, to assess response to treatment, and to prevent or detect complications.
- Auscultate the lungs frequently, noting the degree of wheezing and quality of air movement.
- Review ABG levels, pulmonary function test results, and SaO$_2$ readings.
- If the patient is taking systemic corticosteroids, observe for complications, such as elevated blood glucose levels and friable skin and bruising.
- Cushingoid effects resulting from long-term use of corticosteroids may be minimized by alternate-day dosage or use of prescribed inhaled corticosteroids.

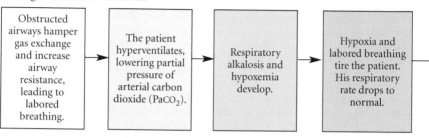

PATHOPHYSIOLOGY

HOW STATUS ASTHMATICUS PROGRESSES

A potentially fatal complication, status asthmaticus arises when impaired gas exchange and heightened airway resistance increase the work of breathing. This flow chart shows the stages of status asthmaticus.

| Obstructed airways hamper gas exchange and increase airway resistance, leading to labored breathing. | → | The patient hyperventilates, lowering partial pressure of arterial carbon dioxide ($PaCO_2$). | → | Respiratory alkalosis and hypoxemia develop. | → | Hypoxia and labored breathing tire the patient. His respiratory rate drops to normal. |

- If the patient is taking corticosteroids by inhaler, watch for signs of candidal infection in the mouth and pharynx. Using an extender device and rinsing the mouth afterward may prevent this.
- Observe the patient's anxiety level. Keep in mind that measures that reduce hypoxemia and breathlessness should help relieve anxiety.
- Keep the room temperature comfortable and use an air conditioner or a fan in hot, humid weather.
- Control exercise-induced asthma by instructing the patient to use a bronchodilator or cromolyn 30 minutes before exercise. Also instruct him to use pursed-lip breathing while exercising.

All patients should know the following:
- Teach the patient and his family to avoid known allergens and irritants.
- Describe to the patient prescribed drugs, including their names, dosages, actions, adverse effects, and special instructions.
- Teach the patient how to use a metered-dose inhaler. If he has difficulty using an inhaler, he may need an extender device to optimize drug delivery and lower the risk of candidal infection with orally inhaled corticosteroids.
- If the patient has moderate to severe asthma, explain how to use a peak flow meter to measure the degree of airway obstruction. Tell him to keep a record of peak flow readings and to bring it to medical appointments. Explain the importance of calling the physician at once if the peak flow drops suddenly (may signal severe respiratory problems).
- Tell the patient to notify the physician if he develops a fever above 100° F (37.8° C), chest pain, shortness of breath without coughing or exercising, or uncontrollable coughing. An uncontrollable asthma attack requires immediate attention.
- Teach the patient diaphragmatic and pursed-lip breathing as well as effective coughing techniques.
- Urge him to drink at least 3 qt (3 L) of fluids daily to help loosen secretions and maintain hydration.

Allergic rhinitis

Allergic rhinitis is a reaction to airborne (inhaled) allergens. Depending on the allergen, the resulting rhinitis and conjunctivitis may occur seasonally (hay fever) or year-round (perennial allergic rhinitis).

Causes and incidence
Hay fever reflects an immunoglobulin (Ig) E-mediated type I hypersensitivity response to an environmental antigen (allergen) in a genetically susceptible individual. In most cases, it's induced by windborne

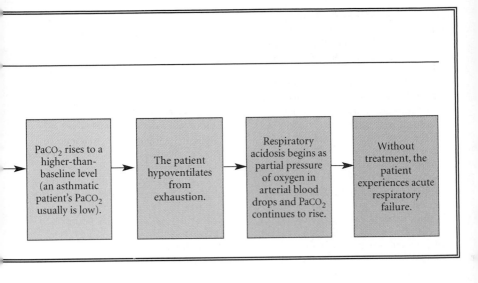

| PaCO$_2$ rises to a higher-than-baseline level (an asthmatic patient's PaCO$_2$ usually is low). | → | The patient hypoventilates from exhaustion. | → | Respiratory acidosis begins as partial pressure of oxygen in arterial blood drops and PaCO$_2$ continues to rise. | → | Without treatment, the patient experiences acute respiratory failure. |

pollens: in the spring by tree pollens (oak, elm, maple, alder, birch, and cottonwood), in the summer by grass pollens (sheep sorrel and English plantain), and in the fall by weed pollens (ragweed). Occasionally, hay fever is induced by allergy to fungal spores. In addition to individual sensitivity and geographical differences in plant population, the amount of pollen in the air can be a factor in determining whether symptoms develop. Hot, dry, windy days have more pollen than cool, damp, rainy days.

In perennial allergic rhinitis, inhaled allergens provoke antigen responses that produce recurring symptoms year-round. The allergens trigger antibody production and histamine release, producing itching, swelling, and mucus. The major perennial allergens and irritants include dust mites, feather pillows, mold, cigarette smoke, upholstery, and animal dander. Seasonal pollen allergy may exacerbate signs and symptoms of perennial rhinitis.

Allergic rhinitis is the most common atopic allergic reaction, affecting more than 20 million Americans. It's most prevalent in young children and adolescents but can occur in all age groups.

Signs and symptoms
In seasonal allergic rhinitis, the key signs and symptoms are paroxysmal sneezing, profuse watery rhinorrhea, nasal obstruc-

tion or congestion, and pruritus of the nose and eyes. It's usually accompanied by pale, cyanotic, edematous nasal mucosa; red and edematous eyelids and conjunctivae; excessive lacrimation; and headache or sinus pain. Some patients also complain of itching in the throat and malaise.

In perennial allergic rhinitis, conjunctivitis and other extranasal effects are rare, but chronic nasal obstruction is common. In many cases, this obstruction extends to eustachian tube obstruction, particularly in children.

In both types of allergic rhinitis, dark circles may appear under the patient's eyes ("allergic shiners") because of venous congestion in the maxillary sinuses. The severity of signs and symptoms may vary from season to season and from year to year.

Diagnosis
Microscopic examination of sputum and nasal secretions reveals large numbers of eosinophils. Blood chemistry shows normal or elevated IgE. A definitive diagnosis is based on the patient's personal and family history of allergies as well as physical findings during a symptomatic phase. Skin testing paired with tested responses to environmental stimuli can pinpoint the responsible allergens given the patient's history. In patients who can't tolerate skin testing, the radioallergosorbent test may be

helpful in determining specific allergen sensitivity.

To distinguish between allergic rhinitis and other nasal mucosa disorders, remember these differences:

- In chronic vasomotor rhinitis, eye symptoms are absent, rhinorrhea is mucoid, and seasonal variation is absent.

- In infectious rhinitis (the common cold), the nasal mucosa is beet red; nasal secretions contain polymorphonuclear, not eosinophilic, exudate; and signs and symptoms include fever and sore throat. This condition isn't a recurrent seasonal phenomenon.

- In rhinitis medicamentosa, which results from excessive use of nasal sprays or drops, nasal drainage and mucosal redness and swelling disappear when such medication is withheld.

- In children, differential diagnosis should rule out a nasal foreign body, such as a bean or a button.

Treatment

Treatment aims to control symptoms by eliminating the environmental antigen, if possible, and providing drug therapy and immunotherapy.

Antihistamines block histamine effects but commonly produce anticholinergic adverse effects (sedation, dry mouth, nausea, dizziness, blurred vision, and nervousness). Antihistamines, such as cetirizine, loratadine, and fexofenadine, produce fewer adverse effects and are less likely to cause sedation.

Inhaled intranasal steroids produce local anti-inflammatory effects with minimal systemic adverse effects. The most commonly used intranasal steroids are fluticasone, mometasone, and triamcinolone. These drugs are effective when symptoms aren't relieved by antihistamines alone.

Advise the patient to use intranasal steroids regularly as prescribed for optimal effectiveness. Cromolyn may be helpful in treating hay fever, but this drug may take up to 4 weeks to produce a satisfactory effect and must be taken regularly during allergy season. Eye drop versions of cromolyn and antihistamines are available for itchy, bloodshot eyes.

Long-term management includes immunotherapy, or desensitization with injections of extracted allergens, administered before or during allergy season or perennially. Seasonal allergies require particularly close dosage regulation.

Special considerations

- Before desensitization injections, assess the patient's symptom status. Afterward, watch for adverse reactions, including anaphylaxis and severe localized erythema.

- Keep epinephrine and emergency resuscitation equipment available, and observe the patient for 30 minutes after the injection. Instruct the patient to call the physician if a delayed reaction should occur.

The following protocol is recommended for allergic rhinitis:

- Monitor the patient's compliance with prescribed drug treatment regimens. Also carefully note any changes in the control of his symptoms or any signs of drug misuse.

- To reduce environmental exposure to airborne allergens, suggest that the patient sleep with the windows closed, avoid the countryside during pollination seasons, use air conditioning to filter allergens and minimize moisture and dust, and eliminate dust-collecting items, such as wool blankets, deep-pile carpets, and heavy drapes, from the home.

- In severe and resistant cases, suggest that the patient consider drastic changes in lifestyle such as relocation to a pollen-free area either seasonally or year-round.

- Be aware that some patients may develop chronic complications, including sinusitis and nasal polyps.

Atopic dermatitis

Atopic dermatitis is a chronic skin disorder that's characterized by superficial skin inflammation and intense itching. Although this disorder may appear at any age, it typically begins during infancy or early childhood. It may then subside spontaneously, followed by exacerbations in late childhood, adolescence, or early adulthood. Atopic dermatitis affects less than 1% of the population.

Causes

The cause of atopic dermatitis is still unknown. However, several theories attempt to explain its pathogenesis. One theory suggests an underlying metabolically or biochemically induced skin disorder that's genetically linked to elevated serum immunoglobulin (Ig) E levels. Another theory suggests defective T-cell function.

Exacerbating factors of atopic dermatitis include irritants, infections (commonly caused by *Staphylococcus aureus*), and some allergens. Although no reliable link exists between atopic dermatitis and exposure to inhalant allergens (such as house dust and animal dander), exposure to food allergens (such as soybeans, fish, or nuts) may coincide with flare-ups of atopic dermatitis.

Signs and symptoms

Scratching the skin causes vasoconstriction and intensifies pruritus, resulting in erythematous, weeping lesions. Eventually, the lesions become scaly and lichenified. Usually, they're located in areas of flexion and extension, such as the neck, antecubital fossa, popliteal folds, and behind the ears. Patients with atopic dermatitis are prone to unusually severe viral infections, bacterial and fungal skin infections, ocular complications, and allergic contact dermatitis.

Diagnosis

Typically, the patient has a history of atopy, such as asthma, hay fever, or urticaria; his family may have a similar history. Laboratory tests reveal eosinophilia and elevated serum IgE levels. A skin biopsy may be performed, but it isn't always required to make the diagnosis.

Treatment

Measures to ease this chronic disorder include meticulous skin care, environmental control of offending allergens, and drug therapy. Because dry skin aggravates itching, frequent application of nonirritating topical lubricants is important, especially after bathing or showering. Minimizing exposure to allergens and irritants, such as wools and harsh detergents, also helps control symptoms.

Drug therapy involves corticosteroids and antipruritics. Active dermatitis responds well to topical corticosteroids, which should be applied immediately after bathing for optimal penetration. Oral antihistamines are commonly used to help control itching. A bedtime dose may reduce involuntary scratching during sleep. If secondary infection develops, antibiotics are necessary. A newer treatment is the use of topical immunomodulators; these agents are steroid-free and have demonstrated an 80% success rate in studies.

Special considerations

- Monitor the patient's compliance with drug therapy.
- Teach the patient when and how to apply topical corticosteroids.
- Emphasize the importance of regular personal hygiene using only water with little soap.
- Be alert for signs and symptoms of secondary infection; teach the patient how to recognize them as well.
- If the patient's diet is modified to exclude food allergens, monitor his nutritional status.
- Offer support to help the patient and his family cope with this chronic disorder.
- Discourage use of laundry additives.
- Dissuade the patient from scratching during urticaria to help prevent an infection.

Latex allergy

Latex is a substance found in an increasing number of products both on the job and in the home environment. Also increasing is the number of latex allergies. Latex allergy is a hypersensitivity reaction to products that contain natural latex, which is derived from the sap of a rubber tree, not synthetic latex. These hypersensitivity reactions range from local dermatitis to a life-threatening anaphylactic reaction.

Causes and incidence

Approximately 1% of the population has a latex allergy. Anyone who is in frequent contact with latex-containing products is at risk for developing a latex allergy. (See *Products that contain latex,* page 358.) The more frequent the exposure, the higher the

PRODUCTS THAT CONTAIN LATEX

Many medical and everyday items contain latex, which can be a threat to the patient with latex allergy. The most common items that contain latex are listed below.

Medical products
- Adhesive bandages
- Airways, nasogastric tubes
- Blood pressure cuff, tubing, and bladder
- Catheters
- Catheter leg straps
- Dental dams
- Elastic bandages
- Electrode pads
- Fluid-circulating hypothermia blankets
- Hand-held resuscitation bag
- Hemodialysis equipment
- I.V. catheters
- Latex or rubber gloves
- Medication vials
- Pads for crutches
- Protective sheets
- Reservoir breathing bags
- Rubber airway and endotracheal tubes
- Tape
- Tourniquets

Nonmedical products
- Adhesive tape
- Balloons (excluding Mylar)
- Cervical diaphragms
- Condoms
- Disposable diapers
- Elastic stockings
- Glue
- Latex paint
- Nipples and pacifiers
- Rubber bands
- Tires

risk. The populations at highest risk are medical and dental professionals, workers in latex companies, and patients with spina bifida.

Other individuals at risk include:
- patients with a history of asthma or other allergies, especially to bananas, avocados, tropical fruits, or chestnuts
- patients with a history of multiple intra-abdominal or genitourinary surgeries
- patients who require frequent intermittent urinary catheterization.

Signs and symptoms
Early signs that a life-threatening hypersensitivity reaction may be occurring include hypotension, tachycardia, and oxygen desaturation. Other clinical findings include urticaria, flushing, bronchospasm, difficulty breathing, pruritus, palpitations, abdominal pain, and syncope. Mild signs and symptoms may include itchy skin, swollen lips, nausea, diarrhea, and red, swollen, teary eyes.

Diagnosis
A patient who describes even the mildest symptoms during a history and physical assessment should be suspected of having a latex allergy. The patient may describe dermatitis or mild respiratory distress when using latex gloves, inflating a balloon, or coming in contact with other latex products.

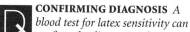 **CONFIRMING DIAGNOSIS** *A blood test for latex sensitivity can confirm the diagnosis. This test, which measures specific immunoglobulin E antibodies against latex, should be used only when latex allergy is suspected; it isn't recommended as a screening tool.*

Treatment
The best treatment of latex allergy is prevention; the more a latex-sensitive person is exposed to latex, the worse his symptoms will become. To avoid exposure, advise the patient to substitute products made of silicone and vinyl for those made of latex.

When a latex allergy is suspected or known, the patient may receive medications before and after surgery or other invasive procedures. Premedications may include prednisone, diphenhydramine, and cimetidine. Postmedications may include hydrocortisone, diphenhydramine, and famotidine.

There's no known treatment for an allergic reaction to latex. Care is supportive in nature. The patient's airway, breathing, and circulation must be monitored. An artificial airway, oxygen therapy, cardiopulmonary resuscitation, and fluid management may be necessary. During an acute reaction, epinephrine, diphenhydramine, and hydrocortisone are commonly administered by I.V. infusion.

Special considerations

- Make sure that items that aren't available in a latex-free form, such as stethoscopes and blood pressure cuffs, are wrapped in cloth before they come in contact with a hypersensitive patient's skin.
- Place the patient in a private room or with another patient who requires a latex-free environment.
- When adding medication to an I.V. bag, inject the drug through the spike port, not the rubber latex port.
- Urge the patient to wear an identification tag mentioning his latex allergy.
- Teach the patient and family members how to use an epinephrine autoinjector.
- Teach the patient to be aware of all latex-containing products and to use vinyl or silicone products instead. Advise him that Mylar balloons don't contain latex.

Anaphylaxis

Anaphylaxis is a dramatic, acute atopic reaction marked by the sudden onset of rapidly progressive urticaria and respiratory distress. A severe reaction may precipitate vascular collapse, leading to systemic shock and, sometimes, death.

Causes and incidence

The source of anaphylactic reactions is ingestion of or other systemic exposure to sensitizing drugs or other substances. Such substances may include serums (usually horse serum), vaccines, allergen extracts, enzymes (L-asparaginase), hormones, penicillin and other antibiotics, sulfonamides, local anesthetics, salicylates, poly-

---

PENICILLIN GUIDELINES

When administering penicillin or its derivatives, such as ampicillin or carbenicillin, follow these recommendations of the World Health Organization to prevent an allergic response:

- Have an emergency kit available to treat allergic reactions.
- Take a detailed patient history, including penicillin allergy and other allergies. In an infant younger than age 3 months, check for penicillin allergy in the mother.
- Never give penicillin to a patient who has had an allergic reaction to it.
- Before giving penicillin to a patient with suspected penicillin allergy, refer the patient for skin and immunologic tests to confirm it.
- Always tell a patient he's going to receive penicillin before he takes the first dose.
- Observe the patient carefully for adverse effects for at least one half-hour after penicillin administration.
- Be aware that penicillin derivatives also elicit an allergic reaction.

---

saccharides, diagnostic chemicals (sulfobromophthalein, sodium dehydrocholate, and radiographic contrast media), foods (especially legumes, nuts, berries, seafood, and egg albumin) and sulfite-containing food additives, insect venom (honeybees, wasps, hornets, yellow jackets, fire ants, mosquitoes, and certain spiders) and, rarely, ruptured hydatid cyst.

A common cause of anaphylaxis is penicillin, which induces anaphylaxis in 1 to 4 of every 10,000 patients treated with it. Penicillin is most likely to induce anaphylaxis after parenteral administration or prolonged therapy and in atopic patients with an allergy to other drugs or foods. (See *Penicillin guidelines*.) An anaphylactic reaction requires previous sensitization or exposure to the specific antigen, resulting in the production of specific immunoglobulin (Ig) E antibodies by plasma cells. This antibody production takes place in the lymph nodes and is enhanced by helper T cells. IgE antibodies then bind to membrane receptors on mast cells (found throughout connective tissue) and basophils.

On re-exposure, the antigen binds to adjacent IgE antibodies or cross-linked IgE receptors, activating a series of cellular reactions that trigger degranulation — the release of powerful chemical mediators (such as histamine, eosinophil chemotactic factor of anaphylaxis, and platelet-activating factor) from mast cell stores. IgG or IgM enters into the reaction and activates the release of complement fractions.

At the same time, two other chemical mediators, bradykinin and leukotrienes, induce vascular collapse by stimulating contraction of certain groups of smooth muscles and by increasing vascular permeability. In turn, increased vascular permeability leads to decreased peripheral resistance and plasma leakage from the circulation to extravascular tissues (which lowers blood volume, causing hypotension, hypovolemic shock, and cardiac dysfunction).

Signs and symptoms

An anaphylactic reaction produces sudden physical distress within seconds or minutes (although a delayed or persistent reaction may occur for up to 24 hours) after exposure to an allergen. The reaction's severity is inversely related to the interval between exposure to the allergen and the onset of symptoms. Usually, the first symptoms include a feeling of impending doom or fright, weakness, sweating, sneezing, shortness of breath, nasal pruritus, urticaria, and angioedema, followed rapidly by symptoms in one or more target organs.

Cardiovascular symptoms include hypotension, shock and, sometimes, cardiac arrhythmias. If untreated, arrhythmia may precipitate circulatory collapse. Respiratory symptoms can occur at any level in the respiratory tract and commonly include nasal mucosal edema, profuse watery rhinorrhea, itching, nasal congestion, and sudden sneezing attacks. Edema of the upper respiratory tract results in hypopharyngeal and laryngeal obstruction (hoarseness, stridor, and dyspnea). This is an early sign of acute respiratory failure, which can be fatal. GI and genitourinary symptoms include severe stomach cramps, nausea, diarrhea, and urinary urgency and incontinence.

Diagnosis

Anaphylaxis can be diagnosed by the rapid onset of severe respiratory or cardiovascular signs and symptoms after ingestion or injection of a drug, vaccine, diagnostic agent, food, or food additive or after an insect sting. If these symptoms occur without a known allergic stimulus, rule out other possible causes of shock (acute myocardial infarction, status asthmaticus, or heart failure).

Treatment

Anaphylaxis is always an emergency. It requires an *immediate* injection of epinephrine 1:1,000 aqueous solution, 0.1 to 0.5 ml, repeated every 5 to 20 minutes as needed.

In the early stages of anaphylaxis, when the patient hasn't lost consciousness and is normotensive, give epinephrine I.M. or subcutaneously and help it move into circulation faster by massaging the injection site. In severe reactions, when the patient has lost consciousness and is hypotensive, give epinephrine I.V.

Maintain airway patency. Observe for early signs of laryngeal edema (hoarseness, stridor, and dyspnea), which will probably require endotracheal tube insertion or a tracheotomy and oxygen therapy.

In case of cardiac arrest, begin cardiopulmonary resuscitation, including closed-chest heart massage, assisted ventilation, and other therapies as indicated by clinical response.

Watch for hypotension and shock, and maintain circulatory volume with volume expanders (plasma, plasma expanders, saline, and albumin) as needed. Stabilize blood pressure with the I.V. vasopressors norepinephrine and dopamine. Monitor blood pressure, central venous pressure, and urine output as a response index.

After the initial emergency, administer other medications as ordered: subcutaneous epinephrine, longer-acting epinephrine, corticosteroids, and I.V. diphenhydramine for long-term management and I.V. aminophylline over 10 to 20 minutes for bronchospasm.

 ALERT *Rapid infusion of aminophylline may cause or aggravate severe hypotension.*

Special considerations

■ To prevent anaphylaxis, teach the patient to avoid exposure to known allergens. A person allergic to certain foods or drugs must learn to avoid the offending food or drug in all its forms. A person allergic to insect stings should avoid open fields and wooded areas during the insect season. An anaphylaxis kit (epinephrine, antihistamine, and tourniquet) should also be carried whenever the patient with known severe allergic reactions goes outdoors. In addition, every patient prone to anaphylaxis should wear a medical identification bracelet identifying his allergies.

■ If a patient must receive a drug to which he's allergic, prevent a severe reaction by making sure he receives careful desensitization with gradually increasing doses of the antigen or advance administration of steroids. Of course, a person with a known allergic history should receive a drug with a high anaphylactic potential only after cautious pretesting for sensitivity. Closely monitor the patient during testing, and make sure you have resuscitative equipment and epinephrine ready. When any patient needs a drug with a high anaphylactic potential (particularly parenteral drugs), make sure he receives each dose under close medical observation.

■ Closely monitor a patient undergoing diagnostic tests that use radiographic contrast media, such as excretory urography, cardiac catheterization, and angiography.

Urticaria and angioedema

Urticaria, commonly known as hives, is an episodic, usually self-limited skin reaction characterized by local dermal wheals surrounded by an erythematous flare. Angioedema is a subcutaneous and dermal eruption that produces deeper, larger wheals (usually on the hands, feet, lips, genitals, and eyelids) and a more diffuse swelling of loose subcutaneous tissue. Urticaria and angioedema can occur simultaneously, but angioedema may last longer.

Causes and incidence

Urticaria and angioedema are common allergic reactions that may occur in 20% of the general population. The causes of these reactions include allergy to drugs, foods, insect bites and stings and, occasionally, inhalant allergens (animal dander and cosmetics) that provoke an immunoglobulin (Ig) E-mediated response to protein allergens. However, certain drugs may cause urticaria without an IgE response. When urticaria and angioedema are part of an anaphylactic reaction, they almost always persist long after the systemic response has subsided. This occurs because circulation to the skin is the last to be restored after an allergic reaction, which results in slow histamine reabsorption at the reaction site.

Nonallergic urticaria and angioedema are also related to histamine release. External physical stimuli, such as cold (usually in young adults), heat, water, or sunlight, may also provoke urticaria and angioedema. *Dermographism urticaria,* which develops after stroking or scratching of the skin, occurs in as much as 20% of the population. Such urticaria develops with varying pressure, usually under tight clothing, and is aggravated by scratching.

Several different mechanisms and underlying disorders may provoke urticaria and angioedema. These include IgE-induced release of mediators from cutaneous mast cells; binding of IgG or IgM to antigen, resulting in complement activation; and such disorders as localized or secondary infections (such as respiratory infection), neoplastic diseases (such as Hodgkin's disease), connective tissue diseases (such as systemic lupus erythematosus), collagen vascular diseases, and psychogenic diseases.

Signs and symptoms

The characteristic features of urticaria are distinct, raised, evanescent (temporary) dermal wheals surrounded by an erythe-

---

HEREDITARY ANGIOEDEMA

A nonallergenic type of angioedema, hereditary angioedema results from an autosomal dominant trait—a hereditary deficiency of an alpha globulin, the normal inhibitor of C1 esterase (a component of the complement system). This deficiency allows uninhibited C1 esterase release, resulting in the vascular changes common to angioedema.

The clinical effects of hereditary angioedema usually appear in childhood with recurrent episodes of subcutaneous or submucosal edema at irregular intervals of weeks, months, or years, in many cases after trauma or stress. Hereditary angioedema is unifocal, without urticarial pruritus, but associated with recurrent edema of the skin and mucosa (especially of the GI and respiratory tracts). GI tract involvement may cause nausea, vomiting, and severe abdominal pain. Laryngeal angioedema may cause fatal airway obstruction.

Treatment of acute hereditary angioedema may require androgens such as danazol. Tracheotomy may be necessary to relieve airway obstruction resulting from laryngeal angioedema.

- drug history, including over-the-counter preparations (vitamins, aspirin, and antacids)
- frequently ingested foods (strawberries, milk products, fish)
- environmental influences (pets, carpet, clothing, soap, inhalants, cosmetics, hair dye, and insect bites and stings).

Diagnosis also requires physical assessment to rule out similar conditions as well as a complete blood count, urinalysis, erythrocyte sedimentation rate, and a chest X-ray to rule out inflammatory infections. Skin testing, an elimination diet, and a food diary (recording time and amount of food eaten and circumstances) can pinpoint provoking allergens. The food diary may also suggest other allergies. For instance, a patient allergic to fish may also be allergic to iodine contrast materials.

Recurrent angioedema without urticaria, along with a familial history, points to hereditary angioedema. (See *Hereditary angioedema*.) Decreased serum levels of complement 4 and complement 1 esterase inhibitors confirm this diagnosis.

Treatment

Treatment aims to prevent or limit contact with triggering factors or, if this is impossible, to desensitize the patient to them and to relieve symptoms. During desensitization, progressively larger doses of specific antigens (determined by skin testing) are injected intradermally. After the triggering stimulus has been removed, urticaria usually subsides in a few days—except for drug reactions, which may persist as long as the drug is in the bloodstream.

Diphenhydramine, hydroxyzine, or another antihistamine can ease itching and swelling in every kind of urticaria. Corticosteroid therapy may be necessary for some patients.

Special considerations

- Inform the patient receiving antihistamines of the possibility of drowsiness.
- Suggest cool compresses to reduce swelling and pain. A cool bath may be used for large areas. Calamine lotion may be soothing as well.
- Advise the patient to avoid tight-fitting clothing.

---

matous flare. These lesions may vary in size. In cholinergic urticaria, the wheals may be tiny and blanched, surrounded by erythematous flares.

Angioedema characteristically produces nonpitted swelling of deep subcutaneous tissue, usually on the eyelids, lips, genitalia, and mucous membranes. These swellings don't usually itch but may burn and tingle.

Diagnosis

An accurate patient history can help determine the cause of urticaria. Such a history should include:

Blood transfusion reaction

Mediated by immune or nonimmune factors, a transfusion reaction accompanies or follows I.V. administration of blood components. Its severity varies from mild (fever and chills) to severe (acute renal failure or complete vascular collapse and death), depending on the amount of blood transfused, the type of reaction, and the patient's general health.

Causes

Hemolytic reactions follow transfusion of mismatched blood. Transfusion of serologically incompatible blood triggers the most serious reaction, marked by intravascular agglutination of red blood cells (RBCs). The recipient's antibodies (immunoglobulin [Ig] G or IgM) attach to the donated RBCs, leading to widespread clumping and destruction of the recipient's RBCs and, possibly, the development of disseminated intravascular coagulation (DIC) and other serious effects.

Transfusion of Rh-incompatible blood triggers a less serious reaction within several days to 2 weeks. Rh reactions are most common in females sensitized to RBC antigens by prior pregnancy or by unknown factors (such as bacterial or viral infection) and in people who have received more than five transfusions. (See *Understanding the Rh system.*)

Allergic reactions are fairly common but only occasionally serious. In this type of reaction, transfused soluble antigens react with surface IgE molecules on mast cells and basophils, causing degranulation and release of allergic mediators. Antibodies against IgA in an IgA-deficient recipient can also trigger a severe allergic reaction (anaphylaxis).

Febrile nonhemolytic reactions, the most common type of reaction, apparently develop when cytotoxic or agglutinating antibodies in the recipient's plasma attack antigens on transfused lymphocytes, granulocytes, or plasma cells.

Although fairly uncommon, *bacterial contamination* of donor blood can occur during donor phlebotomy. Offending organisms are usually gram-negative, especially *Pseudomonas* species, *Citrobacter freundii,* and *Escherichia coli.*

Contamination of donor blood with viruses, such as hepatitis, cytomegalovirus, and malaria, is also possible.

Signs and symptoms

Immediate effects of a hemolytic transfusion reaction develop within a few minutes or hours after the start of the transfusion and may include chills, fever, urticaria, tachycardia, dyspnea, nausea, vomiting, tightness in the chest, chest and back pain, hypotension, bronchospasm, angioedema, and signs and symptoms of anaphylaxis, shock, pulmonary edema, heart failure, and renal failure. In a surgical patient un-

---

UNDERSTANDING THE RH SYSTEM

The Rh system contains more than 30 antibodies and antigens. Eighty-five percent of the world's population is Rh-positive, which means that the red blood cells of most people carry the D or Rh antigen. The remaining 15% of the population, who are Rh-negative, don't carry this antigen.

When Rh-negative people receive Rh-positive blood for the first time, they become sensitized to the D antigen but show no immediate reaction to it. If they receive Rh-positive blood a second time, they then develop a massive hemolytic reaction. For example, an Rh-negative mother who delivers an Rh-positive baby is sensitized by the baby's Rh-positive blood. During her next Rh-positive pregnancy, her sensitized blood would cause a hemolytic reaction in fetal circulation. Thus, the Rh-negative mother should receive Rh_O (D) immune globulin (human) I.M. within 72 hours after delivering an Rh-positive baby to prevent formation of antibodies against Rh-positive blood.

der anesthesia, these symptoms are masked, but blood oozes from mucous membranes or the incision site.

Delayed hemolytic reactions can occur up to several weeks after a transfusion, causing fever, an unexpected fall in serum hemoglobin (Hb) level, and jaundice.

Allergic reactions are typically afebrile and characterized by urticaria and angioedema, possibly progressing to cough, respiratory distress, nausea, vomiting, diarrhea, abdominal cramps, vascular instability, shock, and coma.

The hallmark of febrile nonhemolytic reactions is mild to severe fever that may begin at the start of transfusion or within 2 hours after its completion.

Bacterial contamination produces a high fever, nausea, vomiting, diarrhea, abdominal cramps and, possibly, shock. Symptoms of viral contamination may not appear for several weeks after transfusion.

Diagnosis

CONFIRMING DIAGNOSIS
Confirming a hemolytic transfusion reaction requires proof of blood incompatibility and evidence of hemolysis, such as hemoglobinuria, anti-A or anti-B antibodies in the serum, low serum Hb levels, and elevated bilirubin levels.

If you suspect such a reaction, have the patient's blood retyped and crossmatched with the donor's blood. After a hemolytic transfusion reaction, laboratory tests will show increased indirect bilirubin levels, decreased haptoglobin levels, increased serum Hb levels, and Hb in the urine. As the reaction progresses, tests may show signs of DIC (thrombocytopenia, increased prothrombin time, and decreased fibrinogen level) and acute tubular necrosis (increased blood urea nitrogen and serum creatinine levels).

A blood culture to isolate the causative organism should be done when bacterial contamination is suspected.

Treatment

At the first sign of a hemolytic reaction, *stop the transfusion immediately.* Depending on the nature of the patient's reaction, prepare to:
- monitor vital signs every 15 to 30 minutes, watching for signs of shock

- maintain a patent I.V. line with normal saline solution; insert an indwelling catheter and monitor intake and output
- cover the patient with blankets to ease chills, and explain what's happening
- deliver supplemental oxygen at low flow rates through a nasal cannula or bag-valve-mask (handheld resuscitation bag)
- give drugs as ordered: an I.V. antihypotensive drug and normal saline solution to combat shock, epinephrine to treat dyspnea and wheezing, diphenhydramine to combat cellular histamine released from mast cells, corticosteroids to reduce inflammation, and mannitol or furosemide to maintain urinary function. Administer parenteral antihistamines and corticosteroids for allergic reactions. (Severe reactions such as anaphylaxis may require epinephrine.) Administer antipyretics for nonhemolytic febrile reactions and appropriate I.V. antibiotics for bacterial contamination.

Special considerations
- Remember to fully document the transfusion reaction on the patient's chart, noting the transfusion's duration, the amount of blood absorbed, and a complete description of the reaction and of any interventions.
- To prevent a hemolytic transfusion reaction, make sure you know your hospital's policy about giving blood before you give a blood transfusion. Then make sure you have the right blood and the right patient. Check and double-check the patient's name, hospital number, ABO blood group, and Rh status. If you find even a small discrepancy, don't give the blood. Notify the blood bank immediately and return the unopened unit.

AUTOIMMUNITY

Rheumatoid arthritis

A chronic, systemic, inflammatory disease, rheumatoid arthritis (RA) primarily attacks peripheral joints and surrounding muscles, tendons, ligaments, and blood vessels. Spontaneous remissions and unpredictable exacerbations mark the course of this potentially crippling disease. RA usually requires lifelong treatment and, sometimes, surgery. In most patients, the disease follows an intermittent course and allows normal activity, although 10% suffer total disability from severe articular deformity, associated extra-articular symptoms, or both. The prognosis worsens with the development of nodules, vasculitis, and high titers of rheumatoid factor (RF).

Causes and incidence

RA occurs worldwide, striking three times more females than males. Although it can occur at any age, it begins most often between ages 25 and 55. This disease affects more than 7 million people in the United States alone.

What causes the chronic inflammation characteristic of RA isn't known, but various theories point to infectious, genetic, and endocrine factors. Currently, it's believed that a genetically susceptible individual develops abnormal or altered immunoglobulin (Ig) G antibodies when exposed to an antigen. This altered IgG antibody isn't recognized as "self," and the individual forms an antibody against it — an antibody known as RF. By aggregating into complexes, RF generates inflammation. Eventually, cartilage damage by inflammation triggers additional immune responses, including activation of complement. This in turn attracts polymorphonuclear leukocytes and stimulates release of inflammatory mediators, which enhance joint destruction.

Much more is known about the pathogenesis of RA than about its causes. If unarrested, the inflammatory process within the joints occurs in four stages. First, synovitis develops from congestion and edema of the synovial membrane and joint capsule. Formation of pannus — thickened layers of granulation tissue — marks the second stage's onset. Pannus covers and invades cartilage and eventually destroys the joint capsule and bone. Progression to the third stage is characterized by fibrous ankylosis — fibrous invasion of the pannus and scar formation that occludes the joint space. Bone atrophy and malalignment cause visible deformities and disrupt the articulation of opposing bones, causing

> ## JOINT DEFORMITIES
>
> In advanced rheumatoid arthritis, marked edema and congestion cause spindle-shaped interphalangeal joints and severe flexion deformities.
>
>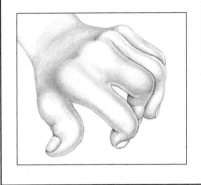

muscle atrophy and imbalance and, possibly, partial dislocations or subluxations. In the fourth stage, fibrous tissue calcifies, resulting in bony ankylosis and total immobility.

Signs and symptoms

RA usually develops insidiously and initially produces nonspecific signs and symptoms, such as fatigue, malaise, anorexia, persistent low-grade fever, weight loss, lymphadenopathy, and vague articular symptoms. Later, more specific localized articular symptoms develop, commonly in the fingers at the proximal interphalangeal, metacarpophalangeal, and metatarsophalangeal joints. These symptoms usually occur bilaterally and symmetrically and may extend to the wrists, knees, elbows, and ankles. The affected joints stiffen after inactivity, especially upon rising in the morning. The fingers may assume a spindle shape from marked edema and joint congestion. The joints become tender and painful, at first only when the patient moves them, but eventually even at rest. They commonly feel hot to the touch. Ultimately, joint function is diminished.

Deformities are common if active disease continues. (See *Joint deformities.*) Proximal interphalangeal joints may develop flexion deformities or become hyperextended. Metacarpophalangeal joints may swell dorsally, and volar subluxation and stretching of tendons may pull the fingers to the ulnar side ("ulnar drift"). The fingers may become fixed in a characteristic "swan's neck" appearance, or "boutonnière" deformity. The hands appear foreshortened, the wrists boggy; carpal tunnel syndrome from synovial pressure on the median nerve causes tingling paresthesia in the fingers.

The most common extra-articular finding is the gradual appearance of rheumatoid nodules—subcutaneous, round or oval, nontender masses—usually on pressure areas such as the elbows. Vasculitis can lead to skin lesions, leg ulcers, and multiple systemic complications. Peripheral neuropathy may produce numbness or tingling in the feet or weakness and loss of sensation in the fingers. Stiff, weak, or painful muscles are common. Other common extra-articular effects include pericarditis, pulmonary nodules or fibrosis, pleuritis, scleritis, and episcleritis.

Another complication is destruction of the odontoid process, part of the second cervical vertebra. Rarely, cord compression may occur, particularly in patients with long-standing deforming disease. Upper motor neuron signs and symptoms, such as a positive Babinski's sign and muscle weakness, may also develop.

RA can also cause temporomandibular joint disease, which impairs chewing and causes earaches. Other extra-articular findings may include infection, osteoporosis, myositis, cardiopulmonary lesions, lymphadenopathy, and peripheral neuritis.

Diagnosis

Typical clinical features suggest this disorder, but a definitive diagnosis is based on laboratory and other test results:

■ X-rays—in early stages, show bone demineralization and soft-tissue swelling; later, loss of cartilage and narrowing of joint spaces; finally, cartilage and bone destruction and erosion, subluxations, and deformities

■ rheumatoid factor test—positive in 75% to 80% of patients as indicated by a titer of 1:160 or higher

■ synovial fluid analysis—reveals increased volume and turbidity but decreased viscosity and complement (C3 and C4) levels; white blood cell count usually exceeds 10,000/µl

■ erythrocyte sedimentation rate—elevated in 85% to 90% of patients (may be useful to monitor response to therapy because elevation commonly parallels disease activity)

■ complete blood count—usually reveals moderate anemia and slight leukocytosis.

A C-reactive protein test can help monitor response to therapy.

Treatment

Salicylates, particularly aspirin, are the mainstay of RA therapy because they decrease inflammation and relieve joint pain. Other useful medications include nonsteroidal anti-inflammatory drugs (such as indomethacin, fenoprofen, and ibuprofen), antimalarials (hydroxychloroquine), gold salts, penicillamine, and corticosteroids (prednisone). Immunosuppressants, such as cyclophosphamide, methotrexate, and azathioprine, are also therapeutic and are being used more commonly in early disease. (See *Drug therapy for arthritis*.)

Supportive measures include 8 to 10 hours of sleep every night, frequent rest periods between daily activities, and splinting to rest inflamed joints. A physical therapy program including range-of-motion exercises and carefully individualized therapeutic exercises forestalls joint function loss; application of heat relaxes muscles and relieves pain. Moist heat usually works best for patients with chronic disease. Ice packs are effective during acute episodes.

Advanced disease may require synovectomy, joint reconstruction, or total joint arthroplasty.

Useful surgical procedures in RA include metatarsal head and distal ulnar resectional arthroplasty, insertion of a Silastic prosthesis between the metacarpophalangeal and proximal interphalangeal joints, and arthrodesis (joint fusion). Arthrodesis sacrifices joint mobility for stability and pain relief. Synovectomy (removal of destructive, proliferating synovium, usually in the wrists, knees, and fingers) may halt or delay the course of this disease. Osteotomy

DRUG THERAPY FOR ARTHRITIS

Drug and adverse effects	Clinical considerations
Aspirin Prolonged bleeding time; GI disturbances, including nausea, dyspepsia, anorexia, ulcers, and hemorrhage; hypersensitivity reactions ranging from urticaria to anaphylaxis; salicylism (mild toxicity: tinnitus, dizziness; moderate toxicity: restlessness, hyperpnea, delirium, marked lethargy; and severe toxicity: coma, seizures, severe hyperpnea)	■ Don't use in patients with GI ulcers, bleeding, or hypersensitivity or in neonates. ■ Tell the patient to take the drug with food, milk, antacid, or a large glass of water to reduce GI adverse effects. ■ Monitor the patient's salicylate level. Remember that toxicity can develop rapidly in febrile, dehydrated children. ■ Teach the patient to reduce the dose, one tablet at a time, if tinnitus occurs. ■ Teach the patient to watch for signs of bleeding, such as bruising, melena, and petechiae.
Fenoprofen, ibuprofen, naproxen, piroxicam, sulindac, and tolmetin Prolonged bleeding time; central nervous system abnormalities (headache, drowsiness, restlessness, dizziness, and tremor); GI disturbances, including hemorrhage and peptic ulcer; increased blood urea nitrogen and liver enzyme levels	■ Don't use in patients with renal disease, in patients with asthma who have nasal polyps, or in children. ■ Use cautiously in patients with GI and cardiac disease or if a patient is allergic to other nonsteroidal anti-inflammatory drugs (NSAIDs). ■ Tell the patient to take the drug with milk or meals to reduce GI adverse effects. ■ Tell the patient that the drug effect may be delayed for 2 to 3 weeks. ■ Monitor the patient's kidney, liver, and auditory functions in long-term therapy. Stop the drug if abnormalities develop. ■ Use cautiously in elderly patients; they may experience severe GI bleeding without warning.
Hydroxychloroquine and sulfasalazine Blood dyscrasias, GI irritation, corneal opacities, and keratopathy or retinopathy	■ Don't use in patients with retinal or visual field changes. ■ Use cautiously in patients with hepatic disease, alcoholism, glucose-6-phosphate dehydrogenase deficiency, or psoriasis. ■ Perform complete blood count (CBC) and liver function tests before therapy and during chronic therapy. The patient should also have regular ophthalmologic examinations. ■ Tell the patient to take the drug with food or milk to minimize GI adverse effects. ■ Warn the patient that dizziness may occur.

(continued)

Note: Other drugs that may be used in resistant cases include prednisone, chloroquine, azathioprine, and cyclophosphamide.

DRUG THERAPY FOR ARTHRITIS (continued)

Drug and adverse effects	Clinical considerations
Gold (oral and parenteral) Dermatitis, pruritus, rash, stomatitis, nephrotoxicity, blood dyscrasias and, with oral form, GI distress and diarrhea	■ Watch for and report adverse effects. Observe for nitritoid reaction (flushing, fainting, and sweating). ■ Check the patient's urine for blood and albumin before giving each dose. If positive, hold the drug and notify the physician. Stress to the patient the need for regular follow-up, including blood and urine testing. ■ To avoid local nerve irritation, mix the drug well and give it via a deep I.M. injection in the buttock. ■ Advise the patient not to expect improvement for 3 to 6 months. ■ Tell the patient to report rash, bruising, bleeding, hematuria, or oral ulcers.
Methotrexate Tubular necrosis, bone marrow depression, leukopenia, thrombocytopenia, pulmonary interstitial infiltrates, hyperuricemia, stomatitis, rash, pruritus, dermatitis, alopecia, diarrhea, dizziness, cirrhosis, and hepatic fibrosis	■ Don't give to women who are pregnant or breast-feeding or to patients who are alcoholic. ■ Monitor the patient's uric acid levels, CBC, and intake and output. ■ Warn the patient to report any unusual bleeding (especially GI) or bruising promptly. ■ Warn the patient to avoid alcohol, aspirin, and NSAIDs. ■ Advise the patient to follow the prescribed regimen.

Note: Other drugs that may be used in resistant cases include prednisone, chloroquine, azathioprine, and cyclophosphamide.

(the cutting of bone or excision of a wedge of bone) can realign joint surfaces and redistribute stresses. Tendons may rupture spontaneously, requiring surgical repair. Tendon transfers may prevent deformities or relieve contractures. (See *When arthritis requires surgery*.)

Special considerations

■ Assess all joints carefully. Look for deformities, contractures, immobility, and inability to perform everyday activities.
■ Monitor the patient's vital signs and note weight changes, sensory disturbances, and level of pain. Administer analgesics as ordered and watch for adverse effects.
■ Provide meticulous skin care. Check for rheumatoid nodules as well as pressure ulcers and breakdowns due to immobility, vascular impairment, corticosteroid treatment, or improper splinting. Use lotion or cleansing oil, not soap, for dry skin.
■ Explain all diagnostic tests and procedures. Tell the patient to expect multiple blood samples to allow firm diagnosis and accurate monitoring of therapy.
■ Monitor the duration, not the intensity, of morning stiffness because duration more accurately reflects the disease's severity. Encourage the patient to take hot showers or baths at bedtime or in the morning to reduce the need for pain medication.
■ Apply splints carefully and correctly. Observe for pressure ulcers if the patient is in traction or wearing splints.
■ Explain the nature of the disease. Make sure the patient and his family understand that RA is a chronic disease that requires major changes in lifestyle. Emphasize that

WHEN ARTHRITIS REQUIRES SURGERY

Arthritis severe enough to necessitate total knee or total hip arthroplasty calls for comprehensive preoperative teaching and postoperative care.

Before surgery

- Explain preoperative and surgical procedures. Show the patient the prosthesis to be used if available.
- Teach the patient postoperative exercises such as isometrics and supervise his practice. Also, teach deep-breathing and coughing exercises that will be necessary after surgery.
- Explain that total hip or knee arthroplasty requires frequent range-of-motion exercises of the leg after surgery; total knee arthroplasty requires frequent leg-lift exercises.
- Show the patient how to use a trapeze to move himself about in bed after surgery, and make sure he has a fracture bedpan handy.
- Tell the patient what kind of dressings to expect after surgery. After total knee arthroplasty, the patient's knee may be placed in a constant-passive-motion device to increase postoperative mobility and prevent emboli. After total hip arthroplasty, he'll have an abduction pillow between the legs to help keep the hip prosthesis in place.

After surgery

- Closely monitor and record vital signs. Watch for complications, such as steroid crisis and shock in patients receiving steroids. Monitor distal leg pulses often, marking them with a waterproof marker to make them easier to find.
- As soon as the patient awakens, have him do active dorsiflexion; if he can't, report this immediately. Supervise isometric exercises every 2 hours. After total hip arthroplasty, check traction for pressure areas and keep the bed's head raised between 30 and 45 degrees.
- Change or reinforce dressings, as needed, using sterile technique. Check wounds for hematoma, excessive drainage, color changes, or foul odor — all possible signs of hemorrhage or infection. (Wounds on rheumatoid arthritis patients may heal slowly.) Avoid contaminating dressings while helping the patient use the urinal or bedpan.
- Administer blood replacement products, antibiotics, and pain medication, as ordered. Monitor serum electrolyte and hemoglobin levels and hematocrit.
- Have the patient turn, cough, and deep-breathe every 2 hours; then percuss his chest.
- After total knee arthroplasty, keep the patient's leg extended and slightly elevated.
- After total hip arthroplasty, keep the patient's hip in abduction to prevent dislocation by using such measures as a wedge pillow. Prevent external rotation and avoid hip flexion greater than 90 degrees. Watch for and immediately report any inability to rotate the hip or bear weight on it, increased pain, or a leg that appears shorter — all may indicate dislocation.
- As soon as allowed, help the patient get out of bed and sit in a chair, keeping his weight on the unaffected side. When he's ready to walk, consult with the physical therapist for walking instruction and aids.

there are no miracle cures, despite claims to the contrary.

- Encourage a balanced diet, but make sure the patient understands that special diets won't cure RA. Stress the need for weight control because obesity adds further stress to joints.
- Urge the patient to perform activities of daily living (ADLs), such as practicing good hygiene and dressing and feeding himself. Suggest ADL aids, such as a long-

handled shoehorn; elastic shoelaces; zipper-pulls; button hooks; easy-to-handle cups, plates, and silverware; elevated toilet seats; and battery-operated toothbrushes. Household cleaning devices such as long-handled dustpans are also available. Patients who have trouble maneuvering fingers into gloves should wear mittens.

■ ADLs that can be done in a sitting position should be encouraged. Allow the patient enough time to calmly perform these tasks.

■ Provide emotional support. Remember that the patient with chronic illness easily becomes depressed, discouraged, and irritable. Encourage the patient to discuss his fears concerning dependency, sexuality, body image, and self-esteem. Refer him to an appropriate social service agency as needed.

■ Discuss sexual aids: alternative positions, pain medication, and moist heat to increase mobility.

■ Before discharge, make sure the patient knows how and when to take prescribed medication and how to recognize possible adverse effects.

■ Teach the patient how to stand, walk, and sit correctly: upright and erect. Tell him to sit in chairs with high seats and armrests; he'll find it easier to get up from a chair if his knees are lower than his hips. If he doesn't own a chair with a high seat, recommend putting blocks of wood under a favorite chair's legs. Suggest an elevated toilet seat.

■ Mobility aids are very helpful. Many medical and commercial stores offer assistive and supportive devices that promote self-care, including an overhead grasping trapeze to get out of bed, easy-to-open drawers, handheld shower nozzles, handrails, and grab bars.

■ Instruct the patient to pace daily activities, resting for 5 to 10 minutes out of each hour and alternating sitting and standing tasks. Adequate sleep and correct sleeping posture are important. He should sleep on his back on a firm mattress and should avoid placing a pillow under his knees, which encourages flexion deformity.

■ Teach the patient to avoid putting undue stress on joints and to use the largest joint available for a given task, to support weak or painful joints as much as possible, to avoid positions of flexion and promote positions of extension, to hold objects parallel to the knuckles as briefly as possible, to always use his hands toward the center of his body, and to slide — not lift — objects whenever possible. Enlist the aid of the occupational therapist to teach how to simplify activities and protect arthritic joints. Stress the importance of shoes with proper support.

 ELDER TIP *Reinforce safety precautions for elderly patients, such as the removal of throw rugs and the use of handrails and adequate night lighting. Recommend a step stool for elderly patients who need to reach in overhead cupboards. Suggest that the patient purchase medication without safety caps, if available, because these caps can be difficult to open. Medication administration should be designed to follow a standard regimen that fits with the patient's lifestyle.*

■ Refer the patient to the Arthritis Foundation for more information on coping with the disease.

Juvenile rheumatoid arthritis

Affecting children younger than age 16, juvenile rheumatoid arthritis (JRA) is an inflammatory disorder of the connective tissues, characterized by joint swelling and pain or tenderness. It may also involve organs such as the skin, heart, lungs, liver, spleen, and eyes, producing extra-articular signs and symptoms.

JRA has three major types: systemic (Still's disease or acute febrile type), polyarticular, and pauciarticular. Depending on the type, this disease can occur as early as age 6 weeks — although rarely before 6 months — with peaks of onset between ages 1 and 3, and 8 and 12.

The prognosis for JRA is generally good, although disabilities can occur. Long periods of spontaneous remission are common. Improvement or remission may occur at puberty.

Causes and incidence

The cause of JRA remains puzzling. Research continues to test several theories, such as those linking the disease to genetic factors or to an abnormal immune response. Viral or bacterial (particularly streptococcal) infection, trauma, and emotional stress may be precipitating factors, but their relationship to JRA remains unclear.

Considered the major chronic rheumatic disorder of childhood, JRA affects an estimated 150,000 to 250,000 children in the United States; overall incidence is twice as high in females, with variation among the types of JRA.

Signs and symptoms

Signs and symptoms vary with the type of JRA. Affecting males and females almost equally, *systemic JRA* accounts for approximately 10% to 30% of cases. The affected children may have mild, transient arthritis or frank polyarthritis associated with fever and rash. Joint involvement may not be evident at first, but the child's behavior may clearly suggest joint pain. Such a child may constantly want to sit in a flexed position, may not walk much, or may refuse to walk at all. Young children with JRA are noticeably irritable and listless.

Fever in systemic JRA occurs suddenly and spikes to 103° F (39.4° C) or higher once or twice daily, usually in the late afternoon, then rapidly returns to normal or subnormal. (This "sawtooth" or intermittent spiking fever pattern helps differentiate JRA from other inflammatory disorders.) When fever spikes, an evanescent rheumatoid rash commonly appears, consisting of small pale or salmon pink macules, usually on the trunk and proximal extremities and occasionally on the face, palms, and soles. Massaging or applying heat intensifies this rash. It's usually most conspicuous where the skin has been rubbed or subjected to pressure such as the areas of skin covered by underclothing.

Other signs and symptoms of systemic JRA may include hepatosplenomegaly, lymphadenopathy, pleuritis, pericarditis, myocarditis, and nonspecific abdominal pain.

Polyarticular JRA accounts for about 40% of cases and is three times more common in females than in males; affected children may be seronegative or seropositive for rheumatoid factor (RF). It involves five or more joints and usually develops insidiously. Most commonly involved joints are the wrists, elbows, knees, ankles, and small joints of the hands and feet. Polyarticular JRA can also affect larger joints, including the temporomandibular joints, cervical spine, hips, and shoulders. These joints become swollen, tender, and stiff. Usually, the arthritis is symmetrical; it may be remittent or indolent. The patient may run a low-grade fever with daily peaks. Listlessness and weight loss can occur, possibly with lymphadenopathy and hepatosplenomegaly. Other signs of polyarticular JRA include subcutaneous nodules on the elbows or heels and noticeable developmental retardation.

Seropositive polyarticular JRA, the more severe type, usually occurs late in childhood and can cause destructive arthritis that mimics adult rheumatoid arthritis.

Pauciarticular JRA involves few joints (usually no more than four), typically affecting the knees and other large joints. This form accounts for 45% of cases and has major subtypes. The first, pauciarticular JRA with chronic iridocyclitis, most commonly strikes females younger than age 6 and involves the knees, elbows, ankles, or iris. Inflammation of the iris and ciliary body is commonly asymptomatic but may produce pain, redness, blurred vision, and photophobia.

The second subtype, pauciarticular JRA with sacroiliitis, usually strikes males (9:1) older than age 8, who tend to test positive for human leukocyte antigen (HLA)-B27. This subtype is characterized by lower extremity arthritis that produces hip, sacroiliac, heel, and foot pain as well as Achilles' tendinitis. These patients may later develop the sacroiliac and lumbar arthritis characteristic of ankylosing spondylitis. Some also experience acute iritis, but not as many as those with the first subtype.

The third subtype includes patients with joint involvement who are antinuclear antibody (ANA) and HLA-B27 negative and don't develop iritis. These patients have a better prognosis than those with the first or second subtype.

Common to all types of JRA is joint stiffness in the morning or after periods of inactivity. Back pain and limited range of motion is common. Growth disturbances may also occur, resulting in uneven length of arms or legs due to overgrowth or undergrowth adjacent to inflamed joints.

Diagnosis

Persistent joint pain and the rash and fever clearly point to JRA. Laboratory tests are useful for ruling out other inflammatory or even malignant diseases that can mimic JRA. Disease activity and response to therapy can also be monitored through laboratory results.

- Complete blood count shows decreased hemoglobin levels, neutrophilia, and thrombocytosis.
- Erythrocyte sedimentation rate and C-reactive protein, haptoglobin, immunoglobulin, and C3 complement levels may be elevated.
- ANA test may be positive in patients who have pauciarticular JRA with chronic iridocyclitis.
- RF is present in 15% of JRA cases, compared with 85% of rheumatoid arthritis cases.
- Positive HLA-B27 antigens may forecast later development of ankylosing spondylitis.
- X-rays in early stages reveal changes, including soft-tissue swelling, effusion, and periostitis in affected joints. Later, osteoporosis and accelerated bone growth may appear, followed by subchondral erosions, joint space narrowing, bone destruction, and fusion.

Treatment

Successful management of JRA usually involves administration of anti-inflammatory drugs, physical therapy, carefully planned nutrition and exercise, and regular eye examinations. Both child and parents must be involved in therapy.

Aspirin is the initial drug of choice, with dosage based on the child's weight. However, other nonsteroidal anti-inflammatory drugs (NSAIDs) may also be used. If these prove ineffective, gold salts, hydroxychloroquine, and penicillamine may be tried. Because of adverse effects, steroids are generally reserved for treatment of systemic complications, such as pericarditis or iritis, that are resistant to NSAIDs. Corticosteroids and mydriatic drugs are commonly used for iridocyclitis. Low-dose cytotoxic drug therapy is currently being investigated. (See *Drug therapy for arthritis*, pages 367 and 368.)

Physical therapy promotes regular exercise to maintain joint mobility and muscle strength, thereby preventing contractures, deformity, and disability. Good posture, gait training, and joint protection are also beneficial. Splints help reduce pain, prevent contractures, and maintain correct joint alignment.

Surgery is usually limited to soft-tissue releases to improve joint mobility. Joint replacement is delayed until the child has matured physically and can handle vigorous rehabilitation. (See *When arthritis requires surgery*, page 369.)

Special considerations

- Parents and health care professionals should encourage the child to be as independent as possible and to develop a positive attitude toward school, social development, and vocational planning.
- Regular slit-lamp examinations help ensure early diagnosis and treatment of iridocyclitis. Children with pauciarticular JRA with chronic iridocyclitis should be checked every 3 months during periods of active disease and every 6 months during remissions.

Psoriatic arthritis

Psoriatic arthritis is a rheumatoid-like joint disease associated with psoriasis of nearby skin and nails. Although the arthritis component of this syndrome may be clinically indistinguishable from rheumatoid arthritis, the rheumatoid nodules are absent, and serologic tests for rheumatoid factor are negative. Psoriatic arthritis is usually mild, with intermittent flare-ups, but in rare cases may progress to crippling arthritis mutilans. This disease affects males and females equally; onset usually occurs between ages 30 and 35.

Causes

Evidence suggests that predisposition to psoriatic arthritis is hereditary; 20% to 50% of patients are human leukocyte antigen-B27 positive. However, onset is usually precipitated by streptococcal infection or trauma.

About 5% to 7% of patients with psoriasis develop psoriatic arthritis. It occurs in up to 1% of the general population.

Signs and symptoms

Psoriatic lesions usually precede the arthritic component; however, after the full syndrome is established, joint and skin lesions recur simultaneously. Arthritis may involve one joint or several joints symmetrically. Spinal involvement occurs in some patients. Peripheral joint involvement is most common in the distal interphalangeal joints of the hands, which have a characteristic sausage-like appearance. Nail changes include pitting, transverse ridges, onycholysis, keratosis, yellowing, and destruction. The patient may experience general malaise, fever, and eye involvement.

Diagnosis

Inflammatory arthritis in a patient with psoriatic skin lesions suggests psoriatic arthritis.

 CONFIRMING DIAGNOSIS
X-rays confirm joint involvement and show:

- *erosion of terminal phalangeal tufts*
- *"whittling" of the distal end of the terminal phalanges*
- *"pencil-in-cup" deformity of the distal interphalangeal joints*
- *relative absence of osteoporosis*
- *sacroiliitis*
- *atypical spondylitis with syndesmophyte formation. Hyperostosis and paravertebral ossification result, which may lead to vertebral fusion.*

Blood studies indicate negative rheumatoid factor and elevated erythrocyte sedimentation rate and uric acid levels.

Treatment

In mild psoriatic arthritis, treatment is supportive and consists of immobilization through bed rest or splints, isometric exercises, paraffin baths, heat therapy, and aspirin and other nonsteroidal anti-inflammatory drugs. Some patients respond well to low-dose systemic corticosteroids; topical steroids may help control skin lesions. Gold salts and, most commonly, methotrexate therapy are effective in treating both the articular and cutaneous effects of psoriatic arthritis. Antimalarials are contraindicated because they can provoke exfoliative dermatitis.

Special considerations

- Explain the disease and its treatment to the patient and his family.
- Encourage exercise, particularly swimming, to maintain strength and range of motion.
- Teach the patient how to apply skin care products and medications correctly; explain possible adverse effects.
- Stress the importance of adequate rest and protection of affected joints.
- Encourage regular, moderate exposure to the sun.
- Refer the patient to the Arthritis Foundation for self-help and support groups.

Ankylosing spondylitis

A chronic, usually progressive inflammatory disease, ankylosing spondylitis primarily affects the sacroiliac, apophyseal, and costovertebral joints, along with adjacent soft tissue. The disease (also known as rheumatoid spondylitis and Marie-Strümpell disease) usually begins in the sacroiliac joints and gradually progresses to the spine's lumbar, thoracic, and cervical regions. Deterioration of bone and cartilage can lead to fibrous tissue formation with eventual fusion of the spine or peripheral joints.

Ankylosing spondylitis may be equally prevalent in both sexes. Progressive disease is well recognized in men, but the diagnosis is commonly overlooked or missed in females, who tend to have more peripheral joint involvement.

Causes and incidence

Evidence strongly suggests a familial tendency in ankylosing spondylitis. The presence of human leukocyte antigen (HLA)-B27 (positive in more than 90% of patients with this disease) and circulating immune complexes suggests immunologic activity.

One out of 10,000 people has ankylosing spondylitis. It affects more males than females and usually emerges between ages 20 and 40, although it may develop in children younger than age 10.

Signs and symptoms

The first indication of ankylosing spondylitis is intermittent low back pain that's usually most severe in the morning or after a period of inactivity. Other signs and symptoms depend on the disease stage and may include:

- hip deformity and associated limited range of motion
- kyphosis in advanced stages, caused by chronic stooping to relieve symptoms
- mild fatigue, fever, anorexia, or weight loss; occasional iritis; aortic insufficiency and cardiomegaly; and upper lobe pulmonary fibrosis (mimics tuberculosis)
- pain and limited expansion of the chest due to involvement of the costovertebral joints
- peripheral arthritis involving shoulders, hips, and knees
- stiffness and limited motion of the lumbar spine
- tenderness over the inflammation site.

These signs and symptoms progress unpredictably, and the disease can go into remission, exacerbation, or arrest at any stage.

Diagnosis

Typical symptoms, family history, and the presence of HLA-B27 strongly suggest ankylosing spondylitis.

 CONFIRMING DIAGNOSIS
Confirmation requires these characteristic X-ray findings:
- *blurring of the bony margins of joints in the early stage*
- *bilateral sacroiliac involvement*
- *patchy sclerosis with superficial bony erosions*
- *eventual squaring of vertebral bodies*
- *bamboo spine with complete ankylosis.*

Erythrocyte sedimentation rate and alkaline phosphatase and serum immunoglobulin A levels may be elevated. A negative rheumatoid factor helps rule out rheumatoid arthritis, which produces similar symptoms.

Treatment

No treatment reliably stops progression of this disease, so management aims to delay further deformity through good posture, stretching and deep-breathing exercises and, in some patients, braces and lightweight supports. Anti-inflammatory analgesics, such as aspirin, indomethacin, sulfasalazine, and sulindac, control pain and inflammation.

Tumor necrosis factor inhibitors have been shown to improve symptoms. Corticosteroid therapy or medication to suppress the immune system may be prescribed to control various symptoms. Cytotoxic drugs that block cell growth have been used in patients who don't respond well to corticosteroids or those who are dependent on high doses of corticosteroids.

Severe hip involvement usually necessitates surgical hip replacement. Severe spinal involvement may require a spinal wedge osteotomy to separate and reposition the vertebrae. This surgery is performed only on selected patients because of the risk of spinal cord damage and the long convalescence involved.

Special considerations

Ankylosing spondylitis can be an extremely painful and crippling disease, so your main responsibility is to promote the patient's comfort. When dealing with such a patient, keep in mind that limited range of motion makes simple tasks difficult. Offer support and reassurance.

- Administer medications as ordered. Apply local heat and provide massage to relieve pain. Assess mobility and degree of discomfort frequently. Teach and assist with daily exercises as needed to maintain strength and function. Stress the importance of maintaining good posture.
- If treatment includes surgery, provide good postoperative nursing care. Because ankylosing spondylitis is a chronic, pro-

gressively crippling condition, a comprehensive treatment plan should also reflect counsel from a social worker, visiting nurse, and dietitian.

■ To minimize deformities, advise the patient to:
– avoid any physical activity that places undue stress on the back such as lifting heavy objects
– stand upright; to sit upright in a high, straight chair; and to avoid leaning over a desk
– sleep in a prone position on a hard mattress and to avoid using pillows under neck or knees
– avoid prolonged walking, standing, sitting, or driving
– perform regular stretching and deep-breathing exercises and to swim regularly, if possible
– have height measured every 3 to 4 months to detect any tendency toward kyphosis
– seek vocational counseling if work requires standing or prolonged sitting at a desk
– contact the local Arthritis Foundation chapter for a support group.

Sjögren's syndrome

The second most common autoimmune rheumatic disorder after rheumatoid arthritis (RA), Sjögren's syndrome is characterized by diminished lacrimal and salivary gland secretion (sicca complex). Sjögren's syndrome may be a primary disorder or it may be associated with connective tissue disorders, such as RA, scleroderma, systemic lupus erythematosus, and polymyositis. In some patients, the disorder is limited to the exocrine glands (glandular Sjögren's syndrome); in others, it also involves other organs, such as the lungs and kidneys (extraglandular Sjögren's syndrome).

Causes and incidence
The cause of Sjögren's syndrome is unknown, but genetic and environmental factors probably contribute to its development. Viral or bacterial infection or perhaps exposure to pollen may trigger Sjögren's syndrome in a genetically susceptible individual. Tissue damage results from infiltration by lymphocytes or from the deposition of immune complexes. Lymphocytic infiltration may be classified as benign, malignant, or pseudolymphoma (nonmalignant, but tumorlike aggregates of lymphoid cells).

This syndrome occurs mainly in females (90% of patients); mean age of onset is 40 to 50.

Signs and symptoms
About 50% of patients with Sjögren's syndrome have confirmed RA and a history of slowly developing sicca complex. However, some patients seek medical help for rapidly progressive and severe oral and ocular dryness, in many cases accompanied by periodic parotid gland enlargement. Ocular dryness (xerophthalmia) leads to foreign body sensation (gritty, sandy eye), redness, burning, photosensitivity, eye fatigue, itching, and mucoid discharge. The patient may also complain of a film across his field of vision.

Oral dryness (xerostomia) leads to difficulty swallowing and talking; abnormal taste or smell sensation or both; thirst; ulcers of the tongue, buccal mucosa, and lips (especially at the corners of the mouth); and severe dental caries. Dryness of the respiratory tract leads to epistaxis, hoarseness, chronic nonproductive cough, recurrent otitis media, and increased incidence of respiratory infections.

Other effects may include dyspareunia and pruritus (associated with vaginal dryness), generalized itching, fatigue, recurrent low-grade fever, and arthralgia or myalgia. Lymph node enlargement may be the first sign of malignant lymphoma or pseudolymphoma.

Specific extraglandular findings in Sjögren's syndrome include interstitial pneumonitis; interstitial nephritis, which results in renal tubular acidosis in 25% of patients; Raynaud's phenomenon (20%); and vasculitis, usually limited to the skin and characterized by palpable purpura on the legs (20%). About 50% of patients show evidence of hypothyroidism related to autoimmune thyroid disease. A few patients develop systemic necrotizing vasculitis.

Diagnosis

Diagnosis of Sjögren's syndrome rests on the detection of two of the following three conditions: xerophthalmia, xerostomia (with salivary gland biopsy showing lymphocytic infiltration), and an associated autoimmune or lymphoproliferative disorder. Diagnosis must rule out other causes of oral and ocular dryness, including sarcoidosis, endocrine disorders, anxiety or depression, and effects of therapy such as radiation to the head and neck. More than 200 commonly used drugs also produce dry mouth as an adverse effect. In patients with salivary gland enlargement and severe lymphoid infiltration, diagnosis must rule out cancer.

Laboratory values include elevated erythrocyte sedimentation rate in most patients, mild anemia and leukopenia in 30%, and hypergammaglobulinemia in 50%. Autoantibodies are also common, including anti-Sjögren's syndrome-A (anti-Ro) and anti-Sjögren's syndrome-B (anti-La), which are antinuclear and antisalivary duct antibodies. From 75% to 90% of patients test positive for rheumatoid factor; 90%, for antinuclear antibodies.

Other tests help support this diagnosis. Schirmer's tearing test and slit-lamp examination with rose bengal dye are used to measure eye involvement. Salivary gland involvement is evaluated by measuring the volume of parotid saliva and by secretory sialography and salivary scintigraphy. Lower-lip biopsy shows salivary gland infiltration by lymphocytes.

Treatment

Treatment is usually symptomatic and includes conservative measures to relieve ocular or oral dryness. Mouth dryness can be relieved by using a methylcellulose swab or spray and by drinking plenty of fluids, especially at mealtime. Meticulous oral hygiene is essential, including regular flossing, brushing, at-home fluoride treatment, and frequent dental checkups.

Instill artificial tears as often as every half hour to prevent eye damage (corneal ulcerations and corneal opacifications) from insufficient tear secretions. Some patients may also benefit from instillation of an eye ointment at bedtime or from twice-a-day use of sustained-release cellulose capsules (Lacrisert). If infection develops, antibiotics should be given immediately; topical steroids should be avoided. Other treatment measures vary with associated extraglandular findings. Parotid gland enlargement requires local heat and analgesics. Pulmonary and renal interstitial disease necessitate corticosteroid use. Accompanying lymphoma is treated with a combination of chemotherapy, surgery, or radiation.

Special considerations

- Stress the need to humidify home and work environments to help relieve respiratory dryness.
- Advise the patient to avoid drugs that decrease saliva production, such as atropine derivatives, antihistamines, anticholinergics, and antidepressants.
- If mouth lesions make eating painful, suggest high-protein, high-calorie liquid supplements to prevent malnutrition.
- Advise the patient to avoid sugar, which contributes to dental caries. Tobacco; alcohol; and spicy, salty, or highly acidic foods, which cause mouth irritation, should also be avoided.
- Suggest normal saline solution drops or aerosolized spray for nasal dryness.
- Advise the patient to avoid prolonged hot showers and baths and to use moisturizing lotions to help ease dry skin. Suggest K-Y lubricating jelly as a vaginal lubricant.
- Suggest the use of sunglasses to protect the patient's eyes from dust, wind, and strong light. Moisture chamber spectacles may also be helpful. Because dry eyes are more susceptible to infection, advise the patient to keep his face clean and to avoid rubbing his eyes.
- Refer the patient to the Sjögren's Syndrome Foundation for additional information and support.

Lupus erythematosus

A chronic inflammatory disorder of the connective tissues, lupus erythematosus appears in two forms. *Discoid lupus erythematosus* affects only the skin. (See *Discoid lupus erythematosus.*) *Systemic lupus ery-*

DISCOID LUPUS ERYTHEMATOSUS

Discoid lupus erythematosus (DLE) is a form of lupus erythematosus marked by chronic skin eruptions that, if untreated, can lead to scarring and permanent disfigurement. About 1 of 20 patients with DLE later develops systemic lupus erythematosus (SLE). The exact cause of DLE is unknown, but some evidence suggests an autoimmune defect. An estimated 60% of patients with DLE are women in their late 20s or older. This disease is rare in children.

DLE lesions are raised, red, scaling plaques, with follicular plugging and central atrophy. The raised edges and sunken centers give them a coinlike appearance. Although these lesions can appear anywhere on the body, they usually erupt on the face, scalp, ears, neck, and arms or on any part of the body that's exposed to sunlight. Such lesions can resolve completely or may cause hypopigmentation or hyperpigmentation, atro-

phy, and scarring. Facial plaques sometimes assume the butterfly pattern characteristic of SLE. Hair tends to become brittle or may fall out in patches.

As a rule, patient history and the appearance of the rash itself are diagnostic. Lupus erythematosus cell test is positive in fewer than 10% of patients. Skin biopsy of lesions reveals immunoglobulins or complement components. SLE must be ruled out.

Patients with DLE should avoid prolonged exposure to the sun, fluorescent lighting, or reflected sunlight. They should wear protective clothing, use sunscreening agents, avoid engaging in outdoor activities during periods of most intense sunlight (between 10 a.m. and 2 p.m.), and report any changes in the lesions. Drug treatment consists of topical, intralesional, or systemic medication, as in SLE.

---

thematosus (SLE) affects multiple organ systems as well as the skin and can be fatal. Like rheumatoid arthritis, SLE is characterized by recurring remissions and exacerbations, especially common during the spring and summer. The prognosis improves with early detection and treatment, but remains poor for patients who develop cardiovascular, renal, or neurologic complications or severe bacterial infections.

Causes and incidence
The exact cause of SLE remains a mystery, but evidence points to interrelated immunologic, environmental, hormonal, and genetic factors. Autoimmunity is thought to be the prime causative mechanism. In autoimmunity, the body produces antibodies against its own cells such as the antinuclear antibody. The formed antigen-antibody complexes can suppress the body's normal immunity and damage tissues. Patients with SLE produce antibodies against many different tissue components, such as red

blood cells (RBCs), neutrophils, platelets, lymphocytes, or almost any organ or tissue in the body.

Certain predisposing factors may make a person susceptible to SLE. Physical or mental stress, streptococcal or viral infections, exposure to sunlight or ultraviolet light, immunization, pregnancy, and abnormal estrogen metabolism may all affect this disease's development.

SLE may also be triggered or aggravated by treatment with certain drugs — for example, procainamide, hydralazine, anticonvulsants and, less commonly, penicillins, sulfa drugs, and hormonal contraceptives.

SLE strikes 8 times more females than men, increasing to 15 times more during childbearing years. It occurs worldwide but is most prevalent among Asians and Blacks.

Signs and symptoms
The onset of SLE may be acute or insidious and produces no characteristic clinical pat-

BUTTERFLY RASH

In the classic butterfly rash, lesions appear on the cheeks and the bridge of the nose, creating a characteristic butterfly pattern. The rash may vary in severity from malar erythema to discoid lesions (plaque).

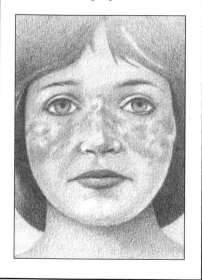

and nontender), abdominal pain, nausea, vomiting, diarrhea, and constipation may occur. Females may experience irregular menstrual periods or amenorrhea during the active phase of SLE.

About 50% of SLE patients develop signs of cardiopulmonary abnormalities, such as pleuritis, pericarditis, and dyspnea. Myocarditis, endocarditis, tachycardia, parenchymal infiltrates, and pneumonitis may occur. Renal effects may include hematuria, proteinuria, urine sediment, and cellular casts, which may progress to total kidney failure. Urinary tract infections may result from heightened susceptibility to infection. Seizure disorders and mental dysfunction may indicate neurologic damage. Central nervous system (CNS) involvement may produce emotional instability, psychosis, and organic mental syndrome. Headaches, irritability, and depression are common. (See *Signs of systemic lupus erythematosus.*)

Diagnosis

Diagnostic tests for patients with SLE include a complete blood count with differential (for signs of anemia and decreased white blood cell [WBC] count); platelet count (may be decreased); erythrocyte sedimentation rate (commonly elevated); and serum electrophoresis (may show hypergammaglobulinemia).

Specific tests for SLE include:

■ antinuclear antibody panel, including anti-deoxyribonucleic acid (DNA) and anti-Smith antibodies — generally positive for lupus alone. (Because the anti-DNA test is rarely positive in other conditions, it's the most specific test for SLE. However, if the patient is in remission, anti-DNA may be reduced or absent [correlates with disease activity, especially renal involvement, and helps monitor response to therapy]. Other tests may be performed as needed to rule out other disorders.)

■ urine studies — may show RBCs and WBCs, urine casts and sediment, and significant protein loss (more than 0.5 g/24 hours)

■ blood studies — decreased serum complement (C3 and C4) levels indicate active disease

tern. However, its symptoms commonly include fever, weight loss, malaise, and fatigue as well as rashes and polyarthralgia. SLE may involve every organ system. In 90% of patients, joint involvement is similar to that in rheumatoid arthritis. Skin lesions are most commonly erythematous rashes in areas exposed to light. The classic butterfly rash over the nose and cheeks occurs in fewer than 50% of the patients. (See *Butterfly rash.*) Ultraviolet rays often provoke or aggravate skin eruptions. Vasculitis can develop (especially in the digits), possibly leading to infarctive lesions, necrotic leg ulcers, or digital gangrene. Raynaud's phenomenon appears in about 20% of patients. Patchy alopecia and painless ulcers of the mucous membranes are common.

Constitutional symptoms of SLE include aching, malaise, fatigue, low-grade or spiking fever, chills, anorexia, and weight loss. Lymph node enlargement (diffuse or local,

- chest X-ray—may show pleurisy or lupus pneumonitis
- electrocardiogram—may show conduction defect with cardiac involvement or pericarditis
- kidney biopsy—determines disease stage and extent of renal involvement.

Some patients show a positive lupus anticoagulant test and a positive anticardiolipin test. Such patients are prone to antiphospholipid syndrome (thrombosis and thrombocytopenia).

Treatment

Patients with mild disease require little or no medication. Nonsteroidal anti-inflammatory drugs, including aspirin, control arthritis symptoms in many patients. Skin lesions need topical treatment. Corticosteroid creams are recommended for acute lesions.

Refractory skin lesions are treated with intralesional corticosteroids or antimalarials such as hydroxychloroquine. Because hydroxychloroquine can cause retinal damage, such treatment requires ophthalmologic examination every 6 months.

Corticosteroids remain the treatment of choice for systemic symptoms of SLE, for acute generalized exacerbations, or for serious disease related to vital organ systems, such as pleuritis, pericarditis, lupus nephritis, vasculitis, and CNS involvement. Initial doses equivalent to 60 mg or more of prednisone often bring noticeable improvement within 48 hours. As soon as symptoms are under control, steroid dosage is tapered slowly. (Rising serum complement levels and decreasing anti-DNA titers indicate patient response.) Diffuse proliferative glomerulonephritis, a major complication of SLE, requires treatment with large doses of steroids. If renal failure occurs, dialysis or kidney transplant may be necessary. In some patients, cytotoxic drugs may delay or prevent deteriorating renal status. Antihypertensive drugs and dietary changes may also be warranted in renal disease.

The photosensitive patient should wear protective clothing (hat, sunglasses, long sleeves, and slacks) and use a screening agent, with a sun protection factor of at least 15, when outdoors. Because SLE usually strikes females of childbearing age,

---

SIGNS OF SYSTEMIC LUPUS ERYTHEMATOSUS

Diagnosing systemic lupus erythematosus (SLE) is difficult because SLE commonly mimics other diseases; symptoms may be vague and vary greatly from patient to patient.

The revised criteria for SLE must include four or more of the following signs:

- abnormal titer of antinuclear antibody
- hemolytic disorder
- malar rash
- discoid rash
- arthritis
- oral ulcerations
- photosensitivity
- serositis
- renal disorder
- neurologic disorder
- immunologic disorder.

---

questions about pregnancy commonly arise. Available evidence indicates that a woman with SLE can have a safe, successful pregnancy if she has no serious renal or neurologic impairment.

Special considerations

Careful assessment, supportive measures, emotional support, and patient education are all important parts of the care plan for patients with SLE.

- Watch for constitutional symptoms: joint pain or stiffness, weakness, fever, fatigue, and chills. Observe for dyspnea, chest pain, and any edema of the extremities. Note the size, type, and location of skin lesions. Check urine for hematuria, scalp for hair loss, and skin and mucous membranes for petechiae, bleeding, ulceration, pallor, and bruising.
- Provide a balanced diet. Renal involvement may mandate a low-sodium, low-protein diet.
- Urge the patient to get plenty of rest. Schedule diagnostic tests and procedures to allow adequate rest. Explain all tests and

procedures. Tell the patient that several blood samples are needed initially, then periodically, to monitor progress.

- Apply heat packs to relieve joint pain and stiffness. Encourage regular exercise to maintain full range of motion (ROM) and prevent contractures. Teach ROM exercises as well as body alignment and postural techniques. Arrange for physical therapy and occupational counseling as appropriate.
- Explain the expected benefit of prescribed medications. Watch for adverse effects, especially when the patient is taking high doses of corticosteroids.
- Advise the patient receiving cyclophosphamide to maintain adequate hydration. If prescribed, give mesna to prevent hemorrhagic cystitis and ondansetron to prevent nausea and vomiting.
- Monitor vital signs, intake and output, weight, and laboratory reports. Check pulse rates and observe for orthopnea. Check stools and GI secretions for blood.
- Observe for hypertension, weight gain, and other signs of renal involvement.
- Assess for signs of neurologic damage: personality change, paranoid or psychotic behavior, ptosis, or diplopia. Take seizure precautions. If Raynaud's phenomenon is present, warm and protect the patient's hands and feet.
- Offer cosmetic tips such as suggesting the use of hypoallergenic makeup and refer the patient to a hairdresser who specializes in scalp disorders.
- Advise the patient to purchase medications in quantity, if possible. Warn against "miracle" drugs for relief of arthritis symptoms.
- Refer the patient to the Lupus Foundation of America and the Arthritis Foundation as needed.

Goodpasture's syndrome

In Goodpasture's syndrome, hemoptysis and rapidly progressive glomerulonephritis follow the deposition of antibody against the alveolar and glomerular basement membrane (GBM). The prognosis improves with aggressive immunosuppressive and antibiotic therapy along with dialysis or renal transplantation.

Causes and incidence

The cause of Goodpasture's syndrome is unknown. Although some cases have been associated with exposure to hydrocarbons or type 2 influenza, many have no precipitating events. The high incidence of human leukocyte antigen DRW2 in these patients suggests a genetic predisposition. Abnormal production and deposition of antibody against GBM and alveolar basement membrane activate the complement and inflammatory responses, resulting in glomerular and alveolar tissue damage.

This syndrome may occur at any age but is most common in males between ages 20 and 30. A second peak incidence occurs between ages 50 and 70, with males and females in this age group affected equally.

Signs and symptoms

Goodpasture's syndrome may initially cause malaise, fatigue, and pallor associated with severe iron deficiency anemia. Pulmonary findings range from slight dyspnea and cough with blood-tinged sputum to hemoptysis and frank pulmonary hemorrhage. Subclinical pulmonary bleeding may precede overt hemorrhage and renal disease by months or years. Usually, renal findings are subtler, although some patients note hematuria and peripheral edema.

Diagnosis

Confirmation of Goodpasture's syndrome requires measurement of circulating anti-GBM antibody by radioimmunoassay and linear staining of GBM and alveolar basement membrane by immunofluorescence.

Immunofluorescence of alveolar basement membrane shows linear deposition of immunoglobulin as well as complement 3 and fibrinogen. Immunofluorescence of GBM also shows linear deposition of immunoglobulin combined with detection of circulating anti-GBM antibody. This finding distinguishes Goodpasture's from other pulmonary-renal syndromes, such as Wegener's granulomatosis, polyarteritis, and systemic lupus erythematosus.

A lung biopsy reveals interstitial and intra-alveolar hemorrhage with hemosiderin-laden macrophages. Chest X-ray reveals pulmonary infiltrates in a diffuse, nodular pattern, and renal biopsy commonly shows focal necrotic lesions and cellular crescents. Creatinine and blood urea nitrogen (BUN) levels typically increase two to three times normal. Urinalysis may reveal red blood cells and cellular casts, which typify glomerular inflammation. Granular casts and proteinuria may also be observed.

Treatment

Treatment aims to remove antibody by plasmapheresis and to suppress antibody production with immunosuppressive drugs, such as cyclophosphamide, to stop attacks by immune cells on the kidneys and lungs. Patients with renal failure may benefit from dialysis or transplantation. Aggressive ultrafiltration helps relieve pulmonary edema that may aggravate pulmonary hemorrhage. High-dose I.V. steroids also help control pulmonary hemorrhage.

Special considerations

■ Promote adequate oxygenation by elevating the bed's head and administering humidified oxygen. Encourage the patient to conserve his energy. Assess respirations and breath sounds regularly; note sputum quantity and quality.

■ Monitor vital signs, arterial blood gases, hematocrit, and coagulation studies.

■ Transfuse blood and administer steroids as ordered. Observe closely for drug adverse effects.

■ Assess renal function by monitoring symptoms, intake and output, daily weights, creatinine clearance, and BUN and creatinine levels.

■ Tell the patient and his family what signs and symptoms to expect and how to relieve them. Carefully describe other treatment measures such as dialysis.

Reiter's syndrome

A self-limiting syndrome associated with polyarthritis (dominant feature), urethritis, balanitis (inflammation of the glans penis), conjunctivitis, and mucocutaneous lesions, Reiter's syndrome appears to be related to infection, either venereal or enteric.

Causes and incidence

The cause of Reiter's syndrome is unknown, but most cases follow venereal or enteric infection. Because 75% to 85% of patients with Reiter's syndrome test positive for the human leukocyte antigen (HLA)-B27, genetic susceptibility is likely. Reiter's syndrome has followed infections caused by *Campylobacter*, *Salmonella*, *Yersinia*, and *Chlamydia* organisms.

This disease usually affects young males (ages 20 to 40); it's rare in females and children. However, due to the uncertainty of diagnosis and variations in the definition of this disorder, incidence is estimated at approximately 3.5 per 100,000 people. About 1% to 3% of all patients with non-specific urethritis develop an episode of arthritis.

Signs and symptoms

The patient with Reiter's syndrome may complain of dysuria, hematuria, urgent and frequent urination, and mucopurulent penile discharge, with swelling and reddening of the urethral meatus. Small painless ulcers may erupt on the glans penis (balanitis). These coalesce to form irregular patches that cover the penis and scrotum. He may also experience suprapubic pain, fever, anorexia with weight loss, and other genitourinary (GU) complications, such as prostatitis and hemorrhagic cystitis.

Arthritic symptoms usually follow GU or enteric symptoms and last from 2 to 4 months. Asymmetrical and extremely variable polyarticular arthritis is most common, with a tendency to develop in weight-bearing joints of the legs and sometimes in the low back or sacroiliac joints. The arthritis is usually acute, with warm, erythematous, and painful joints, but it may be mild, with minimal synovitis. Muscle wasting is common near affected joints. Fingers and toes may swell and appear sausagelike.

Ocular symptoms include mild bilateral conjunctivitis, possibly complicated by keratitis, iritis, retinitis, or optic neuritis. In severe cases, burning, itching, and profuse mucopurulent discharge are possible.

In 30% of patients, skin lesions (keratoderma blennorrhagicum) develop 4 to 6 weeks after onset of other symptoms and may last for several weeks. These macular to hyperkeratotic lesions commonly resemble those of psoriasis. They usually occur on the palms and soles but can develop anywhere on the trunk, extremities, or scalp. Nails become thick, opaque, and brittle; keratic debris accumulates under the nails. In many patients, painless, transient ulcerations erupt on the buccal mucosa, palate, and tongue.

Diagnosis

Nearly all patients with Reiter's syndrome test positive for HLA-B27 and have an elevated white blood cell (WBC) count and erythrocyte sedimentation rate. Mild anemia may develop. Urethral discharge and synovial fluid contain many WBCs, mostly polymorphonuclear leukocytes. Synovial fluid is high in complement and protein and is grossly purulent. Cultures of discharge and synovial fluid rule out other causes such as gonococci.

During the first few weeks, X-rays are normal and may remain so, but some patients may show osteoporosis in inflamed areas. If inflammation persists, X-rays may show erosions of the small joints, periosteal proliferation (new bone formation) of involved joints, and calcaneal spurs.

Treatment

No specific treatment exists for Reiter's syndrome. Most patients recover in 2 to 16 weeks. About 50% of patients have recurring acute attacks, whereas the rest follow a chronic course, experiencing continued synovitis and sacroiliitis. In acute stages, limited weight bearing or complete bed rest may be necessary.

Any underlying infection should be treated with antibiotics. Arthritis is treated with nonsteroidal anti-inflammatory agents and pain relievers. Local administration of corticosteroids may help relieve persistent inflammation in one joint. Physical therapy includes range-of-motion and strengthening exercises and the use of padded or supportive shoes to prevent

contractures and foot deformities. Therapy to suppress the immune system may be considered in severe cases but is limited due to toxic adverse effects.

Special considerations

- Explain Reiter's syndrome. Discuss the medications and their possible adverse effects. Warn the patient to take medications with meals or milk to prevent GI bleeding.
- Encourage normal daily activity and moderate exercise. Suggest a firm mattress and encourage good posture and body mechanics.
- Arrange for occupational counseling if the patient has severe or chronic joint impairment.

Scleroderma

Scleroderma, a systemic sclerosis that's also known as *progressive systemic sclerosis,* is a diffuse connective tissue disease characterized by fibrotic, degenerative, and occasionally inflammatory changes in skin, blood vessels, synovial membranes, skeletal muscles, and internal organs (especially the esophagus, intestinal tract, thyroid, heart, lungs, and kidneys).

This disease occurs in distinctive forms:
- *CREST syndrome* — a benign form characterized by calcinosis, Raynaud's phenomenon, esophageal dysfunction, sclerodactyly, and telangiectasia
- *diffuse systemic sclerosis* — characterized by generalized skin thickening and invasion of internal organ systems
- *localized scleroderma* — characterized by patchy skin changes with a droplike appearance known as morphea
- *linear scleroderma* — characterized by a band of thickened skin on the face or extremities that severely damages underlying tissues, causing atrophy and deformity (most common in childhood).

Other forms include *chemically induced localized scleroderma, eosinophilia myalgia syndrome* (recently associated with ingestion of L-tryptophan), *toxic oil syndrome* (associated with contaminated oil), and *graft-versus-host disease.*

Causes and incidence

The cause of scleroderma is unknown. Known risk factors include exposure to silica dust and polyvinyl chloride.

Scleroderma affects more females than men, especially between ages 30 and 50. Approximately 30% of patients with scleroderma die within 5 years of onset.

Signs and symptoms

Scleroderma typically begins with Raynaud's phenomenon — blanching, cyanosis, and erythema of the fingers and toes in response to stress or exposure to cold. Progressive phalangeal resorption may shorten the fingers.

Compromised circulation, which results from abnormal thickening of the arterial intima, may cause slowly healing ulcerations on the tips of the fingers or toes that may lead to gangrene. Raynaud's phenomenon may precede scleroderma by months or years.

Later symptoms include pain, stiffness, and finger and joint swelling. Skin thickening produces taut, shiny skin over the entire hand and forearm. Facial skin also becomes tight and inelastic, causing a masklike appearance and "pinching" of the mouth. As tightening progresses, contractures may develop.

GI dysfunction causes frequent reflux, heartburn, dysphagia, and bloating after meals. These symptoms may cause the patient to decrease food intake and lose weight. Other GI effects include abdominal distention, diarrhea, constipation, and malodorous floating stools.

In advanced disease, cardiac and pulmonary fibrosis produce arrhythmias and dyspnea. Renal involvement is usually accompanied by malignant hypertension, the main cause of death.

Diagnosis

Typical cutaneous changes provide the first clue to diagnosis. Results of diagnostic tests include:

■ blood studies — slightly elevated erythrocyte sedimentation rate, positive rheumatoid factor in 25% to 35% of patients, and positive antinuclear antibody test
■ chest X-rays — bilateral basilar pulmonary fibrosis

■ electrocardiogram — possible nonspecific abnormalities related to myocardial fibrosis
■ GI X-rays — distal esophageal hypomotility and stricture, duodenal loop dilation, small-bowel malabsorption pattern, and large diverticula
■ hand X-rays — terminal phalangeal tuft resorption, subcutaneous calcification, and joint space narrowing and erosion
■ pulmonary function studies — decreased diffusion and vital capacity and restrictive lung disease
■ skin biopsy — may show changes consistent with the disease's progress, such as marked thickening of the dermis and occlusive vessel changes
■ urinalysis — proteinuria, microscopic hematuria, and casts (with renal involvement).

Treatment

Currently, no cure exists for scleroderma. Treatment aims to preserve normal body functions and minimize complications. Use of an immunosuppressant such as chlorambucil is a common palliative measure. Corticosteroids and colchicine seem to stabilize symptoms; D-penicillamine may be helpful. Blood platelet levels need to be monitored throughout drug therapy.

Other treatments vary according to symptoms:

■ chronic digital ulcerations — a digital plaster cast to immobilize the area, minimize trauma, and maintain cleanliness; possibly surgical debridement
■ esophagitis with stricture — antacids, cimetidine, periodic esophageal dilation, and a soft, bland diet
■ hand debilitation — physical therapy to maintain function and promote muscle strength, heat therapy to relieve joint stiffness, and patient teaching to make performance of daily activities easier
■ Raynaud's phenomenon — various vasodilators and antihypertensive agents (such as methyldopa or calcium channel blockers), intermittent cervical sympathetic blockade or, rarely, thoracic sympathectomy
■ scleroderma kidney (with malignant hypertension and impending renal failure) — dialysis, antihypertensives, and calcium channel blockers

- small-bowel involvement (diarrhea, pain, malabsorption, and weight loss) — broad-spectrum antibiotics, such as erythromycin or tetracycline, to counteract bacterial overgrowth in the duodenum and jejunum related to hypomotility.

Special considerations

- Assess the patient's motion restrictions, pain, vital signs, intake and output, respiratory function, and daily weight.
- Because of compromised circulation, warn against finger-stick blood tests.
- Remember that air conditioning may aggravate Raynaud's phenomenon.
- Help the patient and his family adjust to the patient's new body image and to the limitations and dependence that these changes cause.
- Teach the patient to avoid fatigue by pacing activities and organizing schedules to include necessary rest.
- Stress to the patient and his family the need to accept the fact that this condition is incurable. Encourage them to express their feelings and help them cope with their fears and frustrations by offering information about the disease, its treatment, and relevant diagnostic tests.
- Whenever possible, let the patient participate in treatment by measuring his own intake and output, planning his own diet, assisting in dialysis, giving himself heat therapy, and doing prescribed exercises.
- Direct the patient to seek out support groups, which can be found in every state. Instruct the patient to call 1-800-722-HOPE or go to www.scleroderma.org (if possible) to determine the closest location.

Vasculitis

Vasculitis includes a broad spectrum of disorders characterized by inflammation and necrosis of blood vessels. Its clinical effects, which reflect tissue ischemia caused by blood flow obstruction, and confirming laboratory procedures depend on the vessels involved. The prognosis is variable. For example, hypersensitivity vasculitis is usually a benign disorder limited to the skin, but more extensive polyarteritis nodosa can be rapidly fatal. Vasculitis can occur at any age, except for mucocutaneous lymph node syndrome, which occurs only during childhood. Vasculitis may be a primary disorder or occur secondary to other disorders, such as rheumatoid arthritis or systemic lupus erythematosus.

Causes

How vascular damage develops in vasculitis isn't well understood. It has been associated with a history of serious infectious disease, such as hepatitis B or bacterial endocarditis, and high-dose antibiotic therapy. Current theory holds that it's initiated by excessive circulating antigen, which triggers the formation of soluble antigen-antibody complexes. These complexes can't be effectively cleared by the reticuloendothelial system, so they're deposited in blood vessel walls (type III hypersensitivity). Increased vascular permeability associated with release of vasoactive amines by platelets and basophils enhances such deposition. The deposited complexes activate the complement cascade, resulting in chemotaxis of neutrophils, which release lysosomal enzymes. In turn, these enzymes cause vessel damage and necrosis, which may precipitate thrombosis, occlusion, hemorrhage, and ischemia.

Another mechanism that may contribute to vascular damage is the cell-mediated (T-cell) immune response. In this response, circulating antigen triggers the release of soluble mediators by sensitized lymphocytes, which attracts macrophages. The macrophages release intracellular enzymes, which cause vascular damage. They can also transform into the epithelioid and multinucleated giant cells that typify the granulomatous vasculitides. Phagocytosis of immune complexes by macrophages enhances granuloma formation.

Signs and symptoms

The clinical effects of vasculitis vary according to the blood vessels involved. (See *Types of vasculitis.*)

Diagnosis

Laboratory tests performed to confirm a diagnosis of vasculitis depend on the blood vessels involved. (See *Types of vasculitis.*)

TYPES OF VASCULITIS

Vasculitis occurs in various forms; diagnosis depends on the presenting signs and symptoms.

Type	Vessels involved	Signs and symptoms	Diagnosis
Polyarteritis nodosa	Small to medium arteries throughout the body (Lesions tend to be segmental, occur at bifurcations and branchings of arteries, and spread distally to arterioles. In severe cases, lesions circumferentially involve adjacent veins.)	Hypertension, abdominal pain, myalgias, headache, joint pain, and weakness	History of symptoms; elevated erythrocyte sedimentation rate (ESR); leukocytosis; anemia; thrombocytosis; depressed C3 complement; rheumatoid factor more than 1:60; circulating immune complexes; tissue biopsy showing necrotizing vasculitis
Allergic angiitis and granulomatosis (Churg-Strauss syndrome)	Small to medium arteries (including arterioles, capillaries, and venules), mainly of the lungs but also other organs	Resembles polyarteritis nodosa with hallmark of severe pulmonary involvement	History of asthma; eosinophilia; tissue biopsy showing granulomatous inflammation with eosinophilic infiltration
Polyangiitis overlap syndrome	Small to medium arteries (including arterioles, capillaries, and venules) of the lungs and other organs	Combines symptoms of polyarteritis nodosa, allergic angiitis, and granulomatosis	Possible history of allergy; eosinophilia; tissue biopsy showing granulomatous inflammation with eosinophilic infiltration
Wegener's granulomatosis	Small to medium vessels of the respiratory tract and kidney	Fever, pulmonary congestion, cough, malaise, anorexia, weight loss, and mild to severe hematuria	Tissue biopsy showing necrotizing vasculitis with granulomatous inflammation; leukocytosis; elevated ESR and immunoglobulin (Ig) A and IgG levels; low titer rheumatoid factor; circulating immune complexes; antineutrophil cytoplasmic antibody in more than 90% of patients

(continued)

TYPES OF VASCULITIS *(continued)*

Type	Vessels involved	Signs and symptoms	Diagnosis
Temporal arteritis	Medium to large arteries, most commonly branches of the carotid artery	Fever, myalgia, jaw claudication, visual changes, and headache (associated with polymyalgia rheumatica syndrome)	Decreased hemoglobin (Hb) level; elevated ESR; tissue biopsy showing panarteritis with infiltration of mononuclear cells, giant cells within vessel wall, fragmentation of internal elastic lamina, and proliferation of intima
Takayasu's arteritis (aortic arch syndrome)	Medium to large arteries, particularly the aortic arch, its branches and, possibly, the pulmonary artery	Malaise, pallor, nausea, night sweats, arthralgias, anorexia, weight loss, pain or paresthesia distal to affected area, bruits, loss of distal pulses, syncope and, if a carotid artery is involved, diplopia and transient blindness; may progress to heart failure or stroke	Decreased Hb level; leukocytosis; positive lupus erythematosus cell preparation and elevated ESR; arteriography showing calcification and obstruction of affected vessels; tissue biopsy showing inflammation of adventitia and intima of vessels, and thickening of vessel walls
Hypersensitivity vasculitis	Small vessels, especially of the skin	Palpable purpura, papules, nodules, vesicles, bullae, ulcers, or chronic or recurrent urticaria	History of exposure to antigen, such as a microorganism or drug; tissue biopsy showing leukocytoclastic angiitis, usually in postcapillary venules, with infiltration of polymorphonuclear leukocytes, fibrinoid necrosis, and extravasation of erythrocytes
Mucocutaneous lymph node syndrome (Kawasaki disease)	Small to medium vessels, primarily of the lymph nodes; may progress to involve coronary arteries	Fever; nonsuppurative cervical adenitis; edema; congested conjunctivae; erythema of oral cavity, lips, and palms; and desquamation of fingertips; may progress to arthritis, myocarditis, pericarditis, myocardial infarction, and cardiomegaly	History of symptoms; elevated ESR; tissue biopsy showing intimal proliferation and infiltration of vessel walls with mononuclear cells; echocardiography necessary

TYPES OF VASCULITIS *(continued)*

Type	Vessels involved	Signs and symptoms	Diagnosis
Behçet's disease	Small vessels, primarily of the mouth and genitalia, but also of the eyes, skin, joints, GI tract, and central nervous system	Recurrent oral ulcers, eye lesions, genital lesions, and cutaneous lesions	History of symptoms
Necrotizing vasculitis	Any blood vessel	Red to purple papule skin lesions, pain, infarction, joint pain, numbness, weakness, fever, fatigue, dysmenorrhea, pyrosis, dysphonia, and dysphagia	History of symptoms, muscle biopsy, chest X-ray, and sedimentation rate

Treatment

Treatment of vasculitis aims to minimize irreversible tissue damage associated with ischemia. In primary vasculitis, treatment may involve removal of an offending antigen or use of anti-inflammatory or immunosuppressant drugs. For example, antigenic drugs, food, and other environmental substances should be identified and eliminated, if possible.

Drug therapy in primary vasculitis commonly involves low-dose cyclophosphamide (2 mg/kg orally daily) with daily corticosteroids. In rapidly fulminant vasculitis, cyclophosphamide dosage may be increased to 4 mg/kg daily for the first 2 to 3 days, followed by the regular dose. Prednisone should be given in a dose of 1 mg/kg/day in divided doses for 7 to 10 days, with consolidation to a single morning dose by 2 to 3 weeks. When the vasculitis appears to be in remission or when prescribed cytotoxic drugs take full effect, corticosteroids are tapered down to a single daily dose. Finally, an alternate-day schedule of steroids may continue for 3 to 6 months before slow discontinuation of steroids.

In secondary vasculitis, treatment focuses on the underlying disorder.

Special considerations

■ Assess patients with Wegener's granulomatosis for dry nasal mucosa. Instill nose drops to lubricate the mucosa and help diminish crusting, or irrigate the nasal passages with warm normal saline solution.
■ Monitor vital signs. Use a Doppler ultrasonic flowmeter, if available, to auscultate blood pressure in patients with Takayasu's arteritis, whose peripheral pulses are generally difficult to palpate.
■ Monitor intake and output. Check daily for edema. Keep the patient well hydrated (3 L daily) to reduce the risk of hemorrhagic cystitis associated with cyclophosphamide therapy.
■ Provide emotional support to help the patient and his family cope with an altered body image—the result of the disorder or its therapy. (For example, Wegener's granulomatosis may be associated with saddle nose, steroids may cause weight gain, and cyclophosphamide may cause alopecia.)
■ Teach the patient how to recognize drug adverse effects. Monitor the patient's white blood cell count during cyclophosphamide therapy to prevent severe leukopenia.

Polymyositis and dermatomyositis

Diffuse, inflammatory myopathies of unknown cause, polymyositis and dermatomyositis produce symmetrical weakness of striated muscle — primarily proximal muscles of the shoulder and pelvic girdles, neck, and pharynx. In dermatomyositis, such muscle weakness is accompanied by cutaneous involvement. These diseases usually progress slowly, with frequent exacerbations and remissions. They occur in twice as many females as males (except dermatomyositis with malignant tumor, which is most common in males older than age 40).

The prognosis usually worsens with age. Death commonly occurs from associated cancer, respiratory disease, or heart failure or from the adverse effects of drug therapy. On the other hand, 80% to 90% of affected children regain normal function with proper treatment. However, if untreated, childhood dermatomyositis may progress rapidly to disabling contractures and muscle atrophy.

Causes and incidence

Although the cause of polymyositis remains puzzling, researchers believe that it may result from an autoimmune reaction. Presumably, the patient's T cells inappropriately recognize muscle fiber antigens as foreign and attack muscle tissue, causing diffuse or focal muscle fiber degeneration. (Regeneration of new muscle cells then follows, producing remission.) Polymyositis and dermatomyositis may be associated with other disorders, such as allergic reactions; systemic lupus erythematosus (SLE); scleroderma; rheumatoid arthritis; Sjögren's syndrome; carcinomas of the lung, breast, or other organs; systemic viral infection; or D-penicillamine administration.

Annual incidence is 1 in 100,000 people.

Signs and symptoms

Polymyositis begins acutely or insidiously with muscle weakness, tenderness, and discomfort. It affects proximal muscles more than distal muscles and impairs performance of ordinary activities. The patient may have trouble getting up from a chair, combing his hair, reaching into a high cupboard, climbing stairs, or even raising his head from a pillow. Other muscular symptoms include inability to move against resistance, proximal dysphagia, dysphonia, and difficulty breathing.

In dermatomyositis, an erythematous rash usually erupts on the face, neck, upper back, chest, and arms as well as around the nail beds. A characteristic heliotropic rash appears on the eyelids, accompanied by periorbital edema. Gottron's papules (violet, flat-topped lesions) may appear on the interphalangeal joints.

Diagnosis

CONFIRMING DIAGNOSIS

Diagnosis requires a muscle biopsy that shows necrosis, degeneration, regeneration, and interstitial chronic lymphocytic infiltration. Magnetic resonance imaging and an electrocardiogram, as well as the use of electromyography, aid in diagnosis.

Other tests differentiate polymyositis from diseases that cause similar muscular or cutaneous symptoms, such as muscular dystrophy, advanced trichinosis, psoriasis, seborrheic dermatitis, and SLE.

Typical laboratory results in polymyositis include elevated erythrocyte sedimentation rate, elevated white blood cell count, and elevated muscle enzyme levels (creatine kinase, aldolase, and serum aspartate aminotransferase) not attributable to hemolysis of red blood cells or hepatic or other diseases. Other laboratory results include increased urine creatine level (more than 150 mg/24 hours), decreased creatinine level, and positive antinuclear antibodies. Electromyography shows polyphasic short-duration potentials, fibrillation (positive spike waves), and bizarre high-frequency repetitive changes.

Treatment

High-dose corticosteroid therapy relieves inflammation and lowers muscle enzyme levels. Within 2 to 6 weeks after treatment, serum muscle enzyme levels usually return to normal, and muscle strength improves, permitting a gradual tapering down of corticosteroid dosage. If the patient responds poorly to corticosteroids, treatment may include cytotoxic or immunosuppressant drugs. Supportive therapy includes bed rest during the acute phase, range-of-motion (ROM) exercises to prevent contractures, analgesics and application of heat to relieve painful muscle spasms, and diphenhydramine to relieve itching. Patients older than age 40 need thorough assessment for coexisting cancer.

Special considerations
■ Assess level of pain, muscle weakness, and ROM daily. Give analgesics as needed.
■ If the patient is confined to bed, prevent pressure ulcers by giving good skin care. To prevent footdrop and contractures, apply high-topped sneakers, and assist with passive ROM exercises at least four times daily. Teach the patient's family how to perform these exercises on the patient.
■ If 24-hour urine collection for creatine or creatinine is necessary, make sure your coworkers understand the procedure. When you assist with muscle biopsy, make sure the biopsy isn't taken from an area of recent needle insertion.
■ If the patient has a rash, warn him not to scratch, as it may cause infection. If antipruritic medication doesn't relieve severe itching, apply tepid sponges or compresses.
■ Encourage the patient to feed and dress himself to the best of his ability but to ask for help when needed. Advise him to pace his activities to counteract muscle weakness. Encourage him to express his anxiety. Ease his fear of dependence by reassuring him that muscle weakness is probably temporary.
■ Explain the disease to the patient and his family. Prepare them for diagnostic procedures and possible adverse effects of corticosteroid therapy (weight gain, hirsutism, hypertension, edema, amenorrhea, purplish striae, glycosuria, acne, and easy bruising). Advise a low-sodium diet to prevent fluid retention. Emphatically warn against abruptly discontinuing corticosteroids. Reassure the patient that steroid-induced weight gain will diminish when the drug is discontinued.

IMMUNODEFICIENCY

X-linked infantile hypogammaglobulinemia

X-linked infantile hypogammaglobulinemia is a recessive, congenital disorder in which all five immunoglobulins (Ig) — IgM, IgG, IgA, IgD, and IgE — and circulating B cells are absent or deficient but T cells are intact. It's also called *Bruton's agammaglobulinemia* and *X-linked agammaglobulinemia*. Affecting males almost exclusively, this disorder causes severe, recurrent infections during infancy. Prognosis is good with early treatment, except in infants who develop polio or persistent viral infection. Infection usually causes some permanent damage, especially in the neurologic or respiratory system.

Causes and incidence
In this disease, B cells and B-cell precursors may be present in the bone marrow and peripheral blood, but a mutation in the B-cell protein tyrosine kinase causes failure of the B cells to mature and to secrete immunoglobulin. In the absence of protective immunoglobulins, the affected individual develops repeated infections. Worldwide, malnutrition is the primary cause of antibody disorders.

Humoral immune deficiencies account for 50% of all primary immunodeficiencies. IgA deficiency is the most common antibody deficiency symdrome, followed by common variable immunodeficiency (CVID). The incidence of these two disorders is 1 in 700 persons. Selective IgM deficiency is rare. IgG4 deficiency occurs in 10% to 15% of the population.

Signs and symptoms
Typically, the infant with X-linked hypogammaglobulinemia is asymptomatic until age 6 months, when transplacental maternal immunoglobulins that provided immunity have been depleted. He then develops recurrent bacterial otitis media, pneumonia, dermatitis, bronchitis, and meningitis — usually caused by pneumococci, streptococci, *Haemophilus influ-*

enzae, or other gram-negative organisms. Purulent conjunctivitis, abnormal dental caries, and polyarthritis resembling rheumatoid arthritis may also occur. Severe malabsorption associated with infestation by *Giardia lamblia* may retard development. Despite recurrent infections, lymphadenopathy and splenomegaly are usually absent.

Diagnosis
Diagnosis of X-linked hypogammaglobulinemia can be especially difficult because recurrent infections are common even in normal infants (many of whom don't start producing their own antibodies until age 18 to 20 months). Immunoelectrophoresis and quantitative immunoglobulins (nephelometry) confirm decreased levels, or a total absence, of IgM, IgA, and IgG in the serum. IgG is usually less than 200 mg/dl, and IgA and IgM are almost unmeasurable. However, diagnosis by this method usually isn't possible until the infant is 9 months old. Antigenic stimulation confirms an inability to produce specific antibodies, although cellular immunity remains intact.

Treatment
Treatment aims to prevent or control infections and to boost the patient's immune response. Injection of immune serum globulin (gamma globulin, IV Ig) helps maintain immune response. Because these injections are painful, give them deep into a large muscle mass, such as the gluteal or thigh muscles, and massage well. If the dosage is more than 1.5 ml, divide it and inject it into more than one site; for frequent injections, rotate the injection sites. Because immune globulin is composed primarily of IgG, the patient may also need fresh frozen plasma infusions to provide IgA and IgM. Mucosal secretory IgA can't be replaced by therapy, resulting in crippling pulmonary disease in many patients.

Judicious use of antibiotics also helps combat infection; in some cases, chronic broad-spectrum antibiotics may be indicated. During acute infection, monitor the patient closely. Maintain adequate nutrition and hydration. Perform chest physiotherapy if required.

Special considerations
■ Carefully explain all treatment measures, and make sure the patient and his family understand the disorder.

■ Teach the patient and his family how to recognize early signs of infection and counsel them to report such signs promptly. Advise them to have cuts and scrapes cleaned immediately. Warn them to avoid crowds and people who have active infections.

■ Suggest genetic counseling if parents have questions about vulnerability of future offspring.

Common variable immunodeficiency

Common variable immunodeficiency is characterized by progressive deterioration of B-cell (humoral) immunity, resulting in increased susceptibility to infection. Unlike X-linked hypogammaglobulinemia, this disorder (also known as acquired hypogammaglobulinemia or agammaglobulinemia with immunoglobulin [Ig]-bearing B cells) usually causes symptoms after infancy and childhood, between ages 25 and 40. It affects males and females equally and usually doesn't interfere with normal life span or normal pregnancy and offspring.

Causes
The cause of common variable immunodeficiency is unknown. Most patients have a normal circulating B-cell count but defective synthesis or release of immunoglobulins. Many also exhibit progressive deterioration of T-cell (cell-mediated) immunity revealed by delayed hypersensitivity skin testing.

Signs and symptoms
In common variable immunodeficiency, pyogenic bacterial infections are characteristic but tend to be chronic rather than acute (as in X-linked hypogammaglobulinemia). Recurrent sinopulmonary infections, chronic bacterial conjunctivitis, and malabsorption (commonly associated with infestation by *Giardia lamblia*) are usually the first clues to immunodeficiency.

Common variable immunodeficiency may be associated with autoimmune diseases, such as systemic lupus erythematosus, rheumatoid arthritis, hemolytic anemia, and pernicious anemia, and with cancers, such as leukemia and lymphoma.

Diagnosis

Characteristic diagnostic markers in this disorder are decreased serum IgM, IgA, and IgG levels detected by immunoelectrophoresis, along with a normal circulating B-cell count. Antigenic stimulation confirms an inability to produce specific antibodies; cell-mediated immunity may be intact or delayed. X-rays usually show signs of chronic lung disease or sinusitis.

Treatment

Treatment and care of patients with common variable immunodeficiency are essentially the same as for those with X-linked hypogammaglobulinemia.

Injection of immune globulin (usually weekly to monthly) helps maintain the immune response. Because these injections are painful, give them deep into a large muscle mass, such as the gluteal or thigh muscles, and massage well. If the dosage is more than 1.5 ml, divide the dose and inject it into more than one site; for frequent injections, rotate the injection sites. Because immune globulin is composed primarily of IgG, the patient may also need fresh frozen plasma infusions to provide IgA and IgM.

Antibiotics are the mainstay for combating infection. Regular X-rays and pulmonary function studies help monitor lung infection; chest physiotherapy may be ordered to forestall or help clear such infection.

Special considerations

■ Teach the patient and his family how to recognize early signs of infection and counsel them to report such signs promptly. Advise the patient to avoid crowds and people who have active infections.
■ Stress the importance of good nutrition and regular follow-up care.

IgA deficiency

Total absence or severe deficiency of immunoglobulin (Ig) A, also known as *Janeway Type 3 dysgammaglobulinemia,* is the most common primary immunoglobulin deficiency, appearing in as many as 1 in 400 to 1,000 people. IgA—the major immunoglobulin in human saliva, nasal and bronchial fluids, and intestinal secretions—guards against bacterial and viral reinfections. Consequently, IgA deficiency leads to chronic sinopulmonary infections, allergies, chronic diarrhea, GI diseases, and other disorders. The prognosis is good for patients who receive correct treatment, especially if they have no associated disorders.

Causes

IgA deficiency seems to be linked to autosomal dominant or recessive inheritance. The disorder has familial trends and occurs frequently in immediate relatives of individuals with common variable immunodeficiency. The presence of normal numbers of peripheral blood lymphocytes carrying IgA receptors and of normal amounts of other immunoglobulins suggests that B cells may not be secreting IgA, as they haven't matured into IgA-producing plasma cells. Congenital intrauterine infection with rubella, toxoplasmosis, or cytomegalovirus can result in selective IgA deficiency. Treatment for seizures with phenytoin and hydantoin, as well as Wilson disease (an inherited disorder treated with penicillamine), can result in temporarily acquired selective IgA deficiency. When the medications are stopped, the IgA level returns to normal. Some drugs such as anticonvulsants may cause transient IgA deficiency.

Signs and symptoms

Some IgA-deficient patients have no symptoms, possibly because they have extra amounts of low-molecular-weight IgM. This immunoglobulin takes over IgA function and helps maintain immunologic defenses. Among patients who develop symptoms, chronic sinopulmonary infection is the most common. Other effects are respiratory allergy, often triggered by infection;

GI tract diseases, such as celiac disease, ulcerative colitis, and regional enteritis; autoimmune diseases, such as rheumatoid arthritis, systemic lupus erythematosus, immunohemolytic anemia, and chronic hepatitis; and malignant tumors, such as squamous cell carcinoma of the lungs, reticulum cell sarcoma, and thymoma.

Age of onset varies. Some IgA-deficient children with recurrent respiratory disease and middle ear inflammation may begin to synthesize IgA spontaneously as recurrent infections subside and their condition improves.

Diagnosis

Serum immunoelectrophoresis and quantitative immunologic analyses of patients with IgA-deficiency show serum IgA levels below 7 mg/dl. Although IgA is usually absent from secretions in patients with IgA-deficiency, levels may be normal in rare cases. IgE is normal, whereas IgM may be normal or elevated in serum and secretions. Normally absent low-molecular-weight IgM may be present.

Tests may also indicate autoantibodies and antibodies against IgG (rheumatoid factor), IgM, and bovine milk. Cell-mediated immunity and secretory piece (the glycopeptide that transports IgA) are usually normal, and most circulating B cells appear normal.

Treatment

Selective IgA deficiency has no known cure. Treatment aims to control symptoms of associated diseases, such as respiratory and GI infections, and is generally the same as for a patient with normal IgA.

 ALERT *Don't give an IgA-deficient patient immune globulin (IV Ig) because sensitization may lead to anaphylaxis during future administration of blood products.*

If transfusion with blood products is necessary, minimize the risk of adverse reaction by using washed red blood cells or avoid the reaction completely by crossmatching the patient's blood with that of an IgA-deficient donor.

Special considerations

Because this is a lifelong disorder, teach the patient to prevent infection, to recognize its early signs, and to seek treatment promptly.

DiGeorge syndrome

DiGeorge syndrome, also called *congenital thymic hypoplasia or aplasia,* is a disorder characterized by the partial or total absence of cell-mediated immunity that results from a deficiency of T lymphocytes. It typically produces life-threatening hypocalcemia that may be associated with cardiovascular and facial anomalies. Patients seldom live beyond age 2 without a fetal thymus transplant; the prognosis improves when this transplant, correction of hypocalcemia, and repair of cardiac anomalies are possible.

Causes

DiGeorge syndrome is probably caused by abnormal fetal development (12th week of gestation) of the third and fourth pharyngeal pouches, which interferes with thymus formation. As a result, the thymus is completely absent or partially present in an abnormal location, causing deficient T cell-mediated immunity. (See *Role of the thymus in immune response.*) This syndrome has been associated with maternal alcoholism and resultant fetal alcohol syndrome.

Signs and symptoms

Symptoms are usually obvious at birth or shortly thereafter. An infant with DiGeorge syndrome may have low-set prominent ears, notched ear pinnae, a mouth without the usual bow-shaped lip, an undersized jaw, and abnormally wide-set eyes (hypertelorism) that are low-set and posteriorly angulated. Additionally, an infant may have a bifid uvula and a high, arched palate. Congenital heart anomalies are common. Cardiovascular abnormalities include great blood vessel anomalies (these may also develop soon after birth) and tetralogy of Fallot.

An infant with thymic hypoplasia (rather than aplasia) may experience a spontaneous return of cell-mediated immunity but can develop severe T-cell deficiencies later in life. This allows exaggerated susceptibility to viral, fungal, or bacterial infections, which may be overwhelming. Hypoparathyroidism, usually associated with DiGeorge syndrome, typically causes tetany, hyperphosphatemia, and hypocalcemia. Hypocalcemia (calcium levels less than 7 mg/dl) develops early and is unusually resistant to treatment. It can lead to tetany, seizures, central nervous system damage, and early heart failure.

Rare cases of partial immunoglobulin (Ig) A deficiency have been linked to chromosome 1 and deletions of the IgA1 or IgA2 genes. Alterations in chromosome 6 suggest altered major histocompatibility complex, which is reflected in decreased T-cell responses. Aberrations in chromosome 18 are linked to facial abnormalities, nystagmus, hypotonia, atretic or stenotic ear canals, hearing loss, and mental retardation.

Diagnosis

Immediate diagnosis is difficult unless the infant has typical facial anomalies — normally the first clues to the disorder. A definitive diagnosis depends on successful treatment of hypocalcemia and other life-threatening birth defects during the first few weeks of life. Such diagnosis rests on proof of decreased or absent T lymphocytes (sheep cell test, lymphopenia), partial B-cell immunodeficiency, and of an absent thymus (chest X-ray). Immunoglobulin assays are useless because antibodies present are usually from maternal circulation.

Additional tests showing low serum calcium level, elevated serum phosphorus level, and missing parathyroid hormone confirm hypoparathyroidism.

Treatment

Life-threatening hypocalcemia must be treated immediately, but it's unusually resistant and requires aggressive treatment, for example, with a rapid I.V. infusion of 10% solution of calcium gluconate. During such an infusion, monitor heart rate and watch carefully to avoid infiltration. Remember that calcium supplements *must* be given with vitamin D, or sometimes also with parathyroid hormone, to ensure effective calcium utilization. After hypocalcemia

---

ROLE OF THE THYMUS IN IMMUNE RESPONSE

The thymus provides an environment in which T cells develop and learn to distinguish self from nonself during fetal and early postnatal stages. Most cells that enter the thymus are destroyed. T cell clones that react strongly to self and those that don't recognize self are deleted (negative selection). T-cell clones that recognize self but don't react strongly against self are positively selected.

After early life, mature T cells reside primarily in peripheral lymph organs and recirculate in blood and lymph.

---

is under control, a fetal thymus transplant may restore normal cell-mediated immunity. Cardiac anomalies require surgical repair when possible.

Special considerations

■ Instruct the patient with DiGeorge syndrome to follow a low-phosphorus diet and educate him about measures to prevent infection.

■ Teach the parents of an infant with DiGeorge syndrome to watch for signs of infection and have it treated immediately, to keep the infant away from crowds or any other potential sources of infection, and to provide good hygiene and adequate nutrition and hydration.

■ Advise the parents to schedule and keep regular follow-up visits to the infant's pediatrician.

Acquired immunodeficiency syndrome

Acquired immunodeficiency syndrome (AIDS) is a serious secondary immunodeficiency disorder caused by the human immunodeficiency virus (HIV). Both diseases are characterized by the progressive destruction of cell-mediated (T-cell) immu-

COMMON INFECTIONS AND NEOPLASMS IN HIV AND AIDS

This is a list of commonly seen disorders with human immunodeficiency virus (HIV) and acquired immunodeficiency syndrome (AIDS). AIDS is diagnosed when a patient diagnosed with HIV has a CD4+ T-cell count of less than 200 cells/μl.

- Common infections in a patient with a CD4+ count less than 350 cells/μl include:
  – herpes simplex virus
  – herpes zoster
  – *Mycobacterium tuberculosis*
  – non-Hodgkin's lymphoma
  – oral or vaginal thrush.
- Common infections in a patient with a CD4+ count less than 200 cells/μl include:
  – *Candida esophagitis*
  – *Pneumocystis carinii* pneumonia.
- Common infections in a patient with a CD4+ count less than 100 cells/μl include:
  – AIDS dementia
  – Cryptococcal meningitis
  – progressive multifocal leukoencephalopathy
  – toxoplasmosis encephalitis
  – wasting syndrome.
- Common infections in a patient with a CD4+ count less than 50 cells/μl include:
  – *Cytomegalovirus* infection
  – *Mycobacterium avium.*
- Common neoplasms in patients with HIV and AIDS include:
  – Hodgkin's disease
  – Kaposi's sarcoma
  – malignant lymphoma.

nity with subsequent effects on humoral (B-cell) immunity because of the pivotal role of the CD4+ helper T cells in immune reactions. The resultant immunodeficiency makes the patient susceptible to opportunistic infections, unusual cancers, and other abnormalities. (See *Common infections and neoplasms in HIV and AIDS.*)

The Centers for Disease Control and Prevention (CDC) first described AIDS in 1981. Since then, the CDC has declared a case surveillance definition for AIDS and modified it several times, most recently in January 2000.

Causes and incidence

AIDS results from infection with HIV, which has two forms: HIV-1 and HIV-2. Both forms of HIV have the same modes of transmission and similar opportunistic infections associated with AIDS, but studies indicate that HIV-2 develops more slowly and presents with milder symptoms than HIV-1.

Transmission occurs through contact with infected blood or body fluids and is associated with identifiable high-risk behaviors. It's disproportionately represented in:

- homosexual and bisexual men
- persons who use illicit I.V. drugs
- neonates of infected females
- recipients of contaminated blood or blood products (incidence dramatically decreased since mid-1985)
- heterosexual partners of persons in the former groups.

Signs and symptoms

A person with HIV may remain asymptomatic for months or years. Initially, laboratory evidence or seroconversion to HIV antibodies may be the only clinical evidence of infection. However, as the disease progresses, the patient may develop generalized adenopathy and nonspecific signs and symptoms, such as weight loss, fatigue, night sweats, and fevers. As the patient's T-cell count lowers further, neurologic symptoms, opportunistic infections, and certain normally rare cancers may develop. HIV also destroys lymph nodes and immunologic organs, leading to major dysfunctions of the immunological system. Eventually, HIV advances to AIDS. (Some individuals, termed *nonprogressors,* develop AIDS very slowly or not at all. They seem to have genetic differences that prevent the virus from attaching to certain immune receptors.)

 PEDIATRIC TIP *The clinical course varies slightly in children, who have a shorter incubation time (mean, 17 months.) Signs and symptoms resemble those in adults, except for findings related to sexually transmitted disease (STD). Children show virtually all of the opportunistic infections observed in adults, with a higher incidence of bacterial infections: otitis media, pneumonias other than that caused by* Pneumocystis carinii, *sepsis, chronic salivary gland enlargement, and lymphoid interstitial pneumonia.*

Diagnosis

 CONFIRMING DIAGNOSIS *Signs and symptoms may occur at any time after infection with HIV, but AIDS isn't officially diagnosed until the patient's CD4+ T-cell count falls below 200 cells/µl.*

The most commonly performed tests, antibody tests, indicate HIV infection indirectly by revealing HIV antibodies. The recommended protocol requires initial screening of individuals and blood products with an enzyme-linked immunosorbent assay (ELISA). A positive ELISA should be repeated and then confirmed by an alternate method, usually the Western blot or an immunofluorescence assay. The radioimmunoprecipitation assay is considered more sensitive and specific than the Western blot, but because it requires radioactive materials, it's a poor choice for routine screening. In addition, antibody testing isn't reliable. Because people produce detectable levels of antibodies at different rates — a "window" varying from a few weeks to as long as 35 months in one documented case — an HIV-infected person can test negative for HIV antibodies. Antibody tests are also unreliable in neonates because transferred maternal antibodies persist for 6 to 10 months. To overcome these problems, direct tests are used, including antigen tests (p24 antigen), HIV cultures, nucleic acid probes of peripheral blood lymphocytes, and the polymerase chain reaction. (See *Laboratory tests for diagnosing and tracking HIV and assessing immune status,* page 396.)

Additional tests to support the diagnosis and help evaluate the severity of immunosuppression include CD4+ and CD8+ T-lymphocyte subset counts, erythrocyte sedimentation rate, complete blood cell count, serum beta$_2$-microglobulin, p24 antigen, neopterin levels, and anergy testing. Because many opportunistic infections in AIDS patients are reactivations of previous infections, patients are also tested for associated neoplasms, infections, and STDs.

Treatment

There is no cure for either HIV or AIDS. However, significant advances have been made to help patients control signs and symptoms and impair disease progression. Because HIV can become resistant to any drug, health care professionals use combination treatments and multiple drug regimens to suppress the virus. Patients on medication remain infectious.

An effective method of treatment is highly active antiretroviral therapy (HAART). HAART aims to reduce the number of HIV particles in the blood as measured by viral load, thus increasing T-cell counts and improving the immunologic system's functioning. A regular and vigilant medication regimen is critical or resistance will develop because HIV strains mutate and can become resistant to HAART relatively easily.

The *nucleoside analogues* (sometimes called reverse transcriptase inhibitors) have been the mainstay of AIDS therapy in recent years. These drugs interfere with viral reverse transcriptase, which impairs HIV's ability to turn its ribonucleic acid into deoxyribonucleic acid for insertion into the host cell.

Antiretroviral therapy typically begins when the patient's CD4+ T-cell count drops to less than 500/µl or when the patient develops an opportunistic infection. Most clinicians recommend starting the patient on a combination of these drugs in an attempt to gain the maximum benefit and to inhibit the production of resistant mutant strains of HIV. The drug combinations and dosages are then altered, depending on the patient's response.

LABORATORY TESTS FOR DIAGNOSING AND TRACKING HIV AND ASSESSING IMMUNE STATUS

Test	Findings in HIV infection
HIV antibody tests	
■ Enzyme-linked immunosolvent assay (ELISA)	■ Positive test results must be confirmed by Western blot
■ Western blot	■ Positive
■ Indirect immunofluorescence assay (IFA)	■ Positive test results must be confirmed by Western blot
■ Radioimmunoprecipitation assay (RIPA)	■ Positive, more sensitive and specific than Western blot
■ Home sample collection (dried blood spot, oral mucosa fluid, urine)	■ Findings confirmed with ELISA or Western blot
HIV tracking	
■ P24 antigen	■ Positive for free viral protein
■ Polymerase chain reaction (PCR)	■ Detection of HIV ribonucleic acid (RNA) or DNA
■ Branch deoxyribonucleic acid (bDNA)	■ Detection of HIV RNA
■ Nucleic acid sequence-based amplification (NASBA)	■ Detection of HIV RNA
■ Peripheral blood mononuclear cell (PBMC) culture for HIV-1	■ Positive when two consecutive assays detect reverse transcriptase or p24 antigen in increasing magnitude
■ Quantitative cell culture	■ Measures viral load within cells
■ Quantitative plasma culture	■ Measures viral load by free infectious virus in the plasma
■ β_2 microglobulin	■ Protein is increased with disease progression
■ Serum neopterin	■ Increased levels seen with disease progression
Immune status	
■ Number of CD4+ cells	■ Decreased
■ Percentage of CD4+ cells	■ Decreased
■ CD4+:CD8+ ratio	■ Decreased
■ White blood cell count	■ Normal to decreased
■ Immunoglobulin levels	■ Increased
■ CD4+ cell function tests	■ CD4+ T cells have decreased ability to respond to antigen
■ Skin test sensitivity reaction	■ Decreased to absent

Increasingly, physicians are basing changes in therapy on the patient's viral load rather than on his CD4+ T-cell count. Because the CD4+ count is influenced by the total white blood cell count, changes in the CD4+ count may have nothing to do with changes in the patient's HIV status. Many physicians suggest that patients on antiretroviral therapy have their viral load checked every 3 months.

The increasing use of protease inhibitors (PIs) has greatly increased the life expectancy of patients with AIDS. These drugs block the enzyme protease, which HIV needs to produce virions, the viral particles that spread the virus to other cells. The use of PIs dramatically reduces viral load — sometimes to undetectable levels — while producing a corresponding increase in the CD4+ T-cell count and, because they act at a different site than nucleoside analogues, the PIs don't produce additional adverse effects when added to a patient's regimen.

Antiviral therapy includes the use of multiple combined drug therapies that suppress the replication of the HIV virus in the body. After antiviral therapy is initiated, treatment should be aggressive. Initially, highly active antiviral therapy, consisting of a triple drug therapy regimen—a PI and two non-nucleoside reverse transcriptase inhibitors—is recommended. In addition to these primary treatments, antiinfectives are used to combat opportunistic infections (some are used prophylactically to help patients resist opportunistic infections), and antineoplastic drugs are used to fight associated neoplasms. Supportive treatments help maintain nutritional status and relieve pain and other distressing physical and psychological symptoms.

Special considerations
■ Advise health care workers and the public to use precautions in all situations that risk exposure to blood, body fluids, and secretions. Diligently practicing standard precautions can prevent the inadvertent transmission of AIDS and other infectious diseases that are transmitted by similar routes.
■ Recognize that a diagnosis of AIDS is profoundly distressing because of the disease's social impact and discouraging prognosis. The patient may lose his job and financial security as well as the support of family and friends. Do your best to help him cope with an altered body image, the emotional burden of serious illness, and the threat of death, and encourage and assist the patient in learning about AIDS societies and support programs.

Chronic mucocutaneous candidiasis

Chronic mucocutaneous candidiasis is a form of candidiasis (moniliasis) that usually develops during the first year of life but occasionally occurs as late as the 20s. Affecting males and females, it's characterized by repeated infection with *Candida albicans* that may result from an inherited defect in cell-mediated (T-cell) immunity. (Humoral [B-cell] immunity remains intact and provides a normal antibody response to *C. albicans*.) In some patients, an autoimmune response affecting the endocrine system may induce various endocrinopathies.

Despite chronic candidiasis, these patients seldom die of systemic infection. Instead, they usually die of hepatic or endocrine failure. The prognosis for chronic mucocutaneous candidiasis depends on the severity of the associated endocrinopathy. Patients with associated endocrinopathy seldom live beyond their 30s.

Causes and incidence
No characteristic immunologic defects have been identified in this infection, but many patients have a diminished response to various antigens or to *Candida* alone. In some patients, anergy may result from deficient migration inhibition factor, a mediator normally produced by lymphocytes.

Candida species infections are the most common causes of fungal infections among patients who are immunocompromised. About 3 of every 4 females have at least one bout of vulvovaginal candidiasis during their lifetimes. In individuals who are HIV-positive, more than 90% experience oropharyngeal candidiasis and 10% have at least one episode of esophageal candidiasis.

Signs and symptoms
Chronic candidal infections can affect the skin, mucous membranes, nails, and vagina, usually causing large, circular lesions. These infections seldom produce systemic symptoms but in late stages may be associated with recurrent respiratory tract infections. Other associated conditions include severe viral infections that may precede the onset of endocrinopathy and, sometimes, hepatitis. Involvement of the mouth, nose, and palate may cause speech and eating difficulties.

Symptoms of endocrinopathy are peculiar to the organ involved. Tetany and hypocalcemia are most common and are associated with hypoparathyroidism. Addison's disease, hypothyroidism, diabetes, and pernicious anemia are also connected with chronic mucocutaneous candidiasis. Psychiatric disorders are likely because of disfigurement and multiple endocrine aberrations.

Diagnosis

Laboratory findings usually show a normal circulating T-cell count, although it may be decreased. Skin tests don't usually show delayed hypersensitivity to *Candida,* even during the infectious stage. Migration inhibiting factor that indicates the presence of activated T cells may not respond to *Candida.*

Nonimmunologic abnormalities resulting from endocrinopathy may include hypocalcemia, abnormal hepatic function studies, hyperglycemia, iron deficiency, and abnormal vitamin B_{12} absorption (pernicious anemia). Diagnosis must rule out other immunodeficiency disorders associated with chronic *Candida* infection, especially DiGeorge syndrome, ataxiatelangiectasia, and severe combined immunodeficiency disease, all of which produce severe immunologic defects. After diagnosis, the patient needs evaluation of adrenal, pituitary, thyroid, gonadal, pancreatic, and parathyroid function as well as careful follow-up. The disease is progressive, and most patients eventually develop endocrinopathy.

Treatment

Treatment aims to control infection but isn't always successful. Topical antifungal agents, such as clotrimazole, miconazole, and nystatin, are useful. They may be prescribed as mouthwashes or troches (lozenges) for 5 to 10 days.

Systemic infections may not be fatal, but they're serious enough to warrant vigorous treatment. Ketoconazole and fluconazole have had some positive effect. Oral or I.M. iron replacement may also be necessary. Treatment may also include plastic surgery of the lesions, when possible, and counseling to help patients cope with their disfigurement.

Special considerations

Teach the patient about the disease's progressive manifestations and emphasize the importance of seeing an endocrinologist for regular checkups.

Chronic fatigue syndrome

Sometimes called *chronic Epstein-Barr virus,* or *myalgic encephalomyelitis,* chronic fatigue and immune dysfunction syndrome is typically marked by debilitating fatigue, neurologic abnormalities, and persistent symptoms that suggest chronic mononucleosis. It commonly occurs in adults younger than age 45, primarily in females.

Causes

The cause of chronic fatigue syndrome (CFS) is unknown, but researchers suspect that it may be found in human herpes virus-6 or in other herpesviruses, enteroviruses, or retroviruses. Recent studies have shown that inflammation of nervous system pathways, acting as an immune or autoimmune response, may play a role as well. CFS may also be associated with a reaction to viral illness that's complicated by dysfunctional immune response and by other factors that may include gender, age, genetic disposition, prior illness, stress, and environment.

Signs and symptoms

CFS has specific symptoms and signs, based on the exclusion of other possible causes. Its characteristic symptom is prolonged, often overwhelming fatigue that's commonly associated with a varying complex of other symptoms that are similar to those of many infections, including myalgia and cephalgia. It may develop within a few hours and can last for 6 months or more. Fatigue isn't relieved by rest and is severe enough to restrict activities of daily living by at least 50%. To aid in disease identification, the Centers for Disease Control and Prevention (CDC) uses a "working case definition" to group symptoms and severity.

Diagnosis

Because the cause and nature of CFS are still unknown, no single test unequivocally confirms its presence. Therefore, physicians

CDC CRITERIA FOR DIAGNOSING CHRONIC FATIGUE SYNDROME

To meet the case definition of the Centers for Disease Control and Prevention (CDC), a patient must fulfill 2 major criteria and either 8 of 11 symptom criteria or 6 of the symptom criteria and 2 of 3 physical criteria for chronic fatigue syndrome.

Major criteria
- New onset of persistent or relapsing debilitating fatigue in a person without a history of similar symptoms; fatigue doesn't resolve with bed rest and is severe enough to reduce or impair average daily activity by 50% for 6 months
- Exclusion of other disorders after evaluation through history, physical examination, and laboratory findings

Symptom criteria
Symptom criteria include the initial development of the main symptom complex over a few hours or days, and 10 other symptoms:
- Profound or prolonged fatigue, especially after exercise levels that would have been easily tolerated before
- Low-grade fever
- Painful lymph nodes

- Muscle weakness
- Muscle discomfort or myalgia
- Sleep disturbances (insomnia or hypersomnia)
- Headaches of a new type, severity, or pattern
- Migratory arthralgia without joint swelling or redness
- Photophobia, forgetfulness, irritability, confusion, depression, transient visual scotomata, difficulty thinking, and inability to concentrate

Physical criteria
These criteria must be recorded on at least two occasions, at least 1 month apart:
- Low-grade fever
- Nonexudative pharyngitis
- Palpable or tender nodes

base this diagnosis on the patient's history and the CDC's criteria. (See *CDC criteria for diagnosing chronic fatigue syndrome.*) Because the CDC criteria are admittedly a working concept that may not include all forms of this disease and are based on symptoms that can result from other diseases, diagnosis is difficult and uncertain.

Treatment
No treatment is known to cure CFS. Symptomatic treatment may involve the use of medications to treat depression, anxiety, pain, discomfort, and fever. Hidden yeast infections may be present and should be treated. Antiviral drugs such as acyclovir and selected immunomodulating agents, such as I.V. gamma globulin, ampligen, and transfer factor, may be of assistance.

Special considerations
- Some patients may benefit from avoiding environmental irritants and certain foods.
- Because patients with CFS may benefit from supportive contact with others who share this disease, refer the patient to the CFS Association for information and to local support groups. Patients may also benefit from psychological counseling.

Wiskott-Aldrich syndrome

Also called *immunodeficiency with eczema and thrombocytopenia*, this disease is an X-linked, recessive immunodeficiency disorder characterized by defective B-cell and T-cell functions. Its clinical features include thrombocytopenia with severe bleeding, eczema, recurrent infection, and an increased risk of lymphoid cancers. Symptoms develop in the first year of life. The prognosis is poor. Wiskott-Aldrich syndrome causes early death, usually from massive bleeding during infancy, or from cancer or severe infection in early childhood. The average life span is 4 years; affected children rarely survive to their teens.

Causes and incidence

Because Wiskott-Aldrich syndrome results from an X-linked recessive trait, it affects only males. Children with this genetic defect are born with a normal thymus gland, plasma cells, and lymphoid tissues. However, an inherited defect in both B-cell and T-cell function compromises the child's immune system response and increases his vulnerability to infection. These children also have a metabolic defect in platelet synthesis that causes them to produce only small, short-lived platelets, resulting in thrombocytopenia.

Wiskott-Aldrich syndrome occurs in 4 neonates per 1 million live births.

Signs and symptoms

Characteristically, neonates with Wiskott-Aldrich syndrome develop bloody stools, bleeding from a circumcision site, petechiae, and purpura as a result of thrombocytopenia. As the infants get older, thrombocytopenia subsides. However, beginning at about 6 months, they typically develop recurrent systemic infections, such as chronic pneumonia, sinusitis, otitis media, and herpes simplex of the skin and eyes (which may cause keratitis and vision loss), with hepatosplenomegaly. Usually, *Streptococcus pneumoniae,* meningococci, and *Haemophilus influenzae* are the infecting organisms. Varicella infection can be lethal. At about age 1, eczema develops and becomes progressively more severe; pruritus and persistent scratching commonly lead to skin infections. These children are also highly vulnerable to certain cancers, especially leukemia and lymphoma.

Diagnosis

The most important clues to diagnosis of Wiskott-Aldrich syndrome are thrombocytopenia (demonstrated by coagulation tests showing a platelet count below 100,000/mm^3 and prolonged bleeding time) and bleeding disorders at birth. Laboratory tests may show normal or elevated immunoglobulin (Ig) E and IgA levels, decreased IgM levels, normal IgG levels, and low levels or absence of isohemagglutinins. T-cell immunity may be normal in neonates, but it gradually declines with age.

Treatment

Treatment aims to limit bleeding through the use of fresh, crossmatched platelet transfusions; to prevent or control infection with prophylactic or early and aggressive antibiotic therapy as appropriate; to supply passive immunity with immune globulin infusion; and to control eczema with topical corticosteroids. (Systemic corticosteroids are contraindicated because they further compromise immunity.) An antipruritic may relieve itching.

Treatment with transfer factor has provided some limited success. However, bone marrow transplantation has been remarkably successful in some patients.

Special considerations

■ Provide physical and psychological support and thorough patient education to help children and their families cope with this disorder. As soon as the child is old enough to understand, begin teaching him about his disease and his limitations.

■ Teach the parents of an affected child to watch him for signs of bleeding, such as easy bruising, bloody stools, swollen joints, and tenderness in the trunk area. Help them plan their child's activity levels to ensure normal development. Although the child must avoid contact sports, he's allowed to ride a bike (while wearing protective football gear) and swim.

■ Before giving platelet transfusions, establish the child's baseline platelet count. Be sure to check the platelet count often during therapy; each platelet unit transfused should raise the count by 10,000/mm^3.

■ Instruct parents to observe the child for signs of infection, such as fever, coldlike symptoms, or drainage and redness around any superficial wound. Such signs must be reported promptly. Emphasize the importance of meticulous mouth and skin care (including careful cleaning of all skin wounds, no matter how superficial), good nutrition, and adequate hydration. Stress the need to avoid exposing the child to crowds or to people who have active infections.

■ As appropriate, arrange for the parents of children with Wiskott-Aldrich syndrome to receive genetic counseling to answer any questions they may have about the potential vulnerability of future offspring.

Chronic granulomatous disease

In chronic granulomatous disease (CGD), abnormal neutrophil metabolism impairs phagocytosis — one of the body's chief defense mechanisms — resulting in increased susceptibility to low-virulent or nonpathogenic organisms, such as *Staphylococcus epidermidis, Escherichia coli, Aspergillus,* and *Nocardia.* Phagocytes attracted to sites of infection can engulf these invading organisms but are unable to destroy them. Patients with CGD may develop granulomatous inflammation, which leads to ischemic tissue damage.

Causes
CGD is inherited as a recessive X-linked trait in 50% to 60% of affected patients. Males are more likely to be affected. The genetic defect may be linked to deficiency of the enzyme NADH, NADPH oxidase, or NADH reductase. The inability of phagocytic cells to kill certain bacteria and fungi leads to long-term and repeated infections.

Signs and symptoms
Usually, the patient with CGD displays signs and symptoms associated with infections of the skin, lymph nodes, lung, liver, and bone by age 2. Skin infection is characterized by small, well-localized areas of tenderness. Seborrheic dermatitis of the scalp and axilla is also common. Lymph node infection typically causes marked lymphadenopathy with draining lymph nodes and hepatosplenomegaly. Many patients develop liver abscess, which may be recurrent and multiple; abdominal tenderness, fever,

anorexia, and nausea point to abscess formation. Other common infections include osteomyelitis, which causes localized pain and fever, pneumonia, and gingivitis with severe periodontal disease.

Diagnosis
Clinical features of osteomyelitis, pneumonia, liver abscess, or chronic lymphadenopathy in a young child provide the first clues to CGD diagnosis.

 CONFIRMING DIAGNOSIS *An important tool for confirming this diagnosis is the nitroblue tetrazolium (NBT) test. A clear yellow dye, NBT is normally reduced by neutrophil metabolism, resulting in a color change from yellow to blue. Quantifying this color change estimates the degree of neutrophil metabolism.*

Patients with CGD show impaired NBT reduction, indicating abnormal neutrophil metabolism. Another test measures the rate of intracellular killing by neutrophils; in CGD, killing is delayed or absent.

Other laboratory values may support the diagnosis or help monitor disease activity. Osteomyelitis typically causes elevated white blood cell count and erythrocyte sedimentation rate; bone scans help locate and size such infections. Recurrent liver or lung infection may eventually cause abnormal function studies. Cell-mediated and humoral immunity are usually normal in CGD, although some patients have hypergammaglobulinemia.

Treatment
Early, aggressive treatment of infection is the chief goal in caring for a patient with CGD. Areas of suspected infection should be biopsied or cultured, and broad-spectrum antibiotics are usually started immediately — without waiting for results of cultures. Confirmed abscesses may be drained or surgically removed. Provide meticulous wound care after such treatment, including irrigation or packing.

Many patients with CGD receive a combination of I.V. antibiotics, in many cases extended beyond the usual 10- to 14-day course. However, for fungal infections with *Aspergillus* or *Nocardia,* treatment involves amphotericin B in gradually increasing doses to achieve a maximum cumulative dose. During I.V. drug therapy, monitor vital signs frequently and rotate the I.V. site every 48 to 72 hours.

To help treat antibiotic-resistant or life-threatening infection, or to help localize infection, the patient may receive granulocyte transfusions — usually once daily until the crisis has passed. During such transfusions, watch for fever and chills (these effects can sometimes be prevented by premedication with acetaminophen). Transfusions shouldn't be given for 6 hours before or after amphotericin B to avoid severe pulmonary edema and, possibly, respiratory arrest.

Interferon-gamma may help reduce the number of severe infections. Bone marrow transplantation is also promising.

Special considerations

■ If prophylactic antibiotics are ordered, teach the patient and his family how to administer them properly and how to recognize adverse effects. Advise them to promptly report any signs or symptoms of infection.

■ Stress the importance of good nutrition and hygiene, especially meticulous skin and mouth care.

■ During hospitalizations, encourage the patient to continue his activities of daily living as much as possible.

■ If the patient is a child, arrange for a tutor to help him keep up with his schoolwork.

Severe combined immunodeficiency disease

In severe combined immunodeficiency disease (SCID), both cell-mediated (T-cell) and humoral (B-cell) immunity are deficient or absent, resulting in susceptibility to infection from all classes of microorganisms during infancy. It's the most severe form of T-cell and B-cell deficiency. At least three types of SCID exist: reticular dysgenesis, the most severe type, in which the hematopoietic stem cell fails to differentiate into lymphocytes and granulocytes; Swiss-type agammaglobulinemia, in which the hematopoietic stem cell fails to differ-

entiate into lymphocytes alone; and enzyme deficiency, such as adenosine deaminase (ADA) deficiency, in which the buildup of toxic products in the lymphoid tissue causes damage and subsequent dysfunction.

Causes and incidence

SCID is usually transmitted as an autosomal recessive trait, although it may be X-linked. In most cases, the genetic defect seems associated with failure of the stem cell to differentiate into T and B lymphocytes. Many molecular defects such as mutation of the kinase ZAP-70 can cause SCID. X-linked SCID is due to a mutation of a subunit of the interleukin (IL)-2, IL-4, and IL-7 receptors. Less commonly, it results from an enzyme deficiency.

SCID affects more males than females. Its estimated incidence is 1 in every 100,000 to 500,000 births. Most untreated patients die from infection within 1 year of birth.

Signs and symptoms

An extreme susceptibility to infection becomes obvious in the infant with SCID in the first months of life. The infant fails to thrive and develops chronic otitis; sepsis; watery diarrhea (associated with *Salmonella* or *Escherichia coli*); recurrent pulmonary infections (usually caused by *Pseudomonas,* cytomegalovirus, or *Pneumocystis carinii*); persistent oral candidiasis, sometimes with esophageal erosions; and possibly fatal viral infections such as chickenpox.

P. carinii pneumonia usually strikes a severely immunodeficient infant in the first 3 to 5 weeks of life. Onset is typically insidious, with gradually worsening cough, low-grade fever, tachypnea, and respiratory distress. Chest X-ray characteristically shows bilateral pulmonary infiltrates.

Diagnosis

Diagnosis is generally made clinically because most SCID infants suffer recurrent overwhelming infections within 1 year of birth. Some infants are diagnosed after a severe reaction to vaccination.

Defective humoral immunity is difficult to detect before age 5 months. Before then, even normal infants have very small amounts of serum immunoglobulin (Ig) M and IgA. Normal IgG levels merely reflect maternal IgG.

 CONFIRMING DIAGNOSIS *Severely diminished or absent T-cell number and function, as well as lymph node biopsy showing absence of lymphocytes, can confirm diagnosis of SCID.*

Treatment

Treatment aims to restore the immune response and prevent infection. Histocompatible bone marrow transplantation is the only satisfactory treatment available to correct immunodeficiency. Because bone marrow cells must be human leukocyte antigen and mixed leukocyte culture matched, the most common donors are histocompatible siblings. However, because bone marrow transplant can produce a potentially fatal graft-versus-host (GVH) reaction, newer methods of bone marrow transplant that eliminate GVH reaction (such as lectin separation and the use of monoclonal antibodies) are being evaluated.

Fetal thymus and liver transplants have achieved limited success. Immune globulin administration may also play a role in treatment. Some SCID infants have received long-term protection by being isolated in a completely sterile environment. However, this approach isn't effective if the infant already has had recurring infections.

Gene therapy is being used to treat ADA deficiency.

Special considerations

Patient care is primarily preventive and supportive.

■ Constantly monitor the infant for early signs of infection. If infection develops, provide prompt and aggressive drug therapy as ordered. Watch for adverse effects of any medications given.

■ Avoid vaccinations and give only irradiated blood products if a transfusion is ordered.

■ Although SCID infants must remain in strict protective isolation, try to provide a stimulating atmosphere to promote growth and development. Encourage the parents to visit their child often, to hold him, and to bring him toys that can be easily sterilized. If the parents can't visit, call them of-

ten to report on the infant's condition. Explain all procedures, medications, and precautions to them. Maintain a normal day and night routine for the child and talk to him as much as possible.

■ Because the parents will have questions about the vulnerability of future offspring, refer them for genetic counseling.

■ Arrange for psychological and spiritual support for the parents and siblings to help them cope with the child's inevitable long-term illness and early death.

Complement deficiencies

Complement is a series of circulating enzymatic serum proteins with nine functional components, labeled C1 through C9. (The first four complement components are numbered out of sequence, in order of their discovery — C1, C4, C2, and C3 — but the remaining five are numbered sequentially.) When immunoglobulin (Ig) G or IgM reacts with antigens as part of an immune response, it activates C1, which then combines with C4, initiating the classic complement pathway, or cascade. (An alternative complement pathway involves the direct activation of C3 by the serum protein properdin, bypassing the initial components [C1, C4, and C2] of the classic pathway.) Complement then combines with the antigen-antibody complex and undergoes a sequence of reactions that amplify the immune response against the antigen. This complex process, which is vital to normal immune response, is called *complement fixation;* it's necessary to promote chemotaxis, opsonization, phagocytosis, bacteriolysis, and anaphylaxis reactions.

Complement deficiency or dysfunction may increase susceptibility to infection and also seems related to certain autoimmune disorders. Theoretically, any complement component may be deficient or dysfunctional, and many such disorders are under investigation. Inherited or primary complement deficiencies are rare. The most common are C2, C4, C6, and C8 deficiencies and C5 familial dysfunction. More common secondary complement abnormalities have been confirmed in patients with lupus erythematosus, in some with dermatomyositis, in some with scleroderma, and in a few with gonococcal and meningococcal infections. The prognosis varies with the abnormality and the severity of associated diseases.

Causes and incidence

Primary complement deficiencies are inherited as autosomal recessive traits, except for deficiency of C1 esterase inhibitor, which is autosomal dominant. Secondary deficiencies may follow complement-fixing (complement-consuming) immunologic reactions, such as drug-induced serum sickness, acute streptococcal glomerulonephritis, and acute active systemic lupus erythematosus.

Inherited deficiency is rare in the general population, with an incidence of 0.03%. C2 protein deficiency disorder occurs in 1 in 10,000 persons.

Signs and symptoms

Clinical effects vary with the specific deficiency. C2 and C3 deficiencies and C5 familial dysfunction increase susceptibility to bacterial infection (which may involve several body systems simultaneously). C2 and C4 deficiencies are also associated with collagen vascular disease such as lupus erythematosus and with chronic renal failure. C5 dysfunction, a familial defect in infants, causes failure to thrive, diarrhea, and seborrheic dermatitis. C1 esterase inhibitor deficiency (hereditary angioedema) may cause periodic swelling in the face, hands, abdomen, or throat, with potentially fatal laryngeal edema.

Diagnosis

Diagnosis of a complement deficiency is difficult, requiring careful interpretation of both clinical features and laboratory results. Total serum complement level (CH50) is low in various complement deficiencies. In addition, specific assays may be done to confirm deficiency of specific complement components. For example, detection of complement components and IgG by immunofluorescent examination of glomerular tissues in glomerulonephritis strongly suggests complement deficiency.

Treatment

Primary complement deficiencies have no known cure. Associated infection, collagen vascular disease, or renal disease requires prompt, appropriate treatment. Transfusion of fresh frozen plasma to provide replacement of complement components is controversial because replacement therapy doesn't cure complement deficiencies, and any beneficial effects are transient. A bone marrow transplant may be helpful but can cause a potentially fatal graft-versus-host reaction (GVHR). Anabolic steroids such as danazol and antifibrinolytic agents are often used to reduce acute swelling in patients with C1 esterase inhibitor deficiency.

Special considerations

■ Teach the patient (or his family, if he's a child) the importance of avoiding infection, how to recognize its early signs and symptoms, and the need for prompt treatment if it occurs.
■ After a bone marrow transplant, monitor the patient closely for signs of a transfusion reaction or GVHR.
■ Meticulous patient care can speed recovery and prevent complications. For example, a patient with renal infection needs careful monitoring of intake and output, tests for serum electrolytes and acid-base balance, and observation for signs of renal failure.
■ When caring for a patient with hereditary angioedema, be prepared for emergency management of laryngeal edema; keep airway equipment on hand.

Selected references

Abbas, A.K., and Lichtman, A.H. *Basic Immunology: The Functions of the Immune System*, 2nd ed. Philadelphia: W.B. Saunders Co., 2004.

National Institutes of Health. *Quick Reference: NAEPP Expert Panel Report. Guidelines for the Diagnosis and Management of Asthma. Update on Selected Topics 2002.* NIH Publication No. 02-5075. June 2002. Available at: *www.nhlbi.nih.gov/guidelines/asthma/ execsumm.pdf.*

Ochs, H.D., et al., eds. *Primary Immunodeficiency Disease.* New York: Oxford University Press, 2004.

Porth, C.M. *Pathophysiology: Concepts of Altered Health States*, 6th ed. Philadelphia: Lippincott Williams & Wilkins, 2002.

Stevens, C.D. *Clinical Immunology and Serology: A Laboratory Perspective*, 2nd ed. Philadelphia: F.A. Davis Co., 2003.

Wolf, R., ed. *Essential Pediatric Allergy, Asthma and Immunology*. New York: McGraw-Hill Book Co., 2004.

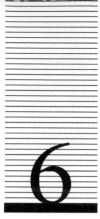

Psychiatric disorders

Introduction *407*

Disorders of infancy, childhood, and adolescence *414*
Mental retardation *414*
Tic disorders *416*
Autistic disorder *418*
Attention deficit hyperactivity disorder *422*
Conduct disorder *424*

Substance-related disorders *426*
Alcohol-related disorder *426*
Substance abuse and induced disorders *431*

Psychotic disorders *439*
Schizophrenia *439*
Delusional disorders *445*

Mood disorders *449*
Bipolar disorders *449*
Major depression *455*

Anxiety disorders *459*
Phobias *459*
Generalized anxiety disorder *461*
Panic disorder *463*
Obsessive-compulsive disorder *465*
Posttraumatic stress disorder *468*

Somatoform disorders *471*
Somatization disorder *471*
Conversion disorder *473*
Pain disorder *475*
Hypochondriasis *476*
Body dysmorphic disorder *478*

Dissociative disorders *479*
Dissociative identity disorder *479*
Dissociative fugue *480*
Dissociative amnesia *481*
Depersonalization disorder *482*
Personality disorders *483*

Eating disorders *490*
Bulimia nervosa *490*
Anorexia nervosa *492*

Sexual and gender identity disorders *495*
Female arousal and orgasmic disorders *495*
Dyspareunia *497*
Vaginismus *498*
Erectile disorder *499*
Premature ejaculation *501*
Gender identity disorders *502*
Paraphilias *503*

Selected references *506*

Introduction

In recent years, a convergence of social, economic, and professional forces has dramatically changed the mental health field. Community and professional organizations, for instance, have established family advocacy programs, substance abuse rehabilitation programs, stress management workshops, bereavement groups, victim assistance programs, and violence shelters. The public education system has established widespread information programs about mental health issues. Mental illness isn't as stigmatizing as it once was. Self-help and coping books have proliferated, and media attention to mental and emotional disorders has increased. Finally, more effective drugs are available to treat many of these illnesses.

Social changes

Today, more people than ever experience mental health problems. Some researchers blame social changes, which have altered the traditional family structure and contributed to the loss of the extended family. The result: more single parents, dysfunctional families, troubled children, and homeless people.

The loss of effective support systems strains a person's ability to cope with even minor problems. For example, a working mother may lack the necessary support to meet the demands of her job, her home, her spouse, and her children. When she views herself as ineffective in these roles, her self-esteem falters and her level of stress intensifies.

Furthermore, alcohol and substance abuse are proliferating and their victims are becoming younger. Up to 7% of adolescents are dependent on alcohol, and 15% to 20% of American teens have experienced a serious episode of depression. Isolation, fear of violent crime, and loneliness have contributed to a similar rise in depression among elderly people. Victims of violence, abuse, and social discord struggle to cope with the trauma they have experienced.

Economic forces

Recent cuts in Federal funding of mental health programs place future control of mental health services in the hands of state and local authorities, drastically reducing the funds available for training and care. One result of decreased funding is increased collaboration between community psychiatric facilities (short-term inpatient, outpatient, and auxiliary services) and long-term inpatient state facilities. Another result is decreased availability of long-term care and reduced length of stay for acute patient care.

Professional changes

Mental health professionals have experienced enormous changes in perspective, focus, and direction, which are reflected in the American Psychiatric Association's *Diagnostic and Statistical Manual of Mental Disorders,* Fourth Edition, Text Revision (*DSM-IV-TR*). With this system of classifying mental disorders, clinicians must consider many aspects of patients' behavior, mental performance, and history, emphasizing observable data rather than subjective and theoretical impressions.

DSM-IV-TR defines a mental disorder as a clinically significant behavioral or psychological syndrome or pattern that's associated with current distress (a painful symptom), disability (impairment in one or more important areas of functioning), or a significantly greater risk of suffering, death, pain, disability, or an important loss of freedom. This syndrome or pattern mustn't be merely an expected response such as grief over the death of a loved one. Whatever its original cause, it must currently be considered a sign of a behavioral, psychological, or biological dysfunction.

To add diagnostic detail, *DSM-IV-TR* uses a multiaxial approach. It specifies that every patient be evaluated on each of these five axes:

■ *Axis I* — clinical disorder, the diagnosis (or diagnoses) that best describes the presenting complaint
■ *Axis II* — personality disorders and mental retardation
■ *Axis III* — general medical conditions, a description of any concurrent medical conditions or disorders

- *Axis IV* — psychosocial and environmental problems
- *Axis V* — global assessment of functioning (GAF), based on a scale of 1 to 100. The GAF scale allows evaluation of the patient's overall psychological, social, and occupational functioning.

The first three axes, which constitute the official diagnostic assessment, encompass the entire spectrum of mental and physical disorders. This system may require multiple diagnoses. For example, on axis I, a patient may have a psychoactive substance abuse disorder and a mood disorder. He may even have multiple diagnoses within the same class, as in major depression superimposed on cyclothymic disorder. A patient also may have a disorder on axes I, II, and III simultaneously.

Axis IV documents the effect of psychosocial and environmental stressors on the patient. Examples of such stressors include marital, familial, interpersonal, occupational, domestic, financial, legal, developmental, and medical concerns as well as environmental factors and natural disasters.

Axis V measures how well the patient has functioned over the past year and includes his current level of functioning.

A patient's diagnosis after being evaluated on these five axes may look like this:

- *Axis I* — adjustment disorder with anxious mood
- *Axis II* — obsessive-compulsive personality
- *Axis III* — Crohn's disease, acute bleeding episode
- *Axis IV* — recent remarriage, death of father
- *Axis V* — GAF = 65 (current).

Related professional forces

An increased emphasis on holistic care has promoted a closer relationship between psychiatry and the rest of medicine. More hospitalized patients benefit from psychiatric consultations, reflecting a growing recognition of the emotional basis of physical disorders. Advances in neurobiology have revolutionized our understanding of the physiologic basis of mental function. The result: better diagnosis and treatment of mental disorders.

Psychosocial assessment

You'll encounter patients with mental and emotional problems in all clinical areas and settings. Begin your care of these patients with a psychosocial assessment.

For this assessment to be effective, you need to establish a therapeutic relationship with the patient that's based on trust. You must communicate to him that his thoughts and behaviors are important. Effective communication involves sending and receiving messages. (See *Communication barriers*.) Words count, as does nonverbal communication — such as eye contact, posture, facial expressions, gestures, clothing, affect, and even silence. All can convey a powerful message.

Choose a quiet, private setting for the assessment interview. Interruptions and distractions threaten confidentiality and interfere with effective listening. If you're meeting the patient for the first time, introduce yourself and explain the interview's purpose. Sit at a comfortable distance from the patient, and give him your undivided attention.

During the interview, adopt a professional but friendly attitude, and maintain eye contact to the level that the patient can tolerate. A calm, nonthreatening tone of voice will encourage the patient to talk more openly. Avoid value judgments. Don't rush through the interview; building a trusting therapeutic relationship takes time.

Patient history

A patient history establishes a baseline and provides clues to the underlying or precipitating cause of the current problem. Remember that the patient may not be a reliable source of information, particularly if he has a mental illness. If possible, verify his responses with family members, friends, or health care personnel. Also check facility records from previous admissions, if possible, and compare his past behavior, symptoms, and circumstances with the current situation.

Explore the patient's chief complaint, current symptoms, psychiatric history, demographic data, socioeconomic data, cultural and religious beliefs, medication history, and physical illnesses.

COMMUNICATION BARRIERS

Ineffective communication can prevent a successful interview.

Language difficulties or differences
If the patient speaks English, try to use language that's appropriate to his educational level and culture. Avoid medical terms that he may not understand.

If the patient speaks a foreign language or an unfamiliar dialect, try to have an interpreter on hand. The presence of a third person, though, may make the patient less willing to share his feelings.

Be aware of words that can have more than one meaning. For instance, the word *bad* also can be used as slang to mean "good."

Inappropriate responses
Your responses to the patient can inadvertently suggest disinterest, anxiety, or annoyance, or they can imply value judgments. Examples include abruptly changing the subject or discounting the patient's feelings.

Hearing loss
If the patient can't hear you clearly, he may misinterpret your responses. If you're interviewing a patient with impaired hearing, check whether he's wearing a hearing aid. If so, is it turned on? If not, can he read lips? If possible, face him and speak clearly and slowly, using common words and keeping your questions short, simple, and direct.

If the patient is elderly, use a low tone of voice. With aging, the ability to hear high-pitched tones deteriorates first. If his hearing impairment is severe, he may have to communicate by writing, or you may need to collect information from his family or friends.

Thought disorders
If the patient's thought patterns are incoherent or irrelevant, he may be unable to interpret messages correctly, focus on

the interview, or provide appropriate responses.

When assessing such a patient, ask simple questions about concrete topics and clarify his responses. Encourage him to express himself clearly.

Paranoid thinking
Deal with a paranoid patient in a nonthreatening way. Avoid touching him because he may misinterpret your touch as an attempt to harm him. Restrict hand motions and maintain physical distance. Accept the patient's statements of paranoid thoughts in a nonjudgmental manner.

Hallucinations
A hallucinating patient experiences imaginary sensory perceptions with no basis in reality. These distortions prevent him from hearing and responding appropriately.

Show concern if the patient is hallucinating, but don't reinforce his perceptions. Be as specific as possible when you give him commands. For instance, if he says he's hearing voices, tell him to stop listening to the voices and to listen to you instead.

Delusions
A deluded patient defends irrational beliefs or ideas despite factual evidence to the contrary. Some delusions may be so bizarre that you'll immediately recognize them; others may be difficult to identify.

Don't condemn or agree with a patient's delusional beliefs and don't dismiss a statement because you think it's delusional. Instead, gently emphasize reality without being argumentative.

Delirium
A delirious patient experiences disorientation, hallucinations, and confusion. Misinterpretation and inappropriate responses commonly result. Talk directly to such a patient and ask simple ques-

(continued)

COMMUNICATION BARRIERS *(continued)*

---

tions. Offer frequent reassurance. Provide protection and appropriate physical care for the underlying cause of the delirium.

Dementia

The patient who suffers dementia — an irreversible deterioration of mental capacity — may experience changes in memory and thought patterns, and his language may become distorted or slurred.

When interviewing such a patient, use simple, concise language and minimize distractions. Don't make statements that he may easily misinterpret. Maintain calm and establish a routine.

■ *Chief complaint.* The patient may not voice his chief complaint directly. Instead, you or others may note that he's having difficulty coping or is exhibiting unusual behavior. If this occurs, determine whether the patient is aware of the problem. When documenting the patient's response, write it verbatim and enclose it in quotation marks.

■ *Current symptoms.* Find out about the onset of symptoms, their severity and persistence, and whether they occurred abruptly or insidiously. Compare the patient's condition with his normal level of functioning.

■ *Psychiatric history.* Discuss past psychiatric disturbances, such as episodes of delusions, violence, depression, attempted suicides, drug or alcohol abuse, and previous psychiatric treatment.

■ *Demographic data.* Determine the patient's age, sex, ethnic origin, primary language, birthplace, religion, and marital status. Use this information to establish a baseline and validate the patient's record.

■ *Socioeconomic data.* Obtain information about the patient's educational level, housing conditions, income, current employment status, and family, because these data may provide clues to his current problem. Determine current stressors from a holistic perspective.

■ *Cultural and religious beliefs.* A patient's background and values affect his response to illness and his adaptation to care. Certain questions and behaviors considered acceptable in one culture may be inappropriate in another. Determine the extent to which the patient may utilize cultural rituals, treatments, and healing practices.

■ *Medication history.* Certain drugs can cause symptoms of mental illness. Review any medications the patient may be taking, including over-the-counter drugs and herbal supplements or remedies, and check for interactions. If he's taking an antipsychotic, antidepressant, anxiolytic, or antimanic drug, ask if his symptoms have improved, if he's taking the medication as prescribed, and if he has had any adverse reactions.

■ *Physical illnesses.* Find out if the patient has a history of medical disorders that may cause distorted thought processes, disorientation, depression, or other symptoms of mental illness. For instance, does he have a history of renal or hepatic failure, infection, thyroid disease, increased intracranial pressure, or a metabolic disorder? Additionally, has the patient suffered recent head trauma, infection, or physical illness?

Patient appearance, behavior, and mental status

Assess the patient's appearance, behavior, mood, thought processes, cognitive function, coping mechanisms, and potential for self-destructive behavior, and record your assessment.

■ *General appearance.* The patient's appearance helps to indicate his emotional and mental status. Specifically, note his dress and grooming. Is his appearance clean and appropriate for his age, sex, and situation?

Is the patient's posture erect or slouched? Is his head lowered? What about his gait? Is it brisk, slow, shuffling, or unsteady? Does he walk normally? Note his facial expression. Does he look alert or does he stare blankly? Does he appear sad or angry? Does the patient maintain direct eye contact? Does he stare at you for long periods?

■ *Behavior.* Note the patient's demeanor and overall attitude as well as any extraordinary behavior such as speaking to a person who isn't present. Also record mannerisms. Does he bite his nails, fidget, or pace? Does he have any tics or tremors? How does he respond to the interviewer? Is he cooperative, friendly, hostile, or indifferent?

Behavior should be evaluated also in light of the patient's culture. For instance, making eye contact is considered respectful and attentive behavior in most Western cultures. However, eye contact may be considered rude and aggressive in several Asian-American and Native American cultures, and avoiding eye contact is considerate and respectful. Blacks may be more actively verbal within their culture group, where oral tradition and multiparty conversations are common. In a traditional medical setting, this patient may be restrained or silent.

■ *Mood.* Does the patient appear excited or depressed? Is he crying, sweating, breathing heavily, or trembling? Ask him to describe his current feelings in concrete terms and to suggest possible reasons for these feelings. Note inconsistencies between body language and mood (such as smiling when discussing an anger-provoking situation).

■ *Thought processes and cognitive function.* Evaluate the patient's orientation to time, place, and person, noting any confusion or disorientation. Look for delusions, hallucinations, obsessions, compulsions, fantasies, and daydreams.

Assess the patient's attention span and ability to recall events in the distant and recent past. For example, to assess immediate recall, ask him to repeat a series of five or six names of objects. Test his intellectual functioning by asking him to add a series of numbers and his sensory perception and

COPING MECHANISMS DEFINED

Coping, or defense, mechanisms help to relieve anxiety. Common ones include:

■ *denial* — avoiding the awareness of truth or reality
■ *displacement* — shifting of an emotion from its original object to a substitute
■ *fantasy* — creation of unrealistic or improbable images to escape from daily pressures and responsibilities
■ *identification* — unconscious adoption of the personality characteristics, attitudes, values, and behavior of another person
■ *projection* — displacement of negative feelings onto another person
■ *rationalization* — substitution of acceptable reasons for the real or actual reasons motivating behavior
■ *reaction formation* — conduct in a manner opposite from the way the person feels
■ *regression* — return to behavior of an earlier, less worrisome time in life
■ *repression* — exclusion of unacceptable thoughts and feelings from the conscious mind, leaving them to operate in the subconscious.

coordination by having him copy a simple drawing. Inappropriate responses to a hypothetical situation ("What would you do if you won the lottery?") can indicate impaired judgment. Keep in mind that the patient's cultural background and personal values will influence his answer.

Note speech characteristics that may indicate altered thought processes, including monosyllabic responses; irrelevant or illogical replies to questions; convoluted or excessively detailed speech; repetitious, accelerated, or slowed speech patterns; flight of ideas; and sudden silence with an obvious reason.

SUICIDE'S WARNING SIGNS

- Withdrawal and social isolation
- Signs and symptoms of depression, which may include crying, fatigue, sadness, helplessness, poor concentration, reduced interest in sex and other activities, constipation, and weight loss
- Farewells to friends and family
- Putting affairs in order
- Giving away prized possessions
- Covert suicide messages and death wishes
- Obvious suicide messages ("I'd be better off dead.")

Finally, assess the patient's insight by asking if he understands the significance of his illness, the plan of treatment, and the effect it will have on his life.
- *Coping mechanisms.* The patient who's faced with a stressful situation will utilize coping, or defense, mechanisms — behaviors that operate on an unconscious level to protect the ego. Examples include denial, regression, displacement, projection, reaction formation, and fantasy. Look for an excessive reliance on these coping mechanisms. (See *Coping mechanisms defined,* page 411.)
- *Potential for self-destructive behavior.* Mentally healthy people may intentionally take death-defying risks such as participating in dangerous sports. The risks taken by self-destructive patients, however, aren't death-defying but rather death-seeking.

Not all self-destructive behavior is suicidal in intent. The patient may engage in self-destructive behavior because it helps him feel alive. A patient who has lost touch with reality may cut or mutilate body parts to focus on physical pain, which may be less overwhelming than emotional distress.

Assess patients for suicidal tendencies, particularly if they report signs and symptoms of depression. (See *Suicide's warning signs.*) Not all such patients want to die; however, the incidence of suicide is higher in depressed patients than in patients with other diagnoses.

Diagnostic tests

The laboratory tests, psychological tests, and EEG and brain imaging studies summarized here provide information about the patient's mental status and possible physical causes of his signs and symptoms.

Laboratory tests

Urinalysis, hemoglobin level, hematocrit, serum electrolyte and serum glucose levels, and liver, kidney, and thyroid function tests screen for physical disorders that can cause psychiatric signs and symptoms. Toxicology studies of blood and urine can detect the presence of many drugs, and current laboratory methods can quantify the blood levels of these drugs. Patients on psychoactive drugs may need routine toxicology screening to ensure that they aren't receiving a toxic dose. (See *Toxicology screening.*)

Psychological and mental status tests

These tests evaluate the patient's mood, personality, and mental status. Commonly used tests include:
- The Mini–Mental Status Examination measures orientation, registration, recall, calculation, language, and graphomotor function.
- The Cognitive Capacity Screening Examination measures orientation, memory, calculation, and language.
- The Cognitive Assessment Scale measures orientation, general knowledge, mental ability, and psychomotor function.
- The Global Deterioration Scale assesses and stages primary degenerative dementia, based on orientation, memory, and neurologic function.
- The Functional Dementia Scale measures orientation, affect, and the ability to perform activities of daily living.
- The Beck Depression Inventory helps diagnose depression, determine its severity, and monitor the patient's response during treatment.
- The Eating Attitudes Test detects patterns that suggest an eating disorder.
- The Minnesota Multiphasic Personality Inventory helps assess personality traits and ego function in adolescents and adults. Test results include information on coping strategies, defenses, strengths, gender iden-

TOXICOLOGY SCREENING

Toxic levels of certain drugs can be detected in blood, urine, or both.

Blood
- Alcohol (ethyl, isopropyl, and methyl)
- Ethchlorvynol

Urine
- Chlorpromazine
- Cocaine
- Desmethyldoxepin (metabolite of doxepin)
- Heroin (metabolized to and detected as morphine)
- Imipramine
- Methadone
- Morphine
- Phencyclidine (PCP)

Blood and urine
- Acetaminophen
- Amitriptyline
- Amobarbital
- Butabarbital
- Butalbital (component in Fiorinal)
- Caffeine
- Carisoprodol
- Chlordiazepoxide
- Codeine
- Desipramine
- Desmethyldiazepam (metabolite of diazepam)
- Diazepam
- Diphenhydramine
- Doxepin
- Flurazepam
- Glutethimide
- Ibuprofen
- Meperidine
- Mephobarbital
- Meprobamate
- Methapyrilene
- Methaqualone
- Methyprylon
- Norpropoxyphene (metabolite of propoxyphene)
- Nortriptyline
- Oxazepam
- Pentazocine
- Pentobarbital
- Phenobarbital
- Propoxyphene
- Salicylates and their conjugates
- Secobarbital

---

tification, and self-esteem. The test pattern may strongly suggest a diagnostic category, point to a suicide risk, or indicate the potential for violence.

EEG and brain imaging studies
To screen for brain abnormalities, the physician may order tests that visualize electrical brain-wave pattern disturbances or anatomic alterations.
- An EEG graphically records the brain's electrical activity. Abnormal results may indicate organic disease, psychotropic drug use, or certain psychological disorders.
- A computed tomography (CT) *scan* combines radiologic and computer analysis of tissue density to produce images of intracranial structures not readily seen on standard X-rays. This test can help detect brain contusions or calcifications, cerebral atrophy, hydrocephalus, inflammation, space-occupying lesions, and vascular abnormalities.
- A magnetic resonance imaging (MRI) scan is a noninvasive imaging technique. MRI localizes atomic nuclei that magnetically align and then fall out of alignment in response to a radio-frequency pulse. The MRI scanner records signals from nuclei as they realign; it then translates the signals into detailed pictures of anatomic structures. Compared with conventional X-rays and CT scans, the MRI scan provides superior contrast of soft tissues and sharper differentiation of normal and abnormal tissues. It also provides images of multiple planes, including sagittal and coronal

views, in regions where bones usually interface.

- A positron emission tomography (PET) scan provides colorimetric information about the brain's metabolic activity by detecting how quickly tissues consume radioactive isotopes. PET scanning is used mainly for diagnosing neuropsychiatric problems, such as Alzheimer's disease, and some mental illnesses.

DISORDERS OF INFANCY, CHILDHOOD, AND ADOLESCENCE

Mental retardation

The American Association on Mental Retardation (AAMR) defines mental retardation as "significantly subaverage general intellectual function existing concurrently with deficits in adaptive behavior manifesting itself during the developmental period (before age 18)." Retardation commonly is accompanied by other physical and emotional disorders that may constitute disabilities in themselves. Mental retardation places a significant burden on patients and their families, resulting in stress, frustration, and family problems.

Causes and incidence

A specific cause is identifiable in only about 25% of people who are mentally retarded, and, of these, only 10% have the potential for cure. (See *Causes of mental retardation*.) In the remaining 75%, predisposing factors, such as deficient prenatal or perinatal care, inadequate nutrition, poor social environment, and poor child-rearing practices, contribute significantly to mental retardation.

Prenatal screening for genetic defects (such as Tay-Sachs disease) and counseling for families at risk for specific defects have reduced the incidence of genetically transmitted mental retardation.

An estimated 1% to 3% of the population is mentally retarded, demonstrating an IQ below 70 and associated difficulty in carrying out tasks required for personal independence.

Signs and symptoms

The observable effects of mental retardation are deviations from normal adaptive behaviors, ranging from learning disabilities and uncontrollable behavior to severe cognitive and motor skill impairment. The earlier a child's adaptive deficit is recognized and he's placed in a special learning program, the more likely he is to achieve age-appropriate adaptive behaviors. If the patient is older, review his adaptation to his environment.

The family of a patient who's mentally retarded may report many problems stemming from frustration, fear, and exhaustion. These problems, such as financial difficulties, abuse, and divorce, can compromise the child's care. Physical examination may reveal signs of abuse or neglect.

People who are mentally retarded may exhibit signs and symptoms of other disorders, such as cleft lip, congenital heart defects, and cerebral palsy as well as a lowered resistance to infection.

Diagnosis

CONFIRMING DIAGNOSIS *A score of less than 70 on a standardized IQ test confirms the diagnosis of mental retardation.*

The IQ test primarily predicts school performance and must be supplemented by other diagnostic evaluations.

For example, the Adaptive Behavior Scale deals with behaviors important to activities of daily living. This test evaluates self-help skills (toileting and eating), physical and social development, language, socialization, and time and number concepts. It also examines inappropriate behaviors, such as violent or destructive acts, withdrawal, and self-abusive or sexually aberrant behavior.

Age-appropriate adaptive behaviors are assessed by using developmental screening tests such as the Denver Developmental Screening test. These tests compare the subject's functional level with the normal level for the same chronologic age. The greater the discrepancy between chronologic and developmental age, the more severe the retardation. In most European and North American cultures, the Vineland Social Maturity Scale, a tool used to determine social competence, is recommended for use when appropriate.

In children, the functional level is based on sensorimotor skills, self-help skills, and socialization. In adolescents and adults, it's based on academic skills, reasoning and judgment skills, and social skills.

Treatment

Effective management requires an interdisciplinary team approach, which continues to assist the patient and his family on primary, secondary, and tertiary levels. A primary goal is to develop the patient's strengths. Another major goal is the development of social adaptive skills.

Children who are mentally retarded require special education and training, ideally beginning in infancy. An individualized, effective education program can optimize the quality of life for even the profoundly retarded.

The prognosis for people who are mentally retarded is related more to timing and aggressive treatment, personal motivation, training opportunities, and associated conditions than to the degree of mental retardation itself. With good support systems, many people who are mentally retarded become productive members of society. Successful management leads to independent functioning and occupational skills for some and a sheltered environment for others.

Special considerations

■ Support the parents of a child diagnosed with mental retardation. They may be overwhelmed by caretaking and financial concerns and may have difficulty accepting and bonding with their child.

■ Remember that a child who's mentally retarded has all the ordinary needs of a healthy child plus those created by his disability. The child especially needs affection, acceptance, stimulation, and prudent, consistent discipline; he's less able to cope if rejected, overprotected, or forced beyond his abilities.

CAUSES OF MENTAL RETARDATION

■ Chromosomal abnormalities (Down syndrome, Klinefelter's syndrome)
■ Disorders resulting from unknown prenatal influences (hydrocephalus, hydranencephaly, microcephaly)
■ Disorders of metabolism or nutrition (phenylketonuria, hypothyroidism, Hurler's syndrome, galactosemia, Tay-Sachs disease)
■ Environmental influences (cultural-familial retardation, poor nutrition, lack of medical care)
■ Gestational disorders (prematurity)
■ Gross brain disorders that develop after birth (neurofibromatosis, intracranial neoplasm)
■ Infection and intoxication (congenital rubella, syphilis, lead poisoning, meningitis, encephalitis, insecticides, drugs, maternal viral infection, toxins)
■ Psychiatric disorders (autism)
■ Trauma or physical conditions (mechanical injury, asphyxia, hyperpyrexia)

■ When caring for a hospitalized patient who's mentally retarded, promote continuity of care by acting as a liaison for parents and other health care professionals.

■ During hospitalization, continue training programs already in place, but remember that illness may bring on some regression.

■ For the parents of a child who's severely retarded, suggest ways to cope with the guilt, frustration, and exhaustion that commonly accompany caring for such a child. The parents may need an extensive teaching and discharge planning program, including physical care procedures, stress reduction techniques, support services, and referral to developmental programs. Ask

---

CLASSIFYING TICS

According to the *Diagnostic and Statistical Manual of Mental Disorders,* Fourth Edition, Text Revision, motor and vocal tics are classified as simple or complex; however, category boundaries remain unclear. Also, combinations of tics may occur simultaneously.

Motor tics

Simple motor tics include eye blinking, neck jerking, shoulder shrugging, head banging, head turning, tongue protrusion, lip or tongue biting, nail biting, hair pulling, and facial grimacing.

Some examples of complex motor tics are facial gestures, grooming behaviors, hitting or biting oneself, jumping, hopping, touching, squatting, deep knee bends, retracing steps, twirling when walking, stamping, smelling an object, and imitating the movements of someone who is being observed (echopraxia).

Vocal tics

Examples of simple vocal tics include coughing, throat clearing, grunting, sniffing, snorting, hissing, clicking, yelping, and barking.

Complex vocal tics may involve repeating words out of context; using socially unacceptable words, many of which are obscene (coprolalia); or repeating the last-heard sound, word, or phrase of another person (echolalia).

---

culty expressing sexual concerns because of limited verbal skills.

Tic disorders

Including Tourette syndrome, chronic motor or vocal tic disorder, and transient tic disorder, tic disorders are similar pathophysiologically but differ in severity and prognosis. All tic disorders, commonly known simply as *tics,* are involuntary, spasmodic, recurrent, and purposeless motor movements or vocalizations. These disorders are classified as motor or vocal and as simple or complex. (See *Classifying tics.*) Tics begin before age 18. Transient tics are usually self-limiting, but Tourette syndrome follows a chronic course with remissions and exacerbations. Some people who have very mild tics don't seek treatment.

Causes and incidence

Although their exact cause is unknown, tic disorders occur more in certain families, suggesting a genetic cause. Tics commonly develop when a child experiences overwhelming anxiety, usually associated with normal maturation. Tics may be precipitated or exacerbated by the use of phenothiazines or central nervous system stimulants or by head trauma.

All tic disorders are three times more common in boys than in girls. About 2% of the population has Tourette syndrome.

Signs and symptoms

Assessment findings vary according to the type of tic disorder. Inspection, coupled with the patient's history, may reveal the specific motor or vocal patterns that characterize the tic as well as the frequency, complexity, and precipitating factors. The patient or his family may report that the tics occur sporadically many times per day. (See *Stress disorders with physical signs.*)

Note whether certain situations exacerbate the tics. All tic disorders may be exacerbated by stress, and they usually diminish markedly during sleep. The patient also may report that they occur during activities that require concentration, such as reading or sewing.

the social services department to look into community resources.

- Teach parents how to care for the special needs of a child who's mentally retarded. Suggest that they contact the AAMR.
- Teach adolescents who are retarded how to deal with physical changes and sexual maturation. Encourage them to participate in appropriate sex education classes. People who are mentally retarded may have diffi-

STRESS DISORDERS WITH PHYSICAL SIGNS

Besides tic disorders, stress-related disorders that produce physical signs in children include stuttering, functional enuresis, functional encopresis, sleepwalking, and sleep terrors.

Stuttering

Characterized by abnormal speech rhythms with repetitions and hesitations at the beginning of words, stuttering may involve movements of the respiratory muscles, shoulders, and face. It may be associated with mental dullness, poor social background, and a history of birth trauma. However, this disorder most commonly occurs in children of average or superior intelligence who fear they can't meet expectations. Related problems may include low self-esteem, tension, anxiety, humiliation, and withdrawal from social situations.

About 80% of stutterers recover after age 16. Evaluation and treatment by a speech pathologist teaches stutterers to place equal weight on each syllable in a sentence, how to breathe properly, and how to control anxiety.

Functional enuresis

This disorder is characterized by intentional or involuntary voiding of urine, usually during the night (nocturnal enuresis). Considered normal in children until age 3 or 4, functional enuresis occurs in about 40% of children at this age. It persists in 10% to age 5, in 5% to age 10, and in 1% of boys to age 18. Enuresis is more common in boys than in girls.

Causes may be related to stress, such as the birth of a sibling, the move to a new home, divorce, separation, hospitalization, faulty toilet training (inconsistent, demanding, or punitive), and unrealistic responsibilities. Associated problems include low self-esteem, social withdrawal from peers because of ostracism and ridicule, and anger, rejection, and punishment by caregivers.

Advise parents that a matter-of-fact attitude helps the child learn bladder control without undue stress. If enuresis persists into late childhood, treatment with imipramine may help. Dry-bed therapy may include the use of an alarm (wet bell pad), social motivation, self-correction of accidents, and positive reinforcement.

Functional encopresis

Denoted by evacuation of feces into the child's clothes or inappropriate receptacles, functional encopresis is associated with low intelligence, cerebral dysfunction, or other developmental symptoms such as language lag. Some children also show inefficient and ineffective gastric motility. Related problems may include repressed anger, withdrawal from peer relationships, and loss of self-esteem.

Treatment involves encouraging the child to come to his parents when he has an "accident." Advise parents to give the child clean clothes without criticism or punishment. Medical examination should rule out any physical disorder. Child, adult, and family therapy may help reduce anger and disappointment over the child's development and improve parenting techniques. Supportive psychotherapy and relaxation therapy techniques may be useful in reducing anxiety and improving self-esteem.

Sleepwalking and sleep terrors

In sleepwalking, the child calmly rises from bed in a state of altered consciousness and walks around with no subsequent recollection of any dreams. In sleep terrors, he awakes terrified, in a state of clouded consciousness, usually unable to recognize parents and familiar surroundings. Visual hallucinations are common.

Sleepwalking is usually a response to an emotional concern. Tell parents to
(continued)

STRESS DISORDERS WITH PHYSICAL SIGNS (*continued*)

gently "talk" the child back to his bed. If he wakes, they should comfort and support him, not tease him.

Sleep terrors are a normal developmental event in 2- and 3-year-old children, usually occurring within 30 minutes to 3½ hours of sleep onset. Tachycardia, tachypnea, diaphoresis, dilated pupils, and piloerection are associated with sleep terrors. The child may also fear being alone.

Tell parents to make sure that the child has access to them at night. Sleep terrors usually are self-limiting and subside within a few weeks.

Determine whether the patient can control the tics. Most patients can do so, with conscious effort, for short periods.

Psychosocial assessment may reveal underlying stressful factors, such as problems with social adjustment, lack of self-esteem, and depression.

Diagnosis
For characteristic findings in patients with this condition, see *Diagnosing tic disorders.*

Treatment
Behavior modification and operant conditioning can help treat certain tic disorders. Psychotherapy can help the patient uncover underlying conflicts and issues as well as deal with the problems caused by the tics. Tourette syndrome is best treated with medications and psychotherapy.

No medications are helpful in treating transient tics. Haloperidol is the drug of choice for treating Tourette syndrome. Pimozide (an oral dopamine-blocking drug) and clonidine are alternative choices. Tetrabenazine has been used but is associated with depression of movement. Antianxiety agents may be useful in dealing with secondary anxiety, but they don't reduce the severity or frequency of the tics.

Special considerations
■ Offer emotional support and help the patient prevent fatigue.
■ Suggest that the patient with Tourette syndrome contact the Tourette Syndrome Association to obtain information and support.

■ Help the patient identify and eliminate any avoidable stress and learn positive new ways to deal with anxiety.
■ Encourage the patient to verbalize his feelings about his disorder. Help him to understand that the movements are involuntary; he shouldn't feel guilty or blame himself for them.

Autistic disorder

A severe, pervasive developmental disorder, autistic disorder is marked by unresponsiveness to social contact, gross deficits in intelligence and language development, ritualistic and compulsive behaviors, restricted capacity for developmentally appropriate activities and interests, and bizarre responses to the environment. Autistic disorder may be complicated by epileptic seizures, depression and, during periods of stress, catatonic phenomena. Autism usually becomes apparent before the child reaches age 36 months but, in some children, the actual onset is difficult to determine. Occasionally, autistic disorder isn't recognized until the child enters school. (See *Other pervasive developmental disorders,* page 420.)

The prognosis for autistic disorder is poor; most patients require a structured environment throughout life.

Causes and incidence
The causes of autistic disorder remain unclear but are thought to include psychological, physiologic, and sociological factors. Much evidence has accumulated to suggest a biological substrate. The parents of a

DIAGNOSING TIC DISORDERS

The diagnosis of a tic disorder is based on criteria from the *Diagnostic and Statistical Manual of Mental Disorders,* Fourth Edition, Text Revision.

Tourette syndrome
- The patient has had multiple motor tics and one or more vocal tics at some time during the illness, although not necessarily concurrently.
- The tics occur many times per day (usually in bouts) nearly every day or intermittently for more than 1 year.
- The disturbance causes marked distress or significant impairment in social, occupational, or other important areas of functioning.
- Onset occurs before age 18.
- The disturbance isn't the direct physiologic effect of a substance or a general medical condition.

Chronic motor or vocal tic disorder
- The patient has had single or multiple motor or vocal tics, but not both, at some time during the illness.
- The tics occur many times per day nearly every day or intermittently for more than 1 year. During this time, the person never had a tic-free period exceeding 3 consecutive months.
- The disturbance causes marked distress or significant impairment in social,

occupational, or other important areas of functioning.
- Onset occurs before age 18.
- The disturbance isn't the direct physiologic effect of a substance or a general medical condition.
- Criteria have never been met for Tourette syndrome.

Transient tic disorder
- The patient has single or multiple motor or vocal tics, or both.
- The tics occur many times per day nearly every day for at least 4 weeks, but for no longer than 12 consecutive months.
- The disturbance causes marked distress or significant impairment in social, occupational, or other important areas of functioning.
- Onset occurs before age 18.
- The disturbance isn't the direct physiologic effect of a substance or a general medical condition.
- Criteria have never been met for Tourette syndrome or chronic motor or vocal tic disorder.

---

child who's autistic may appear distant and unaffectionate. However, because children who are autistic are unresponsive or respond with rigid, screaming resistance to touch and attention, parental remoteness may be merely a frustrated, helpless reaction to this disorder, not its cause.

Some children who are autistic show abnormal but nonspecific EEG findings that suggest brain dysfunction, possibly resulting from trauma, disease, or a structural abnormality. Autistic disorder has also been associated with maternal rubella, untreated phenylketonuria, tuberous sclerosis, anoxia during birth, encephalitis, infantile spasms, and fragile X syndrome. Studies have established a link with abnormalities

in neurotransmitters, including (in some cases) increased dopamine and increased serotonin. There appears to be a genetic component as well; between 2% and 4% of siblings of those with autism also had autistic disorders at a rate higher than the general population.

Autistic disorder is rare, affecting 4 to 5 children per 10,000 births. It affects three to four times more boys than girls.

Signs and symptoms
A primary characteristic of infantile autistic disorder is unresponsiveness to people. Infants with this disorder won't cuddle, avoid eye contact and facial expressions, and are indifferent to affection and physi-

OTHER PERVASIVE DEVELOPMENTAL DISORDERS

Although autistic disorder is the most severe and most typical of the pervasive developmental disorders, recent evidence points to other similar disorders in this class.

For example, the *Diagnostic and Statistical Manual of Mental Disorders,* Fourth Edition, Text Revision category *pervasive developmental disorder not otherwise specified* refers to those patients who don't meet the criteria for autistic disorder but who *do* exhibit impaired development of reciprocal social interaction and of verbal and nonverbal communication skills.

Some patients with this diagnosis exhibit a markedly restricted repertoire of activities and interests, but others don't. Research suggests that these disorders are more common than autistic disorder, occurring in 6 to 10 of every 10,000 children.

cal contact. Parents may report that the child becomes rigid or flaccid when held, cries when touched, and shows little or no interest in human contact.

As the infant grows older, his smiling response is delayed or absent. He doesn't lift his arms in anticipation of being picked up or form an attachment to a specific caregiver. Furthermore, he doesn't show the anxiety about strangers that's typical in the 8-month-old infant.

A child who's autistic fails to learn the usual socialization games (peek-a-boo, pat-a-cake, or bye-bye). He's likely to relate to others only to fill a physical need and then without eye contact or speech. The end result may be mutual withdrawal between parents and child.

Severe language impairment and lack of imaginative play are characteristic. The child may be mute or may use immature speech patterns. For example, he may use a single word to express a series of activities;

he may say "ground" when referring to any step in using a playground slide.

His speech commonly shows echolalia (meaningless repetition of words or phrases addressed to him) and pronoun reversal ("you go walk" when he means, "I want to go for a walk"). When answering a question, he may simply repeat the question to mean yes and remain silent to mean no.

He shows little imagination, seldom acting out adult roles or engaging in fantasy play. In fact, he may insist on lining up an exact number of toys in the same manner over and over or repetitively mimic the actions of someone else.

A child who's autistic shows characteristically bizarre behavior patterns, such as screaming fits, rituals, rhythmic rocking, arm flapping, crying without tears, and disturbed sleeping and eating patterns. His behavior may be self-destructive (hand biting, eye gouging, hair pulling, or head banging) or self-stimulating (playing with his own saliva, feces, and urine). His bizarre responses to his environment include an extreme compulsion for sameness.

In response to sensory stimuli, he may underreact or overreact and he may ignore objects — dropping those he's given or not looking at them — or he may become excessively absorbed in them — continually watching the objects or the movement of his own fingers over the objects. He commonly responds to stimuli by head banging, rocking, whirling, and hand flapping. He tends to avoid using sight and hearing to interact with the environment.

A child who's autistic may exhibit additional behavioral abnormalities, such as:

- cognitive impairment (most have an IQ of 35 to 49)
- eating, drinking, and sleeping problems, for example, limiting his diet to just a few foods, excessive drinking, or repeatedly waking during the night and rocking
- mood disorders, including labile mood, giggling or crying without reason, lack of emotional responses, no fear of real danger but excessive fear of harmless objects, and generalized anxiety.

DIAGNOSING AUTISTIC DISORDER

Autism is diagnosed when the patient meets the criteria in the *Diagnostic and Statistical Manual of Mental Disorders,* Fourth Edition, Text Revision. At least six characteristics from the following three categories must be present, including at least two from the social interaction category and one each from the communication and patterns categories.

Social interaction

Impairment in social interaction, as shown by at least two of the following:
- marked impairment in the use of multiple nonverbal behaviors, such as eye-to-eye gaze, facial expression, body postures, and gestures to regulate social interaction
- failure to develop peer relationships appropriate to developmental level
- no spontaneous sharing of enjoyment, interests, or achievements with others
- lack of social or emotional reciprocity
- gross impairment in ability to make peer friendships.

Communication

Impairment in communication, as shown by at least one of the following:
- delay in, or total lack of, spoken language development
- in individuals with adequate speech, marked impairment in initiating or sustaining a conversation with others
- stereotyped and repetitive use of language or idiosyncratic language
- lack of varied, spontaneous make-believe play or social imitative play appropriate to developmental level.

Patterns

Restricted, repetitive, and stereotyped patterns of behavior, interests, and activities, as manifested by at least one of the following:
- encompassing preoccupation with one or more stereotyped and restricted patterns of interest that's abnormal either in intensity or focus
- apparently inflexible adherence to specific nonfunctional routines or rituals
- stereotyped and repetitive motor mannerisms
- persistent preoccupation with parts of objects.

Additional criteria

Delays or abnormal functioning in at least one of the following before age 3:
- social interaction
- language as used in social communication
- symbolic or imaginative play.

The disturbance isn't better accounted for by Rett's disorder or childhood disintegrative disorder.

Diagnosis

For characteristic findings in patients with this condition, see *Diagnosing autistic disorder.*

Treatment

The difficult and prolonged treatment of autistic disorder must begin early, continue for years (through adolescence), and coordinate efforts to encourage social adjustment and speech development and to reduce self-destructive behavior.

Behavioral techniques are used to decrease symptoms and increase the child's ability to respond. Positive reinforcement, using food and other rewards, can enhance language and social skills. Providing pleasurable sensory and motor stimulation (such as jogging or playing with a ball) encourages appropriate behavior and helps eliminate inappropriate behavior. Drug therapy with an agent, such as haloperidol, may be helpful. Risperidone has been used successfully to diminish aggressiveness and hyperactivity.

Treatment may take place in a psychiatric institution, in a specialized school, or in a day-care program; however, the current trend is toward home treatment. Because family members tend to feel inadequate and guilty, they may need counseling. Until the causes of infantile autism are known, prevention isn't possible.

Special considerations
■ Reduce self-destructive behaviors. Physically stop the child from harming himself, while firmly saying "no." When he responds to your voice, first give a primary reward (such as food); later, substitute verbal or physical reinforcement (such as saying "good" or giving the child a hug or a pat on the back).
■ Foster appropriate use of language. Provide positive reinforcement when the child indicates his needs correctly. Give verbal reinforcement at first (for example, by saying "good" or "great"); later, give physical reinforcement (such as a hug or a pat on the hand or shoulder).
■ Encourage development of self-esteem. Show the child that he's acceptable as a person.
■ Encourage self-care. For example, place a brush in the child's hand and guide his hand to brush his hair. Similarly, teach him to wash his hands and face.
■ Encourage acceptance of minor environmental changes. Prepare the child for the change by telling him about it beforehand. Make initial changes minor; for example, change the color of his bedspread or the placement of food on his plate. When he has accepted minor changes, move on to bigger ones.
■ Provide emotional support to the parents, and refer them to the Autism Society of America.
■ Teach the parents how to physically care for the child's needs.
■ Teach the parents how to identify signs of excessive stress and the coping skills to use under these circumstances. Emphasize that they'll be ineffective caregivers if they don't take the time to meet their own needs in addition to those of their child.

■ Help the parents understand that they aren't responsible for their child's condition and shouldn't feel guilty about it.

Attention deficit hyperactivity disorder

The patient with attention deficit hyperactivity disorder (ADHD) has difficulty focusing his attention; engaging in quiet, passive activities; or both. Although the disorder is present at birth, diagnosis before age 4 or 5 is difficult unless the child shows severe symptoms. In some cases, however, the patient isn't diagnosed until adulthood.

Causes and incidence
ADHD is thought to be a physiologic brain disorder with a familial tendency. Some studies indicate that it may result from disturbances in neurotransmitter levels in the brain due to reduced blood flow in the striated area of the brain. It affects 3% to 5% of school-age children and is three times more common in boys than in girls.

Signs and symptoms
The principal sign of ADHD is hyperactivity that's present over a long period, in at least two settings (such as school and home), and is accompanied by easy distractibility. The patient may be impulsive, emotionally labile, explosive, or irritable. Although he may be highly intelligent, his school or work performance patterns are sporadic. He may jump from one partly completed project, thought, or task to another. The patient may have an attention deficit without hyperactivity; if so, he's less likely to be diagnosed and treated.

In a younger child, signs and symptoms include an inability to wait in line, remain seated, wait his turn, or concentrate on one activity until its completion. An older child or an adult may be described as impulsive and easily distracted by irrelevant thoughts, sounds, or sights. He may also be characterized as emotionally labile, inattentive, or prone to daydreaming. His disorganization becomes apparent as he has difficulty meeting deadlines and keeping

DIAGNOSING ATTENTION DEFICIT HYPERACTIVITY DISORDER

The *Diagnostic and Statistical Manual of Mental Disorders,* Fourth Edition, Text Revision, groups certain signs and symptoms into inattention and hyperactivity-impulsivity categories. The diagnosis of attention deficit hyperactivity disorder is based on the person demonstrating at least six signs or symptoms from the inattention group or at least six from the hyperactivity-impulsivity group. They must have persisted for at least 6 months to a degree that's maladaptive and inconsistent with the person's developmental level.

Symptoms of inattention
The person manifesting *inattention:*
■ often fails to give close attention to details or makes careless mistakes in schoolwork, work, or other activities
■ often has difficulty sustaining attention in tasks or play activities
■ often doesn't seem to listen when spoken to directly
■ often doesn't follow through on instructions and fails to finish schoolwork, chores, or duties in the workplace (not because of oppositional behavior or failure to understand instructions)
■ often has difficulty organizing tasks and activities
■ often avoids, dislikes, or is reluctant to engage in tasks that require sustained mental effort (such as schoolwork or homework)
■ often loses things necessary for tasks or activities (for example, toys, school assignments, pencils, books, or tools)
■ often becomes distracted by extraneous stimuli
■ often demonstrates forgetfulness in daily activities.

Symptoms of hyperactivity-impulsivity
The person manifesting *hyperactivity:*
■ often fidgets with hands or feet or squirms in seat

■ often leaves his seat in the classroom or in other situations in which remaining seated is expected
■ often runs about or climbs excessively in situations in which remaining seated is expected
■ often has difficulty playing or engaging in leisure activities quietly
■ often is characterized as "on the go" or acts as if "driven by a motor"
■ often talks excessively.

Symptoms of impulsivity
The person manifesting *impulsivity:*
■ often blurts out answers before questions have been completed
■ often has difficulty awaiting his turn
■ often interrupts or intrudes on others.

Additional features
■ Some symptoms that caused impairment were evident before age 7.
■ Some impairment from the symptoms is present in two or more settings.
■ Clinically significant impairment in social, academic, or occupational functioning must be clearly evident.
■ The symptoms don't occur exclusively during the course of a pervasive developmental disorder, schizophrenia, or another psychotic disorder and aren't better accounted for by another mental disorder.

---

track of school or work tools and materials.

Diagnosis
The child is usually referred for evaluation by the school. (See *Diagnosing attention deficit hyperactivity disorder.*) Diagnosis of

ADHD usually begins by obtaining data from several sources, including the parents, teachers, and the child himself. Complete psychological, medical, and neurologic evaluations rule out other problems. Then the child undergoes tests that measure impulsiveness, attention, and the ability to sustain a task. The combined findings portray a clear picture of the disorder and of the areas of support the child will need.

Treatment
Education is the first step in effective treatment. The entire treatment team (which ideally includes parents, teachers, and therapists as well as the patient and the physician) must understand the disorder and its effect on the individual's functioning.

Treatment varies, depending on the severity of symptoms and their effects on the child's ability to function. Behavior modification, coaching, external structure, use of planning and organizing systems, and supportive psychotherapy help the patient cope with the disorder.

The patient may benefit from medication to relieve symptoms. Ideally, the treatment team identifies the symptoms to be managed, selects appropriate medication, and then tracks the patient's symptoms carefully to determine the drug's effectiveness. Stimulants are the most commonly used agents. Antipsychotics may sometimes be used in combination with stimulants. However, other drugs, including tricyclic antidepressants, mood stabilizers, and beta-adrenergic blockers, sometimes help control symptoms.

Special considerations
- Work with the individual to develop external structure and controls.
- Set realistic expectations and limits because the patient with ADHD is easily frustrated (which leads to decreased self-control).
- Remain calm and consistent.
- Keep instructions short and simple.
- Provide praise, rewards, and positive feedback whenever possible.

Conduct disorder

Aggressive behavior is the hallmark of conduct disorder. A child with this disorder fights, bullies, intimidates, and assaults others physically or sexually, and is truant from school at an early age. Typically, the patient has poor relationships with peers and adults and violates others' rights and society's rules. Conduct disorder evolves slowly over time until a consistent pattern of behavior is established.

Causes and incidence
Studies have suggested that the disorder has biological (including genetic) and psychosocial components. Roughly 30% to 50% of clinical populations with conduct disorder also have attention deficit hyperactivity disorder (ADHD). Social risk factors that may predispose a child to conduct disorder include socioeconomic deprivation; harsh, punitive parenting with verbal or physical aggression; separation from parents; early institutionalization; family neglect, abuse, or violence; frequent verbal abuse from parents, teachers, or other authority figures; parental psychiatric illness, substance abuse, or marital discord; large family size, crowding, and poverty; and divorce with persistent hostility between the parents. Other risk factors include child abuse and neglect, neurologic damage caused by low birth weight or birth complications, underarousal of the autonomic nervous system, learning impairments, insensitivity to physical pain and punishment, and impaired functioning of the nonadrenergic system.

The prevalence of conduct disorder among people ages 9 to 17 is approximately 1% to 4%. An estimated 6% to 16% of boys and 2% to 9% of girls younger than age 18 have the disorder. The prognosis is worse in children with an earlier onset; these children are more likely to develop antisocial personality disorder as adults.

Signs and symptoms
Signs and symptoms of conduct disorder include:
- abusing others sexually
- cheating in school
- cruelty to animals
- engaging in precocious sexual activity
- fighting with family members and peers
- skipping classes
- smoking cigarettes
- speaking to others in a hostile manner
- stealing or shoplifting
- using drugs or alcohol
- vandalizing or destroying property.

DIAGNOSING CONDUCT DISORDER

A patient with conduct disorder must meet at least three of the criteria from any of the categories below; these criteria must have been noted within the year before the time of examination, and at least one criterion must have been present within the past 6 months.

Aggression to people and animals
- Bullies, threatens, or intimidates others
- Commonly initiates physical fights
- Has used a weapon that can cause serious physical harm to others
- Has been physically cruel to people
- Has stolen while confronting a victim
- Has forced someone into sexual activity

Destruction of property
- Deliberately setting fire with the intention of causing serious damage
- Deliberately destroying others' property

Deceitfulness
- Has broken into someone else's house, car, or building
- Commonly lies to obtain goods or favors or to avoid obligations
- Has stolen items of nontrivial value without confronting a victim

Serious violations of rules
- Often stays out at night despite parental prohibitions, starting before age 13
- Has run away from home overnight at least twice while living in the parents' or surrogate parents' home
- Commonly skips school, beginning before age 13

Additional criteria
- The behavior disturbance must cause clinically significant impairment in social, academic, or occupational functioning.
- The patient is age 18 or older and doesn't meet the criteria for antisocial personality disorder.

Other features
- Conduct disorder is considered mild if the person exhibits few if any conduct problems beyond those required to make the diagnosis and if the conduct problems cause only minor harm to others.
- The disorder is considered moderate if the conduct problems and their effects on others are intermediate between mild and severe.
- The condition is considered severe if the person has many conduct problems beyond those needed to make the diagnosis, or if the conduct problems cause considerable harm to others.

Diagnosis

Medical and psychiatric evaluations, feedback from parents, a school consultant's recommendations, case manager plan, and probation officer reports can assist in a team approach to diagnosis. The diagnosis is made when the patient meets the criteria in the *Diagnostic and Statistical Manual of Mental Disorders,* Fourth Edition, Text Revision. (See *Diagnosing conduct disorder.*)

Treatment

Treatment focuses on coordinating the child's psychological, physiologic, and educational needs. A structured living environment with consistent rules and consequences can help reduce many symptoms. Parents need to be taught how to deal with the child's demands. Juvenile justice interventions may also be used. Medication can be useful as an adjunct to treatment. Overt aggression responds to many medications, such as antipsychotics, lithium, clonidine, and selective serotonin reuptake inhibitors. ADHD, if present, must also be addressed.

Special considerations

- Work to establish a trusting relationship with the child.
- Provide clear behavioral guidelines, including consequences for disruptive and manipulative behavior.
- Teach the child effective coping skills, social skills, and problem-solving skills, and have him demonstrate them in return.
- Teach the child to express anger appropriately through constructive methods to release negative feelings and frustrations.
- Help the child accept responsibility for behavior rather than blaming others, becoming defensive, and wanting revenge.
- Use role-playing to help the child practice handling stress and gain skill and confidence in managing difficult situations.

SUBSTANCE-RELATED DISORDERS

Alcohol-related disorder

The patient with alcohol-related disorder experiences a need for the daily intake of large amounts of alcohol for day-to-day functioning. A regular pattern of heavy drinking limited to weekends, with periods of sobriety between weekends, also suggests a pattern of abuse. People with these patterns of drinking usually show impaired social and occupational functioning.

Causes and incidence

Numerous biological, psychological, and sociocultural factors appear to be involved in alcohol addiction. An offspring of one parent with alcohol-related disorder is seven to eight times more likely to become an alcoholic than is a peer without such a parent. Biological factors may include genetic or biochemical abnormalities, nutritional deficiencies, endocrine imbalances, and allergic responses.

Psychological factors may include the urge to drink alcohol to reduce anxiety or symptoms of mental illness; the desire to avoid responsibility in familial, social, and work relationships; and the need to bolster self-esteem.

Sociocultural factors include the availability of alcoholic beverages, group or peer pressure, an excessively stressful lifestyle, and social attitudes that approve of frequent drinking.

More than 15% of American adults have a problem with alcohol use, and about 5% to 10% of male and 3% to 5% of female drinkers are alcohol dependent, accounting for about 12.5 million people. Alcohol-related disorder cuts across all social and economic groups, involves both sexes, and occurs at all stages of the life cycle, beginning as early as elementary school.

Signs and symptoms

Because the person with alcohol dependence may hide or deny his addiction, and may temporarily manage to maintain a functional life, assessing for alcohol-related disorder can be difficult. Note physical and psychosocial symptoms that suggest alcohol-related disorder. For example, the patient's history may suggest a need for daily or episodic alcohol use to maintain adequate functioning, an inability to discontinue or reduce alcohol intake, episodes of anesthesia or amnesia (blackouts) during intoxication, episodes of violence during intoxication, and interference with social and familial relationships and occupational responsibilities. Many minor complaints may be alcohol-related. The patient may report malaise, dyspepsia, mood swings or depression, and an increased incidence of infection. Observe the patient for poor personal hygiene and untreated injuries, such as cigarette burns, fractures, and bruises, that he can't fully explain. Note any evidence of an unusually high tolerance of sedatives and opioids.

Although each person abusing alcohol may present in his own unique way, secretive or manipulative behavior may be a manifestation of the patient's denial of the severity of his addiction. Suspect alcohol-related disorder if the patient uses inordinate amounts of aftershave or mouthwash.

COMPLICATIONS OF ALCOHOL USE

Alcohol can damage body tissues by its direct irritating effects, by changes that take place in the body during its metabolism, by aggravation of existing disease, by accidents occurring during intoxication, and by interactions between the substance and drugs. Such tissue damage can cause these complications.

Cardiopulmonary complications
- Cardiac arrhythmias
- Cardiomyopathy
- Chronic obstructive pulmonary disease
- Essential hypertension
- Increased risk of tuberculosis
- Pneumonia

GI complications
- Chronic diarrhea
- Esophageal cancer
- Esophageal varices
- Esophagitis
- Gastric ulcers
- Gastritis
- GI bleeding
- Malabsorption
- Pancreatitis

Hematologic complications
- Anemia
- Leukopenia
- Reduced number of phagocytes

Hepatic complications
- Alcoholic hepatitis
- Cirrhosis
- Fatty liver

Neurologic complications
- Alcoholic dementia
- Alcoholic hallucinosis
- Alcohol withdrawal delirium
- Korsakoff's syndrome
- Peripheral neuropathy
- Seizure disorders
- Subdural hematoma
- Wernicke's encephalopathy

Psychiatric complications
- Amotivational syndrome
- Depression
- Fetal alcohol syndrome
- Impaired social and occupational functioning
- Multiple substance abuse
- Suicide

Other complications
- Beriberi
- Hypoglycemia
- Infertility
- Leg and foot ulcers
- Impaired respiratory diffusion
- Increased incidence of pulmonary infections
- Myopathies
- Prostatitis
- Sexual performance difficulties

When confronted, the patient may deny or rationalize the problem. Alternatively, he may be guarded or hostile in his response and may even sign out of the hospital against medical advice. He also may project his anger or feelings of guilt or inadequacy onto others to avoid confronting his illness.

Chronic alcohol abuse brings with it an array of physical complications, including malnutrition, cirrhosis of the liver, peripheral neuropathy, brain damage, and cardiomyopathy. Assess for these complications in a patient with alcohol-related disorder. (See *Complications of alcohol use.*)

After abstinence or reduction of alcohol intake, signs and symptoms of withdrawal — which begin shortly after drinking has stopped and last for 5 to 7 days — may vary. The patient initially experiences anorexia, nausea, anxiety, fever, insomnia, diaphoresis, and tremor, progressing to severe tremulousness, agitation and, possibly, hallucinations and violent behavior. Major motor seizures (alcohol withdrawal seizures) can occur during withdrawal. Suspect alcohol-related disorder in any patient with unexplained seizures. (See *Signs and symptoms of alcohol withdrawal.*)

 ELDER TIP *Remember to consider the possibility of alcohol abuse when evaluating older patients. Research suggests that alcoholism affects 2% to 10% of adults older than age 60. More than half of all elderly hospital admissions are due to alcohol-related problems.*

Diagnosis

For characteristic findings in patients with alcoholism, see *Diagnosing substance dependence and related disorders,* page 430.

Clinical findings may help support the diagnosis of alcohol-related disorder. For example, laboratory tests can confirm alcohol use and complications and document recent alcohol ingestion. A blood alcohol level ranging from 0.08% to 0.10% weight/volume (200 mg/dl) is accepted as the level of intoxication, depending on the state or country. The blood alcohol level in a physically dependent and tolerant drinker may exceed levels that would cause severe dysfunction or death in a nontolerant drinker. For example, a tolerant drinker might have a blood alcohol level of more than 0.5 mg (the usual lethal level) and still be alive, talking, and moving.

In severe hepatic disease, the blood urea nitrogen level is increased, and the serum glucose level is decreased. Further testing may reveal increased serum ammonia and amylase levels. Urine toxicology studies may help determine if the patient with alcohol withdrawal delirium or another acute complication abuses other drugs as well.

Liver function studies revealing increased levels of serum cholesterol, lactate dehydrogenase, alanine aminotransferase, aspartate aminotransferase, and creatine phosphokinase may point to liver damage, and elevated serum amylase and lipase levels point to acute pancreatitis. A hematologic workup can identify anemia, thrombocytopenia, increased prothrombin time, and increased partial thromboplastin time.

Treatment

Total abstinence from alcohol is the only effective treatment. Supportive programs that offer detoxification, rehabilitation, and aftercare, including continued involvement in Alcoholics Anonymous (AA), may produce good long-term results.

Acute intoxication is treated symptomatically by supporting respiration, preventing aspiration of vomitus, replacing fluids, administering I.V. glucose to prevent hypoglycemia, correcting hypothermia or acidosis, and initiating emergency treatment for trauma, infection, or GI bleeding.

Treatment of chronic alcohol abuse requires a varied approach that may include medications to deter alcohol use and treat effects of withdrawal; psychotherapy, consisting of behavior modification techniques, group therapy, and family therapy; and appropriate measures to relieve associated physical problems.

Aversion, or deterrent, therapy involves a daily oral dose of disulfiram to prevent compulsive drinking. This drug interferes with alcohol metabolism and allows toxic levels of acetaldehyde to accumulate in the patient's blood, producing immediate and potentially fatal distress in the event he consumes alcohol up to 2 weeks after taking it. Disulfiram is contraindicated during pregnancy and in the patient with diabetes, heart disease, severe hepatic disease, or any disorder in which such a reaction could be especially dangerous. Another form of aversion therapy attempts to induce aversion by administering alcohol with an emetic.

The first drug approved by the U.S. Food and Drug Administration for the treatment of alcohol-related disorder since disulfiram is naltrexone, an opiate antagonist that effectively reduces the amount of intake, severity of craving, and relapse incidence. It's believed to work by preventing the effects of increased endorphins produced as a product of increased alcohol intake.

For long-term success, the recovering individual must learn to fill the place alcohol once occupied in his life with something constructive. Therapy using disulfiram or naltrexone may only substitute one drug dependence for another, so it should be used prudently.

SIGNS AND SYMPTOMS OF ALCOHOL WITHDRAWAL

Alcohol withdrawal signs and symptoms may vary in degree from mild (morning hangover) to severe (alcohol withdrawal delirium). Formerly known as *delirium tremens*, alcohol withdrawal delirium is marked by acute distress following abrupt withdrawal after prolonged or massive use.

Signs and symptoms	Mild	Moderate	Severe
Anxiety	Mild restlessness	Obvious motor restlessness and anxiety	Extreme restlessness and agitation with intense fearfulness
Appetite	Impaired appetite	Marked anorexia	Rejection of all food and fluid except alcohol
Blood pressure	Normal or slightly elevated systolic	Usually elevated systolic	Elevated systolic and diastolic
Confusion	None	Variable	Marked confusion and disorientation
GI symptoms	Nausea	Nausea and vomiting	Dry heaves and vomiting
Hallucinations	None	Vague, transient visual and auditory hallucinations and illusions (commonly nocturnal)	Visual and occasionally auditory hallucinations, usually of fearful or threatening content; misidentification of people and frightening delusions related to hallucinatory experiences
Seizures	None	Possible	Common
Sleep disturbance	Restless sleep or insomnia	Marked insomnia and nightmares	Total wakefulness
Sweating	Slight	Obvious	Marked hyperhidrosis

Benzodiazepine isn't recommended during rehabilitation due to its addictive nature and the potential for reinforcing the substance abuse behavior.

ELDER TIP *Because the older patient may be more sensitive to these drugs, withdrawal may take longer (weeks or months) and be more severe than in a younger adult.*

Supportive counseling or individual, group, or family psychotherapy may help. Ongoing support groups are helpful. In AA, a self-help group with more than 1 million members worldwide, the alcoholic finds emotional support from others with similar problems. About 40% of AA's members stay sober as long as 5 years, and 30% stay sober longer than 5 years.

DIAGNOSING SUBSTANCE DEPENDENCE AND RELATED DISORDERS

The *Diagnostic and Statistical Manual of Mental Disorders,* Fourth Edition, Text Revision, identifies these diagnostic criteria for substance dependence, abuse, intoxication, and withdrawal.

Substance dependence

A maladaptive pattern of substance use leading to clinically significant impairment or distress, as manifested by three or more of the following, occurring at any time in the same 12-month period:

- Tolerance, as defined by either of the following: the need for increased amounts of the substance to achieve intoxication or desired effect or a markedly diminished effect with continued use of the same amount of the substance.
- Withdrawal, as manifested by either of the following: the characteristic withdrawal syndrome for the substance or the same, or similar, substance is taken to relieve or avoid withdrawal symptoms.
- The person commonly takes the substance in larger amounts or over a longer period than was intended.
- The person experiences a persistent desire or unsuccessful efforts to cut down or control substance use.
- The person spends a lot of time in activities needed to obtain the substance, use the substance, or recover from its effects.
- The person abandons or reduces important social, occupational, or recreational activities because of substance use.
- The person continues using the substance despite knowledge of having a persistent or recurrent physical or psychological problem that's likely to have been caused or exacerbated by the substance.

Substance abuse

A maladaptive pattern of substance use leading to clinically significant impairment or distress, as manifested by one or more of the following, occurring within a 12-month period:

- recurrent substance use resulting in a failure to fulfill major role obligations at work, school, or home
- recurrent substance use in situations in which using the substance is physically hazardous
- recurrent substance-related legal problems
- continued substance use despite having persistent or recurrent social or interpersonal problems caused or exacerbated by the effects of the substance.

The symptoms have never met the criteria for substance dependence for this class of substance.

Substance intoxication

- The development of a reversible substance-specific syndrome resulting from recent ingestion of, or exposure to, a substance.
- Clinically significant maladaptive behavioral or psychological changes, resulting from the effect of the substance on the central nervous system and developing during or shortly after use of the substance.
- Symptoms aren't caused by a general medical condition, and aren't better accounted for by another mental disorder.

Substance withdrawal

- Development of a substance-specific syndrome resulting from the cessation or reduction of substance use that has been heavy and prolonged.
- The substance-specific syndrome causes clinically significant distress or impairment in social, occupational, or other important areas of functioning.
- The symptoms aren't caused by a general medical condition and aren't better accounted for by another mental disorder.

Special considerations

- During acute intoxication or withdrawal, carefully monitor the patient's mental status, heart rate, breath sounds, blood pressure, and temperature every 30 minutes to 6 hours.
- Assess the patient for signs of inadequate nutrition and dehydration. Institute seizure precautions and administer drugs prescribed to treat the signs and symptoms of withdrawal in chronic alcohol abuse.
- During withdrawal, orient the patient to reality because he may have hallucinations and may try to harm himself or others. Maintain a calm environment, minimizing noise and shadows to reduce the incidence of delusions and hallucinations. Avoid restraining the patient unless necessary to protect him or others.
- Approach the patient in a nonthreatening way. Limit sustained eye contact. Even if he's verbally abusive, listen attentively and respond with empathy. Explain all procedures.
- Monitor the patient for signs of depression or impending suicide.
- In chronic alcohol-related disorder, help the patient accept his drinking problem and the necessity for abstinence. Confront him about his behavior, urging him to examine his actions more realistically.
- If the patient is taking disulfiram (or has taken it within the past 2 weeks), warn him of the effects of alcohol ingestion, which may last from 30 minutes to 3 hours or longer. The reaction includes nausea, vomiting, facial flushing, headache, shortness of breath, red eyes, blurred vision, sweating, tachycardia, hypotension, and fainting. Emphasize that even a small amount of alcohol will induce this adverse reaction and that the longer he takes the drug, the greater his sensitivity to alcohol will be. Even medicinal sources of alcohol, such as mouthwash, cough syrups, liquid vitamins, and cold remedies, must be avoided.
- Refer the patient to AA and offer to arrange a visit from an AA member. Stress the effectiveness of this organization.
- For the individual who has lost all contact with his family and friends and who has a long history of unemployment, trouble with the law, or other problems associated with alcohol abuse, rehabilitation may involve job training, sheltered workshops, halfway houses, and other supervised facilities.
- Refer the spouse of an alcoholic to Al-Anon and children of an alcoholic to Alateen. By participating in these self-help groups, family members learn to relinquish responsibility for the individual's drinking. Point out that family involvement in rehabilitation can reduce family tensions.
- Refer adult children of an alcoholic to the National Association for Children of Alcoholics.

Substance abuse and induced disorders

Substance abuse and dependence causes physical, mental, emotional, or social harm. Examples of abused drugs include opioids, stimulants, depressants, antianxiety agents, and hallucinogens. (See *Understanding commonly abused substances,* pages 432 to 436.) Chronic drug abuse, especially I.V. use, can lead to life-threatening complications, such as cardiac and respiratory arrest, intracranial hemorrhage, acquired immunodeficiency syndrome, tetanus, subacute infective endocarditis, hepatitis, vasculitis, septicemia, thrombophlebitis, pulmonary emboli, gangrene, malnutrition and GI disturbances, respiratory infections, musculoskeletal dysfunction, trauma, depression, increased risk of suicide, and psychosis. Materials used to "cut" street drugs also can cause toxic or allergic reactions.

Psychoactive drug abuse can occur at any age. Experimentation with drugs commonly begins in adolescence or even earlier. In many cases, drug abuse leads to addiction, which may involve physical or psychological dependence or both. The most dangerous form of abuse occurs when users mix several drugs simultaneously — including alcohol.

Causes

Psychoactive drug abuse commonly results from a combination of low self-esteem, peer pressure, inadequate coping skills, and curiosity. Most people who are predisposed *(Text continues on page 436.)*

UNDERSTANDING COMMONLY ABUSED SUBSTANCES

Substance	Signs and symptoms	Interventions

Cannabinoids

Marijuana

- *Street names:* pot, grass, weed, Mary Jane, roach, reefer, joint, muggles, Acapulco gold, Texas tea, Yesca, hemp
- *Routes:* ingestion, smoking
- *Dependence:* psychological
- *Duration of effect:* 2 to 3 hours
- *Medical uses:* antiemetic for chemotherapy

- *Of use:* acute psychosis; agitation; amotivational syndrome; anxiety; asthma; bronchitis; conjunctival reddening; decreased muscle strength; delusions; distorted sense of time and self-perception; dry mouth; euphoria; hallucinations; impaired cognition, short-term memory, and mood; incoordination; increased hunger; increased systolic pressure when supine; orthostatic hypotension; paranoia; spontaneous laughter; tachycardia; and vivid visual imagery
- *Of withdrawal:* chills, decreased appetite, increased rapid-eye-movement sleep, insomnia, irritability, nervousness, restlessness, tremors, and weight loss

- Place the patient in a quiet room.
- Monitor his vital signs.
- Give supplemental oxygen for respiratory depression and I.V. fluids for hypotension.
- Give diazepam, as ordered, for extreme agitation and acute psychosis.

Depressants

Alcohol

- *Found in:* beer, wine, and distilled spirits; also contained in cough syrup, aftershave, and mouthwash
- *Route:* ingestion
- *Dependence:* physical and psychological
- *Duration of effect:* varies according to individual and amount ingested; metabolized at rate of 10 ml/hour
- *Medical uses:* neurolysis (absolute alcohol); emergency tocolytic; and treatment of ethylene glycol and methanol poisoning

- *Of acute use:* coma, decreased inhibitions, euphoria followed by depression or hostility, impaired judgment, incoordination, respiratory depression, slurred speech, unconsciousness, and vomiting
- *Of withdrawal:* delirium, hallucinations, seizures, and tremors

- Place the patient in a quiet room.
- If alcohol was ingested within 4 hours, induce vomiting or perform gastric lavage; give activated charcoal and a saline cathartic.
- Monitor his vital signs.
- As ordered, give chlordiazepoxide every 4 hours to prevent withdrawal seizures, tremors, diaphoresis, anxiety, tachycardia, and hypertension. Diazepam may be used if an I.V. route needs to be used.
- Institute seizure precautions.
- Provide I.V. fluid replacement as well as dextrose, thiamine, B-complex vitamins, and vitamin C to treat dehydration, hypoglycemia, and nutritional deficiencies.
- Assess for aspiration pneumonia.
- Prepare the patient for dialysis if his vital functions are severely depressed.

UNDERSTANDING COMMONLY ABUSED SUBSTANCES *(continued)*

Substance	Signs and symptoms	Interventions

Depressants *(continued)*

Barbiturates (amobarbital, phenobarbital, secobarbital)

■ *Street names:* for barbiturates—barbs and downers; for amobarbital—blue angels and blue devils; for phenobarbital—goofballs and purple hearts; and for secobarbital—reds and red devils ■ *Routes:* ingestion and injection ■ *Dependence:* physical and psychological ■ *Duration:* 1 to 16 hours ■ *Medical uses:* anesthetic, anticonvulsant, sedative, hypnotic	■ *Of use:* absent reflexes, blisters or bullous lesions, cyanosis, depressed level of consciousness (LOC) (from confusion to coma), fever, flaccid muscles, hypotension, hypothermia, nystagmus, paradoxical reaction in children and elderly people, poor pupil reaction to light, and respiratory depression ■ *Of withdrawal:* agitation, anxiety, fever, insomnia, orthostatic hypotension, tachycardia, and tremors ■ *Of rapid withdrawal:* anorexia, apprehension, hallucinations, orthostatic hypotension, tonic-clonic seizures, tremors, and weakness	■ If ingestion was recent, induce vomiting or perform gastric lavage. Follow with activated charcoal. ■ Monitor the patient's vital signs and perform frequent neurologic assessments. ■ As ordered, give an I.V. fluid bolus for hypotension and alkalinized urine. ■ Institute seizure precautions. ■ Relieve withdrawal symptoms as ordered. ■ Use a hypothermia or hyperthermia blanket for temperature alterations.

Benzodiazepines (alprazolam, chlordiazepoxide, clonazepam, clorazepate, diazepam, flurazepam, halazepam, lorazepam, midazolam, oxazepam, prazepam, quazepam, temazepam, triazolam)

■ *Street names:* dolls and yellow jackets ■ *Routes:* ingestion and injection ■ *Dependence:* physical and psychological ■ *Duration of effect:* 4 to 8 hours ■ *Medical uses:* antianxiety agent, anticonvulsant, sedative, hypnotic	■ *Of use:* ataxia, drowsiness, hypotension, increased self-confidence, relaxation, and slurred speech ■ *Of overdose:* confusion, coma, drowsiness, and respiratory depression ■ *Of withdrawal:* abdominal cramps, agitation, anxiety, diaphoresis, hypertension, tachycardia, tonic-clonic seizures, tremors, and vomiting	■ If the drug was ingested, induce vomiting or perform gastric lavage. Follow with activated charcoal and a cathartic. ■ Monitor the patient's vital signs. ■ Give supplemental oxygen for hypoxia-induced seizures. ■ As ordered, give I.V. fluids for hypertension, and physostigmine salicylate for respiratory or central nervous system (CNS) depression. Flumazenil, a specific benzodiazepine antagonist, can be used in cases of overdose to reverse the effects of the benzodiazepine.

(continued)

UNDERSTANDING COMMONLY ABUSED SUBSTANCES *(continued)*

Substance	Signs and symptoms	Interventions

Depressants *(continued)*

Opiates (codeine, heroin, morphine, meperidine, and opium)

Substance	Signs and symptoms	Interventions
▪ *Street names:* for heroin — junk, horse, H, smack, Chinese white, and Mexican mud; for morphine — morph, M, and microdots ▪ *Routes:* for codeine, meperidine, and morphine — ingestion, injection, and smoking; for heroin — ingestion, injection, inhalation, and smoking; for opium — ingestion and smoking ▪ *Dependence:* physical and psychological ▪ *Duration of effect:* 3 to 6 hours ▪ *Medical uses:* for codeine — analgesia and antitussive; for heroin — none; for morphine and meperidine — analgesia; for opium — analgesia and antidiarrheal	▪ *Of use:* anorexia, arrhythmias, clammy skin, constipation, constricted pupils, decreased LOC, detachment from reality, drowsiness, euphoria, hypotension, impaired judgment, increased pigmentation over veins, lack of concern, lethargy, nausea, needle marks, respiratory depression, seizures, shallow or slow respirations, skin lesions or abscesses, slurred speech, swollen or perforated nasal mucosa, thrombotic veins, urine retention, and vomiting ▪ *Of withdrawal:* abdominal cramps, anorexia, chills, diaphoresis, dilated pupils, hyperactive bowel sounds, irritability, nausea, panic, piloerection, runny nose, sweating, tremors, watery eyes, and yawning	▪ If the drug was ingested, induce vomiting or perform gastric lavage. ▪ As ordered, give naloxone until CNS effects are reversed. ▪ Give I.V. fluids to increase circulatory volume. ▪ Use extra blankets for hypothermia; if ineffective, use a hyperthermia blanket. ▪ Reorient the patient to time, place, and person. ▪ Assess breath sounds to monitor for pulmonary edema. ▪ Monitor for signs and symptoms of withdrawal. ▪ Naltrexone is an opiate antagonist that reverses the effects of the opiate.

Hallucinogens

Lysergic acid diethylamide

Substance	Signs and symptoms	Interventions
▪ *Street names:* LSD, acid, blue dots, cube, D, owsleys, gel tabs, and microdot ▪ *Routes:* ingestion, smoking ▪ *Dependence:* possibly psychological ▪ *Duration of effect:* 8 to 12 hours ▪ *Medical uses:* none	▪ *Of use:* abdominal cramps, arrhythmias, chills, depersonalization, diaphoresis, diarrhea, distorted visual perception and perception of time and space, dizziness, dry mouth, fever, grandiosity, hallucinations, heightened sense of awareness, hyperpnea, hypertension, illusions, increased salivation, muscle aches, mystical experiences, nausea, palpitations, seizures, tachycardia, and vomiting ▪ *Of withdrawal:* none	▪ Place the patient in a quiet room. ▪ If the drug was ingested, induce vomiting or perform gastric lavage. Follow with activated charcoal and a cathartic. ▪ Monitor his vital signs, and give diazepam for seizures as ordered. ▪ Reorient the patient to time, place, and person, and restrain him as necessary.

UNDERSTANDING COMMONLY ABUSED SUBSTANCES (continued)

Substance	Signs and symptoms	Interventions

Hallucinogens (continued)

Phencyclidine
- *Street names:* PCP, hog, angel dust, peace pill, dummy mist, aurora, bust bee, guerrilla, rocket fuel
- *Routes:* ingestion, injection, and smoking
- *Dependence:* possibly psychological
- *Duration of effect:* 30 minutes to several days
- *Medical uses:* veterinary anesthetic

- *Of use:* amnesia; blank stare; cardiac arrest; decreased awareness of surroundings; delusions; distorted body image; distorted sense of sight, hearing, and touch; drooling; euphoria; excitation and psychoses; fever; gait ataxia; hallucinations; hyperactivity; hypertensive crisis; individualized unpredictable effects; muscle rigidity; nystagmus; panic; poor perception of time and distance; possible chromosomal damage; psychotic behavior; recurrent coma; renal failure; seizures; sudden behavioral changes; tachycardia; and violent behavior
- *Of withdrawal:* none

- Place the patient in a quiet room.
- If the drug was ingested, induce vomiting or perform gastric lavage. Follow with activated charcoal.
- Add ascorbic acid to I.V. solution to acidify urine.
- Monitor the patient's vital signs and urine output.
- If ordered, give a diuretic; propranolol for hypertension or tachycardia; nitroprusside for severe hypertensive crisis; diazepam for seizures; diazepam or haloperidol for agitation or psychotic behavior; and physostigmine, diazepam, chlordiazepoxide, or chlorpromazine for a "bad trip."

Stimulants

Amphetamines
- *Street names:* for amphetamine sulfate — bennies, cartwheels, and grennies; for methamphetamine — speed, meth, and crystal; and for dextroamphetamine sulfate — dexies, hearts, and oranges
- *Routes:* ingestion and injection
- *Dependence:* psychological
- *Duration of effect:* 1 to 4 hours
- *Medical uses:* hyperkinesis, narcolepsy, and weight control

- *Of use:* altered mental status (from confusion to paranoia), coma, diaphoresis, dilated reactive pupils, dry mouth, exhaustion, hallucinations, hyperactive deep tendon reflexes, hypertension, hyperthermia, paradoxical reaction in children, psychotic behavior with prolonged use, seizures, shallow respirations, tachycardia, and tremors
- *Of withdrawal:* abdominal tenderness, apathy, depression, disorientation, irritability, long periods of sleep, and muscle aches, or suicide (with sudden withdrawal)

- Place the patient in a quiet room.
- If the drug was ingested, induce vomiting or perform gastric lavage; give activated charcoal and a saline or magnesium sulfate cathartic.
- Add ammonium chloride or ascorbic acid to I.V. solution to acidify urine to a pH of 5. Also, administer mannitol to induce diuresis, as ordered.
- Monitor the patent's vital signs.
- As ordered, give a short-acting barbiturate, such as pentobarbital, for seizures; haloperidol for assaultive behavior; phentolamine for hypertension; propranolol for tachyarrhythmias; and lidocaine for ventricular arrhythmias.
- Restrain the patient if he's experiencing hallucinations or paranoia.
- Give a tepid sponge bath for fever.
- Institute suicide precautions.

(continued)

UNDERSTANDING COMMONLY ABUSED SUBSTANCES *(continued)*

Substance	Signs and symptoms	Interventions
Stimulants (continued)		

Cocaine

- *Street names:* coke, flake, snow, nose candy, hits, gold dust, toot, crack (hardened form), rock, and crank
- *Routes:* ingestion, injection, sniffing, and smoking
- *Dependence:* psychological
- *Duration of effect:* 15 minutes to 2 hours; with crack, rapid high of short duration followed by down feeling
- *Medical uses:* local anesthetic

- *Of use:* abdominal pain; alternating euphoria and fear; anorexia; cardiotoxicity, such as ventricular fibrillation or cardiac arrest; coma; confusion; diaphoresis; dilated pupils; excitability; fever; grandiosity; hyperpnea; hypotension or hypertension; insomnia; irritability; nausea and vomiting; pallor or cyanosis; perforated nasal septum with prolonged use; pressured speech; psychotic behavior with large doses; respiratory arrest; seizures; spasms; tachycardia; tachypnea; visual, auditory, and olfactory hallucinations; and weight loss
- *Of withdrawal:* anxiety, depression, and fatigue

- Place the patient in a quiet room.
- If cocaine was ingested, induce vomiting or perform gastric lavage. Follow with activated charcoal and a saline cathartic.
- If cocaine was sniffed, remove residual drug from mucous membranes.
- Monitor the patient's vital signs.
- Give propranolol for tachycardia.
- Perform cardiopulmonary resuscitation for ventricular fibrillation and cardiac arrest, as indicated.
- Give a tepid sponge bath for fever.
- Administer an anticonvulsant, as ordered, for seizures.

---

to drug abuse have few mental or emotional resources against stress, an overdependence on others, and a low tolerance for frustration. Taking the drug gives them pleasure by relieving tension, abolishing loneliness, allowing them to achieve a temporarily peaceful or euphoric state, or simply relieving boredom.

Drug dependence may follow experimentation with drugs in response to peer pressure. It also may follow the use of drugs to relieve physical pain, but this is uncommon.

Signs and symptoms

The signs and symptoms of acute intoxication vary, depending on the drug. The drug user seldom seeks treatment specifically for his drug problem. Instead, he may seek emergency treatment for drug-related injuries or complications, such as a motor vehicle accident, burns from freebasing, an overdose, physical deterioration from illness or malnutrition, or symptoms of withdrawal. Friends, family members, or law enforcement officials may bring the patient to the hospital because of respiratory depression, unconsciousness, acute injury, or a psychiatric crisis.

Examine the patient for signs and symptoms of drug use or drug-related complications as well as for clues to the type of drug ingested. For example, fever can result from stimulant or hallucinogen intoxication, from withdrawal, or from infection caused by I.V. drug use.

Inspect the eyes for lacrimation from opiate withdrawal, nystagmus from central nervous system (CNS) depressants or phencyclidine intoxication, and drooping eyelids from opiate or CNS depressant use. Constricted pupils occur with opiate use or withdrawal; dilated pupils, with the use of hallucinogens or amphetamines.

Examine the nose for rhinorrhea from opiate withdrawal and the oral and nasal mucosa for signs of drug-induced irritation. Drug sniffing can result in inflammation, atrophy, or perforation of the nasal mucosa. Dental conditions commonly result from the poor oral hygiene associated with chronic drug use. Also inspect under the tongue for evidence of I.V. drug injection.

Inspect the skin. Sweating, a common sign of intoxication with opiates or CNS stimulants, also accompanies most drug withdrawal syndromes. Drug use sometimes induces a sensation of bugs crawling on the skin, known as formication; as a result, the patient's skin may be excoriated from scratching.

Needle marks or tracks are an obvious sign of I.V. drug abuse. Keep in mind that the patient may attempt to conceal or disguise injection sites with tattoos or by selecting an inconspicuous site such as under the nails. In addition, self-injection can sometimes cause cellulitis or abscesses, especially in the patient who also is a chronic alcoholic. Puffy hands can be a late sign of thrombophlebitis or of fascial infection due to self-injection on the hands or arms.

Auscultation may disclose bilateral crackles and rhonchi caused by smoking and inhaling drugs or by opiate overdose. Other cardiopulmonary signs of overdose include pulmonary edema, respiratory depression, aspiration pneumonia, and hypotension. CNS stimulants and some hallucinogens may precipitate refractory acute-onset hypertension or cardiac arrhythmias. Withdrawal from opiates or depressants also can provoke arrhythmias and, occasionally, hypotension.

During opiate withdrawal, the patient may report abdominal pain, nausea, or vomiting. He may also complain of hemorrhoids, a consequence of the constipating effects of these drugs. Palpation of an enlarged liver, with or without tenderness, may indicate hepatitis.

Neurologic symptoms of drug abuse include tremors, hyperreflexia, hyporeflexia, and seizures. Abrupt withdrawal may precipitate signs of CNS depression (ranging from lethargy to coma), hallucinations, or signs of overstimulation, including euphoria and violent behavior.

Carefully review the patient's medical history. Suspect drug abuse if he reports a painful injury or chronic illness but refuses a diagnostic workup. In his attempt to obtain drugs, the dependent patient may feign illnesses, such as migraine headaches, myocardial infarction, and renal colic; claim an allergy to over-the-counter analgesics; or even request a specific medication. Also be alert for a history of overdose or a high tolerance for potentially addictive drugs. An I.V. drug user may have a history of hepatitis or human immunodeficiency virus (HIV) infection from sharing dirty needles. A female drug user may report a history of amenorrhea.

A patient who abuses drugs may give you a fictitious name and address, be reluctant to discuss previous hospitalizations, or seek treatment at a medical facility across town rather than in his own neighborhood. If possible, interview family members to verify his responses.

If the patient admits to drug use, try to determine the extent to which this behavior interferes with his normal functioning. Note whether he expresses a desire to overcome his dependence on drugs. If possible, obtain a drug history consisting of substances ingested, amount, frequency, and last dose. Expect incomplete or inaccurate responses. Drug-induced amnesia, a depressed level of consciousness, or ignorance may distort the patient's recollection of the facts; he also may fabricate answers to avoid arrest or to conceal a suicide attempt.

The hospitalized drug abuser is likely to be uncooperative, disruptive, or even violent. He may experience mood swings, anxiety, impaired memory, sleep disturbances, flashbacks, slurred speech, depression, and thought disorders. He may resort to plays on sympathy, bribery, or threats to obtain drugs, or he may try to pit one caregiver against another.

Psychoactive substances may be used in cultural practices. For instance, some Native Americans use hallucinatory drugs to help achieve spiritual experiences. Therefore, use and abuse must be carefully distinguished.

Diagnosis

For characteristic findings in patients with this condition, see *Diagnosing substance dependence and related disorders*, page 430. Various tests can confirm drug use, determine the amount and type of drug taken, and reveal complications. For example, a serum or urine drug screen can detect recently ingested substances.

Characteristic findings in other tests include elevated serum globulin levels, hypoglycemia, leukocytosis, liver function abnormalities, positive Venereal Disease Research Laboratory test results, positive rapid plasma reagin test results due to elevated protein fractions, an elevated mean corpuscular hemoglobin level, elevated uric acid levels, and reduced blood urea nitrogen levels.

Treatment

The patient with acute drug intoxication should receive symptomatic treatment based on the drug ingested. Measures include fluid replacement therapy and nutritional and vitamin supplements, if indicated; detoxification with the same drug or a pharmacologically similar drug (exceptions include cocaine, hallucinogens, and marijuana, which aren't used for detoxification); sedatives to induce sleep; anticholinergics and antidiarrheal agents to relieve GI distress; antianxiety drugs for severe agitation, especially in cocaine abusers; and symptomatic treatment of complications. Depending on the dosage and time elapsed before admission, additional treatment may include gastric lavage, induced emesis, activated charcoal, forced diuresis and, possibly, hemoperfusion or hemodialysis.

Treatment of drug dependence commonly involves a triad of care: detoxification, short- and long-term rehabilitation, and aftercare; the latter means a lifetime of abstinence, usually aided by participation in Narcotics Anonymous (NA) or a similar self-help group.

Detoxification, the controlled and gradual withdrawal of an abused drug, is achieved through substituting a drug with a similar action. Such gradual replacement of the abused drug controls the effects of withdrawal, thereby reducing the patient's discomfort and associated risks.

Depending on which drug the patient has abused, detoxification may be managed on an inpatient or outpatient basis. For example, withdrawal from depressants can produce hazardous adverse reactions, such as generalized tonic-clonic seizures, status epilepticus, and hypotension. The severity of these reactions determines whether the patient can be safely treated as an outpatient or if he requires hospitalization. Withdrawal from depressants usually requires detoxification because abrupt or poorly managed withdrawal from barbiturates can cause death.

Opioid withdrawal causes severe physical discomfort and can be life threatening. To minimize these effects, chronic opioid abusers commonly are detoxified with methadone.

To ease withdrawal from opioids, depressants, and other drugs, useful nonchemical measures may include psychotherapy, exercise, relaxation techniques, and nutritional support. Sedatives and tranquilizers may be administered temporarily to help the patient cope with insomnia, anxiety, and depression.

After withdrawal, the patient needs to participate in a rehabilitation program to prevent a recurrence. Rehabilitation programs are available for inpatients and outpatients; they usually last a month or longer and may include individual, group, and family psychotherapy. During and after rehabilitation, participation in a drug-oriented self-help group may be helpful. The largest such group is NA.

Special considerations

Focus on restoring the patient's physical health, educating him and his family about drug abuse and dependence, providing support, and encouraging participation in drug treatment programs and self-help groups.

During an acute episode:
■ Continuously monitor the patient's vital signs, and observe for complications of

overdose and withdrawal, such as cardiopulmonary arrest, seizures, and aspiration.

■ Based on standard hospital policy, institute appropriate measures to prevent suicide attempts.

■ Give medications, as ordered, to decrease withdrawal symptoms; monitor and record their effectiveness.

■ Maintain a quiet, safe environment during withdrawal from any drug because excessive noise may agitate the patient.

■ Remove harmful objects from the patient's room, and use restraints only if you suspect that he might harm himself or others. Institute seizure precautions.

After an acute episode:

■ Learn to control your reactions to the patient's undesirable behaviors — commonly, psychological dependency, manipulation, anger, frustration, and alienation.

■ Set limits for dealing with demanding, manipulative behavior.

■ Promote adequate nutrition and monitor the patient's nutritional intake.

■ Administer medications carefully to prevent hoarding by the patient. Check the patient's mouth to ensure that he has swallowed the medication. Closely monitor visitors who might supply the patient with drugs.

■ Refer the patient for detoxification and rehabilitation, as appropriate. Give him a list of available resources.

■ Encourage family members to seek help whether or not the abuser seeks it. You can suggest private therapy or community mental health clinics.

If the patient refuses to participate in a rehabilitation program, teach him how to minimize the risk of drug-related complications, as follows:

■ Review measures for preventing HIV infection and hepatitis. Stress that these infections are readily transmitted by sharing needles with other drug users and by having unprotected sexual intercourse.

■ Advise the patient to use a new needle for every injection or to clean needles with a solution of chlorine bleach and water.

■ Emphasize the importance of using a condom during intercourse to prevent disease transmission and pregnancy. If necessary, teach the female drug abuser about other methods of birth control. Explain the devastating effects of drugs on the developing fetus.

PSYCHOTIC DISORDERS

Schizophrenia

Schizophrenia is characterized by disturbances (for at least 6 months) in thought content and form, perception, affect, sense of self, volition, interpersonal relationships, and psychomotor behavior. (See *Phases of schizophrenia*, page 440.) The *Diagnostic and Statistical Manual of Mental Disorders*, Fourth Edition, Text Revision (*DSM-IV-TR*), recognizes paranoid, disorganized, catatonic, undifferentiated, and residual schizophrenia. Onset of symptoms usually occurs during adolescence or early adulthood. The disorder produces varying degrees of impairment. Up to one-third of patients with schizophrenia have just one psychotic episode and no more. Some patients have no disability between periods of exacerbation; others need continuous institutional care. The prognosis worsens with each episode.

Causes and incidence

Schizophrenia affects 1% to 2% of the population in the United States and is equally prevalent in both sexes. It may result from a combination of genetic, biological, cultural, and psychological factors. Some evidence supports a genetic predisposition. Close relatives of people with schizophrenia have a greater likelihood of developing schizophrenia; the closer the degree of biological relatedness, the higher the risk.

The most widely accepted biochemical theory holds that schizophrenia results from excessive activity at dopaminergic synapses. Other neurotransmitter alterations, such as serotonin increases, may also contribute to schizophrenic symptoms. In addition, patients with schizophrenia have structural abnormalities of the frontal and temporolimbic systems. Computed tomography scans and magnetic resonance imaging studies show various

PHASES OF SCHIZOPHRENIA

Schizophrenia usually occurs in three phases: prodromal, active, and residual.

Prodromal phase
The *Diagnostic and Statistical Manual of Mental Disorders,* Fourth Edition, Text Revision *(DSM-IV-TR),* characterizes the prodromal phase as clear deterioration in functioning before the active phase of the disturbance that isn't due to a disturbance in mood or to a psychoactive substance use disorder and that involves at least two of the following signs and symptoms:
- marked social isolation or withdrawal
- marked impairment in role functioning as wage-earner, student, or homemaker
- markedly peculiar behavior
- marked impairment in personal hygiene and grooming
- blunted or inappropriate affect
- digressive, vague, overelaborate, or circumstantial speech; poverty of speech; or poverty of content of speech
- odd beliefs or magical thinking influencing behavior and inconsistent with cultural norms
- unusual perceptual experiences
- marked lack of initiative, interests, or energy.

Family members or friends may report personality changes. Typically insidious, this phase may extend over several months or years.

Active phase
During the active phase, the patient exhibits frankly psychotic symptoms. Psychiatric evaluation may reveal delusions, hallucinations, loosening of associations, incoherence, and catatonic behavior. The patient's psychosocial history may also disclose a particular stressor before the onset of this phase.

Residual phase
According to the *DSM-IV-TR,* the residual phase follows the active phase and occurs when at least two of the symptoms noted in the prodromal phase persist. These symptoms don't result from a disturbance in mood or from a psychoactive substance use disorder.

The residual phase resembles the prodromal phase, except that disturbances in affect and role functioning usually are more severe. Delusions and hallucinations may persist.

---

structural brain abnormalities, including frontal lobe atrophy and increased lateral and third ventricles. Positron emission tomography scans substantiate frontal lobe hypometabolism.

Numerous psychological and sociocultural causes, such as disturbed family and interpersonal patterns, also have been proposed. Schizophrenia is more common in lower socioeconomic groups, possibly due to downward social drift, lack of upward socioeconomic mobility, and high stress levels that may stem from poverty, social failure, illness, and inadequate social resources. Higher incidence is also linked to low birth weight and congenital deafness.

Signs and symptoms

Schizophrenia is associated with many abnormal behaviors; therefore, signs and symptoms vary widely, depending on the type and phase (prodromal, active, or residual) of the illness.

Watch for these signs and symptoms:
- ambivalence — coexisting strong positive and negative feelings, leading to emotional conflict
- apathy and other affective abnormalities
- clang associations — words that rhyme or sound alike used in an illogical, nonsensical manner — for instance, "It's the rain, train, pain"
- concrete associations — inability to form or understand abstract thoughts

- delusions — false ideas or beliefs accepted as real by the patient; delusions of grandeur, persecution, and reference (distorted belief regarding the relation between events and one's self — for example, a belief that television programs address the patient on a personal level); feelings of being controlled, somatic illness, and depersonalization
- echolalia — automatic and meaningless repetition of another's words or phrases
- echopraxia — involuntary repetition of movements observed in others
- flight of ideas — rapid succession of incomplete and loosely connected ideas
- hallucinations — false sensory perceptions with no basis in reality; usually visual or auditory, but may also be olfactory (smell), gustatory (taste), or tactile (touch)
- illusions — false sensory perceptions with some basis in reality; for example, a car backfiring mistaken for a gunshot
- loose associations — rapid shifts among unrelated ideas
- magical thinking — belief that thoughts or wishes can control others or events
- neologisms — bizarre words that have meaning only for the patient
- poor interpersonal relationships
- regression — return to an earlier developmental stage
- thought blocking — sudden interruption in the patient's train of thought
- withdrawal — disinterest in objects, people, or surroundings
- word salad — illogical word groupings, such as "She had a star, barn, plant."

Diagnosis

After a complete physical and psychiatric examinations rule out an organic cause of symptoms such as an amphetamine-induced psychosis, a diagnosis of schizophrenia may be considered. A diagnosis is made if the patient's symptoms match those in the *DSM-IV-TR*. (See *Diagnosing schizophrenia*, page 442.)

Treatment

In schizophrenia, treatment focuses on meeting the physical and psychosocial needs of the patient, based on his previous level of adjustment and his response to medical and nursing interventions. Treatment may combine drug therapy, long-term psychotherapy for the patient and his family, psychosocial rehabilitation, vocational counseling, and the use of community resources.

The primary treatment for more than 30 years, antipsychotic drugs (also called neuroleptic drugs) appear to work by blocking postsynaptic dopamine receptors. These drugs reduce the incidence of positive psychotic symptoms, such as hallucinations and delusions, and relieve anxiety and agitation. Newer antipsychotics are effective in relieving positive and negative symptoms of schizophrenia. Other psychiatric drugs, such as antidepressants and anxiolytics, may control associated signs and symptoms.

Certain antipsychotic drugs are associated with numerous adverse reactions, some of which are irreversible. (See *Reviewing adverse effects of antipsychotic drugs,* page 443.) The newer antipsychotic drugs appear to be effective in treating the negative symptoms of schizophrenia (withdrawal, apathy, or blunted affect). Antipsychotic drugs are broken down into two major classes: dopamine receptor antagonists (haloperidol and thorazine) and dopamine-serotonin antagonists, also called *atypical antipsychotics* (risperidone and clozapine). The long-acting medications haloperidol and fluphenazine may be given I.M. every 3 to 4 weeks to improve compliance.

Clozapine may be prescribed for severely ill patients who fail to respond to standard treatment. This agent effectively controls more psychotic signs and symptoms without the usual adverse effects. However, clozapine can cause drowsiness, sedation, excessive salivation, tachycardia, dizziness, and seizures. Agranulocytosis, a potentially fatal blood disorder characterized by a low white blood cell count and pronounced neutropenia, may also occur; therefore, patients on clozapine must be monitored closely with frequent complete blood counts. Risperidone and olanzapine, like clozapine, have reduced the incidence of adverse effects, including extrapyramidal symptoms and anticholinergic adverse effects.

(*Text continues on page 444.*)

DIAGNOSING SCHIZOPHRENIA

The following criteria described in the *Diagnostic and Statistical Manual of Mental Disorders*, Fourth Edition, Text Revision, are used to diagnose a person with schizophrenia.

Characteristic symptoms

A person with schizophrenia has two or more of the following symptoms (each present for a significant time during a 1-month period—or less if successfully treated):

- delusions
- hallucinations
- disorganized speech
- grossly disorganized or catatonic behavior
- negative symptoms (affective flattening, alagia, anhedonia, attention impairment, apathy, and avolition).

The diagnosis requires only one of these characteristic symptoms if the person's delusions are bizarre, or if hallucinations consist of a voice issuing a running commentary on the person's behavior or thoughts or two or more voices conversing.

Social and occupational dysfunction

For a significant period since the onset of the disturbance, one or more major areas of functioning (such as work, interpersonal relations, or self-care) are markedly below the level achieved before the onset.

When the disturbance begins in childhood or adolescence, the dysfunction takes the form of failure to achieve the expected level of interpersonal, academic, or occupational development.

Duration

Continuous signs of the disturbance persist for at least 6 months. The 6-month period must include at least 1 month of symptoms (or less if signs and symptoms have been successfully treated) that match the characteristic symptoms and may include periods of prodromal or residual symptoms.

During the prodromal or residual period, signs of the disturbance may be manifested by only negative symptoms or by two or more characteristic symptoms in a less severe form.

Schizoaffective and mood disorder exclusion

Schizoaffective disorder and mood disorder with psychotic features have been ruled out for these reasons: Either no major depressive, manic, or mixed episodes have occurred concurrently with the active-phase symptoms, *or*, if mood disorder episodes have occurred during active-phase symptoms, their total duration has been brief relative to the duration of the active and residual periods.

Substance and general medical condition exclusion

The disturbance isn't due to the direct physiologic effects of a substance or a general medical condition.

Relationship to a pervasive developmental disorder

If the person has a history of autistic disorder or another pervasive developmental disorder, the additional diagnosis of schizophrenia is appropriate only if prominent delusions or hallucinations are also present for at least 1 month (or less if successfully treated).

REVIEWING ADVERSE EFFECTS OF ANTIPSYCHOTIC DRUGS

The newer atypical agents, such as risperidone, olanzapine, quetiapine, sertindole, and ziprasidone, produce fewer extrapyramidal symptoms than the first, older class of antipsychotics. Risperidone is associated with increases in serum prolactin. Olanzapine, in moderate doses, induces little extrapyramidal symptoms, but has been associated with weight gain and blood glucose abnormalities. Quetiapine can cause weight gain, hypotension, and sedation.

Older classes of antipsychotic drugs (sometimes known as *neuroleptic drugs*) can cause sedative, anticholinergic, or extrapyramidal effects; orthostatic hypotension; and, rarely, neuroleptic malignant syndrome.

Sedative, anticholinergic, and extrapyramidal effects

High-potency drugs (such as haloperidol) are minimally sedative and anticholinergic but cause a high incidence of extrapyramidal adverse effects. Intermediate-potency agents (such as molindone) are associated with a moderate incidence of adverse effects, whereas low-potency drugs (such as chlorpromazine) are highly sedative and anticholinergic but produce few extrapyramidal adverse effects.

The most common extrapyramidal effects are dystonia, parkinsonism, and akathisia. Dystonia usually occurs in young male patients within the first few days of treatment. Characterized by severe tonic contractions of the muscles in the neck, mouth, and tongue, dystonia may be misdiagnosed as a psychotic symptom. Diphenhydramine or benztropine administered I.M. or I.V. provides rapid relief from this symptom.

Drug-induced parkinsonism results in bradykinesia, muscle rigidity, shuffling or propulsive gait, stooped posture, flat facial affect, tremors, and drooling. Parkinsonism may occur from 1 week to several months after the initiation of drug treatment. Drugs prescribed to reverse or prevent this syndrome include benztropine, trihexyphenidyl, and amantadine.

Tardive dyskinesia can occur after only 6 months of continuous therapy and is usually irreversible. No effective treatment is available for this disorder, which is characterized by various involuntary movements of the mouth and jaw; flapping or writhing; purposeless, rapid, and jerky movements of the arms and legs; and dystonic posture of the neck and trunk.

Signs and symptoms of akathisia include restlessness, pacing, and an inability to rest or sit still. Propranolol relieves this adverse effect.

Orthostatic hypotension

Low-potency neuroleptics can cause orthostatic hypotension because they block alpha-adrenergic receptors. If hypotension is severe, the patient is placed in the supine position and given I.V. fluids for hypovolemia. If further treatment is necessary, an alpha-adrenergic agonist, such as norepinephrine or metaraminol, may be ordered to relieve hypotension. Mixed alpha- and beta-adrenergic drugs (such as epinephrine) or beta-adrenergic drugs (such as isoproterenol) shouldn't be given because they can further reduce blood pressure.

Neuroleptic malignant syndrome

Neuroleptic malignant syndrome is a life-threatening syndrome that occurs in up to 1% of patients taking antipsychotic drugs. Signs and symptoms include fever, muscle rigidity, and altered level of consciousness occurring hours to months after initiating drug therapy or increasing the dose. Treatment is symptomatic, largely consisting of dantrolene and other measures to counter muscle rigidity associated with hyperthermia. You'll need to monitor vital signs and mental status continuously.

Routine blood monitoring is essential to detect the estimated 1% to 2% of all patients taking clozapine who develop agranulocytosis. If caught in the early stages, this disorder is reversible.

Clinicians disagree about the effectiveness of psychotherapy in treating schizophrenia. Some consider it a useful adjunct to drug therapy. Others suggest that psychosocial rehabilitation, education, and social skills training are more effective for chronic schizophrenia. In addition to improving understanding of the disorder, these methods teach the patient and his family coping strategies, effective communication techniques, and social skills.

Because schizophrenia typically disrupts the family, family therapy may be helpful to reduce guilt and disappointment as well as improve acceptance of the patient and his bizarre behavior.

Special considerations

■ Assess the patient's ability to carry out activities of daily living, paying special attention to his nutritional status. Monitor his weight if he isn't eating. If he thinks that his food is poisoned, let him fix his own food when possible or offer foods in closed containers that he can open. If you give liquid medication in a unit-dose container, allow the patient to open the container.

■ Maintain a safe environment, minimizing stimuli. Administer prescribed medications to decrease symptoms and anxiety. Use physical restraints according to your hospital's policy to ensure the patient's safety and that of others.

■ Adopt an accepting and consistent approach with the patient. Short, repeated contacts are best until trust has been established.

■ Avoid promoting dependence. Reward positive behavior to help the patient improve his level of functioning.

■ Engage the patient in reality-oriented activities that involve human contact, such as inpatient social skills training groups, outpatient day care, and sheltered workshops. Provide reality-based explanations for distorted body images or hypochondriacal complaints. Explain to the patient that his private language, autistic inventions, or neologisms aren't understood. Set limits on inappropriate behavior.

■ If the patient is hallucinating, explore the content of the hallucinations. If he hears voices, find out if he believes that he must do what they command. Explore the emotions connected with the hallucinations, but don't argue about them. If possible, change the subject.

■ Assist the patient to recognize the nonreality of his hallucinatory experience.

■ Teach the patient techniques that interrupt the hallucinations (listening to an audiocassette player, singing out loud, or reading out loud).

■ Don't tease or joke with a patient with schizophrenia. Choose words and phrases that are unambiguous and clearly understood. For instance, a patient who's told, "That procedure will be done on the floor," may become frightened, thinking he'll need to lie down on the floor.

■ If the patient expresses suicidal thoughts, institute suicide precautions. Document his behavior and your actions.

■ If he's expressing homicidal thoughts (for example, "I have to kill my mother"), institute homicidal precautions. Notify the physician and the potential victim. Document the patient's comments and the names of those who were notified.

■ Don't touch the patient without telling him first exactly what you're going to do — for example, "I'm going to put this cuff on your arm so I can take your blood pressure."

■ If necessary, postpone procedures that require physical contact with hospital personnel until the patient is less suspicious or agitated.

■ Remember, institutionalization may produce symptoms and disabilities that aren't part of the patient's illness, so evaluate symptoms carefully.

■ Mobilize community resources to provide a support system for the patient. Ongoing support is essential to his mastery of social skills.

■ Encourage compliance with the medication regimen to prevent a relapse. Also, monitor the patient carefully for adverse reactions to drug therapy, including acute dystonia, drug-induced parkinsonism, akathisia, tardive dyskinesia, and malignant neuroleptic syndrome. Document and report such reactions promptly.

- Help the patient explore possible connections between anxiety and stress and the exacerbation of symptoms.

For catatonic schizophrenia:

- Assess for physical illness. Remember that the mute patient won't complain of pain or physical symptoms; if he's in a bizarre posture, he's at risk for pressure ulcers or decreased circulation to a body area.

- Meet the patient's physical needs for adequate food, fluid, exercise, and elimination; follow orders with respect to nutrition, urinary catheterization, and enema.

- Provide range-of-motion exercises for the patient or help him ambulate every 2 hours.

- Prevent physical exhaustion and injury during periods of hyperactivity.

- Tell the patient directly, specifically, and concisely which procedures need to be done. For example, you might say to the patient, "It's time to go for a walk. Let's go." Don't offer the negativistic patient a choice.

- Spend some time with the patient even if he's mute and unresponsive. He's acutely aware of his environment even though he seems not to be. Your presence can be reassuring and supportive.

- Verbalize for the patient the message that his nonverbal behavior seems to convey; encourage him to do so as well.

- Offer reality orientation. You might say, "The leaves on the trees are turning colors and the air is cooler. It's fall!" Emphasize reality in all contacts to reduce distorted perceptions.

- Stay alert for violent outbursts; if they occur, get help promptly to ensure the patient's safety and your own.

For paranoid schizophrenia:

- When the patient is newly admitted, minimize his contact with the hospital staff.

- Don't crowd the patient physically or psychologically; he may strike out to protect himself.

- Be flexible; allow the patient some control. Approach him in a calm and unhurried manner. Let him talk about anything he wishes initially, but keep the conversation light and social. Avoid entering into power struggles.

- Respond to the patient's condescending attitudes (arrogance, put-downs, sarcasm, or open hostility) with neutral remarks.

- Don't let the patient put you on the defensive, and don't take his remarks personally. If he tells you to leave him alone, do leave but return soon. Brief contacts with the patient may be most useful at first.

- Don't make attempts to combat the patient's delusions with logic. Instead, respond to feelings, themes, or underlying needs — for example, "It seems you feel you've been treated unfairly."

- Be honest and dependable. Don't threaten the patient or make promises that you can't fulfill.

- If the patient is taking clozapine, stress the importance of returning weekly or biweekly to the hospital or an outpatient setting to have his blood monitored.

- Teach the patient the importance of complying with the medication regimen. Tell him to report any adverse reactions instead of discontinuing the drug. If he takes a slow-release formulation, make sure that he understands when to return to the physician for his next dose.

- Involve the patient's family in his treatment. Teach them how to recognize an impending relapse, and suggest ways to manage symptoms, such as tension, nervousness, insomnia, decreased ability to concentrate, and apathy.

Delusional disorders

According to the *Diagnostic and Statistical Manual of Mental Disorders,* Fourth Edition, Text Revision, delusional disorders are marked by false beliefs with a plausible basis in reality. Formerly referred to as paranoid disorders, delusional disorders involve erotomanic, grandiose, jealous, somatic, or persecutory themes. (See *Delusional themes,* page 446.) Some patients experience several types of delusions, whereas others experience unspecified delusions with no dominant theme. Typically chronic, these disorders commonly interfere with social and marital relationships, but sel-

DELUSIONAL THEMES

In a patient with a delusional disorder, the delusions usually are well systematized and follow a predominant theme. Common delusional themes are discussed below.

Erotomanic delusions

This prevalent delusional theme concerns romantic or spiritual love. The patient believes that he shares an idealized (rather than sexual) relationship with someone of higher status — a superior at work, a celebrity, or an anonymous stranger.

The patient may keep this delusion secret, but more commonly will try to contact the object of his delusion by phone calls, letters (including e-mail), gifts, or even spying. He may attempt to rescue his beloved from imagined danger. Many patients with erotomanic delusions harass public figures and come to the attention of the police.

Grandiose delusions

The patient with grandiose delusions believes that he has great, unrecognized talent, special insights, prophetic power, or has made an important discovery. To achieve recognition, he may contact government agencies such as the Federal Bureau of Investigation. The patient with a religion-oriented delusion of grandeur may become a cult leader. Less commonly, he believes that he shares a special relationship with some well-known personality, such as a rock star or a world leader. He may believe himself to be a famous person, his identity usurped by an imposter.

Jealous delusions

Jealous delusions focus on infidelity. For example, a patient may insist that his spouse or lover has been unfaithful, and may search for evidence to justify the delusion such as spots on bed sheets. He may confront his partner, try to control her movements, follow her, or try to track down her suspected lover. He may physically assault her or, less likely, his perceived rival.

Somatic delusions

Somatic delusions center on an imagined physical defect or deformity. The patient may perceive a foul odor coming from his skin, mouth, rectum, or another body part. Other delusions involve skin-crawling insects, internal parasites, or physical illness.

Persecutory delusions

The patient suffering from persecutory delusions, the most common type of delusion, believes that he's being followed, harassed, plotted against, poisoned, mocked, or deliberately prevented from achieving his long-term goals. These delusions may evolve into a simple or complex persecution scheme, in which even the slightest injustice is interpreted as part of the scheme.

Such a patient may file numerous lawsuits or seek redress from government agencies (querulous paranoia). A patient who becomes resentful and angry may lash out violently against the alleged offender.

---

dom impair intellectual or occupational functioning significantly.

Causes and incidence

Delusional disorders of later life strongly suggest a hereditary predisposition. At least one study has linked the development of delusional disorders to inferiority feelings in the family. Some researchers suggest that delusional disorders are the product of specific early childhood experiences with an authoritarian family structure. Others hold that anyone with a sensitive personality is particularly vulnerable to developing a delusional disorder.

Certain medical conditions — head injury, chronic alcoholism, and deafness — and aging are known to increase the risks of delusional disorders. Predisposing factors linked to aging include isolation, lack of stimulating interpersonal relationships, physical illness, and impaired hearing and vision. In addition, severe stress (such as a move to a foreign country) may precipitate a delusional disorder.

Delusional disorders commonly begin in middle or late adulthood, usually between ages 40 and 55, but they can occur at a younger age. These uncommon illnesses affect less than 1% of the population; the incidence is about equal in men and women.

Signs and symptoms

The psychiatric history of a delusional patient may be unremarkable, aside from behavior related to his delusions. He's likely to report problems with social and marital relationships, including depression or sexual dysfunction. He may describe a life marked by social isolation or hostility. He may deny feeling lonely, relentlessly criticizing or placing unreasonable demands on others.

Gathering accurate information from a delusional patient may prove difficult. He may deny his feelings, disregard the circumstances that lead to his hospitalization, and refuse treatment. However, his responses and behavior during the assessment interview provide clues that can help to identify his disorder. Family members may confirm your observations — for example, by reporting that the patient is chronically jealous or suspicious.

Note how well the patient communicates. He may be evasive or reluctant to answer questions. Conversely, he may be overly talkative, explaining events in great detail and emphasizing what he has achieved, prominent people he knows, or places where he has traveled. Statements that first seem logical may later prove irrelevant. Some of his answers may be contradictory, jumbled, or irrational.

Be alert for expressions of denial, projection, and rationalization. Once delusions become firmly entrenched, the patient will no longer seek to justify his beliefs. However, if he's still struggling to maintain his delusional defenses, he may make statements that reveal his condition, such as "People at work won't talk to me because I'm smarter than them." Accusatory statements are also characteristic of the delusional patient. Record pervasive delusional themes (for example, grandiose or persecutory).

Also watch for nonverbal cues, such as excessive vigilance or obvious apprehension on entering the room. During questions, the patient may listen intently, reacting defensively to imagined slights or insults. He may sit at the edge of his seat or fold his arms as if to shield himself. If he carries papers or money, he may clutch them firmly.

Diagnosis

For characteristic findings in patients with this condition, see *Diagnosing delusional disorders*, page 448. In addition, blood and urine tests, psychological tests, and neurologic evaluation can rule out organic causes of the delusions, such as amphetamine-induced psychoses and Alzheimer's disease. Endocrine function tests rule out hyperadrenalism, pernicious anemia, and thyroid disorders.

Treatment

Effective treatment of delusional disorders, consisting of a combination of drug therapy and psychotherapy, must correct the behavior and mood disturbances that result from the patient's mistaken beliefs. Treatment may also include mobilizing a support system for the isolated elderly patient.

Drug treatment with antipsychotic agents is similar to that used in schizophrenic disorders. Antipsychotics appear to work by blocking postsynaptic dopamine receptors. These drugs reduce the incidence of psychotic symptoms, such as hallucinations and delusions, and relieve anxiety and agitation. Other psychiatric drugs, such as antidepressants and anxiolytics, may be prescribed to control associated symptoms.

A patient's history of medication response is the best guide when selecting

DIAGNOSING DELUSIONAL DISORDERS

In an individual with suspected delusional disorder, psychiatric examination confirms the diagnosis. The examiner bases the diagnosis on the following criteria set forth in the *Diagnostic and Statistical Manual of Mental Disorders*, Fourth Edition, Text Revision:

- Nonbizarre delusions of at least 1 month's duration are present, involving real-life situations, such as being followed, poisoned, infected, loved at a distance, or deceived by one's spouse or lover.
- The patient's symptoms have never met the criteria known as *characteristic symptoms* of schizophrenia. However, tactile and olfactory hallucinations may be present if they're related to a delusional theme.
- Apart from being affected by the delusion or its ramifications, the patient is neither markedly impaired functionally nor is his behavior obviously odd or bizarre.
- If mood disturbances have occurred concurrently with delusions, their total duration has been brief relative to the duration of the delusional disturbance.
- The disturbance isn't due to the direct physiologic effects of a substance or a general medical condition.

Delusional disorder or paranoid schizophrenia?
To distinguish between these two disorders, consider the following characteristics.

Delusional disorder
In a delusional disorder, the patient's delusions reflect reality and are arranged into a coherent system. They're based on misinterpretations of, or elaborations on, reality. The patient doesn't experience hallucinations, and his affect and behavior are normal.

Paranoid schizophrenia
In paranoid schizophrenia, the patient's delusions are scattered, illogical, and incoherently arranged with no direct relation to reality. The patient may have hallucinations, his affect is inappropriate and inconsistent, and his behavior is bizarre.

---

treatment. The lowest dose should be started initially and increased slowly based on the patient's response. If the symptoms don't improve during a 6-week trial, other classes of antipsychotics may be tried. Haloperidol, fluphenazine decanoate, and fluphenazine enanthate are depot formulations that are implanted I.M. to release the drug gradually over a 30-day period, improving compliance. Usually, however, this type of treatment isn't necessary. Pimozide may be particularly effective in delusional disorders.

Clozapine, which differs chemically from other antipsychotic drugs, may be prescribed for severely ill patients who fail to respond to standard treatment. This agent effectively controls a wider range of psychotic symptoms without the usual adverse effects.

However, clozapine can cause drowsiness, sedation, excessive salivation, tachycardia, dizziness, and seizures. Agranulocytosis, a potentially fatal blood disorder characterized by a low white blood cell count and pronounced neutropenia, may also occur. Routine blood monitoring is essential to detect the estimated 1% to 2% of all patients taking clozapine who develop agranulocytosis. If caught in the early stages, this disorder is reversible.

Special considerations
- In dealing with the delusional patient, be direct, straightforward, and dependable. Whenever possible, elicit his feedback. Move slowly and matter-of-factly and re-

spond without anger or defensiveness to his hostile remarks.
- Respect the patient's privacy and space needs. Don't touch him unnecessarily.
- Take steps to reduce social isolation, if the patient allows. Gradually increase social contacts after he has become comfortable with the staff.
- Watch for refusal of medication or food, resulting from the patient's irrational fear of poisoning.
- Monitor the patient carefully for the adverse effects of antipsychotic drugs: drug-induced parkinsonism, acute dystonia, akathisia, tardive dyskinesia, and malignant neuroleptic syndrome.
- If the patient is taking clozapine, stress the importance of returning weekly to the hospital or an outpatient setting to have his blood monitored.
- Involve the patient's family in treatment. Teach them how to recognize an impending relapse, and suggest ways to manage symptoms. These include tension, nervousness, insomnia, decreased concentration ability, and apathy.
- Remember to consider cultural beliefs. Some Chinese men believe that their genitals withdraw into the abdomen as a precursor to death.

MOOD DISORDERS

Bipolar disorders

Marked by severe pathologic mood swings from hyperactivity and euphoria to sadness and depression, bipolar disorders involve various symptom combinations. Type I bipolar disorder is characterized by alternating episodes of mania and depression, whereas type II is characterized by recurrent depressive episodes and occasional mild manic (hypomanic) episodes. In some patients, bipolar disorder assumes a seasonal pattern, marked by a cyclic relation between the onset of the mood episode and a particular 60-day period of the year.

Causes and incidence

The cause of bipolar disorder is unclear, but hereditary, biological, and psychological factors may play a part. For example, the incidence of bipolar disorder among relatives of affected patients is higher than in the general population and highest among maternal relatives. The closer the relationship, the greater the susceptibility. Children with one affected parent have a 25% chance of developing bipolar disorder; children with two affected parents, a 50% chance. The incidence of this illness in siblings is 20% to 25%; in identical twins, the incidence is 66% to 96%.

Although certain biochemical changes accompany mood swings, it isn't clear whether these changes cause the mood swings or result from them. In mania and depression, intracellular sodium concentration increases during illness and returns to normal with recovery.

Patients with mood disorders have a defect in the way the brain handles certain neurotransmitters—chemical messengers that shuttle nerve impulses between neurons. Low levels of the chemicals dopamine and norepinephrine, for example, have been linked to depression, whereas excessively high levels of these chemicals are associated with mania.

Changes in the concentration of acetylcholine and serotonin may also play a role. Although neurobiologists have yet to prove that these chemical shifts cause bipolar disorder, it's widely assumed that most antidepressant medications work by modifying these neurotransmitter systems.

New data suggest that changes in the circadian rhythms that control hormone secretion, body temperature, and appetite may contribute to the development of bipolar disorder.

Emotional or physical trauma, such as bereavement, disruption of an important relationship, or a serious accidental injury, may precede the onset of bipolar disorder; however, bipolar disorder commonly appears without identifiable predisposing factors.

Manic episodes may follow a stressful event, but they're also associated with antidepressant therapy and childbirth. Major depressive episodes may be precipitated by

CYCLOTHYMIC DISORDER

A chronic mood disturbance of at least 2 years' duration, cyclothymic disorder involves numerous episodes of hypomania or depression that aren't of sufficient severity or duration to qualify as a major depressive episode or a bipolar disorder.

Cyclothymia commonly starts in adolescence or early adulthood. Beginning insidiously, this disorder leads to persistent social and occupational dysfunction.

Signs and symptoms
In the hypomanic phase, the patient may experience insomnia; hyperactivity; inflated self-esteem; increased productivity and creativity; overinvolvement in pleasurable activities, including an increased sexual drive; physical restlessness; and rapid speech. Depressive symptoms may include insomnia, feelings of inadequacy, decreased productivity, social withdrawal, loss of libido, loss of interest in pleasurable activities, lethargy, slow speech, and crying.

Diagnosis
Many medical disorders (for example, endocrinopathies, such as Cushing's syndrome, stroke, brain tumors, and head trauma) and drug overdose can produce a similar pattern of mood alteration. These organic causes must be ruled out before making a diagnosis of cyclothymic disorder.

rience bipolar disorder. This disorder affects women and men equally and is more common in higher socioeconomic groups. It can begin any time after adolescence, but onset usually occurs between ages 20 and 35; about 35% of patients experience onset between ages 35 and 60. Before the onset of overt symptoms, many patients with bipolar disorder have an energetic and outgoing personality with a history of wide mood swings.

Bipolar disorder recurs in 80% of patients; as they grow older, the episodes recur more frequently and last longer. This illness is associated with a significant mortality; 20% of patients commit suicide, many just as the depression lifts.

■ **ELDER TIP** *The older adult at highest risk for suicide is at least age 85, is depressed, has high self-esteem, and needs to control his own life. Even a frail nursing home resident with these characteristics may have the strength to kill himself.*

Signs and symptoms
Signs and symptoms vary widely, depending on whether the patient is experiencing a manic or a depressive episode.

During the assessment interview, the *manic* patient typically appears grandiose, euphoric, expansive, or irritable with little control over his activities and responses. He may describe hyperactive or excessive behavior, including elaborate plans for numerous social events, efforts to renew old acquaintances by telephoning friends at all hours of the night, buying sprees, or promiscuous sexual activity. He seldom hesitates to start projects for which he has little aptitude.

The patient's activities may have a bizarre quality, such as dressing in colorful or strange garments, wearing excessive makeup, or giving advice to passing strangers. He commonly expresses an inflated sense of self-esteem, ranging from uncritical self-confidence to marked grandiosity, which may be delusional.

Note the patient's speech patterns and concentration level. Accelerated and pressured speech, frequent changes of topic, and flight of ideas are common features of the manic phase. The patient is easily distracted and responds rapidly to external

chronic physical illness, psychoactive drug dependence, psychosocial stressors, and childbirth. Other familial influences, especially the early loss of a parent, parental depression, incest, or abuse, may predispose a person to depressive illness. (See *Cyclothymic disorder.*)

The American Psychiatric Association estimates that 0.4% to 1.2% of adults expe-

stimuli, such as background noise or a ringing telephone.

Physical examination of the manic patient may reveal signs of malnutrition and poor personal hygiene. He may report sleeping and eating less as well as being more physically active than usual.

Hypomania, more common than acute mania, can be recognized during the assessment interview by three classic symptoms: euphoric but unstable mood, pressured speech, and increased motor activity. The hypomanic patient may appear elated, hyperactive, easily distracted, talkative, irritable, impatient, impulsive, and full of energy but seldom exhibits flight of ideas. Delusions and other symptoms of psychotic intensity are never present.

The patient who experiences a *depressive episode* may report a loss of self-esteem, overwhelming inertia, social withdrawal, and feelings of hopelessness, apathy, or self-reproach. He may believe that he's wicked and deserves to be punished. His growing sadness, guilt, negativity, and fatigue place extraordinary burdens on his family.

During the assessment interview, the depressed patient may speak and respond slowly. He may complain of difficulty concentrating or thinking clearly but is usually not obviously disoriented or intellectually impaired.

Physical examination may reveal reduced psychomotor activity, lethargy, low muscle tonus, weight loss, slowed gait, and constipation. The patient may also report sleep disturbances (falling asleep, staying asleep, or early morning awakening), sexual dysfunction, headaches, chest pains, and a heaviness in the limbs. Typically, symptoms are worse in the morning and gradually subside as the day goes on.

His concerns about his health may become hypochondriacal: He may worry excessively about having cancer or some other serious illness. In an elderly patient, physical symptoms may be the only clues to depression.

Suicide is an ever-present risk, especially as the depression begins to lift. At that point, a rising energy level may strengthen the patient's resolve to carry out suicidal plans.

The suicidal patient may also harbor homicidal ideas—for example, thinking of killing his family either in anger or to spare them pain and disgrace.

Diagnosis

For characteristic findings in patients with this condition, see *Diagnosing bipolar disorders,* pages 452 and 453. Physical examination and laboratory tests, such as endocrine function studies, rule out medical causes of the mood disturbances, including intraabdominal neoplasm, hypothyroidism, heart failure, cerebral arteriosclerosis, parkinsonism, psychoactive drug abuse, brain tumor, and uremia. Moreover, a review of the medications prescribed for other disorders may point to drug-induced depression or mania.

Treatment

Widely used to treat bipolar disorders, lithium has proved to be highly effective in relieving and preventing manic episodes. It curbs the accelerated thought processes and hyperactive behavior without producing the sedating effect of antipsychotic drugs. In addition, it may prevent the recurrence of depressive episodes; however, it's ineffective in treating acute depression.

Because lithium has a narrow therapeutic range, treatment must be initiated cautiously and the dosage must be adjusted slowly. Therapeutic blood levels during the active manic period are 0.4 to 1.4 mEq/L. For safety, the level should never exceed 1.5 mEq/L. Therapeutic blood levels must be maintained for 7 to 10 days before the drug's beneficial effects appear; for this reason, antipsychotic drugs commonly are used in the interim to provide sedation and symptomatic relief. Because lithium is excreted by the kidneys, any renal impairment necessitates withdrawal of the drug.

Anticonvulsants, such as carbamazepine, valproic acid, and clonazepam, are used either alone or with lithium to treat mood disorders. Carbamazepine and divalproex are effective in many patients who are lithium-resistant. Other anticonvulsant drugs have also been used. Electroconvulsive therapy is also effective.

(Text continues on page 454.)

DIAGNOSING BIPOLAR DISORDERS

The diagnosis of a bipolar disorder is confirmed when the patient meets the criteria documented in the *Diagnostic and Statistical Manual of Mental Disorders*, Fourth Edition, Text Revision.

For a manic episode

- A distinct period of abnormally and persistently elevated, expansive, or irritable mood lasting at least 1 week (or any duration if hospitalization is needed).
- During the mood disturbance period, at least three of the following symptoms must have persisted (four, if the mood is only irritable) and have been present to a significant degree:
  - inflated self-esteem or grandiosity
  - decreased need for sleep
  - more talkative than usual or pressured to keep talking
  - flight of ideas or subjective experience that thoughts are racing
  - distractibility
  - increased goal-directed activity or psychomotor agitation
  - excessive involvement in pleasurable activities that have a high potential for painful consequences.
- The symptoms don't meet the criteria for a mixed episode.
- The mood disturbance is sufficiently severe to cause one of the following to occur:
  - marked impairment in occupational functioning or in usual social activities or relationships with others
  - hospitalization to prevent harm to self or others
  - evidence of psychotic features.
- The symptoms aren't due to the direct physiologic effects of a substance or a general medical condition.

For a hypomanic episode

- A distinct period of abnormally and persistently elevated, expansive, or irritable mood lasting at least 4 days that's clearly different from the usual nondepressed mood.
- During the mood disturbance period, at least three of the following symptoms must have persisted (four, if the mood is only irritable) and have been present to a significant degree:
  - inflated self-esteem or grandiosity
  - decreased need for sleep
  - more talkative than usual or pressured to keep talking
  - flight of ideas or subjective experience that thoughts are racing
  - distractibility
  - increased goal-directed activity or psychomotor agitation
  - excessive involvement in pleasurable activities that have a high potential for painful consequences.
- The episode is associated with an unequivocal change in functioning that's uncharacteristic of the person when not symptomatic.
- Others can recognize the disturbance in mood and the change in functioning.
- The episode isn't severe enough to markedly impair social or occupational functioning or to necessitate hospitalization to prevent harm to self or others. No psychotic features are evident.
- The symptoms aren't due to the direct physiologic effects of a substance or a general medical condition.

For a bipolar I single manic episode

- The presence of only one manic episode and no past major depressive episodes.
- The manic episode isn't better accounted for by schizoaffective disorder and isn't superimposed on schizophrenia, schizophreniform disorder, delusional disorder, or psychotic disorder not otherwise specified.

For a bipolar I disorder, most recent episode hypomanic

- The person is currently (or was most recently) in a hypomanic episode.
- The person previously had at least one manic episode or mixed episode.

- The mood symptoms cause clinically significant distress or impairment in social, occupational, or other important areas of functioning.
- The first two exacerbations of the mood episode (above) aren't better accounted for by schizoaffective disorder and aren't superimposed on schizophrenia, schizophreniform disorder, delusional disorder, or psychotic disorder not otherwise specified.

For a bipolar I disorder, most recent episode manic
- The person is currently (or was most recently) in a manic episode.
- The person previously had at least one major depressive episode, manic episode, or mixed episode.
- The first two exacerbations of mood episode (above) aren't better accounted for by schizoaffective disorder and aren't superimposed on schizophrenia, schizophreniform disorder, delusional disorder, or psychotic disorder not otherwise specified.

For a bipolar I disorder, most recent episode mixed
- The person is currently (or was most recently) in a mixed episode.
- The person previously had at least one major depressive episode, manic episode, or mixed episode.
- The first two exacerbations of mood episode (above) aren't better accounted for by schizoaffective disorder and aren't superimposed on schizophrenia, schizophreniform disorder, delusional disorder, or psychotic disorder not otherwise specified.

For a bipolar I disorder, most recent episode depressed
- The person is currently (or was most recently) in a major depressive episode.
- The person previously had at least one manic episode or mixed episode.
- The first two exacerbations of mood episode (above) aren't better accounted for

by schizoaffective disorder and aren't superimposed on schizophrenia, schizophreniform disorder, delusional disorder, or psychotic disorder not otherwise specified.

For a bipolar I disorder, most recent episode unspecified
- Criteria, except for duration, are currently (or most recently) met for a manic, hypomanic, mixed, or major depressive episode.
- The person previously had at least one manic episode or mixed episode.
- The mood symptoms cause clinically significant distress or impairment in social, occupational, or other important areas of functioning.
- The first two exacerbations of mood episode (above) aren't better accounted for by schizoaffective disorder and aren't superimposed on schizophrenia, schizophreniform disorder, delusional disorder, or psychotic disorder not otherwise specified.
- The first two exacerbations of mood episode (above) aren't due to the direct physiologic effects of a substance or a general medical condition.

For a bipolar II disorder
- The presence (or history) of one or more major depressive episodes.
- The presence (or history) of at least one hypomanic episode.
- The patient has never had a manic episode or a mixed episode.
- The first two exacerbations of mood episode (above) aren't better accounted for by schizoaffective disorder and aren't superimposed on schizophrenia, schizophreniform disorder, delusional disorder, or psychotic disorder not otherwise specified.
- The symptoms cause clinically significant distress or impairment in social, occupational, or other important areas of functioning.

Antidepressants are used to treat depressive symptoms, but they may trigger a manic episode.

Special considerations

For the *manic patient:*

▪ Remember the manic patient's physical needs. Encourage him to eat. Alter the diet so that it's high in calories, carbohydrates, and liquids.

▪ As the patient's symptoms subside, encourage him to assume responsibility for personal care.

▪ Provide emotional support, maintain a calm environment, and set realistic goals for behavior.

▪ Provide diversionary activities suited to a short attention span; firmly discourage the patient if he tries to overextend himself. Provide structured activities involving large motor movements to expend surplus energy. Reduce or eliminate group activities during acute manic episodes.

▪ When necessary, reorient the patient to reality. Tactfully divert conversations when they become intimately concerned with other patients or staff members.

▪ Set limits in a calm, clear, and self-confident manner for the manic patient's demanding, hyperactive, manipulative, and acting-out behaviors. Setting limits tells the patient that you'll provide security and protection by refusing inappropriate and possibly harmful requests. Avoid leaving an opening for the patient to test you or argue with you.

▪ Listen to requests attentively and with a neutral attitude. Avoid power struggles if a patient tries to put you on the spot for an immediate answer. Explain that you'll seriously consider the request and will respond later.

▪ Encourage solitary activities such as writing out one's thoughts.

▪ Collaborate with other staff members to provide consistent responses to the patient's manipulative or acting-out behaviors.

▪ Watch for early signs of frustration (when the patient's anger escalates from verbal threats to hitting an object). Tell the patient firmly that threats and hitting are unacceptable. Explain that these behaviors show that he needs help to control his be-

havior. Inform him that the staff will help him move to a quiet area to help him control his behavior so he won't hurt himself or others. Staff members who have practiced as a team can work effectively to prevent acting-out behavior or to remove and confine a patient.

▪ Alert the staff promptly when acting-out behavior escalates. It's safer to have help available before you need it than to try controlling an anxious or frightened patient by yourself.

▪ After the incident is over and the patient is calm and in control, discuss his feelings with him and offer suggestions on how to prevent a recurrence.

▪ If the patient is taking lithium, tell him and his family to temporarily discontinue the drug and notify the physician if signs or symptoms of toxicity, such as diarrhea, abdominal cramps, vomiting, unsteadiness, drowsiness, muscle weakness, polyuria, and tremors, occur.

For the *depressed patient:*

▪ The depressed patient needs continual positive reinforcement to improve his self-esteem. Provide a structured routine, including activities to boost his self-confidence and promote interaction with others (for instance, group therapy). Keep reassuring him that his depression will lift.

▪ Encourage the patient to talk or to write down his feelings if he's having trouble expressing them. Listen attentively and respectfully; allow him time to formulate his thoughts if he seems sluggish. Record your observations and conversations.

▪ To prevent possible self-injury or suicide, remove harmful objects (such as glass, belts, rope, or bobby pins) from the patient's environment, observe him closely, and strictly supervise his medications. Institute suicide precautions as dictated by facility policy.

▪ Don't forget the patient's physical needs. If he's too depressed to take care of himself, help him with personal hygiene measures. Encourage him to eat, or feed him if necessary. If he's constipated, add high-fiber foods to his diet; offer small, frequent meals; and encourage physical activity. To help him sleep, give him back rubs or warm milk at bedtime.

■ If the patient is taking an antidepressant, watch for signs of mania.

Major depression

Also known as *unipolar disorder,* major depression is a syndrome of persistently sad, dysphoric mood, accompanied by disturbances in sleep and appetite, lethargy, and an inability to experience pleasure (anhedonia).

About half of all depressed patients experience a single episode and recover completely; the rest have at least one recurrence. Major depression can profoundly alter social, family, and occupational functioning. However, suicide is the most serious consequence of major depression — feelings of worthlessness, guilt, and hopelessness are so overwhelming that patients no longer consider life worth living. Nearly twice as many women as men attempt suicide, but men are far more likely to succeed.

Causes and incidence
The multiple causes of depression aren't completely understood. Current research suggests possible genetic, familial, biochemical, physical, psychological, and social causes. Psychological causes (the focus of many nursing interventions) may include feelings of helplessness and vulnerability, anger, hopelessness and pessimism, and low self-esteem. They may be related to abnormal character and behavior patterns and troubled personal relationships. In many cases, the history identifies a specific personal loss or severe stressor that probably interacts with the person's predisposition to provoke major depression.

Depression may be secondary to a specific medical condition — for example, metabolic disturbances, such as hypoxia and hypercalcemia; endocrine disorders, such as diabetes and Cushing's syndrome; neurologic diseases, such as Parkinson's and Alzheimer's diseases; cancer (especially of the pancreas); viral and bacterial infections, such as influenza and pneumonia; cardiovascular disorders, such as heart failure; pulmonary disorders, such as chronic obstructive lung disease; musculoskeletal disorders, such as degenerative arthritis; GI disorders, such as irritable bowel syndrome; genitourinary problems, such as incontinence; collagen vascular diseases, such as lupus; and anemias.

Drugs prescribed for medical and psychiatric conditions as well as many commonly abused substances can also cause depression. Examples include antihypertensives, psychotropics, opioid and nonopioid analgesics, antiparkinsonian drugs, numerous cardiovascular medications, oral antidiabetics, antimicrobials, steroids, chemotherapeutic agents, cimetidine, and alcohol. Depression occurs in up to 18 million Americans, affecting all racial, ethnic, and socioeconomic groups. It affects both sexes, but is more common in women.

Signs and symptoms
The primary features of major depression are a predominantly sad mood and a loss of interest or pleasure in daily activities. The patient may complain of feeling "down in the dumps," express doubts about his self-worth or ability to cope, or simply appear unhappy and apathetic. He may also report feeling angry or anxious. Symptoms tend to be more severe than those caused by dysthymic disorder, which is a milder, chronic form of depression. (See *Dysthymic disorder,* page 456.) Other common signs include difficulty concentrating or thinking clearly, distractibility, and indecisiveness. All physiologic and psychologic processes are slowed. Anergia and fatigue are common as are anhedonia (inability to experience pleasure) and insomnia. Take special note if the patient reveals suicidal thoughts, a preoccupation with death, or previous suicide attempts.

The psychosocial history may reveal life problems or losses that can account for the depression. Alternatively, the patient's medical history may implicate a physical disorder or the use of prescription, nonprescription, or illegal drugs that can cause depression.

The patient may report an increase or a decrease in appetite, sleep disturbances (for example, insomnia or early awakening), a lack of interest in sexual activity, constipation, or diarrhea. Other signs that you may note during a physical examination include

DYSTHYMIC DISORDER

Dysthymic disorder is characterized by a chronic dysphoric mood (irritable mood in children), persisting at least 2 years in adults and 1 year in children and adolescents.

Signs and symptoms
During periods of depression, the patient may also experience poor appetite or overeating, insomnia or hypersomnia, low energy or fatigue, low self-esteem, poor concentration or difficulty making decisions, and feelings of hopelessness.

Diagnosis
Dysthymic disorder is confirmed when the patient exhibits at least two of the signs or symptoms listed above nearly every day, with intervening normal moods lasting no more than 2 months during a 2-year period.

The disorder typically begins in childhood, adolescence, or early adulthood and causes only mild social or occupational impairment. In adults, it's more common in women; in children and adolescents, it's equally common in both sexes.

agitation (such as hand wringing or restlessness) and reduced psychomotor activity (for example, slowed speech).

Diagnosis
For characteristic findings in patients with this condition, see *Diagnosing major depression*.

The diagnosis is supported by psychological tests, such as the Beck Depression Inventory, which may help determine the onset, severity, duration, and progression of depressive symptoms. A toxicology screening may suggest drug-induced depression.

Treatment
Depression is difficult to treat, especially in children, adolescents, elderly patients, and those with a history of chronic disease. The primary treatment methods are drug therapy and psychotherapy, particularly cognitive behavioral therapy.

Drug therapy includes tricyclic antidepressants (TCAs) such as amitriptyline, monoamine oxidase (MAO) inhibitors such as isocarboxazid, maprotiline, and trazodone, which has been available for 40 years. A newer class of drugs, the selective serotonin reuptake inhibitors (SSRIs), such as fluoxetine, paroxetine, sertraline, bupropion, venlafaxine, and mirtazapine, are equally effective and have more tolerable adverse effect profiles.

TCAs, the most widely used class of antidepressant drugs, prevent the reuptake of norepinephrine or serotonin (or both) into the presynaptic nerve endings, resulting in increased synaptic concentrations of these neurotransmitters. They also cause a gradual loss in the number of beta-adrenergic receptors.

MAO inhibitors block the enzymatic degradation of norepinephrine and serotonin. These agents commonly are prescribed for patients with atypical depression (for example, depression marked by an increased appetite and need for sleep, rather than anorexia and insomnia) and for some patients who fail to respond to TCAs. MAO inhibitors are associated with a high risk of toxicity; patients treated with one of these drugs must be able to comply with the necessary dietary restrictions.

Maprotiline is a potent blocker of norepinephrine uptake, whereas trazodone is an SSRI. The mechanism of action of bupropion is unknown.

Electroconvulsive therapy (ECT) may be considered in particularly severe or drug-resistant depression. Six to 12 treatments are typically needed, although in many cases improvement is evident after only a few treatments. However, ECT has been associated with later short-term memory loss, heart arrhythmias, and seizure activity. Researchers hypothesize that ECT affects the same receptor sites as antidepressants.

Short-term psychotherapy is also effective in treating major depression. Many

DIAGNOSING MAJOR DEPRESSION

A patient is diagnosed with major depression when he fulfills the following criteria for a single major depressive episode put forth in the *Diagnostic and Statistical Manual of Mental Disorders,* Fourth Edition, Text Revision:

■ At least five of the following symptoms must have been present during the same 2-week period and must represent a change from previous functioning; one of these must be either depressed mood or loss of interest in previously pleasurable activities:
– depressed mood (irritable mood in children and adolescents) most of the day, nearly every day, as indicated by either subjective account or observation by others
– markedly diminished interest or pleasure in all, or almost all, activities most of the day, nearly every day
– significant weight loss or weight gain when not dieting or decrease or increase in appetite nearly every day (in children, consider failure to make expected weight gains)
– insomnia or hypersomnia nearly every day
– psychomotor agitation or retardation nearly every day
– fatigue or loss of energy nearly every day

– feelings of worthlessness or excessive or inappropriate guilt nearly every day
– diminished ability to think or concentrate, or indecisiveness, nearly every day
– recurrent thoughts of death, recurrent suicidal ideation without a specific plan, a suicide attempt, or a specific plan for committing suicide.

■ The symptoms don't meet criteria for a mixed episode.

■ The symptoms cause clinically significant distress or impairment in social, occupational, or other important areas of functioning.

■ The symptoms aren't due to the direct physiologic effects of a substance or a general medical condition.

■ The symptoms aren't better accounted for by bereavement, the symptoms persist for longer than 2 months, or the symptoms are characterized by marked functional impairment, morbid preoccupation with worthlessness, suicidal ideation, psychotic symptoms, or psychomotor retardation.

---

psychiatrists believe that the best results are achieved with a combination of individual, family, or group psychotherapy and medication. After resolution of the acute episode, patients with a history of recurrent depression may be maintained on low doses of antidepressants as a preventive measure.

Depression may be experienced differently by members of different cultures. For instance, in some Asian cultures, there are more somatic manifestations of depression than overt psychologic signs or symptoms.

Special considerations

■ Share your observations of the patient's behavior with him. For instance, you might say, "You're sitting all by yourself, looking very sad. Is that how you feel?" Because the patient may think and react sluggishly, speak slowly and allow ample time for him to respond. Avoid feigned cheerfulness. However, don't hesitate to laugh with the patient and point out the value of humor.

■ Show the patient he's important by listening attentively and respectfully, preventing interruptions, and avoiding judgmental responses.

■ Provide a structured routine, including noncompetitive activities, to build the patient's self-confidence and encourage interaction with others. Urge him to join group activities and to socialize.

SUICIDE PREVENTION GUIDELINES

When the patient is diagnosed with major depression, keep in mind these guidelines.

Assess for clues to suicide
Be alert for the patient's suicidal thoughts, threats, and messages; describing a suicide plan; hoarding medication; talking about death and feelings of futility; giving away prized possessions; and changing behavior, especially as depression begins to lift.

Provide a safe environment
Check patient areas and correct dangerous conditions, such as exposed pipes, windows without safety glass, and access to the roof or balconies.

Remove dangerous objects
Take away potentially dangerous objects, such as belts, razors, suspenders, light cords, glass, knives, nail files and clippers, and metal and hard plastic objects.

Consult with staff
Recognize and document verbal and nonverbal suicidal behaviors, keep the physician informed, share data with all staff members, clarify the patient's specific restrictions, assess risk and plan for observation, and clarify day and night staff responsibilities and the frequency of consultations.

Observe the suicidal patient
Be alert when the patient is using a sharp object (such as a razor), taking medication, or using the bathroom (to prevent hanging or other injury). Assign the patient to a room near the nurses' station and with another patient. Continuously observe the acutely suicidal patient.

Maintain personal contact
Help the suicidal patient feel that he isn't alone or without resources or hope. Encourage continuity of care and consistency of primary nurses. Building emotional ties to others is the ultimate technique for preventing suicide.

■ Inform the patient that he can help ease depression by expressing his feelings, participating in pleasurable activities, and improving grooming and hygiene.

■ Ask the patient if he thinks of death or suicide. Such thoughts signal an immediate need for consultation and assessment. Failure to detect suicidal thoughts early may encourage the patient to attempt suicide. The risk of suicide increases as the depression lifts. (See *Suicide prevention guidelines.*)

■ Tell the patient to inform his primary care physician or other health care professional if he's taking TCAs or MAO inhibitors to prevent possible drug interactions.

■ While tending to the patient's psychological needs, don't forget his physical needs. If he's too depressed to take care of himself, help him with personal hygiene.

Encourage him to eat, or feed him if necessary. If he's constipated, add high-fiber foods to his diet; offer small, frequent meals; and encourage physical activity and fluid intake. Offer warm milk or back rubs at bedtime to improve sleep.

■ Inform the patient that antidepressants may take several weeks to produce an effect.

■ Teach the patient about depression. Emphasize that effective methods are available to relieve his symptoms. Help him to recognize distorted perceptions that may contribute to his depression. After the patient learns to recognize depressive thought patterns, he can consciously begin to substitute self-affirming thoughts.

■ Instruct the patient about prescribed medications. Stress the need for compliance and review adverse effects. For drugs that produce strong anticholinergic effects, such as amitriptyline and amoxapine, suggest sugarless gum or hard candy to relieve dry mouth. Many antidepressants are sedating (for example, amitriptyline and trazodone); warn the patient to avoid activities that require alertness, including driving and operating mechanical equipment until the central nervous system (CNS) effects of the drug are known.

■ Caution the patient taking a TCA to avoid drinking alcoholic beverages or taking other CNS depressants during therapy.

■ If the patient is taking an MAO inhibitor, emphasize that he must avoid foods that contain tyramine, caffeine, or tryptophan. The ingestion of tyramine can cause a hypertensive crisis. Examples of foods that contain these substances include cheese, sour cream, pickled herring, liver, canned figs, raisins, bananas, avocados, chocolate, soy sauce, fava beans, yeast extracts, meat tenderizers, coffee, cola drinks, and beer, Chianti, or sherry.

ANXIETY DISORDERS
Phobias

Defined as a persistent and irrational fear of a specific object, activity, or situation, a phobia results in a compelling desire to avoid the perceived hazard. The patient recognizes that his fear is out of proportion to any actual danger, but he can't control it or explain it away. Three types of phobias exist: agoraphobia, the fear of being alone or of open space; social, the fear of embarrassing oneself in public; and specific, the fear of a single, specific object, such as animals or heights.

A social phobia typically begins in late childhood or early adolescence; a specific phobia usually begins in childhood. Most phobic patients have no family history of psychiatric illness, including phobias.

Agoraphobia and social phobia tend to be chronic, but new treatments are improving the prognosis. A specific phobia usually resolves spontaneously as the child matures.

Causes and incidence
A phobia develops when anxiety about an object or a situation compels the patient to avoid it. The precise cause of most phobias is unknown. Psychoanalytic theory holds that the phobia is actually repression and displacement of an internal conflict. Behavior theorists view phobia as a stimulus-response reflex, avoiding a situation or object that causes anxiety.

Ten percent of Americans suffer from a phobic disorder. In fact, phobias are the most common psychiatric disorders in women and the second most common in men. More men than women experience social phobias, whereas agoraphobia and specific phobias are more common in women.

Signs and symptoms
The phobic patient typically reports signs of severe anxiety when confronted with the feared object or situation. A patient with agoraphobia, for example, may complain of dizziness, a sensation of falling, a feeling of unreality (depersonalization), loss of bladder or bowel control, vomiting, or cardiac distress when he leaves home or crosses a bridge. Similarly, a patient who fears flying may report that he begins to sweat, his heart pounds, and he feels panicky and short of breath when he's on an airplane.

A patient who routinely avoids the object of his phobia may report a loss of self-esteem and feelings of weakness, cowardice, or ineffectiveness. If he hasn't mastered the phobia, he may also exhibit signs of mild depression.

Diagnosis
For characteristic findings in this condition, see *Diagnosing phobias,* pages 460 and 461.

Treatment
The effectiveness of treatment depends on the severity of the patient's phobia. Because phobic behavior may never be completely cured, the goal of treatment is to help the patient function effectively.

Antianxiety medications, tricyclic antidepressants, monoamine oxidase inhibitors, and selective serotonin reuptake inhibitors may help relieve symptoms in

DIAGNOSING PHOBIAS

Phobias are classified as agoraphobia, social phobias, and specific phobias. The diagnosis of all three is based on criteria put forth in the *Diagnostic and Statistical Manual of Mental Disorders*, Fourth Edition, Text Revision.

Agoraphobia

Fear of being in places or situations from which escape might be difficult or embarrassing or in which help might be unavailable if an unexpected or situationally predisposed panic attack or paniclike symptom occurs. Agoraphobic fears typically involve characteristic clusters of situations that include being outside the home alone, being in a crowd or standing in a line, being on a bridge, and traveling in a bus, train, or automobile.

- The situations are avoided or endured with marked distress or with anxiety about having a panic attack or paniclike symptoms, or the person requires the presence of a companion.
- The anxiety or phobic avoidance isn't better accounted for by mental disorder, such as social phobia, specific phobia, obsessive-compulsive disorder, posttraumatic stress disorder, or separation anxiety disorder.

Social phobia

A persistent fear of one or more social or performance situations in which the person is exposed to unfamiliar people or possible scrutiny by others. The person fears that he may act in a way that will be humiliating or embarrassing.

- Exposure to the feared social situation almost invariably provokes anxiety, which may take the form of a situationally bound or situationally predisposed panic attack.
- The person recognizes that the fear is excessive or unreasonable.
- The feared social or performance situations are avoided or endured with intense anxiety or distress.
- The avoidance, anxious anticipation, or distress in the feared social or performance situation interferes with the person's normal routine, occupational functioning, or social activities or relationships. There may be marked distress about having the phobia.
- In individuals younger than age 18, the duration is at least 6 months.
- The fear or avoidance isn't due to the direct physiologic effects of a substance or a general medical condition and isn't better accounted for by another mental disorder.
- If the person has a general medical condition or another mental disorder, the person's social fear is unrelated to the medical or mental condition.

Specific phobia

Marked and persistent fear that's excessive or unreasonable and cued by the presence

---

patients with agoraphobia or social phobias.

Systematic desensitization, a type of behavioral therapy, may be more effective than drugs, especially if it includes encouragement, instruction, and suggestion.

In some cities, phobia clinics and group therapy are available. People who have recovered from phobias can usually help other phobic patients.

Special considerations

- Provide for the patient's safety and comfort, and monitor fluid and food intake, as needed. Certain phobias may inhibit food or fluid intake, disturb hygiene, and disrupt the patient's ability to rest.
- No matter how illogical the patient's phobia seems, avoid the urge to trivialize his fears. Remember that this behavior represents an essential coping mechanism.
- Ask the patient how he normally copes with the fear. When he's able to face the fear, encourage him to verbalize and ex-

or anticipation of a specific object or situation.

■ Exposure to the phobic stimulus almost invariably provokes an immediate anxiety response, which may take the form of a situationally bound or situationally predisposed panic attack.

■ The person recognizes that the fear is excessive or unreasonable.

■ The person avoids the situation or endures it with intense anxiety or distress.

■ The avoidance, anxious anticipation, or distress in the feared situation significantly interferes with the person's normal routine, occupational functioning, or social activities or relationships. There may be marked distress about having the phobia.

■ In individuals younger than age 18, the duration is at least 6 months.

■ The anxiety, panic attacks, or phobic avoidance associated with the specific object or situation isn't better accounted for by another mental disorder, such as obsessive-compulsive disorder, posttraumatic stress disorder, separation anxiety disorder, social phobia, panic disorder with agoraphobia, or agoraphobia without a history of panic disorder.

plore his personal strengths and resources with you.

■ Don't let the patient withdraw completely. If an agoraphobic patient is being treated as an outpatient, suggest small steps to overcome his fears such as planning a brief shopping trip with a supportive family member or friend.

■ In social phobias, the patient fears criticism. Encourage him to interact with others and provide continuous support and positive reinforcement.

■ Support participation in psychotherapy, including desensitization therapy. However, don't force insight. Challenging the patient may aggravate his anxiety or lead to panic attacks.

■ Teach the patient specific relaxation techniques, such as listening to music and meditating.

■ Suggest ways to channel the patient's energy and relieve stress (such as running and creative activities).

Generalized anxiety disorder

Anxiety is a feeling of apprehension that some describe as an exaggerated feeling of impending doom, dread, or uneasiness. Unlike fear — a reaction to danger from a specific external source — anxiety is a reaction to an internal threat, such as an unacceptable impulse or a repressed thought that's straining to reach a conscious level.

A rational response to a real threat, occasional anxiety is a normal part of life. Overwhelming anxiety, however, can result in generalized anxiety disorder — uncontrollable, unreasonable worry that persists for at least 6 months and narrows perceptions or interferes with normal functioning. Recent evidence indicates that the prevalence of generalized anxiety disorder is greater than previously thought and may be even greater than that of depression.

Causes and incidence
Theorists share a common premise: Conflict, whether intrapsychic, sociopersonal, or interpersonal, promotes an anxiety state.

Generalized anxiety disorder has a 1-year prevalence range from 3% to 8%. It's more common in women than in men, and half of all cases begin in childhood or adolescence.

Signs and symptoms
Generalized anxiety disorder can begin at any age but typically has an onset in the 20s and 30s. Psychological or physiologic symptoms of anxiety states vary with the degree of anxiety. Mild anxiety mainly causes psychological symptoms, with unusual self-awareness and alertness to the

DIAGNOSING GENERALIZED ANXIETY DISORDER

When the patient's symptoms match criteria documented in the *Diagnostic and Statistical Manual of Mental Disorders*, Fourth Edition, Text Revision, the diagnosis of generalized anxiety disorder is confirmed. The criteria include:

- Excessive anxiety and worry about numerous events or activities occur more days than not for at least 6 months.
- The person finds it difficult to control the worry.
- The anxiety and worry are associated with at least three of the following six symptoms:
  - restlessness or feeling keyed up or on edge
  - being easily fatigued
  - difficulty concentrating or mind going blank
  - irritability
  - muscle tension
  - sleep disturbances (difficulty falling or staying asleep, or restless, unsatisfying sleep).
- The focus of the anxiety and worry isn't confined to features of an axis I disorder.
- The anxiety, worry, or physical symptoms cause clinically significant distress or impairment in social, occupational, or other important areas of functioning.
- The disturbance isn't due to the direct physiologic effects of a substance or a general medical condition and doesn't occur exclusively during a mood disorder, a psychotic disorder, or a pervasive developmental disorder.

state with acute anxiety causes a complete loss of concentration, typically with unintelligible speech.

Physical examination of the patient with generalized anxiety disorder may reveal signs or symptoms of motor tension, including trembling, muscle aches and spasms, headaches, and an inability to relax. Autonomic signs and symptoms include shortness of breath, tachycardia, sweating, and abdominal complaints.

In addition, the patient may startle easily and complain of feeling apprehensive, fearful, or angry. There may also be difficulty concentrating, eating, and sleeping. The medical, psychiatric, and psychosocial histories fail to identify a specific physical or environmental cause of the anxiety.

Diagnosis

For characteristic findings in patients with this condition, see *Diagnosing generalized anxiety disorder*.

Laboratory tests must exclude organic causes of the patient's signs and symptoms, such as hyperthyroidism, pheochromocytoma, coronary artery disease, supraventricular tachycardia, and Ménière's disease. For example, an electrocardiogram can rule out myocardial ischemia in a patient who complains of chest pain. Blood tests, including complete blood count, white blood cell count and differential, and serum lactate and calcium levels, can rule out hypocalcemia.

Because anxiety is the central feature of other mental disorders, psychiatric evaluation must rule out phobias, obsessive-compulsive disorder, depression, and acute schizophrenia.

Behaviors commonly associated with a diagnosis of anxiety may have cultural origins or acceptance. For example, Hispanics may experience "susto," or a state of anxiety, insomnia, anorexia, and social withdrawal, following a frightening stimulus. Koreans may experience "Hwa-byung" — a state of anxiety and irritability, with various physiologic symptoms, such as headache and palpitations. African-Americans may experience "blockout," involving collapse, dizziness, and reduced physical movement in time of stress.

environment. Moderate anxiety leads to selective inattention but with the ability to concentrate on a single task. Severe anxiety causes an inability to concentrate on more than scattered details of a task. A panic

Treatment

A combination of drug therapy and psychotherapy may help a patient with generalized anxiety disorder. Benzodiazepines may relieve mild anxiety and improve the patient's ability to cope.

 ELDER TIP *A benzodiazepine with a long half-life tends to accumulate in an older patient's system and may cause oversedation. Benzodiazepines are sometimes given along with opioids to add to the analgesic effect or as a preanesthetic. Remember, if the elderly psychiatric patient is scheduled for surgery, he may take longer to recover from anesthesia if these combinations are used.*

Tricyclic antidepressants or higher doses of short-acting benzodiazepines may relieve severe anxiety and panic attacks. Buspirone, an antianxiety drug, causes the patient less sedation and poses less risk of physical and psychological dependence than the benzodiazepines.

Psychotherapy for generalized anxiety disorder has two goals: helping the patient identify and deal with the cause of the anxiety and eliminating environmental factors that precipitate an anxious reaction. In addition, the patient can learn relaxation techniques, such as deep breathing, progressive muscle relaxation, focused relaxation, and visualization.

Special considerations

■ Stay with the patient when he's anxious, and encourage him to discuss his feelings. Reduce environmental stimuli and remain calm.

■ Administer antianxiety drugs or tricyclic antidepressants as prescribed, and evaluate the patient's response. Teach the patient about prescribed medications, including the need for compliance with the medication regimen. Review adverse reactions.

■ Teach the patient effective coping strategies and relaxation techniques. Help him identify stressful situations that trigger his anxiety, and provide positive reinforcement when he uses alternative coping strategies.

Panic disorder

Characterized by recurrent episodes of intense apprehension, terror, and impending doom, panic disorder represents anxiety in its most severe form. Initially unpredictable, panic attacks may become associated with specific situations or tasks. The disorder commonly exists concurrently with agoraphobia. Equal numbers of men and women are affected by panic disorder alone, whereas panic disorder with agoraphobia occurs in about twice as many women.

Panic disorder typically has an onset in late adolescence or early adulthood, typically in response to a sudden loss. It may also be triggered by severe separation anxiety experienced during early childhood. Without treatment, panic disorder can persist for years, with alternating exacerbations and remissions. The patient with panic disorder is at high risk for a psychoactive substance abuse disorder: He may resort to alcohol or anxiolytics in an attempt to relieve his extreme anxiety.

Causes and incidence

Like other anxiety disorders, panic disorder may stem from a combination of physical and psychological factors. For example, some theorists emphasize the role of stressful events or unconscious conflicts that occur early in childhood.

Recent evidence indicates that alterations in brain biochemistry, especially in norepinephrine, serotonin, and gamma-aminobutyric acid activity, may also contribute to panic disorder.

Panic disorder affects about 2% of the population. Symptoms usually develop before age 25.

Signs and symptoms

The patient with panic disorder typically complains of repeated episodes of unexpected apprehension, fear or, rarely, intense discomfort. These panic attacks may last for minutes or hours and leave the patient shaken, fearful, and exhausted. They occur several times a week, sometimes even daily. Because the attacks occur spontaneously, without exposure to a known anxiety-producing situation, the patient generally

DIAGNOSING PANIC DISORDER

The diagnosis of panic disorder is confirmed when the patient meets the criteria put forth in the *Diagnostic and Statistical Manual of Mental Disorders*, Fourth Edition, Text Revision.

Panic attack
A discrete period of intense fear or discomfort in which at least four of the following symptoms develop abruptly and reach a peak within 10 minutes:
- palpitations, pounding heart, or tachycardia
- sweating
- trembling or shaking
- shortness of breath or smothering sensations
- feeling of choking
- chest pain or discomfort
- nausea or abdominal distress
- dizziness or faintness
- depersonalization or derealization
- fear of losing control or going crazy
- fear of dying
- numbness or tingling sensations (paresthesia)
- hot flashes or chills.

Panic disorder without agoraphobia
- The person experiences recurrent unexpected panic attacks and at least one of the attacks has been followed by 1 month (or more) of one (or more) of the following:
  − persistent concern about having additional attacks
  − worry about the implications of the attack or its consequences
  − a significant change in behavior related to the attacks.

- The panic attacks aren't due to the direct physiologic effects of a substance or a general medical condition.
- The panic attacks aren't better accounted for by another mental disorder, such as social phobia, specific phobia, obsessive-compulsive disorder, posttraumatic stress disorder, or separation anxiety disorder.

Panic disorder with agoraphobia
- The person experiences recurrent unexpected panic attacks and at least one of the attacks has been followed by 1 month (or more) of one (or more) of the following:
  − persistent concern about having additional attacks
  − worry about the implications of the attack or its consequences
  − a significant change in behavior related to the attacks.
- The person exhibits agoraphobia.
- The panic attacks aren't due to the direct physiologic effects of a substance or a general medical condition.
- The panic attacks aren't better accounted for by another mental disorder, such as social phobia, specific phobia, obsessive-compulsive disorder, posttraumatic stress disorder, or separation anxiety disorder.

worries between attacks about when the next episode will occur.

Physical examination of the patient during a panic attack may reveal signs of intense anxiety, such as hyperventilation, tachycardia, trembling, and profuse sweating. He may also complain of difficulty breathing, digestive disturbances, and chest pain.

Diagnosis
For characteristic findings in patients with this condition, see *Diagnosing panic disorder*.

Because many medical conditions can mimic panic disorder, additional tests may be ordered to rule out an organic basis for the symptoms. For example, tests for serum glucose levels rule out hypoglycemia; studies of urine catecholamines and vanillylmandelic acid rule out pheochromocytoma; and thyroid function tests rule out hyperthyroidism.

Urine and serum toxicology tests may reveal the presence of psychoactive substances that can precipitate panic attacks, including barbiturates, caffeine, and amphetamines.

Treatment

Panic disorder may respond to behavioral therapy, supportive psychotherapy, or drug therapy, alone or in combination. Behavioral therapy works best when agoraphobia accompanies panic disorder because the identification of anxiety-inducing situations is easier.

Psychotherapy commonly uses cognitive techniques to enable the patient to view anxiety-provoking situations more realistically and to recognize panic symptoms as a misinterpretation of essentially harmless physical sensations.

Drug therapy includes antianxiety drugs, such as diazepam, alprazolam, and clonazepam, and beta blockers, such as propranolol, to provide symptomatic relief. Antidepressants, including tricyclic antidepressants, selective serotonin reuptake inhibitors, and monoamine oxidase inhibitors, are also effective.

Special considerations

■ Stay with the patient until the attack subsides. If left alone, he may become even more anxious.
■ Maintain a calm, serene approach. Statements such as, "I won't let anything here hurt you," and, "I'll stay with you," can assure the patient that you're in control of the immediate situation. Avoid giving him insincere expressions of reassurance.
■ The patient's perceptual field may be narrowed, and excessive stimuli may cause him to feel overwhelmed. Dim bright lights or raise dim lights as necessary.
■ If the patient loses control, move him to a smaller, quieter space.
■ The patient may be so overwhelmed that he can't follow lengthy or complicated instructions. Speak in short, simple sentences, and slowly give one direction at a time. Avoid giving lengthy explanations and asking too many questions.

■ Allow the patient to pace around the room (provided he isn't belligerent) to help expend energy. Show him how to take slow, deep breaths if he's hyperventilating.
■ Avoid touching the patient until you've established a rapport. Unless he trusts you, he may be too stimulated or frightened to find touch reassuring.
■ Administer medication as prescribed.
■ During and after a panic attack, encourage the patient to express his feelings. Discuss his fears and help him identify situations or events that trigger the attacks.
■ Teach the patient relaxation techniques, and explain how he can use them to relieve stress or avoid a panic attack.
■ Review with the patient any adverse effects of the drugs he'll be taking. Caution him to notify the physician before discontinuing the medication because abrupt withdrawal could cause severe symptoms.
■ Encourage the patient and his family to use community resources such as the Anxiety Disorders Association of America.

Obsessive-compulsive disorder

Obsessive thoughts and compulsive behaviors represent recurring efforts to control overwhelming anxiety, guilt, or unacceptable impulses that persistently enter the consciousness. The word *obsession* refers to a recurrent idea, thought, impulse, or image that's intrusive and inappropriate, causing marked anxiety or distress. A compulsion is a ritualistic, repetitive, and involuntary defensive behavior. Performing a compulsive behavior reduces the patient's anxiety and increases the probability that the behavior will recur. Compulsions are commonly associated with obsessions.

Patients with obsessive-compulsive disorder (OCD) are prone to abuse psychoactive substances, such as alcohol and anxiolytics, in an attempt to relieve their anxiety. In addition, other anxiety disorders and major depression commonly coexist with OCD.

OCD is typically a chronic condition with remissions and flare-ups. Mild forms of the disorder are relatively common in the population at large.

Causes and incidence

The cause of OCD is unknown. Some studies suggest the possibility of brain lesions, but the most useful research and clinical studies base an explanation on psychological theories. In addition, major depression, organic brain syndrome, and schizophrenia may contribute to the onset of OCD. Some authorities think that OCD is closely related to some eating disorders.

OCD affects 2% to 3% of Americans — about 7 million people. Symptoms usually are noticed between ages 20 and 30, with 75% of patients displaying symptoms before age 30.

Signs and symptoms

The psychiatric history of a patient with OCD may reveal the presence of obsessive thoughts, words, or mental images that persistently and involuntarily invade the consciousness. Some common obsessions include thoughts of violence (such as stabbing, shooting, maiming, or hitting), thoughts of contamination (images of dirt, germs, or feces), repetitive doubts and worries about a tragic event, and repeating or counting images, words, or objects in the environment. The patient recognizes that the obsessions are a product of his own mind and that they interfere with normal daily activities.

 ELDER TIP *In the older patient, any environmental change, such as transfer to a nursing home or a visit from a stranger in the patient's home, may trigger a need for treatment. A distraction from the patient's ritual activity may provoke anxiety or agitation.*

The patient's history may also reveal the presence of compulsions, irrational and recurring impulses to repeat a certain behavior. Common compulsions include repetitive touching, sometimes combined with counting; doing and undoing (for instance, opening and closing doors or rearranging things); washing (especially hands); and checking (to be sure no tragedy has occurred since the last time he checked). In many cases, the patient's anxiety is so strong that he will avoid the situation or the object that evokes the impulse.

When the obsessive-compulsive phenomena are mental, observation may reveal no behavioral abnormalities. However, compulsive acts may be observed. Feelings of shame, nervousness, or embarrassment may prompt the patient to try limiting these acts to his own private time.

Also evaluate the impact of obsessive-compulsive phenomena on the patient's normal routine. He'll typically report moderate to severe impairment of social and occupational functioning.

Diagnosis

For characteristic findings in patients with this condition, see *Diagnosing obsessive-compulsive disorder.*

Treatment

OCD is tenacious, but improvement occurs in 60% to 70% of patients who obtain treatment. Current treatment usually involves a combination of medication and cognitive behavioral therapy. Other types of psychotherapy may also be helpful.

Effective medications include clomipramine, a tricyclic antidepressant; selective serotonin reuptake inhibitors, such as fluoxetine, paroxetine, sertraline, and fluvoxamine; and the benzodiazepine clonazepam.

Behavioral therapies — aversion therapy, thought stopping, thought switching, flooding, implosion therapy, and response prevention — have also been effective. (See *Behavioral therapies,* page 468.)

Special considerations

- Approach the patient unhurriedly.
- Provide an accepting atmosphere; don't appear shocked, amused, or critical of the ritualistic behavior.
- Keep the patient's physical health in mind. For example, compulsive hand washing may cause skin breakdown; rituals or preoccupations may cause inadequate food and fluid intake and exhaustion. Provide for basic needs, such as rest, nutrition, and grooming, if the patient becomes involved in ritualistic thoughts and behaviors to the point of self-neglect.
- Let the patient know that you're aware of his behavior. For example, you might say, "I noticed you've made your bed three times today; that must be very tiring for you." Help the patient explore feelings associated

DIAGNOSING OBSESSIVE-COMPULSIVE DISORDER

The diagnosis of obsessive-compulsive disorder is made when the patient's signs and symptoms meet the established criteria put forth in the *Diagnostic and Statistical Manual of Mental Disorders,* Fourth Edition, Text Revision.

Either obsessions or compulsions
Obsessions are defined as all of the following:
- Recurrent and persistent thoughts, impulses, or images perceived to be intrusive and inappropriate by the patient, causing anxiety or distress at some point in time during the disturbance.
- The thoughts, impulses, or images are not simply excessive worries about real-life problems.
- The person attempts to ignore or suppress such thoughts or impulses, or to neutralize them with some other thought or action.
- The person recognizes that the obsessions are the products of his mind and not externally imposed.

Compulsions are defined as all of the following:
- Repetitive behaviors or mental acts performed by the person, who feels driven to perform them in response to an obsession or according to rules that must be applied rigidly.
- The behavior or mental acts are aimed at preventing or reducing distress or preventing some dreaded event or situation. However, either the activity isn't connected in a realistic way with what it's

designed to neutralize or prevent or it's clearly excessive.
- The patient recognizes that his behavior is excessive or unreasonable (this may not be true for young children or for patients whose obsessions have evolved into overvalued ideas).

Additional criteria
- At some point, the person recognizes that the obsessions or compulsions are excessive or unreasonable.
- The obsessions or compulsions cause marked distress, are time-consuming (take more than 1 hour per day), or significantly interfere with the person's normal routine, occupational functioning, or usual social activities or relationships.
- If another axis I disorder is present, the content of the obsession is unrelated to it; for example, the ideas, thoughts, or images aren't about food in the presence of an eating disorder, about drugs in the presence of a psychoactive substance abuse disorder, or about guilt in a major depressive disorder.
- The disturbance isn't due to the direct physiologic effects of a substance or a general medical condition.

---

with the behavior. For example, ask him, "What do you think about while you're performing your chores?"
- Make reasonable demands and set reasonable limits, explaining their purpose clearly. Avoid creating situations that increase frustration and provoke anger, which may interfere with treatment.
- Explore patterns leading to the behavior or recurring problems.
- Listen attentively, offering feedback.
- Encourage the use of appropriate defenses to relieve loneliness and isolation.

- Engage the patient in activities to create positive accomplishments and raise his self-esteem and confidence.
- Encourage active diversionary activities, such as whistling or humming a tune, to divert attention from the unwanted thoughts and to promote a pleasurable experience.
- Help the patient develop new ways to solve problems and cultivate more effective coping skills by setting limits on unacceptable behavior (for example, by limiting the number of times per day he may indulge in compulsive behavior). Gradually shorten

BEHAVIORAL THERAPIES

The following behavioral therapies are used to treat the patient with obsessive-compulsive disorder.

Aversion therapy
Application of a painful stimulus creates an aversion to the obsession that leads to undesirable behavior (compulsion).

Flooding
Flooding is frequent, full-intensity exposure (through the use of imagery) to an object that triggers a symptom. It must be used with caution because it produces extreme discomfort.

Implosion therapy
A form of desensitization, implosion therapy calls for repeated exposure to a highly feared object.

Response prevention
Preventing compulsive behavior by distraction, persuasion, or redirection of activity, response prevention may require hospitalization or involvement of the patient's family to be effective.

Thought stopping
Thought stopping breaks the habit of fear-inducing anticipatory thoughts. The patient learns to stop unwanted thoughts by saying the word "stop" and then focusing his attention on achieving calmness and muscle relaxation.

Thought switching
To replace fear-inducing self-instructions with competent self-instructions, the patient learns to replace negative thoughts with positive ones until the positive thoughts become strong enough to overcome the anxiety-provoking ones.

the time allowed. Help him focus on other feelings or problems for the remainder of the time.
- Identify insight and improved behavior (reduced compulsive behavior and fewer obsessive thoughts). Evaluate behavioral changes by your own observations and the patient's reports.
- Identify disturbing topics of conversation that reflect underlying anxiety or terror.
- When interventions don't work, reevaluate them and recommend alternative strategies.
- Help the patient identify progress and set realistic expectations of himself and others.
- Explain how to channel emotional energy to relieve stress (for example, through sports and creative endeavors). In addition, teach the patient relaxation and breathing techniques to help reduce anxiety.
- Work with the patient and other treatment team members to establish behavioral goals and to help the patient tolerate anxiety in pursuing these goals.

Posttraumatic stress disorder

Characteristic psychological consequences that persist for at least 1 month after a traumatic event outside the range of usual human experience are classified as posttraumatic stress disorder (PTSD). This disorder can follow almost any distressing event, including a natural or man-made disaster, physical or sexual abuse, or an assault or a rape. Psychological trauma, which accompanies the physical trauma, is characterized by intense fear and feelings of helplessness and loss of control. PTSD can be acute, chronic, or delayed. When the precipitating event is of human design, the disorder is more severe and more persistent. Onset can occur at any age, even during childhood.

Causes and incidence
PTSD occurs in response to an extremely distressing event, including a serious threat of harm to the patient or his family, such as war, abuse, or violent crime. It may be trig-

gered by sudden destruction of his home or community by a bombing, fire, flood, tornado, earthquake, or similar disaster. It may also follow witnessing the death or serious injury of another person by torture, in a death camp, by natural disaster, or by a motor vehicle or airplane crash.

Preexisting psychopathology can predispose some patients to this disorder, but anyone can develop it, especially if the stressor is extreme.

Any person who has experienced traumatic relocation due to such events as rioting or other civil strife, extreme natural disasters, or war should be assessed for signs of PTSD.

PTSD can occur at any age. Most cases resolve 3 months after the traumatic event, but some cases can last for years.

Signs and symptoms

The psychosocial history of a patient with PTSD may reveal early life experiences, interpersonal factors, military experiences, or other incidents that suggest the precipitating event. Typically, the patient may report that his symptoms began immediately or soon after the trauma, although they may not develop until months or years later. In such a case, avoidance symptoms usually have been present during the latency period.

Symptoms include pangs of painful emotion and unwelcome thoughts; intrusive memories; dissociative episodes (flashbacks); a traumatic reexperiencing of the event; difficulty falling or staying asleep, frequent nightmares of the traumatic event, and aggressive outbursts on awakening; emotional numbing (diminished or constricted response); and chronic anxiety or panic attacks (with physical signs and symptoms).

The patient may display rage and survivor guilt, use of violence to solve problems, depression and suicidal thoughts, phobic avoidance of situations that arouse memories of the traumatic event (such as hot weather and tall grasses for the Vietnam veteran), memory impairment or difficulty concentrating, and feelings of detachment or estrangement that destroy interpersonal relationships. Some have

physical symptoms, fantasies of retaliation, and substance abuse.

Diagnosis

For characteristic findings in patients with this condition, see *Diagnosing posttraumatic stress disorder*, page 470.

Treatment

Treatment of PTSD aims to reduce the target symptoms, prevent chronic disability, and promote occupational and social rehabilitation. Specific treatments may emphasize behavioral techniques (such as relaxation therapy to decrease anxiety and induce sleep or progressive desensitization). Antianxiety and antidepressant drugs or psychotherapy (supportive, insight, or cathartic) may minimize the risks of dependency and chronicity.

Support groups are highly effective and are provided through many Veterans Administration centers and crisis clinics. These groups provide a forum in which victims of this disorder can work through their feelings with others who have had similar conflicts.

Group settings are appropriate for most degrees of symptoms presented. Some group programs include spouses and families in their treatment process. Rehabilitation programs in physical, social, and occupational settings are also available for victims of chronic PTSD.

Many patients need treatment for depression, alcohol or drug abuse, or medical conditions before psychological healing can take place. Treatment of this disorder may be complex, and the prognosis varies.

Special considerations

■ Encourage the patient with PTSD to express his grief, complete the mourning process, and develop coping skills to relieve anxiety and desensitize him to the memories of the traumatic event.

■ Keep in mind that such a patient tends to sharply test your commitment and interest. Therefore, first examine your feelings about the event (war or other trauma) so you won't react with disdain and shock. Such reactions hamper the working relationship with the patient and reinforce his typically poor self-image and sense of guilt.

DIAGNOSING POSTTRAUMATIC STRESS DISORDER

The diagnosis of posttraumatic stress disorder is made when the patient's signs and symptoms meet the following criteria documented in the *Diagnostic and Statistical Manual of Mental Disorders*, Fourth Edition, Text Revision.

■ The person was exposed to a traumatic event in which both of the following occurred:
– The person experienced, witnessed, or was confronted with an event or events that involved actual or threatened death or serious injury or a threat to the physical integrity of self or others.
– The person's response involved intense fear, helplessness, or horror (in children, the response may be expressed by disorganized or agitated behavior).

■ The person persistently reexperiences the traumatic event in at least one of the following ways:
– recurrent and intrusive distressing recollections of the event, including images, thoughts, or perceptions
– recurrent distressing dreams of the event
– acting or feeling as if the traumatic event were recurring (includes a sense of reliving the experience, illusions, hallucinations, and dissociative episodes that occur even when awakening or intoxicated)
– intense psychological distress at exposure to internal or external cues that symbolize or resemble an aspect of the traumatic event.

■ The person persistently avoids stimuli associated with the traumatic event and experiences numbing of general responsiveness (not present before the traumatic event), as indicated by at least three of the following:
– efforts to avoid thoughts or feelings associated with the trauma
– efforts to avoid activities, places, or people that arouse recollections of the trauma
– inability to recall an important aspect of the traumatic event
– markedly diminished interest in significant activities
– feeling of detachment or estrangement from other individuals
– restricted range of affect such as inability to love others
– sense of foreshortened future.

■ The person has persistent symptoms of increased arousal (not present before the trauma), as indicated by at least two of the following:
– difficulty falling or staying asleep
– irritability or outbursts of anger
– difficulty concentrating
– hypervigilance
– exaggerated startle response.

■ The disturbance must be of at least 1 month's duration.

■ The disturbance causes clinically significant distress or impairment in the patient's social, occupational, or other important areas of functioning.

■ Know and practice crisis intervention techniques as appropriate in PTSD.
■ Establish trust by accepting the patient's current level of functioning and assuming a positive, consistent, honest, and nonjudgmental attitude toward the patient.
■ Provide encouragement as the patient shows a commitment to work on his problem.
■ Deal constructively with the patient's displays of anger.

■ Encourage joint assessment of angry outbursts (identify how anger escalates and explore preventive measures that family members can take to regain control).
■ Provide a safe, staff-monitored room in which the patient can safely deal with urges to commit physical violence or self-abuse through displacement (such as pounding clay or destroying selected items).
■ Encourage the patient to move from physical to verbal expressions of anger.

- Help the patient relieve shame and guilt precipitated by real actions (such as killing or mutilation) that violated a consciously held moral code. Help him put his behavior into perspective, recognize his isolation and self-destructive behavior as forms of atonement, learn to forgive himself, and accept forgiveness from others.
- Refer the patient to a member of the clergy, as appropriate.
- Provide for group therapy with other victims for peer support and forgiveness, or refer the patient to such a support group.
- Refer the patient to appropriate community resources.

SOMATOFORM DISORDERS

Somatization disorder

When multiple recurrent signs and symptoms of several years' duration suggest that physical disorders exist without a verifiable disease or pathophysiologic condition to account for them, somatization disorder is present. The patient with somatization disorder usually undergoes repeated medical examinations and diagnostic testing that — unlike the symptoms themselves — can be potentially dangerous or debilitating. However, unlike the hypochondriac, she isn't preoccupied with the belief that she has a specific disease.

Somatization disorder is usually chronic, with exacerbations occurring during times of stress. The patient's signs and symptoms are involuntary, and she consciously wants to feel better. Nonetheless, she's seldom entirely symptom-free. Signs and symptoms usually begin in adolescence; rarely, in the 20s. This disorder primarily affects women; it's seldom diagnosed in men.

Causes and incidence

Genetic and environmental factors contribute to the development of somatization disorder. It usually develops before age 30 and is more common in females than in males.

Signs and symptoms

Examination of a patient with somatization disorder is characterized by physical complaints presented in a dramatic, vague, or exaggerated way, typically as part of a complicated medical history in which many medical diagnoses have been considered. An important clue to this disorder is a history of multiple medical evaluations by different physicians at different institutions — sometimes simultaneously — without significant findings.

The patient usually appears anxious and depressed. Common physical complaints include:

- conversion or pseudoneurologic signs and symptoms (for example, paralysis or blindness)
- GI discomfort (abdominal pain, nausea, or vomiting)
- female reproductive difficulties (such as painful menstruation) or male reproductive difficulties (such as erectile dysfunction)
- psychosexual problems (for example, sexual indifference)
- chronic pain (for example, back pain)
- cardiopulmonary symptoms (chest pain, dizziness, or palpitations).

The patient typically relates her current complaints and previous evaluations in great detail. She may be quite knowledgeable about tests, procedures, and medical jargon. Attempts to explore areas other than her medical history may cause noticeable anxiety. She tends to disparage previous health care professionals and previous treatments, typically with the comment, "Everyone thinks I'm imagining these things." In some cases, this may actually be true. (See *Factitious disorders,* page 472.)

Ongoing assessment should focus on new signs or symptoms or any change in old ones to avoid missing a developing physical disorder.

Diagnosis

For characteristic findings in patients with this condition, see *Diagnosing somatization disorder,* page 473.

Diagnostic tests rule out physical disorders that cause vague and confusing symptoms, such as hyperparathyroidism, porphyria, multiple sclerosis, chronic fatigue

FACTITIOUS DISORDERS

Marked by the irrational, repetitious simulation of a physical or mental illness for the purpose of obtaining medical treatment, factitious disorders are serious psychopathologic conditions. The symptoms are intentionally produced and can be either physical or psychological. These disorders are more common in men than in women.

Factitious disorder with physical symptoms

Also called *Munchausen syndrome,* this is the most common factitious disorder. The patient convincingly presents with intentionally feigned symptoms. These symptoms may be fabricated (acute abdominal pain with no underlying disease), self-inflicted (deliberately infecting an open wound), an exacerbation or exaggeration of a preexisting disorder (taking penicillin despite a known allergy), or a combination of all the above.

The history of a patient with Munchausen syndrome may include:
- multiple admissions to various hospitals, typically across a wide geographic area
- extensive knowledge of medical terminology
- pathologic lying

- evidence of previous treatment such as surgery
- shifting complaints and signs and symptoms
- eagerness to undergo hazardous and painful procedures
- discharge against medical advice to avoid detection
- poor interpersonal relationships
- refusal of psychiatric examination
- psychoactive substance or analgesic abuse.

Factitious disorder with psychological symptoms

Causing severely impaired function, this disorder is characterized by intentional feigning of symptoms, suggesting a mental disorder. However, the symptoms represent how the patient views the mental disorder and seldom coincide with any of the diagnostic categories documented in the *Diagnostic and Statistical Manual of Mental Disorders,* Fourth Edition, Text Revision.

This disorder almost always coexists with a severe personality disorder. Most patients have a history of psychoactive substance use, usually in an attempt to elicit the desired symptoms.

---

syndrome, and systemic lupus erythematosus. In addition, multiple physical signs and symptoms that appear for the first time late in life are usually due to physical disease rather than somatization disorder.

Treatment

The goal of treatment is to help the patient learn to live with her signs and symptoms. After diagnostic evaluation has ruled out organic causes, the patient should be told that she has no serious illness currently but will receive care for her genuine distress and ongoing medical attention for her symptoms.

The most important aspect of treatment is a continuing supportive relationship

with a health care provider who acknowledges the patient's signs and symptoms and is willing to help her live with them. The patient should have regularly scheduled appointments to review her complaints and the effectiveness of her coping strategies. The patient with somatization disorder seldom acknowledges any psychological aspect of her illness and rejects psychiatric treatment.

Special considerations

- Acknowledge the patient's symptoms and her efforts to cope despite distress. Don't characterize her symptoms as imaginary. Tell her test results and their significance.

DIAGNOSING SOMATIZATION DISORDER

The diagnosis of somatization disorder is made when the patient's symptoms match the diagnostic criteria put forth in the *Diagnostic and Statistical Manual of Mental Disorders*, Fourth Edition, Text Revision, as follows:

- A history of many physical complaints, beginning before age 30 and persisting for several years, results in the patient seeking treatment or in the patient experiencing significant social, occupational, or other impairment.
- The patient experiences a selection of symptoms as follows (with individual symptoms occurring at any time during the disturbance):
  – *pain:* a history of pain related to at least *four* different sites or functions (head, abdomen, back, joints, arms and legs, chest, rectum, menstruation, sexual intercourse, or urination)
  – *GI upset:* a history of at least *two* GI symptoms other than pain (vomiting other than during pregnancy, nausea, bloating, diarrhea, and intolerance of different foods)
  – *sexual symptoms:* a history of at least *one* sexual or reproductive symptom other than pain—for example, sexual indifference, erectile or ejaculatory dysfunction, irregular menses, excessive menstrual bleeding, or vomiting throughout pregnancy

- *pseudoneurologic symptoms:* a history of at least *one* symptom or deficit suggesting a neurologic condition not limited to pain (for example, conversion symptoms, such as impaired coordination or balance, paralysis or localized weakness, difficulty swallowing or lump in the throat, aphonia, urine retention, hallucinations, loss of touch or pain sensation, double vision, blindness, deafness, or seizures; dissociative symptoms such as amnesia; or loss of consciousness other than fainting).
- A thorough investigation discloses that either the above symptoms can't be fully explained by a known general medical condition or the direct effects of a substance. If a related general medical condition does exist, the physical complaints or resulting impairments exceed what would be expected from the history, physical examination, and diagnostic findings.
- The symptoms aren't intentionally produced or feigned (as in factitious disorder or malingering).

- Emphasize her strengths, for example, "It's good that you can still work with this pain." Gently point out the time relationship between stress and symptoms.
- Help her manage stress. Typically, her relationships are linked to her symptoms; relieving them can impair her interactions with others.
- Negotiate a plan of care with input from the patient and, if possible, her family. Help them to understand the patient's need for troublesome symptoms.

Conversion disorder

A conversion disorder allows a patient to resolve a psychological conflict through the loss of a specific physical function — for example, by paralysis, blindness, or inability to swallow. Unlike factitious disorders or malingering, conversion disorder results in an involuntary loss of physical function. However, laboratory tests and diagnostic procedures fail to disclose an organic cause. The conversion symptom itself isn't life threatening and usually has a short duration.

DIAGNOSING CONVERSION DISORDER

The diagnosis of conversion disorder is based on the following criteria put forth in the *Diagnostic and Statistical Manual of Mental Disorders,* Fourth Edition, Text Revision:

- The person has one or more symptoms or deficits affecting voluntary motor or sensory function that suggest a neurologic or other general medical condition.
- The person exhibits psychological factors judged to be associated with the symptom or deficit because conflicts or other stressors preceded the symptom's or deficit's manifestation.
- The person's symptom or deficit isn't intentionally produced or feigned.
- The person's symptom or deficit can't, after appropriate investigation, be fully explained by a general medical condi-

tion, by the direct effects of a substance, or as a culturally sanctioned behavior or experience.

- The person's symptom or deficit warrants medical evaluation, causes clinically significant distress, or impairs social, occupational, or other important areas of functioning.
- The person's symptom or deficit isn't limited to pain or sexual dysfunction, doesn't occur exclusively during the course of somatization disorder, and isn't better accounted for by another mental disorder.

Causes and incidence

The patient suddenly develops the conversion symptom soon after experiencing a traumatic conflict that he believes he can't handle. Two theories may explain why this occurs. According to the first, the patient achieves a "primary gain" when the symptom keeps a psychological conflict out of conscious awareness. For example, a person may experience blindness after witnessing a violent crime.

The second theory suggests that the patient achieves "secondary gain" from the symptom by avoiding a traumatic activity. For example, a soldier may develop a "paralyzed" hand that prevents him from entering into combat.

Conversion disorder can occur in either sex at any age. An uncommon disorder, it usually begins in adolescence or early adulthood.

Signs and symptoms

The history of a patient with conversion disorder may reveal the sudden onset of a single, debilitating sign or symptom that prevents normal function of the affected body part such as paralysis of a leg. The pa-

tient may describe a psychologically stressful event that recently preceded the symptom. Oddly, the patient doesn't display the affect and concern that such a severe symptom usually elicits.

Assessment findings obtained during a physical examination are inconsistent with the primary symptom. For instance, tendon reflexes may be normal in a "paralyzed" part of the body, loss of function fails to follow anatomic patterns of innervation, or pupillary responses and evoked potentials are normal in a patient who complains of blindness.

Diagnosis

For characteristic findings in patients with this condition, see *Diagnosing conversion disorder.*

A thorough physical evaluation must rule out a physical cause, especially diseases that typically produce vague physical symptoms (such as multiple sclerosis or systemic lupus erythematosus).

Treatment

Psychotherapy, family therapy, relaxation therapy, behavioral therapy, or hypnosis may be used alone or in combination (two or more).

Special considerations
■ Help the patient maintain integrity of the affected system. Regularly exercise paralyzed limbs to prevent muscle wasting and contractures.

■ Frequently change the bedridden patient's position to prevent pressure ulcers.

■ Ensure adequate nutrition, even if the patient is complaining of GI distress.

■ Provide a supportive environment, and encourage the patient to discuss the stressful event that provoked his disorder.

■ Don't force the patient to talk, but convey a caring attitude to help him share his feelings.

■ Don't insist that the patient use the affected system. This will only anger him and prevent the two of you from forming a therapeutic relationship.

■ Add your support to the recommendation for psychiatric care.

■ Include the patient's family in all care. They may be contributing to the patient's stress, and they're essential to help him regain normal functioning.

Pain disorder

The striking feature of pain disorder is a persistent complaint of pain in the absence of appropriate physical findings. The symptoms are either inconsistent with the normal anatomic distribution of the nervous system or they mimic a disease (such as angina) in the absence of diagnostic validation. Although the pain has no physical cause, it's real to the patient. The pain is usually chronic and may, in many cases, interfere with interpersonal relationships or employment.

Causes and incidence
Pain disorder has no specific cause, but it may be related to severe psychological stress or conflict. The pain provides the patient with a means to cope with upsetting psychological issues. For example, a person with dependency needs may develop this disorder as an acceptable way to receive care and attention. The pain may have spe-

cial significance such as leg pain in the same leg a parent lost through amputation. Pain disorder is more common in women than in men and usually has an onset in the 30s and 40s.

Signs and symptoms
The cardinal feature of pain disorder is a history of chronic, consistent complaints of pain without confirming physical disease. The patient may relate a long history of evaluations and procedures at multiple settings without much pain relief. Because of frequent hospitalizations, the patient may be familiar with pain medications and tranquilizers, ask for a specific drug, and know correct dosages and administration routes. She may openly behave like an invalid.

Physical examination of the painful site reveals that the pain doesn't follow anatomic pathways. The patient may not display typical nonverbal signs of pain, such as grimacing or guarding. (Sometimes such reactions are absent in the patient with chronic organic pain.) Palpation, percussion, and auscultation may not reveal expected associated signs. Psychosocial assessment may reveal a patient who's angry with health care professionals because they've failed to relieve her pain.

Diagnosis
For characteristic findings in patients with this condition, see *Diagnosing pain disorder,* page 476.

Treatment
In pain disorder, treatment aims to ease the pain and help the patient live with it. Thus, long, invasive evaluations and surgical interventions are avoided. Treatment at a comprehensive pain center may be helpful. Supportive measures for pain relief may include hot or cold packs, physical therapy, distraction techniques, and cutaneous stimulation with massage or transcutaneous electrical nerve stimulation. Measures to reduce the patient's anxiety may help, as may an antidepressant medication such as a tricyclic antidepressant.

A continuing, supportive relationship with an understanding health care professional is essential for effective manage-

DIAGNOSING PAIN DISORDER

The diagnosis of pain disorder is difficult because the perception of pain is subjective. Diagnosis is based on fulfillment of the following criteria put forth in the *Diagnostic and Statistical Manual of Mental Disorders*, Fourth Edition, Text Revision:

■ Pain in one or more body sites is the predominant focus of the patient and is sufficiently severe to warrant clinical attention.
■ The pain causes clinically significant distress or impairment in social, occupational, or other important areas of functioning.
■ Psychological factors are judged to have an important role in the onset, severity, exacerbation, and maintenance of the pain.
■ The symptom or deficit isn't intentionally produced or feigned.
■ The pain isn't better accounted for by a mood, anxiety, or psychotic disorder and doesn't meet criteria for dyspareunia.

ment; regularly scheduled follow-up appointments are helpful.

Analgesics become an issue because the patient believes that she has to "fight to be taken seriously." She should clearly be told what medication she will receive in addition to supportive pain-relief measures. Regularly scheduled analgesic doses can be more effective than scheduling medication as needed. Regular doses combat pain by reducing anxiety about asking for medication, and they eliminate unnecessary confrontations. The use of placebos will destroy trust when the patient discovers deceit.

Special considerations
■ Observe and record characteristics of the pain: severity, duration, and any precipitating factors.

■ Provide a caring atmosphere in which the patient's complaints are taken seriously and every effort is made to provide relief. This means communicating to the patient that you'll collaborate on a plan of treatment, clearly stating the limitations. For example, you might say, "I can stay with you now for 15 minutes, but you can't receive another dose until 2 p.m."
■ Don't tell the patient that she's imagining the pain or can wait longer for medication that's due. Assess her complaints and help her understand what's contributing to the pain.
■ Provide other comfort measures, such as repositioning or massage, when possible.
■ Encourage the patient to maintain independence despite her pain.
■ Offer attention at times other than during the patient's complaints of pain to weaken the link to secondary gain.
■ Avoid confronting the patient with the somatoform nature of her pain; this seldom is helpful because such pain is her means of avoiding psychological conflict.
■ Consider psychiatric referrals; however, realize that the patient may resist psychiatric intervention, and don't expect it to replace analgesic measures.
■ Teach the patient noninvasive, drug-free methods of pain control, such as guided imagery, relaxation techniques, and distraction through reading or writing.

Hypochondriasis

The dominant feature of hypochondriasis is an unrealistic misinterpretation of the severity and significance of physical signs or sensations as abnormal. This leads to preoccupation with fear of having a serious disease, which persists despite medical reassurance to the contrary. Hypochondriasis causes severe social and occupational impairment. It isn't due to other mental disorders, such as schizophrenia, mood disorder, or somatization disorder.

The course of hypochondriasis is usually chronic, although the severity of symptoms may vary.

Causes and incidence

Hypochondriasis isn't linked to a specific cause, but it commonly develops in people who have experienced an organic disease or in their relatives. It allows the patient to assume a dependent sick role to ensure that his needs are met. Such a patient is unaware of these unmet needs, and doesn't consciously cause his symptoms. Stress increases the risk of developing hypochondriasis.

Hypochondriasis occurs in men and women with equal frequency. It can begin at any age, but onset usually occurs between ages 20 and 30.

Signs and symptoms

The dominant feature of hypochondriasis is the misinterpretation of symptoms — usually multiple complaints that involve a single organ system — as signs of serious illness. As the medical evaluation proceeds, complaints may shift and change. Symptoms, which can range from specific to general, vague complaints, typically are associated with a preoccupation with normal body functions.

The hypochondriacal patient will relate a chronic history of waxing and waning symptoms. Commonly, he will have undergone multiple evaluations for similar symptoms or complaints of serious illness. His past contacts with health care professionals make him quite knowledgeable about illness, diagnosis, and treatment.

Diagnosis

For characteristic findings in patients with this condition, see *Diagnosing hypochondriasis.*

Treatment

The goal of treatment is to help the patient continue to lead a productive life despite distressing symptoms and fears. After medical evaluation is complete, the patient should be told clearly that he doesn't have a serious disease. Continued medical follow-up, however, will help monitor his symptoms. Providing a diagnosis won't make hypochondriasis disappear, but it may ease the patient's anxiety.

Regular outpatient follow-up can help the patient deal with his symptoms and is

---

DIAGNOSING HYPOCHONDRIASIS

A diagnosis of hypochondriasis is made when the patient's symptoms meet the following criteria put forth in the *Diagnostic and Statistical Manual of Mental Disorders,* Fourth Edition, Text Revision:

- Preoccupation with the fear of having or the belief that one has a serious disease is based on the person's misinterpretation of bodily symptoms.
- The preoccupation persists despite appropriate medical evaluation and reassurance.
- The fear of having or the belief that one has a serious disease isn't of delusional intensity (as in delusional disorder, somatic type) and isn't restricted to a circumscribed concern about appearance (as in body dysmorphic disorder).
- The preoccupation causes clinically significant distress or impairment in social, occupational, or other important areas of functioning.
- The disturbance has persisted for at least 6 months.
- The preoccupation isn't better accounted for by generalized anxiety disorder, obsessive-compulsive disorder, panic disorder, a major depressive episode, separation anxiety, or another somatoform disorder.

---

necessary to detect organic illness. (Up to 30% of these patients develop an organic disease.) Because the patient can be demanding and irritating, consistent follow-up may be difficult.

Most patients don't acknowledge any psychological influence on their symptoms and resist psychiatric treatment.

Special considerations

- Provide a supportive relationship that lets the patient feel cared for and understood. The patient with hypochondriasis

feels real pain and distress, so don't deny his symptoms or challenge his behavior.
- Firmly state that medical test results were normal. Instead of reinforcing his symptoms, encourage him to discuss his other problems, and urge his family to do the same.
- Recognize that the patient will never be symptom-free, and don't become angry when he won't give up his disease. Such anger can drive him to yet another unnecessary medical evaluation.
- Help the patient and his family find new ways to deal with stress other than the development of physical symptoms.

Body dysmorphic disorder

In body dysmorphic disorder, the patient is preoccupied with an imagined or slight defect in physical appearance. He may think he's hideous or grotesque even though others reassure him that he looks fine. The patient with this disorder thinks about the defect for at least 1 hour each day.

Causes and incidence
No cause for body dysmorphic disorder has been identified, although theories have been put forth. The biologic theory holds that some individuals may have a genetic predisposition to psychiatric disorders, making them more likely to develop body dysmorphic disorder. Certain stresses or life events, especially during adolescence, may precipitate the onset of the disorder. It may also be associated with an imbalance of serotonin or other brain chemicals.

The psychological theory holds that low self-esteem and a tendency to judge oneself almost exclusively by appearance may contribute to body dysmorphic disorder. These patients may be perfectionists who strive for an impossible ideal. In such patients, heightened perception about appearance causes increasing focus on every imperfection or slight abnormality.

In the United States, body dysmorphic disorder is estimated to occur in 1% to 2% of the general population, affecting males and females equally. However, its incidence may be underestimated because it fre-

quently goes undiagnosed. It's a chronic condition and usually begins during the late teens. The average age of onset is 17.

Signs and symptoms
Body dysmorphic disorder may be suspected in the patient who reports or exhibits any of these behaviors:
- commonly checks reflection in the mirror, or avoids mirrors
- frequently compares appearance against that of other people
- frequently examines the appearance of other people
- tries to cover the perceived defect with clothing, makeup, or a hat or by changing posture
- seeks corrective treatment, such as surgery or dermatologic therapy, to eradicate the perceived defect, even though physicians, family numbers, and friends think such measures aren't necessary
- constantly seeks reassurance from others about the perceived flaw or, conversely, tries to convince others of its repulsiveness
- performs long grooming rituals, such as repeatedly combing or cutting the hair or applying makeup or cover-up creams
- picks at the skin or squeezes pimples or blackheads for hours
- frequently touches the perceived problem area
- measures the body part that's repulsive
- is anxious and self-conscious
- feels acute distress over appearance, causing functional impairment
- avoids social situations where the perceived defect may be exposed
- has difficulty maintaining relationships with peers, family, and spouses
- performs poorly in school or work, or takes frequent sick days
- has low self-esteem
- has suicidal thoughts or behaviors.

Symptom severity varies. Some patients are able to manage their distress so that they can function, some have severe functional impairment, and still others are so embarrassed or disgusted by their appearance that they avoid some or all social interaction.

Diagnosis

Body dysmorphic disorder shares many of the same symptoms and signs as other psychological illnesses, especially obsessive-compulsive disorder. To assess severity, testing may include diagnostic instruments, such as the Yale-Brown Obsessive-Compulsive Scale modified for body dysmorphic disorder or various others.

The diagnosis of body dysmorphic disorder is confirmed when the patient meets criteria from the *Diagnostic and Statistical Manual of Mental Disorders,* Fourth Edition, Text Revision. Criteria include:
- The patient is preoccupied with an imagined defect in appearance. If a slight physical abnormality actually is present, concern over it is markedly excessive.
- The preoccupation causes clinically significant distress or impairment in social, occupational, or other important areas of functioning.
- The preoccupation isn't better explained by another mental disorder such as anorexia nervosa.

Treatment

The goals of treatment for the patient include enhancement of his self-esteem, reduced preoccupation with the perceived flaw, and elimination of the harmful effects of compulsive behaviors. The patient also needs to improve functional abilities as well as express (and cope with) feelings of anxiety as they arise without resorting to excessive behaviors.

Cognitive-behavioral therapy and group therapies have proven helpful. Behavioral methods, including aversion therapy, thought-stopping, and flooding (also called *implosion therapy*), have proven effective. Other treatments include the use of selective serotonin reuptake inhibitors to help diminish preoccupation, distress, depression, and anxiety. Tricyclic antidepressants have also been effective.

Special considerations

- Provide an accepting, nonjudgmental atmosphere when caring for the patient.
- If the patient becomes involved in ritualistic thoughts and behaviors to the point of self-neglect, provide for basic needs, such

as rest, nutrition, and grooming. Don't block ritualistic behavior, but do set limits.
- Help the patient explore feelings associated with the behavior.
- Engage the patient in activities that create positive accomplishments and raise self-esteem and confidence.
- Suggest active diversions, such as whistling or humming, to divert the patient's attention away from unwanted thoughts.
- Help the patient devise new ways to solve problems and develop more effective coping skills by setting limits on unacceptable behavior.
- Encourage the patient to use appropriate techniques to relieve stress, loneliness, and isolation.
- Monitor for desired and adverse effects of drug therapy, as appropriate.

DISSOCIATIVE DISORDERS

Dissociative identity disorder

A complex disturbance of identity and memory, dissociative identity disorder (formerly referred to as *multiple personality disorder*) is characterized by the existence of two or more distinct, fully integrated personalities in the same person. The personalities alternate in dominance. Each comprises unique memories, behavior patterns, and social relationships; in many cases, rigid and flamboyant personalities are combined. Usually, one personality is unaware of the existence of the others.

Causes and incidence

The cause isn't known. The patient typically has experienced abuse, commonly sexual, or another form of emotional trauma in childhood. A child may evolve multiple personalities to dissociate herself from the traumatic situation. The dissociated contents become linked with one of many possible shaping influences for personality organization.

DIAGNOSING DISSOCIATIVE IDENTITY DISORDER

The diagnosis of dissociative identity disorder is based on fulfillment of the following criteria established in the *Diagnostic and Statistical Manual of Mental Disorders,* Fourth Edition, Text Revision:

- Two or more distinct personalities or personality states (each with its own relatively enduring pattern of perceiving, relating to, and thinking about the environment and self) are present.
- At least two of these personalities or personality states recurrently take full control of the person's behavior.
- The person can't recall important personal information that's too extensive to be explained by ordinary forgetfulness.
- The disturbance isn't due to the direct physiologic effects of a substance or a general medical condition.

Dissociative identity disorder usually begins in childhood, but patients seldom seek treatment until much later in life. The disorder is three to nine times more common in women than in men.

Signs and symptoms

The patient may seek treatment for a concurrent psychiatric disorder present in one of the personalities. She may have a history of unsuccessful psychiatric treatment, or she may report periods of amnesia and disturbances in time perception. Family members may describe incidents that the patient can't recall as well as alterations in facial presentation, voice, and behavior.

Stress or idiosyncratically meaningful social or environmental cues commonly trigger the transition from one personality to another. Although usually sudden, the transition can occur over hours or days. Hypnosis and amobarbital may facilitate transition.

Diagnosis

For characteristic findings in patients with this condition, see *Diagnosing dissociative identity disorder.*

Treatment

Psychotherapy is essential to uniting the personalities and preventing the personality from splitting again. Treatment is usually intensive and prolonged, with success linked to the strength of the patient-therapist relationship with each of the personalities, all of which require equal respect and concern.

Special considerations

- Establish an empathetic relationship with each emerging personality.
- Monitor the patient's actions for evidence of self-directed violence or violence directed at others.
- Recognize even small gains.
- Stress the importance of continuing psychotherapy. Point out that the therapy can be prolonged, with alternating successes and failures, and that one or more of the personalities may resist treatment.

Dissociative fugue

The patient suffering from dissociative fugue wanders or travels while mentally blocking out a traumatic event. During the fugue state, he usually assumes a different personality and later can't recall what happened. The degree of impairment varies, depending on the duration of the fugue and the nature of the personality state it invokes. Dissociative fugue may be related to dissociative identity disorder, narcissistic personality disorder, and sleepwalking.

The age of onset varies. Although the fugue state is usually brief (hours to days), it can last for months and carry the patient far from home. The prognosis for complete recovery is good, and recurrences are rare.

Causes

Dissociative fugue typically follows an extremely stressful event, such as combat experience, a natural disaster, a violent or abusive confrontation, or personal rejection. Heavy alcohol use may constitute a predisposing factor.

Signs and symptoms

Psychiatric examination of the patient with dissociative fugue may reveal that he has assumed a new, more uninhibited identity. If the new personality is still evolving, he may avoid social contact. On the other hand, he may have traveled to a distant location, set up a new residence, and developed a well-integrated network of social relationships that don't suggest any mental alteration.

The psychosocial history of such a patient may include episodes of violent behavior. After recovery, he typically can't remember these and other events that took place during the fugue state.

Diagnosis

For characteristic findings in patients with this condition, see *Diagnosing dissociative fugue.*

Treatment

Psychotherapy aims to help the patient recognize the traumatic event that triggered the fugue state and develop reality-based strategies for coping with anxiety. A trusting, therapeutic relationship is essential for success.

Special considerations

■ When providing care in this disorder, teach the patient effective coping strategies to use in stressful situations rather than strategies that distort reality.
■ Help the patient with dissociative fugue recognize and deal with anxiety-producing experiences.
■ Establish a therapeutic, nonjudgmental relationship with the patient.

Dissociative amnesia

The essential feature of dissociative amnesia is a sudden inability to recall important personal information that can't be explained by ordinary forgetfulness. The patient typically is unable to recall all events that occurred during a specific period, but

DIAGNOSING DISSOCIATIVE FUGUE

The diagnosis of dissociative fugue is made when the patient's symptoms match the following criteria put forth in the *Diagnostic and Statistical Manual of Mental Disorders,* Fourth Edition, Text Revision:

■ The predominant disturbance is sudden, unexpected travel away from home or the patient's customary place of work, with an inability to recall the past.
■ The person experiences confusion about personal identity or assumption of a new partial or complete identity.
■ The disturbance isn't due to dissociative identity disorder, physiologic effects of a substance, or a general medical condition.
■ The symptoms cause clinically significant distress or impairment in social, occupational, or other important areas of functioning.

other types of recall disturbance are also possible.

The *Diagnostic and Statistical Manual of Mental Disorders,* Fourth Edition, Text Revision, recognizes five types of amnesia, based on the time period and amount of information lost to recall:
■ *localized amnesia*—failure to recall all events that occurred during a circumscribed time period
■ *selective amnesia*—failure to recall some of the events that occurred during a circumscribed time period
■ *generalized amnesia*—failure to recall all events over the entire life span
■ *continuous amnesia*—failure to recall events subsequent to a specific time up to and including the present
■ *systematized amnesia*—failure to recall certain categories of information.

This disorder commonly occurs during war and natural disasters. Although it's more common in adolescents and young

DIAGNOSING DISSOCIATIVE AMNESIA

A diagnosis of dissociative amnesia is made when the patient's symptoms meet the following criteria put forth in the *Diagnostic and Statistical Manual of Mental Disorders,* Fourth Edition, Text Revision:

- The predominant disturbance is at least one episode of inability to recall important personal information, usually of a traumatic or stressful nature, that is too extensive to be explained by ordinary forgetfulness.
- The disturbance isn't due to dissociative identity disorder, dissociative fugue, posttraumatic stress disorder, acute stress disorder, or somatization disorder. It's also not due to the direct physiologic effects of a substance or a neurologic or other general medical condition.
- The symptoms cause clinically significant distress or impairment in social, occupational, or other important areas of functioning.

adult women, it's also seen in young men after combat experience. The amnesic event typically ends abruptly, and recovery is complete, with rare recurrences.

Causes
Dissociative amnesia follows severe psychosocial stress, commonly involving a threat of physical injury or death. Amnesia may also occur after thinking about or engaging in unacceptable behavior such as an extramarital affair.

Signs and symptoms
During the assessment interview, the amnesic patient may appear perplexed and disoriented, wandering aimlessly. He won't be able to remember the event that precipitated the episode and probably won't recognize his inability to recall information.

After the episode has ended, the patient is usually unaware that he has suffered what's known as a recall disturbance.

Diagnosis
For characteristic findings in patients with this condition, see *Diagnosing dissociative amnesia.*

Treatment
Psychotherapy aims to help the patient recognize the traumatic event that triggered the amnesia and the anxiety it produced. A trusting, therapeutic relationship is essential to achieving this goal. The therapist subsequently attempts to teach the patient reality-based coping strategies.

Special considerations
- When providing care in this disorder, teach the patient effective coping strategies to use in stressful situations rather than those strategies that distort reality.
- Help the patient with dissociative amnesia recognize and deal with experiences that produce anxiety.
- Establish a therapeutic, nonjudgmental relationship with the patient.

Depersonalization disorder

Persistent or recurrent episodes of detachment characterize depersonalization disorder. During these episodes, self-awareness is temporarily altered or lost; the patient in many cases perceives this alteration in consciousness as a barrier between himself and the outside world. The sense of depersonalization may be restricted to a single body part, such as a limb, or it may encompass the whole self. The patient with this disorder may feel that he's mechanical, in a dream, or detached from his body.

Although the patient seldom loses touch with reality completely, the episodes of depersonalization may cause him severe distress. Depersonalization disorder usually has a sudden onset in adolescence or early in adult life. It follows a chronic course, with periodic exacerbations and remissions, and resolves gradually.

Causes

Depersonalization disorder typically stems from severe stress, including war experiences, accidents, and natural disasters. It may also be due to neurologic or systemic disease.

Signs and symptoms

The patient with depersonalization disorder may complain of feeling detached from his entire being and body, as if he were watching himself from a distance or living in a dream. He may also report sensory anesthesia, a loss of self-control, difficulty speaking, and feelings of derealization and losing touch with reality.

Common findings during the assessment interview include symptoms of depression, obsessive rumination, somatic concerns, anxiety, fear of going insane, a disturbed sense of time, and a prolonged recall time as well as physical complaints such as dizziness.

Diagnosis

For characteristic findings in patients with this condition, see *Diagnosing depersonalization disorder*.

Treatment

Psychotherapy aims to establish a trusting, therapeutic relationship in which the patient recognizes the traumatic event that triggered the disorder and the anxiety it evoked. The therapist subsequently teaches the patient to use reality-based coping strategies rather than to detach himself from the situation.

Special considerations

■ When providing care in this disorder, assist the patient in using reality-based coping strategies under stress rather than those strategies that distort reality.
■ Help the patient who has depersonalization disorder recognize and deal with experiences that produce anxiety.
■ Establish a therapeutic, nonjudgmental relationship with the patient.

DIAGNOSING DEPERSONALIZATION DISORDER

The depersonalization disorder diagnosis is made when the patient's symptoms match the following criteria put forth in the *Diagnostic and Statistical Manual of Mental Disorders*, Fourth Edition, Text Revision:

■ The person has persistent or recurrent experiences of feeling detached from mind or body (as if he were an outside observer) or feeling like an automaton (as if he were in a dream).
■ During the depersonalization experience, reality testing remains intact.
■ The depersonalization causes clinically significant distress or impairment in social, occupational, or other important areas of functioning.
■ The depersonalization experience doesn't occur exclusively during the course of another mental disorder, such as schizophrenia, panic disorder, acute stress disorder, or another dissociative disorder, and isn't due to the direct physiologic effects of a substance or a general medical condition.

Personality disorders

Defined as individual traits that reflect chronic, inflexible, and maladaptive patterns of behavior, personality disorders cause social discomfort and impair social and occupational functioning. The *Diagnostic and Statistical Manual of Mental Disorders*, Fourth Edition, Text Revision, groups personality disorders into three clusters:

■ Cluster A—paranoid, schizoid, and schizotypal personality disorders. These disorders share odd or eccentric behavior.
■ Cluster B—antisocial, borderline, histrionic, and narcissistic personality disorders.

Dramatic, emotional, or erratic behavior highlights these disorders.

■ Cluster C—avoidant, dependent, and obsessive-compulsive personality disorders. These disorders are marked by anxious or fearful behavior.

Each disorder produces characteristic signs and symptoms, which may vary among patients and even with the same patient at different times.

Personality disorders are lifelong conditions with an onset in adolescence or early adulthood. Cluster A and B disorders tend to grow less intense in middle age and late life, whereas cluster C disorders tend to become exaggerated. Patients with cluster B disorders are susceptible to substance abuse, poor impulse control, and suicidal behavior, which may shorten lives.

Personality disorders overlap with other psychiatric disorders, such as substance abuse disorders, mood disorders, and anxiety disorders.

Causes and incidence

Various theories attempt to explain the origin of personality disorders. Genetic factors influence the biological basis of brain function as well as basic personality structure. In turn, personality structure affects how a person responds to life experiences and interacts with the social environment. Over time, each person develops distinctive ways of perceiving the world and of feeling, thinking, and behaving.

Some researchers suspect that poor regulation of the areas controlling emotion within the brain increases the risk of a personality disorder, especially when combined with such factors as abuse, neglect, or separation. For a biologically predisposed person, the major developmental challenges of adolescence and early adulthood may trigger a personality disorder.

Social theories hold that disorders reflect learned responses, having much to do with reinforcement, modeling, and aversive stimuli as contributing factors. According to psychodynamic theories, personality disorders reflect deficiencies in ego and superego development and are related to poor mother-child relationships characterized by unresponsiveness, overprotectiveness, or early separation.

Personality disorders are common and affect 10% to 15% of the population in the United States. Gender influences presence; for example, antisocial and obsessive-compulsive personality disorders are more common in men, whereas borderline, dependent, and histrionic personality disorders are more prevalent in women.

Signs and symptoms

Each specific personality disorder produces characteristic signs and symptoms, which may vary among patients and within the same patient at different times. In general, the history of the patient with a personality disorder will reveal long-standing difficulties in interpersonal relationships, ranging from dependency to withdrawal, and in occupational functioning, with effects ranging from compulsive perfectionism to intentional sabotage.

The patient with a personality disorder may show any degree of self-confidence, ranging from no self-esteem to arrogance. Convinced that his behavior is normal, he avoids responsibility for its consequences, commonly resorting to projections and blame.

Diagnosis

For characteristic findings in patients with this condition, see *Diagnosing personality disorders.*

Treatment

Personality disorders are difficult to treat. Successful therapy requires a trusting relationship in which the therapist can use a direct approach. The type of therapy chosen depends on the patient's symptoms. Family and group therapies are usually effective. Cognitive and self-help groups have also been beneficial.

Drug therapy is effective in some types of personality disorders; for example, pimozide has been successfully used to reduce paranoia ideation in some patients with paranoid personality disorder. Antipsychotic drugs (olanzapine or risperidone) may be used to treat severe agitation or delusional thinking. Selective serotonin reuptake inhibitors, such as fluoxetine, may be used to treat irritability, anger, and ob-
(Text continues on page 488.)

DIAGNOSING PERSONALITY DISORDERS

The diagnosis of a recognized personality disorder is made when a patient's symptoms match the diagnostic criteria put forth in the *Diagnostic and Statistical Manual of Mental Disorders,* Fourth Edition, Text Revision.

Antisocial personality disorder

■ This disorder manifests as a pervasive disregard for and violation of the rights of others occurring since age 15, as indicated by at least three of the following:

– The person fails to conform to social norms with respect to lawful behavior, as demonstrated by repeatedly performing acts that are grounds for arrest.

– The person exhibits deceitfulness, as indicated by repeated lying, using aliases, or conning others for personal profit or pleasure.

– The person demonstrates impulsivity or failure to plan ahead.

– The person is irritable and aggressive, as indicated by repeated physical fights or assaults.

– The person has reckless disregard for the safety of self or others.

– The person shows consistent irresponsibility, as indicated by repeated failure to sustain consistent work behavior or honor financial obligations.

– The person lacks remorse, as indicated by being indifferent to or rationalizing having hurt, mistreated, or stolen from others.

■ The person is at least age 18.

■ The person's history includes evidence of a conduct disorder with an onset before age 15.

■ The antisocial behavior doesn't occur exclusively during the course of schizophrenia or a manic episode.

Avoidant personality disorder

This pervasive pattern of social inhibition, feelings of inadequacy, and hypersensitivity to negative evaluation, beginning by early adulthood and present in a variety of contexts, is indicated by at least four of the following:

■ The person avoids social or occupational activities that involve significant interpersonal contact because of fears of criticism, disapproval, or rejection.

■ The person is unwilling to get involved with people unless he's certain that they will like him.

■ The person shows restraint within intimate relationships because of the fear of being shamed or ridiculed.

■ The person is preoccupied with being criticized or rejected in social situations.

■ The person's feelings of inadequacy inhibit him in new interpersonal situations.

■ The person views himself as socially inept, personally unappealing, or inferior to others.

■ The person is unusually reluctant to take personal risks or to engage in any new activities because they may prove embarrassing.

Borderline personality disorder

This pervasive pattern of instability of interpersonal relationships, self-image and affect, and marked impulsivity, beginning by early adulthood and present in various contexts, is indicated by at least five of the following features:

■ The person makes frantic efforts to avoid real or imagined abandonment (excluding suicidal or self-mutilating behavior).

■ The person has a pattern of unstable and intense interpersonal relationships characterized by alternating extremes of overidealization and devaluation.

■ The person has an identity disturbance characterized by a markedly and persistently unstable self-image or sense of self.

■ The person shows impulsiveness in at least two areas that are potentially self-

(continued)

DIAGNOSING PERSONALITY DISORDERS *(continued)*

damaging, such as spending, sexual activity, substance abuse, shoplifting, reckless driving, and binge eating (excluding suicidal or self-mutilating behavior).
- The person engages in recurrent suicidal threats, gestures, or behavior or in self-mutilating behavior.
- The person has affective instability resulting from marked mood reactivity (for example, depression, irritability, or anxiety, lasting usually a few hours and seldom more than a few days).
- The person has chronic feelings of emptiness or boredom.
- The person has inappropriate intense anger or difficulty controlling anger.
- The person has transient, stress-related paranoid ideation or severe dissociative symptoms.

Dependent personality disorder
This pervasive and excessive need to be taken care of that leads to submissive and clinging behavior and fears of separation, beginning by early adulthood and present in several contexts, is indicated by at least five of the following:
- The person has difficulty making everyday decisions without an excessive amount of advice or reassurance from others.
- The person needs others to assume responsibility for most major areas of his life.
- The person has difficulty expressing disagreement with others because of fear of loss of support or approval (excluding realistic fears of retribution).
- The person has difficulty initiating projects or doing things on his own (because of a lack of self-confidence in his judgment or abilities rather than a lack of motivation or energy).
- The person goes to excessive lengths to obtain nurture and support from others, to the point of volunteering to do things that are unpleasant.

- The person feels uncomfortable or helpless when alone because of exaggerated fears of inability to care for himself.
- The person urgently seeks another relationship as a source of care and support when a close relationship ends.
- The person is unrealistically preoccupied with fears of being left to take care of himself.

Histrionic personality disorder
This pervasive pattern of excessive emotionality and attention-seeking behavior, beginning by early adulthood and present in various contexts, is indicated by at least five of the following:
- The person is uncomfortable in situations in which he isn't the center of attention.
- The person's interaction with others is commonly characterized by inappropriately sexually seductive or provocative behavior.
- The person displays rapidly shifting and shallow expression of emotions.
- The person consistently uses physical appearance to draw attention to self.
- The person has a style of speech that is excessively impressionistic and lacking in detail.
- The person shows self-dramatization, theatricality, and exaggerated emotional expression.
- The person is suggestible (easily influenced by others or circumstances).
- The person considers relationships to be more intimate than they actually are.

Narcissistic personality disorder
This pervasive pattern of grandiosity, need for admiration, and lack of empathy, beginning by early adulthood and present in various contexts, is indicated by at least five of the following:
- The person has a grandiose sense of self-importance.
- The person is preoccupied with fantasies of unlimited success, power, brilliance, beauty, or ideal love.

DIAGNOSING PERSONALITY DISORDERS *(continued)*

- The person believes that he's special and unique and can only be understood by, or should associate with, other special or high-status people (or institutions).
- The person requires excessive admiration.
- The person has a sense of entitlement (an unreasonable expectation of especially favorable treatment or automatic compliance with his expectations).
- The person is interpersonally exploitive, taking advantage of others to achieve his own ends.
- The person lacks empathy.
- The person is typically envious of others or believes that others are envious of him.
- The person shows arrogant, haughty behaviors or attitudes.

Obsessive-compulsive personality disorder
This pervasive pattern of preoccupation with orderliness, perfectionism, and mental and interpersonal control at the expense of flexibility, openness, and efficiency, beginning by early adulthood and present in various contexts, is indicated by at least four of the following:
- The person is preoccupied with details, rules, lists, order, organization, or schedules to the extent that the core point of the activity is lost.
- The person shows perfectionism that interferes with task completion.
- The person is excessively devoted to work and productivity to the exclusion of leisure activities and friendships (not accounted for by obvious economic need).
- The person exhibits overconscientiousness, scrupulousness, and inflexibility about matters of morality, ethics, or values (not accounted for by cultural or religious identification).

- The person can't discard worn-out or worthless objects even when they have no sentimental value.
- The person is reluctant to delegate tasks or to work with others unless they submit exactly to his way of doing things.
- The person adopts a miserly spending style toward self and others; money is viewed as something to be hoarded in preparation for future catastrophes.
- The person shows rigidity and stubbornness.

Paranoid personality disorder
- The person must exhibit a pervasive and unwarranted tendency, beginning by early adulthood and present in various contexts, to interpret the actions of people as deliberately demeaning or threatening, as indicated by at least four of the following:
  – The person suspects, without sufficient basis, that he's being exploited, deceived, or harmed by others.
  – The person questions without justification the loyalty or trustworthiness of friends or associates.
  – The person is reluctant to confide in others because of unwarranted fear that the information will be used against him.
  – The person finds hostile or evil meanings in benign remarks.
  – The person bears grudges or is unforgiving of insults or slights.
  – The person is easily slighted and quick to react with anger or to counterattack.
  – The person questions without justification the fidelity of a spouse or sexual partner.
- The symptoms don't occur exclusively during the course of schizophrenia or other psychotic disorders and aren't the direct physiologic effect of a general medical condition.

(continued)

DIAGNOSING PERSONALITY DISORDERS *(continued)*

Schizoid personality disorder
■ The patient must exhibit a pervasive pattern of indifference to social relationships and a restricted range of emotional experience and expression, beginning by early adulthood and present in various contexts, as indicated by at least four of the following:
– The person neither desires nor enjoys close relationships, including being part of a family.
– The person almost always chooses solitary activities.
– The person seldom, if ever, claims or appears to experience strong emotions, such as anger and joy.
– The person indicates little, if any, desire to have sexual experiences with another person.
– The person is indifferent to the praise and criticism of others.
– The person has no close friends or confidants other than immediate relatives.
– The person displays flat affect.
■ The symptoms don't occur exclusively during the course of schizophrenia, another psychotic disorder, or a pervasive developmental disorder and aren't the direct physiologic effect of a general medical condition.

Schizotypal personality disorder
■ This pervasive pattern of social and interpersonal deficits is marked by acute discomfort with, and reduced capacity for, close relationships as well as by cognitive or perceptual distortions and eccentricities of behavior, beginning by early adulthood and present in various contexts. The person with schizotypal personality disorder has at least five of the following:
– ideas of reference (excluding delusions of reference)
– odd beliefs or magical thinking, influencing behavior and inconsistent with subcultural norms
– unusual perceptual experiences, including bodily illusions
– odd thinking and speech
– suspiciousness or paranoid thinking
– inappropriate or flat affect
– odd behavior or appearance
– no close friends or confidants other than first-degree relatives
– excessive social anxiety that doesn't diminish with familiarity and tends to be associated with paranoid fears rather than negative self-judgment.
■ The symptoms don't occur exclusively during the course of schizophrenia, a mood disorder with psychotic features, another psychotic disorder, or a pervasive developmental disorder.

---

sessional thinking. Antianxiety drugs may be used to treat severe anxiety that interferes with normal thinking.

Hospital inpatient milieu therapy can be effective in crisis situations and possibly for long-term treatment of some disorders. Inpatient treatment is controversial, however, because most patients with personality disorders don't comply with extended therapeutic regimens; for such patients, outpatient therapy may be more helpful.

Special considerations
■ Provide consistent care. Take a direct, involved approach to ensure trust. Keep in mind that many of these patients don't respond well to interviews, whereas others are charming and convincing.
■ Teach the patient social skills, and reinforce appropriate behavior.
■ Encourage expression of feelings, self-analysis of behavior, and accountability for actions.

Specific care measures vary with the particular personality disorder.

For *antisocial personality disorder:*

- Be clear about your expectations and the consequences of failing to meet them.
- Use a straightforward, matter-of-fact approach to set limits on unacceptable behavior. Encourage and reinforce positive behavior.
- Expect the patient to refuse to cooperate so that he can gain control.
- Avoid power struggles and confrontations to maintain the opportunity for therapeutic communication.
- Avoid defensiveness and arguing.
- Observe for physical and verbal signs of agitation.
- Help the patient manage anger.
- Teach the patient social skills and reinforce appropriate behavior.

For *avoidant personality disorder:*

- Assess for signs of depression. Impaired social interaction increases the risk of affective disorders.
- Establish a trusting relationship with the patient. Be aware that he may become dependent on the few staff members whom he believes he can trust.
- Make sure that the patient has plenty of time to prepare for all upcoming procedures. This patient can't handle surprises well.
- Inform the patient when you will and won't be available if he needs assistance.

For *borderline personality disorder:*

- Encourage the patient to take responsibility for himself. Don't attempt to rescue him from the consequences of his actions (except for suicidal and self-mutilating behaviors).
- Don't try to solve problems that the patient can solve himself.
- Maintain a consistent approach in all interactions with the patient, and ensure that other staff members do so as well.
- Recognize behaviors that the patient uses to manipulate people so that you can avoid unconsciously reinforcing them.
- Set appropriate expectations for social interactions, and praise the patient when expectations are met.
- To promote trust, respect the patient's personal space.
- Recognize that the patient may idolize some staff members and devalue others.

- Don't take sides in the patient's disputes with other staff members.

For *dependent personality disorder:*

- Encourage the patient to make decisions. Continue to provide support and reassurance as his decision-making ability improves.
- Give the patient as much opportunity to control treatment as possible. Offer options and allow choice, even if all are chosen.
- Encourage activities that require decision-making to promote autonomy.

For *histrionic personality disorder:*

- Give the patient choices in care strategies, and incorporate his wishes into the plan of treatment as much as possible. By increasing his sense of self-control, you'll reduce his anxiety.
- Be aware that the patient will want to "win over" caregivers and, at least initially, will be responsive and cooperative.

For *narcissistic personality disorder:*

- Convey respect and acknowledge the patient's sense of self-importance so that a coherent sense of self can be reestablished. Don't reinforce either pathologic grandiosity or weakness.
- If the patient makes unreasonable demands or has unreasonable expectations, tell him in a matter-of-fact way that he's being unreasonable. Remain nonjudgmental because a critical attitude may make the patient more demanding and difficult. Don't avoid him as this could increase maladaptive attention-seeking behavior.
- Focus on positive traits, or on feelings of pain, loss, or rejection.

For *obsessive-compulsive personality disorder:*

- Allow the patient to participate in his own treatment plan by offering choices whenever possible.
- Adopt a professional approach in your interactions with the patient. Avoid informality; this patient expects strict attention to detail.

For *paranoid personality disorder:*

- Avoid situations that threaten the patient's autonomy or challenge his beliefs.
- Approach the patient in a straightforward and candid manner, adopting a professional, rather than a casual or friendly,

attitude. Remember that the paranoid patient easily misinterprets remarks intended to be humorous.

■ Encourage the patient to take part in social interactions to expose him to others' perceptions and realities and to promote social skills development.

■ Help the patient identify negative behaviors that interfere with his relationships so that he can see how his behavior affects others.

■ Provide a supportive and nonjudgmental environment in which the patient can safely explore and verbalize his feelings.

For *schizoid personality disorder:*
■ Remember that the schizoid patient needs close human contact but is easily overwhelmed. Respect the patient's need for privacy, and slowly build a trusting, therapeutic relationship, so that he finds more pleasure than fear in relating to you.

■ Give the patient plenty of time to express his feelings. Keep in mind that, if you push him to do so before he's ready, he may retreat.

■ Recognize the patient's need for physical and emotional distance.

■ Remember that the patient needs close human contact but is easily overwhelmed.

For *schizotypal personality disorder:*
■ Recognize that the patient with this disorder is easily overwhelmed by stress. Allow him plenty of time to make difficult decisions.

■ Avoid defensiveness and arguing.

■ Recognize the patient's need for physical and emotional distance.

■ Be aware that the patient may relate unusually well to certain staff members and not at all to others.

EATING DISORDERS

Bulimia nervosa

The essential features of bulimia nervosa include eating binges followed by feelings of guilt, humiliation, and self-deprecation. These feelings cause the patient to engage in self-induced vomiting, use laxatives or diuretics, follow a strict diet, or fast to overcome the effects of the binges. Unless the patient spends an excessive amount of time bingeing and purging, bulimia nervosa seldom is incapacitating. However, electrolyte imbalances (metabolic alkalosis, hypochloremia, and hypokalemia) and dehydration can occur, increasing the risk of physical complications.

Causes and incidence
The cause of bulimia is unknown, but psychosocial factors may contribute to its development. These factors include family disturbance or conflict, sexual abuse, maladaptive learned behavior, struggle for control or self-identity, cultural overemphasis on physical appearance, and parental obesity. Bulimia nervosa is associated with depression, anxiety, phobias, and obsessive-compulsive disorder.

Eating disorders are most prevalent in affluent cultural groups and are essentially unknown in cultural groups where poverty and malnutrition are prevalent. In developing countries, almost no cases of eating disorders have been recognized.

Bulimia nervosa usually begins in adolescence or early adulthood and can occur simultaneously with anorexia nervosa. It affects nine women for every man. Nearly 2% of adult women meet the diagnostic criteria for bulimia nervosa; 5% to 15% have some symptoms of the disorder.

Signs and symptoms
The history of a patient with bulimia nervosa is characterized by episodes of binge eating that may occur up to several times per day. The patient commonly reports a binge-eating episode during which she continues eating until abdominal pain, sleep, or the presence of another person interrupts it. The preferred food is usually sweet, soft, and high in calories and carbohydrate content.

The patient with bulimia may appear thin and emaciated. Typically, however, although her weight frequently fluctuates, it usually stays within normal limits — through the use of diuretics, laxatives, vomiting, and exercise. So, unlike the patient with anorexia, the patient with bulimia can usually hide her eating disorder.

Overt clues to this disorder include hyperactivity, peculiar eating habits or rituals, frequent weighing, and a distorted body image. (See *Characteristics of patients with bulimia*.)

The patient may complain of abdominal and epigastric pain caused by acute gastric dilation. She may also have amenorrhea. Repetitive vomiting may cause painless swelling of the salivary glands, hoarseness, throat irritation or lacerations, and dental erosion. The patient may also exhibit calluses on the knuckles or abrasions and scars on the dorsum of the hand, resulting from tooth injury during self-induced vomiting, although it's common for the patient with bulimia to induce vomiting chemically such as with ipecac.

A patient with bulimia commonly is perceived by others as a "perfect" student, mother, or career woman; an adolescent may be distinguished for participation in competitive activities such as sports. However, the patient's psychosocial history may reveal an exaggerated sense of guilt, symptoms of depression, childhood trauma (especially sexual abuse), parental obesity, or a history of unsatisfactory sexual relationships.

CHARACTERISTICS OF PATIENTS WITH BULIMIA

Recognizing patients with bulimia isn't always easy. Unlike patients with anorexia, patients with bulimia don't deny that their eating habits are abnormal, but they commonly conceal their behavior out of shame. If you suspect bulimia nervosa, watch for these features:

- difficulty with impulse control
- chronic depression
- exaggerated sense of guilt
- low tolerance for frustration
- recurrent anxiety
- feelings of alienation
- self-consciousness
- difficulty expressing feelings such as anger
- impaired social or occupational adjustment.

Diagnosis

For characteristic findings in this condition, see *Diagnosing bulimia nervosa*, page 492.

Additional diagnostic tools include the Beck Depression Inventory, which may identify coexisting depression, and laboratory tests to help determine the presence and severity of complications. Serum electrolyte studies may show elevated bicarbonate, decreased potassium, and decreased sodium levels.

A baseline electrocardiogram may be done if tricyclic antidepressants will be prescribed for the patient.

Treatment

Treatment of bulimia nervosa may continue for several years. Interrelated physical and psychological symptoms must be treated simultaneously. Merely promoting weight gain isn't sufficient to guarantee long-term recovery. A patient whose physical status is severely compromised by inadequate or chaotic eating patterns is difficult to engage in the psychotherapeutic process.

Psychotherapy concentrates on interrupting the binge-purge cycle and helping the patient regain control over her eating behavior. Inpatient or outpatient treatment includes behavior modification therapy, which may take place in highly structured psychoeducational group meetings. Cognitive behavioral therapy, group therapy, and family therapy, which address the eating disorder as a symptom of unresolved conflict, may help the patient understand the basis of her behavior and teach her self-control strategies. Antidepressant drugs may be used as an adjunct to psychotherapy.

The patient may also benefit from participation in self-help groups, such as Overeaters Anonymous, or in a drug rehabilitation program if she has a concurrent substance abuse problem.

Special considerations

- Supervise the patient during mealtimes and for a specified period after meals (usually 1 hour). Set a time limit for each meal.

DIAGNOSING BULIMIA NERVOSA

The diagnosis of bulimia is made when the patient meets criteria put forth in the *Diagnostic and Statistical Manual of Mental Disorders,* Fourth Edition, Text Revision. Both of the behaviors listed below must occur at least twice per week for 3 months:

- recurrent episodes of binge eating (rapid consumption of a large amount of food in a discrete period and a feeling of lack of control over eating behavior during the eating binges)
- recurrent inappropriate compensatory behavior to prevent weight gain (self-induced vomiting; misuse of laxatives, diuretics, enemas, or other medications; fasting; excessive exercise).

Provide a pleasant, relaxed environment for eating.
- Use behavior modification techniques, and reward the patient for satisfactory weight gain.
- Establish a contract with the patient, specifying the amount and type of food to be eaten at each meal.
- Encourage her to recognize and express her feelings about her eating behavior. Maintain an accepting and nonjudgmental attitude, controlling your reactions to her behavior and feelings.
- Encourage the patient to talk about stressful issues, such as achievement, independence, socialization, sexuality, family problems, and control.
- Identify the patient's elimination patterns.
- Assess her suicide potential.
- Refer the patient and her family to the American Anorexia and Bulimia Association and to Anorexia Nervosa and Related Eating Disorders for additional information and support.

- Teach the patient how to keep a food journal to monitor treatment progress.
- Outline the risks of laxative, emetic, and diuretic abuse for the patient.
- Provide assertiveness training to help the patient gain control over her behavior and achieve a realistic and positive self-image.
- If the patient is taking a prescribed tricyclic antidepressant, instruct her to take the drug with food. Warn her to avoid consuming alcoholic beverages; exposing herself to sunlight, heat lamps, or tanning salons; and discontinuing the medication unless she has notified the physician.

Anorexia nervosa

The key feature of anorexia nervosa is self-imposed starvation, resulting from a distorted body image and an intense, irrational fear of gaining weight, even when the patient is obviously emaciated. A patient with anorexia is preoccupied with her body size, describes herself as "fat," and commonly expresses dissatisfaction with a particular aspect of her physical appearance. Although the term *anorexia* suggests that the patient's weight loss is associated with a loss of appetite, this is rare. Anorexia nervosa and bulimia nervosa can occur simultaneously. In anorexia nervosa, the refusal to eat may be accompanied by compulsive exercising, self-induced vomiting, or laxative or diuretic abuse.

Causes and incidence

No causes of anorexia nervosa have been identified; however, genetic, social, and psychological factors have been implicated. Researchers in neuroendocrinology are seeking a physiologic cause, but have found nothing definite. Clearly, social attitudes that equate slimness with beauty play some role in provoking this disorder; family factors are also implicated. Most theorists believe that refusing to eat is a subconscious effort to exert personal control over one's life. Anorexia nervosa has been associated with other psychiatric disorders, such as obsessive-compulsive disorder, depression, and anxiety.

Anorexia occurs in 5% to 10% of the population; about 95% of those affected

COMPLICATIONS OF ANOREXIA NERVOSA

Serious medical complications can result from the malnutrition, dehydration, and electrolyte imbalances caused by prolonged starvation, frequent vomiting, or laxative abuse that's typical in anorexia nervosa.

Malnutrition and related problems
Malnutrition may cause hypoalbuminemia and subsequent edema or hypokalemia, leading to ventricular arrhythmias and renal failure.

Poor nutrition and dehydration, coupled with laxative abuse, produce changes in the bowel similar to those in chronic inflammatory bowel disease.

Frequent vomiting can cause esophageal erosion, ulcers, tears, and bleeding as well as tooth and gum erosion and dental caries.

Cardiovascular consequences
Cardiovascular complications, which can be life-threatening, include decreased left ventricular muscle mass, chamber size, and myocardial oxygen uptake; reduced cardiac output; hypotension; bradycardia; electrocardiographic changes, such as a nonspecific ST interval, T-wave changes, and a prolonged PR interval; heart failure; and sudden death, possibly caused by ventricular arrhythmias.

Infection and amenorrhea
Anorexia nervosa may increase the patient's susceptibility to infection.

In addition, amenorrhea, which may occur when the patient loses about 25% of her normal body weight, usually is associated with anemia. Possible complications of prolonged amenorrhea include estrogen deficiency (increasing the risk of calcium deficiency and osteoporosis) and infertility. Menses usually returns to normal when the patient weighs at least 95% of her normal weight.

---

are women. This disorder occurs primarily in adolescents and young adults but may also affect older women. The occurrence among males is rising. The prognosis varies but improves if the patient is diagnosed early or if she wants to overcome the disorder and seeks help voluntarily. Mortality ranges from 5% to 15% — the highest mortality associated with a psychiatric disturbance. One-third of these deaths can be attributed to suicide.

Signs and symptoms
The patient's history usually reveals a 25% or greater weight loss for no organic reason, coupled with a morbid dread of being fat and a compulsion to be thin. Such a patient tends to be angry and ritualistic. She may report amenorrhea, infertility, loss of libido, fatigue, sleep alterations, intolerance to cold, and constipation.

Hypotension and bradycardia may be present. Inspection may reveal an emaciated appearance, with skeletal muscle atrophy, loss of fatty tissue, atrophy of breast tissue, blotchy or sallow skin, lanugo on the face and body, and dryness or loss of scalp hair. If also bulimic, calluses on the knuckles, and abrasions and scars on the dorsum of the hand may result from tooth injury during self-induced vomiting. Other signs of vomiting include dental caries and oral or pharyngeal abrasions. (See *Complications of anorexia nervosa.*)

Palpation may disclose painless salivary gland enlargement and bowel distention. Slowed reflexes may occur on percussion. Oddly, the patient usually demonstrates hyperactivity and vigor (despite malnourishment). She may exercise avidly without apparent fatigue.

During psychosocial assessment, the patient with anorexia may express a morbid fear of gaining weight and an obsession with her physical appearance. Paradoxically, she may also be obsessed with food,

DIAGNOSING ANOREXIA NERVOSA

A diagnosis of anorexia nervosa is made when the patient meets the following criteria put forth in the *Diagnostic and Statistical Manual of Mental Disorders*, Fourth Edition, Text Revision:

- The patient refuses to maintain body weight over a minimal normal weight for age and height (for instance, weight loss leading to maintenance of body weight 15% below that expected) or failure to achieve expected weight gain during a growth period, leading to body weight 15% below that expected.
- The patient experiences intense fear of gaining weight or becoming fat, despite her underweight status.
- The patient has a distorted perception of body weight, size, or shape (that is, the person claims to feel fat even when emaciated or believes that one body area is too fat even when it's obviously underweight).
- In women, absence of at least three consecutive menstrual cycles when otherwise expected to occur.

sorption syndrome; and other disorders that cause physical wasting.

Abnormal findings that may accompany a weight loss exceeding 30% of normal body weight include:

- low hemoglobin level, platelet count, and white blood cell count
- prolonged bleeding time due to thrombocytopenia
- decreased erythrocyte sedimentation rate
- decreased levels of serum creatinine, blood urea nitrogen, uric acid, cholesterol, total protein, albumin, sodium, potassium, chloride, calcium, and fasting blood glucose (resulting from malnutrition)
- elevated levels of alanine aminotransferase and aspartate aminotransferase in severe starvation states
- elevated serum amylase levels when pancreatitis isn't present
- in females, decreased levels of serum luteinizing hormone and follicle-stimulating hormone
- decreased triiodothyronine levels resulting from a lower basal metabolic rate
- dilute urine caused by the kidneys' impaired ability to concentrate urine
- nonspecific ST interval, prolonged PR interval, and T-wave changes on the electrocardiogram. Ventricular arrhythmias may also be present.

Treatment

Appropriate treatment aims to promote weight gain or control the patient's compulsive binge eating and purging. Malnutrition and the underlying psychological dysfunction must be corrected. Hospitalization in a medical or psychiatric unit may be required to improve the patient's precarious physical condition. The hospital stay may be as brief as 2 weeks or may stretch from a few months to 2 years or longer.

A team approach to care — combining aggressive medical management, nutritional counseling, and individual, group, or family psychotherapy or behavior modification therapy — is most effective in treating anorexia. Treatment results may be discouraging. Many clinical centers are now developing inpatient and outpatient pro-

preparing elaborate meals for others. Social regression, including poor sexual adjustment and fear of failure, is common. Like bulimia nervosa, anorexia nervosa is commonly associated with depression. The patient may report feelings of despair, hopelessness, and worthlessness as well as suicidal thoughts.

Diagnosis

For characteristic findings in patients with this condition, see *Diagnosing anorexia nervosa*.

Laboratory tests help to identify various disorders and deficiencies and help to rule out endocrine, metabolic, and central nervous system abnormalities; cancer; malab-

grams specifically aimed at managing eating disorders.

Treatment may include behavior modification (privileges depend on weight gain); curtailed activity for physical reasons (such as arrhythmias); vitamin and mineral supplements; a reasonable diet with or without liquid supplements; subclavian, peripheral, or enteral hyperalimentation (enteral and peripheral routes carry less risk of infection); and group, family, or individual psychotherapy.

All forms of psychotherapy, from psychoanalysis to hypnotherapy, have been used in treating anorexia nervosa, with varying success. To be successful, psychotherapy should address the underlying problems of low self-esteem, guilt, anxiety, feelings of hopelessness and helplessness, and depression.

Special considerations

- During hospitalization, regularly monitor the patient's vital signs, nutritional status, and intake and output. Weigh the patient daily — before breakfast if possible. Because she fears being weighed, vary the weighing routine. Keep in mind that weight should increase from morning to night.
- Help the patient establish a target weight and support her efforts to achieve this goal.
- Negotiate an adequate food intake with the patient. Make sure she understands that she'll need to comply with this contract or lose privileges. Frequently offer small portions of food or drinks if the patient wants them. Allow the patient to maintain control over the types and amounts of food she eats, if possible.
- Maintain one-on-one supervision of the patient during meals and for 1 hour afterward to ensure compliance with the dietary treatment program. For the hospitalized patient with anorexia, food is considered a medication.
- During an acute anorexic episode, nutritionally complete liquids are more acceptable than solid food because they eliminate the need to choose between foods — something the patient with anorexia may find difficult. If tube feedings or other special feeding measures become necessary, fully explain these measures to the patient and

be ready to discuss her fears or reluctance; limit the discussion about food itself.
- Expect a weight gain of about 1 lb (0.5 kg) per week.
- If edema or bloating occurs after the patient has returned to normal eating behavior, reassure her that this phenomenon is temporary. She may fear that she's becoming fat and stop complying with the plan of treatment.
- Encourage the patient to recognize and express her feelings freely. If she understands that she can be assertive, she may gradually learn that expressing her true feelings won't result in her losing control or love.
- If a patient receiving outpatient treatment must be hospitalized, maintain contact with her treatment team to facilitate a smooth return to the outpatient setting.
- Remember that the patient with anorexia uses exercise, preoccupation with food, ritualism, manipulation, and lying as mechanisms to preserve the only control she thinks that she has in her life.
- Because the patient and her family may need therapy to uncover and correct dysfunctional patterns, refer them to Anorexia Nervosa and Related Eating Disorders, a national information and support organization. This organization may help them understand what anorexia is, convince them that they need help, and help them find a psychotherapist or physician who's experienced in treating this disorder.
- Teach the patient how to keep a food journal, including the types of food eaten, eating frequency, and feelings associated with eating and exercise.
- Advise family members to avoid discussing food with the patient.

SEXUAL AND GENDER IDENTITY DISORDERS

Female arousal and orgasmic disorders

Arousal disorder is an inability to experience sexual pleasure. According to the *Di-*

agnostic and Statistical Manual of Mental Disorders, Fourth Edition, Text Revision (*DSM-IV-TR*), the essential feature is a persistent or recurrent inability to attain, or to maintain until completion of the sexual activity, an adequate lubrication-swelling response of sexual excitement. Orgasmic disorder, according to *DSM-IV-TR,* is a persistent or recurrent delay in or absence of orgasm after a normal sexual excitement phase.

Arousal and orgasmic disorders are considered primary if they exist in a female who has never experienced sexual arousal or orgasm; they're secondary when some physical, mental, or situational condition has inhibited or obliterated a previously normal sexual function. The prognosis is good for temporary or mild disorders resulting from misinformation or situational stress but is guarded for disorders that result from intense anxiety, chronically discordant relationships, psychological disturbances, or drug or alcohol abuse in either partner.

Causes
Any of these factors, alone or in combination, may cause arousal or orgasmic disorder:
- certain drugs, including central nervous system depressants, alcohol, street drugs and, rarely, hormonal contraceptives
- general systemic illnesses, diseases of the endocrine or nervous system, or diseases that impair muscle tone or contractility
- gynecologic factors, such as chronic vaginal or pelvic infection or pain, congenital anomalies, and genital cancers
- stress and fatigue
- inadequate or ineffective stimulation
- psychological factors, such as performance anxiety, guilt, depression, or unconscious conflicts about sexuality
- relationship problems, such as poor communication, hostility or ambivalence toward the partner, fear of abandonment or of independence, or boredom with sex.

All these factors may contribute to involuntary inhibition of the orgasmic reflex. Another crucial factor is the fear of losing control of feelings or behavior. Whether or not these factors produce sexual dysfunction and the type of dysfunction depend

on how well the woman copes with the resulting pressures. Physical factors may also cause arousal or orgasmic disorder.

 ELDER TIP *Female sexual function and responses decline along with estrogen levels in the perimenopausal period. The decrease in estradiol levels during menopause affects nerve transmission and response in the peripheral vascular system. As a result, the timing and degree of vasoconstriction during the sexual response is affected, vasocongestion decreases, muscle tension decreases, and contractions are fewer and less intense during orgasm.*

Signs and symptoms
The female with arousal disorder has limited or absent sexual desire and experiences little or no pleasure from sexual stimulation. Physical signs of this disorder include lack of vaginal lubrication or absence of signs of genital vasocongestion.

Females with orgasmic disorder report an inability to achieve orgasm, either totally or under certain circumstances. Many females experience orgasm through masturbation or other means but not through intercourse alone. Others achieve orgasm with some partners but not with others.

Diagnosis
A thorough physical examination, laboratory tests, and a medical history rule out physical causes of arousal or orgasmic disorder. In the absence of such causes, a complete psychosexual history is the most important tool for assessment. Such a history should include:
- detailed information concerning the patient's level of sex education and previous sexual response patterns
- level of family stress or fatigue
- the patient's feelings during childhood and adolescence about sex in general and, specifically, about masturbation, incest, rape, sexual fantasies, and homosexual or heterosexual practices
- contraceptive practices and reproductive goals
- the patient's present relationship, including her partner's attitude toward sex
- assessment of the patient's self-esteem and body image
- a history of psychotherapy.

When the disorder causes marked distress or interpersonal difficulty, it may fulfill the diagnostic criteria for a *DSM-IV-TR* diagnosis.

Treatment

Arousal disorder is difficult to treat, especially if the female has never experienced sexual pleasure. Therapy is designed to help the patient relax and become aware of her feelings about sex and to eliminate guilt and fear of rejection. Specific measures usually include sensate focus exercises similar to those developed by Masters and Johnson, which emphasize touching and awareness of sensual feelings all over the body — not just genital sensations — and minimize the importance of intercourse and orgasm. Psychoanalytic treatment consists of free association, dream analysis, and discussion of life patterns to achieve greater sexual awareness. One behavioral approach attempts to correct maladaptive patterns through systematic desensitization to situations that provoke anxiety, partially by encouraging the patient to fantasize about these situations.

The goal in treating orgasmic disorder is to decrease or eliminate involuntary inhibition of the orgasmic reflex. Treatment may include experiential therapy, psychoanalysis, or behavior modification.

Treatment of primary orgasmic disorder may involve teaching the patient self-stimulation. Also, the therapist may teach distraction techniques, such as focusing attention on fantasies, breathing patterns, or muscle contractions to relieve anxiety. The patient learns new behavior through exercises she does privately between sessions. Gradually, the therapist involves the patient's sexual partner in the treatment sessions; some therapists treat the couple as a unit from the outset.

Treatment of secondary orgasmic disorder is designed to decrease anxiety and promote the factors necessary for the patient to experience orgasm. Sensate focus exercises are commonly used. The therapist should communicate an accepting attitude and help the patient understand that satisfactory sexual experiences don't always require coital orgasm.

Special considerations

- Be alert for clues to arousal or orgasmic disorder when taking a health history.
- Maintain an open, nonjudgmental attitude toward the patient and her problem.
- Instruct the patient in anatomy and physiology of the reproductive system and in sexual response patterns.
- Refer the patient to a physician, nurse, psychologist, social worker, or counselor trained in sex therapy. Inform the patient that the therapist's certification by the American Association of Sex Educators, Counselors, and Therapists or by the Society for Sex Therapy and Research usually ensures quality treatment.
- If the therapist isn't certified by these organizations, advise the patient to ask about the therapist's credentials.

Dyspareunia

Dyspareunia is genital pain associated with intercourse. It may be mild, or it may be severe enough to affect enjoyment of intercourse. Dyspareunia is commonly associated with physical problems; less commonly, with a psychological disorder. The prognosis is good if the underlying disorder can be treated successfully.

Causes

Physical causes of dyspareunia include an intact hymen; deformities or lesions of the introitus or vagina; marked retroversion of the uterus; genital, rectal, or pelvic scar tissue; acute or chronic infections of the genitourinary tract; and disorders of the surrounding viscera (including residual effects of pelvic inflammatory disease or disease of the adnexal and broad ligaments).

Among the many other possible physical causes are:

- endometriosis
- benign and malignant growths and tumors
- insufficient lubrication
- radiation to the area
- allergic reactions to diaphragms, condoms, or other contraceptives.

Psychological causes include fear of pain or of injury during intercourse, recollection of a previous painful experience, guilty feelings about sex, fear of pregnancy or of injury to the fetus during pregnancy, anxiety caused by a new sexual partner or technique, and mental or physical fatigue. Men and women can suffer pain in the pelvic area during or soon after sexual intercourse.

Signs and symptoms

Dyspareunia produces discomfort, ranging from mild aches to severe pain before, during, or after intercourse. It may also be associated with vaginal itching or burning.

Diagnosis

Physical examination and laboratory tests help determine the underlying disorder. Diagnosis also depends on a detailed sexual history and the answers to such questions as: When does the pain occur? Does it occur with certain positions or techniques or at certain times during the sexual response cycle? Where does the pain occur? What's its quality, frequency, and duration? What factors relieve or aggravate it?

When the disorder causes marked distress or interpersonal difficulty, it may fulfill the diagnostic criteria from the *Diagnostic and Statistical Manual of Mental Disorders,* Fourth Edition, Text Revision.

Treatment

Treatment of physical causes may include creams and water-soluble gels for inadequate lubrication, appropriate medications for infections, excision of hymenal scars, and gentle stretching of painful scars at the vaginal opening. The patient may be advised to change her coital position to reduce pain on deep penetration.

Methods of treating psychologically based dyspareunia vary with the particular patient. Sensate focus exercises deemphasize intercourse itself and teach appropriate foreplay techniques. Education about contraception methods can reduce fear of pregnancy; education about sexual activity during pregnancy can relieve fear of harming the fetus.

Special considerations

■ Provide instruction concerning anatomy and physiology of the reproductive system, contraception, and the human sexual response cycle.

■ When appropriate, provide advice and information on drugs that may affect the patient sexually and on lubricating gels and creams.

■ Listen to the patient's complaints of sex-related pain, and maintain a sympathetic, nonjudgmental attitude toward her, which will encourage her to express her feelings without embarrassment.

Vaginismus

Vaginismus is involuntary spastic constriction of the outer third vaginal muscles. This disorder may coexist with dyspareunia and, if severe, may prevent intercourse (a common cause of unconsummated marriages). Vaginismus affects females of all ages and backgrounds. The prognosis is excellent for a motivated patient who doesn't have untreatable organic abnormalities.

Causes and incidence

Vaginismus may be physical or psychological in origin. It may occur spontaneously as a protective reflex to pain or result from organic causes, such as hymenal abnormalities, genital herpes, obstetric trauma, and atrophic vaginitis.

Psychological causes may include:
■ childhood and adolescent exposure to rigid, punitive, and guilt-ridden attitudes toward sex
■ fears resulting from painful or traumatic sexual experiences, such as incest or rape
■ early traumatic experience with pelvic examinations
■ fear of pregnancy, sexually transmitted disease, or cancer.

Vaginismus is uncommon, affecting less than 2% of women in the United States.

Signs and symptoms

The female with vaginismus typically experiences muscle spasm with constriction and pain on insertion of any object into the vagina, such as a tampon, diaphragm, or speculum. She may profess a lack of sexual interest or a normal level of sexual desire.

Diagnosis

Diagnosis depends on the sexual history and pelvic examination to rule out physical disorders. The sexual history must include early childhood experiences and family attitudes toward sex, previous and current sexual responses, contraceptive practices and reproductive goals, feelings about her sexual partner, and specific details about pain on insertion of any object into the vagina.

 CONFIRMING DIAGNOSIS *A carefully performed pelvic examination confirms the diagnosis by showing involuntary constriction of the musculature surrounding the outer portion of the vagina.*

When the disorder causes marked distress or interpersonal difficulty, it may fulfill diagnostic criteria from the *Diagnostic and Statistical Manual of Mental Disorders,* Fourth Edition, Text Revision.

Treatment

Treatment is designed to eliminate maladaptive muscle constriction and underlying psychological problems. In Masters and Johnson therapy, the patient uses a graduated series of dilators, which she inserts into her vagina while tensing and relaxing her pelvic muscles. The patient controls the amount of time that the dilator is left in place and the movement of the dilator. Together with her sexual partner, she begins sensate focus and counseling therapy to increase sexual responsiveness, improve communication skills, and resolve any underlying conflicts.

Kaplan therapy also uses progressive insertion of dilators or fingers (in vivo or desensitization therapy), with behavior therapy (imagining vaginal penetration until it can be tolerated) and, if necessary, psychoanalysis and hypnosis. Practitioners of both therapies claim a 100% cure rate.

Special considerations

■ Because a pelvic examination may be painful for the patient with vaginismus, proceed gradually, at the patient's own pace. Support her throughout the pelvic examination, explaining each step before it's done. Encourage her to verbalize her feelings, and take plenty of time to answer her questions.

■ Teach the patient about the anatomy and physiology of the reproductive system, contraception, and human sexual response. This can be done quite naturally during the pelvic examination.

■ Ask if the patient is taking medications that may affect her sexual response, such as antihypertensives, tranquilizers, or steroids. If she has insufficient lubrication for intercourse, tell her about lubricating gels and creams.

Erectile disorder

Erectile disorder, or impotence, refers to a male's inability to attain or maintain penile erection sufficient to complete intercourse. The patient with primary impotence has never achieved a sufficient erection; secondary impotence, which is more common and less serious than the primary form, implies that, despite present inability, the patient has succeeded in completing intercourse in the past.

Transient periods of impotence aren't considered dysfunction and probably occur in half of adult males. Erectile disorder affects all age-groups but increases in frequency with age. The prognosis depends on the severity and duration of impotence and the underlying cause.

Causes and incidence

Statistics indicate an organic basis for erectile dysfunction in 20% to 50% of men who have this disorder. In some patients, psychogenic and organic factors coexist, making isolation of the primary cause difficult.

Psychogenic causes may be intrapersonal, reflecting personal sexual anxieties, or interpersonal, reflecting a disturbed sexual relationship. Intrapersonal factors generally involve guilt, fear, depression, or feelings of inadequacy resulting from previous traumatic sexual experience, rejection by parents or peers, exaggerated religious orthodoxy, abnormal mother-son intimacy, or homosexual experiences. Interpersonal factors may stem from differences in sexual preferences between partners, lack of communication, insufficient knowledge of sexual function, or nonsexual personal conflicts. Situational impotence, a temporary condition, may develop in response to stress, as in performance anxiety.

Organic causes may include chronic diseases, such as cardiopulmonary disease, diabetes, multiple sclerosis, or renal failure; spinal cord trauma; complications of surgery; drug- or alcohol-induced dysfunction; and, rarely, genital anomalies or central nervous system defects.

Erection problems are common in adult men, with almost all men experiencing occasional difficulty getting or maintaining an erection.

Signs and symptoms

Secondary erectile disorder is classified as follows:

- *Partial*—The patient is unable to achieve a full erection.
- *Intermittent*—The patient is sometimes potent with the same partner.
- *Selective*—The patient is potent only with certain females.

Some men lose erectile function suddenly; others lose it gradually. If the cause isn't organic, erection may still be achieved through masturbation.

Patients with psychogenic impotence may appear anxious, with sweating and palpitations, or may lose interest in sexual activity. Patients with psychogenic or drug-induced impotence may suffer severe depression, which may cause the impotence or result from it.

Diagnosis

A detailed sexual history helps differentiate between organic and psychogenic factors and between primary and secondary impotence. Questions should include: Does the patient have intermittent, selective, nocturnal, or early-morning erections? Can he achieve erections through other sexual activity? When did his dysfunction begin, and what was his life situation at that time? Did erectile problems occur suddenly or gradually? Is he taking large quantities of prescription or nonprescription drugs?

Diagnosis must rule out chronic diseases, such as diabetes and other vascular, neurologic, or urogenital problems.

When the disorder causes marked distress or interpersonal difficulty, it may fulfill diagnostic criteria from the *Diagnostic and Statistical Manual of Mental Disorders,* Fourth Edition, Text Revision.

Procedures used to differentiate between organic and nonorganic causes of erectile disorder include noninvasive tests, such as monitoring nocturnal penile tumescence, blood pressure measurements in the penis with a Doppler ultrasound, and measuring pudendal nerve latency. Laboratory tests include glucose tolerance tests, plasma hormone assays, liver and thyroid function tests, and prolactin and follicle stimulating hormone levels. Invasive diagnostic studies include penile arteriography and dynamic infusion cavernosonography.

Treatment

Sex therapy, which should include both partners, may effectively cure psychogenic impotence. The course and content of such therapy depend on the specific cause of the dysfunction and the nature of the male-female relationship. Usually, therapy includes sensate focus exercises, which restrict the couple's sexual activity and encourage them to become more attuned to the physical sensations of touching. Sex therapy also includes improving verbal communication skills, eliminating unreasonable guilt, and reevaluating attitudes toward sex and sexual roles.

Treatment of organic impotence focuses on reversing the cause if possible. If not, psychological counseling may help the couple deal realistically with their situation and explore alternatives for sexual expression. Certain patients suffering from organic impotence may benefit from surgically inserted inflatable or noninflatable penile implants. Sildenafil, a recent drug treatment for erectile dysfunction, is also effective and is an alternative to surgery in many male patients.

Special considerations

- When you identify a patient with impotence or with a condition that may cause impotence, help him feel comfortable about discussing his sexuality. Assess his sexual health during your initial nursing history. When appropriate, refer him for further evaluation or treatment.

■ After penile implant surgery, instruct the patient to avoid intercourse until the incision heals, usually in 6 weeks.

To help prevent impotence:

■ Promote establishment of responsible health and sex education programs at primary, secondary, and college levels.

■ Provide information about resuming sexual activity as part of discharge instructions for patients with conditions that require modification of daily activities. Such patients include those with cardiac disease, diabetes, hypertension, and chronic obstructive pulmonary disease and all postoperative patients.

Premature ejaculation

Premature ejaculation refers to a male's inability to control the ejaculatory reflex during intravaginal containment, resulting in persistently early ejaculation. This common sexual disorder affects all age-groups; however, it's more common in younger males and in college-educated males.

Causes

Premature ejaculation may result from anxiety and is typically linked to immature sexual experiences. However, the true cause is undetermined. Other psychological factors may include anxiety or guilt regarding sexual intercourse, unconscious fears about the vagina, and negative cultural conditioning.

However, psychological factors aren't always the cause of premature ejaculation because this disorder can occur in emotionally healthy males with stable, positive relationships. Rarely, premature ejaculation may be linked to an underlying degenerative neurologic disorder, such as multiple sclerosis, or an inflammatory process, such as posterior urethritis or prostatitis.

Signs and symptoms

Premature ejaculation may have a devastating psychological impact on some males, who may exhibit signs of severe inadequacy or self-doubt in addition to general anxiety and guilt.

The patient may be unable to prolong foreplay, or he may have prolonged foreplay capacity but ejaculates as soon as intromission occurs. In other cases, however, premature ejaculation may have little or no psychological impact. In such cases, the complaint lies solely with the sexual partner, who may believe that the male is indifferent to her sexual needs.

Diagnosis

Physical examination and laboratory test results are usually normal because most males with this complaint are quite healthy. However, a detailed sexual history can aid immeasurably in diagnosis. A history of adequate ejaculatory control in the absence of precipitating psychological trauma should suggest an organic cause.

Treatment

Masters and Johnson have developed a highly successful, intensive program synthesizing insight therapy, behavioral techniques, and experiential sessions involving both sexual partners. The program is designed to help the patient focus on sensations of impending orgasm.

The therapy sessions, which continue for 2 weeks or longer, typically include:

■ mutual physical examination, which increases the couple's awareness of anatomy and physiology while reducing shameful feelings about sexual parts of the body

■ sensate focus exercises, which allow each partner to caress the other's body, without intercourse, and to focus on the pleasurable sensations of touch

■ Semans squeeze technique, which helps the patient gain control of ejaculatory tension by having the woman squeeze his penis, with her thumb on the frenulum and her forefinger and middle finger on the dorsal surface, near the coronal ridge. At the male's direction, she applies and releases pressure every few minutes during a touching exercise to delay ejaculation by keeping the male at an earlier phase of the sexual response cycle.

The stop-and-start technique helps delay ejaculation. With the female in the superior position, this method involves pelvic thrusting until orgasmic sensations start and then stopping and restarting to aid in control of ejaculation. Eventually, the couple is allowed to achieve orgasm.

Special considerations
■ Encourage a positive self-image by explaining that premature ejaculation is a common disorder that doesn't reflect on the patient's masculinity.
■ Assure the patient that the condition is reversible.
■ Refer the patient to appropriate resources for therapy.

Gender identity disorders

Sexual disorders that involve gender identity produce persistent feelings of gender discomfort and dissatisfaction. Gender identity is defined as the psychological state reflecting a sense of being male or female. It's based culturally on determined sets of attitude behavior patterns and other attributes usually associated with masculinity or femininity.

Gender identity disorders shouldn't be confused with the more common feelings of inadequacy in fulfilling the expectations normally associated with a particular sex.

Causes and incidence
Current theories about gender identity disorders and their causes suggest a combination of predisposing factors: chromosomal anomaly, hormonal imbalance (occurring particularly during brain formation in utero), and impaired early parent-child bonding and child-rearing practices.

Gender identity disorders, which are rare, may occur in children and adults.

Signs and symptoms
A gender identity disorder may emerge at an early age. A child may express the desire to be — or insist that he or she is — the opposite sex. For example, a male child may express disgust with his genitalia; a female child may wish to be a man when she grows up.

Men with a gender identity disorder may describe a lifelong history of feeling feminine and pursuing feminine activities.

Women report similar propensities for opposite-sex activities and discomfort with the female role. For both sexes, the crisis intensifies during puberty.

Diagnosis
For specific diagnostic criteria from the *Diagnostic and Statistical Manual of Mental Disorders,* Fourth Edition, Text Revision, see *Diagnosing gender identity disorders.*

Treatment
Individual and family therapy is indicated for childhood gender identity disorders. Individual and couples therapy may help adults cope.

Sex reassignment through hormonal and surgical treatment may be an option; however, it's a highly controversial measure that's undergoing much scrutiny. Severe psychological problems may persist after sex reassignment. Furthermore, the patient's gender disorder may be part of a larger depression and personality disorder pattern.

Appropriate psychiatric management, including hospitalization, may be necessary if the patient displays the potential for violent behavior, such as suicide or self-mutilation.

Special considerations
■ Adopt a nonjudgmental approach in facial expression, tone of voice, and choice of words to convey your acceptance of the person's choices.
■ Respect the patient's privacy and sense of modesty, particularly during procedures or examinations.
■ Monitor the patient for related or compounded problems, such as suicidal thought or intent, depression, and anxiety.
■ As needed, refer the patient to a physician, nurse, psychologist, social worker, or counselor trained in sex therapy.
■ As a helpful guideline, inform the patient that the therapist's certification by the American Association of Sex Educators, Counselors, and Therapists or by the Society for Sex Therapy and Research usually ensures quality treatment.

DIAGNOSING GENDER IDENTITY DISORDERS

The diagnosis of gender identity disorder is confirmed when the patient's symptoms meet the following criteria established in the *Diagnostic and Statistical Manual of Mental Disorders,* Fourth Edition, Text Revision:

■ A strong and persistent cross-gender identification (not merely a desire for any perceived cultural advantages of being the other sex).

In children, the disturbance is manifested by at least four of the following:
– repeatedly stated desire to be, or insistence that he or she is, the other sex
– in boys, preference for cross-dressing or simulating female attire; in girls, insistence on wearing only stereotypical masculine clothing
– strong and persistent preferences for cross-sex roles in make-believe play or persistent fantasies of being the other sex
– intense desire to participate in the stereotypical games and pastimes of the other sex
– strong preference for playmates of the other sex.

In adolescents and adults, the disturbance is manifested by such symptoms as a stated desire to be the other sex, frequent passing as the other sex, desire to live or be treated as the other sex, or the conviction that he or she has the typical feelings and reactions of the other sex.

■ Persistent discomfort with his or her sex or sense of inappropriateness in the gender role of that sex.

In children, the disturbance is manifested by any of the following:
– in boys, assertion that his penis or testes are disgusting or will disappear or he'd be better off not to have a penis, rejection of rough-and-tumble play, and rejection of male stereotypical toys, games, and activities
– in girls, rejection of urinating in a sitting position, assertion that she has or will grow a penis, or assertion that she doesn't want to grow breasts or menstruate, or marked aversion toward feminine clothing.

In adolescents and adults, the disturbance is manifested by such symptoms as preoccupation with getting rid of primary and secondary sex characteristics or the belief that he or she was born the wrong sex.

■ The disturbance isn't concurrent with a physical intersex condition.

■ The disturbance causes clinically significant distress or impairment in social, occupational, or other important areas of functioning.

Paraphilias

Characterized by a dependence on unusual behaviors or fantasies to achieve sexual excitement, paraphilias are complex psychosexual disorders. The *Diagnostic and Statistical Manual of Mental Disorders,* Fourth Edition, Text Revision (*DSM-IV-TR*), recognizes eight paraphilias. (See *Diagnosing paraphilias,* pages 504 and 505.) Some paraphilias are considered sex offenses or crimes because they violate social mores or norms. However, everyone has sexual fantasies, and sexual behavior between consenting adults that isn't physically or psychologically harmful isn't considered a paraphilia.

Causes

The cause of paraphilias is unknown, but multiple contributing factors have been identified. Abnormal hormonal values, neurologic disorders, chromosomal abnormalities, seizure disorders, and dyslexia have been identified as contributing factors. For example, many people with these disorders come from dysfunctional families characterized by isolation and sexual, emo-

DIAGNOSING PARAPHILIAS

The most commonly diagnosed paraphilias are exhibitionism, fetishism, frotteurism, pedophilia, sexual masochism, sexual sadism, transvestic fetishism, and voyeurism. Criteria for diagnosis are in the *Diagnostic and Statistical Manual of Mental Disorders*, Fourth Edition, Text Revision.

Exhibitionism

The person with this paraphilia obtains sexual gratification from publicly exposing his genitalia to others — principally female passersby. The problem occurs mostly in men (who may achieve erection while exposing themselves and may masturbate to orgasm at the time).

A diagnosed exhibitionist has had at least 6 months of recurrent, intense, sexually arousing fantasies, urges, or behaviors that involve exposing his genitalia to an unsuspecting stranger.

Fetishism

The term *fetish* describes a recurrent and intense sexual arousal from an inanimate object (usually clothing, such as panties or boots) or from nonsexual body parts. The person typically masturbates while holding, rubbing, or smelling the fetish object — or asks a sexual partner to wear the object during a sexual encounter. Fetishism is usually chronic and occurs primarily in men.

A diagnosed fetishist has had at least 6 months of recurrent, intense, sexually arousing fantasies, urges, or behaviors evoked by inanimate objects. The fetish objects aren't restricted to clothing used in cross-dressing or devices designed for tactile genital stimulation.

Frotteurism

The frotteur achieves sexual arousal by touching or rubbing a nonconsenting person. A male frotteur may rub his genitals against a woman's thigh or fondle her breasts. The behavior may occur in crowded places (for example, buses), where it's easier to avoid detection. It's most common between ages 15 and 25.

A diagnosed frotteur has had at least 6 months of recurrent, intense, sexually arousing fantasies, urges, or behaviors involving touching and rubbing against a nonconsenting person.

Pedophilia

The pedophile (almost always a man) is aroused by, and seeks sexual gratification from, children. This urge forms his preferred or exclusive sexual activity. Prepubescent children are common targets, and attraction to girls is more common than attraction to boys. The pedophile may sexually abuse his own children or those of a friend or relative. Rarely, he may abduct a child. Some pedophiles are also attracted to adults.

A diagnosed pedophile has had at least 6 months of recurrent, intense, sexually arousing fantasies, urges, or behaviors involving a prepubescent child or children (usually age 13 or younger). The pedophile is at least age 16 and at least 5 years older than the desired child. (This excludes a person in late adolescence engaged in an

---

tional, or physical abuse. Others suffer from personality or psychoactive substance use disorders.

Signs and symptoms

The patient's history will reveal the particular pattern of abnormal sexual behaviors associated with one of the eight recognized paraphilias.

Diagnosis

The standard diagnostic criteria for paraphilias, published in the *DSM-IV-TR*, include not only specific criteria for each

ongoing sexual relationship with a child of age 12 or 13.)

Sexual masochism

A sexual masochist achieves sexual gratification by submitting to physical or psychological pain, such as being beaten, tortured, or humiliated.

Infantilism, a form of sexual masochism, is a desire to be treated as a helpless infant, including wearing diapers. A dangerous form of this paraphilia, *sexual hypoxyphilia,* relies on oxygen deprivation to induce sexual arousal. The person uses a noose, mask, plastic bag, or chemical to temporarily reduce cerebral oxygenation. Equipment malfunction or other mistakes can cause accidental death.

A diagnosed sexual masochist has had at least 6 months of recurrent, intense, sexually arousing fantasies, urges, or behaviors involving the act (real, not simulated) of being beaten, humiliated, or otherwise made to suffer.

Sexual sadism

The converse of a sexual masochist, a sadist has recurrent, intense, sexual urges and fantasies that involve inflicting physical or psychological suffering. The sadist derives sexual gratification from this behavior.

A diagnosed sexual sadist has had at least 6 months of recurrent, intense, sexually arousing fantasies, urges, or behaviors involving acts (real, not simulated) that cause another person pain and suffering and that evoke sexual excitement in the sadist.

Transvestic fetishism

The transvestite is a heterosexual man who obtains sexual pleasure from cross-dressing (dressing in women's clothing). He may select a single article of apparel, such as a garter or bra, or he may dress entirely as a woman. This behavior is usually accompanied by masturbation and mental images of other men being attracted to him as a woman.

A diagnosed transvestic fetishist is a heterosexual male who has had at least 6 months of recurrent, intense, sexually arousing fantasies, urges, or behaviors involving cross-dressing.

Voyeurism

The voyeur derives sexual pleasure from looking at sexual objects or situations such as an unsuspecting couple engaged in sexual intercourse. Onset of this disorder, which tends to be chronic, occurs before age 15.

A diagnosed voyeur is a heterosexual male who has had at least 6 months of recurrent, intense, sexually arousing fantasies, urges, or behaviors involving the act of observing an unsuspecting person who's naked, disrobing, or engaging in sexual activity.

paraphilia but also general features. A paraphiliac has ongoing, intense, sexually arousing fantasies, urges, or behaviors involving various aberrant sexual expressions that cause clinically significant distress or impairment in social, occupational, or other important areas of functioning.

Treatment

Paraphilias require mandatory treatment when the patient's sexual preferences result in socially unacceptable, harmful, or criminal behavior. Depending on the paraphilia, treatment may include combinations of psychotherapy, behavior therapy, surgery, or pharmacotherapy. Currently, treatment with selective serotonin reuptake inhibitors is providing better results than previous treatment approaches.

Special considerations

- Use a nonjudgmental approach when dealing with the patient.
- Realize that treating such a patient with empathy doesn't threaten your own sexuality.
- Encourage the patient to express his sexual preferences as well as his feelings about them.
- As needed, refer the patient to a physician, nurse, psychologist, social worker, or counselor trained in sex therapy.
- As a helpful guideline, inform the patient that a therapist's certification by the American Association of Sex Educators, Counselors, and Therapists or by the Society for Sex Therapy and Research usually ensures quality treatment.

Valdivia, I., and Rossy, N. "Brief Treatment Strategies for Major Depressive Disorder: Advice for the Primary Care Clinician," *Topics in Advanced Practice Nursing eJournal* 4(1), 2004. Available at *www.medscape.com.*

Selected references

American Psychiatric Association. *Diagnostic and Statistical Manual of Mental Disorders,* Fourth Edition, Text Revision. Washington, D.C.: American Psychiatric Association, 2000.

Fogel, J. "Dealing with Mental Health Concerns: A Role for the Advanced Practice Nurse in Primary Care," *Topics in Advanced Practice Nursing eJournal* 4(1), 2004. Available at *www.medscape.com.*

Hertzig, M.E. *Annual Progress in Child Psychiatry and Child Development 2002.* New York: Taylor and Francis, 2004.

Millon, T., et al. *Personality Disorders in Modern Life,* 2nd ed. Hoboken, N.J.: Wiley, 2004.

Sadock, B.J., and Sadpock, V.A. *Kaplan & Sadock's Synopsis of Psychiatry,* 9th ed. Philadelphia: Lippincott Williams & Wilkins, 2003.

Seligman, L. *Diagnosis and Treatment Planning in Counseling,* 3rd ed. New York: Kluwer Academic, 2004.

Shives, L.R. *Basic Concepts of Psychiatric-Mental Health Nursing,* 6th ed. Philadelphia: Lippincott Williams & Wilkins, 2005.

Shultz, J.M., and Videbeck, S.L. *Lippincott's Manual of Psychiatric Nursing Care Plans,* 7th ed. Philadelphia: Lippincott Williams & Wilkins, 2004.

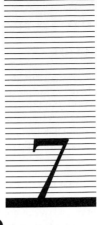

Respiratory disorders

Introduction *508*

Congenital and pediatric disorders *514*
Infant respiratory distress syndrome *514*
Sudden infant death syndrome *516*
Croup *518*
Epiglottiditis *520*

Acute disorders *521*
Acute respiratory distress syndrome *521*
Acute respiratory failure in COPD *524*
Pulmonary edema *526*
Cor pulmonale *527*
Legionnaires' disease *530*
Atelectasis *531*
Respiratory acidosis *533*
Respiratory alkalosis *534*
Pneumothorax *535*
Pneumonia *537*
Idiopathic bronchiolitis obliterans with
  organizing pneumonia *542*
Pulmonary embolism *543*
Sarcoidosis *546*
Severe acute respiratory syndrome *547*
Lung abscess *548*
Hemothorax *549*
Pulmonary hypertension *550*
Pleural effusion and empyema *551*
Pleurisy *553*

Chronic disorders *553*
Chronic obstructive pulmonary
  disease *553*
Bronchiectasis *559*
Idiopathic pulmonary fibrosis *561*
Tuberculosis *563*

Pneumoconioses *565*
Silicosis *565*
Asbestosis *566*
Coal worker's pneumoconiosis *567*

Selected references *569*

Introduction

The respiratory system distributes air to the alveoli, where gas exchange — the addition of oxygen (O_2) and the removal of carbon dioxide (CO_2) from pulmonary capillary blood — takes place. Certain specialized structures within this system play a vital role in preparing air for use by the body. The nose, for example, contains vestibular hairs that filter the air and an extensive vascular network that warms it. The nose also contains a layer of goblet cells and a moist mucosal surface; water vapor enters the airstream from this mucosal surface to saturate inspired air as it's warmed in the upper airways. Ciliated mucosa in the posterior portion of the nose and nasopharynx as well as major portions of the tracheobronchial tree propel particles deposited by impaction or gravity to the oropharynx, where the particles are swallowed.

External respiration

The external component of respiration — ventilation or breathing — delivers inspired air to the lower respiratory tract and alveoli. Contraction and relaxation of the respiratory muscles move air into and out of the lungs. Ventilation begins with the contraction of the inspiratory muscles: the diaphragm (the major muscle of respiration) descends, while external intercostal muscles move the rib cage upward and outward.

Air then enters the lungs in response to the pressure gradient between the atmosphere and the lungs. The lungs adhere to the chest wall and diaphragm because of the vacuum created within the pleural space. As the thorax expands, negative pressure is created in the intrapleural space, causing the lungs to also expand and draw in the warmed, humidified air. The accessory muscles of inspiration, which include the scalene and sternocleidomastoid muscles, raise the clavicles, upper ribs, and sternum. The accessory muscles aren't used in normal inspiration but may be used in some pathologic conditions.

Normal expiration is passive; the inspiratory muscles cease to contract, the diaphragm rises, and the elastic recoil of the lungs causes the lungs to contract. These actions raise the pressure within the lungs above atmospheric pressure, moving air from the lungs to the atmosphere. Active expiration causes pleural pressure to become less negative. (See *What happens in ventilation*.)

An adult lung contains an estimated 300 million alveoli; each alveolus is supplied by many capillaries. To reach the capillary lumen, O_2 must cross the alveolocapillary membrane, which consists of an alveolar epithelial cell, a thin interstitial space, the capillary basement membrane, and the capillary endothelial cell membrane. The O_2 tension of air entering the respiratory tract is approximately 150 mm Hg. In the alveoli, inspired air mixes with CO_2 and water vapor, lowering the O_2 pressure to approximately 100 mm Hg. Because alveolar partial pressure of O_2 is higher than that present in mixed venous blood entering the pulmonary capillaries (approximately 40 mm Hg), O_2 diffuses across the alveolocapillary membrane into the blood.

O_2 and CO_2 transport and internal respiration

Circulating blood delivers O_2 to the cells of the body for metabolism and transports metabolic wastes and CO_2 from the tissues back to the lungs. When oxygenated arterial blood reaches tissue capillaries, O_2 diffuses from the blood into the cells because of the O_2 tension gradient. The amount of O_2 available is determined by the concentration of hemoglobin (Hb; the principal carrier of O_2), the percentage of O_2 saturation of the Hb, regional blood flow, arterial O_2 content, and cardiac output.

Internal (cellular) respiration occurs as a part of cellular metabolism, which can take place with O_2 (aerobic) or without O_2 (anaerobic). The most efficient method for providing fuel (high-energy compounds such as adenosine triphosphate [ATP]) for cellular reactions is aerobic metabolism, which produces CO_2 and water in addition to ATP. Anaerobic metabolism is less efficient because a cell produces only a limited amount of ATP and yields lactic acid as well as CO_2 as a metabolic by-product.

WHAT HAPPENS IN VENTILATION

This illustration shows changes in the intrapleural and intrapulmonary (airway) pressures during inspiration and expiration.

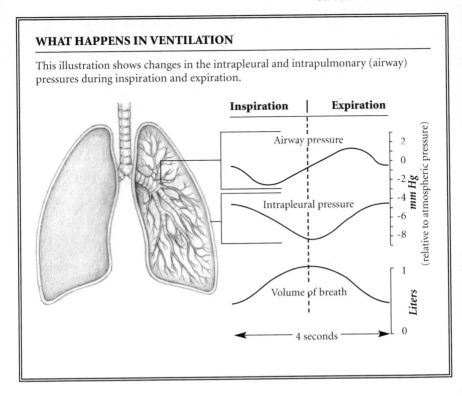

Because circulation is continuous, CO_2 doesn't normally accumulate in tissues. CO_2 produced during cellular respiration diffuses from tissues into regional capillaries and is transported by systemic venous circulation. When CO_2 reaches the alveolar capillaries, it diffuses into the alveoli, where the partial pressure of CO_2 is lower; CO_2 is removed from the alveoli during exhalation.

Mechanisms of control

The central nervous system's (CNS's) control of respiration lies in the respiratory center, located in the lateral medulla oblongata of the brain stem. Impulses travel down the phrenic nerves to the diaphragm, and the intercostal nerves to the intercostal muscles, where the impulses change the rate and depth of respiration. The inspiratory and expiratory centers, located in the posterior medulla, establish the involuntary rhythm of the breathing pattern.

Apneustic and pneumotaxic centers in the pons influence the pattern of breath-ing. Stimulation of the lower pontine apneustic center (by trauma, tumor, or stroke, for example) produces forceful inspiratory gasps alternating with weak expiration. The apneustic center continually excites the medullary inspiratory center and thus facilitates inspiration. Signals from the pneumotaxic center as well as afferent impulses from the vagus nerve inhibit the apneustic center and "turn off" inspiration. The apneustic pattern doesn't occur if vagi are intact.

Partial pressure of arterial oxygen (PaO_2), pH, and pH of cerebrospinal fluid (CSF) influence output from the respiratory center. When CO_2 enters the CSF, the pH of CSF falls, stimulating central chemoreceptors to increase ventilation.

The respiratory center also receives information from peripheral chemoreceptors in the carotid and aortic bodies. These chemoreceptors respond primarily to decreased PaO_2 but also to decreased pH. The peripheral chemoreceptors have little control over respirations until the PaO_2 is less than 60 mm Hg.

During exercise, stretch receptors in lung tissue and the diaphragm prevent overdistention of the lungs. During swallowing, the cortex can interrupt automatic control of ventilation. During sleep, respiratory drive may fluctuate, producing hypoventilation and periods of apnea. External sensations, drugs, chronic hypercapnia, and changes in body temperature can also alter the respiratory pattern.

Diagnostic tests

Diagnostic tests evaluate physiologic characteristics and pathologic states within the respiratory tract.

Noninvasive tests include:
- Chest X-ray shows such conditions as atelectasis, pleural effusion, infiltrates, pneumothorax, lesions, mediastinal shifts, pulmonary edema, and chronic obstructive pulmonary disease (COPD).
- Computed tomography scan provides a three-dimensional picture that's 100 times more sensitive than a chest X-ray.
- Magnetic resonance imaging identifies obstructed arteries and tissue perfusion, but movement of the heart and lungs reduces the image's clarity.
- Sputum specimen analysis assesses sputum quantity, color, viscosity, and odor; microbiological stains and culture of sputum can identify infectious organisms; and cytologic preparations can detect respiratory tract neoplasms. Sensitivity tests determine antibiotic sensitivity and resistance.
- Pulmonary function tests measure lung volume, flow rates, and compliance. Normal values, individualized by body stature and age, are reported in percentage of the normal predicted value. Static measurements are volume measurements that include tidal volume, volume of air contained in a normal breath; functional residual capacity, volume of air remaining in the lungs after normal expiration; vital capacity, volume of air that can be exhaled after maximal inspiration; residual volume, air remaining in the lungs after maximal expiration; and total lung capacity (TLC), volume of air in the lungs after maximal inspiration. Dynamic measurements characterize the movement of air into and out

of the lungs and show changes in lung mechanics. They include measurement of forced expiratory volume in 1 second, maximum volume of air that can be expired in 1 second from total lung capacity; maximal voluntary ventilation, volume of air that can be expired in 1 minute with the patient's maximum voluntary effort; and forced vital capacity, maximal volume of air that the patient can exhale from TLC. (Peak flow rate, which can be obtained at the bedside, is also a dynamic measurement of pulmonary function.)
- Exercise stress test evaluates the ability to transport O_2 and remove CO_2 with increasing metabolic demands.
- Polysomnography can diagnose sleep disorders.
- Lung scan (ventilation-perfusion or scintiphotography scan) demonstrates ventilation and perfusion patterns. It's used primarily to evaluate pulmonary embolus.
- Arterial blood gas (ABG) analysis assesses gas exchange. Decreased PaO_2 may indicate hypoventilation, ventilation-perfusion mismatch, or shunting of blood away from gas exchange sites. Increased partial pressure of arterial carbon dioxide ($PaCO_2$) reflects marked ventilation-perfusion mismatch or hypoventilation; decreased $PaCO_2$ reflects increased alveolar ventilation. Changes in pH may reflect metabolic or respiratory dysfunction.
- Pulse oximetry is a noninvasive assessment of arterial oxygen saturation.
- Capnography may be used either transcutaneously or in ventilator circuit to determine $PaCO_2$ trends.

Invasive tests include:
- Bronchoscopy permits direct visualization of the trachea and mainstem, lobar, segmental, and subsegmental bronchi. It may be used to localize the site of lung hemorrhage, visualize masses in these airways, and collect respiratory tract secretions. Brush biopsy may be used to obtain specimens from the lungs for microbiological stains, culture, and cytology. Lesion biopsies may be performed by using small forceps under direct visualization (when present in the proximal airways) or with the aid of fluoroscopy (when present distal to regions of direct visualization). Bron-

choscopy can also be used to clear secretions and remove foreign bodies.

■ Thoracentesis permits removal of pleural fluid for analysis.

■ Pleural biopsy obtains pleural tissue for histologic examination and culture.

■ Pulmonary artery angiography, the injection of dye into the pulmonary artery, can locate pulmonary embolism. This is considered the gold standard for diagnosing pulmonary emboli.

■ Positron emission tomography scan uses a short-life radionuclide. Increased uptake of the substance is seen in malignant cells.

Assessment

Assessment of the respiratory system begins with a thorough patient history. Ask the patient to describe his respiratory problem. How long has he had it? How long does each attack last? Does one attack differ from another? Does any activity in particular bring on an attack or make it worse? What relieves the symptoms? Always ask whether the patient was or is a smoker, what and how often he smoked or smokes, and how long he smoked or has been smoking. Record this information in "pack years"—the number of packs of cigarettes per day multiplied by the number of smoking years. Remember to ask about the patient's occupation, hobbies, and travel; some of these activities may involve exposure to toxic or allergenic substances.

If the patient has dyspnea, ask if it occurs during activity or at rest. What position is the patient in when dyspnea occurs? How far can he walk? How many flights of stairs can he climb? Has his exercise tolerance been decreasing? Can he relate dyspnea to allergies or environmental conditions? Does it occur only at night, during sleep? If the patient has a cough, ask about its severity, persistence, and duration; ask if it produces sputum and, if so, what kind. Have the patient's cough habits and character of sputum changed recently?

Physical examination

Use inspection skills to check for clues to respiratory disease, beginning with the patient's general appearance. If he's frail or cachectic, he may have a chronic disease that has impaired his appetite. If he's di-aphoretic, restless, or irritable or protective of a painful body part, he may be in acute distress. Also, look for behavior changes that may indicate hypoxemia or hypercapnia. Confusion, lethargy, bizarre behavior, or quiet sleep from which he can't be aroused may point to hypercapnia. Watch for marked cyanosis, indicated by bluish or ashen skin (usually best seen on the lips, tongue, earlobes, and nail beds), which may be due to hypoxemia or poor tissue perfusion.

Assess chest shape and symmetry at rest and during ventilation. Increased anteroposterior diameter ("barrel chest") characterizes emphysema. Kyphoscoliosis also alters chest configuration, which in turn restricts breathing. Assess respiratory excursion and observe for accessory muscle use during breathing. The use of upper chest and neck muscles is normal only during physical stress.

Observe the rate and pattern of breathing because certain disorders produce characteristic changes in breathing patterns. For example, an acute respiratory disorder can produce tachypnea (rapid, shallow breathing) or hyperpnea (increased rate and depth of breathing); intracranial lesions can produce Cheyne-Stokes and Biot's respirations; increased intracranial pressure can result in central hyperventilation and apneustic or ataxic breathing; metabolic disorders can cause Kussmaul's respirations; and airway obstruction can lead to prolonged forceful expiration and pursed-lip breathing.

Also observe posture and carriage. A patient with COPD, for example, usually supports rib cage movement by placing his arms on the sides of a chair to increase expansion and leans forward during exhalation to help expel air.

Palpation of the chest wall detects areas of tenderness, masses, changes in fremitus (palpable vocal vibrations), or crepitus (air in subcutaneous tissues). To assess chest excursion and symmetry, place your hands in a horizontal position, bilaterally on the posterior chest, with your thumbs pressed lightly against the spine, creating folds in the skin. As the patient takes a deep breath, your thumbs should move quickly and equally away from the spine. Repeat this

CHARACTERIZING AND INTERPRETING PERCUSSION SOUNDS

Percussion may produce several kinds of sounds. Known as flat, dull, resonant, hyperresonant, or tympanic, these sounds indicate the location and density of various structures. During percussion, determining other tonal characteristics, such as pitch, intensity, and quality, also will help identify respiratory structure. Use this chart as a guide to interpreting percussion sounds.

Characteristic

Sound	Pitch	Intensity	Quality
Flatness	High	Soft	Extremely dull
Dullness	Medium	Medium	Thudlike
Resonance	Low	Moderate to loud	Hollow
Hyperresonance	Lower than resonance	Very loud	Booming
Tympany	High	Loud	Musical, drumlike

with your hands placed anteriorly, at the costal margins (lower lobes) and clavicles (apices). Unequal movement indicates differences in expansion, seen in atelectasis, diaphragm or chest wall muscle disease, or splinting due to pain.

Percussion should detect resonance over lung fields that aren't covered by bony structures or the heart. A dull sound on percussion may mean consolidation or pleural disease. (See *Characterizing and interpreting percussion sounds.*)

Auscultation normally detects soft, vesicular breath sounds throughout most of the lung fields. Absent or adventitious breath sounds may indicate fluid in small airways or interstitial lung disease (crackles), secretions in moderate and large airways (rhonchi), and airflow obstruction (wheezes).

Special respiratory care

The hospitalized patient with respiratory disease may require an artificial upper airway, chest tubes, chest physiotherapy, and supervision of mechanical ventilation. In cardiopulmonary arrest, establishing an airway always takes precedence. In a patient with this condition, airway obstruction usually results when the tongue slides back and blocks the posterior pharynx. The head-tilt method or, in suspected or confirmed cervical fracture or arthritis, the jaw-thrust maneuver can immediately push the tongue forward, relieving such obstruction. Endotracheal (ET) intubation

Commonly, the chest tube is placed in the sixth or seventh intercostal space, in the axillary region. Occasionally, in pneumothorax, the tube is placed in the second or third intercostal space, in the midclavicular region.

Follow these guidelines when caring for a patient with a chest tube:
- Watch for air bubbling in the water-seal compartment of the drainage system. Bubbling should be intermittent; continuous bubbling may indicate an air leak.
- Monitor changes in suction pressure.
- Make sure that fluid in the drainage tube at the water-seal level fluctuates with breathing when the tube is patent.
- Make sure that all connections in the system are tight and secured with tape.
- Never clamp the chest tube unless checking for air leaks or changing the drainage system.
- Add water to the suction system when necessary.
- Record the amount, color, and consistency of drainage. Watch for signs of shock, such as tachycardia and hypotension, if drainage is excessive.
- Encourage the patient to cough and breathe deeply every hour to enhance lung expansion.

Ventilator methods

Mechanical ventilators are typically used for CNS problems, hypoxemia, or failure of the normal bellows action provided by the diaphragm and rib cage. Volume-cycled ventilators deliver a preset volume of gas. The tidal volume is set at 10 to 15 ml/kg of ideal body weight. Lower volumes are now being advocated to reduce the risk of barotrauma. Positive end-expiratory pressure (PEEP) is used to retain a certain amount of pressure in the lungs at the end of expiration. By keeping small airways and alveoli open with this method, functional residual capacity is increased and oxygenation is improved.

When weaning is an option, several methods can be used to discontinue ventilation. The patient may be taken off the ventilator and supplied with a T-piece (ET tube O_2 adapter) that provides O_2 and humidification. The patient then breathes

---

Implications

These sounds are normal over the sternum. Over the lung, they may indicate atelectasis or pleural effusion.

Normal over the liver, heart, and diaphragm, these sounds over the lung may point to pneumonia, tumor, atelectasis, or pleural effusion.

When percussed over the lung, these sounds are normal.

These are normal findings with percussion over a child's lung. Over an adult's lung, these findings may indicate emphysema, chronic bronchitis, asthma, or pneumothorax.

Over the stomach, these are normal findings; over the lung, they suggest tension pneumothorax.

---

and, sometimes, a tracheotomy may be necessary.

Chest tubes

An important procedure in patients with respiratory disease is chest tube drainage, which removes air or fluid from the pleural space. This allows the collapsed lung to re-expand to fill the evacuated pleural space. Chest drainage also allows removal of pleural fluid for culture. Chest tubes are commonly used after thoracic surgery, penetrating chest wounds, pleural effusion, and empyema. They're also used for evacuation of pneumothorax, hydrothorax, or hemothorax. Sometimes chest tubes are used to instill sclerosing drugs into the pleural space to prevent recurrent malignant pleural effusions.

spontaneously without the ventilator for gradually increasing periods.

With intermittent mandatory ventilation, the ventilator provides a specific number of breaths, and the patient is able to breathe spontaneously between ventilator breaths. The frequency of ventilator breaths is gradually decreased until the patient can breathe on his own. Recently, pressure support ventilation, in which the patient receives a preset pressure boost with each spontaneous breath, has proved effective. Vital signs, ABG levels, physical findings, and subjective symptoms should be monitored periodically during weaning to assess respiratory status.

Chest physiotherapy

In respiratory conditions marked by excessive accumulation of secretions in the lungs, chest physiotherapy may enhance removal of secretions. Chest physiotherapy includes chest assessment, effective breathing and coughing exercises, postural drainage, percussion, vibration, and evaluation of the therapy's effectiveness. Before initiating treatment, review X-rays and physical assessment findings to locate areas of secretions.

■ Deep breathing maintains diaphragm use, increases negative intrathoracic pressure, and promotes venous return; it's especially important when pain or dressings restrict chest movement. An incentive spirometer can provide positive visual reinforcement to promote deep breathing.

■ Pursed-lip breathing is used primarily in obstructive disease to slow expiration and prevent small airway collapse. Such breathing slows air through smaller bronchi, maintaining positive pressure and preventing collapse of small airways and resultant air trapping.

■ Segmental breathing or lateral costal breathing is used after lung resection and for localized disorders. Place your hand over the lung area on the affected side. Instruct the patient to try to push that portion of his chest against your hand on deep inspiration. You should be able to feel this with your hand.

■ Coughing that's controlled and staged gradually increases intrathoracic pressure, reducing pain and bronchospasm of explo-

sive coughing. When wound pain prevents effective coughing, splint the wound with a pillow, towel, or your hand during coughing exercises.

■ Postural drainage uses gravity to drain secretions into larger airways, where they can be expectorated. This technique is used in the patient with copious or tenacious secretions. Before performing postural drainage, auscultate the patient's chest and review chest X-rays to determine the best position for maximum drainage. To prevent vomiting, schedule postural drainage at least 1 hour after meals.

■ Percussion moves air against the chest wall, enhancing the effectiveness of postural drainage by loosening lung secretions. Percussion is contraindicated in severe pain, extreme obesity, cancer that has metastasized to the ribs, crushing chest injuries, bleeding disorders, spontaneous pneumothorax, spinal compression fractures, and in patients with temporary pacemakers.

■ Vibration can be used with percussion or alone when percussion is contraindicated.

■ PEEP therapy maintains positive pressure in airways, preventing small airway collapse.

Before and after chest physiotherapy, auscultate the patient's lung fields and assess for sputum production to evaluate the effectiveness of therapy.

CONGENITAL AND PEDIATRIC DISORDERS

Infant respiratory distress syndrome

Infant respiratory distress syndrome (IRDS), also called *hyaline membrane disease*, is the most common cause of neonatal mortality. In the United States alone, it kills 40,000 neonates every year. IRDS occurs in premature neonates and, if untreated, is fatal within 72 hours of birth in up to 14% of neonates weighing less than 5½ lb

(2.5 kg). Aggressive management using mechanical ventilation can improve the prognosis, but some surviving neonates may develop some degree of bronchopulmonary dysplasia.

Causes and incidence

Although airways and alveoli of a neonate's respiratory system are present by 27 weeks' gestation, the intercostal muscles are weak and the alveolar capillary system is immature. The premature neonate with IRDS develops widespread alveolar collapse due to a lack of surfactant, a lipoprotein present in alveoli and respiratory bronchioles. Surfactant lowers surface tension and helps prevent alveolar collapse. This surfactant deficiency results in widespread atelectasis, which leads to inadequate alveolar ventilation with shunting of blood through collapsed areas of lung, causing hypoxemia and acidosis.

IRDS occurs almost exclusively in neonates born before 37 weeks' gestation (in 60% of those born before the 28th week). The incidence is greatest in the 1,000 to 1,500 g birthweight group. Infants of diabetic mothers, those born by cesarean delivery, second-born twins, infants with perinatal asphyxia, and those delivered suddenly after antepartum hemorrhage are more commonly afflicted.

Signs and symptoms

Although a neonate with IRDS may breathe normally at first, he usually develops rapid, shallow respirations within minutes or hours of birth, with intercostal, subcostal, or sternal retractions, nasal flaring, and audible expiratory grunting. This grunting is a natural compensatory mechanism designed to produce positive end-expiratory pressure (PEEP) and prevent further alveolar collapse.

Severe disease is marked by apnea, bradycardia, and cyanosis (from hypoxemia, left-to-right shunting through the foramen ovale, or right-to-left intrapulmonary shunting through atelectic regions of the lung). Other clinical features include pallor, frothy sputum, and low body temperature as a result of an immature nervous system and the absence of subcutaneous fat.

Diagnosis

 CONFIRMING DIAGNOSIS
Although signs of respiratory distress in a premature neonate during the first few hours of life strongly suggest IRDS, a chest X-ray and arterial blood gas (ABG) analysis are necessary to confirm the diagnosis.
- Chest X-ray may be normal for the first 6 to 12 hours (in 50% of neonates with IRDS), but 24 hours after birth it will show the characteristic ground-glass appearance and air bronchograms.
- ABG analysis shows decreased partial pressure of arterial oxygen; normal, decreased, or increased partial pressure of arterial carbon dioxide; and decreased pH (from respiratory or metabolic acidosis or both).
- Chest auscultation reveals normal or diminished air entry and crackles (rare in early stages).

When a cesarean delivery is necessary before 36 weeks' gestation, amniocentesis enables the determination of the lecithin/sphingomyelin (L/S) ratio and the presence of phosphatidylglycerol. An L/S ratio of more than 2:1 and the presence of phosphatidylglycerol decrease the likelihood of IRDS.

Treatment

Treatment of an infant with IRDS requires vigorous respiratory support. Warm, humidified, oxygen-enriched gases are administered by oxygen hood or, if such treatment fails, by mechanical ventilation. Severe cases may require mechanical ventilation with PEEP or continuous positive airway pressure (CPAP), administered by nasal prongs or, when necessary, endotracheal (ET) intubation. Special ventilation techniques are now used on the patients refractory to conventional mechanical ventilation. These include high-frequency jet ventilation and high-frequency oscillatory ventilation. Extracorporeal membrane oxygenation is the last choice for ventilation and is only available in certain specialized facilities. Treatment of IRDS also includes:
- a radiant warmer or isolette for thermoregulation

■ I.V. fluids and sodium bicarbonate to control acidosis and maintain fluid and electrolyte balance

■ tube feedings or total parenteral nutrition if the neonate is too weak to eat

■ administration of surfactant by an ET tube (Studies show that this treatment can prevent or improve the course of IRDS as well as reduce mortality.)

Special considerations

Neonates with IRDS require continual assessment and monitoring in an intensive care nursery.

■ Closely monitor blood gases as well as fluid intake and output. If the neonate has an umbilical catheter (arterial or venous), check for arterial hypotension or abnormal central venous pressure. Watch for complications, such as infection, thrombosis, or decreased circulation to the legs. If the neonate has a transcutaneous oxygen monitor, change the site of the lead placement every 2 to 4 hours.

■ To evaluate his progress, assess skin color, rate and depth of respirations, severity of retractions, nostril flaring, frequency of expiratory grunting, frothing at the lips, and restlessness.

■ Regularly assess the effectiveness of oxygen or ventilator therapy. Evaluate every change in fraction of inspired oxygen and PEEP or CPAP by monitoring arterial oxygen saturation or ABG levels. Adjust the PEEP or CPAP as indicated, based on findings.

■ Mechanical ventilation in neonates is usually done in a pressure-limited mode rather than the volume-limited mode used in adults.

■ When the neonate is on mechanical ventilation, watch carefully for signs of barotrauma (an increase in respiratory distress and subcutaneous emphysema) and accidental disconnection from the ventilator. Check ventilator settings frequently. Be alert for signs of complications of PEEP or CPAP therapy, such as decreased cardiac output, pneumothorax, and pneumomediastinum. Mechanical ventilation increases the risk of infection in the premature neonate, so preventive measures are essential.

■ As needed, arrange for follow-up care with a neonatal ophthalmologist to check for retinal damage. Premature neonates in an oxygen-rich environment are at increased risk for developing retinopathy of prematurity.

■ Teach the parents about their neonate's condition and, if possible, let them participate in his care (using sterile technique), to encourage normal parent-infant bonding. Advise parents that full recovery may take up to 12 months. When the prognosis is poor, prepare the parents for the neonate's impending death and offer emotional support.

■ Help reduce mortality in the neonate with IRDS by detecting respiratory distress early. Recognize intercostal retractions and grunting, especially in a premature neonate, as signs of IRDS; make sure the neonate receives immediate treatment.

Sudden infant death syndrome

A medical mystery of early infancy, sudden infant death syndrome (SIDS), also called *crib death,* is the unexpected, sudden death of an infant or child younger than age 1 year. Reasons for the death remain unexplained even after an autopsy. Typically, parents put the infant to bed and later find him dead, commonly with no indications of a struggle or distress of any kind. Incidence has decreased with the practice of teaching parents to place an infant on his back to sleep.

Causes and incidence

SIDS is the third leading cause of death in infants between age 1 month and 1 year. It occurs more commonly in winter months. The incidence is higher in males, premature neonates, and those who sleep on their stomachs or in cribs with soft bedding. Incidence is also higher among neonates born in conditions of poverty and to those who were one of a single multiple birth, such as twins and triplets, and to mothers who smoke, take drugs, or failed to seek prenatal care until late in the pregnancy. SIDS may also result from an abnormality in the control of ventilation that allows carbon dioxide to build up in the blood, thereby causing prolonged apneic periods with profound hypoxemia and serious cardiac arrhythmias. It's also thought to be associated with problems in sleep arousal.

Signs and symptoms

Although parents find some victims wedged in crib corners or with blankets wrapped around their heads, autopsies rule out suffocation as the cause of death. Autopsy shows a patent airway, so aspiration of vomitus isn't the cause of death. Typically, SIDS babies don't cry out and show no signs of having been disturbed in their sleep. However, their positions or tangled blankets may suggest movement just before death, perhaps due to terminal spasm.

Depending on how long the infant has been dead, a SIDS baby may have a mottled complexion with extreme cyanosis of the lips and fingertips or pooling of blood in the legs and feet that may be mistaken for bruises. Pulse and respirations are absent, and the diaper is wet and full of stool.

Diagnosis

Diagnosis of SIDS requires an autopsy to rule out other causes of death. Characteristic histologic findings on autopsy include small or normal adrenal glands and petechiae over the visceral surfaces of the pleura, within the thymus, and in the epicardium. Autopsy also reveals extremely well-preserved lymphoid structures and certain pathologic characteristics that suggest chronic hypoxemia such as increased pulmonary artery smooth muscle. Examination also shows edematous, congestive lungs fully expanded in the pleural cavities, liquid (not clotted) blood in the heart, and curd from the stomach inside the trachea.

Treatment

If the parents bring the infant to the emergency department (ED), the physician will decide whether to try to resuscitate him. An "aborted SIDS" infant is one who's found apneic and is successfully resuscitated. Such an infant, or any infant who had a sibling stricken by SIDS, should be tested for infantile apnea. If tests are positive, a home apnea monitor may be recommended. Because the infant usually can't be re-suscitated, however, treatment focuses on providing emotional support for the family.

Special considerations

■ Make sure that parents are present when the child's death is announced. They may lash out at ED personnel, the babysitter, or anyone else involved in the child's care—even each other. Stay calm and let them express their feelings. Reassure them that they weren't to blame.

■ Let the parents see the baby in a private room. Allow them to express their grief in their own way. Stay in the room with them if appropriate. Offer to call clergy, friends, or relatives.

■ After the parents and family have recovered from their initial shock, explain the necessity for an autopsy to confirm the diagnosis of SIDS (in some states, this is mandatory). At this time, provide the family with some basic facts about SIDS and encourage them to give their consent for the autopsy. Make sure that they receive the autopsy report promptly.

■ Find out whether your community has a local counseling and information program for SIDS parents. Participants in such a program will contact the parents, ensure that they receive the autopsy report promptly, put them in touch with a professional counselor, and maintain supportive telephone contact. Also, find out whether there's a local SIDS parents' group; such a group can provide significant emotional support. Contact the National Sudden Infant Death Foundation for information about such local groups.

■ If your facility's policy is to assign a public health nurse to the family, she will provide the continuing reassurance and assistance the parents will need.

■ If the parents decide to have another child, they'll need information and counseling to help them through the pregnancy and the first year of the new infant's life.

■ Infants at high risk for SIDS may be placed on apnea monitoring at home.

■ All new parents should be informed of the American Academy of Pediatrics' recommendation that infants be positioned on their back, not on their stomach or side, for sleeping.

Croup

Croup is a severe inflammation and obstruction of the upper airway, occurring as acute laryngotracheobronchitis (most common), laryngitis, and acute spasmodic laryngitis; it must always be distinguished from epiglottiditis. It's derived from an old German word for "voice box" and refers to swelling around the larynx or vocal cords. Recovery is usually complete.

Causes and incidence

Croup usually results from a viral infection. Parainfluenza viruses cause 75% of such infections; adenoviruses, respiratory syncytial virus (RSV), influenza, and measles viruses account for the rest.

Croup is a childhood disease affecting more boys than girls (typically between ages 3 months and 5 years) that usually occurs during the winter. Up to 15% of patients have a strong family history of croup.

Signs and symptoms

The onset of croup usually follows an upper respiratory tract infection. Clinical features include inspiratory stridor, hoarse or muffled vocal sounds, varying degrees of laryngeal obstruction and respiratory distress, and a characteristic sharp, barking, seal-like cough. These symptoms may last only a few hours or persist for a day or two. As it progresses, croup causes inflammatory edema and, possibly, spasm, which can obstruct the upper airway and severely compromise ventilation. (See *How croup affects the upper airway.*)

Each form of croup has additional characteristics:

In *laryngotracheobronchitis*, the symptoms seem to worsen at night. Inflammation causes edema of the bronchi and bronchioles as well as increasingly difficult expiration that frightens the child. Other characteristic features include fever, diffusely decreased breath sounds, expiratory rhonchi, and scattered crackles.

Laryngitis, which results from vocal cord edema, is usually mild and produces no respiratory distress except in infants. Early signs include a sore throat and cough, which, rarely, may progress to marked hoarseness, suprasternal and intercostal retractions, inspiratory stridor, dyspnea, diminished breath sounds, restlessness and, in later stages, severe dyspnea and exhaustion.

Acute spasmodic laryngitis affects a child between ages 1 and 3, particularly one with allergies and a family history of croup. It typically begins with mild to moderate hoarseness and nasal discharge, followed by the characteristic cough and noisy inspiration (that usually awaken the child at night), labored breathing with retractions, rapid pulse, and clammy skin. The child understandably becomes anxious, which may lead to increasing dyspnea and transient cyanosis. These severe symptoms diminish after several hours but reappear in a milder form on the next one or two nights.

Diagnosis

The clinical picture is very characteristic, so the diagnosis should be suspected immediately. When bacterial infection is the cause, throat cultures may identify the organisms and their sensitivity to antibiotics and rule out diphtheria. On a posterior-anterior X-ray of the chest, narrowing of the upper airway ("steeple sign") may be apparent. Laryngoscopy may reveal inflammation and obstruction in epiglottal and laryngeal areas. In evaluating the patient, assess for foreign body obstruction (a common cause of crouplike cough in a young child) as well as masses and cysts.

Treatment

For most children with croup, home care with rest, cool humidification during sleep, and antipyretics, such as acetaminophen, relieve symptoms. However, respiratory distress that's severe or interferes with oral hydration requires hospitalization and parenteral fluid replacement to prevent dehydration. If bacterial infection is the cause, antibiotic therapy is necessary. Oxygen therapy may also be required. Increasing obstruction of the airway requires intubation and mechanical ventilation.

Inhaled racemic epinephrine and corticosteroids may be used to alleviate respiratory distress.

PATHOPHYSIOLOGY
HOW CROUP AFFECTS THE UPPER AIRWAY

In croup, inflammatory swelling and spasms constrict the larynx, thereby reducing airflow. This cross-sectional drawing (from chin to chest) shows the upper airway changes caused by croup. Inflammatory changes almost completely obstruct the larynx (which includes the epiglottis) and significantly narrow the trachea.

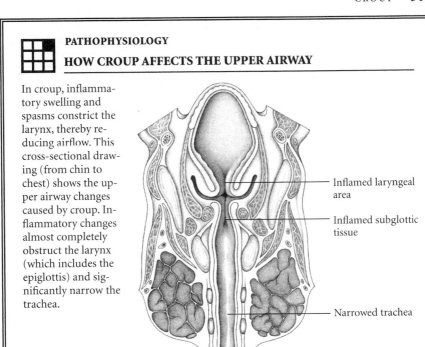

Inflamed laryngeal area

Inflamed subglottic tissue

Narrowed trachea

Special considerations

Monitor and support respiration, and control fever. Because croup is so frightening to the child and his family, you must also provide support and reassurance.

■ Carefully monitor cough and breath sounds, hoarseness, severity of retractions, inspiratory stridor, cyanosis, respiratory rate and character (especially prolonged and labored respirations), restlessness, fever, and cardiac rate.

■ Keep the child as quiet as possible. However, avoid sedation because it may depress respiration. If the patient is an infant, position him in an infant seat or prop him up with a pillow; place an older child in Fowler's position. If an older child requires a cool mist tent to help him breathe, explain why it's needed.

■ Isolate patients suspected of having RSV and parainfluenza infections if possible. Wash your hands carefully before leaving the room, to avoid transmission to other children, particularly infants. Instruct parents and others involved in the care of these children to take similar precautions.

■ Control fever with sponge baths and antipyretics. Keep a hypothermia blanket on hand for temperatures above 102° F (38.9° C). Watch for seizures in infants and young children with high fevers. Give I.V. antibiotics as ordered.

■ Relieve sore throat with soothing, water-based ices, such as fruit sherbet and popsicles. Avoid thicker, milk-based fluids if the child is producing heavy mucus or has great difficulty in swallowing. Apply petroleum jelly or another ointment around the nose and lips to soothe irritation from nasal discharge and mouth breathing.

■ Maintain a calm, quiet environment and offer reassurance. Explain all procedures and answer any questions.

When croup doesn't require hospitalization:

■ Teach the parents effective home care. Suggest the use of a cool humidifier (vaporizer). To relieve croupy spells, tell parents to carry the child into the bathroom, shut the door, and turn on the hot water. Breathing in warm, moist air quickly eases an acute spell of croup.

■ Warn parents that ear infections and pneumonia are complications of croup, which may appear about 5 days after recovery. Stress the importance of immediately reporting earache, productive cough, high fever, or increased shortness of breath.

Epiglottiditis

Acute epiglottiditis is an acute inflammation of the epiglottis that tends to cause airway obstruction. A critical emergency, epiglottiditis can prove fatal unless it's recognized and treated promptly.

Causes and incidence
Epiglottiditis usually results from infection with *Haemophilus influenzae* type B (Hib) and, occasionally, pneumococci and group A streptococci. It typically strikes children between ages 2 and 6 years. (However, immunosuppression can predispose adults to epiglottiditis.) Since the advent of the Hib vaccine, epiglottiditis is becoming more rare.

Signs and symptoms
Sometimes preceded by an upper respiratory infection, epiglottiditis may rapidly progress to complete upper airway obstruction within 2 to 5 hours. Laryngeal obstruction results from inflammation and edema of the epiglottis. Accompanying symptoms include high fever, stridor, sore throat, dysphagia, irritability, restlessness, and drooling. To relieve severe respiratory distress, the child with epiglottiditis may hyperextend his neck, sit up, and lean forward with his mouth open, tongue protruding, and nostrils flaring as he tries to breathe. He may develop inspiratory retractions and rhonchi.

Diagnosis
In acute epiglottiditis, throat examination reveals a large, edematous, bright red epiglottis. Such examination should follow lateral neck X-rays and, generally, *shouldn't* be performed if the suspected obstruction is great. Special equipment (laryngoscope and endotracheal [ET] tubes) should be available because a tongue blade can cause sudden complete airway obstruction. Trained personnel (such as an anesthesiologist) should be on hand during the throat examination to secure an emergency airway. On the lateral soft tissue X-ray of the neck, a large, thick but indistinct ("thumbprint") epiglottis will be seen. Blood on the throat culture may show *H. influenzae* or other bacteria.

Treatment
A child with acute epiglottiditis and airway obstruction requires emergency hospitalization; he may need emergency ET intubation or a tracheotomy with subsequent monitoring in an intensive care unit. Respiratory distress that interferes with swallowing necessitates parenteral fluid administration to prevent dehydration. A patient with acute epiglottiditis should always receive a complete course of parenteral antibiotics — usually a second- or third-generation cephalosporin. (If the child is allergic to penicillin, a quinolone or sulfa drug may be substituted.)

Special considerations
■ Keep equipment available in case of sudden complete airway obstruction to secure an airway. Be prepared to assist with intubation or tracheotomy, as necessary.

○ **ALERT** *Watch for increasing restlessness, rising cardiac rate, fever, dyspnea, and retractions, which may indicate the need for an emergency tracheotomy. Monitor blood gases for hypoxemia and hypercapnia.*

■ After a tracheotomy, anticipate the patient's needs because he won't be able to cry or call out; provide emotional support. Reassure the patient and his family that the tracheotomy is a short-term intervention (usually from 4 to 7 days). Monitor the patient for rising temperature and pulse rate and hypotension — signs of secondary infection.

■ The bacterial infection causing epiglottiditis is contagious and airborne or droplet precautions should be followed. Family members should be screened.

- Discuss immunizations with the Hib vaccine with the family as a preventive measure, as appropriate.

ACUTE DISORDERS

Acute respiratory distress syndrome

A form of noncardiogenic pulmonary edema that causes acute respiratory failure, acute respiratory distress syndrome (ARDS), also called *shock lung* or *adult respiratory distress syndrome*, results from increased permeability of the alveolocapillary membrane. Fluid accumulates in the lung interstitium, alveolar spaces, and small airways, causing the lung to stiffen. Effective ventilation is thus impaired, prohibiting adequate oxygenation of pulmonary capillary blood. Severe ARDS can cause intractable and fatal hypoxemia. However, patients who recover may have little or no permanent lung damage.

Causes and incidence

ARDS results from many respiratory and nonrespiratory insults, such as:
- aspiration of gastric contents
- sepsis (primarily gram-negative), trauma, or oxygen toxicity
- shock
- viral, bacterial, or fungal pneumonia or microemboli (fat or air emboli or disseminated intravascular coagulation)
- drug overdose (barbiturates, glutethimide, or opioids) or blood transfusion
- smoke or chemical inhalation (nitrous oxide, chlorine, or ammonia)
- hydrocarbon and paraquat ingestion
- pancreatitis, uremia, or miliary tuberculosis (rare)
- near drowning.

Altered permeability of the alveolocapillary membrane causes fluid to accumulate in the interstitial space. If the pulmonary lymphatic glands can't remove this fluid, interstitial edema develops. The fluid collects in the peribronchial and peribronchiolar spaces, producing bronchiolar narrowing. Hypoxemia occurs as a result of fluid accumulation in alveoli and subsequent alveolar collapse, causing the shunting of blood through nonventilated lung regions. In addition, alveolar collapse causes a dramatic increase in lung compliance, which makes it more difficult to achieve adequate ventilation. (See *What happens in ARDS,* page 522.)

ARDS affects 10 to 14 people per 100,000, with a mortality rate of 36% to 52%.

Signs and symptoms

ARDS initially produces rapid, shallow breathing and dyspnea within hours to days of the initial injury (sometimes after the patient's condition appears to have stabilized). Hypoxemia develops, causing an increased drive for ventilation. Because of the effort required to expand the stiff lung, intercostal and suprasternal retractions result. Fluid accumulation produces crackles and rhonchi; worsening hypoxemia causes restlessness, apprehension, mental sluggishness, motor dysfunction, and tachycardia (possibly with transient increased arterial blood pressure).

 ELDER TIP *The older patient may appear to do well following an initial episode of ARDS. Symptoms commonly appear 2 to 3 days later.*

Severe ARDS causes overwhelming hypoxemia. If uncorrected, this results in hypotension, decreasing urine output, respiratory and metabolic acidosis, and eventually ventricular fibrillation or standstill.

Diagnosis

On room air, arterial blood gas (ABG) analysis initially shows decreased partial pressure of arterial oxygen (PaO_2; less than 60 mm Hg) and partial pressure of arterial carbon dioxide ($PaCO_2$; less than 35 mm Hg). The resulting pH usually reflects respiratory alkalosis. As ARDS becomes more severe, ABG analysis shows respiratory acidosis (increasing $PaCO_2$ [more than 45 mm Hg]), metabolic acidosis (decreasing bicarbonate [less than 22 mEq/L]), and a decreasing PaO_2 despite oxygen therapy.

Other diagnostic tests include:
- Pulmonary artery catheterization helps identify the cause of pulmonary edema

PATHOPHYSIOLOGY

WHAT HAPPENS IN ARDS

This flowchart shows the process and progress of acute respiratory distress syndrome (ARDS).

Injury reduces normal blood flow to the lungs, allowing platelets to aggregate.

These platelets release substances, such as serotonin, bradykinin and, especially, histamine. These substances inflame and damage the alveolar membrane and later increase capillary permeability. At this early stage, signs and symptoms of ARDS are undetectable.

Histamine and other inflammatory substances increase capillary permeability, allowing fluid to shift into the interstitial space. As a result, the patient may experience tachypnea, dyspnea, and tachycardia.

As capillary permeability increases, proteins and more fluid leak out, increasing interstitial osmotic pressure and causing pulmonary edema. At this stage, the patient may experience increased tachypnea, dyspnea, and cyanosis. Hypoxia (usually unresponsive to increased fraction of inspired air), decreased pulmonary compliance, and crackles and rhonchi may also develop.

Fluid in the alveoli and decreased blood flow damage surfactant in the alveoli, reducing the cells' ability to produce more. Without surfactant, alveoli collapse, impairing gas exchange. Look for thick, frothy sputum and marked hypoxemia with increased respiratory distress.

The patient breathes faster, but sufficient oxygen (O_2) can't cross the alveolocapillary membrane. Carbon dioxide (CO_2), however, crosses more easily and is lost with every exhalation. O_2 and CO_2 levels in the blood decrease. Look for increased tachypnea, hypoxemia, and hypocapnia.

Pulmonary edema worsens. Meanwhile, inflammation leads to fibrosis, which further impedes gas exchange. The resulting hypoxemia leads to metabolic acidosis. At this stage, look for increased partial pressure of arterial carbon dioxide, decreased pH and partial pressure of arterial oxygen, and mental confusion.

(cardiac versus noncardiac) by evaluating pulmonary artery wedge pressure; allows collection of pulmonary artery blood, which shows decreased oxygen saturation, reflecting tissue hypoxia; measures pulmonary artery pressure; measures cardiac output by thermodilution techniques; and provides information to allow calculation of the percentage of blood shunted through the lungs.

■ Serial chest X-rays initially show bilateral infiltrates. In later stages, a ground-glass appearance and eventually (as hypoxemia becomes irreversible), "whiteouts" of both lung fields are apparent. Medical personnel can differentiate ARDS from heart failure by noting the following on serial chest X-rays:

– normal cardiac silhouette
– diffuse bilateral infiltrates that tend to be more peripheral and patchy, as opposed to the usual perihilar "bat wing" appearance of cardiogenic pulmonary edema
– fewer pleural effusions.

Differential diagnosis must rule out cardiogenic pulmonary edema, pulmonary vasculitis, and diffuse pulmonary hemorrhage. To establish the etiology, laboratory work should include sputum Gram stain, culture and sensitivity tests, and blood cultures to detect infections; a toxicology screen for drug ingestion; and, when pancreatitis is a consideration, a serum amylase determination.

Treatment

When possible, treatment is designed to correct the underlying cause of ARDS as well as to prevent progression and the potentially fatal complications of hypoxemia and respiratory acidosis. Supportive medical care consists of administering humidified oxygen with continuous positive airway pressure. Hypoxemia that doesn't respond adequately to these measures requires ventilatory support with intubation, volume ventilation, and positive end-expiratory pressure (PEEP). Other supportive measures include fluid restriction, diuretics, and correction of electrolyte and acid-base abnormalities.

When ARDS requires mechanical ventilation, sedatives, opioids, or neuromuscular blocking agents may be ordered to opti-

mize ventilation. Treatment to reverse severe metabolic acidosis with sodium bicarbonate may be necessary, although in severe cases this may worsen the acidosis if carbon dioxide can't be cleared adequately. Use of fluids and vasopressors may be required to maintain blood pressure. Infections require appropriate anti-infective therapy.

Special considerations

ARDS requires careful monitoring and supportive care.

■ Frequently assess the patient's respiratory status. Be alert for retractions on inspiration. Note the rate, rhythm, and depth of respirations; watch for dyspnea and the use of accessory muscles of respiration. On auscultation, listen for adventitious or diminished breath sounds. Check for clear, frothy sputum, which may indicate pulmonary edema.

■ Observe and document the hypoxemic patient's neurologic status (level of consciousness and mental status).

■ Maintain a patent airway by suctioning, using sterile, nontraumatic technique. Ensure adequate humidification to help liquefy tenacious secretions.

■ Closely monitor heart rate and blood pressure. Watch for arrhythmias that may result from hypoxemia, acid-base disturbances, or electrolyte imbalance. With pulmonary artery catheterization, know the desired pressure levels. Check readings often and watch for decreasing mixed venous oxygen saturation.

■ Monitor serum electrolytes and correct imbalances. Measure intake and output; weigh the patient daily.

■ Check ventilator settings frequently, and empty condensate from tubing promptly to ensure maximum oxygen delivery. Monitor ABG studies and pulse oximetry. The patient with severe hypoxemia may need controlled mechanical ventilation with positive pressure. Give sedatives, as needed, to reduce restlessness.

■ Because PEEP may decrease cardiac output, check for hypotension, tachycardia, and decreased urine output. Suction only as needed to maintain PEEP or use an in-line suctioning apparatus. Reposition the patient often and record an increase in secretions, temperature, or hypotension that may indicate a deteriorating condition. Monitor peak pressures during ventilation. Because of stiff, noncompliant lungs, the patient is at high risk for barotrauma (pneumothorax), evidenced by increased peak pressures, decreased breath sounds on one side, and restlessness.

■ Monitor nutrition, maintain joint mobility, and prevent skin breakdown. Accurately record calorie intake. Give tube feedings and parenteral nutrition, as ordered. Perform passive range-of-motion exercises or help the patient perform active exercises, if possible. Provide meticulous skin care. Plan patient care to allow periods of uninterrupted sleep.

■ Provide emotional support. Warn the patient who's recovering from ARDS that recovery will take some time and that he will feel weak for a while.

■ Watch for and immediately report all respiratory changes in the patient with injuries that may adversely affect the lungs (especially during the 2- to 3-day period after the injury, when the patient may appear to be improving).

Acute respiratory failure in COPD

In patients with essentially normal lung tissue, acute respiratory failure (ARF) usually means partial pressure of arterial carbon dioxide ($PaCO_2$) above 50 mm Hg and partial pressure of arterial oxygen (PaO_2) below 50 mm Hg. These limits, however, don't apply to patients with chronic obstructive pulmonary disease (COPD), who usually have a consistently high $PaCO_2$ and low PaO_2. In patients with COPD, only acute deterioration in arterial blood gas (ABG) values, with corresponding clinical deterioration, indicates ARF.

Causes and incidence

ARF may develop in patients with COPD as a result of any condition that increases the work of breathing and decreases the respiratory drive. Such conditions include respiratory tract infection (such as bronchitis or pneumonia). The most common precipitating factor is bronchospasm, or

accumulating secretions secondary to cough suppression. Other causes of ARF in COPD include:

■ central nervous system (CNS) depression — head trauma or injudicious use of sedatives, opioids, tranquilizers, or oxygen (O_2)

■ cardiovascular disorders — myocardial infarction, heart failure, or pulmonary emboli

■ airway irritants — smoke or fumes

■ endocrine and metabolic disorders — myxedema or metabolic alkalosis

■ thoracic abnormalities — chest trauma, pneumothorax, or thoracic or abdominal surgery.

The incidence of ARF increases markedly with age and is especially high among people age 65 and older.

Signs and symptoms

In patients who have COPD with ARF, increased ventilation-perfusion mismatch and reduced alveolar ventilation decrease PaO_2 (hypoxemia) and increase $PaCO_2$ (hypercapnia). This rise in carbon dioxide (CO_2) lowers the pH. The resulting hypoxemia and acidemia affect all body organs, especially the CNS and the respiratory and cardiovascular systems.

Specific symptoms vary with the underlying cause of ARF but may include these systems:

■ Respiratory — Rate may be increased, decreased, or normal depending on the cause; respirations may be shallow, deep, or alternate between the two; and air hunger may occur. Cyanosis may or may not be present, depending on the hemoglobin (Hb) level and arterial oxygenation. Auscultation of the chest may reveal crackles, rhonchi, wheezing, or diminished breath sounds.

■ CNS — When hypoxemia and hypercapnia occur, the patient may show evidence of restlessness, confusion, loss of concentration, irritability, tremulousness, diminished tendon reflexes, and papilledema; he may slip into a coma.

■ Cardiovascular — Tachycardia, with increased cardiac output and mildly elevated blood pressure secondary to adrenal release of catecholamine, occurs early in response to low PaO_2. With myocardial hypoxia, arrhythmias may develop. Pulmonary hypertension, secondary to pulmonary capillary vasoconstriction, may cause increased pressures on the right side of the heart, elevated jugular veins, an enlarged liver, and peripheral edema. Stresses on the heart may precipitate cardiac failure.

Diagnosis

Progressive deterioration in ABG levels and pH, when compared with the patient's "normal" values, strongly suggests ARF in COPD. (In patients with essentially normal lung tissue, pH below 7.35 usually indicates ARF, but patients with COPD display an even greater deviation from this normal value, as they do with $PaCO_2$ and PaO_2.)

Other supporting findings include:

- Bicarbonate — Increased levels indicate metabolic alkalosis or reflect metabolic compensation for chronic respiratory acidosis.
- Hematocrit (HCT) and Hb — Abnormally low levels may be due to blood loss, indicating decreased oxygen-carrying capacity. Elevated levels may occur with chronic hypoxemia.
- Serum electrolytes — Hypokalemia and hypochloremia may result from diuretic and corticosteroid therapies used to treat ARF.
- White blood cell count — Count is elevated if ARF is due to bacterial infection; Gram stain and sputum culture can identify pathogens.
- Chest X-ray — findings identify pulmonary pathologic conditions, such as emphysema, atelectasis, lesions, pneumothorax, infiltrates, or effusions.
- Electrocardiogram — Arrhythmias commonly suggest cor pulmonale and myocardial hypoxia.

Treatment

ARF in patients with COPD is an emergency that requires cautious O_2 therapy (using nasal prongs or Venturi mask) to raise the PaO_2. In patients with chronic hypercapnia, O_2 therapy can cause hypoventilation by increasing $PaCO_2$ and decreasing the respiratory drive, necessitating mechanical ventilation. The minimum fraction of inspired air (FIO_2) required to maintain ventilation or O_2 saturation

greater than 85% to 90% should be used. If significant uncompensated respiratory acidosis or unrefractory hypoxemia exists, mechanical ventilation (through an endotracheal [ET] or a tracheostomy tube) or noninvasive ventilation (with a face or nose mask) may be necessary. Treatment routinely includes antibiotics for infection, bronchodilators, and possibly steroids.

Special considerations

- Because most patients with ARF are treated in an intensive care unit, orient them to the environment, procedures, and routines to minimize their anxiety.
- To reverse hypoxemia, administer O_2 at appropriate concentrations to maintain PaO_2 at a minimum of 50 to 60 mm Hg. Patients with COPD usually require only small amounts of supplemental O_2. Watch for a positive response — such as improvement in the patient's breathing, color, and ABG levels.
- Maintain a patent airway. If the patient is retaining CO_2, encourage him to cough and to breathe deeply. Teach him to use pursed-lip and diaphragmatic breathing to control dyspnea. If the patient is alert, have him use an incentive spirometer; if he's intubated and lethargic, turn him every 1 to 2 hours. Use postural drainage and chest physiotherapy to help clear secretions.
- In an intubated patient, suction the trachea as needed after hyperoxygenation. Observe for a change in quantity, consistency, and color of sputum. Provide humidification to liquefy secretions.
- Observe the patient closely for respiratory arrest. Auscultate for chest sounds. Monitor ABG levels and report any changes immediately.
- Check the cardiac monitor for arrhythmias.

If the patient requires mechanical ventilation:

- Check ventilator settings, cuff pressures, and ABG values often because the FIO_2 setting depends on ABG levels. Draw specimens for ABG analysis 20 to 30 minutes after every FIO_2 change or oximetry check.
- Prevent infection by using sterile technique while suctioning.
- Stress ulcers are common in the intubated patient. Check gastric secretions for evi-

dence of bleeding if the patient has a naso-gastric tube or if he complains of epigastric tenderness, nausea, or vomiting. Monitor Hb level and HCT; check all stools for occult blood. Administer antacids, histamine-2 receptor antagonists, or sucralfate, as ordered.

■ Prevent tracheal erosion, which can result from artificial airway cuff overinflation. Use the minimal leak technique and a cuffed tube with high residual volume (low-pressure cuff), a foam cuff, or a pressure-regulating valve on the cuff.

■ To prevent oral or vocal cord trauma, make sure that the ET tube is positioned midline or moved carefully from side to side every 8 hours.

■ To prevent nasal necrosis, keep the naso-tracheal tube midline within the nostrils and provide good hygiene. Loosen the tape periodically to prevent skin breakdown. Avoid excessive movement of any tubes; make sure the ventilator tubing is adequately supported.

Pulmonary edema

Pulmonary edema is the accumulation of fluid in the extravascular spaces of the lung. In cardiogenic pulmonary edema, fluid accumulation results from elevations in pulmonary venous and capillary hydrostatic pressures. A common complication of cardiac disorders, pulmonary edema can occur as a chronic condition or it can develop quickly to cause death.

Causes

Pulmonary edema usually results from left-sided heart failure due to arteriosclerotic, hypertensive, cardiomyopathic, or valvular cardiac disease. In such disorders, the compromised left ventricle in unable to maintain adequate cardiac output; increased pressures are transmitted to the left atrium, pulmonary veins, and pulmonary capillary bed. This increased pulmonary capillary hydrostatic force promotes transudation of intravascular fluids into the pulmonary interstitium, decreasing lung compliance and interfering with gas exchange. Other factors that may predispose the patient to pulmonary edema include:

■ excessive infusion of I.V. fluids
■ decreased serum colloid osmotic pressure as a result of nephrosis, protein-losing enteropathy, extensive burns, hepatic disease, or nutritional deficiency
■ impaired lung lymphatic drainage from Hodgkin's disease or obliterative lymphangitis after radiation
■ mitral stenosis, which impairs left atrial emptying
■ pulmonary veno-occlusive disease.

Signs and symptoms

The early symptoms of pulmonary edema reflect interstitial fluid accumulation and diminished lung compliance: dyspnea on exertion, paroxysmal nocturnal dyspnea, orthopnea, and coughing. Clinical features include tachycardia, tachypnea, dependent crackles, jugular vein distention, and a diastolic (S_3) gallop. With severe pulmonary edema, the alveoli and bronchioles may fill with fluid and intensify the early symptoms. Respiration becomes labored and rapid, with more diffuse crackles and coughing that produces frothy, bloody sputum. Tachycardia increases, and arrhythmias may occur. Skin becomes cold, clammy, diaphoretic, and cyanotic. Blood pressure falls and the pulse becomes thready as cardiac output falls.

Symptoms of severe heart failure with pulmonary edema may also include signs of hypoxemia, such as anxiety, restlessness, and changes in the patient's level of consciousness.

Diagnosis

Clinical features of pulmonary edema permit a working diagnosis. Arterial blood gas (ABG) analysis usually shows hypoxia; the partial pressure of arterial carbon dioxide is variable. Profound respiratory alkalosis and acidosis may occur. Chest X-ray shows diffuse haziness of the lung fields and, commonly, cardiomegaly and pleural effusions. Ultrasound (echocardiogram) may show weak heart muscle, leaking or narrow heart valves, and fluid surrounding the heart. Pulmonary artery catheterization helps identify left-sided heart failure by showing elevated pulmonary wedge pressures. This helps to rule out acute respiratory distress syndrome—in which pulmonary wedge pressure is usually normal.

Treatment

Treatment measures for pulmonary edema are designed to reduce extravascular fluid, improve gas exchange and myocardial function and, if possible, correct any underlying pathologic conditions.

Administration of high concentrations of oxygen by a cannula, a face mask and, if the patient fails to maintain an acceptable partial pressure of arterial oxygen level, assisted ventilation improves oxygen delivery to the tissues and usually improves acid-base disturbances. Diuretics—furosemide and bumetanide, for example—promote diuresis, which reduces extravascular fluid.

Treatment of heart failure includes angiotensin-converting enzyme inhibitors, diuretics, inotropic drugs such as digoxin, antiarrhythmic agents, beta-adrenergic blockers, and human B-type natriuretic peptide. Vasodilator drugs, such as nitroprusside, may be used to reduce preload and afterload in acute episodes of pulmonary edema.

Morphine is used to reduce anxiety and dyspnea as well as dilate the systemic venous bed, promoting blood flow from pulmonary circulation to the periphery.

Special considerations

■ Carefully monitor the vulnerable patient for early signs of pulmonary edema, especially tachypnea, tachycardia, and abnormal breath sounds. Report any abnormalities. Assess for peripheral edema and weight gain, which may also indicate that fluid is accumulating in tissue.
■ Administer oxygen as ordered.
■ Monitor the patient's vital signs every 15 to 30 minutes while administering nitroprusside in dextrose 5% in water by I.V. drip. Protect the nitroprusside solution from light by wrapping the bottle or bag with aluminum foil, and discard unused solution after 4 hours. Watch for arrhythmias in the patient receiving cardiac glycosides and for marked respiratory depression in the patient receiving morphine.
■ Assess the patient's condition frequently, and record response to treatment. Monitor ABG levels, oral and I.V. fluid intake, urine

output and, in the patient with a pulmonary artery catheter, pulmonary end-diastolic and wedge pressures. Check the cardiac monitor often. Report changes immediately.
■ Carefully record the time and amount of morphine given.
■ Reassure the patient, who will have be anxious due to hypoxia and respiratory distress. Explain all procedures. Provide emotional support to his family as well.

Cor pulmonale

The World Health Organization defines chronic cor pulmonale as "hypertrophy of the right ventricle resulting from diseases affecting the function or the structure of the lungs, except when these pulmonary alterations are the result of diseases that primarily affect the left side of the heart or of congenital heart disease." Invariably, cor pulmonale follows some disorder of the lungs, pulmonary vessels, chest wall, or respiratory control center. For instance, chronic obstructive pulmonary disease (COPD) produces pulmonary hypertension, which leads to right ventricular hypertrophy and right-sided heart failure. Because cor pulmonale generally occurs late during the course of COPD and other irreversible diseases, the prognosis is generally poor.

Causes and incidence

Approximately 85% of patients with cor pulmonale have COPD, and 25% of patients with COPD eventually develop cor pulmonale.

Other respiratory disorders that produce cor pulmonale include:
■ obstructive lung diseases—for example, bronchiectasis and cystic fibrosis
■ restrictive lung diseases—for example, pneumoconiosis, interstitial pneumonitis, scleroderma, and sarcoidosis
■ loss of lung tissue after extensive lung surgery
■ congenital cardiac shunts—such as a ventricular septal defect
■ pulmonary vascular diseases—for example, recurrent thromboembolism, pri-

mary pulmonary hypertension, schistoso-miasis, and pulmonary vasculitis
■ respiratory insufficiency without pulmonary disease—for example, in chest wall disorders such as kyphoscoliosis, neuromuscular incompetence due to muscular dystrophy and amyotrophic lateral sclerosis, polymyositis, and spinal cord lesions above C6
■ obesity hypoventilation syndrome (pickwickian syndrome) and upper airway obstruction
■ living at high altitudes (chronic mountain sickness).

Pulmonary capillary destruction and pulmonary vasoconstriction (usually secondary to hypoxia) reduce the area of the pulmonary vascular bed. Thus, pulmonary vascular resistance is increased, causing pulmonary hypertension. To compensate for the extra work needed to force blood through the lungs, the right ventricle dilates and hypertrophies. In response to low oxygen content, the bone marrow produces more red blood cells (RBCs), causing erythrocytosis. When the hematocrit (HCT) exceeds 55%, blood viscosity increases, which further aggravates pulmonary hypertension and increases the hemodynamic load on the right ventricle. Right-sided heart failure is the result.

Cor pulmonale accounts for about 25% of all types of heart failure. It's most common in areas of the world where the incidence of cigarette smoking and COPD is high; cor pulmonale affects middle-age to elderly men more often than women, but incidence in women is increasing. In children, cor pulmonale may be a complication of cystic fibrosis, hemosiderosis, upper airway obstruction, scleroderma, extensive bronchiectasis, neurologic diseases affecting respiratory muscles, or abnormalities of the respiratory control center.

Signs and symptoms
As long as the heart can compensate for the increased pulmonary vascular resistance, clinical features reflect the underlying disorder and occur mostly in the respiratory system. They include chronic productive cough, exertional dyspnea, wheezing respirations, fatigue, and weakness. Progression of cor pulmonale is associated with dyspnea (even at rest) that worsens on exertion, tachypnea, orthopnea, edema, weakness, and right upper quadrant discomfort. Chest examination reveals findings characteristic of the underlying lung disease.

Signs of cor pulmonale and right-sided heart failure include dependent edema; distended jugular veins; prominent parasternal or epigastric cardiac impulse; hepatojugular reflux; an enlarged, tender liver; ascites; and tachycardia. Decreased cardiac output may cause a weak pulse and hypotension. Chest examination yields various findings, depending on the underlying cause of cor pulmonale.

In COPD, auscultation reveals wheezing, rhonchi, and diminished breath sounds. When the disease is secondary to upper airway obstruction or damage to central nervous system respiratory centers, chest findings may be normal, except for a right ventricular lift, gallop rhythm, and loud pulmonic component of S_2. Tricuspid insufficiency produces a pansystolic murmur heard at the lower left sternal border; its intensity increases on inspiration, distinguishing it from a murmur due to mitral valve disease. A right ventricular early murmur that increases on inspiration can be heard at the left sternal border or over the epigastrium. A systolic pulmonic ejection click may also be heard. Alterations in the patient's level of consciousness may occur.

Diagnosis
■ Pulmonary artery pressure measurements show increased right ventricular and pulmonary artery pressures, stemming from increased pulmonary vascular resistance. Right ventricular systolic and pulmonary artery systolic pressures will exceed 30 mm Hg. Pulmonary artery diastolic pressure will exceed 15 mm Hg.
■ Echocardiography or angiography indicates right ventricular enlargement; echocardiography can estimate pulmonary artery pressure while also ruling out structural and congenital lesions.
■ Chest X-ray shows large central pulmonary arteries and suggests right ventricular enlargement by rightward enlargement of the heart's silhouette on an anterior chest film.

- Arterial blood gas (ABG) analysis shows decreased partial pressure of arterial oxygen (PaO_2; typically less than 70 mm Hg and usually no more than 90 mm Hg on room air).
- Electrocardiogram frequently shows arrhythmias, such as premature atrial and ventricular contractions and atrial fibrillation during severe hypoxia; it may also show right bundle-branch block, right axis deviation, prominent P waves and inverted T wave in right precordial leads, and right ventricular hypertrophy.
- Pulmonary function tests show results consistent with the underlying pulmonary disease.
- HCT is typically greater than 50%.

Treatment

Treatment of cor pulmonale is designed to reduce hypoxemia, increase the patient's exercise tolerance and, when possible, correct the underlying condition.

In addition to bed rest, treatment may include administration of:
- a cardiac glycoside (digoxin)
- antibiotics when respiratory infection is present; culture and sensitivity of a sputum specimen helps select an antibiotic
- potent pulmonary artery vasodilators (such as diazoxide, nitroprusside, hydralazine, angiotensin-converting enzyme inhibitors, calcium channel blockers, or prostaglandins) in primary pulmonary hypertension
- oxygen by mask or cannula in concentrations ranging from 24% to 40%, depending on PaO_2, as necessary; in acute cases, therapy may also include mechanical ventilation; patients with underlying COPD generally shouldn't receive high concentrations of oxygen because of possible subsequent respiratory depression
- a low-salt diet, restricted fluid intake, and diuretics, such as furosemide, to reduce edema
- phlebotomy to reduce the RBC count
- anticoagulants to reduce the risk of thromboembolism.

Depending on the underlying cause, some variations in treatment may be indicated. For example, a tracheotomy may be necessary if the patient has an upper airway obstruction. Steroids may be used in the patient with a vasculitis autoimmune phenomenon or acute exacerbations of COPD.

Special considerations

- Plan diet carefully with the patient and staff dietitian. Because the patient may lack energy and tire easily when eating, provide small, frequent feedings rather than three heavy meals.
- Prevent fluid retention by limiting the patient's fluid intake to 1 to 2 qt (1 to 2 L)/day and providing a low-sodium diet.
- Monitor serum potassium levels closely if the patient is receiving diuretics. Low serum potassium levels can increase the risk of arrhythmias associated with cardiac glycosides.
- Watch the patient for signs of digoxin toxicity, such as complaints of anorexia, nausea, vomiting, and halos around visual images and color perception shifts. Monitor for cardiac arrhythmias. Teach the patient to check his radial pulse before taking digoxin or any cardiac glycoside. He should be instructed to notify the physician if he detects changes in pulse rate.
- Reposition bedridden patients often to prevent atelectasis.
- Provide meticulous respiratory care, including oxygen therapy and, for the patient with COPD, pursed-lip breathing exercises. Periodically measure ABG levels and watch for signs of respiratory failure: changes in pulse rate, labored respirations, changes in mental status, and increased fatigue after exertion.

Before discharge, maintain the following protocol:
- Make sure that the patient understands the importance of maintaining a low-salt diet, weighing himself daily, and watching for increased edema. Teach him to detect edema by pressing the skin over a shin with one finger, holding it for a second or two, then checking for a finger impression. Increased weight, increased edema, or respiratory difficulty should be reported to the health care provider.
- Instruct the patient to plan for frequent rest periods and to do breathing exercises regularly.
- If the patient needs supplemental oxygen therapy at home, refer him to an

agency that can help obtain the required equipment and, as necessary, arrange for follow-up examinations.

■ If the patient has been placed on anticoagulant therapy, emphasize the need to watch for bleeding (epistaxis, hematuria, bruising) and to report signs to the physician. Also encourage him to return for periodic laboratory tests to monitor partial thromboplastin time, fibrinogen level, platelet count, HCT and hemoglobin, and prothrombin time.

■ Because pulmonary infection commonly exacerbates COPD and cor pulmonale, tell the patient to watch for and immediately report early signs of infection, such as increased sputum production, change in sputum color, increased coughing or wheezing, chest pain, fever, and tightness in the chest. Tell the patient to avoid crowds and persons known to have pulmonary infections, especially during the flu season. The patient should receive pneumovax and annual influenza vaccines.

■ Warn the patient to avoid substances that may depress the ventilatory drive, such as sedatives and alcohol.

Legionnaires' disease

Legionnaires' disease is an acute bronchopneumonia produced by a gram-negative bacillus. It derives its name and notoriety from the peculiar, highly publicized disease that struck 182 people (29 of whom died) at an American Legion convention in Philadelphia in July 1976. This disease may occur epidemically or sporadically, usually in late summer or early fall. Its severity ranges from a mild illness, with or without pneumonitis, to multilobar pneumonia, with a mortality as high as 15%. A milder, self-limiting form (Pontiac syndrome) subsides within a few days but leaves the patient fatigued for several weeks. This form mimics Legionnaires' disease but produces few or no respiratory symptoms, no pneumonia, and no fatalities.

Causes and incidence
The causative agent of Legionnaires' disease, *Legionella pneumophila*, is an aerobic, gram-negative bacillus that's probably

transmitted by an airborne route. In past epidemics, it has spread through cooling towers or evaporation condensers in air-conditioning systems. However, *Legionella* bacilli also flourish in soil and excavation sites. The disease doesn't spread from person to person.

Legionnaires' disease is most likely to affect:

■ middle-age and elderly people
■ immunocompromised patients (particularly those receiving corticosteroids, for example, after a transplant) or those with lymphoma or other disorders associated with delayed hypersensitivity
■ patients with a chronic underlying disease, such as diabetes, chronic renal failure, or chronic obstructive pulmonary disease
■ those with alcoholism
■ cigarette smokers
■ those on a ventilator for extended periods

Signs and symptoms
The multisystem clinical features of Legionnaires' disease follow a predictable sequence, although the onset of the disease may be gradual or sudden. After a 2- to 10-day incubation period, nonspecific, prodromal signs and symptoms appear, including diarrhea, anorexia, malaise, diffuse myalgias and generalized weakness, headache, and recurrent chills. An unremitting fever develops within 12 to 48 hours with a temperature that may reach 105° F (40.6° C). A cough then develops that's nonproductive initially but eventually may produce grayish, nonpurulent, and occasionally blood-streaked sputum.

Other characteristic features include nausea, vomiting, disorientation, mental sluggishness, confusion, mild temporary amnesia, pleuritic chest pain, tachypnea, dyspnea, and fine crackles. Patients who develop pneumonia may also experience hypoxia. Other complications include hypotension, delirium, heart failure, arrhythmias, acute respiratory failure, renal failure, and shock (usually fatal).

Diagnosis
The patient history focuses on possible sources of infection and predisposing conditions. Additional tests reveal:

■ Chest X-ray shows patchy, localized infiltration, which progresses to multilobar consolidation (usually involving the lower lobes), pleural effusion and, in fulminant disease, opacification of the entire lung.

■ Auscultation reveals fine crackles, progressing to coarse crackles as the disease advances.

■ Abnormal findings include leukocytosis, increased erythrocyte sedimentation rate, an increase in liver enzyme levels (alanine aminotransferase, aspartate aminotransferase, and alkaline phosphatase), hyponatremia, decreased partial pressure of arterial oxygen and, initially, decreased partial pressure of arterial carbon dioxide. Bronchial washings and blood, pleural fluid, and sputum tests rule out other infections.

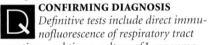

CONFIRMING DIAGNOSIS
Definitive tests include direct immunofluorescence of respiratory tract secretions and tissue, culture of L. pneumophila, and indirect fluorescent antibody testing of serum comparing acute samples with convalescent samples drawn at least 3 weeks later. A convalescent serum showing a fourfold or greater rise in antibody titer for Legionella confirms the diagnosis.

Treatment

Antibiotic treatment begins as soon as Legionnaires' disease is suspected and diagnostic material is collected; it shouldn't await laboratory confirmation. Quinolone (ciprofloxacin, levofloxacin, moxifloxacin, or gatifloxacin) is commonly used, although a macrolide (azithromycin, clarithromycin, or erythromycin) may be prescribed for some patients. Supportive therapy includes administration of antipyretics, fluid replacement, circulatory support with pressor drugs, if necessary, and oxygen administration by mask, cannula, or mechanical ventilation.

Special considerations

■ Closely monitor the patient's respiratory status. Evaluate chest wall expansion, depth and pattern of respirations, cough, and chest pain. Watch for restlessness as a sign of hypoxemia, which requires suctioning, repositioning, or more aggressive oxygen therapy.

■ Continually monitor the patient's vital signs, oximetry or arterial blood gas values, level of consciousness, and dryness and color of lips and mucous membranes. Watch for signs of shock (decreased blood pressure, thready pulse, diaphoresis, and clammy skin).

■ Keep the patient comfortable. Provide mouth care frequently. If necessary, apply soothing cream to the nostrils.

■ Replace fluid and electrolytes, as needed. The patient with renal failure may require dialysis.

■ Provide mechanical ventilation and other respiratory therapy, as needed. Teach the patient how to cough effectively, and encourage deep-breathing exercises. Stress the need to continue these until recovery is complete.

■ Give antibiotic therapy as ordered, and observe carefully for adverse effects.

Atelectasis

Atelectasis is incomplete expansion of lobules (clusters of alveoli) or lung segments, which may result in partial or complete lung collapse. Because parts of the lung are unavailable for gas exchange, unoxygenated blood passes through these areas unchanged, resulting in hypoxemia. Atelectasis may be chronic or acute. Many patients undergoing upper abdominal or thoracic surgery experience atelectasis to some degree. The prognosis depends on prompt removal of any airway obstruction, relief of hypoxemia, and reexpansion of the collapsed lung.

Causes

Atelectasis commonly results from bronchial occlusion by mucus plugs. It's a problem in many patients with chronic obstructive pulmonary disease, bronchiectasis, or cystic fibrosis and in those who smoke heavily. (Smoking increases mucus production and damages cilia.) Atelectasis may also result from occlusion by foreign bodies, bronchogenic carcinoma, and inflammatory lung disease.

Other causes include respiratory distress syndrome of the neonate (hyaline membrane disease), oxygen toxicity, and pulmonary edema, in which alveolar surfactant changes increase surface tension and permit complete alveolar deflation.

External compression, which inhibits full lung expansion, or any condition that makes deep breathing painful, may also cause atelectasis. Such compression or pain may result from abdominal surgical incisions, rib fractures, pleuritic chest pain, tight dressings around the chest, stab wounds, impalement accidents, car accidents in which the driver slams into the steering column, or obesity (which elevates the diaphragm and reduces tidal volume).

Prolonged immobility may also cause atelectasis by producing preferential ventilation of one area of the lung over another. Mechanical ventilation using constant small tidal volumes without intermittent deep breaths may also result in atelectasis. Central nervous system depression (as in drug overdose) eliminates periodic sighing and is a predisposing factor of progressive atelectasis.

Signs and symptoms

Clinical effects vary with the cause of collapse, the degree of hypoxemia, and any underlying disease but generally include some degree of dyspnea. Atelectasis of a small area of the lung may produce only minimal symptoms that subside without specific treatment. However, massive collapse can produce severe dyspnea, anxiety, cyanosis, diaphoresis, peripheral circulatory collapse, tachycardia, and substernal or intercostal retraction. Also, atelectasis may result in compensatory hyperinflation of unaffected areas of the lung, mediastinal shift to the affected side, and elevation of the ipsilateral hemidiaphragm.

Diagnosis

Diagnosis requires an accurate patient history, a physical examination, and a chest X-ray. Auscultation reveals diminished or bronchial breath sounds. When much of the lung is collapsed, percussion reveals dullness. However, extensive areas of "microatelectasis" may exist without abnormalities on the chest X-ray. In widespread atelectasis, the chest X-ray shows characteristic horizontal lines in the lower lung zones. With segmental or lobar collapse,

characteristic dense shadows commonly associated with hyperinflation of neighboring lung zones are also apparent. If the cause is unknown, diagnostic procedures may include bronchoscopy to rule out an obstructing neoplasm or a foreign body.

Treatment

Treatment includes incentive spirometry, frequent coughing, and deep-breathing exercises. If atelectasis is secondary to mucus plugging, mucolytics, chest percussion, and postural drainage may be used. If these measures fail, bronchoscopy may be helpful in removing secretions. Humidity and bronchodilators can improve mucociliary clearance and dilate airways.

Atelectasis secondary to an obstructing neoplasm may require surgery or radiation therapy. Postoperative thoracic and abdominal surgery patients require analgesics to facilitate deep breathing, which minimizes the risk of atelectasis.

Special considerations

- To prevent atelectasis, encourage the postoperative or other high-risk patient to cough and deep-breathe every 1 to 2 hours. To minimize pain during coughing exercises, splint the incision; teach the patient this technique as well. Gently reposition the patient often and encourage ambulation as soon as possible. Administer adequate analgesics.
- If mechanical ventilation is used, tidal volume should be maintained at appropriate levels to ensure adequate expansion of the lungs. Use the sigh mechanism on the ventilator, if appropriate, to intermittently increase tidal volume at the rate of 10 to 15 sighs/hour.
- Use an incentive spirometer to encourage deep inspiration through positive reinforcement. Teach the patient how to use the spirometer, and encourage him to use it every 1 to 2 hours.
- Humidify inspired air and encourage adequate fluid intake to mobilize secretions. To promote loosening and clearance of secretions, encourage deep-breathing and coughing exercises and use postural drainage and chest percussion.
- If the patient is intubated or uncooperative, provide suctioning, as needed. Use

sedatives with discretion because they depress respirations and the cough reflex as well as suppress sighing. However, remember that the patient won't cooperate with treatment if he's in pain.
- Assess breath sounds and ventilatory status frequently; report changes at once.
- Teach the patient about respiratory care, including postural drainage, coughing, and deep breathing.
- Encourage the patient to stop smoking and lose weight, as needed. Refer him to appropriate support groups for help.
- Provide reassurance and emotional support; the patient may be anxious due to hypoxia or respiratory distress.

Respiratory acidosis

An acid-base disturbance characterized by reduced alveolar ventilation and manifested by hypercapnia (partial pressure of arterial carbon dioxide [$PaCO_2$] greater than 45 mm Hg), respiratory acidosis can be acute (due to a sudden failure in ventilation) or chronic (as in long-term pulmonary disease). The prognosis depends on the severity of the underlying disturbance as well as the patient's general clinical condition.

Causes
Some predisposing factors in respiratory acidosis include:
- Drugs — Opioids, anesthetics, hypnotics, and sedatives, including some of the new designer drugs, such as ecstasy, decrease the sensitivity of the respiratory center.
- Central nervous system (CNS) trauma — Medullary injury may impair ventilatory drive.
- Chronic metabolic alkalosis — Respiratory compensatory mechanisms attempt to normalize pH by decreasing alveolar ventilation.
- Ventilation therapy — Use of high-flow oxygen (O_2) in chronic respiratory disorders suppresses the patient's hypoxic drive to breathe.
- Neuromuscular diseases (such as myasthenia gravis, Guillain-Barré syndrome, and poliomyelitis) — Failure of the respiratory muscles to respond properly to respiratory drive decreases alveolar ventilation.
- In addition, respiratory acidosis can result from airway obstruction or parenchymal lung disease, which interferes with alveolar ventilation; chronic obstructive pulmonary disease (COPD); asthma; severe acute respiratory distress syndrome; chronic bronchitis; large pneumothorax; extensive pneumonia; and pulmonary edema.

Hypoventilation compromises elimination of carbon dioxide (CO_2) produced through metabolism. The retained CO_2 then combines with water to form an excess of carbonic acid, decreasing the blood pH. As a result, concentration of hydrogen ions in body fluids, which directly reflects acidity, increases.

Signs and symptoms
Acute respiratory acidosis produces CNS disturbances that reflect changes in the pH of cerebrospinal fluid rather than increased CO_2 levels in cerebral circulation. Effects range from restlessness, confusion, and apprehension to somnolence, with a fine or flapping tremor (asterixis), or coma. The patient may complain of headaches as well as exhibit dyspnea and tachypnea with papilledema and depressed reflexes. Unless the patient is receiving O_2, hypoxemia accompanies respiratory acidosis. This disorder may also cause cardiovascular abnormalities, such as tachycardia, hypertension, atrial and ventricular arrhythmias and, in severe acidosis, hypotension with vasodilation (bounding pulses and warm periphery).

Diagnosis
CONFIRMING DIAGNOSIS
Arterial blood gas (ABG) analysis confirms the diagnosis: $PaCO_2$ exceeds the normal 45 mm Hg; pH is below the normal range of 7.35 to 7.45 unless compensation has occurred; and bicarbonate is normal in the acute stage but elevated in the chronic stage.

Chest X-ray, computed tomography scan, and pulmonary function tests can help determine the cause.

Treatment

Effective treatment of respiratory acidosis requires correction of the underlying source of alveolar hypoventilation.

Significantly reduced alveolar ventilation may require mechanical ventilation until the underlying condition can be treated. In COPD, this includes bronchodilators, O_2, corticosteroids, and antibiotics for infectious conditions; drug therapy for conditions such as myasthenia gravis; removal of foreign bodies from the airway; antibiotics for pneumonia; dialysis or charcoal to remove toxic drugs; and correcting metabolic alkalosis.

Dangerously low blood pH (less than 7.15) can produce profound CNS and cardiovascular deterioration; careful administration of I.V. sodium bicarbonate may be required. In chronic lung disease, elevated CO_2 may persist despite optimal treatment.

Special considerations

■ Be alert for critical changes in the patient's respiratory, CNS, and cardiovascular functions. Report such changes as well as any variations in ABG values or electrolyte status immediately. Also, maintain adequate hydration.

■ Maintain a patent airway and provide adequate humidification if acidosis requires mechanical ventilation. Perform tracheal suctioning regularly and vigorous chest physiotherapy, if ordered. Continuously monitor ventilator settings and respiratory status.

■ To prevent respiratory acidosis, closely monitor patients with COPD and chronic CO_2 retention for signs of acidosis. Also, administer O_2 at low flow rates; closely monitor all patients who receive opioids and sedatives. Instruct patients who have received general anesthesia to turn, cough, and perform deep-breathing exercises frequently to prevent the onset of respiratory acidosis.

Respiratory alkalosis

Respiratory alkalosis is an acid-base disturbance characterized by a decrease in the partial pressure of arterial carbon dioxide ($PaCO_2$) to less than 35 mm Hg, which is due to alveolar hyperventilation. Uncomplicated respiratory alkalosis leads to a decrease in hydrogen ion concentration, which results in elevated blood pH. Hypocapnia occurs when the elimination of carbon dioxide (CO_2) by the lungs exceeds the production of CO_2 at the cellular level.

Causes

Causes of respiratory alkalosis fall into two categories:

■ pulmonary — severe hypoxemia, pneumonia, interstitial lung disease, pulmonary vascular disease, and acute asthma

■ nonpulmonary — anxiety, fever, aspirin toxicity, metabolic acidosis, central nervous system (CNS) disease (inflammation or tumor), sepsis, hepatic failure, and pregnancy.

Signs and symptoms

The cardinal sign of respiratory alkalosis is deep, rapid breathing, possibly exceeding 40 breaths/minute. This pattern of breathing is similar to Kussmaul's respirations that characterize diabetic acidosis. Such hyperventilation usually leads to CNS and neuromuscular disturbances, such as lightheadedness or dizziness (due to below-normal CO_2 levels that decrease cerebral blood flow), agitation, circumoral and peripheral paresthesias, carpopedal spasms, twitching (possibly progressing to tetany), and muscle weakness. Severe respiratory alkalosis may cause cardiac arrhythmias (that may fail to respond to conventional treatment), seizures, or both.

Diagnosis

CONFIRMING DIAGNOSIS
Arterial blood gas (ABG) analysis confirms respiratory alkalosis and rules out respiratory compensation for metabolic acidosis: $PaCO_2$ less than 35 mm Hg; pH elevated in proportion to the fall in $PaCO_2$ in the acute stage, but falling toward normal in the chronic stage; and bicarbonate normal in the acute stage, but below normal in the chronic stage.

Chest X-ray or pulmonary function tests may aid in diagnosing possible lung disease.

Treatment

Treatment is designed to eradicate the underlying condition — for example, removal of ingested toxins, treatment of fever or sepsis, providing oxygen for acute hypoxemia, and treatment of CNS disease. When hyperventilation is caused by severe anxiety, the patient may be instructed to breathe into a paper bag, which increases CO_2 levels and helps relieve anxiety.

Prevention of hyperventilation in patients receiving mechanical ventilation requires monitoring ABG levels and adjusting tidal volume and minute ventilation.

Special considerations

■ Watch for and report any changes in neurologic, neuromuscular, or cardiovascular functions.

■ Remember that twitching and cardiac arrhythmias may be associated with alkalemia and electrolyte imbalances. Monitor ABG and serum electrolyte levels closely, reporting any variations immediately.

■ Explain all diagnostic tests and procedures to reduce anxiety.

Pneumothorax

Pneumothorax is an accumulation of air or gas between the parietal and visceral pleurae. The amount of air or gas trapped in the intrapleural space determines the degree of lung collapse. In tension pneumothorax, the air in the pleural space is under higher pressure than air in adjacent lung and vascular structures. Without prompt treatment, tension or large pneumothorax results in fatal pulmonary and circulatory impairment.

Causes and incidence

Spontaneous pneumothorax usually occurs in otherwise healthy adults ages 20 to 40. It may be caused by air leakage from ruptured congenital blebs adjacent to the visceral pleural surface, near the apex of the lung. Secondary spontaneous pneumothorax is a complication of underlying lung disease, such as chronic obstructive pulmonary disease, asthma, cystic fibrosis, tuberculosis, and whooping cough. Spontaneous pneumothorax may also occur in interstitial lung disease, such as eosinophilic granuloma or lymphangiomyomatosis.

Traumatic pneumothorax may result from insertion of a central venous line, thoracic surgery, or a penetrating chest injury, such as a gunshot or knife wound. It may follow a transbronchial biopsy, or it may also occur during thoracentesis or a closed pleural biopsy. When traumatic pneumothorax follows a penetrating chest injury, it frequently coexists with hemothorax (blood in the pleural space).

In *tension pneumothorax,* positive pleural pressure develops as a result of traumatic pneumothorax. When air enters the pleural space through a tear in lung tissue and is unable to leave by the same vent, each inspiration traps air in the pleural space, resulting in positive pleural pressure. This in turn causes collapse of the ipsilateral lung and marked impairment of venous return, which can severely compromise cardiac output and may cause a mediastinal shift. Decreased filling of the great veins of the chest results in diminished cardiac output and lowered blood pressure.

Pneumothorax can also be classified as open or closed. In *open pneumothorax* (usually the result of trauma), air flows between the pleural space and the outside of the body. In *closed pneumothorax,* air reaches the pleural space directly from the lung.

Signs and symptoms

The cardinal features of pneumothorax are sudden, sharp, pleuritic pain (exacerbated by movement of the chest, breathing, and coughing); asymmetrical chest wall movement; and shortness of breath. Additional signs of tension pneumothorax are weak and rapid pulse, pallor, jugular vein distention, and anxiety. Tracheal deviations may be present with mediastinal shift. Tension pneumothorax produces the most severe respiratory symptoms; a spontaneous pneumothorax that releases only a small amount of air into the pleural space may cause no symptoms. In a nontension pneumothorax, the severity of symptoms is usually related to the size of the pneumothorax and the degree of preexisting respiratory disease.

Diagnosis

Sudden, sharp chest pain and shortness of breath suggest pneumothorax.

 CONFIRMING DIAGNOSIS *Chest X-ray showing air in the pleural space and, possibly, mediastinal shift confirm this diagnosis.*

In the absence of a definitive chest X-ray, the physical examination may reveal:

■ on inspection — overexpansion and rigidity of the affected chest side; in tension pneumothorax, jugular vein distention with hypotension and tachycardia

■ on palpation — crackling beneath the skin, indicating subcutaneous emphysema (air in tissue) and decreased vocal fremitus

■ on percussion — hyperresonance on the affected side

■ on auscultation — decreased or absent breath sounds over the collapsed lung.

If the pneumothorax is significant, arterial blood gas findings include pH less than 7.35, partial pressure of arterial oxygen less than 80 mm Hg, and partial pressure of arterial carbon dioxide above 45 mm Hg.

Treatment

Treatment is conservative for spontaneous pneumothorax in which no signs of increased pleural pressure (indicating tension pneumothorax) appear, lung collapse is less than 30%, and the patient shows no signs of dyspnea or other indications of physiologic compromise. Such treatment consists of bed rest, careful monitoring of blood pressure and pulse and respiratory rates, oxygen administration and, possibly, needle aspiration of air with a large-bore needle attached to a syringe. If more than 30% of the lung is collapsed, treatment to reexpand the lung includes placing a thoracostomy tube in the second or third intercostal space in the midclavicular line (or in the fifth or sixth intercostal space in the midaxillary line), connected to an underwater seal or low suction pressures.

Recurring spontaneous pneumothorax requires thoracotomy and pleurectomy; these procedures prevent recurrence by causing the lung to adhere to the parietal pleura. Traumatic and tension pneumothoraces require chest tube drainage; traumatic pneumothorax may also require surgery.

Special considerations

■ Watch for pallor, gasping respirations, and sudden chest pain. Carefully monitor the patient's vital signs at least every hour for indications of shock, increasing respiratory distress, or mediastinal shift. Listen for breath sounds over both lungs. Falling blood pressure and rising pulse and respiratory rates may indicate tension pneumothorax, which could be fatal without prompt treatment.

■ Urge the patient to control coughing and gasping during thoracotomy. However, after the chest tube is in place, encourage him to cough and breathe deeply (at least once an hour) to facilitate lung expansion.

■ If the patient is undergoing chest tube drainage, watch for continuing air leakage (bubbling), indicating the lung defect has failed to close; this may require surgery. Also watch for increasing subcutaneous emphysema by checking around the neck or at the tube insertion site for crackling beneath the skin. If the patient is on a ventilator, watch for difficulty in breathing in time with the ventilator as well as pressure changes on ventilator gauges.

■ Change dressings around the chest tube insertion site, as necessary and according to your facility's policy. Be careful not to reposition or dislodge the tube. If it dislodges, immediately place a petroleum gauze dressing over the opening to prevent rapid lung collapse.

■ Secure the chest tube drainage apparatus appropriately. Tape connections securely.

■ Monitor the patient's vital signs frequently after thoracotomy. Also, for the first 24 hours, assess respiratory status by checking breath sounds hourly. Observe the chest tube site for leakage, noting the amount and color of drainage. Help the patient walk, as ordered (usually on the first postoperative day), to facilitate deep inspiration and lung expansion.

■ To reassure the patient, explain what pneumothorax is, what causes it, and all diagnostic tests and procedures. Make him as comfortable as possible. (The patient with pneumothorax is usually most comfortable sitting upright.)

Pneumonia

Pneumonia is an acute infection of the lung parenchyma that commonly impairs gas exchange. The prognosis is generally good for people who have normal lungs and adequate host defenses before the onset of pneumonia; however, pneumonia is the sixth leading cause of death in the United States.

Causes and incidence

Pneumonia can be classified in several ways:

■ Microbiologic etiology — Pneumonia can be viral, bacterial, fungal, protozoan, mycobacterial, mycoplasmal, or rickettsial in origin. (See *Types of pneumonia,* pages 538 to 541.)

■ Location — Bronchopneumonia involves distal airways and alveoli; lobular pneumonia, part of a lobe; and lobar pneumonia, an entire lobe.

■ Type — Primary pneumonia results from inhalation or aspiration of a pathogen; it includes pneumococcal and viral pneumonia. Secondary pneumonia may follow initial lung damage from a noxious chemical or other insult (superinfection), or may result from hematogenous spread of bacteria from a distant focus.

Predisposing factors for bacterial and viral pneumonia include chronic illness and debilitation, cancer (particularly lung cancer), abdominal and thoracic surgery, atelectasis, common colds or other viral respiratory infections, such as acquired immunodeficiency syndrome, chronic respiratory disease (chronic obstructive pulmonary disease [COPD], asthma, bronchiectasis, and cystic fibrosis), influenza, smoking, malnutrition, alcoholism, sickle cell disease, tracheostomy, exposure to noxious gases, aspiration, and immunosuppressive therapy.

Predisposing factors for aspiration pneumonia include old age, debilitation, artificial airway use, nasogastric (NG) tube feedings, impaired gag reflex, poor oral hygiene, and decreased level of consciousness.

In elderly patients and patients who are debilitated, bacterial pneumonia may follow influenza or a common cold. Respiratory viruses are the most common cause of pneumonia in children ages 2 to 3. In school-age children, mycoplasma pneumonia is more common.

Signs and symptoms

The main symptoms of pneumonia are coughing, sputum production, pleuritic chest pain, shaking chills, shortness of breath, rapid shallow breathing, and fever. Physical signs vary widely, ranging from diffuse, fine crackles to signs of localized or extensive consolidation and pleural effusion. There may also be associated symptoms of headache, sweating, loss of appetite, excess fatigue, and confusion (in older people).

Complications include hypoxemia, respiratory failure, pleural effusion, empyema, lung abscess, and bacteremia, with spread of infection to other parts of the body, resulting in meningitis, endocarditis, and pericarditis.

Diagnosis

Clinical features, chest X-ray showing infiltrates, and sputum smear demonstrating acute inflammatory cells support the diagnosis. Gram stain and sputum culture may identify the organism. Positive blood cultures in the patient with pulmonary infiltrates strongly suggest pneumonia produced by the organisms isolated from the blood cultures. Pleural effusions, if present, should be tapped and fluid analyzed for evidence of infection in the pleural space. Occasionally, a transtracheal aspirate of tracheobronchial secretions or bronchoscopy with brushings or washings may be done to obtain material for smear and culture. The patient's response to antimicrobial therapy also provides important evidence of the presence of pneumonia.

Treatment

Antimicrobial therapy varies with the causative agent. Therapy should be reevaluated early in the course of treatment. Supportive measures include humidified oxygen therapy for hypoxemia, mechanical ventilation for respiratory failure, a high-calorie diet and adequate fluid intake, bed rest, and an analgesic to relieve pleuritic chest pain. Patients with severe pneumonia (*Text continues on page 540.*)

TYPES OF PNEUMONIA

Type	Signs and symptoms
Aspiration	
Results from vomiting and aspiration of gastric or oropharyngeal contents into trachea and lungs	■ Noncardiogenic pulmonary edema that may follow damage to respiratory epithelium from contact with stomach acid ■ Crackles, dyspnea, cyanosis, hypotension, and tachycardia ■ May be subacute pneumonia with cavity formation; lung abscess may occur if foreign body is present
Bacterial	
Klebsiella	■ Fever and recurrent chills; cough producing rusty, bloody, viscous sputum (currant jelly); cyanosis of lips and nail beds due to hypoxemia; and shallow, grunting respirations ■ Common in patients with chronic alcoholism, pulmonary disease, diabetes, or those at risk for aspiration
Staphylococcus	■ Temperature of 102° to 104° F (38.9° to 40° C), recurrent shaking chills, bloody sputum, dyspnea, tachypnea, and hypoxemia ■ Should be suspected with viral illness, such as influenza or measles, and in patients with cystic fibrosis
Streptococcus (Streptococcus pneumoniae)	■ Sudden onset of single, shaking chills and a sustained temperature of 102° to 104° F (38.9° to 40° C); commonly preceded by upper respiratory tract infection
Protozoan	
Pneumocystis carinii	■ Occurs in immunocompromised persons ■ Dyspnea and nonproductive cough ■ Anorexia, weight loss, and fatigue ■ Low-grade fever
Viral	
Adenovirus (insidious onset; generally affects young adults)	■ Sore throat, fever, cough, chills, malaise, small amounts of mucoid sputum, retrosternal chest pain, anorexia, rhinitis, adenopathy, scattered crackles, and rhonchi

Diagnosis	Treatment
■ *Chest X-ray:* locates areas of infiltrates, which suggest diagnosis	■ *Antimicrobial therapy:* penicillin G or clindamycin ■ *Supportive:* oxygen therapy, suctioning, coughing, deep breathing, and adequate hydration
■ *Chest X-ray:* typically, but not always, consolidation in the upper lobe that causes bulging of fissures ■ *White blood cell (WBC) count:* elevated ■ *Sputum culture and Gram stain:* may show gram-negative *Klebsiella*	■ *Antimicrobial therapy:* an aminoglycoside and a cephalosporin
■ *Chest X-ray:* multiple abscesses and infiltrates; high incidence of empyema ■ *WBC count:* elevated ■ *Sputum culture and Gram stain:* may show gram-positive staphylococci	■ *Antimicrobial therapy:* nafcillin or oxacillin for 14 days if staphylococci are penicillinase producing ■ *Supportive:* chest tube drainage of empyema
■ *Chest X-ray:* areas of consolidation, commonly lobar ■ *WBC count:* elevated ■ *Sputum culture:* may show gram-positive *S. pneumoniae*; this organism not always recovered	■ *Antimicrobial therapy:* penicillin G (or erythromycin, if patient is allergic to penicillin) for 7 to 10 days (Such therapy begins after obtaining culture specimen but without waiting for results.) Resistance to penicillin is becoming much more common and in the patient with risk factors for resistance (extreme age, day care attendance, or immunosuppression), treatment with vancomycin, imipenem, or levofloxacin should be considered.
■ *Fiber-optic bronchoscopy:* obtains specimens for histologic studies ■ *Chest X-ray:* nonspecific infiltrates, nodular lesions, or spontaneous pneumothorax	■ *Antimicrobial therapy:* co-trimoxazole or pentamidine by I.V. administration or inhalation. Prophylactic pentamidine may be used for high-risk patients. ■ *Supportive:* oxygen, improved nutrition, and mechanical ventilation
■ *Chest X-ray:* patchy distribution of pneumonia, more severe than indicated by physical examination ■ *WBC count:* normal to slightly elevated	■ Treat symptoms only ■ Mortality low; usually clears with no residual effects

(continued)

TYPES OF PNEUMONIA *(continued)*

Type	Signs and symptoms
Viral (continued)	
Chicken pox (varicella) (uncommon in children, but present in 30% of adults with varicella)	■ Cough, dyspnea, cyanosis, tachypnea, pleuritic chest pain, hemoptysis, and rhonchi 1 to 6 days after onset of rash
Cytomegalovirus	■ Difficult to distinguish from other nonbacterial pneumonias ■ Fever, cough, shaking chills, dyspnea, cyanosis, weakness, and diffuse crackles ■ Occurs in neonates as devastating multisystemic infection; in normal adults, resembles mononucleosis; in immunocompromised hosts, varies from clinically inapparent to devastating infection
Influenza (prognosis poor even with treatment; 30% mortality)	■ Cough (initially nonproductive; later, purulent sputum), marked cyanosis, dyspnea, high fever, chills, substernal pain and discomfort, moist crackles, frontal headache, and myalgia ■ Death results from cardiopulmonary collapse
Measles (rubeola)	■ Fever, dyspnea, cough, small amounts of sputum, coryza, rash, and cervical adenopathy
Respiratory syncytial virus (most prevalent in infants and children)	■ Listlessness, irritability, tachypnea with retraction of intercostal muscles, wheezing, slight sputum production, fine moist crackles, fever, severe malaise, and cough

on mechanical ventilation may require positive end-expiratory pressure to facilitate adequate oxygenation.

Special considerations
Correct supportive care can increase patient comfort, avoid complications, and speed recovery.

The following protocol should be observed throughout the illness:
■ Maintain a patent airway and adequate oxygenation. Monitor pulse oximetry. Measure arterial blood gas levels, especially in hypoxemic patients. Administer supplemental oxygen if the partial pressure of arterial oxygen is less than 55 to 60 mm Hg. Patients with underlying chronic lung disease should be given oxygen cautiously.

■ Teach the patient how to cough and perform deep-breathing exercises to clear secretions; encourage him to do so often. In severe pneumonia that requires endotracheal intubation or tracheostomy (with or without mechanical ventilation), provide thorough respiratory care. Suction often, using sterile technique, to remove secretions.

■ Obtain sputum specimens as needed, by suction if the patient can't produce specimens independently. Collect specimens in

Diagnosis	Treatment
■ *Chest X-ray:* shows more extensive pneumonia than indicated by physical examination and bilateral, patchy, diffuse, nodular infiltrates ■ *Sputum analysis:* predominant mononuclear cells and characteristic intranuclear inclusion bodies, with characteristic skin rash, confirm diagnosis	■ *Supportive:* adequate hydration, and oxygen therapy in critically ill patients ■ Therapy with I.V. acyclovir
■ *Chest X-ray:* in early stages, variable patchy infiltrates; later, bilateral, nodular, and more predominant in lower lobes ■ *Percutaneous aspiration of lung tissue, transbronchial biopsy, or open lung biopsy:* microscopic examination shows typical intranuclear and cytoplasmic inclusions; the virus can be cultured from lung tissue	■ Generally, benign and self-limiting in mononucleosis-like form ■ *Supportive:* adequate hydration and nutrition, oxygen therapy, and bed rest ■ In immunosuppressed patients, disease is more severe and may be fatal; ganciclovir or foscarnet treatment warranted
■ *Chest X-ray:* diffuse bilateral bronchopneumonia radiating from hilus ■ *WBC count:* normal to slightly elevated ■ *Sputum smears:* no specific organisms	■ *Supportive:* for respiratory failure, endotracheal intubation and ventilator assistance; for fever, hypothermia blanket or antipyretics; and for influenza A, amantadine or rimantadine
■ *Chest X-ray:* reticular infiltrates, sometimes with hilar lymph node enlargement ■ *Lung tissue specimen:* characteristic giant cells	■ *Supportive:* bed rest, adequate hydration, and antimicrobials; assisted ventilation if necessary
■ *Chest X-ray:* patchy bilateral consolidation ■ *WBC count:* normal to slightly elevated	■ *Supportive:* humidified air, oxygen, antimicrobials (commonly given until viral etiology confirmed), and aerosolized ribavirin ■ Usually complete recovery

a sterile container and deliver them promptly to the microbiology laboratory.
■ Administer antibiotics as ordered and pain medication as needed; record the patient's response to medications. Fever and dehydration may require I.V. fluids and electrolyte replacement.
■ Maintain adequate nutrition to offset hypermetabolic state secondary to infection. Ask the dietary department to provide a high-calorie, high-protein diet consisting of soft, easy-to-eat foods. Encourage the patient to eat. As necessary, supplement oral feedings with NG tube feedings or parenteral nutrition. Monitor fluid intake and output. Consider limiting the use of milk products as they may increase sputum production.
■ Provide a quiet, calm environment for the patient, with frequent rest periods.
■ Give emotional support by explaining all procedures (especially intubation and suctioning) to the patient and his family. Encourage family visits. Provide diversionary activities appropriate to the patient's age.
■ To control the spread of infection, dispose of secretions properly. Tell the patient to sneeze and cough into a disposable tissue; tape a lined bag to the side of the bed for used tissues.

Pneumonia can be prevented as follows:
- Advise the patient to avoid using antibiotics indiscriminately during minor viral infections because this may result in upper airway colonization with antibiotic-resistant bacteria. If the patient then develops pneumonia, the organisms producing the pneumonia may require treatment with more toxic antibiotics.
- Encourage pneumovax and annual influenza vaccination for high-risk patients, such as those with COPD, chronic heart disease, or sickle cell disease.
- Urge all bedridden and postoperative patients to perform deep-breathing and coughing exercises frequently. Reposition such patients often to promote full aeration and drainage of secretions. Encourage early ambulation in postoperative patients.
- To prevent aspiration during NG tube feedings, elevate the patient's head, check the tube's position, and administer the formula slowly. Don't give large volumes at one time; this could cause vomiting. Keep the patient's head elevated for at least 30 minutes after the feeding. Check for residual formula at 4- to 6-hour intervals.

Idiopathic bronchiolitis obliterans with organizing pneumonia

Idiopathic bronchiolitis obliterans with organizing pneumonia (BOOP), also known as *cryptogenic organizing pneumonia,* is one of several types of bronchiolitis obliterans. *Organizing pneumonia* refers to unresolved pneumonia, in which inflammatory alveolar exudate persists and eventually undergoes fibrosis. *Bronchiolitis obliterans* is a generic term used to describe an inflammatory disease of the small airways.

Causes and incidence

BOOP has no known cause. However, other forms of bronchiolitis obliterans and organizing pneumonia may be associated with specific diseases or situations, such as bone marrow, heart, or heart-lung transplantation; collagen vascular diseases, such as rheumatoid arthritis and systemic lupus erythematosus; inflammatory diseases, such as Crohn's disease, ulcerative colitis,

and polyarteritis nodosa; bacterial, viral, or mycoplasmal respiratory infections; inhalation of toxic gases; and drug therapy with amiodarone, bleomycin, penicillamine, or lomustine.

Much debate still exists about the various pathologies and classifications of bronchiolitis obliterans. Most patients with BOOP are between ages 50 and 60. Incidence is equally divided between men and women. A smoking history doesn't seem to increase the risk of developing BOOP.

Signs and symptoms

The presenting symptoms of BOOP are usually subacute, with a flulike syndrome of fever, persistent and nonproductive cough, dyspnea (especially with exertion), malaise, anorexia, and weight loss lasting for several weeks to several months. Physical assessment findings may reveal dry crackles as the only abnormality. Less common symptoms include a productive cough, hemoptysis, chest pain, generalized aching, and night sweats.

Diagnosis

Diagnosis begins with a thorough patient history meant to exclude any known cause of bronchiolitis obliterans or diseases with a pathology that includes an organizing pneumonia pattern.
- Chest X-ray usually shows patchy, diffuse airspace opacities with a ground-glass appearance that may migrate from one location to another. High-resolution computed tomography scans show areas of consolidation. Except for the migrating opacities, these findings are nonspecific and present in many other respiratory disorders.
- Pulmonary function tests may be normal or show reduced capacities. The diffusing capacity for carbon monoxide is generally low.
- Arterial blood gas analysis usually shows mild to moderate hypoxemia at rest, which worsens with exercise.
- Blood tests reveal an increased erythrocyte sedimentation rate, an increased C-reactive protein level, an increased white blood cell count with a somewhat an increased proportion of neutrophils, and a minor rise in eosinophils. Immunoglobu-

lin (Ig) G and IgM levels are normal or slightly increased, and the IgE level is normal.

- Bronchoscopy reveals normal or slightly inflamed airways. Bronchoalveolar lavage fluid obtained during bronchoscopy shows a moderate elevation in lymphocytes and, sometimes, elevated neutrophil and eosinophil levels. Foamy-looking alveolar macrophages may also be found.

 CONFIRMING DIAGNOSIS *Lung biopsy, thoracoscopy, or bronchoscopy is required to confirm the diagnosis of BOOP. Pathologic changes in lung tissue include plugs of connective tissue in the lumen of the bronchioles, alveolar ducts, and alveolar spaces.*

These changes may occur in other types of bronchiolitis and in other diseases that cause organizing pneumonia. They also differentiate BOOP from constrictive bronchiolitis (characterized by inflammation and fibrosis that surrounds and may narrow or completely obliterate the bronchiolar airways). Although the pathologic findings in proliferative and constrictive bronchiolitis are different, the causes and presentations may overlap. Any known cause of bronchiolitis obliterans or organizing pneumonia must be ruled out before the diagnosis of BOOP is made.

Treatment

Corticosteroids are the current treatment for BOOP, although the ideal dosage and duration of treatment remain topics of discussion. Relapse is common when steroids are tapered off or stopped. This usually can be reversed when steroids are increased or resumed. Occasionally, a patient may need to continue corticosteroids indefinitely.

Immunosuppressive-cytotoxic drugs, such as cyclophosphamide, have been used in the few cases of intolerance or unresponsiveness.

Oxygen is used to correct hypoxemia. The patient may need either no oxygen or a small amount of oxygen at rest and a greater amount when he exercises.

Other treatments vary, depending on the patient's symptoms, and may include inhaled bronchodilators, cough suppressants, and bronchial hygiene therapies.

BOOP is very responsive to treatment and usually can be completely reversed with corticosteroid therapy. However, a few deaths have been reported, particularly in patients who had more widespread pathologic changes in the lung or patients who developed opportunistic infections or other complications related to steroid therapy.

Special considerations

- Explain all diagnostic tests. The patient may experience anxiety and frustration because of the length of time and number of tests needed to establish the diagnosis.
- Explain the diagnosis to the patient and his family. This uncommon diagnosis may cause confusion and anxiety.
- Monitor the patient for adverse effects of corticosteroid therapy: weight gain, "moon face," glucose intolerance, fluid and electrolyte imbalance, mood swings, cataracts, peptic ulcer disease, opportunistic infections, and osteoporosis leading to bone fractures. In many cases, these effects leave the patient unable to tolerate the treatment. Teach the patient and his family about these adverse effects, emphasizing which reactions should be reported to the physician.
- Teach measures that may help prevent complications related to treatment, such as infection control and improved nutrition.
- Teach breathing, relaxation, and energy conservation techniques to help the patient manage symptoms.
- Monitor oxygenation, both at rest and with exertion. The physician will probably prescribe an oxygen flow rate for use when the patient is at rest and a higher one for exertion. Teach the patient how to increase the oxygen flow rate to the appropriate level for exercise.
- If the patient needs oxygen at home, ensure continuity of care by making appropriate referrals to discharge planners, respiratory care practitioners, and home equipment vendors.

Pulmonary embolism

The most common pulmonary complication in hospitalized patients, pulmonary embolism is an obstruction of the pulmonary arterial bed by a dislodged thrombus, heart valve vegetation, or foreign substance. Although pulmonary infarction that results from embolism may be so mild as to be asymptomatic, massive embolism (more than 50% obstruction of pulmonary arterial circulation) and the accompanying infarction can be rapidly fatal.

Causes

Pulmonary embolism generally results from dislodged thrombi originating in the leg veins. More than half of such thrombi arise in the deep veins of the legs. Other less common sources of thrombi are the pelvic veins, renal veins, hepatic vein, right side of the heart, and upper extremities. Such thrombus formation results directly from vascular wall damage, venostasis, or hypercoagulability of the blood. Trauma, clot dissolution, sudden muscle spasm, intravascular pressure changes, or a change in peripheral blood flow can cause the thrombus to loosen or fragment. Then the thrombus — now called an *embolus* — floats to the heart's right side and enters the lung through the pulmonary artery. There, the embolus may dissolve, continue to fragment, or grow.

By occluding the pulmonary artery, the embolus prevents alveoli from producing enough surfactant to maintain alveolar integrity. As a result, alveoli collapse and atelectasis develops. If the embolus enlarges, it may clog most or all of the pulmonary vessels and cause death.

Rarely, the emboli contain air, fat, bacteria, amniotic fluid, talc (from drugs intended for oral administration, which are injected intravenously by addicts), or tumor cells.

Predisposing factors for pulmonary embolism include long-term immobility, chronic pulmonary disease, heart failure or atrial fibrillation, thrombophlebitis, polycythemia vera, thrombocytosis, autoimmune hemolytic anemia, sickle cell disease, varicose veins, recent surgery, advanced age, pregnancy, lower-extremity fractures or surgery, burns, obesity, vascular injury, cancer, I.V. drug abuse, or hormonal contraceptives.

Signs and symptoms

Total occlusion of the main pulmonary artery is rapidly fatal; smaller or fragmented emboli produce symptoms that vary with the size, number, and location of the emboli. Usually, the first symptom of pulmonary embolism is dyspnea, which may be accompanied by anginal or pleuritic chest pain. Other clinical features include tachycardia, productive cough (sputum may be blood-tinged), low-grade fever, and pleural effusion. Less common signs include massive hemoptysis, chest splinting, leg edema and, with a large embolus, cyanosis, syncope, and distended jugular veins.

In addition, pulmonary embolism may cause pleural friction rub and signs of circulatory collapse (weak, rapid pulse and hypotension) and hypoxia (restlessness and anxiety).

Diagnosis

The patient history should reveal predisposing conditions for pulmonary embolism. A triad of deep vein thrombosis (DVT) formation is stasis, endothelial injury, and hypercoagulability. Risk factors include long car or plane trips, cancer, pregnancy, hypercoagulability, prior DVT, and pulmonary emboli.

■ Chest X-ray helps to rule out other pulmonary diseases; areas of atelectasis, an elevated diaphragm and pleural effusion, aprominent pulmonary artery and, occasionally, the characteristic wedge-shaped infiltrate suggestive of pulmonary infarction, or focal oligemia of blood vessels, are apparent.

■ Lung scan shows perfusion defects in areas beyond occluded vessels; however, it doesn't rule out microemboli.

■ Pulmonary angiography is the most definitive test but requires a skilled angiographer and radiologic equipment; it also poses some risk to the patient. Its use depends on the uncertainty of the diagnosis and the need to avoid unnecessary anticoagulant therapy in a high-risk patient.

■ Electrocardiography may show right axis deviation; right bundle-branch block; tall, peaked P waves; depression of ST segments and T-wave inversions (indicative of right-sided heart strain); and supraventricular tachyarrhythmias in extensive pulmonary embolism. A pattern sometimes observed is S_1, Q_3, and T_3 (S wave in lead I, Q wave in lead III, and inverted T wave in lead III).

■ Auscultation occasionally reveals a right ventricular S_3 gallop and an increased intensity of a pulmonic component of S_2. Also, crackles and a pleural rub may be heard at the embolism site.

■ Arterial blood gas (ABG) analysis showing a decreased partial pressure of arterial oxygen and partial pressure of arterial carbon dioxide are characteristic but don't always occur.

If pleural effusion is present, thoracentesis may rule out empyema, which indicates pneumonia.

Treatment

Treatment is designed to maintain adequate cardiovascular and pulmonary function during resolution of the obstruction and to prevent recurrence of embolic episodes. Because most emboli resolve within 10 to 14 days, treatment consists of oxygen therapy as needed and anticoagulation with heparin to inhibit new thrombus formation, followed by oral warfarin. Heparin therapy is monitored by daily coagulation studies (partial thromboplastin time [PTT]).

Patients with massive pulmonary embolism and shock may need fibrinolytic therapy with thrombolytic therapy (streptokinase, urokinase, or tissue plasminogen activator) to enhance fibrinolysis of the pulmonary emboli and remaining thrombi. Emboli that cause hypotension may require the use of vasopressors. Treatment of septic emboli requires antibiotics — not anticoagulants — and evaluation for the infection's source, particularly endocarditis.

Surgery is performed on patients who can't take anticoagulants, who have recurrent emboli during anticoagulant therapy, or who have been treated with thrombolytic agents or pulmonary thromboendarterectomy. This procedure (which shouldn't be performed without angiographic evidence of pulmonary embolism) consists of vena caval ligation, plication, or insertion of an inferior vena cava device to filter blood returning to the heart and lungs.

Special considerations

■ Give oxygen by nasal cannula or mask. Check ABG levels if the patient develops fresh emboli or worsening dyspnea. Be prepared to provide endotracheal intubation with assisted ventilation if breathing is severely compromised.

■ Administer heparin, as ordered, through I.V. push or continuous drip. Monitor coagulation studies daily. Effective heparin therapy raises the PTT to more than 1½ times normal. Watch closely for nosebleeds, petechiae, and other signs of abnormal bleeding; check stools for occult blood. Patients should be protected from trauma and injury; avoid I.M. injections and maintain pressure over venipuncture sites for 5 minutes, or until bleeding stops, to reduce hematoma.

■ After the patient is stable, encourage him to move about often, and assist with isometric and range-of-motion exercises. Check pedal pulses, temperature, and color of feet to detect venostasis. *Never* massage the patient's legs. Offer diversional activities to promote rest and relieve restlessness.

■ Help the patient walk as soon as possible after surgery to prevent venostasis.

■ Maintain adequate nutrition and fluid balance to promote healing.

■ Report frequent pleuritic chest pain, so that analgesics can be prescribed. Also, incentive spirometry can assist in deep breathing. Provide tissues and a bag for easy disposal of expectorations.

■ Warn the patient not to cross his legs; this promotes thrombus formation.

■ To relieve anxiety, explain procedures and treatments. Encourage the patient's family to participate in his care.

■ Most patients need treatment with an oral anticoagulant (warfarin) for 3 to 6 months after a pulmonary embolism. Advise these patients to watch for signs of bleeding (bloody stools, blood in urine, and large ecchymoses), to take the prescribed medication exactly as ordered, not to change dosages without consulting their physician, and to avoid taking additional medication (including aspirin and vitamins). Stress the importance of follow-up laboratory tests (International Normalized Ratio) to monitor anticoagulant therapy.

- To prevent pulmonary emboli, encourage early ambulation in patients predisposed to this condition. With close medical supervision, low-dose heparin may be useful prophylactically.
- Low-molecular-weight heparin may be given to prevent pulmonary embolism in high-risk patients.

Sarcoidosis

Sarcoidosis is a multisystem, granulomatous disorder that characteristically produces lymphadenopathy, pulmonary infiltration, and skeletal, liver, eye, or skin lesions. Acute sarcoidosis usually resolves within 2 years. Chronic, progressive sarcoidosis, which is uncommon, is associated with pulmonary fibrosis and progressive pulmonary disability.

Causes and incidence
The cause of sarcoidosis is unknown, but these factors may play a role:
- hypersensitivity response (possibly from T-cell imbalance) to such agents as atypical mycobacteria, fungi, and pine pollen
- genetic predisposition (suggested by a slightly higher incidence of sarcoidosis within the same family)
- extreme immune response to infection.
Sarcoidosis occurs most commonly in adults ages 30 to 50. In the United States, sarcoidosis occurs predominantly among blacks, affecting twice as many women as men.

Signs and symptoms
Initial symptoms of sarcoidosis include arthralgia (in the wrists, ankles, and elbows), fatigue, malaise, and weight loss. Other clinical features vary according to the extent and location of the fibrosis:
- respiratory — breathlessness, cough (usually nonproductive), substernal pain; complications in advanced pulmonary disease include pulmonary hypertension and cor pulmonale
- cutaneous — erythema nodosum, subcutaneous skin nodules with maculopapular eruptions, and extensive nasal mucosal lesions

- ophthalmic — anterior uveitis (common), glaucoma, and blindness (rare)
- lymphatic — bilateral hilar and right paratracheal lymphadenopathy and splenomegaly
- musculoskeletal — muscle weakness, polyarthralgia, pain, and punched-out lesions on phalanges
- hepatic — granulomatous hepatitis, usually asymptomatic
- genitourinary — hypercalciuria
- cardiovascular — arrhythmias (premature beats, bundle-branch or complete heart block) and, rarely, cardiomyopathy
- central nervous system — cranial or peripheral nerve palsies, basilar meningitis, seizures, and pituitary and hypothalamic lesions producing diabetes insipidus.

Diagnosis
Typical clinical features with appropriate laboratory data and X-ray findings suggest sarcoidosis. A positive skin lesion biopsy supports the diagnosis.
Other relevant findings include:
- chest X-ray — bilateral hilar and right paratracheal adenopathy with or without diffuse interstitial infiltrates; occasionally large nodular lesions present in lung parenchyma
- lymph node or lung biopsy — noncaseating granulomas with negative cultures for mycobacteria and fungi
- other laboratory data — rarely, increased serum calcium, mild anemia, leukocytosis, and hyperglobulinemia
- pulmonary function tests — decreased total lung capacity and compliance, and decreased diffusing capacity
- arterial blood gas (ABG) analysis — decreased arterial oxygen tension.
Negative tuberculin skin test, fungal serologies, and sputum cultures for mycobacteria and fungi as well as negative biopsy cultures help rule out infection.

Treatment
Sarcoidosis that produces no symptoms requires no treatment. However, those severely affected with sarcoidosis require treatment with corticosteroids. Such therapy is usually continued for 1 to 2 years, but some patients may need lifelong therapy. Immunosuppressive agents, such as

methotrexate, azathioprine, and cyclophosphamide, may also be used. If organ failure occurs (although this is rare), transplantation may be required. Other measures include a low-calcium diet and avoidance of direct exposure to sunlight in patients with hypercalcemia.

Special considerations

■ Watch for and report any complications. Be aware of abnormal laboratory results (anemia, for example) that could alter patient care.

■ For the patient with arthralgia, administer analgesics as ordered. Record signs of progressive muscle weakness.

■ Provide a nutritious, high-calorie diet and plenty of fluids. If the patient has hypercalcemia, suggest a low-calcium diet. Weigh the patient regularly to detect weight loss.

■ Monitor respiratory function. Check chest X-rays for the extent of lung involvement; note and record any bloody sputum or increase in sputum. If the patient has pulmonary hypertension or end-stage cor pulmonale, check ABG levels, observe for arrhythmias, and administer oxygen, as needed.

■ Because steroids may induce or worsen diabetes mellitus, perform fingerstick glucose tests at least every 12 hours at the beginning of steroid therapy. Also, watch for other steroid adverse effects, such as fluid retention, electrolyte imbalance (especially hypokalemia), moon face, hypertension, and personality change. During or after steroid withdrawal (particularly in association with infection or other types of stress), watch for and report vomiting, orthostatic hypotension, hypoglycemia, restlessness, anorexia, malaise, and fatigue. Remember that the patient on long-term or high-dose steroid therapy is vulnerable to infection.

■ When preparing the patient for discharge, stress the need for compliance with prescribed steroid therapy and regular, careful follow-up examinations and treatment. Refer the patient with failing vision to community support and resource groups and the American Foundation for the Blind, if necessary.

Severe acute respiratory syndrome

Severe acute respiratory syndrome (SARS) is a viral respiratory infection that can progress to pneumonia and, eventually, death. The disease was first recognized in 2003 with outbreaks in China, Canada, Singapore, Taiwan, and Vietnam, with other countries — including the United States — reporting smaller numbers of cases.

Causes

SARS is caused by the SARS-associated coronavirus (SARS-CoV). Coronaviruses are a common cause of mild respiratory illnesses in humans, but researchers believe that a virus may have mutated, allowing it to cause this potentially life-threatening disease.

Close contact with a person who's infected with SARS, including contact with infectious aerosolized droplets or body secretions, is the method of transmission. Most people who contracted the disease during the 2003 outbreak contracted it during travel to endemic areas. However, the virus has been found to live on hands, tissues, and other surfaces for up to 6 hours in its droplet form. It has also been found to live in the stool of people with SARS for up to 4 days. The virus may be able to live for months or years in below-freezing temperatures.

Signs and symptoms

The incubation period for SARS is typically 3 to 5 days but may last as long as 14 days. Initial signs and symptoms include fever, shortness of breath and other minor respiratory symptoms, general discomfort, headache, rigors, chills, myalgia, sore throat, and dry cough. Some individuals may develop diarrhea or a rash. Later complications include respiratory failure, liver failure, heart failure, myelodysplastic syndromes, and death.

Diagnosis

Diagnosis of severe respiratory illness is made when the patient has a fever greater than 100.4° F (38° C) or upon clinical findings of lower respiratory illness and a chest

X-ray demonstrating pneumonia or acute respiratory distress syndrome.

Laboratory validation for the virus includes cell culture of SARS-CoV, detection of SARS-CoV ribonucleic acid by the reverse transcription polymerase chain reaction (PCR) test, or detection of serum antibodies to SARS-CoV. Detectable levels of antibodies may not be present until 21 days after the onset of illness, but some individuals develop antibodies within 14 days. A negative PCR, antibody test, or cell culture doesn't rule out the diagnosis.

Treatment
Treatment is symptomatic and supportive and includes maintenance of a patent airway and adequate nutrition. Other treatment measures include supplemental oxygen, chest physiotherapy, or mechanical ventilation. In addition to standard precautions, contact precautions requiring gowns and gloves for all patient contacts and airborne precautions utilizing a negative-pressure isolation room and properly fitted N-95 respirators are recommended for patients who are hospitalized. Quarantine may be used to prevent the spread of infection.

Antibiotics may be given to treat bacterial causes of atypical pneumonia. Antiviral medications have also been used. High doses of corticosteroids have been used to reduce lung inflammation. In some serious cases, serum from individuals who have already recovered from SARS (convalescent serum) has been given. The general benefit of these treatments hasn't been determined conclusively.

Special considerations
- Report suspected cases of SARS to local and national health organizations.
- Frequently monitor the patient's vital signs and respiratory status.
- Maintain isolation as recommended. The patient will need emotional support to deal with anxiety and fear related to the diagnosis of SARS and as a result of isolation.
- Provide patient and family teaching, including the importance of frequent hand washing, covering the mouth and nose when coughing or sneezing, and avoiding close personal contact while infected or potentially infected. Instruct the patient and his family that such items as eating utensils, towels, and bedding shouldn't be shared until they have been washed with soap and hot water and that disposable gloves and household disinfectant should be used to clean any surface that may have been exposed to the patient's body fluids.
- Emphasize to the patient the importance of not going to work, school, or other public places, as recommended by the health care provider.

Lung abscess

Lung abscess is a lung infection accompanied by pus accumulation and tissue destruction. The abscess may be putrid (due to anaerobic bacteria) or nonputrid (due to anaerobes or aerobes) and usually has a well-defined border. The availability of effective antibiotics has made lung abscess much less common than it was in the past.

Causes
Lung abscess is a manifestation of necrotizing pneumonia, generally the result of aspiration of oropharyngeal contents. Poor oral hygiene with dental or gingival (gum) disease is strongly associated with putrid lung abscess. Septic pulmonary emboli commonly produce cavitary lesions. Infected cystic lung lesions and cavitating bronchial carcinoma must be distinguished from lung abscesses.

Signs and symptoms
The clinical effects of lung abscess include a cough that may produce bloody, purulent, or foul-smelling sputum, pleuritic chest pain, dyspnea, excessive sweating, chills, fever, headache, malaise, diaphoresis, and weight loss. Complications include rupture into the pleural space, which results in empyema and, rarely, massive hemorrhage. Chronic lung abscess may cause localized bronchiectasis. Failure of an abscess to improve with antibiotic treatment suggests possible underlying neoplasm or other causes of obstruction.

Diagnosis
- Auscultation of the chest may reveal crackles and decreased breath sounds.

- Chest X-ray shows a localized infiltrate with one or more clear spaces, usually containing air-fluid levels.
- Percutaneous aspiration or bronchoscopy may be used to obtain cultures to identify the causative organism. Bronchoscopy is only used if abscess resolution is eventful and the patient's condition permits it.
- Blood cultures, Gram stain, and sputum culture are also used to detect the causative organism; leukocytosis (white blood cell count greater than 10,000/µl) is commonly present.

Treatment

Treatment consists of prolonged antibiotic therapy, commonly lasting for months, until radiographic resolution or definite stability occurs. Symptoms usually disappear in a few weeks. Postural drainage may facilitate discharge of necrotic material into the upper airways where expectoration is possible; oxygen therapy may relieve hypoxemia. Poor response to therapy requires resection of the lesion or removal of the diseased section of the lung. All patients need rigorous follow-up and serial chest X-rays.

Special considerations

- Help the patient with chest physiotherapy (including coughing and deep breathing), increase fluid intake to loosen secretions, and provide a quiet, restful atmosphere.
- To prevent lung abscess in the unconscious patient and the patient with seizures, first prevent aspiration of secretions. Do this by suctioning the patient and by positioning him to promote drainage of secretions.

Hemothorax

In hemothorax, blood from damaged intercostal, pleural, mediastinal, and (infrequently) lung parenchymal vessels enters the pleural cavity. Depending on the amount of bleeding and the underlying cause, hemothorax may be associated with varying degrees of lung collapse and mediastinal shift. Pneumothorax—air in the pleural cavity—commonly accompanies hemothorax.

Causes

Hemothorax usually results from blunt or penetrating chest trauma; in fact, about 25% of patients with such trauma have hemothorax. In some cases, it results from thoracic surgery, pulmonary infarction, neoplasm, dissecting thoracic aneurysm, or a complication of tuberculosis or anticoagulant therapy.

Signs and symptoms

The patient with hemothorax may experience chest pain, tachypnea, and mild to severe dyspnea, depending on the amount of blood in the pleural cavity and associated pathologic conditions. If respiratory failure results, the patient may appear anxious, restless, possibly stuporous, and cyanotic; marked blood loss produces hypotension and shock. The affected side of the chest expands and stiffens, whereas the unaffected side rises and falls with the patient's breaths.

Diagnosis

Characteristic clinical signs and a history of trauma strongly suggest hemothorax. Percussion and auscultation reveal dullness and decreased to absent breath sounds over the affected side. Thoracentesis yields blood or serosanguineous fluid; chest X-rays show pleural fluid with or without mediastinal shift. Arterial blood gas (ABG) analysis may reveal respiratory failure; hemoglobin may be decreased, depending on the amount of blood lost.

Treatment

Treatment is designed to stabilize the patient's condition, stop the bleeding, evacuate blood from the pleural space, and reexpand the underlying lung. Mild hemothorax usually clears in 10 to 14 days, requiring only observation for further bleeding. In severe hemothorax, thoracentesis not only serves as a diagnostic tool but also removes fluid from the pleural cavity.

After the diagnosis is confirmed, a chest tube is inserted into the sixth intercostal space at the posterior axillary line. Suction may be used; a large-bore tube is used to prevent clot blockage. If the chest tube doesn't improve the patient's condition, he may need a thoracotomy to evacuate blood and clots and to control bleeding.

Special considerations
- Give oxygen by face mask or nasal cannula.
- Give I.V. fluids and blood transfusions, as ordered, to treat shock. Monitor pulse oximetry and ABG levels often.
- Explain all procedures to the patient to allay his fears. Assist with thoracentesis. Warn the patient not to cough during this procedure.
- Carefully observe chest tube drainage and record the volume drained (at least every hour). Milk the chest tube (only if necessary and according to facility and physician protocols) to keep it open and free from clots. If the tube is warm and full of blood and the bloody fluid level in the water-seal bottle is rising rapidly, report this at once. The patient may need immediate surgery.
- Watch the patient closely for pallor and gasping respirations. Monitor his vital signs diligently. Falling blood pressure, rising pulse rate, and rising respiratory rate may indicate shock or massive bleeding.

Pulmonary hypertension

Pulmonary hypertension occurs when pulmonary artery pressure (PAP) rises above normal for reasons other than aging or altitude. No definitive set of values is used to diagnose pulmonary hypertension, but the National Institutes of Health requires a mean PAP of 25 mm Hg or more. The prognosis depends on the cause of the underlying disorder, but the long-term prognosis is poor. Within 5 years of diagnosis, only 25% of patients are still alive.

Causes and incidence
Pulmonary hypertension begins as hypertrophy of the small pulmonary arteries. The medial and intimal muscle layers of these vessels thicken, decreasing distensibility and increasing resistance. This disorder then progresses to vascular sclerosis and obliteration of small vessels.

In most cases, pulmonary hypertension occurs secondary to an underlying disease process, including:
- *alveolar hypoventilation* from chronic obstructive pulmonary disease (most common cause in the United States), sarcoidosis, diffuse interstitial disease, pulmonary metastasis, and certain diseases such as scleroderma (In these disorders, pulmonary vascular resistance occurs secondary to hypoxemia and destruction of the alveolocapillary bed. Other disorders that cause alveolar hypoventilation without lung tissue damage include obesity, kyphoscoliosis, and obstructive sleep apnea.)
- *vascular obstruction* from pulmonary embolism, vasculitis, and disorders that cause obstruction of small or large pulmonary veins, such as left atrial myxoma, idiopathic veno-occlusive disease, fibrosing mediastinitis, and mediastinal neoplasm
- *primary cardiac disease,* which may be congenital or acquired. Congenital defects that cause left-to-right shunting of blood — such as patent ductus arteriosus or atrial or ventricular septal defect — increase blood flow into the lungs and, consequently, raise pulmonary vascular pressure. Acquired cardiac diseases, such as rheumatic valvular disease and mitral stenosis, increase pulmonary venous pressure by restricting blood flow returning to the heart.

Primary (or idiopathic) pulmonary hypertension is rare, occurring most commonly — and with no known cause — in women between ages 20 and 40. Secondary pulmonary hypertension results from existing cardiac, pulmonary, thromboembolic, or collagen vascular diseases or from the use of certain drugs.

Signs and symptoms
Most patients complain of increasing dyspnea on exertion, weakness, syncope, and fatigability. Many also show signs of right-sided heart failure, including peripheral edema, ascites, jugular vein distention, and hepatomegaly. Other clinical effects vary with the underlying disorder.

Diagnosis
Characteristic diagnostic findings include:
- Auscultation reveals abnormalities associated with the underlying disorder.
- Arterial blood gas (ABG) analysis indicates hypoxemia (decreased partial pressure of arterial oxygen).
- Electrocardiography shows right axis deviation and tall or peaked P waves in inferi-

or leads in the patient with right ventricular hypertrophy.

■ Cardiac catheterization reveals pulmonary systolic pressure above 30 mm Hg as well as increased pulmonary artery wedge pressure (PAWP) if the underlying cause is left atrial myxoma, mitral stenosis, or left-sided heart failure (otherwise normal).

■ Pulmonary angiography detects filling defects in pulmonary vasculature such as those that develop in patients with pulmonary emboli.

■ Pulmonary function tests may show decreased flow rates and increased residual volume in underlying obstructive disease and decreased total lung capacity in underlying restrictive disease.

Treatment
Treatment usually includes oxygen therapy to decrease hypoxemia and resulting pulmonary vascular resistance. It may also include vasodilator therapy (nifedipine, diltiazem, or prostaglandin E). For patients with right-sided heart failure, treatment also includes fluid restriction, cardiac glycosides to increase cardiac output, and diuretics to decrease intravascular volume and extravascular fluid accumulation. Treatment also aims to correct the underlying cause.

Some patients with pulmonary hypertension may be candidates for heart-lung transplantation to improve their chances of survival.

Special considerations
Pulmonary hypertension requires keen observation and careful monitoring as well as skilled supportive care.

■ Administer oxygen therapy as ordered, and observe the patient's response. Report any signs of increasing dyspnea to the physician so he can adjust treatment accordingly.

■ Monitor ABG levels for acidosis and hypoxemia. Report any change in the patient's level of consciousness at once.

■ When caring for a patient with right-sided heart failure, especially one receiving diuretics, record his weight daily, carefully measure intake and output, and explain all medications and diet restrictions. Check for worsening jugular vein distention, which may indicate fluid overload.

■ Monitor the patient's vital signs, especially blood pressure and heart rate. Watch for hypotension and tachycardia. If he has a pulmonary artery catheter, check PAP and PAWP, as ordered. Report any changes.

■ Before discharge, help the patient adjust to the limitations imposed by this disorder. Advise against overexertion, and suggest frequent rest periods between activities. Refer the patient to the social services department if he'll need special equipment, such as oxygen equipment, for home use. Make sure that he understands the prescribed medications and diet and the need to weigh himself daily.

Pleural effusion and empyema

Pleural effusion is an excess of fluid in the pleural space. Normally, this space contains a small amount of extracellular fluid that lubricates the pleural surfaces. Increased production or inadequate removal of this fluid results in pleural effusion. Empyema is the accumulation of pus and necrotic tissue in the pleural space. Blood (hemothorax) and chyle (chylothorax) may also collect in this space.

Causes
The balance of osmotic and hydrostatic pressures in parietal pleural capillaries normally results in fluid movement into the pleural space. Balanced pressures in visceral pleural capillaries promote reabsorption of this fluid. Excessive hydrostatic pressure or decreased osmotic pressure can cause excessive amounts of fluid to pass across intact capillaries. The result is a transudative pleural effusion, an ultrafiltrate of plasma containing low concentrations of protein. Such effusions frequently result from heart failure, hepatic disease with ascites, peritoneal dialysis, hypoalbuminemia, and disorders resulting in overexpanded intravascular volume.

Exudative pleural effusions result when capillaries exhibit increased permeability with or without changes in hydrostatic and colloid osmotic pressures, allowing protein-rich fluid to leak into the pleural space. Exudative pleural effusions occur with tuberculosis (TB), subphrenic abscess, pancreatitis, bacterial or fungal pneumonitis or empyema, malignancy, pulmonary embolism with or without infarction, collagen disease (lupus erythematosus [LE] and rheumatoid arthritis), myxedema, and chest trauma.

Empyema is usually associated with infection in the pleural space. Such infection may be idiopathic or may be related to pneumonitis, carcinoma, perforation, or esophageal rupture.

Signs and symptoms

Patients with pleural effusion characteristically display symptoms relating to the underlying pathologic condition. Most patients with large effusions, particularly those with underlying pulmonary disease, complain of dyspnea. Those with effusions associated with pleurisy complain of pleuritic chest pain. Other clinical features depend on the cause of the effusion. Patients with empyema also develop fever and malaise.

Diagnosis

Auscultation of the chest reveals decreased breath sounds; percussion detects dullness over the effused area, which doesn't change with breathing. Chest X-ray shows fluid in dependent regions. However, diagnosis also requires other tests to distinguish transudative from exudative effusions and to help pinpoint the underlying disorder.

The most useful test is thoracentesis, in which pleural fluid is analyzed in the laboratory to show components. Acute inflammatory white blood cells and microorganisms may be evident in empyema.

In addition, if a pleural effusion results from esophageal rupture or pancreatitis, fluid amylase levels are usually higher than serum levels. Aspirated fluid may be tested for LE cells, antinuclear antibodies, and neoplastic cells. It may also be analyzed for color and consistency; acid-fast bacillus, fungal, and bacterial cultures; and triglycerides (in chylothorax). Cell analysis shows leukocytosis in empyema. A negative tuberculin skin test strongly rules against TB as the cause. In exudative pleural effusions in which thoracentesis isn't definitive, pleural biopsy may be done. This is particularly useful for confirming TB or malignancy.

Treatment

Depending on the amount of fluid present, symptomatic effusion may require thoracentesis to remove fluid or careful monitoring of the patient's own reabsorption of the fluid. Hemothorax requires drainage to prevent fibrothorax formation. Pleural effusions associated with lung cancer commonly reaccumulate quickly. If a chest tube is inserted to drain the fluid, a sclerosing agent, such as talc, may be injected through the tube to cause adhesions between the parietal and visceral pleura, thereby obliterating the potential space for fluid to recollect.

Treatment of empyema requires insertion of one or more chest tubes after thoracentesis, to allow drainage of purulent material, and possibly decortication (surgical removal of the thick coating over the lung) or rib resection to allow open drainage and lung expansion. Empyema also requires parenteral antibiotics. Associated hypoxia requires oxygen administration.

Special considerations

- Explain thoracentesis to the patient. Before the procedure, tell him to expect a stinging sensation from the local anesthetic and a feeling of pressure when the needle is inserted. Instruct him to tell you immediately if he feels uncomfortable or has difficulty breathing during the procedure.
- Reassure the patient during thoracentesis. Remind him to breathe normally and avoid sudden movements, such as coughing or sighing. Monitor his vital signs, and watch for syncope. If fluid is removed too quickly, the patient may suffer bradycardia, hypotension, pain, pulmonary edema, or even cardiac arrest. Watch for respiratory distress or pneumothorax (sudden onset of dyspnea and cyanosis) after thoracentesis.
- Administer oxygen and, in empyema, antibiotics, as ordered.
- Encourage the patient to perform deep-breathing exercises to promote lung expansion. Use an incentive spirometer to promote deep breathing.
- Provide meticulous chest tube care, and use sterile technique for changing dressings around the tube insertion site in empyema. Ensure tube patency by watching for fluctuations of fluid or air bubbling in the underwater seal chamber. Continuous bub-

bling may indicate an air leak. Record the amount, color, and consistency of any tube drainage.

■ If the patient has open drainage through a rib resection or intercostal tube, use hand and dressing precautions. Because weeks of such drainage are usually necessary to obliterate the space, make visiting nurse referrals for the patient who will be discharged with the tube in place.

■ If pleural effusion was a complication of pneumonia or influenza, advise prompt medical attention for upper respiratory infections.

Pleurisy

Pleurisy, also known as *pleuritis,* is an inflammation of the visceral and parietal pleurae that line the inside of the thoracic cage and envelop the lungs.

Causes and incidence

Pleurisy develops as a complication of pneumonia, tuberculosis, viruses, systemic lupus erythematosus, rheumatoid arthritis, uremia, Dressler's syndrome, certain cancers, pulmonary infarction, and chest trauma. Pleuritic pain is caused by the inflammation or irritation of sensory nerve endings in the parietal pleura. As the lungs inflate and deflate, the visceral pleura covering the lungs moves against the fixed parietal pleura lining the pleural space, causing pain. This disorder usually begins suddenly.

In the United States, pleural effusions develop in 36% to 66% of hospitalized patients with bacterial pneumonia.

Signs and symptoms

Sharp, stabbing pain that increases with deep breathing may be so severe that it limits movement on the affected side. Dyspnea also occurs. Other symptoms vary according to the underlying pathologic process.

Diagnosis

Auscultation of the chest reveals a characteristic pleural friction rub — a coarse, creaky sound heard during late inspiration and early expiration, directly over the area of pleural inflammation. Palpation over the affected area may reveal coarse vibration. Chest X-ray, ultrasound of the chest, and thoracentesis may aid in diagnosis.

Treatment

Treatment is directed at the underlying cause; bacterial infections are treated with appropriate antibiotics, tuberculosis requires special treatment, and viral infections may be permitted to run their course. Treatment also includes measures to relieve symptoms, such as anti-inflammatory agents, analgesics, and bed rest. Severe pain may require an intercostal nerve block of two or three intercostal nerves. Pleurisy with pleural effusion calls for thoracentesis as a therapeutic and diagnostic measure.

Special considerations

■ Stress the importance of bed rest, and plan your care to allow the patient as much uninterrupted rest as possible.

■ Administer antitussives and pain medication, as ordered, but be careful not to overmedicate. If the pain requires an opioid analgesic, warn the patient who's about to be discharged to avoid overuse because such medication depresses coughing and respiration.

■ Encourage the patient to cough. Tell him to apply firm pressure at the site of the pain during coughing exercises to minimize pain.

CHRONIC DISORDERS

Chronic obstructive pulmonary disease

Chronic obstructive pulmonary disease (COPD) is chronic airway obstruction that results from emphysema, chronic bronchitis, asthma, or any combination of these disorders. (See *Types of chronic obstructive pulmonary disease,* pages 554 to 557. Also see *Three types of emphysema,* page 558.) Usually, more than one of these underlying conditions coexist; in most cases, bronchitis and emphysema occur together. It doesn't always produce symptoms and

(Text continues on page 556.)

TYPES OF CHRONIC OBSTRUCTIVE PULMONARY DISEASE

Disease	Causes and pathophysiology	Clinical features
Asthma • Increased bronchial reactivity to many stimuli, which produces episodic bronchospasm and airway obstruction in conjunction with airway inflammation • Asthma with onset in adulthood: usually without distinct allergies; asthma with onset in childhood: commonly associated with definite allergens. Status asthmaticus is an acute asthma attack with severe bronchospasm that fails to clear with bronchodilator therapy. • *Prognosis:* More than half of children with asthma become asymptomatic as adults; more than half of asthmatics with onset after age 15 have persistent disease, with occasional severe attacks.	• Reversible airway inflammation usually occurs in response to an allergen. Swelling of membranes, bronchoconstriction, and production of mucus obstruct airways. Activated mast cells release chemical mediators, including histamine, bradykinin, prostaglandins, and leukotrienes, which perpetuates the inflammatory response. • Upper airway infection, exercise, anxiety and, rarely, coughing or laughing can precipitate an asthma attack; nocturnal flare-ups are common. • Paroxysmal airway obstruction associated with nasal polyps may be seen in response to aspirin or indomethacin ingestion. • Airway obstruction from spasm of bronchial smooth muscle narrows airways; inflammatory edema of the bronchial wall and inspissation of tenacious mucoid secretions are also important, particularly in status asthmaticus.	• History of intermittent attacks of dyspnea and wheezing • Mild wheezing progresses to severe dyspnea, audible wheezing, chest tightness (a feeling of not being able to breathe), and cough that produces thick mucus. • *Other signs:* prolonged expiration, intercostal and supraclavicular retraction on inspiration, use of accessory muscles of respiration, flaring nostrils, tachypnea, tachycardia, perspiration, and flushing; patients usually have symptoms of eczema and allergic rhinitis (hay fever). • Status asthmaticus, unless treated promptly, can progress to respiratory failure.
Chronic bronchitis • Excessive mucus production with productive cough for at least 3 months per year for 2 successive years • Only a minority of patients with the clinical syndrome of chronic bronchitis develop significant airway obstruction.	• Severity of disease related to the amount and duration of smoking; respiratory infection exacerbates symptoms • Hypertrophy and hyperplasia of bronchial mucous glands, increased goblet cells, damage to cilia, squamous metaplasia of columnar epithelium, and chronic leukocytic and lymphocytic infiltration of bronchial walls; widespread inflammation, distortion, narrowing of airways, and mucus within the airways produce resistance in small airways and cause severe ventilation-perfusion imbalance	• Insidious onset, with productive cough and exertional dyspnea predominant symptoms • *Other signs and symptoms:* upper respiratory infections associated with increased sputum production and worsening dyspnea, which take progressively longer to resolve; copious sputum (gray, white, or yellow); weight gain due to edema; cyanosis; tachypnea; wheezing; prolonged expiratory time; and use of accessory muscles of respiration • Complications include recurrent respiratory tract infections, cor pulmonale, and polycythemia.

Confirming diagnostic measures	Management

- *Physical examination:* usually normal between attacks; auscultation reveals rhonchi and wheezing throughout lung fields on expiration and, at times, inspiration and absent or diminished breath sounds during severe obstruction. Loud bilateral wheezing may be grossly audible; chest is hyperinflated.
- *Chest X-ray:* hyperinflated lungs with air trapping during attack; normal during remission
- *Sputum:* presence of Curschmann's spirals (casts of airways), Charcot-Leyden crystals, and eosinophils
- *Pulmonary function tests (PFTs):* during attacks, decreased forced expiratory volumes that improve significantly after inhaled bronchodilator; increased residual volume and, occasionally, total lung capacity; may be normal between attacks
- *Arterial blood gas (ABG) analysis:* decreased partial pressure of arterial oxygen (PaO_2); decreased, normal, or increased partial pressure of arterial carbon dioxide ($PaCO_2$; in severe attack)
- *Electrocardiogram (ECG):* sinus tachycardia during an attack; severe attack may produce signs of cor pulmonale (right axis deviation, peaked P wave) that resolve after the attack
- *Skin tests:* may identify allergens

- Aerosol containing beta-adrenergic agents, such as metaproterenol or albuterol; also oral beta-adrenergic agents (terbutaline) and oral methylxanthines (theophylline). Many patients require inhaled, oral, or I.V. corticosteroids.
- *Emergency treatment:* oxygen therapy, I.V. corticosteroids, and bronchodilators, such as subcutaneous epinephrine, I.V. theophylline, and inhaled agents (such as metaproterenol, albuterol, or ipratropium bromide).
- Monitor for deteriorating respiratory status and note sputum characteristics; provide adequate fluid intake and oxygen, as ordered.
- *Prevention:* Tell the patient to avoid possible triggers and to use inhaled corticosteroids, antihistamines, decongestants, cromolyn powder by inhalation, leukotriene modifier, and oral or aerosol bronchodilators, as ordered. Explain the influence of stress and anxiety on asthma as well as its frequent association with exercise (particularly running), cold air, and nighttime flare-ups.
- Help the patient identify the triggers and teach him how to use a metered-dose inhaler and a peak flow meter.

- *Physical examination:* barrel chest, rhonchi and wheezes on auscultation, prolonged expiration, jugular vein distention, and pedal edema
- *Chest X-ray:* may show hyperinflation and increased bronchovascular markings
- *PFTs:* increased residual volume, decreased vital capacity and forced expiratory volumes, and normal static compliance and diffusing capacity
- *ABG analysis:* decreased PaO_2, normal or increased $PaCO_2$
- *ECG:* may show atrial arrhythmias; peaked P waves in leads II, III, and aV_F; and, occasionally, right ventricular hypertrophy

- Antibiotics for infections
- Avoidance of smoking and air pollutants
- Bronchodilators to relieve bronchospasm and facilitate mucociliary clearance
- Adequate fluid intake and chest physiotherapy to mobilize secretions
- Ultrasonic or mechanical nebulizer treatments to loosen secretions and aid in mobilization
- Occasionally, corticosteroids
- Diuretics for edema
- Oxygen for hypoxemia or cor pulmonale

(continued)

TYPES OF CHRONIC OBSTRUCTIVE PULMONARY DISEASE *(continued)*

Disease	Causes and pathophysiology	Clinical features
Emphysema ▪ Abnormal, irreversible enlargement of air spaces distal to terminal bronchioles due to destruction of alveolar walls, resulting in decreased elastic recoil properties of lungs ▪ Most common cause of death from respiratory disease in the United States	▪ Cigarette smoking and congenital deficiency of alpha-antitrypsin ▪ Recurrent inflammation associated with release of proteolytic enzymes from cells in lungs causes bronchiolar and alveolar wall damage and, ultimately, destruction. Loss of lung supporting structure results in decreased elastic recoil and airway collapse on expiration. Destruction of alveolar walls decreases surface area for gas exchange.	▪ Insidious onset, with dyspnea the predominant symptom ▪ *Other signs and symptoms of long-term disease:* anorexia, weight loss, malaise, barrel chest, use of accessory muscles of respiration, prolonged expiratory period with grunting, pursed-lip breathing, and tachypnea ▪ *Complications* include recurrent respiratory tract infections, cor pulmonale, and respiratory failure.

causes only minimal disability in many patients. However, COPD tends to worsen with time.

Causes and incidence

Predisposing factors include cigarette smoking, recurrent or chronic respiratory infections, air pollution, occupational exposure to chemicals, and allergies. Smoking is by far the most important of these factors — it impairs ciliary action and macrophage function, inflames airways, increases mucus production, destroys alveolar septae, and causes peribronchiolar fibrosis. Early inflammatory changes may reverse if the patient stops smoking before lung destruction is extensive. Familial and hereditary factors (such as deficiency of alpha$_1$-antitrypsin) may also predispose a person to COPD.

The most common chronic lung disease, COPD (also known as chronic obstructive lung disease) affects an estimated 17 million Americans, and its incidence is rising. It affects more males than females, probably because until recently men were more likely to smoke heavily. COPD occurs mostly in people older than age 40.

Signs and symptoms

The typical patient, a long-term cigarette smoker, has no symptoms until middle age. His ability to exercise or do strenuous work gradually starts to decline and he begins to develop a productive cough. These signs are subtle at first, but become more pronounced as the patient gets older and the disease progresses. Eventually the patient may develop dyspnea on minimal exertion, frequent respiratory infections, intermittent or continuous hypoxemia, and grossly abnormal pulmonary function studies. Advanced COPD may cause severe dyspnea, overwhelming disability, cor pulmonale, severe respiratory failure, and death.

Diagnosis

For specific diagnostic tests used to determine COPD, see *Types of chronic obstructive pulmonary disease.*

Confirming diagnostic measures	Management
■ *Physical examination:* barrel chest, hyperresonance on percussion, decreased breath sounds, expiratory prolongation, and quiet heart sounds ■ *Chest X-ray:* in advanced disease, flattened diaphragm, reduced vascular markings at lung periphery, hyperexpansion of lungs, enlarged anteroposterior chest diameter, and large retrosternal air space ■ *Computed tomography scan:* may show emphysema ■ *PFTs:* increased residual volume, total lung capacity, and compliance; decreased vital capacity, diffusing capacity, and expiratory volumes ■ *ABG analysis:* reduced PaO_2 with normal $PaCO_2$ until late in disease ■ *ECG:* tall, symmetrical P waves in leads II, III, and aV_F; vertical QRS axis; signs of right ventricular hypertrophy late in disease ■ *Red blood cell count:* increased hemoglobin late in disease when persistent severe hypoxia is present	■ Oxygen at low-flow settings to treat hypoxia ■ Avoidance of smoking and air pollutants ■ Breathing techniques to control dyspnea ■ Treatment only slightly helpful for emphysema component of chronic obstructive pulmonary disease ■ Lung volume reduction surgery for selected patients

Treatment

Treatment is designed to relieve symptoms and prevent complications. Because most patients with COPD receive outpatient treatment, they need comprehensive teaching to help them comply with therapy and understand the nature of this chronic, progressive disease. If programs in pulmonary rehabilitation are available, encourage patients to enroll.

Urge the patient to stop smoking. Provide smoking cessation counseling or refer him to a program. Avoid other respiratory irritants, such as secondhand smoke, aerosol spray products, and outdoor air pollution. An air conditioner with an air filter in his home may be helpful.

The patient is usually treated with beta-agonist bronchodilators (albuterol or salmeterol), anticholinergic bronchodilators (ipratropium), and corticosteroids (beclomethasone or triamcinolone). These are usually given by metered-dose inhaler, requiring that the patient be taught the correct administration technique.

Antibiotics are used to treat respiratory infections. Stress the need to complete the prescribed course of antibiotic therapy.

Special considerations

■ Teach the patient and his family how to recognize early signs of infection; warn the patient to avoid contact with people with respiratory infections. Encourage good oral hygiene to help prevent infection. Pneumococcal vaccination and annual influenza vaccinations are important preventive measures.

■ To promote ventilation and reduce air trapping, teach the patient to breathe slowly, prolong expirations to two to three times the duration of inspiration, and to exhale through pursed lips.

■ To help mobilize secretions, teach the patient how to cough effectively. If the patient with copious secretions has difficulty mobilizing secretions, teach his family how to perform postural drainage and chest physiotherapy. If secretions are thick, urge the patient to drink 12 to 15 glasses of fluid per day. A home humidifier may be beneficial, particularly in the winter.

THREE TYPES OF EMPHYSEMA

A Panacinar (panlobular): destroys alveoli and alveolar ducts; associated with aging and alpha$_1$-antitrypsin deficiency
B Paraseptal (distal acinar): commonly causes spontaneous pneumothorax in young adults
C Centriacinar (centrilobular): associated with chronic bronchitis and smoking; destroys respiratory bronchioles

■ Administer low concentrations of oxygen as ordered. Perform blood gas analysis to determine the patient's oxygen needs and to avoid carbon dioxide narcosis. If the patient is to continue oxygen therapy at home, teach him how to use the equipment correctly. The patient with COPD rarely requires more than 2 to 3 L/minute to maintain adequate oxygenation. Higher flow rates will further increase the partial pressure of arterial oxygen, but the patient whose ventilatory drive is largely based on hypoxemia commonly develops markedly increased partial pressure of arterial carbon dioxide tensions. In these cases, chemoreceptors in the brain are relatively insensitive to the increase in carbon dioxide. Teach the patient and his family that excessive oxygen therapy may eliminate the hypoxic respiratory drive, causing confusion and drowsiness, signs of carbon dioxide narcosis.
■ Emphasize the importance of a balanced diet. Because the patient may tire easily when eating, suggest that he eat frequent, small meals and consider using oxygen, administered by nasal cannula, during meals.

■ Help the patient and his family adjust their lifestyles to accommodate the limitations imposed by this debilitating chronic disease. Instruct the patient to allow for daily rest periods and to exercise daily as his physician directs.
■ As COPD progresses, encourage the patient to discuss his fears.
■ To help prevent COPD, advise all patients, especially those with a family history of COPD or those in its early stages, not to smoke.
■ Assist in the early detection of COPD by urging persons to have periodic physical examinations, including spirometry and medical evaluation of a chronic cough, and to seek treatment for recurring respiratory infections promptly.
■ Lung volume reduction surgery is a new procedure for carefully selected patients with primarily emphysema. Nonfunctional parts of the lung (tissue filled with disease and providing little ventilation or perfusion) are surgically removed. Removal allows more functional lung tissue to expand and the diaphragm to return to its normally elevated position.

Bronchiectasis

A condition marked by chronic abnormal dilation of bronchi and destruction of bronchial walls, bronchiectasis can occur throughout the tracheobronchial tree or can be confined to one segment or lobe. However, it's usually bilateral and involves the basilar segments of the lower lobes. This disease has three forms: cylindrical (fusiform), varicose, and saccular (cystic). Bronchiectasis is irreversible once established.

Causes and incidence

Because of the availability of antibiotics to treat acute respiratory tract infections, the incidence of bronchiectasis has dramatically decreased in the past 20 years. Incidence is highest among Eskimos and the Maoris of New Zealand. It affects people of both sexes and all ages.

The different forms of bronchiectasis may occur separately or simultaneously. In *cylindrical bronchiectasis,* the bronchi expand unevenly, with little change in diameter, and end suddenly in a squared-off fashion. In *varicose bronchiectasis,* abnormal, irregular dilation and narrowing of the bronchi give the appearance of varicose veins. In *saccular bronchiectasis,* many large dilations end in sacs. These sacs balloon into pus-filled cavities as they approach the periphery and are then called saccules. (See *Forms of bronchial dilatation,* page 560.)

This disease results from conditions associated with repeated damage to bronchial walls and abnormal mucociliary clearance, which cause a breakdown of supporting tissue adjacent to airways. Such conditions include:

- cystic fibrosis
- immunologic disorders (agammaglobulinemia, for example)
- recurrent, inadequately treated bacterial respiratory tract infections, such as tuberculosis, and complications of measles, pneumonia, pertussis, or influenza
- obstruction (by a foreign body — most common in children, tumor, or stenosis) in association with recurrent infection
- inhalation of corrosive gas or repeated aspiration of gastric juices into the lungs

- congenital anomalies (uncommon), such as bronchomalacia, congenital bronchiectasis, immotile cilia syndrome, and Kartagener's syndrome, a variant of immotile cilia syndrome characterized by situs inversus, bronchiectasis, and either nasal polyps or sinusitis.

In bronchiectasis, hyperplastic squamous epithelium denuded of cilia replaces ulcerated columnar epithelium. Abscess formation involving all layers of the bronchial wall produces inflammatory cells and fibrous tissue, resulting in dilation and narrowing of the airways. Mucus plugs or fibrous tissue obliterates smaller bronchioles, whereas peribronchial lymphoid tissue becomes hyperplastic. Extensive vascular proliferation of bronchial circulation occurs and produces frequent hemoptysis.

Signs and symptoms

Initially, bronchiectasis may be asymptomatic. When symptoms do arise, they're commonly attributed to other illnesses. The patient usually complains of frequent bouts of pneumonia or hemoptysis. The classic symptom, however, is a chronic cough that produces foul-smelling, mucopurulent secretions in amounts ranging from less than 10 ml/day to more than 150 ml/day.

Cough and sputum production are observed in greater than 90% of bronchiectasis patients. Characteristic findings include coarse crackles during inspiration over involved lobes or segments, occasional wheezing, dyspnea, sinusitis, weight loss, anemia, malaise, clubbing, recurrent fever, chills, and other signs of infection.

Advanced bronchiectasis may produce chronic malnutrition as well as right-sided heart failure and cor pulmonale due to hypoxic pulmonary vasoconstriction.

Diagnosis

A history of recurrent bronchial infections, pneumonia, and hemoptysis in a patient whose chest X-rays show peribronchial thickening, areas of atelectasis, and scattered cystic changes suggest bronchiectasis.

In recent years, computed tomography scanning has supplanted bronchography as the most useful diagnostic test for bronch-

FORMS OF BRONCHIAL DILATATION

Dilatations of the air sacs occur due to bronchiectasis, as depicted below.

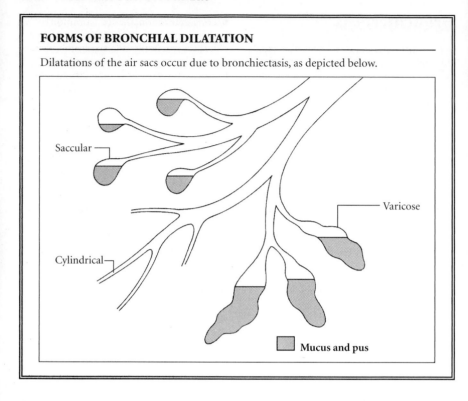

Saccular

Varicose

Cylindrical

■ Mucus and pus

iectasis. It's sometimes used with high-resolution techniques to better determine anatomic changes. Bronchoscopy doesn't establish the diagnosis of bronchiectasis, but it does help to identify the source of secretions. Bronchoscopy can also be instrumental in pinpointing the site of bleeding in hemoptysis.

Other helpful laboratory tests include:
■ sputum culture and Gram stain to identify predominant organisms
■ complete blood count to detect anemia and leukocytosis
■ pulmonary function tests to detect decreased vital capacity, expiratory flow rate, and hypoxemia. These tests also help determine the physiologic severity of the disease and the effects of therapy and help evaluate patients for surgery.

When cystic fibrosis is suspected as the underlying cause of bronchiectasis, a sweat electrolyte test is useful.

Treatment

Treatment includes antibiotics, given orally or I.V., for 7 to 10 days or until sputum production decreases. Bronchodilators, combined with postural drainage and chest percussion, help remove secretions if the patient has bronchospasm and thick, tenacious sputum. Bronchoscopy may be used to remove obstruction and secretions. Hypoxia requires oxygen therapy; severe hemoptysis commonly requires lobectomy, segmental resection, or bronchial artery embolization if pulmonary function is poor. Long-term antibiotic therapy isn't appropriate because it may predispose the patient to serious gram-negative infections and resistant organisms.

Special considerations

Provide supportive care and help the patient adjust to the permanent changes in lifestyle that irreversible lung damage necessitates. Thorough teaching is vital.
■ Administer antibiotics as ordered, and explain all diagnostic tests. Perform chest

physiotherapy, including postural drainage and chest percussion designed for involved lobes, several times a day. The best times to do this are early morning and just before bedtime. Instruct the patient to maintain each position for 10 minutes, and then perform percussion and tell him to cough. Show family members how to perform postural drainage and percussion. Also teach the patient coughing and deep-breathing techniques to promote good ventilation and the removal of secretions.

■ Advise the patient to stop smoking, if appropriate, to avoid stimulating secretions and irritating the airways. Refer him to a local self-help group.

■ Provide a warm, quiet, comfortable environment, and urge the patient to rest as much as possible. Encourage balanced, high-protein meals to promote good health and tissue healing and plenty of fluids (2 to 3 qt [2 to 3 L]) per day to hydrate and thin bronchial secretions). Give frequent mouth care to remove foul-smelling sputum. Teach the patient to dispose of all secretions properly. Instruct him to seek prompt attention for respiratory infections.

■ Tell the patient to avoid air pollutants and people with upper respiratory tract infections. Instruct him to take medications (especially antibiotics) exactly as prescribed.

■ To help prevent this disease, treat bacterial pneumonia vigorously and stress the need for immunization to prevent childhood diseases.

Idiopathic pulmonary fibrosis

Idiopathic pulmonary fibrosis (IPF) is a chronic and usually fatal interstitial pulmonary disease. About 50% of patients with IPF die within 5 years of diagnosis. Once thought to be a rare condition, it's now diagnosed with much greater frequency. IPF has been known by several other names over the years, including cryptogenic fibrosing alveolitis, diffuse interstitial fibrosis, idiopathic interstitial pneumonitis, and Hamman-Rich syndrome.

Causes and incidence

IPF is the result of a cascade of events that involve inflammatory, immune, and fibrotic processes in the lung. However, despite many studies and hypotheses, the stimulus that begins the progression remains unknown. Speculation has revolved around viral and genetic causes, but no good evidence has been found to support either theory. However, it's clear that chronic inflammation plays an important role. Inflammation develops the injury and the fibrosis that ultimately distorts and impairs the structure and function of the alveolocapillary gas exchange surface.

IPF is slightly more common in men than in women and is more common in smokers than in nonsmokers. It usually affects people ages 50 to 70.

Signs and symptoms

The usual presenting symptoms of IPF are dyspnea and a dry, hacking, and typically paroxysmal cough. Most patients have had these symptoms for several months to 2 years before seeking medical help. End-expiratory crackles, especially in the bases of the lungs, are usually heard early in the disease. Bronchial breath sounds appear later, when airway consolidation develops. Rapid, shallow breathing occurs, especially with exertion, and clubbing has been noted in more than 40% of patients. Late in the disease, cyanosis and evidence of pulmonary hypertension (augmented S_2 and S_3 gallop) commonly occur. As the disease progresses, profound hypoxemia and severe, debilitating dyspnea are the hallmark signs.

Diagnosis

Diagnosis begins with a thorough patient history to exclude a more common cause of interstitial lung disease.

CONFIRMING DIAGNOSIS *Lung biopsy is helpful in the diagnosis of IPF. In the past, an open lung biopsy was the only acceptable procedure, but now biopsies may be done through a thoracoscope or bronchoscope.*

Histologic features of the biopsy tissue vary, depending on the stage of the disease and other factors that aren't yet completely understood. The alveolar walls are swollen with chronic inflammatory cellular infiltrate composed of mononuclear cells and polymorphonuclear leukocytes. Intraalveolar inflammatory cells may be found in early stages. As the disease progresses, excessive collagen and fibroblasts fill the interstitium. In advanced stages, alveolar walls are destroyed and are replaced by honeycombing cysts.

Chest X-rays may show one of four distinct patterns: interstitial, reticulonodular, ground-glass, or honeycomb. Although chest X-rays are helpful in identifying the presence of an abnormality, they don't correlate well with histologic findings or pulmonary function tests (PFTs) in determining the severity of the disease. They also don't help distinguish inflammation from fibrosis. However, serial X-rays may help track the progression of the disease.

High-resolution computed tomography scans provide superior views of the four patterns seen on routine X-ray film and are used routinely to help establish the diagnosis of IPF. Research is currently under way to determine whether the four patterns of abnormality seen on these scans correlate with responsiveness to treatment.

PFTs show reductions in vital capacity and total lung capacity and impaired diffusing capacity for carbon monoxide. Arterial blood gas (ABG) analysis and pulse oximetry reveal hypoxemia, which may be mild when the patient is at rest early in the disease but may become severe later in the disease. Oxygenation will always deteriorate, usually to a severe level, with exertion. Serial PFTs (especially carbon monoxide diffusing capacity) and ABG values may help track the course of the disease and the patient's response to treatment.

Treatment

Although it can't change the pathology of IPF, oxygen therapy can prevent the problems related to dyspnea and tissue hypoxia in the early stages of the disease process. The patient may require little or no supplemental oxygen while at rest initially, but he'll need more as the disease progresses and during exertion.

No known cure exists. Corticosteroids and cytotoxic drugs may be given to suppress inflammation but are usually unsuccessful. Recently, interferon-gamma-1B has shown some promise in treating the disease.

Lung transplantation may be successful for younger, otherwise healthy individuals.

Special considerations

- Explain all diagnostic tests to the patient, who may experience anxiety and frustration about the many tests required to establish the diagnosis.
- Monitor oxygenation at rest and with exertion. The physician may prescribe one oxygen flow rate for use when the patient is at rest and a higher one for use during exertion to maintain adequate oxygenation. Instruct the patient to increase his oxygen flow rate to the appropriate level for exercise.
- As IPF progresses, the patient's oxygen requirements will increase. He may need a nonrebreathing mask to supply high oxygen percentages. Eventually, maintaining adequate oxygenation may become impossible despite maximum oxygen flow.
- Most patients will need oxygen at home. Make appropriate referrals to discharge planners, respiratory care practitioners, and home equipment vendors to ensure continuity of care.
- Teach breathing, relaxation, and energy conservation techniques to help the patient manage severe dyspnea.
- Encourage the patient to be as active as possible. Refer him to a pulmonary rehabilitation program.
- Monitor the patient for adverse reactions to drug therapy.
- Teach the patient about prescribed medications, especially adverse effects. Teach the patient and his family members infection prevention techniques.
- Encourage good nutritional habits. Small, frequent meals with high nutritional value may be necessary if dyspnea interferes with eating.
- Provide emotional support for the patient and his family as they deal with the patient's increasing disability, dyspnea, and probable death.

Tuberculosis

An acute or chronic infection caused by *Mycobacterium tuberculosis,* tuberculosis (TB) is characterized by pulmonary infiltrates, formation of granulomas with caseation, fibrosis, and cavitation. People who live in crowded, poorly ventilated conditions and those who are immunocompromised are most likely to become infected. In patients with strains that are sensitive to the usual antitubercular agents, the prognosis is excellent with correct treatment. However, in those with strains that are resistant to two or more of the major antitubercular agents, mortality is 50%.

Causes and incidence

After exposure to *M. tuberculosis,* roughly 5% of infected people develop active TB within 1 year; in the remainder, microorganisms cause a latent infection. The host's immune system usually controls the tubercle bacillus by enclosing it in a tiny nodule (tubercle). The bacillus may lie dormant within the tubercle for years and later reactivate and spread.

Although the primary infection site is the lungs, mycobacteria commonly exist in other parts of the body. Several factors increase the risk of infection reactivation: gastrectomy, uncontrolled diabetes mellitus, Hodgkin's disease, leukemia, silicosis, acquired immunodeficiency syndrome, treatment with corticosteroids or immunosuppressants, and advanced age.

Transmission is by droplet nuclei produced when infected persons cough or sneeze. Persons with a cavitary lesion are particularly infectious because their sputum usually contains 1 to 100 million bacilli per milliliter. If an inhaled tubercle bacillus settles in an alveolus, infection occurs, with alveolocapillary dilation and endothelial cell swelling. Alveolitis results, with replication of tubercle bacilli and influx of polymorphonuclear leukocytes. These organisms spread through the lymph system to the circulatory system and then through the body.

Cell-mediated immunity to the mycobacteria, which develops 3 to 6 weeks later, usually contains the infection and arrests the disease. If the infection reactivates, the body's response characteristically leads to caseation — the conversion of necrotic tissue to a cheeselike material. The caseum may localize, undergo fibrosis, or excavate and form cavities, the walls of which are studded with multiplying tubercle bacilli. If this happens, infected caseous debris may spread throughout the lungs by the tracheobronchial tree. Sites of extrapulmonary TB include the pleurae, meninges, joints, lymph nodes, peritoneum, genitourinary tract, and bowel.

The incidence of TB has been increasing in the United States secondary to homelessness, drug abuse, and human immunodeficiency virus infection. Globally, TB is the leading infectious cause of morbidity and mortality, generating 8 to 10 million new cases each year.

Signs and symptoms

After an incubation period of 4 to 8 weeks, TB is usually asymptomatic in primary infection but may produce nonspecific symptoms, such as fatigue, weakness, anorexia, weight loss, night sweats, and low-grade fever.

 ELDER TIP *Fever and night sweats, the typical hallmarks of TB, may not be present in elderly patients, who instead may exhibit a change in activity or weight. Assess older patients carefully.*

In reactivation, symptoms may include a cough that produces mucopurulent sputum, occasional hemoptysis, and chest pains.

Diagnosis

CONFIRMING DIAGNOSIS *Diagnostic tests include chest X-rays, a tuberculin skin test, and sputum smears and cultures to identify* M. tuberculosis. *The diagnosis must be precise because several other diseases (such as lung cancer, lung abscess, pneumoconiosis, and bronchiectasis) may mimic TB.*

These procedures aid in diagnosis:
■ Auscultation detects crepitant crackles, bronchial breath sounds, wheezing, and whispered pectoriloquy.
■ Chest percussion detects dullness over the affected area, indicating consolidation or pleural fluid.

- Chest X-ray shows nodular lesions, patchy infiltrates (mainly in upper lobes), cavity formation, scar tissue, and calcium deposits; however, it may not be able to distinguish active from inactive TB.
- Tuberculin skin test detects TB infection. Intermediate-strength purified protein derivative or 5 tuberculin units (0.1 ml) are injected intracutaneously on the forearm. The test results are read in 48 to 72 hours; a positive reaction (induration of 5 to 15 mm or more, depending on risk factors) develops 2 to 10 weeks after infection in active and inactive TB. However, severely immunosuppressed patients may never develop a positive reaction.

 CONFIRMING DIAGNOSIS *Stains and cultures (of sputum, cerebrospinal fluid, urine, drainage from abscess, or pleural fluid) show heat-sensitive, nonmotile, aerobic, acid-fast bacilli.*

Treatment

First-line agents for the treatment of TB are isoniazid (INH), rifampin (RIF), ethambutol (EMB), and pyrazinamide. Latent TB is usually treated with daily INH for 9 months. RIF daily for 4 months may be used for people with latent TB whose contacts are INH resistant. For most adults with active TB, the recommended dosing includes the administration of all four drugs daily for 2 months, followed by 4 months of INH and RIF. Drug therapy must be selected according to patient condition and organism susceptibility. Another first-line drug used for TB is rifapentine. Second-line agents, such as cycloserine, ethionamide, p-Aminosalicylic acid, streptomycin, and capreomycin, are reserved for special circumstances or drug-resistant strains. Interruption of drug therapy may require initiation of therapy from the beginning of the regimen or additional treatment.

Directly observed therapy (DOT) may be selected or required. In this therapy, an assigned caregiver directly observes the administration of the drug. The goal of DOT is to monitor the treatment regimen and reduce the development of resistant organisms.

Special considerations

- Initiate acid-fast bacillus (AFB) isolation precautions immediately for all patients suspected or confirmed to have TB. AFB isolation precautions include the use of a private room with negative pressure in relation to surrounding areas and a minimum of six air exchanges per hour (air exhausted should be exhausted directly to the outside).
- Continue AFB isolation until there's clinical evidence of reduced infectiousness (substantially decreased cough, fewer organisms on sequential sputum smears).
- Teach the infectious patient to cough and sneeze into tissues and to dispose of all secretions properly. Place a covered trash can nearby or tape a lined bag to the side of the bed to dispose of used tissues.
- Instruct the patient to wear a mask when outside his room.
- Visitors and staff members should wear particulate respirators that fit closely around the face when they're in the patient's room.
- Remind the patient to get plenty of rest. Stress the importance of eating balanced meals to promote recovery. If the patient is anorexic, urge him to eat small meals frequently. Record weight weekly.
- Be alert for adverse effects of medications. Because INH sometimes leads to hepatitis or peripheral neuritis, monitor aspartate aminotransferase and alanine aminotransferase levels. To prevent or treat peripheral neuritis, give pyridoxine (vitamin B_6), as ordered. If the patient receives EMB, watch for optic neuritis; if it develops, discontinue the drug. If he receives RIF, watch for hepatitis and purpura. Observe the patient for other complications such as hemoptysis.
- Before discharge, advise the patient to watch for adverse effects from the medication and report them immediately. Emphasize the importance of regular follow-up examinations. Instruct the patient and his family concerning the signs and symptoms of recurring TB. Stress the need to follow long-term treatment faithfully.
- Advise staff members and other persons who have been exposed to infected patients to receive tuberculin tests; chest X-rays and prophylactic INH may also be ordered.

■ Emphasize to the patient the importance of taking the medications daily as prescribed. He may enroll in a supervised administration program to avoid the development of drug-resistant organisms.

PNEUMOCONIOSES

Silicosis

Silicosis is a progressive disease characterized by nodular lesions that commonly progress to fibrosis. The most common form of pneumoconiosis, silicosis can be classified according to the severity of pulmonary disease and the rapidity of its onset and progression. It usually occurs as a simple asymptomatic illness.

Acute silicosis develops after 1 to 3 years in workers exposed to very high concentrations of respirable silica (sand blasters and tunnel workers). *Accelerated silicosis* appears after an average of 10 years of exposure to lower concentrations of free silica. *Chronic silicosis* develops after 20 or more years of exposure to lower concentrations of free silica. (Chronic silicosis is further subdivided into simple and complicated forms.)

The prognosis is good unless the disease progresses into the complicated fibrotic form, which causes respiratory insufficiency and cor pulmonale. It's also associated with pulmonary tuberculosis (TB).

Causes and incidence
Silicosis results from the inhalation and pulmonary deposition of respirable crystalline silica dust, mostly from quartz. The danger to the worker depends on the concentration of dust in the atmosphere, the percentage of respirable free silica particles in the dust, and the duration of exposure. Respirable particles are less than 10 microns in diameter, but the disease-causing particles deposited in the alveolar space are usually 1 to 3 microns in diameter.

Industrial sources of silica in its pure form include the manufacture of ceramics (flint) and building materials (sandstone). It occurs in mixed form in the production of construction materials (cement). It's found in powder form (silica flour) in paints, porcelain, scouring soaps, and wood fillers as well as in the mining of gold, coal, lead, zinc, and iron. Foundry workers, boiler scalers, and stonecutters are all exposed to silica dust and, therefore, are at high risk for developing silicosis.

Nodules result when alveolar macrophages ingest silica particles, which they're unable to process. As a result, the macrophages die and release proteolytic enzymes into the surrounding tissue. The subsequent inflammation attracts other macrophages and fibroblasts into the region to produce fibrous tissue and wall off the reaction. The resulting nodule has an onionskin appearance when viewed under a microscope. Nodules develop adjacent to terminal and respiratory bronchioles, concentrate in the upper lobes, and are commonly accompanied by bullous changes in both lobes. If the disease process doesn't progress, minimal physiologic disturbances and no disability occur. Occasionally, however, the fibrotic response accelerates, engulfing and destroying large areas of the lung (progressive massive fibrosis or conglomerate lesions). Fibrosis may continue even after exposure to dust has ended.

The incidence of silicosis has decreased since the Occupational Safety and Health Administration instituted regulations requiring the use of protective equipment that limits the amount of silica dust inhaled.

Signs and symptoms
Initially, silicosis may be asymptomatic or may produce dyspnea on exertion, usually attributed to being "out of shape" or "slowing down." If the disease progresses to the chronic and complicated stage, dyspnea on exertion worsens, and other symptoms—usually tachypnea and an insidious dry cough that's most pronounced in the morning—appear.

Progression to the advanced stage causes dyspnea on minimal exertion, worsening cough, and pulmonary hypertension, which in turn leads to right-sided heart failure and cor pulmonale. Patients with silicosis have a high incidence of active TB, which should be considered when evaluating patients with this disease. Central nervous system changes — confusion, lethargy, and a decrease in the rate and depth of respiration as the partial pressure of arterial carbon dioxide increases — also occur in advanced silicosis.

Other clinical features include malaise, disturbed sleep, and hoarseness. The severity of these symptoms may not correlate with chest X-ray findings or the results of pulmonary function tests.

Diagnosis
The patient history reveals occupational exposure to silica dust. The physical examination is normal in simple silicosis; in chronic silicosis with conglomerate lesions, it may reveal decreased chest expansion, diminished intensity of breath sounds, areas of hyporesonance and hyperresonance, fine to medium crackles, and tachypnea.

In simple silicosis, chest X-rays show small, discrete, nodular lesions distributed throughout both lung fields but typically concentrated in the upper lung zones; the hilar lung nodes may be enlarged and exhibit "eggshell" calcification. In complicated silicosis, X-rays show one or more conglomerate masses of dense tissue.

Pulmonary function tests show:
- Forced vital capacity (FVC) — reduced in complicated silicosis
- Forced expiratory volume in 1 second (FEV_1) — reduced in obstructive disease (emphysematous areas of silicosis); reduced in complicated silicosis, but ratio of FEV_1 to FVC is normal or high
- Maximal voluntary ventilation — reduced in restrictive and obstructive diseases
- Carbon dioxide diffusing capacity — reduced when fibrosis destroys alveolar walls and obliterates pulmonary capillaries or when fibrosis thickens the alveolocapillary membrane.

Treatment
The goal of treatment is to relieve respiratory symptoms, to manage hypoxemia and cor pulmonale, and to prevent respiratory tract irritation and infections. Treatment also includes careful observation for the development of TB. Respiratory symptoms may be relieved through daily use of in-haled bronchodilators and increased fluid intake (at least 3 qt [3 L] daily). Steam inhalation and chest physiotherapy techniques, such as controlled coughing and segmental bronchial drainage with chest percussion and vibration, help clear secretions. In severe cases, it may be necessary to administer oxygen by cannula or mask (1 to 2 L/minute) for the patient with chronic hypoxemia or by mechanical ventilation if arterial oxygen can't be maintained above 40 mm Hg. Respiratory infections require prompt administration of antibiotics.

Special considerations
- Teach the patient to prevent infections by avoiding crowds and persons with respiratory infections and by receiving influenza and pneumococcal vaccines.
- Increase exercise tolerance by encouraging regular activity. Advise the patient to plan his daily activities to decrease the work of breathing. The patient should be instructed to pace himself, rest often, and generally move slowly through his daily routine.

Asbestosis

Asbestosis is a form of pneumoconiosis characterized by diffuse interstitial fibrosis. It can develop as long as 15 to 20 years after regular exposure to asbestos has ended. Asbestos also causes pleural plaques and mesotheliomas of pleura and the peritoneum. A potent co-carcinogen, asbestos increases the risk of lung cancer in cigarette smokers.

Causes and incidence
Asbestosis results from the inhalation of respirable asbestos fibers (50 microns or more in length and 0.5 microns or less in diameter), which assume a longitudinal orientation in the airway and move in the direction of airflow. The fibers penetrate respiratory bronchioles and alveolar walls. Sources include the mining and milling of asbestos, the construction industry, and the fireproofing and textile industries. Asbestos was also used in the production of paints, plastics, and brake and clutch linings.

Asbestos-related diseases develop in families of asbestos workers as a result of exposure to fibrous dust shaken off workers' clothing at home. Such diseases develop in the general public as a result of exposure to fibrous dust or waste piles from nearby asbestos plants, but exposures for occupants of typical buildings are quite low and not in a range associated with asbestosis.

Inhaled fibers become encased in a brown, proteinlike sheath rich in iron (ferruginous bodies or asbestos bodies), found in sputum and lung tissue. Interstitial fibrosis develops in lower lung zones, causing obliterative changes in lung parenchyma and pleurae. Raised hyaline plaques may form in parietal pleura, diaphragm, and pleura contiguous with the pericardium.

Asbestosis occurs in 4 of every 10,000 people.

Signs and symptoms

Clinical features may appear before chest X-ray changes. The first symptom is usually dyspnea on exertion, typically after 10 years' exposure. As fibrosis extends, dyspnea on exertion increases until, eventually, dyspnea occurs even at rest. Advanced disease also causes a dry cough (may be productive in smokers), chest pain (commonly pleuritic), recurrent respiratory infections, and tachypnea.

Cardiovascular complications include pulmonary hypertension, right ventricular hypertrophy, and cor pulmonale. Finger clubbing commonly occurs.

Diagnosis

The patient history reveals occupational, family, or neighborhood exposure to asbestos fibers. Physical examination reveals characteristic dry crackles at lung bases. Chest X-rays show fine, irregular, and linear diffuse infiltrates; extensive fibrosis results in a "honeycomb" or "ground-glass" appearance. X-rays may also show pleural thickening and calcification, with bilateral obliteration of costophrenic angles. In later stages, an enlarged heart with a classic "shaggy" heart border may be evident. Computed tomography scan of the lungs also aids in diagnosis.

Pulmonary function tests show:
- Vital capacity, forced vita capacity, and total lung capacity — decreased
- Forced expiratory volume in 1 second — decreased or normal
- Carbon monoxide diffusing capacity — reduced when fibrosis destroys alveolar walls and thickens alveolocapillary membranes.

Arterial blood gas analysis reveals:
- Partial pressure of arterial oxygen — decreased
- Partial pressure of arterial carbon dioxide — low due to hyperventilation.

Treatment

The goal of treatment is to relieve respiratory symptoms and, in advanced disease, manage hypoxemia and cor pulmonale. Respiratory symptoms may be relieved by chest physiotherapy techniques, such as controlled coughing and segmental bronchial drainage, chest percussion, and vibration. Aerosol therapy, inhaled mucolytics, and increased fluid intake (at least 3 qt [3 L] daily) may also relieve symptoms.

Diuretics, cardiac glycosides, and salt restriction may be indicated for patients with cor pulmonale. Hypoxemia requires oxygen administration by cannula or mask (1 to 2 L/minute) or by mechanical ventilation if arterial oxygen can't be maintained above 40 mm Hg. Respiratory infections require prompt administration of antibiotics.

Special considerations

- Teach the patient to prevent infections by avoiding crowds and persons with infections and by receiving influenza and pneumococcal vaccines.
- Improve the patient's ventilatory efficiency by encouraging physical reconditioning, energy conservation in daily activities, and relaxation techniques.

Coal worker's pneumoconiosis

A progressive nodular pulmonary disease, coal worker's pneumoconiosis (CWP) occurs in two forms. Simple CWP is characterized by small lung opacities; in complicated CWP, also known as *progressive massive fibrosis,* masses of fibrous tissue occasionally develop in the patient's lungs. The risk of developing CWP (also known as black lung disease, coal miner's disease, miner's asthma, anthracosis, and anthracosilicosis) depends upon the duration of exposure to coal dust (usually 15 years or longer), intensity of exposure (dust count and particle size), location of the mine, silica content of the coal (anthracite coal has the highest silica content), and the worker's susceptibility.

The prognosis varies. Simple asymptomatic disease is self-limiting, although progression to complicated CWP is more likely if CWP begins after a relatively short period of exposure. Complicated CWP may be disabling, resulting in severe ventilatory failure and cor pulmonale.

Causes and incidence

CWP is caused by the inhalation and prolonged retention of respirable coal dust particles (less than 5 microns in diameter). Simple CWP results in the formation of macules (accumulations of macrophages laden with coal dust) around the terminal and respiratory bronchioles, surrounded by a halo of dilated alveoli. Macule formation leads to atrophy of supporting tissue, causing permanent dilation of small airways (focal emphysema).

Simple disease may progress to complicated CWP, involving one or both lungs. In this form of the disease, fibrous tissue masses enlarge and coalesce, causing gross distortion of pulmonary structures (destruction of vasculature alveoli and airways).

The incidence of CWP is highest among anthracite coal miners in the eastern United States.

Signs and symptoms

Simple CWP produces no symptoms, especially in nonsmokers. Symptoms of complicated CWP include exertional dyspnea and a cough that occasionally produces inky-black sputum (when fibrotic changes undergo avascular necrosis and their centers cavitate). Other clinical features of CWP include increasing dyspnea and a cough that produces milky, gray, clear, or coal-flecked sputum. Recurrent bronchial and pulmonary infections produce yellow, green, or thick sputum.

Complications include pulmonary hypertension, right ventricular hypertrophy and cor pulmonale, and pulmonary tuberculosis (TB). In cigarette smokers, chronic bronchitis and emphysema may also complicate the disease.

Diagnosis

The patient history reveals exposure to coal dust. Physical examination shows barrel chest, hyperresonant lungs with areas of dullness, diminished breath sounds, crackles, rhonchi, and wheezes. In *simple CWP,* chest X-rays show small opacities (less than 10 mm in diameter). These may be present in all lung zones but are more prominent in the upper lung zones. In *complicated CWP,* one or more large opacities (1 to 5 cm in diameter), possibly exhibiting cavitation, are seen.

Pulmonary function tests show:
- Vital capacity — normal in simple CWP but decreased with complicated CWP
- Forced expiratory volume in 1 second — decreased in complicated disease
- Residual volume and total lung capacity — normal in simple CWP; decreased in complicated CWP.
- Carbon monoxide diffusing capacity — significantly decreased in complicated CWP as alveolar septae are destroyed and pulmonary capillaries obliterated.
- Partial pressure of arterial carbon dioxide — may be increased with concomitant chronic obstructive pulmonary disease.

Treatment

There's no specific treatment. The goal of treatment is to relieve respiratory symptoms, manage hypoxia and cor pulmonale, and avoid respiratory tract irritants and infections. Treatment also includes careful observation for the development of TB. Chest physiotherapy techniques, such as controlled coughing and segmental bronchial drainage combined with chest percussion and vibration, help remove secretions.

Other measures include increased fluid intake (at least 3 qt [3 L] daily) and respiratory therapy techniques, such as aerosol therapy, inhaled mucolytics, and intermittent positive pressure breathing. Diuretics, cardiac glycosides, and salt restriction may be indicated in cor pulmonale. In severe cases, it may be necessary to administer oxygen for hypoxemia by cannula or mask (1 to 2 L/minute) if the patient has chronic hypoxia; mechanical ventilation is utilized if arterial oxygen can't be maintained above 40 mm Hg. Respiratory infections require prompt administration of antibiotics.

Special considerations

■ Teach the patient to prevent infections by avoiding crowds and persons with respiratory infections and by receiving pneumovax and annual influenza vaccines.

■ Encourage the patient to stay active to avoid a deterioration in his physical condition but to pace his activities and practice relaxation techniques.

Selected references

Albert, R.K., et al. *Clinical Respiratory Medicine,* 2nd ed. St. Louis: Mosby–Year Book, Inc., 2004.

Cheng, I.W., et al. "Prognostic Value of Surfactant Proteins A and D in Patients with Acute Lung Injury," *Critical Care Medicine* 31(1):20-27, January 2003.

Diehl, J.L., et al. "Helium/Oxygen Mixture Reduces the Work of Breathing at the End of the Weaning Process in Patients with Severe Chronic Obstructive Pulmonary Disease," *Critical Care Medicine* 31(5):1415-20, May 2003.

Goss, C.H, et al. "Incidence of Acute Lung Injury in the United States,"*Critical Care Medicine* 31(6):1607-11, June 2003.

Hanley, M.E., and Welsh, C.H. *Current Diagnosis and Treatment in Pulmonary Medicine.* New York: McGraw-Hill Book Co., 2004.

Lim, C.M., et al. "Effect of Alveolar Recruitment Maneuver in Early Acute Respiratory Distress Syndrome according to Antiderecruitment Strategy, Etiological Category of Diffuse Lung Injury, and Body Position of the Patient," *Critical Care Medicine* 31(2):411-18, February 2003.

Respiratory Care Made Incredibly Easy. Philadelphia: Lippincott Williams & Wilkins, 2005.

Warren, D.K., et al. "Outcome and Attributable Cost of Ventilator-associated Pneumonia among Intensive Care Unit Patients in a Suburban Medical Center," *Critical Care Medicine* 31(5):1312-17, May 2003.

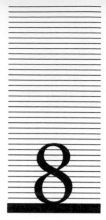

Musculoskeletal disorders

Introduction *571*

Congenital disorders *576*
Clubfoot *576*
Developmental dysplasia of the hip *578*
Muscular dystrophy *581*

Joints *583*
Septic arthritis *583*
Gout *585*
Neurogenic arthropathy *588*
Osteoarthritis *589*

Bones *591*
Osteomyelitis *591*
Osteoporosis *593*
Legg-Calvé-Perthes disease *595*
Osgood-Schlatter disease *596*
Paget's disease *597*
Hallux valgus *599*
Kyphosis *600*
Herniated disk *602*
Scoliosis *604*

Muscle and connective tissue *607*
Tendinitis and bursitis *607*
Epicondylitis *609*
Achilles tendon contracture *610*
Carpal tunnel syndrome *611*
Torticollis *612*
Rhabdomyolysis *614*

Selected references *615*

Introduction

A complex system of bones, muscles, ligaments, tendons, and other connective tissue, the musculoskeletal system gives the body its form and shape. It also protects vital organs, makes movement possible, stores calcium and other minerals, and provides sites for hematopoiesis. A fibrous layer called the *periosteum* covers all bones, except at joints, where they're covered by articular cartilage.

The human skeleton contains 206 bones, which are composed of inorganic salts, such as calcium and phosphate, embedded in a framework of collagen fibers. Bones are classified by shape as long, short, flat, or irregular.

Long bones

Long bones, which are found in the extremities, include the humerus, radius, and ulna of the arm; the femur, tibia, and fibula of the leg; and the phalanges, metacarpals, and metatarsals, which are found in the hands and feet. These bones have a long shaft, or *diaphysis,* and widened, bulbous ends, called *epiphyses.* A long bone is made up mainly of compact bone, which surrounds the medullary cavity (also called the *yellow marrow*), a storage site for fat. The lining of the medullary cavity (the *endosteum*) is a thin layer of connective tissue. The outer layer is the periosteum. (See *Long bone structure,* page 572.)

In children and young adults, lengthwise growth occurs at the epiphyseal cartilage between the diaphysis and epiphysis. In adults, in whom bone growth is complete, this cartilage is ossified and forms the epiphyseal line. The epiphysis also has a surface layer made up of compact bone, but its center is made of spongy or cancellous bone. Cancellous bone contains open spaces between thin threads of bone, called *trabeculae,* which are arranged in various directions to correspond with the lines of maximum stress or pressure. This configuration gives the bone added structural strength.

Unlike cancellous bone, adult compact bone consists of numerous orderly networks of interconnecting canals that run parallel to the bone's long axis. Each of these networks, called a *haversian system,* consists of a central haversian canal surrounded by layers *(lamellae)* of bone. Between adjacent lamellae are small openings *(lacunae),* which contain bone cells *(osteocytes).* All lacunae are joined by an interconnecting network of tiny canals *(canaliculi),* each of which contains one or more capillaries and provides a route for movement of tissue fluids. The haversian system carries blood to the bone through blood vessels that enter the system through channels called *Volkmann's canals.*

Short, flat, or irregular bones

Short bones include the tarsal and carpal bones; flat bones, the frontal and parietal bones of the cranium, ribs, sternum, scapulae, ilium, and pubis; and irregular bones, the bones of the spine (vertebrae, sacrum, and coccyx) and certain bones of the skull (sphenoid, ethmoid, and mandible).

Short, flat, and irregular bones have an outer layer of compact bone and an inner portion of spongy bone. In the sternum and certain areas in the flat bones of the skull, the spongy bone contains red marrow.

Joints

The tissues connecting two bones make up a joint, which permits motion between the bones and provides stability. Joints, like bones, have varying forms.
- Fibrous joints *(synarthroses)* have only minute motion and provide stability when tight union is necessary, as in the seams, called sutures, that join the cranial bones.
- Cartilaginous joints *(amphiarthroses)* have limited motion, as between vertebrae.
- Synovial joints *(diarthroses)* are the most common and have the greatest degree of movement. Such joints include the elbows and knees. Synovial joints have special characteristics: the articulating surfaces of each bone have a smooth hyaline covering (articular cartilage), which is resilient to pressure; their opposing surfaces are congruous and glide smoothly on each other; a fibrous (articular) capsule holds them together. Beneath the capsule and lining the joint cavity, the synovial membrane secretes the clear, viscous synovial fluid. This

LONG BONE STRUCTURE

Long bone composition is depicted below, with an illustrated cross section.

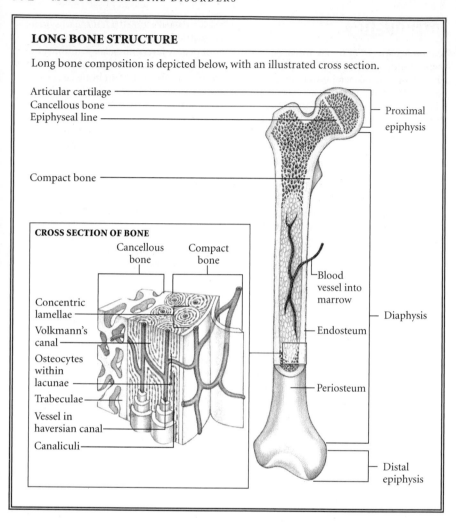

Articular cartilage
Cancellous bone
Epiphyseal line

Proximal epiphysis

Compact bone

CROSS SECTION OF BONE

Cancellous bone
Compact bone

Concentric lamellae
Volkmann's canal
Osteocytes within lacunae
Trabeculae
Vessel in haversian canal
Canaliculi

Blood vessel into marrow
Endosteum
Periosteum

Diaphysis

Distal epiphysis

fluid lubricates the two opposing surfaces during motion and also nourishes the articular cartilage. Surrounding a synovial joint are ligaments, muscles, and tendons, which strengthen and stabilize the joint but allow free movement.

In some synovial joints, the synovial membrane forms two additional structures — bursae and tendon sheaths — which reduce friction that normally accompanies movement. Bursae are small, cushionlike sacs lined with synovial membranes and filled with synovial fluid; most are located between tendons and bones.

Tendon sheaths wrap around the tendon and cushion it as it crosses the joint.

The synovial joints permit angular and circular movements. Angular movements include *flexion* (decrease in joint angle), *extension* (increase in the joint angle), and *hyperextension* (increase in the angle of extension beyond the usual arc). Joints of the knees, elbows, and phalanges permit such movement. Other angular movements are *abduction* (movement away from the body's midline) and *adduction* (movement toward the body's midline).

Circular movements include *rotation* (motion around a central axis), as in the ball-and-socket joints of the hips and shoulders; *pronation* (wrist motion to place palmar surface of the hand down, with the thumb toward the body); *supination* (begging position, with palm up). Other kinds of movement are *inversion* (movement facing inward), *eversion* (movement facing outward), *protraction* (as in forward motion of the mandible), and *retraction* (returning protracted part into place).

Muscles

Muscle tissues' most specialized feature— *contractility*—makes movement of bones and joints possible. Muscles also pump blood through the body, move food through the intestines, and make breathing possible. Muscular activity produces heat, so it's an important component in temperature regulation. Muscles maintain body positions, such as sitting and standing. Muscle mass accounts for about 40% of the body weight of a person of average size.

Muscles are classified in many ways. *Skeletal* muscles are attached to bone, *visceral* muscles permit function of internal organs, and *cardiac* muscles make up the heart wall. Also, muscles may be striated or nonstriated (smooth), depending on their cellular configuration.

Muscles classified according to activity are called *voluntary* or *involuntary*. Voluntary muscles can be controlled at will and are under the influence of the somatic nervous system; these are the skeletal muscles. Involuntary muscles, controlled by the autonomic nervous system, include the cardiac and visceral muscles.

Each skeletal muscle consists of many elongated muscle cells, called *muscle fibers*, through which run slender threads of protein, called *myofibrils*. Muscle fibers are held together in bundles by sheaths of fibrous tissue, called *fascia*. Blood vessels and nerves pass through the fascia to reach the individual muscle fibers.

Skeletal muscles are attached to bone directly or indirectly by fibrous cords called *tendons*. The least movable end of the muscle attachment is called *the point of origin*; the most movable end is *the point of insertion*.

Mechanism of contraction

To stimulate muscle contraction and movement, the brain sends motor impulses through the peripheral motor nerves to motor nerve fibers in the voluntary muscle. These nerve fibers reach membranes of skeletal muscle cells at neuromuscular (*myoneural*) junctions. When an impulse reaches the myoneural junction, it triggers the following sequence: release of the neurochemical acetylcholine, transient release of calcium from the sarcoplasmic reticulum (a membranous network in the muscle fiber), and muscle contraction. The arriving impulse at the myoneural junction also triggers release of adenosine triphosphate, the energy source for muscle contraction. Muscle relaxation is believed to take place by reversal of the above mechanisms.

Musculoskeletal assessment

Most patients with musculoskeletal disorders are elderly, have concurrent medical conditions, or have experienced trauma. Generally, they face prolonged immobilization. These factors make thorough assessment essential. Your assessment should include a complete history and a careful physical examination.

Interview the patient carefully to obtain a complete medical, social, and personal history. Ask about general activity (does he jog daily, or is he sedentary?), which may be significantly altered by musculoskeletal disease or trauma. Obtain information about occupation, diet, sexual activity, and elimination habits, and try to assess how the problem will affect body image. Also, ask how he functions at home. Can he perform activities of daily living? Does he have difficulty getting around? Are there stairs where he lives? Where are the bathroom and bedroom? Does he use any prosthetic devices? Ask if other family members can help with his care.

Get an accurate account of the musculoskeletal problem. Ask the patient if it has caused him to change his everyday routine. When did symptoms begin and how did they progress? Has the patient received treatment for this problem? If he's experienced trauma, find out how he was hurt.

Assess the level of pain. Is the patient in pain at the moment? Ask what makes the discomfort worse or better (movement, position, and so forth). Evaluate past and present responses to treatment. For instance, if the patient has arthritis and uses corticosteroids, ask him about their effectiveness. Does he require more or less medication than before? Did he comply with prescribed treatment?

The physical examination helps to determine the diagnosis and reveals any existing disabilities. (These baseline data will help when the effects of treatment are evaluated.) Observe the patient's appearance. Look for localized edema, pigmentation, redness and tenderness at pressure points, and other deformities such as atrophy. Note mobility, strength, and gait. To check range of motion, ask the patient to abduct, adduct, or flex the muscles in question. Check neurovascular status, including motion sensation and circulation. Measure and record discrepancies in muscle circumference or leg length. Compare one side or extremity to the other. If a neck injury is suspected, don't force range of motion.

Diagnostic tools

- X-rays are a useful diagnostic tool to evaluate musculoskeletal diseases. They can help to identify joint disruption, bone deformities, calcifications, and bone destruction and fractures. X-rays also measure bone density.
- Myelography is an invasive procedure used to evaluate abnormalities of the spinal canal and cord. It entails injection of a radiopaque contrast medium into the subarachnoid space of the spine. Serial X-rays visualize the progress of the contrast medium as it passes through the subarachnoid space. Displacement of the medium indicates a space-occupying lesion, such as a herniated disk or a tumor.
- Magnetic resonance imaging is useful in evaluating soft tissue injuries or ligament tears, such as rotator cuff tears or meniscal tears.
- Computed tomography scan can be used to identify injuries to bones, soft tissue, ligaments, tendons, and muscles.
- Arthroscopy is the visual examination of the interior of a joint with a fiber-optic endoscope.

Other useful tests include bone and muscle biopsies, electromyography, microscopic examination of synovial fluid, and multiple laboratory studies of urine and blood to identify systemic abnormalities.

Patient care

Each patient with musculoskeletal disease needs an individual care plan formulated early in his hospital stay by the entire clinical team, including the physician, physical therapist, and occupational therapist. Develop this plan with short- and long-term goals, during and after hospitalization.

Caring for the patient with a musculoskeletal disease usually includes at least one of the following: traction, casts, braces, splints, crutches, intermittent range-of-motion devices, prolonged immobilization, physical therapy, and occupational therapy.

Traction is the manual or mechanical application of a steady pulling force to reduce a fracture, minimize muscle spasms, or immobilize or align a joint.
- Skin traction is the indirect application of traction to the skeletal system through skin and soft tissues.
- Skeletal traction is the direct application of traction to bones by means of a pin (Steinmann pin) or wire (Kirschner wire) through the affected bone or by calipers or a tonglike device (Gardner-Wells tongs) that grips the bone.
- Manual traction, for emergency use, is the direct application of traction to a body part by hand.

During the use of all types of traction:
- Explain to the patient how traction works, and advise him about permissible amounts of activity and elevation of the head of the bed. Inform him of the anticipated duration of traction and whether or not the traction is removable. Teach active range-of-motion exercises.
- Check neurovascular status to prevent nerve damage. Also, make sure the mattress is firm, that the traction ropes aren't frayed, that they're on the center track of the pulley, and that traction weights are hanging free. Thoroughly investigate any complaint the patient makes.
- Check for signs of infection (odor, local inflammation and drainage, or fever) at pin sites if the patient is in skeletal traction.

Also, check with the physician's or the facility's procedure regarding pin-site care, such as use of peroxide or povidone-iodine.

Ideally, a cast immobilizes without adding too much weight. It's snug-fitting but doesn't constrict and has a smooth inner surface and smooth edges to prevent pressure or skin irritation. Casts require comprehensive patient education.

- A plaster cast takes 24 to 48 hours to dry. To prevent indentations, tell the patient not to squeeze the cast with his fingers, not to cover or walk on the cast until it has dried, and not to bump a damp cast on hard surfaces because dents can cause pressure areas. Warn the patient that while the cast is drying, he'll feel a temporary sensation of heat under the cast.
- If fiberglass is used, the cast may feel dry and the patient may be able to bear weight immediately. Advise the patient, however, not to get the cast wet. Although the fiberglass won't disintegrate as plaster would, the padding will become wet and potentially cause maceration of the skin.
- Emphasize the need to keep the cast above heart level for *24 hours* after its application to reduce swelling in the extremity.
- While the cast is drying and after drying is complete, the patient should watch for and immediately report persistent pain in the extremity inside or distal to the cast as well as edema, changes in skin color, coldness, or tingling or numbness in this area. If any of these signs occur, tell the patient to position the casted body part above heart level and notify his physician.
- The patient should also report drainage through the cast or an odor that may indicate infection. Warn against inserting foreign objects under the cast, getting it wet, pulling out its padding, or scratching inside it. Tell the patient to seek immediate attention for a broken cast.
- Instruct the patient to exercise the joints above and below the cast to prevent stiffness and contracture.

Braces, splints, and slings also provide alignment, immobilization, and pain relief for musculoskeletal diseases. Slings and splints are usually used for short-term immobilization. Explain to the patient and his family why these appliances are necessary, and show them the proper way to apply the sling, splint, or brace for optimal benefit. Tell the patient how long the appliance will have to be worn, and advise him of any activity limitations that must be observed. If the patient has a brace, check with his orthotist (orthopedic appliance specialist) about proper care. Encourage the patient to refer additional questions to his physician. Teach proper crutch walking.

Coping with immobility

Immobilized patients require meticulous care to prevent complications. Without constant care, the bedridden patient becomes susceptible to pressure ulcers, caused by the increased pressure on tissue over bony prominences, and is especially vulnerable to cardiopulmonary complications.

- To prevent pressure ulcers, turn the patient regularly and, if possible, position him in a 30-degree side-lying position for short periods. In addition, place a flotation pad or sheepskin pad under bony prominences, or use an alternating-air-current, convoluted foam, or foam mattress. Show the patient how to use a Balkan frame with a trapeze to move about in bed.
- Keep the patient's skin dry and clean.
- Keep the sheets wrinkle-free.
- Increase fluid intake to minimize risk of renal calculi.
- Provide adequate nutrition; a high-protein diet is preferred, if tolerated.
- Perform passive range-of-motion (ROM) exercises on the affected side, as ordered, to prevent contractures, and instruct the patient in active ROM exercises on the unaffected side. Apply footboards or high-topped sneakers to prevent footdrop. Keep the patient's heels off the bed to prevent heel breakdown. Also, watch for reddened elbows.
- Because most bedridden patients involuntarily perform a Valsalva maneuver when using the upper arms and trunk to move, instruct the patient to exhale (instead of holding his breath) as he turns. This will prevent possible cardiac complications that result from increased intrathoracic pressure.

- Emphasize the importance of coughing and deep breathing, and teach the patient how to use the incentive spirometer if ordered.
- Because constipation is a common problem in bedridden patients, establish a bowel program (fluids, fiber, laxatives, stool softeners), as needed.

Rehabilitation

Restoring the patient to his former state of health isn't always possible. When it isn't, help the patient adjust to a modified lifestyle. During hospitalization, promote independence by letting him finish difficult tasks by himself. If necessary, refer the patient to a community facility for continued rehabilitation.

CONGENITAL DISORDERS

Clubfoot

Clubfoot, or *talipes,* is the most common congenital disorder of the lower extremities. It's marked primarily by a deformed talus and shortened Achilles tendon, which give the foot a characteristic clublike appearance. In talipes equinovarus, the foot points downward (equinus) and turns inward (varus), whereas the front of the foot curls toward the heel (forefoot adduction).

Causes and incidence

A combination of genetic and environmental factors in utero appears to cause clubfoot. Heredity is a definite factor in some cases, although the mechanism of transmission is undetermined. In children without a family history of clubfoot, this anomaly seems linked to arrested development during the 9th and 10th weeks of embryonic life, when the feet are formed. Researchers also suspect muscle abnormalities, leading to variations in length and tendon insertions, as possible causes of clubfoot.

Clubfoot, which has an incidence of approximately 1 per 1,000 live births, usually occurs bilaterally and is twice as common in boys. It may be associated with other birth defects, such as myelomeningocele, spina bifida, and arthrogryposis.

Signs and symptoms

Talipes equinovarus varies greatly in severity. Deformity may be so extreme that the toes touch the inside of the ankle, or it may be only vaguely apparent. In every case, the talus is deformed, the Achilles tendon shortened, and the calcaneus somewhat shortened and flattened. Depending on the degree of the varus deformity, the calf muscles are shortened and underdeveloped, and soft-tissue contractures form at the site of the deformity. The foot is tight in its deformed position and resists manual efforts to push it into normal position. Clubfoot is painless, except in elderly, arthritic patients. In older children, clubfoot may be secondary to paralysis, poliomyelitis, or cerebral palsy, in which case treatment must include management of the underlying disease.

Diagnosis

Early diagnosis of clubfoot is usually possible because the deformity is obvious. In subtle deformity, however, true clubfoot must be distinguished from apparent clubfoot (metatarsus varus or pigeon toe). Apparent clubfoot results when a fetus maintains a position in utero that gives his feet a clubfoot appearance at birth. This can usually be corrected manually. Another form of apparent clubfoot is inversion of the feet, resulting from the peroneal type of progressive muscular atrophy and progressive muscular dystrophy. In true clubfoot, X-rays show superimposition of the talus and the calcaneus and a ladderlike appearance of the metatarsals. (See *Recognizing clubfoot.*)

Treatment

Clubfoot is correctable with prompt treatment, which is performed in three stages: correcting the deformity, maintaining the correction until the foot regains normal muscle balance, and observing the foot closely for several years to prevent the deformity from recurring. In neonates with true clubfoot, corrective treatment should begin at once. An infant's foot contains

RECOGNIZING CLUBFOOT

Clubfoot (*talipes*) may have various names, depending on the orientation of the deformity, as shown in the illustrations at right.

TALIPES EQUINUS

TALIPES CALCANEUS

TALIPES CAVUS

TALIPES VARUS

TALIPES EQUINOVARUS

TALIPES CALCANEOVARUS

TALIPES VALGUS

TALIPES CALCANEOVALGUS

TALIPES EQUINOVALGUS

large amounts of cartilage; the muscles, ligaments, and tendons are supple. The ideal time to begin treatment is during the first few days and weeks of life, when the foot is most malleable.

Clubfoot deformities are usually corrected in sequential order. Several therapeutic methods have been tested and found effective in correcting clubfoot. In all patients, the first procedure should be simple manipulation and casting, whereby the foot is gently manipulated into a partially corrected position and held in place by a cast for several days or weeks. (The skin should be painted with a nonirritating adhesive liquid beforehand to prevent the cast from slipping.) After the cast is removed, the foot is manipulated into an even better position and casted again. This procedure is repeated as many times as necessary. In

some cases, the shape of the cast can be transformed through a series of wedging maneuvers instead of changing the cast each time.

After correction of clubfoot, proper foot alignment should be maintained through exercise, night splints, and orthopedic shoes. With manipulating and casting, correction usually takes about 3 months. The Denis Browne splint, a device that consists of two padded, metal footplates connected by a flat, horizontal bar, is sometimes used as a follow-up measure to help promote bilateral correction and strengthen the foot muscles.

Resistant clubfoot may require surgery. Older children, for example, with recurrent or neglected clubfoot usually need surgery. Tenotomy, tendon transfer, stripping of the plantar fascia, and capsulotomy are some of the surgical procedures that may be used. In severe cases, bone surgery (wedge resections, osteotomy, or astragalectomy) may be appropriate. After surgery, a cast is applied to preserve the correction. Clubfoot severe enough to require surgery is rarely totally correctable; however, surgery can usually ameliorate the deformity.

Special considerations
The primary concern is recognition of clubfoot as early as possible, preferably in neonates.
- Look for any exaggerated attitudes in an infant's feet. Make sure you recognize the difference between true clubfoot and apparent clubfoot. Don't use excessive force in trying to manipulate a clubfoot. The foot with apparent clubfoot moves easily.
- Stress to parents the importance of prompt treatment. Make sure they understand that clubfoot demands immediate therapy and orthopedic supervision until growth is completed.
- After casting, elevate the child's feet with pillows. Check the toes every 1 to 2 hours for temperature, color, sensation, motion, and capillary refill time; watch for edema. Before a child in a clubfoot cast is discharged, teach parents to recognize circulatory impairment.
- Insert plastic petals over the top edges of a new cast while it's still wet to keep urine from soaking and softening the cast. This is done as follows: Cut a plastic sheet into strips long enough to cover the outside of the cast, and tuck them about a finger length beneath the cast edges. Using overlapping strips of tape, tack the corner of each petal to the outside of the cast. When the cast is dry, petal the edges with adhesive tape to keep out plaster crumbs and prevent skin irritation. Perform good skin care under the cast edges every 4 hours, washing and carefully drying the skin. (Don't rub the skin with alcohol, and don't use oils or powders, which tend to macerate the skin.)
- If the child is old enough to walk, caution parents not to let the foot part of the cast get soft and thin from wear. If it does, much of the correction may be lost.
- When the wedging method of shaping the cast is being used, check circulatory

status frequently; it may be impaired by increased pressure on tissues and blood vessels. The equinus (posterior release) correction especially places considerable strain on ligaments, blood vessels, and tendons.
- After surgery, elevate the child's feet with pillows to decrease swelling and pain. Report any signs of discomfort or pain immediately. Try to locate the source of pain; it may result from cast pressure rather than from the incision. If bleeding occurs under the cast, circle the location and mark the time on the cast. If bleeding spreads, report it.
- Explain to the older child and his parents that surgery can improve clubfoot with good function but can't totally correct it; the affected calf muscle will remain slightly underdeveloped.
- Emphasize the need for long-term orthopedic care to maintain correction. Teach parents the prescribed exercises that the child can do at home. Urge them to make the child wear the corrective shoes ordered and the splints during naps and at night. Make sure they understand that treatment for clubfoot continues during the entire growth period. Correcting this defect permanently takes time and patience.

Developmental dysplasia of the hip

Developmental dysplasia of the hip (DDH), an abnormality of the hip joint present from birth, is the most common disorder affecting hip joints of children younger than age 3. DDH can be unilateral or bilateral. This abnormality occurs in three forms of varying severity: *unstable hip dysplasia,* in which the hip is positioned normally but can be dislocated by manipulation; *subluxation or incomplete dislocation,* in which the femoral head rides on the edge of the acetabulum; and *complete dislocation,* in which the femoral head is totally outside the acetabulum.

Developmental hip subluxation or dislocation can cause abnormal acetabular development and permanent disability.

Causes and incidence

Experts are uncertain about the causes of DDH. Dislocation is 10 times more common after breech delivery (malpositioning in utero) than after cephalic delivery, and it's also more common among large neonates and twins. Females are affected more often than males. Genetic factors may also play a role.

Although DDH is found throughout the world, incidence is particularly high among Native Americans.

Signs and symptoms

Clinical effects of hip dysplasia vary with age. In neonates, dysplasia doesn't cause gross deformity or pain. However, in complete dysplasia, the hip rides above the acetabulum, causing the level of the knees to be uneven. As the child grows older and begins to walk, the abduction on the dislocated side is limited. Uncorrected bilateral dysplasia may cause him to sway from side to side, a condition known as "duck waddle"; unilateral dysplasia may produce a limp. If corrective treatment isn't begun until after age 2, DDH may cause degenerative hip changes, lordosis, joint malformation, and soft-tissue damage.

Diagnosis

Several observations during physical examination of the relaxed child strongly suggest DDH. First, place the child on his back, and inspect the folds of skin over his thighs. Usually, a child in this position has an equal number of thigh folds on each side, but a child with subluxation or dislocation may have an extra fold on the affected side (this extra fold is also apparent when the child lies prone). Next, with the child lying prone, check for alignment of the buttock fold. In a child with dysplasia, the buttock fold on the affected side is higher. In addition, abduction of the affected hip is restricted. (See *Complete dysplasia of the hip.*)

CONFIRMING DIAGNOSIS *A positive Ortolani's or Trendelenburg's sign confirms DDH. To elicit Ortolani's sign, place the infant on his back, with his hip flexed and abducted. Adducting the hip while pressing the femur downward will dislocate the hip. Then, abducting the*

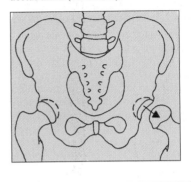

COMPLETE DYSPLASIA OF THE HIP

In complete dislocation, the femoral head is totally displaced outside the acetabulum (see arrow).

hip while moving the femur upward will move the femoral head over the acetabular rim. If you hear a click or feel a jerk as the femoral head moves, the test is positive. This sign indicates subluxation in a neonate younger than 1 month and subluxation or complete dislocation in an older infant.

To elicit Trendelenburg's sign, have the child rest his weight on the side of the dislocation and lift his other knee. His pelvis drops on the normal side because of weak abductor muscles in the affected hip. However, when the child stands with his weight on the normal side and lifts the other knee, the pelvis remains horizontal.

Ultrasound of the hip reveals hip deformity. X-rays show the location of the femur head and a shallow acetabulum. Magnetic resonance imaging may also be used to assess reduction.

Treatment

The earlier the infant receives treatment, the better his chances are for normal development. Treatment varies with the patient's age. In infants younger than 3 months, treatment includes *gentle* manipulation to reduce the dislocation, followed by holding the hips in a flexed and abducted position with a splint-brace or harness to maintain the reduction. The infant must wear this apparatus continuously for 2 to 3 months and then use a night splint for another month so the joint capsule can tighten and stabilize in correct alignment.

If treatment doesn't begin until after age 3 months, it may include bilateral skin traction (in infants) or skeletal traction (in children who have started walking) in an attempt to reduce the dislocation by gradually abducting the hips. In Bryant's traction, or divarication traction, both extremities are placed in traction, even if only one is affected, to help maintain immobilization. This type of traction is used in children who are younger than 3 years and weigh less than 35 lb (16 kg). The length of treatment is 2 to 3 weeks.

If traction fails, gentle closed reduction under general anesthetic can further abduct the hips; the child is then placed in a spica cast for 4 to 6 months. If closed treatment fails, open reduction, followed by immobilization in a spica cast for an average of 6 months, or osteotomy may be considered.

In the child age 2 to 5 years, treatment is difficult and includes skeletal traction and subcutaneous adductor tenotomy. Treatment begun after age 5 rarely restores satisfactory hip function.

Special considerations

The child who must wear a splint, brace, or body cast needs special personal care that requires parent education.

- Teach parents how to correctly splint or brace the hips, as ordered. Stress the need for frequent checkups.
- Listen sympathetically to the parents' expressions of anxiety and fear. Explain possible causes of developmental hip dislocation, and give reassurance that early, prompt treatment will probably result in complete correction.
- During the child's first few days in a cast or splint-brace, he may be prone to irritability due to the unaccustomed restricted movement. Encourage his parents to stay with him as much as possible and to calm and reassure him.
- Assure parents that the child will adjust to this restriction and return to normal

sleeping, eating, and playing behavior in a few days.

- Instruct parents to remove braces and splints while bathing the infant but to replace them immediately afterward. Stress good hygiene; parents should bathe and change the child frequently and wash his perineum with warm water and soap at each diaper change.

If treatment requires a spica cast:

- When transferring the child immediately after casting, use your palms to avoid making dents in the cast. Such dents predispose the patient to pressure sores. Remember that the cast needs 24 to 48 hours to dry naturally. Don't use heat to make it dry faster because heat also makes it more fragile.
- Immediately after the cast is applied, use a plastic sheet to protect it from moisture around the perineum and buttocks. Cut the sheet into strips long enough to cover the outside of the cast, and tuck them about a finger length beneath the cast edges. Using overlapping strips of tape, tack the corner of each petal to the outside of the cast. Remove the plastic under the cast every 4 hours; then wash, dry, and retuck it. Disposable diapers folded lengthwise over the perineum may also be used.
- Position the child either on a Bradford frame elevated on blocks, with a bedpan under the frame, or on pillows to support the child's legs. Be sure to keep the cast dry, and change the child's diapers often.
- Turn the child every 2 hours during the day and every 4 hours at night. Check color, sensation, and motion of the infant's legs and feet. Be sure to examine all his toes. Notify the physician of dusky, cool, or numb toes.
- Check the cast daily for odors, which may herald infection.
- If the child complains of itching, he may benefit from diphenhydramine, or you may aim a hair dryer set on cool at the cast edges to relieve itching. Don't scratch or probe under the cast. Investigate any persistent itching.
- Provide adequate nutrition, and maintain adequate fluid intake to avoid renal calculi and constipation, both complications of inactivity.

- Provide adequate stimuli to promote growth and development.
- Tell parents to watch for signs that the child is outgrowing the cast (cyanosis, cool extremities, or pain).
- Tell parents that treatment may be prolonged and requires patience. The patient in Bryant's traction may be cared for at home if the parents are taught traction application and maintenance.
- Encourage the parents to cuddle and hold the child and encourage him to interact with siblings and friends.
- Maintain skin integrity and check circulation at least every 2 hours.
- Feed the child carefully to avoid aspiration and choking.
- Refer the child and his parents to a child life specialist to ensure continued developmental progress.

Muscular dystrophy

Muscular dystrophy is actually a group of congenital disorders characterized by progressive symmetrical wasting of skeletal muscles without neural or sensory defects. Paradoxically, these wasted muscles tend to enlarge because of connective tissue and fat deposits, giving an erroneous impression of muscle strength. The main types of muscular dystrophy are Duchenne's (pseudohypertrophic), Becker's (benign pseudohypertrophic), facioscapulohumeral (Landouzy-Dejerine), and limb-girdle dystrophy.

The prognosis varies. Duchenne's muscular dystrophy generally strikes during early childhood and usually results in death by age 20. Patients with Becker's muscular dystrophy typically live into their 40s. Facioscapulohumeral and limb-girdle dystrophies usually don't shorten life.

Causes and incidence
Muscular dystrophy is caused by various genetic mechanisms. Duchenne's and Becker's muscular dystrophies are X-linked recessive disorders. Both result from defects in the gene coding for the muscle protein dystrophin; the gene has been mapped to the Xp21 locus.

The incidence muscular dystrophy is about 1 in 651,450 persons in the United States. Duchenne's and Becker's muscular dystrophies affect males almost exclusively.

Facioscapulohumeral dystrophy is an autosomal dominant disorder. Limb-girdle dystrophy is usually autosomal recessive. These two types affect both sexes about equally.

Signs and symptoms
Although all four types of muscular dystrophy cause progressive muscular deterioration, the degree of severity and age of onset vary.

Duchenne's muscular dystrophy begins insidiously, between ages 3 and 5. Initially, it affects leg and pelvic muscles but eventually spreads to the involuntary muscles. Muscle weakness produces a waddling gait, toe walking, and lordosis. Children with this disorder have difficulty climbing stairs, fall down often, can't run properly, and their scapulae flare out (or "wing") when they raise their arms. Calf muscles especially become enlarged and firm. Muscle deterioration progresses rapidly, and contractures develop. Some have abrupt intermittent oscillations of the irises in response to light (Gower's sign). Usually, these children are confined to wheelchairs by ages 9 to 12. Late in the disease, progressive weakening of cardiac muscle causes tachycardia, electrocardiogram abnormalities, and pulmonary complications. Death commonly results from sudden heart failure, respiratory failure, or infection.

Signs and symptoms of Becker's muscular dystrophy resemble those of Duchenne's muscular dystrophy, but they progress more slowly. Although symptoms start around age 5, the patient can still walk well beyond age 15 — sometimes into his 40s.

Facioscapulohumeral dystrophy is a slowly progressive and relatively benign form of muscular dystrophy that commonly occurs before age 10 but may develop during early adolescence. Initially, it weakens the muscles of the face, shoulders, and upper arms but eventually spreads to all voluntary muscles, producing a pendulous lower lip and absence of the nasolabial fold. Early symptoms include the inability to pucker the mouth or whistle, abnormal facial movements, and the absence of facial movements when laughing or crying. Other signs consist of diffuse facial flattening that leads to a masklike expression, winging of the scapulae, the inability to raise the arms above the head and, in infants, the inability to suckle.

Limb-girdle dystrophy follows a similarly slow course and commonly causes only slight disability. Usually, it begins between ages 6 and 10; less commonly, in early adulthood. Muscle weakness first appears in the upper arm and pelvic muscles. Other symptoms include winging of the scapulae, lordosis with abdominal protrusion, waddling gait, poor balance, and the inability to raise the arms.

Diagnosis

Diagnosis depends on typical clinical findings, family history, and diagnostic test findings. If another family member has muscular dystrophy, its clinical characteristics can indicate the type of dystrophy the patient has and how he may be affected.

Electromyography typically demonstrates short, weak bursts of electrical activity or high-frequency, repetitive waxing and waning discharges in affected muscles. Muscle biopsy shows variations in the size of muscle fibers and, in later stages, shows fat and connective tissue deposits; dystrophin is absent in Duchenne's dystrophy and diminished in Becker's dystrophy. Serum creatine kinase is markedly elevated in Duchenne's, but only moderately elevated in Becker's and facioscapulohumeral dystrophies.

Immunologic and molecular biological assays available in specialized medical centers facilitate accurate prenatal and postnatal diagnosis of Duchenne's and Becker's muscular dystrophies and are replacing muscle biopsy and elevated serum creatine kinase levels in diagnosing these dystrophies. These assays can also help to identify carriers.

Treatment

No treatment stops the progressive muscle impairment of muscular dystrophy. However, orthopedic appliances, exercise, physical therapy, and surgery to correct contractures can help preserve the patient's mobility and independence. Prednisone improves muscle strength in patients with Duchenne's.

Special considerations

Comprehensive long-term care and follow-up, patient and family teaching, and psychological support can help the patient and his family deal with this disorder.

- When respiratory involvement occurs in Duchenne's muscular dystrophy, encourage coughing, deep-breathing exercises, and diaphragmatic breathing. Teach parents how to recognize early signs of respiratory complications.
- Encourage and assist with active and passive range-of-motion exercises to preserve joint mobility and prevent muscle atrophy.
- Advise the patient to avoid long periods of bed rest and inactivity; if necessary, limit TV viewing and other sedentary activities.
- Refer the patient for physical therapy. Splints, braces, surgery to correct contractures, trapeze bars, overhead slings, and a wheelchair can help preserve mobility. A footboard or high-topped sneakers and a foot cradle increase comfort and prevent footdrop.
- Because inactivity may cause constipation, encourage adequate fluid intake, increase dietary bulk, and obtain an order for a stool softener. The patient is prone to obesity due to reduced physical activity; help him and his family plan a low-calorie, high-protein, high-fiber diet.
- Always allow the patient plenty of time to perform even simple physical tasks because he's likely to be slow and awkward.
- Encourage communication between the patient's family members to help them deal with the emotional strain this disorder produces. Provide emotional support to help the patient cope with continual changes in body image.

 PEDIATRIC TIP *Help the child with Duchenne's muscular dystrophy maintain peer relationships and realize his intellectual potential by encouraging his parents to keep him in a regular school as long as possible.*

- If necessary, refer adult patients for counseling. Refer those who must acquire new job skills for vocational rehabilitation. (Contact the Department of Labor and Industry in your state for more information.) For information on social services and financial assistance, refer these patients and their families to the Muscular Dystrophy Association.

■ Refer the patient's family members for genetic counseling.

JOINTS

Septic arthritis

Septic, or infectious, arthritis is a medical emergency that occurs when bacterial invasion of a joint causes inflammation of the synovial lining, effusion and pyogenesis, and destruction of bone and cartilage. Septic arthritis can lead to ankylosis and even fatal septicemia. However, prompt antibiotic therapy and joint aspiration or drainage cures most patients.

Causes and incidence

In most cases of septic arthritis, bacteria spread from a primary site of infection — usually in adjacent bone or soft tissue — through the bloodstream to the joint. Common infecting organisms in children are group B *Streptococcus* and *Haemophilus influenzae*. Adults are usually infected by *Staphylococcus, Streptococcus* (pneumonia), and group B *Streptococcus*, whereas chronic septic arthritis is caused by *Mycobacterium tuberculosis* and *Candida albicans.*

Various factors can predispose a person to septic arthritis. Any concurrent bacterial infection (of the genitourinary or the upper respiratory tract, for example) or serious chronic illness (such as malignancy, renal failure, rheumatoid arthritis, systemic lupus erythematosus, diabetes, or cirrhosis) heightens susceptibility. Consequently, elderly people and those who abuse I.V. drugs run a higher risk of developing septic arthritis. Of course, diseases that depress the immune system and immunosuppressive therapy increase susceptibility. Other predisposing factors include recent articular trauma, joint arthroscopy or oth-

er surgery, intra-articular injections, and local joint abnormalities.

Septic arthritis may be seen at any age in children, but it occurs most often in children younger than age 3. It's uncommon from age 3 until adolescence, at which time the incidence increases again.

Signs and symptoms

Acute septic arthritis begins abruptly, causing intense pain, inflammation, and swelling of the affected joint and low-grade fever. It usually affects a single joint. It most commonly develops in the large joints but can strike any joint, including the spine and small peripheral joints. The hip is a frequent site in infants. Systemic signs of inflammation may not appear in some patients. Migratory polyarthritis sometimes precedes localization of the infection. If the bacteria invade the hip, pain may occur in the groin, upper thigh, or buttock or may be referred to the knee.

Diagnosis

CONFIRMING DIAGNOSIS *Identifying the causative organism in a Gram stain or culture of synovial fluid or a biopsy of synovial membrane confirms septic arthritis. When synovial fluid culture is negative, positive blood culture may confirm the diagnosis.*

Joint fluid analysis shows gross pus or watery, cloudy fluid of decreased viscosity, usually with 50,000/μl or more white cells, primarily neutrophils. Synovial fluid glucose is usually more than 40 mg/dl. (See *Other types of arthritis*, page 584.)

Other diagnostic measures include the following:

■ X-rays can show typical changes as early as 1 week after initial infection — distention of joint capsules, for example, followed by narrowing of joint space (indicating cartilage damage) and erosions of bone (joint destruction).

■ White blood cell count may be elevated, with many polymorphonuclear cells; erythrocyte sedimentation rate is increased.

Treatment

Antibiotic therapy should begin as soon as a Gram stain has been done; it may be modified when drug sensitivity of the in-

OTHER TYPES OF ARTHRITIS

Hemophilic arthrosis

Hemophilic arthrosis produces transient or permanent joint changes. Often precipitated by trauma, hemophilic arthrosis usually arises between ages 1 and 5 and tends to recur until about age 10. It usually affects only one joint at a time—most commonly the knee, elbow, or ankle—and tends to recur in the same joint. Initially, the patient may feel only mild discomfort; later, he may experience warmth, swelling, tenderness, and severe pain with adjacent muscle spasm that leads to flexion of the extremity.

Mild hemophilic arthrosis may cause only limited stiffness that subsides within a few days. In prolonged bleeding, however, symptoms may subside after weeks or months or not at all. Severe hemophilic arthrosis may be accompanied by fever and leukocytosis; severe, prolonged, or repeated bleeding may lead to chronic hemophilic joint disease.

Effective treatment includes I.V. infusion of the deficient clotting factor, bed rest with the affected extremity elevated, application of ice packs, analgesics, and joint aspiration. Physical therapy includes progressive range-of-motion and muscle-strengthening exercises to restore motion and to prevent contractures and muscle atrophy.

Intermittent hydrarthrosis

Intermittent hydrarthrosis is a rare, benign condition characterized by regular, recurrent joint effusions. It most commonly affects the knee. The patient may have difficulty moving the affected joint but have no other arthritic symptoms. The cause of intermittent hydrarthrosis is unknown; onset is usually at or soon after puberty and may be linked to familial tendencies, allergies, or menstruation. No effective treatment exists.

Schönlein-Henoch purpura

Schönlein-Henoch purpura—a vasculitic syndrome—is marked by palpable purpura, abdominal pain, and arthralgia that most commonly affects the knees and ankles, producing swollen, warm, and tender joints without joint erosion or deformity. Renal involvement is also common. Most patients have microscopic hematuria and proteinuria 4 to 8 weeks after onset. Incidence is highest in children and young adults, occurring most often in the spring after a respiratory infection. Treatment may include corticosteroids.

Traumatic arthritis

Traumatic arthritis results from blunt, penetrating, or repeated trauma or from forced inappropriate motion of a joint or ligament. Clinical effects may include swelling, pain, tenderness, joint instability, and internal bleeding. Treatment includes analgesics, nonsteroidal antiinflammatory drugs, application of cold followed by heat and, if needed, compression dressings, splinting, joint aspiration, casting, or possibly surgery.

---

fecting organism is known. Bioassays or bactericidal assays of synovial fluid and bioassays of blood may confirm clearing of the infection.

Rest, immobilization, elevation, and warm compresses help with pain relief. Analgesics are given for pain, if needed. The affected joint can be immobilized with a splint or put into traction until the patient can tolerate movement.

In severe cases, needle aspiration (arthrocentesis) or surgery may be done under sterile conditions to remove grossly purulent or infected joint fluid. Late reconstructive surgery is warranted only for severe joint damage and only after all signs of active infection have disappeared, which usually takes several months. Recommended procedures include arthroplasty and joint fusion. Prosthetic replacement remains controversial because it may exacerbate the infection, but it has helped patients with damaged femoral heads or acetabula.

Special considerations

Management of septic arthritis demands meticulous supportive care, close observation, and control of infection.

- Practice strict sterile technique for all procedures. Wash hands carefully before and after giving care. Dispose of soiled linens and dressings properly. Prevent contact between immunosuppressed patients and infected patients.
- Watch for signs of joint inflammation: heat, redness, swelling, pain, or drainage. Monitor vital signs and fever pattern. Remember that corticosteroids mask signs of infection.
- Check splints or traction regularly. Keep the joint in proper alignment, but avoid prolonged immobilization. Start passive range-of-motion exercises immediately, and progress to active exercises as soon as the patient can move the affected joint and put weight on it.
- Monitor pain levels and medicate accordingly, especially before exercise, remembering that the pain of septic arthritis is easy to underestimate. Administer analgesics and opioids for acute pain and heat or ice packs for moderate pain.

ELDER TIP *Prolonged use of opioids in an older adult necessitates particular vigilance because these drugs can impair mental status and may contribute to falls and other accidents.*
- Warn the patient before the first aspiration that it will be *extremely* painful. Carefully evaluate the patient's condition after joint aspiration.

Gout

Gout, also called *gouty arthritis,* is a metabolic disease marked by urate deposits, which cause painfully arthritic joints. It can strike any joint but favors those in the feet and legs. Gout follows an intermittent course and typically leaves patients totally free from symptoms for years between attacks. It can cause chronic disability or incapacitation and, rarely, severe hyperten-

sion and progressive renal disease. The prognosis is good with treatment.

Causes and incidence

Although the exact cause of primary gout remains unknown, it appears to be linked to a genetic defect in purine metabolism, which causes elevated blood levels of uric acid (hyperuricemia) due to overproduction of uric acid, retention of uric acid, or both. In secondary gout, which develops during the course of another disease (such as obesity, diabetes mellitus, hypertension, sickle cell anemia, and renal disease), hyperuricemia results from the breakdown of nucleic acids. Myeloproliferative and lymphoproliferative diseases, psoriasis, and hemolytic anemia are the most common causes. Primary gout usually occurs in men and in postmenopausal women; secondary gout occurs in elderly people.

Secondary gout can also follow drug therapy that interferes with uric acid excretion. Increased concentration of uric acid leads to urate deposits (*tophi*) in joints or tissues and consequent local necrosis or fibrosis. The risk is greater in men, postmenopausal women, and those who use alcohol.

Signs and symptoms

Gout develops in four stages: asymptomatic, acute, intercritical, and chronic. In asymptomatic gout, serum urate levels rise but produce no symptoms. As the disease progresses, it may cause hypertension or nephrolithiasis, with severe back pain. The first acute attack strikes suddenly and peaks quickly. Although it generally involves only one or a few joints, this initial attack is extremely painful. Affected joints are hot, tender, inflamed, and appear dusky-red or cyanotic. The metatarsophalangeal joint of the great toe usually becomes inflamed first (*podagra*), followed by the instep, ankle, heel, knee, or wrist joints. Sometimes a low-grade fever is present. Mild acute attacks usually subside quickly but tend to recur at irregular intervals. Severe attacks may persist for days or weeks.

Intercritical periods are the symptom-free intervals between gout attacks. Most patients have a second attack within 6 months to 2 years, but in some the second attack doesn't occur for 5 to 10 years.

GOUTY DEPOSITS

The final stage of gout is marked by painful polyarthritis, with large, subcutaneous, tophaceous deposits in cartilage, synovial membranes, tendons, and soft tissue. The skin over the tophus is shiny, thin, and taut.

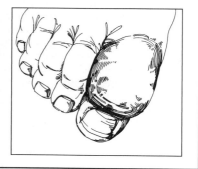

Delayed attacks are more common in untreated patients and tend to be longer and more severe than initial attacks. Such attacks are also polyarticular, invariably affecting joints in the feet and legs, and are sometimes accompanied by fever. A migratory attack sequentially strikes various joints and the Achilles tendon and is associated with either subdeltoid or olecranon bursitis.

Eventually, chronic polyarticular gout sets in. This final, unremitting stage of the disease is marked by persistent painful polyarthritis, with large, subcutaneous tophi in cartilage, synovial membranes, tendons, and soft tissue. Tophi form in fingers, hands, knees, feet, ulnar sides of the forearms, helix of the ear, Achilles tendons and, rarely, internal organs, such as the kidneys and myocardium. The skin over the tophus may ulcerate and release a chalky, white exudate or pus. Chronic inflammation and tophaceous deposits precipitate secondary joint degeneration, with eventual erosions, deformity, and disability. Kidney involvement, with associated tubular damage, leads to chronic renal dysfunction. Hypertension and albuminuria occur in some pa-

tients; urolithiasis is common. (See *Gouty deposits*.)

Diagnosis

CONFIRMING DIAGNOSIS *The presence of monosodium urate monohydrate crystals in synovial fluid taken from an inflamed joint or tophus establishes the diagnosis.*

Aspiration of synovial fluid (arthrocentesis) or of tophaceous material reveals needlelike intracellular crystals of sodium urate. Although hyperuricemia isn't specifically diagnostic of gout, serum uric acid is above normal. Urinary uric acid is usually higher in secondary gout than in primary gout. In acute attacks, erythrocyte sedimentation rate and white blood cell (WBC) count may be elevated, and WBC count shifts to the left.

Initially, X-rays are normal. However, in chronic gout, X-rays show "punched out" erosions, sometimes with periosteal overgrowth. Outward displacement of the overhanging margin from the bone contour characterizes gout. X-rays rarely show tophi. (See *Understanding pseudogout.*)

Treatment

Correct management seeks to terminate an acute attack, reduce hyperuricemia, and prevent recurrence, complications, and the formation of renal calculi. Colchicine is effective in reducing pain, swelling, and inflammation; pain often subsides within 12 hours of treatment and is completely relieved in 48 hours. Treatment for the patient with acute gout consists of bed rest; immobilization and protection of the inflamed, painful joints; and local application of heat or cold, whichever works for the patient. Maximal doses of nonsteroidal anti-inflammatory drugs (NSAIDs) usually provide excellent relief for patients who can tolerate them; doses should be gradually reduced after several days.

ELDER TIP *Older patients are at risk for GI bleeding associated with NSAID use. Encourage the elderly patient to take these drugs with meals, and monitor the patient's stools for occult blood.*

Resistant inflammation may require oral corticosteroids or intra-articular corticosteroid injection to relieve pain. Treatment for chronic gout aims to decrease serum uric acid level. Continuing maintenance dosage of allopurinol may be given to suppress uric acid formation or control uric acid levels, preventing further attacks. However, this powerful drug should be used cautiously in patients with renal failure. Uricosuric agents promote uric acid excretion and inhibit accumulation of uric acid, but their value is limited in patients with renal impairment. These medications shouldn't be given to patients with renal calculi.

Adjunctive therapy emphasizes a few dietary restrictions, primarily the avoidance of alcohol and purine-rich foods (organ meats, beer, wine, and certain types of fish are high in purines). Obese patients should try to lose weight because obesity puts additional stress on painful joints.

In some cases, surgery may be necessary to improve joint function or correct deformities. Tophi must be excised and drained if they become infected or ulcerated. They can also be excised to prevent ulceration, improve the patient's appearance, or make it easier for him to wear shoes or gloves.

Special considerations

Patient care for gout includes these interventions:

■ Encourage bed rest but use a bed cradle to keep bedcovers off extremely sensitive, inflamed joints.

■ Give pain medication, as needed, especially during acute attacks. Apply hot or cold packs to inflamed joints according to what the patient finds effective. Administer anti-inflammatory medication and other drugs, as ordered. Watch for adverse effects. Be alert for GI disturbances with colchicine.

■ Watch for acute gout attacks 24 to 96 hours after surgery. Even minor surgery can precipitate an attack. Before and after surgery, administer colchicine as ordered, to help prevent gout attacks.

■ Tell the patient to avoid high-purine foods, such as anchovies, liver, sardines, kidneys, sweetbreads, lentils, and alcoholic beverages — especially beer and wine — which raise the urate level. Explain the principles of a gradual weight-reduction diet to obese patients.

UNDERSTANDING PSEUDOGOUT

Also known as *calcium pyrophosphate disease,* pseudogout results when calcium pyrophosphate crystals collect in periarticular joint structures.

Signs and symptoms
Like true gout, pseudogout causes sudden joint pain and swelling, most commonly of the knee, wrist, and ankle or other peripheral joints.

Pseudogout attacks are self-limiting and triggered by stress, trauma, surgery, severe dieting, thiazide therapy, or alcohol abuse. Associated symptoms resemble those of rheumatoid arthritis.

Establishing a diagnosis
Diagnosis of pseudogout hinges on joint aspiration and synovial biopsy to detect calcium pyrophosphate crystals. X-rays show calcium deposits in the fibrocartilage and linear markings along the bone ends. Blood tests may detect an underlying endocrine or metabolic disorder.

Relief for pressure and inflammation
Management of pseudogout may include aspirating the joint to relieve pressure; instilling cortocosteroids and administering analgesics, salicylates, phenylbutazone, or other nonsteroidal anti-inflammatory drugs to treat inflammation and, if appropriate, treating the underlying disorder. Without treatment, pseudogout leads to permanent joint damage in about half of those it affects, most of whom are older adults.

■ Advise the patient to report any adverse effects of allopurinol, such as drowsiness, dizziness, nausea, vomiting, urinary frequency, or dermatitis.

Neurogenic arthropathy

Neurogenic arthropathy, also called *Charcot's arthropathy,* is a progressively degenerative disease of peripheral and axial joints, resulting from impaired sensory innervation. The loss of sensation in the joints causes progressive deterioration, resulting from trauma or primary disease, which leads to laxity of supporting ligaments and eventual disintegration of the affected joints.

Causes

Neurogenic arthropathy is most common in men older than 40 years. In adults, the most common cause of neurogenic arthropathy is diabetes mellitus. Other causes include tabes dorsalis (especially among patients age 40 to 60), syringomyelia (progresses to neurogenic arthropathy in about 25% of patients), myelopathy of pernicious anemia, spinal cord trauma, paraplegia, hereditary sensory neuropathy, and Charcot-Marie-Tooth disease. Amyloidosis, peripheral nerve injury, myelomeningocele (in children), leprosy, and alcoholism may cause neurogenic arthropathy, but only in rare occurrences.

Frequent intra-articular injection of corticosteroids has also been linked to neurogenic arthropathy. The analgesic effect of the corticosteroids may mask symptoms and allow continuous stress to accelerate joint destruction.

Signs and symptoms

Neurogenic arthropathy begins insidiously with swelling, warmth, decreased mobility, and instability in a single joint or in many joints. It can progress to deformity. The first clue to vertebral neuroarthropathy, which progresses to gross spinal deformity, may be nothing more than a mild, persistent backache. Characteristically, pain is minimal despite obvious deformity.

The specific joint affected varies according to the underlying cause. Diabetes usually attacks the joints and bones of the feet; tabes dorsalis attacks the large weight-bearing joints, such as the knee, hip, ankle, or lumbar and dorsal vertebrae (Charcot spine); syringomyelia causes occurrence in the shoulder, elbow, or cervical interverte-bral joint. Neurogenic arthropathy caused by intra-articular injection of corticosteroids usually develops in the hip or knee joint.

Diagnosis

Patient history of painless joint deformity and underlying primary disease suggests neurogenic arthropathy. Physical examination may reveal bone fragmentation in advanced disease. X-rays confirm diagnosis and assess severity of joint damage. In the early stage of the disease, soft-tissue swelling or effusion may be the only overt effect; in the advanced stage, articular fracture, subluxation, erosion of articular cartilage, periosteal new bone formation, and excessive growth of marginal loose bodies (osteophytosis) or resorption may be seen. Computed tomography scan helps define the extent of disease.

Other diagnostic measures include:
- vertebral examination: narrowing of disk spaces, deterioration of vertebrae, and osteophyte formation, leading to ankylosis and deforming kyphoscoliosis
- synovial biopsy: bony fragments and bits of calcified cartilage.

Treatment

Effective management relieves pain with analgesics and immobilization using crutches, splints, braces, and restriction of weight bearing to the affected joint.

In severe disease, surgery may include arthrodesis or, in severe diabetic neuropathy, amputation. However, surgery risks further damage through nonunion and infection.

Special considerations

Assess the pattern of pain and give analgesics, as needed. Check sensory perception, range of motion, alignment, joint swelling, and the status of underlying disease.
- Teach the patient to use joint protection techniques, to avoid physically stressful actions that may cause pathologic fractures, and to take safety precautions, such as removing throw rugs and other objects over which the patient may trip.
- Advise the patient to report severe joint pain, swelling, or instability. Warm com-

presses may be applied to relieve local pain and tenderness.
- Instruct the patient in the proper technique for crutches or other orthopedic devices. Stress the importance of proper fitting and regular professional readjustment of such devices. Warn the patient that impaired sensation might allow damage from these aids to occur and progress without discomfort.
- Emphasize the need to continue regular treatment of the underlying disease.

Osteoarthritis

Osteoarthritis, the most common form of arthritis, is a chronic disease that causes deterioration of the joint cartilage and formation of reactive new bone at the margins and subchondral areas of the joints. This degeneration results from a breakdown of chondrocytes, most commonly in the distal interphalangeal and proximal interphalangeal joints, but also in the hip and knee joints.

Osteoarthritis is widespread, occurring equally in both sexes. Its earliest symptoms typically begin after age 40 and may progress with advancing age.

Disability depends on the site and severity of involvement and can range from minor limitation of the dexterity of the fingers to severe disability in persons with hip or knee involvement. The rate of progression varies, and joints may remain stable for years in an early stage of deterioration.

Causes and incidence

Studies indicate that osteoarthritis is acquired and probably results from a combination of metabolic, genetic, chemical, and mechanical factors. Secondary osteoarthritis usually follows an identifiable predisposing event — most commonly trauma, congenital deformity, or obesity — and leads to degenerative changes.

Osteoarthritis may first appear between ages 30 and 40, and is present in almost everyone by age 70. Before age 55, it affects men and women equally, but after age 55 the incidence is higher in women.

 ELDER TIP *Primary osteoarthritis is strongly associated with aging, and indeed aging may predispose to the cartilage degeneration common in persons with osteoarthritis.*

Signs and symptoms

The most common symptom of osteoarthritis is a deep, aching joint pain, particularly after exercise or weight bearing, usually relieved by rest. Other symptoms include stiffness in the morning and after exercise (relieved by rest), aching during changes in weather, "grating" of the joint during motion, altered gait contractures, and limited movement. These symptoms increase with poor posture, obesity, and stress to the affected joint.

Osteoarthritis of the interphalangeal joints produces irreversible joint changes and node formation. The nodes eventually become red, swollen, and tender, causing numbness and loss of dexterity. (See *What happens in osteoarthritis,* page 590.)

Diagnosis

A thorough physical examination confirms typical symptoms, and absence of systemic symptoms rules out an inflammatory joint disorder. X-rays of the affected joint help confirm diagnosis of osteoarthritis but may be normal in the early stages. X-rays may require many views and typically show:
- narrowing of joint space or margin
- cystlike bony deposits in joint space and margins and sclerosis of the subchondral space
- joint deformity due to degeneration or articular damage
- bony growths at weight-bearing areas
- fusion of joints. (See *Digital joint deformities,* page 591.)

Treatment

Treatment is aimed at relieving pain, maintaining or improving mobility, and minimizing disability. Medications include nonsteroidal anti-inflammatory drugs, Cox-2 inhibitors and, in some cases, intra-articular injections of corticosteroids. Studies indicate that glucosamine and chondroitin may be useful in controlling symptoms and reducing functional impairment. Injecting artificial joint fluid into the

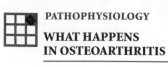

PATHOPHYSIOLOGY

WHAT HAPPENS IN OSTEOARTHRITIS

The characteristic breakdown of articular cartilage is a gradual response to aging or to predisposing factors, such as joint abnormalities or traumatic injury.

Chondrocytes break down.

↓

Cartilage degenerates.

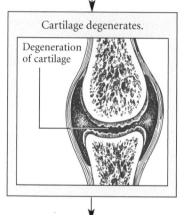

Degeneration of cartilage

↓

Osteophytes (bony spurs) form.

↓

Fragments of bone float freely in joint.

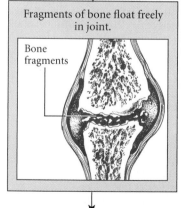

Bone fragments

↓

Stiffness and decreased movement occur.

knee can provide relief of pain for up to 6 months.

Effective treatment also reduces stress by weight loss and supporting or stabilizing the joint with crutches, braces, cane, walker, cervical collar, or traction. Exercise, such as through physical therapy, is integral to maintaining or improving joint mobility. Other supportive measures include massage, moist heat, paraffin dips for hands, protective techniques to prevent undue stress on the joints, and adequate rest (particularly after activity).

Surgical treatment, such as one of the following, is reserved for patients who have severe disability or uncontrollable pain:
- Arthroplasty (partial or total): replacement of deteriorated part of joint with prosthetic appliance
- Arthrodesis: surgical fusion of bones, used primarily in spine (laminectomy)
- Osteoplasty: scraping and lavage of deteriorated bone from joint
- Osteotomy: change in alignment of bone to relieve stress by excision of wedge of bone or cutting of bone.

Special considerations
Patient care for osteoarthritis includes the following:
- Promote adequate rest, particularly after activity. Plan rest periods during the day, and provide for adequate sleep at night. Moderation is the key — teach the patient to pace daily activities.
- Assist with physical therapy, and encourage the patient to perform gentle, isometric range-of-motion exercises.
- Provide emotional support and reassurance to help the patient cope with limited mobility. Explain that osteoarthritis *isn't* a systemic disease.

Specific patient care depends on the affected joint:
- *Hand:* Apply hot soaks and paraffin dips to relieve pain, as ordered.
- *Spine (lumbar and sacral):* Recommend a firm mattress (or bed board) to decrease morning pain.
- *Spine (cervical):* Check cervical collar for constriction; watch for redness with prolonged use.
- *Hip:* Use moist heat pads to relieve pain and administer antispasmodic drugs, as or-

dered. Assist with range-of-motion and strengthening exercises, always making sure the patient gets the proper rest afterward. Check crutches, cane, braces, and walker for proper fit, and teach the patient to use them correctly. For example, the patient with unilateral joint involvement should use an orthopedic appliance such as a walker, or a cane. Recommend the use of cushions when sitting as well as the use of an elevated toilet seat.

■ *Knee:* Twice daily, assist with prescribed range-of-motion exercises, exercises to maintain muscle tone, and progressive resistance exercises to increase muscle strength. Provide elastic supports or braces if needed.

To minimize the long-term effects of osteoarthritis:
■ Teach the patient to take medication exactly as prescribed, and report adverse effects immediately.
■ Advise the patient to avoid overexertion. He should take care to stand and walk correctly, to minimize weight-bearing activities, and to be especially careful when stooping or picking up objects.
■ Instruct the patient to wear proper-fitting, supportive shoes and not to allow the heels to become worn down.
■ Advise the patient to install safety devices at home such as guard rails in the bathroom.
■ Instruct the patient to maintain proper body weight to lessen strain on joints.

BONES

Osteomyelitis

Osteomyelitis is a pyogenic bone infection that may be chronic or acute. It commonly results from a combination of local trauma, which is usually quite trivial but results in hematoma formation, and an acute infection originating elsewhere in the body. Although osteomyelitis usually remains localized, it can spread through the bone to the marrow, cortex, and periosteum. Acute osteomyelitis is usually a blood-borne disease, which most commonly affects rapidly growing children. Chronic osteomyelitis,

---

DIGITAL JOINT DEFORMITIES

Osteoarthritis of the interphalangeal joints produces irreversible changes in the distal joints (Heberden's nodes, below left) and the proximal joints (Bouchard's nodes, below right). Initially painless, these nodes gradually progress to or suddenly flare up, resulting in redness, swelling, tenderness, and impaired sensation and dexterity.

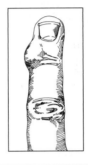 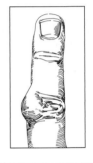

---

which is rare, is characterized by multiple draining sinus tracts and metastatic lesions.

Causes and incidence
Virtually any pathogenic bacteria can cause osteomyelitis under the right circumstances. Typically, these organisms find a culture site in a hematoma from recent trauma or in a weakened area, such as the site of surgery or local infection (for example, furunculosis), and spread directly to bone. As the organisms grow and form pus within the bone, tension builds within the rigid medullary cavity, forcing pus through the haversian canals. This forms a subperiosteal abscess that deprives the bone of its blood supply and may eventually cause necrosis. In turn, necrosis stimulates the periosteum to create new bone *(involucrum);* the old bone *(sequestrum)* detaches and works its way out through an abscess or the sinuses. By the time sequestrum forms, osteomyelitis is chronic.

Osteomyelitis occurs more commonly in children (especially boys) than in adults — usually as a complication of an acute localized infection. The most common sites in children are the lower end of the femur and the upper end of the tibia, humerus, and radius. The most common sites in adults are the pelvis and vertebrae, generally as a result of contamination associated with surgery or trauma. Other common sites are sternoclavicular, sacroiliac, and symphysis pubis. The incidence of both chronic and acute osteomyelitis is declining, except in drug abusers. With prompt treatment, the prognosis for acute osteomyelitis is very good; for chronic osteomyelitis, which is more prevalent in adults, the prognosis is still poor.

Signs and symptoms

Onset of acute osteomyelitis is usually rapid, with sudden pain accompanied by tenderness, heat, swelling, and restricted movement of the affected area. Associated systemic symptoms may include tachycardia, sudden fever, nausea, and malaise. Generally, the clinical features of both chronic and acute osteomyelitis are the same, except that chronic infection can persist intermittently for years, flaring up spontaneously after minor trauma. Sometimes, however, the only symptom of chronic infection is the persistent drainage of pus from an old pocket in a sinus tract.

Diagnosis

Patient history, physical examination, and blood tests help to confirm osteomyelitis:
- White blood cell count shows leukocytosis.
- Erythrocyte sedimentation rate or C-reactive protein is usually elevated but nonspecific in acute cases.
- Cultures of the lesion indicate the source of the organism. Blood cultures help identify causative organism.
- Magnetic resonance imaging is best for detecting spinal infection.
- Computed tomography is best for visualizing islands of dead bone.

X-rays may not show bone involvement until the disease has been active for some time, usually 2 to 3 weeks. Bone scans can detect early infection. Diagnosis must rule

out poliomyelitis, rheumatic fever, myositis, and bone fractures. The gold standard for diagnosing osteomyelitis is histopathologic and microscopic examination of bone.

Treatment

Treatment for acute osteomyelitis should begin before definitive diagnosis. Treatment includes administration of antibiotics after blood cultures are taken; early surgical drainage to relieve pressure buildup and sequestrum formation; immobilization of the affected bone by plaster cast, traction, or bed rest; and supportive measures, such as analgesics and I.V. fluids.

If an abscess forms, treatment includes incision and drainage, followed by a culture of the drained fluid. Intracavitary instillation of antibiotics may be done through closed-system continuous irrigation with low intermittent suction; limited irrigation with blood drainage system with suction; or local application of packed, wet, antibiotic-soaked dressings.

In addition to these therapies, chronic osteomyelitis usually requires surgery to remove dead bone *(sequestrectomy)* and to promote drainage *(saucerization)*. The area may be filled with bone graft or packing material to promote new bone tissue. An infected prosthesis is removed and a new one is implanted the same day or after resolution of the infection.

Some centers use hyperbaric oxygen to increase the activity of naturally occurring leukocytes. Free-tissue transfers and local muscle flaps are also used to fill in dead space and increase blood supply.

Special considerations

Your major concerns are to control infection, protect the bone from injury, and offer meticulous supportive care.
- Use strict sterile technique when changing dressings and irrigating wounds. If the patient is in skeletal traction for compound fractures, cover insertion points of pin tracks with small, dry dressings, and tell him not to touch the skin around the pins and wires.
- Administer I.V. fluids to maintain adequate hydration as necessary. Provide a diet high in protein and vitamin C.

- Assess vital signs, wound appearance, and new pain, which may indicate secondary infection, daily.
- Carefully monitor suctioning equipment, and the amount of solution it instills and suctions.
- Support the affected limb with firm pillows. Keep the limb level with the body; *don't* let it sag. Turn the patient gently every 2 hours and watch for signs of developing pressure ulcers. Report any signs of pressure ulcer formation immediately.
- Support the cast with firm pillows and smooth rough cast edges by petaling with pieces of adhesive tape or moleskin. Check circulation and drainage; if a wet spot appears on the cast, circle it with a marking pen, and note the time of appearance (on the cast). Be aware of how much drainage is expected. Check the circled spot at least every 4 hours. Report any enlargement immediately.
- Protect the patient from mishaps, such as jerky movements and falls, which may threaten bone integrity. Report sudden pain, crepitus, or deformity immediately. Watch for any sudden malposition of the limb, which may indicate fracture.
- Provide emotional support and appropriate diversions. Before discharge, teach the patient how to protect and clean the wound and, most importantly, how to recognize signs of recurring infection (increased temperature, redness, localized heat, and swelling). Stress the need for follow-up examinations. Instruct the patient to seek prompt treatment for possible sources of recurrence — blisters, boils, styes, and impetigo.

Osteoporosis

Osteoporosis is a metabolic bone disorder in which the rate of bone resorption accelerates while the rate of bone formation slows down, causing a loss of bone mass. Bones affected by this disease lose calcium and phosphate salts and thus become porous, brittle, and abnormally vulnerable to fractures. Osteoporosis may be primary or secondary to an underlying disease. Primary osteoporosis is commonly called *postmenopausal osteoporosis* because it typically develops in postmenopausal women.

Causes and incidence

The cause of primary osteoporosis is unknown; however, a mild but prolonged negative calcium balance, resulting from an inadequate dietary intake of calcium, may be an important contributing factor — as may declining gonadal or adrenal function, faulty protein metabolism due to estrogen deficiency, and sedentary lifestyle. Causes of secondary osteoporosis are many: prolonged therapy with steroids or heparin, total immobilization or disuse of a bone (as with hemiplegia, for example), alcoholism, malnutrition, malabsorption, scurvy, lactose intolerance, osteogenesis imperfecta, Sudeck's atrophy (localized to hands and feet, with recurring attacks), and endocrine disorders (hypopituitarism, acromegaly, thyrotoxicosis, long-standing diabetes mellitus, hyperthyroidism).

The incidence of osteoporosis is high, with an estimated 10 million U.S. residents suffering from osteoporosis and another 18 million suffering from low bone mass, or osteopenia. Incidence is higher in women than in men, with women older than age 50 accounting for 20% of cases. Another 30% of women have osteopenia, which can deteriorate into osteoporosis.

Signs and symptoms

Osteoporosis is usually discovered incidentally on roentgenograms; the patient may have been asymptomatic for years. Vertebral collapse, causing a backache with pain that radiates around the trunk, is the most common presenting feature. Any movement or jarring aggravates the backache.

In another common pattern, osteoporosis can develop insidiously, with increasing deformity, kyphosis, and loss of height. Sometimes a dowager hump is present. As bones weaken, spontaneous wedge fractures, pathologic fractures of the neck or femur, Colles' fractures after a minor fall, and hip fractures become increasingly common.

 ELDER TIP *Osteoporosis, usually affecting older people, is a major risk factor in vertebral compression fractures and hip fractures.*

Osteoporosis primarily affects the weight-bearing vertebrae. Only when the condition is advanced or severe, as in Cushing's syndrome or hyperthyroidism, do comparable changes occur in the skull, ribs, and long bones.

Diagnosis

Differential diagnosis must exclude other causes of rarefying bone disease, especially those affecting the spine, such as metastatic cancer and advanced multiple myeloma. The differential diagnosis should also exclude osteomalacia, osteogenesis imperfecta tarda, skeletal hyperparathyroidism, and hyperthyroidism. Initial evaluation attempts to identify the specific cause of osteoporosis through the patient history.

■ Bone mineral density testing is performed in dual-energy X-ray absorptiometry (DEXA) and measures the mineralization of bones. It's the gold standard for evaluating osteoporosis.

■ A spine computed tomography scan shows demineralization. Quantitative computed tomography can evaluate bone density but is less available and more expensive than DEXA.

■ X-rays show fracture or vertebral collapse in severe cases.

■ Urine calcium can provide evidence of bone turnover but is limited in value. Newer tests include urinary N-telopeptide to help diagnose osteoporosis.

Treatment

Treatment aims to slow down or prevent bone loss, prevent additional fractures, and control pain. A physical therapy program that emphasizes gentle exercise and activity is an important part of the treatment. Medications may include bisphosphonates, such as alendronate and risedronate, to prevent bone loss and reduce the risk of fractures. The physician may also recommend adequate calcium and vitamin D intake. Raloxifene and calcitonin have also been prescribed. Weakened vertebrae should be supported, usually with a back brace. Surgery can correct pathologic fractures of the femur by open reduction and internal fixation. Colles' fracture requires reduction with plaster immobilization for 4 to 10 weeks.

The incidence of primary osteoporosis may be reduced through adequate intake of dietary calcium and regular exercise. Fluoride treatments may also offer some preventive benefit. Hormone replacement therapy (HRT) with estrogen and progesterone may retard bone loss and prevent the occurrence of fractures; however, this therapy remains controversial. HRT decreases bone reabsorption and increases bone mass. Secondary osteoporosis can be prevented through effective treatment of the underlying disease as well as corticosteroid therapy, early mobilization after surgery or trauma, careful observation for signs of malabsorption, and prompt treatment of hyperthyroidism. Decreased alcohol consumption and caffeine use, as well as smoking cessation, are also helpful preventive measures.

Special considerations

Your care plan should focus on the patient's fragility, stressing careful positioning, ambulation, and prescribed exercises.

■ Check the patient's skin daily for redness, warmth, and new sites of pain, which may indicate new fractures. Encourage activity; help the patient walk several times daily. As appropriate, perform passive range-of-motion exercises or encourage the patient to perform active exercises. Make sure the patient regularly attends scheduled physical therapy sessions.

■ Impose safety precautions. Keep the side rails of the patient's bed in raised position. Move the patient gently and carefully at all times. Explain to the patient's family and ancillary health care personnel how easily an osteoporotic patient's bones can fracture.

■ Provide a balanced diet, high in nutrients that support skeletal metabolism: vitamin D, calcium, and protein. Administer analgesics and heat to relieve pain.

■ Make sure the patient and her family clearly understand the prescribed drug regimen. Tell them how to recognize significant adverse effects and to report them immediately. The patient should also report any new pain sites immediately, especially after trauma, no matter how slight. Advise the patient to sleep on a firm mattress and avoid excessive bed rest. Make sure she knows how to wear her back brace.

- Thoroughly explain osteoporosis to the patient and her family. If the patient and her family don't understand the nature of this disease, they may feel the fractures could have been prevented if they had been more careful.
- Teach the patient to use good body mechanics — to stoop before lifting anything and to avoid twisting movements and prolonged bending.

Legg-Calvé-Perthes disease

Legg-Calvé-Perthes disease (also called *coxa plana*) is ischemic necrosis that leads to eventual flattening of the head of the femur due to vascular interruption.

The disease occurs in five stages:
- Growth arrest: Avascular phase; may last 6 to 12 months. Early changes include inflammation and synovitis of the hip and ischemic changes in the ossific nucleus of the femoral head.
- Subchondral fracture: Radiographic visualization of the fracture varies with the age of the child at clinical onset and the extent of epiphyseal involvement; may last 3 to 8½ months.
- Reabsorption, also called *fragmentation* or *necrosis:* The necrotic bone beneath the subchondral fracture is gradually and irregularly reabsorbed; lasts 6 to 12 months.
- Reossification, or healing stage: Ossification of the primary bone begins irregularly in the subchondral area and progresses centrally; takes 6 to 24 months.
- Healed stage, also called *residual stage:* Complete ossification of the epiphysis of the femoral head, with or without residual deformity.

Although this disease usually runs its course in 3 to 4 years, it may lead to premature osteoarthritis later in life from misalignment of the acetabulum and flattening of the femoral head.

Causes and incidence
The exact vascular obstructive changes that initiate Legg-Calvé-Perthes disease are unknown. Current etiological theories include venous obstruction with secondary intraepiphyseal thrombosis, trauma to retinacular vessels, vascular irregularities (congenital or developmental), vascular occlusion secondary to increased intracapsular pressure from acute transient synovitis, and increased blood viscosity resulting in stasis and decreased blood flow.

Legg-Calvé-Perthes disease occurs most frequently in boys ages 4 to 10 and tends to occur in families. Although typically unilateral, it occurs bilaterally in 20% of patients.

Signs and symptoms
The first indication of Legg-Calvé-Perthes disease is usually a persistent thigh pain or limp that becomes progressively severe. This symptom appears during the second stage, when bone resorption and deformity begin. Other effects may include mild pain in the hip, thigh, or knee that's aggravated by activity and relieved by rest; muscle spasm; atrophy of muscles in the upper thigh; slight shortening of the leg; and severely restricted abduction and internal rotation of the hip.

Diagnosis
 CONFIRMING DIAGNOSIS *A thorough physical examination and clinical history suggest Legg-Calvé-Perthes disease. Hip X-rays confirm the diagnosis, with findings that vary according to the stage of the disease. Anterior-posterior X-ray and magnetic resonance imaging enhance early diagnosis of necrosis and visualization of articular surface.*

Diagnostic evaluation must also differentiate between Legg-Calvé-Perthes disease (restriction of only the abduction and rotation of the hip) and infection or arthritis (restriction of all motion). Aspiration and culture of synovial fluid rule out joint sepsis.

Treatment
The aim of treatment is to protect the femoral head from further stress and damage by containing it within the acetabulum. After 1 to 2 weeks of bed rest, therapy may include reduced weight bearing by means of bed rest in bilateral split counterpoised traction, then application of hip abduction splint or cast, or weight bearing while a splint, cast, or brace holds the leg in abduction. Braces may remain in place for 6 to 18

months. Analgesics help relieve pain. Physical therapy with passive and active range-of-motion exercises after cast removal helps restore motion.

For a young child in the early stages of the disease, osteotomy and subtrochanteric derotation provide maximum confinement of the epiphysis within the acetabulum to allow return of the femoral head to normal shape and full range of motion. Proper placement of the epiphysis thus allows re-molding with ambulation. Postoperatively, the patient requires a spica cast for about 2 months.

Special considerations
When caring for the hospitalized child:
- Monitor the patient's fluid intake and output. Maintain sufficient fluid balance. Provide a diet sufficient for growth without causing excessive weight gain, which might necessitate cast change and loss of the corrective position.
- Provide cast care. Turn the child every 2 to 3 hours to expose the cast to air. When the cast is still wet, turn the child with your palms because depressions in the plaster may lead to pressure ulcers. After the cast dries, petal it with pieces of adhesive tape or moleskin, changing them as they become soiled. Protect the cast with a plastic covering during each bowel movement.
- Watch for complications. Check toes for color, temperature, swelling, sensation, and motion; report dusky, cool, numb toes immediately. Check the skin under the cast with a flashlight every 4 hours while the patient is awake. Follow a consistent plan of skin care to prevent skin breakdown. *Never* use oils or powders under the cast because they increase skin breakdown and soften the cast. Check under the cast daily for odors, particularly after surgery, to detect skin breakdown or wound problems. Report persistent soreness.
- Relieve itching by using a hair dryer (set on cool) at the cast edges; this also decreases dampness from perspiration. If itching becomes excessive, get an order for an antipruritic. *Never* insert an object under the cast to scratch.
- Provide continuous emotional support. Explain all procedures and the need for bed rest, cast, or braces to the child; encourage him to verbalize his fears and anxiety. Encourage parents to participate in their child's care. Teach them proper cast care and how to recognize signs of skin breakdown. Offer tips for making home management of the bedridden child easier. Tell them what special supplies are needed: pajamas and trousers a size larger (open the side seam, and attach Velcro fasteners to close it), bedpan, adhesive tape, moleskin and, possibly, a hospital bed.
- When the cast is removed, debride dry, scaly skin *gradually* by applying lotion after bathing.
- Stress the need for follow-up care to monitor rehabilitation. Also stress home tutoring and socialization to promote normal mental and emotional growth and development.

Osgood-Schlatter disease

Osgood-Schlatter disease, also called *osteochondrosis,* is a painful, incomplete separation of the epiphysis of the tibial tubercle from the tibial shaft. Severe disease may cause permanent tubercle enlargement.

Causes and incidence
Osgood-Schlatter probably results from trauma before the complete fusion of the epiphysis to the main bone has occurred (between ages 10 and 15). Other causes include locally deficient blood supply and genetic factors. It's most common in active adolescent boys, generally affecting one or both knees.

Signs and symptoms
The patient complains of constant aching and pain and tenderness over the tibial tubercle, which worsens during any activity that causes forceful contraction of the patellar tendon on the tubercle, such as ascending or descending stairs, running, jumping, or forced flexion. The pain may be associated with some obvious soft-tissue swelling and localized heat and tenderness.

Diagnosis
Physical examination supports the diagnosis: the examiner forces the tibia into internal rotation while slowly extending the pa-

tient's knee from 90 degrees of flexion; at about 30 degrees, flexion produces pain that subsides immediately with external rotation of the tibia.

X-rays may be normal or show epiphyseal separation and soft-tissue swelling for up to 6 months after onset; eventually, they may show bone fragmentation. Bone scan may show increased uptake in the area of the tibial tuberosity—even greater than the typical increased uptake in the normal epiphysis of the unaffected side.

Treatment

Osteochondrosis is usually self-limiting, and conservative treatment designed to reduce pain and decrease stress to the affected knee is usually adequate. Avoid strenuous exercises that involve the knee; use frequent ice applications after exercise for pain. Rest and quadriceps strengthening, hip extension, adductor strengthening, and hamstring and quadriceps-stretching exercises are recommended. Knee immobilization in extension for 6 to 8 weeks may be necessary.

Rarely, conservative measures fail, and surgery may be necessary. Such surgery includes removal or fixation of the epiphysis or drilling holes through the tubercle to the main bone to form channels for rapid revascularization.

Special considerations

The following special considerations should be observed for patients with Osgood-Schlatter disease:

■ Monitor the patient's circulation, sensation, and pain, and watch for excessive bleeding after surgery.

■ Assess daily for limitation of motion. Administer analgesics as needed.

■ Make sure knee support or splint isn't too tight. Keep the cast dry and clean, and petal it around the top and bottom margins to avoid skin irritation. Teach proper use of crutches. Tell the patient to protect the injured knee with padding and to avoid trauma and repeated flexion (running, contact sports).

■ Monitor for muscle atrophy.

■ Give reassurance and emotional support because disruption of normal activities is difficult for an active teenager. Emphasize that restrictions are temporary.

Paget's disease

Paget's disease, also called *osteitis deformans*, is a slowly progressive metabolic bone disease characterized by an initial phase of excessive bone resorption (osteoclastic phase), followed by a reactive phase of excessive abnormal bone formation (osteoblastic phase). The new bone structure, which is chaotic, fragile, and weak, causes painful deformities of both external contour and internal structure. Paget's disease usually localizes in one or more areas of the skeleton (most frequently the lower torso), but occasionally skeletal deformity is widely distributed. It can be fatal, particularly when it's associated with heart failure (widespread disease creates a continuous need for high cardiac output), bone sarcoma, or giant-cell tumors.

Causes and incidence

The disease occurs worldwide, but is more common in Europe, Australia, and New Zealand, where it's seen in up to 5% of the elderly population. Although its exact cause is unknown, one theory holds that early viral infection causes a dormant skeletal infection that erupts many years later as Paget's disease. Genetic factors are also suspected.

Signs and symptoms

Clinical effects of Paget's disease vary. Early stages may be asymptomatic, but when pain does develop, it's usually severe and persistent and may coexist with impaired movement resulting from impingement of abnormal bone on the spinal cord or sensory nerve root. Such pain intensifies with weight bearing.

The patient with skull involvement shows characteristic cranial enlargement over frontal and occipital areas (hat size may increase) and may complain of headaches. Other deformities include kyphosis (spinal curvature due to compression fractures of pagetic vertebrae), accompanied by a barrel-shaped chest and asymmetrical bowing of the tibia and femur, which commonly reduces height. Pagetic sites are warm and tender and are susceptible to pathologic fractures after minor trauma. Pagetic fractures heal slowly and usually incompletely.

Bony impingement on the cranial nerves may cause blindness and hearing loss with tinnitus and vertigo. Other complications include hypertension, renal calculi, hypercalcemia, gout, heart failure, and a waddling gait (from softening of pelvic bones).

Diagnosis

X-rays taken before overt symptoms develop show increased bone expansion and density. A bone scan, which is more sensitive than X-rays, clearly shows early pagetic lesions (radioisotope collects around areas of active disease). Computed tomography scan or magnetic resonance imaging shows extra bony extension if sarcomatous degeneration occurs. Bone biopsy reveals characteristic mosaic pattern.

Other laboratory findings include:
■ elevated serum alkaline phosphatase levels (an index of osteoblastic activity and bone formation)
■ elevated serum calcium.

Increasing use of routine chemistry screens (including serum alkaline phosphatase) is making early diagnosis more common. Serum osteocalcin and N-telopeptide are usually increased.

Treatment

Primary treatment consists of drug therapy and includes one of the following:
■ Calcitonin (subcutaneously or intranasally) is used to retard bone resorption (which relieves bone lesions) and reduce levels of serum alkaline phosphate and urinary hydroxyproline secretion. Although calcitonin therapy requires long-term maintenance, improvement is noticeable after the first few weeks of treatment.
■ Bisphosphonates, such as etidronate, alendronate, pamidronate, tiludronate, and risedronate, produce rapid reduction in bone turnover and relieve pain. They also reduce serum alkaline phosphate and urinary hydroxyproline secretion. Therapy produces noticeable improvement after 1 to 3 months.
■ Plicamycin, a cytotoxic antibiotic, is used to decrease calcium, urinary hydrox-

yproline, and serum alkaline phosphatase. It produces remission of symptoms within 2 weeks and biochemical improvement in 1 to 2 months. Plicamycin is used to control the disease and is reserved for severe cases with neurologic compromise and for those resistant to other therapies. However, it may destroy platelets or compromise renal function.

Orthopedic surgery is used to correct specific deformities in severe cases, reduce or prevent pathologic fractures, correct secondary deformities, or relieve neurologic impairment. Joint replacement is difficult because bonding material (methyl methacrylate) doesn't set properly on pagetic bone.

Other treatment varies according to symptoms. Analgesics or nonsteroidal anti-inflammatory drugs may be given to control pain.

Special considerations

Patients with Paget's disease require the following special considerations:
■ To evaluate the effectiveness of analgesics, assess level of pain daily. Watch for new areas of pain or restricted movements, which may indicate new fracture sites, and sensory or motor disturbances, such as difficulty in hearing, seeing, or walking.
■ Monitor serum calcium and alkaline phosphatase levels.
■ If the patient is confined to prolonged bed rest, prevent pressure ulcers by providing good skin care. Reposition the patient frequently, and use a flotation mattress. Provide high-topped sneakers to prevent footdrop.
■ Monitor intake and output. Encourage adequate fluid intake to minimize renal calculi formation.
■ Demonstrate how to inject calcitonin properly and rotate injection sites or how to perform nasal inhalation if that's the form prescribed. Warn the patient that adverse effects may occur (nausea, vomiting, local inflammatory reaction at injection site, facial flushing, itching of hands, and fever). Give reassurance that these adverse effects are usually mild and infrequent.
■ To help the patient adjust to the changes in lifestyle imposed by this disease, teach him how to pace activities and, if necessary, how to use assistive devices. Encour-

age him to follow a recommended exercise program, avoiding both immobilization and excessive activity. Suggest a firm mattress or a bed board to minimize spinal deformities. Warn against imprudent use of analgesics because diminished sensitivity to pain resulting from analgesic use may make patient unaware of new fractures. To prevent falls at home, advise removal of throw rugs and other obstacles.

■ Help the patient and his family make use of community support resources, such as a visiting nurse or home health agency. For more information, refer them to the Paget's Disease Foundation.

Hallux valgus

Hallux valgus is a lateral deviation of the great toe at the metatarsophalangeal joint. It occurs with medial enlargement of the first metatarsal head and bunion formation (bursa and callus formation at the bony prominence).

Causes and incidence

Hallux valgus may be acquired or congenital. Acquired hallux valgus results from degenerative arthritis or prolonged pressure on the foot, especially from narrow-toed or high-heeled shoes that compress the forefoot. Bony alignment is normal at the outset of the disorder. This form typically occurs more frequently in women.

In congenital hallux valgus, abnormal bony alignment — increased space between first and second metatarsal (metatarsus primus varus) — causes bunion formation. This form is usually first observed in childhood.

Signs and symptoms

Hallux valgus characteristically begins as a tender bunion covered by deformed, hard, erythematous skin and palpable bursa, typically distended with fluid. The first indication of hallux valgus may be pain over the bunion from shoe pressure. Pain can also stem from traumatic arthritis, bursitis, or abnormal stresses on the foot because hallux valgus changes the body's weight-bearing pattern. In an advanced stage, a flat, splayed forefoot may occur, with severely curled toes (*hammer toes*) and for-

HAMMER TOE

In hammer toe, the toe assumes a clawlike appearance from hyperextension of the metatarsophalangeal joint, flexion of the proximal interphalangeal joint, and hyperextension of the distal interphalangeal joint, usually under pressure from hallux valgus displacement. A painful corn forms on the back of the interphalangeal joint and on the bone end, and a callus forms on the sole of the foot, both of which make walking painful. Hammer toe may be mild or severe and can affect one toe or all five, as in clawfoot (which also causes a very high arch).

Hammer toe can be congenital (and familial) or acquired from constantly wearing short, narrow shoes, which put pressure on the end of the long toe. Acquired hammer toe is commonly bilateral and often develops in children who rapidly outgrow shoes and socks.

In young children, or adults with early deformity, repeated foot manipulation and splinting of the affected toe relieve discomfort and may correct the deformity. Other treatment includes protection of protruding joints with felt pads, corrective footwear (open-toed shoes and sandals or special shoes that conform to the shape of the foot), the use of a metatarsal arch support, and exercises, such as passive manual stretching of the proximal interphalangeal joint. Severe deformity requires surgical fusion of the proximal interphalangeal joint in a straight position.

mation of a small bunion on the fifth metatarsal. (See *Hammer toe.*)

Diagnosis

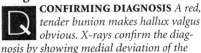 **CONFIRMING DIAGNOSIS** *A red, tender bunion makes hallux valgus obvious. X-rays confirm the diagnosis by showing medial deviation of the*

first metatarsal and lateral deviation of the great toe.

Treatment

In the very early stages of acquired hallux valgus, good foot care and wide-toed shoes may eliminate the need for further treatment. Other useful measures for early management include felt pads to protect the bunion, foam pads or other devices to separate the first and second toes at night, and a supportive pad and exercises to strengthen the metatarsal arch. Early treatment is vital in patients predisposed to foot problems, such as those with rheumatoid arthritis or diabetes mellitus. If the disease progresses to severe deformity with disabling pain, bunionectomy is necessary.

After surgery, the toe is immobilized in its corrected position in one of two ways: with a soft compression dressing that may cover the entire foot or just the great toe and the second toe, thereby serving as a splint, or with a short cast such as a light slipper spica cast.

The patient may need crutches or controlled weight bearing. Depending on the extent of the surgery, some patients walk on their heels a few days after surgery; others must wait 4 to 6 weeks to bear weight on the affected foot. Supportive treatment may include physical therapy, such as warm compresses, soaks, and exercises, and analgesics to relieve pain and stiffness.

Special considerations

Before surgery, obtain a patient history and assess the neurovascular status of the foot (temperature, color, sensation, and blanching sign). If necessary, teach the patient how to walk with crutches.

After bunionectomy:
- Apply ice to reduce swelling. Support the patient's foot with pillows, elevate the foot of the bed, or put the bed in a Trendelenburg position.
- Record the neurovascular status of the toes, including the patient's ability to move the toes (dressing may inhibit movement), every hour for the first 24 hours and then every 4 hours. Report any change in neurovascular status to the surgeon immediately.

- Prepare the patient for walking by having her dangle her foot over the side of the bed for a short time before standing, allowing a gradual increase in venous pressure. If crutches are needed, supervise the patient in using them, and make sure this skill is mastered before discharge. The patient should have a proper cast shoe or boot to protect the cast or dressing.
- Before discharge, instruct the patient to limit activities, to rest frequently with feet elevated, to elevate her feet whenever she feels pain or has edema, and to wear wide-toed shoes and sandals after the dressings are removed. Urge female patients not to resume wearing high-heeled, pointy-toed shoes.
- Teach proper foot care, such as cleanliness, massages, and cutting toenails straight across to prevent ingrown nails and infection.
- Suggest exercises to do at home to strengthen foot muscles, such as standing at the edge of a step on the heel and then raising and inverting the top of the foot.
- Stress the importance of follow-up care and prompt medical attention for painful bunions, corns, and calluses.

Kyphosis

Kyphosis, also called *roundback* or *hunchback,* is an anteroposterior curving of the spine that causes a bowing of the back, commonly at the thoracic, but sometimes at the thoracolumbar or sacral, level. The normal spine displays some convexity, but excessive thoracic kyphosis is pathologic.

Causes and incidence

Kyphosis occurs in children and adults. Although congenital kyphosis is rare, it's usually severe, with resultant cosmetic deformity and reduced pulmonary function.

Adolescent kyphosis (also called *Scheuermann's disease, juvenile kyphosis,* and *vertebral epiphysitis*), the most common form of this disorder, may result from growth retardation or a vascular disturbance in the vertebral epiphysis (usually at the thoracic level) during periods of rapid growth or from congenital deficiency in the thickness of the vertebral plates. Other causes include infection, inflammation, aseptic necrosis, and disk degeneration. The subsequent stress of weight bearing on the compromised vertebrae may result in the thoracic hump commonly seen in adolescents with kyphosis. Symptomatic adolescent kyphosis is more prevalent in girls than in boys and occurs most commonly between ages 12 and 16.

Adult kyphosis (adult roundback) may result from aging and associated degeneration of intervertebral disks, atrophy, and osteoporotic collapse of the vertebrae; from endocrine disorders, such as hyperparathyroidism and Cushing's disease; and from prolonged steroid therapy. Adult kyphosis may also result from conditions such as arthritis, Paget's disease, polio, compression fracture of the thoracic vertebrae, metastatic tumor, plasma cell myeloma, or tuberculosis (TB). In both children and adults, kyphosis may also result from poor posture.

Disk lesions called *Schmorl's nodes* may develop in anteroposterior curving of the spine and are localized protrusions of nuclear material through the cartilage plates and into the spongy bone of the vertebral bodies. If the anterior portions of the cartilage are destroyed, bridges of new bone may transverse the intervertebral space, causing ankylosis.

Signs and symptoms

Development of adolescent kyphosis is usually insidious and may be asymptomatic except for the obvious curving of the back (sometimes more than 90 degrees). In some adolescents, kyphosis may produce mild pain at the apex of the curve (about 50% of patients), fatigue, tenderness or stiffness in the involved area or along the entire spine, and prominent vertebral spinous processes at the lower dorsal and upper lumbar levels, with compensatory increased lumbar lordosis, and hamstring tightness. Rarely, kyphosis may cause neurologic damage: spastic paraparesis secondary to spinal cord compression or herniated nucleus pulposus. In both adolescent and adult forms of kyphosis that aren't due to poor posture alone, the spine won't straighten when the patient assumes a recumbent position.

Adult kyphosis produces a characteristic roundback appearance, possibly associated with pain, weakness of the back, and generalized fatigue. Unlike the adolescent form, adult kyphosis rarely produces local tenderness, except in osteoporosis with a recent compression fracture.

Diagnosis

Physical examination reveals curvature of the thoracic spine in varying degrees of severity. X-rays may show vertebral wedging, Schmorl's nodes, irregular end plates, and possibly mild scoliosis of 10 to 20 degrees. Magnetic resonance imaging should be used to distinguish adolescent kyphosis from TB and other inflammatory or neoplastic diseases that cause vertebral collapse; the severe pain, bone destruction, or systemic symptoms associated with these diseases help rule out a diagnosis of kyphosis. Other sites of bone disease, primary sites of malignancy, and infection must also be evaluated, possibly through vertebral biopsy.

Treatment

For kyphosis caused by poor posture alone, treatment may consist of therapeutic exercises, bed rest on a firm mattress (with or without traction), and a brace to straighten the kyphotic curve until spinal growth is complete. Corrective exercises include pelvic tilt to decrease lumbar lordosis, hamstring stretch to overcome muscle contractures, and thoracic hyperextension to flatten the kyphotic curve. These exercises may be performed in or out of the brace. Lateral X-rays taken every 4 months evaluate correction. Gradual weaning from the brace can begin after maximum correction of the kyphotic curve and after vertebral wedging has decreased and the spine has reached full skeletal maturity. Loss of correction indicates that weaning from the brace has been too rapid, and time out of the brace is decreased accordingly.

Treatment for both adolescent and adult kyphosis also includes appropriate measures for the underlying cause and, possibly, spinal arthrodesis for relief of symptoms. Although rarely necessary, surgery may be recommended when kyphosis causes neurologic damage, a spinal curve greater than 60 degrees, or intractable and disabling back pain in a patient with full skeletal maturity. Preoperative measures may include halo-femoral traction. Corrective surgery includes a posterior spinal fusion with spinal instrumentation, iliac bone grafting, and plaster immobilization. Anterior spinal fusion followed by immobilization in plaster may be necessary when kyphosis produces a spinal curve greater than 70 degrees.

Special considerations

Effective management of kyphosis necessitates first-rate supportive care for patients in traction or a brace, skillful patient teaching, and sensitive emotional support.

■ Teach the patient with adolescent kyphosis caused by poor posture alone the prescribed therapeutic exercises and the fundamentals of good posture. Suggest bed rest when pain is severe. Encourage use of a firm mattress, preferably with a bed board. If the patient needs a brace, explain its purpose and teach him how and when to wear it.

■ Teach good skin care. Tell the patient not to use lotions, ointments, or powders where the brace contacts the skin. Warn him that only the physician or orthotist should adjust the brace.

■ If corrective surgery is needed, explain all preoperative tests thoroughly as well as the need for postoperative traction or casting, if applicable. After surgery, check neurovascular status every 2 to 4 hours for the first 48 hours, and report any changes immediately. Turn the patient often by logrolling and teach the patient how to logroll himself.

■ Provide meticulous skin care. Check the skin at the cast edges several times a day; use heel and elbow protectors to prevent skin breakdown. Remove antiembolism stockings, if ordered, at least three times a day for at least 30 minutes. Change dressings as ordered.

■ Provide emotional support. The adolescent patient is likely to exhibit mood changes and periods of depression. Maintain communication, and offer frequent encouragement and reassurance.

■ Assist during removal of sutures and application of a new cast (usually about 10 days after surgery). Encourage gradual ambulation (usually with the use of a tilt table in the physical therapy department).

■ At discharge, provide detailed, written cast care instructions. Tell the patient to immediately report pain, burning, skin breakdown, loss of feeling, tingling, numbness, or cast odor. Advise him to drink plenty of liquids to avoid constipation and to report any illness immediately. Arrange for home visits by a social worker and a home-care nurse, as needed.

Herniated disk

Herniated disk, also called *ruptured* or *slipped disk* and *herniated nucleus pulposus*, occurs when all or part of the nucleus pulposus — the soft, gelatinous, central portion of an intervertebral disk — is forced through the disk's weakened or torn outer ring (anulus fibrosus). When this happens, the extruded disk may impinge on spinal nerve roots as they exit from the spinal canal or on the spinal cord itself, resulting in back pain and other signs of nerve root irritation.

Causes and incidence

Herniated disks may result from severe trauma or strain or may be related to intervertebral joint degeneration. Although usually occurring in adults (mostly men) less than 45 years old, elderly people are also at risk because minor trauma may cause herniation in disks that have begun to deteriorate due to age. Ninety percent of herniation occurs in the lumbar and lumbosacral regions of the spine; 8% in the cervical region; and 1% to 2% in the thoracic region. Patients with a congenitally small lumbar spinal canal or with osteophyte formation on the vertebrae may be more susceptible to nerve root compression by a herniated disk and more likely to have neurologic symptoms.

Signs and symptoms

The overriding symptom of lumbar herniated disk is severe low-back pain that radiates to the buttocks, legs, and feet, usually unilaterally. When herniation follows trauma, the pain may begin suddenly, subside in a few days, and then recur at shorter intervals and with progressive intensity. Sciatic pain follows, beginning as a dull pain in the buttocks. Valsalva's maneuver, coughing, sneezing, or bending intensifies the pain, which is commonly accompanied by muscle spasms. Herniated disk may also cause paresthesias or hyperthesias, as well as sensory and motor loss in the area innervated by the compressed spinal nerve root and, in later stages, weakness and atrophy of leg muscles.

Diagnosis

Obtaining a careful patient history is vital because the events that intensify disk pain are diagnostically significant. The straight-leg–raising test and its variants are perhaps the best tests for herniated disk, but may still be negative.

For the straight-leg–raising test, the patient lies in a supine position while the examiner places one hand on the patient's ilium, to stabilize the pelvis, and the other hand under the ankle, then slowly raises the patient's leg. The test is positive only if the patient complains of posterior leg (sciatic) pain, not back pain. In Lasègue test, the patient lies flat while the thigh and knee are flexed to a 90-degree angle. Resistance and pain as well as loss of ankle or knee-jerk reflex indicate spinal root compression.

X-rays of the spine are essential to rule out other abnormalities but may not diagnose herniated disk because marked disk prolapse can be present despite a normal X-ray. A thorough check of the patient's peripheral vascular status—including posterior tibial and dorsalis pedis pulses and skin temperature of extremities—helps rule out ischemic disease, another cause of leg pain or numbness. After physical examination and X-rays, myelography, computed tomography scans, and magnetic resonance imaging (MRI) provide the most specific diagnostic information, showing spinal canal compression by herniated disk material. MRI is the method of choice to confirm the diagnosis and determine the exact level of herniation. A myelogram can define the size and location of disk herniation. An electromyogram can determine the exact nerve root involved. A nerve conduction velocity test may also be performed.

Treatment

Unless neurologic impairment progresses rapidly, treatment is initially conservative and consists of several weeks of bed rest (possibly with pelvic traction), administration of nonsteroidal anti-inflammatory drugs, heat applications, and an exercise program. Epidural corticosteroids, short-term oral corticosteroids, nerve root blocks, or physical therapy may be used to decrease pain. Muscle relaxants, such as diazepam, methocarbamol, or cyclobenzaprine, may relieve associated muscle spasms.

A herniated disk that fails to respond to conservative treatment may necessitate surgery. The most common procedure, laminectomy, involves excision of a portion of the lamina and removal of the protruding disk. If laminectomy doesn't alleviate pain and disability, a spinal fusion may be necessary to overcome segmental instability. Laminectomy and spinal fusion are sometimes performed concurrently to stabilize the spine. Microdiskectomy can also be used to remove fragments of nucleus pulposus.

Injection of the enzyme chymopapain into the herniated disk produces a loss of water and proteoglycans from the disk, thereby reducing both the disk's size and the pressure in the nerve root.

Special considerations

Herniated disk requires supportive care, careful patient teaching, and strong emotional support to help the patient cope with the discomfort and frustration of chronic low back pain.

■ If the patient requires myelography, question him carefully about allergies to iodides, iodine-containing substances, or seafood because such allergies may indicate sensitivity to the test's radiopaque dye. Reinforce previous explanations of the need for this test, and tell the patient to expect some pain. Assure him that he'll receive a sedative before the test, if needed, to keep him as calm and comfortable as possible. After the test, urge the patient to remain in bed with his head elevated (especially if metrizamide was used) and to drink plenty of fluids. Monitor intake and output. Watch for seizures and allergic reaction.

■ During conservative treatment, watch for any deterioration in neurologic status (especially during the first 24 hours after admission), which may indicate an urgent need for surgery. Use antiembolism stockings as prescribed, and encourage the patient to move his legs, as allowed. Provide high-topped sneakers to prevent footdrop. Work closely with the physical therapy department to ensure a consistent regimen of leg- and back-strengthening exercises. Give plenty of fluids to prevent renal stasis, and remind the patient to cough, deep breathe, and use blow bottles or an incentive spirometer to preclude pulmonary complications. Provide good skin care. Assess for bowel and bladder functions. Use a fracture bedpan for the patient on complete bed rest.

■ After laminectomy, microdiskectomy, or spinal fusion, enforce bed rest, as ordered. If a blood drainage system (Hemovac or Jackson Pratt drain) is in use, check the tubing frequently for kinks and a secure vacuum. Empty the Hemovac at the end of each shift, and record the amount and color of drainage. Report colorless moisture on dressings (possible cerebrospinal fluid leakage) or excessive drainage immediately. Observe neurovascular status of the legs (color, motion, temperature, and sensation).

■ Monitor vital signs and check for bowel sounds and abdominal distention. Use logrolling technique to turn the patient. Administer analgesics as ordered, especially 30 minutes before initial attempts at sitting or walking. Give the patient assistance during his first attempt to walk. Provide a straight-backed chair for limited sitting.

■ Teach the patient who has undergone spinal fusion how to wear a brace. Assist with straight-leg–raising and toe-pointing exercises, as ordered. Before discharge, teach proper body mechanics — bending at the knees and hips (never at the waist), standing straight, and carrying objects close to the body. Advise the patient to lie down when tired and to sleep on his side (never on his abdomen) on an extra-firm mattress or a bed board. Urge maintenance of proper weight to prevent lordosis caused by obesity.

■ After chemonucleolysis, enforce bed rest as ordered. Administer analgesics and apply heat, as needed. Urge the patient to cough and deep breathe. Assist with physical therapy as necessary and advise the patient to continue these exercises after discharge.

■ Tell the patient who must receive a muscle relaxant of possible adverse effects, especially drowsiness. Warn him to avoid activities that require alertness until he has built up a tolerance to the drug's sedative effects.

■ Provide emotional support. Try to cheer the patient up during periods of frustration and depression. Assure him of his progress, and offer encouragement.

Scoliosis

Scoliosis is a lateral curvature of the spine that may occur in the thoracic, lumbar, or thoracolumbar spinal segment. The curve may be convex to the right (more common in thoracic curves) or to the left (more common in lumbar curves). Rotation of the vertebral column around its axis occurs and may cause rib cage deformity. Scoliosis is commonly associated with kyphosis *(roundback)* and lordosis *(swayback)*.

Causes and incidence

Scoliosis may be functional, structural, or idiopathic. Functional (postural) scoliosis usually results from a discrepancy in leg lengths rather than from a fixed deformity of the spinal column; it corrects when the patient bends toward the convex side. Structural scoliosis results from a deformity of the vertebral bodies, and it doesn't correct when the patient bends to the side. Structural scoliosis may be:

■ *congenital:* usually related to a congenital defect, such as wedge vertebrae, fused ribs or vertebrae, or hemivertebrae; may result from trauma to zygote or embryo

■ *paralytic or musculoskeletal:* develops several months after asymmetrical paralysis of the trunk muscles due to polio, cerebral palsy, or muscular dystrophy

■ *idiopathic (the most common form):* may be transmitted as an autosomal dominant or multifactorial trait. This form appears in a previously straight spine during the growing years. Brain stem dysfunction, possibly due to a lesion of the posterior columns or the inner ear, may be the cause.

Idiopathic scoliosis can be classified as *infantile,* which affects mostly male infants between birth and age 3 and causes left thoracic and right lumbar curves; *juvenile,* which affects both sexes between ages 4 and 10 and causes varying types of curvature; or *adolescent,* which generally affects girls between age 10 and achievement of skeletal maturity and causes varying types of curvature.

Signs and symptoms

The most common curve in functional or structural scoliosis arises in the thoracic segment, with convexity to the right, and compensatory curves (S curves) in the cervical segment above and the lumbar segment below, both with convexity to the left. (See *Cobb method for measuring angle of curvature.*) As the spine curves laterally, compensatory curves develop to maintain body balance and mark the deformity. Scoliosis rarely produces subjective symptoms until it's well established; when symptoms do occur, they include backache, fatigue, and dyspnea. Because many teenagers are shy about their bodies, their parents suspect that something is wrong only after they notice uneven hemlines, pant legs that appear unequal in length, or subtle physical signs like one hip appearing higher than the other. Untreated scoliosis may result in pulmonary insufficiency (curvature may decrease lung capacity), back pain, degenerative arthritis of the spine, disk disease, and sciatica.

Diagnosis

CONFIRMING DIAGNOSIS *Anterior, posterior, and lateral spinal X-rays, taken with the patient standing upright and bending, confirm scoliosis and determine the degree of curvature (Cobb method) and flexibility of the spine.*

A scoliometer can also be used to measure the angle of trunk rotation. Physical examination reveals unequal shoulder

COBB METHOD FOR MEASURING ANGLE OF CURVATURE

The Cobb method measures the angle of curvature in scoliosis. The top vertebra in the curve (T6 in the illustration) is the uppermost vertebra whose upper face tilts toward the curve's concave side. The bottom vertebra in the curve (T12) is the lowest vertebra whose lower face tilts toward the curve's concave side. The angle at which perpendicular lines drawn from the upper face of the top vertebra and the lower face of the bottom vertebra intersect is the angle of the curve.

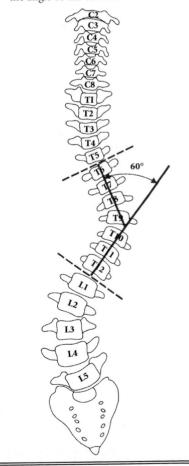

CAST SYNDROME

Cast syndrome is a serious complication that sometimes follows spinal surgery and application of a body cast. Characterized by nausea, abdominal pressure, and vague abdominal pain, cast syndrome probably results from hyperextension of the spine. This hyperextension accentuates lumbar lordosis, compressing the third portion of the duodenum between the superior mesenteric artery anteriorly and the aorta and vertebral column posteriorly. High intestinal obstruction produces nausea, vomiting, and ischemic infarction of the mesentery.

After removal of the cast, treatment includes gastric decompression and I.V. fluids, with nothing by mouth. Antiemetics should be given sparingly because they may mask symptoms of cast syndrome, which, if untreated, may be fatal.

Teach patients who are discharged in body jackets, localizer casts, or high hip spica casts how to recognize cast syndrome, which may manifest several weeks or months after application of the cast.

heights, elbow levels, and heights of the iliac crests. Muscles on the convex side of the curve may be rounded; those on the concave side, flattened, producing asymmetry of paraspinal muscles.

Treatment

Only two treatments effectively treat scoliosis: spinal bracing and surgery. If monitored closely, a properly constructed and fitted brace can successfully halt progression of a curve in approximately 70% of cooperative patients. Most braces should be worn over a long T-shirt or similar article of clothing for 23 hours a day. However, mild curvatures may require less. Exercises must be done daily both in and out of the brace to maintain muscle strength. Patients should be seen for follow-up and brace ad-

justment every 3 months. Radiographs should be repeated at 6-month intervals. As the skeleton matures, as seen radiographically, brace wear should be gradually decreased until it's worn only at night.

The primary indications for surgery are relentless curve progression (usually curves over 40°) or significant curve progression despite bracing. Surgery corrects lateral curvature by posterior spinal fusion and internal stabilization with metal rods. A distraction rod on the concave side of the curve "jacks" the spine into a straight position and provides an internal splint. An alternative procedure, anterior spinal fusion, corrects curvature with vertebral staples and an anterior stabilizing cable. Some spinal fusions may require postoperative immobilization in a brace. Postoperatively, periodic checkups are required for several months to monitor stability of the correction.

Special considerations

It's important to provide emotional support in addition to meticulous skin care and patient teaching.

If the patient needs a brace:
- Enlist the help of a physical therapist, a social worker, and an orthotist. Before the patient goes home, explain what the brace does and how to care for it (how to check the screws for tightness and pad the uprights to prevent excessive wear on clothing). Suggest that loose-fitting, oversized clothes be worn for greater comfort.
- Tell the patient to wear the brace 23 hours per day and to remove it only for bathing and exercise. While he's still adjusting to the brace, tell him to lie down and rest several times per day.
- Suggest a soft mattress if a firm one is uncomfortable.
- To prevent skin breakdown, advise the patient not to use lotions, ointments, or powders on areas where the brace contacts the skin. Tell him to keep the skin dry and clean and to wear a snug T-shirt under the brace.
- Advise the patient to increase activities gradually and avoid vigorous sports. Emphasize the importance of conscientiously performing prescribed exercises.

- Instruct the patient to turn his whole body, instead of just his head, when looking to the side. To make reading easier, tell him to hold the book so he can look straight ahead at it instead of down. If he finds this difficult, help him to obtain prism glasses.

If the patient needs traction or a cast before surgery:
- Explain these procedures to the patient and her family. Remember that application of a body cast can be traumatic because it's done on a special frame and the patient's head and face are covered throughout the procedure.
- Check the skin around the cast edge daily. Keep the cast clean and dry and the edges of the cast petaled. Warn the patient not to insert or let anything get under the cast and to immediately report cracks in the cast, pain, burning, skin breakdown, numbness, or odor.

After corrective surgery:
- Check sensation, movement, color, and blood supply in all extremities every 2 to 4 hours for the first 48 hours and then several times a day, for signs of neurovascular deficit, a serious complication following spinal surgery. Logroll the patient often.
- Measure intake, output, and urine specific gravity to monitor effects of blood loss, which is usually substantial.
- Monitor abdominal distention and bowel sounds.
- Encourage deep-breathing exercises to avoid pulmonary complications.
- Medicate for pain, especially before any activity.
- Promote active range-of-motion arm exercises to help maintain muscle strength. Remember that any exercise, even brushing the hair or teeth, is helpful. Encourage the patient to perform quadriceps-setting, calf-pumping, and active range-of-motion exercises of the ankles and feet.
- Watch for skin breakdown and signs of cast syndrome. Teach the patient how to recognize these signs. (See *Cast syndrome.*)
- Offer emotional support to help prevent depression that may result from altered body image and immobility. Encourage the patient to wear her own clothes, wash her hair, and use makeup.

- If the patient is being discharged with a rod and cast and must have bed rest, arrange for a social worker and a visiting nurse to provide home care. Before discharge, check with the surgeon about activity limitations, and make sure the patient understands them.
- If you work in a school, screen children routinely for scoliosis during physical examinations.

MUSCLE AND CONNECTIVE TISSUE

Tendinitis and bursitis

Tendinitis is a painful inflammation of tendons and of tendon-muscle attachments to bone, usually in the shoulder rotator cuff, hip, Achilles tendon, or hamstring. *Bursitis* is a painful inflammation of one or more of the bursae — closed sacs lubricated with small amounts of synovial fluid that facilitate the motion of muscles and tendons over bony prominences. Bursitis usually occurs in the subdeltoid, olecranon, trochanteric, calcaneal, or prepatellar bursae.

Causes and incidence
Tendinitis commonly results from overuse or injury (such as strain during sports activity), another musculoskeletal disorder (such as rheumatic diseases or congenital defects), or aging.

Bursitis can occur at any age but usually occurs in older individuals due to an inflammatory joint disease (such as rheumatoid arthritis or gout) or recurring trauma that stresses or pressures a joint. Chronic bursitis follows attacks of acute bursitis or repeated trauma and infection. Septic bursitis may result from wound infection or from bacterial invasion of skin over the bursa.

Signs and symptoms
The patient with tendinitis of the shoulder complains of restricted shoulder movement, especially abduction, and localized pain, which is most severe at night and usually interferes with sleep. The pain ex-

tends from the acromion (the shoulder's highest point) to the deltoid muscle insertion, predominantly in the so-called painful arc—that is, when the patient abducts his arm between 50 and 130 degrees. Fluid accumulation causes swelling. In calcific tendinitis, calcium deposits in the tendon cause proximal weakness and, if calcium erodes into adjacent bursae, acute calcific bursitis.

In bursitis, fluid accumulation in the bursae causes irritation, inflammation, sudden or gradual pain, and limited movement. Other symptoms vary according to the affected site. Subdeltoid bursitis impairs arm abduction, prepatellar bursitis (housemaid's knee) produces pain when the patient climbs stairs, and hip bursitis makes crossing the legs painful.

Diagnosis

In tendinitis, X-rays may be normal at first but later show bony fragments, osteophyte sclerosis, or calcium deposits. Arthrography is usually normal, with occasional small irregularities on the undersurface of the tendon. Computed tomography scan and magnetic resonance imaging (MRI) have replaced X-ray and even arthrography of the shoulder as diagnostic tools. An MRI will usually identify tears, partial tears, inflammation, or tumor but cannot reveal irregularities of the tendon sheath itself. Diagnosis of tendinitis must rule out other causes of shoulder pain, such as myocardial infarction, cervical spondylosis, degenerative changes, and tendon tear or rupture. Significantly, in tendinitis, heat aggravates shoulder pain; in other painful joint disorders, heat usually provides relief.

Localized pain and inflammation and a history of unusual strain or injury 2 to 3 days before onset of pain are the bases for diagnosing bursitis. During early stages, X-rays are usually normal, except in calcific bursitis, where X-rays may show calcium deposits.

Treatment

Treatment to relieve pain includes resting the joint (by immobilization with a sling, splint, or cast), nonsteroidal anti-inflammatory drugs (NSAIDs), analgesics, application of cold or heat, ultrasound, or local injection of an anesthetic and cortico-steroids to reduce inflammation. A mixture of a corticosteroid and an anesthetic such as lidocaine generally provides immediate pain relief. Extended-release injections of a corticosteroid, such as triamcinolone or prednisolone, offer longer-term pain relief. Until the patient is free of pain and able to perform range-of-motion exercises easily, treatment also includes oral NSAIDs, such as ibuprofen, naproxen, indomethacin, or oxaprozin. Short-term analgesics include propoxyphene, codeine, acetaminophen with codeine and, occasionally, oxycodone.

Supplementary treatment includes fluid removal by aspiration and heat therapy; for calcific tendinitis, ice packs, physical therapy, ultrasonography, or hydrotherapy generally helps maintain or regain range of motion. It may be necessary to delay treatment until the acute attack is over to ensure maximum patient compliance. Rarely, calcific tendinitis requires surgical removal of calcium deposits. Long-term control of chronic bursitis and tendinitis may require changes in lifestyle to prevent recurring joint irritation.

Special considerations

When treating patients with tendinitis or bursitis, remember to consider the following:

- Assess the severity of pain and the range of motion to determine effectiveness of the treatment.
- Before injecting corticosteroids or local anesthetics, ask the patient about his drug allergies.
- Assist with intra-articular injection. Scrub the patient's skin thoroughly with povidone-iodine or a comparable solution. After the injection, massage the area to ensure penetration through the tissue and joint space. Apply ice intermittently for about 4 hours to minimize pain. Avoid applying heat to the area for 2 days.
- Tell the patient to take anti-inflammatory agents with milk to minimize GI distress and to report any signs of distress immediately.
- Advise the patient to perform strengthening exercises and avoid activities that aggravate the joint.
- Remind the patient to wear a splint or sling during the first few days of an attack of subdeltoid bursitis or tendinitis to sup-

port the arm and protect the shoulder, particularly at night. Demonstrate how to wear the sling so it won't put too much weight on the shoulder.

■ Advise the patient to maintain joint mobility and prevent muscle atrophy by performing exercises or physical therapy when he's free of pain.

 PEDIATRIC TIP *A common form of tendinitis in adolescents (both males and females) is patellar tendinitis associated with inflammation of the tibial epiphysis in Osgood-Schlatter disease.*

Epicondylitis

Lateral epicondylitis of the elbow (tennis elbow) is inflammation of the extensor tendons of the forearm. Medial epicondylitis (golfer's elbow) is inflammation at the origin of the flexor muscles of the wrist.

Causes
Epicondylitis probably begins as a partial tear and is common among tennis players or persons whose activities require a forceful grasp, wrist extension against resistance, or frequent rotation of the forearm such as using a screwdriver. Untreated epicondylitis may become disabling as adherent fibers form between the tendons and the elbow capsule.

Signs and symptoms
The patient's initial symptom is elbow pain that gradually worsens and commonly radiates to the forearm and back of the hand whenever he grasps an object or twists his elbow. Other associated signs and symptoms include tenderness over the involved lateral or medial epicondyle or over the head of the radius and a weak grasp. In rare instances, epicondylitis may cause local heat, swelling, or restricted range of motion.

Diagnosis
Because X-rays are almost always negative, diagnosis typically depends on clinical signs and symptoms and a patient history of playing tennis or engaging in similar activities. The pain can be reproduced by wrist extension and supination with lateral involvement or by flexion and pronation with medial epicondyle involvement.

Treatment
Treatment aims to relieve pain, usually by nonsteroidal anti-inflammatory drugs or local injection of corticosteroids and an anesthetic. Supportive treatment includes an immobilizing splint from the distal forearm to the elbow, which generally relieves pain in 2 to 3 weeks; heat therapy, such as warm compresses, short-wave diathermy, and ultrasound (alone or in combination with diathermy); and physical therapy, such as manipulation and massage to detach the tendon from the chronically inflamed periosteum. A "tennis elbow strap" or counterface brace has helped many patients. This strap, which is wrapped snugly around the forearm approximately 1″ (2.5 cm) below the epicondyle, helps relieve the strain on affected forearm muscles and tendons. If these measures prove ineffective, surgical release of the tendon at the epicondyle may be necessary.

Special considerations
The following special considerations accompany diagnosis and treatment of epicondylitis:

■ Assess the patient's level of pain, range of motion, and sensory function. Monitor heat therapy to prevent burns.

■ Advise the patient to take anti-inflammatory drugs with food to avoid GI irritation.

■ Instruct the patient to rest the elbow until inflammation subsides.

■ Remove the support daily, and gently move the arm to prevent stiffness and contracture.

■ Instruct the patient to follow the prescribed exercise program. For example, he may stretch his arm and flex his wrist to the maximum, then press the back of his hand against a wall until he can feel a pull in his forearm, and hold this position for 1 minute.

■ Advise the patient to warm up for 15 to 20 minutes before beginning any sports activity.

■ Urge the patient to wear an elastic support or splint during any activity that stresses the forearm or elbow.

- Tell the patient to check his equipment. For example, a tennis racquet may not be the right size or weight. Also, changing surfaces may help to reduce stress.

Achilles tendon contracture

Achilles tendon contracture is a shortening of the Achilles tendon *(tendo calcaneus* or *heel cord)* that causes foot pain and strain and limits ankle dorsiflexion.

Causes
Achilles tendon contracture may reflect a congenital structural anomaly or a muscular reaction to chronic poor posture, especially in women who wear high-heeled shoes or joggers who land on the balls of their feet instead of their heels. Other causes include paralytic conditions of the legs, such as poliomyelitis or cerebral palsy.

Signs and symptoms
Sharp, spasmodic pain during dorsiflexion of the foot characterizes the reflex type of Achilles tendon contracture. In footdrop (fixed equinus), contracture of the flexor foot muscle prevents placing the heel on the ground.

Diagnosis
Physical examination and patient history suggest Achilles tendon contracture.

 CONFIRMING DIAGNOSIS *A simple test confirms Achilles tendon contracture: While the patient keeps his knee flexed, the examiner places the foot in dorsiflexion; gradual knee extension forces the foot into plantar flexion.*

Treatment
Conservative treatment aims to correct Achilles tendon contracture by raising the inside heel of the shoe in the reflex type; by gradually lowering the heels of shoes (sudden lowering can aggravate the problem) and stretching exercises if the cause is high heels; or by using support braces or casting to prevent footdrop in a paralyzed patient. Alternative therapy includes using wedged plaster casts or stretching the tendon by

manipulation. Analgesics may be given to relieve pain.

With fixed footdrop, treatment may include surgery. Although this procedure may weaken the tendon, it allows further stretching by cutting the tendon. After surgery, a short leg cast maintains the foot in 90-degree dorsiflexion for 6 weeks. Some surgeons allow partial weight bearing on a walking cast after 2 weeks.

Special considerations
After surgery to lengthen the Achilles tendon:

- Elevate the casted foot to decrease venous pressure and edema by raising the foot of the bed or supporting the foot with pillows.
- Record the neurovascular status of the toes (temperature, color, sensation, capillary refill time, and toe mobility) every hour for the first 24 hours and then every 4 hours. If any changes are detected, increase the elevation of the patient's legs and notify the surgeon immediately.
- Prepare the patient for ambulation by having him dangle his foot over the side of the bed for short periods (5 to 15 minutes) before he gets out of bed, allowing for gradual increase of venous pressure. Assist the patient in walking, as ordered (usually within 24 hours of surgery), using crutches and a non-weight-bearing or touch-down gait.
- Protect the patient's skin with moleskin or by petaling the edges of the cast. Before discharge, teach the patient how to care for the cast, and advise him to elevate his foot regularly when sitting or whenever the foot throbs or becomes edematous. Also, make sure the patient understands how much exercise and walking are recommended after discharge.
- To prevent Achilles tendon contracture in paralyzed patients, apply support braces, universal splints, casts, or high-topped sneakers. Make sure the weight of the sheets doesn't keep paralyzed feet in plantar flexion. For other patients, teach good foot care and urge them to seek immediate medical care for foot problems. Warn women against wearing high heels constantly, and suggest regular foot (dorsiflexion) exercises.

Carpal tunnel syndrome

Carpal tunnel syndrome, a form of repetitive stress injury, is the most common of the nerve entrapment syndromes. It results from compression of the median nerve at the wrist, within the carpal tunnel. This compression neuropathy causes sensory and motor changes in the median distribution of the hand.

Causes and incidence

The carpal tunnel is formed by the carpal bones and the transverse carpal ligament. Inflammation or fibrosis of the tendon sheaths that pass through the carpal tunnel commonly causes edema and compression of the median nerve. Many conditions can cause the contents or structure of the carpal tunnel to swell and press the median nerve against the transverse carpal ligament. Such conditions include rheumatoid arthritis, flexor tenosynovitis (commonly associated with rheumatic disease), nerve compression, pregnancy, renal failure, menopause, diabetes mellitus, acromegaly, edema following Colles' fracture, hypothyroidism, amyloidosis, myxedema, benign tumors, tuberculosis, and other granulomatous diseases. Another source of damage to the median nerve is dislocation or acute sprain of the wrist.

Carpal tunnel injury is five times more common in women than in men. It usually occurs in women between ages 30 and 60 and poses a serious occupational health problem. Assembly-line workers and packers and people who repeatedly use poorly designed tools are most likely to develop this disorder. Any strenuous use of the hands — sustained grasping, twisting, or flexing — aggravates this condition.

Signs and symptoms

The patient with carpal tunnel syndrome usually complains of weakness, pain, burning, numbness, or tingling in one or both hands. This paresthesia affects the thumb, forefinger, middle finger, and half of the fourth finger. The patient is unable to clench his hand into a fist; the nails may be atrophic, the skin dry and shiny. (See *The carpal tunnel.*)

THE CARPAL TUNNEL

The carpal tunnel is clearly visible in this palmar view and cross section of a right hand. Note the median nerve, flexor tendons of fingers, and blood vessels passing through the tunnel on their way from the forearm to the hand.

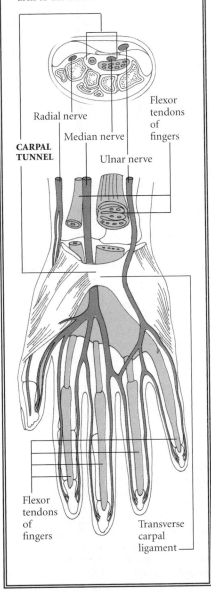

Radial nerve

Flexor tendons of fingers

Median nerve

CARPAL TUNNEL

Ulnar nerve

Flexor tendons of fingers

Transverse carpal ligament

Because of vasodilatation and venous stasis, symptoms are typically worse at night and in the morning. The pain may spread to the forearm and, in severe cases, as far as the shoulder or neck. The patient can usually relieve such pain by shaking or rubbing his hands vigorously or dangling his arms at his side.

Diagnosis

Physical examination reveals decreased sensation to light touch or pinpricks in the affected fingers. Thenar muscle atrophy occurs in about half of all cases of carpal tunnel syndrome, but it's usually a late sign. The patient exhibits a positive Tinel's sign (tingling over the median nerve on light percussion) and responds positively to Phalen's wrist-flexion test (holding the forearms vertically and allowing both hands to drop into complete flexion at the wrists for 1 minute reproduces symptoms of carpal tunnel syndrome). A compression test supports this diagnosis: A blood pressure cuff inflated above systolic pressure on the forearm for 1 to 2 minutes provokes pain and paresthesia along the distribution of the median nerve.

Electromyography and nerve conduction velocity detect a median nerve motor conduction delay of more than 5 milliseconds. Other laboratory tests may identify the underlying disease.

Treatment

Conservative treatment should be tried first, including resting the hands by splinting the wrist in neutral extension for 1 to 2 weeks. Nonsteroidal anti-inflammatory drugs usually provide symptomatic relief. Injection of the carpal tunnel with hydrocortisone and lidocaine may provide significant but temporary relief. If a definite link has been established between the patient's occupation and the development of repetitive stress injury, he may have to seek other work. Effective treatment may also require correction of an underlying disorder. When conservative treatment fails, the only alternative is surgical decompression of the nerve by resecting the entire transverse carpal tunnel ligament or by using endoscopic surgical techniques. Neurolysis

(freeing of the nerve fibers) may also be necessary.

Special considerations

Patient care for carpal tunnel syndrome includes the following:
- Administer mild analgesics as needed. Encourage the patient to use his hands as much as possible. If his dominant hand has been impaired, you may have to help with eating and bathing.
- Teach the patient how to apply a splint. Tell him not to make it too tight. Show him how to remove the splint to perform gentle range-of-motion exercises, which should be done daily. Make sure the patient knows how to do these exercises before he's discharged.
- After surgery, monitor vital signs, and regularly check the color, sensation, and motion of the affected hand.
- Advise the patient who's about to be discharged to occasionally exercise his hands in warm water. If the arm is in a sling, tell him to remove the sling several times a day to do exercises for his elbow and shoulder.
- Suggest occupational counseling for the patient who has to change jobs because of repetitive stress injury.

Torticollis

Torticollis, sometimes called *wryneck,* is a neck deformity in which the sternocleidomastoid neck muscles are spastic or shortened, causing bending of the head to the affected side and rotation of the chin to the opposite side.

Causes and incidence

Torticollis may be congenital or acquired. The three types of acquired torticollis — acute, spasmodic, and hysterical — have differing causes. The acute form results from muscular damage caused by inflammatory diseases, such as myositis, lymphadenitis, or tuberculosis (TB); from cervical spinal injuries that produce scar tissue contracture; and, less commonly, from tumor or medication. The spasmodic form results from rhythmic muscle spasms caused by an organic central nervous system disorder (probably due to irritation of the nerve root by arthritis or osteomyelitis). Hysterical torticollis is due to a psychogenic inability to control neck muscles.

Acquired torticollis usually develops during the first 10 years of life or between ages 30 and 60. Incidence of congenital (muscular) torticollis is highest in infants after difficult delivery (breech presentation), in firstborn infants, and in girls. Possible causes of congenital torticollis include malposition of the head in utero, prenatal injury, fibroma, interruption of blood supply, or fibrotic rupture of the sternocleidomastoid muscle, with hematoma and scar formation.

Signs and symptoms

The first sign of congenital torticollis is commonly a firm, nontender, palpable enlargement of the sternocleidomastoid muscle that's visible at birth and for several weeks afterward. It slowly regresses during a period of 6 months, although incomplete regression can cause permanent contracture. If the deformity is severe, the infant's face and head flatten from sleeping on the affected side; this asymmetry gradually worsens. The infant's chin turns away from the side of the shortened muscle, and his head tilts to the shortened side. His shoulder may elevate on the affected side, restricting neck movement.

The first sign of acquired torticollis is usually recurring unilateral stiffness of neck muscles followed by a drawing sensation and a momentary twitching or contraction that pulls the head to the affected side. This type of torticollis commonly produces severe neuralgic pain throughout the head and neck. (See *Recognizing torticollis.*)

Diagnosis

A history of painless neck deformity from birth suggests congenital torticollis; gradual onset of painful neck deformity suggests acquired torticollis. Diagnosis must rule out TB of the cervical spine, pharyngeal or tonsillar inflammations, spinal accessory nerve damage, ruptured transverse ligaments, subdural hematoma, tumors of soft tissue or bone, dislocations and fractures, scoliosis, congenital abnormalities of the cervical spine and base of the skull,

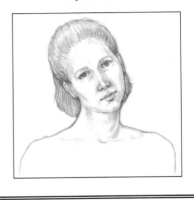

RECOGNIZING TORTICOLLIS

In torticollis, contraction of the sternocleidomastoid neck muscles produces a twisting of the neck and an unnatural position of the head.

rheumatoid arthritis, and osteomyelitis. In acquired torticollis, cervical spine X-rays are negative for bone or joint disease but may reveal an associated disorder (such as TB, scar tissue formation, tumor, deformities, or arthritis). Computed tomography scan or magnetic resonance imaging may help rule out pathogenic causes.

Treatment

Treatment of congenital torticollis aims to stretch the shortened muscle. Nonsurgical treatment includes passive neck stretching and proper positioning during sleep for an infant and active stretching exercises for an older child — for example, touching the ear opposite the affected side to the shoulder and touching the chin to the same shoulder.

Surgical correction involves sectioning the sternocleidomastoid muscle; this should be done during preschool years and only if other therapies fail.

Treatment of acquired torticollis aims to control pain and correct the underlying cause of the disease. In the acute form, application of heat, cervical traction, and gentle massage may help relieve pain; analgesics may also be helpful. Stretching exercises and a neck brace may relieve symptoms of the spasmodic and hysterical forms. Drug treatment includes anticholinergic drugs such as baclofen. Botulinum toxin injections are effective in temporarily relieving torticollis, but injections must be repeated every 3 months.

Special considerations

Patient care for torticollis includes the following:

- To aid early diagnosis of congenital torticollis, observe the infant for limited neck movement, and thoroughly assess his degree of discomfort.
- Teach the parents of an affected child how to perform stretching exercises with him. Suggest placing toys or mobiles on the side of the crib opposite the affected side of the child's neck to encourage the child to move his head and stretch his neck.
- If surgery is necessary, prepare the patient by shaving the neck to the hairline on the affected side.

After corrective surgery:

- Monitor the patient closely for nausea or signs of respiratory complications, especially if he's in cervical traction. Keep suction equipment available to prevent aspiration.
- The patient may be in a cast or in traction day and night or at night only. Monitor the skin around the chin, ears, and back of the head if the patient is in cervical traction. Monitor for problems related to clenching of teeth. If the patient is in a cast, give meticulous cast care, including the monitoring of circulation, sensation, and color around the cast. Protect the cast around the patient's chin and mouth with waterproof material. Check for skin irritation, pressure areas, or softening of cast pad.
- Provide emotional support for the patient and his family to relieve their anxiety due to fear, pain, limitations from the brace or traction, and an altered body image.
- Begin stretching exercises as soon as the patient can tolerate them.
- Before discharge, explain to the patient or his parents the importance of continuing daily heat applications, massages, and stretching exercises, as prescribed, and of keeping the cast clean and dry. Emphasize

that physical therapy is essential for a successful rehabilitation after the cast is removed.

Rhabdomyolysis

Rhabdomyolysis is the breakdown of muscle fibers that results in the release of muscle fiber content into the circulation. It results from the toxicity of destroyed muscle cells, causing kidney damage or failure. Predisposing factors include trauma, ischemia, polymyositis, and drug overdose. Toxins and environmental, infectious, and metabolic factors may induce it. Rhabdomyolysis accounts for 8% to 15% of cases of acute renal failure; about 5% of cases result in death.

Causes and incidence

Rhabdomyolysis follows direct injury to the skeletal muscle fibers, specifically the sarcolemma, which then release myoglobin into the bloodstream. Myoglobin is an oxygen-binding protein pigment found in skeletal muscle. When this muscle is damaged, myoglobin is released into the bloodstream. It's then filtered by the kidneys.

Myoglobin may occlude the structures of the kidney causing damage, such as acute tubular necrosis or kidney failure. Myoglobin can also cause kidney failure because it breaks down into potentially toxic compounds. Necrotic skeletal muscle may cause massive fluid shifts from the bloodstream into the muscle, reducing the relative fluid volume of the body and leading to shock and reduced blood flow to the kidneys.

The disorder may be caused by any condition that results in damage to skeletal muscle. Rhabdomyolysis may result from blunt trauma; extensive burn injury; viral, bacterial, or fungal infection (such as legionnaire's disease or, especially, influenza type A or B); prolonged immobilization; near electrocution or near drowning; metabolic or genetic factors; drug therapy; or toxins. Heavy exercise in children may result in rhabdomyolysis. Other causes include shaken baby syndrome, exposure to extreme cold, heatstroke, and snakebite.

In the United States, rhabdomyolysis affects about 8% to 15% of people with acute renal failure and has a slightly higher incidence in men than in women. The overall mortality rate is 5%. It can occur in infants, toddlers, and adolescents who inherited enzyme deficiencies of carbohydrate and lipid metabolism or those with inherited myopathies, such as Duchenne's muscular dystrophy, and malignant hyperthermia.

Signs and symptoms

Signs and symptoms of rhabdomyolysis include myalgias or muscle pain (especially in the thighs, calves, or lower back), weakness, tenderness, malaise, fever, dark urine, nausea, and vomiting. The patient may also experience weight gain, seizures, joint pain, and fatigue. Symptoms may be subtle initially. Rhabdomyolysis can result in acute renal failure.

Diagnosis

A serum or urine myoglobin test is positive. *Creatine kinase* results 100 times above normal or higher suggest rhabdomyolysis. A urinalysis may reveal casts and may be positive for hemoglobin without evidence of red blood cells on microscopic examination. Serum potassium may be very high (potassium is released from cells into the bloodstream when cell breakdown occurs).

Treatment

Early, aggressive hydration may prevent complications from rhabdomyolysis by rapidly eliminating the myoglobin from the kidneys. I.V. hydration and diuretics promote diuresis. Diuretic medications, such as mannitol or furosemide, may aid in flushing the pigment out of the kidneys. If urine output is sufficient, bicarbonate may be given to maintain an alkaline urine state, thereby helping to prevent the dissociation of myoglobin into toxic compounds. Hyperkalemia should be treated if present. Kidney failure should be treated as appropriate. Dialysis may be necessary and, in severe cases, kidney transplantation.

Special considerations

■ Monitor the patient's intake and output, vital signs, electrolyte levels, daily weight, and laboratory results.

■ Watch for signs of renal failure (such as decreasing urine output and increasing urine specific gravity), fluid overload (such as dyspnea and tachycardia), pulmonary edema, and electrolyte imbalances (such as serum potassium).

■ Provide reassurance and emotional support for the patient and his family.

■ To help prevent rhabdomyolysis from occurring, ensure adequate hydration, monitor the patient for adverse reactions to any of his prescribed drugs, and monitor blood transfusion administration carefully.

Selected references

Engel, A.G., and Armstrong, C.F., eds. *Myology,* 3rd ed. New York: McGraw-Hill Book Co., 2004.

Miller, T., and Schweitzer, M. *Diagnostic Musculoskeletal Imaging.* New York: McGraw-Hill Book Co., 2004.

Prestwood, K.M., and Raisz, L.G. "Prevention and Treatment of Osteoporosis," *Clinical Cornerstone* 4(6):31-41, December 2002.

Puntillo, K., et al. "Accuracy of Emergency Nurses in Assessment of Patients' Pain," *Pain Management Nursing* 4(4):171-75, December 2003.

Saunders, H.D. *Evaluation, Treatment and Prevention of Musculoskeletal Disorders: The Spine,* 4th ed. Philadelphia: W.B. Saunders Co., 2004.

Timby, B.K. *Fundamental Nursing Skills and Concepts,* 8th ed. Philadelphia: Lippincott Williams & Wilkins, 2004.

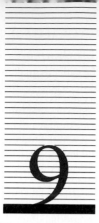

9

Neurologic disorders

Introduction *617*

Congenital anomalies *626*
Cerebral palsy *626*
Hydrocephalus *628*
Cerebral aneurysm *631*
Arteriovenous malformations *635*

Paroxysmal disorders *637*
Headache *637*
Epilepsy *640*

Brain and spinal cord disorders *642*
Stroke *642*
Meningitis *646*
Encephalitis *650*
Brain abscess *654*
Huntington's disease *656*
Parkinson's disease *657*
Myelitis and acute transverse myelitis *659*
Alzheimer's disease *660*
Creutzfeldt-Jakob disease *662*
Reye's syndrome *663*
Guillain-Barré syndrome *666*

Neuromuscular disorders *668*
Myasthenia gravis *668*
Amyotrophic lateral sclerosis *671*
Multiple sclerosis *672*

Cranial nerve disorders *674*
Trigeminal neuralgia *674*
Bell's palsy *676*
Peripheral neuritis *678*

Pain disorders *680*
Complex regional pain syndrome *680*

Selected references *681*

Introduction

The neurologic system, the body's communications network, coordinates and organizes the functions of all body systems. This intricate network has three main divisions:

- *central nervous system (CNS):* the control center, made up of the brain, the brain stem, and the spinal cord
- *peripheral nervous system:* motor and sensory nerves that connect the CNS to remote body parts and relay and receive messages from them
- *autonomic nervous system (part of the peripheral nervous system):* regulates involuntary functioning of the internal organs and vascular system.

Fundamental unit

The fundamental unit of the nervous system is the neuron, a highly specialized conductor cell that receives and transmits electrochemical nerve impulses. Its structure contains delicate, threadlike nerve fibers that extend from the central cell body and transmit signals: *axons,* which carry impulses *away* from the cell body, and *dendrites,* which carry impulses *to* it. Most neurons have multiple dendrites but only one axon. *Sensory (afferent) neurons* transmit impulses from special receptors to the spinal cord or the brain, *motor (efferent) neurons* transmit impulses from the CNS to regulate activity of muscles or glands, and *interneurons (connecting or association neurons)* shuttle signals through complex pathways between sensory and motor neurons. Interneurons account for 99% of all the neurons in the nervous system and include most of the neurons in the brain. (See *Structure of the neuron.*)

Intricate control system

This intricate network of interlocking receptors and transmitters forms, together with the brain and spinal cord, a dynamic control system — a living computer — that controls and regulates every mental and physical function. From birth to death, this astonishing system efficiently organizes the body's affairs — controlling the smallest action, thought, or feeling; monitoring communication and instinct for survival; and

---

STRUCTURE OF THE NEURON

The basic structure of the neuron is composed of the cell body, axon, and dendrites, as depicted below.

---

allowing introspection, wonder, abstract thought, and awareness of one's own intelligence. The brain, the primary center of the CNS, is the large soft mass of nervous tissue housed in the cranium and protected and supported by the meninges and skull bones.

The fragile brain, brain stem, and spinal cord are protected by bone (the skull and vertebrae), cushioning *cerebrospinal fluid (CSF),* and three protective membranes, called *meninges:*

- The *dura mater,* or outer sheath, is made of tough white fibrous tissue.
- The *arachnoid membrane,* the middle layer, is delicate and lacelike.
- The *pia mater,* the inner meningeal layer, is made of fine blood vessels held together by connective tissue. It's thin and transparent and clings to the brain and spinal cord surfaces, carrying branches of the cerebral arteries deep into the brain's fissures and sulci.

Between the dura mater and the arachnoid membrane is the *subdural space;* between the pia mater and the arachnoid membrane is the *subarachnoid space.* The subarachnoid space and the brain's four ventricles contain *CSF,* a clear liquid containing water and traces of organic materials (especially protein), glucose, and minerals.

CSF is formed from blood in capillary networks called *choroid plexus*, which are located primarily in the brain's lateral ventricles. This fluid is eventually reabsorbed into the venous blood through the *arachnoid villi*, in dural sinuses on the brain's surface.

The *cerebrum*, the largest portion of the brain, is the nerve center that controls sensory and motor activities and intelligence. The outer layer of the cerebrum, the *cerebral cortex*, consists of neuron cell bodies *(gray matter)*; the inner layers consist of axons *(white matter)* and basal ganglia, which control motor coordination and steadiness. The cerebral surface is deeply convoluted, furrowed with elevations *(gyri)* and depressions *(sulci)*. A *longitudinal fissure* divides the cerebrum into two hemispheres connected by a wide band of nerve fibers called the *corpus callosum*, through which the hemispheres share information. The hemispheres don't share equally; one always dominates, giving one side control over the other. Because motor impulses descending from the brain through the pyramidal tract cross in the medulla, the right hemisphere controls the left side of the body; the left hemisphere, the right side of the body. Several fissures divide the cerebrum into lobes, each of which is associated with specific functions. (See *A look at the lobes*.)

The *thalamus*, a relay center below the corpus callosum, further organizes cerebral function by transmitting impulses to and from appropriate areas of the cerebrum. In addition to its primary relay function, it's responsible for primitive emotional responses, such as fear, and for distinguishing pleasant stimuli from unpleasant ones.

The *hypothalamus*, which lies beneath the thalamus, is an autonomic center that has connections with the brain, spinal cord, autonomic nervous system, and pituitary gland. It regulates temperature control, appetite, blood pressure, breathing, sleep patterns, and peripheral nerve discharges that occur with behavioral and emotional expression. It also has partial control of pituitary gland secretion and stress reaction.

The base of the brain

Beneath the cerebrum, at the base of the brain, is the *cerebellum*. It's responsible for smooth muscle movements, coordinating sensory impulses with muscle activity, and maintaining muscle tone and equilibrium.

The brain stem houses cell bodies for most of the cranial nerves and includes the *midbrain*, the *pons*, and the *medulla oblongata*. With the thalamus and the hypothalamus, it makes up a nerve network called the *reticular formation*, which acts as an arousal mechanism and controls wakefulness. It also relays nerve impulses between the spinal cord and other parts of the brain. The midbrain is the reflex center for the third and fourth cranial nerves and mediates pupillary reflexes and eye movements. The pons helps regulate respirations; it's also the reflex center for the fifth through eighth cranial nerves and mediates chewing, taste, saliva secretion, hearing, and equilibrium. The medulla oblongata affects cardiac, respiratory, and vasomotor functions.

Bloodline to the brain

Four major arteries — two vertebral and two carotid — supply the brain with oxygenated blood. These arteries originate in or near the aortic arch. The two vertebral arteries (branches of the subclavian) converge to become the basilar artery, which supplies the posterior brain. The common carotids branch into the two internal carotids, which divide further to supply the anterior brain and the middle brain. These arteries interconnect through the *Circle of Willis*, at the base of the brain. This anastomosis usually ensures continual circulation to the brain.

The spinal cord: Conductor pathway

Extending downward from the brain through the vertebrae, to the level of approximately the second lumbar vertebra, is the spinal cord, a two-way conductor pathway between the brain stem and the peripheral nervous system. The spinal cord is also the reflex center for activities that

A LOOK AT THE LOBES

Several fissures divide the cerebrum into hemispheres and lobes; each lobe has a specific function. The *fissure of Sylvius* (lateral sulcus) separates the temporal lobe from the frontal and parietal lobes. The *fissure of Rolando* (central sulcus) separates the frontal lobes from the parietal lobe. The *parieto-occipital fissure* separates the occipital lobe from the two parietal lobes.

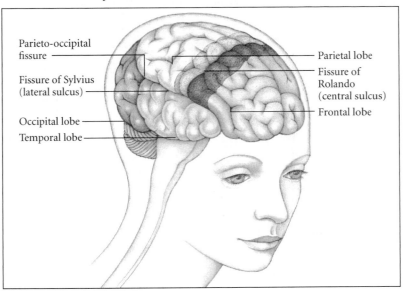

Parieto-occipital fissure

Fissure of Sylvius (lateral sulcus)

Occipital lobe

Temporal lobe

Parietal lobe

Fissure of Rolando (central sulcus)

Frontal lobe

- The *frontal lobe* controls voluntary muscle movements and contains motor areas (including the motor area for speech, or Broca's area). It's the center for personality, behavioral, and intellectual functions, such as judgment, memory, and problem solving; for autonomic functions; and for cardiac and emotional responses.

- The *temporal lobe* is the center for taste, hearing, and smell, and in the brain's dominant hemisphere, it interprets spoken language.
- The *parietal lobe* coordinates and interprets sensory information from the opposite side of the body.
- The *occipital lobe* interprets visual stimuli.

don't require brain control, such as deep tendon reflexes, the jerking reaction elicited by tapping with a reflex hammer.

A cross section of the spinal cord shows an internal H-shaped mass of gray matter divided into horns, which consist primarily of neuron cell bodies. (See *Cross section of the spinal cord,* page 620.) Cell bodies in the posterior, or dorsal, horn primarily relay sensations; those in the anterior, or ventral, horn are needed for voluntary or reflex motor activity. The white matter

surrounding the outer part of these horns consists of myelinated nerve fibers grouped functionally in vertical columns, called *tracts*. The sensory, or ascending, tracts carry sensory impulses up the spinal cord to the brain; the motor, or descending, tracts carry motor impulses down the spinal cord. The brain's motor impulses reach a descending tract and continue through the peripheral nervous system via upper motor neurons. These neurons originate in the brain and form two major systems:

CROSS SECTION OF THE SPINAL CORD

The cross section of the spinal cord below shows the anterior and posterior segments.

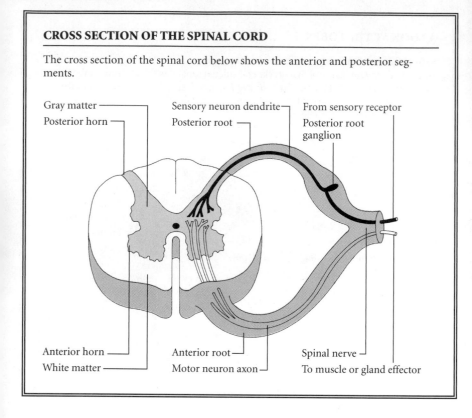

Gray matter — Sensory neuron dendrite — From sensory receptor

Posterior horn — Posterior root — Posterior root ganglion

Anterior horn — Anterior root — Spinal nerve

White matter — Motor neuron axon — To muscle or gland effector

- The *pyramidal system* (corticospinal tract) is responsible for fine, skilled movements of skeletal muscle. An impulse in this system originates in the frontal lobe's motor cortex and travels downward to the pyramids of the medulla, where it crosses to the opposite side of the spinal cord.
- The *extrapyramidal system* (extracorticospinal tract) controls gross motor movements. An impulse traveling in this system originates in the frontal lobe's motor cortex and is mediated by basal ganglia, the thalamus, cerebellum, and reticular formation before descending to the spinal cord.

Outlying areas

Messages transmitted through the spinal cord reach outlying areas through the peripheral nervous system, which originates in 31 pairs of segmentally arranged spinal nerves attached to the spinal cord. Spinal nerves are numbered according to their point of origin in the cord:

- 8 cervical: C1 to C8
- 12 thoracic: T1 to T12
- 5 lumbar: L1 to L5
- 5 sacral: S1 to S5
- 1 coccygeal.

On the cross section of the spinal cord, you'll see that these spinal nerves are attached to the spinal cord by two roots:

- The *anterior,* or *ventral,* root consists of motor fibers that relay impulses from the cord to glands and muscles.
- The *posterior,* or *dorsal,* root consists of sensory fibers that relay sensory information from receptors to the cord. The posterior root has an enlarged area — the posterior root ganglion — which is made up of sensory neuron cell bodies.

After leaving the vertebral column, each spinal nerve separates into *rami* (branches), distributed peripherally, with extensive but organized overlapping. This overlapping reduces the chance of lost sensory or motor function from interruption of a single spinal nerve.

Two functional systems

■ The *somatic (voluntary) nervous system* is activated by will but can also function independently. It's responsible for all conscious and higher mental processes and for subconscious and reflex actions such as shivering.

■ The *autonomic (involuntary) nervous system* regulates unconscious processes to control involuntary body functions, such as digestion, respiration, and cardiovascular function. It's usually divided into two competing systems: The sympathetic nervous system controls energy expenditure, especially in stressful situations, by releasing adrenergic catecholamines. The parasympathetic nervous system helps conserve energy by releasing the cholinergic neurohormone acetylcholine. These systems balance each other to support homeostasis under normal conditions.

Assessing neurologic function

A complete neurologic assessment helps confirm the diagnosis when a neurologic disorder is suspected. It establishes a clinical baseline and can offer lifesaving clues to rapid deterioration. Neurologic assessment includes:

■ *Patient history:* In addition to the usual information, try to elicit the patient's and his family's perception of the disorder. Use the patient interview to make observations that help evaluate mental status and behavior.

■ *Physical examination:* Pay particular attention to obvious abnormalities that may signal serious neurologic problems, for example, fluid draining from the nose or ears. Check for these significant symptoms:
– headaches, especially if they're more severe in the morning, wake the patient, or the pain is unusually intense
– change in visual acuity, especially sudden change
– numbness or tingling in one or more extremities
– clumsiness or complete loss of function in an extremity
– mood swings or personality changes
– any change in seizures.

■ *Neurologic examination:* Determine cerebral, cerebellar, motor, sensory, and cranial nerve function.

Obviously, there isn't always time for a complete neurologic examination during bedside assessment. It's therefore necessary to select priorities; for example, typical bedside assessment focuses on level of consciousness, pupillary response, motor function, reflexes, sensory functions, and vital signs. However, when time permits, a complete neurologic examination can provide valuable information regarding total neurologic function.

Assessing mental status, intellect, and behavior

Mental status and behavior are good indicators of cerebral function, and they're easy to assess. Note the patient's appearance, mannerisms, posture, facial expression, grooming, and tone of voice. Check for orientation to time, place, and person and for memory of recent and past events. To test intellect, ask the patient to count backward from 100 by 7s, to read aloud, or to interpret a common proverb, and see how well he understands and follows commands. If you make such checks frequently, vary the questions to avoid a programmed response.

Assessing level of consciousness

Level of consciousness (LOC) is a valuable indicator of neurologic function. It can vary from alertness (response to verbal stimulus) to coma (failure to respond even to painful stimulus). Document the patient's exact response to the stimulus; for example, write, "Patient pulled away in response to nail bed pressure," rather than a simple adjective like "stuporous."

The Glasgow Coma Scale (GCS), which assesses eye opening as well as verbal and motor responses, provides a quick, standardized account of neurologic status. In this test, each response receives a numerical value. (See *Glasgow Coma Scale,* page 622.) For instance, if the patient readily responds verbally, and is oriented to time, place, and person, he scores a 5; if he's completely unable to respond verbally, he scores a 1. If the patient is intubated or has a tracheostomy, assess and score accordingly, such

GLASGOW COMA SCALE

To quickly assess a patient's level of consciousness and to uncover baseline changes, use the Glasgow Coma Scale. This assessment tool grades consciousness in relation to eye opening and motor and verbal responses. A decreased reaction score in one or more categories warns of an impending neurologic crisis. A patient scoring 7 or less is comatose and probably has severe neurologic damage.

Test	Patient's reaction	Score
Best eye opening response	Open spontaneously	4
	Open to verbal command	3
	Open to pain	2
	No response	1
Best motor response	Obeys verbal command	6
	Localizes painful stimuli	5
	Flexion-withdrawal	4
	Flexion-abnormal (decorticate rigidity)	3
	Extension (decerebrate rigidity)	2
	No response	1
Best verbal response	Oriented and converses	5
	Disoriented and converses	4
	Inappropriate words	3
	Incomprehensible sounds	2
	No response	1
Total		**3 to 15**

as 5/T ('T' meaning tracheostomy). A score of 15 for all three parts is normal; 7 or less indicates coma; 3 — the lowest score possible — generally (but not always) indicates brain death. Although the GCS is useful, it isn't a substitute for a complete neurologic assessment.

Assessing motor function

The inability to perform the following simple tests, or the presence of tics, tremors, or other abnormalities during such testing, suggests cerebellar dysfunction.
- Ask the patient to touch his nose with each index finger, alternating hands. Repeat this test with his eyes closed.
- Instruct the patient to tap the index finger and thumb of each hand together rapidly.
- Have the patient draw a figure eight in the air with his foot.
- To test tandem walk, ask the patient to walk heel to toe in a straight line.
- To test balance, perform the Romberg test: Ask the patient to stand with feet together, eyes closed, and arms outstretched without losing balance.

Motor function is a good indicator of LOC and can also point to central or peripheral nervous system damage. During all tests of motor function, watch for differences between right and left side functions.

■ To check gait, ask the patient to walk while you observe posture, balance, and coordination of leg movement and arm swing.

■ To check muscle tone, palpate muscles at rest and in response to passive flexion. Look for flaccidity, spasticity, and rigidity. Measure muscle size, and look for involuntary movements, such as rapid jerks, tremors, or contractions.

■ To evaluate muscle strength, have the patient grip your hands and squeeze. Then ask him to push against your palm with his foot. Compare muscle strength on each side, using a 5-point scale (5 is normal strength, 0 is complete paralysis). Also test the patient's ability to extend and flex the neck, elbows, wrists, fingers, toes, hips, and knees; to extend the spine; to contract and relax the abdominal muscles; and to rotate the shoulders.

■ Rate reflexes on a 4-point scale (4 is clonus, 0 is absent reflex). Before testing reflexes, make sure that the patient is comfortable and relaxed. Then, to test superficial reflexes, stroke the skin of the abdominal, gluteal, plantar, and scrotal regions with a moderately sharp object that won't puncture the skin. (Don't use the same pin to test another patient.) A normal response to this stimulus is flexion. To test deep reflexes, use a reflex hammer to briskly tap the biceps, the triceps, and the brachioradialis, patellar, and Achilles tendon regions. A normal response is rapid extension and contraction.

Assessing sensory function

Impaired or absent sensation in the trunk or extremities can point to brain, spinal cord, or peripheral nerve damage. Determining the extent of sensory dysfunction is important because it helps locate neurologic damage. For instance, localized dysfunction indicates local peripheral nerve damage, dysfunction over a single dermatome (an area served by 1 of the 31 pairs of spinal nerves) indicates damage to the nerve's dorsal root, and dysfunction extending over more than one dermatome suggests brain or spinal cord damage.

In assessing sensory function, always test both sides of symmetrical areas — for instance, both arms, not just one. Reassure the patient that the test won't be painful.

■ *Superficial pain perception:* Lightly press the point of an open safety pin against the patient's skin. Don't press hard enough to scratch the skin. Discard pin after use.

■ *Thermal sensitivity:* The patient tells what he feels when you place a test tube filled with hot water and one filled with cold water against his skin.

■ *Tactile sensitivity:* Ask the patient to close his eyes and tell you what he feels when touched lightly on hands, wrists, arms, thighs, lower legs, feet, and trunk with a wisp of cotton.

■ *Sensitivity to vibration:* Place the base of a vibrating tuning fork against the patient's wrists, elbows, knees, or other bony prominences. Hold it in place, and ask the patient to tell you when it stops vibrating.

■ *Position sense:* Hold the lateral medial portion of the patient's fingers and toes and move them up, down, and to the side. Ask the patient to tell you the direction of movement.

■ *Discriminatory sensation:* Ask the patient to close his eyes and identify familiar textures (velvet or burlap) or objects placed in his hand or numbers and letters traced on his palm.

■ *Two-point discrimination:* Using calipers or other sharp objects, touch the patient in two different places simultaneously. Ask if he can feel one or two points.

Assessing cranial nerve function

By using the simple tests that follow, you can reliably localize cranial nerve dysfunction.

■ *Olfactory nerve (I):* Have the patient close his eyes and, using each nostril separately, try to identify common nonirritating smells, such as cinnamon, coffee, or peppermint.

■ *Optic nerve (II):* Examine the patient's eyes with an ophthalmoscope, and have him read a Snellen eye chart or a newspaper. To test peripheral vision, ask him to cover one eye and fix his other eye on a point directly in front of him. Then, ask if he can see you wiggle your finger in the four quadrants; you'd expect him to see your finger in all four.

■ *Oculomotor nerve (III):* Compare the size and shape of the patient's pupils and the equality of pupillary response to a small light in a darkened room. Shine the light from a lateral position, not directly in front of the patient's eyes.

■ *Trochlear nerve (IV) and abducens nerve (VI):* To assess for conjugate and lateral eye movement, ask the patient to follow your finger with his eyes as you slowly move it from his far left to his far right.

■ *Trigeminal nerve (V):* To test all three portions of this cranial nerve, test facial sensation by stroking the patient's jaws, cheeks, and forehead with a cotton swab, the point of a pin, or test tubes filled with hot or cold water. Because testing for a blink reflex is irritating to the patient, it's not commonly done. If you must test for this response (it may be decreased in patients who wear contact lenses), touch the cornea lightly with a wisp of cotton or tissue, and avoid repeating the test, if possible. To test for jaw jerk, ask the patient to hold his mouth slightly open, then tap the middle of his chin lightly with a reflex hammer. The jaw should jerk closed.

■ *Facial nerve (VII):* To test upper and lower facial motor function, ask the patient to raise his eyebrows, close his eyes, wrinkle his forehead, and show his teeth. To test sense of taste, ask him to identify the taste of salty, sour, sweet, and bitter substances, which you have placed on his tongue.

■ *Acoustic nerve (VIII):* Ask the patient to identify common sounds such as a ticking clock. With a tuning fork, test for air and bone conduction.

■ *Glossopharyngeal nerve (IX):* To test gag reflex, touch a tongue blade to each side of the patient's pharynx.

■ *Vagus nerve (X):* Observe ability to swallow, and watch for symmetrical movements of soft palate when the patient says, "Ah."

■ *Spinal accessory nerve (XI):* To test shoulder muscle strength, palpate the patient's shoulders, and ask him to shrug against a resistance.

■ *Hypoglossal nerve (XII):* To test tongue movement, ask the patient to stick out his tongue. Inspect it for tremor, atrophy, or lateral deviation. To test for strength, ask the patient to move his tongue from side to side while you hold a tongue blade against it.

Testing for a firm diagnosis

A firm diagnosis of many neurologic disorders usually requires a wide range of diagnostic tests — both noninvasive and invasive. Noninvasive tests are done first and may include the following:

■ Skull X-ray identifies skull malformations, fractures, erosion, or thickening. Changes in landmarks may indicate a space-occupying lesion.

■ Computed tomography (CT) scan produces three-dimensional images that can identify hemorrhage, intracranial tumors, malformation, and cerebral atrophy, edema, calcification, and infarction. If a contrast medium is used, the procedure is invasive.

■ Magnetic resonance imaging (MRI) views the CNS in greater detail than a CT scan and is the procedure of choice for detecting multiple sclerosis; intraluminal clots and blood flow in arteriovenous malformations and aneurysms; brain stem, posterior fossa, and spinal cord lesions; early cerebral infarction; and brain tumors. A noniodinated contrast medium may be used to enhance lesions. Advances in MRI allow visualization of cerebral arteries and venous sinuses without administration of a contrast medium.

■ EEG detects abnormal electrical activity in the brain (for example, from a seizure, metabolic disorder, or drug overdose).

■ Ultrasonography detects carotid lesions or changes in carotid blood flow and velocity. High-frequency sound waves reflect back the velocity of blood flow, which is then reported as a graphic recording of a waveform.

■ Evoked potentials evaluate the visual, auditory, and somatosensory nerve pathways by measuring the brain's electrical response to stimulation of the sensory organs or peripheral nerves.

Invasive tests may include the following:

■ In lumbar puncture, a needle is inserted into the subarachnoid space of the spinal cord, usually between L3 and L4 (or L4 and L5). This allows aspiration of CSF for analysis to detect infection or hemorrhage; to determine cell count and glucose, pro-

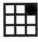

PATHOPHYSIOLOGY

WHAT HAPPENS IN INCREASED INTRACRANIAL PRESSURE

Intracranial pressure (ICP) is the pressure exerted within the intact skull by the intracranial volume—about 10% blood, 10% cerebrospinal fluid (CSF), and 80% brain tissue water. The rigid skull allows very little space for expansion of these substances. When ICP increases to pathologic levels, brain damage can result.

The brain compensates for increases in ICP by regulating the volumes of the three substances in the following ways:
- limiting blood flow to the head
- displacing CSF into the spinal canal
- increasing absorption or decreasing production of CSF—withdrawing water from brain tissue into the blood and excreting it through the kidneys. When compensatory mechanisms become overworked, small changes in volume lead to large changes in pressure.

The chart at right will help you understand the pathophysiology of increased ICP.

Brain insult
Trauma (contusion, laceration, intracranial hemorrhage)
Cerebral edema (following surgery, stroke, infection, hypoxia)
Hydrocephalus
Space-occupying lesion (tumor, abscess)

↓

Slight increase in ICP

↓

Attempt at normal regulation of ICP by decreased blood flow to head

↓

Slight decrease in cerebral perfusion pressure (CPP)

↓

Loss of autoregulatory mechanism of constriction or dilation of cerebral blood vessels if increased ICP persists

↓

Passive dilation

↓

Increased cerebral blood flow; venous congestion

↓

Further increase in ICP

↓

Cellular hypoxia

↓ ↓

Uncal or central herniation | Further decrease in CPP

↓

Brain death

tein, and globulin levels; and to measure CSF pressure. Lumbar puncture is usually contraindicated in hydrocephalus and in increased intracranial pressure (ICP) because a quick pressure reduction may cause brain herniation. (See *What happens in increased intracranial pressure*, page 625.)

■ Myelography follows a lumbar puncture and CSF removal. In this procedure, a radiologic dye is instilled and X-rays show spinal abnormalities and determine spinal cord compression related to back pain or extremity weakness.

■ In cerebral arteriography, also known as *angiography*, a catheter is inserted into an artery — usually the femoral artery — and is threaded up to the carotid artery. Then a radiopaque dye is injected, allowing X-ray visualization of the cerebral vasculature. Sometimes the catheter is threaded directly into the brachial or carotid artery. This test can show cerebrovascular abnormalities and spasms plus arterial changes due to a tumor, arteriosclerosis, hemorrhage, an aneurysm, or blockage. A patient undergoing this procedure is at risk for a stroke and for increased ICP.

■ Digital subtraction angiography visualizes cerebral vessels using contrast medium administered I.V., after which computer-assisted precontrast and postcontrast images are compared. The first image is "subtracted" from the second, which highlights the cerebral vessels.

■ Brain scan measures gamma rays produced by a radioisotope injected I.V. Uptake and distribution of the isotope in the brain highlights intracranial masses, vascular lesions, and other problems.

■ ICP monitoring can be a direct, invasive method of identifying trends in ICP. A subarachnoid screw and an intraventricular catheter convert CSF pressure readings into waveforms that are displayed digitally on an oscilloscope monitor. Another method uses a fiber-optic catheter inserted in the subdural space; with this indirect method, pressure changes are reported digitally or in waveform.

■ Electromyography detects lower motor neuron disorders, neuromuscular disorders, and nerve damage. A needle inserted into selected muscles at rest and during voluntary contraction picks up nerve impulses and measures nerve conduction time.

CONGENITAL ANOMALIES

Cerebral palsy

The most common cause of crippling in children, cerebral palsy (CP) is a group of neuromuscular disorders resulting from prenatal, perinatal, or postnatal CNS damage. Although nonprogressive, these disorders may become more obvious as an affected infant grows older. Three major types of CP occur — spastic, athetoid, and ataxic — sometimes in mixed forms. Motor impairment may be minimal (sometimes apparent only during physical activities such as running) or severely disabling. Associated defects, such as seizures, speech disorders, and mental retardation, are common. The prognosis varies; in cases of mild impairment, proper treatment may make a near-normal life possible.

Causes and incidence

See *Causes of cerebral palsy*, for a more detailed description of the causes of CP. Incidence is slightly higher in premature neonates (anoxia plays the greatest role in contributing to CP) and in neonates who are small for their gestational age. CP is slightly more common in males than in females. For every 1,000 births, 2 to 4 neonates are affected.

Spastic cerebral palsy is the most common type of CP, affecting about 50% of CP patients. Athetoid cerebral palsy affects about 20% of CP patients, ataxic cerebral palsy accounts for another 10% of these patients, and the remaining 20% of patients are mixed, with a combination of symptoms.

Signs and symptoms

Spastic cerebral palsy is characterized by hyperactive deep tendon reflexes, increased stretch reflexes, rapid alternating muscle contraction and relaxation, muscle weakness, underdevelopment of affected limbs, muscle contraction in response to manipulation, and a tendency to contractures. Typically, a child with spastic CP walks on his toes with a scissors gait, crossing one foot in front of the other.

In athetoid cerebral palsy, involuntary movements — grimacing, wormlike writhing, dystonia, and sharp jerks — impair voluntary movement. Usually, these involuntary movements affect the arms more severely than the legs; involuntary facial movements may make speech difficult. These athetoid movements become more severe during stress, decrease with relaxation, and disappear entirely during sleep.

Ataxic cerebral palsy is characterized by disturbed balance, incoordination (especially of the arms), hypoactive reflexes, nystagmus, muscle weakness, tremor, lack of leg movement during infancy, and a wide gait as the child begins to walk. Ataxia makes sudden or fine movements almost impossible.

Some children with CP display a combination of these clinical features. In most, impaired motor function makes eating (especially swallowing) difficult and retards growth and development. Up to 40% of these children are mentally retarded, about 25% have seizure disorders, and about 80% have impaired speech. Many also have dental abnormalities, vision and hearing defects, and reading disabilities.

Diagnosis
Early diagnosis is essential for effective treatment and requires precise neurologic assessment and careful clinical observation during infancy. Computed tomography scan and magnetic resonance imaging can reveal structural or congenital abnormalities. Suspect CP whenever an infant:
- has difficulty sucking or keeping the nipple or food in his mouth
- seldom moves voluntarily or has arm or leg tremors with voluntary movement
- crosses his legs when lifted from behind rather than pulling them up or "bicycling" like a normal infant
- has legs that are difficult to separate, making diaper changing difficult
- persistently uses only one hand or, as he gets older, uses hands well but not legs.

CAUSES OF CEREBRAL PALSY

Conditions that result in cerebral anoxia, hemorrhage, or other damage are probably responsible for cerebral palsy.

- Prenatal conditions that may increase risk of CP: maternal infection (especially rubella), maternal drug ingestion, radiation, anoxia, toxemia, maternal diabetes, abnormal placental attachment, malnutrition, and isoimmunization
- Perinatal and birth difficulties that increase the risk of CP: forceps delivery, breech presentation, placenta previa, abruptio placentae, metabolic or electrolyte disturbances, abnormal maternal vital signs from general or spinal anesthetic, prolapsed cord with delay in delivery of head, premature birth, prolonged or unusually rapid labor, and multiple birth (especially infants born last in a multiple birth)
- Infection or trauma during infancy: poisoning, severe kernicterus resulting from erythroblastosis fetalis, brain infection, head trauma, prolonged anoxia, brain tumor, cerebral circulatory anomalies causing blood vessel rupture, and systemic disease resulting in cerebral thrombosis or embolus

---

Infants at particular risk include those with low birth weight, low Apgar scores at 5 minutes, seizures, and metabolic disturbances. However, all infants should have a screening test for CP as a regular part of their 6-month checkup.

Treatment
CP can't be cured, but proper treatment can help affected children reach their full potential within the limitations set by this disorder. Such treatment requires a comprehensive and cooperative effort involving physicians, nurses, teachers, psychologists, the child's family, and occupational, physi-

cal, and speech therapists. Home care is usually possible. Treatment usually includes interventions that encourage optimum development:

- Braces or splints and special appliances, such as adapted eating utensils and a low toilet seat with arms, help these children perform activities independently.
- An artificial urinary sphincter may be indicated for the incontinent child who can use the hand controls.
- Range-of-motion exercises minimize contractures.
- Orthopedic surgery may be indicated to correct contractures. Botulinum toxin has been shown to reduce or delay the need for surgery.
- Phenytoin, phenobarbital, or another anticonvulsant may be used to control seizures.
- Muscle relaxants or neurosurgery may be required to decrease spasticity.

Children with milder forms of CP should attend a regular school; severely afflicted children may need special classes.

Special considerations

A child with CP may be hospitalized for orthopedic surgery or for treatment of other complications.

- Speak slowly and distinctly. Encourage the child to ask for things he wants. Listen patiently and don't rush him.
- Plan a high-calorie diet that's adequate to meet the child's high-energy needs.
- During meals, maintain a quiet, unhurried atmosphere with as few distractions as possible. The child should be encouraged to feed himself and may need special utensils and a chair with a solid footrest. Teach him to place food far back in his mouth to facilitate swallowing.
- Encourage the child to chew food thoroughly, drink through a straw, and suck on lollipops to develop the muscle control needed to minimize drooling.
- Allow the child to wash and dress independently, assisting only as needed. The child may need clothing modifications.
- Give all care in an unhurried manner; otherwise, muscle spasticity may increase.
- Encourage the child and his family to participate in the plan of care so they can continue it at home.

- Care for associated hearing or visual disturbances, as necessary.
- Give frequent mouth care and dental care, as necessary.
- Reduce muscle spasms that increase postoperative pain by moving and turning the child carefully after surgery; provide analgesics as needed.
- After orthopedic surgery, provide cast care. Reposition the child often, check for foul odor, and ventilate under the cast with a cool air blow-dryer. Use a flashlight to check for skin breakdown beneath the cast. Help the child relax, perhaps by giving a warm bath, before reapplying a bivalved cast.

To help the parents:

- Encourage them to set realistic individual goals.
- Assist in planning crafts and other activities.
- Stress the child's need to develop peer relationships; warn the parents against being overprotective.
- Identify and deal with family stress. The parents may feel unreasonable guilt about their child's handicap and may need psychological counseling.
- Refer the parents to supportive community organizations. For more information, tell them to contact the United Cerebral Palsy Association or their local chapter.

Hydrocephalus

Hydrocephalus is an excessive accumulation of cerebrospinal fluid (CSF) within the ventricular spaces of the brain. In infants, hydrocephalus enlarges the head; in infants and adults, resulting compression can damage brain tissue. With early detection and surgical intervention, the prognosis improves but remains guarded. Even after surgery, such complications as mental retardation, impaired motor function, and vision loss can persist. Without surgery, the prognosis is poor: Mortality may result from increased intracranial pressure (ICP); infants may also die prematurely of infection and malnutrition.

NORMAL CIRCULATION OF CSF

Cerebrospinal fluid (CSF) is produced from blood in a capillary network (choroid plexus) in the brain's lateral ventricles. From the lateral ventricles, CSF flows through the interventricular foramen (foramen of Monro) to the third ventricle. From there, it flows through the aqueduct of Sylvius to the fourth ventricle and through the foramina of Luschka and Magendie to the cisterna of the subarachnoid space.

Then, the fluid passes under the base of the brain, upward over the brain's upper surfaces, and down around the spinal cord. Eventually, CSF reaches the arachnoid villi, where it's reabsorbed into venous blood at the venous sinuses.

Normally, the amount of fluid produced (about 500 ml/day) equals the amount absorbed. The average amount circulated at one time is 150 to 175 ml.

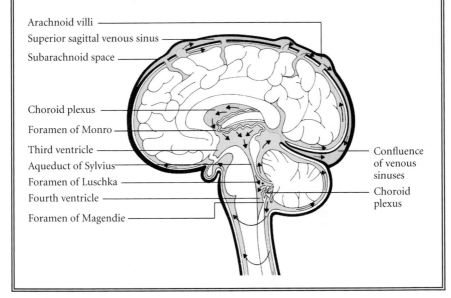

Arachnoid villi
Superior sagittal venous sinus
Subarachnoid space

Choroid plexus
Foramen of Monro

Third ventricle
Aqueduct of Sylvius
Foramen of Luschka
Fourth ventricle

Foramen of Magendie

Confluence of venous sinuses

Choroid plexus

Causes and incidence

Hydrocephalus may result from an obstruction in CSF flow (noncommunicating hydrocephalus) or from faulty absorption of CSF (communicating hydrocephalus). (See *Normal circulation of CSF.*)

In noncommunicating hydrocephalus, the obstruction occurs most frequently between the third and fourth ventricles, at the aqueduct of Sylvius, but it can also occur at the outlets of the fourth ventricle (foramina of Luschka and Magendie) or, rarely, at the foramen of Monro. This obstruction may result from faulty fetal development, infection (syphilis, granulomatous diseases, meningitis), a tumor, cerebral

aneurysm, or a blood clot (after intracranial hemorrhage).

In communicating hydrocephalus, faulty absorption of CSF may result from surgery to repair a myelomeningocele, adhesions between meninges at the base of the brain, or meningeal hemorrhage. Rarely, a tumor in the choroid plexus causes overproduction of CSF, producing hydrocephalus.

Hydrocephalus occurs most commonly in neonates but can also occur in adults as a result of injury or disease. It affects 1 of every 1,000 people.

SIGNS OF HYDROCEPHALUS

In infants, characteristic changes of hydrocephalus include marked enlargement of the head; distended scalp veins; thin, shiny, and fragile-looking scalp skin; and weak muscles that can't support the head.

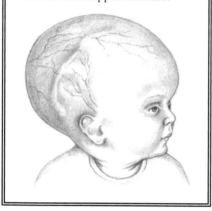

Signs and symptoms

In infants, the unmistakable sign of hydrocephalus is rapidly increasing head circumference, clearly disproportionate to the infant's growth. Other characteristic changes include widening and bulging of the fontanels; distended scalp veins; thin, shiny, and fragile-looking scalp skin; and underdeveloped neck muscles. (See *Signs of hydrocephalus.*) In severe hydrocephalus, the roof of the orbit is depressed, the eyes are displaced downward, and the sclerae are prominent. Sclera seen above the iris is called the "setting-sun sign." A high-pitched, shrill cry, abnormal muscle tone of the legs, irritability, anorexia, and projectile vomiting commonly occur. In adults and older children, indicators of hydrocephalus include decreased level of consciousness (LOC), ataxia, incontinence, and impaired intellect.

Diagnosis

In infants, abnormally large head size for the patient's age strongly suggests hydrocephalus. Measurement of head circumference is a most important diagnostic technique. Skull X-rays show thinning of the skull with separation of sutures and widening of fontanels.

Other diagnostic tests for hydrocephalus, including arteriography, computed tomography scan, and magnetic resonance imaging, can differentiate between hydrocephalus and intracranial lesions and can also demonstrate the Arnold-Chiari deformity, which may occur in an infant with hydrocephalus. (See *Arnold-Chiari syndrome.*)

Treatment

Surgical correction is the only treatment for hydrocephalus. Surgery typically consists of insertion of a ventriculoperitoneal shunt, which transports excess fluid from the lateral ventricle into the peritoneal cavity. A less common procedure is insertion of a ventriculoatrial shunt, which drains fluid from the brain's lateral ventricle into the right atrium of the heart, where the fluid makes its way into the venous circulation.

Complications of surgery include shunt infection, septicemia (after ventriculoatrial shunt), adhesions and paralytic ileus, migration, peritonitis, and intestinal perforation (with peritoneal shunt).

Special considerations

On initial assessment, obtain a complete history from the patient or his family. Note general behavior, especially irritability, apathy, or decreased LOC. Perform a neurologic assessment. Examine the eyes: pupils should be equal and reactive to light. In adults and older children, evaluate movements and motor strength in extremities. Watch especially for ataxia, confusion, and incontinence. Ask the patient if he has headaches, and watch for projectile vomiting; both are signs of increased ICP. Also watch for seizures. Note changes in vital signs.

Before surgery to insert a shunt:
■ Encourage maternal-infant bonding when possible. When caring for the infant yourself, hold him on your lap for feeding; stroke and cuddle him, and speak soothingly.
■ Check fontanels for tension or fullness, and measure and record head circumference. On the patient's chart, draw a picture

showing where to measure the head so that other staff members measure it in the same place, or mark the forehead with ink.

■ To prevent postfeeding aspiration and hypostatic pneumonia, place the infant on his side and reposition every 2 hours, or prop him up in an infant seat.

■ To prevent skin breakdown, make sure his earlobe is flat, and place a sheepskin or rubber foam under his head.

■ When turning the infant, move his head, neck, and shoulders with his body to reduce strain on his neck.

■ Feed the infant slowly. To lessen strain from the weight of the infant's head on your arm while holding him during feeding, place his head, neck, and shoulders on a pillow.

After surgery:

■ Place the infant on the side opposite the operative site with his head level with his body unless the physician's orders specify otherwise.

■ Check temperature, pulse rate, blood pressure, and LOC. Also check fontanels for fullness daily. Watch for vomiting, which may be an early sign of increased ICP and shunt malfunction.

■ Watch for signs of infection, especially meningitis: fever, stiff neck, irritability, or tense fontanels. Also watch for redness, swelling, or other signs of local infection over the shunt tract. Check dressing often for drainage.

■ Listen for bowel sounds after ventriculoperitoneal shunt.

■ Check the infant's growth and development periodically, and help the parents set goals consistent with ability and potential. Help parents focus on their child's strengths, not his weaknesses. Discuss special education programs, and emphasize the infant's need for sensory stimulation appropriate for his age. Teach parents to watch for signs of shunt malfunction, infection, and paralytic ileus. Tell them that surgery for lengthening the shunt will be required periodically as the child grows older. Surgery may also be required to correct shunt malfunctioning or to treat infection. Emphasize that hydrocephalus is a lifelong problem and that the child will require regular, continuing evaluation.

ARNOLD-CHIARI SYNDROME

Arnold-Chiari syndrome frequently accompanies hydrocephalus, especially when a myelomeningocele is also present. In this condition, an elongation or tonguelike downward projection of the cerebellum and medulla extends through the foramen magnum into the cervical portion of the spinal canal, impairing cerebrospinal fluid drainage from the fourth ventricle.

In addition to signs and symptoms of hydrocephalus, infants with Arnold-Chiari syndrome have nuchal rigidity, noisy respirations, irritability, vomiting, weak sucking reflex, and a preference for hyperextension of the neck.

Treatment requires surgery to insert a shunt like that used in hydrocephalus. Surgical decompression of the cerebellar tonsils at the foramen magnum is sometimes indicated.

Cerebral aneurysm

Cerebral aneurysm is a localized dilation of a cerebral artery that typically results from a congenital weakness in the arterial wall. Its most common form is the berry aneurysm, a saclike outpouching in a cerebral artery. Cerebral aneurysms may arise at an arterial junction in the Circle of Willis, the circular anastomosis forming the major cerebral arteries at the base of the brain. Cerebral aneurysms can rupture and cause subarachnoid hemorrhage. (See *Most common sites of cerebral aneurysm,* page 632.)

The prognosis is guarded. Probably half the patients with subarachnoid hemorrhages die immediately; of those who survive untreated, 40% die from the effects of hemorrhage; another 20% die later from recurring hemorrhage. New treatments are improving the prognosis, however.

MOST COMMON SITES OF CEREBRAL ANEURYSM

Cerebral aneurysms usually arise at arterial bifurcations in the Circle of Willis and its branches. The illustration below shows the most common aneurysm sites around this circle.

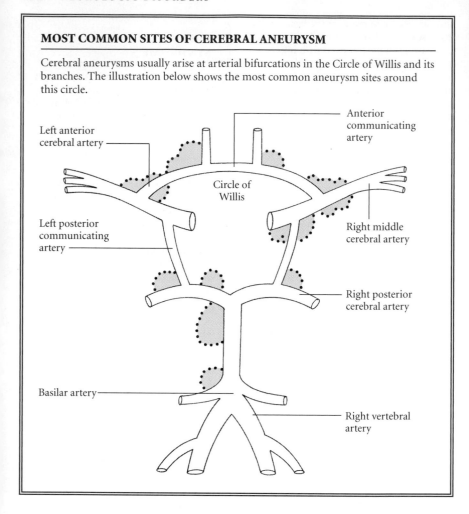

Causes and incidence

Cerebral aneurysm may result from a congenital defect, a degenerative process, or a combination of both. For example, hypertension and atherosclerosis may disrupt blood flow and exert pressure against a congenitally weak arterial wall, stretching it like an overblown balloon and making it likely to rupture. After such rupture, blood spills into the space normally occupied by cerebrospinal fluid (CSF), resulting in subarachnoid hemorrhage. Blood may also spill into the brain tissue and form a clot, which can result in potentially fatal increased intracranial pressure (ICP) and brain-tissue damage.

Incidence is slightly higher in women than in men, especially those in their late 40s or early to mid-50s, but cerebral aneurysm may occur at any age, in both women and men.

Signs and symptoms

Occasionally, rupture of a cerebral aneurysm causes premonitory symptoms that last several days, such as headache, nuchal rigidity, stiff back and legs, and intermittent nausea. Usually, however, onset is abrupt and without warning, causing a sudden severe headache, nausea, vomiting and, depending on the severity and location of bleeding, altered consciousness (including deep coma).

Bleeding causes meningeal irritation, resulting in nuchal rigidity, back and leg pain, fever, restlessness, irritability, occasional seizures, and blurred vision. Bleeding into the brain tissues causes hemiparesis, hemisensory defects, dysphagia, and visual defects. If the aneurysm is near the internal carotid artery, it compresses the oculomotor nerve and causes diplopia, ptosis, dilated pupil, and inability to rotate the eye.

The severity of symptoms varies considerably from patient to patient, depending on the site and amount of bleeding. To better describe their conditions, patients with ruptured cerebral aneurysms are grouped as follows:

- *Grade I (minimal bleed):* Patient is alert with no neurologic deficit; he may have a slight headache and nuchal rigidity.
- *Grade II (mild bleed):* Patient is alert, with a mild to severe headache, nuchal rigidity and, possibly, third-nerve palsy.
- *Grade III (moderate bleed):* Patient is confused or drowsy, with nuchal rigidity and, possibly, a mild focal deficit.
- *Grade IV (severe bleed):* Patient is stuporous, with nuchal rigidity and, possibly, mild to severe hemiparesis.
- *Grade V (moribund; commonly fatal):* If nonfatal, patient is in deep coma or decerebrate.

Generally, cerebral aneurysm poses three major threats:

- *Death from increased ICP:* Increased ICP may push the brain downward, impair brain stem function, and cut off blood supply to the part of the brain that supports vital functions.
- *Rebleed:* Generally, after the initial bleeding episode, a clot forms and seals the rupture, which reinforces the wall of the aneurysm for 7 to 10 days. However, after the 7th day, fibrinolysis begins to dissolve the clot and increases the risk of rebleeding. Signs and symptoms are similar to those accompanying the initial hemorrhage. Rebleeds during the first 24 hours after initial hemorrhage aren't uncommon, and they contribute to cerebral aneurysm's high mortality.

- *Vasospasm:* Why this occurs isn't clearly understood. Usually, vasospasm occurs in blood vessels adjacent to the cerebral aneurysm, but it may extend to major vessels of the brain, causing ischemia and altered brain function.

Other complications of cerebral aneurysm include pulmonary embolism (a possible adverse effect of deep vein thrombosis or aneurysm treatment) and acute hydrocephalus, occurring as CSF accumulates in the cranial cavity because of blockage by blood or adhesions.

Diagnosis

Diagnosis of cerebral aneurysm is based on the patient history and a neurologic examination; computed tomography scan, which reveals subarachnoid or ventricular blood; or magnetic resonance imaging, which can identify a cerebral aneurysm as a flow void.

Cerebral angiography remains the procedure of choice for diagnosing cerebral aneurysm. Lumbar puncture may be used to identify blood in CSF if other studies are negative and the patient has no signs of increased ICP. Lumbar puncture should be performed if no contraindication is present and you strongly suspect a bleed, as imaging studies may miss a bleed.

Other baseline laboratory studies include complete blood count, urinalysis, arterial blood gas (ABG) analysis, coagulation studies, serum osmolality, and electrolyte and glucose levels.

Treatment

Treatment aims to reduce the risk of vasospasm and cerebral infarction by repairing the aneurysm. Usually, surgical repair (by clipping, ligation, or wrapping the aneurysm neck with muscle) takes place 7 to 10 days after the initial bleed; however, surgery performed within 1 to 2 days after hemorrhage has also shown promise in grades I and II. (See *Aneurysm clip,* page 634.)

When surgical correction is risky, for example, when the aneurysm is in a dangerous location, or when surgery is delayed because of vasospasm, treatment includes:

- bed rest in a quiet, darkened room; if immediate surgery isn't possible, such bed rest may continue for 4 to 6 weeks

ANEURYSM CLIP

Clipping is a method of surgical repair for a cerebral aneurysm. The neurosurgeon grasps the clip, opens the jaw, and then slides the clip over the hemorrhaging blood vessel. He then closes the clip over the blood vessel, and the applied pressure stems the hemorrhaging without compromising vessel integrity.

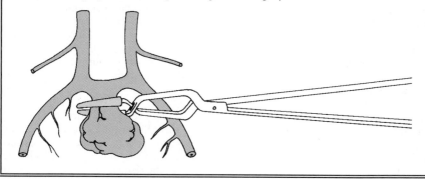

- avoidance of coffee, other stimulants, and aspirin
- codeine or another analgesic, as needed
- antihypertensive agents if the patient is hypertensive
- calcium channel blockers to decrease spasm
- corticosteroids to reduce edema
- phenytoin or another anticonvulsant
- sedatives
- a fibrinolytic inhibitor, to minimize the risk of rebleed by delaying blood clot lysis.

After surgical repair, the patient's condition depends on the extent of damage from the initial bleed and the success of treatment for any resulting complications. Surgery can't improve the patient's neurologic condition unless it removes a hematoma or reduces the compression effect.

Special considerations

An accurate neurologic assessment, good patient care, patient and family teaching, and psychological support can speed recovery and reduce complications.

- During initial treatment after hemorrhage, establish and maintain a patent airway if the patient needs supplementary oxygen. Position the patient to promote pulmonary drainage and prevent upper airway obstruction. If he's intubated, administering 100% oxygen before suction-

ing to remove secretions will prevent hypoxia and vasodilation from carbon dioxide accumulation. Suction no longer than 20 seconds to avoid increased ICP. Give frequent nose and mouth care.

- Impose aneurysm precautions to minimize the risk of rebleed and to avoid increased ICP. Such precautions include bed rest in a quiet, darkened room (keep the head of the bed flat or under 30 degrees, as ordered); limited visitors; avoiding strenuous physical activity and straining with bowel movements; and restricted fluid intake. Be sure to explain why these restrictive measures are necessary.

Preventive measures and good patient care can minimize other complications:
- Turn the patient often. Encourage occasional deep breathing and leg movement. Warn the patient to avoid all unnecessary physical activity. Assist with active range-of-motion exercises; if the patient is paralyzed, perform regular passive range-of-motion exercises.
- Monitor ABG levels, LOC, and vital signs often, and accurately measure intake and output. Avoid taking temperature rectally because vagus nerve stimulation may cause cardiac arrest.
- Watch for these danger signals, which may indicate an enlarging aneurysm, rebleeding, intracranial clot, vasospasm, or

other complication: decreased LOC, unilateral enlarged pupil, onset or worsening of hemiparesis or motor deficit, increased blood pressure, slowed pulse, worsening of headache or sudden onset of a headache, renewed or worsened nuchal rigidity, and renewed or persistent vomiting. Intermittent signs such as restlessness, extremity weakness, and speech alterations can also indicate increasing ICP.

■ Give fluids as ordered, and monitor I.V. infusions to avoid increased ICP.

■ If the patient has facial weakness, assess the gag reflex and assist him during meals, placing food in the unaffected side of his mouth. If he can't swallow, insert a nasogastric tube as ordered, and give all tube feedings slowly. Prevent skin breakdown by taping the tube so it doesn't press against the nostril. If the patient can eat, provide a high-fiber diet to prevent straining at stool, which can increase ICP. Obtain an order for a stool softener, such as dioctyl sodium sulfosuccinate, or a mild laxative, and administer as ordered. Don't force fluids. Implement a bowel program based on previous habits. If the patient is receiving steroids, check the stool for blood.

■ With third or facial nerve palsy, administer artificial tears or ointment to the affected eye, and tape the eye shut at night to prevent corneal damage.

■ To minimize stress, encourage relaxation techniques. If possible, avoid using restraints because these can cause agitation and raise ICP.

■ Administer antihypertensives as ordered. Carefully monitor blood pressure and immediately report *any* significant change, but especially a rise in systolic pressure.

■ Prevent deep vein thrombosis by applying antiembolism stockings or sequential compression sleeves.

■ If the patient can't speak, establish a simple means of communication, or use cards or a notepad. Try to limit conversation to topics that won't frustrate the patient. Encourage his family to speak to him in a normal tone, even if he doesn't seem to respond.

■ Provide emotional support, and include the patient's family in his care as much as possible. Encourage family members to adopt a realistic attitude, but don't discourage hope.

■ Before discharge, make a referral to a visiting nurse or a rehabilitation center when necessary, and teach the patient and his family how to recognize signs of rebleeding.

Arteriovenous malformations

Cerebral arteriovenous malformation (AVM) is a disorder of the blood vessels consisting of an abnormal connection between the arteries and the veins in the brain. It's a congenital disorder commonly resulting in tangled masses of thin-walled, dilated blood vessels between arteries and veins that aren't connected by capillaries. AVM primarily occurs in the posterior portion of the cerebral hemispheres. Adequate perfusion of brain tissue is prevented due to abnormal channels between the arterial and venous systems that allow mixing of oxygenated and unoxygenated blood. AVMs range in size from a few millimeters to large malformations that extend from the cerebral cortex to the ventricles. Patients typically present with multiple AVMs.

Complications of AVM include development of aneurysm and subsequent rupture, hemorrhage (intracerebral, subarachnoid, or subdural, depending on the location of the AVM), and hydrocephalus.

Causes and incidence
Although some AVMs occur as a result of penetrating injuries such as trauma, most are present at birth. However, symptoms typically don't occur until between the ages 10 and 20. Very large AVMs may short-circuit blood flow enough to cause cardiac decompensation, in which the heart can't pump enough blood to compensate for bleeding in the brain. This typically occurs in infants and young children.

The vessels of an AVM are very thin and one or more arteries feed into it, causing it to appear dilated and tortuous. Typically, high-pressured arterial flow moves into the venous system through the connecting channels to increase venous pressure, engorging and dilating the venous structures. If the AVM is large enough, the shunting can deprive the surrounding tissue of adequate blood flow. Thin-walled vessels may ooze small amounts of blood — they may even rupture — causing hemorrhage into the brain or subarachnoid space.

Cerebral arteriovenous malformations occur in approximately 3 out of 10,000 people. Although the lesion is present at birth, symptoms may occur at any time. Two-thirds of cases occur before age 40. Evidence suggests that AVMs run in families. Males and females are affected equally.

Signs and symptoms

An AVM may be asymptomatic until complications occur; these may include rupture and a resulting sudden bleed in the brain, known as a hemorrhagic stroke. Arteriovenous malformations vary in size and location within the brain. Systolic bruit may be auscultated over the carotid artery, mastoid process, or orbit on examination.

Symptoms that occur prior to an AVM rupture are related to smaller and slower bleeding from the abnormal vessels, which are usually fragile because their structure is abnormal.

In more than half of patients with AVM, hemorrhage from the malformation is the first symptom. Depending on the location and the severity of the bleed, the hemorrhage can be profoundly disabling or fatal. The risk of bleeding from an AVM is approximately 2% to 4% per year.

The first symptoms often include headache, seizure, or other sudden neurological problems, such as vision problems, weakness, inability to move a limb or a side of the body, lack of sensation in part of the body, or abnormal sensations, such as ringing and numbness. Symptoms are the same as for stroke. The individual with an AVM may complain of chronic mild headache, a sudden and severe headache, or a localized or general headache. The headache may resemble migraine and vomiting may occur. Seizures may result from focal neurologic deficits (depending on the location of the AVM) resulting from compression and diminished perfusion. Symptoms of intracranial (intracerebral, subarachnoid, or subdural) hemorrhage result. Muscle weakness and decreased sensation can occur in any part of the body. Mental status change can occur where the individual appears sleepy, stuporous, lethargic, confused, disoriented, or irritable. Additional symptoms may include stiff neck, speech or sense of smell impairment, dysfunctional movement, fainting, facial paralysis, eyelid drooping, tinnitus, dizziness, and decreased level of consciousness (LOC).

If an AVM bleeds once, the risk is greater that it will bleed again in the future. Intracerebral or subarachnoid hemorrhages are the most common first symptoms of cerebral arteriovenous malformation. In some cases, symptoms may also occur due to lack of blood flow to an area of the brain (ischemia), compression or distortion of brain tissue by large AVMs, or abnormal brain development in the area of the malformation. Progressive loss of nerve cells in the brain may occur, caused by mechanical (pressure) and ischemic (lack of blood supply) factors.

Diagnosis

Tests used to diagnose AVM include head computed tomography scan, cranial magnetic resonance imaging, and magnetic resonance angiography. An EEG may be performed if symptoms include seizures, but this test isn't diagnostic of the specific area of the lesion.

Cerebral arteriogram confirms the presence of AVMs and evaluates blood flow. Doppler ultrasonography of cerebrovascular system indicates abnormal, turbulent blood flow.

Treatment

General support measures include aneurysm precautions to prevent possible rupture. This involves placing the patient on bed rest or with limited activity and maintaining a quiet atmosphere. Analgesics may be given for headache, and sedatives may be given to help calm the patient and prevent rupture. Stool softeners may be given to prevent straining at stool, which increases intracranial pressure.

A bleeding AVM is a medical emergency requiring immediate hospitalization. The goal of treatment is to prevent further complications by limiting bleeding, controlling seizures and, if possible, removing the AVM. Surgery for correction may include block dissection, laser, or ligation to repair the communicating channels and remove the feeding vessels. Embolization or radiation therapy may be done, if surgery isn't possible, to close the communicating channels and feeder vessels, thereby reducing blood flow to the AVM. Open brain surgery, endovascular treatment, and radiosurgery may be used separately or in any combination, depending upon the physician and the patient's individual situation. Surgery is dependent upon the accessibility and size of the lesion and the patient's status. Open brain surgery involves the actual removal of the malformation in the brain through an opening made in the skull. This surgery is particularly risky because the surgery itself may cause the AVM to bleed uncontrollably.

Embolization (injecting a gluelike substance into the abnormal vessels to stop aberrant blood flow into the AVM) may be an alternative if surgery isn't feasible due to the size or location of the lesion. Stereotactic radiosurgery may also be an alternative for patients with inoperable arteriovenous malformations. It's particularly useful for small, deep lesions, which are difficult to remove by surgery.

Anticonvulsant medications such as phenytoin are usually prescribed if seizures occur.

Special considerations

■ Monitor vital signs and titrate medications to control hypertension
■ Monitor neurologic status.
■ Monitor for seizure activity and institute seizure precautions.
■ Maintain a quiet atmosphere and provide relaxation techniques.
■ Discuss the importance of reporting any signs of intracranial bleeding immediately (sudden severe headache, vision changes, decreased movement in extremities, and change in LOC).
■ Refer to social service for support services if neurological deficits have occurred from a ruptured AVM.

PAROXYSMAL DISORDERS

Headache

The most common patient complaint, headache usually occurs as a symptom of an underlying disorder. Ninety percent of all headaches are vascular, muscle contraction, or a combination; 10% are due to underlying intracranial, systemic, or psychological disorders. Migraine headaches, probably the most intensively studied, are throbbing, vascular headaches that usually begin to appear in childhood or adolescence and recur throughout adulthood.

Causes and incidence

Most chronic headaches result from tension (muscle contraction), which may be caused by emotional stress, fatigue, menstruation, or environmental stimuli (noise, crowds, or bright lights). Other possible causes include glaucoma; inflammation of the eyes or mucosa of the nasal or paranasal sinuses; diseases of the scalp, teeth, extracranial arteries, or external or middle ear; muscle spasms of the face, neck, or shoulders; and cervical arthritis. In addition, headaches may be caused by vasodilators (nitrates, alcohol, and histamine), systemic disease, hypoxia, hypertension, head trauma and tumor, intracranial bleeding, abscess, or aneurysm.

The cause of migraine headache is unknown, but it's associated with constriction and dilation of intracranial and extracranial arteries. Certain biochemical abnormalities are thought to occur during a migraine attack. These include local leakage of a vasodilator polypeptide called neurokinin through the dilated arteries and a decrease in the plasma level of serotonin.

Headache pain may emanate from the pain-sensitive structures of the skin, scalp, muscles, arteries, and veins; cranial nerves V, VII, IX, and X; or cervical nerves 1, 2, and 3. Intracranial mechanisms of headaches include traction or displacement of arteries, venous sinuses, or venous tributaries and inflammation or direct pressure on the cranial nerves with afferent pain fibers.

Affecting up to 10% of Americans, headaches are more common in females and have a strong familial incidence.

Signs and symptoms

Initially, migraine headaches usually produce unilateral, pulsating pain, which later becomes more generalized. They're commonly preceded by a scintillating scotoma, hemianopsia, unilateral paresthesia, or speech disorders. The patient may experience irritability, anorexia, nausea, vomiting, and photophobia. (See *Clinical features of migraine headaches.*)

Both muscle contraction and traction-inflammatory vascular headaches produce a dull, persistent ache, tender spots on the head and neck, and a feeling of tightness around the head, with a characteristic "hatband" distribution. The pain is usually severe and unrelenting. If caused by intracranial bleeding, these headaches may result in neurologic deficits, such as paresthesia and muscle weakness; narcotics may fail to relieve pain in these cases. If caused by a tumor, pain is most severe when the patient awakens.

Diagnosis

Diagnosis requires a history of recurrent headaches and physical examination of the head and neck. Such examination includes percussion, auscultation for bruits, inspection for signs of infection, and palpation for defects, crepitus, or tender spots (especially after trauma). Firm diagnosis also requires a complete neurologic examination, assessment for other systemic diseases—such as hypertension—and a psychosocial evaluation, when such factors are suspected.

Diagnostic tests include cervical spine and sinus X-rays, EEG, computed tomography scan—performed before lumbar puncture to rule out increased intracranial pressure (ICP)—or magnetic resonance imaging. A lumbar puncture isn't done if there's evidence of increased ICP or if a brain tumor is suspected because rapidly reducing pressure by removing spinal fluid can cause brain herniation.

Treatment

Depending on the type of headache, analgesics—ranging from aspirin to codeine or meperidine—may provide symptomatic relief. Other measures include identification and elimination of causative factors and, possibly, psychotherapy for headaches caused by emotional stress. Chronic tension headaches may also require muscle relaxants.

For migraine headaches, ergotamine alone or with caffeine may be an effective treatment. The Food and Drug Administration allows labeling of various analgesic preparations that include caffeine to state that they're for the treatment of migraine headaches. Remember that these medications can't be taken by pregnant women because they stimulate uterine contractions. These drugs and others, such as metoclopramide or naproxen, work best when taken early in the course of an attack. If nausea and vomiting make oral administration impossible, drugs may be given as rectal suppositories.

Drugs in the class of sumatriptan are considered by many clinicians to be the drug of choice for acute migraine attacks or cluster headaches. Drugs that can help prevent migraine headaches include antidepressants (such as nortriptyline or fluoxetine), beta blockers (propranolol), and calcium-channel blockers (verapamil). Corticosteroids provide short-term relief for some patients with cluster headaches.

Special considerations

Headaches seldom require hospitalization unless caused by a serious disorder. If that's the case, direct your care to the underlying problem.

■ Obtain a complete patient history: duration and location of the headache; time of day it usually begins; nature of the pain; concurrence with other symptoms such as blurred vision; precipitating factors, such as tension, menstruation, loud noises, menopause, or alcohol; medications taken such as oral contraceptives; or prolonged fasting. Exacerbating factors can also be assessed through ongoing observation of the patient's personality, habits, activities of daily living, family relationships, coping mechanisms, and relaxation activities.

CLINICAL FEATURES OF MIGRAINE HEADACHES

Type	Signs and symptoms
Common migraine (most prevalent) Usually occurs on weekends and holidays	■ Prodromal symptoms (fatigue, nausea, vomiting, and fluid imbalance) precede headache by about 1 day. ■ Sensitivity to light and noise (most prominent feature) ■ Headache pain (unilateral or bilateral, aching or throbbing)
Classic migraine Usually occurs in compulsive personalities and within families	■ Prodromal symptoms include visual disturbances, such as zigzag lines and bright lights (most common), sensory disturbances (tingling of face, lips, and hands), or motor disturbances (staggering gait). ■ Recurrent and periodic headaches
Hemiplegic and ophthalmoplegic migraine (rare) Usually occurs in young adults	■ Severe, unilateral pain ■ Extraocular muscle palsies (involving third cranial nerve) and ptosis ■ With repeated headaches, possible permanent third cranial nerve injury ■ In hemiplegic migraine, neurologic deficits (hemiparesis, hemiplegia) may persist after the headache subsides.
Basilar artery migraine Occurs in young women before their menstrual periods	■ Prodromal symptoms usually include partial vision loss followed by vertigo, ataxia, dysarthria, tinnitus and, sometimes, tingling of the fingers and toes, lasting from several minutes to almost an hour. ■ Headache pain, severe occipital throbbing, vomiting
Cluster headaches Occur in men more commonly than women and occur at all ages, but more commonly in adolescents and middle-age people.	■ Episodic type (more common) and involves one to three short-lived attacks of periorbital pain per day over a 4- to 8-week period followed by a pain-free interval averaging 1 year. Chronic type occurs after an episodic pattern is established. ■ Unilateral pain occurs without warning, reaching a crescendo within 5 minutes, and described as excruciating and deep, with attacks lasting from 30 minutes to 2 hours. ■ Associated symptoms may include tearing, reddening of the eye, nasal stuffiness, lid ptosis, and nausea.

■ Using the history as a guide, help the patient avoid exacerbating factors. Advise him to lie down in a dark, quiet room during an attack and to place ice packs on his forehead or a cold cloth over his eyes.

■ Instruct the patient to take the prescribed medication at the onset of migraine symptoms, to prevent dehydration by drinking plenty of fluids after nausea and vomiting subside, and to use other headache relief measures.

■ The patient with a migraine headache usually needs to be hospitalized only if nausea and vomiting are severe enough to induce dehydration and possible shock.

■ Avoid repeated use of narcotics if possible.

Epilepsy

Epilepsy, also called *seizure disorder,* is a condition of the brain marked by a susceptibility to recurrent seizures—paroxysmal events associated with abnormal electrical discharges of neurons in the brain.

Causes and incidence
In about half the cases of epilepsy, the cause is unknown. However, some possible causes of epilepsy include:

■ birth trauma (inadequate oxygen supply to the brain, blood incompatibility, or hemorrhage)

■ perinatal infection

■ anoxia (after respiratory or cardiac arrest)

■ infectious diseases (meningitis, encephalitis, or brain abscess)

■ ingestion of toxins (mercury, lead, or carbon monoxide)

■ tumors of the brain

■ inherited disorders or degenerative disease, such as phenylketonuria or tuberous sclerosis

■ head injury or trauma

■ metabolic disorders, such as hypoglycemia or hypoparathyroidism

■ stroke (hemorrhage, thrombosis, or embolism).

Alcohol withdrawal can cause nonepileptic seizures.

Epilepsy affects 1% to 2% of the population. However, 80% of patients have good seizure control if they strictly adhere to the prescribed treatment regimen.

Signs and symptoms
The hallmarks of epilepsy are recurring seizures, which can be classified as partial or generalized (some patients may be affected by more than one type).

Partial seizures arise from a localized area of the brain, causing specific symptoms. In some patients, partial seizure activity may spread to the entire brain, causing a generalized seizure. Partial seizures include simple partial (jacksonian) and complex partial seizures (psychomotor or temporal lobe).

A simple partial motor-type seizure begins as a localized motor seizure characterized by a spread of abnormal activity to adjacent areas of the brain. It typically produces stiffening or jerking in one extremity, accompanied by a tingling sensation in the same area. For example, it may start in the thumb and spread to the entire hand and arm. The patient seldom loses consciousness, although the seizure may progress to a generalized seizure.

A simple partial sensory-type seizure involves perceptual distortion, which can include hallucinations.

The symptoms of a complex partial seizure vary but usually include purposeless behavior. The patient experiences an aura immediately before the seizure. An aura represents the beginning of abnormal electrical discharges within a focal area of the brain and may include a pungent smell, GI distress (nausea or indigestion), a rising or sinking feeling in the stomach, a dreamy feeling, an unusual taste, or a visual disturbance. Overt signs of a complex partial seizure include a glassy stare, picking at one's clothes, aimless wandering, lip-smacking or chewing motions, and unintelligible speech; these signs may last for just a few seconds or as long as 20 minutes. Mental confusion may last several minutes after the seizure; as a result, an observer may mistakenly suspect intoxication with alcohol or drugs or psychosis.

Generalized seizures, as the term suggests, cause a generalized electrical abnormality within the brain and include several distinct types:

■ Absence *(petit mal)* seizures occur most commonly in children, although they may affect adults as well. They usually begin with a brief change in level of consciousness, indicated by blinking or rolling of the eyes, a blank stare, and slight mouth movements. There's little or no tonic-clonic movement. The patient retains his posture and continues preseizure activity without difficulty. Typically, each seizure lasts from 1 to 10 seconds. If not properly treated, seizures can recur as often as 100 times per day. An absence seizure may progress to generalized tonic-clonic seizures.

- A myoclonic *(bilateral massive epileptic myoclonus)* seizure is characterized by brief, involuntary muscular jerks of the body or extremities, which may occur in a rhythmic fashion and may precede generalized tonic-clonic seizures by months or years.
- A generalized tonic-clonic *(grand mal)* seizure typically begins with a loud cry, precipitated by air rushing from the lungs through the vocal cords. The patient then falls to the ground, losing consciousness. The body stiffens (tonic phase) and then alternates between episodes of muscular spasm and relaxation (clonic phase). Tongue-biting, incontinence, labored breathing, apnea, and subsequent cyanosis may also occur. The seizure stops in 2 to 5 minutes, when abnormal electrical conduction of the neurons is completed. The patient then regains consciousness but is somewhat confused and may have difficulty talking. If he can talk, he may complain of drowsiness, fatigue, headache, muscle soreness, and arm or leg weakness. He may fall into deep sleep after the seizure. These seizures may start as facial seizures and spread to become generalized.

An akinetic seizure is characterized by a general loss of postural tone (the patient falls in a flaccid state) and a temporary loss of consciousness. It occurs in young children and is sometimes called a "drop attack" because it causes the child to fall.

Status epilepticus is a continuous seizure state that can occur in all seizure types. The most life-threatening example is generalized tonic-clonic status epilepticus, a continuous generalized tonic-clonic seizure without intervening return of consciousness. Status epilepticus is accompanied by respiratory distress. It can result from abrupt withdrawal of anticonvulsant medications, hypoxic encephalopathy, acute head trauma, metabolic encephalopathy, or septicemia secondary to encephalitis or meningitis.

Diagnosis

Clinically, the diagnosis of epilepsy is based on the occurrence of one or more seizures and proof or the assumption that the condition that led to them is still present.

Diagnostic information is obtained from the patient's history and description of seizure activity and from family history, physical and neurologic examinations, and computed tomography scan or magnetic resonance imaging. These scans offer density readings of the brain and may indicate abnormalities in internal structures. Paroxysmal abnormalities on the EEG confirm the diagnosis by providing evidence of the continuing tendency to have seizures. A negative EEG doesn't rule out epilepsy because the paroxysmal abnormalities occur intermittently. Other tests may include serum glucose and calcium studies, skull X-rays, lumbar puncture, brain scan, and cerebral angiography.

Treatment

Generally, treatment of epilepsy consists of anticonvulsant therapy to reduce the number of future seizures. The most commonly prescribed drugs include phenytoin, carbamazepine, phenobarbital, gabapentin, or primidone administered individually for generalized tonic-clonic seizures and complex partial seizures. Valproic acid, clonazepam, and ethosuximide are commonly prescribed for absence seizures. Gabapentin and felbamate are also anticonvulsant drugs.

A patient taking anticonvulsant medications requires monitoring for toxic signs: nystagmus, ataxia, lethargy, dizziness, drowsiness, slurred speech, irritability, nausea, and vomiting.

If drug therapy fails, treatment may include surgical removal of a demonstrated focal lesion to attempt to stop seizures. Emergency treatment of status epilepticus usually consists of diazepam (or lorazepam), phenytoin, or phenobarbital; dextrose 50% I.V. (when seizures are secondary to hypoglycemia); and thiamine I.V. (in chronic alcoholism or withdrawal).

Special considerations

A key to support is a true understanding of the nature of epilepsy and of the misconceptions that surround it.

■ Encourage the patient and his family to express their feelings about the patient's condition. Answer their questions, and help them cope by dispelling some of the myths about epilepsy, for example, the myth that epilepsy is contagious. Assure them that epilepsy is controllable for most patients who follow a prescribed regimen of medication and that most patients maintain a normal lifestyle.

Because drug therapy is the treatment of choice for most people with epilepsy, information about medications is invaluable.

■ Stress the need for compliance with the prescribed drug schedule. Reinforce dosage instructions and stress the importance of taking medication regularly, at scheduled times. Caution the patient to monitor the quantity of medication he has so he doesn't run out of it.

■ Warn against possible adverse effects — drowsiness, lethargy, hyperactivity, confusion, and visual and sleep disturbances — all of which indicate the need for dosage adjustment. Phenytoin therapy may lead to hyperplasia of the gums, which may be relieved by conscientious oral hygiene. Instruct the patient to report adverse effects immediately.

■ When administering phenytoin I.V., use a large vein and monitor vital signs frequently. Avoid I.M. administration and mixing with dextrose solutions.

■ Emphasize the importance of having anticonvulsant blood levels checked at regular intervals, even if the seizures are under control.

■ Warn the patient against drinking alcoholic beverages.

■ Know which social agencies in your community can help epileptic patients. Refer the patient to the Epilepsy Foundation of America for general information and to the state motor vehicle department for information about a driver's license.

The primary goals of the health care professional and family members caring for a patient having a seizure are protection from injury, protection from aspiration, and observation of the seizure activity.

Generalized tonic-clonic seizures may necessitate first aid. Show the patient's family members how to administer first aid correctly:

■ Avoid restraining the patient during a seizure. Help the patient to a lying position, loosen any tight clothing, and place something flat and soft, such as a pillow, jacket, or hand, under his head. Clear the area of hard objects. *Don't* force anything into the patient's mouth if his teeth are clenched — a tongue blade or spoon could lacerate a mouth and lips or displace teeth, precipitating respiratory distress. However, if the patient's mouth is open, protect his tongue by placing a soft object (such as a folded cloth) between his teeth. Turn his head to provide an open airway. After the seizure subsides, reassure the patient that he's all right, orient him to time and place, and inform him that he's had a seizure.

■ *Don't* restrain the patient during a complex partial seizure. Clear the area of any hard objects. Protect him from injury by gently calling his name and directing him away from the source of danger. After the seizure passes, reassure him and tell him that he has just had a seizure.

BRAIN AND SPINAL CORD DISORDERS

Stroke

A stroke, also called *cerebrovascular accident* or *brain attack,* is a sudden impairment of cerebral circulation in one or more of the blood vessels supplying the brain. A stroke interrupts or diminishes oxygen supply and commonly causes serious damage or necrosis in brain tissues. The sooner circulation returns to normal after a stroke, the better chances are for complete recovery. However, about half of those who survive a stroke remain permanently disabled and experience a recurrence within weeks, months, or years.

Causes and incidence

A stroke results from obstruction of a blood vessel, typically in extracerebral vessels, but occasionally in intracerebral vessels. Factors that increase the risk of stroke include history of transient ischemic attacks (TIAs), atherosclerosis, hypertension, kidney disease, arrhythmias (specifically atrial fibrillation), electrocardiogram changes, rheumatic heart disease, diabetes mellitus, postural hypotension, cardiac or myocardial enlargement, high serum triglyceride levels, lack of exercise, use of oral contraceptives, cigarette smoking, and family history of stroke. (See *Transient ischemic attack.*)

The major causes of stroke are thrombosis, embolism, and hemorrhage. Thrombosis is the most common cause in middle-age and elderly people, who have a higher incidence of atherosclerosis, diabetes, and hypertension. Thrombosis causes ischemia in brain tissue supplied by the affected vessel as well as congestion and edema; the latter may produce more clinical effects than thrombosis itself, but these symptoms subside with the edema. Thrombosis may develop while the patient sleeps or shortly after he awakens; it can also occur during surgery or after a myocardial infarction. The risk increases with obesity, smoking, or the use of oral contraceptives. Cocaine-induced ischemic stroke is now being seen in younger patients.

Embolism, the second most common cause of stroke, is an occlusion of a blood vessel caused by a fragmented clot, a tumor, fat, bacteria, or air. It can occur at any age, especially among patients with a history of rheumatic heart disease, endocarditis, posttraumatic valvular disease, myocardial fibrillation and other cardiac arrhythmias, or after open-heart surgery. It usually develops rapidly — in 10 to 20 seconds — and without warning. When an embolus reaches the cerebral vasculature, it cuts off circulation by lodging in a narrow portion of an artery, most commonly the middle cerebral artery, causing necrosis and edema. If the embolus is septic and infection extends beyond the vessel wall, encephalitis or an abscess may develop.

Hemorrhage, the third most common cause of stroke, may, like embolism, occur suddenly, at any age, and affects more women than men. Hemorrhage results from chronic hypertension or aneurysms,

TRANSIENT ISCHEMIC ATTACK

A transient ischemic attack (TIA) is a recurrent episode of neurologic deficit, lasting from seconds to hours, that clears within 12 to 24 hours. It's usually considered a warning sign of an impending thrombotic stroke. In fact, TIAs have been reported in 50% to 80% of patients who have had a cerebral infarction from such thrombosis. The age of onset varies. Incidence rises dramatically after age 50 and is highest among blacks and men.

Causes
In TIA, microemboli released from a thrombus probably temporarily interrupt blood flow, especially in the small distal branches of the arterial tree in the brain. Small spasms in those arterioles may impair blood flow and also precede TIA. Predisposing factors are the same as for thrombotic strokes. The most distinctive characteristics of TIAs are the transient duration of neurologic deficits and complete return of normal function. The symptoms of TIA easily correlate with the location of the affected artery. These symptoms include double vision, speech deficits (slurring or thickness), unilateral blindness, staggering or uncoordinated gait, unilateral weakness or numbness, falling because of weakness in the legs, and dizziness.

Treatment
During an active TIA, treatment aims to prevent a completed stroke and consists of aspirin or anticoagulants to minimize the risk of thrombosis. After or between attacks, preventive treatment includes carotid endarterectomy or cerebral microvascular bypass.

which cause sudden rupture of a cerebral artery, thereby diminishing blood supply to the area served by the artery. In addition, blood accumulates deep within the brain, further compressing neural tissue and causing even greater damage.

Strokes are classified according to their course of progression. The least severe is the TIA, or "little stroke," which results from a temporary interruption of blood flow, most commonly in the carotid and vertebrobasilar arteries. A progressive stroke, or stroke-in-evolution (thrombus-in-evolution), begins with slight neurologic deficit and worsens in a day or two. In a completed stroke, neurologic deficits are maximal at onset.

Stroke is the third most common cause of death in most developed countries today and the most common cause of neurologic disability. It occurs in 1 out of 15 deaths in the United States each year.

Signs and symptoms

Clinical features of stroke vary with the artery affected (and, consequently, the portion of the brain it supplies), the severity of damage, and the extent of collateral circulation that develops to help the brain compensate for decreased blood supply. If the stroke occurs in the left hemisphere, it produces symptoms on the right side; if in the right hemisphere, symptoms are on the left side. However, a stroke that causes cranial nerve damage produces signs of cranial nerve dysfunction on the same side as the hemorrhage.

Symptoms are usually classified according to the artery affected:
- *Middle cerebral artery:* aphasia, dysphasia, visual field cuts, and hemiparesis on affected side (more severe in the face and arm than in the leg)
- *Carotid artery:* weakness, paralysis, numbness, sensory changes, and visual disturbances on affected side; altered level of consciousness (LOC), bruits, headaches, aphasia, and ptosis
- *Vertebrobasilar artery:* weakness on affected side, numbness around lips and mouth, visual field cuts, diplopia, poor coordination, dysphagia, slurred speech, dizziness, amnesia, and ataxia

- *Anterior cerebral artery:* confusion, weakness, and numbness (especially in the leg) on affected side, incontinence, loss of coordination, impaired motor and sensory functions, and personality changes
- *Posterior cerebral arteries:* visual field cuts, sensory impairment, dyslexia, coma, and cortical blindness; typically, paralysis is absent.

Symptoms can also be classified as premonitory, generalized, and focal. Premonitory symptoms, such as drowsiness, dizziness, headache, and mental confusion, are rare. Generalized symptoms, such as headache, vomiting, mental impairment, seizures, coma, nuchal rigidity, fever, and disorientation, are typical. Focal symptoms, such as sensory and reflex changes, reflect the site of hemorrhage or infarct and may worsen.

Diagnosis

Diagnosis of stroke is based on observation of clinical features, a history of risk factors, and the results of diagnostic tests:
- Computed tomography scan shows evidence of hemorrhagic stroke immediately but may not show evidence of thrombotic infarction for 48 to 72 hours.
- Magnetic resonance imaging may help identify ischemic or infarcted areas and cerebral swelling.
- Electrocardiogram can help diagnose underlying heart disorders.
- Carotid duplex may detect carotid artery stenosis.
- Angiography outlines blood vessels and pinpoints occlusion or rupture site. It's mainly used if surgery is considered.
- EEG helps to localize damaged area.

Other baseline laboratory studies may be done to exclude immune conditions or abnormal clotting that can lead to clot formation.

Treatment

Surgery performed to improve cerebral circulation for patients with thrombotic or embolic stroke includes endarterectomy (removal of atherosclerotic plaques from the inner arterial wall) and microvascular bypass (surgical anastomosis of an extracranial vessel to an intracranial vessel).

Medications useful in stroke include:

- Tissue plasminogen activator has been used successfully in clot dissolution when administered within 3 hours of the onset of symptoms. In other circumstances, heparin and Coumadin may be used, as well as aspirin and other antiplatelet drugs.
- Ticlopidine, an antiplatelet drug, may be more effective than aspirin in preventing stroke and reducing the risk of recurrent stroke after therapy has begun.
- Anticonvulsants may be used to treat or prevent seizures.
- Stool softeners may be used to prevent straining, which increases intracranial pressure (ICP).
- Corticosteroids may be indicated to minimize associated cerebral edema.
- Analgesics may be used to relieve the headache that typically follows hemorrhagic stroke.

Special considerations

During the acute phase, efforts focus on survival needs and prevention of further complications. Effective care emphasizes continuing neurologic assessment, support of respiration, continuous monitoring of vital signs, careful positioning to prevent aspiration and contractures, management of GI problems, and careful monitoring of fluid, electrolyte, and nutritional status. Patient care must also include measures to prevent complications such as infection.

- Maintain patent airway and oxygenation. Loosen constricting clothes. Watch for ballooning of the cheek with respiration. The side that balloons is the side affected by the stroke. If the patient is unconscious, he could aspirate saliva, so keep him in a lateral position to allow secretions to drain naturally or suction secretions, as needed. Insert an artificial airway, and start mechanical ventilation or supplemental oxygen, if necessary.
- Check vital signs and neurologic status, record observations, and report any significant changes to the physician. Monitor blood pressure, LOC, pupillary changes, motor function (voluntary and involuntary movements), sensory function, speech, skin color, temperature, signs of increased ICP, and nuchal rigidity or flaccidity. Remember, if stroke is impending, blood pressure rises suddenly, pulse is rapid and

bounding, and the patient may complain of a headache. Also, watch for signs of pulmonary emboli, such as chest pains, shortness of breath, dusky color, tachycardia, fever, and changed sensorium. If the patient is unresponsive, monitor his blood gases often and alert the physician to increased partial pressure of carbon dioxide or decreased partial pressure of oxygen.

- Maintain fluid and electrolyte balance. If the patient can take liquids orally, offer them as often as fluid limitations permit. Administer I.V. fluids as ordered; never give too much too fast because this can increase ICP. Offer the urinal or bedpan every 2 hours. If the patient is incontinent, he may need an indwelling urinary catheter, but this should be avoided, if possible, because of the risk of infection.
- Ensure adequate nutrition. Check for gag reflex before offering small oral feedings of semisolid foods. Place the food tray within the patient's visual field because loss of peripheral vision is common. If oral feedings aren't possible, insert a nasogastric tube.
- Manage GI problems. Be alert for signs that the patient is straining at elimination because this increases ICP. Modify diet, administer stool softeners, as ordered, and give laxatives, if necessary. If the patient vomits (usually during the first few days), keep him positioned on his side to prevent aspiration.
- Provide careful mouth care. Clean and irrigate the patient's mouth to remove food particles. Care for his dentures as needed.
- Provide meticulous eye care. Remove secretions with a cotton ball and sterile normal saline solution. Instill eyedrops as ordered. Patch the patient's affected eye if he can't close the lid.
- Position the patient and align his extremities correctly. Use high-topped sneakers to prevent footdrop and contracture and convoluted foam, flotation, or pulsating mattresses, or sheepskin, to prevent pressure ulcers. To prevent pneumonia, turn the patient at least every 2 hours. Elevate the affected hand to control dependent edema, and place it in a functional position.
- Assist the patient with exercise. Perform range-of-motion exercises for both the af-

fected and unaffected sides. Teach and encourage the patient to use his unaffected side to exercise his affected side.
- Give medications as ordered, and watch for and report adverse effects.
- Establish and maintain communication with the patient. If he is aphasic, set up a simple method of communicating basic needs. Then, remember to phrase your questions so he'll be able to answer using this system. Repeat yourself quietly and calmly, and use gestures if necessary to help him understand. Even an unresponsive patient may be able to hear, so don't say anything in his presence you wouldn't want him to hear and remember.
- Provide psychological support. Set realistic short-term goals. Involve the patient's family in his care when possible, and explain his deficits and strengths.

Begin your rehabilitation of the patient who has had a stroke on admission. The amount of teaching you'll have to do depends on the extent of neurologic deficit.
- If necessary, teach the patient to comb his hair, dress, and wash. With the aid of a physical therapist and an occupational therapist, obtain appliances, such as walking frames, hand bars by the toilet, and ramps, as needed. The patient may fail to recognize that he has a paralyzed side (called unilateral neglect) and must be taught to inspect that side of his body for injury and to protect it from harm. If speech therapy is indicated, encourage the patient to begin as soon as possible and follow through with the speech pathologist's suggestions. To reinforce teaching, involve the patient's family in all aspects of rehabilitation. With their cooperation and support, devise a realistic discharge plan, and let them help decide when the patient can return home.
- Before discharge, warn the patient or his family to report any premonitory signs of a stroke, such as severe headache, drowsiness, confusion, and dizziness. Emphasize the importance of regular follow-up visits.
- If aspirin has been prescribed to minimize the risk of embolic stroke, tell the patient to watch for possible GI bleeding. Make sure the patient and his family realize that acetaminophen isn't a substitute for aspirin.

To help prevent stroke:
- Stress the need to control diseases, such as diabetes or hypertension.
- Teach all patients (especially those at high risk) the importance of following a low-cholesterol, low-salt diet; watching their weight; increasing activity; avoiding smoking and prolonged bed rest; and minimizing stress.
- Ensure that the patient understands that if symptoms develop, he should go to the emergency department immediately.

Meningitis

In meningitis, the brain and the spinal cord meninges become inflamed, usually as a result of a viral or, less commonly, a bacterial infection. Such inflammation may involve all three meningeal membranes — the dura mater, the arachnoid, and the pia mater. The prognosis is good and complications are rare — *if* the disease is recognized early and the infecting organism responds to antibiotics; however, mortality in untreated meningitis is 70% to 100%. The prognosis is worse for infants and the elderly, particularly if antibiotic therapy isn't started within hours of symptom onset.

Causes and incidence

Meningitis is almost always a complication of another bacterial infection — bacteremia (especially from pneumonia, empyema, osteomyelitis, or endocarditis), sinusitis, otitis media, encephalitis, myelitis, or brain abscess — usually caused by *Neisseria meningitidis, Haemophilus influenzae* (in children and young adults), or *Streptococcus pneumoniae* (in adults). In some cases, a virus is suspected. (See *Lymphocytic choriomeningitis.*) Meningitis may also follow skull fracture, a penetrating head wound, lumbar puncture, or ventricular shunting procedure. Aseptic meningitis may result from a virus or other organism. Sometimes, no causative organism can be found. Meningitis commonly begins as an inflammation of the pia-arachnoid, which may progress to congestion of adjacent tissues and destruction of some nerve cells.

Incidence of meningitis is high among Blacks and Native Americans. Male infants

LYMPHOCYTIC CHORIOMENINGITIS

Lymphocytic choriomeningitis (LCM) is a mild, biphasic, febrile illness lasting about 2 weeks. Human infection occurs through inhalation of the LCM virus or arenavirus from infectious aerosolized particles of the host (rodents such as mice or hamsters) or its excreta (urine, feces, or saliva) 1 to 3 weeks before the onset of symptoms. It can also result from contact with food contaminated with the virus or by contamination of mucous membranes, skin lesions, or cuts with infected body fluids. Handlers of infected animals or their excreta are at risk for this disease. Most cases occur in the northeast and eastern seaboard areas of the United States. LCM is more common during fall and winter.

The incubation period is 8 to 13 days after exposure. Early characteristics include fever, malaise, anorexia, weakness, muscle aches, retro-orbital headache, nausea, and vomiting. Sore throat, nonproductive cough, joint pain, chest pain, testicular pain, and parotid (salivary gland) pain may occur. Meningeal symptoms appear in 15 to 21 days, with signs and symptoms of meningitis (fever, increased headache, and stiff neck) or encephalitis (drowsiness, confusion, sensory disturbances, and motor abnormalities such as paralysis). Alopecia may also occur.

Complications include temporary or permanent neurologic damage, possible maternal transmission (pregnancy-related infection is associated with spontaneous abortion, congenital hydrocephalus, chorioretinitis, and mental retardation), myelitis, Guillain-Barré-type syndrome, orchitis or parotitis, myocarditis, psychosis, joint pain and arthritis, and prolonged convalescence with continuing dizziness, somnolence, and fatigue.

Diagnosis is made by detection of immunoglobulin M antibodies by enzyme-linked immunosorbent assay from serum or cerebrospinal fluid (CSF) (the preferred diagnostic test). Lumbar-puncture CSF is typically abnormal and reveals increased opening pressure, increased protein levels, and a lymphocytic pleocytosis, usually in the range of several hundred white blood cells. Treatment is generally supportive and includes bed rest, anti-inflammatory drugs, and analgesics. Ribavirin has been shown to be effective against LCM in vitro. Acute hydrocephalus may require surgical shunting to relieve increased intracranial pressure.

Prevention involves teaching rodent control measures, basic hygiene practices, use of a personal respirator, importance of adequate ventilation, and use of a liquid disinfectant, such as a diluted household bleach solution, to clean areas with rodent droppings.

---

have a high incidence of gram-negative neonatal meningitis.

Signs and symptoms

The cardinal signs of meningitis are those of infection (fever, chills, and malaise) and of increased intracranial pressure (ICP; headache, vomiting and, rarely, papilledema). Signs of meningeal irritation include nuchal rigidity, positive Brudzinski's and Kernig's signs, exaggerated and symmetrical deep tendon reflexes, and opisthotonos (a spasm in which the back and extremities arch backward so that the body rests on the head and heels). (See *Two signs of meningitis,* pages 648 and 649.) Other manifestations of meningitis are irritability; sinus arrhythmias; photophobia, diplopia, and other visual problems; and delirium, deep stupor, and coma.

An infant may not show clinical signs of infection but may be fretful and refuse to eat. Such an infant may vomit a great deal, leading to dehydration; this prevents a

TWO SIGNS OF MENINGITIS

Brudzinski's sign: Place the patient in a dorsal recumbent position, put your hands behind her neck, and bend it forward. Pain and resistance may indicate meningeal inflammation, neck injury, or arthritis. If the patient also flexes her hips and knees in response to this manipulation, chances are she has meningitis.

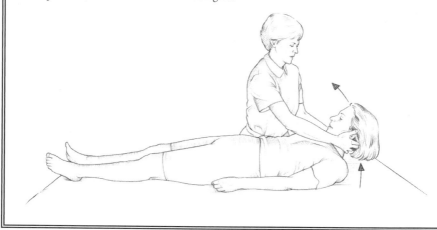

bulging fontanel and thus masks this important sign of increased ICP. As the illness progresses, twitching, seizures (in 30% of infants), or coma may develop. Most older children have the same symptoms as adults. In subacute meningitis, the onset may be insidious.

Diagnosis

A lumbar puncture showing typical cerebrospinal fluid (CSF) findings, when accompanied by positive Brudzinski's and Kernig's signs, usually establishes a diagnosis. The following tests can uncover the primary sites of infection: cultures of blood, urine, and nose and throat secretions; chest X-ray; electrocardiogram; and a physical examination, with special attention to skin, ears, and sinuses. Lumbar puncture usually indicates elevated CSF pressure, from obstructed outflow at the arachnoid villi. The fluid may appear cloudy or milky white, depending on the number of white blood cells present. CSF protein levels tend to be high; glucose levels may be low. (In subacute meningitis, CSF findings may vary.) CSF culture and sensitivity tests usually identify the infecting organism, unless it's a

virus. Leukocytosis and serum electrolyte abnormalities are also common. Computed tomography scan can rule out cerebral hematoma, hemorrhage, or tumor.

Treatment

Treatment of meningitis includes appropriate antibiotic therapy for bacterial meningitis and vigorous supportive care. Usually, I.V. antibiotics are given for at least 2 weeks, followed by oral antibiotics. Dexamethasone has been shown to be effective as adjunctive therapy in the treatment of meningitis caused by *H. influenzae* type B and in pneumococcal meningitis if given before the first dose of antibiotic. It has also been shown to reduce the incidence of deafness, a common complication of meningitis.

Other drugs include mannitol to decrease cerebral edema, an anticonvulsant (usually given I.V.) or sedative to reduce restlessness, and aspirin or acetaminophen to relieve headache and fever. Supportive measures include bed rest, fever reduction, and measures to prevent dehydration. The patient's room is kept darkened and quiet because any increase in sensory stimulation

Kernig's sign: Place the patient in a supine position. Flex her leg at the hip and knee and then straighten the knee. Pain or resistance points to meningitis.

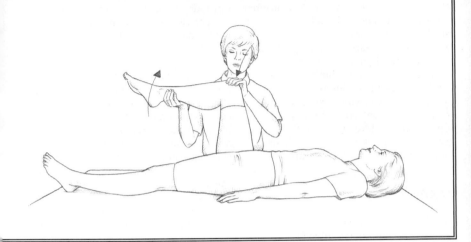

may cause a seizure. Isolation is necessary if nasal cultures are positive. Appropriate therapy for any coexisting conditions, such as endocarditis or pneumonia, is included as well. To prevent meningitis, prophylactic antibiotics are sometimes used after ventricular shunting procedures, skull fracture, or penetrating head wounds, but this use is controversial.

For viral meningitis, treatment is supportive.

Special considerations

Patients must be watched carefully for changes in neurologic function or other signs of worsening condition.

■ Assess neurologic function often. Observe level of consciousness (LOC) and signs of increased ICP (plucking at the bedcovers, vomiting, seizures, and a change in motor function and vital signs). Watch for signs of cranial nerve involvement (ptosis, strabismus, and diplopia).

ALERT *Be especially alert for a temperature increase up to 102° F (38.9° C), deteriorating LOC, onset of seizures, and altered respirations, all of which may signal an impending crisis.*

■ Monitor fluid balance. Maintain adequate fluid intake to avoid dehydration, but avoid fluid overload because of the danger of cerebral edema. Measure central venous pressure and intake and output accurately.
■ Watch for adverse effects of I.V. antibiotics and other drugs. To avoid infiltration and phlebitis, check I.V. site often, and change the site according to hospital policy.
■ Position the patient carefully to prevent joint stiffness and neck pain. Turn him often, according to a planned positioning schedule. Assist with range-of-motion exercises.
■ Maintain adequate nutrition and elimination. It may be necessary to provide small, frequent meals or to supplement meals with nasogastric tube or parenteral feedings. To prevent constipation and minimize the risk of increased ICP resulting from straining at stool, give the patient a mild laxative or stool softener.
■ Ensure the patient's comfort. Provide mouth care regularly. Maintain a quiet environment. Darkening the room may decrease photophobia. Relieve headache with a nonopioid analgesic, such as aspirin or

acetaminophen as ordered. (Opioids interfere with accurate neurologic assessment.)
■ Provide reassurance and support. The patient may be frightened by his illness and frequent lumbar punctures. If he's delirious or confused, attempt to reorient him often. Reassure his family that the delirium and behavior changes caused by meningitis usually disappear. However, if a severe neurologic deficit appears permanent, refer the patient to a rehabilitation program as soon as the acute phase of this illness has passed.
■ To help prevent development of meningitis, teach patients with chronic sinusitis or other chronic infections the importance of proper medical treatment. Follow strict sterile technique when treating patients with head wounds or skull fractures.

Encephalitis

Encephalitis is a severe inflammation of the brain, commonly caused by a mosquito-borne or, in some areas, a tick-borne virus. However, transmission by means other than arthropod bites may occur through ingestion of infected goat's milk and accidental injection or inhalation of the virus. Person to person, airborne transmission of viruses (such as measles or mumps) may also lead to encephalitis in nonimmunized populations. Eastern equine encephalitis may produce permanent neurologic damage and is commonly fatal. (See *Types of encephalitis*.)

In encephalitis, intense lymphocytic infiltration of brain tissues and the leptomeninges causes cerebral edema, degeneration of the brain's ganglion cells, and diffuse nerve cell destruction.

Causes and incidence

Encephalitis generally results from infection with arboviruses specific to rural areas. However, in urban areas, it's most frequently caused by enteroviruses (coxsackievirus, poliovirus, and echovirus). Other causes include herpesvirus, mumps virus, human immunodeficiency virus, adenoviruses, and demyelinating diseases after measles, varicella, rubella, or vaccination.

Between World War I and the Depression, a type of encephalitis known as *lethargic encephalitis, von Economo's disease,* or *sleeping sickness* occurred with some regularity. The causative virus was never clearly identified, and the disease is rare today. Even so, the term *sleeping sickness* persists and is commonly mistakenly used to describe other types of encephalitis as well.

Signs and symptoms

All viral forms of encephalitis have similar clinical features, although certain differences do occur. Usually, the acute illness begins with sudden onset of fever, headache, and vomiting and progresses to include signs and symptoms of meningeal irritation (stiff neck and back) and neuronal damage (drowsiness, coma, paralysis, seizures, ataxia, tremors, nausea, vomiting, and organic psychoses). After the acute phase of the illness, coma may persist for days or weeks.

The severity of arbovirus encephalitis may range from subclinical to rapidly fatal necrotizing disease. Herpes encephalitis also produces signs and symptoms that vary from subclinical to acute and commonly fatal fulminating disease. Associated effects include disturbances of taste or smell.

Diagnosis

During an encephalitis epidemic, diagnosis is readily made on clinical findings and patient history. However, sporadic cases are difficult to distinguish from other febrile illnesses, such as gastroenteritis or meningitis. Diagnosis may be assisted by serologic assays, such as immunoglobulin (Ig) M-capture ELISA (MAC-ELISA) and Ig ELISA. Early in infection, IgM antibody is more specific, whereas later, IgG is more reactive. Monoclonal antibody studies show promise in diagnosis. Polymerase chain reaction is also being investigated.

When possible, identification of the virus in cerebrospinal fluid (CSF) or blood confirms this diagnosis. The common viruses that also cause herpes, measles, and mumps are easier to identify than arboviruses. Both herpesviruses and arbovirus-
(*Text continues on page 654.*)

TYPES OF ENCEPHALITIS

Four main virus agents cause most cases of encephalitis in the United States: eastern equine encephalitis (EEE), western equine encephalitis (WEE), St. Louis encephalitis (SLE), and La Crosse (LAC) encephalitis, all of which are transmitted by mosquitoes. Another virus, Powassan (POW), is a minor cause of encephalitis in the northern United States; this virus is transmitted by ticks. Most cases of arboviral encephalitis occur from June through September, when arthropods are most active. In milder parts of the country, where arthropods are active late into the year, cases can occur into the winter months.

No vaccines are available for these U.S.-based diseases. However, a Japanese encephalitis (JE) vaccine is available for those who will be traveling to Japan, a tick-borne encephalitis vaccine is available for those who will be traveling to Europe, and an equine vaccine is available for EEE, WEE, and Venezuelan equine encephalitis (VEE). Public health measures often require spraying of insecticides to kill larvae and adult mosquitoes as well as controlling standing water that can provide mosquito-breeding sites.

Eastern equine encephalitis
- EEE is caused by an alphavirus virus transmitted to humans and equines by the bite of an infected mosquito.
- Incubation is 4 to 10 days.
- Symptoms begin with a sudden onset of fever, general muscle pains, and a headache of increasing severity; can progress to seizures and coma.
- One-third of those afflicted will die from the disease and of those who recover, many will suffer irreversible brain damage requiring care.
- Human cases are usually preceded by outbreaks in horses.
- The virus occurs in natural cycles involving birds in swampy areas nearly every year during the warm months. The virus doesn't escape from these areas, however, and this mosquito doesn't usually bite humans or other mammals.

Western equine encephalitis
- The alphavirus WEE is the causative agent. The virus is closely related to the EEE and VEE viruses
- The enzootic cycle of WEE involves passerine birds, in which the infection is inapparent, and culicine mosquitoes, principally *Cx. tarsalis*, a species associated with irrigated agriculture and stream drainages.
- Human WEE cases are usually first seen in June or July.
- Most WEE infections are asymptomatic or present as mild, nonspecific illness. Patients with clinically apparent illness usually have a sudden onset with fever, headache, nausea, vomiting, anorexia, and malaise, followed by altered mental status, weakness, and signs of meningeal irritation.
- Children, especially those younger than age 1, are affected more severely than adults and may be left with permanent sequelae, which is seen in 5% to 30% of young patients.
- Mortality is about 3%.

St. Louis encephalitis
- The leading cause of SLE is flaviviral. SLE is the most common mosquito-transmitted human pathogen in the United States.
- Mosquitoes become infected by feeding on birds infected with the SLE virus. Infected mosquitoes then transmit virus to humans and animals during the feeding process. The virus grows both in the infected mosquito and the infected bird, but doesn't make either one sick.
- Less than 1% of SLE viral infections are clinically apparent; the majority are undiagnosed.
- Illness ranges in severity from a simple febrile headache to meningoencephalitis, with an overall case-fatality ratio of 5% to 15%.

(continued)

TYPES OF ENCEPHALITIS *(continued)*

- The incubation period is 5 to 15 days.
- Mild infections present with fever and headache. More severe infection is marked by headache, high fever, neck stiffness, stupor, disorientation, coma, tremors, occasional convulsions (especially in infants), and spastic (but rarely flaccid) paralysis.
- The disease is generally milder in children than in adults, but in those children who do have disease, there's a high rate of encephalitis.
- Elderly people are at highest risk for severe disease and death.
- During the summer season, SLE virus is maintained in a mosquito-bird-mosquito cycle, with periodic amplification by peridomestic birds and *Culex* mosquitoes.

La Crosse encephalitis
- The LAC virus, a Bunyavirus, is a zoonotic pathogen cycled between the daytime-biting tree hole mosquito, *Aedes triseriatus*, and vertebrate amplifier hosts (chipmunks, tree squirrels) in deciduous forest habitats. The virus is maintained over the winter by transmission in mosquito eggs. If the female mosquito is infected, she may lay eggs that carry the virus. Vector uses artificial containers (tires, buckets, and so forth) in addition to tree holes.
- LAC encephalitis initially presents as a nonspecific summertime illness with fever, headache, nausea, vomiting, and lethargy.
- Severe disease occurs most commonly in children younger than age 16 and is characterized by seizures, coma, paralysis, and a variety of neurological sequelae after recovery.
- Death occurs in less than 1% of clinical cases.
- Cases are often reported as aseptic meningitis or viral encephalitis of unknown etiology.
- During an average year, about 75 cases of LAC encephalitis are reported to the Centers for Disease Control and Prevention.

Powassan encephalitis
- The POW virus is a flavivirus.
- Recently a Powassan-like virus was isolated from the deer tick, *Ixodes scapularis.* The virus has been recovered from ticks (*Ixodes marxi* and *Dermacentor andersoni*) and from the tissues of a skunk (*Spiligale putorius*).
- It's a rare cause of acute viral encephalitis.
- Patients who recover may have residual neurologic problems.

Venezuelan equine encephalitis
- Like EEE and WEE viruses, VEE is an alphavirus that causes encephalitis in horses and humans. VEE is a significant veterinary and public health problem in Central and South America.
- Infection of humans with the VEE virus is less severe than with EEE and WEE viruses, and fatalities are rare.
- Adults usually develop only an influenza-like illness; overt encephalitis is usually confined to children.
- Effective VEE virus vaccines are available for equines.

Japanese encephalitis
- JE virus, which is related to SLE, is a flavivirus. It's widespread throughout Asia.
- Epidemics occur in late summer in temperate regions, but the infection is enzootic and occurs throughout the year in many tropical areas of Asia.
- The virus is maintained in a cycle involving culicine mosquitoes and waterbirds. It's transmitted to humans by Culex mosquitoes, primarily *Cx. tritaeniorhynchus,* which breed in rice fields.
- Mosquitoes become infected by feeding on domestic pigs and wild birds infected with the JE virus. Infected mosquitoes then transmit the virus to humans and animals during the feeding

TYPES OF ENCEPHALITIS *(continued)*

process. The virus is amplified in domestic pigs and wild birds.

- The incubation period is 5 to 14 days.
- Mild infections occur without apparent symptoms other than fever with headache. More severe infection is marked by quick onset, headache, high fever, neck stiffness, stupor, disorientation, coma, tremors, occasional seizures (especially in infants), and spastic (but rarely flaccid) paralysis.
- The illness resolves in 5 to 7 days if there's no central nervous system involvement.
- The mortality is less than 10%, but is higher in children and can exceed 30%. Neurologic sequelae in patients who recover are reported in up to 30% of cases.
- A vaccine is currently available for human use in the United States for individuals who might be traveling to endemic countries.

Tick-borne encephalitis

- Tick-borne encephalitis (TBE) is caused by two closely related flaviviruses. The eastern subtype causes Russian spring-summer encephalitis (RSSE) and is transmitted by *Ixodes persulcatus,* whereas the western subtype is transmitted by *Ixodes ricinus* and causes Central European encephalitis (CEE).
- RSSE is the more severe infection, having a mortality of up to 25% in some outbreaks, whereas mortality in CEE seldom exceeds 5%.
- The incubation period is 7 to 14 days.
- Infection usually presents as a mild, influenza-type illness or as benign, aseptic meningitis, but may result in fatal meningoencephalitis.
- Fever is often biphasic, and there may be severe headache and neck rigidity, with transient paralysis of the limbs, shoulders or, less commonly, the respiratory musculature. A few patients are left with residual paralysis.
- Although the great majority of TBE infections follow exposure to ticks, infection has occurred through the ingestion of infected cows' or goats' milk.

- An inactivated TBE vaccine is currently available in Europe and Russia.

West Nile encephalitis

- West Nile virus (WNV) is a flavivirus belonging to the Japanese encephalitis serocomplex that includes the closely related SLE virus, Kunjin, and Murray Valley encephalitis viruses, as well as others.
- SLE and WNE viruses are related.
- WNV can infect a wide range of vertebrates; in humans it usually produces either asymptomatic infection or mild febrile disease, but can cause severe and fatal infection in a small percentage of patients.
- The incubation period is thought to range from 3 to 14 days.
- Symptoms generally last 3 to 6 days.
- Like SLE virus, WNV is transmitted principally by *Culex* species mosquitoes, but also can be transmitted by *Aedes, Anopheles*, and other species.
- The mild form of WNV infection has presented as a febrile illness of sudden onset often accompanied by malaise, anorexia, nausea, vomiting, eye pain, headache, myalgia, rash, and lymphadenopathy.
- A minority of patients with severe disease develop a maculopapular or morbilliform rash involving the neck, trunk, arms, or legs. Some patients experience severe muscle weakness and flaccid paralysis. Neurological presentations include ataxia, cranial nerve abnormalities, myelitis, optic neuritis, polyradiculitis, and seizures. Although not observed in recent outbreaks, myocarditis, pancreatitis, and fulminant hepatitis have been described.

Murray Valley encephalitis

- MVE is endemic in New Guinea and in parts of Australia.
- It's related to the SLE, WN, and JE viruses.
- Infections are common, and the small number of fatalities have mostly been in children.

es can be isolated by inoculating young mice with a specimen taken from the patient. In herpes encephalitis, serologic studies may show rising titers of complement-fixing antibodies.

In all forms of encephalitis, CSF pressure is elevated and despite inflammation, the fluid is usually clear. White blood cell and protein levels in CSF are slightly elevated, but the glucose level remains normal. An EEG reveals abnormalities. Occasionally, a computed tomography scan or magnetic resonance imaging may be ordered to rule out cerebral hematoma.

Treatment

The antiviral agent acyclovir may be prescribed for herpes encephalitis. Antibiotics may be prescribed if the infection is caused by bacteria. Treatment of all other forms of encephalitis is entirely supportive. Drug therapy includes phenytoin or another anticonvulsant, usually given I.V.; steroids such as dexamethasone may be used to reduce cerebral inflammation and edema; corticosteroids; mannitol to reduce cerebral swelling; sedatives for restlessness; and aspirin or acetaminophen to relieve headache and reduce fever. Ribavirin and interferon alpha-2b were found to have some effect on West Nile encephalitis. Other supportive measures include adequate fluid and electrolyte intake to prevent dehydration and antibiotics for an associated infection such as pneumonia. Isolation is unnecessary.

Special considerations

During the acute phase of the illness:
- Assess neurologic function often. Observe level of consciousness and signs of increased intracranial pressure (ICP) (increasing restlessness, plucking at the bedcovers, vomiting, seizures, and changes in pupil size, motor function, and vital signs — such as rising blood pressure, widening pulse pressure, and slowly falling pulse). Watch for cranial nerve involvement (ptosis, strabismus, and diplopia), abnormal sleep patterns, and behavior changes.
- Maintain adequate fluid intake to prevent dehydration, but avoid fluid overload, which may increase cerebral edema. Measure and record intake and output accurately and assess daily weights.
- Carefully position the patient to prevent joint stiffness and neck pain, and turn him often. Assist with range-of-motion exercises.
- Maintain adequate nutrition. It may be necessary to give the patient small, frequent meals or to supplement meals with nasogastric tube or parenteral feedings.
- To prevent constipation and minimize the risk of increased ICP resulting from straining at stool, give a mild laxative or stool softener.
- Provide mouth care.
- Maintain a quiet environment. Darkening the room may decrease photophobia and headache. If the patient naps during the day and is restless at night, plan daytime activities to minimize napping and promote sleep at night.
- Provide emotional support and reassurance because the patient is apt to be frightened by the illness and frequent diagnostic tests.
- If the patient is delirious or confused, attempt to reorient him often. Providing a calendar or a clock in the patient's room may be helpful.
- Reassure the patient and his family that behavior changes caused by encephalitis usually disappear. If a neurologic deficit is severe and appears permanent, refer the patient to a rehabilitation program as soon as the acute phase has passed.
- Discuss prevention through personal protective measures (proper clothing, insect repellent with N,N-diethyl-meta-toluamide [DEET]) and suggest reducing time outdoors in early evening hours.

Brain abscess

Brain abscess, also known as an *intracranial abscess,* is a free or encapsulated collection of pus usually in the temporal lobe, cerebellum, or frontal lobes. It can vary in size and may occur singly or in more than one location.

Untreated brain abscess is usually fatal; even with treatment, the prognosis is only fair, and about 30% of patients develop focal seizures. Multiple metastatic abscesses secondary to systemic or other infections have the poorest prognosis.

Causes and incidence

Brain abscess is usually secondary to some other infection, especially otitis media, sinusitis, dental abscess, and mastoiditis. Other causes include subdural empyema; bacterial endocarditis; human immunodeficiency virus infection; bacteremia; pulmonary or pleural infection; pelvic, abdominal, and skin infections; and cranial trauma, such as a penetrating head wound or compound skull fracture. Brain abscess also occurs in those with congenital heart disease and congenital blood vessel abnormalities of the lungs such as Osler-Weber-Rendu disease. These disorders carry a high risk of infection of the heart or lungs, which can then spread to the brain. Penetrating head trauma or bacteremia usually leads to staphylococcal infection; pulmonary disease, to streptococcal infection.

Brain abscess usually begins with localized inflammatory necrosis and edema, septic thrombosis of vessels, and suppurative encephalitis. This is followed by thick encapsulation of accumulated pus and adjacent meningeal infiltration by neutrophils, lymphocytes, and plasma cells.

Brain abscess has a relatively low incidence. It has a 10% mortality rate.

Signs and symptoms

Onset varies according to cause, but generally brain abscess produces clinical effects similar to those of a brain tumor. Early symptoms result from increased intracranial pressure (ICP) and include constant intractable headache, worsened by straining; nausea; vomiting; and focal or generalized seizures. Typical later symptoms include ocular disturbances, such as nystagmus, decreased vision, and unequal pupil size.

Other features differ with the site of the abscess:

- *temporal lobe abscess:* auditory-receptive dysphasia, central facial weakness, and hemiparesis
- *cerebellar abscess:* dizziness, coarse nystagmus, gaze weakness on lesion side, tremor, and ataxia

- *frontal lobe abscess:* expressive dysphasia, hemiparesis with unilateral motor seizure, drowsiness, inattention, and mental function impairment.

Signs of infection, such as fever, pallor, and bradycardia, are absent until late stages unless they result from the predisposing condition. If the abscess is encapsulated, they may never appear. Depending on abscess size and location, level of consciousness (LOC) varies from drowsiness to deep stupor.

Diagnosis

A history of infection — especially of the middle ear, mastoid, nasal sinuses, heart, or lungs — or a history of congenital heart disease, along with a physical examination showing such characteristic clinical features as increased ICP, points to brain abscess. A computed tomography (CT) scan or magnetic resonance imaging (MRI) and, occasionally, arteriography (which highlights brain abscess by a halo) help locate the site. Blood culture will reveal any bacteria in the blood stream. Chest X-ray may reveal lung infection.

Examination of cerebrospinal fluid can help confirm infection, but lumbar puncture is too risky because it can release the increased ICP and provoke cerebral herniation. A CT-guided stereotactic biopsy may be performed to drain and culture the abscess. Other tests include culture and sensitivity of drainage to identify the causative organism, skull X-rays, and a radioisotope scan.

Treatment

Management of patients with brain abscess has become increasingly challenging because of the proliferation of unusual bacterial, fungal, and parasitic infections, particularly in immunocompromised patients. Therapy consists of antibiotics to combat the underlying infection and surgical aspiration or drainage of the abscess. Surgical drainage or excision may be performed (CT scan or MRI can help determine the need for these procedures). Antimicrobials may be injected directly into the mass. Administration of antibiotics for at least 2 weeks before surgery can reduce the risk of spreading infection.

Other treatments during the acute phase are palliative and supportive and include mechanical ventilation, administration of I.V. fluids with diuretics (urea or mannitol), and glucocorticoids (dexamethasone) to combat increased ICP and cerebral edema. Anticonvulsants, such as phenytoin and phenobarbital, help prevent seizures.

Special considerations

The patient with an acute brain abscess requires intensive monitoring.

■ Frequently assess neurologic status, especially LOC, speech, and sensorimotor and cranial nerve functions. Watch for signs of increased ICP (decreased LOC, vomiting, abnormal pupil response, and depressed respirations), which may lead to cerebral herniation with such signs as fixed and dilated pupils, widened pulse pressure, bradycardia or tachycardia, and absent respirations.

■ Assess and record vital signs at least every hour.

■ Monitor fluid intake and output carefully because fluid overload can contribute to cerebral edema.

If surgery is necessary, explain the procedure to the patient and answer his questions. After surgery:

■ Continue frequent neurologic assessment. Monitor vital signs, and intake and output.

■ Watch for signs of meningitis (nuchal rigidity, headaches, chills, and sweats), an ever-present threat.

■ Be sure to change a damp dressing often, using sterile technique and noting the amount of drainage. Never allow bandages to remain damp. To promote drainage and prevent reaccumulation of purulent material in the abscess, position the patient on the operative side.

■ If the patient remains stuporous or comatose for an extended period, give meticulous skin care to prevent pressure ulcers, and position him to preserve function and prevent contractures.

■ Encourage the patient to ambulate as soon as possible to prevent immobility and encourage independence.

■ To prevent brain abscess, stress the need for treatment of otitis media, mastoiditis, dental abscess, and other infections. Give prophylactic antibiotics, as ordered, after compound skull fracture or penetrating head wound.

Huntington's disease

Also called *Huntington's chorea,* hereditary chorea, chronic progressive chorea, or adult chorea, Huntington's disease is a hereditary disease in which degeneration in the cerebral cortex and basal ganglia causes chronic progressive chorea and mental deterioration, ending in dementia.

Causes and incidence

Huntingdon's disease is inherited as a single faulty gene on chromosome #4 whereby part of the gene is repeated in multiple copies. It's transmitted as an autosomal dominant trait; either sex can transmit and inherit it. Each child of a parent with this disease has a 50% chance of inheriting it.

The disease usually strikes people between ages 35 and 55; however, 2% of cases occur in children, and 5% of cases occur as late as age 60. Death usually results 10 to 15 years after onset, from suicide, heart failure, or pneumonia. Genetic testing is available for persons with a family history of the disease.

Signs and symptoms

Onset is insidious. The patient eventually becomes totally dependent—emotionally and physically—through loss of musculoskeletal control, and he develops progressively severe choreic movements. Such movements are rapid, usually violent, and purposeless. Initially, they're unilateral and more prominent in the face and arms than in the legs, progressing from mild fidgeting to grimacing, tongue smacking, dysarthria (indistinct speech), athetoid movements (especially of the hands) related to emotional state, and torticollis.

Ultimately, the patient with Huntington's disease develops progressive dementia, although the dementia doesn't always progress at the same rate as the chorea. Dementia can be mild at first, but eventually causes severe disruption of the personality. Personality changes include obstinacy, carelessness, untidiness, moodiness, apathy, inappropriate behavior, loss of memory and concentration and, occasionally, paranoia.

Diagnosis

Huntington's disease can be detected by positron emission tomography and deoxyribonucleic acid analysis. Diagnosis is based on a characteristic clinical history: progressive chorea and dementia, onset in early middle age (35 to 40), and confirmation of a genetic link. Computed tomography scan and magnetic resonance imaging demonstrate brain atrophy. Molecular genetics may detect the gene for Huntington's disease in people at risk while they're still asymptomatic.

Treatment

Because Huntington's disease has no known cure, treatment is supportive, protective, and symptomatic. Dopamine blockers, such as phenothiazine or haloperidol, help control choreic movements and reduce abnormal behaviors. Reserpine and other drugs have been used with varying success with choreic movements and reduced abnormal behavior. Drugs, such as tetrabenazine and amantadine, are used to control extra movements. Some evidence suggests that co-enzyme Q10 may minimally decrease progression of the disease. Institutionalization may be necessary because of mental deterioration, which can't be halted or managed by drugs.

Special considerations

Patient comfort and support are the primary considerations.

■ Provide physical support by attending to the patient's basic needs, such as hygiene, skin care, bowel and bladder care, and nutrition. Increase this support as mental and physical deterioration make him increasingly immobile.

■ Offer emotional support to the patient and his family. Teach them about the disease, and listen to their concerns and special problems. Keep in mind the patient's dysarthria, and allow him extra time to express himself, thereby decreasing frustration. Teach the family to participate in the patient's care.

■ Stay alert for possible suicide attempts. Control the patient's environment to protect him from suicide or other self-inflicted injury. Pad the side rails of the bed, but avoid restraints, which may cause the patient to injure himself with violent, uncontrolled movements.

■ If the patient has difficulty walking, provide a walker to help him maintain his balance.

■ Make sure affected families receive genetic counseling. All affected family members should realize that each of their offspring has a 50% chance of inheriting this disease.

■ Refer people at risk who desire genetic testing to centers specializing in Huntington's care, where psychosocial support is available.

■ Refer the patient and his family to the appropriate community organizations.

■ For more information about this degenerative disease, refer the patient and his family to the Huntington's Disease Society of America.

Parkinson's disease

Named for James Parkinson, the English physician who wrote the first accurate description of the disease in 1817, Parkinson's disease characteristically produces progressive muscle rigidity, akinesia, involuntary tremor, and dementia. Death may result from aspiration pneumonia or an infection.

Causes and incidence

Although the cause of Parkinson's disease is unknown, study of the extrapyramidal brain nuclei (corpus striatum, globus pallidus, and substantia nigra) has established that a dopamine deficiency prevents affected brain cells from performing their normal inhibitory function within the central nervous system. Parkinson's disease occurs in families in some cases; in others, it's secondary to external factors such as medications used to treat schizophrenia.

Parkinson's disease, also called *parkinsonism*, paralysis agitans, and shaking palsy, is one of the most common crippling diseases in the United States. Parkinson's disease strikes 2 in every 1,000 people, most often developing in those older than age 50; however, it also occurs in children and young adults. Because of increased longevity, this amounts to roughly 60,000 new cases diagnosed annually in the United States alone. Incidence increases in persons with repeated brain injury, including professional athletes, and persons using psychoactive substances, whether prescribed or illicit.

Signs and symptoms

The cardinal symptoms of Parkinson's disease are muscle rigidity and akinesia and an insidious resting tremor that begins in the fingers (unilateral pill-roll tremor), increases during stress or anxiety, and decreases with purposeful movement and sleep. Muscle rigidity results in resistance to passive muscle stretching, which may be uniform (lead-pipe rigidity) or jerky (cogwheel rigidity). Akinesia causes the patient to walk with difficulty (gait lacks normal parallel motion and may be retropulsive or propulsive) and produces a high-pitched, monotone voice; drooling; a masklike facial expression; loss of posture control (the patient walks with body bent forward); and dysarthria, dysphagia, or both. Occasionally, akinesia may also cause oculogyric crises (eyes are fixed upward, with involuntary tonic movements) or blepharospasm (eyelids are completely closed). Parkinson's disease itself doesn't impair the intellect, but a coexisting disorder, such as arteriosclerosis, may do so.

Diagnosis

Generally, laboratory data are of little value in identifying Parkinson's disease; consequently, diagnosis is based on the patient's age, history, and characteristic clinical picture.

Conclusive diagnosis is possible only after ruling out other causes of tremor, involutional depression, cerebral arteriosclerosis and, in patients younger than age 30, intracranial tumors, Wilson's disease, or phenothiazine or other drug toxicity.

Treatment

Because Parkinson's disease has no cure, the primary aim of treatment is to relieve symptoms and keep the patient functional as long as possible. Treatment consists of drugs, physical therapy and, in severe disease states unresponsive to drugs, stereotactic neurosurgery or the controversial treatment called fetal cell transplantation. In this treatment, fetal brain tissue is injected into the patient's brain. If the injected cells grow within the recipient's brain, they will allow the brain to process dopamine, thereby either halting or reversing disease progression. Neurotransplantation techniques, including the use of nerve cells from other parts of the patient's body, have been attempted with varying results.

Drug therapy usually includes levodopa, a dopamine replacement that's most effective during early stages. It's given in increasing doses until symptoms are relieved or adverse effects appear. Because adverse effects can be serious, levodopa is frequently given in combination with carbidopa to halt peripheral dopamine synthesis. Occasionally, levodopa proves ineffective, producing dangerous adverse effects that include postural hypotension, hallucinations, and increased libido leading to inappropriate sexual behavior. In that case, alternative drug therapy includes anticholinergics such as trihexyphenidyl, antihistamines such as diphenhydramine, and amantadine, an antiviral agent.

Research on the oxidative stress theory has caused a controversy in drug therapy for Parkinson's disease. Traditionally, levodopa-carbidopa has been a first-line drug in management; however, it has also been associated with an acceleration of disease process. Inclusion of entacapone potentiates the effects of levodopa-carbidopa treatment so that less frequent doses are required.

Selegiline, an enzyme-inhibiting agent, allows conservation of dopamine and enhances the therapeutic effect of levodopa. Selegiline used with tocopherols delays the time when the patient with Parkinson's disease becomes disabled.

ELDER TIP *Elderly patients may need smaller doses of antiparkinsonian drugs because of reduced tolerance. Be alert for and report orthostatic hypotension, irregular pulse, blepharospasm, and anxiety or confusion.*

When drug therapy fails, stereotactic neurosurgery, such as subthalamotomy and pallidotomy, may be an alternative. In these procedures, electrical coagulation, freezing, radioactivity, or ultrasound destroys the ventrolateral nucleus of the thalamus to prevent involuntary movement. This is most effective in young, otherwise healthy people with unilateral tremor or muscle rigidity. Neurosurgery can only relieve symptoms. Brain stimulator implantation alters the activity of the area where Parkinson's disease symptoms originate. A pacemaker is implanted into the chest wall, and the electrode is threaded (using magnetic resonance imaging for guidance) to the thalamus, pallidum, or subthalamic nucleus. A successful procedure reduces the need for medication, thus reducing the medication-related adverse effects experienced by the patient.

Individually planned physical therapy complements drug treatment and neurosurgery to maintain normal muscle tone and function. Appropriate physical therapy includes both active and passive range-of-motion exercises, routine daily activities, walking, and baths and massage to help relax muscles.

Special considerations

Effectively caring for the patient with Parkinson's disease requires careful monitoring of drug treatment, emphasis on teaching self-reliance, and generous psychological support.

■ Monitor drug treatment and adjust dosage, if necessary, to minimize adverse effects.

■ If the patient has surgery, watch for signs of hemorrhage and increased intracranial pressure by frequently checking level of consciousness and vital signs.

■ Encourage independence. The patient with excessive tremor may achieve partial control of his body by sitting on a chair and using its arms to steady himself. Advise the patient to change position slowly and dangle his legs before getting out of bed. Remember that fatigue may cause him to depend more on others.

■ Help the patient overcome problems related to eating and elimination. For example, if he has difficulty eating, offer supplementary or small, frequent meals to increase caloric intake. Help establish a regular bowel routine by encouraging him

to drink at least 2 qt (2 L) of liquids daily and eat high-fiber foods. He may need an elevated toilet seat to assist him from a standing to a sitting position.

■ Give the patient and his family emotional support. Teach them about the disease, its progressive stages, and drug adverse effects. Show the family how to prevent pressure ulcers and contractures by proper positioning. Inform them of the dietary restrictions levodopa imposes, and explain household safety measures to prevent accidents. Help the patient and his family express their feelings and frustrations about the progressively debilitating effects of the disease. Establish long- and short-term treatment goals, and be aware of the patient's need for intellectual stimulation and diversion. Refer the patient and his family to the National Parkinson Foundation or the United Parkinson Foundation for more information.

Myelitis and acute transverse myelitis

Myelitis, or inflammation of the spinal cord, can result from several diseases. Poliomyelitis affects the cord's gray matter and produces motor dysfunction; leukomyelitis affects only the white matter and produces sensory dysfunction. These types of myelitis can attack any level of the spinal cord, causing partial destruction or scattered lesions. Acute transverse myelitis, which affects the entire thickness of the spinal cord, produces both motor and sensory dysfunctions. It has a rapid onset and is the most devastating form of myelitis.

The prognosis depends on the severity of cord damage and prevention of complications. If spinal cord necrosis occurs, prognosis for complete recovery is poor. Even without necrosis, residual neurologic deficits usually persist after recovery. Patients who develop spastic reflexes early in the course of the illness are more likely to recover than those who don't.

Causes and incidence

Acute transverse myelitis has a variety of causes. It commonly follows acute infectious diseases, such as measles or pneumonia (the inflammation occurs after the infection has subsided), and primary infections of the spinal cord itself, such as syphilis or acute disseminated encephalomyelitis. Acute transverse myelitis can accompany demyelinating diseases, such as acute multiple sclerosis, and inflammatory and necrotizing disorders of the spinal cord such as hematomyelia.

Certain toxic agents (carbon monoxide, lead, and arsenic) can cause a type of myelitis in which acute inflammation (followed by hemorrhage and possible necrosis) destroys the entire circumference (myelin, axis cylinders, and neurons) of the spinal cord. Other forms of myelitis may result from poliovirus, herpes zoster, herpesvirus B, or rabies virus; disorders that cause meningeal inflammation, such as syphilis, abscesses and other suppurative conditions, and tuberculosis; smallpox or polio vaccination; parasitic and fungal infections; and chronic adhesive arachnoiditis.

Peak incidence occurs between ages 10 and 19, then again between ages 30 and 39. Approximately 1,400 new cases are diagnosed each year in the United States. About 33,000 Americans have some type of disability from this disorder.

Signs and symptoms

In acute transverse myelitis, onset is rapid, with motor and sensory dysfunctions below the level of spinal cord damage appearing in 1 to 2 days.

Patients with acute transverse myelitis develop flaccid paralysis of the legs (sometimes beginning in just one leg) with loss of sensory and sphincter functions. Such sensory loss may follow pain in the legs or trunk. Reflexes disappear in the early stages but may reappear later. The extent of damage depends on the level of the spinal cord affected; transverse myelitis seldom involves the arms. If spinal cord damage is severe, it may cause shock (hypotension and hypothermia).

Diagnosis

Paraplegia of rapid onset usually points to acute transverse myelitis. In such patients, neurologic examination confirms paraplegia or neurologic deficit below the level of the spinal cord lesion and absent (or, in lat-

er stages) hyperactive reflexes. Cerebrospinal fluid may be normal or show increased lymphocytes or elevated protein levels. Diagnostic evaluation must rule out spinal cord tumor and identify the cause of any underlying infection.

Treatment

No effective treatment exists for acute transverse myelitis. However, this condition requires appropriate treatment of any underlying infection. Some patients with postinfectious or multiple sclerosis–induced myelitis have received steroid therapy, but its benefits aren't clear.

Special considerations

Managing symptoms and treating the underlying infection are the primary considerations.

■ Frequently assess vital signs. Watch carefully for signs of spinal shock (hypotension and excessive sweating).
■ Prevent contractures with range-of-motion exercises and proper alignment.
■ Watch for signs of urinary tract infections from indwelling urinary catheters.
■ Prevent skin infections and pressure ulcers with meticulous skin care. Check pressure points often and keep skin clean and dry; use a low-pressure specialty or rotational bed or other pressure-relieving device.
■ Initiate rehabilitation immediately. Assist the patient with physical therapy, bowel and bladder training, and the lifestyle changes his condition requires.

Alzheimer's disease

Alzheimer's disease, also called *primary degenerative dementia*, accounts for more than half of all dementias. It results in memory loss, confusion, impaired judgment, personality changes, disorientation, and loss of language skills; it essentially steals away the patient's mind. Because this is a primary progressive dementia, the prognosis for a patient with this disease is poor.

Causes and incidence

The cause of Alzheimer's disease is unknown; however, several factors are thought to be implicated in this disease. These include *neurochemical factors,* such as deficiencies in the neurotransmitter acetylcholine, somatostatin, substance P, and norepinephrine; *environmental factors;* and *genetic immunologic factors.* Genetic studies show that an autosomal dominant form of Alzheimer's disease is associated with early onset and early death, accounting for about 100,000 deaths a year. A family history of Alzheimer's disease and the presence of Down syndrome are two established risk factors. Alzheimer's disease isn't exclusive to the elder population; its onset begins in middle age in 1% to 10% of cases

The brain tissue of patients with Alzheimer's disease has three hallmark features: neurofibrillary tangles, neuritic plaques, and granulovascular degeneration. Examination of the brain after death also finds that it's atrophic, commonly weighing less than 1,000 g, compared with a normal brain weight of about 1,380 g.

About 360,000 new cases of Alzheimer's are diagnosed each year.

Signs and symptoms
Onset is insidious. Initially, the patient undergoes almost imperceptible changes, such as forgetfulness, recent memory loss, difficulty learning and remembering new information, deterioration in personal hygiene and appearance, and an inability to concentrate. Gradually, tasks that require abstract thinking and activities that require judgment become more difficult. Progressive difficulty in communication and severe deterioration in memory, language, and motor function result in a loss of coordination and an inability to write or speak. Personality changes (restlessness, irritability) and nocturnal awakenings are common.

Patients also exhibit loss of eye contact, a fearful look, wringing of the hands, and other signs of anxiety. When a patient with Alzheimer's disease is overwhelmed with anxiety, he becomes dysfunctional, acutely confused, agitated, compulsive, or fearful.

Eventually, the patient becomes disoriented, and emotional lability and physical and intellectual disability progress. The patient becomes susceptible to infection and

accidents. Usually, death results from infection.

Diagnosis
Early diagnosis of Alzheimer's disease is difficult because the patient's signs and symptoms are subtle. (See *Organic brain syndrome,* page 662.) Diagnosis relies on an accurate history from a reliable family member, mental status and neurologic examinations, and psychometric testing. A positron emission tomography scan measures the metabolic activity of the cerebral cortex and may help in early diagnosis. An EEG and a computed tomography scan may help in later diagnosis. Currently, the disease is diagnosed by exclusion; that is, tests are performed to rule out other disorders. The presence of Alzheimer's can't be confirmed until death, when pathologic findings are revealed at autopsy.

Treatment
Therapy consists of attempts to slow disease progression, manage behavioral problems, modify the home environment, and elicit family support. Some medications have proven helpful. Tacrine, a centrally acting anticholinesterase agent, is given to treat memory deficits. It has slowed progression of the disease and improved cognitive function in some patients. Other agents include donepezil and rivastigmine. Underlying disorders that contribute to the patient's confusion, such as hypoxia, are also identified and treated.

Special considerations
Overall care is focused on supporting the patient's remaining abilities and compensating for those he has lost.
■ Establish an effective communication system with the patient and his family to help them adjust to the patient's altered cognitive abilities.
■ Offer emotional support to the patient and his family members. Behavior problems may be worsened by excess stimulation or change in established routine. Teach them about the disease, and refer them to social service and community resources for legal and financial advice and support.

ORGANIC BRAIN SYNDROME

Although many behavioral disturbances are clearly linked to organic brain dysfunction, the clinical syndromes associated with this type of impairment are sometimes hard to detect because they aren't always determined by the affected area of the brain or even by the extent of tissue damage. Instead, the way the patient's personality interacts with the brain injury determines the specific clinical effects. General symptoms often include impairment of orientation, memory, and intellectual and emotional function. These primary cognitive deficits help to distinguish organic brain syndromes from neurosis and depression.

Diagnosis

Diagnosis of an organic brain syndrome depends on a detailed history of the onset of cognitive and behavioral disturbances; a complete neurologic assessment; and such tests as EEG, computed tomography scans, brain X-rays, cerebrospinal fluid analysis, and psychological studies. Organic brain syndromes are classified by etiology and specific clinical effects. Causes include infection, brain trauma, nutritional deficiency, cerebrovascular disease, degenerative disease, tumor, toxins, and metabolic or endocrine disorders.

Treatment

Effective treatment requires correction of the underlying cause. Special considerations may include reality orientation, emotional support for the patient and his family, a safe environment, mat therapy for an agitated or aggressive patient, and referral for psychological counseling.

■ Anxiety may cause the patient to become agitated or fearful. Intervene by helping him focus on another activity.

■ Provide the patient with a safe environment. Encourage him to exercise, as ordered, to help maintain mobility.

Creutzfeldt-Jakob disease

Creutzfeldt-Jakob disease (CJD) is a rare, rapidly progressive viral disease that attacks the central nervous system, causing dementia and neurologic signs and symptoms, such as myoclonic jerking, ataxia, aphasia, visual disturbances, and paralysis. CJD is always fatal. A new variant of CJD (vCJD) emerged in Europe in 1996. (See *Understanding vCJD.*)

Causes and incidence

The causative organism is difficult to identify because no foreign ribonucleic acid or deoxyribonucleic acid has been linked to the disease. CJD is believed to be caused by a specific protein called a prion, which lacks nucleic acids, resists proteolytic digestion, and spontaneously aggregates in the brain. Most cases are sporadic; 5% to 15% are familial, with an autosomal dominant pattern of inheritance. Although CJD isn't transmitted by normal casual contact, human-to-human transmission can occur as a result of certain medical procedures, such as corneal and cadaveric dura mater grafts. Isolated cases are attributed to treatment during childhood with human growth hormone and to improperly decontaminated neurosurgical instruments and brain electrodes.

CJD generally affects adults ages 40 to 65 and occurs in more than 50 countries. Males and females are affected equally. In people younger than age 30, incidence is 5 in 1,000,000,000; in all other age groups, incidence is 1 in 1,000,000.

Signs and symptoms

Early signs and symptoms of mental impairment may include slowness in thinking, difficulty concentrating, impaired judgment, and memory loss. Dementia is progressive and occurs early. Involuntary movements, such as muscle twitching, trembling, and peculiar body movements, and visual disturbances, appear with disease progression and advancing mental deterioration. Hallucinations are also common. Duration of the typical illness is 4 months.

Diagnosis

CJD must be considered for anyone experiencing signs of progressive dementia. Neurologic examination is the most effective tool in diagnosing CJD. Difficulty with rapid alternating movements and point-to-point movements are typically evident early in the disease.

An EEG may be performed to assess the patient for typical changes in brain wave activity. Computed tomography scan, magnetic resonance imaging of the brain, and lumbar puncture may be useful in ruling out other disorders that cause dementia. Though not diagnostic, presence of the 14-3-3 protein in the spinal fluid is highly suggestive of the disease when it's accompanied by other characteristic symptoms. Definitive diagnosis usually isn't obtained until an autopsy is done and brain tissue is examined.

Treatment

There's no cure for CJD, and its progress can't be slowed. Palliative care is provided to make the patient comfortable and to ease symptoms. Medications may be needed to control aggressive behaviors. These include sedatives and antipsychotics.

The need to provide a safe environment, control aggressive or agitated behavior, and meet physiologic needs may require monitoring and assistance in the home or in an institutionalized setting. Family counseling may help in coping with the changes required for home care.

Behavior modification may be helpful, in some cases, for controlling unacceptable or dangerous behaviors. Reality orientation, with repeated reinforcement of environmental and other cues, may help reduce disorientation.

Legal advice may be appropriate early in the course of the disorder, to form advance directives, power of attorney, and other legal actions that may make it easier to make ethical decisions regarding the care of an individual with CJD.

UNDERSTANDING vCJD

Like conventional Creutzfeldt-Jakob disease (CJD), the variant of the disease (vCJD) is a rare, fatal neurodegenerative disease. Most cases have been reported in the United Kingdom. vCJD is most likely caused by exposure to bovine spongiform encephalopathy (BSE) — a fatal brain disease in cattle also known as *mad cow disease* — via ingestion of beef products from cattle with BSE.

vCJD affects patients at a much younger age (younger than age 55) than CJD, and the duration of the illness is much longer (14 months).

Regulations have been established in Europe to control outbreaks of BSE in cattle and to prevent contaminated meat from entering the food supply. The Centers for Disease Control and Prevention and the World Health Organization are still exploring vCJD and its relationship to BSE.

Special considerations

■ Offer emotional support to the patient and his family. Teach them about the disease, and assist them through the grieving process. Refer the patient and his family to CJD support groups, and encourage participation.

■ Contact social services and hospice, as appropriate, to assist the family with their needs.

■ Encourage the patient and his family to discuss and complete advance directives.

■ To prevent disease transmission, use caution when handling body fluids and other materials from patients suspected of having CJD.

Reye's syndrome

Reye's syndrome is an acute illness affecting children and, less commonly, adults. It causes fatty infiltration of the liver with concurrent hyperammonemia, encephalopathy, and increased intracranial pressure (ICP). In addition, fatty infiltration of the kidneys, brain, and myocardium may occur.

Prognosis depends on the severity of central nervous system depression. Until recently, mortality was as high as 90%. Today, ICP monitoring and, consequently, early treatment of increased ICP, along with other treatment measures, have cut mortality to about 20%. Death is usually a result of cerebral edema or respiratory arrest. Comatose patients who survive may have residual brain damage.

Causes and incidence

Reye's syndrome typically begins within 1 to 3 days of an acute viral infection, such as an upper respiratory tract infection, type B influenza, or varicella (chickenpox). Incidence commonly rises during influenza outbreaks and may be linked to salicylate use. For this reason, use of aspirin for children younger than age 15 isn't recommended. The Reyes Syndrome Foundation warns against the use of salicylates, even in topical preparations, when a viral illness is suspected.

In Reye's syndrome, damaged hepatic mitochondria disrupt the urea cycle, which normally changes ammonia to urea for its excretion from the body. This results in hyperammonemia, hypoglycemia, and an increase in serum short-chain fatty acids, leading to encephalopathy. Simultaneously, fatty infiltration occurs in renal tubular cells, neuronal tissue, and muscle tissue, including the heart.

Reye's syndrome affects children from infancy to adolescence and occurs equally in boys and girls. Peak incidence is at age 6.

Signs and symptoms

The severity of the child's signs and symptoms varies with the degree of encephalopathy and cerebral edema. In any case, Reye's syndrome develops in five stages. After the initial viral infection, a brief recovery period follows when the child doesn't seem seriously ill. A few days later, he develops intractable vomiting; lethargy; rapidly changing mental status (mild to severe agitation, confusion, irritability, and delirium); rising blood pressure, respiratory rate, and pulse rate; and hyperactive reflexes.

Reye's syndrome commonly progresses to coma. As coma deepens, seizures develop, followed by decreased tendon reflexes and, usually, respiratory failure.

Increased ICP, a serious complication, is now considered the result of an increased cerebral blood volume causing intracranial hypertension. Such swelling may develop as a result of acidosis, increased cerebral metabolic rate, and an impaired autoregulatory mechanism.

Diagnosis

A history of a recent viral disorder with typical clinical features strongly suggests Reye's syndrome. An increased serum ammonia level, abnormal clotting studies, and hepatic dysfunction confirm it. Testing serum salicylate level rules out aspirin use. Absence of jaundice despite increased liver aminotransferase levels rules out acute hepatic failure and hepatic encephalopathy.

Abnormal test results may include:
- Liver function studies: aspartate aminotransferase and alanine aminotransferase elevated to twice normal levels; bilirubin level usually normal
- Liver biopsy: fatty droplets uniformly distributed throughout cells
- Cerebrospinal fluid (CSF) analysis: white blood cell count less than 10/µl; with coma, increased CSF pressure.
- Coagulation studies: prothrombin time and partial thromboplastin time prolonged
- Blood values: serum ammonia levels elevated; serum glucose levels normal or, in 15% of cases, low; serum fatty acid and lactate levels increased.

Treatment

For treatment guidelines, see *Stages of treatment for Reye's syndrome.*

Special considerations

Advise parents to give nonsalicylate analgesics and antipyretics such as acetaminophen. For more information, refer parents to the National Reye's Syndrome Foundation.

STAGES OF TREATMENT FOR REYE'S SYNDROME

Signs and symptoms	Baseline treatment	Baseline intervention
Stage I: vomiting, lethargy, hepatic dysfunction	■ To decrease intracranial pressure (ICP) and brain edema, give I.V. fluids at ⅔ maintenance. Also give an osmotic diuretic or furosemide. ■ To treat hypoprothrombinemia, give vitamin K; if vitamin K is unsuccessful, give fresh frozen plasma. ■ Monitor serum ammonia and blood glucose levels and plasma osmolality every 4 to 8 hours to check progress.	■ Monitor the patient's vital signs and check his level of consciousness for increasing lethargy. Take vital signs more often as the patient's condition deteriorates. ■ Monitor fluid intake and output to prevent fluid overload. Maintain urine output at 1.0 ml/kg/hour; plasma osmolality, 290 mOsm; and blood glucose, 150 mg/ml. (*Goal:* Keep glucose level high, osmolality normal to high, and ammonia level low.) Also, restrict protein.
Stage II: hyperventilation, delirium, hepatic dysfunction, hyperactive reflexes	■ Continue baseline treatment.	■ Maintain seizure precautions. ■ Immediately report any signs of coma that require invasive, supportive therapy, such as intubation. ■ Keep the head of the bed at a 30-degree angle.
Stage III: coma, hyperventilation, decorticate rigidity, hepatic dysfunction	■ Continue baseline and seizure treatment. ■ Monitor ICP with a subarachnoid screw or other invasive device. ■ Provide endotracheal intubation and mechanical ventilation to control the partial pressure of arterial carbon dioxide ($PaCO_2$) levels. A paralyzing agent, such as atracurium or pancuronium I.V., may help maintain ventilation. ■ Give mannitol I.V. or glycerol by nasogastric tube.	■ Monitor ICP (should be less than 20 mm Hg before suctioning) or give a barbiturate I.V., as ordered; hyperventilate the patient as necessary. ■ When ventilating the patient, maintain $PaCO_2$ between 25 and 30 mm Hg and the partial pressure of arterial oxygen between 80 and 100 mm Hg. ■ Closely monitor cardiovascular status with a pulmonary artery catheter or central venous pressure line. ■ Give skin and mouth care and perform range-of-motion exercises.
Stage IV: deepening coma; decerebrate rigidity; large, fixed pupils; minimal hepatic dysfunction	■ Continue baseline and supportive care. ■ If all previous measures fail, some pediatric centers use barbiturate coma, decompressive craniotomy, hypothermia, or exchange transfusion.	■ Check the patient for loss of reflexes and signs of flaccidity. ■ Give the patent's family the extra support they need, considering their child's poor prognosis.

(continued)

STAGES OF TREATMENT FOR REYE'S SYNDROME *(continued)*		
Signs and symptoms	**Baseline treatment**	**Baseline intervention**
Stage V: seizures, loss of deep tendon reflexes, flaccidity, respiratory arrest, ammonia level above 300 mg/dl	▪ Continue baseline and supportive care.	▪ Help the patient's family to face his impending death.

Guillain-Barré syndrome

Guillain-Barré syndrome is an acute, rapidly progressive, and potentially fatal form of polyneuritis that causes muscle weakness and mild distal sensory loss. Recovery is spontaneous and complete in about 95% of patients, although mild motor or reflex deficits in the feet and legs may persist. The prognosis is best when symptoms clear between 15 and 20 days after onset.

Causes and incidence
Precisely what causes Guillain-Barré syndrome is unknown, but it may be a cell-mediated immunologic attack on peripheral nerves in response to a virus. The major pathologic effect is segmental demyelination of the peripheral nerves. Because this syndrome causes inflammation and degenerative changes in both the posterior (sensory) and anterior (motor) nerve roots, signs of sensory and motor losses occur simultaneously.

This syndrome (also called infectious polyneuritis, Landry-Guillain-Barré syndrome, and acute idiopathic polyneuritis) can occur at any age but is most common between ages 30 and 50; it affects both sexes equally. In the United States, it has an incidence of 0.6 to 2.4 cases per 100,000 people.

Signs and symptoms
About 50% of patients with Guillain-Barré syndrome have a history of minor febrile illness (10 to 14 days before onset), usually an upper respiratory tract infection or, less commonly, gastroenteritis. When infection precedes onset of Guillain-Barré syndrome, signs of infection subside before neurologic features appear. Other possible precipitating factors include surgery, rabies or swine influenza vaccination, viral illness, Hodgkin's or other malignant disease, and lupus erythematosus.

Symmetrical muscle weakness, the major neurologic sign, usually appears in the legs first (ascending type) and then extends to the arms and facial nerves in 24 to 72 hours. Sometimes, muscle weakness develops in the arms first (descending type) or in the arms and legs simultaneously. (See *Testing for thoracic sensation.*) In milder forms of this disease, muscle weakness may affect only the cranial nerves or may not occur at all.

Another common neurologic sign is paresthesia, which sometimes precedes muscle weakness but tends to vanish quickly. However, some patients with this disorder never develop this symptom. Other clinical features may include facial diplegia (possibly with ophthalmoplegia), dysphagia or dysarthria and, less commonly, weakness of the muscles supplied by cranial nerve XI. Muscle weakness develops so quickly that muscle atrophy doesn't occur, but hypotonia and areflexia do. Stiffness and pain in the form of a severe "charley horse" commonly occur.

The clinical course of Guillain-Barré syndrome is divided into three phases. The initial phase begins when the first definitive symptom appears and ends 1 to 3 weeks later, when no further deterioration manifests. The plateau phase lasts several days to

2 weeks and is followed by the recovery phase, which is believed to coincide with remyelination and axonal process regrowth. The recovery phase extends over a period of 4 to 6 months; patients with severe disease may take up to 2 years to recover, and recovery may not be complete.

Significant complications of Guillain-Barré syndrome include mechanical ventilatory failure, aspiration, pneumonia, sepsis, joint contractures, and deep vein thrombosis. Unexplained autonomic nervous system involvement may cause sinus tachycardia or bradycardia, hypertension, postural hypotension, or loss of bladder and bowel sphincter control.

Diagnosis

A history of preceding febrile illness (usually a respiratory tract infection) and typical clinical features suggest Guillain-Barré syndrome.

Several days after onset of signs and symptoms, cerebrospinal fluid (CSF) protein levels begin to rise, peaking in 4 to 6 weeks, probably as a result of widespread inflammatory disease of the nerve roots. CSF white blood cell count remains normal, but in severe disease CSF pressure may rise above normal. Probably because of predisposing infection, CBC shows leukocytosis and a shift to immature forms early in the illness, but blood studies soon return to normal. Electromyography may show repeated firing of the same motor unit instead of widespread sectional stimulation. Nerve conduction velocities are slowed soon after paralysis develops and show demyelination. Diagnosis must rule out similar diseases such as acute poliomyelitis.

Treatment

Treatment is primarily supportive, including such measures as endotracheal (ET) intubation or tracheotomy if the patient has difficulty clearing secretions. Preventing complications is another goal of treatment.

Plasmapheresis is useful in decreasing severity of symptoms, thereby facilitating a more rapid recovery. I.V. immune globulin is equally effective in reducing the severity and duration of symptoms.

TESTING FOR THORACIC SENSATION

When Guillain-Barré syndrome progresses rapidly, test for ascending sensory loss by touching the patient or pressing his skin lightly with a pin every hour. Move systematically from the iliac crest (T12) to the scapula, occasionally substituting the blunt end of the pin to test the patient's ability to discriminate between sharp and dull.

Mark the level of diminished sensation to measure any change. If diminished sensation ascends to T8 or higher, the patient's intercostal muscle function (and consequently respiratory function) will probably be impaired. As Guillain-Barré syndrome subsides, sensory and motor weakness descends to the lower thoracic segments, heralding a return of intercostal and extremity muscle function.

SEGMENTAL DISTRIBUTION OF SPINAL NERVES TO BACK OF THE BODY

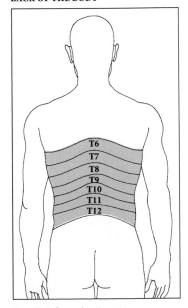

Key: T = thoracic segments

Special considerations

Monitoring the patient for escalation of symptoms is of special concern.

- Watch for ascending sensory loss, which precedes motor loss. Also, monitor vital signs and level of consciousness.
- Assess and treat respiratory dysfunction. If respiratory muscles are weak, take serial vital capacity recordings. Use a respirometer with a mouthpiece or a facemask for bedside testing.
- Obtain arterial blood gas measurements. Because neuromuscular disease results in primary hypoventilation with hypoxemia and hypercapnia, watch for respiratory failure. Be alert for signs of rising partial pressure of carbon dioxide (such as confusion and tachypnea).
- Auscultate breath sounds, turn and position the patient, and encourage coughing and deep breathing. Begin respiratory support at the first sign of dyspnea or with decreasing partial pressure of arterial oxygen.
- If respiratory failure becomes imminent, establish an emergency airway with an ET tube.
- Give meticulous skin care to prevent skin breakdown and contractures. Establish a strict turning schedule; inspect the skin (especially sacrum, heels, and ankles) for breakdown, and reposition the patient every 2 hours. After each position change, stimulate circulation by carefully massaging pressure points. Also, use foam, gel, or alternating pressure pads at points of contact.
- Perform passive range-of-motion exercises within the patient's pain limits. When the patient's condition stabilizes, change to gentle stretching and active assistance exercises.
- To prevent aspiration, test the gag reflex, and elevate the head of the bed before giving the patient anything to eat. If the gag reflex is absent, give nasogastric feedings until this reflex returns. If the patient has severe paralysis and is expected to have a long recovery period, a gastrostomy tube may be necessary to provide adequate nourishment.
- As the patient regains strength and can tolerate a vertical position, be alert for postural hypotension. Monitor blood pressure and pulse during tilting periods and, if necessary, apply toe-to-groin elastic bandages to prevent postural hypotension.
- Inspect the patient's legs regularly for signs of thrombophlebitis (localized pain, tenderness, erythema, edema, and positive Homans' sign), a common complication of Guillain-Barré syndrome. To prevent thrombophlebitis, apply antiembolism stockings and give prophylactic anticoagulants, as ordered.
- If the patient has facial paralysis, give eye and mouth care every 4 hours.
- Watch for urine retention. Measure and record intake and output every 8 hours, and offer the bedpan every 3 to 4 hours. Encourage adequate fluid intake of 2 qt [2 L] per day, unless contraindicated. If urine retention develops, begin intermittent catheterization as ordered. Because the abdominal muscles are weak, the patient may need manual pressure on the bladder (Credé's method) before he can urinate.
- To prevent or relieve constipation, offer the patient plenty of water, prune juice, and a high-bulk diet. If necessary, give daily or alternate-day suppositories (glycerin or bisacodyl) or enemas, as ordered.
- Before discharge, prepare a home care plan. Teach the patient how to transfer from bed to wheelchair, from wheelchair to toilet or tub, and how to walk short distances with a walker or a cane. Teach the family how to help him eat, compensating for facial weakness, and how to help him avoid skin breakdown. Stress the need for a regular bowel and bladder routine. Refer the patient for physical therapy as needed.
- Refer the patient's family to the Guillain-Barré Syndrome Foundation International.

NEUROMUSCULAR DISORDERS

Myasthenia gravis

Myasthenia gravis produces sporadic but progressive weakness and abnormal fatigability of striated (skeletal) muscles, exacerbated by exercise and repeated movement, but improved by anticholinesterase drugs. Usually, this disorder affects muscles inner-

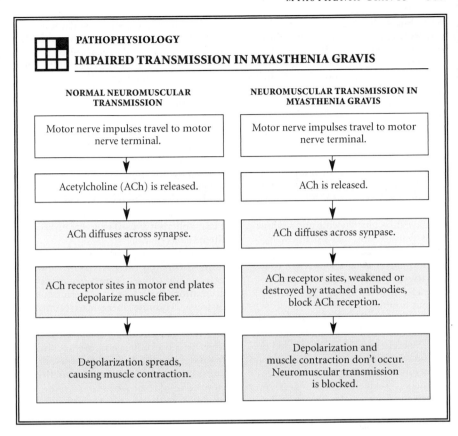

PATHOPHYSIOLOGY

IMPAIRED TRANSMISSION IN MYASTHENIA GRAVIS

NORMAL NEUROMUSCULAR TRANSMISSION	NEUROMUSCULAR TRANSMISSION IN MYASTHENIA GRAVIS
Motor nerve impulses travel to motor nerve terminal.	Motor nerve impulses travel to motor nerve terminal.
Acetylcholine (ACh) is released.	ACh is released.
ACh diffuses across synapse.	ACh diffuses across synpase.
ACh receptor sites in motor end plates depolarize muscle fiber.	ACh receptor sites, weakened or destroyed by attached antibodies, block ACh reception.
Depolarization spreads, causing muscle contraction.	Depolarization and muscle contraction don't occur. Neuromuscular transmission is blocked.

vated by the cranial nerves (face, lips, tongue, neck, and throat), but it can affect any muscle group. Myasthenia gravis follows an unpredictable course of recurring exacerbations and periodic remissions. There's no known cure. Drug treatment has improved prognosis and allows patients to lead relatively normal lives except during exacerbations. When the disease involves the respiratory system, it may be life threatening.

Causes and incidence
Myasthenia gravis causes a failure in transmission of nerve impulses at the neuromuscular junction. Theoretically, such impairment may result from an autoimmune response, ineffective acetylcholine release, or inadequate muscle fiber response to acetylcholine. (See *Impaired transmission in myasthenia gravis*.)

Myasthenia gravis affects 3 of every 10,000 people at any age, but it's more common in young women and older men. About 20% of neonates born to mothers with myasthenia gravis have transient (or occasionally persistent) myasthenia. This disease may coexist with immunologic and thyroid disorders; about 15% of patients with myasthenia gravis have thymomas. Remissions occur in about 25% of patients.

Signs and symptoms
The dominant symptoms of myasthenia gravis are skeletal muscle weakness and fatigability. In the early stages, easy fatigability of certain muscles may appear with no other findings. Later, it may be severe enough to cause paralysis. Typically, myasthenic muscles are strongest in the morning but weaken throughout the day, especially after exercise. Short rest periods temporarily restore muscle function. Mus-

cle weakness is progressive; more and more muscles become weak, and eventually some muscles may lose function entirely. Resulting symptoms depend on the muscle group affected; they become more intense during menses and after emotional stress, prolonged exposure to sunlight or cold, or infections.

Onset may be sudden or insidious. In many patients, weak eye closure, ptosis, and diplopia are the first signs that something is wrong. Patients with myasthenia gravis usually have blank, expressionless faces and nasal vocal tones. They experience frequent nasal regurgitation of fluids and have difficulty chewing and swallowing. Because of this, they usually worry about choking. Their eyelids droop (ptosis), and they may have to tilt their heads back to see. Their neck muscles may become too weak to support their heads without bobbing.

In patients with weakened respiratory muscles, decreased tidal volume and vital capacity make breathing difficult and predispose to pneumonia and other respiratory tract infections. Respiratory muscle weakness (myasthenic crisis) may be severe enough to require an emergency airway and mechanical ventilation.

Diagnosis

Repeated muscle use over a very short time that fatigues and then improves with rest suggests a diagnosis of myasthenia gravis. Tests for this neurologic condition record the effect of exercise and subsequent rest on muscle weakness. Electromyography, with repeated neural stimulation, may help confirm this diagnosis. Acetylcholine receptor antibodies may be present in the blood.

 CONFIRMING DIAGNOSIS *The classic proof of myasthenia gravis is improved muscle function after an I.V. injection of edrophonium or neostigmine (anticholinesterase drugs).*

In patients with myasthenia gravis, muscle function improves within 30 to 60 seconds and lasts up to 30 minutes. Longstanding ocular muscle dysfunction may fail to respond to such testing. This test can differentiate a myasthenic crisis from a cholinergic crisis (caused by acetylcholine

overactivity at the neuromuscular junction). The acetylcholine receptor antibody titer may be elevated in generalized myasthenia. Evaluation should rule out thyroid disease and thymoma.

Treatment

Treatment is symptomatic. Anticholinesterase drugs, such as neostigmine and pyridostigmine, counteract fatigue and muscle weakness and allow about 80% of normal muscle function. However, these drugs become less effective as the disease worsens. Corticosteroids may relieve symptoms. Immunosuppressants are also used. Plasmapheresis is used in severe myasthenic exacerbation.

Patients with thymomas require thymectomy, which may cause remission in some cases of adult-onset myasthenia. Acute exacerbations that cause severe respiratory distress necessitate emergency treatment. Tracheotomy, positive-pressure ventilation, and vigorous suctioning to remove secretions usually produce improvement in a few days. Because anticholinesterase drugs aren't effective in myasthenic crisis, they're stopped until respiratory function improves. Myasthenic crisis requires immediate hospitalization and vigorous respiratory support.

Special considerations

Careful baseline assessment, early recognition and treatment of potential crises, supportive measures, and thorough patient teaching can minimize exacerbations and complications. Continuity of care is essential.

■ Establish an accurate neurologic and respiratory baseline. Thereafter, monitor tidal volume and vital capacity regularly. The patient may need a ventilator and frequent suctioning to remove accumulating secretions.

■ Be alert for signs of an impending crisis (increased muscle weakness, respiratory distress, and difficulty in talking or chewing).

■ To prevent relapses, adhere closely to the ordered drug administration schedule. Be prepared to give atropine for anticholinesterase overdose or toxicity.

- Plan exercise, meals, patient care, and activities to make the most of energy peaks. For example, give medication 20 to 30 minutes before meals to facilitate chewing or swallowing. Allow the patient to participate in his care.
- When swallowing is difficult, give soft, solid foods instead of liquids to lessen the risk of choking.
- Patient teaching is essential because myasthenia gravis is usually a lifelong condition. Help the patient plan daily activities to coincide with energy peaks. Stress the need for frequent rest periods throughout the day. Emphasize that periodic remissions, exacerbations, and day-to-day fluctuations are common.
- Teach the patient how to recognize adverse effects and signs of toxicity of anticholinesterase drugs (headaches, weakness, sweating, abdominal cramps, nausea, vomiting, diarrhea, excessive salivation, and bronchospasm) and corticosteroids (euphoria, insomnia, edema, and increased appetite).
- Warn the patient to avoid strenuous exercise, stress, infection, and needless exposure to the sun or cold. All of these things may worsen signs and symptoms.
- For more information and an opportunity to meet other myasthenia gravis patients who lead full, productive lives, refer the patient to the Myasthenia Gravis Foundation.

Amyotrophic lateral sclerosis

Amyotrophic lateral sclerosis (ALS), also called *Lou Gehrig disease,* is the most common of the motor neuron diseases that cause muscle atrophy. (See *Motor neuron disease.*) Other motor neuron diseases include progressive muscular atrophy and progressive bulbar palsy. Symptoms don't develop until age 50. A chronic, progressively debilitating disease, ALS may be fatal in less than 1 year or continue for 10 years or more, depending on the muscles it affects.

MOTOR NEURON DISEASE

In its final stages, motor neuron disease affects both upper and lower motor neuron cells. However, the site of initial cell damage varies according to the specific disease:

- *progressive bulbar palsy:* degeneration of upper motor neurons in the medulla oblongata
- *progressive muscular atrophy:* degeneration of lower motor neurons in the spinal cord
- *amyotrophic lateral sclerosis:* degeneration of upper motor neurons in the medulla oblongata and lower motor neurons in the spinal cord.

Causes and incidence

ALS affects about 1 of 100,000 people. The exact cause of ALS is unknown, but about 10% of cases have a genetic component. In these patients, it's an autosomal dominant trait and affects men and women equally.

Other than a family member affected with the hereditary form, there are no known risk factors.

Signs and symptoms

Progressive loss of muscle strength and coordination eventually interfere with everyday activities. Patients with ALS develop fasciculations, accompanied by atrophy and weakness, especially in the muscles of the feet and the hands. Other signs include impaired speech; difficulty chewing, swallowing, and breathing and, occasionally, choking and excessive drooling. Mental deterioration doesn't occur, but patients may become depressed as a reaction to the disease.

Diagnosis

Characteristic clinical features indicate a combination of upper and lower motor neuron involvement without sensory impairment. Electromyography and muscle biopsy indicate that the motor nerves aren't functioning, yet sensory nerves are normal. Computed tomography scan and magnetic resonance imaging may help rule out other conditions, such as multiple sclerosis, spinal cord neoplasm, central nervous system syphilis, polyarteritis, syringomyelia, myasthenia gravis, progressive muscular dystrophy, and progressive strokes.

Treatment

Management aims to control symptoms and provide emotional, psychological, and physical support. Riluzole may increase quality of life and survival but doesn't reverse or stop disease progression.

Baclofen or diazepam help control spasticity that interferes with activities of daily living. Trihexyphenidyl or amitriptyline may be used for impaired ability to swallow saliva. Gastrostomy may be needed early to prevent choking; referral to an otolaryngologist is advised. Physical therapy, rehabilitation, and use of appliances or orthopedic intervention may be required to maximize function. Devices to assist in breathing at night or mechanical ventilation should be discussed, but the patient's wishes should be respected.

Special considerations

Because mental status remains intact while progressive physical degeneration takes place, the patient acutely perceives every change. This threatens the patient's relationships, career, income, muscle coordination, sexuality, and energy.

- Implement a rehabilitation program designed to maintain independence as long as possible.
- Help the patient obtain assistive equipment, such as a walker and a wheelchair. Arrange for a visiting nurse to oversee the patient's status, to provide support, and to teach the family about the illness.
- Depending on the patient's muscular capacity, assist with bathing, personal hygiene, and transfers from wheelchair to bed. Help establish a regular bowel and bladder routine.
- To help the patient handle increased accumulation of secretions and dysphagia, teach him to suction himself. He should have a suction machine handy at home to reduce the fear of choking.

- To prevent skin breakdown, provide good skin care when the patient is bedridden. Turn him often, keep his skin clean and dry, and use pressure-reducing devices such as alternating air mattress.
- If the patient has trouble swallowing, give him soft, solid foods and position him upright during meals. Gastrostomy and nasogastric tube feedings may be necessary if he can no longer swallow. Teach the patient (if he's still able to feed himself) or his family how to administer gastrostomy feedings.
- Provide emotional support. A discussion of directives regarding health care decisions should be instituted before the patient becomes unable to communicate his wishes. Prepare the patient and his family members for his eventual death, and encourage the start of the grieving process. Patients with ALS may benefit from a hospice program or the local ALS support group chapter.

Multiple sclerosis

Multiple sclerosis (MS) is a progressive disease caused by demyelination of the white matter of the brain and spinal cord. (See *Demyelination in multiple sclerosis.*) In this disease, sporadic patches of demyelination throughout the central nervous system induce widely disseminated and varied neurologic dysfunction. Characterized by exacerbations and remissions, MS is a major cause of chronic disability in young adults.

The prognosis varies; MS may progress rapidly, disabling some patients by early adulthood or causing death within months of onset. However, 70% of patients lead active, productive lives with prolonged remissions.

Causes and incidence

The exact cause of MS is unknown, but current theories suggest a slow-acting or latent viral infection and an autoimmune response. Other theories suggest that environmental and genetic factors may also be linked to MS. Emotional stress, overwork, fatigue, pregnancy, and acute respiratory tract infections have been known to precede the onset of this illness.

MS usually begins between ages 20 and 40. It affects more women than men. A family history of MS and living in a geographical area with higher incidence of MS (northern Europe, northern United States, southern Australia, and New Zealand) increase the risk.

Signs and symptoms

Clinical findings in MS depend on the extent and site of myelin destruction, the extent of remyelination, and the adequacy of subsequent restored synaptic transmission.

Signs and symptoms in MS may be transient, or they may last for hours or weeks. They may wax and wane with no predictable pattern, vary from day to day, and be bizarre and difficult for the patient to describe.

In most patients, visual problems and sensory impairment, such as numbness and tingling sensations (paresthesia), are the first signs that something may be wrong.

Other characteristic changes include:
- *ocular disturbances:* optic neuritis, diplopia, ophthalmoplegia, blurred vision, and nystagmus
- *muscle dysfunction:* weakness, paralysis ranging from monoplegia to quadriplegia, spasticity, hyperreflexia, intention tremor, and gait ataxia
- *urinary disturbances:* incontinence, frequency, urgency, and frequent infections
- *emotional lability:* characteristic mood swings, irritability, euphoria, and depression.

Associated signs and symptoms include poorly articulated or scanning speech and dysphagia. Clinical effects may be so mild that the patient is unaware of them or so bizarre that he appears hysterical.

Diagnosis

A misdiagnosis of psychiatric problems is common. Because early symptoms may be mild, years may elapse between onset of the first signs and the diagnosis, which typically requires evidence of multiple neurologic attacks and characteristic remissions and exacerbations. Magnetic resonance imaging may detect MS lesions; however, diagnosis still remains difficult. Periodic testing and close observation of the patient

DEMYELINATION IN MULTIPLE SCLEROSIS

Transverse section of cervical spine shows partial loss of myelin, characteristic of multiple sclerosis (MS). This degenerative process is called *demyelination.*

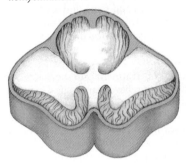

In this illustration, the loss of myelin is nearly complete. Clinical features of MS depend on the extent of demyelination.

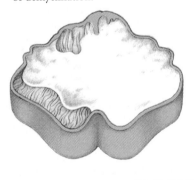

are necessary, perhaps for years, depending on the course of the disease.

Abnormal EEG findings occur in one-third of patients. Lumbar puncture shows elevated gamma globulin fraction of immunoglobulin G but normal total cerebrospinal fluid (CSF) protein levels. Elevated CSF gamma globulin is significant only when serum gamma globulin levels are normal because it reflects hyperactivity of the immune system due to chronic demyelination. Oligoclonal bands of immunoglobulin can be detected when gamma globulin in CSF is examined by electrophoresis, and these bands are present in most patients, even when the percentage of gamma globulin in CSF is normal. In addition, the white blood cell count in CSF may rise. Differential diagnosis must rule out spinal cord compression, foramen magnum tumor (may mimic the exacerbations and remissions of MS), multiple small strokes, syphilis or other infection, and psychological disturbances.

Treatment

The aim of treatment is to shorten exacerbations and relieve neurologic deficits so that the patient can resume a normal lifestyle. Those with relapsing-remitting courses are placed on immune modulating therapy, with interferon or glatiramer acetate. Steroids are used to reduce the associated edema of the myelin sheath during exacerbations.

Other drugs include baclofen, tizanidine, or diazepam to relieve spasticity, cholinergic agents to relieve urine retention and minimize frequency and urgency, amantadine to relieve fatigue, and antidepressants to help with mood or behavioral symptoms. During acute exacerbations, supportive measures include bed rest, comfort measures such as massages, prevention of fatigue, prevention of pressure ulcers, bowel and bladder training (if necessary), administration of antibiotics for bladder infections, physical therapy, and counseling. Physical therapy, speech therapy, occupational therapy, and support groups are also useful. Planned exercise programs help with maintaining muscle tone.

Special considerations

Management considerations focus on educating the patient and his family.
- Assist with physical therapy. Increase patient comfort with massages and relaxing baths. Assist with active, resistive, and stretching exercises to maintain muscle tone and joint mobility, decrease spasticity, improve coordination, and boost morale.
- Educate the patient and his family concerning the chronic course of MS. Emphasize the need to avoid temperature extremes, stress, fatigue, and infections and

other illnesses, all of which can trigger an MS attack. Advise him to maintain independence by developing new ways of performing daily activities.
- Stress the importance of eating a nutritious, well-balanced diet that contains sufficient roughage and adequate fluids to prevent constipation.
- Evaluate the need for bowel and bladder training during hospitalization. Encourage adequate fluid intake and regular urination. Eventually, the patient may require urinary drainage by self-catheterization or, in men, condom drainage. Teach the correct use of suppositories to help establish a regular bowel schedule.
- Promote emotional stability. Help the patient establish a daily routine to maintain optimal functioning. Activity level is regulated by tolerance level. Encourage regular rest periods to prevent fatigue and daily physical exercise.
- Inform the patient that exacerbations are unpredictable, necessitating physical and emotional adjustments in lifestyle.
- For more information, refer him to the National Multiple Sclerosis Society.

CRANIAL NERVE DISORDERS

Trigeminal neuralgia

Trigeminal neuralgia, also called *tic douloureux,* is a painful disorder of one or more branches of the fifth cranial (trigeminal) nerve that produces paroxysmal attacks of excruciating facial pain precipitated by stimulation of a trigger zone. It can subside spontaneously, and remissions may last from several months to years.

Causes and incidence

Although the cause remains undetermined, trigeminal neuralgia may reflect an afferent reflex in the brain stem or in the sensory root of the trigeminal nerve. Such neuralgia may also be related to compression of the nerve root by posterior fossa tumors, middle fossa tumors, or vascular lesions (subclinical aneurysm), although such le-

TRIGEMINAL NERVE FUNCTION AND DISTRIBUTION

Function
- Motor: chewing movements
- Sensory: sensations of face, scalp, and teeth (mouth and nasal chamber)

Distribution
I   ophthalmic
II maxillary
III mandibular

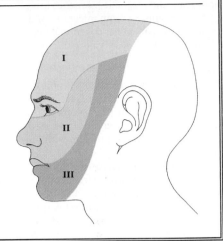

---

sions usually produce simultaneous loss of sensation. Occasionally, trigeminal neuralgia is a manifestation of multiple sclerosis or herpes zoster. Whatever the cause, the pain of trigeminal neuralgia is probably produced by an interaction or short-circuiting of touch and pain fibers.

Trigeminal neuralgia occurs mostly in people older than age 40, in women more commonly than men, and on the right side of the face more commonly than the left. Incidence is 4 to 5 cases per 100,000 people.

Signs and symptoms

Typically, the patient reports a searing or burning pain that occurs in lightninglike jabs and lasts from 1 to 15 minutes (usually 1 to 2 minutes) in an area innervated by one of the divisions of the trigeminal nerve, primarily the superior mandibular or maxillary division. The pain rarely affects more than one division and seldom the first division (ophthalmic) or both sides of the face. It affects the second (maxillary) and third (mandibular) divisions of the trigeminal nerve equally. (See *Trigeminal nerve function and distribution*.)

These attacks characteristically follow stimulation of a trigger zone, usually by a light touch to a hypersensitive area, such as the tip of the nose, the cheeks, or the gums.

Although attacks can occur at any time, they may follow a draft of air, exposure to heat or cold, eating, smiling, talking, or drinking hot or cold beverages. The frequency of attacks varies greatly, from many times a day to several times a month or year. Between attacks, most patients are free from pain, although some have a constant, dull ache. No patient is ever free from the fear of the next attack.

Diagnosis

The patient's pain history is the basis for diagnosis because trigeminal neuralgia produces no objective clinical or pathologic changes. Physical examination shows no impairment of sensory or motor function; indeed, sensory impairment implies a space-occupying lesion as the cause of pain.

Observation during the examination shows the patient favoring (splinting) the affected area. To ward off a painful attack, the patient commonly holds his face immobile when talking. He may also leave the affected side of his face unwashed and unshaven or protect it with a coat or shawl. When asked where the pain occurs, he points to — but never touches — the affected area. Witnessing a typical attack helps to confirm diagnosis. Rarely, a tumor in the posterior fossa can produce pain that's clinically indistinguishable from trigeminal neuralgia. Skull X-rays, computed tomography scan, and magnetic resonance imaging rule out sinus or tooth infections and tumors. If the patient has trigeminal neuralgia, these test results are normal.

Treatment

Oral administration of carbamazepine or phenytoin may temporarily relieve or prevent pain. Narcotics may be helpful during the pain episode. Caution should be used when treating a chronic problem with opioids.

When these medical measures fail or attacks become increasingly frequent or severe, neurosurgical procedures may provide permanent relief. The preferred procedure is percutaneous electrocoagulation of nerve rootlets under local anesthetic. New treatments include a percutaneous radio frequency procedure, which causes partial root destruction and relieves pain, and microsurgery for vascular decompression of the trigeminal nerve.

Special considerations

The focus here is management of pain.

■ Observe and record the characteristics of each attack, including the patient's protective mechanisms.

■ Provide adequate nutrition in small, frequent meals served at room temperature.

■ Avoid jarring the bed and causing increased discomfort.

■ If the patient is receiving carbamazepine, watch for cutaneous and hematologic reactions (erythematous and pruritic rashes, urticaria, photosensitivity, exfoliative dermatitis, leukopenia, agranulocytosis, eosinophilia, aplastic anemia, and thrombocytopenia) and, possibly, urine retention and transient drowsiness. For the first 3 months of carbamazepine therapy, complete blood count and liver function should be monitored weekly, then monthly thereafter. Warn the patient to immediately report fever, sore throat, mouth ulcers, easy bruising, or petechial or purpuric hemorrhage because these may signal thrombocytopenia or aplastic anemia and may require discontinuation of drug therapy.

■ If the patient is receiving phenytoin, also watch for adverse effects, including ataxia, skin eruptions, gingival hyperplasia, and nystagmus.

■ After resection of the first branch of the trigeminal nerve, tell the patient to avoid rubbing his eyes and using aerosol spray. Advise him to wear glasses or goggles outdoors and to blink often.

■ After surgery to sever the second or third branch, tell the patient to avoid hot foods and drinks, which could burn his mouth, and to chew carefully to avoid biting his mouth. It may be necessary for the patient to take pureed food, possibly through a straw. Advise him to place food in the unaffected side of his mouth when chewing, to brush his teeth and rinse his mouth often, and to see the dentist twice a year to detect cavities because he won't experience pain from cavities in the area of the severed nerve.

■ After surgical decompression of the root or partial nerve dissection, check neurologic and vital signs often.

■ Provide emotional support, and encourage the patient to express his feelings. Promote independence through self-care and maximum physical activity. Reinforce natural avoidance of stimulation (air, heat, and cold) of trigger zones (lips, cheeks, and gums).

Bell's palsy

Bell's palsy is a disease of the seventh cranial nerve (facial) that produces unilateral or bilateral facial weakness or paralysis. (See *Recognizing unilateral Bell's palsy*.) Onset is rapid. In 80% to 90% of patients, Bell's palsy subsides spontaneously, with complete recovery in 1 to 8 weeks; however, recovery may be delayed in the elderly. If recovery is partial, contractures may develop on the paralyzed side of the face. Bell's palsy may recur on the same or opposite side of the face.

Causes and incidence

Bell's palsy blocks the seventh cranial nerve, which is responsible for motor innervation of the muscles of the face. The conduction block is due to an inflammatory reaction around the nerve (usually at the internal auditory meatus), which may be

RECOGNIZING UNILATERAL BELL'S PALSY

Bell's palsy usually causes a unilateral facial paralysis. This produces a distorted appearance with an inability to wrinkle the forehead, close the eyelid, smile, show the teeth, or puff out the cheek.

WRINKLING THE FOREHEAD

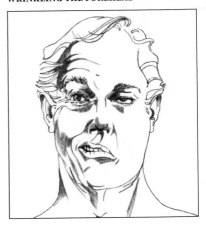

DISTORTED APPEARANCE

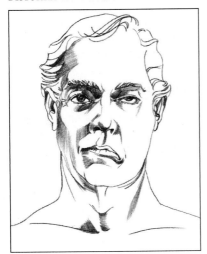

SMILING

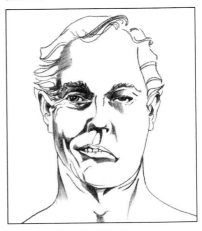

associated with infections or can result from hemorrhage, tumor, meningitis, local trauma, hypertension, sarcoidosis, Lyme disease, or infarction of the nerve.

Bell's palsy affects all age groups and males and females nearly equally, although females are slightly more likely to develop it during their late teens and early 20s. In the United States, incidence is 23 cases per 100,000 people.

Signs and symptoms

Bell's palsy usually produces unilateral facial weakness, occasionally with aching pain around the angle of the jaw or behind the ear. On the weak side, the mouth droops (causing the patient to drool saliva from the corner of his mouth), and taste perception is distorted over the affected anterior portion of the tongue. The forehead appears smooth, and the patient's ability to close his eye on the weak side is markedly impaired. When he tries to close this eye, it rolls upward (Bell's phenomenon) and shows excessive tearing. Although Bell's phenomenon occurs in normal people, it isn't apparent because the eyelids close completely and cover this eye motion. In Bell's palsy, incomplete eye closure makes this upward motion obvious. Other symptoms may include loss of taste and ringing in the ear.

Diagnosis

Diagnosis is based on clinical presentation: distorted facial appearance and the inability to raise the eyebrow, close the eyelid, smile, show the teeth, or puff out the cheek. Electromyography helps determine the severity of nerve damage. Blood tests may be done to rule out acute causes (sarcoidosis or Lyme disease). If no improvement is evident within several weeks of onset, magnetic resonance imaging will rule out other causes of dysfunction.

Treatment

Treatment consists of corticosteroids to reduce facial nerve edema and improve nerve conduction and blood flow. They must be given early — within 24 hours of onset of paralysis — to be most effective. Lubricants or an eye ointment may be needed to protect the eye, as well as patching during sleep.

Special considerations

Patient care includes observation for adverse drug effects, pain relief, and emotional support.

■ During treatment with corticosteroids, watch for adverse effects, such as GI distress and fluid retention. If GI distress is troublesome, a concomitant antacid usually provides relief. If the patient has diabetes, frequent monitoring of serum glucose levels is necessary.

■ To reduce pain, apply moist heat to the affected side of the face, taking care not to burn the skin.

■ To help maintain muscle tone, massage the patient's face with a gentle upward motion two to three times daily for 5 to 10 minutes, or have him massage his face himself. When he's ready for active exercises, teach him to exercise by grimacing in front of a mirror.

■ Advise the patient to protect his eye by covering it with an eye patch, especially when outdoors. Tell him to keep warm and avoid exposure to dust and wind. When exposure is unavoidable, instruct him to cover his face.

■ Instruct the patient to chew on the unaffected side of his mouth. Provide a soft, nutritionally balanced diet, eliminating hot foods and fluids. Give the patient frequent mouth care, being particularly careful to remove residual food that collects between the cheeks and gums.

■ Offer psychological support.

Peripheral neuritis

Peripheral neuritis (also called *multiple neuritis, peripheral neuropathy,* and *polyneuritis*) is the degeneration of peripheral nerves supplying mainly the distal muscles of the extremities. It results in muscle weakness with sensory loss and atrophy and decreased or absent deep tendon reflexes. This syndrome is associated with a noninflammatory degeneration of the axon and myelin sheaths, chiefly affecting the distal muscles of the extremities. Because onset is usually insidious, patients may compensate by overusing unaffected muscles. If the cause can be identified and eliminated, the prognosis is good.

Causes

Causes of peripheral neuritis include:

■ hereditary disorders (Charcot-Marie-Tooth disease or Friedreich's ataxia)

■ exposure to toxic compounds (sniffing glue or toxic compounds, nitrous oxide, industrial agents — especially solvents, and heavy metals, such as lead, arsenic, or mercury)

■ infectious or inflammatory diseases (acquired immunodeficiency syndrome, botulism, Colorado Tick fever, hepatitis, human immunodeficiency virus infection, leprosy, rheumatoid arthritis, sarcoidosis, systemic lupus erythematosus, diphtheria, syphilis, and Guillain-Barré syndrome)

■ systemic or metabolic disorders (diabetes mellitus, dietary deficiencies — especially B_{12}, excessive use of alcohol, uremia, and cancer)

- neuropathy secondary to drugs
- miscellaneous causes (ischemia and prolonged exposure to cold temperature).

Peripheral neuropathy is common. Risk factors include diabetes, heavy alcohol use, and exposure to certain drugs and chemicals. Prolonged pressure on a nerve (such as with a cast, splint, or other device) is another risk factor for developing nerve injury. Although it can occur at any age, incidence is highest in men between ages 30 and 50.

Signs and symptoms

The clinical effects of peripheral neuritis develop slowly, and the disease usually affects the motor and sensory nerve fibers. Symptoms vary according to which type of nerve is affected (sensory, motor, or autonomic). Neuropathy can affect any one or be a combination of all three types.

- *Sensory changes:* Damage to sensory fibers results in changes in sensation, ranging from abnormal sensations, such as burning, nerve pain, or tingling, to numbness or an inability to determine joint position in the area. Sensation changes often begin in the feet and progress toward the center of the body with involvement of other areas as the condition worsens.
- *Motor changes:* Damage to the motor fibers interferes with muscle control and can cause weakness, loss of muscle bulk, and loss of dexterity. Muscle cramping may be a sign of motor nerve involvement. Other muscle-related symptoms include lack of muscle control, difficulty or inability to move a part of the body (paralysis), muscle atrophy, muscle twitching (fasciculation) or cramping, difficulty breathing or swallowing, falling (from legs buckling or tripping over toes), or lack of dexterity (such as the inability to button a shirt).
- *Autonomic changes:* The autonomic nerves control involuntary or semivoluntary functions, such as control of internal organs and blood pressure. Damage to autonomic nerves can cause blurred vision, decreased ability to sweat (anhidrosis), dizziness that occurs when standing up or fainting associated with a fall in blood pressure, heat intolerance with exertion (decreased ability to regulate body temperature), nausea or vomiting after meals, abdominal bloating (swelling), feeling full after eating a small amount (early satiety), diarrhea, constipation, unintentional weight loss (more than 5% of body weight), urinary incontinence, feeling of incomplete bladder emptying, difficulty beginning to urinate (urinary hesitancy), and male impotence.

Diagnosis

Patient history and physical examination delineate characteristic distribution of motor and sensory deficits. Electromyography may show a delayed action potential if this condition impairs motor nerve function. Nerve biopsy and nerve conduction tests can facilitate diagnosis.

Treatment

Effective treatment of peripheral neuritis consists of supportive measures to relieve pain, adequate bed rest, and physical therapy, vocational therapy, occupational therapy, and orthopedic interventions to promote independence, as needed. Most importantly, however, the underlying cause must be identified and corrected. For instance, it's essential to identify and remove the toxic agent, correct nutritional and vitamin deficiencies (the patient needs a high-calorie diet rich in vitamins, especially B-complex), and counsel the patient to avoid alcohol.

Over-the-counter analgesics or prescription pain medications may be needed to control nerve pain. Anticonvulsants (phenytoin, carbamazepine, and gabapentin) or tricyclic antidepressants may be used to reduce the stabbing pains that some patients experience. Whenever possible, medication use should be minimized to avoid adverse effects.

Fludrocortisone or similar medications may be beneficial in reducing postural hypotension for some patients. Medications that increase gastric motility, such as metoclopramide, are helpful for patients with reduced gastric motility.

For patients with bladder dysfunction, manual expression of urine (pressing over the bladder with the hands), intermittent catheterization, or medications such as bethanechol may be necessary.

Special considerations

Patient care includes promoting maximal independence and control of symptoms.

■ Exercises and retraining may be used to increase muscle strength and control. Appliances, such as wheelchairs, braces, and splints, may improve mobility or the ability to use an affected extremity.

■ The patient with decreased sensation should be taught to check his feet or other affected areas frequently for bruises, open skin areas, or other injuries. A podiatrist can usually determine whether special orthotic devices are needed.

■ Discuss safety measures in the home. Safety measures for the patient experiencing difficulty with movement may include railings, specialized appliances, removal of obstacles (such as loose rugs that may slip on the floor), and other measures, as appropriate. Safety measures for the patient with diminished sensation include adequate lighting (including lights left on at night), testing water temperature before bathing or immersing the body in water, and the use of protective shoes (no open toes and no high heels). Shoes should be checked often for grit or rough spots that may cause injury to the feet.

■ The patient with neuropathy (especially the patient with polyneuropathy or mononeuropathy multiplex) is prone to new nerve injury at pressure points, such as the knees and elbows. Caution him to avoid prolonged pressure on these areas from leaning on the elbows, crossing the knees, or similar positions.

■ Advise the patient with orthostatic hypotension to use elastic stockings and sleep with his head elevated.

■ Instruct the patient with reduced gastric motility to eat small, frequent meals and sleep with his head elevated.

■ Assist the patient with bladder dysfunction with manual expression of urine and intermittent catheterization, as necessary.

■ To prevent pressure ulcers, assist in turning and repositioning every 2 hours and apply a food cradle. To prevent contractures, provide range-of-motion exercises as well as arrange for the patient to obtain splints, boards, braces, or other orthopedic appliances.

■ Suggest that the patient's family contact the Neuropathy Association for additional information.

PAIN DISORDERS

Complex regional pain syndrome

Complex regional pain syndrome (CRPS), also known as *reflex sympathetic dystrophy* (CRPS1) or *causalgia* (CRPS2), is a chronic pain disorder that results from abnormal healing after an injury—either minor or major—to a bone, muscle, or nerve. The development of symptoms is commonly disproportionate to the severity of the injury and seems to result from abnormal functioning of the sympathetic nervous system, the part of the nervous system that controls the diameter of blood vessels. One or more extremities and other parts of the body may be affected.

Causes and incidence

The exact cause of CRPS is unknown. Impaired communication between the damaged nerves of the sympathetic nervous system and the brain may cause interference with normal signals for sensations, temperature, and blood flow. This leads to problems in the nerves, blood vessels, skin, bones, and muscles. Infection or injury to an arm or leg may initiate CRPS. It can also occur after heart attacks and strokes. However, the condition can sometimes appear without obvious injury to the affected limb. This condition is more common in people between ages 40 and 60, but has been seen in younger people too. CRPS may also be seen in postoperative patients and in patients with diseases that can cause chronic pain, such as cancer and arthritis. Annual incidence is unknown because CRPS is often misdiagnosed. However, it has been reported in 1% to 2% of patients with various fractures and in 2% to 5% of patients with peripheral nerve injury.

Signs and symptoms

Patients usually report severe and constant pain; severe pain is common with CRPS2 in particular. The affected area may have altered blood flow, feeling either warm or cool to the touch, with discoloration, sweating, or swelling. In time, skin, hair, and nail changes may occur along with impaired mobility and muscle wasting, especially if adequate treatment is delayed.

Diagnosis

There's no laboratory test for CRPS, so the diagnosis is based on the patient's history and clinical findings. A history of injury to an extremity may point to CRPS. Bone X-rays may aid in ruling out other conditions, such as osteomyelitis and stress fractures, which cause similar signs and symptoms. Additional tests may include bone scans, nerve conduction studies, and thermography (a test to show temperature changes and lack of blood supply in the painful area of the affected limb). With early diagnosis, prognosis improves.

Treatment

Treatment typically includes a combination of therapies such as drug therapy, with an anti-inflammatory, antidepressant, vasodilator, and analgesic used singly or in varying combinations, depending on the patient and the severity of symptoms. Steroids may be given in some patients; others may be given bone loss medications such as Actonel. Physical therapy to the injured area, application of heat and cold, the use of a transcutaneous electrical nerve stimulator unit, biofeedback, and psychological support are helpful for some patients.

Treatment may also include techniques for interrupting the hyperactivity of the sympathetic nervous system, such as nerve or regional blocks. Surgical sympathectomy — radical surgery that involves cutting the nerves to destroy the pain — may be done in severe cases; however, this method is rarely used because other sensation may be destroyed in the process.

Special considerations

- Offer emotional support to the patient and his family. Teach them about the disease.
- Monitor effects of prescribed medications.
- In addition to attending physical therapy sessions, the patient may need a home therapy regimen that includes stretching, active and passive exercises, strengthening exercises, compressive stockings or gloves to control edema, and heat or cold pack applications.
- Consult a pain care specialist to provide additional options for the patient, and help manage discomfort.
- Because chronic pain can be an emotional burden to the patient and his family, provide information on resources, such as counseling, support groups, stress-reduction methods, meditation, relaxation training, and hypnosis.

Selected references

Denis, L., et al. "Long-term Treatment Optimization in Individuals with Multiple Sclerosis Using Disease-modifying Therapies: A Nursing Approach," *Journal of Neuroscience Nursing* 36(1):10-22, February 2004.

Mega, M.S. "Difficult Diagnoses of Dementia: Clinical Examination and Laboratory Assessment," *Clinical Cornerstone* 4(6):53-65, 2002.

Saczynski, J.S., and Rebok, G.W. "Strategies for Memory Improvement in Older Adults," *Topics in Advanced Practice Nursing eJournal* 4(1), February 2004. Available at: *www.medscape.com/viewarticle/465740*. Last accessed July 15, 2004.

Smeltzer, S.C., and Bare, B.G. *Brunner and Suddarth's Textbook of Medical-Surgical Nursing*, 10th ed. Philadelphia: Lippincott Williams & Wilkins, 2004.

Weiner, H.L., et al. *Neurology*, 7th ed. Philadelphia: Lippincott Williams & Wilkins, 2004.

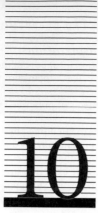

10

Gastrointestinal disorders

Introduction *683*

Mouth and esophagus *687*
Stomatitis and other oral infections *687*
Gastroesophageal reflux *689*
Tracheoesophageal fistula and esophageal
    atresia *691*
Corrosive esophagitis and stricture *695*
Mallory-Weiss syndrome *696*
Esophageal diverticula *697*
Hiatal hernia *699*

Stomach, intestine, and pancreas *701*
Gastritis *701*
Gastroenteritis *703*
Peptic ulcers *704*
Ulcerative colitis *707*
Necrotizing enterocolitis *709*
Crohn's disease *711*
Pseudomembranous enterocolitis *712*
Irritable bowel syndrome *713*
Celiac disease *714*
Diverticular disease *716*
Appendicitis *718*
Peritonitis *719*
Intestinal obstruction *721*
Inguinal hernia *724*
Intussusception *728*
Volvulus *729*

Hirschsprung's disease *730*
Inactive colon *732*
Pancreatitis *734*

Anorectum *736*
Hemorrhoids *736*
Anorectal abscess and fistula *738*
Rectal polyps *739*
Anorectal stricture *741*
Pilonidal disease *741*
Rectal prolapse *742*
Anal fissure *744*
Pruritus ani *744*
Proctitis *745*

Selected references *746*

Introduction

The GI tract, also known as the *alimentary canal,* is a long, hollow, musculomembranous tube consisting of glands and accessory organs (salivary glands, liver, gallbladder, and pancreas). (See *Reviewing GI anatomy and physiology,* page 684, and *Histology of the GI tract,* page 685.) The GI tract breaks down food — carbohydrates, fats, and proteins — into molecules small enough to permeate cell membranes, thus providing cells with the necessary energy to function properly; it prepares food for cellular absorption by altering its physical and chemical composition. (See *Primary source of digestive hormones,* pages 686 and 687.) Consequently, a malfunction along the GI tract can produce far-reaching metabolic effects, eventually threatening life itself.

The GI tract is an unsterile system filled with bacteria and other flora; these organisms can cause superinfection from antibiotic therapy or they can infect other systems when a GI organ ruptures. A common indication of GI problems is referred pain, which makes diagnosis especially difficult.

Accurate assessment vital

Your assessment of the patient with suspected GI disease must begin with a careful history that includes occupation, family history, and recent travel. The medical history should include previous hospital admissions; surgical procedures (including recent tooth extraction); family history of ulcers, colitis, or cancer; and current medications, whether prescribed, over-the-counter, or herbal remedies, with particular attention to aspirin, steroids, or anticoagulants.

Have the patient describe his chief complaint in his own words. Does he have abdominal pain, indigestion, heartburn, or rectal bleeding? How long has he had it? What relieves these symptoms or makes them worse? Has he experienced nosebleeds or difficulty in swallowing recently? Has he had recent weight loss or gain? Is he on a special diet? Does he drink alcoholic beverages or smoke? If yes to either, how much and how often? Ask about bowel habits. Does he regularly use laxatives or enemas? If he experiences nausea and vomiting, what does the vomitus look like? Does changing his position relieve nausea?

Next, try to define and locate any pain. Ask the patient to describe the pain. Is it dull, sharp, burning, aching, spasmodic, or intermittent? Where is it located? Does it radiate? How long does it last? When does it occur? What triggers it? What relieves it?

Visual assessment

Observe how the patient looks and note appropriateness of behavior. Changes in fluid and electrolyte balance, severe infection, drug toxicity, and hepatic disease may cause abnormal behavior. Your visual examination should check:

- *Skin*: loss of turgor, jaundice, cyanosis, pallor, diaphoresis, petechiae, bruises, edema, and texture (dry or oily)
- *Head*: color of sclerae, sunken eyes, dentures, caries, lesions, tongue (color, swelling, dryness), and breath odor
- *Chest*: shape (asymmetrical, barrel, or sunken)
- *Lungs*: rate, rhythm, and quality of respirations
- *Abdomen*: size and shape (distention, contour, visible masses, and protrusions), abdominal scars or fistulae, excessive skin folds (may indicate wasting), and abnormal respiratory movements (inflammation of diaphragm).

Auscultation, palpation, and percussion

Auscultation provides helpful clues to GI abnormalities. For example, absence of bowel sounds over the area to the lower right of the umbilicus may indicate peritonitis. High-pitched sounds that coincide with colicky pain may indicate small bowel obstruction. Less intense, low-pitched rumbling noises may accompany minor irritation.

Palpating the abdomen after auscultation helps detect tenderness, muscle guarding, and abdominal masses. Watch for muscle tone (boardlike rigidity points to peritonitis or hemorrhage; transient rigidity suggests severe pain) and tenderness (rebound tenderness may indicate peritoneal inflammation).

REVIEWING GI ANATOMY AND PHYSIOLOGY

The GI tract includes the mouth, pharynx, esophagus, stomach (fundus, body, and antrum), small intestine (duodenum, jejunum, and ileum), and large intestine (cecum, colon, rectum, and anal canal).

Digestion begins in the mouth through chewing and through the action of an enzyme secreted in saliva — ptyalin (amylase) — which breaks down starch.

Digestion continues in the stomach, where the lining secretes gastric juice that contains hydrochloric acid and the enzymes pepsin (begins protein digestion), lipase (speeds hydrolysis of emulsified fats) and, in infants, rennin (curdles milk).

Through a churning motion, the stomach breaks food into tiny particles, mixes them with gastric juice, and pushes the mass toward the pylorus. The liquid portion (chyme) enters the duodenum in small amounts; any solid material remains in the stomach until it liquefies (usually from 1 to 6 hours). The stomach also produces an intrinsic factor necessary for the absorption of vitamin B_{12}. Although limited amounts of water, alcohol, and some drugs are absorbed in the stomach, chyme passes unabsorbed into the duodenum.

Small intestine's role

Most digestion and absorption occur in the small intestine, where the surface area is increased by millions of villi in the mucous membrane lining. For digestion, the small intestine relies on a vast array of enzymes produced by the pancreas or by the intestinal lining itself. Pancreatic enzymes include trypsin, which digests protein to amino acids; lipase, which digests fat to fatty acids and glycerol; and amylase, which digests starches to sugars. Intestinal enzymes include erepsin, which digests protein to amino acids; lactase, maltase, and sucrase, which digest complex sugars like glucose, fructose, and galactose; and enterokinase, which activates trypsin.

In addition, bile, secreted by the liver and stored in the gallbladder, helps neutralize stomach acid and aids the small intestine to emulsify and absorb fats and fat-soluble vitamins.

Final stages

By the time ingested material reaches the ileocecal valve (where the small intestine joins the large intestine), all its nutritional value has been absorbed through the villi of the small intestine into the bloodstream.

The large intestine, so named because it's larger in diameter than the small intestine, absorbs water from the digestive material before passing it on for elimination. Rectal distention by feces stimulates the defecation reflex, which, when assisted by voluntary sphincter relaxation, permits defecation.

Throughout the GI tract, peristalsis (a coordinated, rhythmic contraction of smooth muscle) propels ingested material along; sphincters prevent its reflux.

Percussion helps detect air, fluid, and solid matter in the abdominal region.

Diagnostic tests

After physical assessment, several tests can identify GI malfunction.

■ A barium or gastrografin swallow is used primarily to examine the esophagus. Gastrografin may be used instead of barium. Like barium, gastrografin facilitates X-ray imaging. However, if gastrografin escapes from the GI tract, it's absorbed by the surrounding tissue, whereas escaped barium isn't absorbed and can cause complications.

- In an upper GI series, swallowed barium sulfate travels through the esophagus, stomach, and duodenum to reveal abnormalities. The barium outlines stomach walls and delineates ulcer craters and defects.
- A small-bowel series, an extension of the upper GI series, visualizes barium flowing through the small intestine to the ileocecal valve.
- A barium enema (lower GI series) allows X-ray visualization of the colon.
- A stool specimen is useful to detect suspected GI bleeding, infection, or malabsorption as well as the presence of parasites. Guaiac test for occult blood, microscopic stool examination for ova and parasites, and tests for fat require several specimens.
- In esophagogastroduodenoscopy, insertion of a fiber-optic scope allows direct visual inspection of the esophagus, stomach, and duodenum. These structures are examined for varices, tumors, inflammation, hernias, polyps, ulcers, and obstruction.
- Proctosigmoidoscopy permits inspection of the rectum and distal sigmoid colon; colonoscopy is used for inspection of the descending, transverse, and ascending colon. These tests help visualize tumors, polyps, hemorrhoids, or ulcers.
- Gastric analysis examines gastric secretions for the presence of high levels of gastrin and the amount of acid produced.
- Endoscopic retrograde cholangiopancreatography directly visualizes the esophagus, stomach, proximal duodenum, and fluoroscopic visualization of the pancreatic, hepatic, and biliary ducts. This test can help visualize duct obstruction, benign structures, cysts, anatomic variations, and malignant tumors.

Intubation

Certain GI disorders require nasogastric (NG) intubation to empty the stomach and intestine, to aid diagnosis and treatment, to decompress obstructed areas, to detect and treat GI bleeding, and to administer medications or feedings. Tubes generally inserted through the nose are the short NG tubes (the Levin, the Salem Sump, and the specialized Sengstaken-Blakemore) and the

---

HISTOLOGY OF THE GI TRACT

The GI tract consists of four tissue layers whose structure varies in different organs:

- *mucous membrane* — innermost layer; secretes gastric juice, protects the tract, and absorbs nutrients
- *submucosa* — connective tissue that contains the major blood vessels and nerves
- *external muscle coat (muscularis externa)* — double layer of smooth-muscle fibers; inner circular and outer longitudinal layers propel gastric contents downward by peristalsis
- *fibroserous coat (serosa)* — outermost protective layer of connective tissue; forms the largest serous membrane of the body — the peritoneum. The peritoneum's parietal layer covers the walls of the abdominal cavity. An extension of the parietal peritoneum, called the mesentery, anchors the small intestine to the abdominal wall. The visceral layer drapes most of the abdominal organs, covering the upper surface of the pelvic organs.

---

long intestinal tubes (Cantor and Miller-Abbott). The larger Ewald tube is usually inserted orally.

When caring for the patient with a tube:
- Explain the procedure before intubation.
- Maintain accurate intake and output records. Measure gastric drainage every 8 hours; record the amount, color, odor, and consistency. When irrigating the tube, note the amount of saline solution instilled and aspirated. Check for fluid and electrolyte imbalances.
- Provide good oral and nasal care. Brush the patient's teeth frequently and provide mouthwash. Make sure that the tube is secure, but isn't causing pressure on the nostrils. Change the tape to the nose every 24

PRIMARY SOURCE OF DIGESTIVE HORMONES

Pyloric mucosa
Gastrin, which originates in the G cells of the pyloric antral mucosa, stimulates secretion of hydrochloric acid by parietal cells and pepsinogen by chief cells.

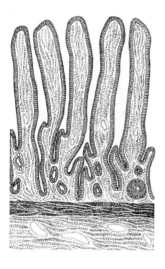

Duodenal mucosa
Secretin, which originates in the duodenal mucosa, stimulates the pancreas to secrete alkaline fluid (water and bicarbonate) into the duodenum, which neutralizes acid from the stomach.

Cholecystokinin-pancreozymin, which originates in the duodenal mucosa, stimulates pancreatic enzyme secretion and contraction and evacuation of the gallbladder.

Motilin, which originates in the duodenal mucosa, slows gastric emptying and stimulates gastric acid and pepsin secretion.

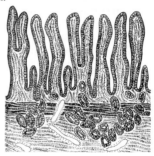

hours. Gently wash the area around the tube, and apply a water-soluble lubricant to soften crusts. These measures help prevent sore throat and nose, dry lips, nasal excoriation, and parotitis.

- Ensure maximum patient comfort. After insertion of a long intestinal tube, instruct the patient to turn from side to side to facilitate its passage through the GI tract. Note the tube's progress. Never attach an intestinal tube to a patient's gown, bed linens, side rails of the bed, and so forth.

- With both types of tubes, tell the patient to expect a feeling of dryness or a lump in the throat; if he's allowed, suggest that he chew gum or eat hard candy to relieve discomfort.

- Always keep scissors taped to the wall near the bed when the patient has a Sengstaken-Blakemore tube in place. If the tube should dislodge and obstruct the bronchus, cut the lumen to the balloons

immediately. Sometimes the tube is taped to the face piece of a football helmet worn by the patient to prevent the tube from dislodging and to put traction on the tube.

- After removing the tube from a patient with GI bleeding, watch for signs and symptoms of recurrent bleeding, such as hematemesis, decreased hemoglobin level, pallor, chills, diaphoresis, hypotension, and rapid pulse.

- Provide emotional support because the patient may panic at the sight of a tube. A calm, reassuring manner can help minimize his fear.

Jejunal mucosa
Gastric inhibitory peptide (GIP), which originates in the jejunal mucosa (also in the duodenal mucosa), stimulates secretion of intestinal juice and insulin and inhibits gastric acid secretion and motility.

Other digestive hormones
Three other digestive hormonelike substances are thought to originate in the hypothalamus, GI tract, and neurons of the brain. These substances include substance P, which increases small bowel motility; bombesin, which increases gastrin secretion and small bowel motility; and somatostatin, which inhibits secretion of gastrin, vasoactive intestinal polypeptide, GIP, secretin, and motilin. Other possible digestive hormones include enterogastrone, enteroglucagon, and somatostatin. More research is needed to confirm and clarify the existence and function of these hormones.

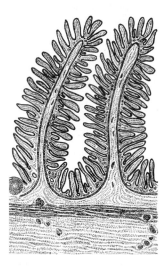

MOUTH AND ESOPHAGUS

Stomatitis and other oral infections

Stomatitis is an inflammation of the oral mucosa that may extend to the buccal mucosa, lips, and palate. It's a common infection that may occur alone or as part of a systemic disease. There are two main types: acute herpetic stomatitis and aphthous stomatitis. Acute herpetic stomatitis is usually self-limiting; however, it may be severe and, in neonates, may be generalized and potentially fatal. Aphthous stomatitis usually heals spontaneously, without a scar, in 10 to 14 days. Other oral infections include gingivitis, periodontitis, and Vincent's angina. (See *Types of oral infections,* page 688.)

Causes and incidence
Acute herpetic stomatitis results from the herpes simplex virus. It's common in children ages 1 to 3. The cause of aphthous stomatitis is unknown, but predisposing factors include stress, fatigue, anxiety, febrile states, trauma, and solar overexposure. This type is common in girls and female adolescents.

Signs and symptoms
Acute herpetic stomatitis begins suddenly with mouth pain, malaise, lethargy, anorexia, irritability, and fever, which may persist for 1 to 2 weeks. Gums are swollen and bleed easily, and the mucous membrane is extremely tender.

Papulovesicular ulcers appear in the mouth and throat and eventually become

TYPES OF ORAL INFECTIONS

Disease and causes	Signs and symptoms	Treatment
Gingivitis (*inflammation of the gingiva*)		
■ Early sign of hypovitaminosis, diabetes, blood dyscrasias ■ Occasionally related to use of hormonal contraceptives	■ Inflammation with painless swelling, redness, change of normal contours, bleeding, and periodontal pocket (gum detachment from teeth)	■ Removal of irritating factors (calculus, faulty dentures) ■ Good oral hygiene, regular dental checkups, vigorous chewing ■ Oral or topical corticosteroids
Glossitis (*inflammation of the tongue*)		
■ Streptococcal infection ■ Irritation or injury; jagged teeth; ill-fitting dentures; biting during seizures; alcohol; spicy foods; smoking; sensitivity to toothpaste or mouthwash ■ Vitamin B deficiency; anemia ■ Skin conditions: lichen planus, erythema multiforme, pemphigus vulgaris	■ Reddened, ulcerated, or swollen tongue (may obstruct airway) ■ Painful chewing and swallowing ■ Speech difficulty ■ Painful tongue without inflammation	■ Treatment of underlying cause ■ Topical anesthetic mouthwash or systemic analgesics (acetaminophen) for painful lesions ■ Good oral hygiene, regular dental checkups, vigorous chewing ■ Avoidance of hot, cold, or spicy foods and alcohol
Periodontitis (*gingival infection and recession, loosening of teeth*)		
■ Early sign of hypovitaminosis, diabetes, blood dyscrasias ■ Occasionally related to use of hormonal contraceptives ■ Dental factors: calculus, poor oral hygiene, malocclusion; major cause of tooth loss after middle age	■ Acute onset of bright red gum inflammation, painless swelling of interdental papillae, easy bleeding ■ Loosening of teeth, typically without inflammatory symptoms, progressing to loss of teeth and alveolar bone ■ Acute systemic infection (fever, chills)	■ Scaling, root planing, and curettage for infection control ■ Periodontal surgery to prevent recurrence ■ Good oral hygiene, regular dental checkups, vigorous chewing
Vincent's angina (*trench mouth, necrotizing ulcerative gingivitis*)		
■ Fusiform bacillus or spirochete infection ■ Predisposing factors: stress, poor oral hygiene, insufficient rest, nutritional deficiency, smoking	■ Sudden onset: painful, superficial bleeding; gingival ulcers (rarely, on buccal mucosa) covered with a gray-white membrane ■ Ulcers become punched-out lesions after slight pressure or irritation ■ Malaise, mild fever, excessive salivation, bad breath, pain on swallowing or talking, enlarged submaxillary lymph nodes	■ Removal of devitalized tissue with ultrasonic cavitron ■ Antibiotics for infection ■ Analgesics, as needed ■ Hourly mouth rinses (with equal amounts of hydrogen peroxide and warm water) ■ Soft, nonirritating diet; rest; no smoking ■ With treatment, improvement common within 24 hours

punched-out lesions with reddened areolae. Submaxillary lymphadenitis is common. Pain usually disappears 2 to 4 days before healing of ulcers is complete. If the child with stomatitis sucks his thumb, these lesions spread to the hand.

A patient with aphthous stomatitis typically reports burning, tingling, and slight swelling of the mucous membrane. Single or multiple shallow ulcers with whitish centers and red borders appear and heal at one site and then reappear at another. (See *Looking at aphthous stomatitis.*)

Diagnosis

Diagnosis is based on the physical examination; in Vincent's angina, a smear of ulcer exudate allows for identification of the causative organism.

Treatment

For acute herpetic stomatitis, treatment is conservative. For local symptoms, supportive measures include warm salt-water mouth rinses (antiseptic mouthwashes are contraindicated because they are irritating) and a topical anesthetic to relieve mouth ulcer pain. Topical antihistamines, antacids, or corticosteroids may also be recommended. Supplementary treatment includes a bland or liquid diet and, in severe cases, I.V. fluids and bed rest.

For aphthous stomatitis, primary treatment is application of a topical anesthetic. Effective long-term treatment requires alleviation or prevention of precipitating factors.

Gastroesophageal reflux

Gastroesophageal reflux, also called *gastroesophageal reflux disease* (GERD), is the backflow of gastric or duodenal contents, or both, into the esophagus and past the lower esophageal sphincter (LES) without associated belching or vomiting. Reflux may cause symptoms or pathologic changes. Persistent reflux may cause reflux esophagitis (inflammation of the esophageal mucosa). Prognosis varies with the underlying cause.

> ### LOOKING AT APHTHOUS STOMATITIS
>
> In aphthous stomatitis, numerous small, round vesicles appear. They soon break and leave shallow ulcers with red areolae.
>
>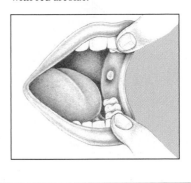

Causes and incidence

The function of the LES — a high-pressure area in the lower esophagus, just above the stomach — is to prevent gastric contents from backing up into the esophagus. Normally, the LES creates pressure, closing the lower end of the esophagus, but relaxes after each swallow to allow food into the stomach. Reflux occurs when LES pressure is deficient or when pressure within the stomach exceeds LES pressure. (See *Influences on LES pressure,* page 690.)

Studies have shown that a patient with symptom-producing reflux can't swallow often enough to create sufficient peristaltic amplitude to clear gastric acid from the lower esophagus. This results in prolonged periods of acidity in the esophagus when reflux occurs.

Predisposing factors include:
- pyloric surgery (alteration or removal of the pylorus), which allows reflux of bile or pancreatic juice
- long-term nasogastric (NG) intubation (more than 4 days)
- any agent that lowers LES pressure, such as food, alcohol, cigarettes; anticholinergics (atropine, belladonna, and propantheline); or other drugs (morphine, diazepam, calcium channel blockers, and meperidine)

INFLUENCES ON LES PRESSURE

Several factors can influence lower esophageal sphincter (LES) pressure, thereby affecting reflux, as noted here.

Factors that increase LES pressure
- Carbohydrates
- Low-dose ethanol
- Nonfat milk
- Protein

Factors that decrease LES pressure
- Antiflatulents (simethicone)
- Chocolate
- Cigarette smoking
- Fat
- High-dose ethanol
- Lying on right or left side
- Orange juice
- Sitting
- Tomatoes
- Whole milk

- hiatal hernia with an incompetent sphincter
- any condition or position that increases intra-abdominal pressure, such as straining, bending, coughing, pregnancy, obesity, and recurrent or persistent vomiting.

About 25% to 40% of Americans experience symptomatic GERD at some point in their lives, while 7% to 10% of Americans experience symptoms on a daily basis. True incidence figures may be even higher because many people with GERD take over-the-counter remedies without reporting their symptoms.

Signs and symptoms

GERD doesn't always cause symptoms, and in patients showing clinical effects, it isn't always possible to confirm physiologic reflux. The most common feature of GERD is heartburn, which may become more severe with vigorous exercise, bending, or lying down, and may be relieved by antacids or sitting upright. The pain of esophageal spasm resulting from reflux esophagitis tends to be chronic and may mimic angina pectoris, radiating to the neck, jaws, and arms.

Other symptoms include odynophagia, which may be followed by a dull substernal ache from severe, long-term reflux; dysphagia from esophageal spasm, stricture, or esophagitis; and bleeding (bright red or dark brown). Rarely, nocturnal regurgitation wakens the patient with coughing, choking, and a mouthful of saliva. Reflux may be associated with hiatal hernia. Direct hiatal hernia becomes clinically significant only when reflux is confirmed.

Pulmonary symptoms result from reflux of gastric contents into the throat and subsequent aspiration; they include chronic pulmonary disease or nocturnal wheezing, bronchitis, asthma, morning hoarseness, and cough. In children, other signs consist of failure to thrive and forceful vomiting from esophageal irritation. Such vomiting sometimes causes aspiration pneumonia.

Diagnosis

CONFIRMING DIAGNOSIS *After a careful history and physical examination, tests to confirm GERD include barium swallow fluoroscopy, esopha-*

geal pH probe, esophageal manometry, and esophagoscopy. In children, barium esophagography under fluoroscopic control can show reflux.
Recurrent reflux after age 6 weeks is abnormal. An acid perfusion (Bernstein) test can show that reflux is the cause of symptoms. Finally, endoscopy and biopsy allow visualization and confirmation of any pathologic changes in the mucosa.

Treatment

Effective management begins by teaching the patient to avoid factors that decrease LES pressure or cause esophageal irritation. The patient should eat a low-fat, high-fiber diet and avoid caffeine, tobacco, and carbonated beverages. He shouldn't eat 2 hours before going to bed and should avoid tight clothing, elevate the head of the bed 6″ to 8″ (15 to 20 cm) and maintain a normal body weight. Promotility agents help increase LES sphincter tone and stimulate upper GI motility. Proton pump inhibitors and histamine-2 (H$_2$) receptor antagonists help reduce gastric acidity. If possible, NG intubation shouldn't be continued for more than 5 days because the tube interferes with sphincter integrity and allows reflux, especially when the patient lies flat.

Positional therapy is especially useful in infants and children who experience GERD without complications.

Surgery may be necessary to control severe and refractory symptoms, such as pulmonary aspiration, hemorrhage, obstruction, severe pain, perforation, an incompetent LES, or associated hiatal hernia. Surgical procedures that create an artificial closure at the gastroesophageal junction may be needed in some patients. These include a procedure that invaginates the esophagus into the stomach and procedures that create a gastric wraparound with or without fixation. The fundoplication procedure can be performed endoscopically. Also, vagotomy or pyloroplasty may be combined with an antireflux regimen to modify gastric contents.

Special considerations

Teach the patient what causes reflux, how to avoid reflux with an antireflux regimen (medication, diet, and positional therapy), and what symptoms to watch for and report.

■ Instruct the patient to avoid circumstances that increase intra-abdominal pressure (such as bending, coughing, vigorous exercise, tight clothing, constipation, and obesity) as well as substances that reduce sphincter control (cigarettes, alcohol, fatty foods, and caffeine).

■ Advise the patient to sit upright, particularly after meals, and to eat small, frequent meals. Tell him to avoid highly seasoned food, acidic juices, alcoholic drinks, bedtime snacks, and foods high in fat or carbohydrates, which reduce LES pressure. He should eat meals at least 2 to 3 hours before lying down.

■ Tell the patient to take antacids, as ordered (usually 1 hour before or 3 hours after meals and at bedtime).

■ Teach the patient correct preparation for diagnostic testing. For example, he shouldn't eat for 6 to 8 hours before a barium swallow or endoscopy.

■ After surgery using a thoracic approach, carefully watch and record chest tube drainage and the patient's respiratory status. If needed, give chest physiotherapy and oxygen. Position the patient with an NG tube in semi-Fowler's position to help prevent reflux. Offer reassurance and emotional support.

Tracheoesophageal fistula and esophageal atresia

Tracheoesophageal fistula is a developmental anomaly characterized by an abnormal connection between the trachea and the esophagus. It usually accompanies esophageal atresia, in which the esophagus is closed off at some point. Although these malformations have numerous anatomic variations, the most common, by far, is esophageal atresia with fistula to the distal segment. (See *Types of tracheoesophageal anomalies*, pages 692 and 693.)

These disorders, two of the most serious surgical emergencies in neonates, require immediate diagnosis and correction. They may coexist with other serious anomalies, such as congenital heart disease, imperfo-

TYPES OF TRACHEOESOPHAGEAL ANOMALIES

Congenital malformations of the esophagus occur in about 1 in 4,000 live births. The American Academy of Pediatrics classifies the anatomic variations of tracheoesophageal anomalies as follows:

- Type A (7.7%): esophageal atresia without fistula
- Type B (0.8%): esophageal atresia with tracheoesophageal fistula to the proximal segment
- Type C (86.5%): esophageal atresia with fistula to the distal segment
- Type D (0.7%): esophageal atresia with fistula to both segments
- Type E (or H-Type) (4.2%): tracheoesophageal fistula without atresia

TYPE A

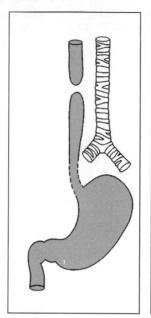

TYPE B

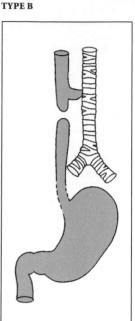

rate anus, genitourinary abnormalities, and intestinal atresia.

Causes and incidence

Tracheoesophageal fistula and esophageal atresia result from failure of the embryonic esophagus and trachea to develop and separate correctly. Respiratory system development begins at about day 26 of gestation. Abnormal development of the septum during this time can lead to tracheoesophageal fistula. The most common abnormality is type C tracheoesophageal fistula with esophageal atresia, in which the upper section of the esophagus terminates in a blind pouch, and the lower section ascends from the stomach and connects with the trachea by a short fistulous tract.

In type A atresia, both esophageal segments are blind pouches, and neither is connected to the airway. In type E (or H-type), tracheoesophageal fistula without atresia, the fistula may occur anywhere between the level of the cricoid cartilage and the midesophagus, but is usually higher in the trachea than in the esophagus. Such a fistula may be as small as a pinpoint. In types B and D, the upper portion of the esophagus opens into the trachea; neonates with this anomaly may experience life-threatening aspiration of saliva or food.

Esophageal atresia occurs in about 1 of every 1,500 to 3,000 live births; about one-third of these neonates are born prematurely.

Signs and symptoms

A neonate with type C tracheoesophageal fistula with esophageal atresia appears to swallow normally but soon after swallowing coughs, struggles, becomes cyanotic, and stops breathing as he aspirates fluids returning from the blind pouch of the esophagus through his nose and mouth. Stomach distention may cause respiratory distress; air and gastric contents (bile and

TYPE C	TYPE D	TYPE E
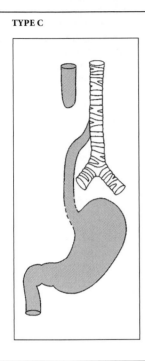	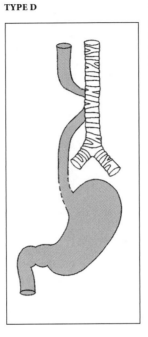	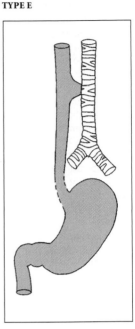

gastric secretions) may reflux through the fistula into the trachea, resulting in chemical pneumonitis.

An infant with type A esophageal atresia appears normal at birth. The infant swallows normally, but as secretions fill the esophageal sac and overflow into the oropharynx, he develops mucus in the oropharynx and drools excessively. When the infant is fed, regurgitation and respiratory distress follow aspiration. Suctioning the mucus and secretions temporarily relieves these symptoms. Excessive secretions and drooling in the neonate strongly suggest esophageal atresia.

Repeated episodes of pneumonitis, pulmonary infection, and abdominal distention may signal type E (or H-type) tracheoesophageal fistula. When a child with this disorder drinks, he coughs, chokes, and becomes cyanotic. Excessive mucus builds up in the oropharynx. Crying forces air from the trachea into the esophagus,

producing abdominal distention. Because such a child may appear normal at birth, this type of tracheoesophageal fistula may be overlooked, and diagnosis may be delayed as long as 1 year.

Type B (proximal fistula) and type D (fistula to both segments) cause immediate aspiration of saliva into the airway and bacterial pneumonitis.

Diagnosis

Respiratory distress and drooling in a neonate suggest tracheoesophageal fistula and esophageal atresia. The following procedures confirm the diagnosis:

- A size 10 or 12 French catheter passed through the nose meets an obstruction (esophageal atresia) approximately 4″ to 5″ (10 to 12.5 cm) distal from the nostrils. Aspirate of gastric contents is less acidic than normal.
- Chest X-ray demonstrates the position of the catheter and can also show a dilated,

air-filled upper esophageal pouch, pneumonia in the right upper lobe, or bilateral pneumonitis. Both pneumonia and pneumonitis suggest aspiration.

- Abdominal X-ray shows gas in the bowel in a distal fistula (type C) but none in a proximal fistula (type B) or in atresia without fistula (type A).
- Cinefluorography allows visualization on a fluoroscopic screen. After a size 10 or 12 French catheter is passed through the patient's nostril into the esophagus, a small amount of contrast medium is instilled to define the tip of the upper pouch and to differentiate between overflow aspiration from a blind end (atresia) and aspiration due to passage of liquid through a tracheoesophageal fistula.

Treatment

Tracheoesophageal fistula and esophageal atresia require surgical correction and are usually surgical emergencies. The type and timing of surgical procedure depend on the nature of the anomaly, the patient's general condition, and the presence of coexisting congenital defects. In premature neonates (nearly 33% of neonates with this anomaly are born prematurely) who are poor surgical risks, correction of combined tracheoesophageal fistula and esophageal atresia is done in two stages: first, gastrostomy (for gastric decompression, prevention of reflux, and feeding) and closure of the fistula; then, 1 to 2 months later, anastomosis of the esophagus.

Before and after surgery, positioning varies with the physician's philosophy and the infant's anatomy: the infant may be placed supine, with his head low to facilitate drainage, or with his head elevated to prevent aspiration.

The infant should receive I.V. fluids, as necessary, and appropriate antibiotics for superimposed infection.

Postoperative complications after correction of tracheoesophageal fistula include recurrent fistulas, esophageal motility dysfunction, esophageal stricture, recurrent bronchitis, pneumothorax, and failure to thrive. Esophageal motility dysfunction or hiatal hernia may develop after surgery to correct esophageal atresia.

Correction of esophageal atresia alone requires anastomosis of the proximal and distal esophageal segments in one or two stages. End-to-end anastomosis commonly produces postoperative stricture; end-to-side anastomosis is less likely to do so. If the esophageal ends are widely separated, treatment may include a colonic interposition (grafting a piece of the colon) or elongation of the proximal segment of the esophagus by bougienage. About 10 days after surgery, and again 1 and 3 months later, X-rays are required to evaluate the effectiveness of surgical repair.

Postoperative treatment includes placement of a suction catheter in the upper esophageal pouch to control secretions and prevent aspiration, maintaining the infant in an upright position to avoid reflux of gastric juices into the trachea, I.V. fluids (nothing by mouth), gastrostomy to prevent reflux and allow feeding, and appropriate antibiotics for pneumonia.

Postoperative complications may include impaired esophageal motility (in one-third of patients), hiatal hernia, and reflux esophagitis.

Special considerations

Postoperative care should include the following:

- Monitor the infant's respiratory status. Administer oxygen and perform pulmonary physiotherapy and suctioning, as needed. Provide a humid environment.
- Administer antibiotics and parenteral fluids, as ordered. Keep accurate intake and output records.
- If the infant has chest tubes postoperatively, check them frequently for patency. Maintain proper suction; measure and mark drainage periodically.
- Observe carefully for signs of complications, such as abnormal esophageal motility, recurrent fistulas, pneumothorax, and esophageal stricture.
- Maintain gastrostomy tube feedings, as ordered. Such feedings initially consist of dextrose and water (not more than 5% solution); later, add a proprietary formula (first diluted and then full strength). If the infant develops gastric atony, use an isoosmolar formula. Oral feedings can usually resume 8 to 10 days postoperatively. If gas-

trostomy feedings and oral feedings are impossible because of intolerance to them or decreased intestinal motility, the infant requires total parenteral nutrition.

■ If the infant can safely handle secretions, he may be given a pacifier to satisfy his sucking needs; however, this is done *only* when he can safely handle secretions because sucking stimulates saliva secretion.

■ Offer the parents support and guidance in dealing with their infant's acute illness. Encourage them to participate in the infant's care and to hold and touch him as much as possible to facilitate bonding.

Corrosive esophagitis and stricture

Corrosive esophagitis is inflammation and damage to the esophagus after ingestion of a caustic chemical. Similar to a burn, this injury may be temporary or may lead to permanent stricture (narrowing or stenosis) of the esophagus that's correctable only through surgery. Severe injury can quickly lead to esophageal perforation, mediastinitis, and death from infection, shock, and massive hemorrhage (due to aortic perforation).

Causes and incidence

The most common chemical injury to the esophagus follows the ingestion of lye or other strong alkali; ingestion of strong acids is less common. The type and amount of chemical ingested determine the severity and location of the damage. In children, household chemical ingestion is accidental; in adults, it's usually a suicide attempt or gesture. The chemical may damage only the mucosa or submucosa or it may damage all layers of the esophagus.

Esophageal tissue damage occurs in three phases: the acute phase, consisting of edema and inflammation; the latent phase, with ulceration, exudation, and tissue sloughing; and the chronic phase, in which there is diffuse scarring.

Gastroesophageal reflux disease accounts for 70% to 80% of all cases of esophageal stricture. Postoperative strictures account for 10% of all cases, and corrosive strictures account for less than 5% of all cases.

Peptic strictures are 10 times more common in Whites than in Blacks and Asians and two to three times more common in men than in women.

Signs and symptoms

Effects vary from none at all to intense pain in the mouth and anterior chest, marked salivation, inability to swallow, and tachypnea. Bloody vomitus containing pieces of esophageal tissue signals severe damage. Signs of esophageal perforation and mediastinitis, especially crepitation, indicate destruction of the entire esophagus. Inability to speak implies laryngeal damage.

The acute phase subsides in 3 to 4 days, enabling the patient to eat again. Fever suggests secondary infection. Symptoms of dysphagia return if stricture develops, usually within weeks; rarely, stricture is delayed and develops several years after the injury.

Diagnosis

CONFIRMING DIAGNOSIS *A history of chemical ingestion and physical examination revealing oropharyngeal burns (including white membranes and edema of the soft palate and uvula) usually confirm the diagnosis.*

The type and amount of the chemical ingested must be identified; this may be done by examining the container of the ingested material or by calling the poison control center.

Two procedures are helpful in evaluating the severity of the injury:

■ Endoscopy (in the first 24 hours after ingestion) delineates the extent and location of the esophageal injury and assesses the depth of the burn. This procedure may also be performed a week after ingestion to assess stricture development.

■ Barium swallow (1 week after ingestion and every 3 weeks thereafter) may identify segmental spasm or fistula, but doesn't always show mucosal injury.

Treatment

Conservative treatment of corrosive esophagitis and stricture includes monitoring the patient's condition; early endoscopy; administering corticosteroids, such as prednisone and hydrocortisone, to control inflammation and inhibit fibrosis; and using a broad-spectrum antibiotic, such as ampicillin, to protect the corticosteroid-immunosuppressed patient against infection by his own mouth flora.

Treatment may also include bougienage, a procedure in which a slender, flexible, cylindrical instrument called a *bougie* is passed into the esophagus to dilate it and minimize stricture. Some physicians begin bougienage immediately and continue it regularly to maintain a patent lumen and prevent stricture; others delay it for a week to avoid the risk of esophageal perforation.

Surgery is necessary immediately for esophageal perforation or later to correct stricture untreatable with bougienage. Corrective surgery may involve transplanting a piece of the colon to the damaged esophagus. However, even after surgery, stricture may recur at the site of the anastomosis.

Supportive treatment includes I.V. therapy to replace fluids or total parenteral nutrition while the patient can't swallow, gradually progressing to clear liquids and a soft diet.

Special considerations

If you're the first health care professional to see the patient who has ingested a corrosive chemical, the quality of your emergency care will be critical. To meet this challenge, follow these important guidelines:

■ *Don't* induce vomiting or lavage because this will expose the esophagus and oropharynx to additional injury.

■ *Don't* perform gastric lavage because the corrosive chemical may cause further damage to the mucous membrane of the GI lining.

■ Provide vigorous support of vital functions, as needed, such as oxygen, mechanical ventilation, administration of I.V. fluids, and treatment for shock, depending on the severity of the injury.

■ Carefully observe and record intake and output.

■ Before X-rays and endoscopy, explain the procedure to the patient to lessen anxiety during the tests and to obtain cooperation.

■ Because the adult who has ingested a corrosive agent has usually done so with

suicidal intent, assist him and his family in seeking psychological counseling. Monitor the patient according to facility protocol if the attempt was a suicide.

■ Provide emotional support for parents whose child has ingested a chemical. They'll be distraught and may feel guilty about the accident. After the emergency and without emphasizing blame, teach appropriate preventive measures, such as locking accessible cabinets and keeping all corrosive agents out of a child's reach.

■ Encourage long-term follow-up because of the increased risk of squamous cell carcinoma.

Mallory-Weiss syndrome

Mallory-Weiss syndrome is mild to massive, usually painless bleeding due to a tear in the mucosa or submucosa of the cardia or lower esophagus. Such a tear, usually singular and longitudinal, results from prolonged or forceful vomiting. Sixty percent of these tears involve the cardia; 15%, the terminal esophagus; and 25%, the region across the esophagogastric junction.

Causes and incidence

Forceful or prolonged vomiting can cause esophageal tearing when the upper esophageal sphincter fails to relax during vomiting; this lack of sphincter coordination seems more common after excessive alcohol intake. Other factors that can increase intra-abdominal pressure and predispose a person to this type of tear include coughing, straining during bowel movements, traumatic injury, seizures, childbirth, hiatal hernia, esophagitis, gastritis, and atrophic gastric mucosa.

Mallory-Weiss syndrome accounts for 1% to 15% of all cases of upper GI bleeding. It's two to four times more common in men than in women. There's no racial predilection. Patients usually present with symptoms during their 40s and 50s, but it can affect people of all ages.

Signs and symptoms

Mallory-Weiss syndrome typically begins with vomiting of blood or passing large amounts of blood rectally a few hours to several days after forceful vomiting. The bleeding, which may be accompanied by epigastric or back pain, may range from mild to massive, but is usually more profuse than in esophageal rupture. In Mallory-Weiss syndrome, the blood vessels are only partially severed, preventing retraction and closure of the lumen. Massive bleeding — most likely when the tear is on the gastric side, near the cardia — may quickly lead to fatal shock.

Diagnosis

 CONFIRMING DIAGNOSIS
Fiber-optic endoscopy (esophagogastroduodenoscopy confirms Mallory-Weiss syndrome by identifying esophageal tears. Recent tears appear as erythematous longitudinal cracks in the mucosa; older tears appear as raised white streaks surrounded by erythema.

Treatment

Treatment varies with the severity of bleeding. GI bleeding usually stops spontaneously, thereafter requiring supportive measures and careful observation but no definitive treatment. However, if bleeding continues, treatment may include:
■ proton pump inhibitors or histamine-2 receptor antagonists to help decrease acidity
■ blood transfusions if blood loss is great
■ endoscopy with electrocoagulation or heater probe for hemostasis
■ transcatheter embolization or thrombus formation with an autologous blood clot or other hemostatic material (such as a shredded adsorbable gelatin sponge)
■ surgery to suture each esophageal laceration.

Special considerations

Observation is necessary to determine whether bleeding is transitory or ongoing.
■ Evaluate the patient's respiratory status, monitor arterial blood gas values, and administer oxygen as necessary.
■ Assess the amount of blood lost and record the color, amount, consistency, and frequency of hematemesis and melena.
■ Draw blood for coagulation studies (prothrombin time, partial thromboplastin

time, and platelet count), and type and crossmatch.
■ Try to keep 3 units of blood available at all times. Insert a 14G to 18G I.V. line, and start an infusion of I.V. solution, as ordered. (If the I.V. infusion is for blood transfusion, use normal saline solution; if the infusion is for fluid replacement, use lactated Ringer's solution or another appropirate solution, depending on the results of laboratory tests.)
■ Monitor the patient's vital signs, central venous pressure, urine output, neurologic status, and overall clinical status.
■ Explain diagnostic tests to the patient.
■ Keep the patient warm and maintain a safe environment.
■ Obtain a detailed history of recent medications taken, dietary habits, and alcohol ingestion.
■ Administer antiemetics, as ordered, to prevent postoperative retching and vomiting.
■ Advise the patient to avoid aspirin, alcohol, and other irritating substances.

Esophageal diverticula

Esophageal diverticula are hollow outpouchings of one or more layers of the esophageal wall. They occur in three main areas: just above the upper esophageal sphincter (Zenker's, or pulsion, diverticulum, the most common type); near the midpoint of the esophagus (traction); and just above the lower esophageal sphincter (epiphrenic). Generally, esophageal diverticula occur later in life — although they can affect infants and children — and are three times more common in men than in women. Epiphrenic diverticula usually occur in middle-aged men, whereas Zenker's diverticula typically affect men older than age 60.

Causes and incidence

Esophageal diverticula are due to primary muscular abnormalities that may be congenital or to inflammatory processes adjacent to the esophagus. Zenker's diverticulum occurs when the pouch results from increased intraesophageal pressure; traction diverticulum occurs when the pouch is pulled out by adjacent inflamed tissue or lymph nodes. Some authorities classify all diverticula as traction diverticula.

Zenker's diverticulum results from developmental muscular weakness of the posterior pharynx above the border of the cricopharyngeal muscle. The pressure of swallowing aggravates this weakness, as does contraction of the pharynx before relaxation of the sphincter. A midesophageal (traction) diverticulum is a response to scarring and pulling on esophageal walls by an external inflammatory process such as tuberculosis. An epiphrenic diverticulum (rare) is generally right-sided and usually accompanies an esophageal motor disturbance, such as esophageal spasm or achalasia. It's thought to be caused by traction and pulsation.

Most diverticula occur in middle-aged and elderly patients. Zenker's diverticula most commonly in patients older than age 50 and are especially prevalent in patients in their 70s and 80s.

Signs and symptoms

Midesophageal and epiphrenic diverticula with an associated motor disturbance (achalasia or spasm) seldom produce symptoms, although the patient may experience dysphagia and heartburn. Zenker's diverticulum, however, produces distinctly staged symptoms, beginning with initial throat irritation followed by dysphagia and near-complete obstruction. In early stages, regurgitation occurs soon after eating; in later stages, regurgitation after eating is delayed and may even occur during sleep, leading to food aspiration and pulmonary infection.

 ELDER TIP *Hoarseness, asthma, and pneumonitis may be the only signs of esophageal diverticula in elderly patients.*

Other signs and symptoms include noise when liquids are swallowed, chronic cough, hoarseness, a bad taste in the mouth or foul breath and, rarely, bleeding.

Diagnosis

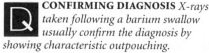 **CONFIRMING DIAGNOSIS** *X-rays taken following a barium swallow usually confirm the diagnosis by showing characteristic outpouching.*

Esophagoscopy can rule out another lesion; however, the procedure risks rupturing the diverticulum by passing the scope into it rather than into the lumen of the esophagus, a special danger with Zenker's diverticulum.

Treatment

Treatment of Zenker's diverticulum is usually palliative and includes a bland diet, thorough chewing, and drinking water after eating to flush out the sac. However, severe symptoms or a large diverticulum necessitates surgery to remove the sac or facilitate drainage. An esophagomyotomy may be necessary to prevent recurrence.

A midesophageal diverticulum seldom requires therapy except when esophagitis aggravates the risk of rupture, in which case treatment includes antacids and an antireflux regimen: keeping the head elevated, maintaining an upright position for 2 hours after eating, eating small meals, controlling chronic coughing, and avoiding constrictive clothing.

Epiphrenic diverticulum requires treatment of accompanying motor disorders. Achalasia is treated by repeated dilations of the esophagus; acute spasm is controlled by anticholinergic administration and diverticulum excision; and dysphagia or severe pain are relieved by surgical excision or suspending the diverticulum to promote drainage. Treatment may also include parenteral feeding to improve the patient's nutritional status.

Special considerations

Care includes documenting the patient's symptoms and nutritional status and educating him about the disorder.

- Regularly assess the patient's nutritional status (weight, calorie intake, and appearance).
- If the patient regurgitates food and mucus, protect against aspiration by positioning him carefully (head elevated or turned to one side). To prevent aspiration, tell the patient to empty any visible outpouching in the neck by massage or postural drainage before retiring.
- If the patient has dysphagia, record well-tolerated foods and what circumstances ease swallowing. Provide a pureed diet,

with vitamin or protein supplements, and encourage thorough chewing.
■ Teach the patient about this disorder. Explain treatment instructions and diagnostic procedures.

Hiatal hernia

Hiatal hernia, also called *hiatus hernia,* is a defect in the diaphragm that permits a portion of the stomach to pass through the diaphragmatic opening into the chest. Hiatal hernia is the most common problem of the diaphragm affecting the alimentary canal. Two types of hiatal hernia can occur: sliding hernia and paraesophageal hernia. (See *Types of hiatal hernia.*) In a sliding hernia, the stomach and the gastroesophageal junction slip up into the chest, so the gastroesophageal junction is above the diaphragmatic hiatus. In paraesophageal hernia, a part of the greater curvature of the stomach rolls through the diaphragmatic defect. Treatment can prevent complications such as strangulation of the herniated intrathoracic portion of the stomach.

Causes and incidence
Hiatal hernia typically results from muscle weakening that's common with aging and may be secondary to esophageal carcinoma, kyphoscoliosis, trauma, or certain surgical procedures. It may also result from certain diaphragmatic malformations that may cause congenital weakness. Obesity and smoking are common risk factors.

In hiatal hernia, the muscular collar around the esophageal and diaphragmatic junction loosens, permitting the lower portion of the esophagus and the stomach to rise into the chest when intra-abdominal pressure increases (possibly causing gastroesophageal reflux). Such increased intra-abdominal pressure may result from ascites, pregnancy, obesity, constrictive clothing, bending, straining, coughing, Valsalva's maneuver, or extreme physical exertion.

Sliding hernias are more common than paraesophageal hernias. The incidence of hiatal hernia increases with age (most occur in people older than age 40), and

TYPES OF HIATAL HERNIA

A hiatal hernia is a displacement of the normal anatomy, as shown in the illustrations below.

NORMAL STOMACH

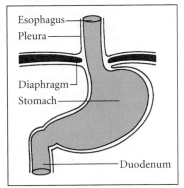

SLIDING HIATAL HERNIA

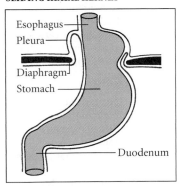

PARAESOPHAGEAL HERNIA

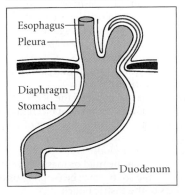

prevalence is higher in women than in men (especially the paraesophageal type). Contributing factors include obesity and trauma. No racial predilection exists.

Signs and symptoms

Typically, a paraesophageal hernia produces no symptoms; it's usually an incidental finding during a barium swallow or when testing for occult blood. Because this type of hernia leaves the closing mechanism of the cardiac sphincter unchanged, it rarely causes acid reflux or reflux esophagitis. Symptoms result from displacement or stretching of the stomach and may include a feeling of fullness in the chest or pain resembling angina pectoris. Even if it produces no symptoms, this type of hernia needs surgical treatment because of the high risk of strangulation that can occur when a large portion of stomach becomes caught above the diaphragm.

A sliding hernia without an incompetent sphincter produces no reflux or symptoms and, consequently, doesn't require treatment. When a sliding hernia causes symptoms, they are typical of gastric reflux, resulting from the incompetent lower esophageal sphincter (LES), and may include:
- Pyrosis (heartburn) occurs 1 to 4 hours after eating (especially overeating) and is aggravated by reclining, belching, and increased intra-abdominal pressure. It may be accompanied by regurgitation or vomiting.
- Retrosternal or substernal chest pain results from reflux of gastric contents, stomach distention, and spasm or altered motor activity. Chest pain usually occurs after meals or at bedtime and is aggravated by reclining, belching, and increased intra-abdominal pressure.

Other common symptoms reflect possible complications:
- Dysphagia occurs when the hernia produces esophagitis, esophageal ulceration, or stricture, especially with ingestion of very hot or cold foods, alcoholic beverages, or a large amount of food.
- Bleeding may be mild or massive, frank or occult; the source may be esophagitis or erosions of the gastric pouch.

- Severe pain and shock result from incarceration, in which a large portion of the stomach is caught above the diaphragm (usually occurs with paraesophageal hernia). Incarceration may lead to perforation of the gastric ulcer and strangulation and gangrene of the herniated portion of the stomach. It requires immediate surgery.

Diagnosis

Diagnosis of hiatal hernia is based on typical clinical features and on the results of these laboratory studies and procedures:
- In barium study, hernia may appear as an outpouching containing barium at the lower end of the esophagus. Small hernias, however, are difficult to recognize. This study also shows diaphragmatic abnormalities.
- Endoscopy (esophagogastroduodenoscopy) and biopsy differentiate among hiatal hernia, varices, and other small gastroesophageal lesions; identify the mucosal junction and the edge of the diaphragm indenting the esophagus; and can rule out malignancy that otherwise may be difficult to detect.
- Esophageal motility studies assess the presence of esophageal motor abnormalities before surgical repair of the hernia.
- pH studies assess for reflux of gastric contents.

Treatment

The primary goals of treatment are to relieve symptoms by minimizing or correcting the incompetent cardia and to manage and prevent complications. Medical therapy is used first because symptoms usually respond to it and because hiatal hernia tends to recur after surgery. Such therapy attempts to modify or reduce reflux by changing the quantity or quality of refluxed gastric contents, by strengthening the LES muscle pharmacologically, or by decreasing the amount of reflux through gravity. These measures include restricting any activity that raises intra-abdominal pressure (coughing, straining, or bending), giving antiemetics, avoiding constrictive clothing, modifying diet, giving stool softeners or laxatives to prevent straining at stool, and discouraging smoking because it stimulates gastric acid production.

Modifying the diet means eating small, frequent, bland meals at least 2 hours before lying down (no bedtime snack), eating slowly, and avoiding spicy foods, fruit juices, alcoholic beverages, and coffee. Antacids also modify the fluid refluxed into the esophagus and are probably the best treatment for intermittent reflux.

To reduce the amount of reflux, the overweight patient should lose weight to decrease intra-abdominal pressure. Elevating the head of the bed 6″ (15 cm) reduces gastric reflux by gravity.

Drug therapy to strengthen cardiac sphincter tone may include a cholinergic agent or a GI stimulant to enhance smooth-muscle contraction, increase cardiac sphincter tone, and decrease reflux after eating.

Surgical repair is necessary when symptoms can't be controlled medically or with the onset of complications, such as stricture, bleeding, pulmonary aspiration, strangulation, or incarceration. Surgery typically involves creating an artificial closing mechanism at the gastroesophageal junction to strengthen the LES's barrier function. The surgeon may use an abdominal or a thoracic approach or he may repair the hernia by laparoscopic surgery, which allows for less dependence on a nasogastric (NG) tube and a shorter hospital stay.

Special considerations

To enhance compliance with treatment, teach the patient about this disorder. Explain treatments, diagnostic tests, and significant symptoms.

■ Prepare the patient for diagnostic tests as needed. After endoscopy, watch for signs of perforation (falling blood pressure, rapid pulse, shock, and sudden pain).

■ If surgery is scheduled, review preoperative and postoperative considerations with the patient.

■ After surgery, carefully record intake and output, including NG tube and wound drainage.

■ While the NG tube is in place, provide meticulous mouth and nose care, but don't manipulate the tube. Give ice chips, if permitted, to moisten oral mucous membranes.

■ If the surgeon used a thoracic approach, the patient may have chest tubes in place. Carefully observe chest tube drainage and the patient's respiratory status, and perform pulmonary physiotherapy.

■ Before discharge, tell the patient what foods he can eat, and recommend small, frequent meals. Warn against activities that cause increased intra-abdominal pressure, and advise a slow return to normal functions (within 6 to 8 weeks).

STOMACH, INTESTINE, AND PANCREAS

Gastritis

Gastritis, an inflammation of the gastric mucosa, may be acute or chronic. Acute gastritis produces mucosal reddening, edema, hemorrhage, and erosion. Chronic gastritis is common among elderly people and people with pernicious anemia. It typically occurs as chronic atrophic gastritis, in which all stomach mucosal layers are inflamed, with reduced numbers of chief and parietal cells. Acute or chronic gastritis can occur at any age.

Causes and incidence

Acute gastritis has numerous causes, including:

■ chronic ingestion of (or an allergic reaction to) irritating foods or beverages, such as hot peppers or alcohol

■ drugs, such as aspirin and other nonsteroidal anti-inflammatory agents (in large doses), cytotoxic agents, corticosteroids, antimetabolites, phenylbutazone, and indomethacin

■ ingestion of poisons, especially DDT, ammonia, mercury, carbon tetrachloride, and corrosive substances

■ endotoxins released from infecting bacteria, such as staphylococci, *Escherichia coli*, or salmonella.

Acute gastritis leading to stress ulcers also may develop in acute illnesses, especially when the patient has had major traumatic injuries; burns; severe infection; hepatic, renal, or respiratory failure; or major surgery.

Chronic gastritis may be associated with peptic ulcer disease or gastrostomy, both of which cause chronic reflux of pancreatic secretions, bile, and bile acids from the duodenum into the stomach. Recurring exposure to irritating substances, such as drugs, alcohol, cigarette smoke, or environmental agents, may also lead to chronic gastritis. Chronic gastritis may occur with pernicious anemia, renal disease, or diabetes mellitus. Pernicious anemia is commonly associated with atrophic gastritis, a chronic inflammation of the stomach resulting from degeneration of the gastric mucosa. In pernicious anemia, the stomach can no longer secrete intrinsic factor, which is needed for vitamin B_{12} absorption.

Bacterial infection with *Helicobacter pylori* is a common cause of nonerosive chronic gastritis. About 35% of adults are infected with *H. pylori*, but the prevalence of *H. pylori* infection in minority groups and in immigrants is much higher. Children ages 2 to 8 in developing nations acquire the infection at a rate of 10% per year; in the United States, the rate of yearly infection is less than 1%.

Signs and symptoms

After exposure to the offending substance, the patient with acute gastritis typically reports a rapid onset of symptoms, such as epigastric discomfort, indigestion, cramping, anorexia, nausea, vomiting, and hematemesis. The symptoms last from a few hours to a few days.

The patient with chronic gastritis may describe similar symptoms or may have only mild epigastric discomfort, or his complaints may be vague, such as an intolerance for spicy or fatty foods or slight pain relieved by eating. The patient with chronic atrophic gastritis may be asymptomatic.

Diagnosis

CONFIRMING DIAGNOSIS
Esophagogastroduodenoscopy or gastroscopy (with biopsy) confirms gastritis when done before lesions heal (usu-

ally within 24 hours). This test is contraindicated after ingestion of a corrosive agent.

Laboratory analyses can detect occult blood in vomitus or stool (or both) if the patient has gastric bleeding. Hemoglobin level and hematocrit are decreased if the patient has developed anemia from bleeding.

Treatment

Treatment for gastritis focuses on eliminating the cause; for example, bacterial gastritis is treated with antibiotics, whereas gastritis caused by ingested poison is treated by neutralizing the poison with the appropriate antidote. Histamine-2 (H_2) receptor antagonists may block gastric secretions. Many over-the-counter preparations are available. Antacids may be used as buffers.

For critically ill patients, antacids administered hourly, with or without H_2-receptor antagonists, may reduce the frequency of gastritis attacks. Some patients also require analgesics. Until healing occurs, patients' oxygen needs, blood volume, and fluid and electrolyte balance must be monitored.

When gastritis causes massive bleeding, treatment includes blood replacement; iced saline lavage, possibly with norepinephrine; angiography with vasopressin infused in normal saline solution; and, sometimes, surgery.

Vagotomy and pyloroplasty achieve limited success when conservative treatments fail. Rarely, partial or total gastrectomy may be required.

Simply avoiding aspirin and spicy foods may prevent exacerbations of chronic gastritis. If symptoms develop or persist, antacids may be taken. If pernicious anemia is the cause, vitamin B_{12} may be administered parenterally. A combination of bismuth and an antibiotic, such as amoxicillin, may relieve *H. pylori* infection, but eradication is difficult.

Special considerations

Patient care includes education and attention to various aspects of nutritional status to control symptoms and prevent their recurrence.

■ For vomiting, give antiemetics and I.V. fluids, as ordered. Monitor fluid intake and output and electrolyte levels.

■ Monitor the patient for recurrent symptoms as food is reintroduced; provide a bland diet.

■ Offer smaller, more frequent meals to reduce irritating gastric secretions. Eliminate foods that cause gastric upset.

■ Administer antacids and other prescribed medications, as ordered.

■ If pain or nausea interferes with the patient's appetite, give analgesics or antiemetics 1 hour before meals.

■ Tell the patient to avoid alcohol, caffeine, and irritating foods such as spicy or highly seasoned foods.

■ If the patient smokes, refer him to a smoking-cessation program.

■ Urge the patient to seek immediate attention for recurring symptoms, such as hematemesis, nausea, or vomiting.

■ Urge the patient to take prophylactic medications, as ordered. To reduce gastric irritation, advise the patient to take steroids with milk, food, or antacids. Instruct him to take antacids between meals and at bedtime and to avoid aspirin-containing compounds.

Gastroenteritis

A self-limiting disorder, gastroenteritis is characterized by diarrhea, nausea, vomiting, and acute or chronic abdominal cramping. Also called *intestinal flu, traveler's diarrhea, viral enteritis,* or *food poisoning,* it occurs in persons of all ages and is a major cause of morbidity and mortality in underdeveloped nations. In the United States, gastroenteritis ranks second to the common cold as a leading cause of lost work time and fifth as the leading cause of death among young children. It also can be life-threatening in elderly or debilitated people.

Causes and incidence

Gastroenteritis has many possible causes, including:

■ bacteria (responsible for acute food poisoning), such as *Staphylococcus aureus, Sal-* *monella, Shigella, Clostridium botulinum, C. perfringens,* and *Escherichia coli*

■ amebae, especially *Entamoeba histolytica*

■ parasites, such as *Ascaris, Enterobius,* and *Trichinella spiralis*

■ viruses (may be responsible for traveler's diarrhea) such as adenoviruses, echoviruses, or coxsackieviruses

■ ingestion of toxins, including plants or toadstools

■ drug reactions; for example, to antibiotics

■ enzyme deficiencies

■ food allergens.

The bowel reacts to any of these enterotoxins with hypermotility, producing severe diarrhea and secondary depletion of intracellular fluid. Chronic gastroenteritis is usually the result of another GI disorder such as ulcerative colitis.

Diarrhea accounts for as many as 3% of pediatric office visits and 10% of hospitalizations for patients younger than age 5. Each year, gastroenteritis affects every adult and accounts for 8 million physician visits and 250,000 hospitalizations. Traveler's diarrhea affects 20% to 25% of people traveling from industrialized countries to developing countries.

Signs and symptoms

Clinical manifestations vary depending on the pathologic organism and on the level of GI tract involved. However, gastroenteritis in adults is usually an acute, self-limiting, nonfatal disease producing diarrhea, abdominal discomfort (ranging from cramping to pain), nausea, and vomiting. Other possible signs and symptoms include fever, malaise, and borborygmi. In children, the elderly, and the debilitated, gastroenteritis produces the same symptoms, but these patients' intolerance to electrolyte and fluid losses leads to a higher mortality.

Diagnosis

Patient history can aid in the diagnosis of gastroenteritis. Stool culture (by direct rectal swab) or blood culture identifies the causative bacteria or parasites.

Treatment

Treatment is usually supportive and consists of bed rest, nutritional support, and increased fluid intake. When gastroenteritis is severe or affects a young child or an elderly or debilitated person, treatment may necessitate hospitalization, specific antimicrobials, I.V. fluid and electrolyte replacement and, possibly, antiemetics (given orally, I.M., or by rectal suppository).

Special considerations

Patient care includes education, administering medications, and assessing symptoms for signs of improvement or worsening.

- Administer medications as ordered; correlate dosages, routes, and times appropriately with the patient's meals and activities (for example, give antiemetics 30 to 60 minutes before meals).
- If the patient can eat, replace lost fluids and electrolytes with broth, ginger ale, and lemonade, as tolerated. Vary the diet to make it more enjoyable, and allow some choice of foods. Warn the patient to avoid milk and milk products, which may provoke recurrence.
- Record intake and output carefully and obtain serial weight measurements. Watch for signs of dehydration, such as dry skin and mucous membranes, fever, and sunken eyes.
- Wash your hands thoroughly after giving care to avoid spreading infection.
- To ease anal irritation, provide warm sitz baths or apply witch hazel compresses.
- If food poisoning is the likely cause of gastroenteritis, contact public health authorities so they can interview patients and food handlers, and take samples of the suspected contaminated food.
- Teach good hygiene to prevent recurrence. Instruct patients to cook foods — especially pork — thoroughly; to refrigerate perishable foods, such as milk, mayonnaise, potato salad, and cream-filled pastry; to always wash hands with warm water and soap before handling food, especially after using the bathroom; to clean utensils thoroughly; to avoid drinking water or eating raw fruit or vegetables when visiting a foreign country; and to eliminate flies and roaches in the home.

Peptic ulcers

Peptic ulcers — circumscribed lesions in the mucosal membrane — can develop in the lower esophagus, stomach, pylorus, duodenum, or jejunum. About 80% of all peptic ulcers are duodenal ulcers, which affect the proximal part of the small intestine.

Gastric ulcers, which affect the stomach mucosa, are most common in middle-aged and elderly men, especially in chronic users of nonsteroidal anti-inflammatory drugs (NSAIDs), alcohol, or tobacco. Duodenal ulcers usually follow a chronic course, with remissions and exacerbations; 5% to 10% of patients develop complications that necessitate surgery.

Causes and incidence

Researchers recognize three major causes of peptic ulcer disease: infection with *Helicobacter pylori* (formerly known as *Campylobacter pylori*), use of NSAIDs, and pathologic hypersecretory disorders such as Zollinger-Ellison syndrome. (See *How peptic ulcers develop.*)

How *H. pylori* produces an ulcer isn't clear. Gastric acid, which was considered a primary cause, now appears mainly to contribute to the consequences of infection. Ongoing studies should soon unveil the full mechanism of ulcer formation.

Salicylates and other NSAIDs encourage ulcer formation by inhibiting the secretion of prostaglandins (the substances that suppress ulceration). Certain illnesses, such as pancreatitis, hepatic disease, Crohn's disease, preexisting gastritis, and Zollinger-Ellison syndrome, are also known causes.

Besides peptic ulcer's main causes, several predisposing factors are acknowledged. They include blood type (gastric ulcers tend to strike people with type A blood; duodenal ulcers tend to afflict people with type O blood) and other genetic factors. Exposure to irritants, such as alcohol, coffee, and tobacco, may contribute by accelerating gastric acid emptying and promoting mucosal breakdown. Ulceration occurs when the acid secretion exceeds the buffering factors. Physical trauma, emotional stress, and normal aging are additional predisposing conditions.

PATHOPHYSIOLOGY
HOW PEPTIC ULCERS DEVELOP

Peptic ulcers can result from factors that increase gastric acid production or from factors that impair mucosal barrier protection.

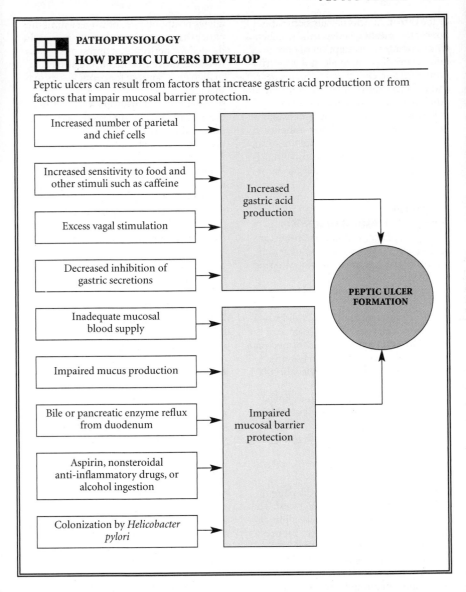

In the United States, about 1.6 million people acquire peptic ulcers yearly. Males and females are affected equally, and incidence increases with age. A higher percentage of *H. pylori* infection occurs in people older than age 50.

Signs and symptoms

Heartburn and indigestion usually signal the beginning of a gastric ulcer attack. Eat-ing stretches the gastric wall and may cause or, in some cases, relieve pain and feelings of fullness and distention. Other typical ef-fects include weight loss and repeated episodes of massive GI bleeding.

Duodenal ulcers produce heartburn, well-localized midepigastric pain (relieved by food), weight gain (because the patient eats to relieve discomfort), and a peculiar sensation of hot water bubbling in the back of the throat. Attacks usually occur about 2 hours after meals, whenever the stomach is empty, or after consumption of orange juice, coffee, aspirin, or alcohol. Exacerbations tend to recur several times per year and then fade into remission. Vomiting and other digestive disturbances are rare.

Ulcers may penetrate the pancreas and cause severe back pain. Other complications of peptic ulcers include perforation, hemorrhage, and pyloric obstruction. Ulcers may, on occasion, produce no symptoms.

Diagnosis

CONFIRMING DIAGNOSIS
Esophagogastroduodenoscopy confirms the presence of an ulcer and permits cytologic studies and biopsy to rule out H. pylori or cancer.

Diagnosis may be confirmed by the following tests:

- Barium swallow or upper GI and small-bowel series may reveal the presence of the ulcer. This is the initial test performed on a patient whose symptoms aren't severe.
- Laboratory analysis may detect occult blood in stools.
- Serologic testing may disclose clinical signs of infection such as an elevated white blood cell count.
- Carbon 13 (^{13}C) urea breath test results reflect activity of *H. pylori*.

Treatment

Experts recommend treating the patient with antibiotics to eradicate *H. pylori*. The patient taking NSAIDs may take a prostaglandin analog (misoprostol) to suppress ulceration (or the patient may take the analog with NSAIDs to prevent ulceration). Histamine-2 (H_2) receptor antagonists or proton pump inhibitors may reduce acid secretion. A coating agent or bismuth may be administered to the patient with a duodenal ulcer to protect the lining.

If GI bleeding occurs, emergency treatment begins with passage of a nasogastric (NG) tube to allow for iced saline lavage, possibly containing norepinephrine. Gastroscopy allows visualization of the bleeding site and coagulation by laser or cautery to control bleeding. This type of therapy

allows postponement of surgery until the patient's condition stabilizes. Surgery is indicated for perforation, unresponsiveness to conservative treatment, and suspected malignancy. Surgery for peptic ulcers may include:

- vagotomy and pyloroplasty: severing one or more branches of the vagus nerve to reduce hydrochloric acid secretion and refashioning the pylorus to create a larger lumen and facilitate gastric emptying
- distal subtotal gastrectomy (with or without vagotomy): excising the antrum of the stomach, thereby removing the hormonal stimulus of the parietal cells, followed by anastomosis of the rest of the stomach to the duodenum or the jejunum
- pyloroplasty: surgical enlargement of the pylorus to provide drainage of gastric secretions.

Special considerations

Management of peptic ulcers requires careful administration of medications, thorough patient teaching, and skillful postoperative care.

- Watch for adverse reactions to H_2-receptor antagonists and omeprazole (dizziness, fatigue, rash, and mild diarrhea).
- Advise any patient who uses antacids, who has a history of cardiac disease, or who follows a sodium-restricted diet to take only those antacids that contain low amounts of sodium.
- Warn the patient to avoid NSAIDs because they irritate the gastric mucosa. For the same reason, advise the patient to stop smoking and to avoid stressful situations, excessive intake of coffee, and drinking alcoholic beverages during exacerbations of peptic ulcer disease.

After gastric surgery:
- Keep the NG tube patent. If the tube isn't functioning, don't reposition it; you might damage the suture line or anastomosis. Notify the surgeon promptly.
- Monitor intake and output, including NG tube drainage. Check for bowel sounds, and allow the patient nothing by mouth until peristalsis resumes and the NG tube is removed or clamped.
- Replace fluids and electrolytes. Assess the patient for signs of dehydration, sodi-

um deficiency, and metabolic alkalosis, which may occur secondary to gastric suction.

- Monitor the patient for possible complications: hemorrhage; shock; iron, folate, or vitamin B_{12} deficiency anemia from malabsorption (pernicious anemia) due to lack of intrinsic factor causing malabsorption of vitamin B_{12}; and dumping syndrome (a rapid gastric emptying, causing distention of the duodenum or jejunum produced by a bolus of food). Signs and symptoms of dumping syndrome include diaphoresis, weakness, nausea, flatulence, explosive diarrhea, distention, and palpitations within 30 minutes after a meal.
- To avoid dumping syndrome, advise the patient to lie down after meals, to drink fluids *between* meals rather than with meals, to avoid eating large amounts of carbohydrates, and to eat four to six small, high-protein, low-carbohydrate meals during the day.

Ulcerative colitis

Ulcerative colitis is an inflammatory, usually chronic disease that affects the mucosa of the colon. It invariably begins in the rectum and sigmoid colon and commonly extends upward into the entire colon; it rarely affects the small intestine, except for the terminal ileum. Ulcerative colitis produces edema (leading to mucosal friability) and ulcerations. Severity ranges from a mild, localized disorder to a fulminant disease that may cause a perforated colon, progressing to potentially fatal peritonitis and toxemia.

Causes and incidence
Although the etiology of ulcerative colitis is unknown, it's thought to be related to abnormal immune response in the GI tract, possibly associated with food or bacteria such as *Escherichia coli*. Stress was once thought to be a cause of ulcerative colitis, but studies show that although it isn't a cause, it does increase the severity of the attack.

Ulcerative colitis occurs primarily in young adults, especially in women. It's also more prevalent among those of Jewish ancestry, indicating a possible familial tendency. The incidence of the disease is unknown; however, some studies indicate as many as 10 to 15 out of 100,000 persons have the disease. Onset of symptoms seems to peak between ages 15 and 30; another peak occurs between ages 50 and 70.

Signs and symptoms
The hallmark of ulcerative colitis is recurrent attacks of bloody diarrhea, in many cases containing pus and mucus, interspersed with asymptomatic remissions. The intensity of these attacks varies with the extent of inflammation. It isn't uncommon for a patient with ulcerative colitis to have as many as 15 to 20 liquid, bloody stools daily. Other symptoms include spastic rectum and anus, abdominal pain, irritability, weight loss, weakness, anorexia, nausea, and vomiting.

Ulcerative colitis may lead to complications, such as hemorrhage, stricture, or perforation of the colon. Other complications include joint inflammation, ankylosing spondylitis, eye lesions, mouth ulcers, liver disease, and pyoderma gangrenosum. Scientists think that these complications occur when the immune system triggers inflammation in other parts of the body. These disorders are usually mild and disappear when the colitis is treated.

Patients with ulcerative colitis have an increased risk of developing colorectal cancer; children with ulcerative colitis may experience impaired growth and sexual development.

Diagnosis
CONFIRMING DIAGNOSIS
Sigmoidoscopy showing increased mucosal friability, decreased mucosal detail, and thick inflammatory exudate suggests this diagnosis. Biopsy can help confirm it.

Colonoscopy may be required to determine the extent of the disease and to evaluate strictured areas and pseudopolyps. (Biopsy would then be done during colonoscopy.) Barium enema can assess the extent of the disease and detect complications, such as strictures and carcinoma.

A stool sample should be cultured and analyzed for leukocytes, ova, and parasites.

Other supportive laboratory values include decreased serum levels of potassium, magnesium, hemoglobin, and albumin as well as leukocytosis and increased prothrombin time. An elevated erythrocyte sedimentation rate correlates with the severity of the attack.

Treatment

The goals of treatment are to control inflammation, replace nutritional losses and blood volume, and prevent complications. Supportive treatment includes bed rest, I.V. fluid replacement, and a clear-liquid diet. For patients awaiting surgery or showing signs of dehydration and debilitation from excessive diarrhea, total parenteral nutrition (TPN) rests the intestinal tract, decreases stool volume, and restores positive nitrogen balance. Blood transfusions or iron supplements may be needed to correct anemia.

Immunomodulators or 5-aminosalicylates may be used to decrease the frequency of attacks. Drug therapy to control inflammation includes steroids. Antispasmodics and antidiarrheals are used only in patients whose ulcerative colitis is under control but who have frequent, loose stools.

ALERT *Antispasmodics and antidiarrheals may precipitate massive dilation of the colon (toxic megacolon) and are generally contraindicated.*

Surgery is the last resort if the patient has toxic megacolon, fails to respond to drugs and supportive measures, or finds symptoms unbearable. A common surgical technique is proctocolectomy with ileostomy. Another procedure, the ileoanal pull-through, is being performed in more cases. This procedure entails performing a total proctocolectomy and mucosal stripping, creating a pouch from the terminal ileum, and anastomosing the pouch to the anal canal. A temporary ileostomy is created to divert stool and allow the rectal anastomosis to heal. The ileostomy is closed in 2 to 3 months, and the patient can then evacuate stool rectally. This procedure removes all the potentially malignant epithelia of the rectum and colon. Total colectomy and ileorectal anastomosis isn't as common because of its mortality rate (2% to 5%). This procedure removes the entire colon and

anastomoses the terminal ileum to the rectum; it requires observation of the remaining rectal stump for any signs of cancer or colitis.

Pouch ileostomy (Kock pouch or continent ileostomy), in which the surgeon creates a pouch from a small loop of the terminal ileum and a nipple valve from the distal ileum, may be an option. The resulting stoma opens just above the pubic hairline and the pouch is emptied periodically through a catheter inserted in the stoma. In ulcerative colitis, a colectomy may be performed after 10 years of active disease because of the increased incidence of colon cancer in these cases. Performing a partial colectomy to prevent colon cancer is controversial.

Special considerations

Patient care includes close monitoring for changes in status.

- Accurately record intake and output, particularly the frequency and volume of stools. Watch for signs of dehydration and electrolyte imbalances, especially signs and symptoms of hypokalemia (muscle weakness and paresthesia) and hypernatremia (tachycardia, flushed skin, fever, and dry tongue). Monitor hemoglobin level and hematocrit, and give blood transfusions as ordered. Provide good mouth care for the patient who's allowed nothing by mouth.
- After each bowel movement, thoroughly clean the skin around the rectum. Provide an air mattress or sheepskin to help prevent skin breakdown.
- Administer medications, as ordered. Watch for adverse effects of prolonged corticosteroid therapy (moon face, hirsutism, edema, and gastric irritation). Be aware that corticosteroid therapy may mask infection.
- If the patient needs TPN, change dressings as ordered, assess for inflammation at the insertion site, and check capillary blood glucose levels every 4 to 6 hours.
- Take precautionary measures if the patient is prone to bleeding. Watch closely for signs of complications, such as a perforated colon and peritonitis (fever, severe abdominal pain, abdominal rigidity and tenderness, and cool, clammy skin) and toxic

megacolon (abdominal distention and decreased bowel sounds).

For the patient requiring surgery:
- Carefully prepare the patient for surgery, and inform him about ileostomy.
- Do a bowel preparation, as ordered.
- After surgery, provide meticulous supportive care and continue teaching correct stoma care.
- Keep the nasogastric tube patent. After removal of the tube, provide a clear-liquid diet and gradually advance to a low-residue diet, as tolerated.
- After a proctocolectomy and ileostomy, teach good stoma care. Wash the skin around the stoma with soapy water and dry it thoroughly. Apply karaya gum around the stoma's base to avoid irritation, and make a watertight seal. Attach the pouch over the karaya ring. Cut an opening in the ring to fit over the stoma, and secure the pouch to the skin. Empty the pouch when it's one-third full.
- After a pouch ileostomy, uncork the catheter every hour to allow contents to drain. After 10 to 14 days, gradually increase the length of time the catheter is left corked until it can be opened every 3 hours. Then remove the catheter and reinsert it every 3 to 4 hours for drainage. Teach the patient how to insert the catheter and how to take care of the stoma.
- Encourage the patient to have regular physical examinations.

Necrotizing enterocolitis

Necrotizing enterocolitis (NEC) is characterized by diffuse or patchy intestinal necrosis, accompanied by sepsis in about one-third of cases. Sepsis usually involves *Escherichia coli, Clostridia, Salmonella, Pseudomonas,* or *Klebsiella.* Initially, necrosis is localized, occurring anywhere along the intestine, but usually in the ileum, ascending colon, or rectosigmoid. If diffuse bleeding occurs, NEC usually results in disseminated intravascular coagulation (DIC).

Causes and incidence
The exact cause of NEC is unknown. Suggested predisposing factors include birth asphyxia, postnatal hypotension, respiratory distress, hypothermia, umbilical vessel catheterization, exchange transfusion, or patent ductus arteriosus. NEC may also be a response to significant prenatal stress, such as premature rupture of membranes, placenta previa, maternal sepsis, toxemia of pregnancy, or breech or cesarean birth.

NEC may develop when the infant suffers perinatal hypoxemia due to shunting of blood from the gut to more vital organs. Subsequent mucosal ischemia provides an ideal medium for bacterial growth. Hypertonic formula may increase bacterial activity because — unlike maternal breast milk — it doesn't provide protective immunologic activity and it contributes to the production of hydrogen gas. As the bowel swells and breaks down, gas-forming bacteria invade damaged areas, producing free air in the intestinal wall. This may result in fatal perforation and peritonitis.

NEC usually occurs in premature infants (less than 34 weeks' gestation) and those of low birth weight (less than 5 lb [2.3 kg]). NEC is more common in some geographic areas, possibly due to the higher incidence and survival of premature neonates and neonates who have low birth weights in these areas. Although the outcome is improved with aggressive, early treatment, it's a serious disease with a death rate of 25%.

Signs and symptoms
Neonates who have suffered from perinatal hypoxemia have the potential for developing NEC. A distended (especially tense or rigid) abdomen with gastric retention is the earliest and most common sign of oncoming NEC, which usually appears 1 to 10 days after birth. Other clinical features are increasing residual gastric contents (which may contain bile), bile-stained vomitus, and occult blood in the stool. About 25% of patients have bloody diarrhea. A red or shiny, taut abdomen may indicate peritonitis.

Nonspecific signs and symptoms include thermal instability, lethargy, metabolic acidosis, jaundice, and DIC. The major complication is perforation, which requires surgery. Recurrence of NEC and mechanical and functional abnormalities of the intestine, especially stricture, are the usual cause of residual intestinal malfunction in any infant who survives acute NEC; this complication may develop as late as 3 months postoperatively.

Diagnosis

Successful treatment of NEC relies on early recognition.

 CONFIRMING DIAGNOSIS Abdominal X-rays confirm the diagnosis, showing nonspecific intestinal dilation and, in later stages of NEC, pneumatosis cystoides intestinalis (gas or air in the intestinal wall).

Blood studies show several abnormalities. Platelet count may fall below 50,000/μl. Serum sodium levels are decreased, and arterial blood gas levels indicate metabolic acidosis (a result of sepsis). Infection-induced red blood cell breakdown elevates bilirubin levels. Blood and stool cultures identify the infecting organism, clotting studies and the hemoglobin level reveal associated DIC, and the guaiac test detects occult blood in the stool.

Treatment

The first signs of NEC necessitate removal of the umbilical catheter (arterial or venous) and discontinuation of oral intake for 7 to 10 days to rest the injured bowel. I.V. fluids, including total parenteral nutrition, maintain fluid and electrolyte balance and nutrition during this time; passage of a nasogastric (NG) tube aids bowel decompression. If coagulation studies indicate a need for transfusion, the infant usually receives dextran to promote hemodilution, increase mesenteric blood flow, and reduce platelet aggregation. Antibiotic therapy consists of parenteral agents — administered through an NG tube, if necessary — to suppress bacterial flora and prevent bowel perforation. Anteroposterior and lateral X-rays are repeated to monitor disease progression.

Surgery is indicated if the patient shows any of these signs or symptoms: signs of perforation (free intraperitoneal air on X-ray or symptoms of peritonitis), respiratory insufficiency (caused by severe abdominal distention), progressive and intractable acidosis, or DIC. Surgery removes all necrotic and acutely inflamed bowel

and creates a temporary colostomy or ileostomy. At least 12″ (30.5 cm) of bowel must remain or the infant may suffer from malabsorption or chronic vitamin B_{12} deficiency.

Special considerations

ALERT Be alert for signs or symptoms of gastric distention and perforation: apnea, cardiovascular shock, sudden drop in temperature, bradycardia, sudden listlessness, rag-doll limpness, increasing abdominal tenderness, edema, erythema, or involuntary abdominal rigidity.

■ To avoid perforating the bowel, don't take rectal temperatures.

■ Prevent cross-contamination by disposing of soiled diapers properly and washing your hands after diaper changes.

■ After surgery, the infant needs mechanical ventilation. Gently suction secretions, and assess his breathing often.

■ Replace fluids lost through NG tube and stoma drainage. Include drainage losses in output records. Weigh the infant daily. A daily weight gain of 10 to 20 g indicates a good response to therapy.

■ An infant with a temporary colostomy or ileostomy needs special care. Explain to the parents what a colostomy or ileostomy is and why it's necessary. Encourage them to participate in their infant's physical care after his condition is no longer critical.

■ Because of the infant's small abdomen, the suture line is near the stoma; as a result, keeping the suture line clean can be a problem. Good skin care is essential because the immature infant's skin is fragile and vulnerable to excoriation and the active enzymes in bowel secretions are corrosive. Improvise premature-sized colostomy bags from urine collection bags, medicine cups, or condoms. Karaya gum is helpful in making a seal. Watch for wound disruption, infection, and excoriation — potential dangers because of severe catabolism.

■ Watch for intestinal malfunction from stricture or short-gut syndrome. Such complications usually develop 1 month after the infant resumes normal feedings.

■ To help prevent NEC, encourage mothers to breast-feed because breast milk contains live macrophages that fight infection and has a low pH that inhibits the growth of many organisms. Also, colostrum — fluid secreted before the milk — contains high concentrations of immunoglobulin A, which directly protects the gut from infection and which the neonate lacks for several days postpartum. Tell mothers that they may refrigerate their milk for 48 hours but shouldn't freeze or heat it because this destroys antibodies. Tell them to use plastic — not glass — containers because leukocytes adhere to glass.

Crohn's disease

Crohn's disease, also known as *regional enteritis* and *granulomatous colitis,* is an inflammation of any part of the GI tract (usually the proximal portion of the colon or, less commonly, the terminal ileum) that extends through all layers of the intestinal wall. It may also involve regional lymph nodes and the mesentery. Granulomas are usually surrounded by normal mucosa; when these lesions are present in multiples, they're commonly referred to as *skip lesions.* The surface of the inflamed GI tract usually has a cobblestone appearance, which is different from alternating areas of inflammation and fissure crevices.

Causes and incidence
In Crohn's disease, lacteal blockage in the intestinal wall leads to edema and, eventually, inflammation, ulceration, and stenosis. Abscesses and fistulas may also occur.

Although the exact cause of Crohn's disease is unknown, autoimmune and genetic factors are thought to play a role. Up to 5% of those with the disease have one or more affected relatives; Jewish ancestry is also a risk factor. However, a pattern of Mendelian inheritance hasn't been identified.

The incidence of Crohn's disease has risen steadily over the past 50 years; it now affects 7 out of every 100,000 people. Crohn's disease is most prevalent in adults ages 20 to 40. It's two to three times more common in those of Jewish ancestry and least common in blacks.

Signs and symptoms
Clinical effects may be mild and nonspecific initially; they vary according to the location and extent of the lesion. Acute inflammatory signs and symptoms mimic appendicitis and include steady, colicky pain in the right lower quadrant, cramping, tenderness, flatulence, nausea, fever, and diarrhea. Bleeding may occur and, although usually mild, may be massive. Bloody stools may also occur.

Chronic symptoms, which are more typical of the disease, are more persistent and less severe; they include diarrhea (four to six stools per day) with pain in the right lower abdominal quadrant, steatorrhea (excess fat in feces), marked weight loss and, rarely, clubbing of fingers. The patient may complain of weakness and fatigue. Complications include intestinal obstruction, fistula formation between the small bowel and the bladder, perianal and perirectal abscesses and fistulas, intra-abdominal abscesses, and perforation.

Diagnosis
Barium enema showing the string sign (segments of stricture separated by normal bowel) supports a diagnosis of Crohn's disease. (See *The "string sign,"* page 712.) Sigmoidoscopy and colonoscopy may show patchy areas of inflammation, thus helping to rule out ulcerative colitis. However, biopsy is required for a definitive diagnosis.

Laboratory findings commonly indicate increased white blood cell count and erythrocyte sedimentation rate, hypokalemia, hypocalcemia, hypomagnesemia, and a decreased hemoglobin level.

Treatment
To control the inflammatory process, medications, such as 5-aminosalicylate, may be prescribed. Corticosteroids and immunomodulators may be prescribed if 5-aminosalicylate isn't effective or in patients with severe Crohn's disease. In debilitated patients, therapy includes total parenteral nutrition to maintain nutritional status while resting the bowel. If abscesses or fistulas occur, antibiotics may be prescribed. Infliximab (an antibody to tumor necrosis factor-alpha, an immune chemical that

THE "STRING SIGN"

The characteristic "string sign" (marked narrowing of the bowel), resulting from inflammatory disease and scarring, strengthens the diagnosis of Crohn's disease.

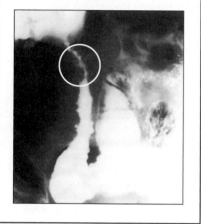

promotes inflammation) may also be prescribed.

Effective treatment requires important changes in lifestyle: physical rest, restricted diet (specific foods vary from person to person), and elimination of dairy products for lactose intolerance.

Surgery may be necessary to correct bowel perforation, massive hemorrhage, fistulas, or acute intestinal obstruction. Colectomy with ileostomy is necessary in many patients with extensive disease of the large intestine and rectum.

Special considerations

Although treatment is based largely on symptoms, you should monitor the patient's status carefully for signs of worsening.

- Record fluid intake and output (including the amount of stool), and weigh the patient daily. Watch for dehydration and maintain fluid and electrolyte balance. Be alert for signs of intestinal bleeding (bloody stools); check stools daily for occult blood.

- Check hemoglobin level and hematocrit regularly. Give iron supplements and blood transfusions, as ordered.
- Provide good patient hygiene and mouth care if the patient is restricted to nothing by mouth. After each bowel movement, give good skin care. Always keep a clean, covered bedpan within the patient's reach. Ventilate the room to eliminate odors.
- Observe the patient for fever and pain or pneumaturia, which may signal bladder fistula. Abdominal pain and distention and fever may indicate intestinal obstruction. Watch for stools from the vagina and an enterovaginal fistula.
- Before ileostomy, arrange for a visit by an enterostomal therapist.
- After surgery, frequently check the patient's I.V. and nasogastric tube for proper functioning. Monitor his vital signs and fluid intake and output. Watch for wound infection. Provide meticulous stoma care, and teach it to the patient and his family. Realize that ileostomy changes the patient's body image, so offer reassurance and emotional support.
- Stress the need for a severely restricted diet and bed rest, which may be trying, particularly for the young patient. Encourage him to try to reduce tension. If stress is clearly an aggravating factor, refer him for counseling.
- Refer the patient to a support group such as the Crohn's and Colitis Foundation of America.

Pseudomembranous enterocolitis

Pseudomembranous enterocolitis is an acute inflammation and necrosis of the small and large intestines, which usually affects the mucosa but may extend into submucosa and, rarely, other layers. Marked by severe diarrhea, this rare condition is generally fatal in 1 to 7 days due to severe dehydration and toxicity, peritonitis, or perforation.

Causes and incidence

The exact cause of pseudomembranous enterocolitis is unknown; however, *Clostridi-*

um difficile is thought to produce a toxin that may play a role in its development. Pseudomembranous enterocolitis has occurred postoperatively in debilitated patients who undergo abdominal surgery and in patients treated with broad-spectrum antibiotics. Whatever the cause, necrotic mucosa is replaced by a pseudomembrane filled with staphylococci, leukocytes, mucus, fibrin, and inflammatory cells.

Incidence of antibiotic-associated diarrhea varies from 5% to 39%, depending on the antibiotic. Pseudomembranous enterocolitis complicates 10% of these cases.

 PEDIATRIC TIP *Ampicillin is the most common antibiotic associated with pseudomembranous enterocolitis in children.*

Signs and symptoms

Pseudomembranous enterocolitis begins suddenly with copious watery or bloody diarrhea, abdominal pain, and fever. Serious complications, including severe dehydration, electrolyte imbalance, hypotension, shock, and colonic perforation, may occur in this disorder.

Diagnosis

Diagnosis is difficult in many cases because of the abrupt onset of enterocolitis and the emergency situation it creates, so consideration of patient history is essential. A rectal biopsy through sigmoidoscopy confirms pseudomembranous enterocolitis. Stool cultures can identify *C. difficile*.

Treatment

A patient receiving broad-spectrum antibiotic therapy must discontinue antibiotics at once. Effective treatment usually includes metronidazole. Oral vancomycin is usually given for severe or resistant cases. A patient with mild pseudomembranous enterocolitis may receive anion exchange resins, such as cholestyramine, to bind the toxin produced by *C. difficile*. Supportive treatment must maintain fluid and electrolyte balance and combat hypotension and shock with pressors, such as dopamine and levarterenol.

Special considerations

Careful observation for signs of worsening is essential.

■ Monitor the patient's vital signs, skin color, and level of consciousness. Immediately report signs of shock.

■ Record fluid intake and output, including fluid lost in stools. Watch for dehydration (poor skin turgor, sunken eyes, and decreased urine output).

■ Check serum electrolyte levels daily, and watch for clinical signs of hypokalemia, especially malaise, and a weak, rapid, irregular pulse.

Irritable bowel syndrome

Irritable bowel syndrome (IBS), also called *spastic colon* and *spastic colitis,* is a common condition marked by chronic or periodic diarrhea, alternating with constipation, and accompanied by straining and abdominal cramps. The prognosis is good. Supportive treatment or avoidance of a known irritant usually relieves symptoms.

Causes and incidence

This functional disorder is generally associated with psychological stress; however, it may result from physical factors, such as diverticular disease, ingestion of irritants (coffee, raw fruits or vegetables), lactose intolerance, laxative abuse, food poisoning, or colon cancer. Some patients may experience a disturbance in the movement of the intestine or a lower tolerance for stretching and movement of the intestine.

IBS affects 10% to 20% of U.S. residents and has a yearly incidence rate of 1% to 2%. The condition occurs most commonly in women ages 20 to 30.

Signs and symptoms

IBS characteristically produces lower abdominal pain (usually relieved by defecation or passage of gas) and diarrhea that typically occurs during the day. These symptoms alternate with constipation or normal bowel function. Stools are commonly small and contain visible mucus. Dyspepsia and abdominal distention may occur.

Diagnosis

Diagnosis of IBS requires a careful history to determine contributing psychological factors such as a recent stressful life change. Diagnosis must also rule out other disorders, such as amebiasis, diverticulitis, colon cancer, and lactose intolerance. Appropriate diagnostic procedures include sigmoidoscopy, colonoscopy, barium enema, rectal biopsy, and stool examination for blood, parasites, and bacteria.

Treatment

Therapy aims to relieve symptoms and includes counseling to help the patient understand the relationship between stress and his illness. Strict dietary restrictions aren't beneficial, but food irritants should be investigated and the patient should be instructed to avoid them. Rest and heat applied to the abdomen are helpful, as is judicious use of sedatives and antispasmodics. However, with chronic use, the patient may become dependent on these drugs. If the cause of IBS is chronic laxative abuse, bowel training may help correct the condition. Tegaserad may be prescribed for the patient with constipation-predominant IBS.

Special considerations

Because the patient with IBS isn't hospitalized, focus your care on patient teaching.
- Tell the patient to avoid irritating foods, and encourage him to develop regular bowel habits.
- Help the patient deal with stress, and warn against dependence on sedatives or antispasmodics.
- Encourage regular checkups because IBS is associated with a higher-than-normal incidence of diverticulitis and colon cancer. For patients older than age 40, emphasize the need for an annual sigmoidoscopy and rectal examination.

Celiac disease

Celiac disease (also known as *idiopathic steatorrhea, nontropical sprue, gluten enteropathy,* and *celiac sprue*) is characterized by poor food absorption and intolerance of gluten, a protein in wheat and wheat products. Malabsorption in the small bowel results from atrophy of the villi and a decrease in the activity and amount of enzymes in the surface epithelium. The prognosis is good with treatment (eliminating gluten from the patient's diet), but residual bowel changes may persist in adults.

Causes and incidence

In celiac disease, an intramucosal enzyme defect produces an inability to digest gluten. Resulting tissue toxicity produces rapid cell turnover, increases epithelial lymphocytes, and damages surface epithelium of the small bowel.

Celiac disease affects 1 of every 133 people in the United States and results from environmental factors and a genetic predisposition, but the exact mechanism is unknown. A strong association exists between the disease and two human leukocyte antigen haplotypes, DR3 and DQw2. It may also be autoimmune in nature. It affects twice as many females as males and occurs more commonly among relatives, especially siblings. This disease primarily affects whites and those of European ancestry.

Many diseases and conditions are associated with celiac disease, including:
- anemia
- lactose intolerance
- skin disorders such as dermatitis herpetiformis (a burning, itching, blistering rash)
- type 1 diabetes mellitus
- thyroid disease
- Down syndrome
- unexplained infertility or miscarriage
- osteoporosis or osteopenia
- autoimmune disorders, such as rheumatoid arthritis and systemic lupus erythematosus.

Signs and symptoms

Celiac disease produces clinical effects on many body systems:
- GI symptoms include recurrent attacks of diarrhea, steatorrhea, abdominal distention due to flatulence, stomach cramps, weakness, anorexia and, occasionally, in-

creased appetite without weight gain. Atrophy of intestinal villi leads to malabsorption of fat, carbohydrates, and protein as well as loss of calories, fat-soluble vitamins (A, D, and K), calcium, and essential minerals and electrolytes. In adults, celiac disease produces multiple nonspecific ulcers in the small bowel, which may perforate or bleed.

- Hematologic effects include normochromic, hypochromic, or macrocytic anemia due to poor absorption of folate, iron, and vitamin B_{12} and to hypoprothrombinemia from jejunal loss of vitamin K.
- Osteomalacia, osteoporosis, tetany, and bone pain (especially in the lower back, rib cage, and pelvis) are some of the musculoskeletal symptoms of celiac disease. These signs and symptoms are due to calcium loss and vitamin D deficiency, which weakens the skeleton, causing rickets in children and compression fractures in adults.
- Neurologic effects may include peripheral neuropathy, seizures, or paresthesia.
- Dry skin, eczema, psoriasis, dermatitis herpetiformis, and acne rosacea are some of the dermatologic effects of celiac disease. Deficiency of sulfur-containing amino acids may cause generalized fine, sparse, prematurely gray hair; brittle nails; and localized hyperpigmentation on the face, lips, or mucosa.
- Endocrine symptoms include amenorrhea, hypometabolism and, possibly, with severe malabsorption, adrenocortical insufficiency.
- Psychosocial effects include mood changes and irritability.

Symptoms may develop during the first year of life, when gluten is introduced into the child's diet as cereal. Clinical effects may disappear during adolescence and reappear in adulthood. One theory proposes that the age at which symptoms first appear depends on the strength of the genetic factor: A strong factor produces symptoms during the child's first 4 years; a weak factor, in late childhood or adulthood.

Diagnosis

 CONFIRMING DIAGNOSIS
Histologic changes seen on small-bowel biopsy specimens obtained with an esophagogastroduodenoscopy confirm the diagnosis: a mosaic pattern of alternating flat and bumpy areas on the bowel surface due to an almost total absence of villi and an irregular, blunt, and disorganized network of blood vessels. These changes appear most prominently in the jejunum.

An elevated alkaline phosphatase level may indicate bone loss, which is commonly experienced before diagnosis. Low cholesterol and albumin levels may reflect malabsorption and malnutrition. Mildly elevated liver enzymes and abnormal blood clotting may also be noted as well as anemia.

Antibody blood tests useful in screening for celiac disease include antiendomysial antibody (IgA), antitransglutaminase (IgA), antigliadin (IgA and IgG), and total serum IgA. Combined, these antibodies provide a sensitive and specific indicator for the presence of celiac disease.

Treatment

Treatment requires elimination of gluten from the patient's diet for life. Even with this exclusion, a full return to normal absorption and bowel histology may not occur for months or may never occur.

Supportive treatment may include supplemental iron, vitamin B_{12}, and folic acid; reversal of electrolyte imbalance (by I.V. infusion, if necessary); I.V. fluid replacement for dehydration; corticosteroids to treat accompanying adrenal insufficiency; and vitamin K for hypoprothrombinemia.

Special considerations

Explain the necessity of a gluten-free diet to the patient (and to his parents, if the patient is a child). Advise eliminating wheat, barley, rye, and oats as well as foods made from these grains, such as breads and baked goods; suggest substituting corn or rice. Consult a dietitian for nutritional instruction on a gluten-free diet. Depending on individual tolerance, the diet initially consists of proteins and gradually expands to include other foods. Assess the patient's acceptance and understanding of the disease, and encourage regular reevaluation.

ALERT *Because many foods contain hidden sources of gluten, food labels must be read carefully.*

■ Observe the patient's nutritional status and progress by daily calorie counts and weight checks. Also, evaluate his tolerance to new foods. In the early stages, offer small, frequent meals to counteract anorexia.

■ Assess the patient's fluid status: record intake, urine output, and number of stools (may exceed 10 per day). Watch for signs of dehydration, such as dry skin and mucous membranes, and poor skin turgor.

■ Check serum electrolyte levels. Watch for signs of hypokalemia (weakness, lethargy, rapid pulse, nausea, and diarrhea) and low calcium levels (impaired blood clotting, muscle twitching, and tetany).

■ Monitor prothrombin time, hemoglobin level, and hematocrit. Protect the patient from bleeding and bruising. Use the Z-track method to give iron I.M. If the patient can tolerate oral iron, give it between meals, when absorption is best. Dilute oral iron preparations, and give them through a straw to prevent staining teeth.

■ Protect the patient with osteomalacia from injury by keeping the bed side rails up and assisting with ambulation, as necessary.

■ Advise the patient to contact the Gluten Intolerance Group or the Associated Celiac Disease Foundation for information and support.

Diverticular disease

In diverticular disease, bulging pouches (diverticula) in the GI wall push the mucosal lining through the surrounding muscle. The most common site for diverticula is in the sigmoid colon, but they may develop anywhere, from the proximal end of the pharynx to the anus. Other typical sites are the duodenum, near the pancreatic border or the ampulla of Vater, and the jejunum. Diverticular disease of the stomach is rare and is usually a precursor of peptic or neoplastic disease. Diverticular disease

of the ileum (Meckel's diverticulum) is the most common congenital anomaly of the GI tract. (See *Meckel's diverticulum.*)

Diverticular disease has two clinical forms. In *diverticulosis,* diverticula are present but don't cause symptoms. In *diverticulitis,* diverticula are inflamed and may cause potentially fatal obstruction, infection, or hemorrhage.

Causes and incidence

In diverticulitis, retained undigested food mixed with bacteria accumulates in the diverticular sac, forming a hard mass (fecalith). This substance cuts off the blood supply to the thin walls of the sac, making them more susceptible to attack by colonic bacteria. Inflammation follows, possibly leading to perforation, abscess, peritonitis, obstruction, or hemorrhage. Occasionally, the inflamed colon segment may produce a fistula by adhering to the bladder or other organs.

Diverticula probably result from high intraluminal pressure on areas of weakness in the GI wall, where blood vessels enter. Diet may also be a contributing factor because insufficient fiber reduces fecal residue, narrows the bowel lumen, and leads to higher intra-abdominal pressure during defecation. The prevalence of diverticulosis in Western industrialized nations, where processing removes much of the roughage from foods, supports this theory. Diverticular disease is most prevalent in those older than age 40.

The incidence of diverticular disease increases with age, but 20% of patients are younger than age 50. Right-sided diverticulitis is most common in Asians, accounting for 75% of cases in that ethnic group. Left-sided diverticulitis is more common in Western countries, where it accounts for 70% of cases.

 ELDER TIP *About 50% of older adults develop diverticulosis. In elderly patients, a rare complication of diverticulosis (without diverticulitis) is hemorrhage from colonic diverticula. Such hemorrhage is usually mild to moderate and easily controlled, but may occasionally be massive and life-threatening.*

Signs and symptoms

Diverticulosis usually produces no symptoms, but may cause recurrent left lower quadrant pain, which is commonly accompanied by alternating constipation and diarrhea and is relieved by defecation or the passage of flatus. Symptoms resemble irritable bowel syndrome (IBS) and suggest that both disorders may coexist.

Mild diverticulitis produces moderate left lower abdominal pain, mild nausea, gas, irregular bowel habits, low-grade fever, and leukocytosis. In severe diverticulitis, the diverticula can rupture and produce abscesses or peritonitis, which occurs in up to 20% of such patients. Symptoms of rupture include abdominal rigidity and left lower quadrant pain. Peritonitis follows release of fecal material from the rupture site and causes signs of sepsis and shock (high fever, chills, and hypotension). Rupture of the diverticulum near a vessel may cause microscopic or massive hemorrhage, depending on the vessel's size.

Chronic diverticulitis may cause fibrosis and adhesions that narrow the bowel's lumen and lead to bowel obstruction. Symptoms of incomplete obstruction are constipation, ribbonlike stools, intermittent diarrhea, and abdominal distention. Increasing obstruction causes abdominal rigidity and pain, diminishing or absent bowel sounds, nausea, and vomiting.

Diagnosis

In many cases, diverticular disease produces no symptoms and is found during an upper GI series performed as part of a differential diagnosis.

 CONFIRMING DIAGNOSIS *Tests showing diverticular disease include computed tomography (reveals areas of inflammation), colonoscopy, sigmoidoscopy, and barium enema.*

Barium-filled diverticula can be single, multiple, or clustered and may have a wide or narrow mouth. Barium outlines — but doesn't fill — diverticula blocked by impacted feces. In patients with acute diverticulitis, a barium enema may rupture the bowel, so this procedure requires caution. If IBS accompanies diverticular disease, X-rays may reveal colonic spasm.

MECKEL'S DIVERTICULUM

In Meckel's diverticulum, a congenital abnormality — a blind tube, like the appendix — opens into the distal ileum near the ileocecal valve. This disorder results from failure of the intra-abdominal portion of the yolk sac to close completely during fetal development. It occurs in 2% of the population, mostly in males.

Uncomplicated Meckel's diverticulum produces no symptoms, but complications cause abdominal pain, especially around the umbilicus, and dark red melena or hematochezia. The lining of the diverticulum is gastric mucosa. This disorder may lead to peptic ulceration, perforation, and peritonitis and may resemble acute appendicitis.

Meckel's diverticulum may also cause bowel obstruction when a fibrous band that connects the diverticulum to the abdominal wall, the mesentery, or other structures snares a loop of the intestine. This may cause intussusception into the diverticulum or volvulus near the diverticular attachment to the back of the umbilicus or another intra-abdominal structure. Meckel's diverticulum should be considered in cases of GI obstruction or hemorrhage, especially when routine GI X-rays are negative.

Treatment consists of surgical resection of the inflamed bowel and antibiotic therapy if infection is present.

Biopsy rules out cancer; however, a colonoscopic biopsy isn't recommended during acute diverticular disease because of the strenuous bowel preparation it requires. Blood studies may show an elevated erythrocyte sedimentation rate in diverticulitis, especially if the diverticula are infected.

Treatment

Diverticulosis that doesn't produce symptoms generally doesn't necessitate treatment. Intestinal diverticulosis with pain, mild GI distress, constipation, or difficult defecation may respond to a liquid or bland diet, stool softeners, and occasional doses of mineral oil. These measures relieve symptoms, minimize irritation, and lessen the risk of progression to diverticulitis. After pain subsides, patients also benefit from a high-residue diet and bulk medication such as psyllium.

Treatment of mild diverticulitis without signs of perforation must prevent constipation and combat infection. It may include bed rest, a liquid diet, stool softeners, and a broad-spectrum antibiotic.

If diverticulitis is refractory to medical treatment, a colon resection is necessary to remove the involved segment. Perforation, peritonitis, obstruction, or fistula that accompanies diverticulitis may require a temporary colostomy to drain abscesses and rest the colon, followed by later reanastomosis 6 weeks to 3 months after initial surgery.

Special considerations

Management of uncomplicated diverticulosis chiefly involves thorough patient education about fiber and dietary habits.

■ Make sure that the patient understands the importance of dietary fiber and the harmful effects of constipation and straining during defecation. Encourage increased intake of foods high in indigestible fiber, including fresh fruits and vegetables, whole grain bread, and wheat or bran cereals. Warn that a high-fiber diet may temporarily cause flatulence and discomfort. Advise the patient to relieve constipation with stool softeners or bulk-forming cathartics. However, caution the patient against taking bulk-forming cathartics without plenty of water; if swallowed dry, they may absorb enough moisture in the mouth and throat to swell and obstruct the esophagus or trachea.

■ If the patient with diverticular disease is hospitalized, observe his stools carefully for frequency, color, and consistency, and keep accurate pulse and temperature charts because changes may signal developing inflammation or complications.

After surgery to resect the colon:
■ Watch for signs of infection.
■ Provide meticulous wound care because perforation may already have infected the area.
■ Check drain sites frequently for signs of infection (purulent drainage or foul odor) or fecal drainage.
■ Change dressings as necessary.
■ Encourage coughing and deep breathing to prevent atelectasis.
■ Watch for signs of postoperative bleeding (hypotension and decreased hemoglobin level and hematocrit).
■ Record intake and output accurately.
■ Keep the nasogastric tube patent.
■ Teach ostomy care as needed.
■ Arrange for a visit by an enterostomal therapist.

Appendicitis

Appendicitis is inflammation of the vermiform appendix due to an obstruction.

Causes and incidence

Appendicitis probably results from an obstruction of the appendiceal lumen caused by a fecal mass, stricture, barium ingestion, or viral infection. This obstruction sets off an inflammatory process that can lead to infection, thrombosis, necrosis, and perforation. If the appendix ruptures or perforates, the infected contents spill into the abdominal cavity, causing peritonitis, the most common and most perilous complication of appendicitis.

Appendicitis occurs more commonly in men than in women, with a peak incidence in the late teens and early 20s. About 250,000 cases are reported annually. It's a common cause of surgical emergency in children, with 4 appendectomies per 1,000 admissions for appendicitis annually in the United States.

Signs and symptoms

Typically, appendicitis begins with generalized or localized abdominal pain in the right upper abdomen, followed by anorexia, nausea, and vomiting (rarely profuse).

Pain eventually localizes in the right lower abdomen (McBurney's point) with abdominal "boardlike" rigidity, retractive respirations, increasing tenderness, increasingly severe abdominal spasms and, almost invariably, rebound tenderness. (Rebound tenderness on the opposite side of the abdomen suggests peritoneal inflammation.) Later signs and symptoms include constipation or diarrhea, slight fever, and tachycardia. The patient may walk bent over or lie with his right knee flexed to reduce pain. Sudden cessation of abdominal pain indicates perforation or infarction of the appendix.

Diagnosis

Diagnosis of appendicitis is based on physical findings and characteristic clinical symptoms. Supportive findings include a temperature of 99° to 102° F (37.2° to 38.9° C) and a moderately elevated white blood cell count (12,000 to 15,000/µl), with increased immature cells.

Diagnosis must rule out illnesses with similar symptoms: gastritis, gastroenteritis, ileitis, colitis, diverticulitis, pancreatitis, renal colic, bladder infection, ovarian cyst, and uterine disease. It may be strongly suspected based on abdominal sonography or computed tomography scan. Appendicitis can be confirmed by exploratory laparoscopy.

Treatment

Appendectomy is the only effective treatment. Laparoscopic appendectomies decrease the recovery time and thus the hospital stay. If peritonitis develops, treatment involves GI intubation, parenteral replacement of fluids and electrolytes, and administration of antibiotics.

Special considerations

If appendicitis is suspected, or during preparation for appendectomy:
- Administer I.V. fluids to prevent dehydration. *Never* administer cathartics or enemas, which may rupture the appendix. Give the patient nothing by mouth, and administer analgesics judiciously because they may mask symptoms.
- To lessen pain, place the patient in Fowler's position. *Never* apply heat to the

right lower abdomen; this may cause the appendix to rupture. An ice bag may be used for pain relief.

After appendectomy:
- Monitor the patient's vital signs and intake and output. Give analgesics, as ordered.
- Encourage the patient to cough, breathe deeply, and turn frequently to prevent pulmonary complications.
- Document bowel sounds, passing of flatus, and bowel movements. In a patient whose nausea and abdominal rigidity have subsided, these signs indicate readiness to resume oral fluids.
- Watch closely for possible surgical complications. Continuing pain and fever may signal an abscess. The complaint that "something gave way" may mean wound dehiscence. If an abscess or peritonitis develops, incision and drainage may be necessary. Frequently assess the dressing for wound drainage.
- Help the patient ambulate as soon as possible after surgery.
- In appendicitis complicated by peritonitis, a nasogastric tube may be needed to decompress the stomach and reduce nausea and vomiting. If so, record drainage and provide mouth and nose care.

Peritonitis

Peritonitis is an acute or chronic inflammation of the peritoneum, the membrane that lines the abdominal cavity and covers the visceral organs. Inflammation may extend throughout the peritoneum or may be localized as an abscess. Peritonitis commonly decreases intestinal motility and causes intestinal distention with gas. Mortality is 10%, with death usually a result of bowel obstruction; mortality was much higher before the introduction of antibiotics.

Causes

Although the GI tract normally contains bacteria, the peritoneum is sterile. When bacteria invade the peritoneum due to inflammation and perforation of the GI tract, peritonitis results. Bacterial invasion of the peritoneum typically results from appendicitis, diverticulitis, peptic ulcer, ulcerative colitis, volvulus, strangulated obstruction, abdominal neoplasm, or a stab wound. Peritonitis may also occur following chemical inflammation, as in the rupture of a fallopian or ovarian tube or the bladder, perforation of a gastric ulcer, or released pancreatic enzymes. It may also be associated with peritoneal dialysis.

In chemical and bacterial inflammation, accumulated fluids containing protein and electrolytes make the transparent peritoneum opaque, red, inflamed, and edematous. Because the peritoneal cavity is so resistant to contamination, infection is commonly localized as an abscess instead of disseminated as a generalized infection.

Signs and symptoms

The key symptom of peritonitis is sudden, severe, and diffuse abdominal pain that tends to intensify and localize in the area of the underlying disorder. For instance, if appendicitis causes the rupture, pain eventually localizes in the right lower quadrant. Many patients display weakness, pallor, excessive sweating, and cold skin as a result of excessive loss of fluid, electrolytes, and protein into the abdominal cavity. Decreased intestinal motility and paralytic ileus result from the effect of bacterial toxins on the intestinal muscles. Intestinal obstruction causes nausea, vomiting, and abdominal rigidity.

Other clinical characteristics include hypotension, tachycardia, signs and symptoms of dehydration (oliguria, thirst, dry swollen tongue, and pinched skin), an acutely tender abdomen associated with rebound tenderness, temperature of 103° F (39.4° C) or higher, and hypokalemia. Inflammation of the diaphragmatic peritoneum may cause shoulder pain and hiccups. Abdominal distention and resulting upward displacement of the diaphragm may decrease respiratory capacity. Typically, the patient with peritonitis tends to breathe shallowly and move as little as possible to minimize pain. He may lie on his back, with his knees flexed, to relax abdominal muscles.

Diagnosis

Severe abdominal pain in a person with direct or rebound tenderness suggests peritonitis. Abdominal X-rays or computed tomography scan showing edematous and gaseous distention of the small and large bowel support the diagnosis. In the case of perforation of a visceral organ, the X-ray shows air lying under the diaphragm in the abdominal cavity. Other appropriate tests include the following:

■ Chest X-ray may show elevation of the diaphragm.
■ Blood studies show leukocytosis (more than 20,000/μl).
■ Paracentesis reveals bacteria, exudate, blood, pus, or urine.
■ Laparotomy may be necessary to identify the underlying cause.

Treatment

Early treatment of GI inflammatory conditions and preoperative and postoperative antibiotic therapy help prevent peritonitis. After peritonitis develops, emergency treatment must combat infection, restore intestinal motility, and replace fluids and electrolytes.

Antibiotic therapy depends on the infecting organisms. If peritonitis is associated with peritoneal dialysis, antibiotics may be infused through the dialysis catheter; however, if the infection is severe, the catheter must be removed. To decrease peristalsis and prevent perforation, the patient should receive nothing by mouth; he should receive supportive fluids and electrolytes parenterally.

Other supplementary treatment measures include preoperative and postoperative administration of an analgesic, nasogastric (NG) intubation to decompress the bowel and, possibly, using a rectal tube to facilitate passage of flatus. When peritonitis results from perforation, surgery is necessary as soon as possible. Surgery aims to eliminate the source of infection by evacuating the spilled contents and inserting drains.

Special considerations

Patient care includes monitoring and measures to prevent complications and the spread of infection.

- Monitor the patient's vital signs, fluid intake and output, and amount of NG drainage or vomitus.
- Place the patient in semi-Fowler's position to help him deep-breathe with less pain and thus prevent pulmonary complications and to help localize purulent exudate in his lower abdomen or pelvis.

After surgery to evacuate the peritoneum:

- Maintain parenteral fluid and electrolyte administration, as ordered. Accurately record fluid intake and output, including NG tube and any drain output.
- Place the patient in semi-Fowler's position to promote drainage (through drainage tube) by gravity. Move him carefully because the slightest movement will intensify the pain.
- Implement other safety measures if fever and pain disorient the patient.
- Encourage and assist ambulation, as ordered, usually on the first postoperative day.
- Watch for signs of dehiscence (the patient may complain that "something gave way") and abscess formation (continued abdominal tenderness and fever).
- Frequently assess for peristaltic activity by listening for bowel sounds and checking for gas, bowel movements, and a soft abdomen.
- Gradually decrease parenteral fluids and increase oral fluids.

Intestinal obstruction

Intestinal obstruction is the partial or complete blockage of the lumen in the small or large bowel. Small-bowel obstruction is far more common (90% of patients) and usually more serious. Complete obstruction in any part of the bowel, if untreated, can cause death within hours from shock and vascular collapse. Intestinal obstruction usually occurs after abdominal surgery or in persons with congenital bowel deformities.

Causes

Adhesions and strangulated hernias usually cause small-bowel obstruction; large-bowel obstruction is typically due to carcinomas.

Mechanical intestinal obstruction results from foreign bodies (fruit pits, gallstones, or worms) or compression of the bowel wall due to stenosis, intussusception, volvulus of the sigmoid or cecum, tumors, or atresia. Nonmechanical obstruction results from physiologic disturbances, such as paralytic ileus, electrolyte imbalances, toxicity (uremia or generalized infection), neurogenic abnormalities (spinal cord lesions), and thrombosis or embolism of mesenteric vessels. (See *Paralytic ileus,* page 722.)

Intestinal obstruction develops in three forms:

- *Simple:* Blockage prevents intestinal contents from passing, with no other complications.
- *Strangulated:* The blood supply to part or all of the obstructed section is cut off, in addition to blockage of the lumen.
- *Close-looped:* Both ends of a bowel section are occluded, isolating it from the rest of the intestine.

The physiologic effects are similar in all three forms of obstruction: When intestinal obstruction occurs, fluid, air, and gas collect near the site. Peristalsis increases temporarily as the bowel tries to force its contents through the obstruction, injuring intestinal mucosa and causing distention at and above the site of the obstruction. Distention blocks the flow of venous blood and halts normal absorptive processes; as a result, the bowel begins to secrete water, sodium, and potassium into the fluid pooled in the lumen.

Obstruction in the small intestine results in metabolic alkalosis from dehydration and loss of gastric hydrochloric acid; lower bowel obstruction causes slower dehydration and loss of intestinal alkaline fluids, resulting in metabolic acidosis. Ultimately, intestinal obstruction may lead to ischemia, necrosis, and death. (See *Symptom progression in intestinal obstruction,* pages 724 and 725.)

ELDER TIP *Watch for air-fluid lock syndrome in older adults who remain recumbent for extended periods. In this syndrome, fluid first collects in the dependent bowel loops. Then peristalsis is too weak to push fluid "uphill." The resulting*

PARALYTIC ILEUS

Paralytic ileus is a physiologic form of intestinal obstruction that usually develops in the small bowel after abdominal surgery. It causes decreased or absent intestinal motility that usually disappears spontaneously after 2 to 3 days. Clinical effects of paralytic ileus include severe abdominal distention, extreme distress and, possibly, vomiting. The patient may be severely constipated or may pass flatus and small, liquid stools.

Causes

This condition can develop as a response to trauma, toxemia, or peritonitis or as a result of electrolyte deficiencies (especially hypokalemia) and the use of certain drugs, such as ganglionic blocking agents and anticholinergics. It can also result from vascular causes, such as thrombosis or embolism. Excessive air swallowing may contribute to it, but paralytic ileus brought on by this factor alone seldom lasts more than 24 hours.

Treatment

Paralytic ileus lasting longer than 48 hours requires intubation for decompression and nasogastric suctioning. Because of the absence of peristaltic activity, a long, weighted intestinal tube — called a *Miller-Abbott tube* — may be necessary in the patient with extraordinary abdominal distention. However, such procedures must be used with extreme caution because additional trauma to the bowel can aggravate ileus. When paralytic ileus results from surgical manipulation of the bowel, treatment may also include cholinergic agents, such as neostigmine or bethanechol.

When caring for patients with paralytic ileus, warn those receiving cholinergic agents to expect certain paradoxical adverse effects, such as intestinal cramps and diarrhea. Remember that neostigmine produces cardiovascular adverse effects, usually bradycardia and hypotension. Check frequently for returning bowel sounds.

---

obstruction primarily occurs in the large bowel.

Signs and symptoms

Colicky pain, nausea, vomiting, constipation, and abdominal distention characterize small-bowel obstruction. It may also cause drowsiness, intense thirst, malaise, and aching and may dry up oral mucous membranes and the tongue. Auscultation reveals bowel sounds, borborygmi, and rushes; occasionally, these are loud enough to be heard without a stethoscope. Palpation elicits abdominal tenderness, with moderate distention; rebound tenderness occurs when obstruction has caused strangulation with ischemia. In late stages, signs of hypovolemic shock result from progressive dehydration and plasma loss.

In complete small-bowel obstruction, vigorous peristaltic waves propel bowel contents toward the mouth instead of the rectum. Spasms may occur every 3 to 5 minutes and last about 1 minute each, with persistent epigastric or periumbilical pain. Passage of small amounts of mucus and blood may occur. The higher the obstruction, the earlier and more severe the vomiting. Vomitus initially contains gastric juice, then bile, and finally contents of the ileum.

Symptoms of large-bowel obstruction develop more slowly because the colon can absorb fluid from its contents and distend well beyond its normal size. Constipation may be the only clinical effect for days. Colicky abdominal pain may then appear suddenly, producing spasms that last less than 1 minute each and recur every few minutes. Continuous hypogastric pain and nausea may develop, but vomiting is usually absent at first. Large-bowel obstruction can cause dramatic abdominal distention; loops of the large bowel may become visible on the abdomen. Eventually, complete large-bowel obstruction may cause fecal vomiting, continuous pain, or localized peritonitis.

Patients with partial obstruction may display any of the previously discussed signs and symptoms in a milder form. However, leakage of liquid stool around the obstruction is common in partial obstruction.

Diagnosis

Progressive, colicky, abdominal pain and distention, with or without nausea and vomiting, suggest bowel obstruction.

CONFIRMING DIAGNOSIS *Tests that show obstruction include barium enema, abdominal computed tomography, upper GI and small bowel series, and abdominal films. Abdominal films show the presence and location of intestinal gas or fluid. In small-bowel obstruction, a typical "stepladder" pattern emerges, with alternating fluid and gas levels apparent in 3 to 4 hours. In large-bowel obstruction, barium enema reveals a distended, air-filled colon or a closed loop of sigmoid with extreme distention (in sigmoid volvulus).*

Laboratory results supporting this diagnosis include:
- decreased sodium, chloride, and potassium levels (due to vomiting)
- a slightly elevated white blood cell count (with necrosis, peritonitis, or strangulation)
- an increased serum amylase level (possibly from irritation of the pancreas by bowel loop).

Treatment

Preoperative therapy consists of correction of fluid and electrolyte imbalances, decompression of the bowel to relieve vomiting and distention, and treatment of shock and peritonitis. Strangulated obstruction usually necessitates blood replacement as well as I.V. fluid administration. Decompression of the intestine may be accomplished with the use of a nasogastric (NG) tube inserted into the stomach or intestine to relieve distension and vomiting.

Close monitoring of the patient's condition determines the duration of treatment; if he fails to improve or if his condition deteriorates, surgery is necessary. In large-bowel obstruction, surgical resection with anastomosis, colostomy, or ileostomy commonly follows decompression with an NG tube.

Total parenteral nutrition may be appropriate if the patient suffers a protein deficit from chronic obstruction, postoperative or paralytic ileus, or infection. Drug therapy includes analgesics, sedatives, and antibiotics for peritonitis due to bowel strangulation or infarction.

Special considerations

Effective management of intestinal obstruction, a life-threatening condition that commonly causes overwhelming pain and distress, requires skillful supportive care and keen observation.
- Monitor the patient's vital signs frequently. A drop in blood pressure may indicate reduced circulating blood volume due to blood loss from a strangulated hernia. Observe the patient closely for signs of shock (pallor, rapid pulse, and hypotension).
- Stay alert for signs and symptoms of metabolic alkalosis (changes in sensorium; slow, shallow respirations; hypertonic muscles; and tetany) or acidosis (shortness of breath on exertion, disorientation and, later, deep, rapid breathing, weakness, and malaise).
- Watch for signs and symptoms of secondary infection, such as fever and chills.
- Monitor the patient's urine output carefully to assess renal function, circulating blood volume, and possible urine retention caused by bladder compression by the distended intestine. If you suspect bladder compression, catheterize the patient for residual urine immediately after he has voided. Also, measure abdominal girth frequently to detect progressive distention.
- Provide mouth and nose care if the patient has vomited or undergone decompression by intubation. Look for signs of dehydration (thick, swollen tongue; dry, cracked lips; and dry oral mucous membranes).
- Record the amount and color of drainage from the decompression tube. Irrigate the tube with normal saline solution to maintain patency. If a weighted tube has been inserted, check periodically to make

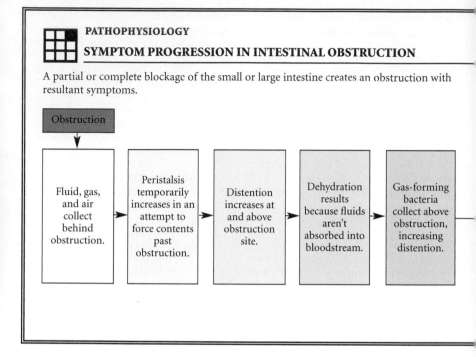

PATHOPHYSIOLOGY

SYMPTOM PROGRESSION IN INTESTINAL OBSTRUCTION

A partial or complete blockage of the small or large intestine creates an obstruction with resultant symptoms.

Obstruction →

| Fluid, gas, and air collect behind obstruction. | → | Peristalsis temporarily increases in an attempt to force contents past obstruction. | → | Distention increases at and above obstruction site. | → | Dehydration results because fluids aren't absorbed into bloodstream. | → | Gas-forming bacteria collect above obstruction, increasing distention. |

sure it's advancing. Help the patient turn from side to side (or walk around, if he can) to facilitate passage of the tube.

■ Keep the patient in Fowler's position as much as possible to promote pulmonary ventilation and ease respiratory distress from abdominal distention. Listen for bowel sounds, and watch for signs of returning peristalsis (passage of flatus and mucus through the rectum).

■ Explain all diagnostic and therapeutic procedures to the patient, and answer any questions he may have. Make sure that he understands that these procedures are necessary to relieve the obstruction and reduce pain. Tell him to lie on his left side for about a half hour before X-rays are taken.

■ Prepare the patient and his family for the possibility of surgery, and provide emotional support and positive reinforcement afterward. Arrange for an enterostomal therapist to visit the patient who has had an ostomy.

Inguinal hernia

A hernia occurs when part of an internal organ protrudes through an abnormal opening in the containing wall of its cavity. Hernias typically occur in the abdominal cavity. Although many kinds of abdominal hernias are possible, inguinal hernias (also called *ruptures*) are most common. (See *Common sites of hernia*, page 726.) In an inguinal hernia, the large or small intestine, omentum, or bladder protrudes into the inguinal canal. Hernias can be reduced (if the hernia can be manipulated back into place with relative ease), incarcerated (if the hernia can't be reduced because adhesions have formed, obstructing the intestinal flow), or strangulated (part of the herniated intestine becomes twisted or edematous, seriously interfering with normal blood flow and peristalsis, and possibly leading to intestinal obstruction and necrosis).

Causes and incidence

An inguinal hernia may be indirect or direct. An indirect inguinal hernia, the more

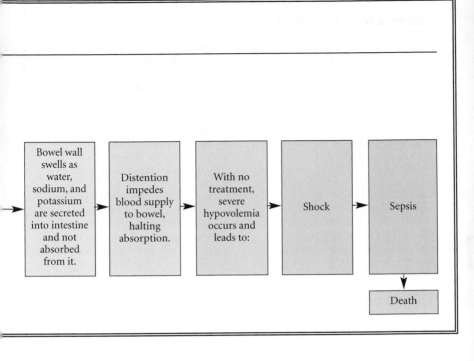

| Bowel wall swells as water, sodium, and potassium are secreted into intestine and not absorbed from it. | Distention impedes blood supply to bowel, halting absorption. | With no treatment, severe hypovolemia occurs and leads to: | Shock | Sepsis |

Death

common form, results from weakness in the fascial margin of the internal inguinal ring. In an indirect hernia, abdominal viscera leave the abdomen through the inguinal ring and follow the spermatic cord (in males) or round ligament (in females); they emerge at the external ring and extend down the inguinal canal, commonly into the scrotum or labia. An indirect inguinal hernia may develop at any age, is more common in males, and is especially prevalent in infants younger than age 1. According to the American Academy of Pediatrics, about 5 out of 100 children have inguinal hernias.

A direct inguinal hernia results from a weakness in the fascial floor of the inguinal canal. Instead of entering the canal through the internal ring, the hernia passes through the posterior inguinal wall, protrudes directly through the transverse fascia of the canal (in an area known as *Hesselbach's triangle*), and comes out at the external ring.

In males, during the seventh month of gestation, the testicle normally descends into the scrotum, preceded by the peri-toneal sac. If the sac closes improperly, it leaves an opening through which the intestine can slip. In either sex, a hernia can result from weak abdominal muscles (caused by congenital malformation, trauma, or aging) or increased intra-abdominal pressure (due to heavy lifting, pregnancy, obesity, or straining).

About 10% of people develop some type of hernia during their lifetime, and more than 500,000 hernia operations are performed in the United States each year. Hernias are seven times more common in males than in females.

Signs and symptoms

Inguinal hernia usually causes a lump to appear over the herniated area when the patient stands or strains. The lump disappears when the patient is supine. Tension on the herniated contents may cause a sharp, steady pain in the groin, which fades when the hernia is reduced. Strangulation produces severe pain and may lead to partial or complete bowel obstruction and even intestinal necrosis. Partial bowel obstruction may cause anorexia, vomiting,

COMMON SITES OF HERNIA

Femoral hernia occurs where the femoral artery passes into the femoral canal. Typically, a fatty deposit within the femoral canal enlarges and eventually creates a hole big enough to accommodate part of the peritoneum and bladder. A femoral hernia appears as a swelling or bulge at the pulse point of the large femoral artery. It's usually a soft, pliable, reducible, nontender mass, but commonly becomes incarcerated or strangulated.

Umbilical hernia results from abnormal muscular structures around the umbilical cord. This hernia is quite common in neonates, but also occurs in women who are obese or who have had several pregnancies. Because most umbilical hernias in infants close spontaneously, surgery is warranted only if the hernia persists for more than 4 or 5 years. Taping or binding the affected area or supporting it with a truss may relieve symptoms until the hernia closes. Severe congenital umbilical hernia allows the abdominal viscera to protrude

outside the body. This condition necessitates immediate repair.

Incisional (ventral) hernia develops at the site of previous surgery, usually along vertical incisions. This hernia may result from a weakness in the abdominal wall, perhaps as a result of an infection or impaired wound healing. Inadequate nutrition, extreme abdominal distention, or obesity also predispose the patient to incisional hernia. Palpation of an incisional hernia may reveal several defects in the surgical scar. Effective repair requires pulling the layers of the abdominal wall together without creating tension. If this isn't possible, surgical reconstruction uses Teflon, Marlex mesh, or tantalum mesh to close the opening.

Inguinal hernia can be direct or indirect. Indirect inguinal hernia causes the abdominal viscera to protrude through the inguinal ring and follow the spermatic cord (in males) or round ligament (in females). Direct inguinal hernia results from a weakness in the fascial floor of the inguinal canal.

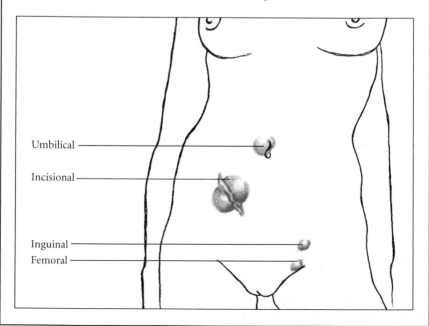

Umbilical

Incisional

Inguinal

Femoral

pain and tenderness in the groin, an irreducible mass, and diminished bowel sounds. Complete obstruction may cause shock, high fever, absent bowel sounds, and bloody stools. In an infant, an inguinal hernia commonly coexists with an undescended testicle or a hydrocele.

Diagnosis

In a patient with a large hernia, physical examination reveals an obvious swelling or lump in the inguinal area. In the patient with a small hernia, the affected area may simply appear full. Palpation of the inguinal area while the patient is performing Valsalva's maneuver confirms the diagnosis. To detect a hernia in a male patient, the patient is asked to stand with his ipsilateral leg slightly flexed and his weight resting on the other leg. The examiner inserts an index finger into the lower part of the scrotum and invaginates the scrotal skin so the finger advances through the external inguinal ring to the internal ring (about 1½″ to 2″ [4 cm to 5 cm] through the inguinal canal). The patient is then told to cough. If the examiner feels pressure against the fingertip, an indirect hernia exists; if pressure is felt against the side of the finger, a direct hernia exists.

A patient history of sharp or "catching" pain when lifting or straining may help confirm the diagnosis. Suspected bowel obstruction requires X-rays and a white blood cell count (may be elevated).

Treatment

If the hernia is reducible, the pain may be temporarily relieved by pushing the hernia back into place. A truss may keep the abdominal contents from protruding into the hernial sac; however, this won't cure the hernia. This device is especially beneficial for an elderly or debilitated patient for whom surgery might be hazardous.

For infants, adults, and otherwise healthy elderly patients, herniorrhaphy is the treatment of choice. Herniorrhaphy replaces the contents of the hernial sac into the abdominal cavity and closes the opening. In many cases, this procedure is performed under local anesthesia in a short-term unit or as a single-day admission. Another effective surgical procedure for re-

pairing hernia is hernioplasty, which reinforces the weakened area with steel mesh, fascia, or wire.

A strangulated or necrotic hernia necessitates bowel resection. Rarely, an extensive resection may require temporary colostomy. In either case, bowel resection lengthens postoperative recovery and requires antibiotics, parenteral fluids, and electrolyte replacement.

Special considerations

Care includes managing symptoms to increase patient comfort and prevent worsening.

- Apply a truss only after a hernia has been reduced. For best results, apply it in the morning, before the patient gets out of bed.
- To prevent skin irritation, tell the patient to bathe daily and apply cornstarch or baby powder. Warn against applying the truss over clothing because this reduces the effectiveness of the truss and may make it slip.
- If incarceration and strangulation occur, don't try to reduce the hernia because this may perforate the bowel. If severe intestinal obstruction develops because of hernial strangulation, inform the physician immediately. A nasogastric tube may be inserted promptly to empty the stomach and relieve pressure on the hernial sac.
- Before surgery for an incarcerated hernia, closely monitor the patient's vital signs. Administer I.V. fluids and analgesics, as ordered. Place the patient in Trendelenburg's position to reduce pressure on the hernia site.
- Give special reassurance and emotional support to a child and parents when hernia repair is scheduled. Encourage him to ask questions, and answer them as simply as possible. Offer appropriate diversions to distract him from the impending surgery.
- After outpatient surgery, make sure that the patient voids before he leaves the hospital. Teach him to check his incision and dressing for drainage, inflammation, or swelling and to watch for fever. If any of these occur, he should notify the physician.
- To reduce scrotal swelling, have the patient support the scrotum with a rolled towel and apply an ice bag.

- Instruct the patient to drink plenty of fluids to maintain hydration and prevent constipation.
- Before discharge, warn the patient against lifting heavy objects or straining during bowel movements. In addition, tell him to watch for signs and symptoms of infection (oozing, tenderness, warmth, and redness) at the incision site and to keep the incision clean and covered until the sutures are removed.
- Advise the patient not to resume normal activity or return to work without the surgeon's permission.

Intussusception

Intussusception is a telescoping (invagination) of a portion of the bowel into an adjacent distal portion. Intussusception may be fatal, especially if treatment is delayed for more than 24 hours.

Causes and incidence
When a bowel segment (the intussusceptum) invaginates, peristalsis propels it along the bowel, pulling more bowel along with it; the receiving segment is the intussuscipiens. This invagination produces edema, hemorrhage from venous engorgement, incarceration, and obstruction. If treatment is delayed for longer than 24 hours, strangulation of the intestine usually occurs, with gangrene, shock, and perforation.

Seasonal peaks — in the spring-summer, coinciding with peak incidence of enteritis, and in the midwinter, coinciding with peak incidence of respiratory tract infections — have been noted in the incidence of intussusception, suggesting a connection to viral infections. Other potential causes include a mass, such as a lymph node, polyp, or tumor that telescopes the gut and leads to intussusception.

Although it can affect adults, intussusception is most common in infants ages 6 months to 1 year. It occurs twice as often in male infants than in female infants.

Signs and symptoms
In an infant or child, intussusception produces four cardinal clinical effects:

- Intermittent attacks of colicky pain cause the child to scream, draw his legs up to his abdomen, turn pale and diaphoretic and, possibly, display grunting respirations.
- Vomiting of stomach contents may occur initially, followed by further vomiting of bile-stained or fecal material.
- "Currant-jelly" stools, containing a mixture of blood and mucus, may be observed.
- The patient will have a tender, distended abdomen, with a palpable, sausage-shaped abdominal mass; the viscera are usually absent from the right lower quadrant.

In adults, intussusception produces nonspecific, chronic, and intermittent symptoms, including colicky abdominal pain and tenderness, vomiting, diarrhea (occasionally constipation), bloody stools, and weight loss. Abdominal pain usually localizes in the right lower quadrant, radiates to the back, and increases with eating. Adults with severe intussusception may develop strangulation with excruciating pain, abdominal distention, and tachycardia.

Diagnosis
CONFIRMING DIAGNOSIS
Barium enema confirms colonic intussusception when it shows the characteristic coiled spring sign; it also delineates the extent of intussusception.

Upright abdominal X-rays may show a soft-tissue mass and signs of complete or partial obstruction, with dilated loops of bowel. Signs of dehydration or shock support the diagnosis, as does the presence of a palpable mass in the abdomen.

Treatment
In children, therapy may include hydrostatic reduction or surgery. Surgery is indicated for children with recurrent intussusception, for those who show signs of shock or peritonitis, and for those in whom symptoms have been present longer than 24 hours. In adults, surgery is always the treatment of choice.

During hydrostatic reduction, the radiologist drips a barium solution into the rectum from a height of no more than 3′ (1 m); fluoroscopy traces the progress of the barium. If the procedure is successful, the barium backwashes into the ileum, and the mass disappears. If not, the procedure is stopped, and the patient is prepared for surgery.

During surgery, manual reduction is attempted first. After compressing the bowel above the intussusception, the physician attempts to milk the intussusception back through the bowel. However, if manual reduction fails or if the bowel is gangrenous or strangulated, the physician will perform a resection of the affected bowel segment.

Special considerations

Care focuses on changes in the patient's condition that might indicate worsening.

■ Monitor the patient's vital signs before and after surgery. A change in temperature may indicate sepsis; infants may become hypothermic at the onset of infection. Rising pulse rate and falling blood pressure may be signs of peritonitis.

■ Check the patient's intake and output. Watch for signs of dehydration and bleeding.

■ A nasogastric (NG) tube is inserted to decompress the intestine and minimize vomiting. Monitor tube drainage and replace volume lost, as ordered.

■ Monitor the patient who has undergone hydrostatic reduction for passage of stools and barium, a sign that the reduction was successful. Keep in mind that the patient may have a recurrence of intussusception, usually within the first 36 to 48 hours after the reduction.

■ After surgery, administer antibiotics, as ordered. Closely check the incision for inflammation, drainage, or suture separation.

■ Encourage the patient to deep-breathe and cough productively. Be sure to splint the incision when he coughs, or teach him to do so himself.

■ The NG tube may be removed when bowel sounds and peristalsis resume. The patient's diet can be advanced as tolerated.

■ Check for abdominal distention after the patient resumes a normal diet and monitor his general condition.

■ Offer special reassurance and emotional support to the child and parents. This condition is considered a pediatric emergency, and parents are generally unprepared for their child's hospitalization and possible surgery; they may feel guilty for not seeking medical aid sooner. Similarly, the child is unprepared for a separation from his parents and home.

To minimize the stress of hospitalization, encourage parents to participate in their child's care as much as possible.

Volvulus

Volvulus is a twisting of the intestine at least 180 degrees on its mesentery, which results in blood vessel compression and ischemia.

Causes and incidence

Twisting in volvulus may result from an anomaly of rotation, an ingested foreign body, or an adhesion; in some cases, however, the cause is unknown. Volvulus usually occurs in a bowel segment with a mesentery long enough to twist. The most common area, particularly in adults, is the sigmoid; the small bowel is a common site in children. Other common sites include the stomach and cecum. Volvulus secondary to meconium ileus may occur in patients with cystic fibrosis.

Acute gastric volvulus has a mortality rate of 42% to 56%. There's no racial predilection, and it affects males and females equally. Peak incidence occurs in people ages 40 to 50, but about 20% of cases occur in infants younger than age 1.

Signs and symptoms

Vomiting and rapid, marked abdominal distention follow sudden onset of severe abdominal pain. Nausea, vomiting, bloody stools, constipation, and shock may occur. Without immediate treatment, volvulus can lead to strangulation of the twisted bowel loop, ischemia, infarction, perforation, and fatal peritonitis.

Diagnosis

The sudden onset of severe abdominal pain and physical examination that may reveal a palpable mass suggest volvulus. Appropriate tests include the following:

■ X-rays — Abdominal X-rays may show obstruction and abnormal air-fluid levels in the sigmoid and cecum; in midgut volvulus, abdominal X-rays may be normal.

- Computed tomography scan — may show evidence of intestinal obstruction.
- Barium enema — In cecal volvulus, barium fills the colon distal to the section of cecum; in sigmoid volvulus in children, barium may twist to a point and, in adults, it may take on an "ace of spades" configuration.
- Upper GI series (with small bowel follow-through) — In midgut volvulus, obstruction and possibly a twisted contour show in a narrow area near the duodenojejunal junction, where barium won't pass.
- White blood cell count — In strangulation, the count is greater than 15,000/µl; in bowel infarction, greater than 20,000/µl.

Treatment
Treatment varies according to the severity and location of the volvulus. For children with midgut volvulus, treatment is surgical. For adults with sigmoid volvulus, a proctoscopic examination is performed to check for infarction, and nonsurgical treatment includes reduction by careful insertion of a sigmoidoscope or a long rectal tube to deflate the bowel.

Success of nonsurgical reduction is indicated by expulsion of gas and immediate relief from abdominal pain. If the bowel is distended but viable, surgery consists of detorsion (untwisting); if the bowel is necrotic, surgery includes resection and anastomosis.

Special considerations
After surgical correction of volvulus:
- Monitor the patient's vital signs, watching for temperature changes (a sign of sepsis) and a rapid pulse rate and falling blood pressure (signs of shock and peritonitis). Carefully monitor fluid intake and output (including stools), electrolyte values, and complete blood count. Be sure to measure and record drainage from the nasogastric (NG) tube and drains.
- Encourage frequent coughing and deep breathing with splinting of the incision.
- Reposition the patient often and perform suction as needed.
- Record excessive or unusual drainage.
- Check for incisional inflammation and separation of sutures.

- When bowel sounds and peristalsis return, remove the NG tube and begin oral feedings with clear liquids, as ordered. When solid food can be tolerated, gradually expand the diet. Reassure the patient and his family appropriately, and explain all diagnostic procedures. If the patient is a child, encourage parents to participate in their child's care to minimize the stress of hospitalization.

Hirschsprung's disease

Hirschsprung's disease, also called *congenital megacolon* and *congenital aganglionic megacolon*, is a disorder of the large intestine characterized by an absence or a marked reduction of parasympathetic ganglion cells in the colorectal wall. This congenital disorder impairs intestinal motility and causes severe, intractable constipation. Without prompt treatment, an infant with colonic obstruction may die within 24 hours from enterocolitis that leads to severe diarrhea and hypovolemic shock. With prompt treatment, prognosis is good.

Causes and incidence
In Hirschsprung's disease, the aganglionic bowel segment contracts without the reciprocal relaxation needed to propel feces forward. In 90% of patients, this aganglionic segment is in the rectosigmoid area, but it occasionally extends to the entire colon and parts of the small intestine.

Hirschsprung's disease is believed to be a familial, congenital defect. It's up to 5 times more common in males than in females. The disease typically coexists with other congenital anomalies, particularly trisomy 21 and anomalies of the urinary tract such as megaloureter.

Signs and symptoms
Clinical effects usually appear shortly after birth, but mild symptoms may not be recognized until later in childhood or during adolescence (usually) or adulthood (rarely). The neonate with Hirschsprung's disease commonly fails to pass meconium within 24 to 48 hours, shows signs of obstruction (bile-stained or fecal vomiting and abdominal distention), irritability,

feeding difficulties (poor sucking and refusal to take feedings), failure to thrive, dehydration (pallor, loss of skin turgor, dry mucous membranes, and sunken eyes), and overflow diarrhea. The infant may also exhibit abdominal distention that causes rapid breathing and grunting. Rectal examination, which may temporarily relieve GI symptoms, reveals a rectum empty of stool and, when the examining finger is withdrawn, an explosive gush of malodorous gas and liquid stool. In infants, the main cause of death is enterocolitis, caused by fecal stagnation that leads to bacterial overgrowth, production of bacterial toxins, intestinal irritation, profuse diarrhea, hypovolemic shock, and perforation.

The older child has intractable constipation (usually requiring laxatives and enemas), abdominal distention, and easily palpated fecal masses. In severe cases, failure to grow is characterized by wasted extremities and loss of subcutaneous tissue, with a large protuberant abdomen.

Adult megacolon, although rare, usually affects men. Patients have abdominal distention, rectal bleeding (rare), and a history of chronic intermittent constipation. They're generally in poor physical condition.

Diagnosis

 CONFIRMING DIAGNOSIS *Rectal biopsy provides a definitive diagnosis by showing the absence of ganglion cells. Suction aspiration using a small tube inserted into the rectum may be performed initially. If this test yields inconclusive findings, diagnosis requires full-thickness surgical biopsy under general anesthesia. In older infants, barium enema showing a narrowed segment of distal colon with a sawtooth appearance and a funnel-shaped segment above it confirms the diagnosis and assesses the extent of intestinal involvement.*

Significantly, infants with Hirschsprung's disease retain barium longer than the usual 12 to 24 hours, so delayed films are usually helpful when other characteristic signs are absent. Other tests include rectal manometry, which detects failure of the internal anal sphincter to relax and contract, and upright plain films of the abdomen, which show marked colonic distention.

Treatment

Surgical treatment involves pulling the normal ganglionic segment through to the anus. However, corrective surgery is usually delayed until the infant is about 6 months old so that he's better able to withstand surgery. Postsurgical management should focus on reestablishing normal fluid and electrolyte balance, preventing bowel distention, and managing complications such as sepsis. Treatment measures include I.V. hydration, nasogastric decompression, and I.V. antibiotics as indicated. Management until the infant is old enough for surgery may consist of daily colonic lavage to empty the bowel. Physiologic saline solution should be used rather than tap water to prevent water intoxication. If total obstruction is present in the neonate, a temporary colostomy or ileostomy is necessary to decompress the colon. Antibiotics are given if the bowel has been perforated or if the infant has enterocolitis.

Special considerations

Before emergency decompression surgery:
- Maintain fluid and electrolyte balance, and prevent shock.
- Provide adequate nutrition, and hydrate with I.V. fluids, as needed. Transfusions may be necessary to correct shock or dehydration.
- Relieve respiratory distress by keeping the patient in an upright position (place an infant in an infant seat).

After colostomy or ileostomy:
- Monitor the patient's vital signs, watching for sepsis and enterocolitis (increased respiratory rate with abdominal distention).
- Monitor and record fluid intake and output (including drainage from ileostomy or colostomy) and electrolytes. Ileostomy is especially likely to cause excessive electrolyte loss. Also, measure and record nasogastric (NG) tube drainage and replace fluids and electrolytes, as ordered. Check stools carefully for excess water — a sign of fluid loss.
- If the infant is receiving hyperalimentation, check urine for specific gravity and

glucose (hyperalimentation may lead to osmotic diuresis).

■ To prevent aspiration pneumonia and skin breakdown, turn and reposition the patient often. Also, suction the nasopharynx frequently.

■ Keep the area around the stoma clean and dry, and cover it with dressings or a colostomy or ileostomy appliance to collect drainage. Use aseptic technique until the wound heals. Watch for prolapse, discoloration, or excessive bleeding. (Slight bleeding is common.) To prevent excoriation, use a powder, such as karaya gum, or a protective stoma disk.

■ Oral feeding can begin when bowel sounds return. An infant may tolerate predigested formulas best.

■ Teach parents to recognize the signs of fluid loss and dehydration (decreased urine output, sunken eyes, and poor skin turgor) and of enterocolitis (sudden marked abdominal distention, vomiting, diarrhea, fever, and lethargy).

■ Before discharge, if possible, make sure the parents consult with an enterostomal therapist for information on ostomy care.

Before corrective surgery:

■ As ordered, perform colonic lavage with normal saline solution to evacuate the colon. Keep accurate records of how much lavage solution is instilled. Repeat lavage until the return solution is completely free from fecal particles.

■ Administer antibiotics for bowel preparation, as ordered.

After corrective surgery:

■ Keep the wound clean and dry, and check for significant inflammation (some inflammation is normal). Don't use a rectal thermometer or suppository until the wound has healed. After 3 to 4 days, the infant will have a first bowel movement, a liquid stool, which will probably create discomfort. Record the number of stools.

■ Check urine for blood, especially in a boy; extensive surgical manipulation may cause bladder trauma.

■ Watch for signs of possible anastomotic leaks (sudden development of abdominal distention unrelieved by gastric aspiration, temperature spike, and extreme irritability), which may lead to pelvic abscess.

■ Begin oral feedings when active bowel sounds begin and NG tube drainage decreases. As an additional check, clamp the NG tube for brief, intermittent periods, as ordered. If abdominal distention develops, the patient isn't ready to begin oral feedings. Begin oral feedings with clear fluids, increasing bulk as tolerated.

■ Instruct parents to withhold foods that have increased the number of stools previously. Reassure them that their child will probably gain sphincter control and be able to eat a normal diet, but warn that complete continence may take several years to develop and that constipation may recur at times.

■ Because an infant with Hirschsprung's disease needs surgery and hospitalization so early in life, parents have difficulty establishing an emotional bond with their child. To promote bonding, encourage them to participate in their child's care as much as possible.

Inactive colon

Inactive colon, also known as *lazy colon, colonic stasis,* or *atonic constipation,* is a state of chronic constipation that, if untreated, may lead to fecal impaction.

Causes

Inactive colon usually results from some deficiency in the three elements necessary for normal bowel activity: dietary bulk, fluid intake, and exercise. It's common in bedridden people because of their inactivity and is generally relieved with diet and exercise. Other possible causes can include habitual disregard of the impulse to defecate, emotional conflicts, chronic use of laxatives, or prolonged dependence on enemas, which dull rectal sensitivity to the presence of feces.

Signs and symptoms

The primary symptom of inactive colon is chronic constipation. The patient commonly strains to produce hard, dry stools accompanied by mild abdominal discomfort. Straining can aggravate other rectal conditions such as hemorrhoids.

Diagnosis

A patient history of dry, hard, infrequent stools suggests inactive colon. A digital rectal examination reveals stool in the lower portion of the rectum and a palpable colon. Proctoscopy may show an unusually small colon lumen, prominent veins, and an abnormal amount of mucus. Diagnostic tests to rule out other causes include upper GI series, barium enema, and examination of stool for occult blood from neoplasms.

Treatment

Treatment varies according to the patient's age and condition. A higher-bulk diet, sufficient exercise, and increased fluid intake commonly relieve constipation. Treatment for severe constipation may include bulk-forming laxatives, such as psyllium, or well-lubricated glycerin suppositories; for fecal impaction, manual removal of feces is necessary. Administration of an oil-retention enema usually precedes removal; an enema is also necessary afterward. For lasting relief from constipation, the patient with inactive colon must modify bowel habits.

Special considerations

In many cases, patient education can help break the constipation habit.
- Advise the patient to drink at least 8 to 10 glasses (2 qt [2 L]) of liquid every day because fluids help keep the intestinal contents in a semisolid state for easier passage. This is particularly important for an older patient. Stimulate the bowel with a drink of hot coffee, warm lemonade, iced liquids — plain or with lemon — or prune juice before breakfast or in the evening.
- The patient should add fiber to the diet with foods such as whole grain cereals (rolled oats, bran, shredded wheat, brown rice, whole wheat bread, and oatmeal) to contribute bulk and induce peristalsis. However, too much bran can create an irritable bowel, so check labels on foods for fiber content (low fiber — 0.3 to 1 g; moderate fiber — 1.1 to 2 g; high fiber — 2.1 to 4.2 g). Increase the bulk content of the diet slowly to prevent flatulence, which can be a transient effect of a high-bulk diet. Include fresh fruits with skins as well as raw and coarse vegetables (broccoli, brussels sprouts, cabbage, cauliflower, cucumbers, lettuce, and turnips) in the diet for additional bulk.

- The patient should moderate his consumption of fat-containing foods, such as bacon, butter, cream, and oil; although these foods will help to soften intestinal contents, they sometimes cause diarrhea.
- Instruct the patient to avoid highly refined foods, such as white rice, cream of wheat, farina, white pastries, pie or cake, macaroni, spaghetti, noodles, candy, cookies, and ice cream.
- The patient should incorporate moderate exercise, such as walking, into his daily routine.
- Advise the patient to avoid overusing laxatives and to maintain a regular time for bowel movements (usually after breakfast). Autosuggestion, relaxation, pleasant reading material, privacy, and use of a small footstool to promote thigh flexion while sitting on the toilet may be helpful. The patient should respond promptly to the urge to defecate. If he worries about constipation, explain that a 2- to 3-day interval between bowel movements can be normal.
- The patient should take bulk-forming laxatives, such as psyllium, with at least 8 oz (240 ml) of liquid. Juices, soft drinks, or other pleasant-tasting liquids help mask the gritty texture of these laxatives.
- Advise the patient against overusing enemas. Frequent use of sodium biphosphate, in particular, is to be avoided because its hypertonic solution can absorb as much as 10% of the colon's sodium content or draw intestinal fluids into the colon, thereby causing dehydration.

ELDER TIP *If an older patient with inactive colon is hospitalized, help him move to a bedside commode for bowel movements because using a bedpan causes additional strain. However, if he must use a bedpan, have him sit in Fowler's position or sit on the pan at the side of his bed to facilitate elimination. Occasional digital rectal stimulation or abdominal massage near the sigmoid area may help stimulate a bowel movement.*

ALERT *If the patient has a history of arteriosclerosis, heart failure, or hypertension, constipation and straining may induce Valsalva's maneuver, thereby causing a vagal effect, in which the heart rate slows or stops entirely.*

CHRONIC PANCREATITIS

Chronic pancreatitis is associated with alcoholism in over 50% of patients, but can also follow hyperparathyroidism (causing hypercalcemia), hyperlipidemia or, infrequently, gallstones, trauma, or peptic ulcer. Inflammation and fibrosis cause progressive pancreatic insufficiency and eventually destroy the pancreas.

Symptoms of chronic pancreatitis include constant dull pain with occasional exacerbations, malabsorption, severe weight loss, and hyperglycemia (leading to diabetic symptoms). Diagnosis is based on the patient history, X-rays showing pancreatic calcification, an elevated erythrocyte sedimentation rate, and examination of stool for steatorrhea.

In many cases, the severe pain of chronic pancreatitis requires large doses of analgesics or opioids, making addiction a serious problem. Treatment also includes a low-fat diet and oral administration of pancreatic enzymes, such as pancreatin or pancrelipase, to control steatorrhea; insulin or oral hypoglycemics to curb hyperglycemia; and, occasionally, surgical repair of biliary or pancreatic ducts or the sphincter of Oddi to reduce pressure and promote the flow of pancreatic juice. The prognosis is good if the patient can avoid alcohol, but poor if he can't.

Pancreatitis

Pancreatitis, inflammation of the pancreas, occurs in acute and chronic forms and may be due to edema, necrosis, or hemorrhage. In men, this disease is commonly associated with alcoholism, trauma, or peptic ulcer; in women, it's linked to biliary tract disease. The prognosis is good when pancreatitis follows biliary tract disease, but poor when it follows alcoholism. Mortality rises as high as 60% when pancreatitis is associated with necrosis and hemorrhage. (See *Chronic pancreatitis.*)

Causes and incidence

The most common causes of pancreatitis are biliary tract disease and alcoholism, but it can also result from pancreatic cancer, trauma, or use of certain drugs, such as glucocorticoids, sulfonamides, chlorothiazide, and azathioprine. This disease also may develop as a complication of peptic ulcer, mumps, or hypothermia. Rarer causes are stenosis or obstruction of the sphincter of Oddi, hyperlipidemia, metabolic endocrine disorders (hyperparathyroidism and hemochromatosis), vasculitis or vascular disease, viral infections, mycoplasmal pneumonia, and pregnancy.

Diabetes, pancreatic insufficiency, and calcification occur in young people, probably from malnutrition and alcoholism, and lead to pancreatic atrophy. Regardless of the cause, pancreatitis involves autodigestion: The enzymes normally excreted by the pancreas digest pancreatic tissue. (See *Anatomy of the pancreas.*)

The incidence of acute pancreatitis varies with age. In the United States, it affects 270 of every 100,000 people ages 15 to 44 and 540 of every 100,000 people age 65 and older. It's uncommon in children. Blacks have a higher incidence than Whites. Males and females are affected equally. Among people with acquired immunodeficiency syndrome, it affects 4 to 22 people out of every 100.

Signs and symptoms

In many patients, the first and only symptom of mild pancreatitis is steady epigastric pain centered close to the umbilicus, radiating between the tenth thoracic and sixth lumbar vertebrae, and unrelieved by vomiting. However, a severe attack causes extreme pain, persistent vomiting, abdominal rigidity, diminished bowel activity (suggesting peritonitis), crackles at lung bases, and left pleural effusion. Progression produces extreme malaise and restlessness, with mottled skin, tachycardia, low-grade fever (100° to 102° F [37.7° to 38.8° C]), and cold, sweaty extremities. The proximi-

ANATOMY OF THE PANCREAS

Pancreatitis is an inflammation of the pancreas, involving irritation and infection of the organ. Obstruction or overdistention of the pancreatic duct can initiate the inflammation that occurs with pancreatitis. Exposure to toxins and other underlying causes can also initiate it. The overall effect is a release of activated pancreatic destructive enzymes into the pancreas and surrounding tissue.

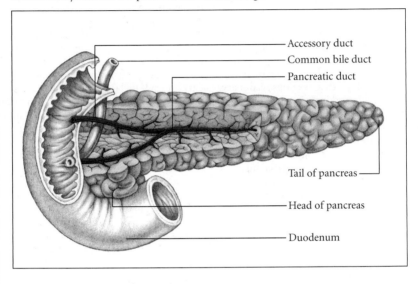

Accessory duct
Common bile duct
Pancreatic duct
Tail of pancreas
Head of pancreas
Duodenum

ty of the inflamed pancreas to the bowel may cause ileus.

If pancreatitis damages the islets of Langerhans, complications may include diabetes mellitus. Fulminant pancreatitis causes massive hemorrhage and total destruction of the pancreas, resulting in diabetic acidosis, shock, or coma.

Diagnosis

A thorough patient history (especially for alcoholism) and physical examination are the first steps in diagnosis, but the retroperitoneal position of the pancreas makes physical assessment difficult.

Dramatically elevated serum amylase levels — in many cases over 500 U/L — confirm pancreatitis and rule out perforated peptic ulcer, acute cholecystitis, appendicitis, and bowel infarction or obstruction. Similarly, dramatic elevations of amylase also occur in urine, ascites, or

pleural fluid. Characteristically, amylase levels return to normal 48 hours after the onset of pancreatitis, despite continuing symptoms.

Supportive laboratory values include:
- increased serum lipase levels, which rise more slowly than serum amylase
- low serum calcium levels (hypocalcemia) from fat necrosis and formation of calcium soaps
- white blood cell counts ranging from 8,000 to 20,000/µl, with increased polymorphonuclear leukocytes
- elevated glucose levels — as high as 500 to 900 mg/dl, indicating hyperglycemia.

Tests used to diagnose pancreatitis may include the following:
- Abdominal X-rays or computed tomography (CT) scans show dilation of the small or large bowel or calcification of the pancreas.

- Ultrasound or CT scan reveals an increased pancreatic diameter and helps distinguish acute cholecystitis from acute pancreatitis.

Treatment
The goal of therapy is to maintain circulation and fluid volume. Treatment measures must also relieve pain and decrease pancreatic secretions.

Emergency treatment of shock (which is the most common cause of death in early-stage pancreatitis) consists of vigorous I.V. replacement of electrolytes and proteins. Metabolic acidosis that develops secondary to hypovolemia and impaired cellular perfusion requires vigorous fluid volume replacement.

Drug treatment may include meperidine for pain, diazepam for restlessness and agitation, and antibiotics for bacterial infections. Morphine and codeine are usually avoided as pain medications because of their effect on the sphincter of Oddi. If the patient has hypocalcemia, he'll need an infusion of 10% calcium gluconate; if he has elevated serum glucose levels, he may require insulin therapy.

After the emergency phase, continuing I.V. therapy should provide adequate electrolytes and protein solutions that don't stimulate the pancreas for 5 to 7 days. If the patient isn't ready to resume oral feedings by then, total parenteral nutrition (TPN) may be necessary. Nonstimulating elemental gavage feedings may be safer because of the decreased risk of infection and overinfusion. In extreme cases, laparotomy to debride the pancreatic bed, partial pancreatectomy, or a combination of both and feeding jejunostomy may be necessary.

Special considerations
Acute pancreatitis is a life-threatening emergency, requiring meticulous supportive care and continuous monitoring of vital systems.
- Monitor the patient's vital signs and pulmonary artery pressure or central venous pressure closely. Give plasma or albumin, if ordered, to maintain blood pressure. Record fluid intake and output; check urine output hourly, and monitor electrolyte levels. Assess for crackles, rhonchi, or decreased breath sounds.
- For bowel decompression, maintain constant nasogastric suctioning, and give nothing by mouth. Perform good mouth and nose care.
- Watch for signs and symptoms of calcium deficiency—tetany, cramps, carpopedal spasm, and seizures. If you suspect hypocalcemia, keep airway and suction apparatus handy and pad side rails.
- Administer analgesics as needed to relieve the patient's pain and anxiety. Remember that anticholinergics reduce salivary and sweat gland secretions. Warn the patient that he may experience dry mouth and facial flushing. *Caution:* Narrow-angle glaucoma contraindicates the use of atropine or its derivatives.
- Monitor glucose levels.
- Watch for complications due to TPN, such as sepsis, hypokalemia, overhydration, and metabolic acidosis. Watch for fever, cardiac irregularities, changes in arterial blood gas measurements, and deep respirations. Use strict aseptic technique when caring for the catheter insertion site.

ANORECTUM

Hemorrhoids

Hemorrhoids are varicosities in the superior or inferior hemorrhoidal venous plexus. Dilation and enlargement of the superior plexus produce internal hemorrhoids; dilation and enlargement of the inferior plexus produce external hemorrhoids that may protrude from the rectum. (See *Types of hemorrhoids.*) Hemorrhoids occur in both sexes; incidence is usually highest between ages 20 and 50.

Causes and incidence
Hemorrhoids probably result from increased venous pressure in the hemorrhoidal plexus. Predisposing factors include occupations that require prolonged standing or sitting; straining due to constipation, diarrhea, coughing, sneezing, or vomiting; heart failure; hepatic disease,

TYPES OF HEMORRHOIDS

Covered by mucosa, *internal hemorrhoids* bulge into the rectal lumen and may prolapse during defecation. Covered by skin, *external hemorrhoids* protrude from the rectum and are more likely to thrombose than internal hemorrhoids. The illustrations below show frontal and cross-sectional views.

INTERNAL HEMORRHOIDS

EXTERNAL HEMORRHOIDS

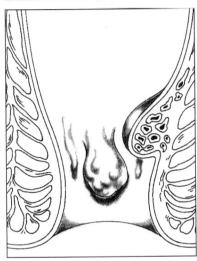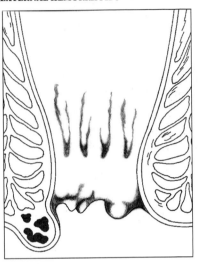

such as cirrhosis, amebic abscesses, or hepatitis; alcoholism; anorectal infections; loss of muscle tone due to old age, rectal surgery, or episiotomy; anal intercourse; and pregnancy.

Hemorrhoids are more common in whites, in persons of higher socioeconomic classes, and in persons who live in rural areas. However, actual incidence figures are unknown because many patients with hemorrhoids self-medicate.

Signs and symptoms

Although hemorrhoids may be asymptomatic, they characteristically cause painless, intermittent bleeding, which occurs on defecation. Bright red blood appears on stool or on toilet paper due to injury of the fragile mucosa covering the hemorrhoid. These first-degree hemorrhoids may itch because of poor anal hygiene. When second-degree hemorrhoids prolapse,

they're usually painless and spontaneously return to the anal canal following defecation. Third-degree hemorrhoids cause constant discomfort and prolapse in response to any increase in intra-abdominal pressure. They must be manually reduced. Thrombosis of external hemorrhoids produces sudden rectal pain and a subcutaneous, large, firm lump that the patient can feel. If hemorrhoids cause severe or recurrent bleeding, they may lead to secondary anemia with significant pallor, fatigue, and weakness; however, such systemic complications are rare.

Diagnosis

Physical examination confirms external hemorrhoids. Proctoscopy confirms internal hemorrhoids and rules out rectal polyps.

Treatment

Treatment depends on the type and severity of the hemorrhoid and on the patient's overall condition. Generally, treatment includes measures to ease pain, combat swelling and congestion, and regulate bowel habits. The patient can relieve constipation by increasing the amount of raw vegetables, fruit, and whole grain cereal in the diet or by using stool softeners. Venous congestion can be prevented by avoiding prolonged sitting; local swelling and pain can be decreased with local anesthetic agents (lotions, creams, or suppositories), astringents, or cold compresses, followed by warm sitz baths or thermal packs. Rarely, the patient with chronic, profuse bleeding may require a blood transfusion. Other nonsurgical treatments are injection of a sclerosing solution to produce scar tissue that decreases prolapse, manual reduction, and hemorrhoid ligation or laser ablation.

Hemorrhoidectomy, the most effective treatment, is necessary for patients with severe bleeding, intolerable pain and pruritus, and large prolapse. This procedure is contraindicated in patients with blood dyscrasias (acute leukemia, aplastic anemia, or hemophilia) or GI carcinoma and during the first trimester of pregnancy.

Special considerations

Patient care includes preoperative and postoperative support.

■ To prepare the patient for hemorrhoidectomy, administer an enema, as ordered (usually 2 to 4 hours before surgery), and record results. Prepare the area as ordered.

■ Postoperatively, check for signs of prolonged rectal bleeding, administer adequate analgesics, and provide sitz baths as ordered.

■ As soon as the patient can resume oral feedings, administer a bulk medication, such as psyllium, about 1 hour after the evening meal, to ensure a daily stool. Warn against using stool-softening medications soon after hemorrhoidectomy because a firm stool acts as a natural dilator to prevent anal stricture from the scar tissue. (The patient may need repeated digital dilation to prevent such narrowing.)

■ Keep the wound site clean to prevent infection and irritation.

■ Before discharge, stress the importance of regular bowel habits and good anal hygiene. Warn against too-vigorous wiping with washcloths and using harsh soaps. Encourage the use of medicated astringent pads and white toilet paper (the fixative in colored paper can irritate the skin).

Anorectal abscess and fistula

Anorectal abscess is a localized collection of pus due to inflammation of the soft tissue near the rectum or anus. Inflammation may produce an anal fistula — an abnormal opening in the anal skin — that may communicate with the rectum.

Causes and incidence

The inflammatory process that leads to abscess may begin with an abrasion or tear in the lining of the anal canal, rectum, or perianal skin and subsequent infection by *Escherichia coli*, staphylococci, or streptococci. Trauma may result from injections for treatment of internal hemorrhoids, enema-tip abrasions, puncture wounds from ingested eggshells or fish bones, or insertion of foreign objects. Other preexisting lesions include infected anal fissure, infections from the anal crypt through the anal gland, ruptured anal hematoma, prolapsed thrombosed internal hemorrhoids, and septic lesions in the pelvis, such as acute appendicitis, acute salpingitis, and diverticulitis. Systemic illnesses that may cause abscesses include ulcerative colitis and Crohn's disease. However, many abscesses develop without preexisting lesions.

As the abscess produces more pus, a fistula may form in the soft tissue beneath the muscle fibers of the sphincters (especially the external sphincter), usually extending into the perianal skin. The internal (primary) opening of the abscess or fistula is usually near the anal glands and crypts; the external (secondary) opening, in the perianal skin.

The peak incidence of anorectal abscess occurs in people in their 30s and 40s, but there's also a high occurrence in infants.

Men are affected two to three times more often than women. About 30% of patients have a previous history of abscess.

Signs and symptoms

Characteristics are throbbing pain and tenderness at the site of the abscess. A hard, painful lump develops on one side, preventing comfortable sitting. Discharge of pus may occur from the rectum, and there may be constipation or pain associated with bowel movements.

Diagnosis

Anorectal abscess is detectable on physical examination. If the abscess drains by forming a fistula, the pain usually subsides and the major signs become pruritic drainage and subsequent perianal irritation. The external opening of a fistula generally appears as a pink or red, elevated, discharging sinus or ulcer on the skin near the anus. Depending on the infection's severity, the patient may have chills, fever, nausea, vomiting, and malaise. Digital examination may reveal a palpable indurated tract and a drop or two of pus on palpation. The internal opening may be palpated as a depression or ulcer in the midline anteriorly or at the dentate line posteriorly. Examination with a probe may require an anesthetic. A proctosigmoidoscopy may be performed to exclude associated diseases.

Treatment

Anorectal abscesses require surgical incision under caudal anesthesia to promote drainage. Fistulas require a fistulotomy — removal of the fistula and associated granulation tissue — under caudal anesthesia. If the fistula tract is epithelialized, treatment requires fistulectomy — removal of the fistulous tract — followed by insertion of drains, which remain in place for 48 hours. Warm sitz baths are useful to relieve inflammation; however, pain medication and antibiotics may be needed.

Special considerations

After incision to drain anorectal abscess, follow these guidelines:
- Provide adequate medication for pain relief, as ordered.

- Examine the wound frequently to assess proper healing, which should progress from the inside out. Healing should be complete in 4 to 5 weeks for perianal fistulas; in 12 to 16 weeks for deeper wounds.
- Inform the patient that complete recovery takes time, and offer encouragement.
- Stress the importance of perianal cleanliness.
- Be alert for the first postoperative bowel movement. The patient may suppress the urge to defecate because of anticipated pain; the resulting constipation increases pressure at the wound site. Such a patient benefits from a stool-softening laxative.

Rectal polyps

Rectal polyps are masses of tissue that rise above the mucosal membrane and protrude into the GI tract. Types of polyps include common polypoid adenomas, villous adenomas, hereditary polyposis, focal polypoid hyperplasia, and juvenile polyps (hamartomas). Most rectal polyps are benign; however, villous and hereditary polyps show a marked inclination to become malignant. Indeed, a striking feature of familial polyposis is that it's commonly associated with rectosigmoid adenocarcinoma.

Causes and incidence

Formation of polyps results from unrestrained cell growth in the upper epithelium. Predisposing factors include heredity, age, infection, and diet.

Villous adenomas are most prevalent in men older than age 55; common polypoid adenomas, in white women between ages 45 and 60. Incidence in both sexes rises after age 70. Juvenile polyps usually occur among children younger than age 10 and are characterized by rectal bleeding.

Signs and symptoms

Because rectal polyps don't generally cause symptoms, they're usually discovered incidentally during a digital examination or rectosigmoidoscopy. Rectal bleeding is a common sign; high rectal polyps leave a streak of blood on the stool, whereas low rectal polyps bleed freely.

Rectal polyps vary in appearance. Common polypoid adenomas are small, multiple lesions that are redder than normal mucosa. They're commonly pedunculated (attached to rectal mucosa by a long, thin stalk) and granular, with a red, lobular, or eroded surface.

Villous adenomas are usually sessile (attached to the mucosa by a wide base) and vary in size from 0.5 to 12 cm. They are soft, friable, and finely lobulated. They may grow large and cause painful defecation; however, because adenomas are soft, they rarely cause bowel obstruction. Sometimes adenomas prolapse outside the anus, expelling parts of the adenoma with feces. These polyps may cause diarrhea, bloody stools, and subsequent fluid and electrolyte depletion, with hypotension and oliguria.

In hereditary polyposis, rectal polyps resemble benign adenomas but occur as hundreds of small (0.5 cm) lesions carpeting the entire mucosal surface. Associated signs include diarrhea, bloody stools, and secondary anemia. In patients with hereditary polyposis, changes in bowel habits with abdominal pain usually signal rectosigmoid cancer.

Juvenile polyps are large, inflammatory lesions, commonly without an epithelial covering. Mucus-filled cysts cover their usually smooth surface.

Focal polypoid hyperplasia produces small (less than 3 mm), granular, sessile lesions, similar to the colon in color, or gray or translucent. They usually occur at the rectosigmoid junction.

Diagnosis

CONFIRMING DIAGNOSIS *Firm diagnosis of rectal polyps requires identification of the polyps through proctosigmoidoscopy or colonoscopy and rectal biopsy.*

Barium enema can help identify polyps that are located high in the colon. Supportive laboratory findings include occult blood in the stools, low hemoglobin level and hematocrit (with anemia) and, possibly, serum electrolyte imbalances in patients with villous adenomas.

Treatment

Treatment varies according to the type and size of the polyps and their location in the colon. Common polypoid adenomas less than 1 cm require polypectomy, usually by fulguration (destruction by high-frequency electricity) during endoscopy. For common polypoid adenomas over 4 cm and all invasive villous adenomas, treatment usually consists of abdominoperineal resection or low anterior resection.

Focal polypoid hyperplasia can be obliterated by biopsy. Depending on GI involvement, hereditary polyps necessitate total abdominoperineal resection with a permanent ileostomy, subtotal colectomy with ileoproctostomy, or ileoanal anastomosis. Juvenile polyps are prone to autoamputation; if this doesn't occur, snare removal during colonoscopy is the treatment of choice.

Special considerations

During diagnostic evaluation:
- Check sodium, potassium, and chloride levels daily in the patient with fluid imbalances; adjust fluid and electrolytes, as necessary. Administer normal saline solution with potassium I.V., as ordered. Weigh the patient daily, and record the amount of diarrhea. Watch for signs of dehydration (decreased urine and increased blood urea nitrogen levels).
- Tell the patient to watch for and report evidence of rectal bleeding.

After biopsy and fulguration:
- Check for signs of perforation and hemorrhage, such as sudden hypotension, a decrease in hemoglobin level or hematocrit, shock, abdominal pain, and passage of red blood through the rectum.
- Have the patient walk as soon as possible after the procedure.
- Watch for and record the first bowel movement, which may not occur for 2 to 3 days.
- Provide sitz baths for 3 days.
- If the patient has benign polyps, stress the need for routine follow-up studies to check the polypoid growth rate.
- Prepare the patient with precancerous or familial lesions for abdominoperineal resection. Provide emotional support and preoperative instruction.

After ileostomy or subtotal colectomy with ileoproctostomy:
- Properly care for abdominal dressings, I.V. lines, and indwelling urinary catheters. Record intake and output, and check the patient's vital signs for hypotension and surgical complications. Administer pain medication, as ordered.
- To prevent embolism, have the patient walk as soon as possible, and apply antiembolism stockings; encourage range-of-motion exercises.
- Provide enterostomal therapy and teach the patient stoma care.

Anorectal stricture

In anorectal stricture, also known as *anorectal stenosis* or *contracture,* the anorectal lumen size decreases and stenosis prevents dilation of the sphincter.

Causes
Anorectal stricture results from scarring after anorectal surgery or inflammation, inadequate postoperative care, or laxative abuse.

Signs and symptoms
The patient with anorectal stricture strains excessively when defecating and is unable to completely evacuate his bowel. Other clinical effects include pain, bleeding, and pruritus ani.

Diagnosis
Visual inspection reveals narrowing of the anal canal. Digital examination reveals tenderness and tightness.

Treatment
Surgical removal of scar tissue is the most effective treatment. Digital or instrumental dilatation may be beneficial; however, this procedure may need to be repeated frequently and may cause additional tears and splits. If the cause of stricture is inflammation, correction of the underlying inflammatory process is necessary.

Special considerations
Patient care consists of preoperative and postoperative support.

- Prepare the patient for the digital examination and testing by explaining procedures thoroughly.
- After surgery, check the patient's vital signs often until he's stable. Watch for signs of hemorrhage (excessive bleeding on rectal dressing).
- If surgery was performed under spinal anesthesia, record the first leg motion, and keep the patient lying flat for 6 to 8 hours after surgery.
- When the patient's condition is stable, resume his normal diet, and record the time of his first bowel movement. Administer stool softeners, as ordered. Give analgesics, provide sitz baths, and change the perianal dressing, as ordered.

Pilonidal disease

In pilonidal disease, a coccygeal cyst forms in the intergluteal cleft on the posterior surface of the lower sacrum. It usually contains hair and becomes infected, producing an abscess, a draining sinus, or a fistula. Incidence is highest among hirsute white men ages 18 to 30.

Causes and incidence
Pilonidal disease may develop congenitally from a tendency to hirsutism, or it may be acquired from stretching or irritation of the sacrococcygeal area (intergluteal fold) from prolonged rough exercise (such as horseback riding), heat, excessive perspiration, or constrictive clothing.

The incidence rate of pilonidal disease is 0.7%. It affects males two to four times more often than females, but the onset is earlier in females, possibly because they begin puberty at an earlier age.

Signs and symptoms
Generally, a pilonidal cyst produces no symptoms until it becomes infected, causing local pain, tenderness, swelling, or heat. Other clinical features include continuous or intermittent purulent drainage, followed by development of an abscess, chills, fever, headache, and malaise.

Diagnosis

Physical examination confirms the diagnosis and may reveal a series of openings along the midline, with thin, brown, foul-smelling drainage or a protruding tuft of hair. Pressure on the sinus tract may produce purulent drainage. Passing a probe back through the sinus tract toward the sacrum shouldn't reveal a perforation between the anterior sinus and anal canal. Cultures of discharge from the infected sinus may show staphylococci or skin bacteria, but don't usually contain bowel bacteria.

Treatment

Conservative treatment of pilonidal disease consists of incision and drainage of abscesses, regular extraction of protruding hairs, and sitz baths (four to six times daily). However, persistent infections may necessitate surgical excision of the entire affected area.

After excision of a pilonidal abscess, the patient requires regular follow-up care to monitor wound healing. The surgeon may periodically palpate the wound during healing with a cotton-tipped applicator, curette excess granulation tissue, and extract loose hairs to promote wound healing from the inside out and to prevent dead cells from collecting in the wound. Complete healing may take several months.

Special considerations

Care includes preoperative and postoperative support and patient education.
- Before incision and drainage of a pilonidal abscess, assure the patient that he'll receive adequate pain relief.
- After surgery, check the compression dressing for signs of excessive bleeding, and change the dressing as directed.
- Encourage the patient to walk as soon as possible after the procedure.
- Tell the patient to place a gauze pad over the wound site after the dressing is removed to allow ventilation and prevent friction from clothing. Advise him to continue taking sitz baths and to let the area air-dry instead of rubbing or patting it dry with a towel.
- After healing, the patient should briskly wash the area daily with a washcloth to remove loose hairs. Encourage the obese patient to establish a weight loss plan.

Rectal prolapse

Rectal prolapse is the circumferential protrusion of one or more layers of the mucous membrane through the anus. Prolapse may be complete (with displacement of the anal sphincter or bowel herniation) or partial (mucosal layer). (See *Types of rectal prolapse*.)

Causes and incidence

Rectal prolapse usually occurs in children younger than age 6 and in adults in their 40s and 70s. It's commonly associated with other conditions, such as pinworms (enterobiasis), whipworm infection (trichuriasis), cystic fibrosis, malnutrition and malabsorption (such as celiac disease), constipation, and previous trauma to the anus or pelvic area.

True incidence figures are unavailable because many cases go unreported. Females are affected more often than males, accounting for 80% to 90% of reported cases.

Signs and symptoms

In rectal prolapse, protrusion of tissue from the rectum may occur during defecation or walking. Other symptoms include a persistent sensation of rectal fullness, bloody diarrhea, and pain in the lower abdomen due to ulceration. Hemorrhoids or rectal polyps may coexist with a prolapse.

Diagnosis

Typical clinical features and visual examination confirm the diagnosis. In complete prolapse, examination reveals the full thickness of the bowel wall and, possibly, the sphincter muscle protruding and mucosa falling into bulky, concentric folds. In partial prolapse, examination reveals only partially protruding mucosa and a smaller mass of radial mucosal folds. Straining during examination may disclose the full extent of prolapse.

TYPES OF RECTAL PROLAPSE

Partial rectal prolapse involves only the rectal mucosa and a small mass of radial mucosal folds. However, in complete rectal prolapse (also known as *procidentia*), the full rectal wall, sphincter muscle, and a large mass of concentric mucosal folds protrude. Ulceration is possible after complete prolapse.

PARTIAL RECTAL PROLAPSE

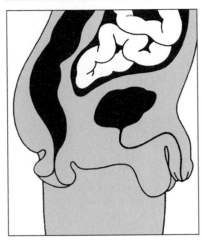

COMPLETE RECTAL PROLAPSE

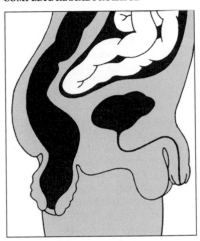

Treatment

In some cases, eliminating the underlying cause is the only treatment necessary. The rectal mucosa can be returned to the rectum manually. While the patient is in a knee-chest position, a soft, warm, wet cloth may be used to apply gentle pressure to the mass to push it back through the anal opening, thereby allowing gravity to help return the prolapse into place. In a child, prolapsed tissue usually diminishes as the child grows. In an older patient, injection of a sclerosing agent to cause a fibrotic reaction fixes the rectum in place. Severe or chronic prolapse requires surgical repair by strengthening or tightening the sphincters with wire or by anterior or rectal resection of prolapsed tissue.

Special considerations

Provide the patient with education regarding underlying causes and preoperative and postoperative support.

■ Help the patient prevent constipation by teaching her the correct diet and stool-softening regimen. Advise the patient with severe prolapse and incontinence to wear a perineal pad.

■ Before surgery, explain possible complications, including permanent rectal incontinence.

■ After surgery, watch for immediate complications (hemorrhage) and later ones (pelvic abscess, fever, pus drainage, pain, rectal stenosis, constipation, or pain on defecation). Teach perineal strengthening exercises: Have the patient lie down, with her back flat on the mattress; then ask her to pull in her abdomen and squeeze while taking a deep breath; or have the patient repeatedly squeeze and relax her buttocks while sitting on a chair.

Anal fissure

Anal fissure is a laceration or crack in the lining of the anus that extends to the circular muscle. Most fissures heal on their own and don't require treatment, aside from good diaper hygiene. However, some fissures may require medical treatment. The prognosis is very good, especially with fissurectomy and good anal hygiene.

Causes and incidence

Anal fissure results from passage of large, hard stools that stretch the lining beyond its limits. It may also be due to prolonged diarrhea, strain on the perineum during childbirth and, rarely, from scar stenosis. Occasionally, anal fissure is secondary to proctitis, anal tuberculosis, cancer, or Crohn's disease.

Anal fissures are common in young infants but may occur at any age, with incidence decreasing rapidly with age. Studies suggest that 80% of infants will have had an anal fissure by age 1. Fissures are less common among school-age children than infants. They affect males and females equally.

Signs and symptoms

Onset of an acute anal fissure is characterized by tearing, cutting, or burning pain during or immediately after a bowel movement. A few drops of blood may streak toilet paper or underclothes. Painful anal sphincter spasms result from ulceration of a "sentinel pile" (swelling at the lower end of the fissure). A fissure may heal spontaneously and completely or it may partially heal and break open again. Chronic fissure produces scar tissue that hampers normal bowel evacuation.

Diagnosis

Anoscopy showing a longitudinal tear and typical clinical features help establish the diagnosis. Digital examination that elicits pain and bleeding supports the diagnosis. Gentle traction on perianal skin can create sufficient eversion to visualize the fistula directly.

Treatment

Treatment varies according to the severity of the tear. Conservative treatment measures include stool softeners, dietary adjustment (addition of bulk to absorb water while in the intestinal tract), use of petroleum jelly and sitz baths, and cleaning more gently. Anesthetic ointment may be useful if pain interferes with normal bowel movements. Topical muscle relaxants may also be soothing. These measures generally heal more than 90% of anal fissures. For fissures that don't heal with these treatments, injection of botulinum toxin into the anal sphincter will temporarily paralyze the anal sphincter muscle, thereby promoting healing. Another option for nonhealing fissures is a minor surgical procedure to relax the sphincter.

For superficial fissures without hemorrhoids, forcible digital dilatation of the anal sphincter under local anesthesia stretches the lower portion of the sphincter. For complicated fissures, treatment includes surgical excision of tissue, adjacent skin, and mucosal tags and division of hypertrophied internal sphincter muscle to release tension.

Special considerations

Care consists of patient education and support.
- Prepare the patient for rectal examination; explain the necessity for the procedure.
- Provide warm sitz baths, warm soaks, and local anesthetic ointment to relieve pain. A low-residue diet, adequate fluid intake, and stool softeners prevent straining during defecation.
- Give diphenoxylate or other antidiarrheals to control diarrhea.

Pruritus ani

Pruritus ani is perianal itching, irritation, or superficial burning. This disorder is more common in males than in females and occurs in adults and children.

Causes

Factors that contribute to pruritus ani include overcleaning of the perianal area (harsh soap, vigorous rubbing with a washcloth or toilet paper); minor trauma caused by straining to defecate; poor hygiene; sensitivity to spicy foods, coffee, alcohol, food preservatives, perfumed or colored toilet paper, detergents, or certain fabrics; specific medications (antibiotics, antihypertensives, or antacids that cause diarrhea); excessive sweating (in occupations associated with physical labor or high stress levels); anal skin tags; systemic disease, especially diabetes; certain skin lesions, such as those associated with squamous cell carcinoma, basal cell carcinoma, Bowen's disease, Paget's disease, melanoma, syphilis, and tuberculosis; fungal or parasitic infection; and local anorectal disease (fissure, hemorrhoids, and fistula).

Signs and symptoms

The key symptom of pruritus ani is perianal itching or burning after a bowel movement, during stress, or at night. In acute pruritus ani, scratching produces reddened skin, with weeping excoriations; in chronic pruritus ani, skin becomes thick and leathery, with excessive pigmentation.

Diagnosis

A detailed patient history is essential. Rectal examination rules out fissures and fistulas; biopsy rules out cancer. Allergy testing may also be helpful.

Treatment

After elimination of the underlying cause, treatment is symptomatic, such as advising the patient to avoid scratching or rubbing the itchy areas. Lukewarm baths and a skin-soothing oatmeal or cornstarch bath may be comforting. Temporary relief may be obtained with cold compresses. Topical antihistamines are also useful.

Special considerations

■ Make sure that the patient understands his condition and the causes.
■ Recommend keeping fingernails short to avoid skin damage from inadvertent scratching. Suggest using cool, light, loose bedclothes and avoiding wearing rough clothing, particularly wool, over the irritated area.

■ Advise the patient to avoid prolonged exposure to excessive heat and humidity.
■ Advise the patient to avoid self-prescribed creams or powders, perfumed soaps, colored toilet paper, and moistened wipes because they may be irritating.
■ Teach the patient to keep the perianal area clean and dry. Suggest witch hazel pads for wiping and cotton balls tucked between the buttocks to absorb moisture.

Proctitis

Proctitis is an acute or chronic inflammation of the rectal mucosa. It can result in discomfort, bleeding, and possibly a discharge of mucus or pus.

Causes

Proctitis caused by sexually transmitted disease (STD) occurs with high frequency among individuals who engage in anal intercourse. STDs that can cause proctitis include gonorrhea, herpes, chlamydia, and lymphogranuloma venereum. Amebiasis can also cause proctitis and can be transmitted by anal-oral sex.

In children, beta-hemolytic streptococcus may cause proctitis. Autoimmune proctitis is associated with such diseases as ulcerative colitis or Crohn's disease. Proctitis may also be caused by medications, radiation, or noxious agents such as chemicals inserted into the rectum.

Other contributing factors include chronic constipation, habitual laxative use, emotional upset, radiation (especially for cancer of the cervix or uterus), endocrine dysfunction, rectal injury, rectal medications, bacterial infections, allergies (especially to milk), vasomotor disturbance that interferes with normal muscle control, and food poisoning.

Signs and symptoms

Key symptoms include tenesmus, constipation, a feeling of rectal fullness, and abdominal cramps on the left side. The patient feels an intense urge to defecate, which produces a small amount of stool that may contain blood and mucus.

Diagnosis

A detailed patient history is essential. In acute proctitis, sigmoidoscopy or proctoscopy reveal edematous, bright red or pink rectal mucosa that's thick, shiny, friable and, possibly, ulcerated. In chronic proctitis, sigmoidoscopy shows thickened mucosa, loss of vascular pattern, and stricture of the rectal lumen. Other supportive tests include biopsy to rule out cancer as well as rectal culture and examination of a stool sample.

Treatment

Primary treatment eliminates the underlying cause (fecal impaction, laxatives, or other medications). Proctitis caused by infection is treated with antibiotics specific for the causative organism. Corticosteroids or mesalamine suppositories may relieve symptoms in Crohn's disease or ulcerative colitis. Soothing enemas or steroid (hydrocortisone) suppositories or enemas may be helpful if proctitis is due to radiation. Tranquilizers may be appropriate for the patient with emotional stress.

Special considerations

- Tell the patient to watch for and report bleeding and other persistent symptoms.
- Fully explain proctitis and its treatment to the patient to help him understand the disorder and prevent its recurrence.
- Offer explanations, emotional support, and reassurance during rectal examinations and treatment.

Selected references

Buchler, M.W., et al. *Diseases of the Pancreas: Acute Pancreatitis, Chronic Pancreatitis, Neoplasms of the Pancreas.* Farmington, Conn.: S. Karger Publishers, 2004.

Charabaty-Pishvaian, A., and Al-Kawas, F. "Endoscopic Treatment of Duodenal Perforation Using a Clipping Device: Case Report and Review of the Literature," *Southern Medical Journal* 97(2):190-93, February 2004.

Fielding, J.W., and Hallissey, M.T., eds. *Hepatobiliary and Upper GI Surgery.* New York: Springer Publishing Co., 2004.

Joneja, J.M. *Digestion, Diet, and Disease: Irritable Bowel Syndrome and Gastrointestinal Function.* New Brunswick, N.J.: Rutgers University Press, 2004.

Kim, K.E. *Acute Gastrointestinal Bleeding: Diagnosis and Treatment.* Totowa, N.J.: Humana Press, Inc., 2003.

Meiner, S., ed. *Care of Gastrointestinal Problems in the Older Adult.* New York: Springer Publishing Co., 2004.

Tierney, L.M., et al. *Current Medical Diagnosis and Treatment 2004,* 43rd ed. New York: McGraw-Hill Book Co., 2004.

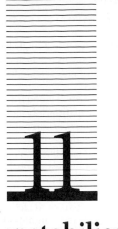

11

Hepatobiliary disorders

Introduction 747

Liver disorders 752
Viral hepatitis 752
Nonviral hepatitis 755
Cirrhosis and fibrosis 756
Liver abscess 759
Fatty liver 760
Wilson's disease 762
Hepatic encephalopathy 764

Gallbladder and duct disorders 765
Cholelithiasis and related disorders 765

Selected references 769

Introduction

The liver is the largest internal organ in the human body, weighing slightly more than 3 lb (1,200 to 1,600 g) in the average adult. It's also one of the busiest, performing well over 100 separate functions. The most important of these are the formation and secretion of bile; detoxification of harmful substances; storage of vitamins; metabolism of carbohydrates, fats, and proteins; and production of plasma proteins. This remarkably resilient organ serves as the body's warehouse and is absolutely essential to life.

Lobular structure
Located above the right kidney, stomach, pancreas, and intestines and immediately below the diaphragm, the liver divides into a left and a right lobe separated by the falciform ligament. The right lobe is six times larger than the left. Glisson's capsule, a network of connective tissue, covers the entire organ and extends into the parenchyma along blood vessels and bile ducts. Within the parenchyma, cylindrical lobules comprise the basic functional units of the liver, consisting of cellular plates that radiate from a central vein, somewhat like spokes in a wheel. Small bile canaliculi fit between the cells in the plates and empty into terminal bile ducts, which join two larger

ones that merge into a single hepatic duct upon leaving the liver. The hepatic duct then joins the cystic duct to form the common bile duct.

The liver receives blood from two major sources: the hepatic artery and the portal vein. The two vessels carry approximately 1,500 ml of blood to the liver per minute, nearly 75% of which is supplied by the portal vein. Sinusoids — offshoots of the hepatic artery and portal vein — run between each row of hepatic cells. Phagocytic Kupffer's cells, part of the reticuloendothelial system, line the sinusoids, destroying old or defective red blood cells and detoxifying harmful substances. The liver has a large lymphatic supply; consequently, cancer frequently metastasizes there.

Liver function

One of the liver's most important functions is the conversion of bilirubin, a breakdown product of hemoglobin, into bile. Liberated by the spleen into plasma and bound loosely to albumin, bilirubin reaches the liver in an unconjugated (water-insoluble) state. The liver then conjugates or dissociates it, converting it to a water-soluble derivative before excreting it as bile. All hepatic cells continually form bile.

The liver also detoxifies many substances through inactivation or through conjugation. Inactivation involves reduction, oxidation, and hydroxylation. An important liver function is the inactivation of many drugs that are metabolized primarily in the liver. Such drugs must be used with caution in hepatic disease because their effects may be markedly prolonged.

ELDER TIP *In elderly people, the blood supply to the liver decreases, and certain liver enzymes become less active. As a result, the liver loses some of its ability to metabolize drugs and higher levels of drugs remain in the circulation, causing more intense drug effects. This increases the risk of drug toxicity.*

As still another example of its amazing versatility, the liver forms vitamin A from certain vegetables and stores vitamins K, D, and B_{12}. It also stores iron in the form of ferritin.

Metabolic functions

The liver figures indispensably in the metabolism of the three major food groups: carbohydrates, fats, and proteins. In carbohydrate metabolism, the liver plays one of its most vital roles by extracting excess glucose from the blood and reserving it for times when blood glucose levels fall below normal, when it releases glucose into the circulation, and then replenishes the supply by a process called glyconeogenesis. To prevent dangerously low blood glucose levels, the liver can also convert galactose or amino acids into glucose (gluconeogenesis). The liver also forms many critical chemical compounds from the intermediate products of carbohydrate metabolism.

The liver performs more than half the body's preliminary breakdown of fats because liver cells metabolize fats more quickly and efficiently than do other body cells. Liver cells break fats down into glycerol and fatty acids and convert the fatty acids into small molecules that can be oxidized. The liver also produces substantial quantities of cholesterol and phospholipids, manufactures lipoproteins, and synthesizes fat from carbohydrates and proteins to be transported in lipoproteins for eventual storage in adipose tissue.

Like so many of its functions, the liver's role in protein metabolism is essential to life. The liver deaminates amino acids so they can be used for energy or converted into fats or carbohydrates. It forms urea to remove ammonia from body fluids and all plasma proteins (as much as 50 to 100 g/day) except gamma globulin. The liver is such an effective synthesizer of protein that it can replenish as much as half its plasma proteins in 4 to 7 days. The liver also synthesizes nonessential amino acids and forms other important chemical compounds from amino acids.

Production of plasma proteins

The liver synthesizes most of the body's large molecules of plasma proteins, including all of the albumin, which binds many substances in plasma and maintains colloid osmotic pressure.

Normally, plasma proteins and amino acid levels maintain equilibrium in the blood. When amino acid levels decrease, the plasma proteins split into amino acids to restore this equilibrium. Reacting to decreased levels of amino acids, the liver steps up production of the plasma proteins. The liver may synthesize approximately 400 g of protein daily; for this reason, significant liver damage leads to hyperproteinemia, which in turn disrupts the colloid osmotic pressure and amino acid levels.

The liver also produces most of the plasma proteins necessary for blood coagulation, including prothrombin and fibrinogen, which are the most abundant. The liver forms prothrombin in a process dependent on vitamin K and the production of bile. Fibrinogen, a large-molecule protein formed entirely by the liver, is an essential factor in the coagulation cascade.

Together, the plasma proteins maintain colloid osmotic pressure throughout the capillaries. Because the plasma protein molecules are too large to cross the capillary membrane, they concentrate at the capillary line and produce an osmotic pressure of pull. This constant colloid osmotic pressure at the arteriolar and venular sections of the capillary provides the major osmotic force regulating the return of fluid to the intravascular compartment.

Because of their large molecular size, the plasma proteins don't easily cross into the interstitial spaces. Their only route for return to the bloodstream is through lymphatic drainage. The lymphatic vessels drain into the lymphatic and thoracic ducts, which drain directly into the superior vena cava.

Assessing for liver disease

In many cases, a careful physical examination and patient history can detect hepatic disease. Watch especially for its cardinal signs: jaundice (a result of increased serum bilirubin levels), ascites (commonly with hemoconcentration, edema, and oliguria), and hepatomegaly. Other signs and symptoms may include right upper quadrant abdominal pain, lassitude, anorexia, nausea, and vomiting. To detect hepatomegaly, palpate the liver's left lobe in the epigastrium between the xiphoid process and the umbilicus. Another primary sign is portal hypertension (portal vein pressure greater than 6 to 12 cm H_2O) revealed by auscultation of a venous hum over the patient's abdomen. Surgical insertion of a catheter into the portal vein allows measurement of portal vein pressure.

Carefully assess the patient's neurologic status because neurologic symptoms, such as those associated with hepatic encephalopathy (confusion, muscle tremors, and asterixis), may signal the onset of life-threatening hepatic failure. Other common signs of hepatic disease include pallor (commonly linked to cirrhosis or carcinoma), parotid gland enlargement (in alcohol-induced liver damage), Dupuytren's contracture, gynecomastia, testicular atrophy, decreased axillary or pubic hair, bleeding disorders (ecchymosis and purpura), spider angiomas, and palmar erythema.

Careful abdominal palpation and auscultation can also detect hepatocellular carcinoma or metastasis, which turn the liver rock-hard and cause abdominal bruits. In hepatitis, the liver is usually enlarged; palpation may elicit tenderness at the liver's edge. In cirrhosis, the atrophic liver is difficult to palpate. In neoplastic disease or hepatic abscess, auscultation may detect a pleural friction rub.

Comprehensive history essential

Ask if the patient has ever had jaundice, anemia, or a splenectomy. Ask about occupational or other exposure him to toxins (carbon tetrachloride, beryllium, or vinyl chloride), which may predispose him to hepatic disease. Consider recent travel or contact with persons who have traveled to areas where hepatic disease is endemic.

Make sure to ask about alcohol consumption, a significant factor in suspected hepatic disease. Remember, an alcoholic may deliberately underestimate his alcohol intake, so interview the patient's family as well. Ask about recent contact with a jaundiced person and about any recent blood or plasma transfusions, blood tests, tattoos, or dental work. Find out if the patient takes any drugs that may cause liver damage, such as sedatives, tranquilizers, analgesics, and diuretics that cause potassium loss. Ask if the onset of symptoms was abrupt or insidious or if it followed abdominal injury that could have damaged the liver. Ask if the patient bruises or bleeds easily. Check the color of stools and urine, and ask about any change in bowel habits. Also ask if the patient's weight has fluctuated recently.

Liver function studies

Numerous tests are available to detect hepatic disease. Perhaps the most useful tests are liver function studies, which measure serum enzymes and other substances. Typical findings in hepatic disease include:

- increased bilirubin levels
- increased alkaline phosphatase and 5'-nucleotidase levels
- elevated levels of aspartate aminotransferase (AST) and alanine aminotransferase (ALT): possible hepatocellular damage, viral hepatitis, or acute hepatic necrosis
- elevated gamma-glutamyltransferase levels: especially helpful because this enzyme level rises even when hepatic damage is still minimal
- hypoalbuminemia: subacute or massive hepatic necrosis or cirrhosis
- hyperglobulinemia: chronic inflammatory disorders
- prolonged prothrombin time or partial thromboplastin time: hepatitis or cirrhosis
- elevated serum ammonia levels: hepatic encephalopathy
- decreased serum total cholesterol levels: liver disease
- positive lupus erythematosus cell test (in chronic active hepatitis and the presence of hepatitis B antigen).

Liver function studies are less reliable after liver trauma. For instance, tests done long after the injury might miss an initial rise in serum AST and ALT levels. Several less specific blood tests for detecting hepatic disease are urine urobilinogen, lactate dehydrogenase, and ornithine carbamoyltransferase.

Other useful diagnostic tests include the following:

- Plain abdominal X-rays may indicate gross hepatomegaly and hepatic masses by elevation or distortion of the diaphragm and may show calcification in the gallbladder, biliary tree, pancreas, and liver.
- Barium studies may indicate an elevated left hepatic lobe by displacing the barium-filled stomach laterally and posteriorly.

- Oral cholecystography is useful because parenchymal dysfunction and impaired bile excretion decrease the excretion of the contrast material and prevent visualization of the gallbladder.
- Percutaneous transhepatic cholangiography distinguishes mechanical biliary obstruction from intrahepatic cholestasis.
- Angiography demonstrates hepatic arterial circulation (altered in cirrhosis) and helps diagnose primary or secondary hepatic tumor masses.
- Radioisotope liver scans (scintiscans) may show an area of decreased uptake (a "hole") using a colloidal or bengal scan or an area of increased uptake (a "hot spot") using a gallium scan in hepatoma or hepatic abscess.
- Computed tomography scan produces in-depth, three-dimensional images of the biliary tract (the liver as well as the pancreas) that help distinguish between obstructive and nonobstructive jaundice and also helps identify space-occupying hepatic lesions.
- Portal and hepatic vein manometry localizes obstructions in the extrahepatic portion of the portal vein and portal inflow system or increased pressure in the presinusoidal vessels.
- Percutaneous or transvenous liver biopsy can determine the cause of unexplained hepatomegaly, hepatosplenomegaly, cholestasis, or persistently abnormal liver function tests; it's also useful when systemic infiltrative disease (such as sarcoidosis) or primary or metastatic hepatic tumors are suspected.
- Laparoscopy visualizes the serosal lining, liver, gallbladder, spleen, and other organs and is useful in unexplained hepatomegaly, ascites, or an abdominal mass.

Gallbladder anatomy

The gallbladder is a pear-shaped organ that lies in the fossa on the underside of the liver and is capable of holding 50 ml of bile. Attached to the large organ above by connective tissue, the peritoneum, and blood vessels, the gallbladder is divided into four parts: the fundus, or broad inferior end; the body, which is funnel-shaped and bound to the duodenum; the neck, which empties into the cystic duct; and the infundibulum, which lies between the body and the neck and sags to form Hartmann's pouch. The hepatic artery supplies the cystic and hepatic ducts with blood, which drains out of the gallbladder through the cystic vein. Rich lymph vessels in the submucosal layer also drain the gallbladder as well as the head of the pancreas.

The biliary duct system provides a passage for bile from the liver to the intestine and regulates bile flow. The gallbladder itself collects, concentrates, and stores bile. The normally functioning gallbladder also removes water and electrolytes from hepatic bile, increases the concentration of the larger solutes, and reduces its pH to less than 7. In gallbladder disease, bile becomes more alkaline, altering bile salts and cholesterol and predisposing the organ to stone formation.

Mechanisms of contraction

The gallbladder responds to sympathetic and parasympathetic innervation. Sympathetic stimulation inhibits muscle contraction, mild vagal stimulation causes the gallbladder to contract and the sphincter of Oddi to relax, and stronger stimulation causes the sphincter to contract. The gallbladder also responds to substances released by the intestine. For instance, after chyme (semiliquid, partially digested food) enters the duodenum from the stomach, the duodenum releases cholecystokinin (CCK) and pancreozymin (PCZ) into the bloodstream and stimulates the gallbladder to contract. The gallbladder also produces secretin, which stimulates the liver to secrete bile and CCK-PCZ. The gallbladder may also respond to some type of hormonal control, a theory based in part on the fact that the gallbladder empties more slowly during pregnancy.

Assessing for gallbladder disease

During your physical examination of a patient with suspected gallbladder disease, look for its telltale signs and symptoms: pain, jaundice (a result of blockage of the common bile duct), fever, chills, indigestion, nausea, and intolerance of fatty foods. Pain may range from vague discomfort (as when pressure within the common bile duct gradually increases) to deep visceral pain (as when the gallbladder suddenly distends). Abrupt onset of pain with epigastric distress indicates gallbladder inflammation or obstruction of bile outflow by a stone or spasm.

The onset of jaundice also varies. If the gallbladder is healthy, jaundice may be delayed several days after bile duct blockage; if the gallbladder is absent or diseased, jaundice may appear within 24 hours after the blockage. Other effects of obstruction—pruritus, steatorrhea, and bleeding tendencies—may accompany jaundice. Gallbladder disorders rarely cause internal bleeding, but when they do—as in cholecystitis or obstructive clots in the biliary tree from GI bleeding—they can be fatal.

Diagnostic tests

After taking a thorough patient history and carefully assessing the clinical features, the next step in accurate diagnosis of gallbladder disease is cholecystography, in which X-rays are taken of the gallbladder after the patient has ingested radiopaque dye. However, visualization depends on absorption of the dye from the small intestine, the liver's capacity to remove the dye from the blood and excrete it in bile, the patency of the ductal system, and the ability of the gallbladder to concentrate and store the dye. Normally, the gallbladder fills about 13 hours after ingestion of the dye. Presence of stones or failure to visualize the gallbladder is significant.

Other diagnostic tests for gallbladder disease include the following:

■ Percutaneous transhepatic cholangiography differentiates extrahepatic from intrahepatic obstructive jaundice and helps detect biliary masses and calculi. Needle insertion in a bile duct permits withdrawal of bile and injection of dye. Fluoroscopic tests evaluate the filling of the hepatic and biliary trees. The test also permits palliative internal or external placement of biliary catheters for free flow of bile.

■ Duodenal drainage diagnoses cholelithiasis, choledocholithiasis, biliary obstruction, hepatic cirrhosis, and pancreatic disease and differentiates types of jaundice. A tube is passed through the GI tract into the duodenum, and CCK-PCZ is given to stimulate the gallbladder, permitting measurement of bile flow and also specimen collection, which is examined for mucus, blood, cholesterol crystals, pancreatic enzymes, cancer cells, bacteria, or calcium bilirubinate. Duodenal drainage is especially useful when gallbladder function is poor or absent, when cholecystography fails to visualize the gallbladder or yields negative results despite continuing symptoms, or when cholecystography is contraindicated because of the patient's condition.

■ In endoscopic retrograde cholangiopancreatography, duodenal endoscopy with dye injection and fluoroscopy are used to cannulate and visualize biliary and pancreatic ducts. This test is useful in locating obstruction, calculi, carcinoma, or stricture and for obtaining bile or pancreatic juice for analysis. Internal stents can be inserted to allow free flow of bile or pancreatic juice.

■ In gallbladder ultrasound, sound waves are used to visualize the gallbladder and locate obstruction, stones, and tumors. This test is 95% accurate in detecting stones.

Other appropriate tests for biliary disease are the same as those for hepatic disease.

LIVER DISORDERS
Viral hepatitis

Viral hepatitis is a fairly common systemic disease, marked by hepatic cell destruction, necrosis, and autolysis, leading to anorexia, jaundice, and hepatomegaly. In most patients, hepatic cells eventually regenerate with little or no residual damage. However, old age and serious underlying disorders make complications more likely. The prognosis is poor if edema and hepatic encephalopathy develop.

Hepatitis occurs in these forms:

■ Type A (infectious or short-incubation hepatitis) is rising among homosexuals and in people with immunosuppression related to human immunodeficiency virus (HIV) infection.

■ Type B (serum or long-incubation hepatitis) also is increasing among HIV-positive individuals. Routine screening of

donor blood for the hepatitis B surface antigen (HBsAg) has decreased the incidence of posttransfusion cases, but transmission by needles shared by drug abusers remains a major problem.

■ Type C accounts for about 20% of all viral hepatitis cases and for most posttransfusion cases.

■ Type D (delta hepatitis) is responsible for about 50% of all cases of fulminant hepatitis, which has a high mortality. Developing in 1% of patients, fulminant hepatitis causes unremitting liver failure with encephalopathy. It progresses to coma and commonly leads to death within 2 weeks. In the United States, type D is confined to people who are frequently exposed to blood and blood products, such as I.V. drug users and patients with hemophilia.

■ Type E (formerly grouped with type C under the name non-A, non-B hepatitis) occurs primarily among patients who have recently returned from an endemic area (such as India, Africa, Asia, or Central America); it's more common in young adults and more severe in pregnant women.

■ Hepatitis G is a newly discovered form of hepatitis. Transmission is by the bloodborne route and it's more common in those who receive blood transfusions.

Causes and incidence

The major forms of viral hepatitis result from infection with the causative viruses: A, B, C, D, E, or G.

Type A hepatitis is highly contagious and is usually transmitted by the fecal-oral route. However, it may also be transmitted parenterally. Hepatitis A usually results from ingestion of contaminated food, milk, or water. Many outbreaks of this type are traced to ingestion of seafood from polluted water. In 2001, there were more than 10,000 acute cases of hepatitis A infection reported in the United States.

Type B hepatitis, once thought to be transmitted only by the direct exchange of contaminated blood, is now known to be transmitted also by contact with human secretions and feces. As a result, nurses, physicians, laboratory technicians, and dentists are frequently exposed to type B hepatitis, in many cases as a result of wearing defective gloves. Transmission also occurs during intimate sexual contact as well as through perinatal transmission. An estimated 200,000 new cases of hepatitis B virus (HBV) and 5,000 deaths from HBV occur annually in the United States.

Although specific type C hepatitis viruses have been isolated, only a small percentage of patients have tested positive for them — perhaps reflecting the test's poor specificity. Usually, this type of hepatitis is transmitted through transfused blood from asymptomatic donors. Hepatitis C accounts for 30,000 new infections and 8,000 to 10,000 deaths each year in the United States. Most exposures (60%) occur through the use of illicit I.V. drugs. However, sexual transmission is responsible for 20% of cases. More than 170 million people have the hepatitis C virus worldwide.

Type D hepatitis is found only in patients with an acute or chronic episode of hepatitis B and requires the presence of HBsAg. The type D virus depends on the double-shelled type B virus to replicate. For this reason, type D infection can't outlast a type B infection. About 15 million people are infected with hepatitis D worldwide. It's more common in adults than in children. People with a history of illicit I.V. drug use and people who live in the Mediterranean basin have a higher incidence.

Type E hepatitis is transmitted enterically, much like type A. Because this virus is inconsistently shed in feces, detection is difficult. In the United States, the prevalence of hepatitis E is less than 2%. It's typically found in developing countries that lie near the equator. Incidence is highest among people ages 15 to 40.

Type G may be transmitted in a manner similar to that of hepatitis C. It may also be transmitted by sexual contact, and its incidence may be higher than previously suspected. It's associated with acute and chronic liver disease, but studies haven't clearly implicated the hepatitis G virus as an etiologic agent.

Other proposed causative factors, such as non-ABCDE viral hepatitis and type F, are under investigation.

Signs and symptoms

Assessment findings are similar for the different types of hepatitis. Typically, signs and symptoms progress in several stages.

In the prodromal (preicteric) stage, the patient typically complains of easy fatigue and anorexia (possibly with mild weight loss), generalized malaise, depression, headache, weakness, arthralgia, myalgia, photophobia, and nausea with vomiting. He also may describe changes in his senses of taste and smell.

Assessment of the patient's vital signs may reveal a fever of 100° to 102° F (37.8° to 38.9° C). As the prodromal stage ends, usually 1 to 5 days before the onset of the clinical jaundice stage, inspection of urine and stool specimens may reveal dark-colored urine and clay-colored stools.

If the patient has progressed to the clinical jaundice stage, he may report pruritus, abdominal pain or tenderness, and indigestion. Early in this stage, he may complain of anorexia; later, his appetite may return. Inspection of the sclerae, mucous membranes, and skin may reveal jaundice, which can last for 1 to 2 weeks. Jaundice indicates that the damaged liver is unable to remove bilirubin from the blood; however, its presence doesn't indicate the severity of the disease. Occasionally, hepatitis occurs without jaundice.

During the clinical jaundice stage, inspection of the skin may detect rashes, erythematous patches, or urticaria, especially if the patient has hepatitis B or C. Palpation may disclose abdominal tenderness in the right upper quadrant, an enlarged and tender liver and, in some cases, splenomegaly and cervical adenopathy.

During the recovery (posticteric) stage, most of the patient's symptoms decrease or subside. On palpation, a decrease in liver enlargement may be noted. The recovery phase commonly lasts from 2 to 12 weeks, although sometimes this phase lasts longer in the patient with hepatitis B, C, or E. Little is known about hepatitis G.

Diagnosis

A hepatitis profile, which identifies antibodies specific to the causative virus and establishes the type of hepatitis, is routine in suspected viral hepatitis.

- Type A: Detection of an antibody to hepatitis A confirms the diagnosis.
- Type B: The presence of HBsAg and hepatitis B antibodies confirms the diagnosis.
- Type C: Diagnosis depends on serologic testing for the specific antibody 1 or more months after the onset of acute hepatitis. Until then, the diagnosis is established primarily by obtaining negative test results for hepatitis A, B, and D.
- Type D: Detection of intrahepatic delta antigens or immunoglobulin (Ig) antidelta antigens in acute disease (or IgM and IgG in chronic disease) establishes the diagnosis.
- Type E: Detection of hepatitis E antigens supports the diagnosis; however, the diagnosis may also be determined by ruling out hepatitis C.
- Type G: Detection of hepatitis G antigen supports the diagnosis but doesn't clearly implicate infection; the patient may be otherwise asymptomatic.

Additional findings from liver function studies support the diagnosis:

- Serum aspartate aminotransferase and serum alanine aminotransferase levels are increased in the prodromal stage of acute viral hepatitis.
- Serum alkaline phosphatase levels are slightly increased.
- Serum bilirubin levels are elevated. Levels may continue to be high late in the disease, especially in severe cases.
- Prothrombin time is prolonged (more than 3 seconds longer than normal indicates severe liver damage).
- White blood cell counts commonly reveal transient neutropenia and lymphopenia followed by lymphocytosis.
- Liver biopsy is performed if chronic hepatitis is suspected; however, it's performed for acute hepatitis only if the diagnosis is questionable.

Treatment

No specific drug therapy has been developed for hepatitis, with the exception of hepatitis C, which has been treated somewhat successfully with interferon alpha. Instead, patients are advised to rest in the early stages of the illness and to combat anorexia by eating small, high-calorie, high-protein meals. (Protein intake should be reduced if signs or symptoms of precoma—lethargy, confusion, and mental changes—develop.) Large meals are usually better tolerated in the morning because many patients experience nausea late in the day.

In acute viral hepatitis, hospitalization usually is required only for the patient with severe symptoms or complications. Parenteral nutrition may be required if the patient experiences persistent vomiting and is unable to maintain oral intake.

Antiemetics may be given 30 minutes before meals to relieve nausea and prevent vomiting; phenothiazines have a cholestatic effect and should be avoided. For severe pruritus, the resin cholestyramine may be given.

Special considerations

Use enteric precautions when caring for patients with type A or E hepatitis. Practice standard precautions for all patients.

- Inform visitors about isolation precautions.
- Provide rest periods throughout the day. Schedule treatments and tests so that the patient can rest between bouts of activity.
- Because inactivity may make the patient anxious, include diversionary activities as part of his care. Gradually add activities to his schedule as he begins to recover.
- Encourage the patient to eat. Don't overload his meal tray or overmedicate him because this will diminish his appetite.
- Encourage fluids (at least 4 qt [4 L] per day). Encourage the anorectic patient to drink fruit juice. Also offer chipped ice and effervescent soft drinks to maintain hydration without inducing vomiting.
- Administer supplemental vitamins and commercial feedings, as ordered. If symptoms are severe and the patient can't tolerate oral intake, provide I.V. therapy and parenteral nutrition, as ordered by the physician.
- Record the patient's weight daily, and keep intake and output records. Observe stools for color, consistency, and amount and record the frequency of bowel movements.
- Watch for signs of fluid shift, such as weight gain and orthostasis.

- Watch for signs of hepatic coma, dehydration, pneumonia, vascular problems, and pressure ulcers.
- In fulminant hepatitis, maintain electrolyte balance and a patent airway, prevent infections, and control bleeding. Correct hypoglycemia and other complications while awaiting liver regeneration and repair.
- Before discharge, emphasize the importance of having regular medical checkups for at least 1 year. The patient will have an increased risk of developing hepatoma. Warn the patient against using alcohol or over-the-counter drugs during this period. Teach him to recognize the signs of a recurrence.
- Inform the patient about the availability of support groups for people with all types of hepatitis and provide contact information if he's interested.

Nonviral hepatitis

Nonviral inflammation of the liver (toxic or drug-induced hepatitis) is a form of hepatitis that usually results from exposure to certain chemicals or drugs. Most patients recover from this illness, although a few develop fulminating hepatitis or cirrhosis.

Causes

Various hepatotoxins — carbon tetrachloride, acetaminophen, trichloroethylene, poisonous mushrooms, and vinyl chloride — can cause the toxic form of this disease. Following exposure to these agents, liver damage usually occurs within 24 to 48 hours, depending on the size of the dose or degree of exposure. Alcohol, anoxia, and preexisting liver disease exacerbate the toxic effects of some of these agents.

Drug-induced (idiosyncratic) hepatitis may stem from a hypersensitivity reaction unique to the affected individual, unlike toxic hepatitis, which appears to affect all people indiscriminately. Among the drugs that may cause this type of hepatitis are niacin, halothane, sulfonamides, isoniazid, methyldopa, and phenothiazines (cholestasis-induced hepatitis). In hypersensitive people, symptoms of hepatic dysfunction may appear at any time during or after exposure to these drugs but usually emerge after 2 to 5 weeks of therapy. Not all adverse drug reactions are toxic. Hormonal contraceptives, for example, may impair liver function and produce jaundice without causing necrosis, fatty infiltration of liver cells, or hypersensitivity.

Signs and symptoms

Clinical features of toxic and drug-induced hepatitis vary with the severity of the liver damage and the causative agent. In most patients, signs and symptoms resemble those of viral hepatitis: anorexia, nausea, vomiting, jaundice, dark urine, hepatomegaly, possible abdominal pain (with acute onset and massive necrosis), and clay-colored stools or pruritus with the cholestatic form of hepatitis. Carbon tetrachloride poisoning also produces headache, dizziness, drowsiness, and vasomotor collapse; halothane-related hepatitis produces fever, moderate leukocytosis, and eosinophilia; chlorpromazine toxicity produces abrupt fever, rash, arthralgia, lymphadenopathy, and epigastric or right upper quadrant pain.

Diagnosis

Diagnostic findings include elevations in serum aspartate aminotransferase and alanine aminotransferase, total and direct bilirubin (with cholestasis), alkaline phosphatase, white blood cell (WBC) count, and eosinophil count (possible in drug-induced type). Liver biopsy may help identify the underlying pathology, especially infiltration with WBCs and eosinophils. Liver function tests have limited value in distinguishing between nonviral and viral hepatitis.

Treatment

Effective treatment must remove the causative agent by lavage, catharsis, or hyperventilation, depending on the route of exposure. Acetylcysteine may serve as an antidote for toxic hepatitis caused by acetaminophen poisoning but doesn't prevent drug-induced hepatitis caused by other substances. Corticosteroids may be ordered for patients with the drug-induced type.

Special considerations
■ Monitor laboratory studies and note trends.

■ Monitor the patient's vital signs and provide support to maintain vital functioning, depending on the severity of his symptoms.

■ Preventive measures should include instructing the patient about the proper use of drugs and the proper handling of cleaning agents and solvents.

Cirrhosis and fibrosis

Cirrhosis is a chronic hepatic disease characterized by diffuse destruction and fibrotic regeneration of hepatic cells. As necrotic tissue yields to fibrosis, this disease alters liver structure and normal vasculature, impairs blood and lymph flow, and ultimately causes hepatic insufficiency. The prognosis is better in noncirrhotic forms of hepatic fibrosis, which cause minimal hepatic dysfunction and don't destroy liver cells.

Causes and incidence
These clinical types of cirrhosis reflect its diverse etiology:

■ Portal, nutritional, or alcoholic (Laennec's) cirrhosis, the most common type, occurs in 30% to 50% of cirrhotic patients, up to 90% of whom have a history of alcoholism. Liver damage results from malnutrition, especially of dietary protein, and chronic alcohol ingestion. Fibrous tissue forms in portal areas and around central veins.

■ Biliary cirrhosis (15% to 20% of patients) results from injury or prolonged obstruction.

■ Postnecrotic (posthepatic) cirrhosis (10% to 30% of patients) stems from various types of hepatitis.

■ Pigment cirrhosis (5% to 10% of patients) may result from disorders such as hemochromatosis.

■ Cardiac cirrhosis (rare) refers to liver damage caused by right-sided heart failure.

■ Idiopathic cirrhosis (about 10% of patients) has no known cause.

Noncirrhotic fibrosis may result from schistosomiasis or congenital hepatic fibrosis or may be idiopathic.

Signs and symptoms
Clinical manifestations of cirrhosis and fibrosis are similar for all types, regardless of the cause. Early indications are vague, but usually include GI signs and symptoms (anorexia, indigestion, nausea, vomiting, constipation, or diarrhea) and a dull abdominal ache. Major and late signs and symptoms develop as a result of hepatic insufficiency and portal hypertension:

■ Respiratory—pleural effusion and limited thoracic expansion due to abdominal ascites, interfering with efficient gas exchange and leading to hypoxia

■ Central nervous system—progressive signs or symptoms of hepatic encephalopathy—lethargy, mental changes, slurred speech, asterixis (flapping tremor), peripheral neuritis, paranoia, hallucinations, extreme obtundation, and coma

■ Hematologic—bleeding tendencies (nosebleeds, easy bruising, and bleeding gums) and anemia

■ Endocrine—testicular atrophy, menstrual irregularities, gynecomastia, and loss of chest and axillary hair

■ Skin—severe pruritus, extreme dryness, poor tissue turgor, abnormal pigmentation, spider angiomas, palmar erythema, and possibly jaundice

■ Hepatic—jaundice, hepatomegaly, ascites, edema of the legs, hepatic encephalopathy, and hepatorenal syndrome comprise the other major effects of full-fledged cirrhosis

■ Miscellaneous—musty breath, enlarged superficial abdominal veins, muscle atrophy, pain in the right upper abdominal quadrant that worsens when the patient sits up or leans forward, palpable liver or spleen, and temperature of 101° to 103° F (38.3° to 39.4° C). Bleeding from esophageal varices results from portal hypertension.

Diagnosis

 CONFIRMING DIAGNOSIS *Liver biopsy, the definitive test for cirrhosis, detects destruction and fibrosis of hepatic tissue.*

Liver scan shows abnormal thickening and a liver mass. Cholecystography and cholangiography visualize the gallbladder and the biliary duct system, respectively;

splenoportal venography visualizes the portal venous system. Percutaneous transhepatic cholangiography differentiates extrahepatic from intrahepatic obstructive jaundice and discloses hepatic pathology and the presence of gallstones.

Laboratory findings that are characteristic of cirrhosis include:

- decreased white blood cell count, hemoglobin level and hematocrit, albumin, serum electrolyte levels (sodium, potassium, chloride, and magnesium), and cholinesterase
- elevated levels of globulin, serum ammonia, total bilirubin, alkaline phosphatase, serum aspartate aminotransferase, serum alanine aminotransferase, and lactate dehydrogenase and increased thymol turbidity
- anemia, neutropenia, and thrombocytopenia, characterized by prolonged prothrombin and partial thromboplastin times
- deficiencies of folic acid, iron, and vitamins A, B_{12}, C, and K.

Treatment

Treatment is designed to remove or alleviate the underlying cause of cirrhosis or fibrosis, prevent further liver damage, and prevent or treat complications. The patient may benefit from a high-calorie and moderate- to high-protein diet, but developing hepatic encephalopathy mandates restricted protein intake. In addition, sodium is usually restricted to 200 to 500 mg/day and fluids to 1 to 1½ qt (1 to 1.5 L)/day.

If the patient's condition continues to deteriorate, he may need tube feedings or total parenteral nutrition. He may also need supplemental vitamins—A, B complex, D, and K—to compensate for the liver's inability to store them and vitamin B_{12}, folic acid, and thiamine for deficiency anemia. Rest, moderate exercise, and avoidance of exposure to infections and toxic agents are essential.

Drug therapy requires special caution because the cirrhotic liver can't detoxify harmful substances efficiently. When absolutely necessary, vasopressin may be prescribed for esophageal varices, and diuretics may be given for edema. However, diuretics require careful monitoring because fluid and electrolyte imbalance may

precipitate hepatic encephalopathy. Encephalopathy is treated with lactulose. Antibiotics are used to decrease intestinal bacteria and reduce ammonia production, which causes encephalopathy. Coagulopathy may be treated with blood products or vitamin K.

Low-protein diets are controversial. They aid in managing acute hepatic encephalopathy but are rarely necessary in chronic conditions because of the underlying protein-calorie malnutrition.

Paracentesis and infusions of salt-poor albumin, in addition to fluid and salt restriction, may alleviate ascites. Surgical procedures include treatment of varices by upper endoscopy with banding or sclerosis, splenectomy, esophagogastric resection, and splenorenal or portacaval anastomosis to relieve portal hypertension. (See *Portal hypertension and esophageal varices,* page 758, and *Circulation in portal hypertension,* page 759.)

 ALERT *If cirrhosis progresses and becomes life-threatening, a liver transplant should be considered.*

Special considerations

The patient with cirrhosis needs close observation, first-rate supportive care, and sound nutritional counseling.

- Check the patient's skin, gums, stools, and vomitus regularly for bleeding. Apply pressure to injection sites to prevent bleeding. Warn him against taking nonsteroidal anti-inflammatory drugs, straining at stool, and blowing his nose or sneezing too vigorously. Suggest using an electric razor and soft toothbrush.
- Observe the patient closely for signs of behavioral or personality changes. Report increasing stupor, lethargy, hallucinations, or neuromuscular dysfunction. Awaken him periodically to determine his level of consciousness. Watch for asterixis, a sign of developing hepatic encephalopathy.
- To assess fluid retention, weigh the patient and measure abdominal girth at least daily, inspect his ankles and sacrum for dependent edema, and accurately record intake and output. Carefully evaluate the patient before, during, and after paracentesis; this drastic loss of fluid may induce shock.

PORTAL HYPERTENSION AND ESOPHAGEAL VARICES

Portal hypertension — elevated pressure in the portal vein — occurs when blood flow meets increased resistance. The disorder is a common result of cirrhosis, but may also stem from mechanical obstruction and occlusion of the hepatic veins (Budd-Chiari syndrome). As portal pressure rises, blood backs up into the spleen and flows through collateral channels to the venous system, bypassing the liver. Consequently, portal hypertension produces splenomegaly with thrombocytopenia, dilated collateral veins (esophageal varices, hemorrhoids, or prominent abdominal veins), and ascites. Nevertheless, in many patients, the first sign of portal hypertension is bleeding from esophageal varices — dilated tortuous veins in the submucosa of the lower esophagus. Bleeding esophageal varices commonly cause massive hematemesis, requiring emergency treatment to control hemorrhage and prevent hypovolemic shock.

Diagnosis and treatment

These procedures help diagnose and correct esophageal varices.

■ Endoscopy identifies the ruptured varix as the bleeding site and excludes other potential sources in the upper GI tract.

■ Angiography may aid diagnosis, but is less precise than endoscopy.

■ Vasopressin infused into the superior mesenteric artery may temporarily stop bleeding. When angiography is unavailable, vasopressin may be infused by I.V. drip or diluted with 5% dextrose in water (except in patients with coronary vascular disease), but this route is usually less effective.

■ A Sengstaken-Blakemore or Minnesota tube may also help control hemorrhage by applying pressure on the bleeding site. Iced saline lavage through the tube may help control bleeding.

The use of vasopressin or a Minnesota or Sengstaken-Blakemore tube is a temporary measure, especially in the patient with a severely deteriorated liver. Fresh blood and fresh frozen plasma, if available, are preferred for blood transfusions to replace clotting factors. Treatment with lactulose promotes elimination of old blood from the GI tract, which combats excessive ammonia production and accumulation.

Appropriate surgical bypass procedures include portosystemic anastomosis, splenorenal shunt, and mesocaval shunt. A portacaval or a mesocaval shunt decreases pressure within the liver and reduces ascites, plasma loss, and the risk of hemorrhage by directing blood from the liver into collateral vessels. Emergency shunts carry a mortality of 25% to 50%. Clinical evidence suggests that portosystemic bypass doesn't prolong the patient's survival time; however, he will eventually die of hepatic coma rather than of hemorrhage.

Patient care

Care for the patient who has portal hypertension with esophageal varices focuses on careful monitoring for signs and symptoms of hemorrhage and subsequent hypotension, compromised oxygen supply, and altered level of consciousness (LOC).

■ Monitor the patient's vital signs, urine output, and central venous pressure to determine fluid volume status.

■ Assess the patient's LOC often.

■ Provide emotional support and reassurance in the wake of massive GI bleeding, which is always a frightening experience.

■ Keep the patient as quiet and comfortable as possible, but remember that tolerance of sedatives and tranquilizers may be decreased because of liver damage.

■ Clean the patient's mouth, which may be dry and flecked with dried blood.

■ Carefully monitor the patient with a Minnesota or Sengstaken-Blakemore tube in place for persistent bleeding in gastric drainage, signs of asphyxiation from tube displacement, proper inflation of balloons, and correct traction to maintain tube placement.

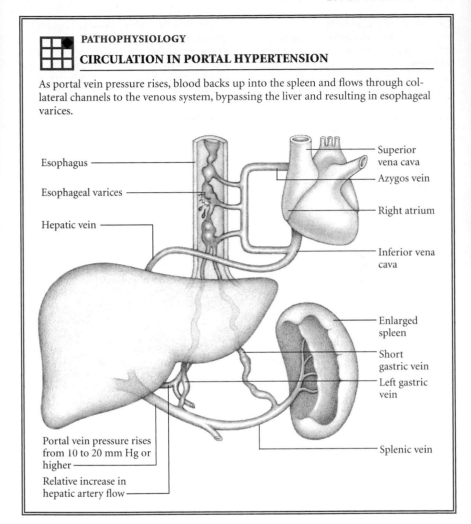

PATHOPHYSIOLOGY
CIRCULATION IN PORTAL HYPERTENSION

As portal vein pressure rises, blood backs up into the spleen and flows through collateral channels to the venous system, bypassing the liver and resulting in esophageal varices.

Esophagus

Esophageal varices

Hepatic vein

Superior vena cava

Azygos vein

Right atrium

Inferior vena cava

Enlarged spleen

Short gastric vein

Left gastric vein

Portal vein pressure rises from 10 to 20 mm Hg or higher

Relative increase in hepatic artery flow

Splenic vein

- To prevent skin breakdown associated with edema and pruritus, avoid using soap when you bathe the patient; instead, use lubricating lotion or moisturizing agents. Handle him gently, and turn and reposition him often to keep his skin intact.
- Tell the patient that rest and good nutrition will conserve his energy and decrease metabolic demands on the liver. Urge him to eat frequent, small meals. Stress the need to avoid infections and abstain from alcohol. Refer him to Alcoholics Anonymous, if necessary.

Liver abscess

A liver abscess occurs when bacteria or protozoa destroy hepatic tissue, producing a cavity, which fills with infectious organisms, liquefied liver cells, and leukocytes. Necrotic tissue then walls off the cavity from the rest of the liver.

Although liver abscess is relatively uncommon, it carries a mortality of 30%. Complications include rupture into the peritoneum, pleura, or pericardium, significantly increasing mortality.

Causes and incidence

In pyogenic liver abscesses, the common infecting organisms are *Escherichia coli, Klebsiella, Staphylococcus, Streptococcus, Bacteroides,* and enterococcus. The infecting organisms may invade the liver directly after a liver wound or they may spread from the lungs, skin, or other organs by the hepatic artery, portal vein, or biliary tract. Pyogenic abscesses are generally multiple and commonly follow cholecystitis, peritonitis, pneumonia, and bacterial endocarditis.

An amebic abscess results from infection with the protozoa *Entamoeba histolytica,* the organism that causes amebic dysentery. Amebic liver abscesses usually occur singly, in the right lobe.

There are 8 to 16 cases of liver abscess for every 100,000 people hospitalized, and there is a 5% to 30% mortality rate. Most cases occur in people in their 60s and 70s.

Signs and symptoms

The clinical manifestations of a liver abscess depend on the degree of involvement. Some patients are acutely ill; in others, the abscess is recognized only at autopsy, after death from another illness. The onset of symptoms of a pyogenic abscess is usually sudden; in an amebic abscess, the onset is more insidious. Common signs and symptoms include right abdominal and shoulder pain, weight loss, fever, chills, diaphoresis, nausea, vomiting, and anemia. Signs of right pleural effusion, such as dyspnea and pleural pain, develop if the abscess extends through the diaphragm. Liver damage may cause jaundice.

Diagnosis

CONFIRMING DIAGNOSIS *A liver scan showing filling defects (at the area of the abscess) more than ¾″ (2 cm) in diameter, together with characteristic clinical features, confirms the diagnosis. A computed tomography scan also confirms the diagnosis.*

A liver ultrasound may indicate defects caused by the abscess, but it's less definitive than a liver scan. Relevant laboratory values include elevated serum aspartate aminotransferase, alanine aminotransferase, alkaline phosphatase, and bilirubin levels; increased white blood cell count; and decreased serum albumin levels. In pyogenic abscess, a blood culture can identify the bacterial agent; in amebic abscess, a stool culture and serologic and hemagglutination tests can assist in diagnosis.

Treatment

If the organism causing the liver abscess is unknown, long-term antibiotic therapy begins immediately. When culture results are obtained, antibiotics are prescribed specific to treat the organism. Therapy usually continues for 2 to 4 months. Surgery is usually avoided, but it may be done for a single pyogenic abscess or for an amebic abscess that fails to respond to antibiotics. In acutely toxic patients, percutaneous needle aspiration and decompression may be needed to remove the abscess.

Special considerations

- Provide supportive care, monitor the patient's vital signs (especially temperature), and maintain fluid and nutritional intake.
- Administer anti-infectives and antibiotics as ordered, and watch for possible adverse effects. Stress the importance of compliance with therapy.
- Explain diagnostic and surgical procedures.
- Watch carefully for complications of abdominal surgery, such as hemorrhage or sepsis.

Fatty liver

Fatty liver, also known as *steatosis,* is a common clinical finding consisting of accumulated triglycerides and other fats in liver cells. In severe fatty liver, fat comprises as much as 40% of the liver's weight (as opposed to 5% in a normal liver), and the weight of the liver may increase from 3.31 lb (1.5 kg) to as much as 11 lb (4.9 kg). Minimal fatty changes are temporary and asymptomatic; severe or persistent changes may cause liver dysfunction. Fatty liver is usually reversible by simply eliminating the cause; however, this disorder may result in recurrent infection or sudden death from fat emboli in the lungs.

Causes

Chronic alcoholism is the most common cause of fatty liver in the United States and in Europe, with the severity of hepatic disease directly related to the amount of alcohol consumed. (Fatty liver can occur in people who consume as little as 10 oz of alcohol per week.) Other causes include malnutrition (especially protein deficiency), obesity, diabetes mellitus, jejunoileal bypass surgery, Cushing's syndrome, Reye's syndrome, pregnancy, large doses of hepatotoxins such as I.V. tetracycline, carbon tetrachloride intoxication, prolonged parenteral nutrition, and DDT poisoning. Whatever the cause, fatty infiltration of the liver probably results from mobilization of fatty acids from adipose tissues or altered fat metabolism.

Signs and symptoms

Clinical features of fatty liver vary with the degree of lipid infiltration, and many patients are asymptomatic. The most typical sign is a large, tender liver (hepatomegaly). Common signs and symptoms include right upper quadrant pain (with massive or rapid infiltration), ascites, edema, jaundice, and fever (all with hepatic necrosis or biliary stasis). (See *Massive ascites in fatty liver.*) Nausea, vomiting, and anorexia are less common. Splenomegaly usually accompanies cirrhosis. Rarer changes are spider angiomas, varices, transient gynecomastia, and menstrual disorders.

Diagnosis

Typical clinical features — especially in patients with chronic alcoholism, malnutrition, poorly controlled diabetes mellitus, or obesity — suggest fatty liver.

 CONFIRMING DIAGNOSIS *A liver biopsy confirms excessive fat in the liver. These liver function tests support this diagnosis:*

- *Albumin: somewhat low*
- *Globulin: usually elevated*
- *Cholesterol: usually elevated*
- *Total bilirubin: elevated*
- *Alkaline phosphatase: elevated*
- *Transaminase: usually low (less than 300 U)*
- *Prothrombin time: possibly prolonged.*

MASSIVE ASCITES IN FATTY LIVER

Massive ascites may result from fatty liver. Emaciated extremities and upper thorax are also typical of ascites.

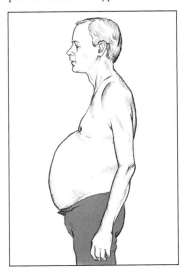

Other findings may include anemia, leukocytosis, elevated white blood cell count, albuminuria, hyperglycemia or hypoglycemia, and iron, folic acid, and vitamin B_{12} deficiencies.

Treatment

Treatment of fatty liver is essentially supportive and consists of correcting the underlying condition or eliminating its cause. For instance, when fatty liver results from parenteral nutrition, decreasing the rate of carbohydrate infusion may correct the disease. In alcoholic fatty liver, abstinence from alcohol and a proper diet can begin to correct liver changes within 4 to 8 weeks. Such correction requires comprehensive patient teaching.

Special considerations

Providing support to the patient and his family is an important element in the care of the patient with steatosis.

■ Suggest counseling for the alcoholic patient and provide emotional support for his family.

■ Teach the patient with diabetes—and his family—about proper care, such as the purpose of insulin injections, diet, and exercise. Refer him to home health nurses or to group classes, as necessary, to promote compliance with treatment. Emphasize the need for long-term medical supervision and urge him to report any changes in his health immediately.

■ Instruct an obese patient and his family about proper diet. Warn against fad diets, which are usually nutritionally inadequate. Recommend medical supervision for a patient who's more than 20% overweight. Encourage attendance at group diet and exercise programs and, if necessary, suggest behavior modification programs to correct eating habits. Be sure to follow up on his progress and provide positive reinforcement for any weight loss.

■ Assess for malnutrition, especially protein deficiency, in the patient with chronic illness. Suggest dietary changes and refer the patient to a dietitian.

■ Advise patients receiving hepatotoxins and those who risk occupational exposure to DDT to watch for and immediately report signs of toxicity.

■ Inform the patient that fatty liver is reversible *only* if he strictly follows the therapeutic program; otherwise, he risks permanent liver damage.

Wilson's disease

Wilson's disease, also called *hepatolenticular degeneration,* is a rare, inherited metabolic disorder characterized by excessive copper retention in the liver, brain, kidneys, and corneas. These deposits eventually lead to tissue necrosis and fibrosis, causing a variety of clinical effects, especially hepatic disease and neurologic changes. Wilson's disease is progressive and, if untreated, leads to fatal hepatic failure.

Causes and incidence
Wilson's disease is inherited as an autosomal recessive trait only when both parents carry the abnormal gene. There is a 25%

chance that carrier parents will transmit Wilson's disease (and a 50% chance that they will transmit the carrier state) to each of their offspring. The disease usually occurs among eastern Europeans, Sicilians, and other southern Italians.

Wilson's disease causes excessive intestinal absorption of copper and subsequent decreased excretion of copper in the stool. Copper accumulates first in the liver. As liver cells die, they release copper into the bloodstream, which carries it to other tissues. For example, in the kidneys, excretion of excessive amounts of unbound copper in urine (hypercupriuria) results from ceruloplasmin deficiency, a serum enzyme normally bound to copper. The deposit of copper in the tissue decreases serum copper (hypocupremia).

Signs and symptoms
Clinical manifestations of Wilson's disease usually appear between ages 6 and 20, although signs and symptoms can occur as late as age 40. Symptoms result from damage to the body tissues caused by progressive copper deposition and vary according to the patient and the state of his disease. The characteristic symptom of Wilson's disease is Kayser-Fleischer ring—a rusty brown ring of pigment at the periphery of the corneas. (See *Kayser-Fleischer ring.*) Fever may also occur in acute disease or with intercurrent infection. Other clinical features depend on the area affected.

■ Liver (including spleen): hepatomegaly, splenomegaly, ascites, jaundice, hematemesis, spider angiomas, and thrombocytopenia, eventually leading to cirrhosis or subacute necrosis of the liver

■ Blood: anemia and leukopenia

■ Central nervous system: "wing-flapping" tremors in arms, pill-rolling tremors in hands, facial and muscular rigidity, dysarthria, unsteady gait, and emotional and behavioral changes

■ Genitourinary tract: aminoaciduria, proteinuria, uricosuria, glycosuria, and phosphaturia

■ Musculoskeletal system (in severe disease): muscle wasting, contractures, deformities, osteomalacia, and pathologic fractures.

Diagnosis

Several tests suggest Wilson's disease:
- Serum ceruloplasmin: less than 20 mg/dl
- Serum copper: less than 80 mcg/dl
- Urine copper: more than 100 mcg/24 hours (may be as high as 1,000 mcg)
- Liver biopsy: excessive copper deposits (250 mcg/g dry weight), tissue changes indicative of chronic active hepatitis, fatty liver, or cirrhosis.

 CONFIRMING DIAGNOSIS
Revelation of Kayser-Fleischer rings during slit-lamp ophthalmic examination confirms the diagnosis. However, rings are present only when the disease has progressed beyond the liver.

Treatment

Treatment aims to reduce the amount of copper in the tissues, prevent additional accumulation, and manage hepatic disease. The most effective treatment for Wilson's disease consists of lifetime therapy with pyridoxine (vitamin B_6) in conjunction with penicillamine, a copper-chelating agent that mobilizes copper from the tissues and promotes its excretion in urine. The patient may require treatment with corticosteroids, such as prednisone, if he can't tolerate penicillamine. Treatment also includes potassium and sodium supplements before meals to prevent GI absorption of copper. Exercises or physical therapy may be needed, and protective measures for the patient who's confused or unable to care for himself. In some cases, a liver transplant may be the treatment of choice.

Special considerations

Patient care is supportive and focuses on education.
- Because penicillamine is chemically related to penicillin, ask whether the patient is allergic to penicillin before administering the first dose. Watch closely for allergic reactions, such as fever, rash, adenopathy, severe leukopenia, and thrombocytopenia.
- Tell the patient and his family which foods to avoid on a low-copper diet (mushrooms, nuts, chocolate, dried fruit, liver, and shellfish). Suggest the use of distilled water because most tap water flows through copper pipes. Copper cooking utensils should be avoided.

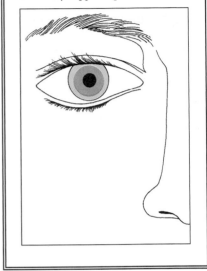

KAYSER-FLEISCHER RING

Wilson's disease produces a characteristic rust-colored ring around the cornea (Kayser-Fleischer ring) caused by copper deposits.

- Make sure to emphasize the necessity of lifetime therapy. Help the patient and his family make arrangements for continuing education, physical or vocational rehabilitation, and community nursing services, as needed.
- Provide emotional support. The neurologic changes Wilson's disease produces commonly lead to its misdiagnosis as a psychiatric disorder. Reassure the patient that his condition has a treatable physical basis.
- For a patient in an advanced stage of the disease, encourage as much self-care as possible to prevent further mental and physical deterioration. Plan an exercise schedule. Avoid sensory deprivation or overload. Prevent injuries that could occur as a result of neurologic deficits.
- If the patient is in a terminal stage, provide end-of-life care, including support to the family in their bereavement.
- Suggest genetic counseling for couples who are blood relatives or who have a relative with Wilson's disease. Explain that the

chance of their having a child with Wilson's disease is 25% with each pregnancy. Teach parents the disease's early symptoms so that they can seek prompt treatment for their child; stress regular pediatric examinations.

Hepatic encephalopathy

Hepatic encephalopathy, also known as *portosystemic encephalopathy* or *hepatic coma*, is a neurologic syndrome that develops as a complication of chronic liver disease. Most common in patients with cirrhosis, this syndrome is due primarily to ammonia intoxication of the brain. It may be acute and self-limiting or chronic and progressive. Treatment requires correction of the precipitating cause and reduction of blood ammonia levels. In advanced stages, the prognosis is extremely poor despite vigorous treatment.

Causes

Hepatic encephalopathy follows rising blood ammonia levels. Normally, the ammonia produced by protein breakdown in the bowel is metabolized to urea in the liver. When portal blood shunts past the liver, ammonia directly enters the systemic circulation and is carried to the brain. Such shunting may result from the collateral venous circulation that develops in portal hypertension or from surgically created portosystemic shunts. Cirrhosis further compounds this problem because impaired hepatocellular function prevents conversion of ammonia that reaches the liver.

Other factors that predispose rising ammonia levels include excessive protein intake, sepsis, excessive accumulation of nitrogenous body wastes (from constipation or GI hemorrhage), and bacterial action on protein and urea to form ammonia. Certain other factors heighten the brain's sensitivity to ammonia intoxication: hypoxia, azotemia, impaired glucose metabolism, infection, and administration of sedatives, narcotics, and general anesthetics. Depletion of the intravascular volume, from bleeding or diuresis, reduces hepatic and renal perfusion and leads to contraction alkalosis. In turn, hypokalemia and alkalosis increase ammonia production and impair its excretion.

Signs and symptoms

Clinical manifestations of hepatic encephalopathy vary (depending on the severity of neurologic involvement) and develop in four stages:

- In the *prodromal* stage, early signs and symptoms are commonly overlooked because they're so subtle: slight personality changes (disorientation, forgetfulness, and slurred speech) and a slight tremor.
- During the *impending* stage, tremor progresses into asterixis (liver flap and flapping tremor), the hallmark of hepatic encephalopathy. Asterixis is characterized by quick, irregular extensions and flexions of the wrists and fingers, when the wrists are held out straight and the hands flexed upward. Lethargy, aberrant behavior, and apraxia also occur.
- At the *stuporous* stage, hyperventilation occurs; the patient is typically stuporous, but becomes noisy and abusive when aroused.
- In the *comatose* stage, the patient has hyperactive reflexes, a positive Babinski's sign, fetor hepaticus (musty, sweet odor to the breath), and coma.

Diagnosis

CONFIRMING DIAGNOSIS
Clinical features, a history of liver disease, and elevated serum ammonia levels in venous and arterial samples confirm hepatic encephalopathy.

Other supportive laboratory values include an EEG that slows as the disease progresses, an increase in spinal fluid glutamine, elevated bilirubin, and prolonged prothrombin time. Recently, evoked potential testing has been advocated as a more specific indicator of encephalopathy, but its benefit over an EEG isn't yet clear.

Treatment

Effective treatment stops progression of encephalopathy by reducing blood ammonia levels. Treatment includes eliminating ammonia-producing substances from the GI tract by administering neomycin to suppress bacterial flora (preventing them from converting amino acids into ammonia), performing sorbitol-induced catharsis to produce osmotic diarrhea and continuous aspiration of blood from the stomach, and reducing dietary protein intake.

Lactulose, which traps ammonia in the bowel and promotes its excretion, is administered to reduce blood ammonia levels. Bacterial enzymes change lactulose to lactic acid, thereby rendering the colon too acidic for bacterial growth. At the same time, the resulting increase in free hydrogen ions prevents diffusion of ammonia through the mucosa; lactulose promotes conversion of systemically absorbable ammonia to ammonium, which is poorly absorbed and can be excreted. It's usually given orally. However, if the patient is in a coma, it may be administered by retention enema.

Treatment may also include potassium supplements to correct alkalosis due to increased ammonia levels, especially if the patient is taking diuretics. Hemodialysis may sometimes be used to clear toxic blood temporarily. Salt-poor albumin may be used to maintain fluid and electrolyte balance, replace depleted albumin levels, and restore plasma. Sedatives, tranquilizers, and other medications metabolized or excreted by the liver should be avoided if possible. Medications containing ammonium (including certain antacids) should also be avoided.

Special considerations
Patient care includes monitoring symptoms and support.
- Assess and record the patient's level of consciousness frequently. Continually orient him to place and time. Keep a daily record of his handwriting to monitor the progression of neurologic involvement.
- Monitor the patient's intake, output, and fluid and electrolyte balance. Check daily weight and measure abdominal girth. Watch for, and immediately report, signs of anemia (decreased hemoglobin level), infection, alkalosis (increased serum bicarbonate), and GI bleeding (melena and hematemesis).
- If the encephalopathy is acute, ask the dietary department to provide the specified low-protein diet, with carbohydrates supplying most of the calories.

- Promote rest, comfort, and a quiet atmosphere. Discourage stressful exercise.
- Use restraints, if necessary, but avoid sedatives. Protect the comatose patient's eyes from corneal injury by using artificial tears or eye patches.
- Provide emotional support for the patient's family in the terminal stage of encephalopathy.

GALLBLADDER AND DUCT DISORDERS

Cholelithiasis and related disorders

Diseases of the gallbladder and biliary tract are common and, in many cases, painful conditions that usually require surgery and may be life-threatening. They are generally associated with deposition of calculi and inflammation. (See *Common sites of calculi formation,* page 766.)

Causes and incidence
Cholelithiasis, stones or calculi (gallstones) in the gallbladder, results from changes in bile components. Gallstones are made of cholesterol, calcium bilirubinate, or a mixture of cholesterol and bilirubin pigment. They arise during periods of sluggishness in the gallbladder due to pregnancy, hormonal contraceptives, diabetes mellitus, celiac disease, cirrhosis of the liver, and pancreatitis. Cholelithiasis is a common health problem, affecting about 1 out of every 1,000 people. The prognosis is usually good with treatment unless infection occurs, in which case the prognosis depends on its severity and response to antibiotics.

One out of every 10 patients with gallstones develops *choledocholithiasis,* or gallstones in the common bile duct (sometimes called "common duct stones"). This occurs when stones passed out of the gallbladder lodge in the hepatic and common bile ducts and obstruct the flow of bile into the duodenum. Prognosis is good unless infection occurs.

COMMON SITES OF CALCULI FORMATION

The illustration below shows sites where calculi typically collect. Calculi vary in size; small calculi may travel.

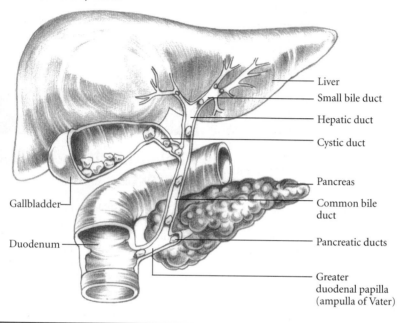

- Liver
- Small bile duct
- Hepatic duct
- Cystic duct
- Pancreas
- Common bile duct
- Pancreatic ducts
- Greater duodenal papilla (ampulla of Vater)
- Gallbladder
- Duodenum

Cholangitis, infection of the bile duct, is commonly associated with choledocholithiasis and may follow percutaneous transhepatic cholangiography or occlusion of endoscopic stents. Predisposing factors may include bacterial or metabolic alteration of bile acids. Widespread inflammation may cause fibrosis and stenosis of the common bile duct. The prognosis for this rare condition is poor without stenting or surgery.

Cholecystitis, acute or chronic inflammation of the gallbladder, is usually associated with a gallstone impacted in the cystic duct, causing painful distention of the gallbladder. Cholecystitis accounts for 10% to 25% of all patients requiring gallbladder surgery. The acute form is most common during middle age; the chronic form usually occurs among elderly patients. The prognosis is good with treatment.

Cholesterolosis, polyps or crystal deposits of cholesterol in the gallbladder's submucosa, may result from bile secretions containing high concentrations of cholesterol and insufficient bile salts. The polyps may be localized or speckle the entire gallbladder. Cholesterolosis, the most common pseudotumor, isn't related to widespread inflammation of the mucosa or lining of the gallbladder. The prognosis is good with surgery.

Biliary cirrhosis, ascending infection of the biliary system, sometimes follows viral destruction of liver and duct cells, but the primary cause is unknown. This condition usually leads to obstructive jaundice and involves the portal and periportal spaces of the liver. It's nine times more common among women ages 40 to 60 than among men. The prognosis is poor without liver transplantation.

Gallstone ileus results from a gallstone lodging at the terminal ileum; it's more common in the elderly. The prognosis is good with surgery.

Postcholecystectomy syndrome commonly results from residual gallstones or stricture of the common bile duct. It occurs in 1% to 5% of all patients whose gallbladders have been surgically removed and may produce right upper quadrant abdominal pain, biliary colic, fatty food intolerance, dyspepsia, and indigestion. The prognosis is good with selected radiologic procedures, endoscopic procedures, or surgery.

Acalculous cholecystitis is more common in critically ill patients, accounting for about 5% of cholecystitis cases. It may result from primary infection with such organisms as *Salmonella typhi, Escherichia coli,* or *Clostridium* or from obstruction of the cystic duct due to lymphadenopathy or a tumor. It appears that ischemia, usually related to a low cardiac output, also has a role in the pathophysiology of this disease. Signs and symptoms of acalculous cholecystitis include unexplained sepsis, right upper quadrant pain, fever, leukocytosis, and a palpable gallbladder.

Each of these disorders produces its own set of complications. Cholelithiasis may lead to any of the disorders associated with gallstone formation: cholangitis, cholecystitis, choledocholithiasis, and gallstone ileus. Cholecystitis can progress to gallbladder complications, such as empyema, hydrops or mucocele, or gangrene. Gangrene may lead to perforation, resulting in peritonitis, fistula formation, pancreatitis, limy bile, and porcelain gallbladder. Other complications include chronic cholecystitis and cholangitis.

Choledocholithiasis may lead to cholangitis, obstructive jaundice, pancreatitis, and secondary biliary cirrhosis. Cholangitis, especially in the suppurative form, may progress to septic shock and death. Gallstone ileus may cause bowel obstruction, which can lead to intestinal perforation, peritonitis, septicemia, secondary infection, and septic shock.

In most cases, gallbladder and bile duct diseases occur in people who are older than age 40 and are more prevalent in women and Native Americans.

Signs and symptoms

Although gallbladder disease may produce no symptoms, acute cholelithiasis, acute cholecystitis, choledocholithiasis, and cholesterolosis produce the symptoms of a classic gallbladder attack. Attacks usually follow meals rich in fats or may occur at night, suddenly awakening the patient. They begin with acute abdominal pain in the right upper quadrant that may radiate to the back, between the shoulders, or to the front of the chest; the pain may be so severe that the patient seeks emergency department care. Other features may include recurring fat intolerance, biliary colic, belching, flatulence, indigestion, diaphoresis, nausea, vomiting, chills, low-grade fever, jaundice (if a stone obstructs the common bile duct), and clay-colored stools (with choledocholithiasis).

Clinical features of cholangitis include a rise in eosinophils, jaundice, abdominal pain, high fever, and chills; biliary cirrhosis may produce jaundice, related itching, weakness, fatigue, slight weight loss, and abdominal pain. Gallstone ileus produces signs and symptoms of small-bowel obstruction — nausea, vomiting, abdominal distention, and absent bowel sounds if the bowel is completely obstructed. Its most telling symptom is intermittent recurrence of colicky pain over several days.

Diagnosis

Echography and X-rays detect gallstones. Other tests may include the following:

■ Abdominal computed tomography scan or ultrasound reflects stones in the gallbladder.

■ Percutaneous transhepatic cholangiography, done under fluoroscopic control, distinguishes between gallbladder or bile duct disease and cancer of the pancreatic head in patients with jaundice.

■ Endoscopic retrograde cholangiopancreatography visualizes the biliary tree after insertion of an endoscope down the esophagus into the duodenum, cannulation of the common bile and pancreatic ducts, and injection of contrast medium.

■ HIDA scan of the gallbladder detects obstruction of the cystic duct.

■ Oral cholecystography shows stones in the gallbladder and biliary duct obstruction.

An elevated icteric index and total bilirubin, urine bilirubin, and alkaline phosphatase levels support the diagnosis. The white blood cell count is slightly elevated during a cholecystitis attack. Differential diagnosis is essential because gallbladder disease can mimic other diseases (myocardial infarction, angina, pancreatitis, pancreatic head cancer, pneumonia, peptic ulcer, hiatal hernia, esophagitis, and gastritis). Serum amylase levels distinguish gallbladder disease from pancreatitis. With suspected heart disease, serial cardiac enzyme tests and electrocardiography should precede gallbladder and upper GI diagnostic tests.

Treatment

Surgery, usually elective, is the treatment of choice for gallbladder and bile duct diseases and may include open or laparoscopic cholecystectomy, cholecystectomy with operative cholangiography, and possibly exploration of the common bile duct. Electrohydraulic shock wave lithotripsy can be used to fragment gallstones if they're few in number; it may be used with ursodeoxycholic acid to improve dissolution. Other treatments include a low-fat diet to prevent attacks and vitamin K for itching, jaundice, and bleeding tendencies due to vitamin K deficiency. Treatment during an acute attack may include insertion of a nasogastric tube and an I.V. line and, possibly, antibiotic administration.

A nonsurgical treatment for choledocholithiasis involves placement of a catheter through the percutaneous transhepatic cholangiographic route. Guided by fluoroscopy, the catheter is directed toward the stone. A basket is threaded through the catheter, opened, twirled to entrap the stone, closed, and withdrawn. This procedure can be performed endoscopically.

Chenodeoxycholic acid, which dissolves radiolucent stones, provides an alternative for patients who are poor surgical risks or who refuse surgery.

Special considerations

Patient care for gallbladder and bile duct diseases focuses on supportive care and close postoperative observation.

■ Before surgery, teach the patient to deep-breathe, cough, expectorate, and perform leg exercises that are necessary after surgery. Also teach splinting, repositioning, and ambulation techniques. Explain the procedures that will be performed before, during, and after surgery to help ease the patient's anxiety and to help ensure his cooperation.

■ After surgery, monitor the patient's vital signs for signs of bleeding, infection, or atelectasis.

■ Evaluate the incision site for bleeding. Serosanguineous drainage is common during the first 24 to 48 hours if the patient has a wound drain. If, after a choledochostomy, a T-tube drain is placed in the duct and attached to a drainage bag, make sure that the drainage tube has no kinks. Also check that the connecting tubing from the T tube is well secured to the patient to prevent dislodgment.

■ Measure and record T-tube drainage daily (200 to 300 ml is normal).

■ Teach patients who will be discharged with a T tube how to perform dressing changes and routine skin care.

■ Monitor the patient's intake and output. Allow him nothing by mouth for 24 to 48 hours or until bowel sounds return and nausea and vomiting cease (postoperative nausea may indicate a full bladder).

■ If the patient doesn't void within 8 hours (or if the amount voided is inadequate based on I.V. fluid intake), percuss over the symphysis pubis for bladder distention (especially in the patient receiving anticholinergics). The patient who has had a laparoscopic cholecystectomy may be discharged the same day or within 24 hours after surgery. He should have minimal pain, be able to tolerate a regular diet within 24 hours after surgery, and be able to return to normal activity within a few days to a week.

■ Encourage deep-breathing and leg exercises every hour. The patient should ambulate after surgery. Provide elastic stockings to support the leg muscles and promote venous blood flow, thus preventing stasis and clot formation.

■ Evaluate the location, duration, and character of any pain. Administer adequate medication to relieve pain, especially before such activities as deep breathing and ambulation, which increase pain.

■ At discharge, advise the patient against heavy lifting or straining for 6 weeks. Urge him to walk daily. Tell him that food restrictions are unnecessary unless he has an intolerance to a specific food or some underlying condition (such as diabetes, atherosclerosis, or obesity) that requires such restriction.

■ Instruct the patient to notify the surgeon if he has pain for more than 24 hours or notices any jaundice, anorexia, nausea or vomiting, fever, or tenderness in the abdominal area because these may indicate a biliary tract injury from cholestectomy, requiring immediate attention.

Selected references

Der, G. "An Overview of Proton Pump Inhibitors," *Gastroenterology Nursing* 26(5):182-90, September-October 2003.

Fielding, J.W., and Hallissey, M.T., eds. *Hepatobiliary and Upper GI Surgery*. New York: Springer Publishing Co., 2004.

Flynn, M. "Noninfectious Liver Disorders: Adult Autoimmune Hepatitis," *The Nurse Practitioner* 28(12):28-31, December 2003.

Jorgensen, R.A. "Nonalcoholic Fatty Liver Disease," *Gastroenterology Nursing* 26(4):150-54, July-August 2003.

Newton, S.E. "Relationship Between Depression and Work Outcomes following Liver Transplantation: The Nursing Perspective," *Gastroenterology Nursing* 26(2):68-72, March-April 2003.

Thames, G. "Drug-induced Liver Injury: What You Need to Know," *Gastroenterology Nursing* 27(1):31-33, January-February 2004.

Tierney, L.M., et al. *Current Medical Diagnosis and Treatment 2004*, 43rd ed. New York: McGraw-Hill Book Co., 2004.

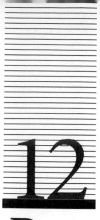

Renal and urologic disorders

Introduction   *771*

Congenital anomalies   *779*
Medullary sponge kidney   *779*
Polycystic kidney disease   *780*

Acute renal disorders   *782*
Acute renal failure   *782*
Acute pyelonephritis   *784*
Acute poststreptococcal
   glomerulonephritis   *786*
Acute tubular necrosis   *787*
Renal infarction   *789*
Renal calculi   *790*
Renal vein thrombosis   *794*

Chronic renal disorders   *795*
Nephrotic syndrome   *795*
Chronic glomerulonephritis   *798*
Renovascular hypertension   *799*
Hydronephrosis   *800*
Renal tubular acidosis   *801*
Chronic renal failure   *802*

Lower urinary tract disorders   *808*
Lower urinary tract infection   *808*
Vesicoureteral reflux   *810*
Neurogenic bladder   *812*
Congenital anomalies of the ureter,
   bladder, and urethra   *814*

Prostate and epididymis disorders   *818*
Prostatitis   *818*
Epididymitis   *819*
Benign prostatic hyperplasia   *821*

Selected references   *823*

STRUCTURE OF THE KIDNEYS

The major components of the kidneys are depicted below.

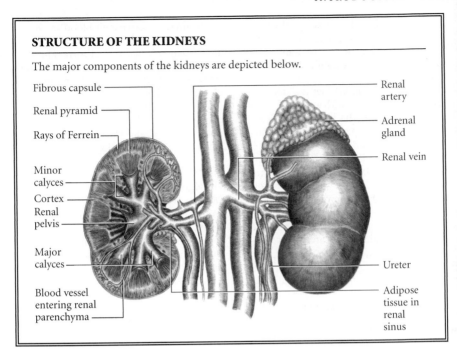

Fibrous capsule

Renal pyramid

Rays of Ferrein

Minor calyces

Cortex

Renal pelvis

Major calyces

Blood vessel entering renal parenchyma

Renal artery

Adrenal gland

Renal vein

Ureter

Adipose tissue in renal sinus

Introduction

The kidneys are located retroperitoneally in the lumbar area, with the right kidney a little lower than the left because of the liver mass above it. The left kidney is slightly longer than the right and closer to the midline. The kidneys assume different locations as the body position changes. They are covered by the fibrous capsule, perirenal fat, renal fascia, and pararenal fat. (See *Structure of the kidneys.*)

Renal arteries branch into five segmental arteries that supply different areas of the kidneys. The segmental arteries then branch into several divisions from which the afferent arterioles and vasa recta arise. Renal veins follow a similar branching pattern, characterized by stellate vessels and segmental branches, and empty into the inferior vena cava. The tubular system receives its blood supply from a peritubular capillary network of vessels.

The gross structure of each kidney includes the lateral and medial margins, the hilus, the renal sinus, and renal parenchyma. The hilus, located at the medial margin, is the indentation where the blood and lymph vessels enter the kidney and the ureter emerges. The hilus leads to the renal sinus, which is a spacious cavity filled with adipose tissue, branches of the renal vessels, calyces, the renal pelvis, and the ureter. The renal sinus is surrounded by parenchyma, which consists of a cortex and a medulla.

The cortex (outermost layer of the kidney) contains glomeruli (parts of the nephron), cortical arches (areas that separate the medullary pyramids from the renal surface), columns of Bertin (areas that separate the pyramids from one another), and medullary rays of Ferrein (long, delicate processes from the bases of the pyramids that mix with the cortex). The medulla contains pyramids (cone-shaped structures of parenchymal tissue), papillae (apical ends of the pyramids through which urine oozes into the minor calyces), and papillary ducts of Bellini (collecting ducts in the pyramids that empty into the papillae).

Ureters

The ureters are a pair of retroperitoneally located, mucosa-lined, fibromuscular tubes that transport urine from the renal pelvis to the urinary bladder. Although the ureters have no sphincters, their oblique entrance into the bladder creates a mucosal fold that may produce a sphincterlike action.

The adult urinary bladder is a spherical, hollow muscular sac, with a normal capacity of 300 to 600 ml. It's located anterior and inferior to the peritoneal cavity, and posterior to the pubic bones. The gross structure of the bladder includes the fundus (large central, posterosuperior portion of the bladder), the apex (anterosuperior region), the body (posteroinferior region containing the ureteral orifices), and the urethral orifice, or neck (most inferior portion of the bladder). The three orifices comprise a triangular area called the *trigone*.

Nephrons

The functional units of each kidney are its 1 to 3 million nephrons. Each nephron is composed of the renal corpuscle and the tubular system. The renal corpuscle includes the glomerulus (a network of minute blood vessels) and Bowman's capsule (an epithelial sac surrounding the glomerulus that's part of the tubular system). The renal corpuscle has a vascular pole, where the afferent arteriole enters and the efferent arteriole emerges, and a urinary pole that narrows to form the beginning of the tubular system. The tubular system includes the proximal convoluted tubule, the loop of Henle, and the distal convoluted tubule. The last portion of the nephron consists of the collecting duct.

Innervation and vasculature

The kidneys are innervated by sympathetic branches from the celiac plexus, upper lumbar splanchnic and thoracic nerves, and the intermesenteric and superior hypogastric plexuses, which form a plexus around the kidneys. Similar numbers of sympathetic and parasympathetic nerves from the renal plexus, superior hypogastric plexus, and intermesenteric plexus innervate the ureters. Nerves that arise from the inferior hypogastric plexuses innervate the bladder. The parasympathetic nerve supply to the bladder controls micturition.

The ureters receive their blood supply from the renal, vesical, gonadal, and iliac arteries, and the abdominal aorta. The ureteral veins follow the arteries and drain into the renal vein. The bladder receives blood through vesical arteries. Vesical veins unite to form the pudendal plexus, which empties into the iliac veins. A rich lymphatic system drains the renal cortex, the kidneys, the ureters, and the bladder.

Homeostasis

Through the production and elimination of urine, the kidneys maintain homeostasis. These vital organs regulate the volume, electrolyte concentration, and acid-base balance of body fluids; detoxify the blood and eliminate wastes; regulate blood pressure; and aid in erythropoiesis. The kidneys eliminate wastes from the body through urine formation (by glomerular filtration, tubular reabsorption, and tubular secretion) and excretion. Glomerular filtration, the process of filtering the blood flowing through the kidneys, depends on the permeability of the capillary walls, vascular pressure, and filtration pressure. The normal glomerular filtration rate (GFR) is about 120 ml/minute.

Clearance measures function

Clearance is the volume of plasma that can be cleared of a given substance per unit of time, and depends on how renal tubular cells handle the substance that has been filtered by the glomerulus:

- If the tubules don't reabsorb or secrete the substance, clearance equals the GFR.
- If the tubules reabsorb it, clearance is less than the GFR.
- If the tubules secrete it, clearance is greater than the GFR.
- If the tubules reabsorb and secrete it, clearance is less than, equal to, or greater than the GFR.

The most accurate measure of glomerular function is creatinine clearance, because this substance is filtered only by the glomerulus and isn't reabsorbed by the tubules.

The transport of filtered substances in tubular reabsorption or secretion may be active (requiring the expenditure of energy) or passive (requiring none). For example, energy is required to move sodium across tubular cells (active transport), but none is required to move urea (passive transport). The amount of reabsorption or secretion of a substance depends on the maximum tubular transport capacity for that substance; that is, the greatest amount of a substance that can be reabsorbed or secreted per minute without saturating the system.

 ELDER TIP *After age 40, a person's renal function begins to diminish; if he lives to age 90, it may have decreased by as much as 50%. This change is reflected in a decreased GFR; it's caused by age-related changes in the renal vasculature that disturb glomerular hemodynamics as well as by reduced cardiac output and atherosclerotic changes that reduce renal blood flow by more than 50%.*

Water regulation

Hormones partially control water regulation by the kidneys. Hormonal control depends on the response of osmoreceptors to changes in osmolality. The two hormones involved are antidiuretic hormone (ADH), produced by the pituitary gland, and aldosterone, produced by the adrenal cortex. ADH alters the collecting tubules' permeability to water. When plasma concentration of ADH is high, the tubules are very permeable to water, so a greater amount of water is reabsorbed, creating a high concentration but small volume of urine. The reverse is true if ADH concentration is low.

Aldosterone regulates sodium and water reabsorption from the distal tubules. High plasma aldosterone concentration promotes sodium and water reabsorption from the tubules and decreases sodium and water excretion in the urine; low plasma aldosterone concentration promotes sodium and water excretion. Aldosterone also helps control the distal tubular secretion of potassium. Other factors that determine potassium secretion include the amount of potassium ingested, number of hydrogen ions secreted, level of intracellular potassium, amount of sodium in the distal tubule, and the GFR.

The countercurrent mechanism — composed of a multiplication system and an exchange system that occur in the renal medulla via the limbs of the loop of Henle

and the vasa recta — is the method by which the kidneys concentrate urine. It achieves active transport of sodium and chloride between the loop of Henle and the medullary interstitial fluid. Failure of the countercurrent mechanism produces polyuria and nocturia.

To regulate acid-base balance, the kidneys secrete hydrogen ions, reabsorb sodium and bicarbonate ions, acidify phosphate salts, and synthesize ammonia — which keep the blood at its normal pH of 7.37 to 7.43.

The kidneys assist in regulating blood pressure by synthesizing and secreting renin in response to an actual, or perceived, decrease in the volume of extracellular fluid. Renin, in turn, acts on a substrate to form angiotensin I, which is converted to angiotensin II. Angiotensin II increases arterial blood pressure by peripheral vasoconstriction and stimulation of aldosterone secretion. The resulting increase in the aldosterone level promotes the reabsorption of sodium and water to correct the fluid deficit and renal ischemia.

The kidneys secrete erythropoietin in response to decreased oxygen tension in the renal blood supply. Erythropoietin then acts on the bone marrow to increase the production of red blood cells (RBCs).

Renal tubular cells synthesize active vitamin D and help regulate calcium balance and bone metabolism.

Clinical assessment

Assessment of the renal and urologic systems begins with an accurate patient history and requires a thorough physical examination and certain laboratory data and test results from invasive and noninvasive procedures. When obtaining a patient history, ask about symptoms that pertain specifically to the pathology of the renal and urologic systems, such as frequency or urgency, and about the presence of any systemic diseases that can produce renal or urologic dysfunction, such as hypertension, diabetes mellitus, or bladder infections. Family history may also suggest a genetic predisposition to certain renal diseases, such as glomerulonephritis or polycystic kidney disease. Also, ask what medications the pa-

COMMON RENAL SYMPTOMS

Symptom	Possible cause
Dribbling	Prostatic enlargement, strictures
Dysuria	Infection, inflammation of bladder or urethra
Edema	Nephrotic syndrome, failure
Frequency	Infection, diabetes, bladder tumors, medications
Hematuria	Glomerular diseases, trauma, neoplasms, renal calculi
Hesitancy	Neurogenic bladder, infection
Incontinence	Infection, neoplasms, prolapsed uterus
Nocturia	Infection, nephrotic syndrome, diabetes, medications
Oliguria	Failure, insufficiency, neoplasms
Proteinuria	Glomerular diseases, infection
Pyuria	Infection
Renal colic	Calculi
Urgency	Infection, prostatic disease, medications

mucous membranes for color, secretions, odor, and intactness; eyes for periorbital edema and vision; general activity for motion, gait, and posture; muscle movement for motor function and general strength; and mental status for level of consciousness, orientation, and response to stimuli. (See *Common renal symptoms.*)

Renal disease causes distinctive changes in vital signs: hypertension due to fluid and electrolyte imbalances and hyperactivity of the renin-angiotensin system; a strong, fast, irregular pulse due to fluid and electrolyte imbalances; hyperventilation to compensate for metabolic acidosis; and an increased susceptibility to infection due to overall decreased resistance. Palpation and percussion may reveal little because the kidneys and bladder are difficult to palpate unless they are enlarged or distended.

Noninvasive tests and monitoring
Laboratory tests analyze serum levels of chemical substances such as uric acid, creatinine, and blood urea nitrogen; tests also determine urine characteristics, including the presence of RBCs, white blood cells, casts, or bacteria; specific gravity and pH; and physical properties, such as clarity, color, and odor. (See *Serum and urine values in renal disease.*)

■ Intake and output assessment: Fluid intake and output measurement helps determine the patient's hydration status but isn't a reliable method of evaluating renal function because urine output varies with different types of renal disorders. To provide the most useful and accurate information, use calibrated containers, establish baseline values for each patient, compare measurement patterns, and validate intake and output measurements by checking the patient's weight daily. Monitor all fluid losses—including blood, vomitus, and diarrhea. Also assess wound and stoma drainage daily.

■ Specimen collection: Meticulous specimen collection is vital for valid laboratory data. If the patient is collecting the specimen, explain the importance of cleaning the meatal area thoroughly. The culture specimen should be caught midstream, in a sterile container; a specimen for urinalysis, in a clean container, preferably at the first

tient has been taking; abuse of analgesics or antibiotics may cause nephrotoxicity.

Physical examination for renal disease
The first step in physical examination is careful observation of the patient's overall appearance, because renal disease affects all body systems. Examine the patient's skin for color, turgor, intactness, and texture;

SERUM AND URINE VALUES IN RENAL DISEASE

	Normal serum value	Deviation	Normal urine value	Deviation
Sodium	135 to 145 mEq/L	↑ or N	30 to 280 mEq/L	V
Potassium	3.8 to 5.5 mEq/L	↑	25 to 100 mEq/L	↓
Chloride	100 to 108 mEq/L	↑	110 to 250 mEq/24 hrs	↓
Calcium	8.9 to 10.1 mg/dl	↓	Female: < 250 mg/ 24 hrs Male: < 275 mg/24 hrs	↓
Phosphorus	2.5 to 4.5 mg/dl	↑ or N	1 g/24 hrs	V
Magnesium	1.7 to 2.1 mEq/L	↑	< 150 mg/ 24 hrs	↓
Carbon dioxide combining power	22 to 34 mEq/L	↓		
Specific gravity			1.005 to 1.035	↓
pH			4.5 to 8	↑
Blood urea nitrogen	8 to 20 mg/dl	↑	10 to 20 g/L	↓
Creatinine	Female: 0.6 to 0.9 mg/dl Male: 0.8 to 1.2 mg/dl	↑	Female: 0 to 80 mg/ 24 hrs Male: 0 to 40 mg/24 hrs	↓
Osmolality	280 to 295 mOsm/kg	V	500 to 1,400 mOsm/kg	↓
Uric acid	Female: 2.3 to 6 mg/dl Male: 4.3 to 8 mg/dl	↑		
Glucose	70 to 100 mg/dl	N	0	N
Protein	6.9 to 7.9 g/dl	↓ or N	0	V

KEY: ↑ = increased; ↓ = decreased; N = normal; V = varies

(continued)

SERUM AND URINE VALUES IN RENAL DISEASE *(continued)*

	Normal serum value	Deviation	Normal urine value	Deviation
Hematocrit	Female: 38% to 46% Male: 42% to 54%	↓		
Hemoglobin	Female: 12 to 16 g/dl Male: 14 to 18 g/dl	↓		
White blood cells	4,000 to 10,000/μl		none	V
Red blood cells			none	V
Casts			none	V
Bacteria			none	V
Alkaline phosphatase	Female ages 24 to 65: 82 to 282 U/L Male ≥ age 19: 98 to 251 U/L	↑		

KEY: ↑ = increased; ↓ = decreased; N = normal; V = varies

voiding of the day. Begin a 24-hour specimen collection after discarding the first voiding; such specimens often necessitate special handling or preservatives. When obtaining a urine specimen from a catheterized patient, remember to avoid taking the specimen from the collection bag; instead, aspirate a sample through the collection port in the catheter, with a sterile needle and a syringe.
■ Kidney-ureter-bladder radiography: This test assesses size, shape, position, and areas of calcification of these organs.
■ Ultrasonography: This safe, painless procedure allows for visualization of the renal parenchyma, calyces, pelvis, ureters, and bladder. Because the test doesn't depend on renal function, it's useful in patients with renal failure and in detecting complications after kidney transplantation.

■ Invasive tests: See *Invasive diagnostic tests for assessing the renal and urologic systems.*

Treatment methods
Treatment of intractable renal or urinary system dysfunction may require urinary diversion, dialysis, or kidney transplantation. Urinary diversion is the surgical creation of an outlet for excreting urine. The types of urinary diversion include ileal conduit, cutaneous ureterostomy, ureterosigmoidostomy, and creation of a rectal bladder.
In dialysis, a semipermeable membrane, osmosis, and diffusion imitate normal renal function by eliminating excess body fluids, maintaining or restoring plasma electrolyte and acid-base balance, and removing waste products and dialyzable poisons from the blood. Dialysis is most often used for patients with acute or chronic re-

INVASIVE DIAGNOSTIC TESTS FOR ASSESSING THE RENAL AND UROLOGIC SYSTEMS

Several invasive tests are available to assist in diagnosis of renal and urologic problems. The most serious complication which occurs with many of these procedures is hypersensitivity to the contrast media. Symptoms may include increased pulse rate, itching, hives, chills, fever, dyspnea, and shock.

Procedure	Purpose	Special considerations
Computed tomography scan (CT) or magnetic resonance imaging (MRI)	Although CT scan and MRI can be noninvasive, I.V. contrast material is often given to enhance the views obtained. These tests are especially helpful in evaluating renal or bladder mass lesions.	*After:* After using I.V. contrast medium, observe for hypersensitivity reaction and hematoma at injection site.
Cystoscopy	A fiber-optic scope is used to visualize the inside of the bladder in cystoscopy.	*Before:* Give sedatives as ordered. *After:* Offer increased fluids; administer analgesics; watch for hematuria and signs of perforation, hemorrhage, and infection (chills, fever, increased pulse rate, shock).
Cystourethrography	In cystourethrography, X-rays and I.V. contrast material are used to determine size and shape of the bladder and urethra.	*During:* Catheterize the patient. *After:* Offer increased fluids; observe for hypersensitivity reaction.
Cystometry	Cystometry is used to evaluate bladder pressure, sensation, and capacity. A catheter is introduced into the bladder, and saline solution is instilled. Results are shown on a computer at the time of testing.	*Before:* Observe voiding; catheterize for residual urine. *After:* Remove catheter; watch for stress incontinence when patient coughs; watch voiding; catheterize for residual urine.
Excretory urography	Excretory urography uses X-rays and I.V. contrast material to allow visualization of renal parenchyma, calyces, pelves, ureters, and bladder.	*After:* Observe for hypersensitivity reaction; watch for hematomas at injection site.

(continued)

INVASIVE DIAGNOSTIC TESTS FOR ASSESSING THE RENAL AND UROLOGIC SYSTEMS *(continued)*

Procedure	Purpose	Special considerations
Nephrotomography	In nephrotomography, I.V. contrast material and tomography are used to visualize parenchymia, calyces, and pelves in layers.	*After:* Observe for hypersensitivity reaction.
Renal angiography	Renal angiography uses contrast material injected into a catheter in the femoral artery or vein to allow visualization of the arterial tree and capillaries as well as venous drainage of the kidney.	*After:* Observe for hypersensitivity reaction, hematomas and hemorrhage at injection site, and nephrotoxicity. Offer increased fluids.
Renal scan	In renal scan, radioisotopes are administered I.V., and images of the kidney are taken at intervals to determine renal function.	*After:* Observe for hypersensitivity reaction.
Renal biopsy	The specimen obtained in renal biopsy is used to develop histologic diagnosis and determine therapy and prognosis.	*Before:* Make sure the patient's clotting times, prothrombin times, and platelet count are recorded on his chart. *After:* Apply gentle pressure to the bandage site. Watch for hemorrhage and hematoma at the biopsy site and look for hematuria.

nal failure. The two most common types of dialysis are peritoneal dialysis and hemodialysis.

In peritoneal dialysis, a dialysate solution is infused into the peritoneal cavity. Substances then diffuse through the peritoneal membrane. Waste products remain in the dialysate solution and are removed.

Hemodialysis separates solutes by differential diffusion through a cellophane membrane placed between the blood and the dialysate solution, in an external receptacle. Because the blood must actually pass out of the body into a dialysis machine, hemodialysis requires an access route to the blood supply by an arteriovenous fistula or cannula or by a bovine or synthetic graft. When caring for a patient with such an access route, monitor the patency of the access route, prevent infection, and promote safety and adequate function. After dialysis, watch for such complications as headache, vomiting, agitation, and twitching.

Patients with end-stage renal disease may benefit from kidney transplantation, despite its limitations: a shortage of donor kidneys, the chance of transplant rejection, and the need for lifelong medications and follow-up care. After kidney transplantation, maintain fluid and electrolyte balance, prevent infection, monitor for rejection, and promote psychological well-being.

CONGENITAL ANOMALIES

Medullary sponge kidney

In medullary sponge kidney, the collecting ducts in the renal pyramids dilate, and cavities, clefts, and cysts form in the medulla. This disease may affect only a single pyramid in one kidney or all pyramids in both kidneys. The kidneys are usually somewhat enlarged but may be of normal size; they appear spongy.

Because this disorder is usually asymptomatic and benign, it's often overlooked until the patient reaches adulthood. The prognosis is generally very good. Medullary sponge kidney is unrelated to medullary cystic disease; these conditions are similar only in the presence and location of the cysts.

Causes and incidence

Medullary sponge kidney may be transmitted as an autosomal dominant trait, but this remains unproven. Most nephrologists consider it a congenital abnormality.

Although medullary sponge kidney may be found in both sexes and in all age groups, it primarily affects males ages 40 to 70. It occurs in about 1 in every 5,000 to 20,000 persons.

Signs and symptoms

Symptoms usually appear only as a result of complications and are seldom present before adulthood. Complications include formation of calcium oxalate stones, which lodge in the dilated cystic collecting ducts or pass through a ureter, and infection secondary to dilation of the ducts. These complications, which occur in about 30% of patients, are likely to produce severe colic, hematuria, lower urinary tract infection ([UTI]; burning on urination, urgency, frequency), and pyelonephritis. Secondary impairment of renal function from obstruction and infection occurs in only about 10% of patients.

Diagnosis

Excretory urography is usually the key to diagnosis, often showing a characteristic flowerlike appearance of the pyramidal cavities when they fill with contrast material. It may also show renal calculi. Urinalysis is generally normal unless complications develop; however, it may show a slight reduction in concentrating ability or hypercalciuria. Diagnosis must distinguish medullary sponge kidney from renal tuberculosis, renal tubular acidosis, and papillary necrosis.

Treatment

Treatment focuses on preventing or treating complications caused by stones and infection. Specific measures include increasing fluid intake and monitoring renal function and urine. New symptoms necessitate immediate evaluation.

Because medullary sponge kidney is a benign condition, surgery is seldom necessary, except to remove stones during acute obstruction. Only serious, uncontrollable infection or hemorrhage requires nephrectomy.

Special considerations

Patient care includes explaining the disease to the patient and his family and reassuring them that the condition is benign and the prognosis good.

■ To prevent infection, instruct the patient to bathe often and use proper toilet hygiene; this is especially important for a female patient because the proximity of the urinary meatus and the anus increases the risk of infection.

■ If infection occurs, stress the importance of completing the prescribed course of antibiotic therapy.

■ Emphasize the need for adequate fluid intake.

■ Explain all diagnostic procedures, and provide emotional support. Teach the patient how to collect a clean-catch urine specimen for culture. Check for allergy to excretory urography dye.

■ When the patient is hospitalized for a stone, strain all urine, administer analgesics as ordered, and force fluids. Before discharge, tell the patient to watch for and report any signs of stone passage and UTI.

POLYCYSTIC KIDNEY

In polycystic kidney disease, cysts are seen in grapelike clusters, as shown below.

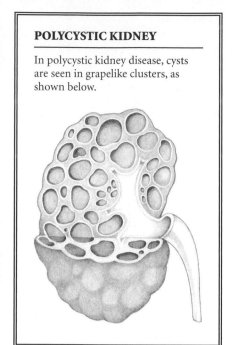

Polycystic kidney disease

Polycystic kidney disease is an inherited disorder characterized by multiple, bilateral, grapelike clusters of fluid-filled cysts that grossly enlarge the kidneys, compressing and eventually replacing functioning renal tissue. (See *Polycystic kidney.*) The disease appears in two distinct forms: The infantile form typically causes stillbirth or early neonatal death, although some infants may survive for 2 years, then develop fatal renal, cardiac, or respiratory failure. The adult form begins insidiously but usually becomes obvious between ages 30 and 50; rarely, it causes no symptoms until the patient is in his 70s. In the adult form, renal deterioration is more gradual but, as in the infantile form, progresses relentlessly to fatal uremia.

The prognosis in adults is extremely variable. Progression may be slow, even after symptoms of renal insufficiency appear. However, after uremic symptoms develop, polycystic kidney disease is usually fatal within 4 years, unless the patient receives treatment with dialysis, kidney transplantation, or both.

Causes and incidence

While both types of polycystic kidney disease are genetically transmitted, the incidence in two distinct age groups and different inheritance patterns suggest two unrelated disorders. The infantile type appears to be inherited as an autosomal recessive trait, whereas the adult type seems to be an autosomal dominant trait. The gene has been located on chromosome 6, supporting the premise that this is a single genetic disease with variable phenotype presentation.

Polycystic kidney disease reportedly affects 1 in every 1,000 Americans; yet that number may be even higher because some cases from patients who aren't symptomatic go unreported. Both types of polycystic kidney disease affect males and females equally.

Signs and symptoms

The neonate with infantile polycystic disease often has pronounced epicanthal folds, a pointed nose, a small chin, and floppy, low-set ears (Potter facies). At birth, he has huge bilateral masses on the flanks that are symmetrical, tense, and can't be transilluminated. He characteristically shows signs of respiratory distress and heart failure. Eventually, he develops uremia and renal failure. Accompanying hepatic fibrosis may cause portal hypertension and bleeding varices to develop, requiring sclerotherapy or portacaval shunting.

Adult polycystic kidney disease is commonly asymptomatic through the patient's 40s, but may induce nonspecific symptoms, such as hypertension, polyuria, and recurrent urinary tract infections (UTIs). Later, the patient develops overt symptoms related to the enlarging kidney mass, such as lumbar pain, widening girth, and swollen or tender abdomen. Abdominal pain is usually worsened by exertion and relieved by lying down. In advanced stages, this disease may cause recurrent hematuria, life-threatening retroperitoneal bleeding resulting from cyst rupture, proteinuria, and colicky abdominal pain from the ureteral passage of clots or calculi. Generally, about 10 years after symptoms appear, progressive compression of kidney structures by the enlarging mass produces renal failure and uremia. Hypertension is found in about 20% to 30% of children and up to 75% of adults due to intrarenal ischemia, which activates the renin-angiotensin system.

Diagnosis

A family history and a physical examination revealing large bilateral, irregular masses in the flanks strongly suggest polycystic kidney disease. In advanced stages, grossly enlarged and palpable kidneys make the diagnosis obvious. In patients with these findings, the following laboratory results are typical:

■ Excretory urography reveals enlarged kidneys, with elongation of pelvis, flattening of the calyces, and indentations caused by cysts. Excretory urography of the neonate shows poor excretion of contrast medium.

■ Ultrasound and computed tomography scan show kidney enlargement and the presence of cysts; tomography demonstrates multiple areas of cystic damage. Ultrasonography is the preferred imaging technique because it's less expensive, doesn't require contrast or radiation exposure, and is easily and safely performed on children and pregnant females.

■ Urinalysis and creatinine clearance tests are nonspecific tests that evaluate renal function and reveal urine protein or blood in the urine.

Diagnosis must rule out the presence of renal tumors.

Treatment

Polycystic kidney disease can't be cured. The primary goal of treatment is preserving renal parenchyma and preventing infectious complications. Management of secondary hypertension will also help prevent rapid deterioration in function. Progressive renal failure requires treatment similar to that for other types of renal disease, including dialysis or, rarely, kidney transplantation.

When adult polycystic kidney disease is discovered in the asymptomatic stage, care-ful monitoring is required, including urine cultures and creatinine clearance tests every 6 months. Prompt and vigorous antibiotic treatment is needed when a urine culture reveals infection — even when the patient is asymptomatic. As renal impairment progresses, selected patients may undergo dialysis, transplantation, or both. Cystic abscess or retroperitoneal bleeding may require surgical drainage; intractable pain (a rare symptom) may also require surgery. However, because this disease affects both kidneys, nephrectomy usually isn't recommended because it increases the risk of infection in the remaining kidney.

Special considerations

Because polycystic kidney disease is usually relentlessly progressive, comprehensive patient teaching and emotional support are essential.

■ Refer the young adult patient or the parents of infants with polycystic kidney disease for genetic counseling. Parents will probably have many questions about the risk to other offspring.

■ Provide supportive care to minimize any associated symptoms. Carefully assess the patient's lifestyle and his physical and mental status; determine how rapidly the disease is progressing. Use this information to plan individualized patient care.

■ Acquaint yourself with all aspects of end-stage renal disease, including dialysis and transplantation, so you can provide appropriate care and patient teaching as the disease progresses.

■ Explain all diagnostic procedures to the patient or to his family if the patient is an infant. Before beginning excretory urography or other procedures that use an iodine-based contrast medium, determine whether the patient has ever had an allergic reaction to iodine or shellfish. Even if the patient has no history of allergy, watch for an allergic reaction after performing the procedures.

■ Administer antibiotics as ordered for UTI. Stress to the patient the need to take the medication exactly as prescribed, even if symptoms are minimal or absent.

ACUTE RENAL DISORDERS

Acute renal failure

Acute renal failure is the sudden interruption of kidney function due to obstruction, reduced circulation, or renal parenchymal disease. It's usually reversible with medical treatment; otherwise, it may progress to end-stage renal disease, uremic syndrome, and death.

Causes and incidence

The causes of acute renal failure are classified as prenal, intrinsic (or parenchymal), and postrenal. Prerenal failure is associated with diminished blood flow to the kidneys, possibly resulting from hypovolemia, shock, severe anaphylaxis, embolism, blood loss, sepsis, pooling of fluid in ascites or burns, or from cardiovascular disorders, such as heart failure, arrhythmias, and tamponade.

Intrinsic renal failure results from damage to the kidneys themselves, usually due to acute tubular necrosis, but possibly due to acute poststreptococcal glomerulonephritis, systemic lupus erythematosus, periarteritis nodosa, vasculitis, sickle-cell disease, bilateral renal vein thrombosis, nephrotoxins, chronic misuse of nonsteroidal anti-inflammatory drugs, radiopaque contrast agents, ischemia, renal myeloma, acute pyelonephritis, and exposure to heavy metals, such as lead or mercury.

Postrenal failure results from bilateral obstruction of urinary outflow. Its multiple causes include kidney stones, blood clots, papillae from papillary necrosis, tumors, benign prostatic hyperplasia, strictures, and urethral edema from catheterization.

In the United States, the annual incidence of acute renal failure is 100 cases for every million people. It's diagnosed in 1% of hospital admissions. Hospital-acquired acute renal failure occurs in 4% of all admitted patients and 20% of patients who are admitted to critical care units.

Signs and symptoms

Acute renal failure is a critical illness. Its early signs are oliguria, azotemia and, rarely, anuria. Electrolyte imbalance, metabolic acidosis, and other severe effects follow, as the patient becomes increasingly uremic and renal dysfunction disrupts other body systems:

- *GI:* anorexia, nausea, vomiting, diarrhea or constipation, stomatitis, bleeding, hematemesis, dry mucous membranes, uremic breath
- *Central nervous system (CNS):* headache, drowsiness, irritability, confusion, peripheral neuropathy, seizures, coma
- *Cutaneous:* dryness, pruritus, pallor, purpura and, rarely, uremic frost
- *Cardiovascular:* early in the disease, hypotension; later, hypertension, arrhythmias, fluid overload, heart failure, systemic edema, anemia, altered clotting mechanisms
- *Respiratory:* pulmonary edema, Kussmaul's respirations.

Fever and chills indicate infection, a common complication.

Diagnosis

The patient's history may include a disorder that can cause renal failure. Blood test results indicating intrinsic acute renal failure include elevated blood urea nitrogen, serum creatinine, and potassium levels and low blood pH, bicarbonate, hematocrit (HCT), and hemoglobin (Hb) level. Urine specimens show casts, cellular debris, decreased specific gravity and, in glomerular diseases, proteinuria and urine osmolality close to serum osmolality. Urine sodium level is less than 20 mEq/L if oliguria is due to decreased perfusion; more than 40 mEq/L if due to an intrinsic problem. Other studies include renal ultrasonography, kidney-ureter-bladder X-rays, cautious use of excretory urography, renal scan, and nephrotomography.

Treatment

The goal of treatment is to correct or eliminate any reversible causes of kidney failure, such as obstructive uropathy, volume depletion, or the use of kidney-toxic medications. Supportive measures include a diet high in calories and low in protein, sodium, and potassium, with supplemental vitamins and restricted fluids. Meticulous electrolyte monitoring is essential to detect hyperkalemia. If hyperkalemia occurs, acute therapy may include dialysis, I.V. administration of hypertonic glucose, insulin infusion, and sodium bicarbonate, and administration of a potassium exchange resin (orally by enema) to remove potassium from the body.

If measures fail to control uremic symptoms, hemodialysis or peritoneal dialysis may be necessary. Continuous arteriovenous hemodiafiltration and continuous venovenous hemodiafiltration are alternative hemodialysis techniques for the treatment of acute renal failure. They're generally reserved for when intermittent dialysis fails to control hypervolemia or uremia, or for patients for whom peritoneal dialysis isn't possible.

Special considerations
Patient care includes careful monitoring and dietary education.
- Measure and record intake and output, including all body fluids, such as wound drainage, nasogastric output, and diarrhea. Weigh the patient daily.
- Assess Hb levels and HCT and replace blood components, as ordered. *Don't* use whole blood if the patient is prone to heart failure and can't tolerate extra fluid volume. Packed red blood cells deliver the necessary blood components without added volume.
- Monitor vital signs. Watch for and report any signs of pericarditis (pleuritic chest pain, tachycardia, pericardial friction rub), inadequate renal perfusion (hypotension), and acidosis.
- Maintain proper electrolyte balance. Strictly monitor potassium levels. Watch for symptoms of hyperkalemia (malaise, anorexia, paresthesia, or muscle weakness) and electrocardiogram changes (tall, peaked T waves, widening QRS segment, and disappearing P waves), and report them immediately. Avoid administering medications containing potassium.
- Assess the patient frequently, especially during emergency treatment to lower potassium levels. If the patient receives hypertonic glucose and insulin infusions,

monitor potassium levels. If you give sodium polystyrene sulfonate rectally, make sure the patient doesn't retain it and become constipated, to prevent bowel perforation.
- Maintain nutritional status. Provide a high-calorie, low-protein, low-sodium, and low-potassium diet, with vitamin supplements. Give the anorectic patient small, frequent meals.
- Use sterile technique, because the patient with acute renal failure is highly susceptible to infection. Personnel with upper respiratory tract infections shouldn't provide care for the patient.
- Prevent complications of immobility by encouraging frequent coughing and deep breathing and by performing passive range-of-motion exercises. Help the patient walk as soon as possible.
- Provide good mouth care frequently because mucous membranes are dry. If stomatitis occurs, an antibiotic solution may be ordered. Have the patient swish the solution around in his mouth before swallowing.
- Monitor for GI bleeding by guaiac testing all stools for blood. Administer medications carefully, especially antacids and stool softeners. Use aluminum-hydroxide–based antacids; magnesium-based antacids can cause serum magnesium levels to rise to critical levels.
- Use appropriate safety measures, such as side rails and restraints, because the patient with CNS involvement may be dizzy or confused.
- Provide emotional support to the patient and his family. Reassure them by clearly explaining all procedures.
- If the patient requires hemodialysis, check the blood access site (arteriovenous fistula, subclavian or femoral catheter) as per facility protocol or every 2 hours for patency and signs of clotting. Don't use the arm with the shunt or fistula for taking blood pressures or drawing blood. Weigh the patient before beginning dialysis. During dialysis, monitor vital signs, clotting times, blood flow, the function of the vascular access site, and arterial and venous pressures. Watch for complications, such as septicemia, embolism, hepatitis, and rapid fluid and electrolyte loss. After dialysis,

monitor vital signs and the vascular access site; weigh the patient; watch for signs of fluid and electrolyte imbalances.
■ During peritoneal dialysis, position the patient carefully. Elevate the head of the bed to reduce pressure on the diaphragm and aid respiration. Be alert for signs of infection (cloudy drainage, elevated temperature) and, rarely, bleeding. If pain occurs, reduce the amount of dialysate. Monitor the diabetic patient's blood glucose periodically, and administer insulin as ordered. Watch for complications, such as peritonitis, atelectasis, hypokalemia, pneumonia, and shock.
■ Use standard precautions when handling all blood and body fluids.

Acute pyelonephritis

Acute pyelonephritis (also known as *acute infective tubulointerstitial nephritis*) is a sudden inflammation caused by bacteria that primarily affects the interstitial area and the renal pelvis or, less often, the renal tubules. It's one of the most common renal diseases. With treatment and continued follow-up care, the prognosis is good, and extensive permanent damage is rare.

Causes and incidence
Acute pyelonephritis results from bacterial infection of the kidneys. Infecting bacteria usually are normal intestinal and fecal flora that grow readily in urine. The most common causative organism is *Escherichia coli,* but *Proteus, Pseudomonas, Staphylococcus aureus,* and *Enterococcus faecalis* (formerly *Streptococcus faecalis*) may also cause this infection.

Typically, the infection spreads from the bladder to the ureters, then to the kidneys, as in vesicoureteral reflux due to congenital weakness at the junction of the ureter and the bladder. Bacteria refluxed to intrarenal tissues may create colonies of infection within 24 to 48 hours. Infection may also result from instrumentation (such as catheterization, cystoscopy, or urologic surgery), from a hematogenic infection (as in septicemia or endocarditis), or possibly from lymphatic infection.

Pyelonephritis may also result from an inability to empty the bladder (for example, in patients with neurogenic bladder), urinary stasis, or urinary obstruction due to tumors, strictures, or benign prostatic hyperplasia.

Pyelonephritis occurs more commonly in females, probably because of a shorter urethra and the proximity of the urinary meatus to the vagina and the rectum — both conditions allow bacteria to reach the bladder more easily — and a lack of the antibacterial prostatic secretions produced in the male. Incidence increases with age and is higher in the following groups:
■ *Sexually active females:* Intercourse increases the risk of bacterial contamination.
■ *Pregnant females:* About 5% develop asymptomatic bacteriuria; if untreated, about 40% develop pyelonephritis.
■ *Diabetics:* Neurogenic bladder causes incomplete emptying and urinary stasis; glycosuria may support bacterial growth in the urine.
■ *Persons with other renal diseases:* Compromised renal function aggravates susceptibility.

Signs and symptoms
Typical clinical features include urgency, frequency, burning during urination, dysuria, nocturia, and hematuria (usually microscopic but may be gross). Urine may appear cloudy and have an ammonia-like or fishy odor. Other common symptoms include a temperature of 102° F (38.9° C) or higher, shaking chills, flank pain, anorexia, and general fatigue.

These symptoms characteristically develop rapidly over a few hours or a few days. Although these symptoms may disappear within days, even without treatment, residual bacterial infection is likely and may cause symptoms to recur later.

 ELDER TIP *Elderly patients may exhibit altered mental status or GI or pulmonary symptoms rather than the usual febrile responses to pyelonephritis.*

PEDIATRIC TIP *In children younger than age 2, fever, vomiting, nonspecific abdominal complaints, or failure to thrive may be the only signs of acute pyelonephritis.*

Diagnosis

Diagnosis requires urinalysis and culture. Typical findings include:

- Pyuria (pus in urine): Urine sediment reveals the presence of leukocytes singly, in clumps, and in casts; and, possibly, a few red blood cells.
- Significant bacteriuria: Urine culture reveals more than 100,000 organisms/µl of urine.
- Low specific gravity and osmolality: These findings result from a temporarily decreased ability to concentrate urine.
- Slightly alkaline urine pH.
- Proteinuria, glycosuria, and ketonuria: These conditions are less common.

Excretory urography or computed tomography (CT) scan of the kidneys, ureters, and bladder also help in the evaluation of acute pyelonephritis by revealing calculi, tumors, or cysts in the kidneys and the urinary tract. In addition, excretory urography may show asymmetrical kidneys.

Treatment

Treatment centers on antibiotic therapy appropriate to the specific infecting organism after identification by urine culture and sensitivity studies. When the infecting organism can't be identified, therapy usually consists of a broad-spectrum antibiotic. Urinary analgesics are also appropriate.

 ALERT *If the patient is pregnant, antibiotics must be prescribed cautiously.*

Symptoms may disappear after several days of antibiotic therapy. Although urine usually becomes sterile within 48 to 72 hours, the course of such therapy is 10 to 14 days. Follow-up treatment may include reculturing urine 1 week after drug therapy stops, then periodically for the next year to detect residual or recurring infection. Most patients with uncomplicated infections respond well to therapy and don't suffer reinfection.

In infection from obstruction or vesicoureteral reflux, antibiotics may be less effective; treatment may then necessitate surgery to relieve the obstruction or correct the anomaly. Patients at high risk of recurring urinary tract and kidney infections, such as those with prolonged use of

an indwelling catheter or maintenance antibiotic therapy, require long-term follow-up. Recurrent episodes of acute pyelonephritis can eventually result in chronic pyelonephritis. (See *Chronic pyelonephritis.*)

Special considerations

Patient care is supportive during antibiotic treatment of the underlying infection.

- Administer antipyretics for fever.
- Encourage fluids to achieve urine output of more than 2,000 ml/day. This helps to empty the bladder of contaminated urine.

CHRONIC PYELONEPHRITIS

Chronic pyelonephritis is a persistent kidney inflammation that can scar the kidneys and may lead to chronic renal failure. Its etiology may be bacterial, metastatic, or urogenous. This disease is most common in patients who are predisposed to recurrent acute pyelonephritis, such as those with urinary obstructions or vesicoureteral reflux.

Patients with chronic pyelonephritis may have a childhood history of unexplained fevers or bedwetting. Clinical effects may include flank pain, anemia, low urine specific gravity, proteinuria, leukocytes in urine and, especially in late stages, hypertension. Uremia rarely develops from chronic pyelonephritis unless structural abnormalities exist in the excretory system. Bacteriuria may be intermittent. When no bacteria are found in the urine, diagnosis depends on excretory urography (renal pelvis may appear small and flattened) and renal biopsy.

Effective treatment of chronic pyelonephritis requires control of hypertension, elimination of the existing obstruction (when possible), and long-term antimicrobial therapy.

Don't encourage intake of more than 2 to 3 qt (2 to 3 L) because this may decrease the effectiveness of the antibiotics.

■ Provide an acid-ash diet to prevent stone formation.

■ Teach proper technique for collecting a clean-catch urine specimen. Be sure to refrigerate or culture a urine specimen within 30 minutes of collection to prevent overgrowth of bacteria.

■ Stress the need to complete prescribed antibiotic therapy, even after symptoms subside. Encourage long-term follow-up care for high-risk patients.

To prevent acute pyelonephritis:

■ Observe strict sterile technique during catheter insertion and care.

■ Instruct females to prevent bacterial contamination by wiping the perineum from front to back after defecation.

■ Advise routine checkups for patients with a history of urinary tract infections. Teach them to recognize signs of infection, such as cloudy urine, burning on urination, urgency, and frequency, especially when accompanied by a low-grade fever.

Acute poststreptococcal glomerulonephritis

Acute poststreptococcal glomerulonephritis (APSGN), also known as *acute glomerulonephritis,* is a relatively common bilateral inflammation of the glomeruli. It usually follows a streptococcal infection of the respiratory tract or, less often, a skin infection such as impetigo.

Causes and incidence

APSGN results from the entrapment and collection of antigen-antibody (produced as an immunologic mechanism in response to streptococcus) in the glomerular capillary membranes, inducing inflammatory damage and impeding glomerular function. Sometimes, the immune complement further damages the glomerular membrane. The damaged and inflamed glomerulus loses the ability to be selectively permeable, and allows red blood cells (RBCs) and proteins to filter through as the glomerular filtration rate (GFR) falls. Uremic poisoning may result.

APSGN is most common in males ages 3 to 7, but it can occur at any age. Incidence is rising in the United States and Europe, with epidemics occurring in developing countries in Africa, the West Indies, and the Middle East.

Up to 95% of children and up to 70% of adults with APSGN recover fully; the rest may progress to chronic renal failure within months.

Signs and symptoms

APSGN begins within 1 to 3 weeks after untreated pharyngitis. Symptoms include mild to moderate edema, oliguria (less than 400 ml/24 hours), proteinuria, azotemia, hematuria, and fatigue. Mild to severe hypertension may result from either sodium or water retention (due to decreased GFR) or inappropriate renin release. Heart failure from hypervolemia leads to pulmonary edema.

 PEDIATRIC TIP *The presenting features of APSGN in children may be encephalopathy with seizures and focal neurological deficits.*

Diagnosis

Diagnosis requires a detailed patient history and assessment of clinical symptoms and laboratory tests.

Urinalysis typically reveals proteinuria and hematuria. RBCs, white blood cells, and mixed cell casts are common in urinary sediment. Elevated serum creatinine levels and low creatinine clearance accompany impaired glomerular filtration. Elevated antistreptolysin-O titers (in 80% of patients), elevated streptozyme and anti-DNase B titers, and low serum complement levels verify recent streptococcal infection. A throat culture may also show group A beta-hemolytic streptococcus. Renal ultrasound may show a normal or slightly enlarged kidney. A renal biopsy may confirm the diagnosis or assess renal tissue status.

Treatment

The goals of treatment are relief of symptoms and prevention of complications. Vigorous supportive care includes bed rest, fluid and dietary sodium restrictions, and correction of electrolyte imbalances (possibly with dialysis, although this is rarely necessary). Therapy may include diuretics to reduce extracellular fluid overload and an antihypertensive. The use of antibiotics is recommended for 7 to 10 days if staphylococcal infection is documented. Otherwise, antibiotic use is controversial.

Special considerations

APSGN usually resolves within 2 weeks, so patient care is primarily supportive.

■ Check vital signs and electrolyte values. Monitor intake and output and daily weight. Assess renal function daily through serum creatinine, blood urea nitrogen, and urine creatinine clearance levels. Watch for and immediately report signs of acute renal failure (oliguria, azotemia, and acidosis).

■ Consult the dietitian to provide a diet high in calories and low in protein, sodium, potassium, and fluids.

■ Protect the debilitated patient against secondary infection by providing good nutrition, using good hygienic technique, and preventing contact with infected persons.

■ Bed rest is necessary during the acute phase. Allow the patient to *gradually* resume normal activities as symptoms subside.

■ Provide emotional support for the patient and his family. If the patient is on dialysis, explain the procedure fully.

■ Advise the patient with a history of chronic upper respiratory tract infections to immediately report signs of infection (fever, sore throat).

■ Tell the patient that follow-up examinations are necessary to detect chronic renal failure. Stress the need for regular blood pressure, urinary protein, and renal function assessments during the convalescent months to detect recurrence. After APSGN, gross hematuria may recur during nonspecific viral infections; abnormal urinary findings may persist for years.

■ Encourage pregnant females with a history of APSGN to have frequent medical evaluations because pregnancy further stresses the kidneys and increases the risk of chronic renal failure.

RISE IN NEPHROTOXIC INJURY

Incidence of acute tubular necrosis (ATN) due to ingestion or inhalation of toxic substances is rising. ATN may occur in hospitalized patients following exposure to toxic agents, such as antibiotics, chemotherapeutic agents, or contrast material. Other nephrotoxic agents include pesticides, fungicides, heavy metals (for example, mercury, arsenic, lead, bismuth, uranium), and organic solvents containing carbon tetrachloride or ethylene glycol, such as cleaning fluids or industrial solvents. Ingestion of these substances may be accidental or intentional.

Acute tubular necrosis

Acute tubular necrosis (ATN), also known as *acute tubulointerstitial nephritis*, accounts for about 75% of all cases of acute renal failure and is the most common cause of acute renal failure in critically ill patients. ATN injures the tubular segment of the nephron, causing renal failure and uremic syndrome. Mortality ranges from 40% to 70%, depending on complications from underlying diseases. Nonoliguric forms of ATN have a better prognosis.

Causes and incidence

ATN results from ischemic or nephrotoxic injury, most commonly in debilitated patients, such as the critically ill or those who have undergone extensive surgery. In ischemic injury, disruption of blood flow to the kidneys may result from circulatory collapse, severe hypotension, trauma, hemorrhage, dehydration, cardiogenic or septic shock, surgery, anesthetics, or reactions to transfusions. Nephrotoxic injury may follow ingestion of certain chemical agents or result from a hypersensitive reaction of the kidneys. (See *Rise in nephrotoxic injury.*) Because nephrotoxic ATN doesn't damage the basement membrane of the nephron, it's potentially reversible. However, ischemic ATN can damage the epithelial and basement membranes and can cause lesions in the renal interstitium. ATN may result from:

- diseased tubular epithelium that allows leakage of glomerular filtrate across the membranes and reabsorption of filtrate into the blood
- obstruction of urine flow by the collection of damaged cells, casts, red blood cells (RBCs), and other cellular debris within the tubular walls
- ischemic injury to glomerular epithelial cells, resulting in cellular collapse and decreased glomerular capillary permeability
- ischemic injury to vascular endothelium, eventually resulting in cellular swelling and obstruction.

Signs and symptoms

Nephrotoxic injury causes multiple symptoms similar to those of renal failure, particularly azotemia, anemia, acidosis, overhydration, and hypertension. Some patients may also experience fever, rash, and eosinophilia. However, ATN is usually difficult to recognize in its early stages because effects of the critically ill patient's primary disease may mask the symptoms of ATN. The first recognizable effect may be decreased urine output. Generally, hyperkalemia and the characteristic uremic syndrome soon follow, with oliguria (or, rarely, anuria) and confusion, which may progress to uremic coma. Other possible complications may include heart failure, uremic pericarditis, pulmonary edema, uremic lung, anemia, anorexia, intractable vomiting, and poor wound healing due to debilitation.

 ALERT *Fever and chills may signal the onset of an infection, which is the leading cause of death in ATN.*

Diagnosis

Diagnosis is usually delayed until the condition has progressed to an advanced stage. The most significant laboratory clues are urinary sediment containing RBCs and casts, and dilute urine of a low specific gravity (1.010), low osmolality (less than 400 mOsm/kg), and high sodium level (40 to 60 mEq/L). Blood studies reveal elevated blood urea nitrogen and serum creatinine levels, anemia, defects in platelet adherence, metabolic acidosis, and hyperkalemia. An electrocardiogram may show arrhythmias (due to electrolyte imbalances) and, with hyperkalemia, widening QRS segment, disappearing P waves, and tall, peaked T waves.

Treatment

Treatment consists of identifying the nephrotoxic substance, eliminating its use, and removing it from the body, possibly by hemodialysis or hemoperfusion in extreme cases. Initial treatment may include administration of diuretics and infusion of a large volume of fluids to flush tubules of cellular casts and debris and to replace fluid loss. However, this treatment carries a risk of fluid overload. Long-term fluid management requires daily replacement of projected and calculated losses (including insensible loss). Diet may be high in carbohydrates and low in protein, sodium, and potassium to minimize their build up in the body. During the course of acute renal failure, treatment is supportive.

Other appropriate measures to control complications include transfusion of packed RBCs for anemia and administration of antibiotics for infection. Epogen may be given to stimulate RBC production as an alternative to blood transfusion. Hyperkalemia may require emergency I.V. administration of 50% glucose, regular insulin, and sodium bicarbonate. Sodium polystyrene sulfonate with sorbitol may be given by mouth or by enema to reduce extracellular potassium levels. Peritoneal dialysis or hemodialysis may be needed if the patient is catabolic.

Special considerations

Patient care is largely supportive.
- Maintain fluid balance. Watch for fluid overload, a common complication of therapy. Accurately record intake and output, including wound drainage, nasogastric output, and hemodialysis and peritoneal dialysis balances. Weigh the patient daily.
- Monitor hemoglobin (Hb) levels and hematocrit, and administer blood products as needed. Use fresh packed cells instead of

whole blood to prevent fluid overload and heart failure.

■ Maintain electrolyte balance. Monitor laboratory results, and report imbalances. Enforce dietary restriction of foods containing sodium and potassium, such as bananas, orange juice, and baked potatoes. Check for potassium content in prescribed medications (for example, potassium penicillin). Provide adequate calories and essential amino acids, while restricting protein intake to maintain an anabolic state. Total parenteral nutrition may be indicated in the severely debilitated or catabolic patient.

■ Use sterile technique, particularly when handling catheters because the debilitated patient is vulnerable to infection. Immediately report fever, chills, delayed wound healing, or flank pain if the patient has an indwelling catheter in place.

■ Watch for complications. If anemia worsens (pallor, weakness, lethargy with decreased Hb level), administer RBCs as ordered. For acidosis, give sodium bicarbonate or assist with dialysis in severe cases, as ordered. Watch for signs of diminishing renal perfusion (hypotension and decreased urine output). Encourage coughing and deep breathing to prevent pulmonary complications.

■ Perform passive range-of-motion exercises. Provide good skin care; apply lotion or bath oil for dry skin. Help the patient to walk as soon as possible, but guard against exhaustion.

■ Provide reassurance and emotional support. Encourage the patient and his family to express their fears. Fully explain each procedure; repeat the explanation each time the procedure is done. Help the patient and his family set realistic goals according to individual prognosis.

■ To prevent ATN, make sure patients are well hydrated before surgery or after X-rays that use a contrast medium. Administer mannitol, as ordered, to high-risk patients before and during these procedures. Carefully monitor patients receiving blood transfusions to detect early signs of transfusion reaction (fever, rash, chills), and discontinue such transfusion immediately.

SITES OF RENAL INFARCTION

The most common sites of renal infarction are illustrated below.

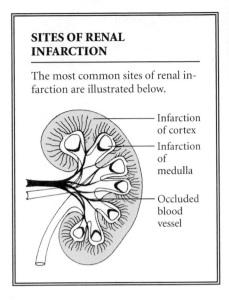

Infarction of cortex

Infarction of medulla

Occluded blood vessel

Renal infarction

Renal infarction is the formation of a coagulated, necrotic area in one or both kidneys that results from renal blood vessel occlusion. The location and size of the infarction depend on the site of vascular occlusion; most often, infarction affects the renal cortex, but it can extend into the medulla. (See *Sites of renal infarction.*) Residual renal function after infarction depends on the extent of the damage from the infarction.

Causes

In 75% of patients, renal infarction results from renal artery embolism secondary to mitral stenosis, infective endocarditis, atrial fibrillation, microthrombi in the left ventricle, rheumatic valvular disease, or recent myocardial infarction. The embolism reduces the rate of blood flow to renal tissue and leads to ischemia. The rate and degree of blood flow reduction determine whether or not the insult will be acute or chronic as arterial narrowing progresses. Less common causes of renal infarction are atherosclerosis, with or without thrombus formation, and thrombus from flank trauma, sickle cell anemia, scleroderma, polyarteritis nodosa, and arterionephrosclerosis.

Signs and symptoms

Although renal infarction may be asymptomatic, typical symptoms include severe upper abdominal pain or gnawing flank pain and tenderness, costovertebral tenderness, fever, anorexia, nausea, and vomiting. Gross hematuria may be present. When arterial occlusion causes infarction, the affected kidney is small and not palpable. Renovascular hypertension, a frequent complication that may occur several days after infarction, results from reduced blood flow, which stimulates the renin-angiotensin mechanism.

Diagnosis

A history of predisposing cardiovascular disease or other factors in a patient with typical clinical features strongly suggests renal infarction. Firm diagnosis requires appropriate laboratory tests:

- Urinalysis reveals proteinuria and microscopic hematuria.
- Urine enzyme levels, especially lactate dehydrogenase (LD) and alkaline phosphatase, are often elevated as a result of tissue destruction.
- Serum enzyme levels, especially aspartate aminotransferase, alkaline phosphatase, and LD, are elevated. Blood studies may also reveal leukocytosis and increased erythrocyte sedimentation rate.
- Excretory urography shows diminished or absent excretion of contrast dye, indicating vascular occlusion or urethral obstruction.
- Isotopic renal scan, a benign, noninvasive technique, demonstrates absent or reduced blood flow to the kidneys.

CONFIRMING DIAGNOSIS *Renal arteriography provides absolute proof of infarction but is used as a last resort because it's a high-risk procedure.*

Treatment

Infection in the infarcted area or significant hypertension may require surgical repair of the occlusion or nephrectomy. Surgery to establish collateral circulation to the area can relieve renovascular hypertension. Persistent hypertension may respond to antihypertensives and a low-sodium diet. Additional treatments may include administration of intra-arterial streptoki-

nase, lysis of blood clots, and heparin therapy. For bilateral emboli, intra-arterial streptokinase or transluminal angioplasty is recommended. If effective renal blood flow is obtained, long-term anticoagulation is recommended.

Special considerations

Assess the degree of renal function and offer supportive care to maintain homeostasis.

- Monitor intake and output, vital signs (particularly blood pressure), electrolytes, and daily weight. Watch for signs of fluid overload, such as dyspnea, tachycardia, pulmonary edema, and electrolyte imbalances.
- Carefully explain all diagnostic procedures.
- Provide reassurance and emotional support for the patient and his family.
- Encourage the patient to return for follow-up examination, which usually includes excretory urography or a renal scan to assess regained renal function.

Renal calculi

Renal calculi or nephrolithiasis (commonly called *kidney stones*) may form anywhere in the urinary tract but usually develop in the renal pelvis or the calyces of the kidneys. Calculi formation follows precipitation of substances normally dissolved in the urine, such as calcium oxalate, calcium phosphate, magnesium ammonium phosphate or, occasionally, urate or cystine. (See *How urine pH affects calculi formation.*) Renal calculi vary in size and may be solitary or multiple. They may remain in the renal pelvis or enter the ureter and may damage renal parenchyma; large calculi cause pressure necrosis. In certain locations, calculi cause obstruction, with resultant hydronephrosis, and tend to recur.

Causes and incidence

Although the exact cause of renal calculi is unknown, predisposing factors include:

- *Dehydration:* Decreased urine production concentrates calculus-forming substances.

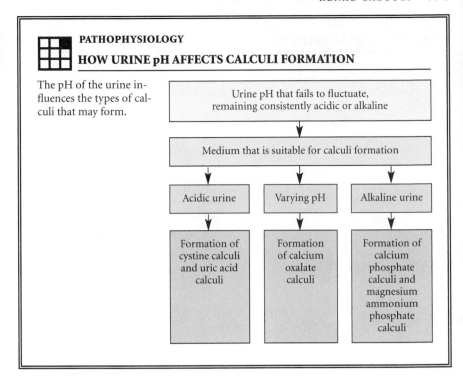

PATHOPHYSIOLOGY

HOW URINE pH AFFECTS CALCULI FORMATION

The pH of the urine influences the types of calculi that may form.

Urine pH that fails to fluctuate, remaining consistently acidic or alkaline

↓

Medium that is suitable for calculi formation

↓

| Acidic urine | Varying pH | Alkaline urine |

↓

Formation of cystine calculi and uric acid calculi

Formation of calcium oxalate calculi

Formation of calcium phosphate calculi and magnesium ammonium phosphate calculi

■ *Infection:* Infected, damaged tissue serves as a site for calculus development; pH changes provide a favorable medium for calculus formation (especially for magnesium ammonium phosphate or calcium phosphate calculi); or infected calculi (usually magnesium ammonium phosphate or staghorn calculi) may develop if bacteria serve as the nucleus in calculus formation. Infections may promote destruction of renal parenchyma.

■ *Obstruction:* Urinary stasis (as in immobility from spinal cord injury) allows calculus constituents to collect and adhere, forming calculi. Obstruction also promotes infection, which, in turn, compounds the obstruction.

■ *Metabolic factors:* These factors may predispose to renal calculi: hyperparathyroidism, renal tubular acidosis, elevated uric acid (usually with gout), defective metabolism of oxalate, genetic defect in metabolism of cystine, and excessive intake of vitamin D or dietary calcium.

Among Americans, renal calculi develop in 2% to 10% of the population, with peo-ple living in southeastern states having an increased risk. They're more common in males (especially those ages 30 to 40) than in females by a 3:1 ratio. They're rare in children.

Some types of calculi tend to be familial; some are associated with other conditions, such as bowel disease, ileal bypass for obesity, or renal tubule defects. Calcium calculi are most common, accounting for over 75% of all calculi, and are two to three times more common in males, usually appearing between ages 20 and 30. The calcium may combine with other substances, such as oxalate (the most common substance), phosphate, or carbonate, to form the stone. Oxalate is present in certain foods. Diseases of the small intestine increase the tendency to form calcium oxalate calculi. Recurrence is likely.

Uric acid calculi are also more common in males and make up about 6% of all calculi. These calculi are associated with gout and chemotherapy. Cystine calculi, which make up about 2% of all calculi, may form in people with cystinuria, a hereditary dis-

TYPES OF RENAL CALCULI

Multiple small calculi may vary in size; they may remain in the renal pelvis or pass down the ureter.

A staghorn calculus (a cast of the calyceal and pelvic collecting system) may form from a stone that stays in the kidney.

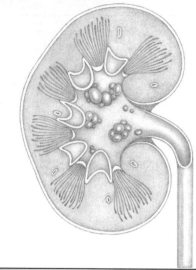

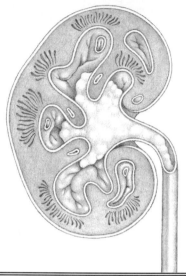

order affecting both males and females. Struvite calculi, accounting for about 15% of all calculi, are mainly found in females as a result of a urinary tract infection (UTI). They can grow very large and may obstruct the kidney, ureter, or bladder.

Indavir stones appear in patients with human immunodeficiency virus who are treated with the protease inhibitor indinavir.

Signs and symptoms

Clinical effects vary with size, location, and etiology of the calculi. Pain, the key symptom, usually results from obstruction; large, rough calculi occlude the opening to the ureter and increase the frequency and force of peristaltic contractions. The pain of classic renal colic travels from the costovertebral angle to the flank, to the suprapubic region and external genitalia. The intensity of this pain fluctuates and may be excruciating at its peak. If calculi are in the renal pelvis and calyces, pain may be more constant and dull. Back pain (from calculi that produce an obstruction within a kidney) and severe abdominal pain (from calculi traveling down a ureter) may also occur. (See *Types of renal calculi.*) Nausea and vomiting usually accompany severe pain.

Other associated signs include fever, chills, hematuria (when calculi abrade a ureter), abdominal distention, pyuria and, rarely, anuria (from bilateral obstruction, or unilateral obstruction in the patient with one kidney).

Diagnosis

Diagnosis is based on the clinical picture and the following tests:
- Computed tomography scan or magnetic resonance imaging are highly sensitive for identifying hydronephrosis and detecting small renal and urethral stones.
- Excretory urography may be used for diagnosis of obstruction by urinary calculus.
- Kidney-ureter-bladder X-rays reveal most renal calculi.
- Calculus analysis shows mineral content.

CONFIRMING DIAGNOSIS
Excretory urography confirms the diagnosis and determines size and location of calculi.

- Kidney ultrasonography is an easily performed, noninvasive, nontoxic test to detect obstructive changes such as hydronephrosis.
- Urine culture of midstream sample may indicate UTI.
- Urinalysis may be normal, or may show increased specific gravity and acid or alkaline pH suitable for different types of stone formation. Other urinalysis findings include hematuria (gross or microscopic), crystals (urate, calcium, or cystine), casts, and pyuria with or without bacteria and white blood cells.
- A 24-hour urine collection is evaluated for calcium oxalate, phosphorus, and uric acid excretion levels.
- Serial blood calcium and phosphorus levels detect hyperparathyroidism and show increased calcium level in proportion to normal serum protein.

Increased blood uric acid levels may indicate gout as the cause. Diagnosis must rule out appendicitis, cholecystitis, peptic ulcer, and pancreatitis as potential sources of pain.

Treatment

Because 90% of renal calculi are smaller than 5 mm in diameter, treatment usually consists of measures to promote their natural passage. Along with vigorous hydration, such treatment includes antimicrobial therapy (varying with the cultured organism) for infection, analgesics such as meperidine for pain, and diuretics to prevent urinary stasis and further calculus formation (thiazides decrease calcium excretion into the urine). Prophylaxis to prevent calculus formation includes a low-calcium diet for absorptive hypercalciuria, parathyroidectomy for hyperparathyroidism, allopurinol for uric acid calculi, and daily administration of ascorbic acid by mouth to acidify the urine.

Calculi too large for natural passage may require surgical removal. When a calculus is in the ureter, a cystoscope may be inserted through the urethra and the calculus manipulated with catheters or retrieval in-

struments. Extraction of calculi from other areas (kidney calyx, renal pelvis) may necessitate a flank or lower abdominal approach. Percutaneous ultrasonic lithotripsy and extracorporeal shock wave lithotripsy shatter the calculus into fragments for removal by suction or natural passage.

Special considerations

Patient care includes confirming the diagnosis, facilitating passage of the stone, and prevention of future occurrences.

- To aid diagnosis, maintain a 24- to 48-hour record of urine pH, with nitrazine pH paper; strain all urine through gauze or a tea strainer, and save all solid material recovered for analysis.
- To facilitate spontaneous passage, encourage the patient to walk if possible. Also promote sufficient intake of fluids to maintain a urine output of 3 to 4 L/day (urine should be very dilute and colorless). To help acidify urine, offer fruit juices, particularly cranberry juice. If the patient can't drink the required amount of fluid, supplemental I.V. fluids may be given. Record intake and output and daily weight to assess fluid status and renal function.
- Stress the importance of proper diet and compliance with drug therapy. For example, if the patient's stone is caused by a hyperuricemic condition, advise him (or whoever prepares his meals) to avoid foods high in purine. Restrict protein to 60 g/day to decrease calcium and uric acid, and limit sodium to 3 to 4 g/day. Oxalate foods are restricted.
- If surgery is necessary, give reassurance by supplementing and reinforcing what the surgeon has told the patient about the procedure. The patient is apt to be fearful, especially if surgery includes removal of a kidney, so emphasize the fact that the body can adapt well to one kidney. If he's to have an abdominal or flank incision, teach deep-breathing and coughing exercises.
- After surgery, the patient will probably have an indwelling catheter or a nephrostomy tube. Unless one of his kidneys was removed, expect bloody drainage from the catheter. Never irrigate the catheter without a physician's order. Check dressings regularly for bloody drainage, and know how much drainage to expect. Immediately

report suspected hemorrhage (excessive drainage, rising pulse rate). Use sterile technique when changing dressings or providing catheter care.

■ Watch for signs of infection (rising fever, chills), and give antibiotics as ordered. To prevent pneumonia, encourage frequent position changes, and ambulate the patient as soon as possible. Have him hold a small pillow over the operative site to splint the incision and thereby facilitate deep-breathing and coughing exercises.

■ Before discharge, teach the patient and his family the importance of following the prescribed dietary and medication regimens to prevent recurrence of calculi. Encourage increased fluid intake. If appropriate, show the patient how to check his urine pH, and instruct him to keep a daily record. Tell him to immediately report symptoms of acute obstruction (pain, inability to void).

Renal vein thrombosis

Renal vein thrombosis — clotting in the renal vein — results in renal congestion, engorgement and, possibly, infarction. Thrombosis may affect both kidneys and may occur in an acute or a chronic form. Chronic thrombosis usually impairs renal function, causing nephrotic syndrome. Abrupt onset of thrombosis that causes extensive damage may precipitate rapidly fatal renal infarction. If thrombosis affects both kidneys, the prognosis is poor. However, less severe thrombosis that affects only one kidney, or gradual progression that allows development of collateral circulation, may preserve partial renal function.

Causes

Renal vein thrombosis often results from a tumor that obstructs the renal vein (usually hypernephroma). Other causes include thrombophlebitis of the inferior vena cava (may result from abdominal trauma) or blood vessels of the legs, heart failure, and periarteritis.

 PEDIATRIC TIP *In infants, renal vein thrombosis usually follows diarrhea that causes severe dehydration. Chronic renal vein thrombosis is often a complication of other glomerulopathic diseases, such as amyloidosis, systemic lupus erythematosus, diabetic nephropathy, and membranoproliferative glomerulonephritis.*

Signs and symptoms

Clinical features of renal vein thrombosis vary with speed of onset. Rapid onset of venous obstruction produces severe lumbar pain and tenderness in the epigastric region and the costovertebral angle. Other characteristic features include fever, leukocytosis, pallor, hematuria, proteinuria, peripheral edema and, when the obstruction is bilateral, oliguria and other uremic signs. The kidneys enlarge and become easily palpable. Hypertension is unusual but may develop.

Gradual onset causes symptoms of nephrotic syndrome. Peripheral edema is possible but pain is generally absent. Other clinical signs include proteinuria, hypoalbuminemia, and hyperlipidemia.

Infants with this disease have enlarged kidneys, oliguria, and renal insufficiency that may progress to acute or chronic renal failure.

Diagnosis

A variety of tests are used to confirm diagnosis of renal vein thrombosis.

■ Computed tomography scan with contrast is the procedure of choice because it reveals enlargement and distention of the affected renal vein with visualization of the clots within the vein.

■ Excretory urography provides reliable diagnostic evidence. In acute renal vein thrombosis, the kidneys appear enlarged and excretory function diminishes. Contrast medium seems to "smudge" necrotic renal tissue. In chronic thrombosis, it may show ureteral indentations that result from collateral venous channels.

CONFIRMING DIAGNOSIS *Renal arteriography and biopsy may also confirm the diagnosis. Venography confirms thrombosis.*

■ Urinalysis reveals gross or microscopic hematuria, proteinuria (more than 2 g/day in chronic disease), casts, and oliguria.

■ Blood studies show leukocytosis, hypoalbuminemia, and hyperlipidemia.

- Magnetic resonance imaging, abdominal X-ray, or abdominal ultrasound may show occlusion of the renal vein.

Treatment

Treatment is most effective for gradual thrombosis that affects only one kidney. Anticoagulation therapy reduces the incidence of new thrombus formation and often reverses the deterioration of renal function. Heparin is the initial therapy of choice. After 5 to 7 days, warfarin (Coumadin) therapy can be instituted for long-term care. Streptokinase or urokinase infusion may be successful in early resolution of acute renal vein thrombosis. Surgery is rarely used; it must be performed within 24 hours of thrombosis but even then has limited success because thrombi often extend into the small veins. Extensive intrarenal bleeding may necessitate nephrectomy.

Patients who survive abrupt thrombosis with extensive renal damage develop nephrotic syndrome and require treatment for renal failure, such as dialysis and, possibly, transplantation.

Some infants with renal vein thrombosis recover completely following heparin therapy or surgery; others suffer irreversible kidney damage.

Special considerations

Patient care includes careful monitoring of symptoms for signs of improvement or worsening.

- Assess renal function regularly. Monitor vital signs, intake and output, daily weight, and electrolytes.
- Administer diuretics for edema as ordered, and enforce dietary restrictions of sodium and potassium intake.
- Monitor closely for signs of pulmonary emboli (chest pain, dyspnea).
- If heparin is given by constant I.V. infusion, frequently monitor partial thromboplastin time to determine the patient's response. Dilute the drug; administer it by infusion pump or controller, so the patient receives the least amount necessary.
- During anticoagulant therapy, watch for and report signs of bleeding, such as tachycardia, hypotension, hematuria, bleeding from nose or gums, ecchymoses, petechiae,

and tarry stools. Instruct the patient on maintenance warfarin therapy to use an electric razor and a soft toothbrush, and to avoid trauma. Suggest that he wear a medical identification bracelet, and tell him to avoid aspirin, which aggravates bleeding tendencies. Stress the need for close follow-up.

CHRONIC RENAL DISORDERS

Nephrotic syndrome

Nephrotic syndrome is a condition characterized by marked proteinuria, hypoalbuminemia, hyperlipidemia, and edema. (See *What happens in nephrotic syndrome,* page 796.) Although nephrotic syndrome isn't a disease itself, it results from a specific glomerular defect and indicates renal damage. The prognosis is highly variable, depending on the underlying cause. Some forms may progress to end-stage renal failure.

Causes and incidence

About 75% of nephrotic syndrome cases result from primary (idiopathic) glomerulonephritis. Classifications include:

- In *lipid nephrosis (nil lesions),* the main cause of nephrotic syndrome in children, the glomerulus looks normal by light microscopy. Some tubules may contain increased lipid deposits.
- *Membranous glomerulonephritis,* the most common lesion in adult idiopathic nephrotic syndrome, is characterized by uniform thickening of the glomerular basement membrane containing dense deposits and eventually progresses to renal failure.
- *Focal glomerulosclerosis* can develop spontaneously at any age, follow renal transplantation, or result from heroin abuse. Reported incidence of this condition is 10% in children with nephrotic syndrome and up to 20% in adults. Lesions initially affect the deeper glomeruli, causing hyaline sclerosis, with later involvement of the superficial glomeruli. These lesions

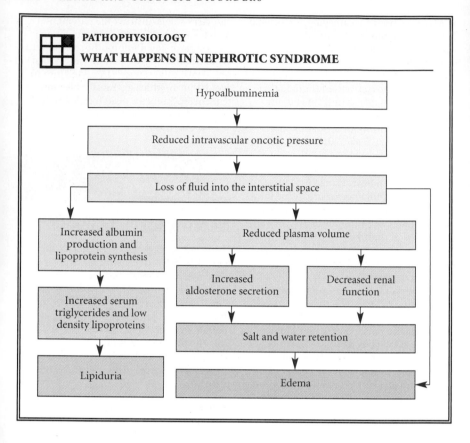

PATHOPHYSIOLOGY
WHAT HAPPENS IN NEPHROTIC SYNDROME

Hypoalbuminemia

↓

Reduced intravascular oncotic pressure

↓

Loss of fluid into the interstitial space

Increased albumin production and lipoprotein synthesis

↓

Increased serum triglycerides and low density lipoproteins

↓

Lipiduria

Reduced plasma volume

Increased aldosterone secretion

Decreased renal function

Salt and water retention

Edema

---

generally cause slowly progressive deterioration in renal function. Remissions occur occasionally.

■ In *membranoproliferative glomerulonephritis,* slowly progressive lesions develop in the subendothelial region of the basement membrane. Lesions may follow infection, particularly streptococcal infection. This disease occurs primarily in children and young adults.

Other causes of nephrotic syndrome include metabolic diseases such as diabetes mellitus; collagen-vascular disorders, such as systemic lupus erythematosus and periarteritis nodosa; circulatory diseases, such as heart failure, sickle cell anemia, and renal vein thrombosis; nephrotoxins, such as mercury, gold, and bismuth; allergic reactions; and infections, such as tuberculosis or enteritis. Other possible causes are pregnancy, hereditary nephritis, multiple myeloma, and other neoplastic diseases.

These diseases increase glomerular protein permeability, leading to increased urinary excretion of protein, especially albumin, and subsequent hypoalbuminemia.

Nephrotic patients have an increased risk of infection, particularly of peritonitis.

 PEDIATRIC TIP *Black children appear to be at greater risk for peritonitis.*

Signs and symptoms

The dominant clinical feature of nephrotic syndrome is mild to severe dependent edema of the ankles or sacrum, or periorbital edema, especially in children. Edema may lead to ascites, pleural effusion, and swollen external genitalia. Accompanying symptoms may include orthostatic hypotension, lethargy, anorexia, depression, and pallor. Major complications are malnutrition, infection, coagulation disorders, thromboembolic vascular occlusion, and accelerated atherosclerosis.

Diagnosis

Consistent proteinuria in excess of 3.5 g/24 hours strongly suggests nephrotic syndrome; examination of urine also reveals increased number of hyaline, granular, and waxy, fatty casts, and oval fat bodies. Serum values that support the diagnosis are increased cholesterol, phospholipids, and triglycerides and decreased albumin levels. Histologic identification of the lesion requires kidney biopsy. Other tests may be done to rule out metabolic causes.

Treatment

The goals of treatment of nephrotic syndrome are to relieve symptoms, prevent complications, and delay progressive kidney damage. Treatment of the causative disorder — possibly lifelong — is necessary to control nephrotic syndrome. Corticosteroid, immunosuppressive, antihypertensive, and diuretic medications may help control symptoms. Antibiotics may be needed to control infections. Angiotensin-converting enzyme inhibitors may significantly reduce the degree of protein loss in urine and are therefore typically prescribed for the treatment of nephrotic syndrome.

Treatment of hypertension and of high cholesterol and triglyceride levels are also recommended to reduce the risk of atherosclerosis and complications. Dietary limitation of cholesterol and saturated fats may be of little benefit because the high levels that accompany this condition seem to result from overproduction by the liver rather than from excessive fat intake. High-protein diets are of debatable value. In many patients, reducing the amount of protein in the diet produces a decrease in urine protein. In most cases, a moderate-protein diet (1 g/kg of body weight per day) is usually recommended. Sodium may be restricted to help control edema. Vitamin D may need to be replaced if nephrotic syndrome is chronic and unresponsive to therapy. Blood thinners may be required to treat or prevent clot formation.

Supportive treatment consists of protein replacement with infusion of salt-poor albumin or with a nutritional diet of 1.5 g protein/kg of body weight, with restricted sodium intake of 0.5 to 1 g/day; diuretics for edema; and antibiotics for infection.

Some patients respond to an 8-week course of corticosteroid therapy (such as prednisone), followed by a maintenance dose. Others respond better to a combination course of prednisone and azathioprine or cyclophosphamide.

Special considerations

Patient care includes identification and treatment of the underlying cause accompanied by supportive care during treatment.

- Frequently check urine protein. (Urine containing protein appears frothy.)
- Measure blood pressure while the patient is supine and also while he's standing; immediately report a drop in blood pressure that exceeds 20 mm Hg.
- After kidney biopsy, watch for bleeding and shock.
- Monitor intake and output and check weight at the same time each morning — after the patient voids and before he eats — and while he's wearing the same kind of clothing. Ask the dietitian to plan a high-protein, low-sodium diet.
- Provide good skin care because the patient with nephrtic syndrome usually has edema.
- To avoid thrombophlebitis, encourage activity and exercise, and provide antiembolism stockings as ordered.
- Watch for and teach the patient and his family how to recognize adverse drug effects, such as bone marrow toxicity from cytotoxic immunosuppressants and cushingoid symptoms (muscle weakness, mental changes, acne, moon face, hirsutism, girdle obesity, purple striae, amenorrhea) from long-term steroid therapy. Other steroid complications include masked infections, increased susceptibility to infections, ulcers, GI bleeding, and steroid-induced diabetes; a steroid crisis may occur if the drug is discontinued abruptly. To prevent GI complications, administer steroids with an antacid or with cimetidine or ranitidine. Explain that steroid adverse effects will subside when therapy stops.

■ Offer the patient and his family reassurance and support, especially during the acute phase, when edema is severe and the patient's body image changes.

Chronic glomerulonephritis

A slowly progressive disease, chronic glomerulonephritis is characterized by inflammation of the glomeruli, which results in sclerosis, scarring, and eventual renal failure. This condition usually remains subclinical until the progressive phase begins, marked by proteinuria, cylindruria (presence of granular tube casts), and hematuria. By the time it produces symptoms, chronic glomerulonephritis is usually irreversible.

Causes and incidence

Common causes of chronic glomerulonephritis include primary renal disorders, such as membranoproliferative glomerulonephritis, membranous glomerulopathy, focal glomerulosclerosis, rapidly progressive glomerulonephritis and, less often, poststreptococcal glomerulonephritis. Systemic disorders that may cause chronic glomerulonephritis include lupus erythematosus, Goodpasture's syndrome, or hemolytic-uremic syndrome.

Chronic glomerulonephritis is twice as common in males as it is in females.

Signs and symptoms

Chronic glomerulonephritis typically develops insidiously and asymptomatically, usually over many years. At any time, however, it may suddenly become progressive, producing nephrotic syndrome, hypertension, proteinuria, and hematuria. In late stages of progressive chronic glomerulonephritis, it may accelerate to uremic symptoms, such as azotemia, nausea, vomiting, pruritus, dyspnea, malaise, and fatigability. Mild to severe edema and anemia may accompany these symptoms. Severe hypertension may cause cardiac hypertrophy, leading to heart failure, and may accelerate the development of advanced renal failure, eventually necessitating dialysis or transplantation.

Diagnosis

Patient history and physical assessment seldom suggest glomerulonephritis. Suspicion develops from urinalysis revealing proteinuria, hematuria, cylindruria, and red blood cell casts. Rising blood urea nitrogen and serum creatinine levels indicate advanced renal insufficiency. X-ray or ultrasound shows smaller kidneys. Kidney biopsy identifies the underlying disease and provides data needed to guide therapy.

Treatment

Treatment is essentially nonspecific and symptomatic, with its goals to control hypertension with antihypertensives and a sodium-restricted diet, to correct fluid and electrolyte imbalances through restrictions and replacement, to reduce edema with diuretics such as furosemide, and to prevent heart failure. Treatment may also include antibiotics (for symptomatic urinary tract infections [UTIs]), dialysis, or transplantation.

Special considerations

Patient care is primarily supportive, focusing on continual observation and sound patient teaching.

■ Accurately monitor vital signs, intake and output, and daily weight to evaluate fluid retention. Observe for signs of fluid, electrolyte, and acid-base imbalances.

■ Ask the dietitian to plan low-sodium, high-calorie meals with adequate protein.

■ Administer medications as ordered, and provide good skin care (because of pruritus and edema) and oral hygiene. Instruct the patient to continue taking prescribed antihypertensives as scheduled, even if he's feeling better, and to report any adverse effects. Advise him to take diuretics in the morning, so he won't have to disrupt his sleep to void. Teach him how to assess ankle edema.

■ Warn the patient to report signs of infection, particularly UTI, and to avoid contact with persons who have infections. Urge follow-up examinations to assess renal function.

■ Help the patient adjust to this illness by encouraging him to express his feelings. Explain all necessary procedures beforehand, and answer the patient's questions about them.

Renovascular hypertension

Renovascular hypertension is a rise in systemic blood pressure resulting from stenosis of the major renal arteries or their branches or from intrarenal atherosclerosis. This narrowing or sclerosis may be partial or complete, and the resulting blood pressure elevation, benign or malignant.

Causes and incidence
Stenosis or occlusion of the renal artery stimulates the affected kidney to release the enzyme renin, which converts angiotensinogen — a plasma protein — to angiotensin I. As angiotensin I circulates through the lungs and liver, it converts to angiotensin II, which causes peripheral vasoconstriction, increased arterial pressure and aldosterone secretion and, eventually, hypertension.

Atherosclerosis (especially in older males) and fibromuscular diseases of the renal artery wall layers — such as medial fibroplasia and, less commonly, intimal and subadventitial fibroplasia — are the primary causes in 95% of all patients with renovascular hypertension. Other causes include arteritis, anomalies of the renal arteries, embolism, trauma, tumor, and dissecting aneurysm. Less than 5% of patients with high blood pressure display renovascular hypertension; it's most common in persons younger than age 30 or older than age 50.

 PEDIATRIC TIP *Fibromuscular dysplasia is the most common cause of renovascular hypertension in children. The surgical cure rate is very high.*

Signs and symptoms
In addition to elevated systemic blood pressure, renovascular hypertension usually produces symptoms common to hypertensive states, such as headache, palpitations, tachycardia, anxiety, lightheadedness, decreased tolerance of temperature extremes, retinopathy, and mental sluggishness. Significant complications include heart failure, myocardial infarction, stroke and, occasionally, renal failure.

Diagnosis
Diagnosis is confirmed by the following tests:

 CONFIRMING DIAGNOSIS
Arterial digital subtraction angiography with assays of venous renin is the definitive diagnostic procedure. When stenosis is significant, transluminal angioplasty can be done during the same procedure.

■ Gadolinium enhanced magnetic resonance angiography can identify turbulent blood flow indicative of renal stenosis.

■ Duplex Doppler ultrasonography scans the renal artery and will reveal stenosis but results vary.

■ Oral captopril renography is the simplest, noninvasive test for detection of renovascular hypertension but has a relatively high false-positive rate.

Treatment
Surgery, the treatment of choice, is performed to restore adequate circulation and to control severe hypertension or severely impaired renal function by renal artery bypass, endarterectomy, arterioplasty or, as a last resort, nephrectomy. Balloon catheter renal artery dilation is used in selected cases to correct renal artery stenosis without the risks and morbidity of surgery. Symptomatic measures include antihypertensives, diuretics, and a sodium-restricted diet.

Medications that may be used in an attempt to control blood pressure include diuretics, beta-adrenergic blockers, calcium channel blockers, angiotensin-converting enzyme inhibitors, angiotensin-receptor blockers, and alpha-adrenergic blockers. Diazoxide or nitroprusside may be given in the hospital if symptoms are acute. Response to medications is highly individual and the dosage or specific drug used may need frequent adjustment.

Lifestyle changes may be recommended, including weight, exercise, dietary adjustments, smoking cessation, and avoidance of alcohol. These habits add to the effects of hypertension in causing complications.

Special considerations

The care plan must emphasize helping the patient and his family understand renovascular hypertension and the importance of following the prescribed treatment.

■ Accurately monitor intake and output and daily weight. Check blood pressure in both arms regularly, with the patient lying down and standing. A drop of 20 mm Hg or more on arising may necessitate an adjustment in antihypertensive medications. Assess renal function daily.

■ Maintain fluid and sodium restrictions. Explain the purpose of a low-sodium diet.

■ Explain the diagnostic tests, and prepare the patient appropriately; for example, adequately hydrate the patient before tests that use contrast media. Make sure the patient isn't allergic to the dye used in diagnostic tests. After excretory urography or arteriography, watch for complications.

■ If a nephrectomy is necessary, reassure the patient that the remaining kidney is adequate for renal function.

■ Postoperatively, watch for bleeding and hypotension. If the sutures around the renal vessels slip, the patient can quickly go into shock because kidneys receive 25% of cardiac output.

■ Provide a quiet, stress-free environment if possible. Urge the patient and his family members to have regular blood pressure screenings.

Hydronephrosis

Hydronephrosis is an abnormal dilation of the renal pelvis and the calyces of one or both kidneys, caused by an obstruction of urine flow in the genitourinary tract. Although partial obstruction and hydronephrosis may not produce symptoms initially, the pressure built up behind the area of obstruction eventually results in symptomatic renal dysfunction.

Causes and incidence

Almost any type of obstructive uropathy can result in hydronephrosis. The most common causes are benign prostatic hyperplasia, urethral strictures, and calculi; less common causes include strictures or stenosis of the ureter or bladder outlet, congenital abnormalities, abdominal tumors, blood clots, and neurogenic bladder.

If obstruction is in the urethra or bladder, hydronephrosis is usually bilateral; if obstruction is in a ureter, it's usually unilateral. Obstructions distal to the bladder cause the bladder to dilate and act as a buffer zone, delaying hydronephrosis. Total obstruction of urine flow with dilation of the collecting system ultimately causes complete cortical atrophy and cessation of glomerular filtration.

Hydronephrosis occurs in 1 out of every 100 people.

Signs and symptoms

Clinical features of hydronephrosis vary with the cause of the obstruction. In some patients, hydronephrosis produces no symptoms or only mild pain and slightly decreased urinary flow; in others, it may produce severe, colicky renal pain or dull flank pain that may radiate to the groin, and gross urinary abnormalities, such as hematuria, pyuria, dysuria, alternating oliguria and polyuria, or complete anuria. Other symptoms of hydronephrosis include nausea, vomiting, abdominal fullness, pain on urination, dribbling, or hesitancy. Unilateral obstruction may cause pain on only one side, usually in the flank area.

The most common complication of an obstructed kidney is infection (pyelonephritis) due to stasis that exacerbates renal damage and may create a life-threatening crisis. Paralytic ileus frequently accompanies acute obstructive uropathy.

Diagnosis

CONFIRMING DIAGNOSIS *While the patient's clinical features may suggest hydronephrosis, excretory urography, isotope renography (radioisotope scan of the kidneys), computed tomography scan of the kidneys or abdomen, abdominal magnetic resonance imaging, renal ultrasound, and renal function studies are necessary to confirm it.*

Treatment

The goals of treatment are to preserve renal function and prevent infection through surgical removal of the obstruction, such as dilation for stricture of the urethra or prostatectomy for benign prostatic hyperplasia.

If renal function has already been affected, therapy may include a diet low in protein, sodium, and potassium. This diet is designed to stop the progression of renal failure before surgery. Inoperable obstructions may necessitate decompression and drainage of the kidney using a nephrostomy tube placed temporarily or permanently in the renal pelvis or placement of a ureteral stent to allow the ureter to drain. Concurrent infection requires appropriate antibiotic therapy.

Special considerations

Explain hydronephrosis as well as the purpose of excretory urography and other diagnostic procedures. Check the patient for allergy to excretory urography dye.
- Administer medication for pain, as needed and prescribed.
- Postoperatively, closely monitor intake and output, vital signs, and fluid and electrolyte status. Watch for a rising pulse rate and cold, clammy skin, which indicate possible impending hemorrhage and shock. Monitor renal function studies daily.
- If a nephrostomy tube has been inserted, check it frequently for bleeding and patency. Irrigate the tube only as ordered, and don't clamp it.
- If the patient is to be discharged with a nephrostomy tube in place, teach him how to care for it properly.
- To prevent progression of hydronephrosis to irreversible renal disease, urge older males (especially those with family histories of benign prostatic hyperplasia or prostatitis) to have routine medical checkups. Teach them to recognize and report symptoms of hydronephrosis (colicky pain, hematuria) or urinary tract infection.

Renal tubular acidosis

Renal tubular acidosis (RTA) — a syndrome of persistent dehydration, hyperchloremia, hypokalemia, metabolic acidosis, and nephrocalcinosis — results from the kidneys' inability to conserve bicarbonate. This disorder occurs as distal RTA (Type I, or classic RTA) or proximal RTA (Type II). The prognosis is usually good but depends on the severity of renal damage that precedes treatment.

Causes

Metabolic acidosis usually results from renal excretion of bicarbonate. However, metabolic acidosis associated with RTA results from a defect in the kidneys' normal tubular acidification of urine.

Distal RTA results from an inability of the distal tubule to secrete hydrogen ions against established gradients across the tubular membrane. This results in decreased excretion of titratable acids and ammonium, increased loss of potassium and bicarbonate in the urine, and systemic acidosis. Prolonged acidosis causes mobilization of calcium from bone and, eventually, hypercalciuria, predisposing the kidney to the formation of renal calculi. Distal RTA may be classified as primary or secondary.
- *Primary distal RTA* may occur sporadically or through a hereditary defect and is most prevalent in females, older children, adolescents, and young adults.
- *Secondary distal RTA* has been linked to many renal or systemic conditions, such as starvation, malnutrition, hepatic cirrhosis, and several genetically transmitted disorders.

Proximal RTA results from defective reabsorption of bicarbonate in the proximal tubule. This causes bicarbonate to flood the distal tubule, which normally secretes hydrogen ions, and leads to impaired formation of titratable acids and ammonium for excretion. Ultimately, metabolic acidosis results. Proximal RTA occurs in two forms:
- In *primary proximal RTA,* the reabsorptive defect is idiopathic and is the only disorder present.
- In *secondary proximal RTA,* the reabsorptive defect may be one of several defects and is due to proximal tubular cell damage from a disease such as Fanconi's syndrome.

Signs and symptoms

In infants, RTA produces anorexia, vomiting, occasional fever, polyuria, dehydration, growth retardation, apathy, weakness, tissue wasting, constipation, nephrocalcinosis, and rickets.

In children and adults, RTA may lead to urinary tract infection, rickets, and growth problems. Possible complications of RTA include nephrocalcinosis and pyelonephritis.

Diagnosis

CONFIRMING DIAGNOSIS
Demonstration of impaired acidification of urine with systemic metabolic acidosis confirms distal RTA. Demonstration of bicarbonate wasting due to impaired reabsorption confirms proximal RTA.

Other relevant laboratory results show:
- decreased serum bicarbonate, pH, potassium, and phosphorus
- increased serum chloride and alkaline phosphatase
- alkaline pH, with low titratable acids and ammonium content in urine; increased urinary bicarbonate and potassium; low specific gravity.

In later stages, X-rays may show nephrocalcinosis.

Treatment

Supportive treatment for patients with RTA requires replacement of those substances being abnormally excreted, especially bicarbonate, and may include sodium bicarbonate tablets or solution to control acidosis. Potassium may be given by mouth for dangerously low potassium levels. Vitamins D and calcium supplements are usually avoided because the tendency toward nephrocalcinosis persists even after bicarbonate therapy. If pyelonephritis occurs, treatment may include antibiotics as well.

Treatment for renal calculi secondary to nephrocalcinosis varies and may include supportive therapy until the calculi pass or until surgery for severe obstruction is performed.

Special considerations

Urge compliance with all medication instructions. Inform the patient and his family that the prognosis for RTA and bone le-

sion healing is directly related to the adequacy of treatment.
- Monitor laboratory values, especially potassium, for hypokalemia.
- Test urine for pH, and strain it for calculi.
- If rickets develops, explain the condition and its treatment to the patient and his family.
- Teach the patient how to recognize signs and symptoms of calculi (hematuria, low abdominal or flank pain). Advise him to immediately report any such signs and symptoms.
- Instruct the patient with low potassium levels to eat foods with a high potassium content, such as bananas, leafy green vegetables, and baked potatoes. Orange juice is also high in potassium.
- Because RTA may be caused by a genetic defect, encourage family members to seek genetic counseling or screening for this disorder.

Chronic renal failure

Chronic renal failure is usually the end result of a gradually progressive loss of renal function; occasionally, it's the result of a rapidly progressive disease of sudden onset. Few symptoms develop until after more than 75% of glomerular filtration is lost; then the remaining normal parenchyma deteriorates progressively, and symptoms worsen as renal function decreases.

If this condition continues unchecked, uremic toxins accumulate and produce potentially fatal physiologic changes in all major organ systems. If the patient can tolerate it, maintenance dialysis or kidney transplantation can sustain life.

Causes and incidence

Diabetes and hypertension are the primary causes of chronic renal failure, accounting for two-thirds of cases. Other causes of chronic renal failure include:
- chronic glomerular disease such as glomerulonephritis
- chronic infections, such as chronic pyelonephritis or tuberculosis
- congenital anomalies such as polycystic kidneys

- vascular diseases such as renal nephrosclerosis
- obstructive processes such as calculi
- collagen diseases such as systemic lupus erythematosus
- nephrotoxic agents such as long-term aminoglycoside therapy.

These conditions gradually destroy the nephrons and eventually cause irreversible renal failure. Similarly, acute renal failure that fails to respond to treatment becomes chronic renal failure.

This syndrome may progress through the following stages:

- reduced renal reserve (creatinine clearance glomerular filtration rate [GFR] is 40 to 70 ml/minute)
- renal insufficiency (GFR 20 to 40 ml/minute)
- renal failure (GFR 10 to 20 ml/minute)
- end-stage renal disease (GFR less than 10 ml/minute).

Chronic renal failure and end-stage renal disease affect about 2 out of 1,000 people in the United States.

Signs and symptoms

Chronic renal failure produces major changes in all body systems:

- *Renal and urologic:* Initially, salt-wasting and consequent hyponatremia produce hypotension, dry mouth, loss of skin turgor, listlessness, fatigue, and nausea; later, somnolence and confusion develop. As the number of functioning nephrons decreases, so does the kidneys' capacity to excrete sodium, resulting in salt retention and overload. Accumulation of potassium causes muscle irritability, then muscle weakness as the potassium level continues to rise. Fluid overload and metabolic acidosis also occur. Urinary output decreases; urine is very dilute and contains casts and crystals.
- *Cardiovascular:* Renal failure leads to hypertension, arrhythmias (including life-threatening ventricular tachycardia or fibrillation), cardiomyopathy, uremic pericarditis, pericardial effusion with possible cardiac tamponade, heart failure, and periorbital and peripheral edema.
- *Respiratory:* Pulmonary changes include reduced pulmonary macrophage activity with increased susceptibility to infection, pulmonary edema, pleuritic pain, pleural

friction rub and effusions, crackles, thick sputum, uremic pleuritis and uremic lung (or uremic pneumonitis), dyspnea due to heart failure, and Kussmaul's respirations as a result of acidosis.

- *GI:* Inflammation and ulceration of GI mucosa cause stomatitis, gum ulceration and bleeding and, possibly, parotitis, esophagitis, gastritis, duodenal ulcers, lesions on the small and large bowel, uremic colitis, pancreatitis, and proctitis. Other GI symptoms include a metallic taste in the mouth, uremic fetor (ammonia smell to breath), anorexia, nausea, and vomiting.
- *Cutaneous:* Typically, the skin is pallid, yellowish bronze, dry, and scaly. Other cutaneous symptoms include severe itching; purpura; ecchymoses; petechiae; uremic frost (most often in critically ill or terminal patients); thin, brittle fingernails with characteristic lines; and dry, brittle hair that may change color and fall out easily.
- *Neurologic:* Restless leg syndrome, one of the first signs of peripheral neuropathy, causes pain, burning, and itching in the legs and feet, which may be relieved by voluntarily shaking, moving, or rocking them. Eventually, this condition progresses to paresthesia and motor nerve dysfunction (usually bilateral footdrop) unless dialysis is initiated. Other signs and symptoms include muscle cramping and twitching, shortened memory and attention span, apathy, drowsiness, irritability, confusion, coma, and seizures. EEG changes indicate metabolic encephalopathy.
- *Endocrine:* Common endocrine abnormalities include stunted growth patterns in children (even with elevated growth hormone levels), infertility and decreased libido in both sexes, amenorrhea and cessation of menses in females, and impotence, decreased sperm production, and testicular atrophy in males. Increased aldosterone secretion (related to increased renin production) and impaired carbohydrate metabolism (increased blood glucose levels similar to diabetes mellitus) may also occur.
- *Hematopoietic:* Anemia, decreased red blood cell (RBC) survival time, blood loss from dialysis and GI bleeding, mild thrombocytopenia, and platelet defects occur. Other problems include increased bleeding and clotting disorders, demonstrated by

purpura, hemorrhage from body orifices, easy bruising, ecchymoses, and petechiae.

■ *Skeletal:* Calcium-phosphorus imbalance and consequent parathyroid hormone imbalances cause muscle and bone pain, skeletal demineralization, pathologic fractures, and calcifications in the brain, eyes, gums, joints, myocardium, and blood vessels. Arterial calcification may produce coronary artery disease. In children, renal osteodystrophy (renal rickets) may develop.

Diagnosis

Diagnosis of chronic renal failure is based on clinical assessment, a history of chronic progressive debilitation, and gradual deterioration of renal function as determined by creatinine clearance tests. The following laboratory findings also aid in diagnosis:

■ Blood studies show elevated blood urea nitrogen, serum creatinine, and potassium levels; decreased arterial pH and bicarbonate; and low hemoglobin (Hb) level and hematocrit (HCT).

■ Urine specific gravity becomes fixed at 1.010; urinalysis may show proteinuria, glycosuria, erythrocytes, leukocytes, and casts, depending on the etiology.

■ X-ray studies include kidney-ureter-bladder films, excretory urography, nephrotomography, renal scan, and renal arteriography.

■ Renal or abdominal computed tomography scan, magnetic resonance imaging, or ultrasound indicate changes associated with chronic renal failure, including abnormally small size in both kidneys.

■ Kidney biopsy allows histologic identification of the underlying pathology.

Treatment

Treatment focuses on controlling the symptoms, minimizing complications, and slowing the progression of the disease. Associated diseases that cause or result from chronic renal failure must be controlled such as hypertension. Conservative treatment aims to correct specific symptoms. A low-protein diet reduces the production of end products of protein metabolism that the kidneys can't excrete. (A patient receiving continuous peritoneal dialysis should have a high-protein diet.) A high-calorie diet prevents ketoacidosis and the negative

nitrogen balance that results in catabolism and tissue atrophy, and restricts sodium and potassium.

Maintaining fluid balance requires careful monitoring of vital signs, weight changes, and urine volume (if present). If some renal function remains, administration of loop diuretics such as furosemide, and fluid restriction can reduce fluid retention. Cardiac glycosides may be used to mobilize edema fluids; antihypertensives, to control blood pressure and associated edema. Antiemetics taken before meals may relieve nausea and vomiting; cimetidine or ranitidine may decrease gastric irritation. Methylcellulose or docusate can help prevent constipation.

Treatment may also include regular stool analysis (guaiac test) to detect occult blood and, as needed, cleaning enemas to remove blood from the GI tract. Anemia necessitates iron and folate supplements; severe anemia requires infusion of fresh frozen packed cells or washed packed cells. However, transfusions relieve anemia only temporarily. Epoetin alpha (erythropoietin) increases RBC production.

Drug therapy often relieves associated symptoms: an antipruritic, such as trimeprazine or diphenhydramine, for itching and aluminum hydroxide gel to lower serum phosphate levels. The patient may also benefit from supplementary vitamins (particularly B vitamins and vitamin D) and essential amino acids.

Careful monitoring of serum potassium levels is necessary to detect hyperkalemia. Emergency treatment for severe hyperkalemia includes dialysis therapy and administration of 50% hypertonic glucose I.V., regular insulin, calcium gluconate I.V., sodium bicarbonate I.V., and cation exchange resins such as sodium polystyrene sulfonate.

 ALERT *Cardiac tamponade resulting from pericardial effusion may require emergency pericardial tap or surgery.*

Blood gas measurements may indicate acidosis; intensive dialysis and thoracentesis can relieve pulmonary edema and pleural effusions.

Hemodialysis or peritoneal dialysis (particularly continuous ambulatory peritoneal dialysis and continuous cyclic peritoneal dialysis) can help control most manifestations of end-stage renal disease; altering dialyzing bath fluids can correct fluid and electrolyte disturbances. (See *Comparing peritoneal dialysis and hemodialysis,* page 806. Also see *Continuous ambulatory peritoneal dialysis,* page 807.) But anemia, peripheral neuropathy, cardiopulmonary and GI complications, sexual dysfunction, and skeletal defects may persist. Maintenance dialysis itself may produce complications, such as protein wasting, refractory ascites, and dialysis dementia. Kidney transplantation may eventually be the treatment of choice for some patients with end-stage renal disease.

 PEDIATRIC TIP *Children require more dialysis in relation to their body weight than adults because their metabolic rates and, therefore, food intake, are higher.*

Special considerations

Because chronic renal failure has such widespread clinical effects, it requires meticulous and carefully coordinated supportive care.

- Good skin care is important. Bathe the patient daily, using superfatted soaps, oatmeal baths, and skin lotion without alcohol to ease pruritus. Don't use glycerin-containing soaps because they'll cause skin drying. Give good perineal care, using mild soap and water. Pad the side rails to guard against ecchymoses. Turn the patient often, and use a convoluted foam mattress to prevent skin breakdown.
- Provide good oral hygiene. Brush the patient's teeth often with a soft brush or sponge tip to reduce breath odor. Sugarless hard candy and mouthwash minimize bad taste in the mouth and alleviate thirst.
- Offer small, palatable meals that are also nutritious; try to provide favorite foods within dietary restrictions. Encourage intake of high-calorie foods. Instruct the outpatient to avoid high-sodium foods and high-potassium foods. Encourage adherence to fluid and protein restrictions. To prevent constipation, stress the need for exercise and sufficient dietary bulk.
- Watch for hyperkalemia. Observe for cramping of the legs and abdomen, and di-

arrhea. As potassium levels rise, watch for muscle irritability and a weak pulse rate. Monitor the electrocardiogram for tall, peaked T waves, widening QRS segment, prolonged PR interval, and disappearance of P waves, indicating hyperkalemia.

- Assess hydration status carefully. Check for jugular vein distention, and auscultate the lungs for crackles. Measure daily intake and output carefully, including all drainage, emesis, diarrhea, and blood loss. Record daily weight, presence or absence of thirst, axillary sweat, dryness of tongue, hypertension, and peripheral edema.
- Monitor for bone or joint complications. Prevent pathologic fractures by turning the patient carefully and ensuring his safety. Provide passive range-of-motion exercises for the bedridden patient.
- Encourage deep breathing and coughing to prevent pulmonary congestion. Listen often for crackles, rhonchi, and decreased breath sounds. Be alert for clinical effects of pulmonary edema (dyspnea, restlessness, crackles). Administer diuretics and other medications, as ordered.
- Maintain strict sterile technique. Use a micropore filter during I.V. therapy. Watch for signs of infection (listlessness, high fever, and leukocytosis). Urge the outpatient to avoid contact with infected persons during the cold and flu season.
- Carefully observe and document seizure activity. Infuse sodium bicarbonate for acidosis, and sedatives or anticonvulsants for seizures, as ordered. Pad the side rails and keep an oral airway and suction setup at bedside. Assess neurologic status periodically, and check for Chvostek's and Trousseau's signs, indicators of low serum calcium levels.
- Observe for signs of bleeding. Watch for prolonged bleeding at puncture sites and at the vascular access site used for hemodialysis. Monitor Hb levels and HCT, and check stool, urine, and vomitus for blood.
- Report signs of pericarditis, such as a pericardial friction rub and chest pain.

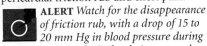 **ALERT** *Watch for the disappearance of friction rub, with a drop of 15 to 20 mm Hg in blood pressure during inspiration (paradoxical pulse) — an early sign of pericardial tamponade.*

(Text continues on page 808.)

COMPARING PERITONEAL DIALYSIS AND HEMODIALYSIS

Advantages, disadvantages, and complications of peritoneal dialysis and hemodialysis are described below.

Type	Advantages	Disadvantages	Possible complications
Peritoneal dialysis	■ Can be performed immediately ■ Requires less complex equipment and less specialized personnel than hemodialysis ■ Requires small amounts of heparin or none at all ■ No blood loss; minimal cardiovascular stress ■ Can be performed by patient anywhere (continuous ambulatory peritoneal dialysis), without assistance and with minimal patient teaching ■ Allows patient independence without long interruptions in daily activities because exchange may be done at night while he sleeps ■ Lower infection rate ■ Lower cost	■ Contraindicated within 72 hours of abdominal surgery ■ Requires 48 to 72 hours for significant response to treatment ■ Severe protein loss necessitates high-protein diet (up to 100 g/day) ■ High risk of peritonitis; repeated bouts may cause scarring, preventing further treatments with peritoneal dialysis ■ Urea clearance less than with hemodialysis (60%)	■ Bacterial or chemical peritonitis ■ Pain (abdominal, low back, shoulder) ■ Shortness of breath, or dyspnea ■ Atelectasis and pneumonia ■ Severe loss of protein into the dialysis solution in the abdominal cavity (10 to 20 g/day) ■ Fluid overload ■ Excessive fluid loss ■ Constipation ■ Catheter site inflammation, infection, or leakage ■ Anorexia ■ Hypertriglyceridemia ■ Abdominal hernias
Hemodialysis	■ Takes only 3 to 5 hours per treatment ■ Faster results in an acute situation ■ Total number of hours of maintenance treatment that's only half that of peritoneal dialysis ■ In an acute situation, can use an I.V. route without a surgical access route	■ Requires surgical creation of a vascular access between circulation and dialysis machine ■ Requires complex water treatment, dialysis equipment, and highly trained personnel ■ Requires administration of larger amounts of heparin ■ Confines patient to special treatment unit	■ Septicemia ■ Air emboli ■ Rapid fluid and electrolyte imbalance (disequilibrium syndrome) ■ Hemolytic anemia ■ Metastatic calcification ■ Increased risk of hepatitis ■ Hypotension or hypertension ■ Itching ■ Pain (generalized or in chest) ■ Heparin overdose, possibly causing hemorrhage ■ Leg cramps ■ Nausea and vomiting ■ Headache

CONTINUOUS AMBULATORY PERITONEAL DIALYSIS

Continuous ambulatory peritoneal dialysis is a useful alternative to hemodialysis in patients with renal failure. Using the peritoneum as a dialysis membrane, it allows almost uninterrupted exchange of dialysis solution. With this method, four to six exchanges of fresh dialysis solution are infused each day. The approximate dwell-time for daytime exchanges is 5 hours; for overnight exchanges, the dwell-time is 8 to 10 hours. After each dwell-time, the patient removes the dialyzing solution by gravity drainage. This form of dialysis offers the unique advantages of a simple, easily taught procedure and patient independence from a special treatment center.

In this procedure, a Tenckhoff catheter is surgically implanted in the abdomen, just below the umbilicus. A bag of dialysis solution is attached using sterile technique to the tube, and the fluid is allowed to flow into the peritoneal cavity (this takes about 10 minutes).

The fluid is then drained out of the peritoneal cavity through gravity flow by unrolling the bag and suspending it below the pelvis (drainage takes about 20 minutes). After the fluid drains, the patient uses sterile technique to connect a new bag of dialyzing solution and fills the peritoneal cavity again. He repeats this procedure four to six times per day.

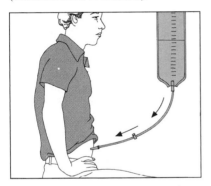

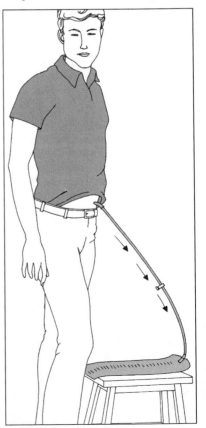

The dialyzing fluid remains in the peritoneal cavity for 4 to 6 hours. During this time, the bag may be rolled up and placed under a shirt or blouse, and the patient can go about normal activities while dialysis takes place.

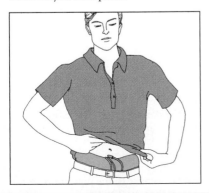

■ Schedule medications carefully. Give iron before meals, aluminum hydroxide gels after meals, and antiemetics, as necessary, a half hour before meals. Administer antihypertensives at appropriate intervals. If the patient requires a rectal infusion of sodium polystyrene sulfonate for dangerously high potassium levels, apply an emollient to soothe the perianal area. Be sure the sodium polystyrene sulfonate enema is expelled; otherwise, it will cause constipation and won't lower potassium levels. Recommend antacid cookies as an alternative to aluminum hydroxide gels needed to bind GI phosphate.

If the patient requires dialysis:
■ Prepare the patient by fully explaining the procedure. Be sure that he understands how to protect and care for the arteriovenous shunt, fistula, or other vascular access. Check the vascular access site per facility protocol or every 2 hours for patency and the extremity for adequate blood supply and intact nervous function (temperature, pulse rate, capillary refill, and sensation). If a fistula is present, feel for a thrill and listen for a bruit. Use a gentle touch to avoid occluding the fistula. Report signs of possible clotting. Don't use the arm with the vascular access site to take blood pressure readings, draw blood, or give injections as these procedures may rupture the fistula or occlude blood flow.
■ Withhold the 6 a.m. (or morning) dose of antihypertensive on the morning of dialysis, and instruct the outpatient to do the same.
■ Use standard precautions when handling body fluids and needles.
■ Monitor Hb levels and HCT. Assess the patient's tolerance of his levels. Some individuals are more sensitive to lower levels than others. Instruct the anemic patient to conserve energy and to rest frequently.
■ After dialysis, check for disequilibrium syndrome, a result of sudden correction of blood chemistry abnormalities. Symptoms range from a headache to seizures. Also, check for excessive bleeding from the dialysis site. Apply pressure dressing or absorbable gelatin sponge, as indicated. Monitor blood pressure carefully after dialysis.
■ A patient undergoing dialysis is under a great deal of stress, as is his family. Refer them to appropriate counseling agencies for assistance in coping with chronic renal failure.

LOWER URINARY TRACT DISORDERS

Lower urinary tract infection

Cystitis and urethritis, the two forms of lower urinary tract infection (UTI), are nearly 10 times more common in females than in males and affect approximately 10% to 20% of all females at least once. Lower UTI is also a prevalent bacterial disease in children, with females again most commonly affected. In males and children, lower UTIs are frequently related to anatomic or physiologic abnormalities and therefore require extremely close evaluation. UTIs often respond readily to treatment but recurrence and resistant bacterial flare-up during therapy are possible.

 PEDIATRIC TIP *All children with proven UTI should receive a workup to exclude an abnormality of the urinary tract that would predispose them to renal damage.*

Causes and incidence
Most lower UTIs result from ascending infection by a single, gram-negative, enteric bacterium, such as *Escherichia coli, Klebsiella, Proteus, Enterobacter, Pseudomonas,* or *Serratia.* However, in a patient with neurogenic bladder, an indwelling catheter, or a fistula between the intestine and bladder, lower UTI may result from simultaneous infection with multiple pathogens. Recent studies suggest that infection results from a breakdown in local defense mechanisms in the bladder that allow bacteria to invade the bladder mucosa and multiply. These bacteria can't be readily eliminated by normal micturition.

Bacterial flare-up during treatment is generally caused by the pathogenic organism's resistance to the prescribed antimicrobial therapy. The presence of even a small number (less than 10,000/µl) of bacteria in a midstream urine sample obtained during treatment casts doubt on the effectiveness of treatment.

In 99% of patients, recurrent lower UTI results from reinfection by the same organism or from some new pathogen; in the remaining 1%, recurrence reflects persistent infection, usually from renal calculi, chronic bacterial prostatitis, or a structural anomaly that may become a source of infection.

The high incidence of lower UTI among females may result from the shortness of the female urethra (1¼″ to 2″ [3 to 5 cm]), which predisposes females to infection caused by bacteria from the vagina, perineum, rectum, or a sexual partner. Males are less vulnerable because their urethras are longer (7¼″ [18.4 cm]) and because prostatic fluid serves as an antibacterial shield. However, in men older than age 60, incidence rates match those of women. In both males and females, infection usually ascends from the urethra to the bladder.

 ELDER TIP *As a person ages, his bladder muscles weaken, which may result in incomplete bladder emptying and chronic urine retention — factors that predispose the older person to bladder infections.*

Signs and symptoms

Lower UTI usually produces urgency, frequency, dysuria, cramps or spasms of the bladder, itching, a feeling of warmth during urination, nocturia, and possibly urethral discharge in males. Inflammation of the bladder wall also causes hematuria and fever. Other common features include low back pain, malaise, nausea, vomiting, abdominal pain or tenderness over the bladder area, chills, and flank pain.

 ELDER TIP *The most common initial symptoms of lower UTI in elderly patients are lethargy and a change in mental status.*

Diagnosis

Characteristic clinical features and a microscopic urinalysis showing red blood cells and white blood cells greater than 10/high-power field suggest lower UTI.

 CONFIRMING DIAGNOSIS *A clean-catch midstream urine specimen revealing a bacterial count above 100,000/µl confirms the diagnosis.*

Lower counts don't necessarily rule out infection, especially if the patient is voiding frequently because bacteria require 30 to 45 minutes to reproduce in urine. Careful midstream, clean-catch collection is preferred to catheterization, which can reinfect the bladder with urethral bacteria.

Sensitivity testing determines the appropriate therapeutic antimicrobial agent. If patient history and physical examination warrant, a blood test or a stained smear of the discharge rules out venereal disease. Voiding cystoureterography or excretory urography may detect congenital anomalies that predispose the patient to recurrent UTIs.

Treatment

Appropriate antimicrobials are the treatment of choice for most initial lower UTIs. A course of antibiotic therapy lasting from 7 to 10 days is standard, but recent studies suggest that a single dose of an antibiotic or an antibiotic regimen of 3 to 5 days length may be sufficient to render the urine sterile. After 3 days of antibiotic therapy, urine culture should show no organisms. If the urine isn't sterile, bacterial resistance has probably occurred, making the use of a different antimicrobial necessary. Single-dose antibiotic therapy with amoxicillin or co-trimoxazole may be effective in females with acute noncomplicated UTI. A urine culture taken 1 to 2 weeks later indicates whether or not the infection has been eradicated.

Recurrent infections due to infected renal calculi, chronic prostatitis, or structural abnormality may necessitate surgery; prostatitis also requires long-term antibiotic therapy. In patients without these predisposing conditions, long-term, low-dosage antibiotic therapy is the treatment of choice.

 PEDIATRIC TIP *Fluoroquinolones aren't used for children because of possible adverse effects on developing cartilage.*

Special considerations

The care plan should include careful patient teaching, supportive measures, and proper specimen collection.

- Explain the nature and purpose of antimicrobial therapy. Emphasize the importance of completing the prescribed course of therapy or, with long-term prophylaxis, of adhering strictly to the ordered dosage. Urge the patient to drink plenty of water (at least eight glasses a day). Stress the need to maintain a consistent fluid intake of about 2 qt (2 L)/day. More or less than this amount may alter the effect of the prescribed antimicrobial. Fruit juices, especially cranberry juice, and oral doses of vitamin C may help acidify the urine and enhance the action of the medication.
- Watch for GI disturbances from antimicrobial therapy. Nitrofurantoin macrocrystals, taken with milk or a meal, prevent such distress. If therapy includes phenazopyridine, warn the patient that this drug may turn urine red-orange.
- Suggest warm sitz baths for relief of perineal discomfort. If baths aren't effective, apply heat sparingly to the perineum but be careful not to burn the patient. Apply topical antiseptics, such as povidone-iodine ointment, on the urethral meatus as necessary.
- Collect all urine samples for culture and sensitivity testing carefully and promptly. Teach the female patient how to clean the perineum properly and keep the labia separated during voiding. A noncontaminated midstream specimen is essential for accurate diagnosis.
- To prevent recurrent lower UTIs, teach the female patient to carefully wipe the perineum from front to back and to clean it thoroughly with soap and water after defecation. Advise an infection-prone woman to void immediately after sexual intercourse. Stress the need to drink plenty of fluids routinely and to avoid postponing urination. Recommend frequent comfort stops during long car trips. Also stress the need to completely empty the bladder. To prevent recurrent infections in males, urge prompt treatment of predisposing conditions such as chronic prostatitis. Have the patient use a commode rather than a bedpan to promote sitting up, which assists in emptying the bladder.

Vesicoureteral reflux

In vesicoureteral reflux, urine flows from the bladder back into the ureters and eventually into the renal pelvis or the parenchyma. Because the bladder empties poorly, urinary tract infection (UTI) may result, possibly leading to acute or chronic pyelonephritis with renal damage.

Vesicoureteral reflux is most common during infancy in males and during early childhood (ages 3 to 7) in females. Primary vesicoureteral reflux that results from congenital anomalies is most prevalent in females and is rare in blacks. Up to 25% of asymptomatic siblings of children with diagnosed primary vesicoureteral reflux also show reflux.

Causes and incidence

In patients with vesicoureteral reflux, incompetence of the ureterovesical junction and shortening of intravesical ureteral musculature allow backflow of urine into the ureter when the bladder contracts during voiding. Incompetence may result from congenital anomalies of the ureters or bladder, including short or absent intravesical ureter, ureteral ectopia lateralis (greater-than-normal lateral placement of ureters), and gaping ureteral orifice; inadequate detrusor muscle buttress in the bladder, stemming from congenital paraureteral bladder diverticulum; acquired diverticulum (from outlet obstruction); flaccid neurogenic bladder; and high intravesical pressure from outlet obstruction or an unknown cause. Vesicoureteral reflux may also result from cystitis, with inflammation of the intravesical ureter, which causes edema and fixation of the intramural ureter and usually leads to reflux in persons with congenital ureteral or bladder anomalies or other predisposing conditions.

Reflux nephropathy occurs in about 4 out of 1,000 asymptomatic people. However, in infants and children who experience UTIs, its prevalence approaches 40% to 50%. Reflux nephropathy may lead to chronic renal failure and end-stage renal disease.

Signs and symptoms

Vesicoureteral reflux typically manifests itself as the signs and symptoms of UTI: frequency, urgency, burning on urination, hematuria, foul-smelling urine and, in infants, dark, concentrated urine. With upper urinary tract involvement, signs and symptoms usually include high fever, chills, flank pain, vomiting, and malaise.

 PEDIATRIC TIP *In children, fever, nonspecific abdominal pain, and diarrhea may be the only clinical effects. Rarely, children with minimal symptoms remain undiagnosed until puberty or later, when they begin to exhibit clear signs of renal impairment (anemia, hypertension, and lethargy).*

Diagnosis

Symptoms of UTI provide the first clues to diagnosis of vesicoureteral reflux. In infants, hematuria or strong-smelling urine may be the first indication; palpation may reveal a hard, thickened bladder (hard mass deep in the pelvis) if posterior urethral valves are causing an obstruction in male infants.

Cystoscopy, with instillation of a solution containing methylene blue or indigo carmine dye, may confirm the diagnosis. After the bladder is emptied and refilled with clear sterile water, color-tinged efflux from either ureter positively confirms reflux.

Other pertinent laboratory studies include the following:

■ Clean-catch urinalysis shows a bacterial count greater than 100,000/µl. Microscopic examination may reveal white blood cells, red blood cells, and an increased urine pH in the presence of infection. Specific gravity less than 1.010 demonstrates inability to concentrate urine.

■ Laboratory studies reveal elevated creatinine levels (more than 1.2 mg/dl) and elevated blood urea nitrogen levels (more than 18 mg/dl), indicating advanced renal dysfunction.

■ Excretory urography may show dilated lower ureter, ureter visible for its entire length, hydronephrosis, calyceal distortion, and renal scarring.

■ Voiding cystourethrography (either fluoroscopic or radionuclide) identifies and determines the degree of reflux and shows when reflux occurs. It may also pinpoint the causative anomaly. In this procedure, contrast material is instilled into the bladder, and X-rays are taken before, during, and after voiding. Nuclear cystography and renal ultrasound may also be used to detect reflux.

■ Abdominal computed tomography scan or ultrasound of the kidneys or abdomen shows hydronephrosis, reflux, a small kidney, or scarring.

■ Catheterization of the bladder after the patient voids determines the amount of residual urine.

Treatment

The goal of treatment in a patient with vesicoureteral reflux is to prevent pyelonephritis and renal dysfunction with antibiotic therapy and, when necessary, vesicoureteral reimplantation. Appropriate surgical procedures create a normal valve effect at the junction by reimplanting the ureter into the bladder wall at a more oblique angle.

Antimicrobial therapy is usually effective for reflux that's secondary to infection, reflux related to neurogenic bladder and, in children, reflux related to a short intravesical ureter (which abates spontaneously with growth). Reflux related to infection generally subsides after the infection is cured. However, 80% of females with vesicoureteral reflux will have recurrent UTIs within a year. Recurrent infection requires long-term prophylactic antibiotic therapy and careful patient follow-up (cystoscopy and excretory urography every 4 to 6 months) to track the degree of reflux.

UTI that recurs despite adequate prophylactic antibiotic therapy necessitates vesicoureteral reimplantation or reconstructive repair. Bladder outlet obstruction in neurogenic bladder requires surgery only if renal dysfunction is present. After surgery, as after antibiotic therapy, close medical follow-up is necessary (excretory urography every 2 to 3 years and urinalysis once per month for 1 year), even if symptoms haven't recurred.

Special considerations
Patient care includes education and postoperative support.

■ To ensure complete emptying of the bladder, teach the patient with vesicoureteral reflux to double void (void once and then try to void again in a few minutes). Because his natural urge to urinate may be impaired, advise him to void every 2 to 3 hours whether or not he feels the urge.

 PEDIATRIC TIP *Because the diagnostic tests may frighten the child, encourage one of his parents to stay with him during all procedures. Explain the procedures to the parents and to the child, if he's old enough to understand.*

■ If surgery is necessary, explain postoperative care: suprapubic catheter in the male, indwelling catheter in the female; and, in both, one or two ureteral catheters or splints brought out of the bladder through a small abdominal incision. The suprapubic or indwelling catheter keeps the bladder empty and prevents pressure from stressing the surgical wound; ureteral catheters drain urine directly from the renal pelvis. After complicated reimplantations, all catheters remain in place for 7 to 10 days. Explain that the child will be able to move and walk with the catheters but must be very careful not to dislodge them.

■ Postoperatively, closely monitor fluid intake and output. Give analgesics and antibiotics, as ordered. Make sure the catheters are patent and draining well. Maintain sterile technique during catheter care. Watch for fever, chills, and flank pain, which suggest a blocked catheter.

■ Before discharging the patient, stress the importance of close follow-up care and adequate fluid intake throughout childhood.

■ Instruct parents to watch for and report recurring signs of UTI (painful, frequent, burning urination; foul-smelling urine).

■ If the child is taking antimicrobial drugs, make sure his parents understand the importance of completing the prescribed therapy or maintaining low-dose prophylaxis.

Neurogenic bladder

Neurogenic bladder (also known as *neuromuscular dysfunction of the lower urinary tract, neurologic bladder dysfunction,* and *neuropathic bladder*) refers to all types of bladder dysfunction caused by an interruption of normal bladder innervation. Subsequent complications include incontinence, residual urine retention, urinary infection, stone formation, and renal failure. A neurogenic bladder can be spastic (hypertonic, reflex, or automatic) or flaccid (hypotonic, atonic, nonreflex, or autonomous).

Causes
At one time, neurogenic bladder was thought to result primarily from spinal cord injury; now, it appears to stem from a host of underlying conditions:

■ cerebral disorders, such as stroke, brain tumor (meningioma and glioma), Parkinson's disease, multiple sclerosis, dementia, and incontinence caused by aging

■ spinal cord disease or trauma, such as herniated vertebral disks, spina bifida, myelomeningocele, spinal stenosis (causing cord compression) or arachnoiditis (causing adhesions between the membranes covering the cord), cervical spondylosis, myelopathies from hereditary or nutritional deficiencies and, rarely, tabes dorsalis

■ disorders of peripheral innervation, including autonomic neuropathies resulting from endocrine disturbances such as diabetes mellitus (most common)

■ metabolic disturbances, such as hypothyroidism, porphyria, or uremia (infrequent)

■ acute infectious diseases such as transverse myelitis

■ heavy metal toxicity

■ chronic alcoholism

■ collagen diseases such as systemic lupus erythematosus

■ vascular diseases such as atherosclerosis

■ distant effects of cancer such as primary oat cell carcinoma of the lung

■ herpes zoster

■ sacral agenesis.

An upper motor neuron lesion (above S2 to S4) causes spastic neurogenic bladder, with spontaneous contractions of detrusor muscles, elevated intravesical voiding pressure, bladder wall hypertrophy with trabeculation, and urinary sphincter spasms. A lower motor neuron lesion (below S2 to S4) causes flaccid neurogenic bladder, with decreased intravesical pressure, increased bladder capacity and large residual urine retention, and poor detrusor contraction.

Signs and symptoms

Neurogenic bladder produces a wide range of clinical effects, depending on the underlying cause and its effect on the structural integrity of the bladder. Usually, this disorder causes some degree of incontinence, changes in initiation or interruption of micturition, and the inability to empty the bladder completely. Other effects of neurogenic bladder include vesicoureteral reflux, deterioration or infection in the upper urinary tract, and hydroureteral nephrosis.

Depending on the site and extent of the spinal cord lesion, spastic neurogenic bladder may produce involuntary or frequent scanty urination, without a feeling of bladder fullness, and possibly spontaneous spasms of the arms and legs. Anal sphincter tone may be increased. Tactile stimulation of the abdomen, thighs, or genitalia may precipitate voiding and spontaneous contractions of the arms and legs. With cord lesions in the upper thoracic (cervical) level, bladder distention can trigger hyperactive autonomic reflexes, resulting in severe hypertension, bradycardia, and headaches.

Flaccid neurogenic bladder may be associated with overflow incontinence, diminished anal sphincter tone, and a greatly distended bladder (evident on percussion or palpation), but without the accompanying feeling of bladder fullness due to sensory impairment.

Diagnosis

The patient's history may include a condition or disorder that can cause neurogenic bladder, incontinence, and disruptions of micturition patterns. Voiding cystourethrography evaluates bladder neck function, vesicoureteral reflux, and continence.

Urodynamic studies help evaluate how urine is stored in the bladder, how well the bladder empties, and the rate of movement of urine out of the bladder during voiding. These studies consist of four components:

- Urine flow study (uroflow) shows diminished or impaired urine flow.
- Cystometry evaluates bladder nerve supply, detrusor muscle tone, and intravesical pressures during bladder filling and contraction.
- Urethral pressure profile determines urethral function with respect to the length of the urethra and the outlet pressure resistance.
- Sphincter electromyelography correlates the neuromuscular function of the external sphincter with bladder muscle function during bladder filling and contraction. This evaluates how well the bladder and urinary sphincter muscles work together.
- Retrograde urethrography reveals the presence of strictures and diverticula. This test may not be performed on a routine basis.

Treatment

The goals of treatment are to maintain the integrity of the upper urinary tract, control infection, and prevent urinary incontinence through evacuation of the bladder, drug therapy, surgery or, less commonly, neural blocks and electrical stimulation.

Techniques of bladder evacuation include Credé's method, Valsalva's maneuver, and intermittent self-catheterization. Credé's method — application of manual pressure over the lower abdomen — promotes complete emptying of the bladder. After appropriate instruction, most patients can perform this maneuver themselves. Even when patients perform this maneuver properly, however, Credé's method isn't always successful and doesn't always eliminate the need for catheterization.

Intermittent self-catheterization — more effective than either Credé's method or Valsalva's maneuver — has proved to be a major advance in the treatment of neurogenic bladder because it allows complete emptying of the bladder without the risks that an indwelling catheter poses. Generally, a male can perform this procedure more easily but a female can learn self-catheterization with the help of a mirror. Intermittent self-catheterization, in conjunction with a bladder-retraining program, is especially useful for patients with flaccid neurogenic bladder.

Drug therapy for neurogenic bladder may include bethanechol and phenoxybenzamine to facilitate bladder emptying and propantheline, methantheline, flavoxate, dicyclomine, and imipramine to facilitate urine storage.

When conservative treatment fails, surgery may correct the structural impairment through transurethral resection of the bladder neck, urethral dilatation, external sphincterotomy, or urinary diversion procedures. Implantation of an artificial urinary sphincter may be necessary if permanent incontinence follows surgery for neurogenic bladder.

Special considerations
Care for patients with neurogenic bladder varies according to the underlying cause and method of treatment.

■ Explain all diagnostic tests clearly so the patient understands the procedure, time involved, and possible results. Assure the patient that the lengthy diagnostic process is necessary to identify the most effective treatment plan. After the treatment plan is chosen, explain it to the patient in detail.

■ Use strict sterile technique during insertion of an indwelling catheter (a temporary measure to drain the incontinent patient's bladder). Don't interrupt the closed drainage system for any reason. Obtain urine specimens with a syringe and small-bore needle inserted through the aspirating port of the catheter itself (below the junction of the balloon instillation site). Irrigate in the same manner if ordered.

■ Clean the catheter insertion site with soap and water at least twice a day. Don't allow the catheter to become encrusted. Use a sterile applicator to apply antibiotic ointment around the meatus after catheter care. Keep the drainage bag below the tubing, and don't raise the bag above the level of the bladder. Clamp the tubing, or empty the bag before transferring the patient to a wheelchair or stretcher to prevent accidental urine reflux. If urine output is considerable, empty the bag more frequently than once every 8 hours because bacteria can multiply in standing urine and migrate up the catheter and into the bladder.

■ Watch for signs of infection (fever, cloudy or foul-smelling urine). Encourage the patient to drink plenty of fluids to prevent calculus formation and infection from urinary stasis. Try to keep the patient as mobile as possible. Perform passive range-of-motion exercises if necessary.

■ If urinary diversion procedure is to be performed, arrange for consultation with an enterostomal therapist, and coordinate the care plans.

■ Before discharge, teach the patient and his family evacuation techniques as necessary (Credé's method, intermittent catheterization). Counsel him regarding sexual activities. Remember, the incontinent patient feels embarrassed and distressed. Provide emotional support.

Congenital anomalies of the ureter, bladder, and urethra

The most common congenital malformations of the ureter, bladder, and urethra include duplicated ureter, retrocaval ureter, ectopic orifice of the ureter, stricture or stenosis of the ureter, ureterocele, exstrophy of the bladder, congenital bladder diverticulum, hypospadias, and epispadias. Some of these abnormalities are obvious at birth; others aren't apparent and are recognized only after they produce symptoms. (See *Congenital urologic anomalies.*)

Causes
Congenital anomalies of the ureter, bladder, and urethra are among the most common birth defects, occurring in about 5% of all births. Their causes are unknown; diagnosis and treatment vary.

Special considerations
PEDIATRIC TIP *Because these anomalies aren't always obvious at birth, carefully evaluate the newborn's urogenital function. Document the amount and color of urine, voiding pattern, strength of stream, and any indications of infection, such as fever and urine odor. Tell*
(Text continues on page 818.)

CONGENITAL UROLOGIC ANOMALIES

Duplicated ureter	Retrocaval ureter (preureteral vena cava)	Ectopic orifice of ureter
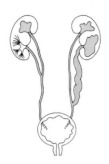	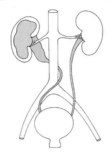	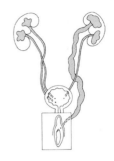

Duplicated ureter

Pathophysiology
- Most common ureteral anomaly
- *Complete*, a double collecting system with two separate pelves, each with its own ureter and orifice
- *Incomplete* (y type), two separate ureters join before entering bladder

Clinical features
- Persistent or recurrent infection
- Frequency, urgency, or burning on urination
- Diminished urine output
- Flank pain, fever, and chills

Diagnosis and treatment
- Excretory urography
- Voiding cystoscopy
- Cystoureterography
- Retrograde pyelography
- Surgery for obstruction, reflux, or severe renal damage

Retrocaval ureter (preureteral vena cava)

Pathophysiology
- The right ureter passes behind the inferior vena cava before entering the bladder. Compression of the ureter between the vena cava and the spine causes dilation and elongation of the pelvis; hydroureter and hydronephrosis; and fibrosis and stenosis of the ureter in the compressed area.
- Relatively uncommon; higher incidence in males

Clinical features
- Right flank pain
- Recurrent urinary tract infection
- Renal calculi
- Hematuria

Diagnosis and treatment
- Excretory urography demonstrates superior ureteral enlargement with spiral appearance
- Surgical resection and anastomosis of ureter with renal pelvis, or reimplantation into bladder

Ectopic orifice of ureter

Pathophysiology
- Ureters single or duplicated in females, ureteral orifice usually inserts in urethra or vaginal vestibule, beyond external urethral sphincter; in males, in prostatic urethra, or in seminal vesicles or vas deferens

Clinical features
- Symptoms rare when ureteral orifice opens between trigone and bladder neck
- Obstruction, reflux, and incontinence (dribbling) in 50% of females
- In males, flank pain, frequency, urgency

Diagnosis and treatment
- Excretory urography
- Urethroscopy, vaginoscopy
- Voiding cystourethrography
- Resection and ureteral reimplantation into bladder for incontinence

(continued)

CONGENITAL UROLOGIC ANOMALIES *(continued)*

Strictures or stenosis of ureter	Ureterocele	Exstrophy of bladder
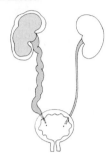	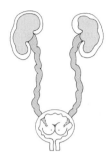	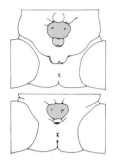

Strictures or stenosis of ureter

Pathophysiology
- Most common site, the distal ureter above ureterovesical junction; less common, uretero-pelvic junction; rare, the midureter
- Discovered during infancy in 25% of patients; before puberty in most
- More common in males

Clinical features
- Megaloureter or hy-droureter (enlarged ureter), with hydro-nephrosis when stenosis occurs in distal ureter
- Hydronephrosis alone when stenosis occurs at ureteropelvic junction

Diagnosis and treatment
- Ultrasound
- Excretory urography
- Voiding cystography
- Surgical repair of stric-ture; nephrectomy for se-vere renal damage

Ureterocele

Pathophysiology
- Bulging of submucosal ureter into bladder can be 1 or 2 cm, or can almost fill entire bladder
- Unilateral, bilateral, ec-topic with resulting hy-droureter and hydro-nephrosis

Clinical features
- Obstruction
- Persistent or recurrent infection

Diagnosis and treatment
- Voiding cystourethrog-raphy
- Excretory urography and cystoscopy show thin, translucent mass
- Surgical excision or re-section of ureterocele, with reimplantation of ureter

Exstrophy of bladder

Pathophysiology
- Absence of anterior ab-dominal and bladder wall allows the bladder to pro-trude onto abdomen
- In males, associated undescended testes and epispadias; in females, cleft clitoris, separated labia, or absent vagina
- Skeletal or intestinal anomalies possible

Clinical features
- Obvious at birth, with urine seeping onto ab-dominal wall from abnor-mal ureteral orifices
- Surrounding skin exco-riated; exposed bladder mucosa ulcerated; infec-tion; related abnormali-ties

Diagnosis and treatment
- Excretory urography
- Surgical closure of de-fect, and bladder and ure-thra reconstruction dur-ing infancy to allow pubic bone fusion; alternative treatment: protective dressing and diapering; urinary diversion eventu-ally necessary for most patients

CONGENITAL UROLOGIC ANOMALIES *(continued)*

Congenital bladder diverticulum	Hypospadias	Epispadias
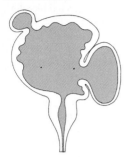	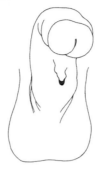	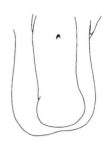

Congenital bladder diverticulum

Pathophysiology
- Circumscribed pouch or sac (diverticulum) of bladder wall
- Can occur anywhere in bladder, usually lateral to ureteral orifice. Large diverticulum at orifice can cause reflux.

Clinical features
- Fever, frequency, and painful urination
- Urinary tract infection
- Cystitis, particularly in males

Diagnosis and treatment
- Excretory urography shows diverticulum
- Retrograde cystography shows vesicoureteral reflux in ureter
- Surgical correction for reflux

Hypospadias

Pathophysiology
- Urethral opening on ventral surface of penis or, in females (rare), within vagina
- Occurs in 1 in 300 live male births; genetic factor suspected in less severe cases

Clinical features
- Usually associated with chordee, making normal urination with penis elevated impossible
- Absence of ventral prepuce
- Vaginal discharge in females

Diagnosis and treatment
- Mild disorder requires no treatment
- Surgical repair of severe anomaly usually necessary before child reaches school age

Epispadias

Pathophysiology
- Urethral opening on dorsal surface of penis; in females, a fissure of the upper wall of urethra
- A rare anomaly; usually more common in males; often accompanies bladder exstrophy

Clinical features
- In mild cases, orifice appears along dorsum of glans; in severe cases, along dorsum of penis
- In females, bifid clitoris and short, wide urethra

Diagnosis and treatment
- Surgical repair, in several stages, almost always necessary

parents to watch for these signs at home. In all children, watch for signs of obstruction, such as dribbling, oliguria or anuria, abdominal mass, hypertension, fever, bacteriuria, or pyuria.

- Monitor renal function daily; record intake and output accurately.
- Follow strict sterile technique in handling cystostomy tubes or indwelling urinary catheters.
- Make sure that ureteral, suprapubic, or urethral catheters remain in place and don't become contaminated. Document the type, color, and amount of drainage.
- Apply sterile saline pads to protect the exposed mucosa of the newborn with bladder exstrophy. Don't use heavy clamps on the umbilical cord, and avoid dressing or diapering the infant. Place the infant in an incubator, and direct a stream of saline mist onto the bladder to keep it moist. Use warm water and mild soap to keep the surrounding skin clean. Rinse well, and keep the area as dry as possible to prevent excoriation.
- Provide reassurance and emotional support to the parents. When possible, allow them to participate in their child's care to promote normal bonding. As appropriate, suggest or arrange for genetic counseling.

PROSTATE AND EPIDIDYMIS DISORDERS

Prostatitis

Prostatitis, inflammation of the prostate gland, may be acute or chronic. Acute prostatitis most often results from gram-negative bacteria and is easy to recognize and treat. However, chronic prostatitis, the most common cause of recurrent urinary tract infections (UTIs) in males, is less easy to recognize.

Causes and incidence

About 80% of bacterial prostatitis cases result from infection by *Escherichia coli;* the rest are due to infection by *Klebsiella, En-* terobacter, *Proteus, Pseudomonas, Streptococcus,* or *Staphylococcus.* These organisms probably spread to the prostate by the bloodstream or from ascending urethral infection, invasion of rectal bacteria via lymphatics, reflux of infected bladder urine into the prostate ducts or, less commonly, infrequent or excessive sexual intercourse or such procedures as cystoscopy or catheterization. Chronic prostatitis usually results from bacterial invasion from the urethra.

It's estimated that 2 of every 10,000 people who seek outpatient care do so because of prostatitis. As many as 35% of males older than age 50 have chronic prostatitis; about 50% of males will be diagnosed with prostatitis at some point in their lives.

Signs and symptoms

Acute prostatitis begins with fever, chills, low back pain, myalgia, perineal fullness, and arthralgia. Urination is frequent and urgent. Dysuria, nocturia, and urinary obstruction may also occur. The urine may appear cloudy. When palpated rectally, the prostate is tender, indurated, swollen, firm, and warm.

Chronic bacterial prostatitis sometimes produces no symptoms but usually elicits the same urinary symptoms as the acute form but to a lesser degree. UTI is a common complication. Other possible signs include painful ejaculation, hemospermia, persistent urethral discharge, and sexual dysfunction.

Diagnosis

Characteristic rectal examination findings suggest prostatitis. In many cases, a urine culture can identify the causative infectious organism.

CONFIRMING DIAGNOSIS *A firm diagnosis depends on a comparison of urine cultures of specimens obtained by the Meares and Stamey technique. This test requires four specimens: one collected when the patient starts voiding (voided bladder one); another midstream; another after the patient stops voiding and the physician massages the prostate to produce secretions (expressed prostate secretions; and a final voided specimen. A significant increase* *in colony count in the prostatic specimens confirms prostatitis.*

Treatment

Systemic antibiotic therapy chosen according to the infecting organism is the treatment of choice for acute prostatitis. If sepsis is likely, I.V. antibiotics may be given until sensitivity test results are known. If test results and clinical response are favorable, parenteral therapy continues for 48 hours to 1 week, after which an oral agent is substituted for 30 days. For infections caused by a sexually transmitted disease, injection of ceftriaxone followed by a 10-day course of doxycycline or floxacin is effective.

Supportive therapy includes bed rest, adequate hydration, and administration of analgesics, antipyretics, sitz baths, and stool softeners as necessary. Diet therapy includes avoiding substances that irritate the bladder, such as alcohol, caffeinated food and beverages, citrus juices, and hot or spicy foods. Increasing the intake of fluids (1,893 to 3,785 ml/day) encourages frequent urination that will help flush the bacteria from the bladder. In symptomatic chronic prostatitis, regular massage of the prostate is most effective. Regular ejaculation may help promote drainage of prostatic secretions. Anticholinergics and analgesics may help relieve nonbacterial prostatitis symptoms.

If drug therapy is unsuccessful, treatment may include transurethral resection of the prostate, which requires removal of all infected tissue. However, this procedure usually isn't performed on young adults because it may cause retrograde ejaculation and sterility. Total prostatectomy is curative but may cause impotence and incontinence.

Special considerations

Patient care is primarily supportive.
■ Ensure bed rest and adequate hydration. Provide stool softeners and administer sitz baths, as ordered.
■ As necessary, prepare to assist with suprapubic needle aspiration of the bladder or a suprapubic cystostomy.
■ Emphasize the need for strict adherence to the prescribed drug regimen. Instruct

ORCHITIS

Orchitis, an infection of the testicles, is a serious complication of epididymitis. It may also result from mumps, which may lead to sterility. Orchitis may, rarely, result from other systemic infections, testicular torsion, or severe trauma. Its typical effects include unilateral or bilateral tenderness, sudden onset of pain, and swelling of the scrotum and testicles. The affected testicle may be red. Nausea and vomiting also occur. Sudden cessation of pain indicates testicular ischemia, which may result in permanent damage to one or both testicles.

Treatment consists of immediate antibiotic therapy; in orchitis due to mumps, diethylstilbestrol may be given to relieve pain, swelling, and fever. Severe orchitis may require surgery to incise and drain the hydrocele and improve testicular circulation. Other treatment is similar to that for epididymitis. To prevent orchitis due to mumps, stress the need for prepubertal males to receive mumps vaccine (or gamma globulin injection after contracting mumps).

the patient to drink at least 8 glasses of water a day. Have him report adverse drug reactions (rash, nausea, vomiting, fever, chills, and GI irritation).

Epididymitis

This infection of the epididymis, the testicle's cordlike excretory duct, is one of the most common infections of the male reproductive tract. It usually affects adults and is rare before puberty. Epididymitis may spread to the testicle itself, causing orchitis; bilateral epididymitis may cause sterility. (See *Orchitis*.)

Causes and incidence

Epididymitis is usually a complication of pyogenic bacterial infection of the urinary tract (urethritis or prostatitis). The pyogenic organisms, such as staphylococci, *Escherichia coli*, streptococci, *Chlamydia trachomatis*, and *Neisseria gonorrhoeae*, reach the epididymis through the lumen of the vas deferens. Rarely, epididymitis is secondary to a distant infection, such as pharyngitis or tuberculosis, that spreads through the lymphatics or, less commonly, the bloodstream. Other causes include trauma, gonorrhea, syphilis, or a chlamydial infection. Trauma may reactivate a dormant infection or initiate a new one. Epididymitis may be a complication of prostatectomy and may also result from chemical irritation by extravasation of urine through the vas deferens. The incidence is about 600,000 cases per year, with the highest prevalence in young males ages 19 to 35.

Signs and symptoms

The key symptoms are pain, extreme tenderness, and swelling in the groin and scrotum with erythema, high fever, malaise, and a characteristic waddle—an attempt to protect the groin and scrotum during walking. An acute hydrocele may also result from inflammation.

Diagnosis

Clinical features suggest epididymitis but diagnosis is actually made with the aid of laboratory tests:
- urinalysis: increased white blood cell (WBC) count indicates infection
- urine culture and sensitivity tests: may identify causative organism
- serum WBC count: more than 10,000/µl in infection.

 ALERT *Scrotal ultrasonography may help differentiate acute epididymitis from other conditions, such as testicular torsion, which is a surgical emergency.*

Testicular scan (nuclear medicine scan) may be done to rule out torsion. In epididymitis, increased blood flow is also demonstrated.

Treatment

The goal of treatment is to reduce pain and swelling and combat infection. Therapy must begin immediately, particularly in the patient with bilateral epididymitis because sterility is always a threat. During the acute phase, treatment consists of bed rest, scrotal elevation with towel rolls or adhesive strapping, broad-spectrum antibiotics, and analgesics. An ice bag applied to the area may reduce swelling and relieve pain (heat is contraindicated because it may damage germinal cells, which are viable only at or below normal body temperature). When pain and swelling subside and allow walking, an athletic supporter may prevent pain. Occasionally, corticosteroids may be prescribed to help counteract inflammation but their use is controversial.

 ELDER TIP *In the older patient undergoing open prostatectomy, bilateral vasectomy may be necessary to prevent epididymitis as a postoperative complication; however, antibiotic therapy alone may prevent it. When epididymitis is refractory to antibiotic therapy, epididymectomy under local anesthetic is necessary.*

Special considerations

Patient care includes support and monitoring for worsening of symptoms.
- Watch closely for abscess formation (localized, hot, red, tender area) or extension of infection into the testes. Closely monitor temperature, and ensure adequate fluid intake.
- Because the patient is usually very uncomfortable, administer analgesics as necessary. During bed rest, check often for proper scrotum elevation.
- Before discharge, emphasize the importance of completing the prescribed antibiotic therapy, even after symptoms subside. Educate the patient regarding preventing the transmission of sexually transmitted diseases, as appropriate.
- If the patient faces the possibility of sterility, suggest supportive counseling as necessary.

Benign prostatic hyperplasia

Although most males older than age 50 have some prostatic enlargement, in benign prostatic hyperplasia (BPH), also known as *benign prostatic hypertrophy,* the prostate gland enlarges sufficiently to compress the urethra and cause some overt urinary obstruction. Depending on the size of the enlarged prostate, the age and health of the patient, and the extent of obstruction, BPH is treated symptomatically or surgically.

Causes and incidence

Evidence suggests a link between BPH and hormonal activity. As males age, production of androgenic hormones decreases, causing an imbalance in androgen and estrogen levels, and high levels of dihydrotestosterone, the main prostatic intracellular androgen. Other causes include neoplasm, arteriosclerosis, diabetes, inflammation, and metabolic or nutritional disturbances.

Whatever the cause, BPH begins with changes in periurethral glandular tissue. As the prostate enlarges, it may extend into the bladder and obstruct urinary outflow by compressing or distorting the prostatic urethra. BPH may also cause a pouch to form in the bladder that retains urine when the rest of the bladder empties. This retained urine may lead to calculus formation or cystitis.

The likelihood of developing an enlarged prostate increases with age. A small amount of prostate enlargement is present in many males older than age 40 and more than 90% of males older than age 80. It's estimated that by 2006, 115 million men age 50 and older will develop BPH. Blacks, with an incidence rate of 224.3 cases per 100,000 people, are at the greatest risk, present with more advanced disease, and have a poorer diagnosis. Whites, by comparison, have an incidence of 150.3 cases per 100,000 people while Asians have an incidence of 82.2 cases per 100,000 people.

Signs and symptoms

Clinical features of BPH depend on the extent of prostatic enlargement and the lobes affected. Characteristically, the condition starts with a group of symptoms known as *prostatism:* reduced urinary stream caliber and force, urinary hesitancy, and difficulty starting micturition (resulting in straining, feeling of incomplete voiding, and an interrupted stream). As the obstruction increases, it causes frequent urination with nocturia, dribbling, urine retention, incontinence, and possibly hematuria. Physical examination indicates a visible midline mass above the symphysis pubis that represents an incompletely emptied bladder; rectal palpation discloses an enlarged prostate. Examination may detect secondary anemia and, possibly, renal insufficiency secondary to obstruction.

As BPH worsens, complete urinary obstruction may follow infection or use of decongestants, tranquilizers, alcohol, antidepressants, or anticholinergics. Complications include infection, renal insufficiency, hemorrhage, and shock.

Diagnosis

Clinical features and a rectal examination are usually sufficient for diagnosis. Other findings help to confirm it:

- Excretory urography may indicate urinary tract obstruction, hydronephrosis, calculi or tumors, and filling and emptying defects in the bladder.
- Elevated blood urea nitrogen and serum creatinine levels suggest renal dysfunction.
- Urinalysis and urine culture show hematuria, pyuria and, when the bacterial count exceeds 100,000/µl, urinary tract infection (UTI).

When symptoms are severe, a cystourethroscopy is definitive, but this test is performed only immediately before surgery to help determine the best procedure. It can show prostate enlargement, bladder wall changes, and a raised bladder.

Treatment

Conservative therapy includes prostate massages, sitz baths, fluid restriction for bladder distention, and antimicrobials for infection. If symptoms are mild, methods for relief may include avoiding alcohol and caffeine, especially after dinner; urinating when the urge is initially felt; avoiding over-the-counter cold and sinus medications that contain decongestants or antihistamines because they can increase BPH symptoms; keeping warm and exercising regularly as cold weather and lack of physical activity may worsen symptoms; performing pelvic strengthening exercises (Kegel exercises); reducing stress because nervousness and tension can lead to more frequent urination. Some males have had success taking extracts of saw palmetto berries, an herb that has been used to ease prostate symptoms. Fat-soluble saw palmetto extract that has been standardized to contain 85% to 95% fatty acids and sterols is more effective. Regular ejaculation may help relieve prostatic congestion.

Urine flow rates can be improved with alpha$_1$-adrenergic blockers, which relieve bladder outlet obstruction by preventing contractions of the prostatic capsule and bladder neck. Finasteride lowers levels of hormones produced by the prostate, reduces the size of the prostate gland, increases urine flow rate, and decreases symptoms of BPH. It may take 3 to 6 months before a significant improvement in symptoms occurs. Potential adverse effects related to finasteride include decreased sex drive and impotence.

Surgery is the only effective therapy to relieve acute urine retention, hydronephrosis, severe hematuria, recurrent UTIs, and other intolerable symptoms. A transurethral resection may be performed if the prostate weighs less than 2 oz (56.7 g). In this procedure, a resectoscope removes tissue with a wire loop and electric current. In high-risk patients, continuous drainage with an indwelling urinary catheter alleviates urine retention. Transurethral needle ablation may be used to heat and destroy prostate tissue by radiofrequency; this helps spare surrounding tissue.

The following procedures involve open surgical removal:
- *suprapubic (transvesical) resection:* most common and useful when prostatic enlargement remains within the bladder
- *retropubic (extravesical) resection:* allows direct visualization; potency and continence are usually maintained.

Balloon dilatation of the prostate is still being investigated. Balloon dilatation or balloon urethroplasty involves passing a flexible balloon catheter through the urethra at the level of the prostate while being guided by fluoroscope. The balloon is inflated for a short time to distend the prostatic urethra.

Special considerations

Prepare the patient for diagnostic tests and surgery, as appropriate.
- Monitor and record the patient's vital signs, intake and output, and daily weight. Watch closely for signs of postobstructive diuresis (such as increased urine output and hypotension), which may lead to serious dehydration, lowered blood volume, shock, electrolyte loss, and anuria.
- Administer antibiotics, as ordered, for UTI, urethral instrumentation, and cystoscopy.
- If urine retention is present, insert an indwelling urinary catheter (although this is usually difficult in a patient with BPH). If the catheter can't be passed transurethrally, assist with suprapubic cystostomy (under local anesthetic). Watch for rapid bladder decompression.

After prostatic surgery:
- Maintain patient comfort, and watch for and prevent postoperative complications. Observe for immediate dangers of prostatic bleeding (shock and hemorrhage). Check the catheter often (every 15 minutes for the first 2 to 3 hours) for patency and urine color; check dressings for bleeding.
- Postoperatively, many urologists insert a three-way catheter and establish continuous bladder irrigation. Keep the catheter open at a rate sufficient to maintain returns that are clear and light pink. Watch for fluid overload from absorption of the irrigating fluid into systemic circulation. If a regular catheter is used, observe it closely. If drainage stops because of clots, irrigate the catheter, as ordered, usually with 80 to 100 ml of normal saline solution, while maintaining *strict* sterile technique.

 ALERT *Watch for septic shock, the most serious complication of prostatic surgery. Immediately report severe chills, sudden fever, tachycardia, hypotension, or other signs of shock. Start rapid infusion of antibiotics I.V. as ordered. Watch for pulmonary embolus, heart failure, and renal shutdown. Monitor vital signs, central venous pressure, and arterial pressure con-*

tinuously. The patient may need intensive supportive care in the intensive care unit.

■ Administer anticholinergics, as ordered, to relieve painful bladder spasms that often occur after transurethral resection.

■ Take patient comfort measures after an open procedure: provide suppositories (except after perineal prostatectomy), analgesic medication to control incisional pain, and frequent dressing changes.

■ Continue infusing I.V. fluids until the patient can drink sufficient fluids (2 to 3 L/day) to maintain adequate hydration.

■ Administer stool softeners and laxatives, as ordered, to prevent straining. *Don't* check for fecal impaction because a rectal examination may precipitate bleeding.

■ After the catheter is removed, the patient may experience frequency, dribbling, and occasional hematuria. Reassure him that he'll gradually regain urinary control.

■ Reinforce prescribed limits on activity. Warn the patient against lifting, strenuous exercise, and long automobile rides because these increase bleeding tendency. Also caution the patient to restrict sexual activity for at least several weeks after discharge from the hospital.

■ Instruct the patient to follow the prescribed oral antibiotic drug regimen, and tell him the indications for using gentle laxatives. Urge him to seek medical care immediately if he can't void, if he passes bloody urine, or if he develops a fever.

Selected references

Brenner, B.M., and Levine, S.A., eds. *Brenner and Rector's The Kidney,* 7th ed. Philadelphia: W.B. Saunders Co., 2004.

Caughey, A.B., et al., eds. *Blueprints Pathophysiology III: Renal, Hematology and Oncology: Notes and Cases.* Cambridge, Mass.: Blackwell Scientific Pubs., 2003.

Gearhart, J.P., ed. *Pediatric Urology.* Totowa, N.J.: Humana Press, 2003.

Kopple, J.D., and Massry, S.G. *Kopple and Massry's Nutrition Management of Renal Disease,* 2nd ed. Philadelphia: Lippincott Williams & Wilkins, 2003.

Potts, J.M., ed. *Essential Urology: A Guide to Clinical Practice.* Totowa, N.J.: Humana Press, 2004.

Smeltzer, S.C., et al., eds. *Brunner & Suddarth's Textbook of Medical-Surgical Nursing,* 10th ed. Philadelphia: Lippincott Williams & Wilkins, 2004.

Tanagho, E.A., and McAninch, J.W. *Smith's General Urology,* 16th ed. New York: McGraw-Hill Book Co., 2003.

13

Endocrine disorders

Introduction *824*

Pituitary gland *827*
Hypopituitarism *827*
Acromegaly and gigantism *830*
Diabetes insipidus *832*

Thyroid gland *834*
Hypothyroidism in adults *834*
Hypothyroidism in children *836*
Thyroiditis *837*
Simple goiter *839*
Hyperthyroidism *840*

Parathyroid glands *844*
Hypoparathyroidism *844*
Hyperparathyroidism *847*

Adrenal glands *849*
Adrenal hypofunction *849*
Cushing's syndrome *852*
Hyperaldosteronism *856*
Adrenogenital syndrome *858*
Pheochromocytoma *861*

Pancreatic and multiple disorders *863*
Multiple endocrine neoplasia *863*
Diabetes mellitus *864*

Selected references *868*

Introduction

Together with the nervous system, the endocrine system regulates and integrates the body's metabolic activities. The endocrine system meets the nervous system at the hypothalamus. The hypothalamus, the main integrative center for the endocrine and autonomic nervous systems, controls the function of endocrine organs by neural and hormonal pathways. A hormone is a chemical transmitter released from specialized cells into the bloodstream, which carries it to specialized organ-receptor cells that respond to it.

Neural pathways connect the hypothalamus to the posterior pituitary, or neurohypophysis. Neural stimulation to the posterior pituitary provokes the secretion of two effector hormones: antidiuretic hormone (ADH) and oxytocin, and influences thyroid-stimulating hormone (TSH), corticotropin, prolactin, and gonadotropin-releasing hormone.

Hypothalamic control
The hypothalamus also exerts hormonal control at the anterior pituitary through releasing and inhibiting factors, which arrive by a portal system. Hypothalamic hormones stimulate the pituitary to release trophic hormones, such as corticotropin, TSH, luteinizing hormone (LH), and

follicle-stimulating hormone (FSH), and to release or inhibit effector hormones, such as the growth hormone and prolactin. In turn, secretion of trophic hormones stimulates the adrenal cortex, thyroid, and gonads. In a patient whose clinical condition suggests endocrine pathology, this complex hormonal sequence requires careful evaluation at each level to identify the dysfunction; dysfunction may result from defects of releasing, trophic, or effector hormones or of the target tissue. Hyperthyroidism, for example, may result from an excess of thyrotropin-releasing hormone, TSH, or thyroid hormone.

In addition to hormonal and neural controls, a negative feedback system regulates the endocrine system. (See *Feedback mechanism of the endocrine system*.) The mechanism of feedback may be simple or complex. Simple feedback occurs when the level of one substance regulates secretion of a hormone. For example, low serum calcium levels stimulate parathyroid hormone (PTH) secretion; high serum calcium levels inhibit it. Complex feedback occurs through the hypothalamic-pituitary-target organ axis; for example, secretion of the hypothalamic corticotropin-releasing hormone (CRH) releases pituitary corticotropin, which, in turn, stimulates adrenal cortisol secretion. Subsequently, a rise in serum cortisol level inhibits corticotropin by decreasing CRH secretion. Steroid therapy disrupts the hypothalamic-pituitary-adrenal (HPA) axis by suppressing hypothalamic-pituitary secretion. Because abrupt withdrawal of steroids doesn't allow time for recovery of the HPA axis to stimulate cortisol secretion, it can induce a life-threatening adrenal crisis.

Hormonal effects

In response to the hypothalamus, the *posterior pituitary* secretes oxytocin and ADH. Oxytocin stimulates contraction of the uterus and is responsible for the milk letdown reflex in lactating females. ADH controls the concentration of body fluids by altering the permeability of the distal convoluted tubules and collecting ducts of the kidneys to conserve water. The secretion of ADH depends on plasma volume and osmolality as monitored by hypothalamic

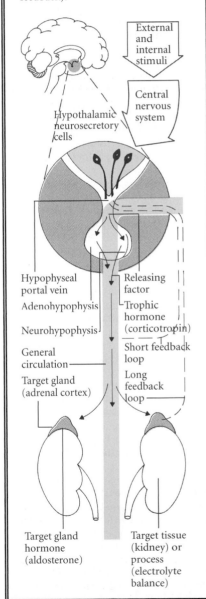

FEEDBACK MECHANISM OF THE ENDOCRINE SYSTEM

The hypothalamus receives regulatory information from its own circulating hormones (short feedback) and also from target glands (long feedback).

External and internal stimuli

Central nervous system

Hypothalamic neurosecretory cells

Hypophyseal portal vein

Adenohypophysis

Neurohypophysis

General circulation

Target gland (adrenal cortex)

Releasing factor

Trophic hormone (corticotropin)

Short feedback loop

Long feedback loop

Target gland hormone (aldosterone)

Target tissue (kidney) or process (electrolyte balance)

neurons. Circulatory shock and severe hemorrhage are the most powerful stimulators of ADH; other stimulators include pain, emotional stress, trauma, morphine, tranquilizers, certain anesthetics, and positive-pressure breathing.

The syndrome of inappropriate ADH secretion is a disorder that produces hyponatremia with water overload. Generally, however, overhydration suppresses ADH secretion (as does alcohol). ADH deficiency causes diabetes insipidus, a condition of high urine output.

The *anterior pituitary* secretes prolactin, which stimulates milk production, and human growth hormone (hGH), which stimulates growth by increasing protein synthesis and fat mobilization and by decreasing carbohydrate utilization. Hyposecretion of hGH results in dwarfism; hypersecretion causes gigantism in children and acromegaly in adults.

The *thyroid gland* secretes the iodinated hormones thyroxine and triiodothyronine. Thyroid hormones, necessary for normal growth and development, act on many tissues to increase metabolic activity and protein synthesis. Deficiency of thyroid hormone causes varying degrees of hypothyroidism, from a mild, clinically insignificant form to life-threatening myxedema coma. Congenital hypothyroidism causes cretinism. Hypersecretion causes hyperthyroidism and, in extreme cases, thyrotoxic crisis. Excessive secretion of TSH causes thyroid gland hyperplasia, resulting in goiter.

The *parathyroid glands* secrete PTH, which regulates calcium and phosphate metabolism. PTH elevates serum calcium levels by stimulating resorption of calcium and phosphate from bone, reabsorption of calcium and excretion of phosphate by the kidneys and, by combined action with vitamin D, absorption of calcium and phosphate from the GI tract. PTH also stimulates conversion of vitamin D to its metabolically active form. Thyrocalcitonin, a secretion from the thyroid, opposes the effect of PTH and therefore decreases serum calcium levels. Hyperparathyroidism results in hypercalcemia, and hypoparathyroidism causes hypocalcemia. Altered calcium levels may also result from nonendocrine causes such as metastatic bone disease.

The *endocrine* part of the *pancreas* produces glucagon from the alpha cells and insulin from the beta cells. Glucagon, the hormone of the fasting state, releases stored glucose to raise the blood glucose level. Insulin, the hormone of the nourished state, facilitates glucose transport, promotes glucose storage, stimulates protein synthesis, and enhances free fatty acid uptake and storage. Absolute or relative insulin deficiency causes diabetes mellitus. Insulin excess can result from an insulinoma (a tumor of the beta cells).

 ELDER TIP *A common and important endocrine change in older people is a decreased ability to tolerate stress, as demonstrated by glucose metabolism. Normally, fasting blood glucose levels aren't significantly different in young and old adults. However, when stress stimulates an older person's pancreas, the blood glucose concentration increases and remains elevated longer than in a young adult.*

The *adrenal cortex* secretes mineralocorticoids, glucocorticoids, and sex steroids. Aldosterone, a mineralocorticoid, regulates the reabsorption of sodium and the excretion of potassium by the kidneys. Although affected by corticotropin, aldosterone is regulated by angiotensin II, which in turn, is regulated by renin and plasma volume. Together, aldosterone, angiotensin, and renin may be implicated in the pathogenesis of hypertension. An excess of aldosterone (aldosteronism) can result primarily from hyperplasia or from adrenal adenoma or secondarily from many conditions, including heart failure and cirrhosis.

Cortisol, a glucocorticoid, stimulates gluconeogenesis, increases protein breakdown and free fatty acid mobilization, suppresses the immune response, and provides for an appropriate response to stress. Hyperactivity of the adrenal cortex results in Cushing's syndrome; hypoactivity of the adrenal cortex causes Addison's disease and, in extreme cases, adrenal crisis. Adrenogenital syndromes may result from overproduction of sex steroids.

The *adrenal medulla* is an aggregate of nervous tissue that produces the catecholamines epinephrine and norepinephrine, both of which cause vasoconstriction. Epinephrine also causes the fight-or-flight response—dilation of bronchioles and increased blood pressure, blood glucose levels, and heart rate. Pheochromocytoma, a tumor of the adrenal medulla, causes hypersecretion of catecholamines and results in characteristic sustained or paroxysmal hypertension.

The *testes* synthesize and secrete testosterone in response to gonadotropic hormones, especially LH, from the anterior pituitary gland; spermatogenesis occurs in response to FSH. The *ovaries* produce sex steroid hormones, primarily estrogen and progesterone, in response to LH and FSH.

Endocrine dysfunction

Chronic endocrine abnormalities are common health problems. For example, deficiencies of cortisol, thyroid hormone, or insulin may require lifelong hormone replacement for survival. Consequently, these conditions make special demands on your skills during ongoing patient assessment, acute illness, and patient teaching.

Common dysfunctions of the endocrine system are classified as hypofunction and hyperfunction, inflammation, and tumor. The source of hypofunction and hyperfunction may originate in the hypothalamus or in the pituitary or effector glands. Inflammation may be acute or subacute, as in thyroiditis, but is usually chronic, commonly resulting in glandular hypofunction. Tumors can occur within a gland—as in thyroid cancer or adrenal pheochromocytoma—or in other areas, resulting in ectopic hormone production. Certain lung tumors, for example, secrete ADH, PTH, or structurally similar substances that have the same effects on target tissues.

The study of endocrine function focuses on measuring the level or effect of a hormone. Radioimmunoassay, for example, measures insulin levels; a fasting blood glucose test measures insulin's effects. Sophisticated techniques of hormone measurement have improved diagnosis of endocrine disorders.

Diagnostic tests confirm endocrine disorders but clinical data usually provide the first clues. Nursing assessment can reveal such signs and symptoms as excessive or delayed growth, wasting, weakness, polydipsia, polyuria, and mental changes. The quality and distribution of hair, skin pigmentation, and the distribution of body fat are also significant.

Nurses are also responsible for patient preparation, including instruction and support during testing, and for specimen collection, particularly of timed blood and urine specimens.

PITUITARY GLAND

Hypopituitarism

Hypopituitarism, which includes panhypopituitarism or dwarfism, is a complex syndrome marked by metabolic dysfunction, sexual immaturity, and growth retardation (when it occurs in childhood), resulting from a deficiency of the hormones secreted by the anterior pituitary gland. Panhypopituitarism refers to a generalized condition caused by partial or total failure of the anterior pituitary's vital hormones—corticotropin, thyroid-stimulating hormone (TSH), luteinizing hormone (LH), follicle-stimulating hormone (FSH), human growth hormone (hGH), and prolactin—plus the posterior pituitary hormone, antidiuretic hormone. Partial hypopituitarism and complete hypopituitarism occur in adults and children; in children, these diseases may cause dwarfism and delayed puberty. The prognosis may be good with adequate replacement therapy and correction of the underlying causes.

Causes

The most common cause of primary hypopituitarism in adults is a tumor. Other causes include congenital defects (hypoplasia or aplasia of the pituitary gland); pituitary infarction (most often from postpartum hemorrhage); or partial or total hypophysectomy by surgery, irradiation, or chemical agents; and, rarely, granulomatous disease (tuberculosis, for example). Occasionally, hypopituitarism may have no identifiable cause, or it may be related to autoimmune destruction of the gland. Secondary hypopituitarism stems from a deficiency of releasing hormones produced by the hypothalamus — either idiopathic or possibly resulting from infection, trauma, or a tumor.

Primary hypopituitarism usually develops in a predictable pattern of hormonal failures. It generally starts with hypogonadism from gonadotropin failure (decreased FSH and LH levels). In adults, it causes cessation of menses in females and impotence in men. Growth hormone (GH) deficiency follows; in children, this causes short stature, delayed growth, and delayed puberty. In adults, it causes osteoporosis, decreased lean-to-fat body mass index, adverse lipid changes, and subtle emotional dysphoria and lethargy. Subsequent failure of thyrotropin (decreased TSH levels) causes hypothyroidism; finally, adrenocorticotropic failure (decreased corticotropin levels) results in adrenal insufficiency. However, when hypopituitarism follows surgical ablation or trauma, the pattern of hormonal events may not necessarily follow this sequence. Sometimes, damage to the hypothalamus or neurohypophysis from one of the above leads to diabetes insipidus.

Signs and symptoms

Clinical features of hypopituitarism develop slowly and vary with the severity of the disorder and the number of deficient hormones. Signs and symptoms of hypopituitarism in adults may include gonadal failure (secondary amenorrhea, impotence, infertility, decreased libido), diabetes insipidus, hypothyroidism (fatigue, lethargy, sensitivity to cold, menstrual disturbances), and adrenocortical insufficiency (hypoglycemia, anorexia, nausea, abdominal pain, orthostatic hypotension).

Postpartum necrosis of the pituitary (Sheehan's syndrome) characteristically causes failure of lactation, menstruation, and growth of pubic and axillary hair; and symptoms of thyroid and adrenocortical failure.

In children, hypopituitarism causes retarded growth or delayed puberty. Dwarfism usually isn't apparent at birth but early signs begin to appear during the first few months of life; by age 6 months, growth retardation is obvious. Although these children generally enjoy good health, pituitary dwarfism may cause chubbiness due to fat deposits in the lower trunk, delayed secondary tooth eruption and, possibly, hypoglycemia. Growth continues at less than half the normal rate — sometimes extending into the patient's 20s or 30s — to an average height of 4' (122 cm), with normal proportions.

When hypopituitarism strikes before puberty, it prevents development of secondary sex characteristics (including facial and body hair). In males, it produces undersized testes, penis, and prostate gland; absent or minimal libido; and the inability to initiate and maintain an erection. In females, it usually causes immature development of the breasts, sparse or absent pubic and axillary hair, and primary amenorrhea.

Panhypopituitarism may induce a host of mental and physiologic abnormalities, including lethargy, psychosis, orthostatic hypotension, bradycardia, anemia, and anorexia. However, clinical manifestations of hormonal deficiencies resulting from pituitary destruction don't become apparent until 75% of the gland is destroyed. Total loss of all hormones released by the anterior pituitary is fatal unless treated.

Neurologic signs associated with hypopituitarism and produced by pituitary tumors include headache, bilateral temporal hemianopia, loss of visual acuity and, possibly, blindness. Acute hypopituitarism resulting from surgery or infection is often associated with fever, hypotension, vomiting, and hypoglycemia — all characteristic of adrenal insufficiency.

Diagnosis

In suspected hypopituitarism, evaluation must confirm hormonal deficiency due to impairment or destruction of the anterior pituitary gland and rule out disease of the target organs (adrenals, gonads, and thyroid) or the hypothalamus. Low serum levels of thyroxine (T_4), for example, indicate diminished thyroid gland function, but further tests are necessary to identify the source of this dysfunction as the thyroid, pituitary, or hypothalamus.

Serum insulin–like growth factor 1 (IGF-1) is decreased. Cranial computed tomography (CT) scan or magnetic resonance imaging (MRI) may reveal a tumor or abnormal mass in the pituitary gland of the hypothalamus. Radioimmunoassay showing decreased plasma levels of some or all pituitary hormones, accompanied by end-organ hypofunction, suggests pituitary failure, and eliminates target gland disease. Failure of thyrotropin-releasing hormone administration to increase TSH or prolactin concentrations rules out hypothalamic dysfunction as the cause of hormonal deficiency.

Provocative tests are helpful in pinpointing the source of low cortisol levels. Oral metyrapone blocks cortisol synthesis, which should stimulate pituitary secretion of corticotropin and the adrenal precursors of cortisol, measured in urine as hydroxycorticosteroids. Insulin-induced hypoglycemia also stimulates corticotropin secretion. Persistently low levels of corticotropin indicate pituitary or hypothalamic failure. These tests require careful medical supervision because they may precipitate an adrenal crisis.

CONFIRMING DIAGNOSIS
Diagnosis of hypopituitarism requires measurement of GH levels in the blood after administration of regular insulin (inducing hypoglycemia) or levodopa (causing hypotension). These drugs should provoke increased secretion of GH. Persistently low GH levels, despite provocative testing, confirm GH deficiency. CT scan, MRI, or cerebral angiography confirms the presence of intrasellar or extrasellar tumors.

Treatment

Replacement of hormones secreted by the target glands is the most effective treatment for hypopituitarism. Hormone replacement therapy includes cortisol, T_4, and androgen or cyclic estrogen. Prolactin need not be replaced. The patient of reproductive age may benefit from administration of FSH and human chorionic gonadotropin to boost fertility. GH replacement is recommended for adults as well as children. Replacement is done by administering daily subcutaneous injections of one of two recombinant deoxyribonucleic acid (DNA) GHs, accompanied by follow-up of serum IGF-1 levels. Lean body mass increases, whereas adipose tissue—particu-

larly in the abdomen—decreases. Risk of cardiovascular disease and osteoporosis also decrease with treatment. Many patients also notice an improved sense of well-being.

Somatrem, which is identical to hGH but is the product of recombinant DNA technology, has replaced GHs derived from human sources. It's effective for treating dwarfism and stimulates growth increases as great as 4″ to 6″ (10 to 15 cm) in the first year of treatment. The growth rate tapers off in subsequent years. After pubertal changes have occurred, the effects of somatrem therapy are limited. Occasionally, a child becomes unresponsive to somatrem therapy, even with larger doses, perhaps because antibodies have formed against it. In such refractory patients, small doses of androgen may again stimulate growth but extreme caution is necessary to prevent premature closure of the epiphyses. Children with hypopituitarism may also need replacement of adrenal and thyroid hormones and, as they approach puberty, sex hormones.

Special considerations

Caring for patients with hypopituitarism requires an understanding of hormonal effects and skilled physical and psychological support.

■ Monitor the results of all laboratory tests for hormonal deficiencies, and know what they mean. Until hormone replacement therapy is complete, check for signs of thyroid deficiency (increasing lethargy), adrenal deficiency (weakness, orthostatic hypotension, hypoglycemia, fatigue, and weight loss), and gonadotropin deficiency (decreased libido, lethargy, and apathy).

■ Watch for anorexia in the patient with panhypopituitarism. Help plan a menu containing favorite foods—ideally, high-calorie foods. Monitor for weight loss or gain.

■ If the patient has trouble sleeping, encourage exercise during the day.

■ Record temperature, blood pressure, and heart rate every 4 to 8 hours. Check eyelids, nail beds, and skin for pallor, which indicates anemia.

■ Prevent infection by giving meticulous skin care. Because the patient's skin is probably dry, use oil or lotion instead of soap. If body temperature is low, provide additional clothing and covers, as needed, to keep the patient warm.

■ Darken the room if the patient has a tumor that's causing headaches and visual disturbances. Help with any activity that requires good vision such as reading the menu. The patient with bilateral hemianopia has impaired peripheral vision, so be sure to stand where he can see you, and advise the family to do the same.

■ During insulin testing, monitor closely for signs of hypoglycemia (initially, slow cerebration, tachycardia, diaphoresis, and nervousness, progressing to seizures). Keep dextrose 50% in water available for I.V. administration to correct hypoglycemia rapidly.

■ To prevent orthostatic hypotension, be sure to keep the patient supine during levodopa testing.

■ Instruct the patient to wear a medical identification bracelet. Teach him and his family members how to administer steroids parenterally in case of an emergency.

■ Refer the family of a child with dwarfism to the appropriate community resources for psychological counseling because the emotional stress caused by this disorder increases as the child becomes more aware of his condition.

Acromegaly and gigantism

Acromegaly and gigantism are chronic, progressive diseases marked by hormonal dysfunction and startling skeletal overgrowth. Acromegaly occurs after epiphyseal closure, causing bone thickening and transverse growth and visceromegaly. Gigantism begins before epiphyseal closure and causes proportional overgrowth of all body tissues. Although the prognosis depends on the causative factor, these disorders usually reduce life expectancy unless treated in a timely fashion.

Causes and incidence

Typically, oversecretion of human growth hormone (hGH) produces changes throughout the body, resulting in acro-

megaly and, when oversecretion occurs before puberty, gigantism. Eosinophilic or mixed-cell adenomas of the anterior pituitary gland may cause this oversecretion but the etiology of the tumors themselves remains unclear. Occasionally, hGH levels are elevated in more than one family member, which suggests the possibility of a genetic cause.

The earliest clinical manifestations of acromegaly include soft-tissue swelling of the extremities and coarsening of facial features. This rare form of hyperpituitarism occurs equally among males and females, usually between ages 30 and 50. Annually, it affects 3 to 4 people per every million.

In gigantism, proportional overgrowth of all body tissues starts before epiphyseal closure. This causes remarkable height increases of as much as 6″ (15 cm) per year. Gigantism affects infants and children, causing them to attain as much as three times the normal height for their age. As adults, they may ultimately reach a height of more than 80″ (203 cm). Gigantism is rare; there have only been 100 reported cases.

Signs and symptoms

Acromegaly develops slowly and typically produces diaphoresis, oily skin, hypermetabolism, and hypertrichosis. Severe headache, central nervous system impairment, bitemporal hemianopia, loss of visual acuity, and blindness may result from the intrasellar tumor compressing the optic chiasm or nerves.

Hypersecretion of hGH produces cartilaginous and connective tissue overgrowth, resulting in a characteristic hulking appearance, with an enlarged supraorbital ridge and thickened ears and nose. Prognathism, projection of the jaw, becomes marked and may interfere with chewing. Laryngeal hypertrophy, paranasal sinus enlargement, and thickening of the tongue cause the voice to sound deep and hollow. Distal phalanges display an arrowhead appearance on X-rays, and the fingers are thickened. Irritability, hostility, and various psychological disturbances may occur.

Prolonged effects of excessive hGH secretion include bowlegs, barrel chest, arthritis, osteoporosis, kyphosis, hypertension, and arteriosclerosis. Both gigantism and acromegaly may also cause signs of glucose intolerance and clinically apparent diabetes mellitus because of the insulin-antagonistic character of hGH. If acromegaly is left untreated, the patient is at risk for premature cardiovascular disease, colon polyps, and colon cancer.

Gigantism develops abruptly, producing some of the same skeletal abnormalities seen in acromegaly. As the disease progresses, the pituitary tumor enlarges and invades normal tissue, resulting in the loss of other trophic hormones, such as thyroid-stimulating hormone, luteinizing hormone, follicle-stimulating hormone, and corticotropin, thus causing the target organ to stop functioning.

Diagnosis
Plasma hGH and somatomedin-C levels measured by radioimmunoassay typically are elevated. Because hGH secretion is pulsatile, the results of random sampling may be misleading. The glucose suppression test offers more reliable information. Glucose normally suppresses hGH secretion; therefore, a glucose infusion that doesn't suppress the hormone level to below the accepted normal value of 5 ng/ml, when combined with characteristic clinical features, strongly suggests hyperpituitarism. The level of insulin-like growth factor 1 is high.

In addition, skull X-rays, computed tomography scan, arteriography, and magnetic resonance imaging determine the presence and extent of the pituitary lesion. Bone X-rays showing a thickening of the cranium (especially of frontal, occipital, and parietal bones) and of the long bones, as well as osteoarthritis in the spine, support this diagnosis.

Treatment
Treatment aims to curb overproduction of hGH through removal of the underlying tumor by cranial or transsphenoidal hypophysectomy or pituitary radiation therapy. In acromegaly, surgery is mandatory when a tumor causes blindness or other severe neurologic disturbances. Postoperative therapy often requires replacement of thyroid, cortisone, and gonadal hormones.

Adjunctive treatment may include administration of bromocriptine or cabergoline and octreotide and postoperative conventional proton beam radiation, which inhibit hGH synthesis. The therapeutic goal is to reach and maintain hGH levels less than 2 ng/dl, because at that level, life expectancy is restored to that of age-matched controls.

Special considerations
The extreme body changes characteristic of this disorder can cause severe psychological stress; therefore, emotional support to help the patient cope with his altered body image is an integral part of patient care.

■ Assess for skeletal manifestations, such as arthritis of the hands and osteoarthritis of the spine. Administer medications as ordered. To promote maximum joint mobility, perform or assist with range-of-motion exercises.

■ Evaluate muscle weakness, especially in the patient with late-stage acromegaly. Check the strength of his handclasp. If it's very weak, help with tasks such as cutting food.

■ Keep the skin dry. Avoid using an oily lotion because the skin is already oily.

■ Test blood for glucose. Check for signs of hyperglycemia (fatigue, polyuria, and polydipsia).

■ Be aware that the tumor may cause visual problems. If the patient has hemianopia, stand where he can see you. Remember, this disease can also cause inexplicable mood changes. Reassure the family that these mood changes result from the disease and can be modified with treatment.

■ Before surgery, reinforce what the surgeon has told the patient, and try to allay the patient's fear with a clear and honest explanation of the scheduled operation.

 PEDIATRIC TIP *If the patient is a child, explain to his parents that such surgery prevents permanent soft-tissue deformities but won't correct bone changes that have already taken place. Arrange for counseling, if necessary, to help the child and his parents cope with these permanent defects.*

 ALERT *After surgery, diligently monitor vital signs and neurologic status. Immediately report increased*

urinary output lasting over 2 hours, alteration in level of consciousness, unequal pupil size, changes in visual acuity, vomiting, falling pulse rate, or rising blood pressure. These changes may signal an increase in intracranial pressure due to intracranial bleeding or cerebral edema.

- Check blood glucose level often. Remember, hGH levels usually fall rapidly after surgery, removing an insulin-antagonist effect in many patients and possibly precipitating hypoglycemia. Measure intake and output hourly, and report large increases. Transient diabetes insipidus, which sometimes occurs after surgery for hyperpituitarism, can cause such increases in urine output.
- If the transsphenoidal approach is used, a large nasal packing is kept in place for several days. Because the patient must breathe through his mouth, give good mouth care. Pay special attention to the mucous membranes — which usually become dry — and the incision site under the upper lip, at the top of the gum line. The surgical site is packed with a piece of tissue generally taken from a midthigh donor site. Watch for cerebrospinal fluid leaks from the packed site, which may necessitate additional surgery to repair the leak. Look for increased external nasal drainage or drainage into the nasopharynx.
- Encourage the patient to walk as soon as possible after surgery.
- Before discharge, emphasize the importance of continuing hormone replacement therapy, if ordered. Make sure the patient and his family understand which hormones are to be taken and why as well as the correct times and dosages. Warn against stopping the hormones suddenly.
- Advise the patient to wear a medical identification bracelet at all times and to bring his hormone replacement schedule with him whenever he returns to the health care facility.
- Instruct the patient to have follow-up examinations for the rest of his life because a slight chance exists that the tumor that caused his condition may recur.

Diabetes insipidus

Diabetes insipidus (also called *pituitary diabetes insipidus*) is a disorder of water metabolism resulting from a deficiency of circulating vasopressin (also called *antidiuretic hormone* [ADH]). It's characterized by excessive fluid intake and hypotonic polyuria. The disorder may start in childhood or early adulthood (the median age of onset is 21) and is more common in males than in females. Incidence is slightly higher today than in the past. In uncomplicated diabetes insipidus, the prognosis is good with adequate water replacement and replacement of ADH by tablet or nasal spray, and patients usually lead normal lives.

Causes and incidence

Diabetes insipidus results centrally from intracranial neoplastic or metastatic lesions, hypophysectomy or other neurosurgery, a skull fracture, or head trauma that damages the neurohypophyseal structures. It can also result nephrogenically from infection, granulomatous disease, and vascular lesions; it may be idiopathic and, rarely, familial. (*Note:* Pituitary diabetes insipidus shouldn't be confused with nephrogenic diabetes insipidus, a rare congenital disturbance of water metabolism that results from renal tubular resistance to vasopressin.)

Normally, the hypothalamus synthesizes vasopressin. The posterior pituitary gland (or neurohypophysis) stores vasopressin and releases it into general circulation, where it causes the kidneys to reabsorb water by making the distal tubules and collecting duct cells water-permeable. The absence of vasopressin in diabetes insipidus allows the filtered water to be excreted in the urine instead of being reabsorbed.

Nephrogenic diabetes insipidus involves a defect in the parts of the kidneys that reabsorb water back into the bloodstream. It occurs less commonly than central diabetes insipidus. Nephrogenic diabetes insipidus may occur as an inherited disorder in which male children receive the abnormal gene that causes the disease on the X chromosome from their mothers. Nephrogenic diabetes insipidus may also be caused by diseases of the kidney (such as polycystic kidney disease) and the effects of certain drugs (such as lithium and amphotericin B). Diabetes insipidus is rare, affecting 1 in 25,000 people. Males and females are affected equally.

Signs and symptoms

The patient's history typically shows an abrupt onset of extreme polyuria (usually 4 to 16 L/day of dilute urine but sometimes as much as 30 L/day). As a result, the patient is extremely thirsty and drinks great quantities of water to compensate for the body's water loss. This disorder may also result in nocturia. In severe cases, it may lead to extreme fatigue from inadequate rest caused by frequent voiding and excessive thirst.

Other characteristic features of diabetes insipidus include signs and symptoms of dehydration (poor tissue turgor, dry mucous membranes, constipation, muscle weakness, dizziness, and hypotension). These symptoms usually begin abruptly, commonly appearing within 1 to 2 days after a basal skull fracture, a stroke, or surgery. Relieving cerebral edema or increased intracranial pressure may cause all of these symptoms to subside just as rapidly as they began.

Diagnosis

Urinalysis reveals almost colorless urine of low osmolality (50 to 200 mOsm/kg, less than that of plasma) and low specific gravity (less than 1.005).

 CONFIRMING DIAGNOSIS
Diagnosis requires evidence of vasopressin deficiency, resulting in the kidneys' inability to concentrate urine during a water deprivation test.

In this test, after baseline vital signs, weight, and urine and plasma osmolalities are obtained, the patient is deprived of fluids and observed to make sure he doesn't drink anything surreptitiously. Hourly measurements then record the total volume of urine output, body weight, urine osmolality or specific gravity, and plasma osmolality. Throughout the test, blood pressure and pulse rate must be monitored for signs of orthostatic hypotension. Fluid deprivation continues until the patient loses 3% of his body weight (indicating severe dehydration). When urine osmolality stops increasing in three consecutive hourly specimens, patients receive 5 units of aqueous vasopressin subcutaneously (S.C.).

Hourly measurements of urine volume and specific gravity continue after S.C. injection of aqueous vasopressin. Patients with pituitary diabetes insipidus respond to exogenous vasopressin with decreased urine output and increased specific gravity. Patients with nephrogenic diabetes insipidus show no response to vasopressin.

Treatment

Mild cases require no treatment other than fluid intake to replace fluid lost. Until the cause of more severe cases of diabetes insipidus can be identified and eliminated, administration of various forms of vasopressin or of a vasopressin stimulant can control fluid balance and prevent dehydration. Vasopressin injection is an aqueous preparation that's administered S.C. or I.M. several times a day because it's effective for only 2 to 6 hours; this form of the drug is used in acute disease and as a diagnostic agent.

Desmopressin acetate can be given by nasal spray that's absorbed through the mucous membranes, or by injection given S.C. or I.V.; this drug is effective for 8 to 20 hours, depending on the dosage. It's also available in tablet form, to be given at bedtime or in divided doses. Hydrochlorothiazide can be used in both central and nephrogenic diabetes insipidus. Indomethacin and amiloride are also used for nephrogenic diabetes insipidus. If nephrogenic diabetes insipidus is caused by medication (such as lithium), stopping the medicine leads to kidney recovery.

Special considerations

Patient care includes monitoring symptoms to ensure that fluid balance is restored and maintained.
■ Record fluid intake and output carefully. Maintain fluid intake that's adequate to prevent severe dehydration. Watch for signs

of hypovolemic shock, and monitor blood pressure and heart and respiratory rates regularly, especially during the water deprivation test. Check the patient's weight daily.

- If the patient is dizzy or has muscle weakness, keep the side rails up and assist him with walking.
- Monitor urine specific gravity between doses. Watch for a decrease in specific gravity accompanied by increasing urine output, indicating the recurrence of polyuria and necessitating administration of the next dose of medication or a dosage increase.
- Institute safety precautions for the patient who's dizzy or who has muscle weakness.
- If constipation develops, add more high-fiber foods and fruit juices to the patient's diet. If necessary, obtain an order for a mild laxative such as milk of magnesia.
- Provide meticulous skin and mouth care; apply petroleum jelly, as needed, to cracked or sore lips.
- Before discharge, teach the patient how to monitor intake and output.
- Instruct the patient to administer desmopressin by nasal spray only after the onset of polyuria — not before — to prevent excess fluid retention and water intoxication.
- Tell the patient to report weight gain, which may indicate that his medication dosage is too high. Recurrence of polyuria, as reflected on the intake and output sheet, indicates that the dosage is too low.
- Teach the parents of a child with diabetes insipidus about normal growth and development. Discuss how their child may differ from others at his developmental stage.
- Encourage the parents to help identify the child's strengths and to use them in developing coping strategies.
- Refer the family for counseling if necessary.
- Advise the patient with diabetes insipidus to wear a medical identification bracelet and to carry his medication with him at all times.

THYROID GLAND
Hypothyroidism in adults

Hypothyroidism, a state of low serum thyroid hormone, results from hypothalamic, pituitary, or thyroid insufficiency. The disorder can progress to life-threatening myxedema coma.

Causes and incidence

Hypothyroidism results from inadequate production of thyroid hormone — usually because of dysfunction of the thyroid gland due to surgery (thyroidectomy), irradiation therapy (particularly with ^{131}I), inflammation, chronic autoimmune thyroiditis (Hashimoto's disease) or, rarely, conditions such as amyloidosis and sarcoidosis. It may also result from pituitary failure to produce thyroid-stimulating hormone (TSH), hypothalamic failure to produce thyrotropin-releasing hormone, inborn errors of thyroid hormone synthesis, the inability to synthesize thyroid hormone because of iodine deficiency (usually dietary), or the use of antithyroid medications such as propylthiouracil. In patients with hypothyroidism, infection, exposure to cold, and sedatives may precipitate myxedema coma.

Hypothyroidism is more prevalent in females than males, and frequency increases with age; in the United States, incidence is rising significantly in people ages 40 to 50.

Signs and symptoms

Typically, the early clinical features of hypothyroidism are vague: fatigue, menstrual changes, hypercholesterolemia, forgetfulness, sensitivity to cold, unexplained weight gain, and constipation. As the disorder progresses, characteristic myxedematous signs and symptoms appear: decreasing mental stability; dry, flaky, inelastic skin; puffy face, hands, and feet; hoarseness; periorbital edema; upper eyelid droop; dry, sparse hair; and thick, brittle nails. (See *Facial signs of myxedema*.)

Cardiovascular involvement leads to decreased cardiac output, slow pulse rate, signs of poor peripheral circulation and, occasionally, an enlarged heart. Other common effects include anorexia, abdominal distention, menorrhagia, decreased libido, infertility, ataxia, intention tremor, and nystagmus. Reflexes show delayed relaxation time (especially in the Achilles tendon).

 ALERT *Progression to myxedema coma is usually gradual but when stress (such as hip fracture, infection, or myocardial infarction) aggravates severe or prolonged hypothyroidism, coma may develop abruptly. Clinical effects include progressive stupor, hypoventilation, hypoglycemia, hyponatremia, hypotension, and hypothermia.*

Diagnosis

CONFIRMING DIAGNOSIS *Radioimmunoassay confirms hypothyroidism with low triiodothyronine (T_3) and thyroxine (T_4) levels.* Supportive laboratory findings include:
- increased TSH level when hypothyroidism is due to thyroid insufficiency; decreased TSH level when hypothyroidism is due to hypothalamic or pituitary insufficiency
- elevated levels of serum cholesterol, alkaline phosphatase, and triglycerides
- normocytic normochromic anemia.

In myxedema coma, laboratory tests may also show low serum sodium levels, and decreased pH and increased partial pressure of carbon dioxide, indicating respiratory acidosis.

Treatment

Therapy for hypothyroidism consists of gradual thyroid replacement with levothyroxine (for low T_4 levels) and, occasionally, liothyronine (for inadequate T_3 levels).

During myxedema coma, effective treatment supports vital functions while restoring euthyroidism. To support blood pressure and pulse rate, treatment includes I.V. administration of levothyroxine and hydrocortisone to correct possible pituitary or adrenal insufficiency. Hypoventilation requires oxygenation and respiratory support. Other supportive measures include fluid replacement and antibiotics for infection.

FACIAL SIGNS OF MYXEDEMA

Characteristic myxedematous signs in adults include dry, flaky, inelastic skin; puffy face; and upper eyelid droop.

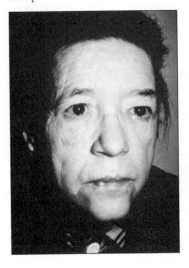

Special considerations

To manage the hypothyroid patient:
- Provide a high-bulk, low-calorie diet and encourage activity to combat constipation and promote weight loss. Administer cathartics and stool softeners, as needed.
- After thyroid replacement therapy begins, watch for symptoms of hyperthyroidism, such as restlessness, sweating, and excessive weight loss.
- Tell the patient to report any signs of aggravated cardiovascular disease, such as chest pain and tachycardia.
- To prevent myxedema coma, tell the patient to continue his course of thyroid medication even if his symptoms subside.
- Warn the patient to report infection immediately and to make sure any physician who prescribes drugs for him knows about the underlying hypothyroidism.

Treatment of myxedema coma requires supportive care:

- Check frequently for signs of decreasing cardiac output such as falling urine output.
- Monitor temperature until stable. Provide extra blankets and clothing and a warm room to compensate for hypothermia. Rapid rewarming may cause vasodilation and vascular collapse.
- Record intake and output and daily weight. As treatment begins, urine output should increase and body weight decrease; if not, report this immediately.
- Turn the edematous bedridden patient every 2 hours, and provide skin care, particularly around bony prominences.
- Avoid sedation when possible or reduce dosage because hypothyroidism delays metabolism of many drugs.
- Maintain a patent I.V. line. Monitor serum electrolyte levels carefully when administering I.V. fluids.

ALERT *Monitor vital signs carefully when administering levothyroxine because rapid correction of hypothyroidism can cause adverse cardiac effects. Report chest pain or tachycardia immediately. Watch for hypertension and heart failure in the elderly patient.*

- Check arterial blood gas values for hypercapnia and hypoxia to determine whether the patient who's severely myxedematous requires ventilatory assistance.
- Because myxedema coma may have been precipitated by an infection, check possible sources of infection, such as blood or urine, and obtain sputum cultures.

Hypothyroidism in children

Deficiency of thyroid hormone secretion during fetal development or early infancy results in infantile cretinism (congenital hypothyroidism). Untreated hypothyroidism is characterized in infants by respiratory difficulties, persistent jaundice, and hoarse crying; in older children, by stunted growth (dwarfism), bone and muscle dystrophy, and mental deficiency.

Cretinism is three times more common in females than in males. Early diagnosis and treatment allow the best prognosis; infants treated before age 3 months usually grow and develop normally. However,

athyroid children who remain untreated beyond age 3 months and children with acquired hypothyroidism who remain untreated beyond age 2 suffer irreversible mental retardation; their skeletal abnormalities are reversible with treatment.

Causes

In infants, cretinism usually results from defective embryonic development that causes congenital absence or underdevelopment of the thyroid gland. The next most common cause can be traced to an inherited enzymatic defect in the synthesis of thyroxine (T_4) caused by an autosomal recessive gene. Less frequently, antithyroid drugs taken during pregnancy produce cretinism in infants. In children older than age 2, cretinism usually results from chronic autoimmune thyroiditis.

Signs and symptoms

The weight and length of an infant with infantile cretinism appear normal at birth, but characteristic signs of hypothyroidism develop by the time he's 3 to 6 months old. In a breast-fed infant the onset of most symptoms may be delayed until weaning because breast milk contains small amounts of thyroid hormone.

Typically, an infant with cretinism sleeps excessively, seldom cries (except for occasional hoarse crying), and is inactive. Because of this, his parents may describe him as a "good baby—no trouble at all." However, such behavior actually results from lowered metabolism and progressive mental impairment. The infant with cretinism also exhibits abnormal deep tendon reflexes, hypotonic abdominal muscles, a protruding abdomen, and slow, awkward movements. He has feeding difficulties, develops constipation and, because his immature liver can't conjugate bilirubin, becomes jaundiced.

His large, protruding tongue obstructs respiration, making breathing loud and noisy and forcing him to open his mouth to breathe. He may have dyspnea on exertion, anemia, abnormal facial features—such as a short forehead; puffy, wide-set eyes (periorbital edema); wrinkled eyelids; and a broad, short, upturned nose—and a dull expression, resulting from mental retardation. His skin is cold and mottled because of poor circulation, and his hair is dry, brittle, and dull. Teeth erupt late and tend to decay early; body temperature is below normal; and pulse rate is slow.

In the child who acquires hypothyroidism after age 2, appropriate treatment can prevent mental retardation. However, growth retardation becomes apparent in short stature (due to delayed epiphyseal maturation, particularly in the legs), obesity, and a head that appears abnormally large because the arms and legs are stunted. An older child may show delayed or accelerated sexual development.

Diagnosis

A high serum level of thyroid-stimulating hormone (TSH), associated with low triiodothyronine and T_4 levels, points to cretinism. Because early detection and treatment can minimize the effects of cretinism, many states require measurement of infant thyroid hormone levels at birth.

Thyroid scan and radioactive iodine uptake tests show decreased uptake levels and confirm the absence of thyroid tissue in athyroid children. Increased gonadotropin levels are compatible with sexual precocity in older children and may coexist with hypothyroidism. Electrocardiogram shows bradycardia and flat or inverted T waves in untreated infants. Hip, knee, and thigh X-rays reveal absence of the femoral or tibial epiphyseal line and delayed skeletal development that's markedly inappropriate for the child's chronological age. A low T_4 level associated with a normal TSH level suggests hypothyroidism secondary to hypothalamic or pituitary disease, a rare condition.

Treatment

Early detection is mandatory to prevent irreversible mental retardation and permit normal physical development. Treatment of infants younger than age 1 consists of replacement therapy with oral levothyroxine, beginning with moderate doses. Dosage gradually increases to levels sufficient for lifelong maintenance. (Rapid increase in dosage may precipitate thyrotoxicity.) Doses are proportionately higher in children than in adults because children metabolize thyroid hormone more quickly. Therapy in older children includes levothyroxine.

Special considerations

Prevention, early detection, comprehensive parent teaching, and psychological support are essential. Know the early signs. Be especially wary if parents emphasize how good and how quiet their new baby is.

■ During early management of infantile cretinism, monitor blood pressure and pulse rate; report hypertension and tachycardia immediately. But remember — normal infant heart rate is approximately 120 beats per minute. If the infant's tongue is unusually large, position him on his side and observe him frequently to prevent airway obstruction. Check rectal temperature every 2 to 4 hours. Keep the infant warm and his skin moist.

■ Inform parents that the child will require lifelong treatment with thyroid supplements. Teach them to recognize signs of overdose: rapid pulse rate, irritability, insomnia, fever, sweating, and weight loss. Stress the need to comply with the treatment regimen to prevent further mental impairment.

■ Provide support to help parents deal with a child who may be mentally retarded. Help them adopt a positive but realistic attitude and focus on their child's strengths rather than his weaknesses. Encourage them to provide stimulating activities to help the child reach his maximum potential. Refer them to the appropriate community resources for support.

■ To prevent infantile cretinism, emphasize the importance of adequate nutrition during pregnancy, including iodine-rich foods and the use of iodized salt or, in case of sodium restriction, an iodine supplement.

Thyroiditis

Inflammation of the thyroid gland occurs as autoimmune thyroiditis (long-term inflammatory disease), subacute granulomatous thyroiditis (self-limiting inflammation), Riedel's thyroiditis (rare, invasive fibrotic process), and miscellaneous thyroiditis (acute suppurative, chronic infective, and chronic noninfective).

Causes and incidence

Autoimmune thyroiditis is due to antibodies to thyroid antigens in the blood. It may cause inflammation and lymphocytic infiltration (Hashimoto's thyroiditis). Glandular atrophy (myxedema) and Graves' disease are linked to autoimmune thyroiditis.

Subacute granulomatous thyroiditis usually follows mumps, influenza, coxsackievirus, or adenovirus infection. Riedel's thyroiditis is a rare condition of unknown etiology.

Miscellaneous thyroiditis results from bacterial invasion of the gland in acute suppurative thyroiditis; tuberculosis, syphilis, actinomycosis, or other infectious agents in the chronic infective form; and sarcoidosis and amyloidosis in chronic noninfective thyroiditis. Postpartum thyroiditis (silent thyroiditis) is another autoimmune disorder associated with transient thyroiditis in females within 1 year after delivery.

Thyroiditis is most prevalent among people ages 30 to 50 and is more common in females than in males. Incidence is highest in the Appalachian region of the United States.

Signs and symptoms

Autoimmune thyroiditis is usually asymptomatic and commonly occurs in females, with peak incidence in middle age. It's the most prevalent cause of spontaneous hypothyroidism.

In subacute granulomatous thyroiditis, moderate thyroid enlargement may follow an upper respiratory tract infection or a sore throat. The thyroid may be painful and tender, and dysphagia may occur.

In Riedel's thyroiditis, the gland enlarges slowly as it's replaced by hard, fibrous tissues. This fibrosis may compress the trachea or the esophagus. The thyroid feels firm.

Clinical effects of miscellaneous thyroiditis are characteristic of pyogenic infection: fever, pain, tenderness, and reddened skin over the gland.

Diagnosis

Precise diagnosis depends on the type of thyroiditis:

- *Autoimmune:* high titers of thyroglobulin and microsomal antibodies present in serum
- *Subacute granulomatous:* elevated erythrocyte sedimentation rate, increased thyroid hormone levels, decreased thyroidal radioiodine uptake
- *Chronic infective and noninfective:* varied findings, depending on underlying infection or other disease.

Treatment

Appropriate treatment varies with the type of thyroiditis. Drug therapy includes levothyroxine for accompanying hypothyroidism, analgesics and anti-inflammatory drugs for mild subacute granulomatous thyroiditis, propranolol for transient hyperthyroidism, and steroids for severe episodes of acute inflammation. Suppurative thyroiditis requires antibiotic therapy. A partial thyroidectomy may be necessary to relieve tracheal or esophageal compression in Riedel's thyroiditis.

Special considerations

Before treatment, obtain a patient history to identify underlying diseases that may cause thyroiditis, such as tuberculosis or a recent viral infection.

- Check the patient's vital signs, and examine her neck for unusual swelling, enlargement, or redness. Provide a liquid diet if she has difficulty swallowing, especially when due to fibrosis. If the neck is swollen, measure and record the circumference daily to monitor progressive enlargement.
- Administer antibiotics as ordered, and report and record elevations in temperature.
- Instruct the patient to watch for and report signs of hypothyroidism (lethargy, restlessness, sensitivity to cold, forgetfulness, and dry skin), especially if she has Hashimoto's thyroiditis, which often causes hypothyroidism.
- Check for signs of hyperthyroidism (nervousness, tachycardia, tremor, and weakness), which commonly occurs in subacute thyroiditis.

- After thyroidectomy, check vital signs every 15 to 30 minutes until the patient's condition stabilizes. Stay alert for signs of tetany secondary to accidental parathyroid injury during surgery. Keep 10% calcium gluconate available for I.V. use if needed. Assess dressings frequently for excessive bleeding. Watch for signs of airway obstruction, such as difficulty in talking or increased swallowing; keep tracheotomy equipment handy.
- Explain to the patient that she'll need lifelong thyroid hormone replacement therapy if hypothyroidism occurs. Tell her to watch for signs of overdosage, such as nervousness and palpitations.

Simple goiter

Simple (or nontoxic) goiter is a thyroid gland enlargement that isn't caused by inflammation or a neoplasm, and is commonly classified as endemic or sporadic. Endemic goiter usually results from inadequate dietary intake of iodine associated with such factors as iodine-depleted soil or malnutrition. Sporadic goiter follows ingestion of certain drugs or foods.

Simple goiter affects more females than males, especially during adolescence, pregnancy, and menopause, when the body's demand for thyroid hormone increases. Sporadic goiter affects no particular population segment. With appropriate treatment, the prognosis is good for either type of goiter.

Causes and incidence

Simple goiter occurs when the thyroid gland can't secrete enough thyroid hormone to meet metabolic requirements. As a result, the thyroid gland enlarges to compensate for inadequate hormone synthesis, a compensation that usually overcomes mild to moderate hormonal impairment. Because thyroid-stimulating hormone (TSH) levels are generally within normal limits in patients with simple goiter, goitrogenicity probably results from impaired intrathyroidal hormone synthesis and depletion of glandular iodine, which increases the thyroid gland's sensitivity to TSH.

However, increased levels of TSH may be transient and therefore missed.

Endemic goiter usually results from inadequate dietary intake of iodine, which leads to inadequate secretion of thyroid hormone. Since the introduction of iodized salt in the United States, cases of endemic goiter have virtually disappeared.

Sporadic goiter commonly results from the ingestion of large amounts of goitrogenic foods or the use of goitrogenic drugs. Goitrogenic foods, such as rutabagas, cabbage, soybeans, peanuts, peaches, peas, strawberries, spinach, and radishes, contain agents that decrease thyroxine (T_4) production. Goitrogenic drugs include propylthiouracil, iodides, phenylbutazone, para-aminosalicylic acid, cobalt, and lithium. In a pregnant woman, these substances may cross the placenta and affect the fetus.

Inherited defects may be responsible for insufficient T_4 synthesis or impaired iodine metabolism. Because families tend to congregate in a single geographic area, this familial factor may contribute to the incidence of both endemic and sporadic goiters.

Females are more commonly affected than males. Incidence increases after age 40.

Signs and symptoms

Thyroid enlargement may range from a mildly enlarged gland to a massive, multinodular goiter. (See *Massive goiter,* page 840.) Because simple goiter doesn't alter the patient's metabolic state, clinical features arise solely from enlargement of the thyroid gland. The patient may complain of respiratory distress and dysphagia from compression of the trachea and esophagus, and swelling and distention of the neck. In addition, large goiters may obstruct venous return, produce venous engorgement and, in rare cases, induce development of collateral venous circulation in the chest. Obstruction may cause dizziness or syncope (Pemberton's sign) when the patient raises her arms above her head.

Diagnosis

Diagnosis of simple goiter requires a thorough patient history and physical examination to rule out disorders with similar clin-

MASSIVE GOITER

Massive multinodular goiter causes gross distention and swelling of the neck.

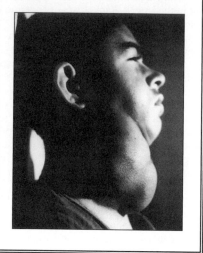

ical effects, such as Graves' disease, Hashimoto's thyroiditis, and thyroid carcinoma. A detailed patient history may also reveal goitrogenic medications or foods or endemic influence. The results of diagnostic laboratory tests include the following:
- TSH: high or normal levels
- Serum T_4 concentrations: low normal or normal
- Thyroid scan and uptake: normal or increased (50% of the dose at 24 hours)
- Ultrasound of thyroid: nodules may be present, necessitating biopsy for further evaluation.

Treatment
The goal of treatment is to reduce thyroid hyperplasia. Exogenous thyroid hormone replacement with levothyroxine is the treatment of choice; it inhibits TSH secretion and allows the gland to rest. Small doses of iodide (Lugol's or potassium iodide solution) commonly relieve goiter that's due to iodine deficiency. Sporadic goiter requires avoidance of known goitrogenic drugs and foods. A large goiter that's unresponsive to treatment may require subtotal thyroidectomy.

Special considerations
Patient care includes measuring the patient's neck circumference daily to check for progressive thyroid gland enlargement, and checking for the development of hard nodules in the gland, which may indicate carcinoma.
- To maintain constant hormone levels, instruct the patient to take the prescribed thyroid hormone preparations at the same time each day. Advise her to avoid taking the medicine at the same time as any calcium or iron-containing supplements (including prenatal vitamins), or with Metamucil, grapefruit, or grapefruit juice. Teach the patient and her family to identify and immediately report signs of thyrotoxicosis, including increased pulse rate, palpitations, diarrhea, sweating, tremors, agitation, and shortness of breath.
- Instruct the patient with endemic goiter to use iodized salt to supply the daily 150 to 300 mcg of iodine necessary to prevent goiter.
- Monitor the patient taking goitrogenic drugs for signs of sporadic goiter.

Hyperthyroidism

Hyperthyroidism (also known as *Graves' disease, Basedow's disease,* or *thyrotoxicosis*) is a metabolic imbalance that results from thyroid hormone overproduction. The most common form of hyperthyroidism is Graves' disease, which increases thyroxine (T_4) production, enlarges the thyroid gland (goiter), and causes multiple system changes.

With treatment, most patients can lead normal lives. However, *thyroid storm* — an acute exacerbation of hyperthyroidism — is a medical emergency that may lead to life-threatening cardiac, hepatic, or renal failure.

Causes and incidence
Hyperthyroidism may result from both genetic and immunologic factors. An increased incidence of this disorder in monozygotic twins, for example, points to an in-

herited factor, probably an autosomal recessive gene. This disease occasionally coexists with abnormal iodine metabolism and other endocrine abnormalities, such as diabetes mellitus, hyperparathyroidism, and thyroiditis. Hyperthyroidism is also associated with autoantibody production (thyroid-stimulating immunoglobulin and thyroid-stimulating hormone [TSH]-binding inhibitory immunoglobulin), possibly due to a defect in suppressor–T-lymphocyte function that allows the formation of autoantibodies.

In latent hyperthyroidism, excessive dietary intake of iodine and, possibly, stress can precipitate clinical hyperthyroidism. In a person with inadequately treated hyperthyroidism, stress — including surgery, infection, toxemia of pregnancy, and diabetic ketoacidosis — can precipitate thyroid storm. (See *Other forms of hyperthyroidism.*)

Incidence of Graves' disease is highest between ages 30 and 40, especially in people with family histories of thyroid abnormalities; only 5% of hyperthyroid patients are younger than age 15.

Signs and symptoms

The classic features of hyperthyroidism are an enlarged thyroid (goiter), nervousness, heat intolerance, weight loss despite increased appetite, sweating, diarrhea, tremor, and palpitations. Exophthalmos is considered most characteristic but is absent in many patients with hyperthyroidism. Many other symptoms are common because hyperthyroidism profoundly affects virtually every body system:

■ *Central nervous system:* difficulty in concentrating because increased T_4 secretion accelerates cerebral function; excitability or nervousness due to increased basal metabolic rate; fine tremor, shaky handwriting, and clumsiness from increased activity in the spinal cord area that controls muscle tone; emotional instability and mood swings, ranging from occasional outbursts to overt psychosis

■ *Skin, hair, and nails:* smooth, warm, flushed skin (patient sleeps with minimal covers and little clothing); fine, soft hair; premature graying and increased hair loss in both sexes; friable nails and onycholysis

OTHER FORMS OF HYPERTHYROIDISM

■ *Toxic adenoma* — a small, benign nodule in the thyroid gland that secretes thyroid hormone — is the second most common cause of hyperthyroidism. The cause of toxic adenoma is unknown; incidence is highest in the elderly. Clinical effects are essentially similar to those of Graves' disease, except that toxic adenoma doesn't induce ophthalmopathy, pretibial myxedema, or acropachy. Presence of adenoma is confirmed by radioactive iodine (^{131}I) uptake and thyroid scan, which show a single hyperfunctioning nodule suppressing the rest of the gland. Treatment includes ^{131}I therapy, or surgery to remove adenoma after antithyroid drugs achieve a euthyroid state.

■ *Thyrotoxicosis factitia* results from chronic ingestion of thyroid hormone for thyrotropin suppression in patients with thyroid carcinoma, or from thyroid hormone abuse by people who are trying to lose weight.

■ *Functioning metastatic thyroid carcinoma* is a rare disease that causes excess production of thyroid hormone.

■ *Thyroid-stimulating hormone–secreting pituitary tumor* causes overproduction of thyroid hormone.

■ *Subacute thyroiditis* is a virus-induced granulomatous inflammation of the thyroid, producing transient hyperthyroidism associated with fever, pain, pharyngitis, and tenderness in the thyroid gland.

■ *Silent thyroiditis* is a self-limiting, transient form of hyperthyroidism, with histologic thyroiditis but no inflammatory symptoms.

(distal nail separated from the bed); pretibial myxedema (dermopathy), producing thickened skin, accentuated hair follicles, raised red patches of skin that are itchy and sometimes painful, with occasional nodule formation (Microscopic examination shows increased mucin deposits.)

■ *Cardiovascular system:* tachycardia; full, bounding pulse; wide pulse pressure; cardiomegaly; increased cardiac output and blood volume; visible point of maximal impulse; paroxysmal supraventricular tachycardia and atrial fibrillation (especially in the elderly); and occasionally, systolic murmur at the left sternal border

■ *Respiratory system:* dyspnea on exertion and at rest, possibly from cardiac decompensation and increased cellular oxygen utilization

■ *GI system:* possible anorexia; nausea and vomiting due to increased GI mobility and peristalsis; increased defecation; soft stools or, with severe disease, diarrhea; and liver enlargement

■ *Musculoskeletal system:* weakness, fatigue, and muscle atrophy; rare coexistence with myasthenia gravis; generalized or localized paralysis associated with hypokalemia may occur; and occasional acropachy — soft-tissue swelling, accompanied by underlying bone changes where new bone formation occurs

■ *Reproductive system:* in females, oligomenorrhea or amenorrhea, decreased fertility, higher incidence of spontaneous abortions; in males, gynecomastia due to increased estrogen levels; in both sexes, diminished libido

■ *Eyes:* exophthalmos (from the combined effects of accumulation of mucopolysaccharides and fluids in the retro-orbital tissues that force the eyeball outward, and of lid retraction that produces the characteristic staring gaze); occasional inflammation of conjunctivae, corneas, or eye muscles; diplopia; and increased tearing.

ALERT *When hyperthyroidism escalates to thyroid storm, these symptoms can be accompanied by extreme irritability, hypertension, tachycardia, vomiting, temperature up to 106° F (41.1° C), delirium, and coma.*

Diagnosis

The diagnosis of hyperthyroidism is usually straightforward and depends on a careful clinical history and physical examination, a high index of suspicion, and routine hormone determinations.

 CONFIRMING DIAGNOSIS *The following tests confirm the disorder:*
■ *Radioimmunoassay shows increased serum T_4 and triiodothyronine (T_3) concentrations.*

■ *Thyroid scan reveals increased uptake of radioactive iodine (^{131}I). This test is contraindicated if the patient is pregnant.*

■ *TSH levels are decreased.*

■ *Ultrasonography confirms subclinical ophthalmopathy.*

■ *Antithyroglobulin antibody is positive in Grave's disease.*

Treatment

A number of approaches are used to treat hyperthyroidism, primarily antithyroid drugs, ^{131}I, and surgery. Appropriate treatment depends on the size of the goiter, the causes, the patient's age and parity, and how long surgery will be delayed (if the patient is an appropriate candidate for surgery).

Antithyroid drug therapy is used for children, young adults, pregnant females, and patients who refuse surgery or ^{131}I treatment. Thyroid hormone antagonists are given to block thyroid hormone synthesis. Although hypermetabolic symptoms subside within 4 to 8 weeks after such therapy begins, the patient must continue the medication for 6 months to 2 years, depending on the clinical circumstances. Beta-adrenergic blockers may be given concomitantly to manage tachycardia and other peripheral effects of excessive hypersympathetic activity.

During pregnancy, antithyroid medication should be kept at the minimum dosage required to keep maternal thyroid function within the high-normal range until delivery and to minimize the risk of fetal hypothyroidism — even though most infants of hyperthyroid mothers are born with mild and transient hyperthyroidism. (Neonatal hyperthyroidism may even necessitate treatment with antithyroid medications and propranolol for 2 to 3 months.) Because hyperthyroidism is sometimes exacerbated in the puerperal period, continuous control of maternal thyroid function is essential. Approximately 3 to 6 months postpartum, antithyroid drug administration can be gradually tapered and thyroid function reassessed. The mother receiving low-dose antithyroid treatment may breast-feed as long as the infant's thyroid function is checked periodically. Small amounts of the drug can be found in breast milk.

A single oral dose of ^{131}I is the treatment of choice for patients not planning to have children. (Patients of reproductive age must not be pregnant and should give informed consent for this treatment because small amounts of ^{131}I concentrate in the gonads. However, there have been no reports of damage to subsequently conceived children in more than 50 years of ^{131}I use.) During treatment with ^{131}I, the thyroid gland picks up the radioactive element as it would regular iodine. Subsequently, the radioactivity destroys some of the cells that normally concentrate iodine and produce T_4, thus decreasing thyroid hormone production and normalizing thyroid size and function. In most patients, hypermetabolic symptoms diminish from 6 to 8 weeks after such treatment. However, some patients may require a second dose.

Subtotal (partial) thyroidectomy, which decreases the thyroid gland's capacity for hormone production, is indicated for patients with a large goiter whose hyperthyroidism has repeatedly relapsed after drug therapy or patients who refuse or aren't candidates for ^{131}I treatment. Preoperatively, the patient may receive iodides (Lugol's solution or saturated solution of potassium iodide), antithyroid drugs, or high doses of propranolol, to help prevent thyroid storm. If euthyroidism isn't achieved, surgery should be delayed and propranolol administered to decrease the systemic effects (cardiac arrhythmias) caused by hyperthyroidism. After ablative treatment with ^{131}I or surgery, patients require regular medical supervision for the rest of their lives because they usually develop hypothyroidism, sometimes as long as several years after treatment.

Therapy for hyperthyroid ophthalmopathy includes local applications of topical medications but may require high doses of corticosteroids. A patient with severe exophthalmos that causes pressure on the optic nerve may require external beam radiation therapy or surgical decompression to lessen pressure on the orbital contents.

Treatment of thyroid storm includes administration of an antithyroid drug, propranolol I.V. to block sympathetic effects, a corticosteroid to inhibit the conversion of T_4 to T_3 and to replace depleted cortisol levels, and an iodide to block the release of thyroid hormone. Supportive measures include administration of nutrients, vitamins, fluids, and sedatives.

Special considerations

Patients with hyperthyroidism require vigilant care to prevent acute exacerbations and complications.

- Record vital signs and weight.
- Monitor serum electrolyte levels, and check periodically for hyperglycemia and glycosuria.
- Carefully monitor cardiac function if the patient is elderly or has coronary artery disease. If the heart rate is more than 100 beats/minute, check blood pressure and pulse rate often.
- Check level of consciousness and urine output.

 ALERT *If the patient is pregnant, tell her to watch closely during the first trimester for signs of spontaneous abortion and to report such signs immediately.*

- Encourage bed rest, and keep the patient's room cool, quiet, and dark. The patient with dyspnea will be most comfortable sitting upright or in high Fowler's position.
- Remember, extreme nervousness may produce bizarre behavior. Reassure the patient and his family that such behavior will probably subside with treatment. Provide sedatives as necessary.
- To promote weight gain, provide a balanced diet, with six meals a day. If the patient has edema, suggest a low-sodium diet.
- If iodide is part of the treatment, mix it with milk, juice, or water to prevent GI dis-

tress, and administer it through a straw to prevent tooth discoloration.

 ALERT *Watch for signs of thyroid storm, such as tachycardia, hyperkinesis, fever, vomiting, and hypertension.*

■ Check intake and output carefully to ensure adequate hydration and fluid balance.
■ Closely monitor blood pressure, cardiac rate and rhythm, and temperature. If the patient has a high fever, reduce it with appropriate hypothermic measures. Maintain an I.V. line and give drugs, as ordered.
■ If the patient has exophthalmos or other ophthalmopathy, suggest sunglasses or eye patches to protect his eyes from light. Moisten the conjunctivae often with isotonic eye drops. Warn the patient with severe lid retraction to avoid sudden physical movements that might cause the lid to slip behind the eyeball. He should avoid cigarette smoke.
■ Avoid excessive palpation of the thyroid to avoid precipitating thyroid storm.

Thyroidectomy necessitates meticulous postoperative care to prevent complications:
■ Watch for evidence of hemorrhage into the neck, such as a tight dressing with no blood on it. Change dressings and perform wound care, as ordered; check the *back* of the dressing for drainage. Keep the patient in semi-Fowler's position, and support his head and neck with sandbags to ease tension on the incision.
■ Check for dysphagia or hoarseness from possible laryngeal nerve injury.
■ Watch for signs of hypoparathyroidism (tetany, numbness), a complication that results from accidental removal of the parathyroid glands during surgery.
■ Stress the importance of regular medical follow-up after discharge because hypothyroidism may develop from 2 to 4 weeks postoperatively.

 ALERT *Check often for respiratory distress, and keep a tracheotomy tray at bedside.*

Drug therapy and ^{131}I therapy require careful monitoring and comprehensive patient teaching:
■ After ^{131}I therapy, tell the patient not to expectorate or cough freely because his saliva will be radioactive for 24 hours.

Stress the need for repeated measurement of serum T_4 levels.
■ If the patient is taking propylthiouracil and methimazole, monitor complete blood count periodically to detect leukopenia, thrombocytopenia, and agranulocytosis. Instruct him to take these medications with meals to minimize GI distress and to avoid over-the-counter cough preparations because many contain iodine.
■ Tell him to report fever, enlarged cervical lymph nodes, sore throat, mouth sores, and other signs of blood dyscrasias and any rash or skin eruptions — signs of hypersensitivity.
■ Watch the patient taking propranolol for signs of hypotension (dizziness, decreased urine output). Tell him to rise slowly after sitting or lying down to prevent orthostatic syncope.
■ Instruct the patient receiving antithyroid drugs or ^{131}I therapy to report any symptoms of hypothyroidism.

PARATHYROID GLANDS

Hypoparathyroidism

Hypoparathyroidism is a deficiency of parathyroid hormone (PTH) caused by disease, injury (usually surgical), or congenital malfunction of the parathyroid glands. Because the parathyroid glands primarily regulate calcium balance, hypoparathyroidism causes hypocalcemia, producing neuromuscular symptoms ranging from paresthesia to tetany. The clinical effects of hypoparathyroidism are usually correctable with replacement therapy. However, some complications of this disorder, such as cataracts and basal ganglion calcifications, are irreversible.

Causes and incidence

Hypoparathyroidism may be acute or chronic and is classified as idiopathic or acquired. The acquired form may also be reversible. *Idiopathic hypoparathyroidism* may result from an autoimmune genetic disorder or the congenital absence of the

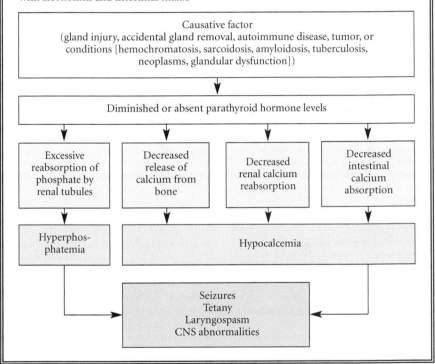

PATHOPHYSIOLOGY
WHAT HAPPENS IN ACUTE HYPOPARATHYROIDISM

Causes of acute hypoparathyroidism include injury to the glands, accidental removal of the parathyroid glands during thyroidectomy or other neck surgery, autoimmune disease, tumor, tuberculosis, sarcoidosis, hemochromatosis, and severe magnesium deficiency associated with alcoholism and intestinal malabsorption. These disorders and conditions cause a cascade of effects that result in severe hypocalcemia and hyperphosphatemia, which can lead to seizures, tetany, laryngospasm, and central nervous system (CNS) abnormalities, as shown in the flow chart below.

Causative factor
(gland injury, accidental gland removal, autoimmune disease, tumor, or conditions [hemochromatosis, sarcoidosis, amyloidosis, tuberculosis, neoplasms, glandular dysfunction])

Diminished or absent parathyroid hormone levels

Excessive reabsorption of phosphate by renal tubules

Decreased release of calcium from bone

Decreased renal calcium reabsorption

Decreased intestinal calcium absorption

Hyperphosphatemia

Hypocalcemia

Seizures
Tetany
Laryngospasm
CNS abnormalities

parathyroid glands. *Acquired hypoparathyroidism* commonly results from accidental removal of or injury to one or more parathyroid glands during thyroidectomy or other neck surgery; rarely it results from massive thyroid irradiation. It may also result from ischemic infarction of the parathyroids during surgery or from hemochromatosis, sarcoidosis, amyloidosis, tuberculosis, neoplasms, or trauma. An *acquired, reversible hypoparathyroidism* may result from hypomagnesemia-induced impairment of hormone synthesis, from suppression of normal gland function due to hypercalcemia, or from delayed maturation of parathyroid function. (See *What happens in acute hypoparathyroidism.*)

PTH isn't regulated by the pituitary or hypothalamus. It normally maintains blood calcium levels by increasing bone resorption and GI absorption of calcium. It also maintains an inverse relationship between serum calcium and phosphate levels by inhibiting phosphate reabsorption in the renal tubules. Abnormal PTH production disrupts this balance. The incidence is

4 out of 100,000 people. Incidence of the idiopathic and reversible forms is highest in children; that of the irreversible acquired form, in older patients who have undergone surgery for hyperthyroidism or other head and neck conditions.

Signs and symptoms

Although mild hypoparathyroidism may be asymptomatic, it usually produces hypocalcemia and high serum phosphate levels that affect the central nervous system (CNS) as well as other body systems. Chronic hypoparathyroidism typically causes neuromuscular irritability, increased deep tendon reflexes, Chvostek's sign (hyperirritability of the facial nerve, producing a characteristic spasm when it's tapped), dysphagia, organic mental syndrome, psychosis, mental deficiency in children, and tetany.

Acute (overt) tetany begins with a tingling in the fingertips, around the mouth and, occasionally, in the feet. This tingling spreads and becomes more severe, producing muscle tension and spasms and consequent adduction of the thumbs, wrists, and elbows. Pain varies with the degree of muscle tension but seldom affects the face, legs, and feet. Chronic tetany is usually unilateral and less severe; it may cause difficulty in walking and a tendency to fall. Both forms of tetany can lead to laryngospasm, stridor and, eventually, cyanosis. They may also cause seizures. These CNS abnormalities tend to be exaggerated during hyperventilation, pregnancy, infection, withdrawal of thyroid hormone, therapy with diuretics, and before menstruation.

Other clinical effects include abdominal pain; dry, lusterless hair; spontaneous hair loss; brittle fingernails that develop ridges or fall out; dry, scaly skin; cataracts; and weakened tooth enamel, which causes teeth to stain, crack, and decay easily. Hypocalcemia may induce cardiac arrhythmias and may eventually lead to heart failure.

Diagnosis

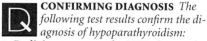 **CONFIRMING DIAGNOSIS** *The following test results confirm the diagnosis of hypoparathyroidism:*
■ *Radioimmunoassay for PTH: decreased PTH concentration*

■ *Serum calcium: decreased*
■ *Serum phosphorus: increased*
■ *Electrocardiogram (ECG): prolonged QT and ST intervals due to hypocalcemia.*

Inflating a blood pressure cuff on the upper arm to between diastolic and systolic blood pressure and maintaining this inflation for 3 minutes elicits Trousseau's sign (carpal spasm), thereby provoking clinical evidence of hypoparathyroidism.

Treatment

Because calcium absorption from the small intestine requires the presence of vitamin D, treatment includes vitamin D and calcium supplements. Therapy is usually lifelong, except for the reversible form of the disease. If the patient can't tolerate the pure form of vitamin D, alternatives include dihydrotachysterol, if hepatic and renal function is adequate, and calcitriol, if it's severely compromised. In patients with preexisting hypomagnesemia, this condition must be corrected to treat the resulting hypocalcemia. A high-calcium, low-phosphorous diet is recommended.

Acute life-threatening tetany requires immediate I.V. administration of calcium to raise serum calcium levels. The patient who's awake and able to cooperate can help raise serum calcium levels by breathing into a paper bag and then inhaling his own carbon dioxide; this produces hypoventilation and mild respiratory acidosis. Sedatives and anticonvulsants may control spasms until calcium levels rise. Chronic tetany requires maintenance therapy with oral calcium and vitamin D supplements.

Special considerations

While awaiting diagnosis of hypoparathyroidism in a patient with a history of tetany, maintain a patent I.V. line and keep I.V. calcium available. Because the patient is vulnerable to seizures, maintain seizure precautions. Also, keep a tracheotomy tray and endotracheal tube at the bedside because laryngospasm may result from hypocalcemia.
■ Instruct the patient to follow a high-calcium, low-phosphorus diet.
■ When caring for the patient with chronic disease, particularly a child, stay alert for minor muscle twitching and for signs of

laryngospasm because these effects may signal the onset of tetany.

■ For the patient on drug therapy, emphasize the importance of checking serum calcium levels at least three times a year. Instruct the patient to watch for signs of hypercalcemia and to keep medications away from light and heat.

■ Dental changes, cataracts, and brain calcifications are permanent. These can be prevented with early detection and periodic calcium determinations.

 ALERT *Because the patient with chronic disease has prolonged QT intervals on ECG, watch for heart block and signs of decreasing cardiac output. Because calcium potentiates the effect of cardiac glycosides, closely monitor the patient receiving both a cardiac glycoside and calcium. Stay alert for signs of digoxin toxicity, such as arrhythmias, nausea, fatigue, vision changes.*

■ Instruct the patient with scaly skin to use creams to soften his skin. Also, tell him to keep his nails trimmed to prevent them from splitting.

■ Hyperventilation or recent blood transfusions may worsen tetany. (Anticoagulant in stored blood binds calcium.)

■ For the patient with tetany, administer 10% calcium gluconate by slow I.V. infusion (1 ml/minute), and maintain a patent airway. The patient may also require intubation and sedation. Monitor vital signs often after administration sedation to make certain that blood pressure and heart rate return to normal.

Hyperparathyroidism

Hyperparathyroidism is characterized by overactivity of one or more of the four parathyroid glands, resulting in excessive secretion of parathyroid hormone (PTH). Hypersecretion of PTH promotes bone resorption and leads to hypercalcemia and hypophosphatemia, which in turn results in increased renal and GI absorption of calcium.

Causes and incidence

Hyperparathyroidism may be primary or secondary. In primary hyperparathy-roidism, one or more of the parathyroid glands enlarges, increasing PTH secretion and elevating serum calcium levels. The most common cause is a single adenoma. Other causes include a genetic disorder or multiple endocrine neoplasia. Primary hyperparathyroidism usually occurs between ages 30 and 50 but can also occur in children and the elderly. It affects two to three times more females than males. It's a common disorder, affecting 1 in 1,000 people.

In secondary hyperparathyroidism, excessive compensatory production of PTH stems from a hypocalcemia-producing abnormality outside the parathyroid gland, which causes a resistance to the metabolic action of PTH. Some hypocalcemia-producing abnormalities are chronic renal failure, renal absorption disorders, vitamin D deficiency (especially in the housebound elderly), or osteomalacia due to phenytoin or laxative abuse.

Signs and symptoms

Clinical effects of primary hyperparathyroidism result from hypercalcemia and are typically present in several body systems:

■ *Renal system:* nephrocalcinosis due to elevated levels of calcium and, possibly, recurring nephrolithiasis, which may lead to renal insufficiency. Renal manifestations, including polyuria, are the most common effects of hyperparathyroidism.

■ *Skeletal and articular system:* chronic low back pain and easy fracturing due to bone degeneration, bone tenderness, chondrocalcinosis, occasional severe osteopenia, especially on the vertebrae, erosions of the juxta-articular surface, subchondral fractures, traumatic synovitis, and pseudogout

■ *GI system:* pancreatitis, causing constant, severe epigastric pain radiating to the back; peptic ulcers, causing abdominal pain, anorexia, nausea, and vomiting

■ *Neuromuscular system:* marked muscle weakness and atrophy, particularly in the legs

■ *Central nervous system:* psychomotor and personality disturbances, depression, overt psychosis, stupor and, possibly, coma

■ *Other:* skin necrosis, cataracts, calcium microthrombi to lungs and pancreas, polyuria, anemia, and subcutaneous calcification.

BONE RESORPTION IN PRIMARY HYPERPARATHYROIDISM

Erosion and demineralization, which occur with hyperparathyroidism, are illustrated at right.

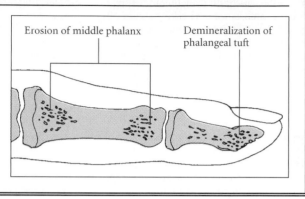

Erosion of middle phalanx

Demineralization of phalangeal tuft

Similarly, in secondary hyperparathyroidism, decreased serum calcium levels may produce the same features of calcium imbalance, with skeletal deformities of the long bones (rickets, for example) as well as symptoms of the underlying disease.

Diagnosis

CONFIRMING DIAGNOSIS *In primary disease, a high concentration of serum PTH on radioimmunoassay with accompanying hypercalcemia confirms the diagnosis.*

In addition, X-rays may show diffuse demineralization of bones, bone cysts, outer cortical bone absorption, and subperiosteal erosion of the phalanges and distal clavicles. (See *Bone resorption in primary hyperparathyroidism.*) Microscopic examination of the bone with tests such as X-ray spectrophotometry typically demonstrates increased bone turnover. Reduced bone mineral density, particularly of the forearm, is seen on bone densitometry.

Laboratory tests reveal elevated urine and serum calcium, chloride, and alkaline phosphatase levels and decreased serum phosphorus levels. Hyperparathyroidism may also raise uric acid and creatinine levels and increase basal acid secretion and serum immunoreactive gastrin. Increased serum amylase levels may indicate acute pancreatitis.

Laboratory findings in secondary hyperparathyroidism show normal or slightly decreased serum calcium levels and variable serum phosphorus levels. Phosphorus can be quite elevated, especially in osteomalacia or renal disease. Patient history may reveal familial renal disease, seizure disorders, or drug ingestion. Other laboratory values and physical examination findings identify the cause of secondary hyperparathyroidism.

Treatment

Treatment varies, depending on the cause of the disease. Treatment of primary hyperparathyroidism may include surgery to remove the adenoma or, depending on the extent of hyperplasia, all but half of one gland (the remaining part of the gland is necessary to maintain normal PTH levels). Surgery may relieve bone pain within 3 days. However, renal damage may be irreversible.

Preoperatively — or if surgery isn't feasible or necessary — other treatments can decrease calcium levels. These include forcing fluids; limiting dietary intake of calcium; promoting sodium and calcium excretion through forced diuresis using normal saline solution (up to 6 L in life-threatening circumstances), furosemide, or ethacrynic acid; and administering oral sodium or potassium phosphate, subcutaneous calcitonin, I.V. plicamycin, or I.V. biphosphonates.

Therapy for potential postoperative magnesium and phosphate deficiencies includes I.V. administration of magnesium and phosphate, or sodium phosphate solution given orally or by retention enema. In addition, during the first 4 to 5 days after surgery, when serum calcium falls to low normal levels, supplemental calcium may be necessary; vitamin D or calcitriol may also be used to raise serum calcium levels.

Treatment of secondary hyperparathyroidism must correct the underlying cause of parathyroid hypertrophy. Vitamin D therapy or, in the patient with renal disease, administration of an oral calcium preparation (calcium acetate, if possible) for hyperphosphatemia, are typically used, although surgical excision may be necessary. In the patient with renal failure, dialysis is necessary to lower calcium levels and may have to continue for the remainder of the patient's life. In the patient with chronic secondary hyperparathyroidism, the enlarged glands may not revert to normal size and function even after calcium levels have been controlled.

Special considerations
Care emphasizes prevention of complications from the underlying disease and its treatment.

■ Obtain pretreatment baseline serum potassium, calcium, phosphate, and magnesium levels because these values may change abruptly during treatment.

■ During hydration to reduce serum calcium level, record intake and output accurately. Strain urine to check for calculi. Provide at least 3 qt (3 L) of fluid a day, including cranberry or prune juice to increase urine acidity and help prevent calculus formation. As ordered, obtain blood and urine samples to measure sodium, potassium, and magnesium levels, especially for the patient taking furosemide.

■ Auscultate for breath sounds often. Listen for signs of pulmonary edema in the patient receiving large amounts of saline solution I.V., especially if he has pulmonary or cardiac disease. Monitor the patient on digitalis glycosides carefully because elevated calcium levels can rapidly produce toxic effects.

■ Because the patient is predisposed to pathologic fractures, take safety precautions to minimize the risk of injury. Assist him with walking, keep the bed at its lowest position, and raise the side rails. Lift the

immobilized patient carefully to minimize bone stress. Schedule care to allow the patient with muscle weakness as much rest as possible.

■ Watch for signs of peptic ulcer and administer antacids, as appropriate.

After parathyroidectomy:

■ Check frequently for respiratory distress, and keep a tracheotomy tray at the bedside. Watch for postoperative complications, such as laryngeal nerve damage or, rarely, hemorrhage. Monitor intake and output carefully.

■ Check for swelling at the operative site. Place the patient in semi-Fowler's position, and support his head and neck with sandbags to decrease edema, which may cause pressure on the trachea.

■ Watch for signs of mild tetany, such as complaints of tingling in the hands and around the mouth. These symptoms should subside quickly but may be prodromal signs of tetany, so keep calcium gluconate or calcium chloride I.V. available for emergency administration. Watch for increased neuromuscular irritability and other signs of severe tetany, and report them immediately. Ambulate the patient as soon as possible postoperatively, even though he may find this uncomfortable, because pressure on bones speeds up bone recalcification.

■ Check laboratory results for low serum calcium and magnesium levels.

■ Monitor mental status and watch for listlessness. In the patient with persistent hypercalcemia, check for muscle weakness and psychiatric symptoms.

■ Before discharge, advise the patient of the possible adverse effects of drug therapy. Emphasize the need for periodic follow-up through laboratory blood tests. If hyperparathyroidism wasn't corrected surgically, warn the patient to avoid calcium-containing antacids and thiazide diuretics.

ADRENAL GLANDS
Adrenal hypofunction
Primary adrenal hypofunction (also called *adrenal insufficiency* or *Addison's disease*)

originates within the adrenal gland itself and is characterized by decreased mineralocorticoid, glucocorticoid, and androgen secretion. Adrenal hypofunction can also occur secondary to a disorder outside the gland (such as pituitary tumor, with corticotropin deficiency), but aldosterone secretion frequently continues intact. A relatively uncommon disorder, adrenal hypofunction can occur at any age and in both sexes. Secondary adrenal hypofunction occurs when a patient abruptly stops taking long-term exogenous steroid therapy. With early diagnosis and adequate replacement therapy, the prognosis for adrenal hypofunction is good.

Adrenal crisis (addisonian crisis), a critical deficiency of mineralocorticoids and glucocorticoids, generally follows acute stress, sepsis, trauma, surgery, or omission of steroid therapy in patients who have chronic adrenal insufficiency. A medical emergency, adrenal crisis necessitates immediate, vigorous treatment.

Causes and incidence
Adrenal hypofunction occurs when more than 90% of both adrenal glands are destroyed, an occurrence that typically results from an autoimmune process in which circulating antibodies react specifically against the adrenal tissue. Other causes include tuberculosis (once the chief cause; now responsible for less than 10% of adult cases), bilateral adrenalectomy, hemorrhage into the adrenal gland, neoplasms, and infections (acquired immunodeficiency syndrome, histoplasmosis, and cytomegalovirus). Rarely, a familial tendency to autoimmune disease predisposes the patient to adrenal hypofunction and other endocrinopathies.

Secondary adrenal hypofunction that results in glucocorticoid deficiency can stem from hypopituitarism (causing decreased corticotropin secretion), abrupt withdrawal of long-term corticosteroid therapy (long-term exogenous corticosteroid stimulation suppresses pituitary corticotropin secretion and results in adrenal gland atrophy), or removal of a nonendocrine, corticotropin-secreting tumor. Adrenal crisis follows when trauma, surgery, or other physiologic stress exhausts the body's stores of glucocorticoids in a person with adrenal hypofunction.

Adrenal hypofunction affects 1 in 16,000 neonates congenitally. In adults, it affects 8 in 100,000 people, and males and females are affected equally. There's no racial predilection.

Signs and symptoms
Adrenal hypofunction typically produces such effects as weakness, fatigue, weight loss, and various GI disturbances, such as nausea, vomiting, anorexia, and chronic diarrhea. When primary, the disorder usually causes a conspicuous bronze coloration of the skin. The patient appears to be deeply suntanned, especially in the creases of the hands and over the metacarpophalangeal joints, the elbows, and the knees. He may also exhibit a darkening of scars, areas of vitiligo (absence of pigmentation), and increased pigmentation of the mucous membranes, especially the buccal mucosa. Abnormal skin and mucous membrane coloration results from decreased secretion of cortisol (one of the glucocorticoids), which causes the pituitary gland to simultaneously secrete excessive amounts of corticotropin and melanocyte-stimulating hormone (MSH).

Associated cardiovascular abnormalities in adrenal hypofunction include orthostatic hypotension, decreased cardiac size and output, and a weak, irregular pulse. Other clinical effects include decreased tolerance for even minor stress, poor coordination, fasting hypoglycemia (due to decreased gluconeogenesis), and a craving for salty food. Adrenal hypofunction may also retard axillary and pubic hair growth in females, decrease the libido (from decreased androgen production) and, in severe cases, cause amenorrhea.

Secondary adrenal hypofunction produces similar clinical effects but without hyperpigmentation because corticotropin and MSH levels are low. Because aldosterone secretion may continue at fairly normal levels in secondary adrenal hypofunction, this condition doesn't necessarily cause accompanying hypotension and electrolyte abnormalities.

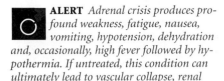 **ALERT** *Adrenal crisis produces profound weakness, fatigue, nausea, vomiting, hypotension, dehydration and, occasionally, high fever followed by hypothermia. If untreated, this condition can ultimately lead to vascular collapse, renal shutdown, coma, and death.*

Diagnosis

Diagnosis requires demonstration of decreased corticosteroid concentrations in plasma and an accurate classification of adrenal hypofunction as primary or secondary. If secondary adrenal hypofunction is suspected, the metyrapone test is indicated. This test requires oral or I.V. administration of metyrapone, which blocks cortisol production and should stimulate the release of corticotropin from the hypothalamic-pituitary system. In adrenal hypofunction, the hypothalamic-pituitary system responds normally, and plasma reveals high levels of corticotropin; however, plasma levels of cortisol precursor and urinary concentrations of 17-hydroxycorticosteroids don't rise.

If either primary or secondary adrenal hypofunction is suspected, a short corticotropin stimulation test may be done. If both corticotropin and cortisol are low, the long corticotropin test may be done. The test involves I.V. administration of corticotropin over 6 to 8 hours, after samples have been obtained to determine baseline plasma cortisol and 24-hour urine cortisol levels. In adrenal hypofunction, plasma and urine cortisol levels fail to rise normally in response to corticotropin; in secondary hypofunction, repeated doses of corticotropin over successive days produce a gradual increase in cortisol levels until normal values are reached.

In a patient with typical addisonian symptoms, the following laboratory findings strongly suggest acute adrenal hypofunction:
- decreased cortisol levels in plasma (less than 10 mcg/dl in the morning, with lower levels in the evening); however, this test is time-consuming, and emergency therapy shouldn't be postponed for test results
- decreased serum sodium and fasting blood glucose levels
- increased serum potassium and blood urea nitrogen levels
- elevated hematocrit and lymphocyte and eosinophil counts
- X-rays showing a small heart and adrenal calcification.

Treatment

For all patients with primary or secondary adrenal hypofunction, corticosteroid replacement, usually with cortisone or hydrocortisone (both of which also have a mineralocorticoid effect), is the primary treatment and must continue throughout life. Adrenal hypofunction may also necessitate treatment with I.V. desoxycorticosterone, a pure mineralocorticoid, or oral fludrocortisone, a synthetic mineralocorticoid; both prevent dangerous dehydration and hypotension.

Adrenal crisis requires prompt I.V. bolus administration of hydrocortisone. Later, doses are given I.M. or are diluted with dextrose in saline solution and given I.V. until the patient's condition stabilizes.

With proper treatment, adrenal crisis usually subsides quickly; the patient's blood pressure should stabilize, and water and sodium levels should return to normal. After the crisis, maintenance doses of hydrocortisone preserve physiologic stability.

Special considerations

In adrenal crisis, monitor vital signs carefully, especially for hypotension, volume depletion, and other signs of shock (decreased level of consciousness and urine output). Watch for hyperkalemia before treatment and for hypokalemia after treatment (from excessive mineralocorticoid effect).
- If the patient also has diabetes, check blood glucose levels periodically because steroid replacement may require adjustment of insulin dosage.
- Record weight and intake and output carefully because the patient may have volume depletion. Until onset of mineralocorticoid effect, force fluids to replace excessive fluid loss.

To manage the patient receiving maintenance therapy:

- Arrange for a diet that maintains sodium and potassium balances.
- If the patient is anorectic, suggest six small meals a day to increase calorie intake. Ask the dietitian to provide a diet high in protein and carbohydrates. Keep a late-morning snack available in case the patient becomes hypoglycemic.
- Observe the patient receiving steroids for cushingoid signs such as fluid retention around the eyes and face. Watch for fluid and electrolyte imbalance, especially if the patient is receiving mineralocorticoids. Monitor weight and check blood pressure to assess body fluid status. Remember, steroids administered in the late afternoon or evening may cause stimulation of the central nervous system and insomnia in some patients. Check for petechiae because the patient bruises easily.
- If the patient receives glucocorticoids alone, observe for orthostatic hypotension or electrolyte abnormalities, which may indicate a need for mineralocorticoid therapy.
- Explain that lifelong steroid therapy is necessary.
- Teach the patient the symptoms of too great or too little a dose.
- Tell the patient that dosage may need to be increased during times of stress (when he has a cold for example).
- Warn that infection, injury, or profuse sweating in hot weather may precipitate adrenal crisis.
- Warn the patient that any stress may necessitate additional cortisone to prevent adrenal crisis.
- Instruct the patient to always carry a medical identification card stating that he takes a steroid and giving the name of the drug and the dosage.
- Tell the patient to keep an emergency kit available containing hydrocortisone in a prepared syringe for use in times of stress.
- Teach the patient how to give himself an injection of hydrocortisone.

Cushing's syndrome

Cushing's syndrome is a cluster of clinical abnormalities caused by excessive levels of adrenocortical hormones (particularly cortisol) or related corticosteroids and, to a lesser extent, androgens and aldosterone. Its unmistakable signs include rapidly developing adiposity of the face (moon face), neck, and trunk and purple striae on the skin. (See *Symptoms of cushingoid syndrome.*) The prognosis depends on the underlying cause; it's poor in untreated people and in those with untreatable ectopic corticotropin-producing carcinoma.

Causes and incidence

In approximately 70% of patients, Cushing's syndrome results from excessive production of corticotropin and consequent hyperplasia of the adrenal cortex. Overproduction of corticotropin may stem from pituitary hypersecretion (Cushing's disease), a corticotropin-producing tumor in another organ (particularly bronchogenic or pancreatic cancer), or excessive administration of exogenous glucocorticoids.

In the remaining 30% of patients, Cushing's syndrome results from a cortisol-secreting adrenal tumor, which is usually benign. In infants, the usual cause of Cushing's syndrome is adrenal carcinoma.

Cushing's syndrome affects 13 of every 1 million people. It's more common in females than in males and occurs primarily between ages between ages 25 and 40.

Signs and symptoms

Like other endocrine disorders, Cushing's syndrome induces changes in multiple body systems, depending on the adrenocortical hormone involved. Clinical effects may include the following:

- *Endocrine and metabolic systems:* diabetes mellitus, with decreased glucose tolerance, fasting hyperglycemia, and glycosuria
- *Musculoskeletal system:* muscle weakness due to hypokalemia or to loss of muscle mass from increased catabolism, pathologic fractures due to decreased bone mineral, and skeletal growth retardation in children
- *Skin:* purplish striae; fat pads above the clavicles, over the upper back (buffalo hump), on the face (moon face), and throughout the trunk, with slender arms and legs; little or no scar formation; poor wound healing; acne and hirsutism in females

SYMPTOMS OF CUSHINGOID SYNDROME

Chronic depression, alcoholism, and long-term treatment with corticosteroids may produce an adverse effect called *cushingoid syndrome* — a condition marked by obvious fat deposits between the shoulders and around the waist, and widespread systemic abnormalities.

Differentiating between cushingoid syndrome and Cushing's syndrome can be difficult, so in addition to the symptoms shown in the illustration at right, observe for signs of hypertension, renal disorders, hyperglycemia, tissue wasting, muscle weakness, and labile emotional state. The patient may also have amenorrhea and glycosuria.

Resolution of the underlying disorder results in disappearance of cushingoid symptoms.

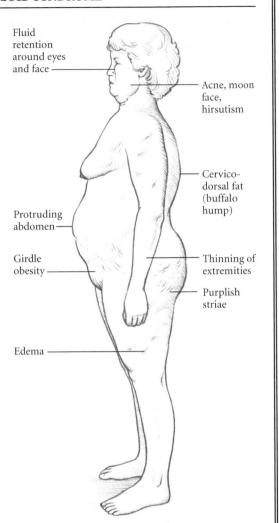

Fluid retention around eyes and face

Acne, moon face, hirsutism

Cervico-dorsal fat (buffalo hump)

Protruding abdomen

Girdle obesity

Thinning of extremities

Purplish striae

Edema

■ *GI system:* peptic ulcer, resulting from increased gastric secretions and pepsin production, and decreased gastric mucus
■ *Central nervous system (CNS):* irritability and emotional lability, ranging from euphoric behavior to depression or psychosis; insomnia
■ *Cardiovascular system:* hypertension due to sodium and water retention; left ventricular hypertrophy; capillary weakness due

to protein loss, which leads to bleeding, petechiae, and ecchymosis
■ *Immune system:* increased susceptibility to infection due to decreased lymphocyte production and suppressed antibody formation; decreased resistance to stress (Suppressed inflammatory response may mask even a severe infection.)
■ *Renal and urologic systems:* sodium and secondary fluid retention, increased potassium excretion, inhibited antidiuretic hor-

mone secretion, ureteral calculi from increased bone demineralization with hypercalciuria

■ *Reproductive system:* increased androgen production with clitoral hypertrophy, mild virilism, and amenorrhea or oligomenorrhea in females. Sexual dysfunction also occurs.

Diagnosis

Initially, diagnosis of Cushing's syndrome requires determination of plasma steroid levels. In people with normal hormone balance, plasma cortisol levels are higher in the morning and decrease gradually throughout the day (diurnal variation). In patients with Cushing's syndrome, cortisol levels don't fluctuate and typically remain consistently elevated; 24-hour urine sample demonstrates elevated free cortisol levels.

CONFIRMING DIAGNOSIS *A low-dose dexamethasone suppression test confirms the diagnosis of Cushing's syndrome. Salivary cortisol levels collected at midnight (usually performed on an outpatient basis) are elevated and are the most sensitive confirmatory test.* (See Diagnosing Cushing's syndrome.)

A high-dose dexamethasone suppression test can determine if Cushing's syndrome results from pituitary dysfunction (Cushing's disease). In this test, dexamethasone suppresses plasma cortisol levels, and urinary 17-hydroxycorticosteroid (17-OHCS) and 17-ketogenic steroid levels fall to 50% or less of basal levels. Failure to suppress these levels indicates that the syndrome results from an adrenal tumor or a nonendocrine, corticotropin-secreting tumor. This test can produce false-positive results.

In a stimulation test, administration of metyrapone, which blocks cortisol production by the adrenal glands, tests the ability of the pituitary gland and the hypothalamus to detect and correct low levels of plasma cortisol by increasing corticotropin production. The patient with Cushing's disease reacts to this stimulus by secreting an excess of plasma corticotropin as measured by levels of urinary 17-OHCS. If the patient has an adrenal or a nonendocrine corticotropin-secreting tumor, the pituitary gland—which is suppressed by the high cortisol levels—can't respond normally, so steroid levels remain stable or fall.

Ultrasound, computed tomography (CT) scan, or angiography localizes adrenal tumors; CT scan and magnetic resonance imaging of the head may identify pituitary tumors.

Treatment

Treatment to restore hormone balance and reverse Cushing's syndrome may necessitate radiation, drug therapy, or surgery. For example, pituitary-dependent Cushing's syndrome with adrenal hyperplasia and severe cushingoid symptoms (such as psychosis, poorly controlled diabetes mellitus, osteoporosis, and severe pathologic fractures) may require partial or complete hypophysectomy or pituitary irradiation. If the patient fails to respond, bilateral adrenalectomy may be performed. Nonendocrine corticotropin-producing tumors require excision of the tumor, followed by drug therapy (for example, with mitotane, metyrapone, or aminoglutethimide) to decrease cortisol levels if symptoms persist.

Aminoglutethimide and ketoconazole decrease cortisol levels and have been beneficial for many cushingoid patients. Aminoglutethimide alone, or in combination with metyrapone, may also be useful in metastatic adrenal carcinoma.

Before surgery, the patient with cushingoid symptoms should have special management to control hypertension, edema, diabetes, and cardiovascular manifestations and to prevent infection. Glucocorticoid administration on the morning of surgery can help prevent acute adrenal hypofunction during surgery.

Cortisol therapy is essential during and after surgery, to help the patient tolerate the physiologic stress imposed by removal of the pituitary or adrenals. If normal cortisol production resumes, steroid therapy may be gradually tapered and eventually discontinued. However, bilateral adrenalectomy or total hypophysectomy mandates lifelong steroid replacement therapy to correct hormonal deficiencies.

DIFFERENTIAL DIAGNOSIS
DIAGNOSING CUSHING'S SYNDROME

The flowchart below aids in differential diagnosis of Cushing's syndrome.

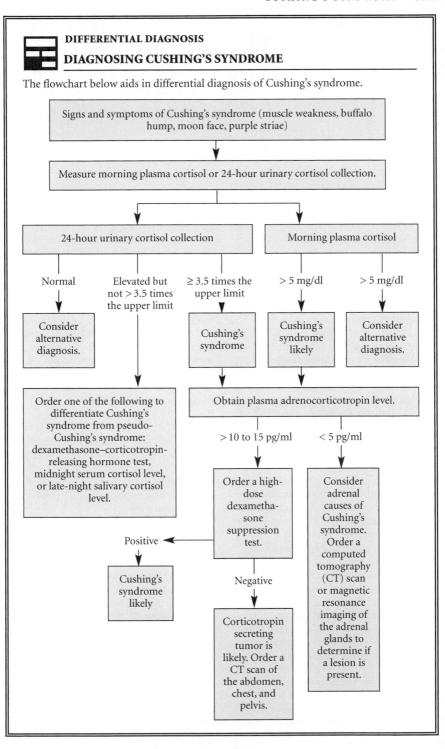

Special considerations

Patients with Cushing's syndrome require painstaking assessment and vigorous supportive care:

- Frequently monitor vital signs, especially blood pressure. Carefully observe the hypertensive patient who also has cardiac disease.
- Check laboratory reports for hypernatremia, hypokalemia, hyperglycemia, and glycosuria.
- Because the cushingoid patient is likely to retain sodium and water, check for edema, and monitor daily weight and intake and output carefully. To minimize weight gain, edema, and hypertension, ask the dietary department to provide a diet that's high in protein and potassium but low in calories, carbohydrates, and sodium.
- Watch for infection—a particular problem in Cushing's syndrome.
- If the patient has osteoporosis and is bedridden, perform passive range-of-motion exercises carefully because of the severe risk for pathologic fractures.
- Remember, Cushing's syndrome produces emotional lability. Record incidents that upset the patient, and try to prevent such situations from occurring if possible. Help him get the physical and mental rest he needs—by sedation if necessary. Offer support to the emotionally labile patient throughout the difficult testing period.

After bilateral adrenalectomy and pituitary surgery:

- Report wound drainage or temperature elevation to the patient's physician immediately. Use strict sterile technique in changing the patient's dressings.
- Administer analgesics and replacement steroids, as ordered.
- Monitor urine output, and check vital signs carefully, watching for signs of shock (decreased blood pressure, increased pulse rate, pallor, and cold, clammy skin). To counteract shock, give vasopressors and increase the rate of I.V. fluids, as ordered. Because mitotane, aminoglutethimide, and metyrapone decrease mental alertness and produce physical weakness, assess neurologic and behavioral status, and warn the patient of adverse CNS effects. Also watch for severe nausea, vomiting, and diarrhea.

- Check laboratory reports for hypoglycemia due to removal of the source of cortisol, a hormone that maintains blood glucose levels.
- Check for abdominal distention and return of bowel sounds after adrenalectomy.
- Check regularly for signs of adrenal hypofunction—orthostatic hypotension, apathy, weakness, fatigue—indicators that steroid replacement is inadequate.
- In the patient undergoing pituitary surgery, check for and immediately report signs of increased intracranial pressure (confusion, agitation, changes in level of consciousness, nausea, and vomiting). Watch for hypopituitarism.

Provide comprehensive teaching to help the patient cope with lifelong treatment:

- Advise the patient to take replacement steroids with antacids or meals, to minimize gastric irritation. (Usually it's helpful to take two-thirds of the dosage in the morning and the remaining third in the early afternoon to mimic diurnal adrenal secretion.)
- Tell the patient to carry a medical identification card and to immediately report physiologically stressful situations such as infections, which necessitate increased dosage.
- Instruct the patient to watch closely for signs of inadequate steroid dosage (fatigue, weakness, dizziness) and of overdosage (severe edema, weight gain). Emphatically warn against abrupt discontinuation of steroid dosage because this may produce a fatal adrenal crisis.

Hyperaldosteronism

In hyperaldosteronism (Conn's syndrome), hypersecretion of the mineralocorticoid aldosterone by the adrenal cortex causes excessive reabsorption of sodium and water, and excessive renal excretion of potassium.

Causes and incidence

Hyperaldosteronism may be primary (uncommon) or secondary. In 70% of patients, hyperaldosteronism results from a benign aldosterone-producing adrenal adenoma. In 15% to 30% of patients, the cause is unknown; rarely, the cause is bilateral adrenocortical hyperplasia (in children) or carcinoma. Incidence is three times higher in females than in males and is highest between ages 30 and 50.

In primary hyperaldosteronism, chronic aldosterone excess is independent of the renin-angiotensin system and, in fact, suppresses plasma renin activity. This aldosterone excess enhances sodium reabsorption by the kidneys, which leads to mild hypernatremia and, simultaneously, hypokalemia and increased extracellular fluid (ECF) volume. Expansion of intravascular fluid volume also occurs and results in volume-dependent hypertension and increased cardiac output. Excessive ingestion of English black licorice or licorice-like substances can produce a syndrome similar to primary hyperaldosteronism due to the mineralocorticoid action of glycyrrhizic acid.

Secondary hyperaldosteronism results from an extra-adrenal abnormality that stimulates the adrenal gland to increase production of aldosterone. For example, conditions that reduce renal blood flow (renal artery stenosis) and ECF volume or produce a sodium deficit activate the renin-angiotensin system and, subsequently, increase aldosterone secretion. Thus, secondary hyperaldosteronism may result from conditions that induce hypertension through increased renin production (such as Wilms' tumor), ingestion of hormonal contraceptives, and pregnancy.

However, secondary hyperaldosteronism may also result from disorders unrelated to hypertension, which may or may not cause edema. For example, nephrotic syndrome, hepatic cirrhosis with ascites, and heart failure commonly induce edema, whereas Bartter's syndrome and salt-losing nephritis don't.

Signs and symptoms

Most clinical effects of hyperaldosteronism result from hypokalemia, which increases neuromuscular irritability and produces muscle weakness; intermittent, flaccid paralysis; fatigue; headaches; paresthesia; and, possibly, tetany (resulting from metabolic alkalosis), which can lead to hypocalcemia.

Diabetes mellitus is common, perhaps because hypokalemia interferes with normal insulin secretion. Hypertension and its accompanying complications are also common. Other characteristic findings include visual disturbances and loss of renal concentrating ability, resulting in nocturnal polyuria and polydipsia. Azotemia indicates chronic potassium depletion nephropathy.

Diagnosis

Persistently low serum potassium levels in a nonedematous patient who isn't taking diuretics, who doesn't have obvious GI losses (from vomiting or diarrhea), and who has a normal sodium intake, suggest hyperaldosteronism. If hypokalemia develops in a hypertensive patient shortly after starting treatment with potassium-wasting diuretics (such as thiazides), and if it persists after the diuretic has been discontinued and potassium replacement therapy has been instituted, evaluation for hyperaldosteronism is necessary.

CONFIRMING DIAGNOSIS *A low plasma renin level that fails to increase appropriately during volume depletion (upright posture, sodium depletion) and a high plasma aldosterone level during volume expansion by salt loading confirm primary hyperaldosteronism in a hypertensive patient without edema.*

The serum bicarbonate level is often elevated, with ensuing alkalosis due to hydrogen and potassium ion loss in the distal renal tubules. Other tests show markedly increased urinary aldosterone levels, increased plasma aldosterone levels and, in secondary hyperaldosteronism, increased plasma renin levels.

A suppression test is useful to differentiate between primary and secondary hyperaldosteronism. During this test, the patient receives oral desoxycorticosterone for 3 days while plasma aldosterone levels and urinary metabolites are continuously measured. These levels decrease in secondary hyperaldosteronism but remain the same in primary hyperaldosteronism. Simultaneously, renin levels are low in primary hyperaldosteronism and high in secondary hyperaldosteronism.

Other helpful diagnostic evidence includes an increase in plasma volume of 30% to 50% above normal, electrocardiogram signs of hypokalemia (ST-segment depression and U waves), chest X-ray showing left ventricular hypertrophy from chronic hypertension, and localization of the tumor by adrenal angiography or computed tomography scan.

Treatment

Although treatment of primary hyperaldosteronism may include unilateral adrenalectomy, administration of a potassium-sparing diuretic — spironolactone — and sodium restriction may control hyperaldosteronism without surgery. For bilateral adrenal hyperplasia, spironolactone is the drug of choice. Treatment of secondary hyperaldosteronism must include correction of the underlying cause.

Special considerations

Patient care includes careful monitoring and recording of urine output, blood pressure, weight, and serum potassium levels.

■ Watch for signs of tetany (muscle twitching, Chvostek's sign) and for hypokalemia-induced cardiac arrhythmias, paresthesia, or weakness. Give potassium replacement, as ordered, and keep calcium gluconate I.V. available.

■ Ask the dietitian to provide a low-sodium, high-potassium diet.

■ After adrenalectomy, watch for weakness, hyponatremia, rising serum potassium levels, and signs of adrenal hypofunction, especially hypotension.

■ If the patient is taking spironolactone, advise him to watch for signs of hyperkalemia. Tell him that impotence and gynecomastia may follow long-term use.

■ Tell the patient who must take steroid hormone replacement to wear a medical identification bracelet.

Adrenogenital syndrome

Adrenogenital syndrome results from disorders of adrenocortical steroid biosynthesis. This syndrome may be inherited (congenital adrenal hyperplasia [CAH]) or acquired, usually as a result of an adrenal tumor (adrenal virilism). Salt-losing CAH may cause fatal adrenal crisis in neonates.

Causes and incidence

CAH is transmitted as an autosomal recessive trait that causes deficiencies in the enzymes needed for adrenocortical secretion of cortisol and, possibly, aldosterone. Compensatory secretion of corticotropin produces varying degrees of adrenal hyperplasia. In simple virilizing CAH, deficiency of the enzyme 21-hydroxylase results in underproduction of cortisol. In turn, this cortisol deficiency stimulates increased secretion of corticotropin, producing large amounts of cortisol precursors and androgens that don't require 21-hydroxylase for synthesis.

In salt-losing CAH, 21-hydroxylase is almost completely absent. Corticotropin secretion increases, causing excessive production of cortisol precursors, including salt-wasting compounds. However, plasma cortisol and aldosterone levels — both dependent on 21-hydroxylase — fall precipitously and, in combination with the excessive production of salt-wasting compounds, precipitate acute adrenal crisis. Corticotropin hypersecretion stimulates adrenal androgens, possibly even more than in simple virilizing CAH, and produces masculinization. Other rare CAH enzyme deficiencies exist and lead to increased or decreased production of affected hormones.

CAH is the most prevalent adrenal disorder in infants and children; simple virilizing CAH and salt-losing CAH are the most common forms. Acquired adrenal virilism is rare and affects twice as many females as males. About 1 in 10,000 to 18,000 are born with CAH.

Signs and symptoms

The neonatal female with simple virilizing CAH has ambiguous genitalia (enlarged clitoris, with urethral opening at the base; some labioscrotal fusion) but normal genital tract and gonads. As she grows older, signs of progressive virilization develop: early appearance of pubic and axillary hair, deep voice, acne, and facial hair. The neonatal male with this condition has no obvious abnormality; however, at prepu-

ACQUIRED ADRENAL VIRILISM

Acquired adrenal virilism results from virilizing adrenal tumors, carcinomas, or adenomas. This rare disorder is twice as common in females as in males. Although acquired adrenal virilism can develop at any age, its clinical effects vary with age at onset:

- Prepubescent females: pubic hair, clitoral enlargement; at puberty, delayed breast development, delayed or absent menses
- Prepubescent males: hirsutism, macrogenitosomia praecox (excessive body development, with marked enlargement of genitalia). Occasionally, the penis and prostate equal those of an adult male in size; however, testicular maturation fails to occur.
- Females (especially middle-aged): dark hair on legs, arms, chest, back, and face; pubic hair extending toward navel; oily skin, sometimes with acne; menstrual irregularities; muscular hypertrophy (masculine resemblance); male pattern baldness; and atrophy of breasts and uterus
- Males: no overt signs; discovery of tumor usually accidental
- All patients: good muscular development; taller than average during childhood and adolescence; short stature as adults due to early closure of epiphyses.

Diagnosis and treatment
Diagnostic tests for this disorder include:

- Urinary total 17-ketosteroids (17-KS): greatly elevated but levels vary daily; dexamethasone P.O. doesn't suppress 17-KS
- Plasma levels of dehydroepiandrosterone: greatly elevated
- Serum electrolyte levels: normal
- X-ray of kidneys: may show downward displacement of kidneys by tumor.

Treatment requires surgical excision of tumor and metastases (if present), when possible, or radiation therapy and chemotherapy. Preoperative treatment may include glucocorticoids. With treatment, the prognosis is very good in patients with slow-growing and nonrecurring tumors. Periodic follow-up urine testing (for increased 17-KS levels) to check for tumor recurrence is essential.

---

berty he shows accentuated masculine characteristics, such as deepened voice and an enlarged phallus, with frequent erections. At puberty, females fail to begin menstruation, and males have small testes. Both males and females with this condition may be taller than other children their age as a result of rapid bone and muscle growth, but because excessive androgen levels hasten epiphyseal closure, abnormally short adult stature results. (See *Acquired adrenal virilism.*)

Salt-losing CAH in females causes more complete virilization than the simple form and results in development of male external genitalia without testes. Because males with this condition have no external genital abnormalities, immediate neonatal diagnosis is difficult, and is commonly delayed until the infant develops severe systemic symptoms. Characteristically, such an infant is apathetic, fails to eat, and has diarrhea; he develops symptoms of adrenal crisis in the first week of life (vomiting, dehydration from hyponatremia, hyperkalemia). Unless this condition is treated promptly, dehydration and hyperkalemia may lead to cardiovascular collapse and cardiac arrest.

Diagnosis
Physical examination revealing pseudohermaphroditism in females or precocious pu-

HERMAPHRODITISM

True hermaphroditism *(hermaphrodism, intersexuality)* is a rare condition characterized by the presence of both ovarian and testicular tissues. External genitalia are usually ambiguous but may be completely male or female, thereby masking hermaphroditism until puberty. The hermaphrodite almost always has a uterus (however, fertility is rare) and ambiguous gonads distributed:

- Bilaterally: testis and ovary on both sides, ovotestes
- Unilaterally: ovary or testis on one side, an ovotestis on the other
- Asymmetrically or laterally: an ovary and a testis on opposite sides.

Causes and diagnosis

Because the Y chromosome is needed to develop testicular tissue, hermaphroditism in infants with XY karyotypes is particularly perplexing but may result from mosaicism (XX/XY, XX/XXY), hidden mosaicism, or hidden gene alterations. In patients with XX karyotype, ovaries are usually better developed than in those with XY karyotype. Fifty percent of hermaphrodites have a 46, XX karyotype, 20% have XY, and 30% are mosaics.

Although ambiguous external genitalia suggest hermaphroditism, chromosomal studies (particularly a buccal smear for Barr bodies, indicating an XX karyotype), a 24-hour urine specimen for 17-ketosteroids to rule out congenital adrenal hyperplasia, and gonadal biopsy are necessary to confirm it.

Early treatment crucial

Sexual assignment, based on the anatomy of the external genitalia, and surgical reconstruction should be done as early as possible to prevent physical and psychological consequences of delayed reassignment. During surgery, inappropriate reproductive organs are removed to prevent incongruous secondary sex characteristics at puberty. Hormonal replacement may be necessary.

Nursing intervention emphasizes psychological support of the parents and reinforcement of their choice about sexual assignment.

---

berty in both sexes strongly suggests CAH. (See *Hermaphroditism.*)

 CONFIRMING DIAGNOSIS *The following laboratory findings confirm the diagnosis: elevated plasma 17-ketosteroids (17-KS), which can be suppressed by administering oral dexamethasone; elevated urinary levels of hormone metabolites, particularly pregnanetriol; elevated plasma 17-hydroxyprogesterone level; and normal or decreased urinary levels of 17-hydroxycorticosteroids. Elevated dehydroepiandrosterone sulfate is present.*

Adrenal hypofunction or adrenal crisis in the first week of life suggests salt-losing CAH. Hyperkalemia, hyponatremia, and hypochloremia with excessive urinary 17-KS and pregnanetriol and decreased urinary aldosterone levels confirm it.

Treatment

Simple virilizing CAH requires correction of the cortisol deficiency and inhibition of excessive pituitary corticotropin production by daily administration of cortisol. Treatment returns androgen production to normal levels. Measurement of urinary 17-KS levels determines the initial dose of cortisone or hydrocortisone; this dose is usually large and is given I.M. Later dosage is modified according to decreasing urinary 17-KS levels. Infants must continue to receive cortisone or hydrocortisone I.M. until age 18 months; after that, they may take it orally.

 PEDIATRIC TIP *The infant with salt-losing CAH in adrenal crisis requires immediate I.V. sodium chloride and glucose infusion to maintain fluid and electrolyte balance and to stabilize vital*

signs. If saline and glucose infusion doesn't control symptoms while the diagnosis is being established, desoxycorticosterone I.M. and hydrocortisone I.V. are necessary. Later, maintenance includes mineralocorticoid (desoxycorticosterone, fludrocortisone, or both) and glucocorticoid (cortisone or hydrocortisone) replacement.

Sex chromatin and karyotype studies determine the genetic sex of patients with ambiguous external genitalia. Females with masculine external genitalia require reconstructive surgery, such as correction of the labial fusion and of the urogenital sinus. Surgery is usually scheduled between ages 1 and 3, after the effect of cortisone therapy has been assessed.

Special considerations

Suspect CAH in infants hospitalized for failure to thrive, dehydration, or diarrhea, as well as in tall, sturdy-looking children with a record of numerous episodic illnesses.

■ When caring for an infant with adrenal crisis, keep the I.V. line patent, infuse fluids, and give steroids, as ordered. Monitor body weight, blood pressure, and serum electrolyte levels carefully, especially sodium and potassium levels. Watch for cyanosis, hypotension, tachycardia, tachypnea, and signs of shock. Minimize external stressors.

■ If the child is receiving maintenance therapy with steroid injections, rotate I.M. injection sites to prevent atrophy; tell parents to do the same. Teach them the possible adverse effects (cushingoid symptoms) of long-term therapy. Explain that maintenance therapy with hydrocortisone, cortisone, or the mineralocorticoid fludrocortisone is essential for life. Warn parents not to withdraw these drugs suddenly because potentially fatal adrenal hypofunction will result. Instruct parents to report stress and infection, which require increased steroid dosages.

■ Monitor the patient receiving desoxycorticosterone or fludrocortisone for edema, weakness, and hypertension. Be alert for significant weight gain and rapid changes in height because normal growth is an important indicator of adequate therapy.

■ Instruct the patient to wear a medical identification bracelet indicating that she's on prolonged steroid therapy and providing information about dosage.

■ Help the parents of a female infant with male genitalia to understand that she's physiologically a female and that this abnormality can be surgically corrected. Arrange for counseling if necessary.

Pheochromocytoma

A pheochromocytoma is a chromaffin-cell tumor of the adrenal medulla that secretes an excess of the catecholamines epinephrine and norepinephrine, resulting in severe hypertension, increased metabolism, and hyperglycemia. This disorder is potentially fatal but the prognosis is generally good with treatment. However, pheochromocytoma-induced kidney damage is irreversible.

Causes and incidence

A pheochromocytoma may result from an inherited autosomal dominant trait. According to some estimates, about 0.5% of newly diagnosed patients with hypertension have pheochromocytoma. While this tumor is usually benign, it may be malignant in as many as 10% of these patients. It affects all races and both sexes, occurring primarily between ages 30 and 40.

Signs and symptoms

The cardinal sign of pheochromocytoma is persistent or paroxysmal hypertension. Common clinical effects include palpitations, tachycardia, headache, diaphoresis, pallor, warmth or flushing, paresthesia, tremor, excitation, fright, nervousness, feelings of impending doom, abdominal pain, tachypnea, nausea, and vomiting. Orthostatic hypotension and paradoxical response to antihypertensive drugs are common, as are associated glycosuria, hyperglycemia, and hypermetabolism. Patients with hypermetabolism may show marked weight loss but some patients with pheochromocytomas are obese. Symptomatic episodes may recur as seldom as once every 2 months or as often as 25 times a day. They may occur spontaneously or may follow certain precipitating events, such as postural change, exercise, laughing, smoking, induction of anesthesia, urination, or a change in environmental or body temperature.

Pheochromocytoma is commonly diagnosed during pregnancy, when uterine pressure on the tumor induces more frequent attacks; such attacks can prove fatal for both mother and fetus as a result of a stroke, acute pulmonary edema, cardiac arrhythmias, or hypoxia. In such patients, the risk of spontaneous abortion is high but most fetal deaths occur during labor or immediately after birth.

Diagnosis

The most common presentation for pheochromocytoma is continuous hypertension with or without orthostatic hypotension. A history of acute episodes of hypertension, headache, sweating, and tachycardia—particularly in a patient with hyperglycemia, glycosuria, and hypermetabolism—strongly suggests pheochromocytoma. A patient who has intermittent attacks may have no symptoms during a latent phase. The tumor is rarely palpable; when it is, palpation of the surrounding area may induce an acute attack and help confirm the diagnosis. Generally, diagnosis depends on laboratory findings.

CONFIRMING DIAGNOSIS *Increased urinary excretion of total free catecholamines and their metabolites, vanillylmandelic acid (VMA) and metanephrine, as measured by analysis of a 24-hour urine specimen, confirms pheochromocytoma.*

Labile blood pressure necessitates urine collection during a hypertensive episode and comparison of this specimen with a baseline specimen. Direct assay of total plasma catecholamines shows levels 10 to 50 times higher than normal.

Provocative tests with glucagon and phentolamine suggest the diagnosis; however, because they may precipitate a hypertensive crisis or induce a false-positive or false-negative result, they're seldom used. The clonidine suppression test will cause decreased plasma catecholamine levels in normal patients but no change in those with pheochromocytoma. After demonstrating biochemical evidence of pheochromocytoma, computed tomography scan or magnetic resonance imaging of the abdomen (where 95% of pheochromocytomas are located) is warranted. If a tumor isn't located—or if there is more than one—a radioactive iodine metaiodobenzylguanidine scintiscan or nuclear scan usually confirms the diagnosis in unclear cases. Angiography and excretory urography are no longer used; adrenal venography is used, but rarely.

Treatment

Surgical removal of the tumor is the treatment of choice. To decrease blood pressure, an alpha-adrenergic blocker or metyrosine is given from 1 to 2 weeks before surgery. A beta-adrenergic blocker (propranolol) may also be used after achieving alpha blockade. Postoperatively, I.V. fluids, plasma volume expanders, vasopressors and, possibly, transfusions may be required for hypotension. Persistent hypertension in the immediate postoperative period can occur. If surgery isn't feasible, alpha-adrenergic blockers and beta-adrenergic blockers—such as phenoxybenzamine and propranolol, respectively—are beneficial in controlling catecholamine effects and preventing attacks. Management of an acute attack or hypertensive crisis requires I.V. phentolamine (push or drip) or nitroprusside to normalize blood pressure.

Special considerations

To ensure the reliability of urine catecholamine measurements, make sure the patient avoids foods high in vanillin (such as coffee, nuts, chocolate, and bananas) for 2 days before urine collection of VMA. Also, be aware of possible drug therapy that may interfere with the accurate determination of VMA (such as guaifenesin and salicylates). Collect the urine in a special container, with hydrochloric acid, that has been prepared by the laboratory.

- Obtain blood pressure readings often because transient hypertensive attacks are possible. Tell the patient to report headaches, palpitations, nervousness, or other symptoms of an acute attack. If hypertensive crisis develops, monitor blood pressure and heart rate every 2 to 5 minutes until blood pressure stabilizes at an acceptable level.
- Check blood for glucose, and watch for weight loss from hypermetabolism.
- After surgery, blood pressure may rise or fall sharply. Keep the patient quiet; provide a private room, if possible, because excitement may trigger a hypertensive episode. Postoperative hypertension is common because the stress of surgery and manipulation of the adrenal gland stimulate secretion of catecholamines. Because this excess secretion causes profuse sweating, keep the room cool, and change the patient's clothing and bedding often. If the patient receives phentolamine, monitor blood pressure closely. Observe and record adverse effects: dizziness, hypotension, and tachycardia. The first 24 to 48 hours immediately after surgery are the most critical because blood pressure can drop drastically.
- If the patient is receiving vasopressors I.V., check blood pressure as per facility protocol or every 15 minutes while titrating, and regulate the drip to maintain a safe pressure. Arterial pressure lines facilitate constant monitoring.
- Watch for abdominal distention and return of bowel sounds.

 ALERT *Check dressings and vital signs for indications of hemorrhage (increased pulse rate, decreased blood pressure, cold and clammy skin, pallor, and unresponsiveness).*

- Give analgesics for pain, as ordered, but monitor blood pressure carefully because many analgesics, especially meperidine, can cause hypotension.
- If autosomal dominant transmission of pheochromocytoma is suspected, the patient's family should also be evaluated for this condition.

PANCREATIC AND MULTIPLE DISORDERS

Multiple endocrine neoplasia

Multiple endocrine neoplasia (MEN) is a hereditary disorder in which two or more endocrine glands develop hyperplasia, adenoma, or carcinoma, concurrently or consecutively. Two of the types that occur are well documented: MEN I (Werner's syndrome) involves hyperplasia and adenomatosis of the pituitary and parathyroid glands, islet cells of the pancreas and, rarely, the thyroid and adrenal glands; MEN II (Sipple's syndrome) involves medullary carcinoma of the thyroid, with hyperplasia and adenomatosis of the adrenal medulla (pheochromocytoma) and parathyroid glands. MEN I is the most common form.

Causes and incidence
MEN usually results from autosomal dominant inheritance. It affects males twice as often as females and may occur at any time from adolescence to old age, but is rare in children. There's no racial predilection.

Signs and symptoms
Clinical effects of MEN may develop in various combinations and orders, depending on the glands involved. The most common manifestation of MEN I is hyperparathyroidism, followed by ulcer due to Zollinger-Ellison syndrome (marked by increased gastrin production from non-beta islet cell tumors of the pancreas). Hypoglycemia may result from pancreatic beta islet cell tumors, with increased insulin production. When MEN I affects the parathyroids, it produces signs of hyperparathyroidism, including hypercalcemia (because the parathyroids are primarily responsible for the regulation of calcium and phosphorus levels). When MEN causes pituitary tumor, it's most commonly a prolactinoma, but can be a growth hormone

or corticotropin, or even a nonsecretory adenoma.

Characteristic features of MEN II with medullary carcinoma of the thyroid include enlarged thyroid mass, with resultant increased calcitonin and, occasionally, ectopic corticotropin, causing Cushing's syndrome. With tumors of the adrenal medulla, symptoms include headache, tachyarrhythmias, and hypertension; with adenomatosis or hyperplasia of the parathyroids, symptoms result from renal calculi.

Diagnosis

Investigating symptoms of pituitary tumor, hypoglycemia, hypercalcemia, or GI hemorrhage may lead to a diagnosis of MEN. Diagnostic tests must be used to carefully evaluate each affected endocrine gland. For example, radioimmunoassay showing increased levels of gastrin in patients with peptic ulceration and Zollinger-Ellison syndrome suggests the need for follow-up studies for MEN I because 50% of patients with Zollinger-Ellison syndrome have MEN. After confirmation of MEN, family members must also be assessed for this inherited syndrome.

Magnetic resonance imaging or computed tomography scan of the abdomen may show pancreatic tumor. Insulin test may show increased levels and fasting blood sugar may be low.

Treatment

Treatment must eradicate the tumors. Subsequent therapy controls residual symptoms. In MEN I, peptic ulceration is usually the most urgent clinical feature, so primary treatment emphasizes control of bleeding or resection of necrotic tissue. In hypoglycemia caused by insulinoma, oral administration of diazoxide or glucose can keep blood glucose levels within acceptable limits. Subtotal (partial) pancreatectomy is required to remove the tumor. Because all parathyroid glands have the potential for neoplastic enlargement, subtotal parathyroidectomy may also be required along with transsphenoidal hypophysectomy. In MEN II, treatment of an adrenal medullary tumor includes antihypertensives and re-

section of the tumor. Bromocriptine may be used for pituitary tumors that secrete prolactin. Hormonal replacement therapy is necessary when glands are removed or secretion is inadequate.

Special considerations

Supportive care depends on the body system involved.

- If MEN involves the pancreas, monitor blood glucose levels frequently. If it affects the adrenal glands, monitor blood pressure closely, especially during drug therapy.
- Manage peptic ulcers, hypoglycemia, and other complications, as needed.
- If pituitary tumor is suspected, watch for signs of pituitary trophic hormone dysfunction, which may affect any of the endocrine glands. Also, be aware that pituitary apoplexy (sudden severe headache, altered level of consciousness, visual disturbances) may occur.

Diabetes mellitus

Diabetes mellitus (DM) is a chronic disease of absolute or relative insulin deficiency or resistance characterized by disturbances in carbohydrate, protein, and fat metabolism. A leading cause of death by disease in the United States, this syndrome is a contributing factor in about 50% of myocardial infarctions and about 75% of strokes as well as in renal failure and peripheral vascular disease. It's also the leading cause of new blindness.

DM occurs in four forms classified by etiology: type 1, type 2, other specific types, and gestational diabetes mellitus (GDM). Type 1 is further subdivided into immune-mediated diabetes and idiopathic diabetes. Those who were previously in the type 1 diabetes group fall into this group. Children and adolescents with type 1 immune-mediated diabetes rapidly develop ketoacidosis, but most adults with this type experience only modest fasting hyperglycemia unless they develop an infection or experience another stressor. Patients with type 1 idiopathic diabetes are prone to ketoacidosis.

Most patients with type 2 diabetes are obese. The "other specific types" category includes people who have diabetes as a result of a genetic defect, endocrinopathies, or exposure to certain drugs or chemicals. GDM occurs during pregnancy. In this type of diabetes, glucose tolerance levels usually return to normal after delivery.

Causes and incidence

DM affects an estimated 6% of the population of the United States, about half of whom are undiagnosed. Incidence is greater in females and rises with age. Type 2 accounts for 90% of cases.

In type 1 diabetes, pancreatic beta-cell destruction or a primary defect in beta-cell function results in failure to release insulin and ineffective glucose transport. Type 1 immune-mediated diabetes is caused by cell-mediated destruction of pancreatic beta cells. The rate of beta-cell destruction is usually higher in children than in adults. The idiopathic form of type 1 diabetes has no known cause. Patients with this form have no evidence of autoimmunity and don't produce insulin.

In type 2 diabetes, beta cells release insulin, but receptors are insulin-resistant and glucose transport is variable and ineffective. Risk factors for type 2 diabetes include:

■ obesity (even an increased percentage of body fat primarily in the abdominal region); risk decreases with weight and drug therapy
■ lack of physical activity
■ history of GDM
■ hypertension
■ Black, Hispanic, Pacific Islander, Asian American, Native American origin
■ strong family history of diabetes
■ older than age 45
■ high-density lipoprotein cholesterol of less than 35 or triglyceride of greater than 250
■ Seriously impaired glucose tolerance (IGT) test.

ELDER TIP *As the body ages, the cells become more resistant to insulin, thus reducing the older adult's ability to metabolize glucose. In addition, the release of insulin from the pancreatic beta*

cells is reduced and delayed. These combined processes result in hyperglycemia. In the older patient, sudden concentrations of glucose cause increased and more prolonged hyperglycemia.

The "other specific types" of DM result from various conditions (such as a genetic defect of the beta cells or endocrinopathies) or from use of or exposure to certain drugs or chemicals. GDM is considered present whenever a patient has any degree of abnormal glucose during pregnancy. This form may result from weight gain and increased levels of estrogen and placental hormones, which antagonize insulin.

Insulin transports glucose into the cell for use as energy and storage as glycogen. It also stimulates protein synthesis and free fatty acid storage in the fat deposits. Insulin deficiency compromises the body tissues' access to essential nutrients for fuel and storage.

Signs and symptoms

Diabetes may begin dramatically with ketoacidosis or insidiously. Its most common symptom is fatigue from energy deficiency and a catabolic state. Insulin deficiency causes hyperglycemia, which pulls fluid from body tissues, causing osmotic diuresis, polyuria, dehydration, polydipsia, dry mucous membranes, poor skin turgor and, in most patients, unexplained weight loss.

 ELDER TIP *Because their thirst mechanism functions less effectively, older adults may not report polydipsia, a hallmark of diabetes in younger adults.*

In ketoacidosis and hyperosmolar hyperglycemic nonketotic syndrome, dehydration may cause hypovolemia and shock. Wasting of glucose in the urine usually produces weight loss and hunger in type 1 diabetes, even if the patient eats voraciously.

Long-term effects of diabetes may include retinopathy, nephropathy, atherosclerosis, and peripheral and autonomic neuropathy. Peripheral neuropathy usually affects the hands and feet and may cause numbness or pain. Autonomic neuropathy may manifest itself in several ways, including gastroparesis (leading to delayed gastric

---

CLASSIFYING BLOOD GLUCOSE LEVELS

The American Diabetes Association classifies blood glucose levels as follows:
- Normal: < 100 mg/dl
- Prediabetes: 100 to 125 mg/dl
- Diabetes: ≥ 126 mg/dl

---

emptying and a feeling of nausea and fullness after meals), nocturnal diarrhea, impotence, and orthostatic hypotension.

Because hyperglycemia impairs the patient's resistance to infection, diabetes may result in skin and urinary tract infections (UTIs) and vaginitis. Glucose content of the epidermis and urine encourages bacterial growth.

Diagnosis

According to the American Diabetes Association (ADA), DM can be diagnosed if any of the following exist:
- symptoms of diabetes (polyuria, polydipsia, and unexplained weight loss) plus a random (non-fasting) blood glucose level greater than or equal to 200 mg/dl accompanied by symptoms of diabetes.
- a fasting blood glucose level (no caloric intake for at least 8 hours) greater than or equal to 126 mg/dl.
- a plasma glucose value in the 2-hour sample of the oral glucose tolerance test greater than or equal to 200 mg/dl. This test should be performed after a glucose load dose of 75 g of anhydrous glucose.

If results are questionable, the diagnosis should be confirmed by a repeat test on a different day. The ADA also recommends the following testing guidelines:
- Test every 3 years: people age 45 or older without symptoms
- Test immediately: people with the classic symptoms
- High-risk groups should be tested frequently: Individuals with impaired glucose tolerance usually have normal blood levels unless challenged by a glucose load, such as

a piece of pie or glass of orange juice. Two hours after a glucose load, the glucose level ranges from 140 to 199 mg/dl. These individuals have an abnormal fasting glucose level between 110 and 125 mg/dl. Because the fasting plasma glucose test is sufficient to make the diagnosis of diabetes, it replaces the oral glucose tolerance test. (See *Classifying blood glucose levels*.)

An ophthalmologic examination may show diabetic retinopathy. Other diagnostic and monitoring tests include urinalysis for acetone and blood testing for glycosylated hemoglobin (Hb A_{1C}), which reflects recent glucose cortisol.

Treatment

Effective treatment normalizes blood glucose and decreases complications using insulin replacement, diet, and exercise. Current forms of insulin replacement include single-dose, mixed-dose, split-mixed dose, and multiple-dose regimens. The multiple-dose regimens may use an insulin pump. Insulin may be rapid acting, intermediate acting, long acting, or a combination of rapid acting and intermediate acting; it may be standard or purified, and it may be derived from beef, pork, or human sources. Purified human insulin is used commonly today. Pancreas transplantation is experimental and requires chronic immunosuppression.

Successful treatment requires an extensive dietary education. The patient's diet is specifically tailored to include the right amount and combination of foods. Almost all foods may be eaten occasionally. The diet should address dietary prescriptions as well as personal and cultural preferences to improve adherence and control. For the obese patient with type 2 diabetes, weight reduction is a goal. In type 1 diabetes, the calorie allotment may be high, depending on growth stage and activity level.

Type 2 diabetes may require oral antidiabetic drugs to stimulate endogenous insulin production, increase insulin sensitivity at the cellular level, and suppress hepatic gluconeogenesis.

Five types of drugs have been used to treat diabetes. Sulfonylureas stimulate pancreatic insulin release, increase tissue sensitivity to insulin, and require insulin's presence to work. Meglitinides cause immediate, brief release of insulin and are taken immediately before meals. Biguanides decrease hepatic glucose production and increase tissue sensitivity to insulin. Alpha-glucosidase inhibitors slow the breakdown of glucose and decrease postprandial glucose peaks. The thiazolidinediones enhance the action of insulin; however, insulin must be present for them to work. These drugs also reduce insulin resistance by decreasing hepatic glucose production and increasing glucose uptake. They have also been shown to lower blood pressure in diabetic hypertensive patients. Cholesterol and triglyceride levels may also be reduced.

Treatment of long-term diabetic complications may include transplantation or dialysis for renal failure, photocoagulation for retinopathy, and vascular surgery for large-vessel disease. Meticulous blood glucose control is essential.

ALERT *Any patient with a wound that has lasted more than 8 weeks and who has tried standard wound care and revascularization without improvement should consider hyperbaric oxygen therapy. This treatment may speed healing by allowing more oxygen to get to the wound and may therefore result in fewer amputations.*

Keeping glucose at near-normal levels for 5 years or more reduces both the onset and progression of retinopathy, nephropathy, and neuropathy. In type 2 diabetes, blood pressure control as well as smoking cessation reduces the onset and progression of complications, including cardiovascular disease.

Special considerations

Stress the importance of complying with the prescribed treatment program. Tailor your teaching to the patient's needs, abilities, and developmental stage. Include diet; purpose, administration, and possible adverse effects of medication; exercise; monitoring; hygiene; and the prevention and recognition of hypoglycemia and hyperglycemia. Stress the effect of blood glucose control on long-term health.

ALERT *Watch for acute complications of diabetic therapy, especially hypoglycemia (vagueness, slow cerebration, dizziness, weakness, pallor, tachycardia, diaphoresis, seizures, and coma); immediately give carbohydrates, ideally in the form of fruit juice, glucose tablets, honey or, if the patient is unconscious, glucagon or dextrose I.V.*

ALERT *Be alert for signs of ketoacidosis (acetone breath, dehydration, weak and rapid pulse, and Kussmaul's respirations) and hyperosmolar coma (polyuria, thirst, neurologic abnormalities, and stupor). These hyperglycemic crises require I.V. fluids, insulin and, usually, potassium replacement.*

■ Monitor diabetes control by obtaining blood glucose, glycohemoglobulin, lipid levels, and blood pressure measurements regularly.

■ Watch for diabetic effects on the cardiovascular system, such as cerebrovascular, coronary artery, and peripheral vascular impairment, and on the peripheral and autonomic nervous systems. Treat all injuries, cuts, and blisters (particularly on the legs or feet) meticulously. Be alert for signs of UTI and renal disease.

■ Urge regular ophthalmologic examinations to detect diabetic retinopathy.

■ Assess for signs of diabetic neuropathy (numbness or pain in hands and feet, footdrop, neurogenic bladder). Stress the need for personal safety precautions because decreased sensation can mask injuries. Minimize complications by maintaining strict blood glucose control.

■ Teach the patient to care for his feet by washing them daily, drying carefully between toes, and inspecting for corns, calluses, redness, swelling, bruises, and breaks in the skin. Urge him to report changes to the physician. Advise him to wear nonconstricting shoes and to avoid walking barefoot. Instruct him to use over-the-counter athlete's foot remedies and seek professional care should athlete's foot not improve.

■ Teach the patient how to manage his diabetes when he has a minor illness, such as a cold, flu, or upset stomach.

■ To delay the clinical onset of diabetes, teach people at high risk to avoid risk factors. Advise genetic counseling for young adult diabetics who are planning families.

■ Further information may be obtained from the Juvenile Diabetes Foundation, the ADA, and the American Association of Diabetes Educators.

Selected references

Bolander, F.F. *Molecular Endocrinology,* 3rd ed. Boston: Elsevier Academic Press, 2004.

Griffin, J.E., and Ojeda, S.R., eds. *Textbook of Endocrine Physiology,* 5th ed. New York: Oxford University Press, 2004.

Martini, L., ed. *Encyclopedia of Endocrine Diseases.* Boston: Elsevier Academic Press, 2004.

Pescovitz, O.H., and Eugster, E.A., eds. *Pediatric Endocrinology: Mechanisms and Management.* Philadelphia: Lippincott Williams & Wilkins, 2004.

Smeltzer, S.C., et al., eds. *Brunner & Suddarth's Textbook of Medical-surgical Nursing,* 10th ed. Philadelphia: Lippincott Williams & Wilkins, 2004.

Speroff, L., and Fritz, M. *Clinical Gynecologic Endocrinology and Infertility,* 7th ed. Philadelphia: Lippincott Williams & Wilkins, 2005.

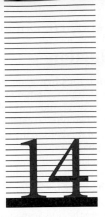

14

Metabolic and nutritional disorders

Introduction   870

Nutritional imbalance   875
Vitamin A deficiency   875
Vitamin B deficiencies   876
Vitamin C deficiency   879
Vitamin D deficiency   881
Vitamin E deficiency   882
Vitamin K deficiency   883
Hypervitaminoses A and D   884
Iodine deficiency   885
Zinc deficiency   886
Obesity   887
Protein-calorie malnutrition   888

Metabolic disorders   890
Galactosemia   890
Glycogen storage diseases   892
Hypoglycemia   895
Hereditary fructose intolerance   898
Hyperlipoproteinemia   898
Gaucher's disease   901
Amyloidosis   902
Porphyrias   904
Metabolic syndrome   904

Homeostatic imbalance   908
Potassium imbalance   908
Sodium imbalance   911

Calcium imbalance   914
Chloride imbalance   919
Magnesium imbalance   921
Phosphorus imbalance   923
Syndrome of inappropriate
   antidiuretic hormone   924
Metabolic acidosis   925
Metabolic alkalosis   927

Selected references   928

Introduction

Metabolism is the physiologic process that allows cells to transform food into energy and continually rebuild body cells. Metabolism has two phases: catabolism and anabolism. In *catabolism*, the energy-producing phase of metabolism, the body breaks down large food molecules into smaller ones; in *anabolism*, the tissue-building phase, the body converts small molecules into larger ones (such as antibodies to keep the body capable of fighting infection). Both phases are accomplished by means of a chemical process using energy. A wide range of nutrients is metabolized to meet the body's needs. (See *Essential nutrients and their functions.*)

 ELDER TIP *A person's protein, vitamin, and mineral requirements usually remain the same as he ages, although calorie needs decline.* Diminished activity may lower energy requirements by almost 200 calories per day for men and women ages 51 to 75, 400 calories per day for women older than age 75, and 500 calories per day for men older than age 75.

Carbohydrates: Primary energy source

The body gets most of its energy by metabolizing carbohydrates, especially glucose. Glucose catabolism proceeds in three phases:

■ *Glycolysis,* a series of chemical reactions, converts glucose molecules into pyruvic or lactic acid.

■ The *citric acid cycle* removes ionized hydrogen atoms from pyruvic acid and produces carbon dioxide.

■ *Oxidative phosphorylation* traps energy from the hydrogen electrons and combines the hydrogen ions and electrons with oxygen to form water and the common form of biologic energy, adenosine triphosphate (ATP).

Other essential processes in carbohydrate metabolism include glycogenesis — the formation of glycogen, a storage form of glucose — which occurs when cells become saturated with glucose-6-phosphate (an intermediate product of glycolysis); glycogenolysis, the reverse process, which converts glycogen into glucose-6-phosphate in muscle cells and liberates free glucose in the liver; and gluconeogenesis, or "new" glucose formation from protein amino acids or fat glycerols.

A complex interplay of hormonal and neural controls regulates glucose metabolism. Hormone secretions of five endocrine glands dominate this regulatory function:

■ Alpha cells of the islets of Langerhans secrete glucagon, which increases the blood glucose level by stimulating phosphorylase activity to accelerate liver glycogenolysis.

■ Beta cells of the islets of Langerhans secrete the glucose-regulating hormone insulin, which assists in glucose transport across cell membranes and storage of excess glucose as fat.

■ The adrenal medulla, as a physiologic response to stress, secretes epinephrine, which stimulates liver and muscle glycogenolysis to increase the blood glucose level.

■ Corticotropin and glucocorticoids also increase blood glucose levels. Glucocorticoids accelerate gluconeogenesis by promoting the flow of amino acids to the liver, where they're synthesized into glucose.

■ Human growth hormone (hGH) limits the fat storage and favors fat catabolism; consequently, it inhibits carbohydrate catabolism and thus raises blood glucose levels.

■ Thyroid-stimulating hormone and thyroid hormone have mixed effects on carbohydrate metabolism and may raise or lower blood glucose levels.

Fats: Catabolism and anabolism

The breaking up of triglycerides — *lipolysis* — yields fatty acids and glycerol. Beta-oxidation breaks down fatty acids into acetyl coenzyme A, which can then enter the citric acid cycle; glycerol can also undergo gluconeogenesis or enter the glycolytic pathways to produce energy. Conversely, *lipogenesis* is the chemical formation of fat from excess carbohydrates and proteins or from the fatty acids and glycerol products of lipolysis. Adipose tissue is the primary storage site for excess fat and thus is the greatest source of energy reserve. Certain unsaturated fatty acids are necessary for synthesis of vital body com-

ESSENTIAL NUTRIENTS AND THEIR FUNCTIONS

Nutrients are required for the body to work properly and avoid disease.

Nutrients	Functions
Carbohydrates	▪ Energy source
Fats and essential fatty acids	▪ Energy source; essential for growth, normal skin, and membranes
Proteins and amino acids	▪ Synthesis of all body proteins, growth, and tissue maintenance

Water-soluble vitamins:

▪ Ascorbic acid (C)	▪ Collagen synthesis, wound healing, antioxidation
▪ Thiamine (B_1)	▪ Coenzyme in carbohydrate metabolism
▪ Riboflavin (B_2)	▪ Coenzyme in energy metabolism
▪ Niacin	▪ Coenzyme in carbohydrate, fat, energy metabolism, and tissue metabolism
▪ Vitamin B_{12}	▪ Deoxyribonucleic acid (DNA) and ribonucleic acid synthesis; erythrocyte formation
▪ Folic acid	▪ Coenzyme in amino acid metabolism; heme and hemoglobin formation; DNA synthesis; lowering homocysteine levels

Fat-soluble vitamins:

▪ Vitamin A	▪ Vision in dim light, mucosal epithelium integrity, tooth development, endocrine function
▪ Vitamin D	▪ Regulation of calcium and phosphate absorption and metabolism; renal phosphate clearance
▪ Vitamin E	▪ Antioxidation; essential for muscle, liver, and red blood cell integrity
▪ Vitamin K	▪ Blood clotting (catalyzes synthesis of prothrombin by liver)

pounds. Because the body can't produce these essential fatty acids, they must be provided through diet. Insulin, hGH, catecholamines, corticotropin, and glucocorticoids control fat metabolism in an inverse relationship with carbohydrate metabolism; large amounts of carbohydrates promote fat storage, and deficiency of available carbohydrates promotes fat breakdown for energy needs.

Proteins: Anabolism

The primary process in protein metabolism is anabolism. Catabolism is relegated to a supporting role in protein metabolism—a reversal of the roles played by these two processes in carbohydrate and fat metabolisms. By synthesizing proteins—the tissue-building foods—the body derives substances essential for life (such as plasma proteins) and can reproduce, control cell growth, and repair itself. However, when carbohydrates or fats are unavailable as energy sources, or when energy demands are exceedingly high, protein catabolism converts protein into an available energy source. Protein metabolism consists of many processes, including:

▪ *Deamination:* a catabolic and energy-producing process occurring in the liver with the splitting off of the amino acid to form ammonia and a keto acid

▪ *Transamination:* anabolic conversion of keto acids to amino acids

▪ *Urea formation:* a catabolic process occurring in the liver, producing urea, the end product of protein catabolism.

The male hormone testosterone and hGH stimulate protein anabolism; corticotropin prompts secretion of glucocorticoids, which, in turn, facilitate protein catabolism. Normally, the rate of protein anabolism equals the rate of protein catabolism—a condition known as *nitrogen balance* (because ingested nitrogen equals nitrogen waste excreted in urine, feces, and sweat). When excessive catabolism causes the amount of nitrogen excreted to exceed the amount ingested, a state of *negative nitrogen balance* exists—usually the result of starvation and cachexia or surgical stress.

Fluid and electrolyte balance

A critical component of metabolism is fluid and electrolyte balance. Water is an essential body substance and constitutes almost 60% of an adult's body weight and more than 75% of a neonate's body weight. In both older and obese adults, the ratio of water to body weight drops; children and lean people have a higher proportion of water in their bodies.

Body fluids can be classified as intracellular (or cellular) or extracellular. Intracellular fluid constitutes about 40% of total body weight and 60% of all body fluid; it contains large quantities of potassium and phosphates but very little sodium and chloride. Conversely, extracellular fluid (ECF) contains mostly sodium and chloride but very little potassium and phosphates. Incorporating interstitial, cerebrospinal, intraocular, and GI fluids and plasma, ECF supplies cells with nutrients and other substances needed for cellular function. The many components of body fluids have the important function of preserving osmotic pressure and acid-base and anion-cation balance.

Homeostasis is a stable state—the equilibrium of chemical and physical properties of body fluid. Body fluids contain two kinds of dissolved substances: those that dissociate in solution (electrolytes) and those that don't. For example, glucose, when dissolved in water, doesn't break down into smaller particles; but sodium chloride dissociates in solution into sodium cations (+) and chloride anions (−). The composition of these electrolytes in body fluids is electrically balanced so the positively charged ions (cations: sodium, potassium, calcium, and magnesium) equal the negatively charged ions (anions: chloride, bicarbonate, sulfate, phosphate, proteinate, and carbonic and other organic acids). Although these particles are present in relatively low concentrations, any deviation from their normal levels can have profound physiologic effects.

ELDER TIP *Institutionalized older people are at particularly high risk for dehydration because of their diminished thirst perception and any combination of physical, cognitive, speech, mobility, and visual impairment.*

In homeostasis—an ever-changing but balanced state—water and electrolytes and other solutes move continually between cellular and extracellular compartments. Such motion is made possible by semipermeable membranes that allow diffusion, filtration, and active transport. Diffusion refers to the movement of particles or molecules from an area of greater concentration to one of lesser concentration. Normally, particles move randomly and constantly until the concentrations within given solutions are equal. Diffusion also depends on permeability, electrical gradient, and pressure gradient. Particles, however, can't diffuse against any of these gradients without energy and a carrier substance (active transport). ATP is released from cells to aid particles needing energy to pass through the cell membrane.

The diffusion of water from a solution of low concentration to one of high concentration is called osmosis. The pressure that develops when a selectively permeable cell membrane separates solutions of different strengths of concentrations is known as *osmotic pressure*, expressed in terms of osmols or milliosmols (mOsm). Osmotic activity is described in terms of *osmolality*—the osmotic pull exerted by all particles per unit of water, expressed in mOsm/kg of water—or *osmolarity*, when expressed in mOsm/L of solution.

The normal range of body fluid osmolality is 285 to 295 mOsm/kg. Solutions of 50 mOsm above or below the high and low points of this normal range exert little or no osmotic effect (isosmolality). A solution below 240 mOsm contains a lower particle concentration than plasma (hypo-osmolar) while a solution over 340 mOsm has a higher particle concentration than plasma (hyperosmolar).

Rapid I.V. administration of isosmolar solutions to patients who are debilitated, are very old or very young, or have cardiac or renal insufficiency could lead to ECF volume overload and induce pulmonary edema and heart failure because particulate concentration is the same as plasma, so fluid shifting into and out of cells will occur.

Continuous I.V. administration of hypo-osmolar solutions decreases serum osmolality and leads to excess intracellular fluid volume (water intoxication), whereas continuous I.V. administration of hyperosmolar solutions results in intracellular dehydration, increased serum osmolality and, eventually, ECF volume deficit due to excessive urinary excretion. These states occur because of fluid diffusion and the cell's attempt to balance the particulate concentrations inside and outside the cell.

Regulation of pH

Primarily through the complex chemical regulation of carbonic acid by the lungs and of base bicarbonate by the kidneys, the body maintains the hydrogen ion concentration to keep the ECF pH between 7.35 and 7.45. Nutritional deficiency or excess, disease, injury, or metabolic disturbance can interfere with normal homeostatic mechanisms and raise pH (acidosis) or lower it (alkalosis).

Assessing homeostasis

The goal of metabolism and homeostasis is to maintain the complex environment of ECF — the plasma — which nourishes and supports every body cell. This special environment is subject to multiple interlocking influences and readily reflects any disturbance in nutrition, chemical or fluid content, and osmotic pressure. Such disturbances can be detected by various laboratory tests. For example, measurements of albumin, prealbumin, and other blood proteins; electrolyte concentration; enzyme and antibody levels; and urine and blood chemistry levels (lipoproteins, glucose, blood urea nitrogen [BUN], creatinine, and creatinine-height index) accurately reflect the state of metabolism, homeostasis, and nutrition throughout the body. (See *Laboratory tests: Assessing nutritional status,* page 874.) Results of such laboratory tests, of course, supplement the information obtained from dietary history and physical examination — which offer gross clinical information about the quality, quantity, and efficiency of metabolic processes. To support clinical information, anthropometry, height-weight ratio, and skin-fold thickness determinations specifically define tissue nutritional status.

The following measures can help you maintain your patient's homeostasis:
- Obtain a complete dietary history and nutritional assessment to determine if carbohydrate, fat, protein, vitamin, mineral, and water intake are adequate for energy production and for tissue repair and growth. Remember that during periods of rapid tissue synthesis (growth, pregnancy, healing), protein needs increase.
- Consult a dietitian about any patient who may be malnourished because of malabsorption syndromes, renal or hepatic disease, clear-liquid diets, or who may possibly receive nothing by mouth for more than 5 days. Planned meals that provide adequate carbohydrates, fats, and protein are necessary for convalescence. Supplementary carbohydrates are often needed to spare protein and achieve a positive nitrogen balance.
- Accurately record intake and output to assess fluid balance (this includes intake of oral liquids or I.V. solutions, and urine, gastric, and stool output).
- Weigh the patient daily — at the same time, with the same-type clothing, and on the same scale. Remember, a weight loss of 2.2 lb (1 kg) is equivalent to the loss of 1 L of fluid.
- Observe the patient closely for insensible water or unmeasured fluid losses (such as through diaphoresis). Remember, fluid loss from the skin and lungs (normally 900 ml/day) can reach as high as 2,000 ml/day from hyperventilation or tachypnea, thus increasing insensible water losses.

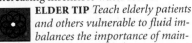 **ELDER TIP** *Teach elderly patients and others vulnerable to fluid imbalances the importance of maintaining adequate fluid intake.*

LABORATORY TESTS: ASSESSING NUTRITIONAL STATUS

Blood and urine tests provide the most precise data about nutritional status, often revealing nutritional problems before they're clinically apparent. The list below explains some common tests and what their results mean.

Serum vitamins and minerals
Vitamin and mineral deficiencies commonly screened for include A, B, B_{12}, folic acid, ascorbic acid, beta carotene, riboflavin and, sometimes, zinc, calcium, magnesium, iron, and other minerals.

Serum nutrients
Glucose levels help assess suspected diabetes or hypoglycemia. Cholesterol and triglyceride levels help differentiate the type of hyperlipoproteinemia.

Nitrogen balance
A negative nitrogen balance indicates inadequate intake of protein or calories.

Hemoglobin and hematocrit
Decreased levels can occur in protein-calorie malnutrition, iron deficiency, overhydration, hemorrhage, and hemolytic disease; elevated levels in dehydration, polycythemia, and folate and B_{12} deficiency.

Serum albumin
Reduced levels may indicate overhydration or visceral protein depletion because of GI disease, liver disease, or nephrotic syndrome. Elevated levels occur in dehydration.

Delayed hypersensitivity skin testing
One or more positive responses, in 24 to 48 hours, to intradermally injected common recall antigens indicates intact cell-mediated immunity. Negative, delayed, or absent response may indicate protein-calorie malnutrition but may also be seen in patients on steroids or with cancer, as well as patients with shock or sepsis.

Creatinine-height index (CHI)
This calculated value reflects muscle mass and estimates muscle protein depletion. Reduced CHI may indicate protein-calorie malnutrition or impaired renal function.

Serum prealbumin
This carrier protein for thyroxine is a sensitive indicator of visceral protein.

Total lymphocyte count
This provides an indication of immune status. Counts are low in malnutrition and acquired immunodeficiency syndrome.

■ Recognize I.V. solutions that are hyposmolar, such as 0.45% NaCl (half-normal saline solution). Isosmolar solutions include normal saline solution (0.9% NaCl), 5% dextrose in 0.2% NaCl, Ringer's solutions, and 5% dextrose in water. (The latter acts like a hypotonic solution because dextrose is quickly metabolized, leaving only free water.) Hyperosmolar solutions include 5% dextrose in normal saline solution, 10% dextrose in water, and 5% dextrose in Ringer's lactate solution.
■ When continuously administering hypoosmolar solutions, watch for signs of water intoxication: headaches, behavior changes (confusion or disorientation), nausea, vomiting, rising blood pressure, and falling pulse rate.
■ When continuously administering hyperosmolar solutions, be alert for signs of hypovolemia: thirst, dry mucous membranes, slightly falling blood pressure, rising pulse rate and respirations, low-grade fever (99° F [37.2° C]), and elevated hematocrit, hemoglobin, and BUN levels.
■ Administer fluid cautiously, especially to the patient with cardiopulmonary or renal disease, and watch for signs of overhydra-

tion: constant and irritating cough, dyspnea, moist crackles, rising central venous pressure, and pitting edema (late sign). When the patient is in an upright position, neck and hand vein engorgement is a sign of fluid overload.

 ELDER TIP *Many older patients take drugs to treat a variety of conditions. Remember that drugs can affect the patient's nutritional status by altering nutrient absorption, metabolism, utilization, or excretion. Likewise, various foods, beverages, and mineral or vitamin supplements can affect the absorption and effectiveness of drugs. Be aware of these potential interactions when evaluating the patient's medication regimen and nutritional status.*

NUTRITIONAL IMBALANCE

Vitamin A deficiency

A fat-soluble vitamin absorbed in the GI tract, vitamin A maintains epithelial tissue and retinal function. Consequently, deficiency of this vitamin may result in night blindness, decreased color adjustment, keratinization of epithelial tissue, and poor bone growth. Healthy adults have adequate vitamin A reserves to last up to a year; children often don't.

Causes and incidence

Vitamin A deficiency usually results from inadequate intake of foods high in vitamin A (liver, kidney, butter, milk, cream, cheese, and fortified margarine) or carotene, a precursor of vitamin A found in dark green leafy vegetables and yellow or orange fruits and vegetables. (Six mg of beta-carotene is equal to 1 mg of vitamin A.) The recommended daily allowance for vitamin A is 1 mg for adult males and 0.8 mg for adult females.

Less common causes include:
- malabsorption due to celiac disease, sprue, cirrhosis, obstructive jaundice, cystic fibrosis, giardiasis, or habitual use of mineral oil as a laxative

- massive urinary excretion caused by cancer, tuberculosis, pneumonia, nephritis, or urinary tract infection
- decreased storage and transport of vitamin A due to hepatic disease.

Each year, more than 80,000 people worldwide—mostly children in underdeveloped countries—lose their sight from severe vitamin A deficiency. This condition is rare in the United States, although many disadvantaged children have substandard levels of vitamin A. With therapy, the chance of reversing symptoms of night blindness and milder conjunctival changes is excellent. When corneal damage is present, emergency treatment is necessary.

Signs and symptoms

Typically, the first symptom of vitamin A deficiency is night blindness (nyctalopia), which usually becomes apparent when the patient enters a dark place or is caught in the glare of oncoming headlights while driving at night. This condition can progress to xerophthalmia, or drying of the conjunctivas, with development of gray plaques (Bitot's spots); if unchecked, perforation, scarring, and blindness may result. Keratinization of epithelial tissue causes dry, scaly skin; follicular hyperkeratosis; and shrinking and hardening of the mucous membranes, possibly leading to infections of the eyes and the respiratory or genitourinary tract. An infant with severe vitamin A deficiency shows signs of failure to thrive and apathy, along with dry skin and corneal changes, which can lead to ulceration and rapid destruction of the cornea.

Diagnosis

Dietary history and typical ocular lesions suggest vitamin A deficiency. Carotene levels less than 40 mcg/dl also suggest vitamin A deficiency, but they vary with seasonal ingestion of fruits and vegetables.

CONFIRMING DIAGNOSIS *A serum level of vitamin A that falls below 10 mcg/dl confirms the diagnosis. Levels between 10 and 19 mcg/dl are also considered low but the patient isn't likely to have developed significant symptoms.*

RECOMMENDED DAILY ALLOWANCE OF B-COMPLEX VITAMINS

Vitamin	Men (23 to 50)	Women (23 to 50)	Infants	Children (1 to 10)
B_1*	1.4 mg	1 mg	0.4 mg	0.7 to 1.2 mg
B_2*	1.6 mg	1.2 mg	0.5 mg	0.8 to 1.4 mg
Niacin*	18 mg	13 mg	5 to 8 mg	9 to 16 mg
B_6	2.2 mg	2 mg	0.4 mg	0.9 to 1.6 mg
B_{12}	3 mcg	3 mcg	0.3 mcg	2 to 3 mcg

*requirements per 1,000 kilocalories of dietary intake

Treatment

Mild conjunctival changes or night blindness requires vitamin A replacement in the form of cod liver oil or halibut liver oil. Acute deficiency requires aqueous vitamin A solution I.M., especially when corneal changes have occurred. Therapy for underlying biliary obstruction consists of administration of bile salts; for pancreatic insufficiency, pancreatin. Dry skin responds well to cream-based or petroleum-based products.

In patients with chronic malabsorption of fat-soluble vitamins, and in those with low dietary intake, prevention of vitamin A deficiency requires aqueous I.V. supplements or an oral water-miscible preparation.

Special considerations

■ Administer oral vitamin A supplements with or after meals or parenterally, as ordered. Watch for signs of hypercarotenemia (orange coloration of the skin and eyes) and hypervitaminosis A (rash, hair loss, anorexia, transient hydrocephalus, and vomiting in children; bone pain, hepatosplenomegaly, diplopia, and irritability in adults). If these signs occur, discontinue supplements and notify the physician immediately. (Hypercarotenemia is relatively harmless; hypervitaminosis A may be toxic.)

■ Because vitamin A deficiency usually results from dietary insufficiency, provide nutritional counseling. Tell the patient that vitamin A comes from animal sources, such as eggs, meat, milk, cheese, cream, liver, kidney, and cod and halibut fish oil, but that healthier choices, such as carrots, pumpkins, sweet potatoes, and most dark green, leafy vegetables are good sources of beta-carotene, vitamin A's precursor form. Instruct the patient that the more intense the color of a fruit or vegetable, the higher its beta-carotene content. Provide referrals to appropriate community agencies if necessary.

Vitamin B deficiencies

Vitamin B complex is a group of water-soluble vitamins essential to normal metabolism, cell growth, and blood formation. (See *Recommended daily allowance of B-complex vitamins.*) The most common deficiencies involve thiamine (B_1), riboflavin (B_2), niacin, pyridoxine (B_6), and cobalamin (B_{12}).

Causes and incidence

Thiamine deficiency results from malabsorption or inadequate dietary intake of vitamin B_1. It also results from alcoholism, prolonged diarrhea, or from increased requirement, which can occur in pregnancy, lactation, and hyperthyroidism. Beriberi, a serious thiamine-deficiency disease, is most prevalent in Asians, who subsist mainly on diets of unenriched rice and wheat. Although this disease is uncommon in the United States, alcoholics may develop cardiac (wet) beriberi with high-output heart failure, neuropathy, and cerebral disturbances. In times of stress (pregnancy, for example), malnourished young adults may develop beriberi; infantile beriberi may appear in infants on low-protein diets or in those breast-fed by thiamine-deficient mothers.

Riboflavin deficiency (ariboflavinosis) results from a diet deficient in milk, meat, fish, legumes, and green, leafy vegetables. Alcoholism or prolonged diarrhea may also induce riboflavin deficiency. Exposure of milk to sunlight or treatment of legumes with baking soda can destroy riboflavin.

Niacin deficiency, in its advanced form, produces pellagra, which affects the skin, central nervous system (CNS), and GI tract. (See *Recognizing pellagra*.) Although this deficiency is now seldom found in the United States, it was once common among Southerners who subsisted mainly on corn and consumed minimal animal protein. (Corn is low in niacin and in available tryptophan, the amino acid from which the body synthesizes niacin.) Niacin deficiency is still common in parts of Egypt, Romania, Africa, Serbia, and Montenegro, where corn is the dominant staple food. Niacin deficiency can also occur secondary to carcinoid syndrome or Hartnup disease.

Pyridoxine deficiency usually results from destruction of pyridoxine in infant formulas by autoclaving. A frank deficiency is uncommon in adults, except in patients taking pyridoxine antagonists, such as isoniazid and penicillamine.

Cobalamin deficiency most commonly results from an absence of intrinsic factor in gastric secretions, or an absence of receptor sites after ileal resection. Other causes include malabsorption syndromes associated with sprue, intestinal worm infestation, regional ileitis, and gluten enteropathy, and a diet low in animal protein.

RECOGNIZING PELLAGRA

This patient with pellagra shows dark, scaly, advanced dermatitis. In advanced niacin deficiency, such dermatitis usually occurs on areas exposed to the sun.

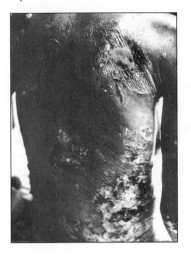

Signs and symptoms

Thiamine deficiency causes polyneuritis and, possibly, Wernicke's encephalopathy and Korsakoff's psychosis. In infants (infantile beriberi), this deficiency produces edema, irritability, abdominal pain, pallor, vomiting, loss of voice and, possibly, seizures. In wet beriberi, severe edema starts in the legs and moves up through the body; dry beriberi causes multiple neurologic symptoms and an emaciated appearance. Thiamine deficiency may also cause cardiomegaly, palpitations, tachycardia, dyspnea, and circulatory collapse. Constipation and indigestion are common; ataxia, nystagmus, and ophthalmoplegia are also possible.

Riboflavin deficiency characteristically causes cheilosis (cracking of the lips and corners of the mouth), sore throat, and glossitis. It may also cause seborrheic dermatitis in the nasolabial folds, scrotum, and vulva and, possibly, generalized dermatitis involving the arms, legs, and trunk.

This deficiency can also affect the eyes, producing burning, itching, light sensitivity, tearing, and vascularization of the corneas. Late-stage riboflavin deficiency causes neuropathy, mild anemia and, in children, growth retardation.

Niacin deficiency in its early stages produces fatigue, anorexia, muscle weakness, headache, indigestion, mild skin eruptions, weight loss, and backache. In advanced stages (pellagra), it produces dark, scaly dermatitis, especially on exposed body parts, that makes the patient appear to be severely sunburned. The mouth, tongue, and lips become red and sore, which may interfere with eating. Common GI symptoms include nausea, vomiting, and diarrhea. Associated CNS aberrations—confusion, disorientation, and neuritis—may become severe enough to induce hallucinations and paranoia. Because of this triad of symptoms, pellagra is sometimes called a "3-D" syndrome—dementia, dermatitis, and diarrhea. If not reversed by therapeutic doses of niacin, pellagra can be fatal.

Pyridoxine deficiency in infants causes a wide range of symptoms: dermatitis, occasional cheilosis or glossitis unresponsive to riboflavin therapy, abdominal pain, vomiting, ataxia, and seizures. This deficiency can also lead to CNS disturbances.

Cobalamin deficiency causes pernicious anemia, which produces anorexia, weight loss, abdominal discomfort, constipation, diarrhea, and glossitis; peripheral neuropathy; and, possibly, ataxia, spasticity, and hyperreflexia.

Diagnosis

The following values confirm vitamin B deficiency:

- Thiamine deficiency: commonly measured as micrograms per deciliter in a 24-hour urine collection. Deficiency levels are age-related: 1 to 3 years, less than 120; 4 to 6 years, less than 85; 7 to 9 years, less than 70; 10 to12 years, less than 60; 13 to 15 years, less than 50; adults, less than 27; pregnant women, less than 23 (second trimester), less than 21 (third trimester).
- Riboflavin deficiency: measured as micrograms per gram of creatinine in a 24-hour urine collection. Deficiency levels are age-related: 1 to 3 years, less than 150; 4 to

6 years, less than 100; 7 to 9 years, less than 85; 10 to 15 years, less than 70; adults, less than 27; pregnant women, less than 39 (second trimester); less than 30 (third trimester).

- Niacin deficiency: measured by N-methyl nicotinamide in a 24-hour urine collection as micrograms per gram of creatinine. Deficiency levels are: adults, less than 0.5; first trimester of pregnancy, less than 0.5; second trimester, less than 0.6; third trimester, less than 0.8.
- Pyridoxine deficiency: xanthurenic acid more than 50 mg/day in 24-hour urine collection after administration of 10 g of L-tryptophan; decreased levels of serum and red blood cell transaminases; reduced excretion of pyridoxic acid in urine.
- Cobalamin deficiency: cobalamin serum levels less than 150 pg/ml. Tests to discover the deficiency's cause include gastric analysis and hemoglobin studies. In addition, the Schilling test measures absorption of radioactive cobalamin with and without intrinsic factor.

Treatment

Diet and supplementary vitamins can correct or prevent vitamin B deficiencies, as follows:

- Thiamine deficiency: a high-protein diet, with adequate calorie intake, possibly supplemented by B-complex vitamins for early symptoms. Thiamine-rich foods include pork, peas, wheat bran, oatmeal, and liver. Alcoholic beriberi may require thiamine supplements or thiamine hydrochloride as part of a B-complex concentrate.
- Riboflavin deficiency: supplemental riboflavin in patients with intractable diarrhea or increased need for riboflavin related to growth, pregnancy, lactation, or wound healing. Good sources of riboflavin are meats, enriched flour, milk and dairy products, green, leafy vegetables, eggs, and cereal. Acute riboflavin deficiency requires daily oral doses of riboflavin alone or with other B-complex vitamins. Riboflavin phosphate can also be administered I.V. or I.M.
- Niacin deficiency: supplemental B-complex vitamins and dietary enrichment in patients at risk because of marginal diets or alcoholism. Meats, fish, peanuts, brew-

er's yeast, enriched breads, and cereals are rich in niacin; milk and eggs, in tryptophan. Confirmed niacin deficiency requires daily doses of niacinamide orally or I.V.

■ Pyridoxine deficiency: prophylactic pyridoxine therapy in infants and in children with a seizure disorder; supplemental B-complex vitamins in patients with anorexia, malabsorption, or those taking isoniazid or penicillamine. Some women who take hormonal contraceptives may have to supplement their diets with pyridoxine. Confirmed pyridoxine deficiencies require oral or parenteral pyridoxine. Children with convulsive seizures stemming from metabolic dysfunction may require daily doses of 200 to 600 mg pyridoxine.

■ Cobalamin deficiency: parenteral cobalamin in patients with reduced gastric secretion of hydrochloric acid, lack of intrinsic factor, some malabsorption syndromes, or ileum resections. Strict vegetarians may have to supplement their diets with oral vitamin B_{12}. Depending on the deficiency's severity, supplementary cyanocobalamin is usually given parenterally for 5 to 10 days, followed by monthly or daily vitamin B_{12} supplements.

Special considerations
An accurate dietary history provides a baseline for effective dietary counseling.
■ Identify and observe patients who are at risk for vitamin B deficiencies — alcoholics, the elderly, pregnant women, and people on limited diets.
■ Administer prescribed supplements. Make sure patients understand how important it is that they adhere strictly to their prescribed treatment for the rest of their lives. Watch for adverse effects from large doses of niacinamide, such as a flushed sensation or hot flashes, in patients with niacin deficiency. Remember, prolonged intake of niacin can cause hepatic dysfunction. Caution patients with Parkinson's disease receiving pyridoxine that this drug can impair response to levodopa therapy.
■ Explain all tests and procedures. Reassure patients that, with treatment, the prognosis is good. Refer patients to appropriate assistance agencies if their diets are inadequate due to adverse socioeconomic conditions.

Vitamin C deficiency

Vitamin C (ascorbic acid) deficiency leads to scurvy or inadequate production of collagen, an extracellular substance that binds the cells of the teeth, bones, and capillaries. It's essential for wound healing and burn recovery. Vitamin C is also an important factor in metabolizing such amino acids as tyrosine and phenylalanine. It also acts as a reductant, activating enzymes in the body, as well as converting folic acid into useful components.

Severe vitamin C deficiency results in scurvy, evident by hemorrhagic tendencies and abnormal osteoid and dentin formation.

Causes and incidence
This deficiency's primary cause is a diet lacking in vitamin C-rich foods, such as citrus fruits, tomatoes, cabbage, broccoli, spinach, and berries. Because the body can't store this water-soluble vitamin in large amounts, the supply needs to be replenished daily. Other causes include:
■ destruction of vitamin C in foods by overexposure to air or by overcooking
■ excessive ingestion of vitamin C during pregnancy, which causes the neonate to require large amounts of the vitamin after birth
■ marginal intake of vitamin C during periods of physiologic stress — caused by infectious disease, for example — which can deplete tissue saturation of vitamin C.

Historically common among sailors and others deprived of fresh fruits and vegetables for long periods of time, vitamin C deficiency is uncommon today in the United States, except in alcoholics, people on restricted-residue diets, and infants weaned from breast milk to cow's milk without a vitamin C supplement.

Signs and symptoms
Clinical features of vitamin C deficiency appear as capillaries become increasingly fragile. In an adult, it produces petechiae, ecchymoses, follicular hyperkeratosis (es-

SCURVY'S EFFECT ON GUMS AND LEGS

In adults, scurvy causes swollen or bleeding gums and loose teeth.

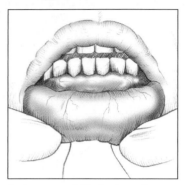

It also causes follicular hyperkeratosis, usually on the legs.

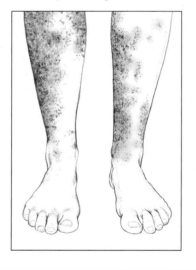

cal disturbances as irritability, depression, hysteria, and hypochondriasis.

In a child, vitamin C deficiency produces tender, painful swelling in the legs, causing the child to lie with his legs partially flexed. Other symptoms include fever, diarrhea, and vomiting.

Diagnosis

 CONFIRMING DIAGNOSIS *Serum ascorbic acid levels less than 0.2 mg/ dl and white blood cell ascorbic acid levels less than 30 mg/dl help confirm the diagnosis.*

Dietary history revealing an inadequate intake of ascorbic acid suggests vitamin C deficiency. A capillary fragility test may be performed on the patient's forearm with a blood pressure cuff; it's positive if more than 10 petechiae form after 5 minutes of pressure.

Treatment

Because scurvy is potentially fatal, treatment begins immediately to restore adequate vitamin C intake by daily doses of 100 to 200 mg vitamin C in synthetic form or in orange juice in mild disease and by doses as high as 500 mg/day in severe disease. Symptoms usually subside in 2 to 3 days; hemorrhages and bone disorders, in 2 to 3 weeks.

To prevent vitamin C deficiency, patients unable or unwilling to consume foods rich in vitamin C or those facing surgery should take daily supplements of ascorbic acid. The recommended daily allowance is 60 mg/day. Vitamin C supplementation may also prevent this deficiency in recently weaned infants or those drinking formula not fortified with vitamin C.

Special considerations

■ Administer ascorbic acid orally or by slow I.V. infusion, as ordered. Avoid moving the patient unnecessarily, to avoid irritating painful joints and muscles. Encourage him to drink orange juice.
■ Explain the importance of supplemental ascorbic acid. Counsel the patient and his family about good dietary sources of vitamin C.
■ Advise against taking too much vitamin C. Explain that excessive doses of ascorbic

pecially on the buttocks and legs), anemia, anorexia, limb and joint pain (especially in the knees), pallor, weakness, swollen or bleeding gums, loose teeth, lethargy, insomnia, poor wound healing, and ocular hemorrhages in the bulbar conjunctivae. (See *Scurvy's effect on gums and legs.*) Vitamin C deficiency can also cause beading, fractures of the costochondral junctions of the ribs or epiphysis, and such psychologi-

acid may cause nausea, diarrhea, and renal calculi formation and may also interfere with anticoagulant therapy.

Vitamin D deficiency

Vitamin D deficiency, commonly called *rickets,* causes failure of normal bone calcification, which occurs through several mechanisms: decreased calcium and phosphorus (the major components of bone) from the intestines, increased excretion of calcium from renal tubules, and increased parathyroid secretion resulting in increased release of calcium from the bone. The deficiency results in rickets in infants and young children and osteomalacia in adults. With treatment, the prognosis is good. However, in rickets, bone deformities usually persist, while in osteomalacia, such deformities may disappear.

Causes and incidence

Vitamin D deficiency results from inadequate dietary intake of preformed vitamin D, malabsorption of vitamin D, or too little exposure to sunlight.

Once a common childhood disease, rickets is now rare in the United States but occasionally appears in breast-fed infants who don't receive a vitamin D supplement or in infants receiving a formula with a nonfortified milk base. This deficiency may also occur in overcrowded urban areas in which smog limits sunlight penetration. Incidence is highest in black children who, because of their skin color, absorb less sunlight. (Solar ultraviolet rays irradiate 7-dehydrocholesterol, a precursor of vitamin D, to form calciferol.)

Osteomalacia, also uncommon in the United States, is most prevalent in Asia, among young multiparas who eat a cereal diet and have minimal exposure to sunlight. Other causes include:

■ vitamin D–resistant rickets (refractory rickets, familial hypophosphatemia) from an inherited impairment of renal tubular reabsorption of phosphate (from vitamin D insensitivity)

■ conditions that lower absorption of fat-soluble vitamin D, such as chronic pancreatitis, celiac disease, Crohn's disease, cystic

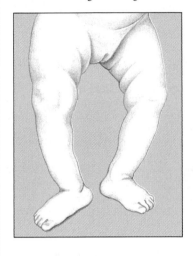

RECOGNIZING BOWLEGS

This infant with rickets shows characteristic bowing of the legs.

fibrosis, gastric or small bowel resections, fistulas, colitis, and biliary obstruction

■ hepatic or renal disease, which interferes with the formation of hydroxylated calciferol, necessary to initiate the formation of a calcium-binding protein in intestinal absorption sites

■ malfunctioning parathyroid gland (decreased secretion of parathyroid hormone), which contributes to calcium deficiency (normally, vitamin D controls calcium and phosphorus absorption through the intestine) and interferes with activation of vitamin D in the kidneys.

Signs and symptoms

Early indications of vitamin D deficiency are profuse sweating, restlessness, and irritability. Chronic deficiency induces numerous bone malformations due to softening of the bones: bowlegs, knock-knees, rachitic rosary (beading of ends of ribs), enlargement of wrists and ankles, pigeon breast, delayed closing of the fontanels, softening of the skull, and bulging of the forehead. (See *Recognizing bowlegs.*)

Other rachitic features are poorly developed muscles (potbelly) and infantile tetany. Bone deformities may cause difficulty in walking and in climbing stairs, spontaneous multiple fractures, and lower back and leg pain.

Diagnosis

Physical examination, dietary history, and laboratory tests establish the diagnosis. Test results that suggest vitamin D deficiency include plasma calcium serum levels less than 7.5 mg/dl, serum inorganic phosphorus levels less than 3 mg/dl, serum citrate levels less than 2.5 mg/dl, and alkaline phosphatase levels less than 4 Bodansky units/dl.

CONFIRMING DIAGNOSIS *X-rays confirm the diagnosis by showing characteristic bone deformities and abnormalities such as Looser's zones (pseudofractures).*

Treatment

For osteomalacia and rickets — except when caused by malabsorption — treatment consists of oral doses of vitamin D or sources such as fish, liver, and processed milk. Exposure to sunlight is encouraged. For rickets refractory to vitamin D or in rickets accompanied by hepatic or renal disease, treatment includes 25-hydroxycholecalciferol, 1, 25-dihydroxycholecalciferol, or a synthetic analogue of active vitamin D. Replacement of deficient calcium and phosphorus also helps to eliminate most symptoms of rickets. Positioning or bracing may be used to reduce or prevent deformities; some skeletal deformities may require corrective surgery.

Special considerations

■ Obtain a dietary history to assess the patient's current vitamin D intake. Encourage him to eat foods high in vitamin D — fortified milk, fish liver oils, herring, liver, and egg yolks — and get sufficient sun exposure. If deficiency is due to socioeconomic conditions, refer the patient to appropriate community agencies.

■ If the patient must take vitamin D for a prolonged period, tell him to watch for signs of vitamin D toxicity (headache, nausea, constipation and, after prolonged use, renal calculi).

■ To prevent rickets, administer supplementary aqueous preparations of vitamin D for chronic fat malabsorption, hydroxylated cholecalciferol for refractory rickets, and supplemental vitamin D for breast-fed infants.

■ Consider genetic counseling for a patient with a family history of inherited disorders that can cause rickets.

Vitamin E deficiency

Vitamin E (tocopherol) appears to act primarily as an antioxidant, preventing intracellular oxidation of polyunsaturated fatty acids and other lipids. It protects body tissue from damage caused by unstable substances called free radicals, which can harm cells, tissues, and organs and are believed to be one of the causes of aging's degenerative process. Vitamin E is also important in the formation of red blood cells (RBCs) and helps the body to use vitamin K. Vitamin E deficiency usually manifests as hemolytic anemia in low-birth-weight or premature neonates. With treatment, prognosis is good.

Causes and incidence

Vitamin E deficiency in infants usually results from consuming formulas high in polyunsaturated fatty acids that are fortified with iron but not vitamin E. Such formulas increase the need for antioxidant vitamin E because the iron supplement catalyzes the oxidation of RBC lipids. A neonate has low tissue concentrations of vitamin E to begin with because only a small amount passes through the placenta; the mother retains most of it. Because vitamin E is a fat-soluble vitamin, deficiency develops in conditions associated with fat malabsorption, such as kwashiorkor, celiac disease, or cystic fibrosis. These conditions may induce megaloblastic or hemolytic anemia and creatinuria, all of which are reversible with vitamin E administration.

Vitamin E deficiency is uncommon in adults but is possible in people whose diets are high in polyunsaturated fatty acids, which increase vitamin E requirements, and in people with vitamin E malabsorption, which impairs RBC survival.

Signs and symptoms

Vitamin E deficiency is difficult to recognize, but its early symptoms include edema and skin lesions in infants and muscle weakness or intermittent claudication in adults. In premature neonates, vitamin E deficiency produces hemolytic anemia, thrombocythemia, and erythematous papular skin eruption, followed by desquamation.

Diagnosis

 CONFIRMING DIAGNOSIS *Dietary and medical histories suggest vitamin E deficiency. Serum alpha-tocopherol levels below 0.5 mg/dl in adults and below 0.2 mg/dl in infants confirm it. Creatinuria, increased creatine kinase levels, hemolytic anemia, and an elevated platelet count generally support the diagnosis.*

Treatment

Replacement of vitamin E with a water-soluble supplement, either oral or parenteral, is the only appropriate treatment.

Special considerations

■ As ordered, prevent deficiency by providing vitamin E supplements for low-birth-weight neonates receiving formulas not fortified with vitamin E and for adults with vitamin E malabsorption. Many commercial multivitamin supplements are easily absorbed by patients with vitamin E malabsorption.

■ Inform new mothers who plan to breast-feed that human milk provides adequate vitamin E.

■ Encourage adult patients to eat foods high in vitamin E; good sources include vegetable oils (corn, safflower, soybean, cottonseed); whole grains; dark green, leafy vegetables; nuts; and legumes. Tell them that heavy consumption of polyunsaturated fatty acids increases the need for vitamin E.

■ If vitamin E deficiency is related to socioeconomic conditions, refer the patient to appropriate community agencies.

Vitamin K deficiency

Deficiency of vitamin K, an element necessary for formation of prothrombin and other clotting factors in the liver, produces abnormal bleeding. If the deficiency is corrected, the prognosis is excellent.

Causes

Vitamin K deficiency is common among neonates in the first few days postpartum due to poor placental transfer of vitamin K and inadequate production of vitamin K-producing intestinal flora. Its other causes include prolonged use of drugs, such as the anticoagulant warfarin and antibiotics that destroy normal intestinal bacteria; decreased flow of bile to the small intestine from obstruction of the bile duct or bile fistula; malabsorption of vitamin K due to sprue, pellagra, bowel resection, ileitis, or ulcerative colitis; chronic hepatic disease, with impaired response of hepatic ribosomes to vitamin K; and cystic fibrosis, with fat malabsorption. Vitamin K deficiency seldom results from insufficient dietary intake of this vitamin.

Signs and symptoms

The cardinal sign of vitamin K deficiency is an abnormal bleeding tendency, accompanied by prolonged prothrombin time (PT); these signs disappear with vitamin K administration. Without treatment, bleeding may be severe and, possibly, fatal.

Diagnosis

 CONFIRMING DIAGNOSIS *A PT that's 25% longer than the normal range of 10 to 20 seconds, measured by the Quick method, confirms the diagnosis of vitamin K deficiency after other causes of prolonged PT (such as anticoagulant therapy or hepatic disease) have been ruled out. The International Normalized Ratio (normal value, 0.8 to 1.2) is the more common method of assessing PT adequacy.*

Repetition of testing in 24 hours (and regularly during treatment) monitors the therapy's effectiveness.

Treatment

Administration of vitamin K I.V. or I.M. corrects abnormal bleeding tendencies.

IMPORTANT FACTS ABOUT VITAMINS A AND D

This table illustrates good sources of vitamins A and D, their recommended daily allowances, and the actions they produce.

Vitamin	Sources	Recommended dietary allowance	Action
Vitamin A	▪ Carrots; sweet potatoes; dark green, leafy vegetables; butter; margarine; liver; egg yolk	▪ Children: 1,400 IU ▪ Adults: 4,000 to 5,000 IU ▪ Lactating women: 6,000 IU	▪ Produces retinal pigment and maintains epithelial tissue
Vitamin D	▪ Ultraviolet light; fortified foods (especially milk)	▪ 400 IU daily	▪ Promotes absorption and regulates metabolism of calcium and phosphorus

---

Special considerations

To prevent vitamin K deficiency:
▪ Administer vitamin K to neonates and patients with fat malabsorption or with prolonged diarrhea due to colitis, ileitis, or long-term antibiotic drug therapy.
▪ Warn against self-medication with or overuse of antibiotics, because these drugs destroy the intestinal bacteria necessary to generate significant amounts of vitamin K.
▪ If the deficiency has a dietary cause, help the patient and his family plan a diet that includes important sources of vitamin K, such as cauliflower, tomatoes, cheese, egg yolks, liver, and green, leafy vegetables.

Hypervitaminoses A and D

Hypervitaminosis A is excessive accumulation of vitamin A; hypervitaminosis D, of vitamin D. Although these are toxic conditions, they usually respond well to treatment. They're most prevalent in infants and children, usually as a result of accidental or misguided overdosage by parents. A related, benign condition called hypercarotenemia results from excessive consumption of carotene, a chemical precursor of vitamin A.

Causes

Vitamins A and D are fat-soluble vitamins that accumulate in the body because they aren't dissolved and excreted in the urine. (See *Important facts about vitamins A and D.*) In most cases, hypervitaminoses A and D result from ingestion of excessive amounts of supplemental vitamin preparations. A single dose of more than 1 million units of vitamin A can cause acute toxicity; daily doses of 15,000 to 25,000 units taken over weeks or months have proven toxic in infants and children. For the same dose to produce toxicity in adults, ingestion over years is necessary. Chronic ingestion of only 1,600 to 2,000 IU daily of vitamin D is sufficient to cause toxicity.

Hypervitaminosis A may occur in patients receiving pharmacologic doses of vitamin A for dermatologic disorders. Hypervitaminosis D may occur in patients receiving high doses of the vitamin as treatment for hypoparathyroidism, rickets, and the osteodystrophy of chronic renal failure, and in infants who consume fortified milk and cereals plus a vitamin supplement. Concentrations of vitamin A in common foods are generally too low to pose a danger of excessive intake. However, a benign condition called *hypercarotenemia* results from excessive consumption of vegetables high in carotene (a protovitamin that the body converts into vitamin A), such as carrots, sweet potatoes, and dark green, leafy vegetables.

Signs and symptoms

Chronic hypervitaminosis A produces anorexia, irritability, headache, hair loss, malaise, itching, vertigo, bone pain, bone fragility, and dry, peeling skin. It may also cause hepatosplenomegaly and emotional lability. Acute toxicity may also produce transient hydrocephalus and vomiting. (Hypercarotenemia produces yellow or orange skin coloration.)

Hypervitaminosis D causes anorexia, headache, nausea, vomiting, weight loss, polyuria, and polydipsia. Because vitamin D promotes calcium absorption, severe toxicity can lead to hypercalcemia, including calcification of soft tissues, as in the heart, aorta, and renal tubules. Lethargy, confusion, and coma may accompany severe hypercalcemia.

Diagnosis

A thorough patient history suggests hypervitaminosis A.

 CONFIRMING DIAGNOSIS *An elevated serum vitamin A level (over 90 mcg/dl) confirms hypervitaminosis A.*

Patient history and an elevated serum calcium level (over 10.5 mcg/dl) suggest hypervitaminosis D.

 CONFIRMING DIAGNOSIS *An elevated serum vitamin D level confirms hypervitaminosis D.*

In children, X-rays showing calcification of tendons, ligaments, and subperiosteal tissues support this diagnosis.

 CONFIRMING DIAGNOSIS *An elevated serum carotene level (over 250 mcg/dl) confirms hypercarotenemia.*

Treatment

Withholding vitamin supplements usually corrects hypervitaminosis A quickly and hypervitaminosis D gradually. Hypercalcemia may persist for weeks or months after the patient stops taking vitamin D. Treatment for severe hypervitaminosis D may include glucocorticoids to control hy-

percalcemia and prevent renal damage. In the acute stage, diuretics or other emergency measures for severe hypercalcemia may be necessary. Hypercarotenemia responds well to a diet free of high-carotene foods.

Special considerations

- Keep the patient comfortable, and reassure him that symptoms will subside after he stops taking the vitamin.
- Make sure the patient or the parents of a child with these conditions understand that vitamins aren't innocuous. Explain the hazards associated with excessive vitamin intake. Point out that vitamin A and D requirements can easily be met with a diet containing dark green, leafy vegetables; fruits; and fortified milk or milk products.
- To prevent hypervitaminosis A or D, monitor serum vitamin A levels in patients receiving doses above the recommended daily allowance and serum calcium levels in patients receiving pharmacologic doses of vitamin D.

Iodine deficiency

Iodine deficiency is the absence of sufficient levels of iodine to satisfy daily metabolic requirements. Because the thyroid gland uses most of the body's iodine stores, iodine deficiency is apt to cause hypothyroidism and thyroid gland hypertrophy (endemic goiter). Other effects of deficiency range from dental caries to cretinism in neonates born to iodine-deficient mothers. Iodine deficiency is most common in pregnant or lactating women due to their exaggerated metabolic need for this element. Iodine deficiency responds readily to treatment with iodine supplements.

Causes

Iodine deficiency usually results from insufficient intake of dietary sources of iodine, such as iodized table salt, seafood, and dark green, leafy vegetables. (Normal iodine requirements range from 35 mcg/day for infants to 150 mcg/day for lactating women; the average adult needs 1 mcg/kg of body weight.) Iodine deficiency may also result from an increase in metabolic demands during pregnancy, lactation, and adolescence.

Signs and symptoms

Clinical features of iodine deficiency depend on the degree of hypothyroidism that develops (in addition to the development of a goiter). Mild deficiency may produce only mild, nonspecific symptoms, such as lassitude, fatigue, and loss of motivation. Severe deficiency usually generates the typically overt and unmistakable features of hypothyroidism: bradycardia; decreased pulse pressure and cardiac output; weakness; hoarseness; dry, flaky, inelastic skin; puffy face; thick tongue; delayed relaxation phase in deep tendon reflexes; poor memory; hearing loss; chills; anorexia; and nystagmus. In women, iodine deficiency may also cause menorrhagia and amenorrhea.

Cretinism — hypothyroidism that develops in utero or in early infancy — is characterized by failure to thrive, neonatal jaundice, and hypothermia. By age 3 to 6 months, the infant may display spastic diplegia and signs and symptoms similar to those seen in infants with Down syndrome.

Diagnosis

CONFIRMING DIAGNOSIS
Abnormal laboratory test results include low thyroxine (T_4) levels with high radioactive iodine (^{131}I) uptake, low 24-hour urine iodine levels, and high thyroid-stimulating hormone levels. Radioiodine uptake test traces ^{131}I in the thyroid 24 hours after administration; triiodothyronine-resin or T_4-resin uptake test shows values 25% below normal.

Treatment

Severe iodine deficiency requires administration of iodine supplements (potassium iodide [SSKI]). Mild deficiency may be corrected by increasing iodine intake through the use of iodized table salt and consumption of iodine-rich foods (seafood and green, leafy vegetables).

Special considerations

■ Administer SSKI preparation in milk or juice to reduce gastric irritation and mask its metallic taste. To prevent tooth discoloration, tell the patient to drink the solution through a straw. Store the solution in a light-resistant container.

■ To prevent iodine deficiency, recommend the use of iodized salt and consumption of iodine-rich foods for high-risk patients — especially adolescents and pregnant or lactating women.

■ Advise pregnant women that severe iodine deficiency may produce cretinism in neonates, and instruct them to watch for early signs of iodine deficiency, such as fatigue, lassitude, weakness, and decreased mental function.

Zinc deficiency

Zinc, an essential trace element that's present in the bones, teeth, hair, skin, testes, liver, and muscles, is also a vital component of many enzymes. Zinc promotes synthesis of deoxyribonucleic acid, ribonucleic acid and, ultimately, protein, and maintains normal blood concentrations of vitamin A by mobilizing it from the liver. The prognosis is good with correction of the deficiency.

Causes and incidence

Zinc deficiency usually results from excessive intake of foods (containing iron, calcium, vitamin D, and the fiber and phytates in cereals) that bind zinc to form insoluble chelates that prevent its absorption. Occasionally, it results from blood loss due to parasitism and low intake of foods containing zinc. Alcohol and corticosteroids increase renal excretion of zinc.

Zinc deficiency is most common in people from underdeveloped countries, especially in the Middle East. Children are most susceptible to this deficiency during periods of rapid growth.

Signs and symptoms

Zinc deficiency produces hepatosplenomegaly, sparse hair growth, soft and misshapen nails, poor wound healing, anorexia, hypogeusesthesia (decreased taste acuity), dysgeusia (unpleasant taste), hyposmia (decreased odor acuity), dysosmia (unpleasant odor in nasopharynx), severe iron deficiency anemia, bone deformities and, when chronic, hypogonadism, dwarfism, and hyperpigmentation.

Diagnosis

 CONFIRMING DIAGNOSIS *Fasting serum zinc levels below 70 mcg/ dl confirm zinc deficiency and indicate altered phosphate metabolism, imbalance between aerobic and anaerobic metabolism, and decreased pancreatic enzyme levels.*

Treatment

Treatment consists of correcting the deficiency's underlying cause and administering zinc supplements, as necessary.

Special considerations

■ Advise the patient to take zinc supplements with milk or meals to prevent gastric distress and vomiting.

■ To prevent zinc deficiency, encourage a balanced diet that includes seafood, oatmeal, bran, meat, eggs, nuts, and dry yeast and the correct use of calcium and iron supplements.

Obesity

Obesity is an excess of body fat, generally 20% above ideal body weight. The prognosis for correction of obesity is poor: Fewer than 30% of patients succeed in losing 20 lb (9 kg), and only half of these maintain the loss over a prolonged period.

Causes and incidence

Obesity results from excessive calorie intake and inadequate expenditure of energy. Theories to explain this condition include hypothalamic dysfunction of hunger and satiety centers, genetic predisposition, abnormal absorption of nutrients, and impaired action of GI and growth hormones and of hormonal regulators such as insulin. An inverse relationship between socioeconomic status and the prevalence of obesity has been documented, especially in women. Obesity in parents increases the probability of obesity in children, from genetic or environmental factors, such as activity levels and learned patterns of eating. Psychological factors, such as stress or emotional eating, may also contribute to obesity. Rates of obesity are climbing, and the percentage of children and adolescents who are obese has doubled in the last 20 years.

Diagnosis

Observation and comparison of height and weight to a standard table indicate obesity. Measurement of the thickness of subcutaneous fat folds with calipers provides an approximation of total body fat. Although this measurement is reliable and isn't subject to daily fluctuations, it has little meaning for the patient in monitoring subsequent weight loss. Obesity may lead to serious complications, such as respiratory difficulties, hypertension, cardiovascular disease, diabetes mellitus, renal disease, gallbladder disease, psychosocial difficulties, and premature death.

Treatment

Successful management of obesity must decrease the patient's daily calorie intake while increasing his activity level. Effective treatment must be based on a balanced, low-calorie diet that eliminates foods high in fat or sugar. Lifelong maintenance of these improved eating and exercise patterns is necessary to achieve long-term benefits.

The popular low-carbohydrate diets offer no long-term advantage; rapid early weight reduction is due to loss of water, not fat. These and other crash or fad diets have the overwhelming drawback that they don't teach the patient long-term modification of eating patterns and often lead to the "yo-yo syndrome" — episodes of repeated weight loss followed by weight gain. This can be more detrimental than the obesity itself because of the severe stress it can place on the body.

Total fasting is an effective method of rapid weight reduction but requires close monitoring and supervision to minimize risks of ketonemia, electrolyte imbalance, hypotension, and loss of lean body mass. Prolonged fasting and very-low-calorie diets have been associated with sudden death, possibly resulting from cardiac arrhythmias caused by electrolyte abnormalities. These methods also neglect patient re-education, which is necessary for long-term weight maintenance.

Treatment may also include hypnosis and behavior modification techniques, which promote fundamental changes in eating habits and activity patterns. In addition, psychotherapy may be beneficial for some patients, because weight reduction may lead to depression or even psychosis. Antidepressants are also helpful in weight loss.

Amphetamines and amphetamine congeners have been used to enhance compliance with a prescribed diet by temporarily suppressing the appetite and creating a feeling of well-being. However, because their value in long-term weight control is questionable, and they have significant potential for dependence and abuse, their use is generally avoided. If these drugs are used at all, they should be prescribed only for short-term therapy and should be monitored carefully.

The drug combination known as *fen-phen* (fenfluramine and phentermine) had been touted as an effective method of suppressing appetite. However, after researchers linked the drug combination to potentially fatal heart valve disease, fenfluramine was withdrawn from the market in September 1997. Phentermine wasn't withdrawn but physicians are no longer allowed to combine the two drugs.

As a last resort, morbid obesity, which is indicated by body weight that's 50% to 100% higher than ideal, body weight that's 100 pounds higher than ideal, or a body mass index greater than 39, may be treated surgically with a variety of restrictive procedures. The two most popular bariatric surgeries are vertical banded gastroplasty and gastric bypass surgery. These procedures decrease the volume of food that the stomach can hold or bypass the stomach, with the goal of producing satiety with small intake. Bypassing the stomach also induces diarrhea when concentrated sweets are ingested. These techniques cause fewer complications than jejunoileal bypass, which induces a permanent malabsorption syndrome. Extended liquid diets are necessary adjuncts to surgery. Psychological counseling is also recommended.

Special considerations

■ Obtain an accurate diet history to identify the patient's eating patterns and the importance of food to his lifestyle. Ask the patient to keep a careful record of what, where, and when he eats to help identify situations that normally provoke overeating.

■ Explain the prescribed diet carefully, and encourage compliance to improve health status.

■ To increase calorie expenditure, promote increased physical activity, including an exercise program. Recommend varying activity levels according to the patient's general condition and cardiovascular status.

■ Watch carefully for signs of dependence or abuse if the patient is taking appetite-suppressing drugs; also watch for adverse effects, such as insomnia, excitability, dry mouth, and GI disturbances.

■ Teach the grossly obese patient the importance of good skin care to prevent breakdown in moist skin folds. Recommend the regular use of powder to keep skin dry.

■ To help prevent obesity in children, teach parents to avoid overfeeding their infants and to familiarize themselves with actual nutritional needs and optimum growth rates. Discourage parents from using food to reward or console their children, from emphasizing the importance of "clean plates," and from allowing eating to prevent hunger rather than to satisfy it.

■ Encourage physical activity and exercise, especially in children and young adults, to establish lifelong patterns. Suggest low-calorie snacks such as raw vegetables.

Protein-calorie malnutrition

One of the most prevalent and serious depletion disorders, protein-calorie malnutrition (PCM) occurs as marasmus (protein-calorie deficiency), characterized by growth failure and wasting, and as kwashiorkor (protein deficiency), characterized by tissue edema and damage. Both forms vary from mild to severe and may be fatal, depending on the accompanying stress (particularly sepsis or injury) and duration of deprivation. PCM increases the risk of death from pneumonia, chickenpox, or measles.

Causes and incidence

Both kwashiorkor (edematous PCM) and marasmus (nonedematous PCM) are common in underdeveloped countries and in areas in which dietary amino acid content is insufficient to satisfy growth requirements. Kwashiorkor typically occurs at about age 1, after infants are weaned from breast milk to a protein-deficient diet of starchy gruels or sugar water, but it can develop at any time during the formative years. Marasmus affects infants ages 6 to 18 months as a result of breast-feeding failure, or a debilitating condition such as chronic diarrhea.

In industrialized countries, PCM may occur secondary to chronic metabolic disease that decreases protein and calorie intake or absorption, or trauma that increases protein and calorie requirements. In the United States, PCM is estimated to occur to some extent in 50% of elderly people in nursing homes. Those who aren't allowed anything by mouth for an extended period are at high risk of developing PCM. Conditions that increase protein-calorie requirements include severe burns and injuries, systemic infections, and cancer (accounts for the largest group of hospitalized patients with PCM). Conditions that cause defective utilization of nutrients include malabsorption syndrome, short-bowel syndrome, and Crohn's disease.

Signs and symptoms

Children with chronic PCM are small for their chronological age and tend to be physically inactive, mentally apathetic, and susceptible to frequent infections. Anorexia and diarrhea are common.

In acute PCM, children are small, gaunt, and emaciated, with no adipose tissue. Skin is dry and "baggy," and hair is sparse and dull brown or reddish-yellow. Temperature is low; pulse rate and respirations are slowed. Such children are weak, irritable, and usually hungry, although they may have anorexia, with nausea and vomiting.

Unlike marasmus, chronic kwashiorkor allows the patient to grow in height, but adipose tissue diminishes as fat metabolizes to meet energy demands. Edema often masks severe muscle wasting; dry, peeling skin and hepatomegaly are common. Patients with secondary PCM show signs similar to marasmus, primarily loss of adipose tissue and lean body mass, lethargy, and edema. Severe secondary PCM may cause loss of immunocompetence.

Diagnosis

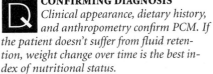

CONFIRMING DIAGNOSIS
Clinical appearance, dietary history, and anthropometry confirm PCM. If the patient doesn't suffer from fluid retention, weight change over time is the best index of nutritional status.

The following factors support the diagnosis:

- height and weight less than 80% of standard for the patient's age and sex, and below-normal arm circumference and triceps skinfold
- serum albumin level less than 2.8 g/dl (normal: 3.3 to 4.3 g/dl)
- urinary creatinine (24-hour) level used to show lean body mass status by relating creatinine excretion to height and ideal body weight, to yield creatinine-height index.

Treatment

The aim of treatment is to provide sufficient proteins, calories, and other nutrients for nutritional rehabilitation and maintenance. When treating severe PCM, restoring fluid and electrolyte balance parentally is the initial concern. A patient who shows normal absorption may receive enteral nutrition after anorexia has subsided. When possible, the preferred treatment is oral feeding. Foods are introduced slowly. Carbohydrates are given first to supply energy, and then high-quality protein foods, especially milk, and protein-calorie supplements, are given. A patient who's unwilling or unable to eat may require supplementary feedings through a nasogastric tube or total parenteral nutrition (TPN), which is given through a central venous catheter because of its higher osmolality. Peripheral parenteral nutrition, which has a lower osmolality than TPN and can be given through a peripheral I.V. line, is an alternative to TPN, but it's given less commonly.

Accompanying infection must also be treated, preferably with antibiotics that don't inhibit protein synthesis. Cautious realimentation is essential to prevent complications from overloading the compromised metabolic system.

Special considerations

■ Encourage the patient with PCM to consume as much nutritious food and beverage as possible (it's often helpful to "cheer him on" as he eats). Assist the patient with eating if necessary. Cooperate closely with the dietitian to monitor intake, and provide acceptable meals and snacks.

■ If TPN is necessary, observe strict sterile technique when handling catheters, tubes, and solutions and during dressing changes.

■ Watch for PCM in patients who have been hospitalized for a prolonged period, have had no oral intake for several days, or have cachectic disease.

■ To help eradicate PCM in developing countries, encourage prolonged breast-feeding, educate mothers about their children's needs, and provide supplementary foods, as needed.

 ELDER TIP *If the older patient is anorectic, consider asking family members and other visitors to bring in special foods from home that may improve the patient's appetite. In addition, encouraging the family to collaborate on feeding a dependent patient can help promote his recovery, enhance his feelings of well-being, and stimulate him to eat more.*

METABOLIC DISORDERS

Galactosemia

Galactosemia is any disorder of galactose metabolism. It produces symptoms ranging from cataracts and liver damage to mental retardation and occurs in two forms: classic galactosemia and galactokinase-deficiency galactosemia. Although a galactose-free diet relieves most symptoms, galactosemia-induced mental impairment is irreversible; some residual vision impairment may also persist.

Causes and incidence

Both forms of galactosemia are inherited as autosomal recessive defects and occur in about 1 in 60,000 births in the United States. Up to 1.25% of the population is heterozygous for the classic galactosemia gene. Classic galactosemia results from a defect in the enzyme galactose-1-phosphate uridyl transferase. (See *Metabolic pathway in galactosemia.*) Galactokinase-deficiency galactosemia, the rarer form of this disorder, stems from a deficiency of the enzyme galactokinase. In both forms of galactosemia, the inability to normally metabolize the sugar galactose (which is mainly formed by digestion of the disaccharide lactose that's present in milk) causes galactose accumulation.

Signs and symptoms

In children who are homozygous for the classic galactosemia gene, signs are evident at birth or begin within a few days after milk ingestion, and include failure to thrive, vomiting, and diarrhea. Other clinical effects include liver damage (which causes jaundice, hepatomegaly, cirrhosis, and ascites), splenomegaly, galactosuria, proteinuria, and aminoaciduria. Cataracts may also be present at birth or develop later. Pseudotumor cerebri may occur.

Continued ingestion of galactose- or lactose-containing foods may cause mental retardation, malnourishment, progressive hepatic failure, and death — from the still-unknown process of galactose metabolites accumulating in body tissues. Although treatment may prevent mental impairment, galactosemia can produce a short attention span, difficulty with spatial and mathematical relationships, and apathetic, withdrawn behavior. Cataracts may be the only sign of galactokinase deficiency, resulting from the accumulation of galactitol, a metabolic by-product of galactose, in the lens.

Diagnosis

 CONFIRMING DIAGNOSIS *Deficiency of the enzyme galactose-1-phosphate uridyl transferase in*

red blood cells (RBCs) confirms classic galactosemia; decreased RBC levels of galactokinase confirm galactokinase deficiency. Prenatal diagnosis may be made by direct measurement of galactose-1-phosphate uridyl transferase.

Related laboratory results include increased galactose levels in blood (normal value in children is less than 20 mg/dl) and urine (must use galactose oxidase to avoid confusion with other reducing sugars). Galactose measurements in blood and urine must be interpreted carefully because some children who consume large amounts of milk have elevated plasma galactose concentrations and galactosuria but aren't galactosemic. Also, neonates excrete galactose in their urine for about a week after birth; premature infants, even longer.

Other test results include:
- liver biopsy: typical acinar formation
- liver enzymes (aspartate aminotransferase, alanine aminotransferase levels): elevated
- urinalysis: albumin in urine
- ophthalmoscopy: punctate lesions in the fetal lens nucleus (with treatment, cataracts regress)
- amniocentesis: prenatal diagnosis of galactosemia (recommended for heterozygous and homozygous parents).

Treatment

Elimination of galactose and lactose from the diet causes most effects to subside. The infant is fed soy formula, meat-base formula, protein hydrolysate formula, or another lactose-free formula. The infant gains weight; liver anomalies, nausea, vomiting, galactosemia, proteinuria, and aminoaciduria disappear; and cataracts regress. As the child grows, a balanced, galactose-free diet must be maintained. A pregnant woman who's heterozygous or homozygous for galactosemia should also follow a galactose-restricted diet. Such a diet supports normal growth and development and may delay symptoms in the neonate.

Special considerations

- To eliminate galactose and lactose from an infant's diet, replace cow's milk formula

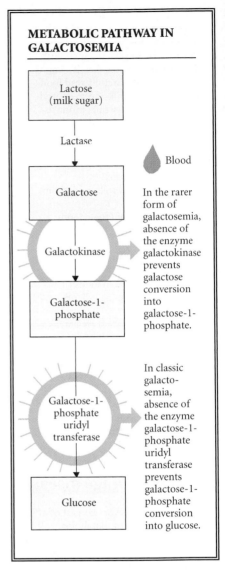

METABOLIC PATHWAY IN GALACTOSEMIA

Lactose (milk sugar)

Lactase

Blood

Galactose

In the rarer form of galactosemia, absence of the enzyme galactokinase prevents galactose conversion into galactose-1-phosphate.

Galactokinase

Galactose-1-phosphate

Galactose-1-phosphate uridyl transferase

In classic galactosemia, absence of the enzyme galactose-1-phosphate uridyl transferase prevents galactose-1-phosphate conversion into glucose.

Glucose

or breast milk with a meat-base or soybean formula.
- Teach the parents about dietary restrictions and stress the importance of compliance. (See *Diet for galactosemia*, page 892.) Warn them to read medication labels carefully and avoid giving any medication that contains lactose fillers.
- If the child has a learning disability, help parents secure educational assistance. Refer parents who want to have other children

---

DIET FOR GALACTOSEMIA

A patient with galactosemia must follow a lactose-free diet. It's important for him to carefully read food labels to avoid milk and milk products, including dry milk products.

He may eat these foods:
- fish and animal products (except brains and mussels)
- fresh fruits and vegetables (except peas and lima beans)
- only bread and rolls made from cracked wheat.

He should avoid these foods:
- dairy products
- puddings, cookies, cakes, pies
- food coloring
- instant potatoes
- canned and frozen foods (if lactose is listed as an ingredient).

---

for genetic counseling. In some states, screening of all neonates for galactosemia is required by law.
- Instruct the parents to contact support groups, such as Parents of Galactosemic Children, for further information and support if appropriate.

Glycogen storage diseases

Glycogen storage diseases consist of at least eight distinct errors of metabolism, all inherited, that alter the synthesis or degradation of glycogen, the form in which glucose is stored in the body. Normally, muscle and liver cells store glycogen. Muscle glycogen is used in muscle contraction; liver glycogen can be converted into free glucose, which can then diffuse out of the liver cells to increase blood glucose levels. Glycogen storage diseases manifest as dysfunctions of the liver, heart, or musculoskeletal system. Symptoms vary from mild and easily controlled hypoglycemia to severe organ involvement that may lead to heart failure and respiratory failure.

Causes

Almost all glycogen storage diseases (Types I through V and Type VII) are transmitted as autosomal recessive traits. The transmission mode of Type VI is unknown; Type VIII may be an X-linked trait.

The most common glycogen storage disease is Type I — von Gierke's, or hepatorenal glycogen storage disease — which results from a deficiency of the liver enzyme glucose-6-phosphatase. This enzyme converts glucose-6-phosphate into free glucose and is necessary for the release of stored glycogen and glucose into the bloodstream, to relieve hypoglycemia. Infants may die of acidosis before age 2; if they survive past this age, with proper treatment, they may grow normally and live to adulthood, with only minimal hepatomegaly. However, there's a danger of adenomatous liver nodules, which may be premalignant.

Signs and symptoms

Primary clinical features of the liver glycogen storage diseases (Types I, III, IV, VI, and VIII) are hepatomegaly and rapid onset of hypoglycemia and ketosis when food is withheld. Symptoms of the muscle glycogen storage diseases (Types II, V, and VII) include poor muscle tone; Type II may result in death from heart failure. (See *Rare forms of glycogen storage disease.*)

In addition, Type I may produce these symptoms:
- infants: acidosis, hyperlipidemia, GI bleeding, coma
- children: low resistance to infection and, without proper treatment, short stature
- adolescents: gouty arthritis and nephropathy; chronic tophaceous gout; bleeding (especially epistaxis); small superficial vessels visible in skin due to impaired platelet function; fat deposits in cheeks, buttocks, and subcutaneous tissues; poor muscle tone; enlarged kidneys; xanthomas over extensor surfaces of arms and legs; steatorrhea; multiple, bilateral, yellow lesions in fundi; and osteoporosis, probably secondary to negative calcium balance. Correct treatment of glycogen storage disease should prevent all of these effects.

RARE FORMS OF GLYCOGEN STORAGE DISEASE

Type	Clinical features	Diagnostic test results
II (Pompe's) Absence of alpha-1,4-glucosidase (acid maltase)	■ *Infants:* cardiomegaly, profound hypotonia and, occasionally, endocardial fibroelastosis (usually fatal before age 1 due to cardiac or respiratory failure) ■ *Some infants and young children:* muscle weakness and wasting, variable organ involvement (slower progression, usually fatal by age 19) ■ *Adults:* muscle weakness without organomegaly (slowly progressive but not fatal)	■ *Muscle biopsy:* increased concentration of glycogen with normal structure; alpha-1,4-glucosidase deficiency ■ *Electrocardiogram (in infants):* large QRS complexes in all leads; inverted T waves; shortened PR interval ■ *Electromyography (in adults):* muscle fiber irritability; myotonic discharges ■ *Amniocentesis:* alpha-1,4-glucosidase deficiency ■ *Placenta or umbilical cord examination:* alpha-1,4-glucosidase deficiency
III (Cori's) Absence of debranching enzyme (amylo-1,6-glucosidase) (*Note:* predominant cause of glycogen storage disease in Israel)	■ *Young children:* massive hepatomegaly, which may disappear by puberty; growth retardation; moderate splenomegaly; hypoglycemia ■ *Adults:* progressive myopathy ■ Occasionally, moderate cardiomegaly, cirrhosis, muscle wasting, hypoglycemia	■ *Liver biopsy:* deficient debranching activity; increased glycogen concentration ■ *Laboratory tests (in children only):* elevated aspartate aminotransferase or alanine aminotransferase levels; increased erythrocyte glycogen levels
IV (Andersen's) Deficiency of branching enzyme (amylo-1,4-1,6-transglucosidase) (*Note:* extremely rare)	■ *Infants:* hepatosplenomegaly, ascites, muscle hypotonia; usually fatal before age 2 from progressive cirrhosis	■ *Liver biopsy:* deficient branching enzyme activity; glycogen molecule has longer outer branches
V (McArdle's) Deficiency of muscle phosphorylase	■ *Children:* mild or no symptoms ■ *Adults:* muscle cramps and pain during strenuous exercise, possibly resulting in myoglobinuria and renal failure ■ *Older patients:* significant muscle weakness and wasting	■ *Serum lactate:* no increase in venous levels in sample drawn from extremity after ischemic exercise ■ *Muscle biopsy:* lack of phosphorylase activity; increased glycogen content
VI (Hers') Possible deficiency of hepatic phosphorylase	■ Mild symptoms (similar to those of Type I), requiring no treatment	■ *Liver biopsy:* decreased phosphorylase b activity, increased glycogen concentration *(continued)*

RARE FORMS OF GLYCOGEN STORAGE DISEASE *(continued)*

Type	Clinical features	Diagnostic test results
VII Deficiency of muscle phosphofructokinase	■ Muscle cramps during strenuous exercise, resulting in myoglobinuria and possible renal failure ■ Reticulocytosis	■ *Serum lactate:* no increase in venous levels in sample drawn from extremity after ischemic exercise ■ *Muscle biopsy:* deficient phosphofructokinase; marked rise in glycogen concentration ■ *Blood studies:* low erythrocyte phosphofructokinase activity; reduced half-life of red blood cells
VIII Deficiency of hepatic phosphorylase kinase	■ Mild hepatomegaly ■ Mild hypoglycemia	■ *Liver biopsy:* deficient phosphorylase *b* kinase activity; increased glycogen concentration ■ *Blood study:* deficient phosphorylase *b* kinase in leukocytes

Diagnosis

CONFIRMING DIAGNOSIS *Liver biopsy confirms the diagnosis by showing normal glycogen synthetase and phosphorylase enzyme activities but reduced or absent glucose-6-phosphatase activity. Glycogen structure is normal but amounts are elevated. Spectroscopy may be used to show abnormal muscle metabolism with the use of magnetic resonance imaging in specialized centers.*

■ Laboratory studies of plasma demonstrate low glucose levels but high levels of free fatty acids, triglycerides, cholesterol, and uric acid. Serum analysis reveals high pyruvic acid levels and high lactic acid levels. Prenatal diagnoses are available for Types II, III, and IV.

■ Injection of glucagon or epinephrine increases pyruvic and lactic acid levels but doesn't increase blood glucose levels. Glucose tolerance test curve typically shows depletional hypoglycemia and reduced insulin output. Intrauterine diagnosis is possible.

Treatment

For Type I, treatment aims to maintain glucose homeostasis and prevent secondary consequences of hypoglycemia through frequent feedings and constant nocturnal nasogastric (NG) drip with Polycose, dextrose, or Vivonex. Treatment includes a low-fat diet, with normal amounts of protein and calories; carbohydrates should contain glucose or glucose polymers only.

Therapy for Type III includes frequent feedings and a high-protein diet. Type IV requires a high-protein, high-calorie diet; bed rest; diuretics; sodium restriction; and paracentesis, if necessary, to relieve ascites. Types V and VII require no treatment except avoidance of strenuous exercise. No treatment is necessary for Types VI and VIII; no effective treatment exists for Type II.

Special considerations

When managing Type I disease:

■ Advise the patient or his parents to include carbohydrate foods containing mainly starch in his diet and to sweeten foods with glucose only.

■ Before discharge, teach the patient or his family member how to pass an NG tube, use a pump with alarm capacity, monitor blood glucose levels with glucose reagent strips, and recognize symptoms of hypoglycemia.

■ Watch for and report signs of infection (fever, chills, myalgia) and of hepatic encephalopathy (mental confusion, stupor, asterixis, coma) due to increased blood ammonia levels.

When managing other types:

- *Type II:* Explain test procedures, such as electromyography and EEG, thoroughly.
- *Type III:* Instruct the patient to eat a high-protein diet (eggs, nuts, fish, meat, poultry, and cheese).
- *Type IV:* Watch for signs of hepatic failure (nausea, vomiting, irregular bowel function, clay-colored stools, right upper quadrant pain, jaundice, dehydration, electrolyte imbalance, edema, and changes in mental status, progressing to coma).

When caring for patients with Types II, III, and IV glycogen storage disease, offer the patient and his parents reassurance and emotional support. Recommend and arrange for genetic counseling, if appropriate.

- *Types V through VIII:* Care for these patients is minimal. Explain the disorder to the patient and his family, and help them accept the limitations imposed by his particular type of glycogen storage disease.

Hypoglycemia

Hypoglycemia is an abnormally low glucose level in the bloodstream. It occurs when glucose burns up too rapidly, when the glucose release rate falls behind tissue demands, or when excessive insulin enters the bloodstream. Hypoglycemia is classified as reactive or fasting. *Reactive hypoglycemia* results from the reaction to the disposition of meals or the administration of excessive insulin. *Fasting hypoglycemia* causes discomfort during long periods of abstinence from food, for example, in the early morning before breakfast. Although hypoglycemia is a specific endocrine imbalance, its symptoms are often vague and depend on how quickly the patient's glucose levels drop. If not corrected, severe hypoglycemia may result in coma and irreversible brain damage.

Causes and incidence

Reactive hypoglycemia may take several forms. In a diabetic patient, it may result from administration of too much insulin or, less commonly, too much oral antidiabetic medication. In a mildly diabetic patient (or one in the early stages of diabetes mellitus), reactive hypoglycemia may result from delayed and excessive insulin production after carbohydrate ingestion. Similarly, a nondiabetic patient may suffer reactive hypoglycemia from a sharp increase in insulin output after a meal. Sometimes called *postprandial hypoglycemia*, this type of reactive hypoglycemia usually disappears when the patient eats something sweet. In some patients, reactive hypoglycemia has no known cause (idiopathic reactive) or may result from gastric dumping syndrome and from impaired glucose tolerance.

Fasting hypoglycemia usually results from an excess of insulin or insulin-like substance or from a decrease in counterregulatory hormones. It can be *exogenous,* resulting from such external factors as alcohol or drug ingestion, or *endogenous,* resulting from organic problems. Endogenous hypoglycemia may result from tumors or liver disease. Insulinomas, small islet cell tumors in the pancreas, secrete excessive amounts of insulin, which inhibit hepatic glucose production. They're generally benign (in 90% of patients). Extrapancreatic tumors, though uncommon, can also cause hypoglycemia by increasing glucose utilization and inhibiting glucose output. Such tumors occur primarily in the mesenchyma, liver, adrenal cortex, GI system, and lymphatic system. They may be benign or malignant. Among nonendocrine causes of fasting hypoglycemia are severe liver diseases, including hepatitis, cancer, cirrhosis, and liver congestion associated with heart failure. All of these conditions reduce the uptake and release of glycogen from the liver. Some endocrine causes include adrenocortical insufficiency, which contributes to hypoglycemia by reducing the production of cortisol and cortisone needed for gluconeogenesis; and pituitary insufficiency, which reduces corticotropin and growth hormone levels.

Hypoglycemia is at least as common in neonates and children as it is in adults and affects 1 out of 1,000 people. Usually, infants develop hypoglycemia because of an increased number of cells per unit of body weight and because of increased demands on stored liver glycogen to support respirations, thermoregulation, and muscular activity. In full-term neonates, hypoglycemia may occur 24 to 72 hours after birth and is usually transient. In neonates who are premature or small for gestational age, onset of hypoglycemia is much more rapid (it can occur as soon as 6 hours after birth) because of their small, immature livers, which produce much less glycogen. Maternal disorders that can produce hypoglycemia in neonates within 24 hours after birth include diabetes mellitus, toxemia, erythroblastosis, and glycogen storage disease.

Signs and symptoms

Signs and symptoms of reactive hypoglycemia include fatigue, malaise, nervousness, irritability, trembling, tension, headache, hunger, cold sweats, and rapid heart rate. These same clinical effects usually characterize fasting hypoglycemia. In addition, fasting hypoglycemia may also cause central nervous system (CNS) disturbances; for example, blurry or double vision, confusion, motor weakness, hemiplegia, seizures, or coma.

In infants and children, signs and symptoms of hypoglycemia are vague. A neonate's refusal to feed may be the primary clue to underlying hypoglycemia. Associated CNS effects include tremors, twitching, weak or high-pitched cry, sweating, limpness, seizures, and coma.

Diagnosis

A blood glucose monitor or glucose reagent strips provide quick screening methods for determining the blood glucose level. A reading less than 45 mg/dl indicates the need for a venous blood sample.

CONFIRMING DIAGNOSIS
Laboratory testing confirms the diagnosis by showing decreased blood glucose levels. The following values indicate hypoglycemia:
- *Full-term infants:*
  - less than 30 mg/dl before feeding
  - less than 40 mg/dl after feeding
- *Preterm infants:*
  - less than 20 mg/dl before feeding
  - less than 30 mg/dl after feeding

- *Children and adults:*
  - less than 40 mg/dl before meal
  - less than 50 mg/dl after meal.

In addition, a 5-hour glucose tolerance test may be administered to provoke reactive hypoglycemia. Following a 12-hour fast, laboratory testing to detect plasma insulin and plasma glucose levels may identify fasting hypoglycemia. (See *Diagnosing hypoglycemia.*)

Treatment

Effective treatment of reactive hypoglycemia requires dietary modification to help delay glucose absorption and gastric emptying. Usually this includes small, frequent meals; ingestion of complex carbohydrates, fiber, and fat; and avoidance of simple sugars, alcohol, and fruit drinks. The patient may also receive anticholinergic drugs to slow gastric emptying and intestinal motility and to inhibit vagal stimulation of insulin release.

For fasting hypoglycemia, surgery and drug therapy are usually required. In patients with insulinoma, tumor removal is the treatment of choice. Drug therapy may include nondiuretic thiazides such as diazoxide to inhibit insulin secretion; streptozocin; and hormones, such as glucocorticoids and long-acting glycogen.

Therapy for neonates who have hypoglycemia or who are at risk of developing it includes preventive measures. A hypertonic solution of 10% dextrose, calculated at 5 to 10 ml/kg of body weight administered I.V. over 10 minutes and followed by 4 to 8 mg/kg/minute for maintenance, should correct a severe hypoglycemic state in neonates. To reduce the chance of hypoglycemia in high-risk neonates, they should receive feedings (either breast milk or a solution of 5% to 10% glucose and water) as soon after birth as possible.

Special considerations

- Watch for and report signs of hypoglycemia, such as poor feeding, in high-risk neonates.
- Monitor infusion of hypertonic glucose in the neonate to avoid hyperglycemia, circulatory overload, and cellular dehydration. Terminate glucose solutions gradually

DIFFERENTIAL DIAGNOSIS

DIAGNOSING HYPOGLYCEMIA

This flowchart lists possible diagnostic findings and interpretations to assist with treatment of the patient with hypoglycemia.

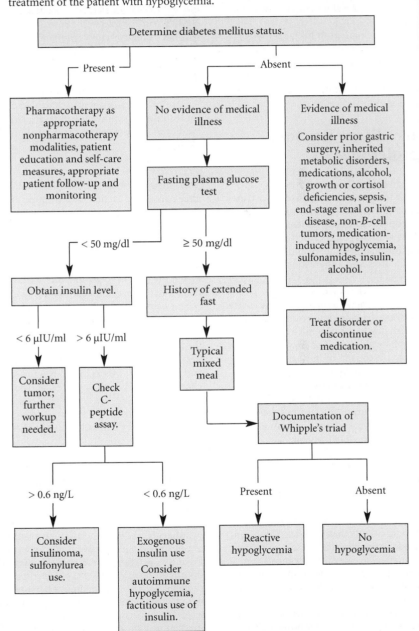

to prevent hypoglycemia caused by hyper-insulinemia.

■ Explain the purpose and procedure for any diagnostic tests. Collect blood samples at the appropriate times, as ordered.

■ Monitor the effects of drug therapy and watch for the development of any adverse effects.

■ Teach the patient or his family which foods to include in his diet (complex carbohydrates, fiber, fat) and which foods to avoid (simple sugars, alcohol). Refer the patient and his family for dietary counseling as appropriate.

Hereditary fructose intolerance

Hereditary fructose intolerance is an inability to metabolize fructose. After fructose is eliminated from the diet, symptoms subside within weeks. Older children and adults with hereditary fructose intolerance have normal intelligence and apparently normal liver and kidney function.

Causes and incidence
Transmitted as an autosomal recessive trait, hereditary fructose intolerance results from a deficiency in the enzyme fructose-1-phosphate aldolase. The enzyme operates at only 1% to 10% of its normal biological activity, thus preventing rapid uptake of fructose by the liver after ingestion of fruit or foods containing cane sugar.

In some European countries, hereditary fructose intolerance may have an incidence as high as 1 in 20,000 people.

Signs and symptoms
Typically, clinical features of hereditary fructose intolerance appear shortly after dietary introduction of foods containing fructose or sucrose. Symptoms are more severe in infants than in older people and include hypoglycemia, nausea, vomiting, pallor, excessive sweating, cyanosis, and tremor. In neonates and young children, continuous ingestion of foods containing fructose may result in failure to thrive, hypoglycemia, jaundice, hyperbilirubinemia, ascites, hepatomegaly, vomiting, dehydration, hypophosphatemia, albuminuria,

aminoaciduria, seizures, coma, febrile episodes, substernal pain, and anemia.

Diagnosis
A dietary history often suggests hereditary fructose intolerance.

 CONFIRMING DIAGNOSIS *A fructose tolerance test (using glucose oxidase or paper chromatography to measure glucose levels) usually confirms the diagnosis. However, liver biopsy showing a deficiency in fructose-1-phosphate aldolase may be necessary for a definitive diagnosis.*

Supportive values may include decreased serum inorganic phosphorus levels. Urine studies may show fructosuria and albuminuria.

Treatment
Treatment of hereditary fructose intolerance consists of exclusion of fructose and sucrose (cane sugar or table sugar) from the diet. Otherwise, treatment is supportive as the patient's progress is monitored.

Special considerations
■ Tell the patient to avoid fruits containing fructose and vegetables containing sucrose (sugar beets, sweet potatoes, and peas), because sucrose is digested to glucose and fructose in the intestine. Fruits containing the least amount of fructose include strawberries, blackberries, blueberries, oranges, and grapefruits; others low in fructose are cherries, pears, bananas, grapes, and apples.

■ Refer the patient and his family for genetic and dietary counseling as appropriate.

Hyperlipoproteinemia

Hyperlipoproteinemia occurs as five distinct metabolic disorders, all of which may be inherited. Types I and III are transmitted as autosomal recessive traits; Types II, IV, and V are transmitted as autosomal dominant traits. (See *Types of hyperlipoproteinemia.*) About one in five persons with elevated plasma lipid and lipoprotein levels has hyperlipoproteinemia. It's marked by increased plasma concentrations of one or more lipoproteins. Hyper-

TYPES OF HYPERLIPOPROTEINEMIA

Type	Causes and incidence	Diagnostic findings
I (Frederickson's hyperlipoproteinemia, fat-induced hyperlipemia, idiopathic familial)	■ Deficient or abnormal lipoprotein lipase, resulting in decreased or absent post-heparin lipolytic activity ■ Relatively rare ■ Present at birth	■ Chylomicrons (very-low-density lipoprotein [VLDL], low-density lipoprotein [LDL], high-density lipoprotein), in plasma 14 hours or more after last meal ■ Highly elevated serum chylomicrons and triglyceride levels; slightly elevated serum cholesterol levels ■ Lower serum lipoprotein lipase levels ■ Leukocytosis
II (familial hyperbetalipoproteinemia, essential familial hypercholesterolemia)	■ Deficient cell surface receptor that regulates LDL degradation and cholesterol synthesis, resulting in increased levels of plasma LDL over joints and pressure points ■ Onset between ages 10 and 30	■ Increased plasma concentrations of LDL ■ Increased serum LDL and cholesterol levels ■ Amniocentesis shows increased LDL levels
III (familial broad-beta disease, dysbetalipoproteinemia, remnant removal disease, xanthoma tuberosum)	■ Unknown underlying defect results in deficient conversion of triglyceride-rich VLDL to LDL ■ Uncommon; usually occurs after age 20 but can occur earlier in men	■ Abnormal serum beta-lipoprotein ■ Elevated cholesterol and triglyceride levels ■ Slightly elevated glucose tolerance ■ Hyperuricemia
IV (endogenous hypertriglyceridemia, hyperbetalipoproteinemia)	■ Usually occurs secondary to obesity, alcoholism, diabetes, or emotional disorders ■ Relatively common, especially in middle-age men	■ Elevated VLDL levels ■ Abnormal levels of triglycerides in plasma; variable increase in serum ■ Normal or slightly elevated serum cholesterol levels ■ Mildly abnormal glucose tolerance ■ Family history ■ Early coronary artery disease
V (mixed hypertriglyceridemia, mixed hyperlipidemia)	■ Defective triglyceride clearance causes pancreatitis; usually secondary to another disorder, such as obesity or nephrosis ■ Uncommon; onset usually occurs in late adolescence or early adulthood	■ Chylomicrons in plasma ■ Elevated plasma VLDL levels ■ Elevated serum cholesterol and triglyceride levels

lipoproteinemia may also occur secondary to other conditions, such as diabetes, pancreatitis, hypothyroidism, or renal disease. This disorder affects lipid transport in serum and produces varied clinical changes, from relatively mild symptoms that can be corrected by dietary management to potentially fatal pancreatitis.

Signs and symptoms

- *Type I:* recurrent attacks of severe abdominal pain similar to pancreatitis, usually preceded by fat intake; abdominal spasm, rigidity, or rebound tenderness; hepatosplenomegaly, with liver or spleen tenderness; papular or eruptive xanthomas (pinkish-yellow cutaneous deposits of fat) over pressure points and extensor surfaces; lipemia retinalis (reddish-white retinal vessels); malaise; anorexia; and fever
- *Type II:* tendinous xanthomas (firm masses) on the Achilles tendons and tendons of the hands and feet, tuberous xanthomas, xanthelasma, juvenile corneal arcus (opaque ring surrounding the corneal periphery), accelerated atherosclerosis and premature coronary artery disease, and recurrent polyarthritis and tenosynovitis
- *Type III:* peripheral vascular disease manifested by claudication or tuboeruptive xanthomas (soft, inflamed, pedunculated lesions) over the elbows and knees; palmar xanthomas on the hands, particularly the fingertips; premature atherosclerosis
- *Type IV:* predisposition to atherosclerosis and early coronary artery disease, exacerbated by excessive calorie intake, obesity, diabetes, and hypertension
- *Type V:* abdominal pain (most common), pancreatitis, peripheral neuropathy, eruptive xanthomas on extensor surfaces of the arms and legs, lipemia retinalis, and hepatosplenomegaly.

Treatment

The first goal is to identify and treat any underlying problem such as diabetes. If no underlying problem exists, the primary treatment of Types II, III, and IV is dietary management, especially restriction of cholesterol intake, possibly supplemented by drug therapy (cholestyramine, clofibrate, niacin) to lower plasma triglyceride or cholesterol level when diet alone is ineffective.

Type I hyperlipoproteinemia requires long-term weight reduction, with fat intake restricted to less than 20 g/day. A 20- to 40-g/day medium-chain triglyceride diet may be ordered to supplement calorie intake. The patient should also avoid alcoholic beverages, to decrease plasma triglyceride levels. The prognosis is good with treatment; without treatment, death can result from pancreatitis.

For Type II, dietary management to restore normal lipid levels and decrease the risk of atherosclerosis includes restriction of cholesterol intake to less than 300 mg/day for adults and less than 150 mg/day for children; triglycerides must be restricted to less than 100 mg/day for children and adults. Diet should also be high in polyunsaturated fats. In familial hypercholesterolemia, nicotinic acid with a bile acid usually normalizes low-density lipoprotein levels. For severely affected children, a portacaval shunt is a last resort to reduce plasma cholesterol levels. The prognosis remains poor regardless of treatment; in homozygotes, myocardial infarction usually causes death before age 30.

For Type III, dietary management includes restriction of cholesterol intake to less than 300 mg/day; carbohydrates must also be restricted, while polyunsaturated fats are increased. Clofibrate and niacin help lower blood lipid levels. Weight reduction is helpful. With strict adherence to prescribed diet, the prognosis is good.

For Type IV, weight reduction may normalize blood lipid levels without additional treatment. Long-term dietary management includes restricted cholesterol intake, increased polyunsaturated fats, and avoidance of alcoholic beverages. Clofibrate and niacin may lower plasma lipid levels. The prognosis remains uncertain, however, because of predisposition to premature coronary artery disease.

The most effective treatment for Type V is weight reduction and long-term maintenance of a low-fat diet. Alcoholic beverages must be avoided. Niacin, clofibrate, gemfibrozil, and a 20- to 40-g/day medium-chain triglyceride diet may prove helpful. The prognosis is uncertain because of the risk of pancreatitis. Increased fat intake may cause recurrent bouts of illness, possibly leading to pseudocyst formation, hemorrhage, and death.

Special considerations

Nursing care for hyperlipoproteinemia emphasizes careful monitoring for adverse drug effects and teaching the importance of long-term dietary management.

- Administer cholestyramine before meals or before bedtime. This drug must not be given with other medications. (See *Using bile acid sequestrants.*) Watch for adverse effects, such as nausea, vomiting, constipation, steatorrhea, rashes, and hyperchloremic acidosis. Also watch for malabsorption of other medications and fat-soluble vitamins.
- Give clofibrate as ordered. Watch for adverse effects, such as cholelithiasis, cardiac arrhythmias, intermittent claudication, thromboembolism, nausea, weight gain (from fluid retention), and myositis.

ALERT *Don't administer niacin to patients with active peptic ulcers or hepatic disease. Use with caution in patients with diabetes. In other patients, watch for adverse effects, such as flushing, pruritus, hyperpigmentation, and exacerbation of inactive peptic ulcers.*

- Urge the patient to adhere to the ordered diet (usually 1,000 to 1,500 calories/day) and to avoid excess sugar and alcoholic beverages, to minimize his intake of saturated fats (higher in meats, coconut oil), and to increase his intake of polyunsaturated fats (vegetable oils).
- Instruct the patient, for the 2 weeks preceding serum cholesterol and serum triglyceride tests, to maintain a steady weight and to adhere strictly to the prescribed diet. He should also fast for 12 hours preceding the test.
- Instruct women with elevated serum lipid levels to avoid hormonal contraceptives or drugs that contain estrogen.

Gaucher's disease

Gaucher's disease, the most common lysosomal storage disease, causes an abnormal accumulation of glucocerebrosides in reticuloendothelial cells. It occurs in three forms: Type I (adult); Type II (infantile);

USING BILE ACID SEQUESTRANTS

Before giving the patient a bile acid sequestrant, such as cholestyramine, to lower cholesterol levels, make certain he isn't taking a drug whose absorption is affected by bile acid sequestrants. For example, bile acid sequestrants decrease the absorption of diuretics such as chlorothiazide. Other drugs affected besides diuretics include:

- beta-adrenergic blockers
- digitoxin
- fat-soluble vitamins
- folic acid
- thiazides
- thyroxine
- warfarin.

---

and Type III (juvenile). Type II can prove fatal within 9 months of onset, usually from pulmonary involvement.

Causes and incidence

Gaucher's disease results from an autosomal recessive inheritance, which causes decreased activity of the enzyme glucocerebrosidase. Glucocerebrosidase deficiency leads to an accumulation of glucosylceramide in the storage compartments (lysosomes) of certain body cells. Glucosylceramide buildup occurs in the liver, spleen, bones, and bone marrow, eventually leading to decreased production of red blood cells (anemia) and thinning of the bones (osteopenia).

There are three forms of Gaucher's disease, classified by age of onset and the presence or absence of neurologic involvement. Type I, characterized by lack of neurologic involvement, is the most common form affecting both children and adults and is most prevalent in the Ashkenazi Jewish population, affecting anywhere from 1 of 500 to 1,000 births. Type II usually presents in infancy with severe neurologic involvement, resulting in seizures and central nervous system damage. Type II also presents with spleen and bone marrow damage. Type III typically has mild neurologic involvement and runs a slower, more favorable course. The incidence of Types II and III is 1 of 50,000 to 100,000 births. The juvenile form can begin in childhood, typically in the teenage years, and cause spleen, bone marrow, and neurologic damage.

Signs and symptoms

The key signs of all types of Gaucher's disease are hepatosplenomegaly and bone lesions. In Type I, bone lesions lead to thinning of cortices, pathologic fractures, collapsed hip joints and, eventually, vertebral compression. Severe episodic pain may develop in the legs, arms, and back but usually not until adolescence. (The adult form of Gaucher's disease is generally diagnosed while the patient is in his teens; the word "adult" is used loosely here.) Other clinical effects of Type I are fever, abdominal distention (from hypotonicity of the large bowel), respiratory problems (pneumonia or, rarely, cor pulmonale), easy bruising and bleeding, anemia and, rarely, pancytopenia. Older patients may develop a yellow pallor and brown-yellow pigmentation on the face and legs.

In Type II, motor dysfunction and spasticity occur at age 6 to 7 months. Other signs of the infantile form of Gaucher's disease include abdominal distention, strabismus, muscle hypertonicity, retroflexion of the head, neck rigidity, dysphagia, laryngeal stridor, hyperreflexia, seizures, respiratory distress, and easy bruising and bleeding.

Clinical effects of Type III after infancy include seizures, hypertonicity, strabismus, poor coordination and mental ability and, possibly, easy bruising and bleeding.

Diagnosis

CONFIRMING DIAGNOSIS *Bone marrow aspiration showing Gaucher's cells and direct assay of glucocerebrosidase activity, which can be performed on venous blood, confirms this diagnosis.*

Supportive laboratory results include increased serum acid phosphatase level, decreased platelets and serum iron level and, in Type III, abnormal EEG after infancy.

Treatment

Treatment is mainly supportive and consists of vitamins, supplemental iron or liver extract to prevent anemia caused by iron deficiency and to alleviate other hematologic problems, blood transfusions for anemia, splenectomy for thrombocytopenia, and strong analgesics for bone pain. Injections of a replacement synthetic enzyme have proven helpful. Gene therapy is an experimental approach. An oral treatment with N-butyl deoxynojirimycin (OGT 918), which inhibits glucocerebrosidase formation, is being evaluated. Clinical trials have shown improvement in the key clinical features of Gaucher's disease, including liver and spleen size and, to a lesser degree, blood counts.

Special considerations

■ In the patient confined to bed, prevent pathologic fractures by turning him carefully. If he's ambulatory, make sure that he's assisted when getting out of bed or walking.

■ Observe closely for changes in pulmonary status.

■ Explain all diagnostic tests and procedures to the patient or his parents. Help the patient accept the limitations imposed by this disorder.

■ Recommend genetic counseling for patients with a family history of Gaucher's disease. Prenatal testing can determine if a fetus has the syndrome.

Amyloidosis

Amyloidosis is a rare, chronic disease resulting in the accumulation of an abnormal fibrillar scleroprotein (amyloid), which infiltrates body organs and soft tissues. Amyloidosis is classified in two ways, based on histologic findings: *perireticular type,* which affects the inner coats of blood vessels, and *pericollagen type,* which affects the outer coats of blood vessels and also involves the parenchyma.

Although prognosis varies with type and with the site and extent of involvement, amyloidosis sometimes results in permanent — usually life-threatening — organ damage.

Causes and incidence

Amyloidosis is sometimes familial, especially in people of Portuguese ancestry. It may occur in conjunction with tuberculosis, chronic infection, rheumatoid arthritis, multiple myeloma, Hodgkin's disease, paraplegia, and brucellosis. It may also accompany Alzheimer's disease.

In amyloidosis, accumulation and infiltration of amyloid produces pressure and causes atrophy of nearby cells. Reticuloendothelial cell dysfunction and abnormal immunoglobulin synthesis occur in some types of amyloidosis. In the United States, evidence of amyloidosis on autopsy is 0.5%, but true incidence is difficult to determine.

Signs and symptoms

Amyloidosis produces dysfunction of the kidneys, heart, GI tract, peripheral nerves, and liver.

■ *Kidneys:* The primary sign of renal involvement is proteinuria, leading to nephrotic syndrome and, eventually, renal failure.

■ *Heart:* Amyloidosis often causes intractable heart failure, due to amyloid deposits in the subendocardium, endocardium, and myocardium.

■ *GI tract:* GI amyloidosis may produce stiffness and enlargement of the tongue, hindering enunciation. In addition, it may decrease intestinal motility and produce malabsorption, bleeding, infiltration of blood vessel walls, abdominal pain, constipation, and diarrhea. Tumorlike amyloid deposits may occur in all portions of this system. Chronic malabsorption may lead to malnutrition and predispose to infection.

■ *Peripheral nervous system:* The appearance of peripheral neuropathy indicates peripheral nerve involvement.

■ *Liver:* Hepatic amyloidosis is rare and usually coexists with other forms of this disease. It generally produces liver enlargement, often with azotemia, anemia, albuminuria and, rarely, jaundice.

Diagnosis

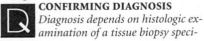 **CONFIRMING DIAGNOSIS**
Diagnosis depends on histologic examination of a tissue biopsy speci-
men, using a polarizing or electron microscope. Rectal mucosa biopsy and abdominal fat pad aspiration are the best screening tests because they're less hazardous than kidney or liver biopsy. Other biopsy sites include the gingiva, skin, and nerves.

In cardiac amyloidosis, other findings include faint heart sounds and an electrocardiogram showing low voltage and conduction or rhythm abnormalities resembling those characteristic of myocardial infarction. In hepatic amyloidosis, liver function studies are generally normal, except for a slightly elevated serum alkaline phosphatase level.

Treatment

Treatment is directed at eliminating the underlying cause and is mainly supportive. Transplantation may be useful for amyloidosis-induced renal failure, although the donor kidney may also develop amyloidosis. Patients with cardiac amyloidosis require conservative treatment to prevent dangerous arrhythmias. Malnutrition caused by malabsorption in end-stage GI involvement may require total parenteral nutrition.

Special considerations

■ Maintain nutrition and fluid balance; give analgesics to relieve intestinal pain; control constipation or diarrhea; and manage infection and fever.

■ Provide good mouth care for the patient with tongue involvement. Refer him for speech therapy if needed; provide an alternate method of communication if he can't talk.

■ Regularly assess airway patency when the tongue is involved and prevent respiratory tract compromise by gentle and adequate suctioning, when indicated. Keep a tracheostomy tray at the bedside.

■ When long-term bed rest is necessary, properly position the patient and turn him often to prevent pressure ulcers. Perform range-of-motion exercises to prevent contractures.

■ Provide psychological support. Exercise patience and understanding to help the patient cope with this chronic illness.

Porphyrias

Porphyrias are metabolic disorders that affect the biosynthesis of heme (a component of hemoglobin) and cause excessive production and excretion of porphyrins or their precursors. Porphyrins, which are present in all protoplasm, figure prominently in energy storage and utilization.

Classification of porphyrias depends on the site of excessive porphyrin production; they may be erythropoietic (erythroid cells in bone marrow), hepatic (in the liver), or erythrohepatic (in bone marrow and liver). (See *Types of porphyria.*) An acute episode of intermittent hepatic porphyria may cause fatal respiratory paralysis. In the other forms of porphyrias, the prognosis is good with proper treatment.

Causes

Porphyrias are inherited as autosomal dominant traits, except for Günther's disease (autosomal recessive trait) and toxic-acquired porphyria (usually from ingestion of or exposure to lead). Menstruation often precipitates acute porphyria in premenopausal women.

Signs and symptoms

Porphyrias are generally marked by photosensitivity, acute abdominal pain, and neuropathy. Hepatic porphyrias may produce a complex syndrome marked by distinct neurologic and hepatic dysfunction:
- Neurologic symptoms include chronic brain syndrome, peripheral neuropathy and autonomic effects, tachycardia, labile hypertension, severe colicky lower abdominal pain, and constipation.
- During an acute attack, fever, leukocytosis, and fluid and electrolyte imbalance may occur.
- Structural hepatic effects include fatty infiltration of the liver, hepatic siderosis, and focal hepatocellular necrosis.
- Skin lesions may cause itching and burning, erythema, and altered pigmentation and edema in areas exposed to light. Some chronic skin changes include milia (white papules on the hands' dorsal aspects) and hirsutism on the upper cheeks and periorbital areas.

Diagnosis

CONFIRMING DIAGNOSIS *Generally, diagnosis requires screening tests for porphyrins or their precursors (such as aminolevulinic acid [ALA] and porphobilinogen [PBG]) in urine, stool, blood or, occasionally, skin biopsy. A urinary lead level of 0.2 mg/L confirms toxic-acquired porphyria.*

Other laboratory values may include increased serum iron levels in porphyria cutanea tarda; leukocytosis, syndrome of inappropriate antidiuretic hormone, and elevated bilirubin and alkaline phosphatase levels in acute intermittent porphyria.

Treatment

Treatment for porphyrias includes avoiding overexposure to the sun and using beta-carotene to reduce photosensitivity, as well as support for acute and long-term management. Hemin (an enzyme-inhibitor derived from processed red blood cells) is given to control recurrent attacks of acute intermittent porphyria, Günther's disease, variegate porphyria, and hereditary coproporphyria. A high-carbohydrate diet decreases urinary excretion of ALA and PBG, with restricted fluid intake to inhibit release of antidiuretic hormone.

Special considerations

- Warn the patient to avoid excessive sun exposure, use a sunscreen when outdoors, and take a beta-carotene supplement to reduce photosensitivity.
- Encourage a high-carbohydrate diet.
- Administer beta-carotene and hemin, as ordered.

Metabolic syndrome

Metabolic syndrome—also called *syndrome X, insulin resistance syndrome, dysmetabolic syndrome,* and *multiple metabolic syndrome*—is a cluster of conditions characterized by abdominal obesity, high blood glucose (Type 2 diabetes mellitus), insulin resistance, high blood cholesterol and triglycerides, and high blood pressure. More than 22% of people in the United States meet three or more of these criteria, raising their risk of heart disease and stroke

TYPES OF PORPHYRIA

Porphyria	Signs and symptoms	Treatment
Erythropoietic porphyria		

Günther's disease
- Usual onset before age 5

- Red urine (earliest, most characteristic sign); severe cutaneous photosensitivity, leading to vesicular or bullous eruptions on exposed areas and, eventually, scarring and ulceration
- Hypertrichosis
- Brown-stained or red-stained teeth
- Splenomegaly, hemolytic anemia

- Oral beta-carotene to prevent photosensitivity reactions
- Anti-inflammatory ointments
- Prednisone to reverse anemia
- Packed red cells to inhibit erythropoiesis and excreted porphyrins
- Hemin for recurrent attacks
- Splenectomy for hemolytic anemia
- Topical dihydroxyacetone and lawsone sunscreen filter

Erythrohepatic porphyria

Protoporphyria
- Usually affects children
- Occurs most often in males

- Photosensitive dermatitis
- Hemolytic anemia
- Chronic hepatic disease

- Avoidance of causative factors
- Beta-carotene to reduce photosensitivity

Toxic-acquired porphyria
- Usually affects children
- Significant mortality

- Acute colicky pain
- Anorexia, nausea, vomiting
- Neuromuscular weakness
- Behavioral changes
- Seizures, coma

- Chlorpromazine I.V. to relieve pain and GI symptoms
- Avoidance of lead exposure

Hepatic porphyria

Acute intermittent porphyria
- Most common form
- Affects females most often, usually between ages 15 and 40

- Colicky abdominal pain with fever, general malaise, and hypertension
- Peripheral neuritis, behavioral changes, possibly leading to frank psychosis
- Possible respiratory paralysis

- Chlorpromazine I.V. to relieve abdominal pain and control psychic abnormalities
- Avoidance of barbiturates, infections, alcohol, and fasting
- Hemin for recurrent attacks
- High-carbohydrate diet

(continued)

TYPES OF PORPHYRIA *(continued)*

Porphyria	Signs and symptoms	Treatment
Hepatic porphyria (continued)		
Variegate porphyria ■ Usual onset between ages 30 and 50 ■ Occurs almost exclusively among South African whites ■ Affects males and females equally	■ Skin lesions, extremely fragile skin in exposed areas ■ Hypertrichosis ■ Hyperpigmentation ■ Abdominal pain during acute attack ■ Neuropsychiatric manifestations	■ High-carbohydrate diet ■ Avoidance of sunlight, or wearing protective clothing when avoidance isn't possible ■ Hemin for recurrent attacks
Porphyria cutanea tarda ■ Most frequent in men ages 40 to 60 ■ Highest incidence in South Africans	■ Facial pigmentation ■ Red-brown urine ■ Photosensitive dermatitis ■ Hypertrichosis	■ Avoidance of precipitating factors, such as alcohol and estrogens ■ Phlebotomy at 2-week intervals to lower serum iron level
Hereditary coproporphyria ■ Rare ■ Affects males and females equally	■ Asymptomatic or mild neurologic, abdominal, or psychiatric symptoms	■ High-carbohydrate diet ■ Avoidance of barbiturates ■ Hemin for recurrent attacks

and placing them at high risk for dying of myocardial infarction.

In the normal digestion process, the intestines break down food into its basic components, one of which is glucose. Glucose provides energy for cellular activity, while excess glucose is stored in cells for future use. Insulin, a hormone secreted in the pancreas, guides glucose into storage cells. However, in people with metabolic syndrome, glucose is insulin-resistant and doesn't respond to insulin's attempt to guide it into storage cells. Excess insulin is then required to overcome this resistance. This excess in quantity and force of insulin causes damage to the lining of the arteries, promotes fat storage deposits, and prevents fat breakdown. This series of events can lead to diabetes, blood clots, and coronary events.

Causes

Abdominal obesity is a strong predictor of metabolic syndrome because intra-abdominal fat tends to be more resistant to insulin than fat in other areas. This increases the release of free fatty acid into the portal system, leading to increased apolipoprotein B, increased low-density lipoprotein (LDL), decreased high-density lipoprotein (HDL), and increased triglycerides. As a result, the risk of cardiovascular disease is increased.

Type 2 diabetes mellitus is a risk factor because a hallmark for metabolic syndrome is a fasting glucose level greater than 110 mg/dl. People with diabetes develop atherosclerotic heart disease at a younger age than other people. They're also at increased risk of macrovascular disease (ischemic heart disease, stroke, and peripheral vascular disease). Diabetes is a coronary heart disease risk equivalent.

Insulin resistance and dyslipidemia are also risk factors because insulin resistance leads to hyperinsulinemia, hyperglycemia, abnormal glucose and lipid metabolism, damaged endothelium, and cardiovascular disease. Insulin is also responsible for reducing the amount of free fatty acids in the liver. However, people with insulin resistance have an increased amount of free fatty acids reaching the liver, resulting in high triglycerides and LDLs and producing an abnormal endothelium and atherosclerosis.

High blood pressure is a risk factor because the combination of insulin resistance, hyperinsulinemia, and abdominal obesity leads to hypertension and its harmful cardiovascular effects. Moreover, insulin resistance promotes salt sensitivity in people with high blood pressure.

Research also indicates that there may be a genetic predisposition to metabolic syndrome.

Signs and symptoms

Assessment commonly reveals a history of hypertension, abdominal obesity, sedentary lifestyle, poor diet, and a family history of metabolic syndrome. Physical findings include abdominal obesity (evidenced by a waist of more than 40″ [101.6 cm] in men and 35″ [88.9 cm] in women), blood pressure 130/85 mm Hg or higher, and a fasting blood glucose level that's 100 mg/dl or higher. The patient may feel tired, especially after eating, and may have difficulty losing weight. If left untreated, such complications as coronary artery disease, diabetes, hyperlipidemia, and premature death may develop.

Diagnosis

Blood studies commonly indicate elevated blood glucose levels, hyperinsulinemia, and elevated serum uric acid. Use of lipid profile studies reveal elevated LDL levels, low HDL levels, and elevated triglycerides. Further diagnostic procedures are nonspecific, but may be performed to detect hypertension, diabetes, hyperlipidemia, and hyperinsulinemia.

Treatment

Lifestyle modification, focusing on weight reduction and exercise, is an important part of the treatment regimen. Modest weight reduction through diet and exercise considerably improves hemoglobin A_{1c} levels, reduces insulin resistance, improves blood lipid levels, and decreases blood pressure — all elements of metabolic syndrome. Recent studies have shown that in patients with impaired glucose tolerance, losing an average of 7% of body weight reduced the risk of developing Type 2 diabetes by 58%.

To improve cardiovascular health, a diet rich in vegetables, fruits, whole grains, fish, and low-fat dairy products combined with regular exercise is recommended. Moreover, nutrient-dense, low-energy foods should replace low-nutrient, high-calorie foods. Meal replacements and shakes may also reduce risk factors for metabolic syndrome and improve weight loss. (See *Therapeutic lifestyle change diet*, page 908.)

A regular exercise program of moderate physical activity, in addition to dietary modifications, promotes weight loss, improves insulin sensitivity, and reduces blood glucose levels. According to the Surgeon General's Report on Physical Activity and Health, a person should exercise moderately for a minimum of 30 minutes on most (if not all) days of the week. The selected exercise program should improve cardiovascular conditioning, increase strength through resistance training, and improve flexibility.

Medications may be used in the treatment of metabolic syndrome for patients who have a body mass index (BMI) of 27 kg/m² or greater in the presence of other risk factors (such as diabetes, hypertension, and hyperlipidemia) or for patients with a BMI of 30 kg/m² or greater without other risk factors. Weight loss medications may also be added to lifestyle changes if the patient hasn't achieved significant weight loss after 12 weeks.

Pharmacologic treatment may also be indicated. Phentermine is used for short-term treatment of obesity in conjunction with diet and exercise. The only two medications that have been approved for long-term weight loss are orlistat and sibutramine. Orlistat works by decreasing the absorption of dietary fat by inhibiting pancreatic lipase, which is needed for fat breakdown and absorption. However, because absorption of fat-soluble vitamins is reduced, the patient may require vitamin supplementation. Studies show that when obese patients take orlistat in conjunction with dieting, they achieve greater weight

THERAPEUTIC LIFESTYLE CHANGE DIET

The therapeutic lifestyle change diet is low in saturated fats and cholesterol to reduce blood cholesterol levels and prevent development of heart disease and its complications.

Nutrient	Recommended intake
Saturated fat*	< 7% of total calories
Polyunsaturated fat	Up to 10% of total calories
Monounsaturated fat	Up to 20% of total calories
Total fat	25% to 35% of total calories
Carbohydrate**	50% to 60% of total calories
Fiber	20 to 30 gm/day
Protein	Approximately 15% of total calories
Cholesterol	< 200 mg/day
Total calories***	Balance energy intake and expenditure to maintain desirable body weight and prevent weight gain

*Trans fatty acids are another low-density lipoprotein-raising fat that should be kept at a low intake.

**Carbohydrates should be derived predominantly from foods rich in complex carbohydrates, including grains — especially whole grains, fruits, and vegetables.

***Daily expenditure should include at least moderate physical activity (contributing approximately 200 kcal/day).

Source: The National Heart, Blood, and Lung Institute. Available at: *www.nhlbi. nih.gov/chd/lifestyles.htm.*

loss and serum glucose control than by dieting alone. Sibutramine promotes weight loss by inhibiting the reuptake of serotonin, norepinephrine, and dopamine and increases the satiety-producing effects of serotonin. Further, it reduces the drop in metabolic rate that commonly occurs with weight loss.

Surgical treatment of obesity, such as through gastric bypass procedures, produces a greater degree and duration of weight loss than other therapies and improves or resolves most of the factors of metabolic syndrome. Candidates for surgical intervention include patients with a BMI greater than 40 kg/m² or those with a BMI greater than 35 kg/m² with obesity-related medical conditions. Gastric bypass procedures produce permanent weight loss in the majority of patients.

Special considerations
■ Monitor the patient's blood pressure, blood glucose, blood cholesterol, and insulin levels.
■ Because research indicates that longer lifestyle modification programs are associated with improved weight loss maintenance, encourage patients with metabolic syndrome to begin an exercise and weight loss program with a friend or family member. Assist him in exploring options and support his efforts.
■ To improve compliance, schedule frequent follow-up appointments with the patient. At that time, review his food diaries and exercise logs. Be positive and promote his active participation and partnership in his treatment plan.

HOMEOSTATIC IMBALANCE

Potassium imbalance

Potassium, a cation that's the dominant cellular electrolyte, facilitates contraction of both skeletal and smooth muscles — including myocardial contraction — and figures prominently in nerve impulse conduction, acid-base balance, enzyme action, and

CLINICAL EFFECTS OF POTASSIUM IMBALANCE

Dysfunction	Hypokalemia	Hyperkalemia
Acid-base balance	▪ Metabolic alkalosis	▪ Metabolic acidosis
Cardiovascular	▪ Dizziness, hypotension, arrhythmias, electrocardiogram (ECG) changes (flattened T waves, elevated U waves, depressed ST segment), cardiac arrest (with serum potassium levels < 2.5 mEq/L)	▪ Tachycardia and later bradycardia, ECG changes (tented and elevated T waves, widened QRS complex, prolonged PR interval, flattened or absent P waves, depressed ST segment), cardiac arrest (with levels > 7 mEq/L)
GI	▪ Nausea, vomiting, anorexia, diarrhea, abdominal distention, paralytic ileus or decreased peristalsis	▪ Nausea, diarrhea, abdominal cramps
Genitourinary	▪ Polyuria	▪ Oliguria, anuria
Musculoskeletal	▪ Muscle weakness and fatigue, leg cramps	▪ Muscle weakness, flaccid paralysis
Neurologic	▪ Malaise, irritability, confusion, mental depression, speech changes, decreased reflexes, respiratory paralysis	▪ Hyperreflexia progressing to weakness, numbness, tingling, flaccid paralysis

cell membrane function. Because serum potassium level has such a narrow range (3.5 to 5 mEq/L), a slight deviation in either direction can produce profound clinical consequences. Paradoxically, both hypokalemia (potassium deficiency) and hyperkalemia (potassium excess) can lead to muscle weakness and flaccid paralysis, because both create an ionic imbalance in neuromuscular tissue excitability. Both conditions also diminish excitability and conduction rate of the heart muscle, which may lead to cardiac arrest. (See *Clinical effects of potassium imbalance.*)

Causes

Because many foods contain potassium, hypokalemia seldom results from a dietary deficiency. Instead, potassium loss may result from:

▪ excessive GI losses, such as diarrhea, dehydration, anorexia, or chronic laxative abuse (Vomiting and gastric suction cause dehydration, resulting in hyperaldostero-nism [sodium retention and potassium excretion occur.])

▪ trauma (injury, burns, or surgery), in which damaged cells release potassium, which enters serum or extracellular fluid, to be excreted in the urine

▪ chronic renal disease, with tubular potassium wasting

▪ certain drugs, especially potassium-wasting diuretics, steroids, and certain sodium-containing antibiotics (carbenicillin)

▪ acid-base imbalances, which cause potassium shifting into cells without true depletion in alkalosis

▪ prolonged potassium-free I.V. therapy

▪ hyperglycemia, causing osmotic diuresis and glycosuria

▪ Cushing's syndrome, primary hyperaldosteronism, excessive licorice ingestion, and severe serum magnesium deficiency.

Hyperkalemia results from the kidneys' inability to excrete excessive amounts of potassium infused I.V. or administered orally; from decreased urine output, renal dysfunction or failure; or the use of potassium-sparing diuretics, such as triamterene, by patients with renal disease. It may also result from any injuries or conditions that release cellular potassium or favor its retention, such as burns, crushing injuries, failing renal function, adrenal gland insufficiency, dehydration, or diabetic acidosis.

Diagnosis

CONFIRMING DIAGNOSIS *Serum potassium levels less than 3.5 mEq/L confirm hypokalemia; serum levels greater than 5 mEq/L confirm hyperkalemia.* Additional tests may be necessary to determine the imbalance's underlying cause. Hypokalemia is also associated with hypomagnesemia, so further study of other electrolytes is warranted.

Treatment

For hypokalemia, replacement therapy with potassium chloride (I.V. or orally) is the primary treatment. When diuresis is necessary, spironolactone, a potassium-sparing diuretic, may be administered concurrently with a potassium-wasting diuretic to minimize potassium loss. Hypokalemia can be prevented by giving a maintenance dose of potassium I.V. to patients who may not take anything by mouth and to others predisposed to potassium loss.

For hyperkalemia, rapid infusion of 10% calcium gluconate decreases myocardial irritability and temporarily prevents cardiac arrest but doesn't correct serum potassium excess; it's also contraindicated in patients receiving cardiac glycosides. As an emergency measure, sodium bicarbonate I.V. increases pH and causes potassium to shift back into the cells. Insulin and 10% to 50% glucose I.V. also move potassium back into cells. Infusions should be followed by dextrose 5% in water because infusion of 10% to 15% glucose will stimulate endogenous insulin secretion. Sodium polystyrene sulfonate with 70% sorbitol produces exchange of sodium ions for potassium ions in the intestine. Hemodialysis or peritoneal dialysis also aids in removal of excess potassium.

Special considerations

For hypokalemia:
- Check serum potassium and other electrolyte levels in patients apt to develop potassium imbalance and in those requiring potassium replacement; they risk overcorrection to hyperkalemia.
- Assess intake and output carefully. Remember, the kidneys excrete 80% to 90% of ingested potassium. Never give supplementary potassium to a patient whose urine output is below 600 ml/day. Also, measure GI loss from suctioning or vomiting.
- Administer slow-release potassium or dilute oral potassium supplements in 4 oz (118 ml) or more of water or other fluid to reduce gastric and small-bowel irritation. Determine the patient's chloride level. As ordered, give a potassium chloride supplement if the level is low; potassium gluconate if it's normal.
- Give potassium I.V. only after it's diluted in solution (usually, 10 mEq/100 ml of fluid); potassium is very irritating to vascular, subcutaneous, and fatty tissues and may cause phlebitis or tissue necrosis if it infiltrates. Infuse slowly (no more than 20 mEq/L/hour through central administration or 10 mEq/hour through peripheral administration) to prevent hyperkalemia.

 ALERT *Never administer by I.V. push or bolus; it may cause cardiac arrest.*

- Carefully monitor patients receiving cardiac glycosides because hypokalemia enhances the action of these drugs and may produce signs of digoxin toxicity (anorexia, nausea, vomiting, blurred vision, and arrhythmias).
- To prevent hypokalemia, instruct patients (especially those predisposed to hypokalemia due to long-term diuretic therapy) to include in their diet foods rich in potassium — oranges, bananas, tomatoes, milk, dried fruits, apricots, peanuts and dark green, leafy vegetables.
- Monitor cardiac rhythm and report any irregularities immediately.

For hyperkalemia:
- As in hypokalemia, frequently monitor serum potassium and other electrolyte levels, and carefully record intake and output.

■ Administer sodium polystyrene sulfonate orally or rectally (by retention enema) in patients with significant potassium elevations because of intravascular sodium shifting. Watch for signs of hypokalemia with prolonged use and for clinical effects of hypoglycemia (muscle weakness, syncope, hunger, diaphoresis) with repeated insulin and glucose treatment.

■ Watch for signs of hyperkalemia in predisposed patients, especially those with poor urine output or those receiving potassium supplements orally or I.V. Administer no more than 10 to 20 mEq/L of potassium chloride per hour; check the I.V. infusion site for signs of phlebitis or infiltration of potassium into tissues. Also, before giving a blood transfusion, check to see how long ago the blood was donated; cell hemolysis in older blood releases potassium. Infuse only *fresh* blood for patients with average to high serum potassium levels.

■ Monitor for and report cardiac arrhythmias.

Sodium imbalance

Sodium is the major cation (90%) in extracellular fluid (ECF); potassium, the major cation in intracellular fluid. During repolarization, the sodium-potassium pump continually shifts sodium into the cells and potassium out of the cells; during depolarization, it does the reverse. Sodium cation functions include maintaining tonicity and concentration of ECF, acid-base balance (reabsorption of sodium ion and excretion of hydrogen ion), nerve conduction and neuromuscular function, glandular secretion, and water balance. Although the body requires only 2 to 4 g of sodium daily, most Americans consume 6 to 10 g daily (mostly sodium chloride, as table salt), excreting excess sodium through the kidneys and skin.

A low-sodium diet or excessive use of diuretics may induce hyponatremia (decreased serum sodium concentration); dehydration may induce hypernatremia (increased serum sodium concentration).

Causes

Hyponatremia can result from:

■ excessive GI loss of water and electrolytes due to vomiting, suctioning, or diarrhea; excessive perspiration or fever; use of potent diuretics; or tap-water enemas (When such losses decrease circulating fluid volume, increased secretion of antidiuretic hormone [ADH] promotes maximum water reabsorption, which further dilutes serum sodium. These factors are especially likely to cause hyponatremia when combined with excessive intake of free water.)

■ excessive drinking of water, infusion of I.V. dextrose in water without other solutes, malnutrition or starvation, or a low-sodium diet, usually in combination with one of the other causes

■ trauma, surgery (wound drainage), or burns, which cause sodium to shift into damaged cells

■ adrenal gland insufficiency (Addison's disease) or hypoaldosteronism

■ cirrhosis of the liver with ascites

■ syndrome of inappropriate antidiuretic hormone (SIADH), resulting from brain tumor, stroke, pulmonary disease, or neoplasm with ectopic ADH production. Certain drugs, such as chlorpropamide and clofibrate, may produce a SIADH-like syndrome.

Causes of hypernatremia include:

■ decreased water intake (When severe vomiting and diarrhea cause water loss that exceeds sodium loss, serum sodium levels rise, but overall extracellular fluid volume decreases.)

■ excess adrenocortical hormones, as in Cushing's syndrome

■ ADH deficiency (diabetes insipidus)

■ salt intoxication (less common), which may be produced by excessive ingestion of table salt.

Signs and symptoms

Sodium imbalance has profound physiologic effects and can induce severe central nervous system, cardiovascular, and GI abnormalities. For example, hyponatremia may cause renal dysfunction or, if serum sodium loss is abrupt or severe, seizures; hypernatremia may produce pulmonary edema, circulatory disorders, and decreased level of consciousness. (See *Clinical effects of sodium imbalance*, page 912.)

CLINICAL EFFECTS OF SODIUM IMBALANCE

Dysfunction	Hyponatremia	Hypernatremia
Cardiovascular	▪ Hypotension; tachycardia; with severe deficit, vasomotor collapse, thready pulse	▪ Hypertension, tachycardia, pitting edema, excessive weight gain
Cutaneous	▪ Cold, clammy skin; decreased skin turgor	▪ Flushed skin; dry, sticky mucous membranes
Gastrointestinal	▪ Nausea, vomiting, abdominal cramps	▪ Rough, dry tongue; intense thirst
Genitourinary	▪ Oliguria or anuria	▪ Oliguria
Neurologic	▪ Anxiety, headaches, muscle twitching and weakness, seizures	▪ Fever, agitation, restlessness, seizures
Respiratory	▪ Cyanosis with severe deficiency	▪ Dyspnea, respiratory arrest, and death (from dramatic rise in osmotic pressure)

Diagnosis

Hyponatremia is defined as a serum sodium level less than 135 mEq/L; hypernatremia, as a serum sodium level greater than 145 mEq/L. However, additional laboratory studies are necessary to determine etiology and to differentiate between a true deficit and an apparent deficit due to sodium shift or to hypervolemia or hypovolemia. In true hyponatremia, supportive values include urine sodium greater than 100 mEq/24 hours, with low serum osmolality; in true hypernatremia, urine sodium level is less than 40 mEq/24 hours, with high serum osmolality. (See *Diagnosing hyponatremia.*)

Treatment

Therapy for mild hyponatremia usually consists of restricted free-water intake when it's due to hemodilution, SIADH, or such conditions as heart failure, cirrhosis of the liver, and renal failure. If fluid restriction alone fails to normalize serum sodium levels, demeclocycline or lithium, which blocks ADH action in the renal tubules, can be used to promote water excretion. In extremely rare instances of severe symptomatic hyponatremia, when serum sodium levels fall below 110 mEq/L, treatment may include infusion of 3% or 5% saline solution.

Treatment with saline infusion requires careful monitoring of venous pressure to prevent potentially fatal circulatory overload. The aim of treatment of secondary hyponatremia is to correct the underlying disorder.

Primary treatment of hypernatremia is administration of salt-free solutions (such as dextrose in water) to return serum sodium levels to normal, followed by infusion of half-normal saline solution to prevent hyponatremia. Other measures include a sodium-restricted diet and discontinuation of drugs that promote sodium retention.

Special considerations

When managing the patient with hyponatremia:

▪ Watch for and report extremely low serum sodium and accompanying serum chloride levels. Monitor urine specific gravity and other laboratory results. Record fluid intake and output accurately, and weigh the patient daily.

▪ During administration of isosmolar or hyperosmolar saline solution, watch closely for signs of hypervolemia (dyspnea, crackles, engorged jugular or hand veins). Re-

DIFFERENTIAL DIAGNOSIS

DIAGNOSING HYPONATREMIA

This flowchart lists possible diagnostic findings and interpretations to assist with treatment of the patient with hyponatremia.

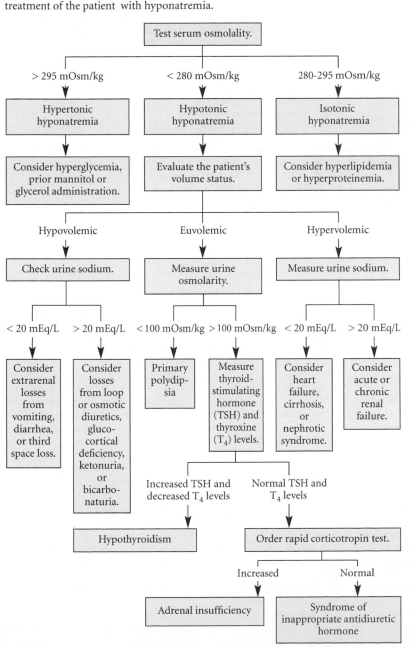

CLINICAL EFFECTS OF CALCIUM IMBALANCE

Dysfunction	Hypocalcemia	Hypercalcemia
Cardiovascular	▪ Arrhythmias, hypotension	▪ Signs of heart block, cardiac arrest in systole, hypertension
Gastrointestinal	▪ Increased GI motility, diarrhea	▪ Anorexia, nausea, vomiting, constipation, dehydration, polydipsia
Musculoskeletal	▪ Paresthesia (tingling and numbness of the fingers), tetany or painful tonic muscle spasms, facial spasms, abdominal cramps, muscle cramps, spasmodic contractions	▪ Weakness, muscle flaccidity, bone pain, pathologic fractures
Neurologic	▪ Anxiety, irritability, twitching around mouth, laryngospasm, seizures, Chvostek's sign, Trousseau's sign	▪ Drowsiness, lethargy, headaches, depression or apathy, irritability, confusion
Other	▪ Blood-clotting abnormalities	▪ Renal polyuria, flank pain and, eventually, azotemia

port conditions that may cause excessive sodium loss (diaphoresis or prolonged diarrhea or vomiting, and severe burns).
▪ Refer the patient on maintenance dosage of diuretics to a dietitian for instruction about dietary sodium intake.
▪ To prevent hyponatremia, administer isosmolar solutions.

When managing the patient with hypernatremia:
▪ Measure serum sodium levels at least every 6 hours until stabilized. Monitor vital signs for changes, especially for rising pulse rate. Watch for signs of hypervolemia, especially in the patient receiving I.V. fluids.
▪ Record fluid intake and output accurately, checking for body fluid loss. Weigh the patient daily.
▪ Obtain a drug history to check for drugs that promote sodium retention.
▪ Explain the importance of sodium restriction and teach the patient how to plan a low-sodium diet. Closely monitor the serum sodium levels of high-risk patients.

Calcium imbalance

Calcium plays an indispensable role in cell permeability, bone and teeth formation, blood coagulation, transmission of nerve impulses, and normal muscle contraction. Nearly all (99%) of the body's calcium is found in the bones. The remaining 1% exists in the blood, with 50% of the remainder bound to plasma proteins and 40% ionized or free. The ionized calcium in the serum is critical to healthy neurologic function. The parathyroid glands regulate ionized calcium and determine its resorption into bone, absorption from the GI mucosa, and excretion in urine and feces. Severe calcium imbalance requires emergency treatment because a deficiency (hypocalcemia) can lead to tetany and seizures; an excess (hypercalcemia), to cardiac arrhythmias and coma. (See *Clinical effects of calcium imbalance.*)

Causes

Common causes of hypocalcemia include:

- inadequate intake of calcium and vitamin D, in which inadequate levels of vitamin D inhibit intestinal absorption of calcium
- hypoparathyroidism as a result of injury, disease, or surgery that decreases or eliminates secretion of parathyroid hormone (PTH), which is necessary for calcium absorption and normal serum calcium levels
- malabsorption or loss of calcium from the GI tract, caused by increased intestinal motility from severe diarrhea or laxative abuse; can also result from inadequate levels of vitamin D or PTH, or a reduction in gastric acidity, decreasing the solubility of calcium salts
- severe infections or burns, in which diseased and burned tissue traps calcium from the extracellular fluid
- overcorrection of acidosis, resulting in alkalosis, which causes decreased ionized calcium and induces symptoms of hypocalcemia
- pancreatic insufficiency, which may cause malabsorption of calcium and subsequent calcium loss in feces. In pancreatitis, participation of calcium ions in saponification contributes to calcium loss
- renal failure, resulting in excessive excretion of calcium secondary to increased retention of phosphate
- hypomagnesemia, which causes decreased PTH secretion and blocks the peripheral action of that hormone.

Causes of hypercalcemia include the following:
- hyperparathyroidism, which increases serum calcium levels by promoting calcium absorption from the intestine, resorption from bone, and reabsorption from the kidneys
- hypervitaminosis D, which can promote increased absorption of calcium from the intestine
- tumors, which raise serum calcium levels by destroying bone or by releasing PTH or a PTH-like substance, osteoclast-activating factor, prostaglandins and, perhaps, a vitamin D-like sterol
- multiple fractures and prolonged immobilization, which release bone calcium and raise the serum calcium level
- multiple myeloma, which promotes loss of calcium from bone.

TROUSSEAU'S SIGN

To check for Trousseau's sign, apply a blood pressure cuff to the patient's arm. A carpopedal spasm that causes thumb adduction and phalangeal extension, as shown, confirms tetany.

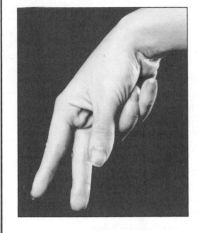

Other causes include milk-alkali syndrome, sarcoidosis, hyperthyroidism, adrenal insufficiency, thiazide diuretics, and loss of serum albumin secondary to renal disease.

Signs and symptoms
Calcium deficit causes nerve fiber irritability and repetitive muscle spasms. Consequently, characteristic symptoms of hypocalcemia include perioral paresthesia, twitching, carpopedal spasm, tetany, seizures and, possibly, cardiac arrhythmias. Chvostek's sign and Trousseau's sign are reliable indicators of hypocalcemia. (See *Trousseau's sign.* Also see *Chvostek's sign,* page 918.)

Clinical effects of hypercalcemia include muscle weakness, decreased muscle tone, lethargy, anorexia, constipation, nausea, vomiting, dehydration, polydipsia, and polyuria. Severe hypercalcemia (serum levels that exceed 15 mg/dl) may produce cardiac arrhythmias and, eventually, coma.

(*Text continues on page 918.*)

DIFFERENTIAL DIAGNOSIS

DIAGNOSING HYPERCALCEMIA

This flowchart lists possible diagnostic findings and interpretations to assist with treatment of the patient with hypercalcemia:

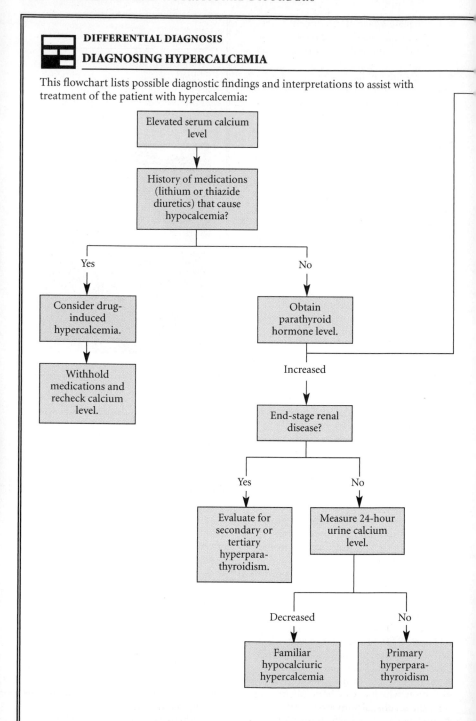

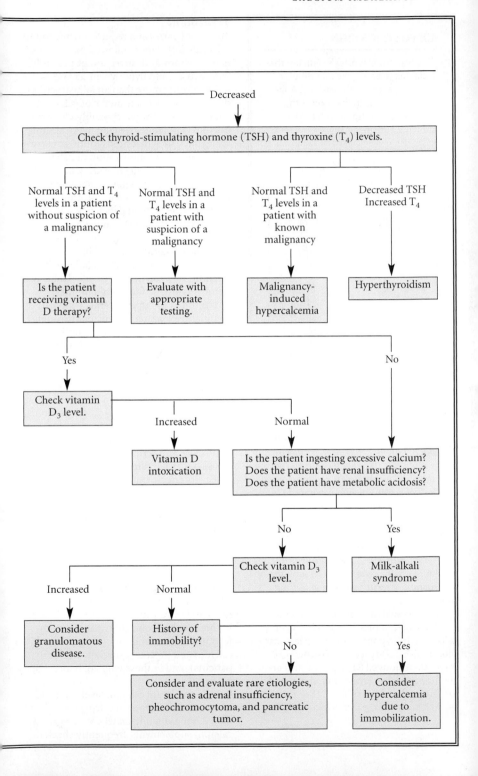

CHVOSTEK'S SIGN

To check for Chvostek's sign, tap the facial nerve above the mandibular angle, adjacent to the earlobe. A facial muscle spasm that causes the patient's upper lip to twitch, as shown, confirms tetany.

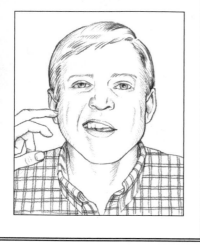

Diagnosis

CONFIRMING DIAGNOSIS
A serum calcium level less than 8.5 mg/dl confirms hypocalcemia; a level more than 10.5 mg/dl confirms hypercalcemia. (However, because approximately one-half of serum calcium is bound to albumin, changes in serum protein must be considered when interpreting serum calcium levels. A common conversion formula is calcium corrected = calcium actual + 0.8 × [4.0 – albumin level]. Ionized calcium levels are 4.65 to 5.28 mg/dl and are a measure of the fraction of serum calcium in ionized form.)

The Sulkowitch urine test shows increased calcium precipitation in hypercalcemia. In hypocalcemia, an electrocardiogram (ECG) reveals lengthened QT interval, prolonged ST segment, and arrhythmias; in hypercalcemia, shortened QT interval and heart block. (See *Diagnosing hypercalcemia,* pages 916 and 917.)

Treatment

Treatment varies and requires correction of the acute imbalance, followed by maintenance therapy and correction of the underlying cause. Mild hypocalcemia may require nothing more than an adjustment in diet to allow adequate intake of calcium, vitamin D, and protein, possibly with oral calcium supplements. Acute hypocalcemia is an emergency that needs immediate correction by I.V. administration of calcium gluconate or calcium chloride. Chronic hypocalcemia also requires vitamin D supplements to facilitate GI absorption of calcium. To correct mild deficiency states, the amounts of vitamin D in most multivitamin preparations are adequate. For severe deficiency, vitamin D is used in four forms: ergocalciferol (vitamin D_2), cholecalciferol (vitamin D_3), calcitriol, and dihydrotachysterol, a synthetic form of vitamin D_2.

Treatment of hypercalcemia primarily eliminates excess serum calcium through hydration with normal saline solution, which promotes calcium excretion in the urine. Loop diuretics, such as ethacrynic acid and furosemide, also promote calcium excretion. (Thiazide diuretics are contraindicated in hypercalcemia because they inhibit calcium excretion.) Corticosteroids, such as prednisone and hydrocortisone, are helpful in treating sarcoidosis, hypervitaminosis D, and certain tumors. Plicamycin can also lower serum calcium levels and is especially effective against hypercalcemia secondary to certain tumors. Calcitonin may also be helpful in certain instances. Sodium phosphate solution administered orally or by retention enema promotes calcium deposition in bone and inhibits its absorption from the GI tract.

Special considerations

Watch for hypocalcemia in patients receiving massive transfusions of citrated blood; in those with chronic diarrhea, severe infections, and insufficient dietary intake of calcium and protein (especially in elderly patients); and in those who are hyperventilating.

■ Monitor serum calcium levels every 12 to 24 hours and report a calcium level less than 8.5 mg/dl immediately. When giving calcium supplements, frequently check the

pH level because a pH lower than 7.45 inhibits calcium ionization. Check for Trousseau's and Chvostek's signs.
■ Administer calcium gluconate slow I.V. in 5% dextrose in water (*never* in saline solution, which encourages renal calcium loss). Don't add calcium gluconate I.V. to solutions containing bicarbonate; it will precipitate. When administering calcium solutions, watch for anorexia, nausea, and vomiting—possible signs of overcorrection to hypercalcemia. Never infuse more than 1g/hour, except in an emergency. Use a volume-control device to ensure proper flow rate.
■ If the patient is receiving calcium chloride, watch for abdominal discomfort.

 ALERT *Don't confuse calcium chloride with calcium gluconate in administration; 1 gm of calcium chloride has three times the calcium as 1 gm of calcium gluconate.*

■ Monitor the patient closely for a possible drug interaction if he's receiving cardiac glycosides with large doses of oral calcium supplements; watch for signs of digoxin toxicity (anorexia, nausea, vomiting, yellow vision, and cardiac arrhythmias). Administer oral calcium supplements 1 to 1½ hours after meals or with milk.
■ Provide a quiet, stress-free environment for the patient with tetany. Observe seizure precautions for patients with severe hypocalcemia.
■ To prevent hypocalcemia, advise all patients—especially elderly patients—to eat foods rich in calcium, vitamin D, and protein, such as fortified milk and cheese. Explain how important calcium is for normal bone formation and blood coagulation. Discourage chronic use of laxatives. Also, warn hypocalcemic patients not to overuse antacids, because these may aggravate the condition.
   If the patient has hypercalcemia:
■ Monitor serum calcium levels frequently. Watch for cardiac arrhythmias if serum calcium levels exceed their normal values of 8.5 to 10.5 mg/dl. Increase fluid intake to dilute calcium in serum and urine, and to prevent renal damage and dehydration. Watch for signs of heart failure in patients receiving normal saline diuresis.

■ Administer loop diuretics (not thiazide diuretics), as ordered. Monitor intake and output, and check urine for renal calculi and acidity. Provide acid-ash drinks, such as cranberry or prune juice, because calcium salts are more soluble in acid than in alkali.
■ Check ECG and vital signs frequently. In the patient receiving cardiac glycosides, watch for signs of toxicity, such as anorexia, nausea, vomiting, and bradycardia (often with arrhythmia).
■ Ambulate the patient as soon as possible. Handle the patient with chronic hypercalcemia *gently* to prevent pathologic fractures. If the patient is bedridden, reposition him frequently and encourage range-of-motion exercises to promote circulation and prevent urinary stasis and calcium loss from bone.
■ To prevent recurrence, suggest a low-calcium diet, with increased fluid intake.

Chloride imbalance

Hypochloremia and hyperchloremia are, respectively, conditions of deficient or excessive serum levels of the chloride anion. A predominantly extracellular anion, chloride accounts for two-thirds of all serum anions. Secreted by stomach mucosa as hydrochloric acid, it provides an acid medium that aids digestion and activation of enzymes. Chloride also participates in maintaining acid-base and body water balances, influences the osmolality or tonicity of extracellular fluid (ECF), plays a role in the exchange of oxygen and carbon dioxide in red blood cells, and helps activate salivary amylase (which, in turn, activates the digestive process).

Causes
Hypochloremia may result from:
■ decreased chloride intake or absorption, as in low dietary sodium intake, sodium deficiency, potassium deficiency, metabolic alkalosis; prolonged use of mercurial diuretics; or administration of dextrose I.V. without electrolytes
■ excessive chloride loss resulting from prolonged diarrhea or diaphoresis; loss of hydrochloric acid in gastric secretions due

to vomiting, gastric suctioning, or gastric surgery.

Hyperchloremia may result from:
- excessive chloride intake or absorption—as in hyperingestion of ammonium chloride, or ureterointestinal anastomosis—allowing reabsorption of chloride by the bowel
- hemoconcentration due to dehydration
- compensatory mechanisms for other metabolic abnormalities, as in metabolic acidosis, brain stem injury causing neurogenic hyperventilation, and hyperparathyroidism.

Signs and symptoms

Hypochloremia is usually associated with hyponatremia and its characteristic muscle weakness and twitching because renal chloride loss always accompanies sodium loss, and sodium reabsorption isn't possible without chloride. However, if chloride depletion results from metabolic alkalosis secondary to loss of gastric secretions, chloride is lost independently from sodium; typical symptoms are muscle hypertonicity, tetany, and shallow, depressed breathing.

Because of the natural affinity of sodium and chloride ions, hyperchloremia usually produces clinical effects associated with hypernatremia and resulting ECF volume excess (agitation, tachycardia, hypertension, pitting edema, dyspnea). Hyperchloremia associated with metabolic acidosis is due to excretion of base bicarbonate by the kidneys, and induces deep, rapid breathing; weakness; diminished cognitive ability; and, ultimately, coma.

Diagnosis

CONFIRMING DIAGNOSIS *A serum chloride level below 98 mEq/L confirms hypochloremia. (Supportive values in metabolic alkalosis include serum pH above 7.45 and serum carbon dioxide [CO_2] level above 32 mEq/L.) A serum chloride level above 108 mEq/L confirms hyperchloremia; with metabolic acidosis, serum pH is below 7.35 and serum CO_2 level is below 22 mEq/L.*

Treatment

Hypochloremia therapy aims to correct the condition that causes excessive chloride loss and to give oral replacement such as salty broth. When oral therapy isn't possible, or when emergency measures are necessary, treatment may include normal saline solution I.V. (if hypovolemia is present) or chloride-containing drugs, such as ammonium chloride, to increase serum chloride levels, and potassium chloride for metabolic alkalosis. For severe hyperchloremic acidosis, treatment consists of sodium bicarbonate I.V. to raise the serum bicarbonate level and permit renal excretion of the chloride anion, because bicarbonate and chloride compete for combination with sodium. For mild hyperchloremia, Ringer's lactate solution is administered; it converts to bicarbonate in the liver, thus increasing base bicarbonate to correct acidosis.

In either kind of chloride imbalance, treatment must correct the underlying disorder.

Special considerations

When managing the patient with hypochloremia:
- Monitor serum chloride levels frequently, particularly during I.V. therapy.
- Watch for signs of hyperchloremia or hypochloremia. Be alert for respiratory difficulty.
- To prevent hypochloremia, monitor laboratory results (serum electrolyte levels and blood gas values) and fluid intake and output of patients who are vulnerable to chloride imbalance, particularly those recovering from gastric surgery. Record and report excessive or continuous loss of gastric secretions. Also report prolonged infusion of dextrose in water without saline.

When managing the patient with hyperchloremia:
- Check serum electrolyte levels every 3 to 6 hours. If the patient is receiving high doses of sodium bicarbonate, watch for signs of overcorrection (metabolic alkalosis, respiratory depression) or lingering signs of hyperchloremia, which indicate inadequate treatment.
- To prevent hyperchloremia, check laboratory results for elevated serum chloride

levels or potassium imbalance if the patient is receiving I.V. solutions containing sodium chloride, and monitor fluid intake and output. Also, watch for signs of metabolic acidosis. When administering I.V. fluids containing Ringer's lactate solution, monitor flow rate according to the patient's age, physical condition, and bicarbonate level. Report any irregularities promptly.

Magnesium imbalance

Magnesium is the second most common cation in intracellular fluid. Although its major function is to enhance neuromuscular integration, it also stimulates parathyroid hormone (PTH) secretion, thus regulating intracellular fluid calcium levels. Therefore, magnesium deficiency (hypomagnesemia) may result in transient hypoparathyroidism or interference with the peripheral action of PTH. Magnesium may also regulate skeletal muscles through its influence on calcium utilization by depressing acetylcholine release at synaptic junctions. In addition, magnesium activates many enzymes for proper carbohydrate and protein metabolism, aids in cell metabolism and the transport of sodium and potassium across cell membranes, and influences sodium, potassium, calcium, and protein levels.

Approximately one-third of magnesium taken into the body is absorbed through the small intestine and is eventually excreted in the urine; the remaining unabsorbed magnesium is excreted in the stool.

Because many common foods contain magnesium, a dietary deficiency is rare. Hypomagnesemia generally follows impaired absorption, too-rapid excretion, or inadequate intake during total parenteral nutrition. It frequently coexists with other electrolyte imbalances, especially low calcium and potassium levels. Magnesium excess (hypermagnesemia) is common in patients with renal failure and excessive intake of magnesium-containing antacids.

Causes

Hypomagnesemia usually results from impaired absorption of magnesium in the intestines or excessive excretion in urine or stool. Possible causes include:

- decreased magnesium intake or absorption, as in malabsorption syndrome, chronic diarrhea, or postoperative complications after bowel resection; chronic alcoholism; prolonged diuretic therapy, nasogastric suctioning, or administration of parenteral fluids without magnesium salts; and starvation or malnutrition
- excessive loss of magnesium, as in severe dehydration and diabetic acidosis; hyperaldosteronism and hypoparathyroidism, which result in hypokalemia and hypocalcemia; hyperparathyroidism and hypercalcemia; excessive release of adrenocortical hormones; and diuretic therapy.

Hypermagnesemia results from the kidneys' inability to excrete magnesium that was either absorbed from the intestines or infused. Common causes of hypermagnesemia include:

- chronic renal insufficiency
- use of laxatives (magnesium sulfate, milk of magnesia, and magnesium citrate solutions), especially with renal insufficiency
- overuse of magnesium-containing antacids
- severe dehydration (resulting oliguria can cause magnesium retention)
- overcorrection of hypomagnesemia.

Signs and symptoms

Hypomagnesemia causes neuromuscular irritability and cardiac arrhythmias. Hypermagnesemia causes central nervous system and respiratory depression, in addition to neuromuscular and cardiac effects. (See *Signs and symptoms of magnesium imbalance*, page 922.)

Diagnosis

CONFIRMING DIAGNOSIS *Serum magnesium levels less than 1.5 mEq/L confirm hypomagnesemia; levels greater than 2.5 mEq/L confirm hypermagnesemia.*

Low levels of other serum electrolytes (especially potassium and calcium) often coexist with hypomagnesemia. In fact, unresponsiveness to correct treatment for hypokalemia strongly suggests hypomagnesemia. Similarly, elevated levels of other

SIGNS AND SYMPTOMS OF MAGNESIUM IMBALANCE

Dysfunction	Hypomagnesemia	Hypermagnesemia
Cardiovascular	■ Arrhythmias (such as torsade de pointes), vasomotor changes (vasodilation and hypotension) and, occasionally, hypertension	■ Bradycardia, weak pulse, hypotension, heart block, cardiac arrest (common with serum levels of 25 mEq/L)
Neurologic	■ Confusion, delusions, hallucinations, seizures	■ Drowsiness, flushing, lethargy, confusion, diminished sensorium
Neuromuscular	■ Hyperirritability, tetany, leg and foot cramps, Chvostek's sign (facial muscle spasms induced by tapping the branches of the facial nerve)	■ Diminished reflexes, muscle weakness, flaccid paralysis, respiratory muscle paralysis that may cause respiratory insufficiency

serum electrolytes are associated with hypermagnesemia.

Treatment
Therapy for magnesium imbalance aims to identify and correct the underlying cause.

Treatment of mild hypomagnesemia consists of daily magnesium supplements I.M. or orally; of severe hypomagnesemia, magnesium sulfate I.V. (10 to 40 mEq/L diluted in I.V. fluid). Magnesium intoxication (a possible adverse effect) requires calcium gluconate I.V.

Therapy for hypermagnesemia includes increased fluid intake and loop diuretics (such as furosemide) with impaired renal function; calcium gluconate (10%), a magnesium antagonist, for temporary relief of symptoms in an emergency; and peritoneal dialysis or hemodialysis if renal function fails or if excess magnesium can't be eliminated.

Special considerations
For patients with hypomagnesemia:
■ Monitor serum electrolyte levels (including magnesium, calcium, and potassium) daily for mild deficits and every 6 to 12 hours during replacement therapy.
■ Measure intake and output frequently. (Urine output shouldn't fall below 0.5 to 1 ml/kg/day in patients with healthy body weight; in heavier patients, less than

50 ml/hour is a cause for concern.) Remember, the kidneys excrete excess magnesium, and hypermagnesemia could occur with renal insufficiency.
■ Monitor vital signs during I.V. therapy. Infuse magnesium replacement slowly and watch for bradycardia, heart block, and decreased respiratory rate. Have calcium gluconate I.V. available to reverse hypermagnesemia from overcorrection. In patients with torsade de pointes, elevated magnesium levels are therapeutic.
■ Advise patients to eat foods high in magnesium, such as fish and green vegetables.
■ Watch for and report signs of hypomagnesemia in patients with predisposing diseases or conditions, especially those not permitted anything by mouth or who receive I.V. fluids without magnesium.

For patients with hypermagnesemia:
■ Frequently assess level of consciousness, muscle activity, and vital signs.
■ Keep accurate intake and output records. Provide sufficient fluids for adequate hydration and maintenance of renal function.
■ Report abnormal serum electrolyte levels immediately.
■ Monitor and report electrocardiogram changes (peaked T waves, increased PR intervals, widened QRS complex).
■ Watch patients receiving cardiac glycosides and calcium gluconate simultaneously, because calcium excess enhances digoxin

action, predisposing the patient to digoxin toxicity.

■ Advise patients, particularly elderly patients and patients with compromised renal function, not to abuse laxatives and antacids containing magnesium.

■ Watch for signs of hypermagnesemia in predisposed patients. Observe closely for respiratory distress if magnesium serum levels rise above 10 mEq/L.

Phosphorus imbalance

Phosphorus exists primarily in inorganic combination with calcium in teeth and bones. In extracellular fluid, the phosphate ion supports several metabolic functions: utilization of B vitamins, acid-base homeostasis, bone formation, nerve and muscle activity, cell division, transmission of hereditary traits, and metabolism of carbohydrates, proteins, and fats. Renal tubular reabsorption of phosphate is inversely regulated by calcium levels — an increase in phosphorus causes a decrease in calcium. An imbalance causes hypophosphatemia or hyperphosphatemia. Incidence of hypophosphatemia varies with the underlying cause; hyperphosphatemia occurs most often in children, who tend to consume more phosphorus-rich foods and beverages than adults, and in children and adults with renal insufficiency. The prognosis for both conditions depends on the underlying cause.

Causes

Hypophosphatemia is usually the result of inadequate dietary intake; it's often related to malnutrition resulting from a prolonged catabolic state or chronic alcoholism. It may also stem from intestinal malabsorption, chronic diarrhea, hyperparathyroidism with resultant hypercalcemia, hypomagnesemia, or deficiency of vitamin D, which is necessary for intestinal phosphorus absorption. Other causes include chronic use of antacids containing aluminum hydroxide, use of parenteral nutrition solution with inadequate phosphate content, renal tubular defects, tissue damage in which phosphorus is released by injured cells, and diabetic acidosis.

Hyperphosphatemia is generally secondary to hypocalcemia, hypervitaminosis D, hypoparathyroidism, or renal failure (often due to stress or injury). It may also result from overuse of laxatives with phosphates or phosphate enemas.

Signs and symptoms

Hypophosphatemia produces anorexia, muscle weakness, tremor, paresthesia and, when persistent, osteomalacia, causing bone pain. Impaired red blood cell functions may occur in hypophosphatemia due to alterations in oxyhemoglobin dissociation, which may result in peripheral hypoxia. Hyperphosphatemia usually remains asymptomatic unless it results in hypocalcemia, with tetany and seizures.

Diagnosis

CONFIRMING DIAGNOSIS
Serum phosphorus levels less than 1.7 mEq/L or 2.5 mg/dl confirm hypophosphatemia. Urine phosphorus levels above 1.3 g/24 hours support this diagnosis. Serum phosphorus levels above 2.6 mEq/L or 4.5 mg/dl confirm hyperphosphatemia. Supportive values include decreased levels of serum calcium (less than 9 mg/dl) and urine phosphorus (less than 0.9 g/24 hours).

Treatment

Treatment aims to correct the underlying cause of phosphorus imbalance. Until this is done, management of hypophosphatemia consists of phosphorus replacement with a high-phosphorus diet and oral administration of phosphate salt tablets or capsules. (See *Foods high in phosphorus,* page 924.) Severe hypophosphatemia requires I.V. infusion of potassium phosphate. Severe hyperphosphatemia may require peritoneal dialysis or hemodialysis to lower the serum phosphorus level.

Special considerations

■ Carefully monitor serum electrolyte, calcium, magnesium, and phosphorus levels. Report any changes immediately.
To manage hypophosphatemia:
■ Record intake and output accurately. Administer potassium phosphate slow I.V. to prevent overcorrection to hyperphosphatemia. Assess renal function and be

FOODS HIGH IN PHOSPHORUS

Food	Portion	Amount (mg)
Almonds	⅔ cup	475
Beef liver (fried)	3½ oz	476
Broccoli (cooked)	⅔ cup	62
Carbonated beverages	12 oz	Up to 500
Milk (whole)	8 oz	93
Turkey (roasted)	3½ oz	251

alert for hypocalcemia when giving phosphate supplements. If phosphate salt tablets cause nausea, use capsules instead.

■ To prevent recurrence, advise the patient to follow a high-phosphorus diet containing milk and milk products, kidney, liver, turkey, and dried fruits.

To manage hyperphosphatemia:

■ Monitor intake and output. If urine output falls below 25 ml/hour or 600 ml/day, notify the physician immediately, because decreased output can seriously affect renal clearance of excess serum phosphorus.

■ Watch for signs of hypocalcemia, such as muscle twitching and tetany, which often accompany hyperphosphatemia.

■ To prevent recurrence, advise the patient to eat foods with low phosphorus content such as vegetables. Obtain dietary consultation if the condition results from chronic renal insufficiency.

Syndrome of inappropriate antidiuretic hormone

Syndrome of inappropriate antidiuretic hormone (SIADH), also known as *dilutional hyponatremia,* is marked by excessive release of antidiuretic hormone (ADH), which disturbs fluid and electrolyte balance. Such disturbances result from the inability to excrete dilute urine, free water retention, extracellular fluid volume expansion, and hyponatremia. SIADH occurs secondary to diseases that affect the osmoreceptors (supraoptic nucleus) of the hypothalamus. The prognosis depends on the underlying disorder and response to treatment.

Causes

The most common cause of SIADH (80% of patients) is oat cell carcinoma of the lung, which secretes excessive ADH or vasopressor-like substances. Other neoplastic diseases, such as pancreatic and prostatic cancer, Hodgkin's disease, and thymoma, may also trigger SIADH.

Less common causes include:

■ central nervous system disorders: brain tumor or abscess, stroke, head injury, Guillain-Barré syndrome, and lupus erythematosus

■ pulmonary disorders: pneumonia, tuberculosis, lung abscess, and positive-pressure ventilation

■ drugs: chlorpropamide, vincristine, cyclophosphamide, carbamazepine, clofibrate, and morphine

■ miscellaneous conditions: myxedema and psychosis.

Signs and symptoms

SIADH may produce weight gain despite anorexia, nausea, and vomiting; muscle weakness; restlessness; and, possibly, coma and seizures. Edema is rare unless water overload exceeds 4 L because much of the free water excess is within cellular boundaries.

Diagnosis

A complete medical history revealing positive water balance may suggest SIADH.

CONFIRMING DIAGNOSIS *Serum osmolality less than 280 mOsm/kg of water and a serum sodium level below 123 mEq/L confirm the diagnosis (normal urine osmolality is 1½ times serum values).*

Supportive laboratory values include high urine sodium secretion (more than

20 mEq/L) without diuretics and high urine osmolality. In addition, diagnostic studies show normal renal function and no evidence of dehydration.

Treatment

Treatment for SIADH is symptomatic and begins with restricted water intake (500 to 1,000 ml/day). Some patients who continue to have symptoms are given a high-salt, high-protein diet or urea supplements to enhance water excretion. They may also receive demeclocycline or lithium to help block the renal response to ADH. With severe water intoxication, administration of 200 to 300 ml of 5% saline may be necessary to raise the serum sodium level. When possible, treatment should include correction of the underlying cause of SIADH. If SIADH is due to cancer, success in alleviating water retention may be obtained by surgical resection, irradiation, or chemotherapy.

Special considerations

■ Closely monitor and record intake and output, vital signs, and daily weight. Watch for hyponatremia.
■ Observe for restlessness, irritability, seizures, heart failure, and unresponsiveness due to hyponatremia and water intoxication.
■ To prevent water intoxication, explain to the patient and his family why he must restrict his intake.

Metabolic acidosis

Metabolic acidosis is a physiologic state of excess acid accumulation and deficient base bicarbonate produced by an underlying pathologic disorder. Symptoms result from the body's attempts to correct the acidotic condition through compensatory mechanisms in the lungs, kidneys, and cells. Metabolic acidosis is more prevalent among children, who are vulnerable to acid-base imbalance because their metabolic rates are faster and their ratios of water to total-body weight are lower. Severe or untreated metabolic acidosis can be fatal.

Causes

Metabolic acidosis usually results from excessive fat burning in the absence of usable carbohydrates. This can be caused by diabetic ketoacidosis, chronic alcoholism, malnutrition, or a low-carbohydrate, high-fat diet — all of which produce more keto acids than the metabolic process can handle. Other causes include:
■ anaerobic carbohydrate metabolism: a decrease in tissue oxygenation or perfusion (as occurs with pump failure after myocardial infarction, or with pulmonary or hepatic disease, shock, or anemia) forces a shift from aerobic to anaerobic metabolism, causing a corresponding rise in lactic acid level
■ renal insufficiency and failure (renal acidosis): underexcretion of metabolized acids or inability to conserve base
■ diarrhea and intestinal malabsorption: loss of sodium bicarbonate from the intestines, causing the bicarbonate buffer system to shift to the acidic side. For example, ureteroenterostomy and Crohn's disease can also induce metabolic acidosis.

Less frequently, metabolic acidosis results from salicylate intoxication (overuse of aspirin), exogenous poisoning, or Addison's disease with an increased excretion of sodium and chloride, and retention of potassium ions.

Signs and symptoms

In mild acidosis, the underlying disease's symptoms may obscure any direct clinical evidence. Metabolic acidosis typically begins with headache and lethargy, progressing to drowsiness, central nervous system depression, Kussmaul's respirations (as the lungs attempt to compensate by "blowing off" carbon dioxide), stupor and, if the condition is severe and goes untreated, coma and death. Associated GI distress usually produces anorexia, nausea, vomiting, and diarrhea, and may lead to dehydration. Underlying diabetes mellitus may cause fruity breath from catabolism of fats and excretion of accumulated acetone through the lungs.

ANION GAP

The anion gap is the difference between concentrations of serum cations and anions — determined by measuring one cation (sodium) and two anions (chloride and bicarbonate). The normal concentration of sodium is 140 mEq/L; of chloride, 102 mEq/L; and of bicarbonate, 26 mEq/L. Thus, the anion gap between *measured* cations (actually sodium alone) and *measured* anions is about 12 mEq/L (140 minus 128).

Concentrations of potassium, calcium, and magnesium (*unmeasured* cations), or proteins, phosphate, sulfate, and organic acids (*unmeasured* anions) aren't needed to measure the anion gap. Added together, the concentration of unmeasured cations would be about 11 mEq/L; of unmeasured anions, about 23 mEq/L. Thus, the normal anion gap between unmeasured cations and anions is about 12 mEq/L (23 minus 11) — plus or minus 2 mEq/L for normal variation. An anion gap over 14 mEq/L indicates *metabolic acidosis*. It may result from accumulation of excess organic acids or from retention of hydrogen ions, which chemically bond with bicarbonate and decrease bicarbonate levels.

Diagnosis

CONFIRMING DIAGNOSIS *Arterial pH below 7.35 confirms metabolic acidosis. In severe acidotic states, pH may fall to 7.10, and the partial pressure of arterial carbon dioxide may be normal or below 34 mm Hg as compensatory mechanisms take hold. Bicarbonate may be below 22 mEq/L.*

A metabolic panel can help reveal the cause and severity of metabolic acidosis. A complete blood count can be done to help assess possible causes as well. Supportive findings include:

- urine pH: below 4.5 in the absence of renal disease
- serum potassium levels: above 5.5 mEq/L from chemical buffering
- glucose levels: above 150 mg/dl in diabetes
- serum ketone bodies: elevated levels in diabetes mellitus
- serum osmolarity: increased levels, as in hyperosmolar hyperglycemic nonketotic acidosis or dehydration
- plasma lactic acid: elevated levels in lactic acidosis
- anion gap: greater than 14 mEq/L indicating metabolic acidosis (diabetic ketoacidosis, aspirin overdose, alcohol poisoning). (See *Anion gap.*)

Treatment

In metabolic acidosis, treatment consists of administration of sodium bicarbonate I.V. for severe cases, evaluation and correction of electrolyte imbalances and, ultimately, correction of the underlying cause. For example, in diabetic ketoacidosis, a low-dose continuous I.V. infusion of insulin is recommended.

Special considerations

- Keep sodium bicarbonate ampules handy for emergency administration. Monitor vital signs, laboratory results, and level of consciousness frequently because changes can occur rapidly.
- In diabetic acidosis, watch for secondary changes due to hypovolemia, such as decreasing blood pressure.
- Record intake and output accurately to monitor renal function. Watch for signs of excessive serum potassium — weakness, flaccid paralysis, and arrhythmias, possibly leading to cardiac arrest. After treatment, check for overcorrection to hypokalemia.
- Because metabolic acidosis commonly causes vomiting, position the patient to prevent aspiration. Prepare for possible seizures with seizure precautions.
- Provide good oral hygiene. Use sodium bicarbonate washes to neutralize mouth acids, and lubricate the patient's lips with lemon and glycerin swabs as indicated.
- To prevent metabolic acidosis, carefully observe patients receiving I.V. therapy or who have intestinal tubes in place as well as

those suffering from shock, hyperthyroidism, hepatic disease, circulatory failure, or dehydration. Teach the patient with diabetes how to routinely test urine for glucose and acetone, and encourage strict adherence to insulin or oral hypoglycemic therapy.

Metabolic alkalosis

A clinical state marked by decreased amounts of acid or increased amounts of base bicarbonate, metabolic alkalosis causes metabolic, respiratory, and renal responses, producing characteristic symptoms (most notably hypoventilation). This condition is always secondary to an underlying cause. With early diagnosis and prompt treatment, prognosis is good; however, untreated metabolic alkalosis may lead to coma and death.

Causes

Metabolic alkalosis results from loss of acid, retention of base, or renal mechanisms associated with decreased serum levels of potassium and chloride.

Causes of critical acid loss include vomiting, nasogastric (NG) tube drainage or lavage without adequate electrolyte replacement, fistulas, and the use of steroids and certain diuretics (furosemide, thiazides, and ethacrynic acid). Hyperadrenocorticism is another cause of severe acid loss. Cushing's disease, primary hyperaldosteronism, and Bartter's syndrome, for example, all lead to retention of sodium and chloride, and urinary loss of potassium and hydrogen.

Excessive base retention can result from excessive intake of bicarbonate of soda or other antacids (usually for treatment of gastritis or peptic ulcer), excessive intake of absorbable alkali (as in milk-alkali syndrome, often seen in patients with peptic ulcers), administration of excessive amounts of I.V. fluids with high concentrations of bicarbonate or lactate, or respiratory insufficiency—all of which cause chronic hypercapnia from high levels of plasma bicarbonate.

Signs and symptoms

Clinical features of metabolic alkalosis result from the body's attempt to correct the acid-base imbalance, primarily through hypoventilation. Other manifestations include irritability, picking at bedclothes (carphology), twitching, confusion, nausea, vomiting, and diarrhea (which aggravates alkalosis). Cardiovascular abnormalities (such as atrial tachycardia) and respiratory disturbances (such as cyanosis and apnea) also occur. In the alkalotic patient, diminished peripheral blood flow during repeated blood pressure checks may provoke carpopedal spasm in the hand—a possible sign of impending tetany (Trousseau's sign). Uncorrected metabolic alkalosis may progress to seizures and coma.

Diagnosis

 CONFIRMING DIAGNOSIS *Blood pH level greater than 7.45 and bicarbonate levels above 29 mEq/L confirm the diagnosis. A partial pressure of carbon dioxide above 45 mm Hg indicates attempts at respiratory compensation. Serum electrolyte studies show low potassium, calcium, and chloride levels.*

Other characteristic findings include:
- Urine pH is usually about 7.0.
- Urinalysis reveals alkalinity after the renal compensatory mechanism begins to excrete bicarbonate.
- Electrocardiogram may show low T wave, merging with a U wave (secondary to hypocalcemia from metabolic alkalosis), and atrial or sinus tachycardia.

Treatment

Treatment aims to correct the underlying cause of metabolic alkalosis. Therapy for severe alkalosis may include cautious administration of ammonium chloride I.V. or hydrochloric acid to release hydrogen chloride and restore concentration of extracellular fluid and chloride levels. Potassium chloride and normal saline solution (except in the presence of heart failure) are usually sufficient to replace losses from gastric drainage. Electrolyte replacement with potassium chloride and discontinuing diuretics correct metabolic alkalosis resulting from potent diuretic therapy.

Oral or I.V. acetazolamide, which enhances renal bicarbonate excretion, may be prescribed to correct metabolic alkalosis without rapid volume expansion. Because acetazolamide also enhances potassium excretion, potassium may have to be administered before giving this drug.

Special considerations

Structure the care plan around cautious I.V. therapy, keen observation, and strict monitoring of the patient's status.

- Dilute potassium when giving I.V. containing potassium salts. Monitor the infusion rate to prevent damage to blood vessels; watch for signs of phlebitis. When administering ammonium chloride 0.9%, limit the infusion rate to 1 L in 4 hours; faster administration may cause hemolysis of red blood cells. Avoid overdosage because it may cause overcorrection to metabolic acidosis. Don't give ammonium chloride with signs of hepatic or renal disease; instead, use hydrochloric acid.
- Watch closely for signs of muscle weakness, tetany, or decreased activity. Monitor vital signs frequently and record intake and output to evaluate respiratory, fluid, and electrolyte status. Remember, respiratory rate usually decreases in an effort to compensate for alkalosis. Hypotension and tachycardia may indicate electrolyte imbalance, especially hypokalemia.
- Observe seizure precautions.
- To prevent metabolic alkalosis, warn patients against overusing alkaline agents. Irrigate NG tubes with isotonic saline solution instead of plain water to prevent loss of gastric electrolytes. Monitor I.V. fluid concentrations of bicarbonate or lactate. Teach patients with ulcers to recognize signs of milk-alkali syndrome: a distaste for milk, anorexia, weakness, and lethargy.

Selected references

Bales, C.W., and Ritchie, C.S., eds. *Handbook of Clinical Nutrition and Aging.* Totowa, N.J.: Humana Press, 2004.

Birmingham, C.L., and Beumont, P. *The Medical Management of Eating Disorders: A Textbook with Manuals for Health Care Professionals.* New York: Cambridge University Press, 2004.

Escott-Stump, S. *Nutrition and Diagnosis-Related Care,* 5th ed. Philadelphia: Lippincott Williams & Wilkins, 2002.

Farthing, M.J., and Mahalanabis, D. *The Control of Food and Fluid Intake in Health and Disease.* Philadelphia: Lippincott Williams & Wilkins, 2004.

Houston, S.M., et al., eds. *Nutrition and the IGF System.* Totowa, N.J.: Humana Press, 2004.

Lavin, N. *Manual of Endocrinology and Metabolism,* 3rd ed. Philadelphia: Lippincott Williams & Wilkins, 2003.

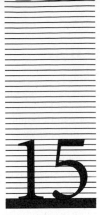

15

Obstetric and gynecologic disorders

Introduction *930*

Gynecologic disorders *936*
Premenstrual syndrome *936*
Dysmenorrhea *937*
Vulvovaginitis *939*
Ovarian cysts *940*
Endometriosis *942*
Uterine leiomyomas *943*
Precocious puberty *944*
Menopause *945*
Female infertility *947*
Pelvic inflammatory disease *950*

Uterine bleeding disorders *951*
Amenorrhea *951*
Abnormal premenopausal bleeding *952*
Dysfunctional uterine bleeding *954*
Postmenopausal bleeding *955*

Disorders of pregnancy *956*
Abortion *956*
Ectopic pregnancy *959*
Hyperemesis gravidarum *961*
Pregnancy-induced hypertension *962*
Hydatidiform mole *964*
Placenta previa *965*
Abruptio placentae *967*

Cardiovascular disease in pregnancy *969*
Adolescent pregnancy *970*
Diabetic complications during
  pregnancy *972*

Abnormalities of parturition *974*
Premature labor *974*
Premature rupture of membranes *976*
Cesarean birth *978*

Postpartum disorders *979*
Puerperal infection *979*
Mastitis and breast engorgement *981*
Galactorrhea *983*

Hemolytic diseases of the neonate *984*
Hyperbilirubinemia *984*
Erythroblastosis fetalis *987*

Selected references *991*

Introduction

Medical care of the obstetric or gynecologic patient reflects a growing interest in improving the quality of health care for females. Today, you must be able to assess, counsel, teach, and refer these patients, while weighing such relevant factors as the desire to have children, sexual adjustment problems, and self-image. Frequently, the situation is further complicated by the fact that multiple obstetric and gynecologic abnormalities often occur simultaneously. For example, a patient with dysmenorrhea may also have trichomonal vaginitis, dysuria, and unsuspected infertility. Her condition may be further complicated by associated urologic disorders, due to the proximity of the urinary and reproductive systems. This tendency to multiple and complex disorders is readily understandable upon review of the female genitalia's anatomic structure. (See *External and internal female genitalia.*)

External structures

Female genitalia include the following external structures, collectively known as the *vulva:* mons pubis (or mons veneris), labia majora, labia minora, clitoris, and the vestibule. The perineum is the external region between the vulva and the anus. The size, shape, and color of these structures — as well as pubic hair distribution and skin texture and pigmentation — vary greatly among individuals. Furthermore, these external structures undergo distinct changes during the life cycle.

The mons pubis is the pad of fat over the symphysis pubis (pubic bone), which is usually covered by the base of the inverted triangular patch of pubic hair that grows over the vulva after puberty.

The labia majora are the two thick, longitudinal folds of fatty tissue that extend from the mons pubis to the posterior aspect of the perineum. The labia majora protect the perineum and contain large sebaceous glands that help maintain lubrication. Virtually absent in the young child, their development is a characteristic sign of puberty's onset. The skin of the more prominent parts of the labia majora is pigmented and darkens after puberty.

The labia minora are the two thin, longitudinal folds of skin that border the vestibule. Firmer than the labia majora, they extend from the clitoris to the fourchette.

The clitoris is the small, protuberant organ located just beneath the arch of the mons pubis. The clitoris contains erectile tissue, venous cavernous spaces, and specialized sensory corpuscles that are stimulated during coitus.

The vestibule is the oval space bordered by the clitoris, labia minora, and fourchette. The urethral meatus is located in the anterior portion of the vestibule; the vaginal meatus, in the posterior portion. The hymen is the elastic membrane that partially obstructs the vaginal meatus in virgins.

Several glands lubricate the vestibule. Skene's glands open on both sides of the urethral meatus; Bartholin's glands, on both sides of the vaginal meatus.

The fourchette is the posterior junction of the labia majora and labia minora. The perineum, which includes the underlying muscles and fascia, is the external surface of the floor of the pelvis, extending from the fourchette to the anus.

Internal structures

The following internal structures are included in the female genitalia: vagina, cervix, uterus, fallopian tubes (or oviducts), and ovaries.

The vagina occupies the space between the bladder and the rectum. A muscular, membranous tube that's approximately 3″ (7.5 cm) long, the vagina connects the uterus and the vestibule of the external genitalia. It serves as a passageway for sperm to the fallopian tubes, for the discharge of menstrual fluid, and for childbirth.

The cervix, or neck of the uterus, protrudes at least ¾″ (2 cm) into the proximal end of the vagina. A rounded, conical structure, the cervix joins the uterus and the vagina at a 45- to 90-degree angle.

The uterus is the hollow, pear-shaped organ in which the conceptus grows during pregnancy. The part of the uterus above the junction of the fallopian tubes is called

EXTERNAL AND INTERNAL FEMALE GENITALIA

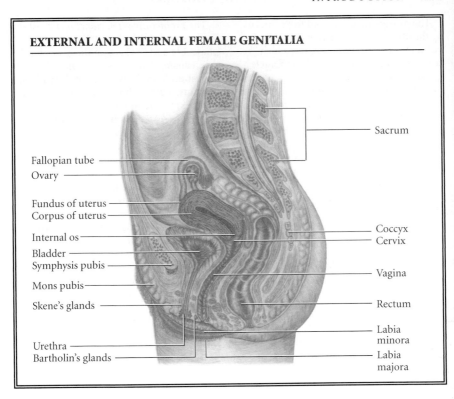

Fallopian tube
Ovary
Fundus of uterus
Corpus of uterus
Internal os
Bladder
Symphysis pubis
Mons pubis
Skene's glands
Urethra
Bartholin's glands

Sacrum
Coccyx
Cervix
Vagina
Rectum
Labia minora
Labia majora

the *fundus;* the part below this junction is called the *corpus.* The junction of the corpus and cervix forms the lower uterine segment.

The thick uterine wall consists of mucosal, muscular, and serous layers. The inner mucosal lining — the endometrium — undergoes cyclic changes to facilitate and maintain pregnancy.

The smooth muscular middle layer — the myometrium — interlaces the uterine and ovarian arteries and veins that circulate blood through the uterus. During pregnancy, this vascular system expands dramatically. After abortion or childbirth, the myometrium contracts to constrict the vasculature and control blood loss.

The outer serous layer — the parietal peritoneum — covers all of the fundus, part of the corpus, but none of the cervix. This incompleteness allows surgical entry into the uterus without incision of the peritoneum, thereby reducing the risk of peritonitis.

The fallopian tubes extend from the sides of the fundus and terminate near the ovaries. Through ciliary and muscular action, these small tubes (3¼″ to 5½″ [8 to 14 cm] long) carry ova from the ovaries to the uterus and facilitate the movement of sperm from the uterus toward the ovaries. Fertilization of the ovum normally occurs in a fallopian tube. The same ciliary and muscular action helps move a zygote (fertilized ovum) down to the uterus, where it implants in the blood-rich inner uterine lining, the endometrium.

The ovaries are two almond-shaped organs, one on either side of the fundus, that are situated behind and below the fallopian tubes. The ovaries produce ova and two primary hormones — estrogen and progesterone — in addition to small amounts of androgen. These hormones, in turn, produce and maintain secondary sex characteristics, prepare the uterus for pregnancy, and stimulate mammary gland development.

The ovaries are connected to the uterus by the utero-ovarian ligament and are divided into two parts: the cortex, which contains primordial and graafian follicles in various stages of development, and the medulla, which consists primarily of vasculature and loose connective tissue.

A normal female is born with at least 400,000 primordial follicles in her ovaries. At puberty, these ova precursors become graafian follicles, in response to the effects of pituitary gonadotropic hormones — follicle-stimulating hormone (FSH) and luteinizing hormone (LH). In the life cycle of a female, however, less than 500 ova eventually mature and develop the potential for fertilization.

The menstrual cycle

Maturation of the hypothalamus and the resultant increase in hormone levels initiate puberty. In the young girl, breast development — the first sign of puberty — is followed by the appearance of pubic and axillary hair and the characteristic adolescent growth spurt. The reproductive system begins to undergo a series of hormone-induced changes that result in menarche, onset of menstruation (or menses). In North American females, menarche usually occurs at about age 13 but may occur between ages 9 and 18. Menstrual periods initially are irregular and anovulatory, but after a year or so, they become more regular. (See *Menstrual cycle.*)

The menstrual cycle consists of three different phases: menstrual, proliferative (estrogen-dominated), and secretory (progesterone-dominated). These phases correspond to the phases of ovarian function. The menstrual and proliferative phases correspond to the follicular ovarian phase; the secretory phase corresponds to the luteal ovarian phase.

The *menstrual phase* begins with day 1 of menstruation. During this phase, low estrogen and progesterone levels stimulate the hypothalamus to secrete gonadotropin-releasing hormone (Gn-RH). This substance, in turn, stimulates pituitary secretion of FSH and LH. When the FSH level rises, LH output increases.

The *proliferative (follicular) phase* lasts from cycle day 6 to day 14. During this phase, LH and FSH act on the ovarian follicle, causing estrogen secretion, which in turn stimulates the buildup of the endometrium. Late in this phase, estrogen levels peak, FSH secretion declines, and LH secretion increases, surging at midcycle (around day 14). Then estrogen production decreases, the follicle matures, and ovulation occurs.

During the *secretory phase*, FSH and LH levels drop. Estrogen levels decline initially, then increase along with progesterone levels as the corpus luteum begins functioning. During this phase, the endometrium responds to progesterone stimulation by becoming thick and secretory in preparation for implantation of a fertilized ovum. About 10 to 12 days after ovulation, the corpus luteum begins to diminish, as do estrogen and progesterone levels, until hormone levels are insufficient to sustain the endometrium in a fully developed secretory state. Then the endometrial lining is shed (menses). Subsequently decreasing estrogen and progesterone levels stimulate the hypothalamus to produce Gn-RH, which in turn begins the cycle again.

In the nonpregnant female, LH controls the secretions of the corpus luteum; in the pregnant female, human chorionic gonadotropin (hCG) controls them. At the end of the secretory phase, the uterine lining is ready to receive and nourish a zygote. If fertilization doesn't occur, increasing estrogen and progesterone levels decrease LH and FSH production. Because LH is necessary to maintain the corpus luteum, a decrease in LH production causes the corpus luteum to atrophy and stop secreting estrogen and progesterone. The thickened uterine lining then begins to slough off, and menstruation begins again.

If fertilization and pregnancy do occur, the endometrium grows even thicker. After implantation of the zygote (about 5 or 6 days after fertilization), the endometrium becomes the decidua. Chorionic villi produce hCG soon after implantation, stimulating the corpus luteum to continue secreting estrogen and progesterone, which prevents further ovulation and menstruation.

MENSTRUAL CYCLE

The menstrual cycle is divided into three distinct phases:

The *menstrual phase* starts on the first day of menstruation. The top layer of the endometrium (the material lining the uterus) breaks down and flows out of the body. This flow, called the *menses,* consists of blood, mucus, and unneeded tissue.

During *the proliferative phase,* the endometrium begins to thicken, and the estrogen level in the blood rises.

In the *secretory phase,* the endometrium continues to thicken to nourish an embryo should fertilization occur. Without fertilization, the top layer of the endometrium breaks down, and the menstrual phase of the cycle begins again.

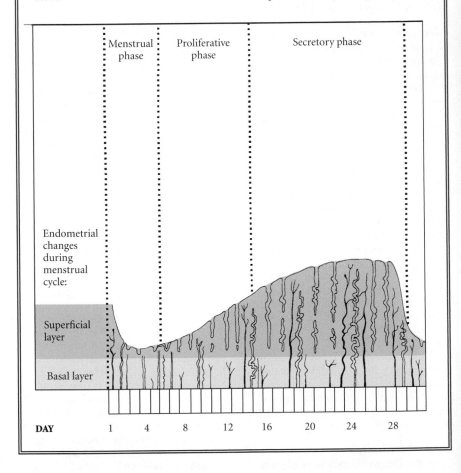

Menstrual phase | Proliferative phase | Secretory phase

Endometrial changes during menstrual cycle:

Superficial layer

Basal layer

DAY   1   4   8   12   16   20   24   28

HCG continues to stimulate the corpus luteum until the placenta—the vascular organ that develops to transport materials to and from the fetus—forms and starts producing its own estrogen and progesterone. After the placenta takes over hormonal production, secretions of the corpus luteum are no longer needed to maintain the pregnancy, and the corpus luteum gradually decreases its function and begins to degenerate.

Pregnancy

Cell multiplication and differentiation begin in the zygote at the moment of conception. By about 17 days after conception, the placenta has established circulation to what is now an *embryo* (the term used for the conceptus between the 2nd and 7th weeks of pregnancy). By the end of the embryonic stage, fetal structures are formed. Further development now consists primarily of growth and maturation of already formed structures. From this point until birth, the conceptus is called a *fetus.*

First trimester

Normal pregnancies last an average of 280 days. Although pregnancies vary in duration, they're conveniently divided into three trimesters.

During the first trimester, a female usually experiences physical changes, such as amenorrhea, urinary frequency, nausea and vomiting (more severe in the morning or when the stomach is empty), breast swelling and tenderness, fatigue, increased vaginal secretions, and constipation.

Within 7 to 10 days after conception, pregnancy tests, which detect hCG in the urine and serum, are usually positive. A pelvic examination at this stage can yield various findings, such as Hegar's sign (cervical and uterine softening), Chadwick's sign (a bluish coloration of the vagina and cervix resulting from increased venous circulation), and enlargement of the uterus. A pelvic examination will help estimate gestational age but vaginal sonography is more accurate.

The first trimester is a critical time during pregnancy. Rapid cell differentiation makes the developing embryo or fetus highly susceptible to the teratogenetic effects of viruses, alcohol, cigarettes, caffeine, and other drugs.

Second trimester

From the 13th to the 28th week of pregnancy, uterine and fetal size increase substantially, causing weight gain, a thickening waistline, abdominal enlargement and, possibly, reddish streaks as abdominal skin stretches (striation). In addition, pigment changes may cause skin alterations, such as linea nigra, melasma (mask of pregnancy), and a darkening of the areolae of the nipples.

Other physical changes may include diaphoresis, increased salivation, indigestion, continuing constipation, hemorrhoids, nosebleeds, and some dependent edema. The breasts become larger and heavier, and approximately 19 weeks after the last menstrual period, they may secrete colostrum. By about the 18th to the 20th week of pregnancy, the fetus is large enough for the mother to feel it move (quickening).

Third trimester

During this period, the mother feels Braxton Hicks contractions — sporadic episodes of painless uterine tightening — which help strengthen uterine muscles in preparation for labor. Increasing uterine size may displace pelvic and intestinal structures, causing indigestion, protrusion of the umbilicus, shortness of breath, and insomnia. The mother may experience backaches because she walks with a swaybacked posture to counteract her frontal weight. By lying down, she can help minimize the development of varicose veins, hemorrhoids, and ankle edema.

Labor and delivery

About 2 to 4 weeks before birth, lightening — the descent of the fetal head into the pelvis — shifts the uterine position. This relieves pressure on the diaphragm and enables the mother to breathe more easily.

Onset of labor characteristically produces low back pain and passage of a small amount of bloody "show." A brownish or blood-tinged plug of cervical mucus may be passed up to 2 weeks before labor. As labor progresses, the cervix becomes soft, then effaces and dilates; the amniotic membranes may rupture spontaneously, causing a gush or leakage of amniotic fluid. Uterine contractions become increasingly regular, frequent, intense, and long.

Labor is usually divided into four stages:

■ *Stage I,* the longest stage, lasts from onset of regular contractions until full cervical dilation (4″ [10 cm]). Average duration of this stage is about 12 hours for a primigravida and 6 hours for a multigravida.

■ *Stage II* lasts from full cervical dilation until delivery of the infant — about 1 to

3 hours for a primigravida, 30 to 60 minutes for a multigravida.

■ *Stage III,* the time between delivery and expulsion of the placenta, usually lasts several minutes (duration varies widely) but may last up to 30 minutes.

■ *Stage IV* is a period of recovery during which homeostasis is re-established. This final stage lasts 1 to 4 hours after the placenta is expelled.

Sources of pathology

In no other body part do so many interrelated physiologic functions occur so close together as in the area of the female reproductive tract. Besides the internal genitalia, the female pelvis contains the organs of the urinary and the GI systems (bladder, ureters, urethra, sigmoid colon, and rectum). The reproductive tract and its surrounding area are thus the site of urination, defecation, menstruation, ovulation, copulation, impregnation, and parturition. It's easy to understand how an abnormality in one pelvic organ can readily induce abnormality in another.

When conducting a pelvic examination, therefore, you must consider all possible sources of pathology. Remember that some serious abnormalities of the pelvic organs can be asymptomatic. Remember, too, that some abnormal findings in the pelvic area may result from pathologic changes in other organ systems, such as the upper urinary and GI tracts, the endocrine glands, and the neuromusculoskeletal system. Pain symptoms are often associated with the menstrual cycle; therefore, in many common diseases of the female reproductive tract, such pain follows a cyclic pattern. A patient with pelvic inflammatory disease, for example, may complain of increasing premenstrual pain that's relieved by onset of menstruation.

Pelvic examination

A pelvic examination and a thorough patient history are essential for any patient with symptoms related to the reproductive tract or adjacent body systems. Document any history of pregnancy, miscarriage, and abortion. Ask the patient if she has experienced any recent changes in her urinary habits or menstrual cycle. If she practices birth control, find out what method she uses and whether she has experienced any adverse effects.

Then prepare the patient for the pelvic examination as follows:

■ Ask the patient if she has douched within the last 24 hours. Explain that douching washes away cells or organisms that the examination is designed to evaluate.

■ Check weight and blood pressure.

■ For the patient's comfort, instruct her to empty her bladder before the examination. Provide a urine specimen container if needed.

■ To help the patient relax, which is essential for a thorough pelvic examination, explain what the examination entails and why it's necessary.

■ If the patient is scheduled for a Papanicolaou (Pap) test, inform her that another smear may have to be taken later if there are abnormal findings with the first test. Reassure her that this is done to confirm the first test's results. If she has never had a Pap test before, tell her it may be uncomfortable.

■ After the Pap test, a bimanual examination is performed to assess the size and location of the ovaries and uterus.

■ After the examination, offer the patient premoistened tissues to clean the vulva.

Other diagnostic tests

Diagnostic measures for gynecologic disorders also include the following tests, which can be performed in the physician's office:

■ wet smear to examine vaginal secretions for specific organisms, such as *Trichomonas vaginalis* and *Candida albicans,* or to evaluate semen specimens collected in connection with rape or infertility cases

■ endometrial biopsy to assess hormonal secretions of the corpus luteum, to determine whether normal ovulation is occurring, and to check for neoplasia

■ dilatation and curettage with hysteroscopy to evaluate atypical bleeding and to detect carcinoma.

Laparoscopy, used to evaluate infertility, dysmenorrhea, and pelvic pain, and as a means of sterilization, is usually performed in a health care facility while the patient is under anesthesia. Increasingly, however, it's being performed as a less invasive procedure under conscious sedation in an office setting using microlaparoscopic technique.

GYNECOLOGIC DISORDERS

Premenstrual syndrome

Also designated "late luteal phase dysphoric disorder" (LLPD) in *the Diagnostic and Statistical Manual of Mental Disorders,* Fourth Edition, Text Revision, premenstrual syndrome (PMS) is characterized by varying symptoms that appear 7 to 14 days before menses and usually subside with its onset. The effects of PMS range from minimal discomfort to severe, disruptive symptoms and can include nervousness, irritability, depression, and multiple somatic complaints.

Causes and incidence
The list of biological theories offered to explain the cause of PMS is impressive. It includes such conditions as a progesterone deficiency in the menstrual cycle's luteal phase and vitamin deficiencies. Although there's no evidence that PMS is hormonally mediated, failure to identify a specific disorder with a specific mechanism suggests that PMS represents a variety of manifestations triggered by normal physiologic hormonal changes. Researchers believe that 70% to 90% of women experience PMS at some time during their childbearing years, usually between ages 25 and 45.

Signs and symptoms
Clinical effects vary widely among patients and may include any combination of the following:
- *behavioral* — mild to severe personality changes, nervousness, hostility, irritability, agitation, sleep disturbances, fatigue, lethargy, and depression
- *somatic* — breast tenderness or swelling, abdominal tenderness or bloating, joint pain, headache, edema, diarrhea or constipation, and exacerbations of skin problems (such as acne or rashes), respiratory problems (such as asthma), or neurologic problems (such as seizures).

PMS may need to be differentiated from premenstrual dysphoric disorder, which is a more severe form of PMS that's marked by severe depression, irritability, and tension before menstruation. (See *Premenstrual dysphoric disorder.*)

Diagnosis
The patient history shows typical symptoms related to the menstrual cycle. To help ensure an accurate history, the patient may be asked to record menstrual symptoms and body temperature on a calendar for 2 to 3 months prior to diagnosis. Estrogen and progesterone blood levels may be evaluated to help rule out hormonal imbalance. A psychological evaluation is also recommended to rule out or detect an underlying psychiatric disorder.

Treatment
Educating and reassuring patients that PMS is a real physiologic syndrome are important parts of treatment. Because treatment is predominantly symptomatic, each patient must learn to cope with her own individual set of symptoms. Treatment may include calcium and magnesium supplementation, vitamins (such as B complex), prostaglandin inhibitors, and nonsteroidal anti-inflammatory drugs. Diuretics may be prescribed for patients who experience significant weight gain due to fluid retention. Psychiatric medications and therapy may be prescribed for women who develop anxiety, irritability, or depression. Hormonal therapy may include a trial on hormonal contraceptives, which may either decrease or increase PMS symptoms. The use of progesterone vaginal suppositories during the second half of the menstrual cycle is still controversial.

For treatment to be effective, the patient may have to maintain a diet that's low in simple sugars, caffeine, and salt.

Special considerations
- Inform the patient that self-help groups exist for women with PMS; help her contact such a group if appropriate.
- Obtain a complete patient history to help identify any emotional problems that

PREMENSTRUAL DYSPHORIC DISORDER

Premenstrual dysphoric disorder (PMDD) is a severe form of premenstrual syndrome (PMS) that has a cyclical occurrence of psychiatric symptoms that starts after ovulation (usually the week before the onset of menstruation) and ends within the first day or two of menses. Its underlying cause and pathophysiology remain unclear. However, researchers theorize that normal cyclic changes in the body cause abnormal responses to neurotransmitters, such as serotonin, resulting in physical and behavioral signs and symptoms.

PMDD affects as many as 1 in 20 American women who have regular menstrual periods. It's unclear why some women are affected while others aren't.

How PMDD and PMS differ

PMDD is characterized by severe monthly mood swings and physical signs and symptoms that interfere with everyday life. Compared to PMS, its signs and symptoms are abnormal and unmanageable. Although depression, anxiety, and sadness are common with PMS, in PMDD, these symptoms are extreme. Some women may feel the urge to hurt or kill themselves or others.

The Diagnostic and Statistical Manual of Mental Disorders, Fourth Edition, Text Revision, sets these criteria for diagnosing PMDD:

- functional impairment
- predominant mood symptoms, with one being affective
- symptoms beginning 1 week before the onset of menstruation
- symptoms that aren't due to any underlying primary mood disorder.

In addition, at least five of the following symptoms must be present:

- appetite changes
- decreased interests
- difficulty concentrating
- fatigue
- feelings of being overwhelmed
- insomnia or hypersomnia
- irritability
- "low mood"
- mood swings
- physical symptoms
- tension.

---

may contribute to PMS. Refer the patient for psychological counseling if necessary.

- If possible, discuss ways in which the patient can modify her lifestyle, such as making changes in her diet and avoiding stimulants and alcohol.
- Suggest that the patient seek further medical consultation if symptoms are severe and interfere with her normal lifestyle.

Dysmenorrhea

Dysmenorrhea — painful menstruation — is the most common gynecologic complaint and a leading cause of absenteeism from school (affecting 10% of high school girls each month) and work (causing about 140 million lost work hours annually). Dysmenorrhea can occur as a primary disorder or secondary to an underlying disease. Because primary dysmenorrhea is self-limiting, the prognosis is generally good. The prognosis for secondary dysmenorrhea depends on the underlying disorder.

Causes and incidence

Although primary dysmenorrhea has no known single cause, possible contributing factors include hormonal imbalances and psychogenic factors. The pain of dysmenorrhea probably results from increased prostaglandin secretion, which intensifies normal uterine contractions. (See *Causes of pelvic pain,* page 938.) Dysmenorrhea may also be secondary to such gynecologic disorders as endometriosis, cervical stenosis, uterine leiomyomas, uterine malposition, pelvic inflammatory disease, pelvic tumors, or adenomyosis.

CAUSES OF PELVIC PAIN

The characteristic pelvic pain of dysmenorrhea must be distinguished from the acute pain caused by many other disorders, such as:

- *GI disorders:* appendicitis, acute diverticulitis, acute or chronic cholecystitis, chronic cholelithiasis, acute pancreatitis, peptic ulcer perforation, intestinal obstruction
- *pregnancy disorders:* impending abortion (pain and bleeding early in pregnancy), ectopic pregnancy, abruptio placentae, uterine rupture, leiomyoma degeneration, toxemia
- *reproductive disorders:* acute salpingitis, chronic inflammation, degenerating fibroid, ovarian cyst torsion
- *urinary tract disorders:* cystitis, renal calculi.

Other conditions that may mimic dysmenorrhea include ovulation and normal uterine contractions experienced in pregnancy. Emotional conflicts can cause psychogenic (functional) pain.

Because dysmenorrhea almost always follows an ovulatory cycle, both the primary and secondary forms are rare during the anovulatory cycles of menses. After age 20, dysmenorrhea is generally secondary.

Signs and symptoms

Dysmenorrhea produces sharp, intermittent, cramping, lower abdominal pain, which usually radiates to the back, thighs, groin, and vulva. Such pain — sometimes compared to labor pains — typically starts with or immediately before menstrual flow and peaks within 24 hours. Dysmenorrhea may also be associated with the characteristic signs and symptoms of premenstrual syndrome (urinary frequency, nausea, vomiting, diarrhea, headache, chills, abdominal bloating, painful breasts, depression, and irritability).

Diagnosis

Pelvic examination and a detailed patient history may help suggest the cause of dysmenorrhea.

Primary dysmenorrhea is diagnosed when secondary causes are ruled out. Appropriate tests (such as laparoscopy, dilatation and curettage, and pelvic ultrasound) are used to diagnose underlying disorders in secondary dysmenorrhea.

Treatment

Initial treatment aims to relieve pain. Pain-relief measures may include:

- analgesics (such as aspirin) for mild to moderate pain (most effective when taken 24 to 48 hours before onset of menses; are especially effective for treating dysmenorrhea because they also inhibit prostaglandin synthesis; stronger anti-inflammatories may be used.
- opioids if pain is severe (infrequently used)
- prostaglandin inhibitors (such as mefenamic acid and ibuprofen) to relieve pain by decreasing the severity of uterine contractions
- cox-2 inhibitors (such as celecoxib, rofecoxib, and valdecoxib) to promote comfort
- heat applied locally to the lower abdomen (may relieve discomfort in mature women but isn't recommended in young adolescents because appendicitis may mimic dysmenorrhea).

For primary dysmenorrhea, administration of sex steroids is an effective alternative to treatment with antiprostaglandins or analgesics. Such therapy usually consists of hormonal contraceptives to relieve pain by suppressing ovulation. However, patients who are attempting pregnancy should rely on antiprostaglandin therapy instead of hormonal contraceptives to relieve symptoms of primary dysmenorrhea.

Because persistently severe dysmenorrhea may have a psychogenic cause, psychological evaluation and appropriate counseling may be helpful.

In secondary dysmenorrhea, treatment is designed to identify and correct the underlying cause. This may include surgical treatment of underlying disorders, such as endometriosis or uterine leiomyomas. However, surgical treatment is recommended only after conservative therapy fails.

Special considerations

Effective management of the patient with dysmenorrhea focuses on relief of symptoms, emotional support, and appropriate patient teaching, especially for the adolescent.

■ Obtain a complete history, focusing on the patient's gynecologic complaints, including detailed information on any signs and symptoms of pelvic disease, such as excessive bleeding, changes in bleeding pattern, vaginal discharge, and dyspareunia.
■ Provide thorough patient teaching. Explain normal female anatomy and physiology to the patient, as well as the nature of dysmenorrhea. This may be a good opportunity, depending on circumstances, to provide the adolescent patient with information on pregnancy and contraception.
■ Encourage the patient to keep a detailed record of her menstrual symptoms and to seek medical care if her symptoms persist.
■ Instruct the patient on some home care remedies that may be helpful in relieving discomfort, such as applying a heating pad to the lower abdomen, taking warm showers or baths, drinking warm beverages, and performing circular massage with the fingertips around the lower abdomen.
■ Encourage the patient to walk or exercise regularly. Recommend pelvic rocking exercises and relaxation techniques, such as meditation or yoga. Let her know that keeping her legs elevated while lying down or lying on her side with her knees bent may also increase comfort.
■ Instruct the patient to eat light but frequent meals and to follow a diet rich in foods high in complex carbohydrates, such as whole grains, fruits, and vegetables. Tell her to avoid alcohol and foods high in salt, sugar, and caffeine.

Vulvovaginitis

Vulvovaginitis is inflammation of the vulva (vulvitis) and vagina (vaginitis). Because of the proximity of these two structures, inflammation of one occasionally causes inflammation of the other. Vulvovaginitis may occur at any age and affects most females at some time. The prognosis is excellent with treatment.

Causes and incidence

Common causes include:
■ infection with *Trichomonas vaginalis,* a protozoan flagellate usually transmitted through sexual intercourse
■ infection with *Candida albicans,* a fungus that requires glucose for growth. Incidence rises during the menstrual cycle's secretory phase (Such infection occurs twice as often in pregnant females as in nonpregnant females. It also commonly affects users of hormonal contraceptives, patients who are diabetic, and patients receiving systemic therapy with broad-spectrum antibiotics [incidence may reach 75%.])
■ infection with *Gardnerella vaginalis,* a gram-negative bacillus
■ parasitic infection (*Phthirus pubis* [crab louse])
■ trauma (skin breakdown may lead to secondary infection)
■ poor personal hygiene
■ chemical irritations, or allergic reactions to hygiene sprays, douches, detergents, clothing, or toilet paper
■ vulval atrophy in menopausal women due to decreasing estrogen levels
■ retention of a foreign body, such as a tampon or diaphragm.

Signs and symptoms

In trichomonal vaginitis, vaginal discharge is thin, bubbly, green-tinged, and malodorous. This infection causes marked irritation and itching, and urinary symptoms, such as burning and frequency. Candidal vaginitis produces a thick, white, cottage cheese-like discharge and red, edematous mucous membranes, with white flecks adhering to the vaginal wall, and is often accompanied by intense itching. *G. vaginalis* produces a gray, foul, "fishy" smelling discharge.

Acute vulvitis causes a mild to severe inflammatory reaction, including edema, erythema, burning, and pruritus. Severe pain on urination and dyspareunia may necessitate immediate treatment. Herpes infection may cause painful ulceration or vesicle formation during the active phase.

Diagnosis

Diagnosis of vulvovaginitis requires identification of the infectious organism during microscopic examination of vaginal exudate on a wet slide preparation (a drop of vaginal exudate placed in normal saline solution). In some cases, a culture of the vaginal discharge may identify the organism causing the infection.

Diagnosis of vulvitis or suspected venereal disease may require complete blood count, urinalysis, cytology screening, biopsy of chronic lesions to rule out malignancy, culture of exudate from acute lesions, and possible human immunodeficiency virus testing.

Treatment

The cause of vulvovaginitis determines the appropriate treatment. It may include oral or topical antibiotics, antifungal creams, antibacterial creams, or similar medications. An antihistamine may be prescribed for allergic reactions. Cold compresses or cool sitz baths may provide relief from pruritus in acute vulvitis; severe inflammation may require warm compresses. Other therapy includes avoiding drying soaps, wearing loose clothing to promote air circulation, and applying topical corticosteroids to reduce inflammation. Chronic vulvitis may respond to topical hydrocortisone or antipruritics and good hygiene (especially in elderly or incontinent patients). Topical estrogen ointments may be used to treat atrophic vulvovaginitis. No cure exists for herpes-virus infections; however, oral and topical acyclovir decreases the duration and symptoms of active lesions.

If a sexually transmitted disease (STD) is diagnosed, it's very important that partners also receive treatment, even if there are no symptoms. Failure of partners to receive treatment can lead to continual reinfection, which may eventually lead to infertility and affect the patient's overall health.

Special considerations

- Ask the patient if she has any drug allergies. Stress the importance of taking the medication for the length of time prescribed, even if symptoms subside.
- Teach the patient how to insert vaginal ointments and suppositories. Tell her to remain prone for at least 30 minutes after insertion to promote absorption (insertion at bedtime is ideal). Suggest she wear a pad to prevent staining her underclothing.
- Encourage good hygiene. Advise the patient with a history of recurrent vulvovaginitis to wear all-cotton underpants. Advise her to avoid wearing tight-fitting pants and panty hose, which encourage the growth of the infecting organisms. Removing underpants at night is also helpful.
- Report notifiable cases of STDs to local public health authorities.
- Tell the patient that persistent, recurring candidiasis may suggest diabetes or undiagnosed pregnancy.

Ovarian cysts

Ovarian cysts are usually nonneoplastic sacs on an ovary that contain fluid or semisolid material. Although these cysts are usually small and produce no symptoms, they generally require thorough investigation as possible sites of malignant change. Common ovarian cysts include follicular cysts, lutein cysts (granulosa-lutein [corpus luteum] and theca-lutein cysts), and polycystic ovarian disease. Ovarian cysts can develop at any time between puberty and menopause, including during pregnancy. Granulosa-lutein cysts occur infrequently, usually during early pregnancy. The prognosis for nonneoplastic ovarian cysts is excellent.

Causes

Follicular cysts are generally very small and arise from follicles that overdistend. When such cysts persist into menopause, they secrete excessive amounts of estrogen in response to the hypersecretion of follicle-stimulating hormone and luteinizing hormone that normally occurs during menopause. (See *Follicular cyst.*)

Granulosa-lutein cysts, which occur within the corpus luteum, are functional, nonneoplastic enlargements of the ovaries caused by excessive accumulation of blood during the hemorrhagic phase of the menstrual cycle. Theca-lutein cysts are commonly bilateral and filled with clear, straw-colored fluid; they're often associated with hydatidiform mole, choriocarcinoma, or hormone therapy (with human chorionic gonadotropin [hCG] or clomiphene citrate).

Polycystic ovarian disease is part of the Stein-Leventhal syndrome and stems from endocrine abnormalities.

Signs and symptoms

Small ovarian cysts (such as follicular cysts) usually don't produce symptoms unless torsion or rupture causes signs of an acute abdomen (abdominal tenderness, distention, and rigidity). Large or multiple cysts may induce mild pelvic discomfort, low back pain, dyspareunia, or abnormal uterine bleeding secondary to a disturbed ovulatory pattern. Ovarian cysts with torsion induce acute abdominal pain similar to that of appendicitis.

Granulosa-lutein cysts that appear early in pregnancy may grow as large as 2″ to 2½″ (5 to 6 cm) in diameter and produce unilateral pelvic discomfort and, if rupture occurs, massive intraperitoneal hemorrhage. In nonpregnant women, these cysts may cause delayed menses, followed by prolonged or irregular bleeding. Polycystic ovarian disease may also produce secondary amenorrhea, oligomenorrhea, or infertility.

Diagnosis

Generally, characteristic clinical features suggest ovarian cysts.

 CONFIRMING DIAGNOSIS
Visualization of the ovary through ultrasound, computed tomography scan, laparoscopy, or surgery (often for another condition) confirms ovarian cysts.

Extremely elevated hCG titers strongly suggest theca-lutein cysts. Pregnancy, including molar pregnancy, must be ruled out.

In polycystic ovarian disease, physical examination demonstrates bilaterally enlarged polycystic ovaries. Tests reveal slight elevation of urinary 17-ketosteroids and anovulation (shown by basal body temperature graphs and endometrial biopsy). Direct visualization must rule out paraovarian cysts of the broad ligament,

FOLLICULAR CYST

A common type of ovarian cyst, a follicular cyst is usually semitransparent and overdistended with watery fluid that's visible through its thin walls.

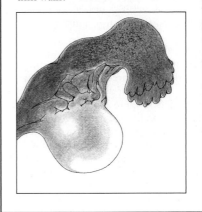

salpingitis, endometriosis, and neoplastic cysts.

Treatment

Follicular cysts generally don't require treatment because they tend to disappear spontaneously within 60 days. However, if they interfere with daily activities, clomiphene citrate by mouth for 5 days or progesterone I.M. (also for 5 days) reestablishes the ovarian hormonal cycle and induces ovulation. Hormonal contraceptives haven't been proven to accelerate involution of functional cysts (including both types of lutein cysts and follicular cysts).

Treatment for granulosa-lutein cysts that occur during pregnancy is aimed at relieving symptoms because these cysts diminish during the third trimester and rarely require surgery. Theca-lutein cysts disappear spontaneously after elimination of the hydatidiform mole, destruction of choriocarcinoma, or discontinuation of hCG or clomiphene citrate therapy.

Treatment of polycystic ovarian disease may include the administration of such drugs as clomiphene citrate to induce ovulation, medroxyprogesterone acetate for 10 days of every month for the patient who doesn't want to become pregnant, or low-dose hormonal contraceptives for the patient who needs reliable contraception.

Surgery, in the form of laparoscopy or exploratory laparotomy with possible ovarian cystectomy or oophorectomy, may become necessary if an ovarian cyst is found to be persistent or suspicious.

Special considerations

Thorough patient teaching is a primary consideration. Carefully explain the cyst's nature, the type of discomfort — if any — the patient is apt to experience, and how long the condition is expected to last.

■ Preoperatively, watch for signs of cyst rupture, such as increasing abdominal pain, distention, and rigidity. Monitor vital signs for fever, tachypnea, or hypotension, which may indicate peritonitis or intraperitoneal hemorrhage. Administer sedatives, as ordered, to ensure adequate rest before surgery.

■ Postoperatively, encourage frequent movement in bed and early ambulation, as ordered. Early ambulation prevents pulmonary embolism.

■ Provide emotional support. Offer appropriate reassurance if the patient fears cancer or infertility.

■ Before discharge, advise the patient to increase her activities at home gradually — preferably over 4 to 6 weeks. Tell her to abstain from sexual intercourse and not to use tampons and douches during this period.

Endometriosis

Endometriosis is the presence of endometrial tissue outside the lining of the uterine cavity. Such ectopic tissue is generally confined to the pelvic area, most commonly around the ovaries, uterovesical peritoneum, uterosacral ligaments, and cul-de-sac, but it can appear anywhere in the body. This ectopic endometrial tissue responds to normal stimulation in the same way that the endometrium does. During menstruation, the ectopic tissue bleeds, which causes inflammation of the sur-

rounding tissues. This inflammation causes fibrosis, leading to adhesions that produce pain and infertility.

Active endometriosis usually occurs between ages 20 and 40; it's uncommon before age 20. Severe symptoms of endometriosis may have an abrupt onset or may develop over many years. This disorder usually becomes progressively severe during the menstrual years; after menopause, it may subside.

Causes and incidence

The mechanisms by which endometriosis causes symptoms, including infertility, are unknown. The main theories to explain this disorder are:

■ transtubal regurgitation of endometrial cells and implantation at ectopic sites

■ coelomic metaplasia (repeated inflammation may induce metaplasia of mesothelial cells to the endometrial epithelium)

■ lymphatic or hematogenous spread to explain extraperitoneal disease.

Endometriosis occurs in 10% of women during the reproductive years. Prevalence may be as high as 25% to 35% among infertile women. A woman with a mother or sister with endometriosis is six times more likely to develop endometriosis than a woman without this familial history.

Signs and symptoms

The classic symptom of endometriosis is acquired dysmenorrhea, which may produce constant pain in the lower abdomen and in the vagina, posterior pelvis, and back. This pain usually begins from 5 to 7 days before menses reaches its peak and lasts for 2 to 3 days. It differs from primary dysmenorrheal pain, which is more cramp-like and concentrated in the abdominal midline. However, the pain's severity doesn't necessarily indicate the extent of the disease.

Other clinical features depend on the location of the ectopic tissue:

■ ovaries and oviducts: infertility and profuse menses

■ ovaries or cul-de-sac: deep-thrust dyspareunia

■ bladder: suprapubic pain, dysuria, hematuria

- small bowel and appendix: nausea and vomiting, which worsen before menses, and abdominal cramps
- cervix, vagina, and perineum: bleeding from endometrial deposits in these areas during menses.

The primary complications of endometriosis are infertility and chronic pelvic pain.

Diagnosis

Pelvic examination may suggest endometriosis. Palpation may detect multiple tender nodules on uterosacral ligaments or in the rectovaginal septum in one-third of patients. These nodules enlarge and become more tender during menses. Palpation may also uncover ovarian enlargement in the presence of endometrial cysts on the ovaries or thickened, nodular adnexa (as in pelvic inflammatory disease). Laparoscopy must confirm the diagnosis and determine the disease's stage before treatment is initiated. Endometriosis is classified in stages: Stage I, mild; Stage II, moderate; Stage III, severe; and Stage IV, extensive.

Treatment

Treatment varies according to the disease's stage and the patient's age and desire to have children. Conservative therapy for young women who want to have children includes androgens, such as danazol, which produce a temporary remission in Stages I and II. Progestins and hormonal contraceptives also relieve symptoms. Gonadotropin-releasing hormone agonists, by inducing a pseudomenopause and, thus, a "medical oophorectomy," may cause a remission of disease and are commonly used. However, medical therapy remains inadequate.

When ovarian masses are present, surgery must rule out cancer. Conservative surgery includes laparoscopic removal of endometrial implants with conventional or laser techniques and presacral neurectomy for severe dysmenorrhea. The treatment of choice for women who don't want to bear children or for extensive disease is a total abdominal hysterectomy with bilateral salpingo-oophorectomy.

Special considerations

- Because infertility is a possible complication, advise the patient who wants children not to postpone childbearing.
- Recommend an annual pelvic examination and Papanicolaou test to all patients.

Uterine leiomyomas

The most common benign tumors in women, uterine leiomyomas, also known as *myomas, fibromyomas,* or *fibroids,* are smooth-muscle tumors. They usually occur in multiples in the uterine corpus, although they may appear on the cervix or on the round or broad ligament. Though uterine leiomyomas are often called *fibroids,* this term is misleading because they consist of muscle cells and not fibrous tissue.

Causes and incidence

The cause of uterine leiomyomas is unknown, but steroid hormones, including estrogen and progesterone, and several growth factors, including epidermal growth factor, have been implicated as regulators of leiomyoma growth. Leiomyomas typically arise after menarche and regress after menopause, implicating estrogen as a promoter of leiomyoma growth.

Uterine leiomyomas occur in 20% to 25% of women of reproductive age and reportedly affect three times as many black women as white women. The tumors become malignant (leiomyosarcoma) in only 0.1% or less of patients.

Signs and symptoms

Leiomyomas may be located within the uterine wall or may protrude into the endometrial cavity or from the serosal surface of the uterus. Most leiomyomas produce no symptoms. The most common symptom is abnormal bleeding, which typically presents clinically as menorrhagia. Uterine leiomyomas probably don't cause pain directly except when associated with torsion of a pedunculated subserous tumor. Pelvic pressure and impingement on adjacent viscera are common indications for treatment. Various reproductive disorders, including infertility, recurrent spontaneous abortion, and preterm labor, have been attributed to uterine leiomyomas. Infertility, however, is rarely due to leiomyomas.

Diagnosis

Clinical findings and patient history may suggest uterine leiomyomas. Bimanual examination may reveal an enlarged, firm, nontender, and irregularly contoured uterus. Ultrasound (transvaginal or pelvic) or magnetic resonance imaging allows accurate assessment of the dimensions, number, and location of tumors. Other diagnostic procedures include hysterosalpingography, dilatation and curettage, endometrial biopsy, and laparoscopy.

Treatment

Treatment depends on the symptoms' severity, the tumors' size and location, and the patient's age, parity, pregnancy status, desire to have children, and general health.

Treatment options include nonsurgical as well as surgical procedures. Nonsurgical methods include taking serial histories and performing physical assessments at clinically indicated intervals and administering gonadotropin-releasing hormone (Gn-RH) analogues, which are capable of rapidly suppressing pituitary gonadotropin release, leading to profound hypoestrogenemia and a 50% reduction in uterine volume. The peak effects of these Gn-RH analogues occur in the 12th week of therapy. The benefits are reduction in tumor size before surgery, reduction in intraoperative blood loss, and an increase in preoperative hematocrit. Gn-RH analogues aren't curative.

Surgical procedures include abdominal, laparoscopic, or hysteroscopic myomectomy—for patients who want to preserve fertility. Myolysis can successfully treat fibroids without hysterectomy or major surgery. Performed on an outpatient basis, this laparoscopic procedure coagulates the fibroids and preserves the uterus and the patient's childbearing potential. Hysterectomy is the definitive treatment for symptomatic women who have completed childbearing, but uterine artery embolization may be an alternative in some situations.

Special considerations

- Tell the patient to report any abnormal bleeding or pelvic pain immediately.
- If a hysterectomy or oophorectomy is indicated, explain the operation's effects on menstruation, menopause, and sexual activity to the patient.
- Reassure the patient that she most likely won't experience premature menopause if her ovaries are left intact.
- If it's necessary for the patient to have a multiple myomectomy, make sure she understands pregnancy is still possible. Explain that a cesarean delivery may be indicated.

Precocious puberty

In females, precocious puberty is the early onset of pubertal changes: breast development, pubic and axillary hair development, and menarche before age 9. (Normally, the mean age for menarche is 13.) In true precocious puberty, the ovaries mature and pubertal changes progress in an orderly manner. In pseudoprecocious puberty, pubertal changes occur without corresponding ovarian maturation.

Causes

About 85% of all cases of true precocious puberty in females are constitutional, resulting from early development and activation of the endocrine glands without corresponding abnormality. Other causes of true precocious puberty are pathologic and include central nervous system (CNS) disorders resulting from tumors, trauma, infection, or other lesions. These CNS disorders include hypothalamic tumors, intracranial tumors (pinealoma, granuloma, hamartoma), hydrocephaly, degenerative encephalopathy, tuberous sclerosis, neurofibromatosis, encephalitis, skull injuries, meningitis, and peptic arachnoiditis. Albright's syndrome, Silver's syndrome, and juvenile hypothyroidism are conditions often associated with female precocity.

Pseudoprecocious puberty may result from increased levels of sex hormones due to ovarian and adrenocortical tumors, adrenal cortical virilizing hyperplasia, or ingestion of estrogens or androgens. It may also result from increased end-organ sensitivity to low levels of circulating sex hormones, whereby estrogens promote premature breast development and androgens promote premature pubic and axillary hair growth.

Signs and symptoms

The usual pattern of precocious puberty in females is a rapid growth spurt, thelarche (breast development), pubarche (pubic hair development), and menarche—all before age 9. These changes may occur independently or simultaneously.

Diagnosis

Diagnosis requires a complete patient history, a thorough physical examination, and special tests to differentiate between true and pseudoprecocious puberty and to indicate what treatment may be necessary. X-rays of the hands, wrists, knees, and hips determine bone age and possible premature epiphyseal closure. Other tests detect abnormally high hormonal levels for the patient's age: vaginal smear for estrogen secretion, urinary tests for gonadotropic activity and excretion of 17-ketosteroids, and radioimmunoassay for both luteinizing and follicle-stimulating hormones.

As indicated, ultrasound, laparoscopy, or exploratory laparotomy may verify a suspected abdominal lesion; EEG, ventriculography, pneumoencephalography, computed axial tomography scan, or angiography can detect CNS disorders.

Treatment

Treatment of constitutional true precocious puberty may include medroxyprogesterone to reduce secretion of gonadotropins and prevent menstruation. Other therapy depends on the cause of precocious puberty and its stage of development:
- Adrenogenital syndrome necessitates cortical or adrenocortical steroid replacement.
- Abdominal tumors necessitate surgery to remove ovarian and adrenal tumors. Regression of secondary sex characteristics may follow such surgery, especially in young children.

- Choriocarcinomas require surgery and chemotherapy.
- Hypothyroidism requires thyroid extract or levothyroxine to decrease gonadotropic secretions.
- Drug ingestion requires that the medication be discontinued.

In precocious thelarche and pubarche, no treatment is necessary.

Special considerations

The dramatic physical changes produced by precocious puberty can be upsetting and alarming for the child and her family. Provide a calm, supportive atmosphere, and encourage the patient and her family to express their feelings about these changes. Explain all diagnostic procedures and tell the patient and her family that surgery may be necessary.
- Explain the condition to the child in terms she can understand to prevent feelings of shame and loss of self-esteem. Provide appropriate sex education, including information on menstruation and related hygiene.
- Tell parents that, although their daughter seems physically mature, she isn't psychologically mature, and the discrepancy between physical appearance and psychological and psychosexual maturation may create problems. Warn them against expecting more of her than they would expect of other children her age.
- Suggest that parents continue to dress their daughter in clothes that are appropriate for her age and that don't call attention to her physical development.
- Reassure parents that precocious puberty doesn't usually precipitate precocious sexual behavior.

Menopause

Menopause is the cessation of menstruation. It results from a complex syndrome of physiologic changes—the climacteric—caused by declining ovarian function. The climacteric produces various body changes, the most dramatic being menopause.

Causes and incidence

■ Physiologic menopause, the normal decline in ovarian function due to aging, begins in most women between ages 45 and 55, on average 51, and results in infrequent ovulation, decreased menstrual function and, eventually, cessation of menstruation.

■ Pathologic (premature) menopause, the gradual or abrupt cessation of menstruation before age 40, occurs idiopathically in about 5% of women in the United States. However, certain diseases, especially severe infections and reproductive tract tumors, may cause pathologic menopause by seriously impairing ovarian function. Other factors that may precipitate pathologic menopause include malnutrition, debilitation, extreme emotional stress, excessive radiation exposure, and surgical procedures that impair ovarian blood supply.

Signs and symptoms

Many menopausal women are asymptomatic but some have severe symptoms. The decline in ovarian function and consequent decreased estrogen level produce menstrual irregularities: a decrease in the amount and duration of menstrual flow, spotting, and episodes of amenorrhea and polymenorrhea (possibly with hypermenorrhea). Irregularities may last a few months or persist for several years before menstruation ceases permanently.

The following body system changes may occur (usually after the permanent cessation of menstruation):

■ Reproductive system: Menopause may cause shrinkage of vulval structures and loss of subcutaneous fat, possibly leading to atrophic vulvitis; atrophy of vaginal mucosa and flattening of vaginal rugae, possibly causing bleeding after coitus or douching; vaginal itching and discharge from bacterial invasion; and loss of capillaries in the atrophying vaginal wall, causing the pink, rugal lining to become smooth and white. Menopause may also produce excessive vaginal dryness and dyspareunia due to decreased lubrication from the vaginal walls and decreased secretion from Bartholin's glands; smaller ovaries and oviducts; and progressive pelvic relaxation as the supporting structures lose their tone due to the absence of estrogen.

ELDER TIP *As a woman ages, atrophy causes the vagina to shorten and the mucous lining to become thin, dry, less elastic, and pale as a result of decreased vascularity. In addition, the pH of vaginal secretions increases, making the vaginal environment more alkaline. The type of flora also changes, increasing the older woman's chance of vaginal infections.*

■ Urinary system: Atrophic cystitis due to the effects of decreased estrogen levels on bladder mucosa and related structures may cause pyuria, dysuria, and urinary frequency, urgency, and incontinence. Urethral carbuncles from loss of urethral tone and mucosal thinning may cause dysuria, meatal tenderness, and hematuria.

■ Mammary system: Breast size decreases.

n Integumentary system: The patient may experience loss of skin elasticity and turgor due to estrogen deprivation, loss of pubic and axillary hair and, occasionally, slight alopecia.

■ Autonomic nervous system: The patient may exhibit hot flashes and night sweats (in 60% of women), vertigo, syncope, tachycardia, dyspnea, tinnitus, emotional disturbances (irritability, nervousness, crying spells, fits of anger), and exacerbation of pre-existing depression, anxiety, and compulsive, manic, or schizoid behavior.

Menopause may also induce atherosclerosis, and a decrease in estrogen level contributes to osteoporosis.

Ovarian activity in younger women is believed to provide a protective effect on the cardiovascular system, and the loss of this function at menopause may partly explain the increased death rate from myocardial infarction in older women. Also, estrogen has been found to increase levels of high-density lipoprotein cholesterol.

Diagnosis

Patient history and typical clinical features suggest menopause. A Papanicolaou (Pap) test may show the influence of estrogen deficiency on vaginal mucosa. Radioimmunoassay (RIA) may be performed, but because of the expense involved, it isn't necessary to confirm a diagnosis of menopause. If done, RIA shows the following blood hormone levels:

■ estrogen: 0 to 14 ng/dl

- plasma estradiol: 15 to 40 pg/ml
- estrone: 25 to 50 pg/ml.

RIA also shows the following urine values:

- estrogen: 6 to 28 µg/24 hours
- pregnanediol (urinary secretion of progesterone): 0.3 to 0.9 mg/24 hours.

Follicle-stimulating hormone production may increase as much as 15 times its normal level; luteinizing hormone production, as much as 5 times.

Pelvic examination, endometrial biopsy, and dilatation and curettage may rule out organic disease in patients with abnormal menstrual bleeding.

Treatment

Menopause is a natural process that doesn't require treatment unless menopausal symptoms, such as hot flashes or vaginal dryness, are particularly bothersome. Hormonal agents for patients with a uterus include estrogen with progesterone to prevent endometrial cancer. If the patient doesn't have a uterus, progesterone isn't necessary.

The Women's Health Initiative has led physicians to revise their recommendations regarding hormone replacement therapy (HRT). Health risks (increased incidence of breast cancer, heart attacks, strokes, and blood clots) outweigh the health benefits (decreased osteoporosis) for women taking both estrogen and progesterone. If symptoms are severe, HRT may be considered for short-term use (2 to 4 years) to reduce vaginal dryness, hot flashes, and other symptoms. If this is used, frequent pelvic examinations, Pap smears, physical examinations, breast examinations, and mammograms are indicated to reduce the risks of estrogen replacement therapy while still gaining the treatment's benefits.

Medications may be prescribed to help with mood swings, hot flashes, and other symptoms. These include low doses of antidepressants, such as paroxetine, venlafaxine, and fluoxetine, or clonidine, which is normally used to control high blood pressure.

Special considerations

- Provide the patient with all the facts about HRT, if used. Make sure she realizes the need for regular monitoring.
- Before HRT begins, have the patient undergo a baseline physical examination, Pap test, and mammogram.
- Advise the patient not to discontinue contraceptive measures until cessation of menstruation has been confirmed.
- Tell the patient to immediately report vaginal bleeding or spotting after menstruation has ceased.
- Discuss alternatives to HRT, which can help with the discomforting symptoms of menopause:
  – Advise the patient to dress lightly and in layers.
  – Tell the patient to avoid caffeine, alcohol, and spicy foods. Encourage soy-based foods.
  – Instruct the patient to practice slow, deep breathing whenever a hot flash starts to come on, or to try other relaxation techniques, such as yoga, tai chi, or meditation. Tell her that acupuncture may also be helpful.
  – If the patient is in a sexually active relationship, tell her to remain sexually active to preserve vaginal elasticity. Water-based lubricants can be used during sexual intercourse to decrease dryness.
  – Instruct the patient that Kegel exercises may be performed daily to strengthen the vaginal and pelvic muscles.

Female infertility

Primary infertility is the inability to conceive after regular intercourse for at least 1 year without contraception. Secondary infertility occurs in couples who have previously been pregnant at least once, but are unable to achieve another pregnancy. About 30% to 40% of all infertility is attributed to the male, and 40% to 50% to the female; about 10% to 30% is due to a combination of male and female factors. Following extensive investigation and treatment, approximately 50% of these infertile couples achieve pregnancy. Of the 50% who don't, 10% have no pathologic basis for infertility; the prognosis for this group becomes extremely poor if pregnancy isn't achieved within 3 years.

Causes and incidence

The causes of female infertility may be functional, anatomic, or psychosocial:

■ Functional causes: complex hormonal interactions determine the normal function of the female reproductive tract and require an intact hypothalamic-pituitary-ovarian axis — the system that stimulates and regulates the hormone production necessary for normal sexual development and function. Any defect or malfunction of this axis can cause infertility due to insufficient gonadotropin secretions (both luteinizing hormone [LH] and follicle-stimulating hormone). The ovary controls, and is controlled by, the hypothalamus through a system of negative and positive feedback mediated by estrogen production. Insufficient gonadotropin levels may result from infections, tumors, or neurologic disease of the hypothalamus or pituitary gland. Hypothyroidism also impairs fertility.

■ Anatomic causes include the following:

– Ovarian factors are related to anovulation and oligo-ovulation (infrequent ovulation) and are a major cause of infertility. Pregnancy or direct visualization provides irrefutable evidence of ovulation. Presumptive signs of ovulation include regular menses, cyclic changes reflected in basal body temperature readings, postovulatory progesterone levels, and endometrial changes due to the presence of progesterone. Absence of presumptive signs suggests anovulation. Ovarian failure, in which no ova are produced by the ovaries, may result from ovarian dysgenesis or premature menopause. Amenorrhea is often associated with ovarian failure. Oligo-ovulation may be due to a mild hormonal imbalance in gonadotropin production and regulation and may be caused by polycystic disease of the ovary or abnormalities in the adrenal or thyroid gland that adversely affect hypothalamic-pituitary functioning.

– Uterine fibroids or uterine abnormalities rarely cause infertility; however, uterine abnormalities may include congenitally absent uterus, bicornuate or double uterus, leiomyomas, or Asherman's syndrome, in which the anterior and posterior uterine walls adhere because of scar tissue formation.

– Tubal and peritoneal factors are due to faulty tubal transport mechanisms and unfavorable environmental influences affecting the sperm, ova, or recently fertilized ovum. Tubal loss or impairment may occur secondary to ectopic pregnancy.

Frequently, tubal and peritoneal factors result from anatomic abnormalities: bilateral occlusion of the tubes due to salpingitis (resulting from gonorrhea, tuberculosis, or puerperal sepsis), peritubal adhesions (resulting from endometriosis, pelvic inflammatory disease [PID], diverticulosis, or childhood rupture of the appendix), and uterotubal obstruction (due to tubal spasm).

– Cervical factors may include malfunctioning cervix that produces deficient or excessively viscous mucus and is impervious to sperm, preventing entry into the uterus. In cervical infection, viscous mucus may contain spermicidal macrophages. Cervical antibodies have also been found to immobilize sperm.

■ Psychosocial problems probably account for relatively few cases of infertility. Occasionally, ovulation may stop under stress due to failure of LH release. The frequency of intercourse may be related. More often, however, psychosocial problems result from, rather than cause, infertility.

About 10% to 20% of couples will be unable to conceive after 1 year of attempting to become pregnant. Healthy couples who are younger than age 30 and having intercourse regularly only have a 25% to 30% change of getting pregnant each month. A woman's peak fertility is in her early 20s. As a woman ages beyond 35 (and particularly beyond 40), the likelihood of conception is less than 10% per month.

Diagnosis

Inability to achieve pregnancy after having regular intercourse without contraception for at least 1 year suggests infertility. (In women older than age 35, many clinicians use 6 months rather than 1 year as a cutoff point.)

Diagnosis requires a complete physical examination and health history, including specific questions on the patient's reproductive and sexual function, past diseases, mental state, previous surgery, types of contraception used in the past, and family history. Irregular, painless menses may indicate anovulation. A history of PID may suggest fallopian tube blockage. Sometimes PID is silent, and no history may be known.

The following tests assess ovulation:
■ Basal body temperature graph shows a sustained elevation in body temperature postovulation until just before the onset of menses, indicating the approximate time of ovulation.
■ Endometrial biopsy, done on or about day 26, provides histologic evidence that ovulation has occurred. However, endometrial biopsy is retrospective, which diminishes its utility.
■ Progesterone blood levels, measured when they should be highest, can show a luteal phase deficiency or presumptive evidence of ovulation.

The following procedures assess structural integrity of the fallopian tubes, the ovaries, and the uterus:
■ Urinary LH kits, available without a prescription, can sensitively detect the LH surge about 24 hours preovulation, allowing couples to time coitus.
■ Hysterosalpingography provides radiologic evidence of tubal obstruction and uterine cavity abnormalities by injecting radiopaque contrast fluid through the cervix.

Male-female interaction studies include the following:
■ Postcoital test (Sims'-Huhner test) examines the cervical mucus for motile sperm cells following intercourse that takes place at midcycle (as close to ovulation as possible).
■ Immunologic or antibody testing detects spermicidal antibodies in the female's sera.

Treatment
Treatment depends on identifying the underlying abnormality or dysfunction within in the hypothalamic-pituitary-ovarian complex. In hyperactivity or hypoactivity of the adrenal or thyroid gland, hormone therapy is necessary; progesterone deficiency requires progesterone replacement.

Anovulation necessitates treatment with clomiphene, human menopausal gonadotropins, or human chorionic gonadotropin; ovulation usually occurs several days after such administration. If mucus production decreases (an adverse effect of clomiphene), small doses of estrogen to improve the quality of cervical mucus may be given concomitantly; however, such intervention remains unproven.

Surgical restoration may correct certain anatomic causes of infertility such as fallopian tube obstruction. Surgery may also be necessary to remove tumors located within or near the hypothalamus or pituitary gland. Endometriosis requires drug therapy (danazol or medroxyprogesterone, or noncyclic administration of hormonal contraceptives), surgical removal of areas of endometriosis, or a combination of both.

Other options, often controversial and involving emotional and financial cost, include surrogate mothering, frozen embryos, or in vitro fertilization (IVF). In view of the good success rate of IVF (about 20%), IVF may be used instead of surgery in many cases.

Special considerations
Management includes providing the infertile couple with emotional support and information about diagnostic and treatment techniques.
■ An infertile couple may suffer loss of self-esteem; they may feel angry, guilty, or inadequate, and the diagnostic procedures for this disorder may intensify their fear and anxiety. You can help by explaining these procedures thoroughly. Above all, encourage the patient and her partner to talk about their feelings, and listen to what they have to say with a nonjudgmental attitude.
■ If the patient requires surgery, tell her what to expect postoperatively; this, of course, depends on which procedure is to be performed.

Pelvic inflammatory disease

Pelvic inflammatory disease (PID) is any acute, subacute, recurrent, or chronic infection of the oviducts and ovaries, with adjacent tissue involvement. It includes inflammation of the fallopian tubes (salpingitis) and ovaries (oophoritis), which can extend to the connective tissue lying between the broad ligaments (parametritis). Early diagnosis and treatment prevent damage to the reproductive system. Untreated PID may cause infertility and may lead to potentially fatal septicemia and shock.

Causes and incidence

PID can result from infection with aerobic or anaerobic organisms. The organisms *Neisseria gonorrhoeae* and *Chlamydia trachomatis* are the most common cause because they most readily penetrate the bacteriostatic barrier of cervical mucus.

Normally, cervical secretions have a protective and defensive function. Therefore, conditions or procedures that alter or destroy cervical mucus impair this bacteriostatic mechanism and allow bacteria present in the cervix or vagina to ascend into the uterine cavity; such procedures include conization or cauterization of the cervix.

Uterine infection can also follow the transfer of contaminated cervical mucus into the endometrial cavity by instrumentation. Consequently, PID can follow insertion of an intrauterine device, use of a biopsy curet or an irrigation catheter, or tubal insufflation. Other predisposing factors include abortion, pelvic surgery, and infection during or after pregnancy.

Bacteria may also enter the uterine cavity through the bloodstream or from drainage from a chronically infected fallopian tube, a pelvic abscess, a ruptured appendix, diverticulitis of the sigmoid colon, or other infectious foci.

Common bacteria found in cervical mucus are staphylococci, streptococci, diphtheroids, chlamydiae, and coliforms, including *Pseudomonas* and *Escherichia coli*. Uterine infection can result from any one or several of these organisms or may follow the multiplication of normally nonpatho-genic bacteria in an altered endometrial environment. Bacterial multiplication is most common during parturition because the endometrium is atrophic, quiescent, and not stimulated by estrogen.

In the United States, nearly 1 million people develop PID each year; many cases go undiagnosed. About 1 in 8 active adolescents will develop PID before age 21.

Signs and symptoms

Clinical features of PID vary with the affected area but generally include a profuse, purulent vaginal discharge, sometimes accompanied by low-grade fever and malaise (particularly if gonorrhea is the cause). The patient experiences lower abdomen pain; movement of the cervix or palpation of the adnexa may be extremely painful. Frequent, painful urination is also commonly reported.

Diagnosis

Diagnostic tests generally include:
- Gram stain of secretions from the endocervix or cul-de-sac. Culture and sensitivity testing aids selection of the appropriate antibiotic. Urethral and rectal secretions may also be cultured.
- Ultrasonography to identify an adnexal or uterine mass.

In addition, patient history is significant. In general, PID is associated with recent sexual intercourse, insertion of an intrauterine device, childbirth, abortion, or a sexually transmitted disease.

Treatment

To prevent progression of PID, antibiotic therapy begins immediately after culture specimens are obtained. Such therapy can be re-evaluated as soon as laboratory results are available (usually after 24 to 48 hours). Infection may become chronic if treated inadequately.

Development of a pelvic abscess necessitates adequate drainage. A ruptured abscess is life-threatening. If this complication develops, the patient may need a total abdominal hysterectomy with bilateral salpingo-oophorectomy. Alternatively, laparoscopic drainage with preservation of the ovaries and uterus may be done.

Concurrent treatment of sexual partners and condom use throughout the course of treatment are necessary.

Special considerations
- After establishing that the patient has no drug allergies, administer antibiotics and analgesics, as ordered.
- Check for fever. If it persists, carefully monitor fluid intake and output for signs of dehydration.
- Watch for abdominal rigidity and distention, possible signs of developing peritonitis. Provide frequent perineal care if vaginal drainage occurs.
- To prevent a recurrence, explain the nature and seriousness of PID, and encourage the patient to comply with the treatment regimen.
- Stress the need for the patient's sexual partner to be examined and, if necessary, treated for infection.
- Because PID may cause painful intercourse, advise the patient to consult with her physician about sexual activity.
- To prevent infection after minor gynecologic procedures, such as dilatation and curettage, tell the patient to immediately report any fever, increased vaginal discharge, or pain. After such procedures, instruct her to avoid douching and intercourse for at least 7 days.

UTERINE BLEEDING DISORDERS

Amenorrhea

Amenorrhea is the abnormal absence or suppression of menstruation. Primary amenorrhea is the absence of menarche in an adolescent (by age 18). Secondary amenorrhea is the failure of menstruation for at least 3 months after normal onset of menarche.

Causes and incidence
Amenorrhea is normal before puberty, after menopause, or during pregnancy and lactation; it's pathologic at any other time. It usually results from anovulation due to hormonal abnormalities, such as decreased secretion of estrogen, gonadotropins, luteinizing hormone, and follicle-stimulating hormone; lack of ovarian response to gonadotropins; or constant presence of progesterone or other endocrine abnormalities.

Amenorrhea may also result from the absence of a uterus, endometrial damage, or from ovarian, adrenal, or pituitary tumors. It's also linked to emotional disorders and is common in patients with severe disorders, such as depression and anorexia nervosa. Mild emotional disturbances tend merely to distort the ovulatory cycle, while severe psychic trauma may abruptly change the bleeding pattern or may completely suppress one or more full ovulatory cycles. Amenorrhea may also result from malnutrition, intense exercise, and prolonged hormonal contraceptive use. The incidence of primary amenorrhea in the United States is less than 1%. The incidence of secondary amenorrhea (due to some other cause than pregnancy) is about 4%.

Diagnosis
CONFIRMING DIAGNOSIS *A history of failure to menstruate in a female older than age 18 confirms primary amenorrhea.*

Secondary amenorrhea can be diagnosed when a change is noted in a previously established menstrual pattern (absence of menstruation for 3 months). A thorough physical and pelvic examination rules out pregnancy, as well as anatomic abnormalities such as cervical stenosis that may cause false amenorrhea (cryptomenorrhea), in which menstruation occurs without external bleeding.

Onset of menstruation within 1 week after administration of pure progestational agents, such as medroxyprogesterone and progesterone, indicates a functioning uterus. If menstruation doesn't occur, special diagnostic studies are appropriate.

Blood and urine studies may reveal hormonal imbalances, such as lack of ovarian response to gonadotropins (elevated pituitary gonadotropins), failure of gonadotropin secretion (low pituitary gonadotropin levels), and abnormal thyroid levels. Tests for identification of dominant or

DIFFERENTIAL DIAGNOSIS

DIAGNOSING AMENORRHEA

The flowchart lists possible diagnostic findings and interpretations to assist with the treatment of the patient with amenorrhea.

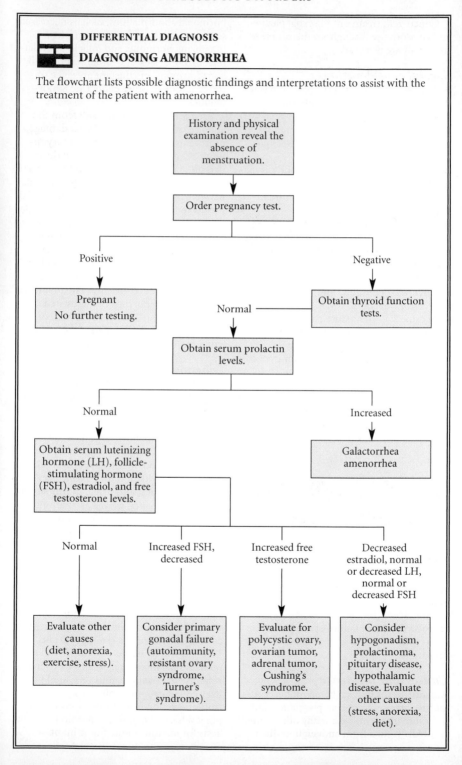

missing hormones include cervical mucus ferning, vaginal cytologic examinations, basal body temperature, endometrial biopsy (during dilatation and curettage), urinary 17-ketosteroids, and plasma progesterone, testosterone, and androgen levels. A complete medical workup, including appropriate X-rays, laparoscopy, and a biopsy, may detect ovarian, adrenal, and pituitary tumors. (See *Diagnosing amenorrhea.*)

Treatment

Appropriate hormone replacement reestablishes menstruation. Treatment of amenorrhea not related to hormone deficiency depends on the cause. For example, amenorrhea that results from a tumor usually requires surgery.

Special considerations

- Explain all diagnostic procedures.
- Provide reassurance and emotional support. Psychiatric counseling may be necessary if amenorrhea results from emotional disturbances.
- After treatment, teach the patient how to keep an accurate record of her menstrual cycles to aid early detection of recurrent amenorrhea.

Abnormal premenopausal bleeding

Abnormal premenopausal bleeding refers to any bleeding that deviates from the normal menstrual cycle before menopause. These deviations include menstrual bleeding that's abnormally infrequent (oligomenorrhea), abnormally frequent (polymenorrhea), excessive (menorrhagia or hypermenorrhea), deficient (hypomenorrhea), or irregular (metrorrhagia [uterine bleeding between menses]). Rarely, menstrual symptoms aren't accompanied by external bleeding (cryptomenorrhea). Premenopausal bleeding may merely be troublesome or can result in severe hemorrhage; the prognosis depends on the underlying cause. Abnormal bleeding patterns often respond to hormonal or other therapy.

Causes and incidence

Causes of abnormal premenopausal bleeding vary with the type of bleeding:

- Oligomenorrhea and polymenorrhea usually result from anovulation due to an endocrine or systemic disorder.
- Menorrhagia usually results from local lesions, such as uterine leiomyomas, endometrial polyps, and endometrial hyperplasia. It may also result from endometritis, salpingitis, and anovulation.
- Hypomenorrhea results from local, endocrine, or systemic disorders, or from blockage due to partial obstruction by the hymen or to cervical obstruction.
- Cryptomenorrhea may result from an imperforate hymen or cervical stenosis.
- Metrorrhagia usually results from slight physiologic bleeding from the endometrium during ovulation but may also result from local disorders, such as uterine malignancy, cervical erosions, polyps (which tend to bleed after intercourse), or inappropriate estrogen therapy. Complications of pregnancy can also cause premenopausal bleeding. Such bleeding may be as mild as spotting or as severe as menorrhagia. (See *Causes of abnormal premenopausal bleeding,* page 954.)

Signs and symptoms

Bleeding not associated with abnormal pregnancy is usually painless, but it may be severely painful. When bleeding is associated with abnormal pregnancy, other symptoms include nausea, breast tenderness, bloating, and fluid retention. Severe or prolonged bleeding causes anemia, especially in patients with underlying disease such as blood dyscrasia and in patients receiving anticoagulants.

Diagnosis

The typical clinical picture confirms abnormal premenopausal bleeding. Special tests identify the underlying cause:

- Serum hormone levels reflect adrenal, pituitary, or thyroid dysfunction.
- Urinary 17-ketosteroids reveal adrenal hyperplasia, hypopituitarism, or polycystic ovarian disease.
- Endometrial sampling rules out malignant tumors and should be performed in all patients with premenopausal bleeding who are older than age 35.

CAUSES OF ABNORMAL PREMENOPAUSAL BLEEDING

Premenopausal bleeding can take several forms and may be due to a number of causes.

	Hypomenorrhea	Oligomenorrhea	Metrorrhagia	Polymenorrhea	Menorrhagia	Menometrorrhagia
Malnutrition	◆	◆				
Hyperthyroidism	◆	◆				
Hypothyroidism					◆	◆
Severe psychic trauma	◆	◆				◆
Blood dyscrasias			◆	◆	◆	
Severe infections	◆	◆				
Endometritis				◆		
Drugs (such as cardiac glycosides, corticosteroids, anticoagulants)				◆		
Uterine tumors				◆		◆

- Pelvic examination, Papanicolaou (Pap) test, and patient history rule out local or malignant causes.
- Complete blood count rules out anemia.

If testing rules out pelvic and hormonal causes of abnormal bleeding, a complete hematologic survey (including platelet count and bleeding time) is appropriate to determine clotting abnormalities.

Treatment

Treatment depends on the type of bleeding abnormality and its cause. Menstrual irregularity alone may not require therapy unless it interferes with the patient's attempt to achieve or avoid conception or leads to anemia. When it requires treatment, clomiphene induces ovulation. Electrocautery, chemical cautery, or cryosurgery can remove cervical polyps; dilatation and curettage, uterine polyps. Organic disorders (such as cervical or uterine malignancy) may necessitate hysterectomy, radium or X-ray therapy, or both of these treatments, depending on the disease's site and extent. Of course, anemia and infections require appropriate treatment.

Special considerations

- If the patient complains of abnormal bleeding, tell her to record the dates of the bleeding and the number of tampons or pads used per day. This helps to assess the cyclic pattern and the amount of bleeding.
- Instruct the patient to report abnormal bleeding immediately to help rule out major hemorrhagic disorders, such as occur in abnormal pregnancy.
- To prevent abnormal bleeding due to organic causes, and for early detection of malignancy, encourage the patient to have a Pap smear and a pelvic examination annually.
- Offer reassurance and support. The patient may be particularly anxious about excessive or frequent blood loss and passage of clots. Suggest that she minimize blood flow by avoiding strenuous activity and occasionally lying down with her feet elevated.

Dysfunctional uterine bleeding

Dysfunctional uterine bleeding (DUB) refers to abnormal endometrial bleeding without recognizable organic lesions. The prognosis varies with the cause. DUB is the indication for almost 25% of gynecologic surgical procedures.

Causes and incidence

DUB usually results from an imbalance in the hormonal-endometrial relationship, where persistent and unopposed stimulation of the endometrium by estrogen occurs. Disorders that cause sustained high estrogen levels are polycystic ovary syndrome, obesity, immaturity of the hypothalamic-pituitary-ovarian mechanism (in postpubertal teenagers), and anovulation (in women in their late 30s or early 40s).

In most cases of DUB, the endometrium shows no pathologic changes. However, in chronic unopposed estrogen stimulation (as from a hormone-producing ovarian tumor), the endometrium may show hyperplastic or malignant changes. DUB occurs in 20% of adolescents and in 40% of women older than age 40.

Signs and symptoms

DUB usually occurs as metrorrhagia (episodes of vaginal bleeding between menses); it may also occur as hypermenorrhea (heavy or prolonged menses, longer than 8 days) or chronic polymenorrhea (menstrual cycle of less than 18 days). Such bleeding is unpredictable and can cause anemia.

Diagnosis

Diagnostic studies must rule out other causes of excessive vaginal bleeding, such as organic, systemic, psychogenic, and endocrine causes, including certain cancers, polyps, incomplete abortion, pregnancy, and infection.

 CONFIRMING DIAGNOSIS *Dilatation and curettage (D & C) and biopsy results confirm the diagnosis by revealing endometrial hyperplasia.*

Hemoglobin levels and hematocrit determine the need for blood or iron replacement.

Treatment

High-dose estrogen-progestogen combination therapy (hormonal contraceptives), the primary treatment, is designed to control endometrial growth and re-establish a normal cyclic pattern of menstruation. (The patient's age and the cause of bleeding help determine the drug choice and dosage.) In patients older than age 35, endometrial biopsy is necessary before the start of estrogen therapy to rule out endometrial adenocarcinoma. Progestogen therapy is a necessary alternative in some women such as those susceptible to estrogen's adverse effects (thrombophlebitis, for example).

If drug therapy is ineffective, D & C serves as a supplementary treatment, through removal of a large portion of the bleeding endometrium. Also, D & C can help determine the original cause of hormonal imbalance and can aid in planning further therapy. Regardless of the primary treatment, the patient may need iron replacement or transfusions of packed cells or whole blood, as indicated, because of anemia caused by recurrent bleeding.

Special considerations

- Explain the importance of adhering to the prescribed hormonal therapy. If D & C is ordered, explain this procedure and its purpose.
- Stress the need for regular checkups to assess the effectiveness of treatment.

Postmenopausal bleeding

Postmenopausal bleeding is defined as bleeding from the reproductive tract that occurs 1 year or more after cessation of menses. Sites of bleeding include the vulva, vagina, cervix, and endometrium. The prognosis varies with the cause.

Causes

Postmenopausal bleeding may result from:
- exogenous estrogen, when administration is excessive or prolonged or when small amounts are given in the presence of a hypersensitive endometrium
- endogenous estrogen production, especially when levels are high, as in persons with estrogen-producing ovarian tumor; however, in some persons, even a slight fluctuation in estrogen levels may cause bleeding
- atrophic endometrium due to low estrogen levels
- atrophic vaginitis, usually triggered by trauma during coitus in the absence of estrogen production
- aging, which increases vascular vulnerability by thinning epithelial surfaces, increasing vascular fragility, producing degenerative tissue changes, and decreasing resistance to infections
- cervical or endometrial cancer (more common after age 60)

- adenomatous hyperplasia or atypical adenomatous hyperplasia (usually considered a premalignant lesion).

Signs and symptoms
Vaginal bleeding, the primary symptom, ranges from spotting to outright hemorrhage; its duration also varies. Other symptoms depend on the cause. Excessive estrogen stimulation, for example, may also produce copious cervical mucus; estrogen deficiency may cause vaginal mucosa to atrophy.

Diagnosis
Diagnostic evaluation of the patient with postmenopausal bleeding should include physical examination (especially pelvic examination), a detailed history, standard laboratory tests (such as complete blood count), and cytologic examination of smears from the cervix and the endocervical canal. An endometrial biopsy or dilatation and curettage (D & C) with hysteroscopy reveals pathologic findings in the endometrium.

Diagnosis must rule out underlying degenerative or systemic disease. For instance, evidence of elevated levels of endogenous estrogen may suggest an ovarian tumor. Before testing for estrogen levels, the patient must stop all sources of exogenous estrogen intake—including face and body creams that contain estrogen—to rule out excessive exogenous estrogen as a cause.

Treatment
Emergency treatment to control massive hemorrhage is rarely necessary, except in advanced cancer. Treatment may include D & C to relieve bleeding. Other therapy varies according to the underlying cause. Estrogen creams and suppositories are usually effective in correcting estrogen deficiency because they're rapidly absorbed. Hysterectomy is indicated for repeated episodes of postmenopausal bleeding from the endometrial cavity. Such bleeding may indicate endometrial cancer.

Special considerations
Obtain a detailed patient history to rule out excessive exogenous estrogen as a cause

of bleeding. Ask the patient about use of cosmetics (especially face and body creams), drugs, and other products that may contain estrogen. Discuss the risks and benefits of estrogen replacement therapy with her.

- Provide emotional support. The patient will probably be afraid that the bleeding indicates cancer.
- To prevent disorders that cause postmenopausal bleeding, stress the fact that periodic gynecologic examinations are as important after menopause as they were before.

DISORDERS OF PREGNANCY

Abortion

Abortion is the spontaneous or induced (therapeutic) expulsion of the products of conception from the uterus. Up to 15% of all pregnancies and approximately 30% of first pregnancies end in spontaneous abortion (miscarriage). At least 75% of miscarriages occur during the first trimester. (See *Types of spontaneous abortion.*)

Causes
Spontaneous abortion may result from fetal, placental, or maternal factors. Fetal factors, which usually cause such abortions at up to 12 weeks' gestation, include the following:

- defective embryologic development resulting from abnormal chromosome division (most common cause of fetal death)
- faulty implantation of the fertilized ovum
- failure of the endometrium to accept the fertilized ovum.

Placental factors usually cause abortion around the 14th week of gestation, when the placenta takes over the hormone production necessary to maintain the pregnancy. These factors include:

- premature separation of the normally implanted placenta
- abnormal placental implantation.

Maternal factors usually cause abortion between the 11th and 19th week of gestation and include:
- maternal infection, abnormalities of the reproductive organs (especially an incompetent cervix, in which the cervix dilates painlessly in the second trimester)
- endocrine problems, such as thyroid dysfunction or a luteal phase defect
- trauma
- phospholipid antibody disorder
- blood group incompatibility
- drug ingestion (particularly uterotonic agents).

The goal of therapeutic abortion is to preserve the mother's mental or physical health in cases of rape, unplanned pregnancy, or medical conditions such as moderate or severe cardiac dysfunction.

Signs and symptoms
Prodromal signs of spontaneous abortion may include a pink discharge for several days or a scant brown discharge for several weeks before the onset of cramps and increased vaginal bleeding. For a few hours, the cramps intensify and occur more frequently; then the cervix dilates to expel uterine contents. If the entire contents are expelled, cramps and bleeding subside. However, if any contents remain, cramps and bleeding continue.

Diagnosis
Diagnosis of spontaneous abortion is based on clinical evidence of expulsion of uterine contents, pelvic examination, and laboratory studies. Human chorionic gonadotropin (hCG) in the blood or urine confirms pregnancy; decreased hCG levels suggest spontaneous abortion or tubal pregnancy. Pelvic examination determines the uterus' size and whether this size is consistent with the pregnancy's length. Tissue histology indicates evidence of products of conception. Laboratory tests reflect decreased hemoglobin levels and hematocrit due to blood loss. However, blood loss is rarely excessive in spontaneous abortion. It's critical that ectopic pregnancy be ruled out in a woman who's pregnant with vaginal bleeding.

TYPES OF SPONTANEOUS ABORTION

- *Threatened abortion*: Bloody vaginal discharge occurs during the first half of pregnancy. Approximately 20% of pregnant women have vaginal spotting or actual bleeding early in pregnancy; of these, about 50% abort.
- *Inevitable abortion*: Membranes rupture and the cervix dilates. As labor continues, the uterus expels the products of conception.
- *Incomplete abortion*: The uterus retains part or all of the placenta. Before the 10th week of gestation, the fetus and placenta usually are expelled together; after the 10th week, separately. Because part of the placenta may adhere to the uterine wall, bleeding continues. Hemorrhage is possible because the uterus doesn't contract and seal the large vessels that fed the placenta.
- *Complete abortion*: The uterus passes all the products of conception. Minimal bleeding usually accompanies complete abortion because the uterus contracts and compresses maternal blood vessels that feed the placenta.
- *Missed abortion*: The uterus retains the products of conception for 2 months or more after the fetus' death. Uterine growth ceases; uterine size may even seem to decrease. Prolonged retention of the dead products of conception may cause coagulation defects, such as disseminated intravascular coagulation, usually after at least 1 month in utero.
- *Habitual abortion*: Spontaneous loss of three or more consecutive pregnancies constitutes habitual abortion.
- *Septic abortion*: Infection accompanies abortion. This may occur with spontaneous abortion but usually results from an illegal abortion.

Treatment

An accurate evaluation of uterine contents is necessary before a plan of treatment can be formulated. The progression of spontaneous abortion can't be prevented, except possibly in cases caused by an incompetent cervix. The patient must be hospitalized to control severe hemorrhage. If bleeding is severe, a transfusion with packed red blood cells or whole blood is required. Initially, I.V. administration of oxytocin stimulates uterine contractions (if given above 20 weeks' gestation — receptors are absent before this gestational age). If any remnants remain in the uterus, dilatation and curettage or dilatation and evacuation (D & E) should be performed.

D & E is also performed in first- and second-trimester therapeutic abortions. In second-trimester therapeutic abortions, the insertion of a prostaglandin vaginal suppository induces labor and the expulsion of uterine contents. When performed competently, second-trimester D & E is a very safe procedure and allows for termination of pregnancy without the need for a lengthy induction of labor. Early first-trimester abortion may also be accomplished pharmacologically with mifepristone (RU-486) an antiprogestin, followed by a dose of a prostaglandin analogue 2 days later, or surgically, using vacuum aspiration.

After an abortion, spontaneous or induced, an Rh-negative female with a negative indirect Coombs' test should receive $Rh_o(D)$ immune globulin (human) to prevent future Rh isoimmunization.

In a habitual aborter, spontaneous abortion can result from an incompetent cervix (a clinical retrospective diagnosis suggested by a history of previous second-trimester losses accompanied by membrane rupture or painless cervical dilation). Treatment involves surgical reinforcement of the cervix (cerclage) 12 to 24 weeks after the last menstrual period. A few weeks before the estimated delivery date, the sutures are removed, and the patient awaits the onset of labor. An alternative procedure is to leave the sutures in place and to deliver the infant by cesarean birth. Cerclage hasn't been shown to be more effective than bed rest.

Special considerations

Elective abortion is a controversial issue. The decision to have an elective abortion is a personal decision that requires competent counseling. Many women believe they can't share their feelings with others, therefore it's important for a woman contemplating an abortion to examine her existing support system and identify those people capable of helping her through a difficult time. A reputable provider or clinic where the woman can obtain adequate counseling regarding all options for pregnancy resolution, have the procedure performed, and obtain support and follow-up care should be identified ahead during the decision-making process.

Before possible abortion:
■ Be sure to inform the patient who desires an elective abortion of all the available alternatives. She needs to know what the procedure involves, what the risks are, and what to expect during and after the procedure, both emotionally and physically. Be sure to ascertain whether the patient is comfortable with her decision to have an elective abortion.
■ The patient *shouldn't* have bathroom privileges, because she may expel uterine contents without knowing it. After she uses the bedpan, inspect the contents carefully for intrauterine material.

After spontaneous or elective abortion:
■ Note the amount, color, and odor of vaginal bleeding. Save all the pads the patient uses, for evaluation.
■ Administer analgesics and oxytocin, as ordered.
■ Provide good perineal care.
■ Obtain vital signs as indicated.
■ Monitor urine output.

Care of the patient who has had a spontaneous abortion includes emotional support and counseling during the grieving process. Stress to the patient that she isn't responsible for a spontaneous abortion, as this generally can't be prevented. Encourage the patient and her partner to express their feelings. Some couples may want to talk to a clergy member or, depending on their religion, may wish to have the fetus baptized.

The patient who has had a therapeutic abortion also benefits from support. Encourage her to verbalize her feelings. Remember, she may feel ambivalent about the procedure; intellectual and emotional acceptance of abortion aren't the same. If you identify an inappropriate coping response, refer the patient for professional counseling.

To prepare the patient for discharge:
- Tell the patient to expect vaginal bleeding or spotting and to report bleeding that lasts longer than 8 to 10 days or excessive, bright-red blood immediately.
- Advise the patient to watch for signs of infection, such as a temperature higher than 100.5° F (38° C) and foul-smelling vaginal discharge.
- Encourage the gradual increase of daily activities to include whatever tasks the patient feels comfortable doing, as long as these activities don't increase vaginal bleeding or cause fatigue. Most patients return to work after 24 hours.
- Urge 1 to 2 weeks' abstinence from intercourse, and encourage the use of a contraceptive.
- Instruct the patient to avoid using tampons for 1 to 2 weeks.
- Tell the patient to see her physician in 2 to 4 weeks for a follow-up examination.

To help prevent future elective abortions, medical and nursing personnel need to make contraceptive information available. An educated population motivated to utilize contraception would have less need for elective abortion.

To minimize the risk of future spontaneous abortions, emphasize to the pregnant woman the importance of good nutrition and the need to avoid alcohol, cigarettes, and drugs. If the patient has a history of habitual spontaneous abortions, suggest that she and her partner have thorough examinations. For the woman, this includes premenstrual endometrial biopsy, a hormone assessment (estrogen; progesterone; and thyroid, follicle-stimulating, and luteinizing hormones), and hysterosalpingography and laparoscopy to detect anatomic abnormalities. Genetic counseling may also be indicated.

Ectopic pregnancy

Ectopic pregnancy is the implantation of the fertilized ovum outside the uterine cavity. The most common site is the fallopian tube (more than 90% of ectopic implantations occur in the fimbria, ampulla, or isthmus), but other possible sites include the interstitium, tubo-ovarian ligament, ovary, abdominal viscera, and internal cervical os. (See *Implantation sites of ectopic pregnancy*, page 960.) The prognosis is good with prompt diagnosis, appropriate surgical intervention, and control of bleeding; rarely, in cases of abdominal implantation, the fetus may survive to term. Usually, a subsequent intrauterine pregnancy is achieved.

Causes and incidence
Conditions that prevent or retard the fertilized ovum's passage through the fallopian tube and into the uterine cavity include:
- diverticula, the formation of blind pouches that cause tubal abnormalities
- endometriosis, the presence of endometrial tissue outside the lining of the uterine cavity
- endosalpingitis, an inflammatory reaction that causes folds of the tubal mucosa to agglutinate, narrowing the tube
- pelvic inflammatory disease (PID), an infection of the oviducts and ovaries with adjacent tissue involvement
- previous surgery (tubal ligation or resection, or adhesions from previous abdominal or pelvic surgery)
- tumors pressing against the tube.

Ectopic pregnancy may result from congenital defects in the reproductive tract or ectopic endometrial implants in the tubal mucosa. The increased prevalence of sexually transmitted tubal infection may also be a factor. In whites, it occurs in 1 in 200 pregnancies; in nonwhites, in 1 in 120.

Signs and symptoms
Ectopic pregnancy sometimes produces symptoms of normal pregnancy or no symptoms other than mild abdominal pain, making diagnosis difficult. Characteristic clinical effects after fallopian tube implantation include amenorrhea or abnormal menses, followed by slight vaginal bleeding, and unilateral pelvic pain over

IMPLANTATION SITES OF ECTOPIC PREGNANCY

In 90% of patients with ectopic pregnancy, the ovum implants in the fallopian tube, either in the fimbria, ampulla, or isthmus. Other possible sites include the interstitium, tubo-ovarian ligament, ovary, abdominal viscera, and internal cervical os.

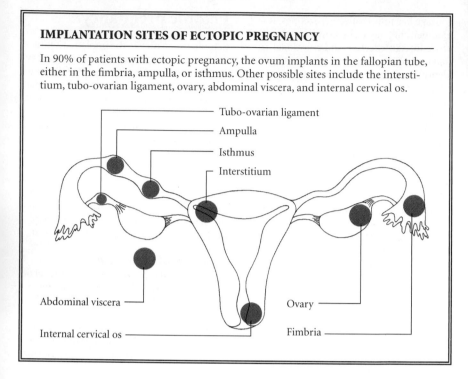

Tubo-ovarian ligament
Ampulla
Isthmus
Interstitium
Abdominal viscera
Internal cervical os
Ovary
Fimbria

---

the mass. Rupture of the tube causes life-threatening complications, including hemorrhage, shock, and peritonitis. The patient experiences sharp lower abdominal pain, possibly radiating to the shoulders and neck, often precipitated by activities that increase abdominal pressure, such as a bowel movement; she feels extreme pain upon motion of the cervix and palpation of the adnexa during a pelvic examination.

Diagnosis

Clinical features, patient history, and the results of a pelvic examination suggest ectopic pregnancy. The following tests help confirm it:

■ Serum pregnancy test shows presence of human chorionic gonadotropin.
■ Real time ultrasonography determines extrauterine pregnancy (performed if serum pregnancy test is positive).
■ In culdocentesis, fluid is aspirated from the pouch of Douglas through the posterior vaginal fornix to detect free or nonclotting blood in the peritoneum (sometimes

performed if ultrasonography fails to detect a gestational sac in the uterus).
■ Laparoscopy or laparotomy is used to diagnose as well as to treat an ectopic pregnancy by either removal of the tube (salpingectomy) or removal of the pregnancy with preservation of the tube (salpingostomy).

Decreased hemoglobin levels and hematocrit due to blood loss support the diagnosis. Differential diagnosis must rule out uterine abortion, appendicitis, ruptured corpus luteum cyst, salpingitis, and torsion of the ovary.

Treatment

If culdocentesis is positive or the patient has peritoneal signs consistent with a surgical abdomen, laparoscopy and laparotomy are indicated. The ovary is preserved as a rule; however, ovarian pregnancy may necessitate oophorectomy. Interstitial pregnancy may rarely require hysterectomy; abdominal pregnancy requires a laparotomy to remove the fetus, except in rare cases, when the fetus survives to term or calcifies undetected in the abdominal cavity.

Supportive treatment includes transfusion with whole blood or packed red cells to replace excessive blood loss, administration of broad-spectrum antibiotics I.V. for septic infection, and administration of supplemental iron by mouth or I.M.

Methotrexate I.M. is also a therapeutic option in stable patients, avoiding surgery in most cases.

Special considerations

Patient care measures include careful monitoring and assessment of vital signs and vaginal bleeding, preparing the patient with excessive blood loss for emergency surgery, and providing blood replacement and emotional support and reassurance.

- Record the pain's location and character, and administer analgesics as ordered. (Remember, however, that analgesics may mask the symptoms of intraperitoneal rupture of the ectopic pregnancy.)
- Check the amount, color, and odor of vaginal bleeding. Ask the patient the date of her last menstrual period and to describe this period's character.
- Observe for signs of pregnancy (enlarged breasts, soft cervix).
- Provide a quiet, relaxing environment, and encourage the patient to freely express her feelings of fear, loss, and grief.

To prevent ectopic pregnancy:
- Advise prompt treatment of pelvic infections to prevent diseases of the fallopian tube. Inform patients who have undergone surgery involving the fallopian tubes or those with confirmed PID that they're at increased risk of ectopic pregnancy.
- Tell the patient who's vulnerable to ectopic pregnancy to delay using an intrauterine device until after she has completed her family.

Hyperemesis gravidarum

Unlike the transient nausea and vomiting normally experienced between the 6th and 12th weeks of pregnancy, hyperemesis gravidarum is severe and unremitting nausea and vomiting that persists after the first trimester. If untreated, it produces substan-tial weight loss; starvation; dehydration, with subsequent fluid and electrolyte imbalance (hypokalemia); and acid-base disturbances (acidosis and alkalosis). This syndrome occurs in approximately 1 in 200 pregnancies. The prognosis is good with appropriate treatment.

Causes and incidence

Although its cause is unknown, hyperemesis gravidarum often affects pregnant females with conditions that produce high levels of human chorionic gonadotropin, such as hydatidiform mole or multiple pregnancies. Its other possible causes include pancreatitis (elevated serum amylase levels are common), biliary tract disease, drug toxicity, inflammatory obstructive bowel disease, and vitamin deficiency (especially of B_6). In some patients, it may be related to psychological factors such as ambivalence toward pregnancy.

This disorder occurs in 0.5 to 10 of every 1,000 pregnancies. The incidence increases in molar and multiple pregnancies.

Signs and symptoms

The cardinal symptoms of hyperemesis gravidarum are unremitting nausea and vomiting. The vomitus initially contains undigested food and mucus as well as small amounts of bile; later, only bile and mucus; and finally, blood and material that resembles coffee grounds. Persistent vomiting causes substantial weight loss and eventual emaciation. Associated effects may include pale, dry, waxy, and possibly jaundiced skin; subnormal or elevated temperature; rapid pulse; a fetid, fruity breath odor from acidosis; and central nervous system symptoms, such as confusion, delirium, headache, lassitude, stupor and, possibly, coma.

Diagnosis

Diagnosis depends on a history of uncontrolled nausea and vomiting that persists beyond the first trimester, evidence of substantial weight loss, and other characteristic clinical features. Serum analysis shows decreased protein, chloride, sodium, and potassium levels, and increased blood urea nitrogen levels. Other laboratory tests reveal ketonuria, slight proteinuria, and elevated hemoglobin and white blood cell levels. Diagnosis must rule out other conditions with similar clinical effects.

Treatment
Hyperemesis gravidarum may necessitate hospitalization to correct electrolyte imbalance and prevent starvation. I.V. infusions maintain nutrition until the patient can tolerate oral feedings. She progresses slowly to a clear liquid diet, then a full liquid diet and, finally, small, frequent meals of high-protein solid foods. A midnight snack helps stabilize blood glucose levels; vitamin B supplements help correct vitamin deficiency.

When vomiting stops and electrolyte balance has been restored, the pregnancy usually continues without recurrence of hyperemesis gravidarum. Most patients feel better as they begin to regain normal weight, but some continue to vomit throughout the pregnancy, requiring extended treatment. If appropriate, some patients may benefit from consultations with clinical nurse specialists, psychologists, or psychiatrists.

Special considerations
- Encourage the patient to eat. Suggest dry foods and decreased liquid intake during meals.
- Instruct the patient to remain upright for 45 minutes after eating to decrease reflux.
- Provide reassurance and a calm, restful atmosphere. Encourage the patient to discuss her feelings regarding her pregnancy.
- Before discharge, provide good nutritional counseling.

Pregnancy-induced hypertension

Pregnancy-induced hypertension (PIH), also known as *gestational hypertension,* is a potentially life-threatening disorder that usually develops late in the second trimester or in the third trimester. *Preeclampsia,* the nonconvulsive form of PIH, may be mild or severe. *Eclampsia* is the convulsive form of PIH.

Causes and incidence
The cause of pregnancy-induced hypertension is unknown, but geographic, ethnic, racial, nutritional, immunologic, and familial factors and pre-existing vascular disease may contribute to its development. Age is also a factor. Primiparas who are older than age 35 are at higher risk for preeclampsia.

Preeclampsia develops in about 7% of pregnancies. Incidence is significantly higher in low socioeconomic groups. About 5% of females with preeclampsia develop eclampsia; of these, about 15% die from PIH itself or its complications. Fetal mortality is high due to the increased incidence of premature delivery and uteroplacental insufficiency.

Signs and symptoms
Mild preeclampsia generally produces the following clinical effects: hypertension, proteinuria (less than 5 g/24 hours), generalized edema, and sudden weight gain of more than 3 lb (1.4 kg) per week during the second trimester or more than 1 lb (0.5 kg) a week during the third trimester.

Severe preeclampsia is marked by increased hypertension and proteinuria, eventually leading to the development of oliguria. Hemolysis, elevated liver enzymes, and low platelets (the HELLP syndrome) is a severe variant. Other symptoms that may indicate worsening preeclampsia include blurred vision due to retinal arteriolar spasms, epigastric pain or heartburn, and severe frontal headache.

In eclampsia, all the clinical manifestations of preeclampsia are magnified and are associated with seizures and, possibly, coma, premature labor, stillbirth, renal failure, and hepatic damage.

Diagnosis
The following findings suggest preeclampsia:
- elevated blood pressure readings: 140 systolic, measured on two occasions, 6 hours apart; 90 diastolic, measured on two occasions, 6 hours apart
- proteinuria: at least 300 mg/24 hours.

The following findings suggest severe preeclampsia:

- higher blood pressure readings: 160/110 mm Hg or higher on two occasions, 6 hours apart, on bed rest
- increased proteinuria: 5 g/24 hours or more
- presence of pulmonary edema
- ultrasound: may reveal oligohydraminos
- oliguria: urine output less than or equal to 400 ml/24 hours.

Seizures strongly suggest eclampsia. Rarely, ophthalmoscopic examination may reveal vascular spasm, papilledema, retinal edema or detachment, and arteriovenous nicking or hemorrhage.

Real-time ultrasonography, stress and nonstress tests, and biophysical profiles evaluate fetal status. In the stress test, oxytocin stimulates contractions; fetal heart tones are then monitored electronically. In the nonstress test, fetal heart tones are monitored electronically during periods of fetal activity, without oxytocin stimulation. Electronic monitoring reveals stable or increased fetal heart tones during periods of fetal activity.

Ultrasonography aids evaluation of fetal health by assessing fetal breathing movements, gross body movements, fetal tone, reactive fetal heart rate, and qualitative amniotic fluid volume.

Treatment

Therapy for preeclampsia is designed to halt the disorder's progress—specifically, the early effects of eclampsia, such as seizures, residual hypertension, and renal shutdown—and to ensure fetal survival. Some physicians advocate the prompt induction of labor, especially if the patient is near term; others follow a more conservative approach. Therapy may include complete bed rest to increase placental perfusion, reduce hypertension, and evaluate response to therapy. Antihypertensive therapy doesn't alter the potential for developing eclampsia. Diuretics aren't appropriate during pregnancy.

If the patient's blood pressure fails to respond to bed rest and sedation and persistently rises above 160/100 mm Hg, or if central nervous system irritability increases, magnesium sulfate may produce general sedation, promote diuresis, and prevent seizures. Cesarean birth or oxytocin induc-

tion may be required to terminate the pregnancy.

Emergency treatment of eclamptic seizures consists of immediate administration of magnesium sulfate (I.V. drip), oxygen administration, and electronic fetal monitoring. After the seizures subside and the patient's condition stabilizes, delivery should proceed with induction of labor or cesarean birth, depending upon the circumstances.

Adequate nutrition, good prenatal care, and control of pre-existing hypertension during pregnancy decrease the incidence and severity of preeclampsia. Early recognition and prompt treatment of preeclampsia can prevent progression to eclampsia.

Special considerations

- Monitor regularly for changes in blood pressure, pulse rate, respiration, fetal heart tones, vision, level of consciousness, and deep tendon reflexes and for headache unrelieved by medication. Report changes immediately. Assess these signs before administering medications. Absence of patellar reflexes may indicate magnesium sulfate toxicity.
- Assess fluid balance by measuring intake and output and by checking daily weight.
- Observe for signs of fetal hypoxemia by closely monitoring the results of stress and nonstress tests.
- Instruct the patient to lie in a left lateral position to increase venous return, cardiac output, and renal blood flow.
- Keep emergency resuscitative equipment and drugs available in case of seizures and cardiac or respiratory arrest. Also keep calcium gluconate at the bedside because it counteracts magnesium sulfate's toxic effects.
- To protect the patient from injury, maintain seizure precautions. Don't leave an unstable patient unattended.
- Assist with emergency medical treatment for the convulsive patient. Provide a quiet, darkened room until the patient's condition stabilizes, and enforce absolute bed rest. Carefully monitor administration of magnesium sulfate; give oxygen as ordered. Don't administer anything by mouth. Insert an indwelling urinary

catheter for accurate measurement of intake and output.

■ Inform the patient about the tests that are done to evaluate fetal status. The baby's welfare is of prime concern to the parents.

■ Provide emotional support for the patient and her family. If the patient's condition necessitates premature delivery, point out that infants of mothers with PIH are usually small for gestational age but sometimes fare better than other premature babies of the same weight, possibly because they have developed adaptive responses to stress in utero.

Hydatidiform mole

Hydatidiform mole is an uncommon chorionic tumor of the placenta. Its early signs — amenorrhea and uterine enlargement — mimic normal pregnancy; however, it eventually causes vaginal bleeding. With prompt diagnosis and appropriate treatment, the prognosis is excellent; however, approximately 15% of patients with hydatidiform mole develop gestational trophoblastic neoplasm. Recurrence is possible in about 2% of cases.

Causes and incidence

The cause of hydatidiform mole is unknown. Abnormal genetic events upon fusion of the oocyte with one or more sperm play a role. It occurs in 1 in 1,500 to 2,000 pregnancies, most commonly in women older than age 45. Incidence is highest in Asian women.

Signs and symptoms

The early stages of a pregnancy in which a hydatidiform mole develops typically seem normal, except that the uterus may grow more rapidly than usual. The first obvious signs of trouble — absence of fetal heart tones, vaginal bleeding (from spotting to hemorrhage), and lower abdominal cramps — mimic those of spontaneous abortion. The blood may contain hydatid vesicles; hyperemesis is possible, and signs and symptoms of preeclampsia are also possible. Other complications of hydatidiform mole may include anemia, infection, trophoblast embolism, uterine rupture, and choriocarcinoma.

Diagnosis

Persistent bleeding and an abnormally enlarged uterus suggest hydatidiform mole. Diagnosis is based on a typical sonographic "snowstorm" pattern. Confirmation of hydatidiform mole requires dilatation and curettage.

The following findings also support a diagnosis of hydatidiform mole:

■ absence of a gestational sac, by ultrasound assessment, or absence of fetal heart tones, by Doppler, after 12 weeks

■ pregnancy test showing elevated human chorionic gonadotropin (hCG) serum levels greater than 100,000 IU

■ development of preeclampsia prior to 20 weeks

■ uterine size greater than estimated gestational size

■ vaginal bleeding.

Treatment

Hydatidiform mole necessitates uterine evacuation via suction curettage. Oxytocin I.V. may be used to promote uterine contractions.

Postoperative treatment varies, depending on the amount of blood lost and complications. If no complications develop, hospitalization is usually brief, and normal activities can be resumed quickly, as tolerated.

Because of the possibility of choriocarcinoma development following hydatidiform mole, scrupulous follow-up care is essential. HCG levels initially are checked on a weekly basis, until they're repeatedly negative; then on a monthly basis for one year. A baseline chest X-ray is used to rule out pulmonary involvement, and a head computed tomography scan may be performed to rule out cranial metastases. Another pregnancy should be postponed until at least 1 year after hCG levels return to normal.

Special considerations

■ Preoperatively, observe for signs of complications, such as hemorrhage and uterine infection, and vaginal passage of hydatid vesicles. Save any expelled tissue for laboratory analysis.

■ Postoperatively, monitor vital signs, especially blood pressure, and check blood loss.

■ Provide the patient and her family teaching, and give emotional support. Encourage the patient to express her feelings, and help her through the grieving process for her lost infant.

■ Instruct the patient to promptly report any new symptoms (for example, hemoptysis, cough, suspected pregnancy, nausea, vomiting, and vaginal bleeding).

■ Stress the need for regular follow-up by hCG and chest X-ray monitoring, for early detection of possible malignant changes.

■ Explain to the patient that she must use contraceptives to prevent pregnancy for at least 1 year after hCG levels return to normal, and regular ovulation and menstrual cycles are re-established.

Placenta previa

In placenta previa, the placenta is implanted in the lower uterine segment, where it encroaches on the internal cervical os. Generally, termination of pregnancy is necessary when placenta previa is diagnosed in the presence of life-threatening maternal bleeding. Maternal prognosis is good if hemorrhage can be controlled; fetal prognosis depends on gestational age and amount of blood lost. Anemia may be managed by blood transfusion to permit the pregnancy to continue in utero.

Causes and incidence

In placenta previa, the placenta may cover all (total, complete, or central), part (partial or incomplete), or a fraction (marginal or low-lying) of the internal cervical os. The degree of placenta previa depends largely on the extent of cervical dilation at the time of examination because the dilating cervix gradually uncovers the placenta. (See *Three types of placenta previa.*) Although the specific cause of placenta previa is unknown, factors that may affect the site of the placenta's attachment to the uterine wall include:

■ defective vascularization of the decidua

THREE TYPES OF PLACENTA PREVIA

Low marginal implantation—A small placental edge can be felt through the internal os.

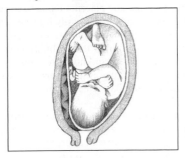

Partial placenta previa—The placenta partially caps the internal os.

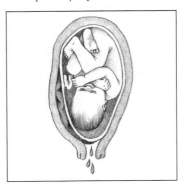

Total placenta previa—The internal os is covered entirely.

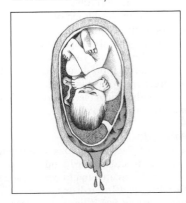

- multiple pregnancy (the placenta requires a larger surface for attachment)
- previous uterine surgery
- multiparity
- advanced maternal age.

In placenta previa, the uterus' lower segment fails to provide as much nourishment as the fundus. The placenta tends to spread out, seeking the blood supply it needs, and becomes larger and thinner than normal. Eccentric insertion of the umbilical cord often develops, for unknown reasons. Hemorrhage occurs as the internal cervical os effaces and dilates, tearing the uterine vessels.

This disorder, one of the most common causes of bleeding during the second half of pregnancy, occurs in approximately 1 in 200 pregnancies, more commonly in multigravidas than in primigravidas.

Signs and symptoms
Placenta previa usually produces painless third-trimester bleeding (often the first complaint). Various malpresentations occur because of the placenta's location and interfere with proper descent of the fetal head. (The fetus remains active, however, with good heart tones.) Complications of placenta previa include shock or maternal and fetal death.

Diagnosis
Special diagnostic measures that confirm placenta previa include:
- transvaginal ultrasound scanning for placental position
- pelvic examination (under a double set-up because of the likelihood of hemorrhage), performed only immediately before delivery to confirm the diagnosis. In most cases, only the cervix is visualized.

Digital examination should be deferred in any pregnant woman in the third trimester with vaginal bleeding, until ultrasound rules out placenta previa.

Treatment
Treatment of placenta previa is designed to assess, control, and restore blood loss; to deliver a viable infant; and to prevent coagulation disorders. Immediate therapy includes starting an I.V. line using a large-bore catheter; drawing blood for hemoglobin levels and hematocrit as well as type and crossmatching; initiating external electronic fetal monitoring; monitoring maternal blood pressure, pulse rate, and respirations; and assessing the amount of vaginal bleeding.

If the fetus is premature, following determination of the degree of placenta previa and necessary fluid and blood replacement, treatment consists of careful observation to allow the fetus more time to mature. If clinical evaluation confirms complete placenta previa, the patient may be hospitalized because of the increased risk of hemorrhage. As soon as the fetus is sufficiently mature, or in case of intervening severe hemorrhage, immediate delivery by cesarean birth may be necessary. Vaginal delivery is considered only when the bleeding is minimal and the placenta previa is marginal, or when the labor is rapid. Because of the possibility of fetal blood loss through the placenta, a pediatric team should be on hand during such delivery to immediately assess and treat neonatal shock, blood loss, and hypoxia.

Complications of placenta previa necessitate appropriate and immediate intervention.

Special considerations
- If the patient shows active bleeding because of placenta previa, a primary nurse should be assigned for continuous monitoring of maternal blood pressure, pulse rate, respirations, central venous pressure, intake and output, amount of vaginal bleeding, and fetal heart tones. Electronic monitoring of fetal heart tones is recommended.
- Prepare the patient and her family for a possible cesarean birth and the birth of a premature infant. Thoroughly explain postpartum care, so the patient and her family know what measures to expect.
- Provide emotional support during labor. Because of the infant's prematurity, the patient may not be given analgesics, so labor pain may be intense. Reassure her of her progress throughout labor and keep her informed of the fetus' condition. Although neonatal death is a possibility, continued monitoring and prompt management reduce this prospect.

■ Placenta previa, especially in women who have had one or more cesarean births, is associated with placenta accreta, a dangerous condition in which the placenta grows into the myometrium.

Abruptio placentae

In abruptio placentae, also called *placental abruption*, the placenta separates from the uterine wall prematurely, usually after the 20th week of gestation, producing hemorrhage. Abruptio placentae is a common cause of bleeding during the second half of pregnancy. Firm diagnosis, in the presence of heavy maternal bleeding, may necessitate termination of pregnancy. Fetal prognosis depends on the gestational age and amount of blood lost; maternal prognosis is good if hemorrhage can be controlled.

Causes
The cause of abruptio placentae is often unknown. Predisposing factors include trauma, such as a direct blow to the uterus, placental site bleeding from a needle puncture during amniocentesis, chronic or pregnancy-induced hypertension (which raises pressure on the placenta's maternal side), multiparity, smoking, and cocaine abuse.

In abruptio placentae, blood vessels at the placental bed rupture spontaneously owing to a lack of resiliency or to abnormal changes in uterine vasculature. Hypertension complicates the situation, as does an enlarged uterus, which can't contract sufficiently to seal off the torn vessels. Consequently, bleeding continues unchecked, possibly shearing off the placenta partially or completely. Typically, such bleeding is external or marginal (in about 80% of patients) if a peripheral portion of the placenta separates from the uterine wall; it is internal or concealed (in about 20%) if the central portion of the placenta becomes detached and the still-intact peripheral portions trap the blood. As blood enters the muscle fibers, complete relaxation of the uterus becomes impossible, increasing uterine tone and irritability. If bleeding into the muscle fibers is profuse, the uterus turns blue or purple, and the accumulated

blood prevents its normal contractions after delivery (Couvelaire uterus, or uteroplacental apoplexy).

Signs and symptoms
Abruptio placentae produces a wide range of clinical effects, depending on the extent of placental separation and the amount of blood lost from maternal circulation. (See *Degrees of placental separation in abruptio placentae*, page 968.) Mild abruptio placentae (marginal separation) develops gradually and produces mild to moderate bleeding, vague lower abdominal discomfort, mild to moderate abdominal tenderness, and uterine irritability. Fetal heart tones remain strong and regular.

Moderate abruptio placentae (about 50% placental separation) may develop gradually or abruptly and produces continuous abdominal pain, moderate dark red vaginal bleeding, a tender uterus that remains firm between contractions, barely audible or irregular and bradycardiac fetal heart tones and, possibly, signs of shock. Labor usually starts within 2 hours and often proceeds rapidly.

Severe abruptio placentae (70% placental separation) develops abruptly and causes agonizing, unremitting uterine pain (described as tearing or knifelike); a boardlike, tender uterus; moderate vaginal bleeding; rapidly progressive shock; and absence of fetal heart tones.

In addition to hemorrhage and shock, complications of abruptio placentae may include renal failure, disseminated intravascular coagulation (DIC), and maternal and fetal death.

Diagnosis
Diagnostic measures for abruptio placentae include observation of clinical features, speculum examination, and ultrasonography to rule out placenta previa. Decreased hemoglobin (Hb) levels and platelet counts support the diagnosis. Periodic assays for fibrin split products aid in monitoring the progression of abruptio placentae and detect the development of DIC.

Treatment
Treatment of abruptio placentae is designed to assess, control, and restore the

DEGREES OF PLACENTAL SEPARATION IN ABRUPTIO PLACENTAE

Mild separation with internal bleeding between the placenta and uterine wall.

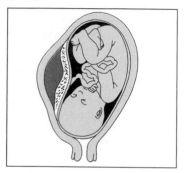

Moderate separation with external hemorrhage through the vagina.

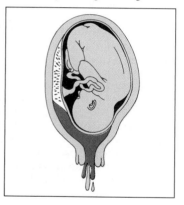

Severe separation.

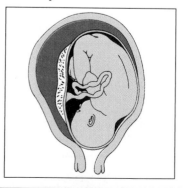

amount of blood lost; to deliver a viable infant; and to prevent coagulation disorders. Immediate measures for abruptio placentae include starting I.V. infusion (via large-bore catheter) of appropriate fluids (lactated Ringer's solution) to combat hypovolemia; placement of a central venous pressure line and urinary catheter to monitor fluid status; drawing blood for Hb levels and hematocrit determination, for coagulation studies, and for type and crossmatching; external electronic fetal monitoring; and monitoring of maternal vital signs and vaginal bleeding.

After determination of the severity of abruption and appropriate fluid and blood replacement, prompt delivery by cesarean birth is necessary if the fetus is in distress. If the fetus isn't in distress, monitoring continues; delivery is usually performed at the first sign of fetal distress. Because of possible fetal blood loss through the placenta, a pediatric team should be ready at delivery to assess and treat the neonate for shock, blood loss, and hypoxia. If placental separation is severe and there are no signs of fetal life, vaginal delivery may be performed unless uncontrolled hemorrhage or other complications contraindicate it.

Complications of abruptio placentae require appropriate treatment. For example, DIC requires immediate intervention with heparin, platelets, and whole blood to prevent exsanguination.

Special considerations
■ Check maternal blood pressure, pulse rate, respirations, central venous pressure, intake and output, and amount of vaginal bleeding every 10 to 15 minutes. Monitor fetal heart tones electronically.
■ Prepare the patient and her family for cesarean birth. Thoroughly explain postpartum care so the patient and her family will know what to expect.
■ If vaginal delivery is elected, provide emotional support during labor. Because of the infant's prematurity, the mother may not receive analgesics during labor and may experience intense pain. Reassure the patient of her progress through labor and keep her informed of the fetus' condition.

- Provide emotional support. In the case of fetal demise, encourage the patient to seek counseling as appropriate.

Cardiovascular disease in pregnancy

Cardiovascular disease ranks fourth (after infection, pregnancy-induced hypertension, and hemorrhage) among the leading causes of maternal death. The physiologic stress of pregnancy and delivery is often more than a compromised heart can tolerate and often leads to maternal and fetal mortality.

The prognosis for the pregnant patient with cardiovascular disease is good, with careful management. Decompensation is the leading cause of maternal death. Infant mortality increases with decompensation because uterine congestion, insufficient oxygenation, and the elevated carbon dioxide content of the blood not only compromise the fetus, but also commonly cause premature labor and delivery.

Causes and incidence

Approximately 1% to 2% of pregnant females have cardiac disease, but the incidence is rising because medical treatment today allows more females with rheumatic heart disease (present in more than 80% of patients who develop cardiovascular complications) and congenital defects (present in 10% to 15% of patients) to reach childbearing age. Coronary artery disease accounts for about 2% of cardiovascular complications.

The diseased heart is sometimes unable to meet the normal demands of pregnancy: 25% increase in cardiac output, 40% to 50% increase in plasma volume, increased oxygen requirements, retention of salt and water, weight gain, and alterations in hemodynamics during delivery. This physiologic stress often leads to the heart's failure to maintain adequate circulation (decompensation). The degree of decompensation depends on the patient's age, the duration of cardiac disease, and the heart's functional capacity at the pregnancy's outset.

Signs and symptoms

Typical clinical features of cardiovascular disease during pregnancy include distended jugular veins, diastolic murmurs, moist basilar pulmonary crackles, cardiac enlargement (discernible on percussion or as a cardiac shadow on chest X-ray), and cardiac arrhythmias (other than sinus or paroxysmal atrial tachycardia). Other characteristic abnormalities may include cyanosis, pericardial friction rub, pulse delay, and pulsus alternans.

Decompensation may develop suddenly or gradually, with persistent crackles at the lung bases. As it progresses, edema, increasing dyspnea on exertion, palpitations, a smothering sensation, and hemoptysis may occur.

Diagnosis

A diastolic murmur, cardiac enlargement, a systolic murmur of grade $^3/_6$ intensity, and severe arrhythmia suggest cardiovascular disease. Determination of the disease's extent and cause may necessitate electrocardiography, echocardiography (for valvular disorders such as rheumatic heart disease), or other studies. X-rays show cardiac enlargement and pulmonary congestion. Cardiac catheterization should be postponed until after delivery, unless surgery is necessary.

Treatment

The goal of antepartum management is to prevent complications and minimize the strain on the mother's heart, primarily through rest. This may require periodic hospitalization for patients with moderate cardiac dysfunction or with symptoms of decompensation, toxemia, or infection. Older women or those with previous decompensation may require hospitalization and bed rest throughout the pregnancy.

Drug therapy is often necessary and should always include the safest possible drug in the lowest possible dosage to minimize harmful effects to the fetus. Diuretics and drugs that increase blood pressure, blood volume, or cardiac output should be used with extreme caution. If an anticoagulant is needed, heparin is the drug of choice. Cardiac glycosides and common antiarrhythmics, such as quinidine and procainamide, are often required. The prophylactic use of antibiotics is reserved for patients who are susceptible to endocarditis.

A therapeutic abortion should be considered for patients with severe cardiac dysfunction, especially if decompensation occurs during the first trimester. Patients hospitalized with heart failure usually follow a regimen of cardiac glycosides, oxygen, rest, sedation, diuretics, and restricted intake of sodium and fluids. Patients in whom symptoms of heart failure don't improve after treatment with bed rest and cardiac glycosides may require cardiac surgery, such as valvotomy and commissurotomy. During labor, the patient may require oxygen and an analgesic, such as meperidine or morphine, for relief of pain and apprehension without undue depression of the fetus or herself. Depending on which procedure promises to be less stressful for the patient's heart, delivery may be vaginal or by cesarean birth. Forceps may augment vaginal delivery to minimize the need to push, which strains the heart.

Bed rest and medications already instituted should continue for at least 1 week after delivery because of a high incidence of decompensation, cardiovascular collapse, and maternal death during the early puerperal period. These complications may result from the sudden release of intraabdominal pressure at delivery and the mobilization of extracellular fluid for excretion, which increase the strain on the heart, especially if excessive interstitial fluid has accumulated. Breast-feeding is undesirable for patients with severely compromised cardiac dysfunction because it increases fluid and metabolic demands on the heart.

Special considerations
■ During pregnancy, stress the importance of rest and weight control to decrease the strain on the heart. Suggest a diet of limited fluid and sodium intake to prevent vascular congestion. Encourage the patient to take supplementary folic acid and iron to prevent anemia.
■ During labor, watch for signs of decompensation, such as dyspnea and palpitations. Monitor pulse rate, respirations, and blood pressure. Auscultate for crackles every 30 minutes during the first phase of labor and every 10 minutes during the active and transition phases. Check carefully for edema and cyanosis, and assess intake and output. Administer oxygen for respiratory difficulty.
■ Use electronic fetal monitoring to watch for the earliest signs of fetal distress.
■ Keep the patient in a semirecumbent position. Limit her efforts to bear down during labor, which significantly raise blood pressure and stress the heart.
■ After delivery, provide reassurance and encourage the patient to adhere to her program of treatment. Emphasize the need to rest during her hospital stay.

Adolescent pregnancy

Adolescent pregnancy can pose a major health risk to both the mother and the child because up to 70% of adolescents who become pregnant don't receive adequate prenatal care. Pregnant adolescents develop special problems and are known to have a significantly higher incidence of anemia, pregnancy-induced hypertension, and perinatal mortality. For example, they're more likely to have babies who are premature or of low birth weight, with a higher neonatal mortality, and who are predisposed to injury at birth, childhood illness, and retardation or other neurologic defects. These risks are aggravated if the mother has abused drugs during the pregnancy. (See *How maternal drug use affects infants*.)

As a rule, the younger the mother, the greater the health risk for both mother and infant. Adolescents account for one-third of all abortions performed in the United States.

Causes and incidence
Adolescent pregnancy is prevalent in all socioeconomic levels, and its contributing factors vary. Such factors may include ignorance about sexuality and contraception, increasing sexual activity at a young age, rebellion against parental influence, and a desire to escape an unhappy family

PATHOPHYSIOLOGY
HOW MATERNAL DRUG USE AFFECTS INFANTS

An infant born to a drug-dependent mother risks developing certain medical problems during the first 8 months of life. These problems range from mild to severe withdrawal symptoms, to a host of complications that affect virtually every body system.

The onset and severity of adverse reactions vary with the type and amount of drugs the mother has been taking and for how long. However, *any* drug the mother takes, including over-the-counter products, alcohol, and illicit drugs, may cross the placenta and enter the fetal circulation, where its concentration is 50% to 100% higher than the maternal drug concentration. This chart lists fetal body systems affected by drugs and some common adverse reactions that may result.

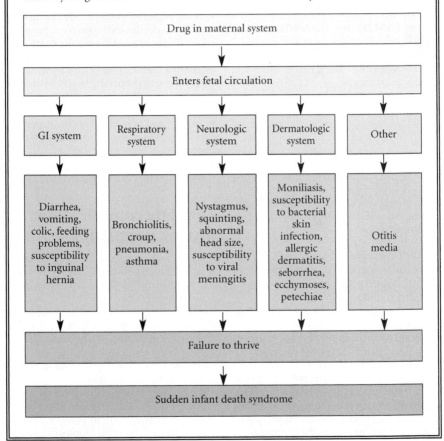

situation and to fulfill emotional needs unmet by the family.

In the United States, an estimated 1 million adolescents become pregnant each year.

Signs and symptoms
Clinical manifestations of adolescent pregnancy are the same as those of adult pregnancy (amenorrhea, nausea, vomiting, breast tenderness, fatigue). However, the

pregnant adolescent is much more likely to develop complications, such as poor weight gain during pregnancy, premature labor, and pregnancy-induced hypertension. In addition, the neonate is more likely to be of low birth weight. Some of these complications are related to the pregnant adolescent's physical immaturity, rapid growth, interest in fad diets, and generally poor nutrition; other complications may stem from the adolescent's need to deny her condition or to her ignorance of early signs of pregnancy, which often delays initiation of prenatal care.

Diagnosis

 CONFIRMING DIAGNOSIS *A positive pregnancy test that shows human chorionic gonadotropin in the blood or urine and a pelvic examination confirm pregnancy.*

Auscultation of fetal heart sounds with a Doppler ultrasonic flowmeter or fetoscope and ultrasonography assess fetal gestational age.

Treatment

The pregnant adolescent requires the standard prenatal care that's appropriate for an adult. However, she also needs psychological support and close observation for signs of complications.

Special considerations

■ Because you may be the first health care professional the pregnant adolescent encounters, you must help motivate her to follow sound medical advice without being judgmental, condescending, or threatening. Emphasize the importance of adhering to the prescribed diet, getting plenty of rest, and taking prescribed vitamin and iron supplements. Your understanding and support can ensure proper health care during the pregnancy for both mother and infant. Encourage her to ask questions and to express her feelings about the pregnancy. Answer her questions fully. It's also important to ascertain if the patient wishes to place the child up for adoption or is considering abortion. Any decision should be accepted in a nonjudgmental way.
■ Try to help the pregnant adolescent identify her own strengths and support systems for coping with pregnancy, birth, and parenting.
■ Prepare the patient and her partner for the physical and psychological process of labor and birth. Encourage attendance at prenatal classes: The use of educational films, tours of the health care facility, and role-playing techniques will facilitate her cooperation with care providers.
■ Following birth, encourage the patient to set realistic goals for the future. If she opts for adoption, make sure she clearly understands her legal rights and responsibilities. Allow the patient to care for the infant, as she desires.
■ If the patient decides to raise the infant, help her make the transition from pregnancy to parenthood during the postpartum period. Facilitate bonding. Help her establish a realistic plan regarding childcare, parenting, returning to school or work, and her relationship with the infant's father.
■ In the event of stillbirth or the neonate's death, help the patient through the grieving process.
■ Before the patient is discharged, provide information on contraception.

Diabetic complications during pregnancy

Pregnancy places special demands on carbohydrate metabolism and causes the insulin requirement to increase, even in a healthy female. Consequently, pregnancy may lead to a prediabetic state, to the conversion of an asymptomatic subclinical diabetic state to a clinical one (gestational diabetes occurs in about 1% to 2% of all pregnancies), or to complications in a previously stable diabetic state.

The incidence of diabetes mellitus increases with age. Maternal and fetal prognoses can be equivalent to those in nondiabetic females if maternal blood glucose is well controlled and ketosis and other complications are prevented. Infant morbidity and mortality depend on recognizing and successfully controlling hypoglycemia, which may develop within hours after delivery. Preconceptual counseling is helpful in optimizing pregnancy outcomes.

Causes

In diabetes mellitus, glucose is inadequately utilized either because insulin isn't synthesized or because tissues are resistant to the hormonal action of endogenous insulin. During pregnancy, the fetus relies on maternal glucose as a primary fuel source.

Pregnancy triggers protective mechanisms that have anti-insulin effects: increased hormone production (placental lactogen, estrogen, and progesterone), which antagonizes insulin's effects; degradation of insulin by the placenta; and prolonged elevation of stress hormones (cortisol, epinephrine, and glucagon), which raise blood glucose levels.

In a normal pregnancy, an increase in anti-insulin factors is counterbalanced by an increase in insulin production to maintain normal blood glucose levels. However, females who are prediabetic or diabetic are unable to produce sufficient insulin to overcome the insulin antagonist mechanisms of pregnancy, or their tissues are insulin-resistant. As insulin requirements rise toward term, the patient who's prediabetic may develop gestational diabetes, necessitating dietary management and, possibly, exogenous insulin to achieve glycemic control, whereas the patient who's insulin-dependent may need increased insulin dosage.

Signs and symptoms

Indications for diagnostic screening for maternal diabetes mellitus during pregnancy include obesity, excessive weight gain, excessive hunger or thirst, polyuria, recurrent monilial infections, glycosuria, previous delivery of a large neonate, polyhydramnios, maternal hypertension, and a family history of diabetes.

Uncontrolled diabetes in a pregnant female can cause stillbirth, fetal anomalies, premature delivery, and birth of a neonate who's large or small for gestational age. Such neonates are predisposed to severe episodes of hypoglycemia shortly after birth and may also develop hypocalcemia, hyperbilirubinemia, and respiratory distress syndrome.

Diagnosis

The prevalence of gestational diabetes makes careful screening for hyperglycemia appropriate in all pregnancies. A screening 50-gram 1-hour glucose tolerance test is normally performed at 24 to 28 weeks. In addition, women with a history of fetal macrosomia or who may have nongestational diabetes should be formally tested for diabetes with a 3-hour glucose tolerance test.

 CONFIRMING DIAGNOSIS *A 100-gram 3-hour glucose tolerance test confirms diabetes mellitus when two or more values are above normal.*

Procedures to assess fetal status include stress and nonstress tests; ultrasonography to determine fetal age and growth; measurement of phosphatidyl-glycerol; and determination of the lecithin-sphingomyelin (L/S) ratio from amniotic fluid to predict pulmonary maturity. The L/S ratio is less useful in diabetic pregnancies and generally requires a ratio of 3.5:1 to confirm fetal lung maturity.

Treatment

Treatment of both the newly diagnosed and the established diabetic is designed to maintain blood glucose levels within acceptable limits through dietary management and insulin administration. Many females with overt diabetes mellitus require hospitalization at the beginning of pregnancy to assess physical status, check for cardiac and renal disease, and regulate diabetes.

For pregnant patients with diabetes, therapy includes:

- bimonthly visits to the obstetrician and the internist during the first 6 months of pregnancy; weekly visits may be necessary during the third trimester
- maintenance of fasting blood glucose levels at or below 100 mg/dl and 2-hour postprandial blood glucose levels at or below 120 mg/dl during the pregnancy
- frequent monitoring for glycosuria and ketonuria (ketosis presents a grave threat to the fetal central nervous system)
- weight control (gain not to exceed 3 to 3½ lb [1.4 to 1.6 kg] per month during the last 6 months of pregnancy)

- high-protein diet of 2 g/day/kg of body weight, or a minimum of 80 g/day during the second half of pregnancy; daily calorie intake of 30 to 40 calories/kg of body weight; daily carbohydrate intake of 200 g; and enough fat to provide 36% of total calories (however, vigorous calorie restriction can cause starvation ketosis)
- exogenous insulin if diet doesn't control blood glucose levels. Be alert for changes in insulin requirements from one trimester to the next and immediately postpartum. Oral antidiabetic drugs are contraindicated during pregnancy because they may cause fetal hypoglycemia and congenital anomalies.

Generally, the optimal time for delivery is between 37 and 39 weeks' gestation, although with reassuring antenatal testing and no evidence of macrosomia, 40 weeks or later is also feasible. The insulin-dependent diabetic may require hospitalization before delivery for frequent monitoring of blood glucose levels and prompt intervention if complications develop.

Depending on fetal status and maternal history, the obstetrician may induce labor or perform a cesarean delivery. During labor and delivery, the patient with diabetes should receive continuous I.V. infusion of dextrose with regular insulin in water. Maternal and fetal status must be monitored closely throughout labor. The patient may benefit from half her prepregnancy dosage of insulin before a cesarean delivery. Her insulin requirement will fall markedly after delivery.

Special considerations

- Teach the newly diagnosed patient about diabetes, including dietary management, insulin administration, home monitoring of blood glucose or urine testing for glucose and ketones, and skin and foot care. Instruct her to report ketonuria immediately.
- Evaluate the patient who's diabetic for her knowledge about this disease and provide supplementary patient teaching, as she requires. Inform the patient that frequent monitoring and adjustment of insulin dosage are necessary throughout the course of her pregnancy.

- Give reassurance that strict compliance to prescribed therapy should ensure a favorable outcome.
- Refer the patient to appropriate social service agencies if financial assistance is necessary because of prolonged hospitalization.
- Encourage medical counseling regarding the prognosis of future pregnancies.

ABNORMALITIES OF PARTURITION

Premature labor

Premature labor, also called *preterm labor,* is the onset of rhythmic uterine contractions that produce cervical change after fetal viability but before fetal maturity. It usually occurs between the 20th and 37th weeks of gestation. Approximately 5% to 10% of pregnancies end prematurely; about 75% of neonatal deaths and a great many birth defects stem from this disorder. Fetal prognosis depends on birth weight and length of gestation: Neonates weighing less than 1 lb 10 oz (737 g) and of less than 26 weeks' gestation have a survival rate of 40% to 50%; neonates weighing 1 lb 10 oz to 2 lb 3 oz (737 to 992 g) and of 27 to 28 weeks' gestation have a survival rate of 70% to 80%; those weighing 2 lb 3 oz to 2 lb 11 oz (992 to 1,219 g) and of 28 weeks' gestation have an 85% to 97% survival rate.

Causes and incidence

The possible causes of premature labor are many; they may include premature rupture of the membranes (occurs in 30% to 50% of premature labors), preeclampsia, chronic hypertensive vascular disease, hydramnios, multiple pregnancy, placenta previa, abruptio placentae, incompetent cervix, abdominal surgery, trauma, structural anomalies of the uterus, infections (such as rubella or toxoplasmosis), congenital adrenal hyperplasia, and fetal death.

Other important provocative factors include:

- Fetal stimulation: Genetically imprinted information tells the fetus that nutrition is inadequate and that a change in environment is required for well-being; this provokes onset of labor.
- Oxytocin sensitivity: Labor begins because the myometrium becomes hypersensitive to oxytocin, the hormone that normally induces uterine contractions.
- Myometrial oxygen deficiency: The fetus becomes increasingly proficient in obtaining oxygen, depriving the myometrium of the oxygen and energy it needs to function normally, thus making the myometrium irritable.
- Maternal genetics: A genetic defect in the mother shortens gestation and precipitates premature labor.

Signs and symptoms

Like labor at term, premature labor produces rhythmic uterine contractions, cervical dilation and effacement, possible rupture of the membranes, expulsion of the cervical mucus plug, and a bloody discharge.

Diagnosis

Premature labor is confirmed by the combined results of prenatal history, physical examination, presenting signs and symptoms, and ultrasonography (if available) showing the fetus' position in relation to the mother's pelvis. Vaginal examination confirms progressive cervical effacement and dilation.

Treatment

Treatment is intended to suppress premature labor when tests show immature fetal pulmonary development, cervical dilation is less than 1½″ (4 cm), and the absence of factors that contraindicate continuation of pregnancy. Such treatment consists of bed rest and, when necessary, drug therapy, but neither has been proven beneficial in all patients.

The following pharmacologic agents can suppress premature labor for up to 48 hours:

- Beta-adrenergic stimulants (terbutaline, isoxsuprine, or ritodrine): Stimulation of the beta$_2$-adrenergic receptors inhibits contractility of uterine smooth muscle. Adverse effects include maternal tachycardia and hypotension, and fetal tachycardia.
- Magnesium sulfate: Direct action on the myometrium relaxes the muscle. It also produces maternal adverse effects, such as drowsiness, slurred speech, flushing, decreased reflexes, decreased GI motility, and decreased respirations. Fetal and neonatal adverse effects may include central nervous system (CNS) depression, decreased respirations, and decreased sucking reflex.

Maternal factors that jeopardize the fetus, making premature delivery the lesser risk, include intrauterine infection, abruptio placentae, placental insufficiency, and severe preeclampsia. Among the fetal problems that become more perilous as pregnancy nears term are severe isoimmunization and congenital anomalies.

Ideally, treatment for active premature labor should take place in a regional perinatal intensive care center, where the staff is specially trained to handle this situation. In such settings, the neonate can remain close to his parents. (Community health care facilities commonly lack the equipment necessary for special neonatal care and transfer the neonate alone to a perinatal center.)

Treatment and delivery require an intensive team effort, focusing on:
- continuous assessment of the neonate's health through fetal monitoring
- administration of antenatal steroids to assist fetal lung development, unless contraindicated
- maintenance of adequate hydration through I.V. fluids.

Prevention of premature labor requires good prenatal care, adequate nutrition, and proper rest. Insertion of a purse-string suture (cerclage) to reinforce an incompetent cervix at 14 to 18 weeks' gestation may prevent premature labor in patients with histories of this disorder. However, this can be dangerous if an incompetent cervix is misdiagnosed and premature labor is the true cause.

Special considerations

A patient in premature labor requires close observation for signs of fetal or maternal distress, and comprehensive supportive care.

■ During attempts to suppress premature labor, maintain bed rest and administer medications, as ordered. Give sedatives and analgesics sparingly, because they can have potentially harmful effects on the fetus. Minimize the need for these drugs by providing comfort measures, such as frequent repositioning and good perineal and back care.

■ When administering beta-adrenergic stimulants, sedatives, and opioids, monitor blood pressure, pulse rate, respirations, fetal heart rate, and uterine contraction pattern. Minimize adverse effects by keeping the patient in a lateral recumbent position as much as possible. Provide adequate hydration.

■ Tocolytic therapy has never been shown to benefit fetal morbidity and mortality; it's best used to delay delivery for 48 hours while allowing antenatal steroids to effect lung development in the fetus.

■ When administering magnesium sulfate, monitor neurologic reflexes. Watch the neonate for signs of magnesium toxicity, including neuromuscular and respiratory depression.

■ Offer emotional support to the patient and her family. Encourage the parents to express their fears concerning the neonate's survival and health.

■ During active premature labor, remember that the premature neonate has a lower tolerance for the stress of labor and is much more likely to become hypoxic than the term neonate. If necessary, administer oxygen to the patient through a nasal cannula. Encourage the patient to lie on her left side or sit up during labor; this position prevents caval compression, which can cause supine hypotension and subsequent fetal hypoxia. Observe fetal response to labor through continuous fetal monitoring. Prevent maternal hyperventilation; a rebreathing bag may be necessary. Continually reassure the patient throughout labor to help ease her anxiety.

■ Help the patient get through labor with as little analgesic medication and anesthetic as possible. To minimize fetal CNS depression, avoid administering analgesics when delivery seems imminent. Monitor fetal and maternal response to local and regional anesthetics.

■ Explain all procedures. Throughout labor, keep the patient informed of her progress and the fetus' condition. If the father is present during labor, allow the parents some time together to share their feelings.

■ A prepared resuscitation team, consisting of a physician, nurse, respiratory therapist, and an anesthesiologist or anesthetist, should be in attendance to take care of the neonate immediately. Have resuscitative equipment available in case of neonatal respiratory distress.

■ Inform the parents of their child's condition. Describe his appearance and explain the purpose of any supportive equipment. Help them gain confidence in their ability to care for their child. Provide privacy and encourage them to hold and feed the neonate, when possible.

■ As necessary, before the parents leave the facility with the neonate, refer them to a community health nurse who can help them adjust to caring for a premature neonate.

Premature rupture of membranes

Premature rupture of membranes (PROM) is a spontaneous break or tear in the amniochorial sac before onset of regular contractions, resulting in progressive cervical dilation. Labor usually starts within 24 hours; more than 80% of these neonates are mature. The latent period (between membrane rupture and onset of labor) is generally brief when the membranes rupture near term; when the neonate is premature, this period is prolonged, which increases the risk of mortality from maternal infection (amnionitis, endometritis), fetal infection (pneumonia, septicemia), and prematurity.

Causes and incidence

Although the cause of PROM is unknown, malpresentation and contracted pelvis commonly accompany the rupture. Predisposing factors may include:

■ poor nutrition and hygiene, and lack of proper prenatal care

- incompetent cervix (perhaps as a result of abortions)
- increased intrauterine tension due to hydramnios or multiple pregnancies
- defects in the amniochorial membranes' tensile strength
- uterine infection.

PROM occurs in nearly 10% of all pregnancies over 20 weeks' gestation.

Signs and symptoms

Typically, PROM causes blood-tinged amniotic fluid containing vernix particles to gush or leak from the vagina. Maternal fever, fetal tachycardia, and foul-smelling vaginal discharge indicate infection.

Diagnosis

Characteristic passage of amniotic fluid confirms PROM. Physical examination shows amniotic fluid in the vagina. Examination of this fluid helps determine appropriate management. For example, aerobic and anaerobic cultures and a Gram stain from the cervix reveal pathogenic organisms and indicate uterine or systemic infection.

CONFIRMING DIAGNOSIS
Alkaline pH of fluid collected from the posterior fornix turns Nitrazine paper deep blue. (The presence of blood can give a false-positive result.) If a smear of fluid is placed on a slide and allowed to dry, it takes on a fernlike pattern due to the high sodium and protein content of amniotic fluid.

Staining the fluid with Nile blue sulfate reveals two categories of cell bodies. Blue-stained bodies represent shed fetal epithelial cells, while orange-stained bodies originate in sebaceous glands. Incidence of prematurity is low when more than 20% of cells stain orange.

Physical examination also determines the presence of multiple pregnancies. Fetal presentation and size should be assessed by abdominal palpation (Leopold's maneuvers).

Other data determine the fetus's gestational age:
- historical: date of last menstrual period, quickening
- physical: initial detection of unamplified fetal heart sound, measurement of fundal

height above the symphysis, ultrasound measurements of fetal biparietal diameter
- chemical: tests on amniotic fluid, such as the lecithin-sphingomyelin (L/S) ratio (an L/S ratio greater than 2 indicates pulmonary maturity); foam stability (shake test) also indicates fetal pulmonary maturity. Presence of phosphatidylglycerol (PG) in the fluid indicates that respiratory distress is unlikely.

Treatment

Treatment for PROM depends on fetal age and the risk of infection. In a term pregnancy, if spontaneous labor and vaginal delivery aren't achieved within a relatively short time (usually within 24 hours after the membranes rupture), induction of labor with oxytocin is usually required; if induction fails, cesarean delivery is usually necessary. Cesarean hysterectomy is recommended with gross uterine infection.

Management of a preterm pregnancy of less than 34 weeks is controversial. However, with advances in technology, a conservative approach to PROM has now been proven effective. With a preterm pregnancy of 28 to 34 weeks, treatment includes hospitalization and observation for signs of infection (maternal leukocytosis or fever, and fetal tachycardia) while awaiting fetal maturation. If clinical status suggests infection, baseline cultures and sensitivity tests are appropriate. If these tests confirm infection, labor must be induced, followed by I.V. administration of antibiotics. A culture should also be made of gastric aspirate or a swabbing from the neonate's ear because antibiotic therapy may be indicated for him as well. At such delivery, have resuscitative equipment available to treat neonatal distress.

Special considerations

- Teach the patient in the early stages of pregnancy how to recognize PROM. Make sure she understands that amniotic fluid doesn't always gush; it may leak slowly.
- Stress that the patient *must* report PROM immediately because prompt treatment may prevent dangerous infection.
- Warn the patient not to engage in sexual intercourse or to douche after the membranes rupture.

■ Before physical examination in suspected PROM, explain all diagnostic tests and clarify any misunderstandings the patient may have. During the examination, stay with the patient and provide reassurance. Such examination requires sterile gloves and sterile lubricating jelly. Don't use iodophor antiseptic solution, because it discolors Nitrazine paper and makes pH determination impossible.

■ After the examination, provide proper perineal care. Send fluid samples to the laboratory promptly because bacteriologic studies need immediate evaluation to be valid. If labor starts, observe the mother's contractions and monitor vital signs every 2 hours. Watch for signs of maternal infection (fever, abdominal tenderness, and changes in amniotic fluid, such as foul odor or purulence) and fetal tachycardia. (Fetal tachycardia may precede maternal fever.) Report such signs immediately.

■ The L/S ratio isn't useful if obtained from a vaginal pool of amniotic fluid, because vaginal epithelium secretes lecithin. The PG level is accurate, however.

Cesarean birth

Cesarean birth, also known as *cesarean section,* is delivery of a neonate by surgical incision through the abdomen and uterus. It can be performed as elective surgery or as an emergency procedure when conditions prohibit vaginal delivery.

Causes and incidence
The most common reasons for cesarean birth are malpresentation (such as shoulder or face presentation), fetal intolerance of labor distress, cephalopelvic disproportion ([CPD] the pelvis is too small to accommodate the fetal head), certain cases of toxemia, previous cesarean birth, and inadequate progress in labor (failure of induction).

Conditions causing fetal distress that indicate a need for cesarean birth include prolapsed cord with a live fetus, fetal hypoxia, abnormal fetal heart rate patterns, unfavorable intrauterine environment (from infection), and moderate to severe Rh isoimmunization. Less common maternal conditions that may necessitate cesarean birth include complete placenta previa, abruptio placentae, placenta accreta, malignant tumors, and chronic diseases in which delivery is indicated before term.

Cesarean birth may also be necessary if induction is contraindicated or difficult or if advanced labor increases the risk of morbidity and mortality.

In the case of a previous cesarean delivery, some physicians allow a subsequent vaginal delivery if the cesarean wasn't classic or if the original reason for the cesarean no longer exists. However, vaginal delivery risks uterine rupture if the uterus is scarred.

The rising incidence of cesarean birth coincides with recent medical and technologic advances in fetal and placental surveillance and care. In the United States, 9% to 16% of all pregnancies terminate in cesarean births, rising to 17% to 25% in perinatal centers that handle high-risk deliveries.

Diagnosis
Special tests and monitoring procedures provide early indications of the need for cesarean birth:

■ Magnetic resonance imaging or clinical pelvimetry reveals CPD and malpresentation.

■ Ultrasonography shows pelvic masses that interfere with vaginal delivery and fetal position.

■ Auscultation of fetal heart rate (by fetoscope, Doppler unit, or electronic fetal monitor) determines acute fetal intolerance of labor.

Treatment
The most common type of cesarean birth is the *lower segment cesarean,* in which a transverse incision across the lower abdomen opens the visceral peritoneum over the uterus. The lower anterior uterine wall is then incised (transversely or longitudinally) behind the bladder.

The *classic cesarean* — in which a longitudinal incision is made into the body of the uterus, extending into the fundus and opening the top of the uterus — is rarely performed because it exaggerates the risk of infection and of uterine rupture in subsequent pregnancies. *Cesarean hysterectomy* removes the entire uterus and is reserved for such cases as malignant tumors, severe infection, and placenta accreta.

Patients may have general or regional anesthetic for surgery, depending on the extent of maternal or fetal distress. Possible maternal complications of cesarean delivery include respiratory tract infection, wound dehiscence, thromboembolism, paralytic ileus, hemorrhage, and genitourinary tract infection.

Special considerations

Before cesarean delivery:
- Explain cesarean birth to the patient and her partner, and answer any questions they may have. Provide reassurance and emotional support. Cesarean birth is often performed after hours of labor have exhausted the patient.
- Administer preoperative medications as ordered.
- Prepare the patient by shaving her from below the breasts to the pubic region and the upper quarter of the anterior thighs. Make sure her bladder is empty, using an indwelling urinary catheter as ordered. Insert an I.V. line for fluid replacement therapy as ordered. Assess maternal temperature, pulse rate, respirations, and blood pressure and fetal heart rate.
- In the operating room, place the patient in a slight lateral position. Use of a 15-degree wedge reduces caval compression (supine hypotension) and subsequent fetal hypoxia.

After cesarean delivery:
- Check vital signs every 15 minutes until they stabilize. Maintain a patent airway. If general anesthetic was used, remain with the patient until she's responsive. If regional anesthetic was used, monitor the return of sensation to the legs.
- Encourage parent-infant bonding as soon as practical.
- Gently assess the fundus. Check the incision and lochia for signs of infection such as a foul odor. Check frequently for bleeding and report it immediately. Keep the incision clean and dry.
- Observe the neonate for signs of respiratory distress (tachypnea, retractions, and cyanosis) until there's evidence of physiologic stability. Keep resuscitative equipment available.
- Assess intake and output (some patients have indwelling urinary catheters in place up to 48 hours postoperative). Observe the patient closely for indications of bladder fullness or urinary tract infection.
- Administer pain medication, as ordered, and provide comfort measures for breast engorgement as appropriate. Offer reassurance and reduce anxiety by answering any questions. If the mother wishes to breast-feed, offer encouragement and help. Recognize afterpains in multiparas.
- Promote early ambulation to prevent cardiovascular and pulmonary complications.
- Provide psychological support. If the patient seems anxious about having had a cesarean delivery, encourage her to share her feelings with you. If appropriate, suggest that she participate in a cesarean birth sharing group. Encourage support from her family members as well.

POSTPARTUM DISORDERS

Puerperal infection

A common cause of childbirth-related death, puerperal infection is a postpartum infection of the uterus and higher structures, with a characteristic fever pattern. It can result in endometritis, parametritis, pelvic and femoral thrombophlebitis, and peritonitis. The prognosis is good with treatment.

Causes and incidence

Microorganisms that commonly cause puerperal infection include group B streptococci, coagulase-negative staphylococci, *Clostridium perfringens*, *Bacteroides fragilis*, and *Escherichia coli*. Most of these organisms are considered normal vaginal flora but are known to cause puerperal infection in the presence of certain predisposing factors:
- prolonged and premature rupture of the membranes

- prolonged (more than 24 hours) labor
- frequent or unsanitary vaginal examinations or unsanitary delivery
- retained products of conception
- hemorrhage
- maternal conditions, such as anemia or debilitation from malnutrition
- cesarean birth (20-fold increase in risk for puerperal infection).

In the United States, puerperal infection develops in about 6% of maternity patients.

Signs and symptoms

A characteristic sign of puerperal infection is fever (at least 100.4° F [38° C]) that occurs in the first 24 hours in the first 9 days postpartum. This fever can spike as high as 105° F (40.6° C) and is commonly associated with chills, headache, malaise, restlessness, and anxiety. Abortion or miscarriage isn't usually associated with this infection and fever.

Accompanying signs and symptoms depend on the infection's extent and site and may include:

- endometritis: heavy, sometimes foul-smelling lochia; tender, enlarged uterus; backache; severe uterine contractions persisting after childbirth
- parametritis (pelvic cellulitis): vaginal tenderness and abdominal pain and tenderness (pain may become more intense as infection spreads).

The inflammation may remain localized, may lead to abscess formation, or may spread through the blood or lymphatic system. Widespread inflammation may cause:

- pelvic thrombophlebitis: severe, repeated chills and dramatic swings in body temperature; lower abdominal or flank pain; and, possibly, a palpable tender mass over the affected area, which usually develops near the second postpartum week
- femoral thrombophlebitis: pain, stiffness, or swelling in a leg or the groin; inflammation or shiny, white appearance of the affected leg; malaise; fever; and chills, usually beginning 10 to 20 days postpartum (these signs may precipitate pulmonary embolism)
- peritonitis: body temperature usually elevated, accompanied by tachycardia (greater than 140 beats/minute), weak pulse, hiccups, nausea, vomiting, and diarrhea; constant and possibly excruciating abdominal pain.

Diagnosis

Development of the typical clinical features, especially fever within 48 hours after delivery, suggests a diagnosis of puerperal infection. Uterine tenderness is also highly suggestive.

A culture of lochia, incisional exudate (from cesarean incision or episiotomy), uterine tissue, or material collected from the vaginal cuff that reveals the causative organism may confirm the diagnosis, but such cultures are generally contaminated with vaginal flora and aren't considered helpful.

Within 36 to 48 hours, white blood cell count usually demonstrates leukocytosis (15,000 to 30,000/µl).

Typical clinical features usually suffice for diagnosis of endometritis and peritonitis. In parametritis, pelvic examination shows induration without purulent discharge.

Diagnosis of pelvic or femoral thrombophlebitis is suggested by characteristic clinical signs, venography, Doppler ultrasonography, palpable veins inside the thigh and calf, pain in the calf when pressure is applied on the inside of the foot, and pain on passive dorsiflexion of the foot with the knee extended (Homans' sign). Homans' sign should be elicited passively by asking the patient to dorsiflex the foot. Active dorsiflexion could lead to embolization of a clot.

Treatment

Treatment of puerperal infection usually begins with I.V. infusion of a broad-spectrum antibiotic to control the infection and prevent its spread while awaiting culture results. After identification of the infecting organism, a more specific antibiotic should be administered. (An oral antibiotic may be prescribed after hospital discharge.)

Ancillary measures include analgesics for pain; antiseptics for local lesions; and antiemetics for nausea and vomiting from peritonitis. Isolation or transfer from the maternity unit generally isn't appropriate.

Supportive care includes bed rest, adequate fluid intake, I.V. fluids when necessary, and measures to reduce fever. Sitz baths and heat lamps may relieve discomfort from local lesions.

Surgery may be necessary to remove any remaining products of conception or to drain local lesions such as an abscess in parametritis.

Management of septic pelvic thrombophlebitis consists of heparinization for about 10 days in conjunction with broad-spectrum antibiotic therapy.

Special considerations

■ Monitor vital signs every 4 hours (more frequently if peritonitis has developed) and intake and output. Enforce strict bed rest.
■ Frequently inspect the perineum. Assess the fundus and palpate for tenderness (subinvolution may indicate endometritis). Note the amount, color, and odor of vaginal drainage, and document your observations.
■ Administer antibiotics and analgesics, as ordered. Assess and document the type, degree, and location of pain as well as the patient's response to analgesics. Give the patient an antiemetic to relieve nausea and vomiting, as necessary.
■ Provide sitz baths and a heat lamp for local lesions. Change bed linen and perineal pads and under pads frequently. Keep the patient warm.
■ Elevate the thrombophlebitic leg about 30 degrees. Provide warm soaks. Watch for signs of pulmonary embolism, such as cyanosis, dyspnea, and chest pain.

■ **ALERT** *Don't rub or manipulate the thrombophlebitic leg or compress it with bed linen.*

■ Offer reassurance and emotional support. Thoroughly explain all procedures to the patient and her family.
■ If the mother is separated from her neonate, provide her with frequent reassurance about his progress. Encourage the father to reassure the mother about the neonate's condition as well.

To prevent puerperal infection:
■ Maintain sterile technique when performing a vaginal examination. Limit the number of vaginal examinations performed during labor. Take care to wash your hands thoroughly after each patient contact.
■ Instruct all pregnant patients to call their physicians immediately when their membranes rupture. Warn them to avoid intercourse after rupture or leak of the amniotic sac.
■ Keep the episiotomy site clean and teach the patient how to maintain good perineal hygiene.
■ Screen personnel and visitors to keep persons with active infections away from maternity patients.

Mastitis and breast engorgement

Mastitis (parenchymatous inflammation of the mammary glands) and breast engorgement (congestion) are disorders that may affect lactating females. The prognosis for both disorders is good.

Causes and incidence

Mastitis develops when a pathogen that typically originates in the nursing infant's nose or pharynx invades breast tissue through a fissured or cracked nipple and disrupts normal lactation. The most common pathogen of this type is *Staphylococcus aureus;* less frequently, it's *S. epidermidis* or beta-hemolytic streptococci. Rarely, mastitis may result from disseminated tuberculosis or the mumps virus. Predisposing factors include a fissure or abrasion on the nipple; blocked milk ducts; and an incomplete let-down reflex, usually due to emotional trauma. Blocked milk ducts can result from a tight bra or prolonged intervals between breast-feedings. Causes of breast engorgement include venous and lymphatic stasis, and alveolar milk accumulation. (See *Physiology of lactation,* page 982.)

Mastitis occurs postpartum in about 1% of pregnant women, mainly in primiparas who are breast-feeding. It occurs occasionally in nonlactating females and rarely in males. All breast-feeding mothers develop some degree of engorgement, which isn't an infectious process.

PHYSIOLOGY OF LACTATION

During pregnancy, progesterone and estrogen normally interact to suppress milk secretion while developing the breasts for lactation. Estrogen causes the breasts to grow by increasing their fat content; progesterone causes lobule growth and develops the alveolar cells' secretory capacity.

After childbirth, the mother's anterior pituitary gland secretes prolactin (suppressed during pregnancy), which helps the alveolar epithelium produce and release colostrum. Usually, within 3 days of prolactin release, the breasts secrete large amounts of milk rather than colostrum. The infant's sucking stimulates nerve endings at the nipple, initiating the let-down reflex that allows the expression of milk from the mother's breasts. Sucking also stimulates the release of another pituitary hormone, oxytocin, into the mother's bloodstream. This hormone causes alveolar contraction, which forces milk into the ducts and the lactiferous sinuses beneath the alveolar surface, making milk available to the infant. (It also promotes normal involution of the uterus.)

The infant's suckling provides the stimulus for both milk production and milk expression. Consequently, the more the infant breast-feeds, the more milk the breast produces. Conversely, the less sucking stimulation the breast receives, the less milk it produces.

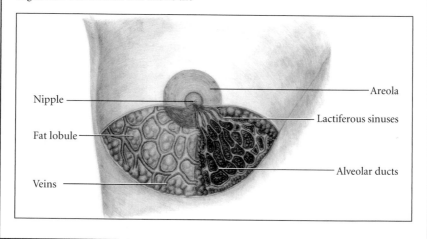

Nipple
Fat lobule
Veins
Areola
Lactiferous sinuses
Alveolar ducts

Signs and symptoms

Mastitis may develop anytime during lactation but usually begins 1 to 2 weeks postpartum with fever (101° F [38.3° C] or higher in acute mastitis), malaise, and flu-like symptoms. The breast (or, occasionally, both breasts) becomes tender, hard, swollen, and warm. Unless mastitis is treated adequately, it may progress to breast abscess.

Breast engorgement generally starts with onset of lactation (day 2 to day 5 postpartum). The breasts undergo changes similar to those in mastitis, and body temperature may be elevated. Engorgement may be mild, causing only slight discomfort, or severe, causing considerable pain. A severely engorged breast can interfere with the infant's capacity to feed because of his inability to position his mouth properly on the swollen, rigid breast.

Diagnosis

 CONFIRMING DIAGNOSIS
Diagnosis is usually easily made if pus is expressed from the nipple; culture may be helpful in confirming mastitis.

Treatment

Antibiotic therapy, the primary treatment for mastitis, generally consists of oral cephalosporins, cloxacillin, or dicloxacillin to combat staphylococcus; azithromycin may be used in patients allergic to penicillin. Although symptoms usually subside 2 to 3 days after treatment begins, antibiotic therapy should continue for 10 days. Other appropriate measures include analgesics for pain and, rarely, when antibiotics fail to control the infection and mastitis progresses to breast abscess, incision and drainage of the abscess.

The goal of treatment of breast engorgement is to relieve discomfort and control swelling, and may include analgesics to alleviate pain, and ice packs and an uplift support bra to minimize edema. Rarely, oxytocin nasal spray may be necessary to release milk from the alveoli into the ducts. To facilitate breast-feeding, the mother may manually express excess milk before a feeding so the infant can grasp the nipple properly.

Special considerations

If the patient has mastitis:
- Isolate the patient and her infant to prevent the spread of infection to other nursing mothers. Explain mastitis to the patient and why isolation is necessary.
- Obtain a complete patient history, including a drug history, especially allergy to penicillin.
- Assess and record the cause and amount of discomfort. Give analgesics as needed.
- Reassure the mother that breast-feeding during mastitis won't harm her infant, because he's the source of the infection. Tell her to offer the infant the affected breast first to promote complete emptying of it and prevent clogged ducts. However, if an open abscess develops, she must stop breast-feeding with this breast and use a breast pump until the abscess heals. She should continue to breast-feed on the unaffected side. Suggest applying a warm, wet towel to the affected breast or taking a warm shower to relax and improve her ability to breast-feed.
- To prevent mastitis and relieve its symptoms, teach the patient good health care, breast care, and breast-feeding habits. Advise her to always wash her hands before touching her breasts.
- Instruct the patient to combat fever by getting plenty of rest, drinking sufficient fluids, and following the prescribed antibiotic therapy.

If the patient has breast engorgement:
- Assess and record the level of discomfort. Give analgesics, and apply ice packs and a compression binder, as needed.
- Teach the patient how to express excess breast milk manually. She should do this just before nursing to enable the infant to get the swollen areola into his mouth. Caution against excessive milk expression between feedings because this stimulates milk production and prolongs engorgement.
- Explain that because breast engorgement is due to the physiologic processes of lactation, breast-feeding is the best remedy for engorgement. Suggest breast-feeding every 2 to 3 hours and at least once during the night.
- Ensure that the mother wears a well-fitted nursing bra, usually a size larger than she normally wears.

Galactorrhea

Galactorrhea, also known as *hyperprolactinemia*, is inappropriate breast milk secretion. It generally occurs 3 to 6 months after the discontinuation of breast-feeding (usually after a first delivery). It may also follow an abortion or may develop in a female who hasn't been pregnant; it rarely occurs in males.

Causes

Galactorrhea usually develops in a person with increased prolactin secretion from the anterior pituitary gland, with possible abnormal patterns of secretion of growth, thyroid, and adrenocorticotropic hormones. However, increased prolactin serum concentration doesn't always cause galactorrhea.

Additional factors that may precipitate this disorder include the following:

■ endogenous: pituitary (high incidence with chromophobe adenoma), ovarian, or adrenal tumors and hypothyroidism; in males, pituitary, testicular, or pineal gland tumors

■ idiopathic: possibly from stress or anxiety, which causes neurogenic depression of the prolactin-inhibiting factor

■ exogenous: breast stimulation, genital stimulation, or drugs (such as hormonal contraceptives, meprobamate, and phenothiazines).

Signs and symptoms

In the female with galactorrhea, milk continues to flow after the 21-day period that's normal after weaning. Galactorrhea may also be spontaneous and unrelated to normal lactation, or it may be caused by manual expression. Such abnormal flow is usually bilateral and may be accompanied by amenorrhea.

Diagnosis

Characteristic clinical features and the patient history (including drug and sex histories) confirm galactorrhea.

Laboratory tests to help determine the cause include measurement of serum levels of prolactin, cortisol, thyroid-stimulating hormone, triiodothyronine, and thyroxine. A computed tomography scan and, possibly, mammography may also be indicated.

Treatment

Treatment varies according to the underlying cause and ranges from simple avoidance of precipitating exogenous factors such as drugs to treatment of tumors with surgery, radiation, or chemotherapy.

Therapy for idiopathic galactorrhea depends on whether the patient plans to have more children. If she does, treatment usually consists of bromocriptine; if she doesn't, oral estrogens such as ethinyl estradiol and progestins such as progesterone effectively treat this disorder. Idiopathic galactorrhea may recur after discontinuation of drug therapy.

Special considerations

■ Watch for central nervous system abnormalities, such as headache, failing vision, and dizziness.

■ Maintain adequate fluid intake, especially if the patient has a fever. However, advise the patient to avoid tea, coffee, and certain tranquilizers that may aggravate engorgement.

■ Instruct the patient to keep her breasts and nipples clean.

■ Tell the patient who's taking bromocriptine to report nausea, vomiting, dyspepsia, appetite loss, dizziness, fatigue, numbness, and hypotension. To prevent GI upset, advise her to eat small meals frequently and to take this drug with dry toast or crackers. After treatment with bromocriptine, milk secretion usually stops in 1 to 2 months, and menstruation recurs after 6 to 24 weeks.

HEMOLYTIC DISEASES OF THE NEONATE

Hyperbilirubinemia

Hyperbilirubinemia, also called *neonatal jaundice,* is the result of hemolytic processes in the neonate. It's marked by elevated serum bilirubin levels and mild jaundice and can be physiologic (with jaundice the only symptom) or pathologic (resulting from an underlying disease). Physiologic jaundice tends to be more common and more severe in certain ethnic groups (Chinese, Japanese, Koreans, Native Americans), whose mean peak of unconjugated bilirubin is approximately twice that of the rest of the population. Physiologic jaundice is self-limiting; the prognosis for pathologic jaundice varies, depending on the cause.

Untreated, severe hyperbilirubinemia may result in kernicterus, a neurologic syndrome resulting from deposition of unconjugated bilirubin in the brain cells and characterized by severe neural symptoms. Survivors may develop cerebral palsy, epilepsy, or mental retardation or have only minor sequelae, such as perceptual-motor handicaps and learning disorders.

Causes

As erythrocytes break down at the end of their neonatal life cycle, hemoglobin (Hb) separates into globin (protein) and heme (iron) fragments. Heme fragments form unconjugated (indirect) bilirubin, which binds with albumin for transport to liver cells to conjugate with glucuronide, forming direct bilirubin. Because unconjugated bilirubin is fat-soluble and can't be excreted in the urine or bile, it may escape to extravascular tissue, especially fatty tissue and the brain, resulting in hyperbilirubinemia.

This pathophysiologic process may develop when:

- certain factors disrupt conjugation and usurp albumin-binding sites, including drugs (such as aspirin, tranquilizers, and sulfonamides) and conditions (such as hypothermia, anoxia, hypoglycemia, and hypoalbuminemia)
- decreased hepatic function results in reduced bilirubin conjugation
- increased erythrocyte production or breakdown results from hemolytic disorders, or Rh or ABO incompatibility
- biliary obstruction or hepatitis results in blockage of normal bile flow
- maternal enzymes present in breast milk inhibit the neonate's glucuronyltransferase conjugating activity. (See *Causes of hyperbilirubinemia*, page 986.)

Signs and symptoms

The primary sign of hyperbilirubinemia is jaundice, which doesn't become clinically apparent until serum bilirubin levels reach about 7 mg/dl. Physiologic jaundice develops 24 hours after delivery in 50% of term neonates (usually day 2 to day 3) and 48 hours after delivery in 80% of premature neonates (usually day 3 to day 5). It generally disappears by day 7 in term neonates and by day 10 in premature neonates. Throughout physiologic jaundice, serum unconjugated bilirubin levels don't exceed 12 mg/dl. Pathologic jaundice may appear anytime after the first day of life and persists beyond 7 days with serum bilirubin levels greater than 12 mg/dl in a term neonate, 15 mg/dl in a premature neonate, or increasing more than 5 mg/dl in 24 hours.

Diagnosis

 CONFIRMING DIAGNOSIS
Jaundice and elevated levels of serum bilirubin confirm the diagnosis of hyperbilirubinemia.

Inspection of the neonate in a well-lit room (without yellow or gold lighting) reveals yellowish skin coloration, particularly in the sclerae. Jaundice can be verified by pressing the skin on the cheek or abdomen lightly with one finger, then releasing pressure and observing skin color immediately. Signs of jaundice necessitate measuring and charting serum bilirubin levels every 4 hours. Testing may include direct and indirect bilirubin levels, particularly for pathologic jaundice. Bilirubin levels that are excessively elevated or vary daily suggest a pathologic process.

Identifying the underlying cause of hyperbilirubinemia requires a detailed patient history (including prenatal history), family history (paternal Rh factor, inherited red cell defects), present neonate status (immaturity, infection), and blood testing of the neonate and mother (blood group incompatibilities, Hb levels, direct Coombs' test, hematocrit).

Treatment

Depending on the underlying cause, treatment may include phototherapy, exchange transfusions, albumin infusion and, possibly, drug therapy. Phototherapy is the treatment of choice for physiologic jaundice, and pathologic jaundice due to erythroblastosis fetalis (after the initial exchange transfusion). Phototherapy uses fluorescent light to decompose bilirubin in the skin by oxidation and is usually discontinued after bilirubin levels fall below 10 mg/dl and continue to decrease for 24 hours. However, phototherapy is rarely the only treatment for jaundice due to a pathologic cause.

An exchange transfusion replaces the neonate's blood with fresh blood (less than 48 hours old), removing some of the unconjugated bilirubin in serum. Possible indications for exchange transfusions include hydrops fetalis, polycythemia, erythroblastosis fetalis, marked reticulocytosis, drug toxicity, and jaundice that develops within the first 6 hours after birth.

CAUSES OF HYPERBILIRUBINEMIA

The neonate's age at onset of hyperbilirubinemia may provide clues to the sources of this jaundice-causing disorder.

Day 1
- Blood type incompatibility (Rh, ABO, other minor blood groups)
- Intrauterine infection (rubella, cytomegalic inclusion body disease, toxoplasmosis, syphilis and, occasionally, bacteria such as *Escherichia coli, Staphylococcus, Pseudomonas, Klebsiella, Proteus,* and *Streptococcus*)

Day 2 or 3
- Infection (usually from gram-negative bacteria)
- Polycythemia
- Enclosed hemorrhage (skin bruises, subdural hematoma)
- Respiratory distress syndrome (hyaline membrane disease)
- Heinz body anemia from drugs and toxins (vitamin K_3, sodium nitrate)
- Transient neonatal hyperbilirubinemia
- Abnormal red blood cell morphology

- Red cell enzyme deficiencies (glucose-6-phosphate dehydrogenase, hexokinase)
- Physiologic jaundice
- Blood group incompatibilities

Days 4 and 5
- Breast-feeding, respiratory distress syndrome, maternal diabetes
- Crigler-Najjar syndrome (congenital nonhemolytic icterus)
- Gilbert syndrome

Day 7 and later
- Herpes simplex
- Pyloric stenosis
- Hypothyroidism
- Neonatal giant cell hepatitis
- Infection (usually acquired in neonatal period)
- Bile duct atresia
- Galactosemia
- Choledochal cyst

Other therapy for excessive bilirubin levels may include albumin administration (1 g/kg of 25% salt-poor albumin), which provides additional albumin for binding unconjugated bilirubin. This may be done 1 to 2 hours before exchange or as a substitute for a portion of the plasma in the transfused blood.

Drug therapy, which is rare, usually consists of phenobarbital administered to the mother before delivery and to the neonate several days after delivery. This drug stimulates the hepatic glucuronide-conjugating system.

Special considerations
- Assess and record the neonate's jaundice, and note the time it began. Report the jaundice and serum bilirubin levels immediately.
- Reassure parents that most neonates experience some degree of jaundice. Explain hyperbilirubinemia, its causes, diagnostic tests, and treatment. Also, explain that the neonate's stool contains some bile and may be greenish.

For the neonate receiving phototherapy:
- Keep a record of how long each bilirubin light bulb is in use because these bulbs require frequent changing for optimum effectiveness.
- Undress the neonate, so his entire body surface is exposed to the light rays. Keep him 18″ to 30″ (46 to 76 cm) from the light source. Protect his eyes with shields that filter the light.
- Monitor and maintain the neonate's body temperature; high and low temperatures predispose him to kernicterus. Remove the neonate from the light source every 3 to 4 hours and take off the eye shields. Allow his parents to visit and feed him.

■ The neonate usually shows a decrease in serum bilirubin level 1 to 12 hours after the start of phototherapy. When the neonate's bilirubin level is less than 10 mg/dl and has been decreasing for 24 hours, discontinue phototherapy as ordered. Resume therapy, as ordered, if serum bilirubin increases several milligrams per deciliter, as it often does because of a rebound effect.

For the exchange transfusions:
■ Prepare the neonate warmer and tray before the transfusion. Try to keep the neonate quiet. Give him nothing by mouth for 3 to 4 hours before the procedure.
■ Check the blood to be used for the exchange — type, Rh, age. Keep emergency equipment (resuscitative and intubation equipment, and oxygen) available. During the procedure, monitor respiratory and heart rates every 15 minutes; check the neonate's temperature every 30 minutes. Continue to monitor vital signs every 15 to 30 minutes for 2 hours.
■ Measure intake and output. Observe for cord bleeding and complications, such as hemorrhage, hypocalcemia, sepsis, and shock. Report serum bilirubin and Hb levels. Bilirubin levels may rise, as a result of a rebound effect, within 30 minutes after transfusion, necessitating repeat transfusions.

To prevent hyperbilirubinemia:
■ Maintain oral intake. Don't skip any feedings, because fasting stimulates the conversion of heme to bilirubin.
■ Administer $Rh_o(D)$ immuneglobulin (human), as ordered, to an Rh-negative mother after amniocentesis, or — to prevent hemolytic disease in subsequent infants — to an Rh-negative mother during the third trimester, after the birth of an Rh-positive neonate, or after spontaneous or elective abortion.

Erythroblastosis fetalis

Erythroblastosis fetalis, a hemolytic disease of the fetus and neonate, stems from an incompatibility of fetal and maternal blood, resulting in maternal antibody activity against fetal red cells. Intrauterine transfusions can save 40% of fetuses with erythroblastosis. However, in severe, untreated erythroblastosis fetalis, the prognosis is poor, especially if kernicterus develops. About 70% of these neonates die, usually within the first week of life; survivors inevitably develop pronounced neurologic damage — sensory impairment, mental deficiencies, and cerebral palsy. Severely affected fetuses that develop hydrops fetalis (the most severe form of this disorder, associated with profound anemia and edema) are commonly stillborn; even if they're delivered live, they rarely survive longer than a few hours.

Causes and incidence

Although more than 60 red cell antigens can stimulate antibody formation, erythroblastosis fetalis usually results from Rh isoimmunization — a condition that develops in approximately 7% of all pregnancies in the United States. Before the development of $Rh_o(D)$ immuneglobulin, this condition was an important cause of kernicterus and neonatal death. (See *ABO incompatibility,* page 988.)

During her first pregnancy, an Rh-negative female becomes sensitized (during delivery or abortion) by exposure to Rh-positive fetal blood antigens inherited from the father. A female may also become sensitized from receiving blood transfusions with alien Rh antigens, causing agglutinins to develop; from inadequate doses of $Rh_o(D)$; or from failure to receive $Rh_o(D)$ after significant fetal-maternal leakage from abruptio placentae. Subsequent pregnancy with an Rh-positive fetus provokes increasing amounts of maternal agglutinating antibodies to cross the placental barrier, attach to Rh-positive cells in the fetus, and cause hemolysis and anemia. To compensate for this, the fetus steps up the production of red blood cells (RBCs), and erythroblasts (immature RBCs) appear in the fetal circulation. Extensive hemolysis results in the release of large amounts of unconjugated bilirubin, which the liver is unable to conjugate and excrete, causing hyperbilirubinemia and hemolytic anemia. (See *What happens in Rh isoimmunization,* page 989.)

ABO INCOMPATIBILITY

ABO incompatibility, a form of fetomaternal incompatibility, occurs between mother and fetus in about 25% of all pregnancies, with highest incidence among blacks. In about 1% of this number, it leads to hemolytic disease of the neonate. Although ABO incompatibility is more common than Rh isoimmunization, it's less severe. Low antigenicity of fetal or neonatal ABO factors may account for the milder clinical effects.

Each blood group has specific antigens on red blood cells (RBCs) and specific antibodies in serum. Maternal antibodies form against fetal cells when blood groups differ. Neonates with group A blood, born of group O mothers, account for approximately 50% of all ABO incompatibilities. Unlike Rh isoimmunization, which always follows sensitization in a previous pregnancy, ABO incompatibility is likely to develop in a firstborn neonate.

Blood group	Antigens on RBCs	Antibodies in serum	Most common incompatible groups
A	A	Anti-B	Mother A, neonate B or AB
B	B	Anti-A	Mother B, neonate A or AB
AB	A and B	No antibodies	Mother AB, neonate (no incompatibility)
O	No antigens	Anti-A and anti-B	Mother O, neonate A or B

Clinical effects of ABO incompatibility include jaundice, which usually appears in the neonate in 24 to 48 hours, mild anemia, and mild hepatosplenomegaly.

Diagnosis is based on clinical symptoms in the neonate, the presence of ABO incompatibility, a weak to moderate positive Coombs' test, and elevated serum bilirubin levels. Cord hemoglobin and indirect bilirubin levels indicate the need for an exchange transfusion. This type of transfusion is done with blood of the same group and Rh type as that of the mother. Because infants with ABO incompatibility respond so well to phototherapy, an exchange transfusion is seldom necessary.

Signs and symptoms

Jaundice usually isn't present at birth but may appear as soon as 30 minutes later or within 24 hours. The mildly affected neonate shows mild to moderate hepatosplenomegaly and pallor. In severely affected neonates who survive birth, erythroblastosis fetalis usually produces pallor, edema, petechiae, hepatosplenomegaly, grunting respirations, pulmonary crackles, poor muscle tone, neurologic unresponsiveness, possible heart murmurs, a bile-stained umbilical cord, and yellow or meconium-stained amniotic fluid. Approx-imately 10% of untreated neonates develop kernicterus from hemolytic disease and show symptoms such as anemia, lethargy, poor sucking ability, retracted head, stiff extremities, squinting, a high-pitched cry, and seizures.

Hydrops fetalis causes extreme hemolysis, fetal hypoxia, heart failure (with possible pericardial effusion and circulatory collapse), edema (ranging from mild peripheral edema to anasarca), peritoneal and pleural effusions (with dyspnea and pulmonary crackles), and green- or brown-

PATHOPHYSIOLOGY
WHAT HAPPENS IN RH ISOIMMUNIZATION

Rh isoimmunization occurs when a pregnant woman who's Rh-negative develops antibodies against an RH-positive fetus, as shown at right.

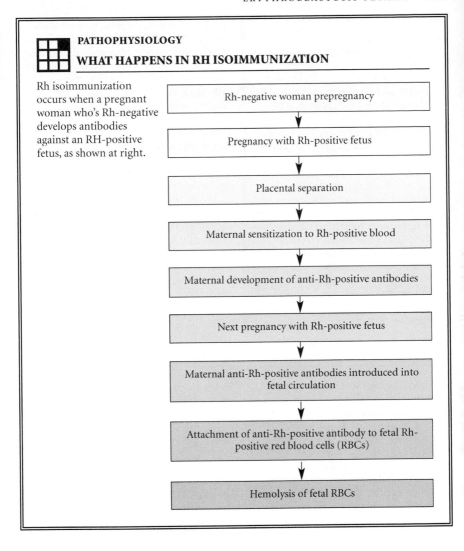

Rh-negative woman prepregnancy

↓

Pregnancy with Rh-positive fetus

↓

Placental separation

↓

Maternal sensitization to Rh-positive blood

↓

Maternal development of anti-Rh-positive antibodies

↓

Next pregnancy with Rh-positive fetus

↓

Maternal anti-Rh-positive antibodies introduced into fetal circulation

↓

Attachment of anti-Rh-positive antibody to fetal Rh-positive red blood cells (RBCs)

↓

Hemolysis of fetal RBCs

---

tinged amniotic fluid (usually indicating a stillbirth).

Other distinctive characteristics of the neonate with hydrops fetalis include enlarged placenta, marked pallor, hepatosplenomegaly, cardiomegaly, and ascites. Petechiae and widespread ecchymoses are present in severe cases, indicating concurrent disseminated intravascular coagulation. This disorder retards intrauterine growth, so the neonate's lungs, kidneys, brain, and thymus are small, and despite edema, his body size is smaller than that of neonates of comparable gestational age.

Diagnosis
Diagnostic evaluation takes into account both prenatal and neonatal findings:
- maternal history (for erythroblastotic stillbirths, abortions, previously affected children, previous anti-Rh titers)
- blood typing and screening (titers should be taken frequently to determine changes in the degree of maternal immunization)
- paternal blood test (for Rh, blood group, and Rh zygosity)
- history of blood transfusion.

PREVENTION OF RH ISOIMMUNIZATION

Administration of Rh_o (D) immune human globulin to an unsensitized Rh-negative mother, as soon as possible after the birth of an Rh-positive neonate or after a spontaneous or elective abortion, prevents complications in subsequent pregnancies.

The following patients should be screened for Rh isoimmunization or irregular antibodies:

- all Rh-negative mothers during their first prenatal visit, and at 28 weeks' gestation
- all Rh-positive mothers with histories of transfusion; a jaundiced baby; stillbirth; cesarean birth; induced abortion; placenta previa; or abruptio placentae.

In addition, amniotic fluid analysis may show an increase in bilirubin (indicating possible hemolysis) and anti-Rh titers. Radiologic studies may show edema and, in hydrops fetalis, the halo sign (edematous, elevated, subcutaneous fat layers) and the Buddha position (fetus' legs are crossed).

Neonatal findings indicating erythroblastosis fetalis include:

- direct Coombs' test of umbilical cord blood to measure RBC (Rh-positive) antibodies in the neonate (positive only when the mother is Rh-negative and the fetus is Rh-positive)
- decreased cord hemoglobin (Hb) level (less than 10 g), signaling severe disease
- many nucleated peripheral RBCs.

Treatment

Treatment depends on the degree of maternal sensitization and hemolytic disease's effects on the fetus or neonate.

- Percutaneous umbilical cord sampling allows for assessment of fetal well-being and direct transfusion, if necessary.
- An intrauterine-intraperitoneal transfusion is performed when amniotic fluid analysis suggests the fetus is severely affected and delivery is inappropriate because of fetal immaturity. A transabdominal puncture under fluoroscopy into the fetal peritoneal cavity allows infusion of group O, Rh-negative blood. This may be repeated every 2 weeks until the fetus is mature enough for delivery. Some facilities can perform percutaneous umbilical blood sampling to provide transfusion.

- Planned delivery is usually done 2 to 4 weeks before term date, depending on maternal history, serologic tests, and amniocentesis; labor may be induced from the 34th to 38th week of gestation. During labor, the fetus should be monitored electronically; capillary blood scalp sampling determines acid-base balance. Any indication of fetal distress necessitates immediate cesarean delivery.

- An exchange transfusion removes antibody-coated RBCs and prevents hyperbilirubinemia through removal of the neonate's blood and replacement with fresh group O, Rh-negative blood.

- Albumin infusion aids in the binding of bilirubin, reducing the chances of hyperbilirubinemia.

- Phototherapy by exposure to ultraviolet light reduces bilirubin levels.

Neonatal therapy for hydrops fetalis consists of maintaining ventilation by intubation, oxygenation, and mechanical assistance, when necessary; and removal of excess fluid to relieve severe ascites and respiratory distress. Other appropriate measures include an exchange transfusion and maintenance of the neonate's body temperature.

Gamma globulin that contains anti-Rh-positive antibody (Rh_o[D]) can provide passive immunization, which prevents maternal Rh isoimmunization in Rh-negative females. However, it's ineffective if sensitization has already resulted from a previous pregnancy, abortion, or transfusion. (See *Prevention of Rh isoimmunization*.)

Special considerations

Structure the care plan around close maternal and fetal observation, explanations of diagnostic tests and therapeutic measures, and emotional support.

- Reassure the parents that they aren't to blame for having a child with erythroblastosis fetalis. Encourage them to express their fears concerning possible complications of treatment.
- Before intrauterine transfusion, explain the procedure and its purpose. Before the transfusion, obtain a baseline fetal heart rate through electronic monitoring. Afterward, carefully observe the mother for uterine contractions and fluid leakage from the puncture site. Monitor fetal heart rate for tachycardia or bradycardia.
- During exchange transfusion, maintain the neonate's body temperature by placing him under a heat lamp or overhead radiant warmer. Keep resuscitative and monitoring equipment handy and warm blood before transfusion.
- Watch for complications of transfusion, such as lethargy, muscular twitching, seizures, dark urine, edema, and change in vital signs. Watch for postexchange serum bilirubin levels that are usually 50% of pre-exchange levels (although these levels may rise to 70% to 80% of pre-exchange levels due to rebound effect). Within 30 minutes of transfusion, bilirubin may rebound, requiring repeat exchange transfusions.
- Measure intake and output. Observe for cord bleeding and complications, such as hemorrhage, hypocalcemia, sepsis, and shock. Report serum bilirubin and Hb levels.
- To promote normal parental bonding, encourage parents to visit and to help care for the neonate as often as possible.
- To prevent hemolytic disease in the neonate, evaluate all pregnant females for possible Rh incompatibility. Administer $Rh_o(D)$ I.M., as ordered, to all Rh-negative, antibody-negative females following transfusion reaction or ectopic pregnancy, or during the second and third trimesters to patients with abruptio placentae, placenta previa, or amniocentesis.

Selected references

Hulley, S.B., and Grady, D. "The WHI Estrogen-Alone Trial — Do Things Look Any Better?" *JAMA* 291(14):1769-71, April 2004.

Hurskainen, R., et al. "Clinical Outcomes and Costs With the Levonorgestrel-Releasing Intrauterine System or Hysterectomy for Treatment of Menorrhagia: Randomized Trial 5-Year Follow-up." *JAMA* 291(12):1456-63, March 2004.

Littleton, L.Y., and Engebretson, J.C. *Maternity Nursing Care.* Clifton Park, N.Y.: Thomson Delmar Learning, 2004.

Morgan, M., and Siddighi, S., eds. *Obstetrics and Gynecology,* 5th ed. Philadelphia: Lippincott Williams & Wilkins, 2004.

Scott, J.R., et al., eds. *Danforth's Obstetrics and Gynecology,* 9th ed. Philadelphia: Lippincott Williams & Wilkins, 2003.

Speroff, L., and Fritz, M.A. *Clinical Gynecologic Endocrinology and Infertility,* 7th ed. Philadelphia: Lippincott Williams & Wilkins, 2005.

Sweet, R.L., and Gibbs, R.S. *Atlas of Infectious Diseases of the Female Genital Tract.* Philadelphia: Lippincott Williams & Wilkins, 2004.

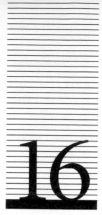

16

Sexual disorders

Introduction *992*

Sexually transmitted diseases *995*
Gonorrhea *995*
Chlamydial infections *997*
Genital herpes *999*
Genital warts *1001*
Syphilis *1002*
Trichomoniasis *1005*
Chancroid *1006*
Nonspecific genitourinary infections
  1007

Male reproductive disorders *1008*
Hypogonadism *1008*
Undescended testes *1010*
Testicular torsion *1011*
Male infertility *1012*
Precocious puberty in males *1013*

Selected references *1014*

Introduction

Sexuality is an integral human function that's inevitably colored and influenced by a host of interrelated factors. Its expression reflects the interaction of all the biological, psychological, and sociologic ingredients that affect a person's self-image and behavior.

Depending on these complex factors, human sexuality can be healthy and enriching, or it can be the source of mental and physical distress. A sexually healthy person is commonly defined as a person who:

■ exhibits behavior that agrees with gender identity (persistent feeling of oneself as male or female)
■ can participate in a potentially loving or committed relationship
■ finds erotic stimulation pleasurable
■ can make decisions about sexual behavior that are compatible with values and beliefs.

Hazards to sexual health
An important group of sex-related disorders results from infection that's transmitted through sexual contact. These disorders include human immunodeficiency virus infection, gonorrhea, syphilis, chlamydial infections, genital herpes, genital warts, tri-

chomoniasis, chancroid, and lympho-granuloma venereum. Sexually transmitted diseases (STDs) are among the most prevalent infections around the world; gonorrhea, chlamydial infections, and genital warts are approaching epidemic proportions in the United States.

Sexual dysfunction disorders, including arousal disorders, orgasmic disorders, and sexual pain disorders (dyspareunia and vaginismus), may be caused by a general medical condition, psychological factors, or a combination of factors, or they may be substance-induced. Other disorders have a definite physical etiology.

Gender identity disorders and paraphilias are sexual disorders whose diagnostic criteria are found in the *Diagnostic and Statistical Manual of Mental Disorders,* Fourth Edition, Text Revision.

Physical assessment

Physical assessment, primarily a diagnostic tool, can also serve as an excellent opportunity for patient teaching.

- During examination of the female, evaluate breast development, pubic hair distribution, and the development of external genitalia. With gloved hands, use a speculum to examine internal genitalia, including the cervix and vagina. Palpate the uterus and ovaries.

 ELDER TIP *Take special care when examining an older woman because atrophic changes of the vaginal mucosa may increase her discomfort during a pelvic examination. Use a small speculum because of the decreased vaginal size. To ease insertion, dampen the speculum with warm water; don't use a lubricant because it may alter Papanicolaou test results. Proceed slowly; abrupt insertion of the speculum may damage sensitive degenerating tissue.*

- During examination of the male, check pubic and axillary hair distribution. With a gloved hand, palpate the penis, scrotum, prostate gland, and rectum. Inspect the penis (shaft, glans, and urethral meatus) for lesions, swelling, inflammation, scars, or discharge. In the uncircumcised male, retract the foreskin to visualize the glans. Examine the scrotum for size, shape, and abnormalities, such as nodules or inflammation. Check for the presence of both testes (the left testis is typically lower than the right).

ELDER TIP *The testes of an older male may be slightly smaller than those of a younger male, but they should be equal in size, smooth, freely moveable, and soft without nodules.*

- Inspect and palpate the inguinal canal; you shouldn't observe any bulging of tissues or organs. (See *Male sexual anatomy,* page 994.)

Sexual history

Careful assessment helps identify the cause of a sexual problem as psychological or physical. A sexual history provides the basis for prevention, diagnosis, and treatment.

- Ensure privacy, as for physical assessment. Allow sufficient time so that the patient doesn't feel rushed.
- Approach a sexual history objectively. Remember, sexual health is relative; avoid making assumptions or judgments about the patient's sexual activities.
- After listening to the patient, determine his level of sexual understanding and phrase your questions in language that he can understand. Avoid technical terms.
- Begin with the least threatening questions. Usually, a menstrual or urologic history helps lead into a sexual history.
- Inquire about what the patient accepts as normal sexual behavior. Ask about sexual needs and priorities and whether the patient can discuss them with a sex partner.
- Assess risk behavior concerning selection of sex partners and specific sexual practices.
- Ask about possible homosexual activity, which can influence the risk and treatment of some STDs.
- Ask the female patient if she has adequate lubrication during intercourse and if she has ever experienced orgasm or pain with sexual contact. Ask the male patient if he has ever had difficulties with erection or ejaculation.
- Ask about current or past contraceptive practices.
- Try to use the history therapeutically by encouraging the patient to express anxiety. Such fears may be alleviated simply by providing factual information and answering questions.

MALE SEXUAL ANATOMY

The *scrotum,* which contains the testes, epididymis, and lower spermatic cords, maintains the proper testicular temperature for spermatogenesis through relaxation and contraction. The penis consists of three cylinders of erectile tissue: two corpora cavernosa and the corpus spongiosum, which contains the urethra.

The *testes* (gonads, testicles) produce sperm in the seminiferous tubules, with complete spermatogenesis developing in most males by age 15 or 16. In the fetus, the testes form in the abdominal cavity and descend into the scrotum during the seventh month of gestation. The testes also secrete hormones, especially testosterone, in the interstitial cells (Leydig's cells). Testosterone affects the development and maintenance of secondary sex characteristics and sex drive. It also regulates metabolism, stimulates protein anabolism (encouraging skeletal growth and muscular development), inhibits pituitary secretion of the gonadotropins (follicle-stimulating hormone and interstitial cell-stimulating hormone), pro-

motes potassium excretion, and mildly influences renal sodium reabsorption.

The *vas deferens* connects the *epididymis,* in which sperm develop and mature for up to 6 weeks, and the *ejaculatory ducts.* (Vasectomy achieves sterilization by severing and interrupting the vas deferens, as both ends are tied off.) The *seminal vesicles,* two convoluted membranous pouches, secrete a viscous liquid of fructose-rich semen and prostaglandins that probably facilitates fertilization. The *prostate gland* secretes the thin alkaline substance that comprises most of the seminal fluid; this fluid also protects sperm from acidity in the male urethra and in the vagina, increasing sperm motility.

The *bulbourethral (Cowper's) glands* secrete an alkaline pre-ejaculatory fluid, probably similar in function to that produced by the prostate gland. The *spermatic cords* are cylindrical fibrous coverings in the inguinal canal, containing the vas deferens, blood vessels, and nerves.

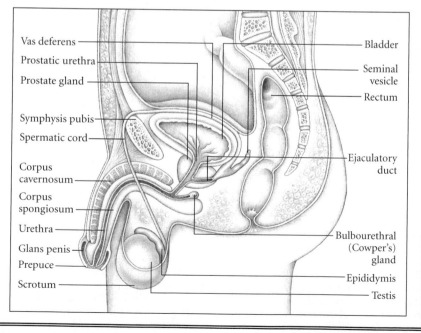

Vas deferens
Prostatic urethra
Prostate gland
Symphysis pubis
Spermatic cord
Corpus cavernosum
Corpus spongiosum
Urethra
Glans penis
Prepuce
Scrotum

Bladder
Seminal vesicle
Rectum
Ejaculatory duct
Bulbourethral (Cowper's) gland
Epididymis
Testis

Types of sex therapy

Sex therapy can be a vital therapeutic tool for treating sexual dysfunction. Before therapy begins, a history, a physical examination, and appropriate treatment must rule out organic causes of sexual dysfunction. The major forms of sex therapy include psychoanalysis, behavioral therapy, group therapy, classic (Masters and Johnson) therapy, and Kaplan's sex therapy. The type of therapy appropriate for the patient depends on his problems, needs, and finances.

SEXUALLY TRANSMITTED DISEASES

Gonorrhea

A common sexually transmitted disease, gonorrhea is an infection of the genitourinary tract (especially the urethra and cervix) and, occasionally, the rectum, pharynx, and eyes. Untreated gonorrhea can spread through the blood to the joints, tendons, meninges, and endocardium; in females, it can also lead to chronic pelvic inflammatory disease (PID) and sterility. After adequate treatment, the prognosis for both males and females is excellent, although reinfection is common. Gonorrhea is especially prevalent among young people and people with multiple partners, particularly those between ages 15 and 29. In these patients, suspect concomitant chlamydia infection.

Causes and incidence

Transmission of *Neisseria gonorrhoeae*, the organism that causes gonorrhea, usually follows sexual contact with an infected person. Children born of infected mothers can contract gonococcal ophthalmia neonatorum during passage through the birth canal. Children and adults with gonorrhea can contract gonococcal conjunctivitis by touching their eyes with contaminated hands.

The Centers for Disease Control and Prevention estimates that there are about 700,000 new cases of gonorrhea each year; only about half of these cases are reported to health care officials.

Signs and symptoms

Although many infected males may be asymptomatic, after a 3- to 6-day incubation period, some develop symptoms of urethritis, including dysuria and purulent urethral discharge, with redness and swelling at the infection site. Most infected females remain asymptomatic but may develop inflammation and a greenish yellow discharge from the cervix—the most common gonorrheal symptoms in females. (See *What happens in gonorrhea,* page 996.)

Other clinical features vary according to the site involved:

- *urethra:* dysuria, urinary frequency and incontinence, purulent discharge, itching, and red and edematous meatus
- *vulva:* occasional itching, burning, and pain due to exudate from an adjacent infected area (symptoms tend to be more severe before puberty or after menopause)
- *vagina* (most common site in children older than age 1): engorgement, redness, swelling, and profuse purulent discharge
- *liver:* right upper quadrant pain in a patient with perihepatitis
- *pelvis:* severe pelvic and lower abdominal pain, muscle rigidity, tenderness, and abdominal distention. As the infection spreads, nausea, vomiting, fever, and tachycardia may develop in a patient with salpingitis or PID.

Other possible symptoms include pharyngitis, tonsillitis, rectal burning and itching, and bloody mucopurulent discharge.

Gonococcal septicemia is more common in females than in males. Its characteristic signs include tender papillary skin lesions on the hands and feet; these lesions may be pustular, hemorrhagic, or necrotic. Gonococcal septicemia may also produce migratory polyarthralgia and polyarthritis and tenosynovitis of the wrists, fingers, knees, or ankles. Untreated septic arthritis leads to progressive joint destruction.

Signs of gonococcal ophthalmia neonatorum include lid edema, bilateral con-

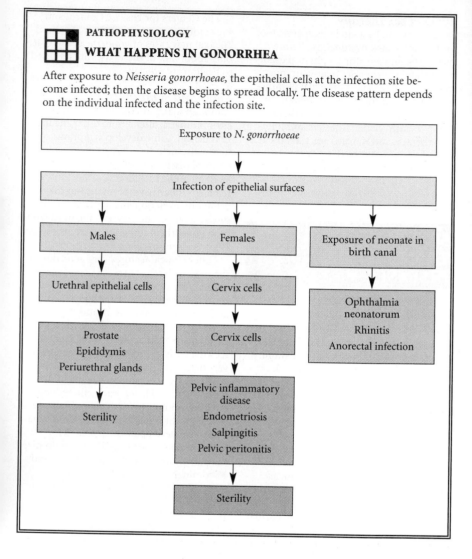

PATHOPHYSIOLOGY
WHAT HAPPENS IN GONORRHEA

After exposure to *Neisseria gonorrhoeae*, the epithelial cells at the infection site become infected; then the disease begins to spread locally. The disease pattern depends on the individual infected and the infection site.

Exposure to *N. gonorrhoeae*

↓

Infection of epithelial surfaces

↓

Males → Urethral epithelial cells → Prostate, Epididymis, Periurethral glands → Sterility

Females → Cervix cells → Cervix cells → Pelvic inflammatory disease, Endometriosis, Salpingitis, Pelvic peritonitis → Sterility

Exposure of neonate in birth canal → Ophthalmia neonatorum, Rhinitis, Anorectal infection

---

junctival infection, and abundant purulent discharge 2 to 3 days after birth. Adult conjunctivitis, most common in men, causes unilateral conjunctival redness and swelling. Untreated gonococcal conjunctivitis can progress to corneal ulceration and blindness.

Diagnosis

CONFIRMING DIAGNOSIS *A culture from the infection site (urethra, cervix, rectum, or pharynx), grown on a Thayer-Martin or Transgrow medium, usually establishes the diagnosis by isolating N. gonorrhoeae. (See Neisseria gonorrhoeae.) A Gram stain showing gram-negative diplococci supports the diagnosis and may be sufficient to confirm gonorrhea in males.*

Lipase chain reaction is an assay that can detect *N. gonorrhoeae* and *Chlamydia trachomatis* from urethral or cervical swabs. It allows for rapid diagnosis and offers improved sensitivity and specificity compared to swab specimen cultures.

Confirmation of gonococcal arthritis requires identification of gram-negative diplococci on smears made from joint fluid and skin lesions. Complement fixation and immunofluorescent assays of serum reveal antibody titers four times the normal rate. Culture of conjunctival scrapings confirms gonococcal conjunctivitis.

Treatment

For adults and adolescents, the recommended treatment for uncomplicated gonorrhea caused by susceptible non-penicillinase-producing *N. gonorrhoeae* is a single dose of ceftriaxone; for presumptive treatment of concurrent *C. trachomatis* infection, doxycycline. Common alternative prescriptions may include ciprofloxacin, ofloxacin, spectinomycin, cefuroxime, cefpodoxime proxetil, or erythromycin. A follow-up visit 7 days after treatment to recheck cultures and confirm the cure of infection is recommended, especially for women who are asymptomatic or may not have symptoms associated with the infection. A single dose of ceftriaxone and erythromycin is recommended for pregnant patients and those allergic to penicillin.

Treatment of gonococcal conjunctivitis requires a single dose of ceftriaxone, and lavage of the infected eye with saline solution once.

Routine instillation of 1% silver nitrate drops or erythromycin ointment into the neonate's eyes soon after delivery has greatly reduced the incidence of gonococcal ophthalmia neonatorum.

Special considerations

- Before treatment, establish whether the patient has any drug sensitivities, and watch closely for adverse drug reactions during therapy.
- Warn the patient that, until cultures prove negative, he's still infectious and can transmit gonococcal infection.
- If the patient has gonococcal arthritis, apply moist heat to ease pain in affected joints.
- Urge the patient to inform sexual contacts of his infection so that they can seek treatment, even if cultures are negative. Advise him to avoid sexual intercourse until treatment is complete.

NEISSERIA GONORRHOEAE

In gonorrhea, microscopic examination reveals gram-negative diplococcus — *N. gonorrhoeae,* the causative organism.

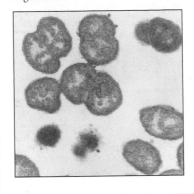

- Report all cases of gonorrhea to local public health authorities for follow-up on sexual contacts. Examine and test all people exposed to gonorrhea as well as children of infected mothers.
- Routinely instill two drops of 1% silver nitrate solution or erythromycin ointment in the eyes of all neonates immediately after birth. Check the neonate of an infected mother for signs of infection. Take specimens for culture from the neonate's eyes, pharynx, and rectum.
- To prevent gonorrhea, tell patients to avoid anyone *suspected* of being infected, to use condoms during intercourse, to wash genitals with soap and water before and after intercourse, and to avoid sharing washcloths or douche equipment. Also tell them that abstinence is the only sure way to prevent gonorrhea.
- Report all cases of gonorrhea in children to child abuse authorities.

Chlamydial infections

Chlamydial infections — including urethritis in men and urethritis and cervicitis in women — are a group of infections that are linked to one organism: *Chlamydia tra-*

LYMPHOGRANULOMA VENEREUM

A rare disease in the United States, lymphogranuloma venereum is caused by serovars L_1, L_2, or L_3 of *Chlamydia trachomatis*. The most common clinical manifestation of LGV among heterosexuals, especially male patients, is enlarged inguinal lymph nodes (usually unilateral). These nodes may become fluctuant, tender masses. Regional nodes draining the initial lesion may enlarge and appear as a series of bilateral buboes. Untreated buboes may rupture and form sinus tracts that discharge a thick, yellow, granular secretion.

Women and homosexually active men may have proctocolitis or inflammatory involvement of perirectal or perianal lymphatic tissues, resulting in fistulas and strictures.

By the time most patients seek treatment, the self-limited genital ulcer that sometimes occurs at the inoculation site is no longer present. The diagnosis usually is made serologically and by excluding other causes of inguinal lymphadenopathy or genital ulcers.

The treatment of choice is doxycycline. Treatment cures infection and prevents ongoing tissue damage, although the patient may develop a scar or an indurated inguinal mass. Buboes may require aspiration or incision and drainage through intact skin.

chomatis. Trachoma inclusion conjunctivitis, a chlamydial infection that seldom occurs in the United States, is a leading cause of blindness in Third World countries. Lymphogranuloma venereum, a rare disease in the United States, is also caused by *C. trachomatis*. (See *Lymphogranuloma venereum*.)

Untreated, chlamydial infections can lead to such complications as acute epididymitis, salpingitis, pelvic inflammatory disease (PID) and, eventually, sterility. Some studies show that a chlamydial infection in a pregnant woman is associated with spontaneous abortion and premature delivery.

Causes and incidence

Transmission of *C. trachomatis* primarily follows vaginal or rectal intercourse or orogenital contact with an infected person. Because symptoms of chlamydial infections commonly appear late in the disease's course, sexual transmission of the organism typically occurs unknowingly. Children born of mothers who have chlamydial infections may contract associated conjunctivitis, otitis media, and pneumonia during passage through the birth canal.

Chlamydial infections are the most common sexually transmitted diseases in the United States, affecting an estimated four million people in the United States each year.

Signs and symptoms

Both men and women with chlamydial infections may be asymptomatic or may show signs of infection on physical examination. Individual signs and symptoms vary with the specific type of chlamydial infection and are determined by the organism's route of transmission to susceptible tissue.

A woman with cervicitis may develop cervical erosion, mucopurulent discharge, pelvic pain, and dyspareunia.

A woman with endometritis or salpingitis may experience signs of PID, such as pain and tenderness of the abdomen, cervix, uterus, and lymph nodes; chills; fever; breakthrough bleeding; bleeding after intercourse; and vaginal discharge. She may also have dysuria.

A woman with urethral syndrome may experience dysuria, pyuria, and urinary frequency.

A man with urethritis may experience dysuria, erythema, tenderness of the urethral meatus, urinary frequency, pruritus, and urethral discharge. In urethritis, such discharge may be copious and purulent or scant and clear or mucoid.

A man with epididymitis may experience painful scrotal swelling and urethral discharge.

A man with *prostatitis* may have lower back pain, urinary frequency, dysuria, nocturia, and painful ejaculation.

A patient with *proctitis* may have diarrhea, tenesmus, pruritus, bloody or mucopurulent discharge, and diffuse or discrete ulceration in the rectosigmoid colon.

Diagnosis

A swab from the site of infection (urethra, cervix, or rectum) establishes a diagnosis of urethritis, cervicitis, salpingitis, endometritis, or proctitis. A culture of aspirated material establishes a diagnosis of epididymitis.

Antigen detection methods, including the enzyme-linked immunosorbent assay and the direct fluorescent antibody test, have long been used for identifying chlamydial infection. Tissue cell cultures, however, are more sensitive and specific. Newer nucleic acid probes using polymerase chain reactions are also commercially available and have become the diagnostic tests of choice.

Treatment

The recommended first-line treatment for adults and adolescents who have chlamydial infections is drug therapy with tetracycline, erythromycin, or azithromycin.

For pregnant women with chlamydial infections, erythromycin (stearate base) or azithromycin may be used.

Special considerations

■ Practice standard precautions when caring for a patient with a chlamydial infection.
■ Make sure that the patient fully understands the dosage requirements of prescribed medications for this infection.
■ Stress the importance of completing the entire course of drug therapy even after the symptoms subside.
■ Teach the patient to follow meticulous personal hygiene measures as recommended.

■ To prevent eye contamination, instruct the patient to avoid touching any discharge and to wash and dry his hands thoroughly before touching his eyes.
■ To prevent reinfection during treatment, urge the patient to abstain from intercourse until he and his partner are cured.
■ Urge the patient to inform sexual contacts of his infection so that they can receive appropriate treatment.
■ If required in your state, report all cases of chlamydial infection to the appropriate local public health authorities, who will then conduct follow-up notification of the patient's sexual contacts.
■ Suggest that the patient and his sex partners receive testing for the human immunodeficiency virus.
■ Tell the patient to return for follow-up testing.
■ Check the neonate of an infected mother for signs of chlamydial infection. Obtain appropriate specimens for diagnostic testing.

Genital herpes

Genital herpes is an acute inflammatory disease of the genitalia. The prognosis varies, depending on the patient's age, the strength of his immune defenses, and the infection site. Primary genital herpes is usually self-limiting but may cause painful local or systemic disease. (See *Understanding the genital herpes cycle,* page 1000.) In neonates and patients who are immunocompromised, such as those with acquired immunodeficiency syndrome, genital herpes is usually severe, resulting in complications and a high mortality.

Causes and incidence

Genital herpes is usually caused by infection with herpes simplex virus Type 2, but some studies report increasing incidence of infection with herpes simplex virus Type 1. This disease is typically transmitted through sexual intercourse, orogenital sexual activity, kissing, and hand-to-body contact. Pregnant women may transmit the infection to neonates during vaginal delivery if an active infection is present. Such transmitted infection may be localized (for

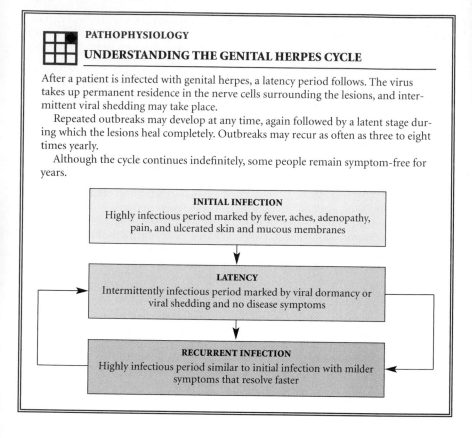

PATHOPHYSIOLOGY

UNDERSTANDING THE GENITAL HERPES CYCLE

After a patient is infected with genital herpes, a latency period follows. The virus takes up permanent residence in the nerve cells surrounding the lesions, and intermittent viral shedding may take place.

Repeated outbreaks may develop at any time, again followed by a latent stage during which the lesions heal completely. Outbreaks may recur as often as three to eight times yearly.

Although the cycle continues indefinitely, some people remain symptom-free for years.

INITIAL INFECTION
Highly infectious period marked by fever, aches, adenopathy, pain, and ulcerated skin and mucous membranes

LATENCY
Intermittently infectious period marked by viral dormancy or viral shedding and no disease symptoms

RECURRENT INFECTION
Highly infectious period similar to initial infection with milder symptoms that resolve faster

instance, in the eyes) or disseminated and may be associated with central nervous system involvement.

An estimated 86 million people worldwide are thought to have genital herpes.

Signs and symptoms

After a 3- to 7-day incubation period, fluid-filled vesicles appear, usually on the cervix (the primary infection site) and possibly on the labia, perianal skin, vulva, or vagina of the female and on the glans penis, foreskin, or penile shaft of the male. Extragenital lesions may appear on the mouth or anus. In both males and females, the vesicles, usually painless at first, will rupture and develop into extensive, shallow, painful ulcers, with redness, marked edema, tender inguinal lymph nodes, and the characteristic yellow, oozing centers.

Other features of initial mucocutaneous infection include fever, malaise, dysuria

and, in females, leukorrhea. Rare complications (generally from extragenital lesions) include herpetic keratitis, which may lead to blindness, and potentially fatal herpetic encephalitis.

Diagnosis

Diagnosis is based on the physical examination and patient history. Helpful (but nondiagnostic) measures include laboratory data showing increased antibody titers, smears of genital lesions showing atypical cells, and cytologic preparations (Tzanck test) that reveal giant cells.

CONFIRMING DIAGNOSIS
Diagnosis can be confirmed by demonstration of the herpes simplex virus in vesicular fluid, using tissue culture techniques, or by antigen tests that identify specific antigens.

Treatment

Acyclovir has proved to be an effective treatment for genital herpes. I.V. administration may be required for patients who are hospitalized with severe genital herpes or for those who are immunocompromised and have a potentially life-threatening herpes infection. Oral acyclovir may be prescribed for the patient with a first-time infection or recurrent outbreak. Other agents include famciclovir, valacyclovir, and penciclovir; these drugs suppress symptoms but don't cure the infection. Daily prophylaxis with acyclovir reduces the frequency of recurrences by at least 50%, but this is only appropriate for a patient with frequent outbreaks and may not decrease transmission rate of the disease.

Foscavir, a powerful antiviral agent, is the treatment of choice for herpes strains that are severe in nature or have become resistant to acyclovir and similar drugs. Administered I.V., foscavir can have several toxic effects, such as reversible impairment of kidney function or induction of seizures. As with other antiviral drugs, this drug doesn't cure herpes.

Special considerations

■ Encourage the patient to get adequate rest and nutrition and to keep the lesions dry.
■ Tell the patient that warm baths may relieve the pain associated with genital lesions.
■ Recommend gentle cleaning of the lesions with soap and water.
■ Secondary infections of skin lesions by bacteria require a topical or oral antibiotic. Tell the patient to report worsening of lesions, indicating possible secondary infection, to the health care provider.
■ Advise the patient to avoid sexual intercourse during the active stage of this disease (while lesions are present) and to use condoms during all sexual exposures. Urge him to have his sex partners seek medical examination.
■ Advise the female patient to have a Papanicolaou test every 6 months.
■ Refer patients to the Herpes Resource Center, which has local chapters nationwide, for support.

Genital warts

Genital warts (also known as *venereal warts* or *condylomata acuminata*) consist of papillomas with fibrous tissue overgrowth from the dermis and thickened epithelial coverings. They're uncommon before puberty or after menopause. Certain types of human papillomavirus (HPV) infections have been strongly associated with genital dysplasia and, over a period of years (depending on the viral strain), with cervical neoplasia.

Causes

Infection with one of the more than 70 known strains of HPV causes genital warts, which are transmitted through sexual contact. The warts grow rapidly in the presence of heavy perspiration, poor hygiene, or pregnancy and commonly accompany other genital infections.

Signs and symptoms

After a 1- to 6-month incubation period (usually 2 months), genital warts develop on moist surfaces: in males, on the subpreputial sac, within the urethral meatus and, less commonly, on the penile shaft; in females, on the vulva and on vaginal and cervical walls. In both sexes, papillomas spread to the perineum and the perianal area. These painless warts start as tiny red or pink swellings that grow (sometimes up to 10 cm) and become pedunculated. Typically, multiple swellings give them a cauliflower-like appearance. If infected, the warts become malodorous.

Most patients report no symptoms; a few complain of itching or pain.

Diagnosis

Dark-field examination of scrapings from wart cells shows marked vascularization of epidermal cells, which helps to differentiate genital warts from condylomata lata associated with second-stage syphilis. Applying 5% acetic acid (white vinegar) to the warts turns them white. Warts usually are diagnosed early by visual inspection; biopsy is indicated only when neoplasia is strongly suspected.

Treatment

Treatment is mostly for cosmetic reasons and should be guided by the patient's preference. Treatment aims to remove exophytic warts and to ameliorate signs and symptoms. Topical drug therapy (10% to 25% podophyllum in compound benzoin tincture, trichloroacetic acid, or dichloroacetic acid) removes small warts. (Podophyllum is contraindicated in pregnancy.) Warts larger than 2.5 cm are generally removed by carbon dioxide laser treatment, cryosurgery, or electrocautery. Other treatments include Podofilox, Imiquimod, interferon, and combined laser and interferon therapy. No therapy has proved effective in eradicating HPV; relapse is common.

Special considerations

- Tell the patient to remove the podophyllum with soap and water 4 to 6 hours after applying it.
- Encourage the patient's sex partners to be examined for HPV, human immunodeficiency virus, and other sexually transmitted diseases (STDs).
- Advise the female patient to have a Papanicolaou test every year.
- Recommend the use of condoms, and tell the patient that abstinence is the only sure way to avoid genital warts and other STDs.

Syphilis

A chronic, infectious, sexually transmitted disease, syphilis begins in the mucous membranes and quickly becomes systemic, spreading to nearby lymph nodes and the bloodstream. This disease, when untreated, is characterized by progressive stages: primary, secondary, latent, and late (formerly called *tertiary*). Untreated syphilis leads to long-term health problems, but the prognosis is excellent with early treatment.

Causes and incidence

Infection from the spirochete *Treponema pallidum* causes syphilis. Transmission occurs primarily through sexual contact during the primary, secondary, and early latent stages of infection. Prenatal transmission from an infected mother to her fetus is also possible. (See *Prenatal syphilis.*)

Incidence is highest in people ages 20 to 29.

Signs and symptoms

Primary syphilis develops after an incubation period that generally lasts about 3 weeks. Initially, one or more chancres (small, fluid-filled lesions) erupt on the genitalia; others may erupt on the anus, fingers, lips, tongue, nipples, tonsils, or eyelids. These chancres, which are usually painless, start as papules and then erode; they have indurated, raised edges and clear bases. Chancres typically disappear after 3 to 6 weeks, even when untreated. They're usually associated with regional lymphadenopathy (unilateral or bilateral). In females, chancres are commonly overlooked because they usually develop on internal structures—the cervix or the vaginal wall.

The development of symmetrical mucocutaneous lesions and general lymphadenopathy signals the onset of *secondary syphilis,* which may develop within a few days or up to 8 weeks after onset of initial chancres. The rash of secondary syphilis can be macular, papular, pustular, or nodular. Lesions are of uniform size, well defined, and generalized. Macules typically erupt between rolls of fat on the trunk and, proximally, on the arms, palms, soles, face, and scalp. In warm, moist areas (perineum, scrotum, vulva, and between rolls of fat), the lesions enlarge and erode, producing highly contagious, pink or grayish white lesions (condylomata lata).

Mild constitutional symptoms of syphilis appear in the second stage and may include headache, malaise, anorexia, weight loss, nausea, vomiting, sore throat and, possibly, slight fever. Alopecia may occur, with or without treatment, and is usually temporary. Nails become brittle and pitted.

Latent syphilis is characterized by an absence of clinical symptoms but a reactive serologic test for syphilis. Because infectious mucocutaneous lesions may reappear when infection is of less than 4 years' duration, early latent syphilis is considered contagious. Approximately two-thirds of patients remain asymptomatic in the late

PRENATAL SYPHILIS

A woman can transmit syphilis transplacentally to her unborn child throughout pregnancy. This type of syphilis is often called congenital, but prenatal is a more accurate term. Approximately 50% of infected fetuses die before or shortly after birth. The prognosis is better for infants who develop overt infection after age 2.

Signs and symptoms

The neonate with prenatal syphilis may appear healthy at birth, but usually develops characteristic lesions — vesicular, bullous eruptions, often on the palms and soles — 3 weeks later. Shortly afterward, a maculopapular rash similar to that in secondary syphilis may erupt on the face, mouth, genitalia, palms, or soles. Condylomata lata typically occur around the anus. Lesions may erupt on the mucous membranes of the mouth, pharynx, and nose. When the infant's larynx is affected, his cry becomes weak and forced. If nasal mucous membranes are involved, he may also develop nasal discharge, which can be slight and mucopurulent or copious with blood-tinged pus. Visceral and bone lesions, liver or spleen enlargement with ascites, and nephrotic syndrome may also occur.

Late prenatal syphilis becomes apparent after age 2; it may be identifiable only through blood studies or may cause unmistakable syphilitic changes: screwdriver-shaped central incisors, deformed molars or cusps, thick clavicles, saber shins, bowed tibias, nasal septum perforation, eighth nerve deafness, and neurosyphilis.

Diagnosis and treatment

In the neonate with prenatal syphilis, the Venereal Disease Research Laboratory titer, if reactive at birth, stays the same or rises, indicating active disease. The infant's titer drops in 3 months if the mother has received effective prenatal treatment. Absolute diagnosis necessitates dark-field examination of umbilical vein blood or lesion drainage.

An infant with abnormal cerebrospinal fluid (CSF) may be treated with aqueous crystalline penicillin G. An infant with normal CSF may be treated with a single injection of penicillin G.

When caring for a child with prenatal syphilis, record the extent of the rash and watch for signs of systemic involvement, especially laryngeal swelling, jaundice, and decreasing urine output.

latent stage; the rest develop characteristic late-stage symptoms.

Late syphilis is the final, destructive but noninfectious stage of the disease. It has three subtypes, any or all of which may affect the patient: late benign syphilis, cardiovascular syphilis, and neurosyphilis. The lesions of *late benign syphilis* develop on the skin, bones, mucous membranes, upper respiratory tract, liver, or stomach between 1 and 10 years after infection. The typical lesion is a gumma — a chronic, superficial nodule or deep, granulomatous lesion that's solitary, asymmetrical, painless, and indurated. Gummas can be found on any bone — particularly the long bones of the legs — and in any organ. If late syphilis involves the liver, it can cause epigastric pain, tenderness, enlarged spleen, and anemia; if it involves the upper respiratory tract, it can cause perforation of the nasal septum or the palate. In severe cases, late benign syphilis results in destruction of bones or organs, which eventually causes death.

Cardiovascular syphilis develops about 10 years after the initial infection in approximately 10% of patients with late, untreated syphilis. It causes fibrosis of elastic tissue of the aorta and leads to aortitis, usually in the ascending and transverse sections of the aortic arch. Cardiovascular syphilis may be asymptomatic or may cause aortic insufficiency or aneurysm.

TREPONEMA PALLIDUM

In syphilis, a dark-field examination that shows spiral-shaped bacterial organisms — *T. pallidum* — confirms the diagnosis.

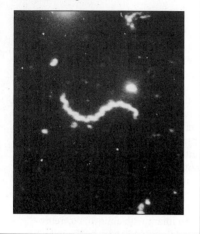

Symptoms of *neurosyphilis* develop in about 8% of patients with late, untreated syphilis and appear from 5 to 35 years after infection. These clinical effects consist of meningitis and widespread central nervous system damage that may include general paresis, personality changes, and arm and leg weakness.

Diagnosis

CONFIRMING DIAGNOSIS
Identifying T. pallidum *from a lesion on dark-field examination confirms the diagnosis of syphilis. This method is most effective when moist lesions are present, as in primary, secondary, and prenatal syphilis. (See* Treponema pallidum.*)*

The fluorescent treponemal antibody-absorption test identifies antigens of *T. pallidum* in tissue, ocular fluid, cerebrospinal fluid (CSF), tracheobronchial secretions, and exudates from lesions. This is the most sensitive test available for detecting syphilis in all stages. Once reactive, it remains so permanently.

Other appropriate procedures include the following:

■ Venereal Disease Research Laboratory (VDRL) slide test and rapid plasma reagin test (RPR) detect nonspecific antibodies. Both tests, if positive, become reactive within 1 to 2 weeks after the primary lesion appears or 4 to 5 weeks after the infection begins.

■ CSF examination identifies neurosyphilis when the total protein level is above 40 mg/dl, the VDRL slide test is reactive, and the cell count exceeds five mononuclear cells/µl.

Treatment

Treatment of choice is administration of penicillin I.M. or I.V. depending on the infection's stage. After therapy, follow-up RPR tests are usually done to check for adequacy of treatment. The nonpregnant patient who is allergic to penicillin may be treated with tetracycline or doxycycline. Nonpenicillin therapy for latent or late syphilis should be used only after neurosyphilis has been excluded. Tetracycline is contraindicated in the pregnant woman because it causes discoloration of the infant's teeth. If a pregnant woman with syphilis is allergic to penicillin, desensitization is recommended to permit the use of penicillin.

Special considerations

■ Stress the importance of completing the full course of antibiotic therapy even after symptoms subside.

■ Check for a history of drug sensitivity before administering the first dose.

■ In secondary syphilis, keep lesions clean and dry. If they're draining, dispose of contaminated materials properly.

■ In late syphilis, provide symptomatic care during prolonged treatment.

■ In cardiovascular syphilis, check for signs of decreased cardiac output (decreased urine output, hypoxia, and decreased sensorium) and pulmonary congestion.

■ In neurosyphilis, regularly check level of consciousness and monitor vital signs. Watch for signs of ataxia.

■ Urge the patient to seek testing after treatment to determine the treatment's effectiveness. A patient treated for latent or late syphilis should be encouraged to continue follow-up care after treatment to determine its effectiveness.

■ Be sure to report all cases of syphilis to local public health authorities. Urge the patient to inform sex partners of his infection so that they can also receive treatment.

■ Remind the patient that safer sex practices and consistent condom use are important measures in syphilis prevention.

■ Screen patients who are pregnant for syphilis to reduce the risk that the disease will be passed on to the fetus.

■ Refer the patient and his sex partners for human immunodeficiency virus testing as appropriate.

Trichomoniasis

A protozoal infection of the lower genitourinary (GU) tract, trichomoniasis affects about 15% of sexually active females and 10% of sexually active males. This infection, which occurs worldwide, may be acute or chronic in females. The risk of recurrence is minimized when sex partners are treated concurrently.

Causes and incidence

Trichomonas vaginalis — a tetraflagellated, motile protozoan — causes trichomoniasis in females by infecting the vagina, the urethra and, possibly, the endocervix, bladder, Bartholin's glands, or Skene's glands; in males, it infects the lower urethra and, possibly, the prostate gland, seminal vesicles, or epididymis.

T. vaginalis grows best when the vaginal mucosa is more alkaline than normal (pH about 5.5 to 5.8). Therefore, factors that raise the vaginal pH — use of hormonal contraceptives, pregnancy, bacterial overgrowth, exudative cervical or vaginal lesions, or frequent douching, which disturbs lactobacilli that normally live in the vagina and maintain acidity — may predispose a woman to trichomoniasis.

Trichomoniasis is usually transmitted by intercourse; less commonly, by contaminated douche equipment or moist washcloths. In the United States, incidence is highest in women ages 16 to 35.

Signs and symptoms

Approximately 70% of females — including those with chronic infections — and most males with trichomoniasis are asymptomatic. In females, acute infection may produce variable signs, such as a gray or greenish yellow and possibly profuse and frothy, malodorous vaginal discharge. Its other effects include severe itching, redness, swelling, tenderness, dysparcunia, dysuria, urinary frequency and, occasionally, postcoital spotting, menorrhagia, or dysmenorrhea.

Such symptoms may persist for 1 week to several months and may be more pronounced just after menstruation or during pregnancy. If trichomoniasis is untreated, symptoms may subside, although *T. vaginalis* infection persists, possibly associated with an abnormal cytologic smear of the cervix.

In males, trichomoniasis may produce mild to severe transient urethritis, possibly with dysuria and frequency.

Diagnosis

CONFIRMING DIAGNOSIS *Direct microscopic examination of vaginal or seminal discharge is decisive when it reveals* T. vaginalis *(a motile, pear-shaped organism) on wet prep. A Papanicolaou test may also detect the organism. Examination of clear urine specimens may also reveal* T. vaginalis.

Physical examination of symptomatic females shows vaginal erythema; edema; frank excoriation; a frothy, malodorous, greenish-yellow vaginal discharge and, rarely, a thin, gray pseudomembrane over the vagina. Cervical examination demonstrates punctate cervical hemorrhages, giving the cervix a strawberry appearance that's almost pathognomonic for this disorder.

Treatment

The treatment of choice for trichomoniasis is metronidazole given to both sex partners. Oral metronidazole hasn't been proven safe during the first trimester of pregnancy but can be considered for use if symptoms are severe. In general, treatment during the first trimester should be avoided if possible. Effective alternatives aren't

CHANCROIDAL LESION

Chancroid produces a soft, painful chancre, similar to that of syphilis. Without treatment, it may progress to inguinal adenitis and formation of buboes (enlarged, inflamed lymph nodes).

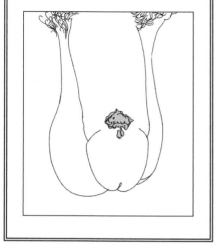

available for patients who are allergic to metronidazole. Sitz baths may be used to help relieve symptoms.

Special considerations
■ Instruct the patient to refrain from douching before being examined for trichomoniasis.
■ Urge abstinence from intercourse until treatment is completed. Refer partners for treatment. Tell the patient to avoid using tampons.
■ Warn the patient to abstain from alcoholic beverages while taking metronidazole because alcohol consumption may provoke a disulfiram-type reaction (confusion, headache, cramps, vomiting, and seizures). Also, tell her this drug may turn urine dark brown.
■ Caution the patient to avoid over-the-counter douches and vaginal sprays because chronic use can alter vaginal pH.
■ Advise the patient to scrub the bathtub with a disinfecting cleaner before and after sitz baths.

■ Tell the patient she can reduce the risk of GU bacterial growth by wearing loose-fitting, cotton underpants, which allows ventilation; bacteria flourish in a warm, dark, moist environment.

Chancroid

Chancroid (also known as *soft chancre*) is a sexually transmitted disease (STD) characterized by painful genital ulcers and inguinal adenitis. Chancroidal lesions may heal spontaneously and usually respond well to treatment in the absence of secondary infections. A high rate of human immunodeficiency virus (HIV) infection has been reported among patients with chancroid.

Causes and incidence
Chancroid results from *Haemophilus ducreyi,* a gram-negative Streptobacillus, and is transmitted through sexual contact. Poor hygiene may predispose males — especially those who are uncircumcised — to this disease.

This infection occurs worldwide but is particularly common in tropical countries; it affects more males than females.

Signs and symptoms
After a 3- to 5-day incubation period, a small papule appears at the entry site, usually the groin or inner thigh; in the male, it may appear on the penis; in the female, on the vulva, vagina, or cervix. (See *Chancroidal lesion.*) Occasionally, this papule may erupt on the tongue, lip, breast, or navel. The papule rapidly ulcerates, becoming painful, soft, and malodorous; it bleeds easily and produces pus. It's gray and shallow, with irregular edges, and measures up to 2.5 cm in diameter. Within 2 to 3 weeks, inguinal adenitis develops, creating suppurated, inflamed nodes that may rupture into large ulcers or buboes. Headache and malaise occur in 50% of patients. During the healing stage, phimosis may develop.

Diagnosis
Gram stain smears of ulcer exudate or bubo aspirate are 50% reliable; blood agar cultures are 75% reliable. Biopsy confirms

the diagnosis but is reserved for resistant cases or cases in which cancer is suspected. Dark-field examination and serologic testing rule out other STDs that cause similar ulcers. Testing for HIV infection should be done at the time of diagnosis.

Treatment

The treatment of choice is azithromycin, erythromycin, ceftriaxone, or ciprofloxacin. The safety of azithromycin for pregnant or lactating women hasn't been established. Aspiration of fluid-filled nodes may be indicated as well.

Special considerations

- Make sure the patient isn't allergic to any drug before giving the first dose.
- Instruct the patient not to apply lotions, creams, or oils on or near the genitalia or on other lesion sites.
- Tell the patient to abstain from sexual contact until healing is complete (usually about 2 weeks after treatment begins) and to wash the genitalia daily with soap and water. Instruct uncircumcised males to retract the foreskin for thorough cleaning.
- To prevent chancroid, advise the patient to avoid sexual contact with infected people, to use condoms during sexual activity, and to wash the genitalia with soap and water after sexual activity. Tell the patient that abstinence is the only sure way to prevent chancroid.

Nonspecific genitourinary infections

Nonspecific genitourinary (GU) infections, including nongonococcal urethritis (NGU) in males and mild vaginitis or cervicitis in females, are a group of infections with similar manifestations that aren't linked to a single organism. These sexually transmitted diseases (STDs) have become more prevalent since the mid-1960s. They're more widespread than gonorrhea and may be the most common STDs in the United States. The prognosis is good if sex partners are treated simultaneously.

Causes

Nonspecific GU infections are spread primarily through sexual intercourse. In males, NGU commonly results from infection with *Chlamydia trachomatis* or *Ureaplasma urealyticum*. Less commonly, infection may be related to pre-existing strictures, neoplasms, and chemical or traumatic inflammation. Some cases remain unexplained.

Although less is known about nonspecific GU infections in females, chlamydial organisms may also cause these infections. A thin vaginal epithelium may predispose prepubertal and postmenopausal females to nonspecific vaginitis.

Signs and symptoms

NGU occurs 1 week to 1 month after coitus, with scant or moderate mucopurulent urethral discharge, variable dysuria, and occasional hematuria. If untreated, NGU may lead to acute epididymitis. Subclinical urethritis may be found on physical examination, especially if the sex partner has a positive diagnosis.

Females with nonspecific GU infections may experience persistent vaginal discharge, acute or recurrent cystitis for which no underlying cause can be found, or cervicitis with inflammatory erosion.

Both males and females with nonspecific GU infections may be asymptomatic but show signs of urethral, vaginal, or cervical infection on physical examination.

Diagnosis

In males, microscopic examination of smears of prostatic or urethral secretions shows excess polymorphonuclear leukocytes but few, if any, specific organisms.

In females, cervical or urethral smears also reveal excess leukocytes and no specific organisms. "Clue cells" (normal epithelial cells covered with bacteria that appear stippled) are diagnostic.

Treatment

Therapy for both sexes consists of azithromycin or doxycycline. If the infection recurs or persists, metronidazole with erythromycin is recommended.

Special considerations

- Tell the female patient to clean the pubic area before applying vaginal medication and to avoid using tampons during treatment.
- Make sure the patient clearly understands and strictly follows the dosage schedule for prescribed medications.

To prevent nonspecific GU infections:

- Tell the patient to abstain from sexual contact with infected partners, to use condoms during sexual activity and follow appropriate hygienic measures afterward, and to void before and after intercourse.
- Encourage the patient to maintain adequate fluid intake.
- Advise the female patient to avoid routinely using douches and feminine hygiene sprays, wearing tight-fitting pants or pantyhose, and inserting foreign objects into the vagina.
- Suggest that the female patient wear cotton underpants and remove them before going to bed.

MALE REPRODUCTIVE DISORDERS

Hypogonadism

Hypogonadism is a condition resulting from decreased androgen production in males, which may impair spermatogenesis (causing infertility) and inhibit the development of normal secondary sex characteristics. (See *Production of sperm.*) The clinical effects of androgen deficiency depend on the patient's age at onset.

Causes and incidence

Primary hypogonadism results directly from interstitial (Leydig's cell) cellular or seminiferous tubular damage due to faulty development or mechanical damage. This causes increased secretion of gonadotropins by the pituitary in an attempt to increase the testicular functional state and is therefore termed *hypergonadotropic hypogonadism.* This form of hypogonadism includes Klinefelter syndrome, Reifenstein's syndrome, Turner syndrome, Sertoli-

cell-only syndrome, anorchism, orchitis, and sequelae of irradiation.

Secondary hypogonadism is due to faulty interaction within the hypothalamic-pituitary axis, resulting in failure to secrete normal levels of gonadotropins, and is therefore termed *hypogonadotropic hypogonadism.* This form of hypogonadism includes hypopituitarism, isolated follicle-stimulating hormone deficiency, isolated luteinizing hormone deficiency, Kallmann's syndrome, and Prader-Willi syndrome. Depending on the patient's age at onset, hypogonadism may cause eunuchism (complete gonadal failure) or eunuchoidism (partial failure).

Medications, such as exogenous testosterone or anabolic steroids, can also cause of hypogonadism, resulting in infertility.

Hypogonadism is rare, and it has no racial predilection.

Signs and symptoms

Although symptoms vary, depending on the specific cause of hypogonadism, some characteristic findings may include delayed closure of epiphyses and immature bone age; delayed puberty; infantile penis and small, soft testes; below-average muscle development and strength; fine, sparse facial hair; scant or absent axillary, pubic, and body hair; and a high-pitched, effeminate voice. In an adult, hypogonadism diminishes sex drive and potency and causes regression of secondary sex characteristics.

Diagnosis

Accurate diagnosis necessitates a detailed patient history, physical examination, and hormonal studies. Serum and urinary gonadotropin levels increase in primary (hypergonadotropic) hypogonadism but decrease in secondary (hypogonadotropic) hypogonadism. Other relevant hormonal studies include assessment of neuroendocrine functions, such as thyrotropin, corticotropin, growth hormone, and vasopressin levels. Chromosomal analysis may determine the specific causative syndrome. Testicular biopsy and semen analysis determine sperm production, identify impaired spermatogenesis, and assess low levels of testosterone.

PRODUCTION OF SPERM

Spermatogenesis, the production of male gametes within the seminiferous tubules of the testes, is basically a five-step process:

1. Diploid spermatogonia, the cells forming the tubule's outer layer, divide mitotically to generate new cells used in spermatozoa production.
2. Some of the spermatogonia move toward the lumen of the tubule and enlarge to primary spermatocytes.
3. Each primary spermatocyte divides meiotically, forming two secondary spermatocytes, one retaining the X chromosome and the other the Y chromosome.
4. Each secondary spermatocyte also divides meiotically, becoming spermatids.
5. After a series of structural changes, the spermatids develop into mature spermatozoa.

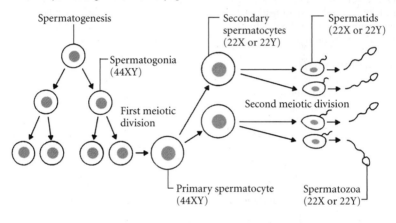

Spermatogenesis

Spermatogonia (44XY)

First meiotic division

Primary spermatocyte (44XY)

Secondary spermatocytes (22X or 22Y)

Second meiotic division

Spermatids (22X or 22Y)

Spermatozoa (22X or 22Y)

Treatment

Treatment depends on the underlying cause and may consist of hormonal replacement, especially with testosterone, methyltestosterone, estrogen, progesterone, or human chorionic gonadotropin (hCG) for primary hypogonadism, and with hCG for secondary hypogonadism. Fertility can't be restored after permanent testicular damage. However, eunuchism that results from hypothalamic-pituitary lesions can be corrected when administration of gonadotropins stimulates normal testicular function.

Special considerations

Because the patient with hypogonadism tends to have multiple associated physical problems, the care plan should be tailored to meet his specific needs.

■ When caring for an adolescent boy with hypogonadism, make every possible effort to promote his self-confidence. If he feels sensitive about his underdeveloped body, provide access to a private bathroom. Explain hypogonadism to his parents. Encourage them to express their concerns about their son's delayed development. Reassure them and the patient that effective treatment is available.
■ Make sure the parents and the patient understand hormonal replacement therapy fully, including expected adverse effects, such as acne and water retention.
■ Encourage counseling as appropriate.

Undescended testes

Undescended testes is a congenital disorder in which one or both testes fail to descend into the scrotum, remaining in the abdomen or inguinal canal or at the external ring. Although this condition, also known as *cryptorchidism,* may be bilateral, it more commonly affects the right testis. True undescended testes remain along the path of normal descent, whereas ectopic testes deviate from that path. If bilateral cryptorchidism persists untreated into adolescence, it may result in sterility, make the testes more vulnerable to trauma, and significantly increase the risk of testicular cancer, presumably due to the higher temperature of the abdominal cavity.

Causes and incidence

The mechanism whereby the testes descend into the scrotum is still unexplained. Some evidence is available to implicate hormonal factors — most likely androgenic hormones from the placenta, maternal or fetal adrenals, or the immature fetal testis and, possibly, maternal progesterone or gonadotropic hormones from the maternal pituitary.

Researchers have linked undescended testes to the development of the gubernaculum, a fibromuscular band that connects the testes to the scrotal floor. In the normal male fetus, testosterone stimulates the formation of the gubernaculum. This band probably helps pull the testes into the scrotum by shortening as the fetus grows. Thus, cryptorchidism may result from inadequate testosterone levels or a defect in the testes or the gubernaculum.

Because the testes normally descend into the scrotum during the eighth month of gestation, cryptorchidism most commonly affects premature neonates. (It occurs in 30% of premature male neonates but in only 3% to 4% of those born at term.) In about 80% of affected infants, the testes descend spontaneously during the first year; in the rest, the testes may descend later.

Signs and symptoms

In the young boy with unilateral cryptorchidism, the testis on the affected side isn't palpable in the scrotum, and the scrotum may appear underdeveloped. On the unaffected side, the scrotum occasionally appears enlarged as a result of compensatory hypertrophy. After puberty, uncorrected bilateral cryptorchidism prevents spermatogenesis and results in infertility, although testosterone levels remain normal.

Diagnosis

CONFIRMING DIAGNOSIS
Physical examination confirms cryptorchidism after the following laboratory tests determine sex:
- *Buccal smear determines genetic sex by showing a male sex chromatin pattern.*
- *Serum gonadotropin confirms the presence of testes by assessing the level of circulating hormone.*

Treatment

If the testes don't descend spontaneously by age 1 year, surgical correction may be indicated. Orchiopexy secures the testes in the scrotum and is commonly performed before the boy reaches age 4 (optimum age is 1 to 2). Orchiopexy prevents sterility and excessive trauma from abnormal positioning. It also prevents harmful psychological effects. Human chorionic gonadotropin (hCG) or testosterone may be given to stimulate descent. However, hormonal therapy with hCG is ineffective if the testes are located in the abdomen.

Special considerations

- Encourage parents of the child with undescended testes to express their concern about his condition. Provide information about causes, available treatments, and the ultimate effect on reproduction. Emphasize that, especially in premature neonates, the testes may descend spontaneously.
- If orchiopexy is necessary, explain the surgery to the child, using terms he understands. Tell him that a rubber band may be taped to his thigh for about 1 week after surgery to keep the testis in place. Explain that his scrotum may swell but shouldn't be painful.

After orchiopexy:
- Monitor vital signs and intake and output. Check dressings. Encourage coughing

and deep breathing. Watch for urine retention.
■ Keep the operative site clean. Tell the child to wipe from front to back after defecating. If a rubber band has been applied to keep the testis in place, maintain tension, but make sure it isn't too tight.
■ Encourage parents to participate in postoperative care, such as bathing or feeding the child. Also urge the child to do as much for himself as possible.

Testicular torsion

Testicular torsion is an abnormal twisting of the spermatic cord due to rotation of a testis or the mesorchium (a fold in the area between the testis and epididymis), which causes strangulation and, if untreated, eventual infarction of the testis. This condition is almost always (90%) unilateral in presentation, but the defect is bilateral, requiring both testicles to be surgically treated. Testicular torsion is most common between ages 12 and 18, but it may occur at any age. The prognosis is good with early detection and prompt treatment.

Causes
Normally, the tunica vaginalis envelops the testis and attaches to the epididymis and spermatic cord. In *intravaginal torsion* (the most common type of testicular torsion in adolescents), testicular twisting may result from an abnormality of the tunica, in which the testis is abnormally positioned, or from a narrowing of the mesentery support. In *extravaginal torsion* (most common in neonates), loose attachment of the tunica vaginalis to the scrotal lining causes spermatic cord rotation above the testis. Typically, there's no history of trauma, and the pain occurs suddenly. A sudden forceful contraction of the cremaster muscle may precipitate this condition. (See *Extravaginal torsion.*)

Signs and symptoms
Torsion produces excruciating pain in the affected testis or iliac fossa. Nausea, vomiting, and light-headedness may also occur.

EXTRAVAGINAL TORSION

In extravaginal torsion, rotation of the spermatic cord above the testis causes strangulation and, eventually, infarction of the testis.

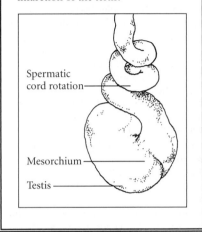

Spermatic cord rotation

Mesorchium

Testis

Diagnosis
Physical examination reveals tense, tender swelling in the scrotum or inguinal canal and hyperemia of the overlying skin. Doppler ultrasonography helps distinguish testicular torsion from strangulated hernia, undescended testes, or epididymitis.

Treatment
Treatment consists of untwisting the testes and immediate surgical repair by orchiopexy (fixation of a viable testis to the scrotum) or orchiectomy (excision of a nonviable testis). Both testes are usually anchored to the scrotum as a preventive measure. As with ovarian torsion in the female, preservation of the organ is the preferred option. If surgery is performed within 6 hours, most testicles can be saved.

Special considerations
■ Promote the patient's comfort before and after surgery.
■ After surgery, administer pain medication as ordered. Monitor voiding, and apply an ice bag with a cover to reduce edema. Protect the wound from contamination. Otherwise, allow the patient to per-

form as many normal daily activities as possible.

Male infertility

Male infertility may be suspected whenever a couple fails to achieve pregnancy after about 1 year of regular, unprotected intercourse.

Causes and incidence

Some factors associated with male infertility include:
- varicocele, a mass of dilated and tortuous varicose veins in the spermatic cord
- semen disorders, such as volume or motility disturbances and inadequate sperm density
- proliferation of abnormal or immature sperm, with variations in the head's size and shape
- systemic disease, such as diabetes mellitus, neoplasms, hepatic and renal diseases, and viral disturbances, especially mumps-related orchitis
- genital infections, such as gonorrhea, tuberculosis, and herpes
- disorders of the testes, such as cryptorchidism, Sertoli-cell-only syndrome, and ductal obstruction (caused by absence or ligation of vas deferens or infection)
- genetic defects, such as Klinefelter's and Reifenstein's syndromes
- immunologic disorders, such as autoimmune infertility and allergic orchitis
- endocrine imbalances that disrupt pituitary gonadotropins, inhibiting spermatogenesis, testosterone production, or both (as in Kallmann's syndrome, panhypopituitarism, hypothyroidism, and congenital adrenal hyperplasia)
- chemicals and drugs that can inhibit gonadotropins or interfere with spermatogenesis, such as arsenic, methotrexate, medroxyprogesterone, nitrofurantoin, monoamine oxidase inhibitors, and some antihypertensives
- sexual problems, such as erectile dysfunction, ejaculatory incompetence, and low libido.

Age, occupation, and traumatic injury to the testes can also contribute to male infertility. Approximately 30% to 40% of infertility problems in the United States are attributed to the male.

Signs and symptoms

The obvious indication of male infertility is failure to impregnate a fertile woman. Clinical features may include atrophied testes; empty scrotum; scrotal edema; varicocele or anteversion of the epididymis; inflamed seminal vesicles; beading or abnormal nodes on the spermatic cord and vas; penile nodes, warts, plaques, or hypospadias; prostatitis, which may be acute or chronic; and prostatic enlargement, nodules, swelling, or tenderness. In addition, male infertility commonly induces troublesome negative emotions in a couple — anger, hurt, disgust, guilt, and loss of self-esteem.

Diagnosis

A detailed patient history may reveal abnormal sexual development, delayed puberty, infertility in previous relationships, and a medical history of prolonged fever, mumps, impaired nutritional status, previous surgery, or trauma to genitalia. After a thorough patient history and physical examination, the most conclusive test for male infertility is semen analysis. The specimen is collected after 2 to 3 days of complete abstinence to determine volume and viscosity as well as sperm count, motility, swimming speed, and shape.

Other laboratory tests include gonadotropin assay to determine the integrity of the pituitary gonadal axis, serum testosterone levels to determine end organ response to luteinizing hormone (LH), urine 17-ketosteroid levels to measure testicular function, and testicular biopsy to help clarify unexplained oligospermia and azoospermia. Vasography and seminal vesiculography may be necessary.

Treatment

When anatomic dysfunction or infection causes infertility, treatment consists of correcting the underlying problem. A varicocele requires surgical repair or removal. For patients with sexual dysfunction, treatment includes education, counseling or therapy (on sexual techniques, coital frequency, and reproductive physiology), and proper nutrition with vitamin supplements. Decreased follicle-stimulating hormone levels may respond to vitamin B therapy; decreased LH levels, to human chorionic gonadotropin (hCG) therapy. Normal or elevated LH level requires low dosages of testosterone. Decreased testosterone levels, decreased semen motility, and volume disturbances may respond to hCG.

A patient with oligospermia who has a normal history and physical examination, normal hormonal assays, and no signs of systemic disease requires emotional support and counseling, adequate nutrition, multivitamins, and selective therapeutic agents, such as clomiphene, hCG, and low dosages of testosterone. Obvious alternatives to such treatment are adoption and artificial insemination.

Special considerations

■ Educate the couple, as necessary, about reproductive and sexual function and about factors that may interfere with fertility such as the use of lubricants and douches.

■ Urge men with oligospermia to avoid habits that may interfere with normal spermatogenesis by elevating scrotal temperature, such as wearing tight underwear and athletic supporters, taking hot tub baths, or habitually riding a bicycle. Explain that cool scrotal temperature is essential for normal spermatogenesis.

■ When possible, advise the infertile couple to join group programs to share their feelings and concerns with other couples who have the same problem.

■ Help prevent male infertility by encouraging the patient to have regular physical examinations, to protect gonads during athletic activity, and to receive early treatment for sexually transmitted diseases and surgical correction for anatomic defects.

Precocious puberty in males

In precocious puberty, boys begin to mature sexually before age 10. This disorder can occur as *true precocious puberty,* which is most common, with early maturation of the hypothalamic-pituitary-gonadal axis,

development of secondary sex characteristics, gonadal development, and spermatogenesis, or as *pseudoprecocious puberty,* with development of secondary sex characteristics without gonadal development. Boys with true precocious puberty reportedly have fathered children as early as age 7.

In most boys with precocious puberty, sexual characteristics develop in essentially normal sequence; these children function normally when they reach adulthood.

Causes

True precocious puberty may be idiopathic (constitutional) or cerebral (neurogenic). In some patients, idiopathic precocity may be genetically transmitted as a dominant trait. Cerebral precocity results from pituitary or hypothalamic intracranial lesions that cause excessive secretion of gonadotropin.

Pseudoprecocious puberty may result from testicular tumors (hyperplasia, adenoma, or carcinoma) or from congenital adrenogenital syndrome. Testicular tumors produce excessive testosterone levels; adrenogenital syndrome produces high levels of adrenocortical steroids.

Signs and symptoms

All boys with precocious puberty experience early bone development, causing an initial growth spurt, early muscle development, and premature closure of the epiphyses, which results in stunted adult stature. Other features are adult hair pattern, penile growth, and bilateral enlarged testes. Symptoms of precocity due to cerebral lesions include nausea, vomiting, headache, vision disturbances, and internal hydrocephalus.

In pseudoprecocity caused by testicular tumors, adult hair patterns and acne develop. A discrepancy in testis size also occurs; the enlarged testis may be hard or may contain a palpable, isolated nodule. Adrenogenital syndrome produces adult skin tone, excessive hair (including beard), and deepened voice. A boy with this syndrome appears stocky and muscular; his penis, scrotal sac, and prostate are enlarged (but not the testes).

Diagnosis

Assessing the cause of precocious puberty requires a complete physical examination. A detailed patient history can help evaluate the patient's recent growth pattern, behavior changes, a family history of precocious puberty, or ingestion of hormones.

In true precocity, laboratory results include the following:

- Serum levels of luteinizing and follicle-stimulating hormones and corticotropin are elevated.
- Plasma tests for testosterone demonstrate elevated levels (equal to those of an adult male).
- Evaluation of ejaculate reveals the presence of live spermatozoa.
- Brain scan, skull X-rays, and EEG can detect possible central nervous system tumors. Abdominal scans can detect testicular tumors.

A child with an initial diagnosis of idiopathic precocious puberty should be reassessed regularly for possible tumors.

In pseudoprecocity, chromosomal karyotype analysis demonstrates an abnormal pattern of autosomes and sex chromosomes. Elevated levels of 24-hour urinary 17-ketosteroids and other steroids also indicate pseudoprecocity.

Treatment

Boys with idiopathic precocious puberty generally require no medical treatment and suffer no physical complications in adulthood. Supportive psychological counseling is the most important therapy.

When precocious puberty is caused by tumors, the outlook is less encouraging. Brain tumors necessitate neurosurgery but may resist treatment and prove fatal. Testicular tumors may be treated by removing the affected testis (orchiectomy). Malignant tumors require chemotherapy and lymphatic radiation therapy. The prognosis is generally good, depending on tumor histology and degree of differentiation.

Adrenogenital syndrome that causes precocious puberty may respond to lifelong therapy with maintenance doses of glucocorticoids (cortisol) to inhibit corticotropin production.

Special considerations

- Emphasize to parents that the child's social and emotional development should remain consistent with his chronological age, not with his physical development. Advise parents not to place unrealistic demands on him.
- Reassure the child that, although his body is changing more rapidly than those of other boys, eventually they will experience the same changes. Help him feel less self-conscious about his changing body. Suggest clothing that de-emphasizes sexual development.
- Provide sex education for the child with true precocity.
- If the child must take glucocorticoids for the rest of his life, explain the medication's adverse effects (cushingoid symptoms) to the family.

Selected references

Emans, S.J., et al. *Pediatric and Adolescent Gynecology,* 5th ed. Philadelphia: Lippincott Williams & Wilkins, 2005.

Morgan, M., and Siddighi, S. *NMS Obstetrics and Gynecology,* 5th ed. Philadelphia: Lippincott Williams & Wilkins, 2004.

Moyer, P. "Long-Term Nightly Sildenafil Promotes Normal Erectile Function," *Medscape Medical News,* May 2004. Available at: *www.medscape.com.*

Patrizio, P., et al. *A Color Atlas for Human Assisted Reproduction: Laboratory and Clinical Insights.* Philadelphia: Lippincott Williams & Wilkins, 2003.

Peck, P. "Testosterone Patch Increases Sexual Function in Women," *Medscape Medical News,* May 2004. Available at *www.medscape.com.*

Scott, J.R., et al., eds. *Danforths' Obstetrics and Gynecology,* 9th ed. Philadelphia: Lippincott Williams & Wilkins, 2003.

Siroky, M.B., et al., eds. *Handbook of Urology: Diagnosis and Therapy,* 3rd ed. Philadelphia: Lippincott Williams & Wilkins, 2004.

Speroff, L., and Fritz, M. *Clinical Gynecology Endocrinology and Infertility,* 7th ed. Philadelphia: Lippincott Williams & Wilkins, 2005.

Sweet, R.L., and Gibbs, R.S. *Atlas of Infectious Diseases of the Female Genital Tract.* Philadelphia: Lippincott Williams & Wilkins, 2005.

Tierney, L.M., et al. *Current Medical Diagnosis and Treatment,* 43rd ed. New York: McGraw-Hill Book Co., 2004.

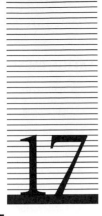

Hematologic disorders

Introduction   *1015*

Anemias   *1020*
Pernicious anemia   *1020*
Folic acid deficiency anemia   *1024*
Aplastic anemias   *1025*
Sideroblastic anemias   *1028*
Thalassemia   *1030*
Iron deficiency anemia   *1031*

Polycythemias   *1035*
Polycythemia vera   *1035*
Spurious polycythemia   *1038*
Secondary polycythemia   *1039*

Hemorrhagic disorders   *1040*
Allergic purpuras   *1040*
Hereditary hemorrhagic
   telangiectasia   *1042*
Thrombocytopenia   *1043*
Idiopathic thrombocytopenic
   purpura   *1046*
Platelet function disorders   *1047*
Von Willebrand's disease   *1049*
Disseminated intravascular
   coagulation   *1050*

Miscellaneous disorders   *1053*
Granulocytopenia and
   lymphocytopenia   *1053*
Hyperslenism   *1055*

Selected references   *1056*

Introduction

Blood, one of the body's major fluid tissues, continuously circulates through the heart and blood vessels, carrying vital elements to every part of the body.

Blood basics

Blood performs several vital functions through its special components: the liquid portion (plasma) and the formed constituents (erythrocytes, leukocytes, and thrombocytes) that are suspended in it. Erythrocytes (red blood cells [RBCs]) carry oxygen to the tissues and remove carbon dioxide from them. Leukocytes (white blood cells [WBCs]) act in inflammatory and immune responses. Plasma (a clear, straw-colored fluid) carries antibodies and nutrients to tissues and carries waste away; plasma coagulation factors and thrombocytes (platelets) control clotting. (See *Coagulation factors,* page 1016.)

Typically, the average person has 5 to 6 L of circulating blood, which constitute 5% to 7% of body weight (as much as 10% in premature neonates). Blood is three to five times more viscous than water, with an alkaline pH of 7.35 to 7.45, and is either bright red (arterial blood) or dark red (venous blood), depending on the degree of oxygen saturation and the hemoglobin (Hb) level.

1015

COAGULATION FACTORS

Factor	Synonym	Location
Factor I	Fibrinogen	Plasma
Factor II	Prothrombin	Plasma
Factor III	Tissue thromboplastin	Tissue cells
Factor IV	Calcium ion	Plasma
Factor V	Labile factor	Plasma
Factor VII	Stable factor	Plasma
Factor VIII	Antihemophilic globulin or antihemophilic factor A	Plasma
Factor IX	Plasma thromboplastin component, Christmas factor	Plasma
Factor X	Stuart-Prower factor	Plasma
Factor XI	Plasma thromboplastin antecedent	Plasma
Factor XII	Hageman factor	Plasma
Factor XIII	Fibrin stabilizing factor	Plasma

Formation and characteristics

Hematopoiesis, the process of blood formation, occurs primarily in the bone marrow, where primitive blood cells (stem cells) produce the precursors of erythrocytes (normoblasts), leukocytes, and thrombocytes. During embryonic development, blood cells are derived from mesenchyma and form in the yolk sac. As the fetus matures, blood cells are produced in the liver, the spleen, and the thymus; by the fifth month of gestation, blood cells also begin to form in bone marrow. After birth, blood cells are usually produced only in the marrow.

Blood's function

The most important function of blood is to *transport oxygen* (bound to RBCs inside Hb) from the lungs to the body tissues and to *return carbon dioxide* from these tissues to the lungs. Blood also performs the following functions:

- production and delivery of antibodies (by WBCs) formed by plasma cells and lymphocytes
- transportation of granulocytes and monocytes to defend the body against pathogens by phagocytosis
- immunity against viruses and cancer cells through sensitized lymphocytes
- provision of complement, a group of immunologically important protein substances in plasma.

Blood's other functions include control of hemostasis by platelets, plasma, and coagulation factors that repair tissue injuries and prevent or halt bleeding; acid-base and fluid balance; regulation of body temperature by carrying off excess heat generated by the internal organs for dissipation through the skin; and transportation of nutrients and regulatory hormones to body tissues and of metabolic wastes to the organs of excretion (kidneys, lungs, and skin).

Blood dysfunction

Because of the rapid reproduction of bone marrow cells and the short life span and minimal storage in the bone marrow of circulating cells, bone marrow cells and their precursors are particularly vulnerable to physiologic changes that can affect cell production. Resulting blood disorders may be primary or secondary, quantitative or qualitative, or both; they may involve some or all blood components. Quantitative blood disorders result from increased or decreased cell production or cell destruction; qualitative blood disorders stem from intrinsic cell abnormalities or plasma component dysfunction. Specific causes of blood disorders include trauma, chronic disease, surgery, malnutrition, drugs, exposure to toxins and radiation, and genetic and congenital defects that disrupt production and function. For example, depressed bone marrow production or mechanical destruction of mature blood cells can reduce the number of RBCs, platelets, and granulocytes, resulting in pancytopenia (anemia, thrombocytopenia, and granulocytopenia). Increased production of multiple bone marrow components can follow myeloproliferative disorders.

Erythropoiesis

The tissues' demand for oxygen and the blood cells' ability to deliver it regulate RBC production. Consequently, hypoxia (or tissue anoxia) stimulates RBC production by triggering the formation and release of erythropoietin, a hormone (probably produced by the kidneys) that activates bone marrow to produce RBCs. Erythropoiesis may also be stimulated by androgens (which accounts for higher RBC counts in men). RBCs have a life span of approximately 120 days.

The actual formation of an erythrocyte begins with an uncommitted stem cell that may eventually develop into an RBC or a WBC. Such formation requires certain vitamins — B_{12} and folic acid — and minerals, such as copper, cobalt, and especially iron, which is vital to hemoglobin's oxygen-carrying capacity. Iron is obtained from various foods and is absorbed in the duodenum and upper jejunum, leaving the excess for temporary storage in reticuloendothelial cells, especially those in the liver. Iron excess is stored as ferritin and hemosiderin until it's released for use in the bone marrow to form new RBCs.

ELDER TIP *In older adults, fatty bone marrow replaces some active cell-forming marrow — first in the long bones and later in the flat bones. The altered bone marrow can't increase erythrocyte production as readily as before in response to such stimuli as hormones, anoxia, hemorrhage, and hemolysis.*

RBC disorders

RBC disorders include quantitative and qualitative abnormalities. Deficiency of RBCs (anemia) can follow any condition that destroys or inhibits the formation of these cells. Common factors leading to this deficiency include:

- chronic illnesses, such as renal disease, cancer, and chronic infections
- congenital or acquired defects that cause bone marrow aplasia and suppress general hematopoiesis (aplastic anemia) or erythropoiesis
- deficiencies of vitamins (vitamin B_{12} deficiency or pernicious anemia) or minerals (iron, folic acid, copper, and cobalt deficiency anemias) that cause inadequate RBC production
- drugs, toxins, and ionizing radiation
- excessive chronic or acute blood loss (posthemorrhagic anemia)
- intrinsically or extrinsically defective red cells (sickle cell anemia and hemolytic transfusion reaction)
- metabolic abnormalities (sideroblastic anemia).

Comparatively few conditions lead to excessive numbers of RBCs:

- abnormal proliferation of all bone marrow elements (polycythemia vera), especially RBC mass
- a single-element abnormality (for instance, an increase in RBCs that results from erythropoietin excess, which in turn results from hypoxemia, hypertension, or pulmonary disease)
- decreased plasma cell volume, which produces a corresponding relative increase in RBC concentration (such as through the use of drugs).

Function of WBCs

WBCs, or leukocytes, protect the body against harmful bacteria and infection and are classified as granular leukocytes (basophils, neutrophils, and eosinophils) or nongranular leukocytes (lymphocytes, monocytes, and plasma cells). (See *Two types of leukocytes.*) Usually, WBCs are produced in bone marrow; lymphocytes and plasma cells are produced in lymphoid tissue as well. Neutrophils have a circulating half-life of less than 6 hours; some lymphocytes may survive for weeks or months. Normally, WBCs number between 5,000 and 10,000/µl.

There are six types of WBCs:
- *Neutrophils,* the predominant form of granulocyte, make up about 60% of WBCs; they help devour invading organisms by phagocytosis.
- *Eosinophils,* minor granulocytes, may defend against parasites and lung and skin infections and act in allergic reactions. They account for 1% to 5% of the total WBC count.
- *Basophils,* minor granulocytes, may release heparin and histamine into the blood and participate in delayed hypersensitivity reactions. They account for 0% to 1% of the total WBC count.
- *Monocytes,* along with neutrophils, help devour invading organisms by phagocytosis. They help process antigens for lymphocytes and form macrophages in the tissues; they account for 1% to 6% of the total WBC count.
- *Lymphocytes* occur as B cells and T cells. B cells aid antibody synthesis; T cells regulate cell-mediated immunity. They account for 20% to 40% of the total WBC count.
- *Plasma cells* develop from lymphocytes, reside in the tissue, and produce antibodies.

A temporary increase in production and release of mature WBCs (leukemic reaction) is a normal response to infection. However, an excessive number of immature WBC precursors and their accumulation in bone marrow or lymphoid tissue is characteristic of leukemia. These nonfunctioning WBCs (blasts) provide no protection against infection; crowd out RBCs, platelets, and mature WBCs; and spill into the bloodstream, sometimes infiltrating organs and impairing function.

WBC deficiencies may reflect inadequate cell production, drug reactions, ionizing radiation, infiltrated bone marrow (cancer), congenital defects, aplastic anemia, folic acid deficiency, or hypersplenism. The major WBC deficiencies are granulocytopenia, lymphocytopenia, and monocytopenia.

Platelets, plasma, and clotting

Platelets are small (2 to 4 microns in diameter), colorless, disk-shaped cytoplasmic fragments split from cells in bone marrow called megakaryocytes. The normal platelet concentration is 150,000 to 400,000/µl. These fragments, which have a life span of approximately 10 days, perform three vital functions:
- initiate vasoconstriction of damaged blood vessels to minimize blood loss
- form hemostatic plugs in injured blood vessels
- with plasma, provide materials that accelerate blood coagulation — notably platelet factor 3.

Plasma consists mainly of proteins (chiefly albumin, globulin, and fibrinogen) held in aqueous suspension. Other components of plasma include glucose, lipids, amino acids, electrolytes, pigments, hormones, respiratory gases (oxygen and carbon dioxide), and products of metabolism, such as urea, uric acid, creatinine, and lactic acid. Its fluid characteristics — including osmotic pressure, viscosity, and suspension qualities — depend on its protein content. Plasma components regulate acid-base balance and immune responses and mediate coagulation and nutrition.

In a complex process called *hemostasis,* platelets, plasma, and coagulation factors interact to control bleeding.

Hemostasis and the clotting mechanism

Hemostasis is the complex process by which the body controls bleeding. When a blood vessel ruptures, local vasoconstriction and platelet clumping (aggregation) at the injury site initially help prevent hemorrhage. This activation of the coagulation system, called *extrinsic cascade,* requires re-

TWO TYPES OF LEUKOCYTES

Leukocytes vary in size, shape, and number. Granular leukocytes (granulocytes) are the most numerous and include basophils, containing cytoplasmic granules that stain readily with alkaline dyes; eosinophils, which stain with acidic dyes; and neutrophils, which are finely granular and recognizable by their multinucleated appearance. Lymphocytes and monocytes have few, if any, granulated particles in the cytoplasm.

GRANULAR LEUKOCYTES

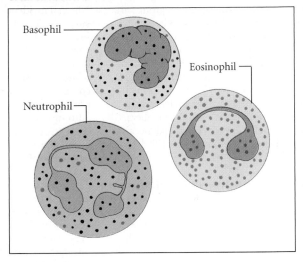

Basophil

Eosinophil

Neutrophil

NONGRANULAR LEUKOCYTES

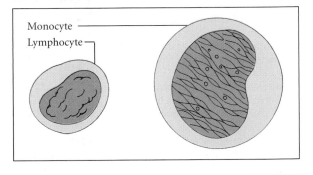

Monocyte

Lymphocyte

---

lease of tissue thromboplastin from the damaged cells. However, formation of a more stable clot requires initiation of the complex clotting mechanism known as the *intrinsic cascade system.* When endothelial vessel injury or a foreign body in the bloodstream activates this system, *activating factor XII* triggers clotting. In the final common pathway, prothrombin is converted to thrombin and fibrinogen to fibrin, which is necessary for creation of a fibrin clot.

Therapy with blood components

Because of improved methods of collection, component separation, and storage, blood transfusions are being used more effectively than ever. Separating blood into components permits a single unit of blood to benefit several patients with different hematologic abnormalities. Component therapy allows replacement of a specific blood component without risking reactions from other components.

Blood typing, crossmatching, and human leukocyte antigen (HLA) typing are compatibility tests used to ensure safe, effective replacement therapy and minimize the risk of transfusion reactions. Blood typing determines the antigens present in the patient's RBCs by reaction with standardized sera. (Critical antigen groups are those of ABO and Rh factor.) Crossmatching the patient's blood with transfusion blood provides some assurance that the patient doesn't have antibodies against donor red cells. HLA typing may be helpful for the patient who needs long-term transfusion therapy or frequent platelet transfusions, but usually, only family members can provide an appropriate match because antigenic properties are genetically determined.

Bone marrow transplantation

Bone marrow transplantation is used to treat acute leukemia, aplastic anemia, severe combined immunodeficiency disease, Nezelof syndrome, and Wiskott-Aldrich syndrome. In this procedure, marrow from a twin or another HLA-identical donor (usually a sibling) is transfused in an attempt to repopulate the recipient's bone marrow with normal cells.

A hematologic disorder can affect nearly every aspect of the patient's life, perhaps resulting in life-threatening emergencies that require prompt medical treatment. Astute, sensitive care founded on a firm understanding of hematologic basics can help the patient survive such illnesses. In situations with poor prognoses, the patient may need to make many adjustments to maintain an optimal quality of life.

ANEMIAS

Pernicious anemia

Pernicious anemia, also known as *Addison's anemia*, is a megaloblastic anemia characterized by decreased gastric production of hydrochloric acid and deficiency of intrinsic factor (IF), a substance normally secreted by the parietal cells of the gastric mucosa that's essential for vitamin B_{12} absorption in the ileum. The resulting deficiency of vitamin B_{12} causes serious neurologic, gastric, and intestinal abnormalities.

Untreated pernicious anemia may lead to permanent neurologic disability and death.

Causes and incidence

Familial incidence of pernicious anemia suggests a genetic predisposition. (It may involve an inherited single dominant autosomal factor.) Significantly higher incidence in patients with immunologically related diseases, such as thyroiditis, myxedema, and Graves' disease, seems to support a widely held theory that an inherited autoimmune response causes gastric mucosal atrophy and, therefore, deficiency of hydrochloric acid and IF. IF deficiency impairs vitamin B_{12} absorption. The resultant vitamin B_{12} deficiency inhibits cell growth, particularly of red blood cells (RBCs), leading to insufficient and deformed RBCs with poor oxygen-carrying capacity. It also impairs myelin formation, causing neurologic damage. Iatrogenic induction can follow partial gastrectomy.

 PEDIATRIC TIP *Juvenile pernicious anemia, occurring in children younger than age 10, stems from a congenital stomach disorder that causes secretion of abnormal IF.*

ELDER TIP *With age, vitamin B_{12} absorption may also diminish, resulting in reduced erythrocyte mass and decreased hemoglobin (Hb) levels and hematocrit (HCT).*

Pernicious anemia primarily affects people of northern European ancestry. It's rare in children and infants. Onset typically occurs after age 35, and incidence increases with age. It affects about 2% of people older than age 60.

Signs and symptoms

Characteristically, pernicious anemia has an insidious onset but eventually causes an unmistakable triad of symptoms: weakness, sore tongue, and numbness and tingling in the extremities. The lips, gums, and tongue appear markedly bloodless. Hemolysis-induced hyperbilirubinemia may cause faintly jaundiced sclera and pale to bright yellow skin. In addition, the patient may become highly susceptible to infection, especially of the genitourinary tract.

Other systemic symptoms of pernicious anemia include the following:

■ *GI:* Gastric mucosal atrophy and decreased hydrochloric acid production disturb digestion and lead to nausea, vomiting, anorexia, weight loss, flatulence, diarrhea, and constipation. Gingival bleeding and tongue inflammation may hinder eating and intensify anorexia.

■ *Central nervous system (CNS):* Demyelination caused by vitamin B_{12} deficiency initially affects the peripheral nerves but gradually extends to the spinal cord. Consequently, the neurologic effects of pernicious anemia may include neuritis; weakness in extremities; peripheral numbness and paresthesia; disturbed position sense; lack of coordination; ataxia; impaired fine finger movement; positive Babinski's and Romberg's signs; light-headedness; altered vision (diplopia and blurred vision), taste, and hearing (tinnitus); optic muscle atrophy; loss of bowel and bladder control; and, in males, impotence. Its effects on the nervous system may also produce irritability, poor memory, headache, depression, and delirium. Although some of these symptoms are temporary, irreversible CNS changes may have occurred before treatment.

■ *Cardiovascular:* Increasingly fragile cell membranes induce widespread destruction of RBCs, resulting in low Hb levels. The impaired oxygen-carrying capacity of the blood secondary to lowered Hb leads to weakness, fatigue, and light-headedness. Compensatory increased cardiac output results in palpitations, wide pulse pressure, dyspnea, orthopnea, tachycardia, premature beats and, eventually, heart failure.

■ *Musculoskeletal:* Scissors gait can also occur as a late sign of untreated anemia.

Diagnosis

A positive family history, typical ethnic heritage, and results of blood studies, bone marrow aspiration, gastric analysis, and the Schilling test establish the diagnosis. (See *Tests for blood composition, production, and function,* pages 1022 and 1023.) Laboratory screening must rule out other anemias with similar symptoms, such as folic acid deficiency anemia, because treatment differs. Diagnosis must also rule out vitamin

B_{12} deficiency resulting from malabsorption due to GI disorders, gastric surgery, radiation, or drug therapy.

Blood study results that suggest pernicious anemia include:

■ decreased Hb levels (4 to 5 g/dl) and decreased RBC count

 ELDER TIP *Hb levels drop 1 to 2 g/ dl in elderly men, and HCT may decrease slightly in both men and women. These changes reflect decreased bone marrow and hematopoiesis and (in men) decreased androgen levels; they aren't an indicator of pernicious anemia.*

■ increased mean corpuscular volume (greater than 120/µl); because larger-than-normal RBCs *each* contain increased amounts of Hb, mean corpuscular Hb concentration is also increased

■ possible low white blood cell and platelet counts and large, malformed platelets

■ serum vitamin B_{12} assay levels less than 0.1 mcg/ml

■ elevated serum lactate dehydrogenase levels.

Bone marrow aspiration reveals erythroid hyperplasia (crowded red bone marrow), with increased numbers of megaloblasts but few normally developing RBCs. Gastric analysis shows absence of free hydrochloric acid after histamine or pentagastrin injection.

 CONFIRMING DIAGNOSIS *The Schilling test is the definitive test for pernicious anemia. In this test, the patient receives a small oral dose (0.5 to 2 mcg) of radioactive vitamin B_{12} after fasting for 12 hours. A larger dose (1 mg) of nonradioactive vitamin B_{12} is given I.M. 2 hours later, as a parenteral flush, and the radioactivity of a 24-hour urine specimen is measured. About 7% of the radioactive B_{12} dose is excreted in the first 24 hours; people with pernicious anemia excrete less than 3%. (In pernicious anemia, the vitamin remains unabsorbed and is passed in the stool.) When the Schilling test is repeated with IF added, the test shows normal excretion of vitamin B_{12}.*

Important serologic findings may include IF antibodies and antiparietal cell antibodies.

TESTS FOR BLOOD COMPOSITION, PRODUCTION, AND FUNCTION

Overall composition
- Peripheral blood smear shows maturity and morphologic characteristics of blood elements and determines qualitative abnormalities.
- Complete blood count determines the actual number of blood elements in relation to volume and quantifies abnormalities.
- Bone marrow aspiration or biopsy allows evaluation of hematopoiesis by showing blood elements and precursors, and abnormal or malignant cells.

Red blood cell function
- Hematocrit, or packed cell volume, measures the percentage of red blood cells (RBCs) per fluid volume of whole blood.
- Hemoglobin (Hb) measures the amount (grams) of Hb per deciliter of blood, to determine oxygen-carrying capacity.
- Reticulocyte count assesses RBC production by determining concentration of this erythrocyte precursor.
- Schilling test determines absorption of vitamin B_{12} (necessary for erythropoiesis) by measuring excretion of radioactive B_{12} in the urine.
- Mean corpuscular volume describes the RBC in terms of size.
- Mean corpuscular Hb determines the average amount of Hb per RBC.
- Mean corpuscular Hb concentration establishes the average Hb concentration in 1 dl of packed RBCs.

- Sucrose hemolysis test assesses the susceptibility of RBCs to hemolyze with complement.
- Direct Coombs' test demonstrates the presence of immunoglobulin G (IgG) antibodies (such as antibodies to Rh factor) or, possibly, complement on circulating RBCs.
- Indirect Coombs' test, a two-step test, detects the presence of IgG antibodies in the serum.
- Sideroblast test detects stainable iron (available for Hb synthesis) in normoblastic RBCs.
- Hb electrophoresis demonstrates abnormal Hb such as sickle cell.

Hemostasis
- Platelet count determines the number of platelets.
- Bleeding time (Ivy bleeding time) assesses the capacity for platelets to stop bleeding in capillaries and small vessels.
- Prothrombin time (Quick's test, pro time) assists in evaluation of thrombin generation (extrinsic clotting mechanism).
- Partial thromboplastin time aids evaluation of the adequacy of plasma-clotting factors (intrinsic clotting mechanism).
- International Normalized Ratio normalizes ratios between labs.
- Fibrin degradation products (fibrin split products, FDPs) test the amount of clot breakdown products in serum.
- Thrombin time detects abnormalities in thrombin fibrinogen reaction.

Treatment

Early parenteral vitamin B_{12} replacement can reverse pernicious anemia, minimize complications and, possibly, prevent permanent neurologic damage. An initial high dose of parenteral vitamin B_{12} causes rapid RBC regeneration. Within 2 weeks, Hb levels should rise to normal, and the patient's condition should improve markedly. Because rapid cell regeneration increases the patient's iron and folate requirements, concomitant iron and folic acid replacement is necessary to prevent iron deficiency anemia.

After the patient's condition improves, the vitamin B_{12} dosage can be decreased to maintenance levels and given monthly. Because such injections must be continued for life, the patient should learn self-administration of vitamin B_{12}.

If anemia causes extreme fatigue, the patient may require bed rest until Hb levels rise. If Hb levels are dangerously low, he may need blood transfusions. Digoxin, a

- Fibrinogen (factor I) measures this coagulation factor in plasma.
- D-dimer test determines if FDPs are from normal mechanisms or excessive fibrinolysis and is commonly used to diagnose disseminated intravascular coagulation.

White blood cell function

- White blood cell (WBC) count, differential establishes quantity and maturity of WBC elements (neutrophils [called polymorphonuclear granulocytes or bands], basophils, eosinophils, lymphocytes, monocytes).
- Quantified $CD4^+$:$CD8^+$ T lymphocytes determines helper:suppressor ratio important to immune function with human immunodeficiency virus infection.

Plasma

- Erythrocyte sedimentation rate measures the rate of RBCs settling from plasma and may reflect infection.
- Electrophoresis of serum proteins determines the amount of various serum proteins (classified by mobility in response to an electrical field). It's commonly used to diagnose plasma cell myeloma.
- Immunoelectrophoresis of serum proteins separates and classifies serum antibodies (immunoglobulins) through specific antisera.

diuretic, and a low-sodium diet may be necessary for a patient with heart failure. Most important is the replacement of vitamin B_{12} to control the condition that led to this failure. Antibiotics help combat accompanying infections.

Special considerations

Supportive measures minimize the risk of complications and speed recovery. Patient and family teaching can promote compliance with lifelong vitamin B_{12} replacement.

- If the patient has severe anemia, plan activities, rest periods, and necessary diagnostic tests to conserve his energy. Monitor pulse rate often; tachycardia means his activities are too strenuous.
- To ensure accurate Schilling test results, make sure that all urine over a 24-hour period is collected and that the specimens are uncontaminated.
- Warn the patient to guard against infections and tell him to report signs of infection promptly, especially pulmonary and urinary tract infections, because the patient's weakened condition may increase susceptibility.
- Provide a well-balanced diet, including foods high in vitamin B_{12} (meat, liver, fish, eggs, and milk). Offer between-meal snacks and encourage the family to bring favorite foods from home.
- Because a sore mouth and tongue make eating painful, ask the dietitian to avoid giving the patient irritating foods. If these symptoms make talking difficult, supply a pad and pencil or some other aid to facilitate nonverbal communication; explain this problem to the family. Provide diluted mouthwash or, with severe conditions, swab the patient's mouth with tap water or warm saline solution.
- Warn the patient with a sensory deficit not to use a heating pad, because it may cause burns.
- If the patient is incontinent, establish a regular bowel and bladder routine. After the patient is discharged, a home health care nurse should follow up on this schedule and make adjustments, as needed.
- If neurologic damage causes behavioral problems, assess mental and neurologic status often; if necessary, give tranquilizers, as ordered, and apply a jacket restraint at night.
- Stress that vitamin B_{12} replacement isn't a permanent cure and that these injections *must* be continued for life, even after symptoms subside.
- To prevent pernicious anemia, emphasize the importance of vitamin B_{12} supplements for patients who have had extensive gastric resections or who follow strict vegetarian or vegan diets.

FOODS HIGH IN FOLIC ACID

Folic acid (pteroylglutamic acid, folacin) is found in most body tissues, where it acts as a coenzyme in metabolic processes involving one carbon transfer. It's essential for formation and maturation of red blood cells and for synthesis of deoxyribonucleic acid. Although its body stores are relatively small (about 70 mg), this vitamin is plentiful in most well-balanced diets.

However, because folic acid is water-soluble and heat-labile, it's easily destroyed by cooking. Also, approximately 20% of folic acid intake is excreted unabsorbed. Insufficient daily folic acid intake (less than 50 mcg/ day) usually induces folic acid deficiency within 4 months. Below is a list of foods high in folic acid content.

Food	mcg/100 g
Asparagus spears	109
Beef liver	294
Broccoli spears	54
Collards (cooked)	102
Mushrooms	24
Oatmeal	33
Peanut butter	57
Red beans	180
Wheat germ	305

Folic acid deficiency anemia

Folic acid deficiency anemia is a common, slowly progressive, megaloblastic anemia. It usually occurs in infants, adolescents, pregnant and lactating females, alcoholics, elderly people, and people with malignant or intestinal diseases.

Causes and incidence

Folic acid deficiency anemia may result from:

- alcohol abuse (alcohol may suppress metabolic effects of folate)
- poor diet (common in alcoholics, elderly people living alone, and infants, especially those with infections or diarrhea)
- impaired absorption (due to intestinal dysfunction from disorders such as celiac disease, tropical sprue, regional jejunitis, or bowel resection)
- bacteria competing for available folic acid
- excessive cooking, which can destroy a high percentage of folic acids in foods (See *Foods high in folic acid.*)
- limited storage capacity in infants
- prolonged drug therapy (anticonvulsants and estrogens)
- increased folic acid requirements during pregnancy; during rapid growth in infancy (common because of recent increase in survival of premature infants); during childhood and adolescence (because of general use of folate-poor cow's milk); and in patients with neoplastic diseases and some skin diseases (chronic exfoliative dermatitis).

It's estimated that 10% of the United States population has low folate stores.

Signs and symptoms

Folic acid deficiency anemia gradually produces clinical features characteristic of other megaloblastic anemias, without the neurologic manifestations: progressive fatigue, shortness of breath, palpitations, weakness, glossitis, nausea, anorexia, headache, fainting, irritability, forgetfulness, pallor, and slight jaundice. Folic acid deficiency anemia doesn't cause neurologic impairment unless it's associated with vitamin B_{12} deficiency, as in pernicious anemia.

Diagnosis

The Schilling test and a therapeutic trial of vitamin B_{12} injections distinguish between folic acid deficiency anemia and pernicious anemia. Significant findings include macrocytosis, decreased reticulocyte count, abnormal platelets, and serum folate less than 3 ng/ml.

Treatment

Treatment consists primarily of folic acid supplements and elimination of contributing causes. Folic acid supplements may be given orally or parenterally (to patients who are severely ill, have malabsorption, or are unable to take oral medication). Many patients respond favorably to a well-balanced diet. If the patient has combined B_{12} and folate deficiencies, folic acid replenishment alone may aggravate neurologic dysfunction.

Special considerations

■ Teach the patient to meet daily folic acid requirements by including a food from each food group in every meal. If he has a severe deficiency, explain that diet only reinforces folic acid supplementation and isn't therapeutic by itself. Urge compliance with the prescribed course of therapy. Advise him not to stop taking the supplements when he begins to feel better.

■ If the patient has glossitis, emphasize the importance of good oral hygiene. Suggest regular use of mild or diluted mouthwash and a soft toothbrush.

■ Watch fluid and electrolyte balance, particularly in the patient who has severe diarrhea and is receiving parenteral fluid replacement therapy.

■ Because anemia causes severe fatigue, schedule regular rest periods until the patient is able to resume normal activity.

■ To prevent folic acid deficiency anemia, emphasize the importance of a well-balanced diet high in folic acid. Identify alcoholics with poor dietary habits and try to arrange for appropriate counseling. Tell mothers who aren't breast-feeding to use commercially prepared formulas.

Aplastic anemias

Aplastic, or hypoplastic, anemias result from injury to or destruction of stem cells in bone marrow or the bone marrow matrix, causing pancytopenia (anemia, granulocytopenia, and thrombocytopenia) and bone marrow hypoplasia. Although commonly used interchangeably with other terms for bone marrow failure, aplastic anemias properly refer to pancytopenia resulting from the decreased functional capacity of a hypoplastic, fatty bone marrow. These disorders generally produce fatal bleeding or infection, particularly when they're idiopathic or stem from chloramphenicol or from infectious hepatitis. Mortality for aplastic anemias with severe pancytopenia is 80% to 90%.

Causes and incidence

Aplastic anemias usually develop when damaged or destroyed stem cells inhibit red blood cell (RBC) production. Less commonly, they develop when damaged bone marrow microvasculature creates an unfavorable environment for cell growth and maturation. About one-half of such anemias result from drugs (antibiotics and anticonvulsants), toxic agents (such as benzene and chloramphenicol), or radiation. The rest may result from immunologic factors (unconfirmed), severe disease (especially hepatitis), or preleukemic and neoplastic infiltration of bone marrow.

Idiopathic anemias may be congenital. Two such forms of aplastic anemia have been identified: Congenital hypoplastic anemia (Blackfan-Diamond anemia) develops between ages 2 and 3 months; Fanconi's syndrome, between birth and age 10. In Fanconi's syndrome, chromosomal abnormalities are usually associated with multiple congenital anomalies, such as dwarfism, and hypoplasia of the kidneys and spleen. In the absence of a consistent familial or genetic history of aplastic anemia, researchers suspect that these congenital abnormalities result from an induced change in the fetus' development.

Incidence is 0.6 to 6.1 cases per 1 million people. There is no racial predilection.

Signs and symptoms

Clinical features of aplastic anemias vary with the severity of pancytopenia but develop insidiously in many cases. Anemic symptoms include progressive weakness and fatigue, shortness of breath, headache, pallor and, ultimately, tachycardia and heart failure. Thrombocytopenia leads to ecchymosis, petechiae, and hemorrhage,

BONE MARROW TRANSPLANTATION

In bone marrow transplantation, usually 500 to 700 ml of marrow is aspirated from the pelvic bones of a human leukocyte antigen (HLA)-compatible donor (allogeneic) or of the recipient himself during complete remission (autologous). The aspirated marrow is filtered and then infused into the recipient in an attempt to repopulate the patient's marrow with normal cells. This procedure has effected long-term, healthy survival in about 50% of patients with severe aplastic anemia. Bone marrow transplantation may also be effective in patients with acute leukemia, certain immunodeficiency diseases, and solid tumor neoplasms.

Because bone marrow transplantation carries serious risks, it requires strict adherence to infection control and strict sterile techniques, and a primary nurse to provide consistent care and continuous monitoring of the patient's status.

Before transplantation
- Explain that the success rate depends on the stage of the disease and an HLA-identical match.
- After bone marrow aspiration is completed under local anesthetic, apply pressure dressings to the donor's aspiration sites. Observe the sites for bleeding. Relieve pain with analgesics and ice packs, as needed.
- Assess the patient's understanding of bone marrow transplantation. If necessary, correct any misconceptions about this procedure and provide additional information, as appropriate. Prepare the patient to expect an extended hospital stay. Explain that chemotherapy and possible radiation treatments are necessary to destroy cells that may cause the body to reject the transplant.
- Various treatment protocols are used. For example, I.V. cyclophosphamide may be used with additional chemotherapeutic agents or total body irradiation and requires aggressive hydration to prevent hemorrhagic cystitis. Control nausea and vomiting with an antiemetic, such as ondansetron, prochlorperazine, metoclopramide, or lorazepam, as needed. Give allopurinol, as prescribed, to prevent hyperuricemia resulting from tumor breakdown products. Because alopecia is a common adverse effect of high-dose cyclophosphamide therapy, encourage the patient to choose a wig or scarf before treatment begins.
- Total body irradiation (in one dose or several daily doses) follows chemotherapy, inducing total marrow aplasia. Warn the patient that cataracts, GI disturbances, and sterility are possible adverse effects.

During marrow infusion
- Monitor vital signs every 15 minutes.
- Watch for complications of marrow infusion, such as pulmonary embolus and volume overload.
- Reassure the patient throughout the procedure.

---

especially from the mucous membranes (nose, gums, rectum, and vagina) or into the retina or central nervous system. Neutropenia may lead to infection (fever, oral and rectal ulcers, and sore throat) but without characteristic inflammation.

Diagnosis
Confirmation of aplastic anemia requires a series of laboratory tests:
- RBCs are usually normochromic and normocytic (although macrocytosis [larger-than-normal erythrocytes] and anisocytosis [excessive variation in erythrocyte size] may exist), with a total count of 1 million/μl or less. Absolute reticulocyte count is very low.
- Serum iron level is elevated (unless bleeding occurs), but total iron-binding capacity is normal or slightly reduced. Hemosiderin (a derivative of hemoglobin [Hb]) is present, and tissue iron storage is visible microscopically.

After the infusion

- Continue to monitor the patient's vital signs every 15 minutes for 2 hours after infusion, then every 4 hours. Watch for fever and chills, which may be the only signs of infection. Give prophylactic antibiotics as prescribed. To reduce the possibility of bleeding, don't administer medications rectally or I.M.
- Administer methotrexate or cyclosporine, as prescribed, to prevent graft-versus-host (GVH) reaction, a potentially fatal complication of allogeneic transplantation. Watch for signs or symptoms of GVH reaction, such as maculopapular rash, pancytopenia, jaundice, joint pain, and generalized edema.
- Administer vitamins, steroids, and iron and folic acid supplements, as appropriate. Administration of blood products, such as platelets and packed red blood cells, may also be indicated, depending on the results of daily blood studies.
- Provide good mouth care every 2 hours. Use hydrogen peroxide and nystatin mouthwash or oral fluconazole, for example, to prevent candidiasis and other mouth infections. Also provide meticulous skin care, paying special attention to pressure points and open sites, such as aspiration and I.V.

- Platelet, neutrophil, and white blood cell counts fall.
- Coagulation tests (bleeding time), reflecting decreased platelet count, are abnormal.
- Bone marrow aspiration from several sites may yield a "dry tap," and biopsy will show severely hypocellular or aplastic marrow, with varied amounts of fat, fibrous tissue, or gelatinous replacement; absence of tagged iron (because iron is deposited in the liver rather than bone marrow) and

megakaryocytes (platelet precursors); and depression of erythroid elements.

Differential diagnosis must rule out paroxysmal nocturnal hemoglobinuria and other diseases in which pancytopenia is common.

Treatment

Effective treatment must eliminate any identifiable cause and provide vigorous supportive measures, such as packed RBC, platelet, and experimental histocompatibility locus antigen-matched leukocyte transfusions. Even after elimination of the cause, recovery can take months. Bone marrow transplantation is the treatment of choice for anemia due to severe aplasia and for patients who need constant RBC transfusions. (See *Bone marrow transplantation*.)

Patients with low leukocyte counts need special measures to prevent infection. The infection itself may require specific antibiotics; however, these aren't given prophylactically because they tend to encourage resistant strains of organisms. Patients with low Hb levels may need respiratory support with oxygen in addition to blood transfusions.

For older patients, or for those who don't have a matched bone marrow donor, antithymocyte globulin (ATG) is an alternative treatment. ATG is a horse serum that contains antibodies against human T cells. It may be used in an attempt to suppress the body's immune system, allowing the bone marrow to resume its blood cell-generating function. Other immunosuppressant agents, such as cyclosporine, may also be used.

Other treatments may include corticosteroids to stimulate erythroid production, marrow-stimulating agents such as androgens (which remain controversial), and colony stimulation factors to encourage growth of specific cellular components.

Special considerations

- If the platelet count is low (less than 20,000/µl), prevent bleeding by avoiding I.M. injections, suggesting the use of an electric razor and a soft toothbrush, humidifying oxygen to prevent drying of mucous membranes, avoiding enemas and rectal temperatures, and promoting regular bowel movements through the use of a stool softener and a proper diet to prevent constipation. Also, apply pressure to venipuncture sites until bleeding stops. Detect bleeding early by checking for blood in urine and stool, and assessing skin for petechiae.

- Take safety precautions to prevent falls that could lead to prolonged bleeding or hemorrhage.
- Help prevent infection by washing your hands thoroughly before entering the patient's room, by making sure he's receiving a nutritious diet (high in vitamins and proteins) to improve his resistance, and by encouraging meticulous mouth and perianal care.
- Watch for life-threatening hemorrhage, infection, adverse effects of drug therapy, or blood transfusion reaction. Make sure routine throat, urine, nose, rectal, and blood cultures are done regularly and correctly to check for infection. Teach the patient to recognize signs of infection, and tell him to report them immediately.
- If the patient has a low Hb level, which causes fatigue, schedule frequent rest periods. Administer oxygen therapy as needed. If blood transfusions are necessary, assess for a transfusion reaction by checking the patient's temperature and watching for the development of other signs and symptoms, such as rash, hives, itching, back pain, restlessness, and shaking chills.
- Reassure and support the patient and his family by explaining the disease and its treatment, particularly if he has recurring acute episodes. Explain the purpose of all prescribed drugs and discuss possible adverse effects, including which ones he should report promptly. Encourage the patient who doesn't require hospitalization to continue his normal lifestyle, with appropriate restrictions (such as regular rest periods), until remission occurs.
- To prevent aplastic anemia, monitor blood studies carefully in the patient receiving anemia-inducing drugs.
- Support efforts to educate the public about the hazards of toxic agents. Tell parents to keep toxic agents out of the reach of children. Encourage people who work with radiation to wear protective clothing and a radiation-detecting badge, and to observe plant safety precautions. Those who work with benzene (solvent) should know that 10 parts per million is the highest safe environmental level and that a delayed reaction to benzene may develop.

Sideroblastic anemias

Sideroblastic anemias are a group of heterogenous disorders with a common defect; they fail to use iron in hemoglobin (Hb) synthesis, despite the availability of adequate iron stores. These anemias may be hereditary or acquired; the acquired form, in turn, can be primary or secondary. Hereditary sideroblastic anemia commonly responds to treatment with pyridoxine. Correction of the secondary acquired form depends on the causative disorder; the primary acquired (idiopathic) form, however, resists treatment and usually proves fatal within 10 years after onset of complications or a concomitant disease.

Causes and incidence

Hereditary sideroblastic anemia appears to be transmitted by X-linked inheritance, occurring mostly in young males; females are carriers and usually show no signs of this disorder.

The acquired form may be secondary to ingestion of or exposure to toxins, such as alcohol and lead, or to certain drugs. It can also occur as a complication of other diseases, such as rheumatoid arthritis, lupus erythematosus, multiple myeloma, tuberculosis, and severe infections.

The primary acquired form, known as refractory anemia with ringed sideroblasts, is most common in elderly people. It's commonly associated with thrombocytopenia or leukopenia as part of a myelodysplastic syndrome.

In sideroblastic anemia, normoblasts fail to use iron to synthesize Hb. As a result, iron is deposited in the mitochondria of normoblasts, which are then termed ringed sideroblasts.

Signs and symptoms

Sideroblastic anemias usually produce nonspecific clinical effects, which may exist for several years before being identified.

Such effects include anorexia, fatigue, weakness, dizziness, pale skin and mucous membranes and, occasionally, enlarged lymph nodes. Heart and liver failure may develop due to excessive iron accumulation in these organs, causing dyspnea, exertional angina, slight jaundice, and hepatosplenomegaly. Hereditary sideroblastic anemia is associated with increased GI absorption of iron, causing signs of hemosiderosis. Additional symptoms in secondary sideroblastic anemia depend upon the underlying cause.

Diagnosis

CONFIRMING DIAGNOSIS *Ringed sideroblasts on microscopic examination of bone marrow aspirate, stained with Prussian blue or alizarin red dye, confirm this diagnosis. (See* Ringed sideroblast.*)*

Microscopic examination of blood shows erythrocytes to be hypochromic or normochromic and slightly macrocytic. Red cell precursors may be megaloblastic, with anisocytosis (abnormal variation in red blood cell [RBC] size) and poikilocytosis (abnormal variation in RBC shape). Unlike iron deficiency anemia, sideroblastic anemia lowers Hb levels and raises serum iron and transferrin levels. In turn, faulty Hb production raises urobilinogen and bilirubin levels. Platelets and leukocytes remain normal, but, occasionally, thrombocytopenia or leukopenia occurs.

Treatment

Treatment of sideroblastic anemias depends on the underlying cause. The hereditary form usually responds to several weeks of treatment with high doses of pyridoxine (vitamin B_6). The acquired secondary form generally subsides after the causative drug or toxin is removed, or the underlying condition is adequately treated. Folic acid supplements may also be beneficial when concomitant megaloblastic nuclear changes in RBC precursors are present. Elderly patients with sideroblastic anemia (usually the primary acquired form) are less likely to improve quickly and are more likely to develop serious complications. Deferoxamine may be used to treat chronic iron overload in selected patients.

RINGED SIDEROBLAST

Electron microscopy shows large iron deposits in the mitochondria that surround the nucleus, forming the characteristic ringed sideroblast.

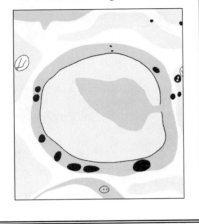

Carefully crossmatched transfusions (providing needed Hb) or high doses of androgens are effective palliative measures for some patients with the primary acquired form of sideroblastic anemia. However, this form is essentially refractory to treatment and usually leads to death from acute leukemia or from respiratory or cardiac complications.

Some patients with sideroblastic anemia may benefit from phlebotomy to prevent hemochromatosis (the accumulation of iron in body tissues). Phlebotomy steps up the rate of erythropoiesis and uses up excess iron stores; thus, it reduces serum and total-body iron levels.

Special considerations

■ Administer medications as ordered. Teach the patient the importance of continuing prescribed therapy, even after he begins to feel better.

■ Provide frequent rest periods if the patient becomes easily fatigued.

■ If phlebotomy is scheduled, explain the procedure thoroughly to help reduce anxiety. If this procedure must be repeated frequently, provide a high-protein diet to help

THALASSEMIA MAJOR

X-rays show a characteristic skull abnormality in thalassemia major: diploetic fibers extending from the internal lamina.

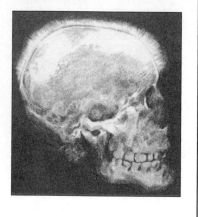

replace the protein lost during phlebotomy. Encourage the patient to follow a similar diet at home.

■ Always inquire about the possibility of exposure to lead in the home (especially for children) or on the job.

■ Identify patients who abuse alcohol; refer them for appropriate therapy.

Thalassemia

Thalassemia, a hereditary group of hemolytic anemias, is characterized by defective synthesis in the polypeptide chains necessary for hemoglobin (Hb) production. Consequently, red blood cell (RBC) synthesis is also impaired.

ß-thalassemia is the most common form of this disorder. It results from defective beta polypeptide chain synthesis and occurs in three clinical forms: major, intermedia, and minor. The resulting anemia's severity depends on whether the patient is homozygous or heterozygous for the thalassemic trait. The prognosis for ß-thalassemia varies. People with thalassemia major seldom survive to adulthood; children with thalassemia intermedia develop normally into adulthood, although puberty is usually delayed; people with thalassemia minor can expect a normal life span.

Causes and incidence

Thalassemia major and *thalassemia intermedia* result from homozygous inheritance of the partially dominant autosomal gene responsible for this trait. *Thalassemia minor* results from heterozygous inheritance of the same gene. In these disorders, total or partial deficiency of beta polypeptide chain production impairs Hb synthesis and results in continual production of fetal Hb, lasting even past the neonatal period.

Thalassemia is most common in people of Mediterranean ancestry (especially Italian and Greek) but also occurs in blacks and people from southern China, southeast Asia, and India.

Signs and symptoms

In thalassemia major (also known as *Cooley's anemia, Mediterranean disease,* and *erythroblastic anemia*), the neonate is well at birth but develops severe anemia, bone abnormalities, failure to thrive, and life-threatening complications. (See *Thalassemia major.*) In many cases, the first signs are pallor and yellow skin and scleras in infants ages 3 to 6 months. Later clinical features, in addition to severe anemia, include splenomegaly or hepatomegaly, with abdominal enlargement, frequent infections, bleeding tendencies (especially toward epistaxis), and anorexia.

Children with thalassemia major typically have small bodies and large heads and may also be mentally retarded. Infants may have mongoloid features because bone marrow hyperactivity has thickened the bone at the base of the nose. As these children grow older, they become susceptible to pathologic fractures as a result of expansion of the marrow cavities with thinning of the long bones. They're also subject to cardiac arrhythmias, heart failure, and other complications that result from iron deposits in the heart and in other tissues from repeated blood transfusions.

Thalassemia intermedia comprises moderate thalassemic disorders in homozygotes. Patients with this condition show some degree of anemia, jaundice, and splenomegaly and, possibly, signs of hemosiderosis due to increased intestinal absorption of iron.

Thalassemia minor may cause mild anemia but usually produces no symptoms and is commonly overlooked. It should be differentiated from iron deficiency anemia.

Diagnosis

In thalassemia major, laboratory results show lowered RBC count and Hb level, microcytosis, and elevated reticulocyte, bilirubin, and urinary and fecal urobilinogen levels. A low serum folate level indicates increased folate utilization by the hypertrophied bone marrow. A peripheral blood smear reveals target cells, microcytes, pale nucleated RBCs, and marked anisocytosis. X-rays of the skull and long bones show thinning and widening of the marrow space because of overactive bone marrow. The bones of the skull and vertebrae may appear granular; long bones may show areas of osteoporosis. The phalanges may also be deformed (rectangular or biconvex). Quantitative Hb studies show a significant rise in HbF and a slight increase in HbA_2. Diagnosis must rule out iron deficiency anemia, which also produces hypochromia (slightly lowered Hb level) and microcytic (notably small) RBCs.

In thalassemia intermedia, laboratory results show hypochromia and microcytic RBCs, but the anemia is less severe than that in thalassemia major. In thalassemia minor, laboratory results show hypochromia and microcytic RBCs. Quantitative Hb studies show a significant increase in HbA_2 levels and a moderate rise in HbF levels.

Treatment

Treatment of thalassemia major is essentially supportive. For example, infections require prompt treatment with appropriate antibiotics. Folic acid supplements help maintain folic acid levels in the face of increased requirements. Transfusions of packed RBCs raise Hb levels but must be used judiciously to minimize iron overload. In addition, patients who receive blood transfusions should avoid iron supplements and oxidative drugs because iron

levels can become toxic. Those who receive significant numbers of blood transfusions may require chelation therapy to remove iron from the body. Bone marrow transplantation is being investigated as a treatment, with success found mostly in children.

Thalassemia intermedia and thalassemia minor generally don't require treatment.

Iron supplements are contraindicated in all forms of thalassemia.

Special considerations

■ During and after RBC transfusions for thalassemia major, watch for adverse reactions — shaking chills, fever, rash, itching, and hives.
■ Stress the importance of good nutrition, meticulous wound care, periodic dental checkups, and other measures to prevent infection.
■ Discuss with the parents of a young patient various options for healthy physical and creative outlets. Such a child must avoid strenuous athletic activity because of increased oxygen demand and the tendency toward pathologic fractures, but he may participate in less stressful activities.
■ Teach parents to watch for signs of hepatitis and iron overload, which are always possible with frequent transfusions.
■ Because parents may have questions about the vulnerability of future offspring, refer them for genetic counseling. Also refer adult patients with thalassemia minor and thalassemia intermedia for genetic counseling; they need to recognize the risk of transmitting thalassemia major to their children if they marry another person with thalassemia. If such people choose to marry and have children, their children should be evaluated for thalassemia by age 1. Be sure to tell people with thalassemia minor that their condition is benign.

Iron deficiency anemia

Iron deficiency anemia is caused by an inadequate supply of iron for optimal formation of red blood cells (RBCs), resulting in smaller (microcytic) cells with less color on staining. Body stores of iron, including plasma iron, decrease, as do levels of trans-

ABSORPTION AND STORAGE OF IRON

Iron, which is essential to erythropoiesis, is abundant throughout the body. Two-thirds of total body iron is found in hemoglobin (Hb); the other third, mostly in the reticuloendothelial system (liver, spleen, bone marrow), with small amounts in muscle, blood serum, and body cells.

Adequate dietary ingestion of iron and recirculation of iron released from disintegrating red cells maintain iron supplies. The duodenum and upper part of the small intestine absorb dietary iron. Such absorption depends on gastric acid content, the amount of reducing substances (ascorbic acid, for example) present in the alimentary canal, and dietary iron intake. If iron intake is deficient, the body gradually depletes its iron stores, causing decreased Hb levels and, eventually, symptoms of iron deficiency anemia.

■ blood loss secondary to drug-induced GI bleeding (from anticoagulants, aspirin, and steroids) or due to heavy menses, hemorrhage from trauma, GI ulcers, esophageal varices, or cancer
■ pregnancy, which diverts maternal iron to the fetus for erythropoiesis
■ intravascular hemolysis-induced hemoglobinuria or paroxysmal nocturnal hemoglobinuria
■ mechanical erythrocyte trauma caused by a prosthetic heart valve or vena cava filters.

A common disease worldwide, iron deficiency anemia affects 10% to 30% of the adult population of the United States. It occurs most commonly in premenopausal women, infants (particularly premature or low-birth-weight neonates), children, and adolescents (especially girls). Persons who are at increased risk for iron deficiency include those of low socioeconomic status who don't get a well-balanced diet that includes iron-rich foods.

Signs and symptoms
Because of the gradual progression of iron deficiency anemia, many patients are initially asymptomatic except for symptoms of any underlying condition. They tend not to seek medical treatment until anemia is severe. At advanced stages, decreased Hb levels and the consequent decrease in the blood's oxygen-carrying capacity cause the patient to develop dyspnea on exertion, fatigue, listlessness, pallor, inability to concentrate, irritability, headache, and a susceptibility to infection. Decreased oxygen perfusion causes the heart to compensate with increased cardiac output and tachycardia.

In chronic iron deficiency anemia, nails become spoon-shaped and brittle, the mouth's corners crack, the tongue turns smooth, and the patient complains of dysphagia or may develop pica. Associated neuromuscular effects include vasomotor disturbances, numbness and tingling of the extremities, and neuralgic pain.

Diagnosis
Blood studies (serum iron levels, total iron-binding capacity, and ferritin levels) and stores in bone marrow may confirm iron

ferrin, which binds with and transports iron. Insufficient body stores of iron lead to a depleted RBC mass and, in turn, to a decreased hemoglobin (Hb) concentration (hypochromia) and decreased oxygen-carrying capacity of the blood. (See *Absorption and storage of iron.*)

Causes and incidence
Iron deficiency anemia may result from:
■ inadequate dietary intake of iron (less than 1 to 2 mg/day), such as in prolonged unsupplemented breast-feeding or bottle-feeding of infants or during periods of stress such as rapid growth in children and adolescents
■ iron malabsorption, such as in chronic diarrhea, partial or total gastrectomy, chronic diverticulosis, and malabsorption syndromes, such as celiac disease and pernicious anemia

deficiency anemia. However, the results of these tests can be misleading because of complicating factors, such as infection, pneumonia, blood transfusion, or iron supplements. Characteristic blood test results include:

- low Hb levels (in males, less than 12 g/dl; in females, less than 10 g/dl)
- low hematocrit (in males, less than 39%; in females, less than 35%)
- low serum iron levels, with high binding capacity
- low serum ferritin levels
- low RBC count, with microcytic and hypochromic cells (in early stages, RBC count may be normal, except in infants and children)
- decreased mean corpuscular Hb in severe anemia.

Bone marrow studies reveal depleted or absent iron stores (done by staining) and normoblastic hyperplasia.

Diagnosis must rule out other forms of anemia, such as those that result from thalassemia minor, cancer, and chronic inflammatory, hepatic, and renal disease.

Treatment

The first priority of treatment is to determine the underlying cause of anemia. Once this is determined, iron replacement therapy can begin. Treatment of choice is an oral preparation of iron or a combination of iron and ascorbic acid (which enhances iron absorption). However, in some cases, iron may have to be administered parenterally — for instance, if the patient is noncompliant to the oral preparation, if he needs more iron than he can take orally, if malabsorption prevents adequate iron absorption, or if a maximum rate of Hb regeneration is desired.

Because total dose I.V. infusion of supplemental iron is painless and requires fewer injections, it's usually preferred to I.M. administration. Pregnant patients and geriatric patients with severe anemia, for example, should receive a total dose infusion of iron dextran in normal saline solution over 8 hours. To minimize the risk of an allergic reaction to iron, an I.V. test dose of 0.5 ml should be given first. For more patient care information, see *Supportive management of patients with anemia,* page 1034.

Special considerations

- Monitor the patient's compliance with the prescribed iron supplement therapy. Advise the patient not to stop therapy even if he feels better, because replacement of iron stores takes time.
- Tell the patient he may take iron supplements with a meal to decrease gastric irritation. Advise him to avoid milk, milk products, and antacids because they interfere with iron absorption; however, vitamin C can increase absorption.
- Warn the patient that iron supplements may result in dark green or black stools and can cause constipation.
- Instruct the patient to drink liquid supplemental iron through a straw to prevent staining his teeth.
- Tell the patient to report reactions, such as nausea, vomiting, diarrhea, constipation, fever, or severe stomach pain, which may require a dosage adjustment.
- If the patient receives I.V. iron, monitor the infusion rate carefully and observe for an allergic reaction. Stop the infusion and begin supportive treatment immediately if the patient shows signs of an adverse reaction. Also, watch for dizziness and headache and for thrombophlebitis around the I.V. site.
- Use the Z-track injection method when administering iron I.M. to prevent skin discoloration, scarring, and irritating iron deposits in the skin. (See *How to inject iron solutions,* page 1035.)
- Because an iron deficiency may recur, advise regular checkups and blood studies.

Health professionals can play a vital role in preventing iron deficiency anemia by:
- teaching the basics of a nutritionally balanced diet — red meats, green vegetables, eggs, whole wheat products, and iron-fortified bread. (However, no food in itself contains enough iron to *treat* iron deficiency anemia; an average-sized person with anemia would have to eat at least 10 lb of steak daily to receive therapeutic amounts of iron.)
- emphasizing the need for high-risk individuals — such as premature infants, children younger than age 2, and pregnant women — to receive prophylactic oral iron, as ordered by a physician. (Children younger than age 2 should also receive sup-

SUPPORTIVE MANAGEMENT OF PATIENTS WITH ANEMIA

To meet the anemic patient's nutritional needs:

- If the patient is fatigued, urge him to eat small, frequent meals throughout the day.
- If the patient has oral lesions, suggest soft, cool, bland foods.
- If the patient has dyspepsia, eliminate spicy foods, and include milk and dairy products in his diet.
- If the patient is anorexic and irritable, encourage his family to bring his favorite foods from home (unless his diet is restricted) and to keep him company during meals, if possible.

To set limitations on activities:

- Assess the effect of a specific activity by monitoring pulse rate during the activity. If the patient's pulse accelerates rapidly and he develops hypotension with hyperpnea, diaphoresis, lightheadedness, palpitations, shortness of breath, or weakness, the activity is too strenuous.
- Tell the patient to pace his activities and to allow for frequent rest periods.

To decrease susceptibility to infection:

- Use strict sterile technique.
- Isolate the patient from infectious persons.
- Instruct the patient to avoid crowds and other sources of infection. Encourage him to practice good hand-washing technique. Stress the importance of receiving necessary immunizations and prompt medical treatment for any sign of infection.

To prepare the patient for diagnostic testing:

- Explain erythropoiesis, the function of blood, and the purpose of diagnostic and therapeutic procedures.
- Tell the patient how he can participate in diagnostic testing. Give him an honest description of the pain or discomfort he will probably experience.
- If possible, schedule all tests to avoid disrupting the patient's meals, sleep, and visiting hours.

To prevent complications:

- Observe for signs of bleeding that may exacerbate anemia. Check stool for occult bleeding. Assess for ecchymoses, gingival bleeding, and hematuria. Monitor vital signs frequently.
- If the patient is confined to strict bed rest, assist with range-of-motion exercises and frequent turning, coughing, and deep breathing.
- If blood transfusions are needed for severe anemia (hemoglobin level less than 5 g/dl), give washed red blood cells, as ordered, in partial exchange if evidence of pump failure is present. Carefully monitor for signs of circulatory overload or transfusion reaction. Watch for a change in pulse rate, blood pressure, or respiratory rate, or onset of fever, chills, pruritus, or edema. If any of these signs develop, stop the transfusion and notify the physician.
- Warn the patient to move about or change positions slowly to minimize dizziness induced by cerebral hypoxia.

plemental cereals and formulas high in iron.)

- assessing a family's dietary habits for iron intake and noting the influence of childhood eating patterns, cultural food preferences, and family income on adequate nutrition.
- encouraging families with deficient iron intake to eat meat, fish, or poultry; whole or enriched grain; and foods high in ascorbic acid.
- carefully assessing a patient's drug history because certain drugs, such as pancreatic enzymes and vitamin E, may interfere with iron metabolism and absorption and because aspirin, steroids, and other drugs may cause GI bleeding. (Teach patients who must take gastric irritants to take these medications with meals.)

HOW TO INJECT IRON SOLUTIONS

For deep I.M. injections of iron solutions, use the Z-track technique to avoid subcutaneous irritation and discoloration from leaking medication.

Choose a 19G to 20G, 2″ to 3″ needle. After drawing up the solution, change to a fresh needle to avoid tracking the solution through to subcutaneous tissue. Draw 0.5 cc of air into the syringe as an "air lock."

Displace the skin and fat at the injection site (in the upper outer quadrant of the buttocks or the ventro-gluteal site only) firmly to one side. Clean the area and insert the needle. Aspirate to check for entry into a blood vessel. Inject the solution slowly, followed by the 0.5 cc of air in the syringe. Wait 10 seconds, then pull the needle straight out, and release tissues.

Apply direct pressure to the site but don't massage it. Caution the patient against vigorous exercise for 15 to 30 minutes.

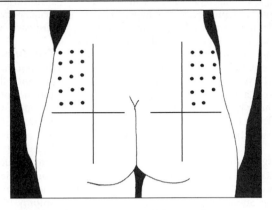

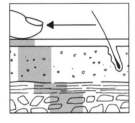

1. Displace tissues.

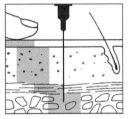

2. Inject solution.

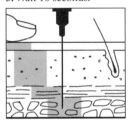

3. Wait 10 seconds.

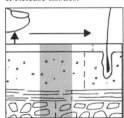

4. Release tissues.

POLYCYTHEMIAS

Polycythemia vera

Polycythemia vera is a chronic, myeloproliferative disorder characterized by increased red blood cell (RBC) mass, leukocytosis, thrombocytosis, and increased hemoglobin concentration, with normal or increased plasma volume. This disease is also known as *primary polycythemia, erythremia, polycythemia rubra vera, splenomegalic polycythemia,* and *Vaquez-Osler disease.*

The prognosis depends on the patient's age at diagnosis, the type of treatment used, and complications. Mortality is high if polycythemia is untreated or is associated with leukemia or myeloid metaplasia.

Causes and incidence

In polycythemia vera, uncontrolled and rapid cellular reproduction and maturation cause proliferation or hyperplasia of all bone marrow cells (panmyelosis). The cause of such uncontrolled cellular activity is unknown but it's probably due to a multipotential stem cell defect.

Polycythemia vera usually occurs between ages 40 and 60, most commonly among males of Jewish ancestry; it seldom affects children or blacks and doesn't appear to be familial.

Signs and symptoms

Increased RBC mass results in hyperviscosity and inhibits blood flow to microcirculation. Subsequently, increased viscosity, diminished velocity, and thrombocytosis promote intravascular thrombosis. In early stages, polycythemia vera usually produces no symptoms. (Increased hematocrit [HCT] may be an incidental finding.) However, as altered circulation secondary to increased RBC mass produces hypervolemia and hyperviscosity, the patient may complain of a feeling of fullness in the head, headache, dizziness, and other symptoms, depending on the body system affected. The patient may also complain of severe itching after a warm or hot shower. Hyperviscosity may lead to thrombosis of smaller vessels with ruddy cyanosis of the nose and clubbing of the digits.

Paradoxically, hemorrhage is a complication of polycythemia vera. It may be due to defective platelet function or to hyperviscosity and the local effects from excess RBCs exerting pressure on distended venous and capillary walls. (See *Clinical features of polycythemia vera.*)

Diagnosis

Laboratory studies confirm polycythemia vera by showing increased RBC mass and normal arterial oxygen saturation in association with splenomegaly or two of the following: thrombocytosis, leukocytosis, elevated leukocyte alkaline phosphatase level, or elevated serum vitamin B_{12} level or unbound B_{12}-binding capacity.

Another common finding is increased uric acid production, leading to hyperuricemia and hyperuricuria. Other laboratory results include increased blood histamine levels, decreased serum iron concentration, and decreased or absent urinary erythropoietin. Bone marrow biopsy reveals panmyelosis.

Treatment

Phlebotomy can reduce RBC mass promptly. The frequency of phlebotomy and the amount of blood removed each time depend on the patient's condition. Typically, 350 to 500 ml of blood can be removed every other day until the HCT is reduced to the low-normal range. After repeated phlebotomies, the patient develops iron deficiency, which stabilizes RBC production and reduces the need for phlebotomy. Pheresis permits the return of plasma to the patient, diluting the blood and reducing hypovolemic symptoms.

Phlebotomy doesn't reduce the white blood cell or platelet count and won't control the hyperuricemia associated with marrow cell proliferation. For severe symptoms, myelosuppressive therapy may be used. Chemotherapeutic agents may be used to suppress the bone marrow, but these agents may cause leukemia and should be reserved for older patients and those with problems uncontrolled by phlebotomy. The current preferred myelosuppressive agent is hydroxyurea, which isn't associated with leukemia. Patients who have had previous thrombotic problems should be considered for myelosuppressive therapy. The use of antiplatelet therapy is controversial because it may cause gastric bleeding. Allopurinol may be given for hyperuricemia.

Special considerations

If the patient requires phlebotomy, explain the procedure, and reassure him that it will relieve distressing symptoms. Check blood pressure, pulse rate, and respiratory rate. During phlebotomy, make sure the patient is lying down comfortably to prevent vertigo and syncope. Stay alert for tachycardia, clamminess, or complaints of vertigo. If these effects occur, the procedure should be stopped.

■ Immediately after phlebotomy, check blood pressure and pulse rate. Have the patient sit up for about 5 minutes before al-

CLINICAL FEATURES OF POLYCYTHEMIA VERA

Signs and symptoms	Causes
Eye, ear, nose, and throat	
■ Visual disturbances (blurring, diplopia, scotoma, engorged veins of fundus and retina) and congestion of conjunctiva, retina, retinal veins, oral mucous membrane	■ Hypervolemia and hyperviscosity
■ Epistaxis or gingival bleeding	■ Engorgement of capillary beds
Central nervous system	
■ Headache or fullness in the head, lethargy, weakness, fatigue, syncope, tinnitus, paresthesia of digits, and impaired mentation	■ Hypervolemia and hyperviscosity
Cardiovascular system	
■ Hypertension	■ Hypervolemia and hyperviscosity
■ Intermittent claudication, thrombosis and emboli, angina, thrombophlebitis	■ Hypervolemia, thrombocytosis, and vascular disease
■ Hemorrhage	■ Engorgement of capillary beds
Skin	
■ Pruritus (especially after hot bath)	■ Basophilia (secondary histamine release)
■ Urticaria	■ Altered histamine metabolism
■ Ruddy cyanosis	■ Hypervolemia and hyperviscosity due to congested vessels, increased oxyhemoglobin, and reduced hemoglobin
■ Night sweats	■ Hypermetabolism
■ Ecchymosis	■ Hemorrhage
GI system	
■ Epigastric distress	■ Hypervolemia and hyperviscosity
■ Early satiety and fullness	■ Hepatosplenomegaly
■ Peptic ulcer pain	■ Gastric thrombosis and hemorrhage
■ Hepatosplenomegaly	■ Congestion, extramedullary hemopoiesis, and myeloid metaplasia
■ Weight loss	■ Hypermetabolism
Respiratory system	
■ Dyspnea	■ Hypervolemia and hyperviscosity
Musculoskeletal system	
■ Joint symptoms	■ Increased urate production secondary to nucleoprotein turnover

lowing him to walk; this prevents vasovagal attack or orthostatic hypotension. Also, have him drink 24 oz (710 ml) of juice or water.

■ Tell the patient to watch for and report signs or symptoms of iron deficiency (pallor, weight loss, asthenia [weakness], and glossitis).

■ Keep the patient active and ambulatory to prevent thrombosis. If bed rest is absolutely necessary, prescribe a daily program of both active and passive range-of-motion exercises.

■ Watch for complications: hypervolemia, thrombocytosis, and signs or symptoms of an impending stroke (decreased sensation, numbness, transitory paralysis, fleeting blindness, headache, and epistaxis).

■ Regularly examine the patient closely for bleeding. Tell him which are the most common bleeding sites (such as the nose, gingiva, and skin) so he can check for bleeding. Advise him to report any abnormal bleeding promptly.

■ To compensate for increased uric acid production, give additional fluids, administer allopurinol, and alkalinize the urine to prevent uric acid calculi.

■ If the patient has symptom-producing splenomegaly, suggest or provide small, frequent meals, followed by a rest period, to prevent nausea and vomiting.

■ Report acute abdominal pain immediately; it may signal splenic infarction, renal calculi, or abdominal organ thrombosis.

During myelosuppressive treatment:

■ Monitor complete blood count and platelet count before and during therapy. Warn the outpatient who develops leukopenia that his resistance to infection is low; advise him to avoid crowds and watch for the symptoms of infection. If leukopenia develops in a hospitalized patient who needs reverse isolation, follow hospital guidelines. If thrombocytopenia develops, tell the patient to watch for signs of bleeding (blood in urine, nosebleeds, and black stool).

■ Tell the patient about possible reactions (nausea, vomiting, and risk of infection) to alkylating agents. Alopecia may follow the use of busulfan, cyclophosphamide, and uracil mustard; sterile hemorrhagic cystitis may follow the use of cyclophosphamide (forcing fluids can prevent it). Watch for and report all reactions. If nausea and vomiting occur, begin antiemetic therapy and adjust the patient's diet.

Spurious polycythemia

Spurious polycythemia, also known as *relative polycythemia, stress erythrocytosis, stress polycythemia, benign polycythemia, Gaisböck's syndrome,* and *pseudopolycythemia,* is characterized by increased hematocrit (HCT) and normal or decreased red blood cell (RBC) total mass; it results from de-

creasing plasma volume and subsequent hemoconcentration.

Causes and incidence

There are three possible causes of spurious polycythemia:

■ Dehydration — Conditions that promote severe fluid loss decrease plasma levels and lead to hemoconcentration. Such conditions include persistent vomiting or diarrhea, burns, adrenocortical insufficiency, aggressive diuretic therapy, decreased fluid intake, diabetic acidosis, and renal disease.

■ Hemoconcentration due to stress — Nervous stress leads to hemoconcentration by some unknown mechanism (possibly by temporarily decreasing circulating plasma volume or vascular redistribution of erythrocytes). This form of erythrocytosis (chronically elevated HCT) is particularly common in the middle-aged man who's a chronic smoker and a type A personality (tense, hard driving, and anxious).

■ High normal RBC mass and low normal plasma volume — In many patients, an increased HCT merely reflects a normally high RBC mass and low plasma volume. This is particularly common in patients who don't smoke, aren't obese, and have no history of hypertension.

Other factors that may be associated with spurious polycythemia include hypertension, thromboembolitic disease, elevated serum cholesterol and uric acid levels, and familial tendency. It usually affects middle-aged people and occurs more commonly in men than in women.

Signs and symptoms

The patient with spurious polycythemia usually has no specific symptoms but may have vague complaints, such as headaches, dizziness, and fatigue. Less commonly, he may develop diaphoresis, dyspnea, and claudication.

Typically, the patient has a ruddy appearance, a short neck, slight hypertension, and a tendency to hypoventilate when recumbent. He shows no associated hepatosplenomegaly but may have cardiac or pulmonary disease.

Diagnosis

Hemoglobin levels, HCT, and RBC count are elevated; RBC mass, arterial oxygen saturation, and bone marrow are normal. Plasma volume may be decreased or normal. Hypercholesterolemia, hyperlipidemia, or hyperuricemia may be present. Spurious polycythemia is distinguishable from true polycythemia vera by its characteristic normal RBC mass, elevated HCT, and the absence of leukocytosis.

Treatment

The principal goals of treatment are to prevent life-threatening thromboembolism and to correct dehydration. Rehydration with appropriate fluids and electrolytes is the primary therapy for spurious polycythemia secondary to dehydration. Therapy must also include appropriate measures to prevent continuing fluid loss.

Special considerations

■ During rehydration, carefully monitor intake and output to maintain fluid and electrolyte balance.

■ To prevent thromboemboli in predisposed patients, suggest regular exercise and a low-cholesterol diet. Antilipemics may also be necessary. Reduced calorie intake may be required for the obese patient.

■ Whenever appropriate, suggest counseling about the patient's work habits and lack of relaxation. If the patient smokes, make sure he understands how important it is that he stop. Refer him to a smoking-cessation program if necessary.

■ Emphasize the need for follow-up examinations every 3 to 4 months after leaving the hospital.

■ Thoroughly explain spurious polycythemia, diagnostic measures, and therapy. The hard-driving person predisposed to spurious polycythemia is likely to be more inquisitive and anxious than the average patient. Answer questions honestly, but take care to reassure him that he can effectively control symptoms by complying with the prescribed treatment.

Secondary polycythemia

Secondary polycythemia (also called *reactive polycythemia*) is a disorder characterized by excessive production of circulating red blood cells (RBCs) due to hypoxia, tumor, or disease.

Causes and incidence

Secondary polycythemia may result from increased production of erythropoietin. This hormone, which is possibly produced and secreted in the kidneys, stimulates bone marrow production of RBCs. Increased production may be a compensatory physiologic response to hypoxemia, which may result from:

■ chronic obstructive pulmonary disease
■ hemoglobin (Hb) abnormalities (such as carboxyhemoglobinemia, which is seen in heavy smokers)
■ heart failure (causing a decreased ventilation-perfusion ratio)
■ right-to-left shunting of blood in the heart (as in transposition of the great vessels)
■ central or peripheral alveolar hypoventilation (as in barbiturate intoxication or pickwickian syndrome)
■ low oxygen content at high altitudes.

Increased production of erythropoietin may also be an inappropriate (pathologic) response to renal disease (such as renal vascular impairment, renal cysts, or hydronephrosis), to central nervous system disease (such as encephalitis and parkinsonism), to neoplasms (such as renal tumors, uterine myomas, or cerebellar hemangiomas), or to endocrine disorders (such as Cushing's syndrome, Bartter's syndrome, or pheochromocytomas). Rarely, secondary polycythemia results from a recessive genetic trait.

Secondary polycythemia occurs in approximately 2 out of every 100,000 people living at or near sea level; incidence rises among those living at high altitudes.

Signs and symptoms

In the hypoxic patient, suggestive physical findings include ruddy cyanotic skin, emphysema, and hypoxemia without hepatosplenomegaly or hypertension. Clubbing of the fingers may occur if the underlying disease is cardiovascular. When secondary polycythemia isn't caused by hypoxemia, it's usually an incidental finding during treatment of an underlying disease.

Diagnosis

CONFIRMING DIAGNOSIS
Laboratory values for secondary polycythemia include increased RBC mass (increased hematocrit, Hb levels, and mean corpuscular volume and mean corpuscular Hb values) and urinary erythropoietin and blood histamine levels, with decreased or normal arterial oxygen saturation. Bone marrow biopsies reveal hyperplasia confined to the erythroid series.

Unlike polycythemia vera, secondary polycythemia isn't associated with leukocytosis or thrombocytosis.

Treatment

The goal of treatment is correction of the underlying disease or environmental condition. In severe secondary polycythemia in which altitude is a contributing factor, relocation may be advisable. If secondary polycythemia has produced hazardous hyperviscosity or if the patient doesn't respond to treatment of the primary disease, reduction of blood volume by phlebotomy or pheresis may be effective. Emergency phlebotomy is indicated for prevention of impending vascular occlusion or before emergency surgery. In the latter case, it's usually advisable to remove excess RBCs and reinfuse the patient's plasma.

Because a patient with polycythemia has an increased risk of hemorrhage during and after surgery, elective surgery should be avoided until polycythemia is controlled. Generally, secondary polycythemia disappears when the primary disease is corrected.

Special considerations

■ Keep the patient as active as possible to decrease the risk of thrombosis due to increased blood viscosity.
■ Reduce calorie and sodium intake to counteract the tendency toward hypertension.
■ Before and after phlebotomy, check blood pressure with the patient lying down. After the procedure, have the patient

drink 24 oz (710 ml) of water or juice. To prevent syncope, have him sit upright for about 5 minutes before walking.
■ Emphasize the importance of regular blood studies (every 2 to 3 months), even after the disease is controlled.
■ Teach the patient and his family about the underlying disorder. Help them understand its relationship to polycythemia and the measures needed to control both.
■ Teach the patient to recognize symptoms of recurring polycythemia and the importance of reporting them promptly.

HEMORRHAGIC DISORDERS

Allergic purpuras

Allergic purpura, a nonthrombocytopenic purpura, is an acute or chronic vascular inflammation affecting the skin, joints, and GI and genitourinary (GU) tracts, in association with allergy symptoms. When allergic purpura primarily affects the GI tract, with accompanying joint pain, it's called *Henoch-Schönlein syndrome,* or *anaphylactoid purpura.* However, the term *allergic purpura* applies to purpura associated with many other conditions such as erythema nodosum. An acute attack of allergic purpura can last for several weeks and is potentially fatal (usually from renal failure); however, most patients do recover.

Fully developed allergic purpura is persistent and debilitating, possibly leading to chronic glomerulonephritis (especially following a streptococcal infection).

Causes and incidence

The most common identifiable cause of allergic purpura is probably an autoimmune reaction directed against vascular walls, triggered by a bacterial infection (particularly streptococcal infection). Typically, upper respiratory tract infection occurs 1 to 3 weeks before the onset of symptoms. Other possible causes include allergic reactions to some drugs and vaccines, to insect bites, and to some foods (such as wheat, eggs, milk, and chocolate).

Allergic purpura affects more males than females and is most prevalent in children ages 3 to 7. The prognosis is more favorable for children than adults.

Signs and symptoms

Characteristic skin lesions of allergic purpura are purple, macular, ecchymotic, and of varying size. They're caused by vascular leakage into the skin and mucous membranes. (See *Purpuric lesions.*) The lesions usually appear in symmetric patterns on the arms, legs, and buttocks and are accompanied by pruritus, paresthesia and, occasionally, angioneurotic edema. In children, skin lesions are generally urticarial and expand and become hemorrhagic. Scattered petechiae may appear on the legs, buttocks, and perineum.

Henoch-Schönlein syndrome commonly produces transient or severe colic, tenesmus (spasmodic contraction of the anal sphincter) and constipation, vomiting, and edema or hemorrhage of the mucous membranes of the bowel, resulting in GI bleeding, occult blood in the stool and, possibly, intussusception. Such GI abnormalities may *precede* overt, cutaneous signs of purpura. Musculoskeletal symptoms, such as rheumatoid pains and periarticular effusions, mostly affect the legs and feet.

In 25% to 50% of patients, allergic purpura is associated with GU signs and symptoms: nephritis; renal hemorrhages that may cause microscopic hematuria and disturb renal function; bleeding from the mucosal surfaces of the ureters, bladder, or urethra; and, occasionally, glomerulonephritis. Also possible are moderate and irregular fever, headache, anorexia, and localized edema of the hands, feet, or scalp.

Diagnosis

No laboratory test clearly identifies allergic purpura (although white blood cell count and erythrocyte sedimentation rate are elevated). Diagnosis therefore necessitates careful clinical observation, in many cases during the second or third attack. Except for a positive tourniquet test (a test to assess the capillaries' ability to withstand increased pressure), coagulation and platelet function tests are usually normal. Small-bowel X-rays may reveal areas of transient

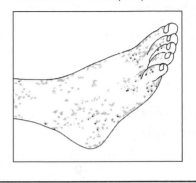

PURPURIC LESIONS

Lesions of allergic purpura, such as those pictured on the foot and leg below, characteristically vary in size.

edema; in many cases, tests for blood in the urine and stool are positive. Increased blood urea nitrogen and creatinine levels may indicate renal involvement. Diagnosis must rule out other forms of nonthrombocytopenic purpura.

Treatment

Treatment is generally symptomatic; for example, severe allergic purpura may require steroids to relieve edema and analgesics to relieve joint and abdominal pain. Some patients with chronic renal disease may benefit from immunosuppressive therapy with azathioprine along with identification of the provocative allergen. *An accurate allergy history is essential.*

Special considerations

■ Encourage maintenance of an elimination diet to help identify specific allergenic foods so these foods can be eliminated from the patient's diet.
■ Monitor skin lesions and level of pain. Provide analgesics as needed.
■ Watch carefully for complications: GI and GU tract bleeding, edema, nausea, vomiting, headache, hypertension (with nephritis), abdominal rigidity and tenderness, and absence of stool (with intussusception).

- To prevent muscle atrophy in the bedridden patient, provide passive or active range-of-motion exercises.
- Provide emotional support and reassurance, especially if the patient is temporarily disfigured by florid skin lesions.
- After the acute stage, stress the need for the patient to *immediately* report *any* recurrence of symptoms (recurrence is most common about 6 weeks after initial onset) and to return for follow-up urinalysis as scheduled.

Hereditary hemorrhagic telangiectasia

Hereditary hemorrhagic telangiectasia (also called *Osler-Weber-Rendu syndrome*) is an inherited vascular disorder in which venules and capillaries dilate to form fragile masses of thin convoluted vessels (telangiectases), resulting in an abnormal tendency to hemorrhage. This disorder affects both sexes but may cause less severe bleeding in females.

Causes

Hereditary hemorrhagic telangiectasia is transmitted by autosomal dominant inheritance. It seldom skips generations. In its homozygous state, it may be lethal.

Signs and symptoms

Signs of hereditary hemorrhagic telangiectasia are present in childhood but increase in severity with age. Localized aggregations of dilated capillaries appear on the skin of the face, ears, scalp, hands, arms, and feet; under the nails; and on the mucous membranes of the nose, mouth, and stomach. These dilated capillaries cause frequent epistaxis, hemoptysis, and GI bleeding, possibly leading to iron deficiency anemia. (In children, epistaxis is usually the first symptom.)

Characteristic telangiectases are violet, bleed spontaneously, may be flat or raised, blanch on pressure, and are nonpulsatile. They may be associated with vascular malformations such as arteriovenous fistulas. Visceral telangiectases are common in the liver, bladder, respiratory tract, and stomach. The type and distribution of these lesions are generally similar among family members.

Generalized capillary fragility, as evidenced by spontaneous bleeding, petechiae, ecchymoses, and spider hemangiomas of varying sizes, may exist without overt telangiectasia. Rarely, vascular malformation may cause pulmonary arteriovenous fistulas; then, shunting of blood through the fistulas may lead to hypoxemia, recurring cerebral embolism, brain abscess, and clubbing of digits.

Diagnosis

Diagnosis is based principally on an established familial pattern of bleeding disorders and on clinical evidence of telangiectasia and hemorrhage. Bone marrow aspiration demonstrating depleted iron stores confirms secondary iron deficiency anemia. Hypochromic, microcytic anemia is common; abnormal platelet function may also be found. Coagulation tests are essentially irrelevant, however, because hemorrhage in telangiectasia results from weakness in the vascular wall.

Treatment

Supportive therapy includes blood transfusions for acute hemorrhage and supplemental iron administration to replace iron lost in repeated mucosal bleeding. Ancillary treatments consist of applying pressure and topical hemostatic agents to bleeding sites, cauterizing bleeding sites not readily accessible, and protecting the patient from trauma and unnecessary bleeding. An interventional radiologist may clot off large collections of abnormal blood vessels in the lungs, called *arteriovenous malformations*, by using a coiling procedure.

Parenteral administration of supplemental iron enhances absorption to maintain adequate iron stores and prevents gastric irritation. Administering antipyretics or antihistamines before blood transfusions, and using saline-washed cells, frozen blood, or other types of leukocyte-poor blood instead of whole blood may prevent febrile transfusion reactions.

The administration of estrogen has proved effective in some patients, especially when used to control epistaxis.

Special considerations

■ During the first 15 minutes of a blood transfusion, stay with the patient to observe for adverse reactions. Afterward, check again every 15 minutes for signs and symptoms of a febrile or an allergic transfusion reaction (flushing, shaking chills, fever, headache, rash, tachycardia, and hypertension) because patients with this disorder are quite susceptible to this type of reaction.

■ Observe the patient for indications of GI bleeding, such as hematemesis and melena. Instruct him to watch for and report such signs as well.

■ If the patient requires an iron supplement, stress the importance of following dosage instructions and of taking oral iron with meals to minimize gastric irritation. Warn him that iron turns stools dark green or black and may cause constipation.

■ Provide emotional and psychological support. Encourage the patient to express concerns he may have about his disease and its treatment. As much as possible, include him in care decisions.

■ Encourage fluid intake, when possible, if the patient is experiencing a bleeding episode or is hypovolemic. Monitor intake and output.

■ Provide good skin care and hygiene, and use sterile technique when caring for the patient. Lesions bleed easily, which may result in infection and skin breakdown.

■ Monitor the patient's organ function through physical examination and the comparison of laboratory tests to detect renal, hepatic, or respiratory failure.

■ Teach the patient and his family how to manage minor bleeding episodes, especially recurrent epistaxis, and how to recognize major episodes that necessitate emergency intervention.

■ Teach the patient and his family about the disease's hereditary nature. Refer him for genetic counseling, as appropriate, and to the Hereditary Hemorrhagic Telangiectasia Foundation International for support and information.

Thrombocytopenia

The most common cause of hemorrhagic disorders, thrombocytopenia is characterized by deficiency of circulating platelets. Because platelets play a vital role in coagulation, this disease poses a serious threat to hemostasis. (See *What happens in thrombocytopenia,* pages 1044 and 1045.) The prognosis is excellent in drug-induced thrombocytopenia if the offending drug is withdrawn; in such cases, recovery may be immediate. In other types, the prognosis depends on the patient's response to treatment of the underlying cause.

Causes

Thrombocytopenia may be congenital or acquired; the acquired form is more common. In either case, it usually results from decreased or defective production of platelets in the marrow (such as occurs in leukemia, aplastic anemia, or toxicity with certain drugs) or from increased destruction outside the marrow caused by an underlying disorder (such as cirrhosis of the liver, disseminated intravascular coagulation, or severe infection). Less commonly, it results from sequestration (hypersplenism and hypothermia) or platelet loss. Acquired thrombocytopenia may result from certain drugs, such as sulfonamides, antibiotics, gold salts, estrogens, or chemotherapeutic agents. (See *Causes of decreased circulating platelets,* page 1046.)

ELDER TIP *In older adults, platelet characteristics change. Granular constituents decrease and platelet-release factors increase. These changes may reflect diminished bone marrow and increased fibrinogen levels.*

An idiopathic form of thrombocytopenia commonly occurs in children. A transient form may follow viral infection (such as Epstein-Barr virus or infectious mononucleosis).

Signs and symptoms

Thrombocytopenia typically produces a sudden onset of petechiae or ecchymoses in the skin or bleeding into any mucous membrane. Nearly all patients are otherwise asymptomatic, although some may complain of malaise, fatigue, and general

PATHOPHYSIOLOGY

WHAT HAPPENS IN THROMBOCYTOPENIA

Thrombocytopenia is the most common cause of bleeding disorders and is characterized by a severe decrease in platelets. This platelet decrease can result from hematologic malignancy, radiation or drug therapy, idiopathic causes, blood transfusions, disseminated intravascular coagulation (DIC), or splenomegaly. Excessive hemorrhaging can lead to shock if interventions are delayed. This chart shows how these conditions and treatments develop into thrombocytopenic hemorrhage.

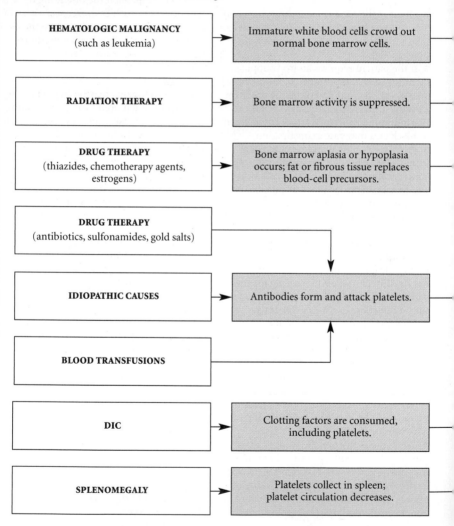

HEMATOLOGIC MALIGNANCY (such as leukemia)	Immature white blood cells crowd out normal bone marrow cells.
RADIATION THERAPY	Bone marrow activity is suppressed.
DRUG THERAPY (thiazides, chemotherapy agents, estrogens)	Bone marrow aplasia or hypoplasia occurs; fat or fibrous tissue replaces blood-cell precursors.
DRUG THERAPY (antibiotics, sulfonamides, gold salts)	
IDIOPATHIC CAUSES	Antibodies form and attack platelets.
BLOOD TRANSFUSIONS	
DIC	Clotting factors are consumed, including platelets.
SPLENOMEGALY	Platelets collect in spleen; platelet circulation decreases.

weakness. In adults, large, blood-filled bullae characteristically appear in the mouth. In severe thrombocytopenia, hemorrhage may lead to tachycardia, shortness of breath, loss of consciousness, and death.

Diagnosis

Diagnosis is based on the results of the patient history (especially a drug history), physical examination, and laboratory tests. Coagulation tests reveal a decreased platelet count (in adults, less than 100,000/µl), prolonged bleeding time, and normal prothrombin time and partial thromboplastin time. If increased destruction of platelets is causing thrombocytopenia, bone marrow studies will reveal a greater number of megakaryocytes (platelet precursors) and shortened platelet survival (several hours or days rather than the usual 7 to 10 days).

Treatment

Treatment varies with the underlying cause and may include corticosteroids or immune globulin to increase platelet production. The treatment of choice is removal of the offending agents in drug-induced thrombocytopenia or treatment of the underlying cause. Platelet transfusions are helpful only in treating complications of severe hemorrhage.

Special considerations

When caring for the patient with thrombocytopenia, take every possible precaution against bleeding.
- Protect the patient from trauma. Keep the side rails up and pad them, if possible. Promote the use of an electric razor and a soft toothbrush. Avoid invasive procedures, such as venipuncture or urinary catheterization, if possible. When venipuncture is unavoidable, be sure to exert pressure on the puncture site for at least 20 minutes or until the bleeding stops.
- Monitor platelet count daily. A 1- to 2-hour postplatelet count will aid assessment of response.
- Test stool for guaiac; dipstick urine and vomitus for blood.

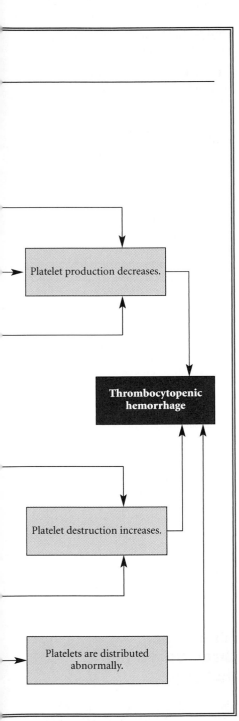

Platelet production decreases.

Thrombocytopenic hemorrhage

Platelet destruction increases.

Platelets are distributed abnormally.

CAUSES OF DECREASED CIRCULATING PLATELETS

Diminished or defective platelet production
Congenital
- Wiskott-Aldrich syndrome
- Maternal ingestion of thiazides
- Neonatal rubella

Acquired
- Aplastic anemia
- Marrow infiltration (acute and chronic leukemias, tumor)
- Nutritional deficiency (B_{12}, folic acid)
- Myelosuppressive agents
- Drugs that directly influence platelet production (thiazides, alcohol, hormones)
- Radiation
- Viral infections (measles, dengue)

Increased peripheral platelet destruction
Congenital
- Nonimmune (prematurity, erythroblastosis fetalis, infection)
- Immune (drug sensitivity, maternal idiopathic thrombocytopenic purpura [ITP]).

Acquired
- Nonimmune (infection, disseminated intravascular coagulation, thrombotic thrombocytopenic purpura)
- Immune (drug-induced, especially with quinine and quinidine; posttransfusion purpura; acute and chronic ITP; sepsis; alcohol)
- Invasive lines and devices
- Intra-aortic balloon pump
- Prosthetic heart valves
- Heparin

Platelet sequestration
- Hypersplenism
- Hypothermia

Platelet loss
- Hemorrhage
- Extracorporeal perfusion

- Watch for bleeding (petechiae, ecchymoses, surgical or GI bleeding, and menorrhagia).
- Warn the patient to avoid aspirin in any form and other drugs that impair coagulation. Teach him how to recognize aspirin or ibuprofen compounds on labels of over-the-counter remedies.
- Advise the patient to avoid straining at stool or coughing, as both can lead to increased intracranial pressure, possibly causing cerebral hemorrhage in the patient with thrombocytopenia. Provide a stool softener to avoid constipation.
- During periods of active bleeding, maintain the patient on strict bed rest if necessary.
- When administering platelet concentrate, remember that platelets are extremely fragile, so infuse them quickly. Don't give platelets to a patient with a fever.
- During platelet transfusion, monitor for febrile reaction (flushing, chills, fever, headache, tachycardia, and hypertension). Histocompatibility locus antigen–typed platelets may be ordered to prevent febrile reaction. A patient with a history of minor reactions may benefit from acetaminophen and diphenhydramine before transfusion.
- If thrombocytopenia is drug-induced, stress the importance of avoiding the offending drug.
- If the patient must receive long-term steroid therapy, teach him to watch for and report cushingoid signs (acne, moon face, hirsutism, buffalo hump, hypertension, girdle obesity, thinning arms and legs, glycosuria, and edema). Emphasize that steroid doses must be discontinued gradually. During steroid therapy, monitor fluid and electrolyte balance, and watch for infection, pathologic fractures, and mood changes.

Idiopathic thrombocytopenic purpura

Idiopathic thrombocytopenic purpura (ITP), thrombocytopenia that results from immunologic platelet destruction, may be acute (postviral thrombocytopenia) or chronic (Werlhof's disease, purpura hemorrhagica, essential thrombocytopenia, and autoimmune thrombocytopenia). The prognosis for acute ITP is excellent; nearly four out of five patients recover without treatment. The prognosis for chronic ITP is good; remissions lasting weeks or years are common, especially among women.

Causes and incidence

ITP may be an autoimmune disorder, because antibodies that reduce the life span of platelets have been found in nearly all patients. The spleen probably helps to remove platelets modified by the antibody. Acute ITP usually follows a viral infection, such as rubella or chickenpox, and can follow immunization with a live virus vaccine. Chronic ITP seldom follows infection and is commonly linked to immunologic disorders such as systemic lupus erythematosus. It's also linked to drug reactions. ITP frequently occurs in patients who have abused alcohol, heroin, or morphine, and in patients with acquired immunodeficiency syndrome who are exposed to the rubella virus.

Acute ITP usually affects children between ages 2 and 6; chronic ITP mainly affects adults younger than age 50, especially women between ages 20 and 40.

Signs and symptoms

Clinical features of ITP common to all forms of thrombocytopenia include petechiae, ecchymoses, and mucosal bleeding from the mouth, nose, or GI tract. Generally, hemorrhage is a rare physical finding. Purpuric lesions may occur in vital organs, such as the lungs, kidneys, or brain, and may prove fatal. In acute ITP, which commonly occurs in children, onset is usually sudden, causing easy bruising, epistaxis, and bleeding gums. Onset of chronic ITP is insidious.

Diagnosis

Platelet count less than 20,000/µl and prolonged bleeding time suggest ITP. Platelet size and morphologic appearance may be abnormal; anemia may be present if bleeding has occurred. As in thrombocytopenia, bone marrow studies show an abundance of megakaryocytes and a shortened circulating platelet survival time (hours or days). Occasionally, platelet antibodies may be found in vitro, but this diagnosis is usually inferred from platelet survival data and the absence of an underlying disease.

Treatment

Acute ITP may be allowed to run its course without intervention or may be treated with glucocorticoids or immune globulin. For chronic ITP, corticosteroids may be the initial treatment of choice. Patients who fail to respond within 1 to 4 months or who need high steroid dosage are candidates for splenectomy, which may be successful in 50% of cases. Alternative treatments include immunosuppression, high-dose gamma globulin injections, and immunoabsorption apheresis using staphylococcal protein-A columns, which filter antibodies out of the bloodstream. Anti-RhD therapy can also be useful in people with specific blood types.

Before splenectomy, the patient may require blood, blood components, and vitamin K to correct anemia and coagulation defects. After splenectomy, he may need blood and component replacement and platelet concentrate. Normally, platelets increase spontaneously after splenectomy.

Special considerations

Patient care for ITP is essentially the same as for other types of thrombocytopenia, with emphasis on teaching the patient to observe for petechiae, ecchymoses, and other signs of recurrence. Monitor patients receiving immunosuppressants for signs of bone marrow depression, infection, mucositis, GI ulcers, and severe diarrhea or vomiting. Tell the patient to avoid aspirin, ibuprofen, and warfarin, as these drugs interfere with platelet function and blood clotting.

Platelet function disorders

Platelet function disorders are similar to thrombocytopenia but result from platelet dysfunction rather than platelet deficiency. They characteristically cause defects in platelet adhesion or procoagulation activity (ability to bind coagulation factors to

---

FACTS ABOUT PLATELET CONCENTRATE

Contents

- Platelets, white blood cells, some plasma
- Random platelets (ABO matched)
- Human leukocyte antigen (HLA) platelets (HLA-typed for multiple transfusions)

Amount

- 30 to 50 ml per donor
- 4 to 8 donor units given each time (each unit should raise the platelet count by 5,000/μl)

Shelf life

- 6 to 72 hours (best used within 24 hours)

Hepatitis risk

- Same as with whole blood

---

their surface to form a stable fibrin clot). Such disorders may also create defects in platelet aggregation and thromboxane A_2 and may produce abnormalities by preventing the release of adenosine diphosphate (defective platelet release reaction). The prognosis varies widely.

Causes

Abnormal platelet function disorders may be inherited (autosomal recessive) or acquired. Inherited disorders cause bone marrow production of platelets that are ineffective in the clotting mechanism. Acquired disorders result from the effects of such drugs as aspirin or carbenicillin; from such systemic diseases as uremia; or from other hematologic disorders.

Signs and symptoms

Generally, the sudden appearance of petechiae or purpura or excessive bruising and bleeding of the nose and gums are the first overt signs of platelet function disorders. More serious signs are external hemorrhage, internal hemorrhage into the muscles and visceral organs, or excessive bleeding during surgery.

Diagnosis

Prolonged bleeding time in a patient with both a normal platelet count and normal clotting factors suggests this diagnosis. Determination of the defective mechanism requires a blood film and a platelet function test to measure platelet release reaction and aggregation. Depending on the type of platelet dysfunction, some or all of the test results may be abnormal.

Other typical laboratory findings are poor clot retraction and decreased prothrombin conversion. Baseline testing includes complete blood count and differential and appropriate tests to determine hemorrhage sites. In platelet function disorders, plasma clotting factors, platelet counts, prothrombin and partial thromboplastin levels, and thrombin times are usually normal.

Treatment

Platelet replacement is the only satisfactory treatment for inherited platelet dysfunction. However, acquired platelet function disorders respond to adequate treatment of the underlying disease or discontinuation of damaging drug therapy. Plasmapheresis effectively controls bleeding caused by a plasma element that's inhibiting platelet function. During this procedure, one or more units of whole blood are removed from the patient; the plasma is removed from the whole blood, and the remaining packed red blood cells are reinfused. (See *Facts about platelet concentrate.*)

Special considerations

- Obtain an accurate patient history, including onset of bleeding, use of drugs (especially aspirin), and family history of bleeding disorders.
- Watch closely for bleeding from skin, nose, gums, GI tract, or an injury site.
- Help the patient avoid unnecessary trauma. Advise him to tell his dentist about this condition before undergoing oral surgery. (Also stress the need for good oral hygiene to help prevent the need for such surgery.)
- Alert other care team members to the patient's hemorrhagic potential, especially

before he undergoes diagnostic tests or surgery that may cause trauma and bleeding.

■ Observe the patient undergoing plasmapheresis for hypovolemia, hypotension, tachycardia, and other signs of volume depletion.

■ If platelet dysfunction is inherited, help the patient and his family understand and accept the disorder's nature. Teach them how to manage potential bleeding episodes. Warn them that petechiae, ecchymoses, and bleeding from the nose, gums, and GI tract signal abnormal bleeding and should be reported immediately.

■ Tell the patient with a known coagulopathy or hepatic disease to avoid aspirin, aspirin compounds, and other agents that impair coagulation.

■ Advise the patient to wear a medical identification bracelet or to carry a card identifying him as a potential bleeder.

Von Willebrand's disease

Von Willebrand's disease is a hereditary bleeding disorder characterized by prolonged bleeding time; moderate deficiency of von Willebrand's factor (vWF), clotting factor VIII (antihemophilic factor) and, possibly, factor VIII coagulant protein (VIII:C); and impaired platelet function. This disease commonly causes bleeding from the skin or mucosal surfaces and, in females, excessive uterine bleeding. Bleeding may range from mild and asymptomatic to severe, potentially fatal hemorrhage. The prognosis, however, is usually good.

Causes and incidence
Unlike hemophilia, von Willebrand's disease is inherited as an autosomal dominant trait that affects males and females equally. One theory of pathophysiology holds that mild to moderate deficiency of factor VIII and defective platelet adhesion prolong coagulation time. Specifically, this results from a deficiency of the vWF, which stabilizes the factor VIII molecule and is needed for proper platelet function.

Defective platelet function is characterized by:

■ decreased agglutination and adhesion at the bleeding site
■ reduced platelet retention when filtered through a column of packed glass beads
■ diminished ristocetin-induced platelet aggregation.

Recently, an acquired form has been identified in patients with cancer and immune disorders.

Von Willebrand's disease, which doesn't have any racial or ethnic associations, affects about 1% of the population.

Signs and symptoms
Von Willebrand's disease produces easy bruising, epistaxis, and bleeding from the gums. Petechiae are rarely seen. Severe forms of this disease may cause hemorrhage after laceration or surgery, menorrhagia, and GI bleeding. Excessive postpartum bleeding is uncommon because factor VIII levels and bleeding time abnormalities become less pronounced during pregnancy. Massive soft-tissue hemorrhage and bleeding into joints seldom occur. Severity of bleeding may lessen with age, and bleeding episodes occur sporadically—a patient may bleed excessively after one dental extraction but not after another.

Diagnosis
Diagnosis is difficult because symptoms are mild, laboratory values are borderline, and factor VIII levels fluctuate. However, a positive family history and characteristic bleeding patterns and laboratory values help establish the diagnosis. Typical laboratory data include:

■ prolonged bleeding time (more than 6 minutes)
■ slightly prolonged partial thromboplastin time (more than 45 seconds)
■ absent or reduced levels of factor VIII-related antigens and low factor VIII activity level
■ defective in vitro platelet aggregation (using the ristocetin coagulation factor assay test)
■ normal platelet count and normal clot retraction.

Treatment
The goals of treatment are to shorten bleeding time by local measures and to re-

place factor VIII (and, consequently, vWF) by infusion of cryoprecipitate or blood fractions that are rich in factor VIII.

During bleeding and before surgery, I.V. infusion of cryoprecipitate or fresh frozen plasma (in quantities sufficient to raise factor VIII levels to 50% of normal) shortens bleeding time. Desmopressin given parenterally or intranasally is effective in raising serum levels of vWF.

Special considerations
The care plan should include local measures to control bleeding and patient teaching to prevent bleeding, unnecessary trauma, and complications.
- After surgery, monitor bleeding time for 24 to 48 hours, and watch for signs of new bleeding.
- During a bleeding episode, elevate and apply cold compresses and gentle pressure to the bleeding site.
- Refer parents of affected children for genetic counseling.
- Advise the patient to consult the physician after even minor trauma and before all surgery to determine if replacement of blood components is necessary.
- Instruct the patient to watch for signs of hepatitis within 6 weeks to 6 months after transfusion.
- Warn the patient against using aspirin and other drugs that impair platelet function.
- Advise the patient who has a severe form to avoid contact sports.

Disseminated intravascular coagulation

Disseminated intravascular coagulation (DIC) occurs as a life-threatening complication of diseases and conditions that accelerate clotting, causing small blood vessel occlusion, organ necrosis, depletion of circulating clotting factors and platelets, and activation of the fibrinolytic system. This, in turn, can provoke severe hemorrhage. (See *Three mechanisms of DIC*.) Clotting in the microcirculation usually affects the kidneys and extremities but may occur in the brain, lungs, pituitary and adrenal glands, and GI mucosa. Other conditions,

such as vitamin K deficiency, hepatic disease, and anticoagulant therapy, may cause a similar hemorrhage. DIC, also called consumption coagulopathy or defibrination syndrome, is generally an acute condition but may be chronic in cancer patients. The prognosis depends on early detection and treatment, the hemorrhage's severity, and treatment of the underlying disease or condition.

Causes
DIC may result from:
- infection — gram-negative or gram-positive septicemia; viral, fungal, or rickettsial infection; protozoal infection
- obstetric complications — abruptio placentae, amniotic fluid embolism, retained dead fetus, septic abortion, and eclampsia
- neoplastic disease — acute leukemia, metastatic carcinoma, and aplastic anemia
- disorders that produce necrosis — extensive burns and trauma, brain tissue destruction, transplant rejection, and hepatic necrosis
- other factors — heatstroke, shock, poisonous snakebite, cirrhosis, fat embolism, incompatible blood transfusion, cardiac arrest, surgery necessitating cardiopulmonary bypass, giant hemangioma, severe venous thrombosis, and purpura fulminans.

It isn't clear why such disorders lead to DIC, nor is it certain that they lead to it through a common mechanism. In many patients, the triggering mechanisms may be the entrance of foreign protein into the circulation and vascular endothelial injury. Regardless of how DIC begins, the typical accelerated clotting results in generalized activation of prothrombin and a consequent excess of thrombin. Excess thrombin converts fibrinogen to fibrin, producing fibrin clots in the microcirculation. This process consumes exorbitant amounts of coagulation factors (especially fibrinogen, prothrombin, platelets, and factor V and factor VIII), causing hypofibrinogenemia, hypoprothrombinemia, thrombocytopenia, and deficiencies in factor V and factor VIII. Circulating thrombin activates the fibrinolytic system, which lyses fibrin clots into fibrin degradation products. The hemorrhage that occurs may be due largely to

PATHOPHYSIOLOGY
THREE MECHANISMS OF DIC

However disseminated intravascular coagulation (DIC) begins, accelerated clotting (characteristic of DIC) usually results in excess thrombin, which in turn causes fibrinolysis with excess fibrin formation and fibrin degradation products (FDP), activation of fibrin-stabilizing factor (factor XIII), consumption of platelet and clotting factors and, eventually, hemorrhage.

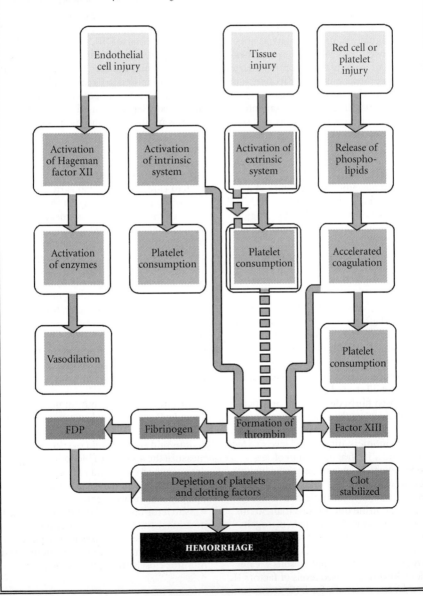

the anticoagulant activity of fibrin degradation products, as well as depletion of plasma coagulation factors.

Signs and symptoms

The most significant feature of DIC is abnormal bleeding, *without* a history of a serious hemorrhagic disorder. Principal signs of such bleeding include cutaneous oozing, petechiae, ecchymoses, and hematomas caused by bleeding into the skin. Bleeding from surgical or I.V. sites and from the GI tract are equally significant signs, as are acrocyanosis (cyanosis of the extremities) and signs of acute tubular necrosis. Related signs, symptoms, and other effects include nausea, vomiting, dyspnea, oliguria, seizures, coma, shock, major organ failure, confusion, epistaxis, hemoptysis, and severe muscle, back, abdominal, and chest pain.

Diagnosis

Abnormal bleeding in the absence of a known hematologic disorder suggests DIC but may be late in the pathophysiologic process. Initial laboratory findings reflect coagulation factor deficiencies.

- decreased platelet count: less than 100,000/µl
- decreased fibrinogen level: less than 150 mg/dl

As the excessive clot breaks down, hemorrhagic diathesis occurs, and test results reflect coagulation abnormalities:

- prolonged prothrombin time: more than 15 seconds
- prolonged partial thromboplastin time: more than 60 seconds
- increased fibrin degradation products: commonly more than 100 mcg/ml.

Other supportive data include positive fibrin monomers, diminished levels of factors V and VIII, fragmentation of red blood cells (RBCs), and decreased hemoglobin (Hb) level (less than 10 g/dl). Assessment of renal status demonstrates reduction in urine output (less than 30 ml/hour) and elevated blood urea nitrogen (more than 25 mg/dl) and serum creatinine (more than 1.3 mg/dl) levels.

A positive D-dimer test (results greater than 500 and decreased levels of factors II, V, and VIII) is specific for DIC. Confirming the diagnosis may be difficult because many of these test results also occur in other disorders (primary fibrinolysis, for example).

Treatment

Successful management of DIC necessitates prompt recognition and adequate treatment of the underlying disorder. Treatment may be supportive when the underlying disorder is self-limiting or highly specific. If the patient isn't bleeding, supportive care alone may reverse DIC. However, bleeding may require administration of blood, fresh frozen plasma, platelets, or packed RBCs to support hemostasis. Cryoprecipitates may also be used if fibrinogen is significantly decreased. Heparin is used in early stages to prevent microclotting and is sometimes used in combination with replacement therapy.

Special considerations

Patient care must focus on early recognition of abnormal bleeding, prompt treatment of the underlying disorders, and prevention of further bleeding.

- To avoid dislodging clots and causing fresh bleeding, don't scrub bleeding areas. Use pressure, cold compresses, and topical hemostatic agents to control bleeding.
- To prevent injury, enforce complete bed rest during bleeding episodes. If the patient is agitated, pad the side rails.
- Check all I.V. and venipuncture sites frequently for bleeding. Apply pressure to injection sites for at least 20 minutes. Alert other personnel to his tendency to hemorrhage.
- Monitor intake and output hourly in acute DIC, especially when administering blood products. Watch for transfusion reactions and signs of fluid overload. To measure the amount of blood lost, weigh dressings and linen, and record drainage. Weigh the patient daily, particularly if there's renal involvement.
- Watch for bleeding from the GI and genitourinary tracts. If you suspect intra-abdominal bleeding, measure the patient's abdominal girth at least every 4 hours, and monitor closely for signs of shock.

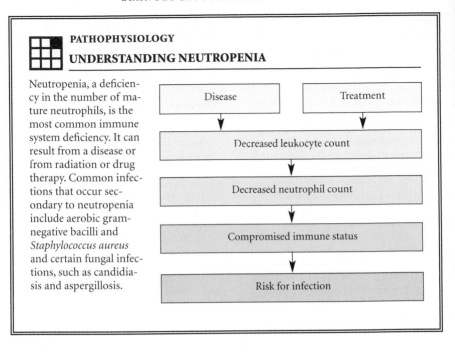

PATHOPHYSIOLOGY
UNDERSTANDING NEUTROPENIA

Neutropenia, a deficiency in the number of mature neutrophils, is the most common immune system deficiency. It can result from a disease or from radiation or drug therapy. Common infections that occur secondary to neutropenia include aerobic gram-negative bacilli and *Staphylococcus aureus* and certain fungal infections, such as candidiasis and aspergillosis.

Disease → Treatment

Decreased leukocyte count

Decreased neutrophil count

Compromised immune status

Risk for infection

- Monitor the results of serial blood studies (particularly hematocrit, Hb levels, and coagulation times).
- Explain all diagnostic tests and procedures. Allow time for questions.
- Inform the patient's family of his progress. Prepare them for his appearance (I.V. lines, nasogastric tubes, bruises, and dried blood). Provide emotional support for the patient and his family. As needed, enlist the aid of a social worker, chaplain, and other members of the health care team in providing such support.

MISCELLANEOUS DISORDERS

Granulocytopenia and lymphocytopenia

Granulocytopenia (also called *agranulocytosis*) is characterized by a marked reduction in the number of circulating granulocytes. Although this implies all the granulocytes (neutrophils, basophils, and eosinophils) are reduced, granulocytopenia usually refers to decreased neutrophils. (See *Understanding neutropenia*.) This disorder, which can occur at any age, is associated with infections and ulcerative lesions of the throat, GI tract, other mucous membranes, and skin. The severest form is known as *agranulocytosis*.

Lymphocytopenia (sometimes called *lymphopenia*), a rare disorder, is a deficiency of circulating lymphocytes (leukocytes produced mainly in lymph nodes).

In both granulocytopenia and lymphocytopenia, the total leukocyte count (white blood cell [WBC] count) may reach dangerously low levels, leaving the body unprotected against infection. The prognosis in both disorders depends on the underlying cause and whether it can be treated. Untreated, severe granulocytopenia can be fatal in 3 to 6 days.

Causes

Granulocytopenia may result from diminished production of granulocytes in bone marrow, increased peripheral destruction of granulocytes, or greater utilization of granulocytes. Diminished production of granulocytes in bone marrow generally stems from radiation or drug therapy; it's a common adverse effect of antimetabolites and alkylating agents and may occur in the patient who is hypersensitive to phenothiazine, sulfonamides (and some sulfonamide derivatives), antibiotics, and antiarrhythmic drugs. Drug-induced granulocytopenia usually develops slowly and typically correlates with the dosage and duration of therapy. Production of granulocytes also decreases in conditions such as aplastic anemia and bone marrow malignancies and in some hereditary disorders (infantile genetic agranulocytosis).

The growing loss of peripheral granulocytes is due to increased splenic sequestration, diseases that destroy peripheral blood cells (viral and bacterial infections), and drugs that act as haptens (carrying antigens that attack blood cells and causing acute idiosyncratic or non-dose-related drug reactions). Infections such as infectious mononucleosis may result in granulocytopenia because of increased utilization of granulocytes.

Similarly, lymphocytopenia may result from decreased production, increased destruction, or loss of lymphocytes. Decreased production of lymphocytes may be secondary to a genetic or a thymic abnormality or to immunodeficiency disorders, such as thymic dysplasia or ataxia-telangiectasia. Increased destruction of lymphocytes may be secondary to radiation, chemotherapy, or human immunodeficiency virus infection. Loss of lymphocytes may follow postsurgical thoracic duct drainage, intestinal lymphangiectasia, or impaired intestinal lymphatic drainage (as in Whipple's disease).

Lymphocyte depletion can also result from elevated plasma corticoid levels (due to stress, corticotropin or steroid treatment, or heart failure). Other disorders associated with lymphocyte depletion include Hodgkin's disease, leukemia, aplastic anemia, sarcoidosis, myasthenia gravis, lupus erythematosus, protein-calorie malnutrition, renal failure, terminal cancer, tuberculosis and, in infants, severe combined immunodeficiency disease (SCID).

Signs and symptoms

Characteristically, patients with granulocytopenia experience slowly progressive fatigue and weakness; if they develop an infection, they can exhibit sudden onset of fever and chills and mental status changes. Overt signs of infection (pus formation) are usually absent. Localized infection can quickly become systemic (bacteremic) or spread throughout an organ (pneumonia). All patients should be meticulously evaluated for even subtle signs of infection because untreated infections can lead to septic shock in 8 to 24 hours. If granulocytopenia results from an idiosyncratic drug reaction, signs of infection develop abruptly, without slowly progressive fatigue and weakness.

Patients with lymphocytopenia may exhibit enlarged lymph nodes, spleen, and tonsils and signs of an associated disease.

Diagnosis

Diagnosis of granulocytopenia necessitates a thorough patient history to check for precipitating factors. Physical examination for clinical effects of underlying disorders is also essential.

CONFIRMING DIAGNOSIS *A markedly decreased neutrophil count (less than 500/µl leads to severe bacterial infections) and a WBC count lower than 2,000/µl, with few observable granulocytes on complete blood count (CBC), confirm granulocytopenia.*

Bone marrow examination shows a scarcity of granulocytic precursor cells beyond the most immature forms, but this may vary, depending on the cause.

A lymphocyte count below 1,500/µl in adults or below 3,000/µl in children indicates lymphocytopenia. Identifying the cause by evaluation of clinical status, bone marrow and lymph node biopsies, or other appropriate diagnostic tests helps establish the diagnosis.

Treatment

Effective management of granulocytopenia must identify and eliminate the cause and control infection until the bone marrow can generate more leukocytes. In many cases, this means drug or radiation therapy must be stopped and antibiotic treatment begun immediately, even while awaiting test results. Treatment may also include antifungal preparations. Administration of granulocyte colony-stimulating factor (CSF) or granulocyte-macrophage CSF is a newer treatment used to stimulate bone marrow production of neutrophils. Spontaneous restoration of leukocyte production in bone marrow generally occurs within 1 to 3 weeks.

Treatment of lymphocytopenia includes eliminating the cause and managing any underlying disorders. For infants with SCID, therapy may include bone marrow transplantation.

Special considerations

- Monitor vital signs frequently. Obtain cultures from blood, throat, urine, mouth, nose, rectum, vagina, and sputum, as ordered. Give antibiotics as scheduled.
- Explain the necessity of infection protection procedures to the patient and his family. Teach proper hand-washing technique and the correct use of gowns and masks. Prevent patient contact with staff or visitors with respiratory infections.
- Maintain adequate nutrition and hydration because malnutrition aggravates immunosuppression. Make sure the patient with mouth ulcerations receives a high-calorie liquid diet. Offer a straw to make drinking less painful.
- Provide warm saline water gargles and rinses, analgesics, and anesthetic lozenges. Good oral hygiene promotes comfort and facilitates healing.
- Ensure adequate rest, which is essential to the mobilization of the body's defenses against infection. Provide good skin and perineal care.
- Monitor CBC and differential, blood culture results, serum electrolyte levels, intake and output, and daily weight.
- To help detect granulocytopenia and lymphocytopenia in the early, most treatable stages, monitor the WBC count of any patient receiving radiation or chemotherapy. After the patient has developed bone marrow depression, he must zealously avoid exposure to infection.
- Advise the patient with known or suspected sensitivity to a drug that may lead to granulocytopenia or lymphocytopenia

---

CAUSES OF SPLENOMEGALY

Infectious
- Acute (abscesses, subacute infective endocarditis), chronic (tuberculosis, malaria, Felty's syndrome)

Congestive
- Cirrhosis, thrombosis

Hyperplastic
- Hemolytic anemia, polycythemia vera

Infiltrative
- Gaucher's disease, Niemann-Pick disease

Cystic or neoplastic
- Cysts, leukemia, lymphoma, myelofibrosis

---

to alert medical personnel to this sensitivity in the future.

Hypersplenism

Hypersplenism is a syndrome marked by exaggerated splenic activity and, possibly, splenomegaly. This disorder results in peripheral blood cell deficiency as the spleen traps and destroys peripheral blood cells.

Causes

Hypersplenism may be idiopathic (primary) or secondary to an extrasplenic disorder, such as chronic malaria, polycythemia vera, or rheumatoid arthritis. (See *Causes of splenomegaly*.) In hypersplenism, the spleen's normal filtering and phagocytic functions accelerate indiscriminately, automatically removing antibody-coated, aging, and abnormal cells, even though some cells may be functionally normal. The spleen may also temporarily sequester normal platelets and red blood cells (RBCs), withholding them from circulation. In this manner, the enlarged spleen may trap as much as 90% of the body's platelets and up to 45% of its RBC mass.

Signs and symptoms

Most patients with hypersplenism develop anemia, leukopenia, or thrombocytopenia, in many cases with splenomegaly. They may contract bacterial infections frequently, bruise easily, hemorrhage spontaneously from the mucous membranes and GI or genitourinary tract, and suffer ulcerations of the mouth, legs, and feet. They commonly develop fever, weakness, and palpitations. Patients with secondary hypersplenism may have other clinical abnormalities, depending on the underlying disease.

Diagnosis

Diagnosis requires evidence of abnormal splenic destruction or sequestration of RBCs or platelets and splenomegaly.

 CONFIRMING DIAGNOSIS *The most definitive test measures erythrocytes in the spleen and liver after I.V. infusion of chromium-labeled RBCs or platelets. A high spleen-liver ratio of radioactivity indicates splenic destruction or sequestration.*

Complete blood count shows decreased hemoglobin level (as low as 4 g/dl), white blood cell count (less than 4,000/µl), and platelet count (less than 125,000/µl) and an elevated reticulocyte count (more than 75,000/µl). Splenic biopsy, scan, and angiography may be useful; biopsy is hazardous and should be avoided if possible. In sequestration, the spleen is palpable. Use abdominal palpation cautiously because it may create injury, bleeding, or rupture.

Treatment

Splenectomy is indicated only in transfusion-dependent patients who are refractory to medical therapy. Splenectomy seldom cures the patient, but it does correct the effects of cytopenia. Postoperative complications may include infection and thromboembolic disease. Occasionally, splenectomy may result in accelerated blood cell destruction in the bone marrow and liver. Secondary hypersplenism necessitates treatment of the underlying disease.

Special considerations

■ If splenectomy is scheduled, administer preoperative transfusions of blood or blood products (fresh frozen plasma and platelets) to replace deficient blood elements. Also treat symptoms or complications of any underlying disorder.

■ Postoperatively, monitor vital signs. Check for any excessive drainage or apparent bleeding. Watch for infection, thromboembolism, and abdominal distention. Keep the nasogastric tube patent; listen for bowel sounds. Instruct the patient to perform deep-breathing exercises, and encourage early ambulation to prevent respiratory complications and venous stasis.

ELDER TIP *Older adults may be at higher risk for infection because of decreased leukocyte and lymphocyte production. Fewer and weaker lymphocytes and immune system changes diminish the antigen-antibody response in older adults.*

Selected references

Anderson, S.C., and Poulsen, K. *Atlas of Hematology.* Philadelphia: Lippincott Williams & Wilkins, 2003.

Chantler, M., et al. *The Washington Manual Hematology and Oncology Subspecialty Consult.* Philadelphia: Lippincott Williams & Wilkins, 2003.

DeVita, V.T., et al. *Cancer: Principles and Practice of Oncology,* 7th ed. Philadelphia: Lippincott Williams & Wilkins, 2005.

Farhi, D.C., et al. *Pathology of Bone Marrow and Blood Cells.* Philadelphia: Lippincott Williams & Wilkins, 2004.

Rodgers, G.P., and Young, N.S. *Bethesda Handbook of Clinical Hematology.* Philadelphia: Lippincott Williams & Wilkins, 2005.

Tierney, L.M., et al. *Current Medical Diagnosis and Treatment,* 43rd ed. New York: McGraw-Hill Book Co., 2004.

Turgeon, M.L. *Clinical Hematology,* 4th ed. Philadelphia: Lippincott Williams & Wilkins, 2004.

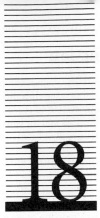

Cardiovascular disorders

Introduction *1058*

Congenital acyanotic defects *1064*
Ventricular septal defect *1064*
Atrial septal defect *1066*
Coarctation of the aorta *1068*
Patent ductus arteriosus *1070*

Congenital cyanotic defects *1072*
Tetralogy of Fallot *1072*
Transposition of the great arteries *1075*

Acquired inflammatory heart disease *1077*
Myocarditis *1077*
Endocarditis *1079*
Pericarditis *1081*
Rheumatic fever and rheumatic heart disease *1084*

Valve disorders *1086*
Valvular heart disease *1086*

Degenerative cardiovascular disorders *1091*
Hypertension *1091*
Coronary artery disease *1095*
Myocardial infarction *1100*
Heart failure *1105*
Dilated cardiomyopathy *1110*
Hypertrophic cardiomyopathy *1113*
Restrictive cardiomyopathy *1114*

Cardiac complications *1115*
Hypovolemic shock *1115*
Cardiogenic shock *1118*
Ventricular aneurysm *1122*
Cardiac tamponade *1123*
Cardiac arrhythmias *1125*

Vascular disorders *1134*
Thoracic aortic aneurysm *1134*
Abdominal aneurysm *1138*
Femoral and popliteal aneurysms *1141*
Thrombophlebitis *1143*
Raynaud's disease *1146*
Buerger's disease *1147*
Arterial occlusive disease *1148*

Selected references *1151*

Introduction

The cardiovascular system begins its activity when the fetus is barely a month old and is the last body system to cease activity at the end of life. This system is so vital that its activity defines the presence of life.

Life-giving transport system

The heart, arteries, veins, and lymphatics form the cardiovascular network that serves as the body's transport system, bringing life-supporting oxygen and nutrients to cells, removing metabolic waste products, and carrying hormones from one part of the body to another. Often called the *circulatory system,* it may be divided into two branches: *pulmonary circulation,* in which blood picks up new oxygen and liberates the waste product carbon dioxide; and *systemic circulation* (including coronary circulation), in which blood carries oxygen and nutrients to all active cells while transporting waste products to the kidneys, liver, and skin for excretion.

Circulation requires normal functioning of the heart, which propels blood through the system by continuous rhythmic contractions. Located behind the sternum, the heart is a muscular organ the size of a man's fist. It has three layers: the *endocardium* — the smooth inner layer; the *myocardium* — the thick, muscular middle layer that contracts in rhythmic beats; and the *epicardium* — the thin, serous membrane, or outer surface of the heart. Covering the entire heart is a saclike membrane called the *pericardium,* which has two layers: a *visceral* layer that's in contact with the heart and a *parietal,* or outer, layer. To prevent irritation when the heart moves against this layer during contraction, fluid lubricates the parietal pericardium.

The heart has four chambers: two thin-walled chambers called *atria* and two thick-walled chambers called *ventricles.* The atria serve as reservoirs during ventricular contraction (systole) and as booster pumps during ventricular relaxation (diastole). The left ventricle propels blood through the systemic circulation. The right ventricle, which forces blood through the pulmonary circulation, is much thinner than the left because it meets only one-sixth the resistance.

 ELDER TIP *As a person's body ages, the ventricular and aortic walls stiffen, decreasing the heart's pumping action.*

Heart valves

Two kinds of valves work inside the heart: *atrioventricular* and *semilunar.* The atrioventricular valve between the right atrium and ventricle has three leaflets, or cusps, and three papillary muscles; hence, it's called the *tricuspid valve.* The atrioventricular valve between the left atrium and ventricle consists of two cusps shaped like a bishop's miter and two papillary muscles and is called the *mitral valve.* The tricuspid and mitral valves prevent blood backflow from the ventricles to the atria during ventricular contraction. The leaflets of both valves are attached to the ventricle's papillary muscles by thin, fibrous bands called *chordae tendineae;* the leaflets separate and descend funnellike into the ventricles during diastole and are pushed upward and together during systole to occlude the mitral and tricuspid orifices. The valves' action isn't entirely passive, because papillary muscles contract during systole and prevent the leaflets from prolapsing into the atria during ventricular contraction.

The two semilunar valves, which resemble half moons, prevent blood backflow from the aorta and pulmonary arteries into the ventricles when those chambers relax and fill with blood from the atria. They're referred to as the *aortic valve* and *pulmonic valve* for their respective arteries.

 ELDER TIP *In elderly people, fibrotic and sclerotic changes thicken heart valves and reduce their flexibility. These changes lead to rigidity and incomplete closure of the valves, which may result in systolic or diastolic murmurs.*

The cardiac cycle

Diastole is the phase of ventricular relaxation and filling. As diastole begins, ventricular pressure falls below arterial pressure, and the aortic and pulmonic valves close. As ventricular pressure continues to fall below atrial pressure, the mitral and tricuspid valves open, and blood flows rapidly into the ventricle. Atrial contraction then increases the volume of ventricular filling by pumping 15% to 25% more blood into the ventricle. When *systole* begins, the ventricular muscle contracts, raising ventricular pressure above atrial pressure and closing the mitral and tricuspid valves. When ventricular pressure finally becomes greater than that in the aorta and pulmonary artery, the aortic and pulmonic valves open, and the ventricles eject blood. Ventricular pressure continues to rise as blood is expelled from the heart. As systole ends, the ventricles relax and stop ejecting blood, and ventricular pressure falls, closing both valves.

S_1 (the first heart sound) is heard as the ventricles contract and the atrioventricular valves close. S_1 is loudest at the heart's apex, over the mitral area. S_2 (the second heart sound), which is normally rapid and sharp, occurs when the aortic and pulmonic valves close. S_2 is loudest at the heart's base (second intercostal space on both sides of the sternum).

Normally, with inspiration, a split S_2 will be auscultated. With expiration, the splitting becomes closer or may become single. However, a fixed split S_2 will be heard if the patient has a right bundle-branch block.

Ventricular distention during diastole, which can occur in heart failure, creates low-frequency vibrations that may be heard as a third heart sound (S_3), or ventricular gallop. An atrial gallop (S_4) may appear at the end of diastole, just before S_1, if atrial filling is forced into a ventricle that has become less compliant or overdistended or has a decreased ability to contract. A pressure rise and ventricular vibrations cause this sound.

Cardiac conduction

The heart's conduction system is composed of specialized cells capable of generating and conducting rhythmic electrical impulses to stimulate heart contraction. This system includes the sinoatrial (SA) node, the atrioventricular (AV) junction, the bundle of His and its bundle branches, and the ventricular conduction tissue and Purkinje fibers.

Normally, the SA node controls the heart rate and rhythm at 60 to 100 beats/minute.

Because the SA node has the lowest resting potential, it's the heart's pacemaker. If it defaults, another part of the system takes over. The AV junction may emerge at 40 to 60 beats/minute; the bundle of His and bundle branches at 30 to 40 beats/minute; and ventricular conduction tissue at 20 to 30 beats/minute.

 ELDER TIP *As the myocardium of the aging heart becomes more irritable, extra systoles may occur along with sinus arrhythmias and sinus bradycardias. In addition, increased fibrous tissue infiltrates the SA nodes and internodal atrial tracts, which may cause atrial fibrillation and flutter.*

Cardiac output

Cardiac output—the amount of blood pumped by the left ventricle into the aorta each minute—is calculated by multiplying the stroke volume (the amount of blood the left ventricle ejects during each contraction) by the heart rate (number of beats/minute). When cellular demands increase, stroke volume or heart rate must increase.

Many factors affect the heart rate, including exercise, pregnancy, and stress. When the sympathetic nervous system releases norepinephrine, the heart rate increases; when the parasympathetic system releases acetylcholine, it slows. As a person ages, the heart rate takes longer to normalize after exercise.

Stroke volume depends on the ventricle's blood volume and pressure at the end of diastole (preload), resistance to ejection (afterload), and the myocardium's contractile strength (inotropy). Changes in preload, afterload, or inotropic state can alter the stroke volume.

 ELDER TIP *Exercise cardiac output declines slightly with age. A decrease in maximum heart rate and contractility may cause this change.*

Circulation and pulses

Blood circulates through three types of vessels: *arteries, veins,* and *capillaries.* The sturdy, pliable walls of the arteries adjust to the volume of blood leaving the heart. The major artery branching out of the left ventricle is the aorta. Its segments and sub-

PULSE POINTS

Peripheral pulse rhythm should correspond exactly to the auscultatory heart rhythm. The pulse's character may offer useful information. For example, *pulsus alternans,* a strong beat followed by a weak one, can mean myocardial weakness. A *water-hammer* (or *Corrigan's*) pulse, a forceful bounding pulse best felt in the carotid arteries or in the forearm, accompanies increased pulse pressure — commonly with capillary pulsations of the fingernails (*Quincke's sign*). This pulse usually indicates patent ductus or aortic insufficiency.

Pulsus biferiens, a double peripheral pulse for every apical beat, can signal aortic stenosis, hyperthyroidism, or some other disease. *Pulsus bigeminus* is a coupled rhythm; you feel its beat in pairs. *Pulsus paradoxus* is exaggerated waxing and waning of the arterial pressure (≥ 15 mm Hg decrease in systolic blood pressure during inspiration).

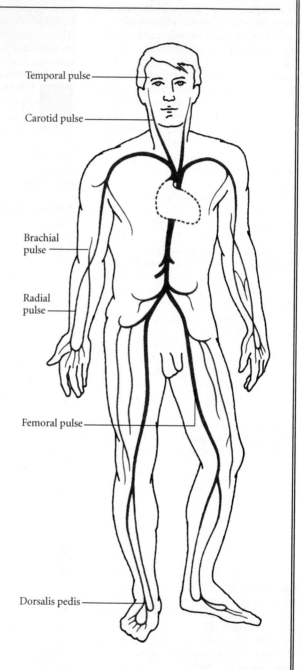

Temporal pulse

Carotid pulse

Brachial pulse

Radial pulse

Femoral pulse

Dorsalis pedis

branches ultimately divide into minute, thin-walled (one-cell thick) capillaries. Capillaries pass the blood to the veins, which return it to the heart. In the veins, valves prevent blood backflow.

ELDER TIP *Aging contributes to arterial and venous insufficiency as the strength and elasticity of blood vessels decrease.*

Pulses are felt best wherever an artery runs near the skin and over a hard structure. (See *Pulse points.*) Easily found pulses are:

- *radial artery*—anterolateral aspect of the wrist
- *temporal artery*—in front of the ear, above and lateral to the eye
- *common carotid artery*—neck (side)
- *femoral artery*—groin.

The lymphatic system also plays a role in the cardiovascular network. Originating in tissue spaces, the lymphatic system drains fluid and other plasma components that build up in extravascular spaces and reroutes them back to the circulatory system as lymph, a plasmalike fluid. Lymphatics also extract bacteria and foreign bodies.

Cardiovascular assessment

Physical assessment provides vital information about cardiovascular status.

- Check for underlying cardiovascular disorders, such as central cyanosis (impaired gas exchange), edema (heart failure or valvular disease), and clubbing (congenital cardiovascular disease).
- Palpate the peripheral pulses bilaterally and evaluate their rate, equality, and quality on a scale of 0 (absent) to +4 (bounding). (See *Pulse amplitude scale.*)
- Inspect the carotid arteries for equal appearance. Auscultate for bruits; then palpate the arteries individually, one side at a time, for thrills (fine vibrations due to irregular blood flow).
- Check for pulsations in the jugular veins (more easily seen than felt). Watch for jugular vein distention—a possible sign of right-sided heart failure, valvular stenosis, cardiac tamponade, or pulmonary embolism. Take blood pressure readings in both arms while the patient is lying, sitting, and standing.

PULSE AMPLITUDE SCALE

To record your patient's pulse amplitude, use this standard scale:

0: pulse isn't palpable.

+1: pulse is thready, weak, difficult to find, may fade in and out, and disappears easily with pressure.

+2: pulse is constant but not strong; light pressure must be applied or pulse will disappear.

+3: pulse considered normal. Is easily palpable, doesn't disappear with pressure.

+4: pulse is strong, bounding, and doesn't disappear with pressure.

- Palpate the precordium for any abnormal pulsations, such as lifts, heaves, or thrills. Use the palms (at the base of the fingertips) or the fingertips. The normal apex will be felt as a light tap and extends over 1″ (2.5 cm) or less.
- Systematically auscultate the anterior chest wall for each of the four heart sounds in the aortic area (second intercostal space at the right sternal border), pulmonic area (second intercostal space at the left sternal border), right ventricular area (lower half of the left sternal border), and mitral area (fifth intercostal space at the midclavicular line). However, don't limit your auscultation to these four areas. Valvular sounds may be heard all over the precordium. Therefore, inch your stethoscope in a Z pattern, from the base of the heart across and down and then over to the apex, or start at the apex and work your way up. For low-pitched sounds, use the bell of the stethoscope; for high-pitched sounds, the diaphragm. Carefully inspect each area for pulsations, and palpate for thrills. Check the location of apical pulsation for deviations in normal size (³⁄₈″ to ³⁄₄″ [1 to 2 cm]) and position (in the mitral area)—possible signs of left ventricular hypertrophy, left-sided valvular disease, or right ventricular disease.

POSITIONING CHEST ELECTRODES

To record the 12-lead electrocardiogram, place electrodes on the patient's arms and legs (with the ground lead on the patient's right leg). The three standard limb leads (I, II, III) and the three augmented leads (aV_R, aV_L, aV_F) are recorded using these electrodes.

To record the precordial (chest) leads, place the electrodes as follows:

- V_1—fourth intercostal space (ICS), right sternal border
- V_2—fourth ICS, left sternal border
- V_3—midway between V_2 and V_4
- V_4—fifth ICS, left mid-clavicular line
- V_5—fifth ICS, left anterior axillary line
- V_6—fifth ICS, left mid-axillary line.

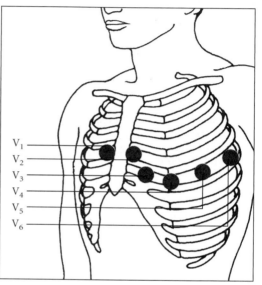

- Listen for the vibrating sound of turbulent blood flow through a stenotic or incompetent valve. Time the murmur to determine where it occurs in the cardiac cycle—between S_1 and S_2 (systolic), between S_2 and the following S_1 (diastolic), or throughout systole (holosystolic). Finally, listen for the scratching or squeaking of a pericardial friction rub.

Special cardiovascular tests

Electrocardiography (ECG) measures electrical activity by recording currents transmitted by the heart. It can detect ischemia, injury, necrosis, bundle-branch blocks, fascicular blocks, conduction delay, chamber enlargement, and arrhythmias. In Holter monitoring, a tape recording tracks as many as 100,000 cardiac cycles over a 12- or 24-hour period. This test may be used to assess the effectiveness of antiarrhythmic drugs or to evaluate arrhythmia symptoms. A signal-averaged ECG will identify after

potentials, which are associated with a risk of ventricular arrhythmias. (See *Positioning chest electrodes.*)

Chest X-rays may reveal cardiac enlargement and aortic dilation. They also assess pulmonary circulation. When pulmonary venous and arterial pressures rise, characteristic changes appear, such as dilation of the pulmonary venous shadows. When pulmonary venous pressure exceeds oncotic pressure of the blood, capillary fluid leaks into lung tissues, causing pulmonary edema. This fluid may settle in the alveoli, producing a butterfly pattern, or the lungs may appear cloudy or hazy; in the interlobular septa, sharp linear densities (Kerley's lines) may appear.

Exercise testing using a bicycle ergometer or treadmill determines the heart's response to physical stress. This test measures blood pressure and ECG changes during increasingly rigorous exercises. Myocardial ischemia, abnormal blood pressure response, or arrhythmias indicate the circulatory system's failure to adapt to exercise.

Cardiac catheterization evaluates chest pain, the need for coronary artery surgery or angioplasty, congenital heart defects, and valvular heart disease and determines the extent of heart failure. Right-sided catheterization involves threading a pulmonary artery thermodilution catheter, which can measure cardiac output, through a vein into the right side of the heart, pulmonary artery, and its branches in the lungs to measure right atrial, right ventricular, pulmonary artery, and pulmonary artery wedge pressures. Left-sided catheterization entails retrograde catheterization of the left ventricle or transseptal catheterization of the left atrium. Ventriculography during left-sided catheterization involves injecting radiopaque dye into the left ventricle to measure ejection fraction and to disclose abnormal heart wall motion or mitral valve incompetence.

In coronary arteriography, radiopaque material injected into coronary arteries allows cineangiographic visualization of coronary arterial narrowing or occlusion.

Digital subtraction angiography evaluates the coronary arteries through the use of X-ray images that are digitally subtracted by computer. Time-based color enhancement shows blood flow in nearby areas.

Echocardiography uses echoes from pulsed high-frequency sound waves (ultrasound) to evaluate cardiac structures. M-mode echocardiography, in which a single, stationary ultrasound beam strikes the heart, produces a vertical view of cardiac structures. Two-dimensional echocardiography (most common), in which an ultrasound beam rapidly sweeps through an arc, produces a cross-sectional or fan-shaped view of cardiac structures. Both M-mode and two-dimensional echocardiography may use contrast agents for enhancement. Doppler echocardiography records blood flow within the cardiovascular system. Color Doppler echocardiography shows the direction of blood flow, which provides information about the degree of valvular insufficiency. Transesophageal echocardiography combines ultrasound with endoscopy to better view the heart's structures.

This procedure allows images to be taken from the heart's posterior aspect.

Echocardiography provides information about valve leaflets, size and dimensions of heart chambers, and thickness and motion of the septum and the ventricular walls. It can also reveal intracardiac masses, detect pericardial effusion, diagnose hypertrophic cardiomyopathy, and estimate cardiac output and ejection fraction. This test can also evaluate possible aortic dissection when it involves the ascending aorta.

In multiple-gated acquisition scanning, a radioactive isotope in the intravascular compartment allows measurement of stroke volume, wall motion, and ventricular ejection fraction. Myocardial imaging usually uses the radioactive agent thallium-201 or Tc-99m sestamibi (Cardiolite) to detect abnormalities in myocardial perfusion. This agent concentrates in normally perfused areas of the myocardium but not in ischemic areas ("cold spots"), which may be permanent (scar tissue) or temporary (from transient ischemia). These tests can be done as exercise studies or can be combined with drugs, such as adenosine or Persantine, in patients unable to exercise.

Acute infarct imaging documents muscle viability (not perfusion) through the use of technetium-labeled pyrophosphate. Unlike thallium, technetium accumulates only in irreversibly damaged myocardial tissue. Areas of necrosis appear as "hot spots" and can be detected only during an acute myocardial infarction (MI). This test determines the size and location of an infarction but can produce false results.

Cardiac enzymes (cellular proteins released into the blood as a result of cell membrane injury) in the blood confirm acute MI or severe cardiac trauma. All cardiac enzymes — creatine kinase (CK), lactate dehydrogenase, and aspartate aminotransferase, for example — are also found in other cells. Fractionation of enzymes can determine the source of damaged cells. For example, three fractions of CK are isolated, one of which (an isoenzyme called CK-MB) is found only in cardiac cells. CK-MB in the blood indicates injury to myocardial cells.

Measurement of a cardiac protein called *troponin* is the most precise way to determine if a patient has experienced an MI. Some 6 hours after an MI, a blood test can detect two forms of troponin: T and I. Troponin T levels peak about 2 days after an MI and return to normal about 16 days later. Troponin I levels reach their peak in less than 1 day after an MI and return to normal in about 7 days.

Peripheral arteriography consists of a fluoroscopic X-ray after arterial injection of a contrast medium. Similarly, phlebography defines the venous system after injection of a contrast medium into a vein. Impedance plethysmography evaluates the venous system to detect pressure changes transmitted to lower leg veins.

Doppler ultrasonography evaluates the peripheral vascular system and assesses arterial occlusive disease.

Endomyocardial biopsy can detect cardiomyopathy, infiltrative myocardial diseases, and transplant rejection.

Electrophysiologic studies help diagnose conduction system disease and serious arrhythmias. Electronic induction and termination of arrhythmias aid drug selection. Endocardial mapping detects an arrhythmia's focus using a finger electrode. Epicardial mapping uses a computer and a fabric sock with electrodes that's slipped over the heart to detect arrhythmias.

Magnetic resonance imaging can investigate cardiac structure and function. Positron emission tomography and magnetic resonance spectroscopy are used to assess myocardial metabolism.

Electron beam computed tomography, also known as ultrafast computed tomography, is used to detect micro-calcifications in the coronary arteries. This test is useful for identifying early coronary artery disease.

Managing cardiovascular disease
Patients with cardiovascular disease pose a tremendous challenge. Their sheer numbers alone compel a thorough understanding of cardiovascular anatomy, physiology, and pathophysiology. Anticipate a high anxiety level in cardiac patients, and provide support and reassurance, especially during procedures such as cardiac catheterization.

Cardiac rehabilitation programs are widely prescribed and offer education and support along with exercise instruction. Rehabilitation programs begin in health care facilities and continue on an outpatient basis. Helping the patient resume a satisfying lifestyle requires planning and comprehensive teaching. Inform the patient about health care facilities and organizations that offer cardiac rehabilitation programs.

CONGENITAL ACYANOTIC DEFECTS

Ventricular septal defect

In ventricular septal defect (VSD), the most common congenital heart disorder, an opening in the septum between the ventricles allows blood to shunt between the left and right ventricles. This disease accounts for up to 30% of all congenital heart defects. The prognosis is good for defects that close spontaneously or are correctable surgically but poor for untreated defects, which are sometimes fatal by age 1, usually from secondary complications.

Causes and incidence
In neonates with VSD, the ventricular septum fails to close completely by the eighth week of gestation, as it would normally. VSD occurs in some neonates with fetal alcohol syndrome, but a causal relationship hasn't been established. Although most children with congenital heart defects are otherwise normal, in some, VSD coexists with additional birth defects, especially Down syndrome and other autosomal trisomies, renal anomalies, and such cardiac defects as patent ductus arteriosus and coarctation of the aorta. VSDs are located in the membranous or muscular portion of the ventricular septum and vary in size. Some defects close spontaneously; in other defects, the entire septum is absent, creating a single ventricle.

VSD isn't readily apparent at birth, because right and left ventricular pressures are approximately equal, so blood doesn't shunt through the defect. As the pulmonary vasculature gradually relaxes, 4 to 8 weeks after birth, right ventricular pressure decreases, allowing blood to shunt from the left to the right ventricle. Less than 1% of neonates are born with VSD. In 80% to 90% of neonates who are born with this disorder, the hole is small and will usually close spontaneously. In the remaining 10% to 20% of neonates, surgery is needed to close the hole.

Signs and symptoms

Clinical features of VSD vary with the defect's size, the shunting's effect on the pulmonary vasculature, and the infant's age. In a small VSD, shunting is minimal, and pulmonary artery pressure and heart size remain normal. Such defects may eventually close spontaneously without ever causing symptoms.

Initially, large VSD shunts cause left atrial and left ventricular hypertrophy. Later, an uncorrected VSD will cause right ventricular hypertrophy due to increasing pulmonary vascular resistance. Eventually, biventricular heart failure and cyanosis (from reversal of shunt direction) occur. Resulting cardiac hypertrophy may make the anterior chest wall prominent. A large VSD increases the risk of pneumonia.

Infants with large VSDs are thin and small and gain weight slowly. They may develop heart failure with dusky skin; liver, heart, and spleen enlargement because of systemic venous congestion; diaphoresis; feeding difficulties; rapid, grunting respirations; and increased heart rate. They may also develop severe pulmonary hypertension. Fixed pulmonary hypertension may occur much later in life with right-to-left shunt (Eisenmenger complex), causing cyanosis and clubbing of the nail beds.

The typical murmur associated with a VSD is blowing or rumbling and varies in frequency. In the neonate, a moderately loud early systolic murmur may be heard along the lower left sternal border. About the second or third day after birth, the murmur may become louder and longer. In infants, the murmur may be loudest near the heart's base and may suggest pulmonary stenosis. A small VSD may produce a functional murmur or a characteristic loud, harsh systolic murmur. Larger VSDs produce audible murmurs (at least a grade 3 pansystolic), loudest at the fourth intercostal space, usually with a thrill. In addition, the pulmonic component of S_2 sounds loud and is widely split. Palpation reveals displacement of the point of maximal impulse to the left. When fixed pulmonary hypertension is present, a diastolic murmur may be audible on auscultation, the systolic murmur becomes quieter, and S_2 is greatly accentuated.

Diagnosis

Diagnostic findings include:

- Chest X-ray is normal in small defects; in large VSDs, it shows cardiomegaly, left atrial and left ventricular enlargement, and prominent pulmonary vascular markings.
- Electrocardiography (ECG) is normal in children with small VSDs; in large VSDs, it shows left and right ventricular hypertrophy, suggesting pulmonary hypertension.
- Echocardiography may detect a large VSD and its location in the septum, estimate the size of a left-to-right shunt, suggest pulmonary hypertension, and identify associated lesions and complications.

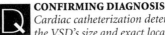 **CONFIRMING DIAGNOSIS**
Cardiac catheterization determines the VSD's size and exact location, calculates the degree of shunting by comparing the blood oxygen saturation in each ventricle, determines the extent of pulmonary hypertension, and detects associated defects.

Treatment

In mild cases, no treatment is needed, although the infant should be closely followed to make sure that the hole closes properly as he grows. Large defects usually require early surgical correction before heart failure and irreversible pulmonary vascular disease develop.

For small defects, surgery consists of simple suture closure. Moderate to large defects require insertion of a patch graft, using cardiopulmonary bypass. In patients with heart failure, digoxin and diuretics may be prescribed to control symptoms. In patients who develop increased pulmonary resistance and irreversible pulmonary vascular changes that produce a reversible right-to-left shunt (Eisenmenger's syndrome), a heart-lung transplant may be required.

If the child has other defects and will benefit from delaying surgery, pulmonary artery banding normalizes pressures and flow distal to the band and prevents pulmonary vascular disease, allowing postponement of surgery. (Pulmonary artery banding is done only when the child has other complications.) A rare complication of VSD repair is complete heart block from interference with the bundle of His during surgery. (Heart block may require temporary or permanent pacemaker implantation.)

Before surgery, treatment consists of:
- digoxin, sodium restriction, and diuretics to prevent heart failure
- careful monitoring by physical examination, X-ray, and ECG to detect increased pulmonary hypertension, which indicates a need for early surgery
- measures to prevent infection (prophylactic antibiotics, for example, to prevent infective endocarditis).

Generally, postoperative treatment includes a brief period of mechanical ventilation. The patient will need analgesics and may also require diuretics to increase urine output, continuous infusions of nitroprusside or adrenergic agents to regulate blood pressure and cardiac output and, in rare cases, a temporary pacemaker.

Special considerations
Although the parents of an infant with VSD often suspect something is wrong with their child before diagnosis, they need psychological support to help them accept the reality of a serious cardiac disorder. Because surgery may take place months after diagnosis, parent teaching is vital to prevent complications until the child is scheduled for surgery or the defect closes. Thorough explanations of all tests are also essential.
- Instruct parents to watch for signs of heart failure, such as poor feeding, sweating, and heavy breathing.
- If the child is receiving digoxin or other medications, tell the parents how to give it and how to recognize adverse effects. Caution them to keep medications out of the reach of all children.

- Teach parents to recognize and report early signs of infection and to avoid exposing the child to people with obvious infections.
- Encourage parents to let the child engage in normal activities.
- Tell parents to follow-up with their pediatrician. Also tell them that child life therapy may be appropriate if their child displays delayed growth and development or failure to thrive.
- Stress the importance of prophylactic antibiotics before and after surgery.

After surgery to correct VSD:
- Monitor vital signs and intake and output. Maintain the infant's body temperature with an overbed warmer. Give catecholamines, nitroprusside, and diuretics, as ordered; analgesics as needed.
- Monitor central venous pressure, intraarterial blood pressure, and left atrial or pulmonary artery pressure readings. Assess heart rate and rhythm for signs of conduction block.
- Check oxygenation, particularly in a child who requires mechanical ventilation. Suction to maintain a patent airway and to prevent atelectasis and pneumonia, as needed.
- Monitor pacemaker effectiveness if needed. Watch for signs of failure, such as bradycardia and hypotension.
- Reassure parents and allow them to participate in their child's care.

Atrial septal defect

In an atrial septal defect (ASD), an opening between the left and right atria allows shunting of blood between the chambers. *Ostium secundum defect* (most common) occurs in the region of the fossa ovalis and, occasionally, extends inferiorly, close to the vena cava; *sinus venosus defect* occurs in the superior-posterior portion of the atrial septum, sometimes extending into the vena cava, and is almost always associated with abnormal drainage of pulmonary veins into the right atrium; *ostium primum defect* occurs in the inferior portion of the septum primum and is usually associated with atrioventricular valve abnormalities (cleft mitral valve) and conduction defects.

ASD accounts for about 10% of congenital heart defects and appears almost twice as often in females as in males, with a strong familial tendency. Although ASD is usually a benign defect during infancy and childhood, delayed development of symptoms and complications makes it one of the most common congenital heart defects diagnosed in adults. The prognosis is excellent in asymptomatic patients but poor in those with cyanosis caused by large, untreated defects.

Causes and incidence

The cause of ASD is unknown. In this condition, blood shunts from left to right because left atrial pressure normally is slightly higher than right atrial pressure; this pressure difference forces large amounts of blood through a defect. The left-to-right shunt results in right heart volume overload, affecting the right atrium, right ventricle, and pulmonary arteries. Eventually, the right atrium enlarges, and the right ventricle dilates to accommodate the increased blood volume. If pulmonary artery hypertension develops because of the shunt (rare in children), increased pulmonary vascular resistance and right ventricular hypertrophy will follow. In some adult patients, irreversible (fixed) pulmonary artery hypertension causes reversal of the shunt direction, which results in unoxygenated blood entering the systemic circulation, causing cyanosis.

ASD is present in 4 of every 100,000 people. Symptoms usually develop before age 30. When no other congenital defect exists, the patient — especially children — may be asymptomatic.

Signs and symptoms

ASD commonly goes undetected in preschoolers; such children may complain about feeling tired only after extreme exertion and may have frequent respiratory tract infections but otherwise appear normal and healthy. However, they may show growth retardation if they have large shunts. Children with ASD seldom develop heart failure, pulmonary hypertension, infective endocarditis, or other complications. However, as adults, they usually manifest pronounced symptoms, such as fatigability and dyspnea on exertion, frequently to the point of severe limitation of activity (especially after age 40).

In children, auscultation reveals an early to midsystolic murmur, superficial in quality, heard at the second or third left intercostal space. In patients with large shunts (resulting from increased tricuspid valve flow), a low-pitched diastolic murmur is heard at the lower left sternal border, which becomes more pronounced on inspiration. Although the murmur's intensity is a rough indicator of the size of the left-to-right shunt, its low pitch sometimes makes it difficult to hear. Other signs include a fixed, widely split S_2, caused by delayed closure of the pulmonic valve, and a systolic click or late systolic murmur at the apex, resulting from mitral valve prolapse, which occasionally affects older children with ASD.

In older patients with large, uncorrected defects and fixed pulmonary artery hypertension, auscultation reveals an accentuated S_2. A pulmonary ejection click and an audible S_4 may also be present. Clubbing and cyanosis become evident; syncope and hemoptysis may occur with severe pulmonary vascular disease.

Diagnosis

A history of increasing fatigue and characteristic physical features suggest ASD. The following findings confirm it:

■ Chest X-ray shows an enlarged right atrium and right ventricle, a prominent pulmonary artery, and increased pulmonary vascular markings.

■ Electrocardiography may be normal but usually shows right axis deviation, prolonged PR interval, varying degrees of right bundle-branch block, right ventricular hypertrophy, atrial fibrillation (particularly in severe cases after age 30) and, in ostium primum defect, left axis deviation.

■ Echocardiography measures right ventricular enlargement, may locate the defect, and shows volume overload in the right side of the heart. (Other causes of right ventricular enlargement must be ruled out.)

 CONFIRMING DIAGNOSIS *Two-dimensional echocardiography with color Doppler flow, contrast echocar-*

diography, or both have supplanted cardiac catheterization as the confirming tests for ASD. Cardiac catheterization is used if inconsistencies exist in the clinical data or if significant pulmonary hypertension is suspected.

Treatment

Operative repair is advised for all patients with uncomplicated ASD with evidence of significant left-to-right shunting. Ideally, this is performed when the patient is between ages 2 and 4. Operative treatment shouldn't be performed on patients with small defects and trivial left-to-right shunts. Because ASD seldom produces complications in infants and toddlers, surgery can be delayed until they reach preschool or early school age. A large defect may need immediate surgical closure with sutures or a patch graft.

Physicians have developed a new procedure, referred to as catheter closure or transcatheter closure of the atrial septal defect, that uses wires or catheters that can close ASD without surgery. In this procedure, the surgeon makes a tiny incision in the groin to introduce the catheters. Then, he advances the catheters into the heart and places the closure device across the ASD. This procedure may not be applicable to all patients.

Special considerations

■ Before cardiac catheterization, explain pretest and posttest procedures to the child and her parents. If possible, use drawings or other visual aids to explain it to the child.

■ As needed, teach the patient about prophylactic antibiotics to prevent infective endocarditis. (They may be administered before dental or other invasive procedures.)

■ If surgery is scheduled, teach the child and her parents about the intensive care unit and introduce them to the staff. Show parents where they can wait during the operation. Explain postoperative procedures, tubes, dressings, and monitoring equipment.

■ After surgery, closely monitor the patient's vital signs, central venous and intraarterial pressures, and intake and output.

Watch for atrial arrhythmias, which may remain uncorrected.

Coarctation of the aorta

Coarctation is a narrowing of the aorta, usually just below the left subclavian artery, near the site where the ligamentum arteriosum (the remnant of the ductus arteriosus, a fetal blood vessel) joins the pulmonary artery to the aorta. Coarctation may occur with aortic valve stenosis (usually of a bicuspid aortic valve) and with severe cases of hypoplasia of the aortic arch, patent ductus arteriosus, and ventricular septal defect. Generally, the prognosis for coarctation of the aorta depends on the severity of associated cardiac anomalies; the prognosis for isolated coarctation is good if corrective surgery is performed before this condition induces severe systemic hypertension or degenerative changes in the aorta.

Causes and incidence

Coarctation of the aorta may develop as a result of spasm and constriction of the smooth muscle in the ductus arteriosus as it closes. Possibly, this contractile tissue extends into the aortic wall, causing narrowing. The obstructive process causes hypertension in the aortic branches above the constriction (arteries that supply the arms, neck, and head) and diminished pressure in the vessels below the constriction.

Restricted blood flow through the narrowed aorta increases the pressure load on the left ventricle and causes dilation of the proximal aorta and ventricular hypertrophy. Untreated, this condition may lead to left-sided heart failure and, rarely, to cerebral hemorrhage and aortic rupture. If ventricular septal defect accompanies coarctation, blood shunts left to right, straining the right side of the heart. This leads to pulmonary hypertension and, eventually, right-sided heart hypertrophy and failure.

Coarctation of the aorta occurs in 1 of every 10,000 people and is usually diagnosed in children or adults younger than age 40. It accounts for about 7% of all congenital heart defects in children and is

RECOGNIZING COARCTATION OF THE AORTA

Collateral circulation develops to bypass the occluded aortic lumen, and can be seen on X-ray as notching of the ribs. By adolescence, palpable, visible pulsations may be evident.

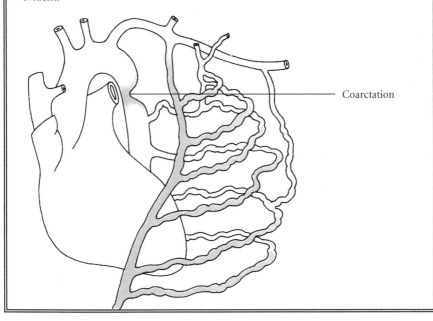

Coarctation

twice as common in males as in females. When it occurs in females, it's commonly associated with Turner's syndrome, a chromosomal disorder that causes ovarian dysgenesis.

Signs and symptoms

Clinical features vary with age. During the first year of life, when aortic coarctation may cause heart failure, the infant displays tachypnea, dyspnea, pulmonary edema, pallor, tachycardia, failure to thrive, cardiomegaly, and hepatomegaly. In most cases, heart sounds are normal unless a coexisting cardiac defect is present. Femoral pulses are absent or diminished.

If coarctation is asymptomatic in infancy, it usually remains so throughout adolescence, as collateral circulation develops to bypass the narrowed segment. During adolescence, this defect may produce dyspnea, claudication, headaches, epistaxis, and hypertension in the upper extremities

despite collateral circulation. It commonly causes resting systolic hypertension and wide pulse pressure; high diastolic pressure readings are the same in both the arms and legs. Coarctation may also produce a visible aortic pulsation in the suprasternal notch, a continuous systolic murmur, an accentuated S_2, and an S_4.

Diagnosis

CONFIRMING DIAGNOSIS *The cardinal signs of coarctation of the aorta are resting systolic hypertension, absent or diminished femoral pulses, and wide pulse pressure.*

The following tests support this diagnosis:

■ Chest X-ray may demonstrate left ventricular hypertrophy, heart failure, a wide ascending and descending aorta, and notching of the undersurfaces of the ribs, due to extensive collateral circulation. (See *Recognizing coarctation of the aorta.*)

- Electrocardiography may eventually reveal left ventricular hypertrophy.
- Echocardiography may show increased left ventricular muscle thickness, coexisting aortic valve abnormalities, and the coarctation site.
- Doppler ultrasound and cardiac catheterization evaluate collateral circulation and measure pressure in the right and left ventricles and in the ascending and descending aortas (on both sides of the obstruction).
- Aortography locates the site and extent of coarctation.

Treatment

For an infant with heart failure caused by coarctation of the aorta, treatment consists of medical management with digoxin, diuretics, oxygen, and sedatives. If medical management fails, surgery may be needed.

The child's condition usually determines the timing of surgery. Signs of heart failure or hypertension may call for early surgery. If these signs don't appear, surgery usually occurs during the preschool years.

Before the operation, the child may require endocarditis prophylaxis or, if he's older and has previously undetected coarctation, antihypertensive therapy. During surgery, the physician uses a flap of the left subclavian artery to reconstruct an unobstructed aorta.

Balloon therapy may be indicated for some patients as an alternative to surgical repair. It uses a technique similar to that used to open the coronary arteries, but is performed on the aorta.

Special considerations

- When coarctation in an infant requires rapid digitalization, monitor vital signs closely and watch for digoxin toxicity (poor feeding and vomiting).
- Balance intake and output carefully, especially if the infant is receiving diuretics with fluid restriction.
- Because the infant may not be able to maintain proper body temperature, regulate environmental temperature with an overbed warmer if needed.
- Monitor blood glucose levels to detect possible hypoglycemia, which may occur as glycogen stores become depleted.

- Offer the parents emotional support and an explanation of the disorder. Also explain diagnostic procedures, surgery, and drug therapy. Tell parents what to expect postoperatively.
- For an older child, assess the blood pressure in his extremities regularly, explain any exercise restrictions, stress the need to take medications properly and to watch for adverse effects, and teach him about tests and other procedures.

After corrective surgery:
- Monitor blood pressure closely, using an intra-arterial line. Take blood pressure in all extremities. Monitor intake and output.
- If the patient develops hypertension and requires nitroprusside or trimethaphan, administer it, as ordered, by continuous I.V. infusion, using an infusion pump. Watch for severe hypotension and regulate the dosage carefully.
- Provide pain relief and encourage a gradual increase in activity.
- Promote adequate respiratory functioning through turning, coughing, and deep breathing.
- Watch for abdominal pain or rigidity and signs of GI or urinary bleeding.
- If an older child needs to continue antihypertensives after surgery, teach him and his parents about them.
- Stress the importance of continued endocarditis prophylaxis.

Patent ductus arteriosus

The ductus arteriosus is a fetal blood vessel that connects the pulmonary artery to the descending aorta. In patent ductus arteriosus (PDA), the lumen of the ductus remains open after birth. This creates a left-to-right shunt of blood from the aorta to the pulmonary artery and results in recirculation of arterial blood through the lungs. Initially, PDA may produce no clinical effects, but in time it can precipitate pulmonary vascular disease, causing symptoms to appear by age 40. The prognosis is good if the shunt is small or surgical repair is effective. Otherwise, PDA may advance to intractable heart failure, which may be fatal.

Causes and incidence

Normally, the ductus closes within days to weeks after birth. Failure to close is most prevalent in premature neonates, probably as a result of abnormalities in oxygenation or the relaxant action of prostaglandin E, which prevents ductal spasm and contracture necessary for closure. PDA commonly accompanies rubella syndrome and may be associated with other congenital defects, such as coarctation of the aorta, ventricular septal defect, and pulmonary and aortic stenoses.

In PDA, relative resistances in pulmonary and systemic vasculature and the size of the ductus determine the amount of left-to-right shunting. The left atrium and left ventricle must accommodate the increased pulmonary venous return, in turn increasing filling pressure and workload on the left side of the heart and possibly causing heart failure. In the final stages of untreated PDA, the left-to-right shunt leads to chronic pulmonary artery hypertension that becomes fixed and unreactive. This causes the shunt to reverse; unoxygenated blood thus enters systemic circulation, causing cyanosis.

PDA is found in 1 of every 2,500 to 5,000 infants and is the most common congenital heart defect found in adults. It affects twice as many females than males.

Signs and symptoms

In neonates, especially those who are premature, a large PDA usually produces respiratory distress, with signs of heart failure due to the tremendous volume of blood shunted to the lungs through a patent ductus and the increased workload on the left side of the heart. Other characteristic features may include heightened susceptibility to respiratory tract infections, slow motor development, and failure to thrive. Most children with PDA have no symptoms except cardiac ones. Others may exhibit signs of heart disease, such as physical underdevelopment, fatigability, and frequent respiratory tract infections. Adults with undetected PDA may develop pulmonary vascular disease and, by age 40, may display fatigability and dyspnea on exertion. About 10% of them also develop infective endocarditis.

Auscultation reveals the classic machinery murmur (Gibson murmur): a continuous murmur (during systole and diastole) best heard at the heart's base, at the second left intercostal space under the left clavicle in 85% of children with PDA. This murmur may obscure S_2. However, with a right-to-left shunt, such a murmur may be absent. Palpation may reveal a thrill at the left sternal border and a prominent left ventricular impulse. Peripheral arterial pulses are bounding (Corrigan's pulse); pulse pressure is widened because of an elevation in systolic blood pressure and, primarily, a drop in diastolic pressure.

Diagnosis

■ Chest X-ray may show increased pulmonary vascular markings, prominent pulmonary arteries, and left ventricle and aorta enlargement.
■ Electrocardiography (ECG) may be normal or may indicate left atrial or ventricular hypertrophy and, in pulmonary vascular disease, biventricular hypertrophy.
■ Echocardiography detects and helps estimate the size of a PDA. It also reveals an enlarged left atrium and left ventricle or right ventricular hypertrophy from pulmonary vascular disease.

CONFIRMING DIAGNOSIS
Cardiac catheterization shows pulmonary arterial oxygen content higher than right ventricular content because of the influx of aortic blood. Increased pulmonary artery pressure indicates a large shunt or, if it exceeds systemic arterial pressure, severe pulmonary vascular disease. Catheterization allows calculation of blood volume crossing the ductus and can rule out associated cardiac defects. Dye injection definitively demonstrates PDA.

Treatment

Asymptomatic infants with PDA require no immediate treatment. Those with heart failure require fluid restriction, diuretics, and cardiac glycosides to minimize or control symptoms. If these measures can't control heart failure, surgery is necessary to ligate the ductus. If symptoms are mild, surgical correction is usually delayed until the infant is between ages 6 months to 3 years, unless problems develop. Before surgery, children with PDA require antibiotics to protect against infective endocarditis.

Other forms of therapy include cardiac catheterization to deposit a plug or coil in the ductus to stop shunting or administration of indomethacin I.V. (a prostaglandin inhibitor that's an alternative to surgery in premature neonates) to induce ductus spasm and closure.

Special considerations

PDA necessitates careful monitoring, patient and family teaching, and emotional support.

■ Watch carefully for signs of PDA in all premature neonates.

■ Be alert for respiratory distress symptoms resulting from heart failure, which may develop rapidly in a premature neonate. Frequently assess vital signs, ECG, electrolyte levels, and intake and output. Record response to diuretics and other therapy. Watch for signs of digoxin toxicity (poor feeding and vomiting).

■ If the infant receives indomethacin for ductus closure, watch for possible adverse effects, such as diarrhea, jaundice, bleeding, and renal dysfunction.

■ Before surgery, carefully explain all treatments and tests to parents. Include the child in your explanations. Arrange for the child and her parents to meet the intensive care unit staff. Tell them about expected I.V. lines, monitoring equipment, and postoperative procedures.

■ Immediately after surgery, the child may have a central venous pressure catheter and an arterial line in place. Carefully assess vital signs, intake and output, and arterial and venous pressures. Provide pain relief as needed.

■ Before discharge, review instructions to the parents about activity restrictions based on the child's tolerance and energy levels. Advise parents not to become overprotective as their child's tolerance for physical activity increases.

■ Stress the need for regular follow-up examinations. Advise parents to inform any physician who treats their child about his history of surgery for PDA — even if the child is being treated for an unrelated medical problem.

CONGENITAL CYANOTIC DEFECTS

Tetralogy of Fallot

Tetralogy of Fallot is a combination of four cardiac defects: ventricular septal defect (VSD), right ventricular outflow tract obstruction (pulmonary stenosis), right ventricular hypertrophy, and dextroposition of the aorta, with overriding of the VSD. Blood shunts right to left through the VSD, permitting unoxygenated blood to mix with oxygenated blood, resulting in cyanosis. Tetralogy of Fallot sometimes coexists with other congenital heart defects, such as patent ductus arteriosus or atrial septal defect.

Causes and incidence

The cause of tetralogy of Fallot is unknown, but it results from embryologic hypoplasia of the outflow tract of the right ventricle. Multiple factors, such as Down syndrome, have been associated with its presence. Prenatal risk factors include maternal rubella or other viral illnesses, poor prenatal nutrition, maternal alcoholism, mother older than age 40, and diabetes.

Tetralogy of Fallot occurs in approximately 5 of every 10,000 infants and accounts for about 10% of all congenital heart diseases. It occurs equally in boys and girls. Before surgical advances made correction possible, about one-third of these children died in infancy.

Signs and symptoms

The degree of pulmonary stenosis, interacting with the VSD's size and location, determines the clinical and hemodynamic effects of this complex defect. The VSD usually lies in the outflow tract of the right ventricle and is generally large enough to permit equalization of right and left ventricular pressures. However, the ratio of systemic vascular resistance to pulmonary stenosis affects the direction and magnitude of shunt flow across the VSD. Severe obstruction of right ventricular outflow produces a right-to-left shunt, causing decreased systemic arterial oxygen saturation, cyanosis, reduced pulmonary blood flow, and hypoplasia of the entire pulmonary vasculature. Increased right ventricular pressure causes right ventricular hypertrophy. Milder forms of pulmonary stenosis result in a left-to-right shunt or no shunt at all.

Generally, the hallmark of the disorder is cyanosis, which usually becomes evident within several months after birth but may be present at birth if the neonate has severe pulmonary stenosis. Between ages 2 months and 2 years, children with tetralogy of Fallot may experience cyanotic or "blue" spells. Such spells result from increased right-to-left shunting, possibly caused by spasm of the right ventricular outflow tract, increased systemic venous return, or decreased systemic arterial resistance.

Exercise, crying, straining, infection, or fever can precipitate blue spells. Blue spells are characterized by dyspnea; deep, sighing respirations; bradycardia; fainting; seizures; and loss of consciousness. Older children may also develop other signs of poor oxygenation, such as clubbing, diminished exercise tolerance, increasing dyspnea on exertion, growth retardation, and eating difficulties. These children habitually squat when they feel short of breath; this is thought to decrease venous return of unoxygenated blood from the legs and increase systemic arterial resistance.

Children with tetralogy of Fallot also risk developing cerebral abscesses, pulmonary thrombosis, venous thrombosis or cerebral embolism, and infective endocarditis.

In females with tetralogy of Fallot who live to childbearing age, incidence of spontaneous abortion, premature births, and low birth weight rises.

Diagnosis

In a patient with tetralogy of Fallot, auscultation detects a loud systolic heart murmur (best heard along the left sternal border), which may diminish or obscure the pulmonic component of S_2. In a patient with a large patent ductus, the continuous murmur of the ductus obscures the systolic murmur. Palpation may reveal a cardiac thrill at the left sternal border and an obvi-

ous right ventricular impulse. The inferior sternum appears prominent.

The results of special tests also support the diagnosis:

- Chest X-ray may demonstrate decreased pulmonary vascular marking, depending on the pulmonary obstruction's severity, and a boot-shaped cardiac silhouette.
- Electrocardiography shows right ventricular hypertrophy, right axis deviation and, possibly, right atrial hypertrophy.
- Echocardiography identifies septal overriding of the aorta, the VSD, and pulmonary stenosis and detects the hypertrophied walls of the right ventricle.
- Laboratory findings reveal diminished arterial oxygen saturation and polycythemia (hematocrit may be more than 60%) if the cyanosis is severe and long-standing, predisposing the patient to thrombosis.

 CONFIRMING DIAGNOSIS
Cardiac catheterization confirms the diagnosis by visualizing pulmonary stenosis, the VSD, and the overriding aorta and ruling out other cyanotic heart defects. This test also measures the degree of oxygen saturation in aortic blood.

Treatment

Effective management of tetralogy of Fallot necessitates prevention and treatment of complications, measures to relieve cyanosis, and palliative or corrective surgery. During cyanotic spells, the knee-chest position and administration of oxygen and morphine improve oxygenation. Propranolol (a beta-adrenergic blocking agent) may prevent blue spells.

Palliative surgery is performed on infants with potentially fatal hypoxic spells. The goal of surgery is to enhance blood flow to the lungs to reduce hypoxia; this is often accomplished by joining the subclavian artery to the pulmonary artery (Blalock-Taussig procedure). Supportive measures include prophylactic antibiotics to prevent infective endocarditis or cerebral abscess administered before, during, and after bowel, bladder, or any other surgery or dental treatments. Management may also include phlebotomy in children with polycythemia.

Complete corrective surgery to relieve pulmonary stenosis and close the VSD, directing left ventricular outflow to the aorta, requires cardiopulmonary bypass with hypothermia to decrease oxygen utilization during surgery, especially in young children. An infant may have this corrective surgery without prior palliative surgery. It's usually done when progressive hypoxia and polycythemia impair the quality of his life, rather than at a specific age. However, most children require surgery before they reach school age.

Special considerations

■ Explain tetralogy of Fallot to the parents. Inform them that their child will set his own exercise limits and will know when to rest. Make sure they understand that their child can engage in physical activity, and advise them not to be overprotective.

■ Teach the parents to recognize serious hypoxic spells, which can cause dramatically increased cyanosis; deep, sighing respirations; and loss of consciousness. Tell them to place their child in the knee-chest position and to report such spells immediately. Emergency treatment may be necessary.

■ Instruct the parents on ways to prevent overexerting their child, such as feeding him slowly and providing smaller and more frequent meals. Tell them that remaining calm may decrease his anxiety and that anticipating his needs may minimize crying. Encourage the parents to recruit other family members in the care of the child to help prevent their own exhaustion.

■ To prevent infective endocarditis and other infections, warn the parents to keep their child away from people with infections. Urge them to encourage good dental hygiene, and tell them to watch for ear, nose, and throat infections and dental caries, all of which necessitate immediate treatment. When dental care, infections, or surgery requires prophylactic antibiotics, tell the parents to make sure the child completes the prescribed regimen.

■ If the child requires medical attention for an unrelated problem, advise the parents to inform the physician immediately of the child's history of tetralogy of Fallot because any treatment must take this serious heart defect into consideration.

■ During hospitalization, alert the staff to the child's condition. Because of the right-to-left shunt through the VSD, treat I.V. lines like arterial lines. A clot dislodged from a catheter tip in a vein can cross the VSD and cause cerebral embolism. The same thing can happen if air enters the venous lines.

After palliative surgery:

■ Monitor oxygenation and arterial blood gas (ABG) values closely in the intensive care unit.

■ If the child has undergone the Blalock-Taussig procedure, don't use the arm on the operative side for measuring blood pressure, inserting I.V. lines, or drawing blood samples, because blood perfusion on this side diminishes greatly until collateral circulation develops. Note this on the child's chart and at his bedside.

After corrective surgery:

■ Watch for right bundle-branch block or more serious disturbances of atrioventricular conduction and for ventricular ectopic beats.

■ Be alert for other postoperative complications, such as bleeding, right-sided heart failure, and respiratory failure. After surgery, transient heart failure is common and may require treatment with digoxin and diuretics.

■ Monitor left atrial pressure directly. A pulmonary artery catheter may also be used to check central venous and pulmonary artery pressures.

■ Frequently check color and vital signs. Obtain ABG measurements regularly to assess oxygenation. Suction to prevent atelectasis and pneumonia, as needed. Monitor mechanical ventilation.

■ Monitor and record intake and output accurately.

■ If atrioventricular block develops with a low heart rate, a temporary external pacemaker may be necessary.

■ If blood pressure or cardiac output is inadequate, catecholamines may be ordered by continuous I.V. infusion. To decrease left ventricular workload, administer nitroprusside, if ordered, and provide analgesics, as needed.

■ Keep the parents informed about their child's progress. After discharge, the child may require digoxin, diuretics, and other drugs. Stress the importance of complying with the prescribed regimen and make sure the parents know how and when to administer these medications. Teach the parents to watch for signs of digoxin toxicity (anorexia, nausea, and vomiting). Prophylactic antibiotics to prevent infective endocarditis will still be required. Advise the parents to avoid becoming overprotective as the child's tolerance for physical activity rises.

Transposition of the great arteries

In this congenital heart defect, the great arteries are reversed: the aorta arises from the right ventricle and the pulmonary artery from the left ventricle, producing two noncommunicating circulatory systems (pulmonary and systemic). Transposition accounts for about 5% of all congenital heart defects and often coexists with other congenital heart defects, such as ventricular septal defect (VSD), VSD with pulmonary stenosis (PS), atrial septal defect (ASD), and patent ductus arteriosus (PDA). It affects two to three times more males than females.

Causes and incidence
Transposition of the great arteries results from faulty embryonic development, but the cause of such development is unknown. In transposition, oxygenated blood returning to the left side of the heart is carried back to the lungs by a transposed pulmonary artery; unoxygenated blood returning to the right side of the heart is carried to the systemic circulation by a transposed aorta.

Communication between the pulmonary and systemic circulations is necessary for survival. In infants with isolated transposition, blood mixes only at the patent foramen ovale and at the PDA, resulting in slight mixing of unoxygenated systemic blood and oxygenated pulmonary blood. In infants with concurrent cardiac defects, greater mixing of blood occurs.

Transposition of the great arteries occurs in approximately 40 of every 100,000 infants.

Signs and symptoms
Within the first few hours after birth, neonates with transposition of the great arteries and no other heart defects generally show cyanosis and tachypnea, which worsen with crying. After several days or weeks, such neonates usually develop signs of heart failure (gallop rhythm, tachycardia, dyspnea, hepatomegaly, and cardiomegaly). S$_2$ is louder than normal because the anteriorly transposed aorta is directly behind the sternum; in many cases, however, no murmur can be heard during the first few days of life. Associated defects (ASD, VSD, or PDA) cause their typical murmurs and may minimize cyanosis but may also cause other complications (especially severe heart failure). VSD with PS produces a characteristic murmur and severe cyanosis.

As infants with this defect grow older, cyanosis is their most prominent abnormality. However, they also develop diminished exercise tolerance, fatigability, coughing, clubbing, and more pronounced murmurs if ASD, VSD, PDA, or PS is present.

Diagnosis
- Chest X-rays are normal in the first days of life. Within days to weeks, right atrial and right ventricular enlargement characteristically cause the heart to appear oblong. X-rays also show increased pulmonary vascular markings, except when pulmonary stenosis coexists.
- Electrocardiography typically reveals right axis deviation and right ventricular hypertrophy but may be normal in a neonate.

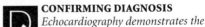 **CONFIRMING DIAGNOSIS**
Echocardiography demonstrates the reversed position of the aorta and pulmonary artery and records echoes from both semilunar valves simultaneously, due to aortic valve displacement. It also detects other cardiac defects. Cardiac catheterization reveals decreased oxygen saturation in left ventricular blood and aortic blood; increased right atrial, right ventricular, and pulmonary artery oxygen saturation; and right ventricular systolic pressure equal to systemic pressure. Dye injection reveals the transposed vessels and the presence of any other cardiac defects.

MUSTARD PROCEDURE

In the Mustard procedure, a Dacron patch (1) is sutured in the excised atrial septum (2) to divert pulmonary venous return to the tricuspid valve and systemic venous return to the mitral valve (3).

1

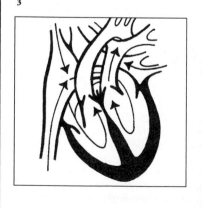

2

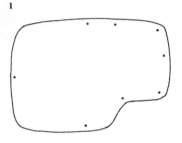

3

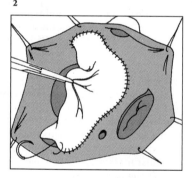

■ Arterial blood gas (ABG) measurements indicate hypoxia and secondary metabolic acidosis.

Treatment

An infant with transposition may undergo atrial balloon septostomy (Rashkind procedure) during cardiac catheterization. This procedure enlarges the patent foramen ovale, which improves oxygenation by allowing greater mixing of the pulmonary and systemic circulations. Atrial balloon septostomy requires passage of a balloon-tipped catheter through the foramen ovale and subsequent inflation and withdrawal across the atrial septum. This procedure alleviates hypoxia to a certain degree. Afterward, digoxin and diuretics can lessen heart failure until the infant is ready to withstand corrective surgery (usually between birth and age 1).

One of three surgical procedures can correct transposition, depending on the defect's physiology. The Mustard procedure replaces the atrial septum with a Dacron or pericardial partition that allows systemic venous blood to be channeled to the pulmonary artery—which carries the blood to the lungs for oxygenation—and oxygenated blood returning to the heart to be channeled from the pulmonary veins into the aorta. (See *Mustard procedure.*) The Senning procedure accomplishes the same result, using the atrial septum to create partitions to redirect blood flow. In the arterial switch, or Jantene procedure, transposed arteries are surgically anastomosed to the correct ventricle. For this procedure to be successful, the left ventricle must be used to pump at systemic pressure, as it does in neonates or in children with a left ventricular outflow obstruction or a large VSD. Surgery also corrects other heart defects.

Special considerations

■ Explain cardiac catheterization and all necessary procedures to the parents. Offer emotional support.
■ Monitor vital signs, ABG values, urine output, and central venous pressure, watching for signs of heart failure. Give digoxin and I.V. fluids, being careful to avoid fluid overload.

- Teach the parents to recognize signs of heart failure and digoxin toxicity (poor feeding and vomiting). Stress the importance of regular checkups to monitor cardiovascular status.
- Teach the parents to protect their infant from infection and to give antibiotics.
- Tell the parents to let their child develop normally. They need not restrict activities; he'll set his own limits.
- If the patient is scheduled for surgery, explain the procedure to the parents and child, if old enough. Teach them about the intensive care unit and introduce them to the staff. Also explain postoperative care.
- Preoperatively, monitor ABG values, acid-base balance, intake and output, and vital signs.

After corrective surgery:
- Monitor cardiac output by checking blood pressure, skin color, heart rate, urine output, central venous and left atrial pressures, and level of consciousness. Report abnormalities or changes.
- Carefully monitor ABG levels and report changes in trends.
- To detect supraventricular conduction blocks and arrhythmias, monitor the patient closely. Watch for signs of atrioventricular blocks, atrial arrhythmias, and faulty sinoatrial function.
- After Mustard or Senning procedures, watch for signs of baffle obstruction such as marked facial edema.
- Encourage parents to help their child assume new activity levels and independence. Teach them about postoperative antibiotic prophylaxis for endocarditis.

ACQUIRED INFLAMMATORY HEART DISEASE

Myocarditis

Myocarditis is focal or diffuse inflammation of the cardiac muscle (myocardium). It may be acute or chronic and can occur at any age. In many cases, myocarditis fails to produce specific cardiovascular symptoms or electrocardiogram (ECG) abnormalities, and recovery is usually spontaneous, without residual defects. Occasionally, myocarditis is complicated by heart failure; in rare cases, it leads to cardiomyopathy.

Causes and incidence
Myocarditis may result from:
- bacterial infections — diphtheria; tuberculosis; typhoid fever; tetanus; and staphylococcal, pneumococcal, and gonococcal infections
- chemical poisons — such as chronic alcoholism
- helminthic infections — such as trichinosis
- hypersensitive immune reactions — acute rheumatic fever and postcardiotomy syndrome
- parasitic infections — especially South American trypanosomiasis (Chagas' disease) in infants and immunosuppressed adults; also toxoplasmosis
- radiation therapy — large doses of radiation to the chest in treating lung or breast cancer
- viral infections (most common cause in the United States and western Europe) — coxsackievirus A and B strains and, possibly, poliomyelitis, influenza, rubeola, rubella, and adenoviruses and echoviruses.

Myocarditis occurs in 1 to 10 of every 100,000 people in the United States. The median age for this disorder is 42, and incidence is equal between males and females. Children, especially neonates, and persons who are immunocompromised or pregnant (especially pregnant black women) are at higher risk for developing this disorder.

Signs and symptoms
Myocarditis usually causes nonspecific symptoms — such as fatigue, dyspnea, palpitations, and fever — that reflect the accompanying systemic infection. Occasionally, it may produce mild, continuous pressure or soreness in the chest (unlike the recurring, stress-related pain of angina pectoris). Although myocarditis is usually self-limiting, it may induce myofibril degeneration that results in right- and left-

sided heart failure, with cardiomegaly, jugular vein distention, dyspnea, persistent fever with resting or exertional tachycardia disproportionate to the degree of fever, and supraventricular and ventricular arrhythmias. Sometimes myocarditis recurs or produces chronic valvulitis (when it results from rheumatic fever), cardiomyopathy, arrhythmias, and thromboembolism.

Diagnosis

Patient history commonly reveals recent febrile upper respiratory tract infection, viral pharyngitis, or tonsillitis. Physical examination shows supraventricular and ventricular arrhythmias, S_3 and S_4 gallops, a faint S_1, possibly a murmur of mitral insufficiency (from papillary muscle dysfunction) and, if pericarditis is present, a pericardial friction rub.

Laboratory tests can't unequivocally confirm myocarditis, but the following findings support this diagnosis:

- cardiac enzymes: elevated creatine kinase (CK), CK-MB, aspartate aminotransferase, and lactate dehydrogenase levels
- increased white blood cell count and erythrocyte sedimentation rate
- elevated antibody titers (such as antistreptolysin-O titer in rheumatic fever).

CONFIRMING DIAGNOSIS
Endomyocardial biopsy is rarely performed to diagnose myocarditis; the procedure is invasive and costly. A negative biopsy doesn't exclude the diagnosis, and a repeat biopsy may be needed.

ECG typically shows diffuse ST-segment and T-wave abnormalities as in pericarditis, conduction defects (prolonged PR interval), and other supraventricular arrhythmias. Echocardiography demonstrates some degree of left ventricular dysfunction, and radionuclide scanning may identify inflammatory and necrotic changes characteristic of myocarditis.

Stool and throat cultures may identify bacteria.

Treatment

Treatment includes antibiotics for bacterial infection, modified bed rest to decrease heart workload, and careful management of complications. Inotropic support of cardiac function with amrinone, dopamine, or dobutamine may be needed. Heart failure requires restriction of activity to minimize myocardial oxygen consumption, supplemental oxygen therapy, sodium restriction, diuretics to decrease fluid retention, and cardiac glycosides to increase myocardial contractility. However, cardiac glycosides should be administered cautiously because some patients with myocarditis may show a paradoxical sensitivity to even small doses. Arrhythmias necessitate prompt but cautious administration of antiarrhythmics because these drugs depress myocardial contractility. Thromboembolism requires anticoagulation therapy. Treatment with corticosteroids or other immunosuppressants may be used to reduce inflammation, but they haven't been shown to change the progression of myocarditis infections. Nonsteroidal anti-inflammatory drugs are contraindicated during the acute phase (first 2 weeks) because they increase myocardial damage.

Surgical treatment may include left ventricular assistive devices and extra corporeal membrane oxygenation for support of cardiogenic shock. Cardiac transplantation has been beneficial for giant cell myocarditis.

Special considerations

- Assess cardiovascular status frequently, watching for signs of heart failure, such as dyspnea, hypotension, and tachycardia. Check for changes in cardiac rhythm or conduction.
- Observe for signs of digoxin toxicity (anorexia, nausea, vomiting, blurred vision, and cardiac arrhythmias) and for complicating factors that may potentiate toxicity, such as electrolyte imbalance or hypoxia.
- Stress the importance of bed rest. Assist with bathing, as necessary; provide a bedside commode because this stresses the heart less than using a bedpan. Reassure the patient that activity limitations are temporary. Offer diversional activities that are physically undemanding.
- During recovery, recommend that the patient resume normal activities slowly and avoid competitive sports.

Endocarditis

Endocarditis (also known as *infective* or *bacterial endocarditis*) is an infection of the endocardium, heart valves, or cardiac prosthesis resulting from bacterial or fungal invasion. This invasion produces vegetative growths on the heart valves, endocardial lining of a heart chamber, or endothelium of a blood vessel that may embolize to the spleen, kidneys, central nervous system, and lungs. In endocarditis, fibrin and platelets aggregate on the valve tissue and engulf circulating bacteria or fungi that flourish and produce friable verrucous vegetations. (See *Degenerative changes in endocarditis.*) Such vegetations may cover the valve surfaces, causing ulceration and necrosis; they may also extend to the chordae tendineae, leading to their rupture and subsequent valvular insufficiency. Untreated endocarditis is usually fatal, but with proper treatment, 70% of patients recover. The prognosis is worst when endocarditis causes severe valvular damage, leading to insufficiency and heart failure, or when it involves a prosthetic valve.

Causes and incidence

Most cases of endocarditis occur in I.V. drug abusers, patients with prosthetic heart valves, and those with mitral valve prolapse (especially males with a systolic murmur). These conditions have surpassed rheumatic heart disease as the leading risk factor. Other predisposing conditions include coarctation of the aorta, tetralogy of Fallot, subaortic and valvular aortic stenosis, ventricular septal defects, pulmonary stenosis, Marfan syndrome, degenerative heart disease (especially calcific aortic stenosis) and, rarely, syphilitic aortic valve. However, some patients with endocarditis have no underlying heart disease.

Infecting organisms differ among these groups. In patients with native valve endocarditis who aren't I.V. drug abusers, causative organisms usually include — in order of frequency — streptococci (especially *Streptococcus viridans),* staphylococci, or enterococci. Although many other bacteria occasionally cause the disorder, fungal causes are rare in this group. The mitral

DEGENERATIVE CHANGES IN ENDOCARDITIS

This illustration shows typical vegetations on the endocardium produced by fibrin and platelet deposits on infection sites.

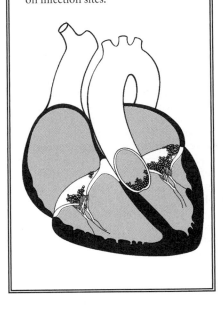

valve is involved most commonly, followed by the aortic valve.

In patients who are I.V. drug abusers, *Staphylococcus aureus* is the most common infecting organism. Less commonly, streptococci, enterococci, gram-negative bacilli, or fungi cause the disorder. The tricuspid valve is involved most commonly, followed by the aortic and then the mitral valve.

In patients with prosthetic valve endocarditis, early cases (those that develop within 60 days of valve insertion) are usually due to staphylococcal infection. However, gram-negative aerobic organisms, fungi, streptococci, enterococci, or diphtheroids may also cause the disorder. The course is usually fulminant and is associated with a high mortality. Late cases (occurring after 60 days) present similarly to native valve endocarditis.

In the United States, endocarditis affects 1.4 to 4.2 people out of every 100,000. Males are twice as likely as females to acquire this infection, and the mean age of onset is 50. Mortality is associated with increased age, infection of the aortic valve, heart failure and underlying heart disease, and central nervous system complications; mortality rates vary with the infecting organism.

Signs and symptoms

Early clinical features of endocarditis are usually nonspecific and include malaise, weakness, fatigue, weight loss, anorexia, arthralgia, night sweats, chills, valvular insufficiency and, in 90% of patients, an intermittent fever that may recur for weeks. A more acute onset is associated with organisms of high pathogenicity such as *S. aureus*. Endocarditis commonly causes a loud, regurgitant murmur typical of the underlying heart lesion. A suddenly changing murmur or the discovery of a new murmur in the presence of fever is a classic physical sign of endocarditis.

In about 30% of patients, embolization from vegetating lesions or diseased valvular tissue may produce typical features of splenic, renal, cerebral, or pulmonary infarction or of peripheral vascular occlusion:

- splenic infarction — pain in the left upper quadrant, radiating to the left shoulder; and abdominal rigidity
- renal infarction — hematuria, pyuria, flank pain, and decreased urine output
- cerebral infarction — hemiparesis, aphasia, or other neurologic deficits
- pulmonary infarction (most common in right-sided endocarditis, which commonly occurs among I.V. drug abusers and after cardiac surgery) — cough, pleuritic pain, pleural friction rub, dyspnea, and hemoptysis
- peripheral vascular occlusion — numbness and tingling in an arm, leg, finger, or toe, or signs of impending peripheral gangrene.

Other signs may include splenomegaly; petechiae of the skin (especially common on the upper anterior trunk) and the buccal, pharyngeal, or conjunctival mucosa; and splinter hemorrhages under the nails. Rarely, endocarditis produces Osler's nodes (tender, raised, subcutaneous lesions on the fingers or toes), Roth's spots (hemor-

rhagic areas with white centers on the retina), and Janeway lesions (purplish macules on the palms or soles).

Diagnosis

CONFIRMING DIAGNOSIS *Three or more blood cultures in a 24- to 48-hour period (each from a separate venipuncture) identify the causative organism in up to 90% of patients. Blood cultures should be drawn from three different sites with 1 hour between each draw.*

The remaining 10% may have negative blood cultures, possibly suggesting fungal infection or infections that are difficult to diagnose such as *Haemophilus parainfluenzae*.

Other abnormal but nonspecific laboratory test results include:

- normal or elevated white blood cell count
- abnormal histiocytes (macrophages)
- elevated erythrocyte sedimentation rate
- normocytic, normochromic anemia (in 70% to 90% of patients)
- proteinuria and microscopic hematuria (in about 50% of patients)
- positive serum rheumatoid factor (in about 50% of patients after endocarditis is present for 3 to 6 weeks).

Echocardiography (particularly, transesophageal) may identify valvular damage; electrocardiography may show atrial fibrillation and other arrhythmias that accompany valvular disease.

Treatment

The goal of treatment is to eradicate the infecting organism with appropriate antimicrobial therapy, which should start promptly and continue over 4 to 6 weeks. Selection of an antibiotic is based on identification of the infecting organism and on sensitivity studies. While awaiting results, or if blood cultures are negative, empiric antimicrobial therapy is based on the likely infecting organism.

Supportive treatment includes bed rest, aspirin for fever and aches, and sufficient fluid intake. Severe valvular damage, especially aortic or mitral insufficiency, may require corrective surgery if refractory heart failure develops, or in cases requiring that an infected prosthetic valve be replaced.

Special considerations

■ Before giving antibiotics, obtain a patient history of allergies. Administer antibiotics on time to maintain consistent antibiotic blood levels.

■ Observe for signs of infiltration or inflammation at the venipuncture site, possible complications of long-term I.V. drug administration. To reduce the risk of these complications, rotate venous access sites.

■ Watch for signs of embolization (hematuria, pleuritic chest pain, left upper quadrant pain, or paresis), a common occurrence during the first 3 months of treatment. Tell the patient to watch for and report these signs, which may indicate impending peripheral vascular occlusion or splenic, renal, cerebral, or pulmonary infarction.

■ Monitor the patient's renal status (blood urea nitrogen levels, creatinine clearance, and urine output) to check for signs of renal emboli or evidence of drug toxicity.

■ Observe for signs of heart failure, such as dyspnea, tachypnea, tachycardia, crackles, jugular vein distention, edema, and weight gain.

■ Provide reassurance by teaching the patient and his family about this disease and the need for prolonged treatment. Tell them to watch closely for fever, anorexia, and other signs of relapse about 2 weeks after treatment stops. Suggest quiet diversionary activities to prevent excessive physical exertion.

■ Make sure susceptible patients understand the need for prophylactic antibiotics before, during, and after dental work, childbirth, and genitourinary, GI, or gynecologic procedures.

■ Teach patients how to recognize symptoms of endocarditis and tell them to notify the physician at once if such symptoms occur.

Pericarditis

Pericarditis is an inflammation of the pericardium, the fibroserous sac that envelops, supports, and protects the heart. It occurs in both acute and chronic forms. Acute pericarditis can be fibrinous or effusive, with purulent serous or hemorrhagic exudate; chronic constrictive pericarditis is characterized by dense fibrous pericardial thickening. The prognosis depends on the underlying cause but is generally good in acute pericarditis, unless constriction occurs.

Causes and incidence

Common causes of this disease include:
■ bacterial, fungal, or viral infection (infectious pericarditis)
■ neoplasms (primary or metastatic from lungs, breasts, or other organs)
■ high-dose radiation to the chest
■ uremia
■ hypersensitivity or autoimmune disease, such as acute rheumatic fever (most common cause of pericarditis in children), systemic lupus erythematosus, and rheumatoid arthritis
■ postcardiac injury such as myocardial infarction (MI), which later causes an autoimmune reaction (Dressler's syndrome) in the pericardium; trauma; or surgery that leaves the pericardium intact but causes blood to leak into the pericardial cavity
■ drugs, such as hydralazine or procainamide
■ idiopathic factors (most common in acute pericarditis).

Less common causes include aortic aneurysm with pericardial leakage, and myxedema with cholesterol deposits in the pericardium.

Pericarditis most commonly affects men ages 20 to 50, but it can also occur in children following infection with an adenovirus or coxsackievirus.

Signs and symptoms

Acute pericarditis typically produces a sharp and often sudden pain that usually starts over the sternum and radiates to the neck, shoulders, back, and arms. However, unlike the pain of MI, pericardial pain is often pleuritic, increasing with deep inspiration and decreasing when the patient sits up and leans forward, pulling the heart away from the diaphragmatic pleurae of the lungs.

Pericardial effusion, the major complication of acute pericarditis, may produce effects of heart failure (such as dyspnea, orthopnea, and tachycardia), ill-defined substernal chest pain, and a feeling of fullness in the chest. (See *Patterns of cardiac pain*.)

ALERT *If the fluid accumulates rapidly, cardiac tamponade may occur, resulting in pallor, clammy skin, hypotension, pulsus paradoxus (a decrease in systolic blood pressure of 15 mm Hg or more during slow inspiration), jugular vein distention and, eventually, cardiovascular collapse and death.*

Chronic constrictive pericarditis causes a gradual increase in systemic venous pressure and produces symptoms similar to those of chronic right-sided heart failure (fluid retention, ascites, and hepatomegaly).

Diagnosis

Because pericarditis commonly coexists with other conditions, diagnosis of acute pericarditis depends on typical clinical features and elimination of other possible causes. The pericardial friction rub, a classic symptom, is a grating sound heard as the heart moves. It can usually be auscultated best during forced expiration, while the patient leans forward or is on his hands and knees in bed. It may have up to three components, corresponding to the timing of atrial systole, ventricular systole, and the rapid-filling phase of ventricular diastole. Occasionally, this friction rub is heard only briefly or not at all. Nevertheless, its presence, together with other characteristic features, is diagnostic of acute pericarditis. In addition, if acute pericarditis has caused very large pericardial effusions, physical examination reveals increased cardiac dullness and diminished or absent apical impulse and distant heart sounds.

Chest X-ray, echocardiogram, chest magnetic resonance imaging (MRI), heart MRI, heart computed tomography scan, and radionuclide scanning can detect fluid that has accumulated in the pericardial sac. They may also show enlargement of the heart and signs of inflammation or scarring, depending on the cause of pericarditis.

In patients with chronic pericarditis, acute inflammation or effusions don't occur—only restricted cardiac filling.

Laboratory results reflect inflammation and may identify its cause:
- normal or elevated white blood cell count, especially in infectious pericarditis
- elevated erythrocyte sedimentation rate
- slightly elevated cardiac enzyme levels with associated myocarditis
- culture of pericardial fluid obtained by open surgical drainage or cardiocentesis (sometimes identifies a causative organism in bacterial or fungal pericarditis)
- electrocardiography showing the following changes in acute pericarditis: elevation of ST segments in the standard limb leads and most precordial leads without significant changes in QRS morphology that occur with MI, atrial ectopic rhythms such as atrial fibrillation and, in pericardial effusion, diminished QRS voltage.

Other pertinent laboratory data include blood urea nitrogen levels to check for uremia, antistreptolysin-O titers to detect rheumatic fever, and a purified protein derivative skin test to check for tuberculosis. In pericardial effusion, echocardiography is diagnostic when it shows an echo-free space between the ventricular wall and the pericardium.

Treatment

The goal of treatment is to relieve symptoms and manage the underlying systemic disease. In acute idiopathic pericarditis and postthoracotomy pericarditis, treatment consists of bed rest as long as fever and pain persist, and nonsteroidal drugs, such as aspirin and indomethacin, to relieve pain and reduce inflammation. Post-MI patients should avoid nonsteroidal anti-inflammatory drugs and steroids because they may interfere with myocardial scar formation. If these drugs fail to relieve symptoms, corticosteroids may be used. Although corticosteroids produce rapid and effective relief, they must be used cautiously because episodes may recur when therapy is discontinued.

Infectious pericarditis that results from disease of the left pleural space, mediastinal abscesses, or septicemia requires antibiotics (possibly by direct pericardial injection), surgical drainage, or both. Cardiac tamponade may require pericardiocentesis. Signs of tamponade include pulsus para-

PATTERNS OF CARDIAC PAIN

Although pain perception is individualistic, specific characteristics are associated with different types of cardiac pain, as shown below.

Pericarditis

Onset and duration
- Sudden onset; continuous pain lasting for days; residual soreness

Location and radiation
- Substernal pain to left of midline; radiation to back or subclavicular area

Quality and intensity
- Mild ache to severe pain, deep or superficial; "stabbing," "knifelike"

Signs and symptoms
- Precordial friction rub; increased pain with movement, inspiration, laughing, coughing; decreased pain with sitting or leaning forward (sitting up pulls heart away from diaphragm)

Precipitating factors
- Myocardial infarction or upper respiratory tract infection; invasive cardiac trauma

Angina

Onset and duration
- Gradual or sudden onset; pain usually lasts less than 15 minutes and not more than 30 minutes (average: 3 minutes)

Location and radiation
- Substernal or anterior chest pain, not sharply localized; radiation to back, neck, arms, jaws, even upper abdomen or fingers

Quality and intensity
- Mild-to-moderate pressure; deep sensation; varied pattern of attacks; "tightness," "squeezing," "crushing," "pressure"

Signs and symptoms
- Dyspnea, diaphoresis, nausea, desire to void, belching, apprehension

Precipitating factors
- Exertion, stress, eating, cold or hot and humid weather

Myocardial infarction

Onset and duration
- Sudden onset; pain lasts 30 minutes to 2 hours; waxes and wanes; residual soreness 1 to 3 days

Location and radiation
- Substernal, midline, or anterior chest pain; radiation to jaws, neck, back, shoulders, or one or both arms

Quality and intensity
- Persistent, severe pressure; deep sensation; "crushing," "squeezing," "heavy," "oppressive"

Signs and symptoms
- Nausea, vomiting, apprehension, dyspnea, diaphoresis, increased or decreased blood pressure; gallop heart sound, "sensation of impending doom"

Precipitating factors
- Occurrence at rest or during physical exertion or emotional stress

---

doxus, jugular vein distention, dyspnea, and shock.

Recurrent pericarditis may necessitate partial pericardectomy, which creates a "window" that allows fluid to drain into the pleural space. In constrictive pericarditis, total pericardectomy to permit adequate filling and contraction of the heart may be necessary. Treatment must also include management of rheumatic fever, uremia, tuberculosis, and other underlying disorders.

Special considerations

A patient with pericarditis needs complete bed rest. In addition, health care includes:
- assessing pain in relation to respiration and body position to distinguish pericardial pain from myocardial ischemic pain.
- placing the patient in an upright position to relieve dyspnea and chest pain; providing analgesics and oxygen; and reassuring the patient with acute pericarditis that his condition is temporary and treatable.

■ monitoring for signs of cardiac compression or cardiac tamponade, possible complications of pericardial effusion. Signs include decreased blood pressure, increased central venous pressure, and pulsus paradoxus. Because cardiac tamponade requires immediate treatment, keep a pericardiocentesis set handy whenever pericardial effusion is suspected.

■ explaining tests and treatments to the patient. If surgery is necessary, he should learn deep-breathing and coughing exercises beforehand. Postoperative care is similar to that given after cardiothoracic surgery.

Rheumatic fever and rheumatic heart disease

Acute rheumatic fever is a systemic inflammatory disease of childhood, in many cases recurrent, that follows a group A beta-hemolytic streptococcal infection. Rheumatic heart disease refers to the cardiac manifestations of rheumatic fever and includes pancarditis (myocarditis, pericarditis, and endocarditis) during the early acute phase and chronic valvular disease later. Long-term antibiotic therapy can minimize the recurrence of rheumatic fever, reducing the risk of permanent cardiac damage and eventual valvular deformity. However, severe pancarditis occasionally produces fatal heart failure during the acute phase. Of the patients who survive this complication, about 20% die within 10 years.

Causes and incidence

Rheumatic fever appears to be a hypersensitivity reaction to a group A beta-hemolytic streptococcal infection, in which antibodies manufactured to combat streptococci react and produce characteristic lesions at specific tissue sites, especially in the heart and joints. Because very few persons (3%) with streptococcal infections ever contract rheumatic fever, altered host resistance must be involved in its development or recurrence. Although rheumatic fever tends to be familial, this may merely reflect contributing environmental factors. For example, in lower socioeconomic groups, incidence is highest in children between ages 5 and 15, probably as a result of

malnutrition and crowded living conditions. This disease strikes generally during cool, damp weather in the winter and early spring. In the United States, it's most common in the northern states.

Signs and symptoms

In 95% of patients, rheumatic fever characteristically follows a streptococcal infection that appeared a few days to 6 weeks earlier. A temperature of at least 100.4° F (38° C) occurs, and most patients complain of migratory joint pain or polyarthritis. Swelling, redness, and signs of effusion usually accompany such pain, which most commonly affects the knees, ankles, elbows, or hips. In 5% of patients (generally those with carditis), rheumatic fever causes skin lesions such as erythema marginatum, a nonpruritic, macular, transient rash that gives rise to red lesions with blanched centers. Rheumatic fever may also produce firm, movable, nontender, subcutaneous nodules about 3 mm to 2 cm in diameter, usually near tendons or bony prominences of joints (especially the elbows, knuckles, wrists, and knees) and less often on the scalp and backs of the hands. These nodules persist for a few days to several weeks and, like erythema marginatum, often accompany carditis.

Later, rheumatic fever may cause transient chorea, which develops up to 6 months after the original streptococcal infection. Mild chorea may produce hyperirritability, a deterioration in handwriting, or an inability to concentrate. Severe chorea (Sydenham's chorea) causes purposeless, nonrepetitive, involuntary muscle spasms; poor muscle coordination; and weakness. Chorea always resolves without residual neurologic damage.

The most destructive effect of rheumatic fever is carditis, which develops in up to 50% of patients and may affect the endocardium, myocardium, pericardium, or the heart valves. Pericarditis causes a pericardial friction rub and, occasionally, pain and effusion. Myocarditis produces characteristic lesions called Aschoff bodies (in the acute stages) and cellular swelling and fragmentation of interstitial collagen, leading to formation of a progressively fibrotic nodule and interstitial scars. Endocarditis causes valve leaflet swelling, erosion along the lines of leaflet closure, and blood, platelet, and fibrin deposits, which form beadlike vegetations. Endocarditis affects the mitral valve most often in females; the aortic, most often in males. In both females and males, endocarditis affects the tricuspid valves occasionally and the pulmonic only rarely.

Severe rheumatic carditis may cause heart failure with dyspnea; right upper quadrant pain; tachycardia; tachypnea; a hacking, nonproductive cough; edema; and significant mitral and aortic murmurs. The most common of such murmurs include:

- a systolic murmur of mitral insufficiency (high-pitched, blowing, holosystolic, loudest at apex, possibly radiating to the anterior axillary line)
- a midsystolic murmur due to stiffening and swelling of the mitral leaflet
- occasionally, a diastolic murmur of aortic insufficiency (low-pitched, rumbling, almost inaudible). Valvular disease may eventually result in chronic valvular stenosis and insufficiency, including mitral stenosis and insufficiency, and aortic insufficiency. In children, mitral insufficiency remains the major sequela of rheumatic heart disease.

Diagnosis

Diagnosis depends on recognition of one or more of the classic symptoms (carditis, rheumatic fever without carditis, polyarthritis, chorea, erythema marginatum, or subcutaneous nodules) and a detailed patient history. Laboratory data support the diagnosis:

- White blood cell count and erythrocyte sedimentation rate may be elevated (during the acute phase); blood studies show slight anemia due to suppressed erythropoiesis during inflammation.
- C-reactive protein is positive (especially during acute phase).
- Cardiac enzyme levels may be increased in severe carditis.
- Antistreptolysin-O titer is elevated in 95% of patients within 2 months of onset.
- Electrocardiogram changes aren't diagnostic; but PR interval is prolonged in 20% of patients.
- Chest X-rays show normal heart size (except with myocarditis, heart failure, or pericardial effusion).

- Echocardiography helps evaluate valvular damage, chamber size, and ventricular function.
- Cardiac catheterization evaluates valvular damage and left ventricular function in severe cardiac dysfunction.

Treatment

Effective management eradicates the streptococcal infection, relieves symptoms, and prevents recurrence, reducing the chance of permanent cardiac damage. During the acute phase, treatment includes penicillin, sulfadiazine, or erythromycin. Salicylates such as aspirin relieve fever and minimize joint swelling and pain; if carditis is present or salicylates fail to relieve pain and inflammation, corticosteroids may be used. Supportive treatment requires strict bed rest for about 5 weeks during the acute phase with active carditis, followed by a progressive increase in physical activity, depending on clinical and laboratory findings and the response to treatment.

After the acute phase subsides, low-dose antibiotics may be used to prevent recurrence. Such preventive treatment usually continues for 5 years or until age 21 (whichever is longer). Heart failure necessitates continued bed rest and diuretics. Severe mitral or aortic valve dysfunction that causes persistent heart failure requires corrective valvular surgery, including commissurotomy (separation of the adherent, thickened leaflets of the mitral valve), valvuloplasty (inflation of a balloon within a valve), or valve replacement (with prosthetic valve). Such surgery is seldom necessary before late adolescence.

Special considerations

Because rheumatic fever and rheumatic heart disease require prolonged treatment, the care plan should include comprehensive patient teaching to promote compliance with the prescribed therapy.

- Before giving penicillin, ask the patient or his parents if he has ever had a hypersensitive reaction to it. If he hasn't, warn that such a reaction is possible. Tell them to stop the drug and call the physician immediately if he develops a rash, fever, chills, or other signs of allergy *at any time* during penicillin therapy.

■ Instruct the patient and his family to watch for and report early signs of heart failure, such as dyspnea and a hacking, nonproductive cough.

■ Stress the need for bed rest during the acute phase and suggest appropriate, physically undemanding diversions. After the acute phase, encourage his family and friends to spend as much time as possible with the patient to minimize boredom. Advise his parents to secure tutorial services to help the child keep up with schoolwork during the long convalescence.

■ Help his parents overcome any guilt feelings they may have about their child's illness. Tell them that failure to seek treatment for streptococcal infection is common because this illness often seems no worse than a cold. Encourage the child and his parents to vent their frustrations during the long, tedious recovery. If the child has severe carditis, help them prepare for permanent changes in his lifestyle.

■ Teach the patient and his family about this disease and its treatment. Warn parents to watch for and immediately report signs of recurrent streptococcal infection — sudden sore throat, diffuse throat redness and oropharyngeal exudate, swollen and tender cervical lymph glands, pain on swallowing, temperature of 101° to 104° F (38.3° to 40° C), headache, and nausea. Urge them to keep the child away from people with respiratory tract infections.

■ Promote good dental hygiene to prevent gingival infection. Make sure the patient and his family understand the need to comply with prolonged antibiotic therapy and follow-up care and the need for additional antibiotics during dental surgery or procedures. Arrange for a home health nurse to oversee home care if necessary.

■ Teach the patient to follow current recommendations of the American Heart Association for prevention of bacterial endocarditis. Antibiotic regimens used to prevent recurrence of acute rheumatic fever are inadequate for preventing bacterial endocarditis.

VALVE DISORDERS

Valvular heart disease

In valvular heart disease, three types of mechanical disruption can occur: stenosis, or narrowing, of the valve opening; incomplete closure of the valve; or prolapse of the valve. They can result from such disorders as endocarditis (most common), congenital defects, and inflammation, and they can lead to heart failure.

Valvular heart disease occurs in varying forms, described below. Additional information is provided in *Types of valvular heart disease.*

■ Mitral insufficiency: In this form, blood from the left ventricle flows back into the left atrium during systole, causing the atrium to enlarge to accommodate the backflow. As a result, the left ventricle also dilates to accommodate the increased volume of blood from the atrium and to compensate for diminishing cardiac output. Ventricular hypertrophy and increased end-diastolic pressure result in increased pulmonary artery pressure, eventually leading to left- and right-sided heart failure.

■ Mitral stenosis: Narrowing of the valve by valvular abnormalities, fibrosis, or calcification obstructs blood flow from the left atrium to the left ventricle. Consequently, left atrial volume and pressure rise and the chamber dilates. Greater resistance to blood flow causes pulmonary hypertension, right ventricular hypertrophy, and right-sided heart failure. Also, inadequate filling of the left ventricle produces low cardiac output.

■ Mitral valve prolapse (MVP): One or both valve leaflets protrude into the left atrium. MVP is the term used when the anatomic prolapse is accompanied by signs and symptoms unrelated to the valvular abnormality.

■ Aortic insufficiency: Blood flows back into the left ventricle during diastole, causing fluid overload in the ventricle, which dilates and hypertrophies. The excess volume causes fluid overload in the left atri-

(Text continues on page 1090.)

TYPES OF VALVULAR HEART DISEASE

Causes and incidence	Clinical features	Diagnostic measures
Aortic insufficiency ■ Results from rheumatic fever, syphilis, hypertension, endocarditis, or may be idiopathic ■ Associated with Marfan syndrome ■ Most common in males ■ Associated with ventricular septal defect, even after surgical closure	■ Dyspnea, cough, fatigue, palpitations, angina, syncope ■ Pulmonary venous congestion, heart failure, pulmonary edema (left-sided heart failure), "pulsating" nail beds ■ Rapidly rising and collapsing pulses (pulsus biferiens), cardiac arrhythmias, wide pulse pressure in severe insufficiency ■ Auscultation reveals S_3 and diastolic blowing murmur at left sternal border ■ Palpation and visualization of apical impulse in chronic disease	■ Cardiac catheterization: reduction in arterial diastolic pressures, aortic insufficiency, other valvular abnormalities, and increased left ventricular end-diastolic pressure ■ X-ray: left ventricular enlargement, pulmonary vein congestion ■ Echocardiography: left ventricular enlargement, alterations in mitral valve movement (indirect indication of aortic valve disease), and mitral thickening ■ Electrocardiography (ECG): sinus tachycardia, left ventricular hypertrophy, and left atrial hypertrophy in severe disease
Aortic stenosis ■ Results from congenital aortic bicuspid valve (associated with coarctation of the aorta), congenital stenosis of valve cusps, rheumatic fever, or atherosclerosis in elderly persons ■ Most common in males	■ Dyspnea on exertion, paroxysmal nocturnal dyspnea, fatigue, syncope, angina, palpitations ■ Pulmonary venous congestion, heart failure, pulmonary edema ■ Diminished carotid pulses, decreased cardiac output, cardiac arrhythmias; may have pulsus alternans ■ Auscultation reveals systolic murmur at base or in carotids and, possibly, S_4	■ Cardiac catheterization: pressure gradient across valve (indicating obstruction), increased left ventricular end-diastolic pressures ■ X-ray: valvular calcification, left ventricular enlargement, and pulmonary venous congestion ■ Echocardiography: thickened aortic valve and left ventricular wall ■ ECG: left ventricular hypertrophy

(continued)

TYPES OF VALVULAR HEART DISEASE *(continued)*

Causes and incidence	Clinical features	Diagnostic measures
Mitral insufficiency ■ Results from rheumatic fever, hypertrophic cardiomyopathy, mitral valve prolapse, myocardial infarction, severe left-sided heart failure, or ruptured chordae tendineae ■ Associated with other congenital anomalies such as transposition of the great arteries ■ Rare in children without other congenital anomalies	■ Orthopnea, dyspnea, fatigue, angina, palpitations ■ Peripheral edema, jugular vein distention (JVD), hepatomegaly (right-sided heart failure) ■ Tachycardia, crackles, pulmonary edema ■ Auscultation reveals holosystolic murmur at apex, possible split S_2, and S_3	■ Cardiac catheterization: mitral insufficiency with increased left ventricular end-diastolic volume and pressure, increased atrial pressure and pulmonary artery wedge pressure (PAWP); and decreased cardiac output X-ray: left atrial and ventricular enlargement, pulmonary venous congestion ■ Echocardiography: abnormal valve leaflet motion, left atrial enlargement ■ ECG: left atrial and ventricular hypertrophy, sinus tachycardia, and atrial fibrillation
Mitral stenosis ■ Results from rheumatic fever (most common cause) ■ Most common in females ■ May be associated with other congenital anomalies	■ Dyspnea on exertion, paroxysmal nocturnal dyspnea, orthopnea, weakness, fatigue, palpitations ■ Peripheral edema, JVD, ascites, hepatomegaly (right-sided heart failure in severe pulmonary hypertension) ■ Crackles, cardiac arrhythmias (atrial fibrillation), signs of systemic emboli ■ Auscultation reveals loud S_1 or opening snap and diastolic murmur at apex	■ Cardiac catheterization: diastolic pressure gradient across valve; elevated left atrial pressure and PAWP (> 15 mm Hg) with severe pulmonary hypertension and pulmonary artery pressures (PAPs); elevated right-sided heart pressure; decreased cardiac output; and abnormal contraction of the left ventricle ■ X-ray: left atrial and ventricular enlargement, enlarged pulmonary arteries, and mitral valve calcification ■ Echocardiography: thickened mitral valve leaflets, left atrial enlargement ■ ECG: left atrial hypertrophy, atrial fibrillation, right ventricular hypertrophy, and right axis deviation

TYPES OF VALVULAR HEART DISEASE *(continued)*

Causes and incidence	Clinical features	Diagnostic measures
Mitral valve prolapse syndrome		
■ Cause unknown; researchers speculate that metabolic or neuroendocrine factors cause constellation of signs and symptoms. ■ Most commonly affects young women but may occur in both sexes and in all age-groups	■ May produce no signs ■ Chest pain, palpitations, headache, fatigue, exercise intolerance, dyspnea, lightheadedness, syncope, mood swings, anxiety, panic attacks ■ Auscultation typically reveals mobile, midsystolic click, with or without mid-to-late systolic murmur	■ Two-dimensional echocardiography: prolapse of mitral valve leaflets into left atrium ■ Color-flow Doppler studies: mitral insufficiency ■ Resting ECG: ST-segment changes, biphasic or inverted T-waves in leads II, III, or AV ■ Exercise ECG: evaluates chest pain and arrhythmias
Pulmonic insufficiency		
■ May be congenital or may result from pulmonary hypertension ■ May rarely result from prolonged use of pressure monitoring catheter in the pulmonary artery	■ Dyspnea, weakness, fatigue, chest pain ■ Peripheral edema, JVD, hepatomegaly (right-sided heart failure) ■ Auscultation reveals diastolic murmur in pulmonic area	■ Cardiac catheterization: pulmonic insufficiency, increased right ventricular pressure, and associated cardiac defects ■ X-ray: right ventricular and pulmonary arterial enlargement ■ ECG: right ventricular or right atrial enlargement
Pulmonic stenosis		
■ Results from congenital stenosis of valve cusp or rheumatic heart disease (infrequent) ■ Associated with other congenital heart defects such as tetralogy of Fallot	■ Asymptomatic or symptomatic with dyspnea on exertion, fatigue, chest pain, syncope ■ May lead to peripheral edema, JVD, hepatomegaly (right-sided heart failure) ■ Auscultation reveals systolic murmur at left sternal border, split S_2 with delayed or absent pulmonic component	■ Cardiac catheterization: increased right ventricular pressure, decreased PAP, and abnormal valve orifice ■ ECG: may show right ventricular hypertrophy, right axis deviation, right atrial hypertrophy, and atrial fibrillation
Tricuspid insufficiency		
■ Results from right-sided heart failure, rheumatic fever and, rarely, trauma and endocarditis ■ Associated with congenital disorders	■ Dyspnea and fatigue ■ May lead to peripheral edema, JVD, hepatomegaly, and ascites (right-sided heart failure) ■ Auscultation reveals possible S_3 and systolic murmur at lower left sternal border that increases with inspiration	■ Right-sided heart catheterization: high atrial pressure, tricuspid insufficiency, decreased or normal cardiac output ■ X-ray: right atrial dilation, right ventricular enlargement ■ Echocardiography: shows systolic prolapse of tricuspid valve, right atrial enlargement ■ ECG: right atrial or right ventricular hypertrophy, atrial fibrillation

(continued)

TYPES OF VALVULAR HEART DISEASE *(continued)*

Causes and incidence	Clinical features	Diagnostic measures
Tricuspid stenosis ■ Results from rheumatic fever ■ May be congenital ■ Associated with mitral or aortic valve disease ■ Most common in women	■ May be symptomatic with dyspnea, fatigue, syncope ■ Possibly peripheral edema, JVD, hepatomegaly, and ascites (right-sided heart failure) ■ Auscultation reveals diastolic murmur at lower left sternal border that increases with inspiration	■ Cardiac catheterization: increased pressure gradient across valve, increased right atrial pressure, decreased cardiac output ■ X-ray: right atrial enlargement ■ Echocardiography: leaflet abnormality, right atrial enlargement ■ ECG: right atrial hypertrophy, right or left ventricular hypertrophy, and atrial fibrillation

um and, finally, the pulmonary system. Left-sided heart failure and pulmonary edema eventually result.

■ Aortic stenosis: Increased left ventricular pressure tries to overcome the resistance of the narrowed valvular opening. The added workload increases the demand for oxygen, whereas diminished cardiac output causes poor coronary artery perfusion, ischemia of the left ventricle, and left-sided heart failure.

■ Pulmonic insufficiency: Blood ejected into the pulmonary artery during systole flows back into the right ventricle during diastole, causing fluid overload in the ventricle, ventricular hypertrophy and, finally, right-sided heart failure.

■ Pulmonic stenosis: Obstructed right ventricular outflow causes right ventricular hypertrophy, eventually resulting in right-sided heart failure.

■ Tricuspid insufficiency: Blood flows back into the right atrium during systole, decreasing blood flow to the lungs and the left side of the heart. Cardiac output also lessens. Fluid overload in the right side of the heart can eventually lead to right-sided heart failure.

■ Tricuspid stenosis: Obstructed blood flow from the right atrium to the right ventricle causes the right atrium to dilate and hypertrophy. Eventually, this leads to right-

sided heart failure and increases pressure in the vena cava.

Treatment
Treatment depends on the nature and severity of associated symptoms. For example, heart failure requires digoxin, diuretics, a sodium-restricted diet and, in acute cases, oxygen. Other measures may include anticoagulant therapy or antiplatelet medications to prevent thrombus formation around diseased or replaced valves, prophylactic antibiotics before and after surgery or dental care, and valvuloplasty. An intra-aortic balloon pump may be used temporarily to reduce backflow by enhancing forward blood flow into the aorta.

If the patient has severe signs and symptoms that can't be managed medically, open heart surgery using cardiopulmonary bypass for valve replacement is indicated.

Special considerations
■ Watch closely for signs of heart failure or pulmonary edema and for adverse effects of drug therapy.

■ Teach the patient about diet restrictions, medications, and the importance of consistent follow-up care.

■ If the patient has surgery, watch for hypotension, arrhythmias, and thrombus formation. Monitor vital signs, arterial blood gas values, intake, output, daily weight, blood chemistries, chest X-rays, and pulmonary artery catheter readings.

DEGENERATIVE CARDIOVASCULAR DISORDERS

Hypertension

Hypertension, an intermittent or sustained elevation in diastolic or systolic blood pressure, occurs as two major types: essential (idiopathic) hypertension, the most common, and secondary hypertension, which results from renal disease or another identifiable cause. Malignant hypertension is a severe, fulminant form of hypertension common to both types. Hypertension is a major cause of stroke, cardiac disease, and renal failure. The prognosis is good if this disorder is detected early and treatment begins before complications develop. Severely elevated blood pressure (hypertensive crisis) may be fatal. (See *What happens in hypertensive crisis*, page 1092 and 1093.)

Causes and incidence
Hypertension affects 25% of adults in the United States. If untreated, it carries a high mortality. Risk factors for hypertension include family history, race (most common in blacks), stress, obesity, a diet high in saturated fats or sodium, tobacco use, sedentary lifestyle, and aging.

Secondary hypertension may result from renal vascular disease; pheochromocytoma; primary hyperaldosteronism; Cushing's syndrome; thyroid, pituitary, or parathyroid dysfunction; coarctation of the aorta; pregnancy; neurologic disorders; and use of hormonal contraceptives or other drugs, such as cocaine, epoetin alfa (erythropoietin), and cyclosporine.

Cardiac output and peripheral vascular resistance determine blood pressure. Increased blood volume, cardiac rate, and stroke volume as well as arteriolar vasoconstriction can raise blood pressure. The link to sustained hypertension, however, is unclear. Hypertension may also result from failure of intrinsic regulatory mechanisms:

- Renal hypoperfusion causes release of renin, which is converted by angiotensinogen, a liver enzyme, to angiotensin I. Angiotensin I is converted to angiotensin II, a powerful vasoconstrictor. The resulting vasoconstriction increases afterload. Angiotensin II stimulates adrenal secretion of aldosterone, which increases sodium reabsorption. Hypertonic-stimulated release of antidiuretic hormone from the pituitary gland follows, increasing water reabsorption, plasma volume, cardiac output, and blood pressure.
- Autoregulation changes an artery's diameter to maintain perfusion despite fluctuations in systemic blood pressure. The intrinsic mechanisms responsible include stress relaxation (vessels gradually dilate when blood pressure rises to reduce peripheral resistance) and capillary fluid shift (plasma moves between vessels and extravascular spaces to maintain intravascular volume).
- When the blood pressure drops, baroreceptors in the aortic arch and carotid sinuses decrease their inhibition of the medulla's vasomotor center, which increases sympathetic stimulation of the heart by norepinephrine. This, in turn, increases cardiac output by strengthening the contractile force, increasing the heart rate, and augmenting peripheral resistance by vasoconstriction. Stress can also stimulate the sympathetic nervous system to increase cardiac output and peripheral vascular resistance.

Signs and symptoms
Hypertension usually doesn't produce clinical effects until vascular changes in the heart, brain, or kidneys occur. Severely elevated blood pressure damages the intima of small vessels, resulting in fibrin accumulation in the vessels, development of local edema and, possibly, intravascular clotting. Symptoms produced by this process depend on the location of the damaged vessels:

- brain — stroke
- retina — blindness
- heart — myocardial infarction

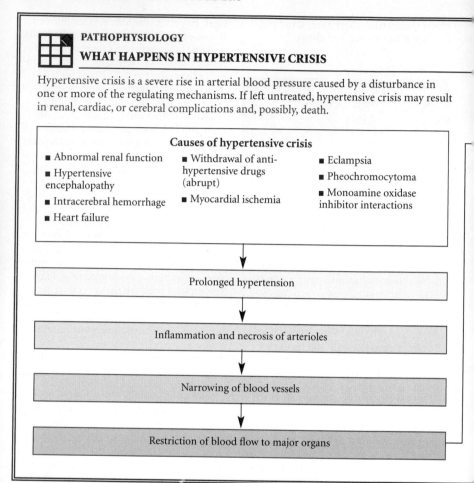

PATHOPHYSIOLOGY

WHAT HAPPENS IN HYPERTENSIVE CRISIS

Hypertensive crisis is a severe rise in arterial blood pressure caused by a disturbance in one or more of the regulating mechanisms. If left untreated, hypertensive crisis may result in renal, cardiac, or cerebral complications and, possibly, death.

Causes of hypertensive crisis

- Abnormal renal function
- Hypertensive encephalopathy
- Intracerebral hemorrhage
- Heart failure

- Withdrawal of antihypertensive drugs (abrupt)
- Myocardial ischemia

- Eclampsia
- Pheochromocytoma
- Monoamine oxidase inhibitor interactions

Prolonged hypertension

↓

Inflammation and necrosis of arterioles

↓

Narrowing of blood vessels

↓

Restriction of blood flow to major organs

- kidneys — proteinuria, edema and, eventually, renal failure.

Hypertension increases the heart's workload, causing left ventricular hypertrophy and, later, left- and right-sided heart failure and pulmonary edema.

Diagnosis

Serial blood pressure measurements are obtained and compared to previous readings and trends to reveal an increase in diastolic and systolic pressures. (See *Classifying blood pressure readings,* page 1094.)

Auscultation may reveal bruits over the abdominal aorta and the carotid, renal, and femoral arteries; ophthalmoscopy reveals arteriovenous nicking and, in hypertensive encephalopathy, papilledema. Patient history and the following additional tests may show predisposing factors and help identify an underlying cause such as renal disease:

- Urinalysis: Protein levels and red and white blood cell counts may indicate glomerulonephritis.
- Excretory urography: Renal atrophy indicates chronic renal disease; one kidney more than ⅝" (1.5 cm) shorter than the other suggests unilateral renal disease.
- Serum potassium: Levels less than 3.5 mEq/L may indicate adrenal dysfunction (primary hyperaldosteronism).
- Blood urea nitrogen (BUN) and serum creatinine: BUN level that's normal or ele-

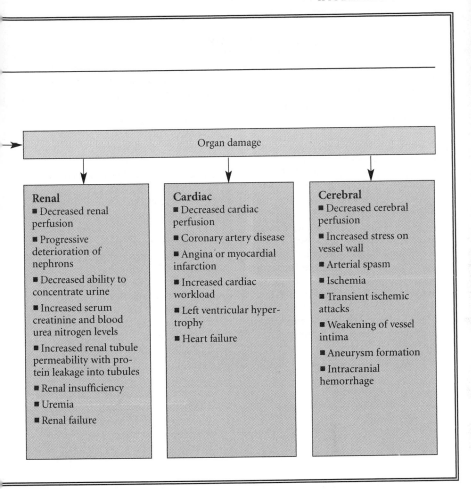

Organ damage

Renal
- Decreased renal perfusion
- Progressive deterioration of nephrons
- Decreased ability to concentrate urine
- Increased serum creatinine and blood urea nitrogen levels
- Increased renal tubule permeability with protein leakage into tubules
- Renal insufficiency
- Uremia
- Renal failure

Cardiac
- Decreased cardiac perfusion
- Coronary artery disease
- Angina or myocardial infarction
- Increased cardiac workload
- Left ventricular hypertrophy
- Heart failure

Cerebral
- Decreased cerebral perfusion
- Increased stress on vessel wall
- Arterial spasm
- Ischemia
- Transient ischemic attacks
- Weakening of vessel intima
- Aneurysm formation
- Intracranial hemorrhage

vated to more than 20 mg/dl and serum creatinine level that's normal or elevated to more than 1.5 mg/dl suggest renal disease.

Other tests help detect cardiovascular damage and other complications:
- Electrocardiography may show left ventricular hypertrophy or ischemia.
- Chest X-ray may show cardiomegaly.
- Echocardiography may show left ventricular hypertrophy.

Treatment

The National Institutes of Health recommend the following approach for treating primary hypertension:
- First, help the patient initiate necessary lifestyle modifications, including weight reduction, moderation of alcohol intake, regular physical exercise, reduction of sodium intake, and smoking cessation.
- If the patient fails to achieve the desired blood pressure or make significant progress, continue lifestyle modifications and begin drug therapy.
- For stage 1 hypertension (systolic [SBP] blood pressure 140 to 159 mm Hg, or diastolic blood pressure [DBP] 90 to 99 mm Hg) in the absence of compelling indications (heart failure, postmyocardial infarction, high coronary disease risk, diabetes, chronic kidney disease, or recurrent stroke prevention), give most patients thiazide-type diuretics. Consider using an angiotensin-converting enzyme (ACE) in-

CLASSIFYING BLOOD PRESSURE READINGS

The National Institutes of Health, which used to classify blood pressure according to severity categories — mild, moderate, severe, and very severe — has replaced this classification system with a system based on stages.

The following revised categories are based on the average of two or more readings taken on separate visits after an initial screening. They apply to adults age 18 and older who aren't taking antihypertensives, aren't acutely ill, and don't have other health conditions, such as diabetes and kidney disease. (If the systolic and diastolic pressures fall into different categories, use the higher of the two pressures to classify the reading. For example, a reading of 160/92 mm Hg should be classified as stage 2.)

Normal blood pressure with respect to cardiovascular risk is a systolic reading below 120 mm Hg and a diastolic reading below 80 mm Hg. In general, hypertension is defined as a systolic blood pressure of 140 mm Hg or higher or a diastolic pressure above 90 mm Hg. (For patients with diabetes or chronic kidney disease, hypertension is defined as a reading of 130/80 mm Hg or higher.)

In addition to classifying stages of hypertension based on average blood pressure readings, clinicians should also take note of target organ disease and any additional risk factors. For example, a patient with diabetes, left ventricular hypertrophy, and a blood pressure reading of 144/98 mm Hg would be classified as "stage I hypertension with target-organ disease (left ventricular hypertrophy) and another major risk factor (diabetes)." This additional information is important to obtain a true picture of the patient's cardiovascular health.

Category	Systolic		Diastolic
Normal	< 120 mm Hg	and	< 80 mm Hg
Pre-hypertension	120 to 139 mm Hg	or	80 to 89 mm Hg
Hypertension			
Stage 1	140 to 159 mm Hg	or	90 to 99 mm Hg
Stage 2	≥ 160 mm Hg	or	≥ 100 mm Hg

hibitor, beta-adrenergic blocker, calcium channel blocker (CCB), angiotensin-receptor blocker (ARB), or a combination.

■ For stage 2 hypertension (SBP ≥ 160 mm Hg, or DBP ≥ 100 mm Hg) in the absence of compelling indications, give most patients a two-drug combination (usually a thiazide-type diuretic and an ACE inhibitor, ARB, CCB, or beta-adrenergic blocker).

■ If the patient has one or more compelling indications, base drug treatment on benefits from outcome studies or existing clinical guidelines. Treatment may include the following, depending on indication:

– Heart failure — diuretic, beta-adrenergic blocker, ACE inhibitor, ARB, or aldosterone antagonist
– High coronary disease risk — diuretic, beta-adrenergic blocker, ACE inhibitor, or CCB
– Diabetes — diuretic, beta-adrenergic blocker, ACE inhibitor, or CCB
– Chronic kidney disease — ACE inhibitor or ARB
– Postmyocardial failure — ACE inhibitor, beta-adrenergic blocker, or aldosterone antagonist
– Recurrent stroke prevention — diuretic or ACE inhibitor.

Give other antihypertensive drugs as needed.

■ If the patient fails to achieve the desired blood pressure, continue lifestyle modifications and optimize drug dosages or add additional drugs until the goal blood pressure is achieved. Also, consider consultation with a hypertension specialist.

Treatment of secondary hypertension focuses on correcting the underlying cause and controlling hypertensive effects.

Typically, hypertensive emergencies require parenteral administration of a vasodilator or an adrenergic inhibitor or oral administration of a selected drug, such as nifedipine, captopril, clonidine, or labetalol, to rapidly reduce blood pressure. The initial goal is to reduce mean arterial blood pressure by no more than 25% (within minutes to hours) then to 160/110 within 2 hours while avoiding excessive falls in blood pressure that can precipitate renal, cerebral, or myocardial ischemia.

Examples of hypertensive emergencies include hypertensive encephalopathy, intracranial hemorrhage, acute left-sided heart failure with pulmonary edema, and dissecting aortic aneurysm. Hypertensive emergencies are also associated with eclampsia or severe gestational hypertension, unstable angina, and acute myocardial infarction.

Hypertension without accompanying symptoms or target-organ disease seldom requires emergency drug therapy.

Special considerations

■ To encourage adherence to antihypertensive therapy, suggest that the patient establish a daily routine for taking his medication. Warn that uncontrolled hypertension may cause stroke and heart attack. Tell him to report adverse drug effects. Also, advise him to avoid high-sodium antacids and over-the-counter cold and sinus medications, which contain harmful vasoconstrictors.

■ Encourage a change in dietary habits. Help the obese patient plan a weight-reduction diet; tell him to avoid high-sodium foods (pickles, potato chips, canned soups, and cold cuts) and table salt.

■ Help the patient examine and modify his lifestyle (for example, by reducing stress and exercising regularly).

■ If a patient is hospitalized with hypertension, find out if he was taking his prescribed medication. If he wasn't, ask why. If he can't afford the medication, refer him to appropriate social service agencies. Tell the patient and his family to keep a record of drugs used in the past, noting especially which ones were or weren't effective. Suggest recording this information on a card so that the patient can show it to his physician.

■ When routine blood pressure screening reveals elevated pressure, first make sure the cuff size is appropriate for the patient's upper arm circumference. Take the pressure in both arms in lying, sitting, and standing positions. Ask the patient if he smoked, drank a beverage containing caffeine, or was emotionally upset before the test. Advise him to return for blood pressure testing at frequent and regular intervals.

■ To help identify hypertension and prevent untreated hypertension, participate in public education programs dealing with hypertension and ways to reduce risk factors. Encourage public participation in blood pressure screening programs. Routinely screen all patients, especially those at risk (blacks and people with family histories of hypertension, stroke, or heart attack).

Coronary artery disease

Coronary artery disease (CAD) occurs when the arteries that supply blood to the heart muscle harden and narrow. The result is the loss of oxygen and nutrients to myocardial tissue because of diminished coronary blood flow. This reduction in blood flow can also lead to coronary syndrome (angina or myocardial infarction).

Causes and incidence

Atherosclerosis is the usual cause of CAD. In this form of arteriosclerosis, fatty, fibrous plaques, possibly including calcium deposits, narrow the lumen of the coronary arteries, reduce the volume of blood that can flow through them, and lead to myocardial ischemia. Plaque formation also

CORONARY ARTERY SPASM

In coronary artery spasm, a spontaneous, sustained contraction of one or more coronary arteries causes ischemia and dysfunction of the heart muscle. This disorder also causes Prinzmetal's angina and even myocardial infarction in patients with unoccluded coronary arteries. Its cause is unknown but possible contributing factors include:
- intimal hemorrhage into the medial layer of the blood vessel
- hyperventilation
- elevated catecholamine levels
- fatty buildup in lumen
- cocaine use.

Signs and symptoms
The major symptom of coronary artery spasm is angina. But unlike classic angina, this pain often occurs spontaneously and may not be related to physical exertion or emotional stress; it's also more severe, usually lasts longer, and may be cyclic, frequently recurring every day at the same time. Such ischemic episodes may cause arrhythmias, altered heart rate, lower blood pressure and, occasionally, fainting due to diminished cardiac output. Spasm in the left coronary artery may result in mitral insufficiency, producing a loud systolic murmur and, possibly, pulmonary edema, with dyspnea, crackles, hemoptysis, or sudden death.

Treatment
After diagnosis by coronary angiography and electrocardiography (ECG), the patient may receive calcium channel blockers (verapamil, nifedipine, or diltiazem) to reduce coronary artery spasm and vascular resistance; and nitrates (nitroglycerin or isosorbide dinitrate) to relieve chest pain.

When caring for a patient with coronary artery spasm, explain all necessary procedures and teach him how to take his medications safely. For calcium antagonist therapy, monitor blood pressure, pulse rate, and ECG patterns to detect arrhythmias. For nifedipine and verapamil therapy, monitor digoxin levels and check for signs of digoxin toxicity. Because nifedipine may cause peripheral and periorbital edema, watch for fluid retention.

Because coronary artery spasm is commonly associated with atherosclerotic disease, advise the patient to stop smoking, avoid overeating, maintain a low-fat diet, use alcohol sparingly, and maintain a balance between exercise and rest.

---

predisposes to thrombosis, which can provoke myocardial infarction (MI).

Atherosclerosis usually develops in high-flow, high-pressure arteries, such as those in the heart, brain, kidneys, and in the aorta, especially at bifurcation points. It has been linked to many risk factors: family history, male gender, age (risk increased in those aged 65 or older), hypertension, obesity, smoking, diabetes mellitus, stress, sedentary lifestyle, high serum cholesterol (particularly high low-density lipoprotein cholesterol) or triglyceride levels, low high-density lipoprotein cholesterol levels, high blood homocysteine levels, menopause and, possibly, infections producing inflammatory responses in the artery walls.

Uncommon causes of reduced coronary artery blood flow include dissecting aneurysms, infectious vasculitis, syphilis, and congenital defects in the coronary vascular system. Coronary artery spasms may also impede blood flow. (See *Coronary artery spasm.*)

Coronary artery disease is the leading cause of death in the United States. According to the American Heart Association, someone in the United States suffers a coronary heart event approximately every 29 seconds, and someone dies from such an event approximately every 60 seconds.

Signs and symptoms

The classic symptom of CAD is angina, the direct result of inadequate oxygen flow to the myocardium. Anginal pain is usually described as a burning, squeezing, or tight feeling in the substernal or precordial chest that may radiate to the left arm, neck, jaw, or shoulder blade. Typically, the patient clenches his fist over his chest or rubs his left arm when describing the pain, which may be accompanied by nausea, vomiting, fainting, sweating, and cool extremities. Anginal episodes most often follow physical exertion but may also follow emotional excitement, exposure to cold, or a large meal.

Angina has four major forms: *stable* (pain is predictable in frequency and duration and can be relieved with nitrates and rest), *unstable* (pain increases in frequency and duration and is more easily induced), *Prinzmetal's* or *variant* (from unpredictable coronary artery spasm), and *microvascular* (in which impairment of vasodilator reserve causes angina-like chest pain in a patient with normal coronary arteries). Severe and prolonged anginal pain generally suggests MI, with potentially fatal arrhythmias and mechanical failure.

Diagnosis

The patient history — including the frequency and duration of angina and the presence of associated risk factors — is crucial in evaluating CAD. Additional diagnostic measures include the following:

■ Electrocardiogram (ECG) during angina may show ischemia and, possibly, arrhythmias such as premature ventricular contractions. ECG is apt to be normal when the patient is pain-free. Arrhythmias may occur without infarction, secondary to ischemia.

■ Treadmill or exercise stress test may provoke chest pain and ECG signs of myocardial ischemia.

■ Coronary angiography reveals coronary artery stenosis or obstruction, possible collateral circulation, and the arteries' condition beyond the narrowing.

■ Myocardial perfusion imaging with thallium-201, Cardiolite, or Myoview during treadmill exercise detects ischemic areas of the myocardium, visualized as "cold spots."

■ Stress echocardiography may show wall motion abnormalities.

■ Electron-beam computed tomography identifies calcium within arterial plaque; the more calcium seen, the higher the likelihood of CAD.

Treatment

The goal of treatment in patients with angina is to either reduce myocardial oxygen demand or increase oxygen supply. Therapy consists primarily of nitrates such as nitroglycerin (given sublingually, orally, transdermally, or topically in ointment form) to dilate coronary arteries and improve blood supply to the heart. Glycoprotein IIb-IIIa inhibitors and antithrombin drugs may be used to reduce the risk of blood clots. Beta-adrenergic blockers may be used to decrease heart rate and lower the heart's oxygen use. Calcium channel blockers may be used to relax the coronary arteries and all systemic arteries, reducing the heart's workload. Angiotensin-converting enzyme inhibitors, diuretics, or other medications may be used to lower blood pressure.

Percutaneous transluminal coronary angioplasty (PTCA) may be performed during cardiac catheterization to compress fatty deposits and relieve occlusion in patients with no calcification and partial occlusion. PTCA carries a certain risk but its morbidity is lower than that for surgery. (See *Relieving occlusions with angioplasty,* pages 1098 and 1099.) Laser angioplasty corrects occlusion by vaporizing fatty deposits. In addition, a stent may be placed in the artery to act as a scaffold to hold the artery open. Another procedure is rotational atherectomy, which removes arterial plaque with a high-speed burr. Obstructive lesions may necessitate coronary artery bypass graft (CABG) surgery and the use of vein grafts.

A surgical technique available as an alternative to traditional CABG surgery is minimally invasive coronary artery bypass surgery, also known as "keyhole" surgery. This procedure requires a shorter recovery period and has fewer postoperative complications. Instead of sawing open the pa-

RELIEVING OCCLUSIONS WITH ANGIOPLASTY

Percutaneous transluminal coronary angioplasty can open an occluded coronary without opening the chest — an important advantage over bypass surgery. First, coronary angiography must confirm the presence and location of the arterial occlusion. Then, the physician threads a guide catheter through the patient's femoral artery into the coronary artery under fluoroscopic guidance, as shown at right.

When angiography shows the guide catheter positioned at the occlusion site, the phyisician carefully inserts a smaller double-lumen balloon catheter through the guide catheter and directs the balloon through the occlusion (opposite page, left). A marked pressure gradient will be obvious.

The physician alternately inflates and deflates the balloon until an angiogram verifies successful arterial dilation (opposite page, right) and the pressure gradient has decreased.

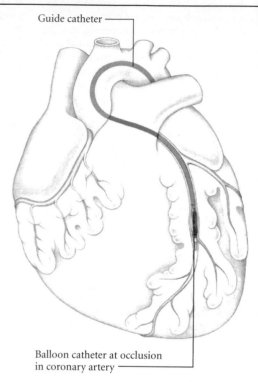

Guide catheter

Balloon catheter at occlusion in coronary artery

---

tient's sternum and spreading the ribs apart, several small cuts are made in the torso through which small surgical instruments and fiber-optic cameras are inserted. This procedure was initially designed to correct blockages in just one or two easily reached arteries; it may not be suitable for more complicated cases.

Coronary brachytherapy, which involves delivering beta or gamma radiation into the coronary arteries, may be used in patients who've undergone stent implantation in a coronary artery but then developed such problems as diffuse in-stent restenosis. Brachytherapy is a promising technique, but its use is restricted to the treatment of stent-related problems because of complications and the unknown long-term effects of the radiation. However-

er, in some facilities, brachytherapy is being studied as a first-line treatment of coronary disease.

Because CAD is so widespread, prevention is of incalculable importance. Dietary restrictions aimed at reducing intake of calories (in obesity) and salt, saturated fats, and cholesterol serve to minimize the risk, especially when supplemented with regular exercise. Abstention from smoking and stress reduction are also beneficial. Other preventive actions include control of hypertension, control of elevated serum cholesterol or triglyceride levels (with antilipemics), and measures to minimize platelet aggregation and the danger of blood clots (with aspirin or other antiplatelet agents).

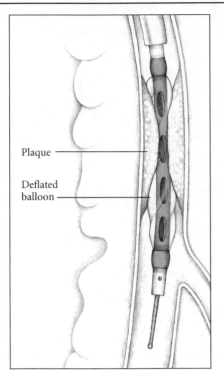

Plaque

Deflated
balloon

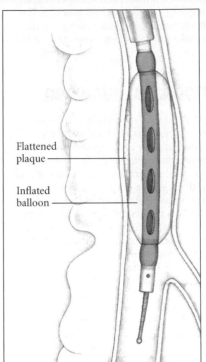

Flattened
plaque

Inflated
balloon

Special considerations

■ During anginal episodes, monitor blood pressure and heart rate. Take an ECG during anginal episodes and before administering nitroglycerin or other nitrates. Record duration of pain, amount of medication required to relieve it, and accompanying symptoms.

■ Keep nitroglycerin available for immediate use. Instruct the patient to call immediately whenever he feels chest, arm, or neck pain.

■ Before cardiac catheterization, explain the procedure to the patient. Make sure he knows why it's necessary, understands the risks, and realizes that it may indicate a need for surgery.

■ After catheterization, review the expected course of treatment with the patient and his family. Monitor the catheter site for bleeding. Also, check for distal pulses. To counter the dye's diuretic effect, make sure the patient drinks plenty of fluids. Assess potassium levels.

■ If the patient is scheduled for surgery, explain the procedure to him and his family. Give them a tour of the intensive care unit and introduce them to the staff.

■ After surgery, monitor blood pressure, intake and output, breath sounds, chest tube drainage, and ECG, watching for signs of ischemia and arrhythmias. Also, observe for and treat chest pain and possible dye reactions. Give vigorous chest physiotherapy and guide the patient in removal of secretions through deep-breathing, coughing, and expectoration of mucus.

■ Before discharge, stress the need to follow the prescribed drug regimen (antihypertensives, nitrates, and antilipemics, for example), exercise program, and diet. Encourage regular, moderate exercise. Refer the patient to a self-help program to stop smoking.

Myocardial infarction

Myocardial infarction (MI), commonly known as a *heart attack* and part of a broader category of disease known as *acute coronary syndrome,* results from prolonged myocardial ischemia due to reduced blood flow through one of the coronary arteries. In cardiovascular disease, the leading cause of death in the United States and western Europe, death usually results from the cardiac damage or complications of MI. (See *Complications of myocardial infarction.*) Mortality is high when treatment is delayed, and almost one-half of sudden deaths due to an MI occur before hospitalization, within 1 hour of the onset of symptoms. The prognosis improves if vigorous treatment begins immediately.

Causes and incidence

Predisposing risk factors include:
■ diabetes mellitus
■ drug use, especially cocaine
■ elevated serum triglyceride, total cholesterol, and low-density lipoprotein levels
■ hypertension
■ obesity or excessive intake of saturated fats, carbohydrates, or salt
■ positive family history
■ sedentary lifestyle
■ smoking
■ stress or a type A personality.

The site of the MI depends on the vessels involved. Occlusion of the circumflex branch of the left coronary artery causes a lateral wall infarction; occlusion of the anterior descending branch of the left coronary artery, an anterior wall infarction. True posterior or inferior wall infarctions generally result from occlusion of the right coronary artery or one of its branches. Right ventricular infarctions can also result from right coronary artery occlusion, can accompany inferior infarctions, and may

cause right-sided heart failure. In Q-wave (transmural) MI, tissue damage extends through all myocardial layers; in non-Q-wave (subendocardial) MI, only in the innermost and possibly the middle layers.

Incidence is high: About 1 million patients visit the hospital each year with an MI and another 200,000 to 300,000 people die from MI-related complications without seeking medical care. Men and postmenopausal women are more susceptible to MI than premenopausal women, although incidence is rising among females, especially those who smoke and take hormonal contraceptives.

Signs and symptoms

The cardinal symptom of MI is persistent, crushing substernal pain that may radiate to the left arm, jaw, neck, or shoulder blades. Such pain is usually described as heavy, squeezing, or crushing, and may persist for 12 hours or more. However, in some MI patients — particularly elderly people or those with diabetes — pain may not occur at all; in others, it may be mild and confused with indigestion. In patients with coronary artery disease, angina of increasing frequency, severity, or duration (especially if not provoked by exertion, a heavy meal, or cold and wind) may signal impending infarction.

Other clinical effects include a feeling of impending doom, fatigue, nausea, vomiting, and shortness of breath. Some patients may have no symptoms. The patient may experience catecholamine responses, such as coolness in extremities, perspiration, anxiety, and restlessness. Fever is unusual at the onset of an MI, but a low-grade temperature elevation may develop during the next few days. Blood pressure varies; hypotension or hypertension may be present.

The most common post-MI complications include recurrent or persistent chest pain, arrhythmias, left-sided heart failure (resulting in heart failure or acute pulmonary edema), and cardiogenic shock. Unusual but potentially lethal complications that may develop soon after infarction include thromboembolism; papillary muscle dysfunction or rupture, causing mitral insufficiency; rupture of the ventricular septum, causing ventricular septal defect; rupture of

COMPLICATIONS OF MYOCARDIAL INFARCTION

Complication	Diagnosis	Treatment
Arrhythmias	■ Electrocardiogram (ECG) shows premature ventricular contractions, ventricular tachycardia, or ventricular fibrillation; in inferior wall myocardial infarction (MI), bradycardia and junctional rhythms or atrioventricular block; in anterior wall MI, tachycardia or heart block.	■ Antiarrhythmics, atropine, and pacemaker; cardioversion for tachycardia
Heart failure	■ In left-sided heart failure, chest X-rays show venous congestion, cardiomegaly, and Kerley's B lines. ■ Catheterization shows increased pulmonary artery pressure (PAP) and central venous pressure.	■ Diuretics, angiotensin-converting enzyme inhibitors, vasodilators, inotropic agents, cardiac glycosides, and beta-adrenergic blockers
Cardiogenic shock	■ Catheterization shows decreased cardiac output and increased PAP and pulmonary artery wedge pressure (PAWP). ■ Signs include hypertension, tachycardia, S_3, S_4, decreased levels of consciousness, decreased urine output, jugular vein distension, and cool, pale skin.	■ I.V. fluids, vasodilators, diuretics, cardiac glycosides, intra-aortic balloon pump (IABP), and beta-adrenergic stimulants
Rupture of left ventricular papillary muscle	■ Auscultation reveals an apical holosystolic murmur. Inspection of jugular vein pulse or hemodynamic monitoring shows increased v waves. ■ Dyspnea is prominent. ■ Color-flow and Doppler echocardiogram show mitral insufficiency. Pulmonary artery catheterization shows increased PAP and PAWP.	■ Nitroprusside ■ IABP ■ Surgical replacement of the mitral valve with possible concomitant myocardial revascularization (in patients with significant coronary artery disease)
Ventricular septal rupture	■ In left-to-right shunt, auscultation reveals a holosystolic murmur and thrill. ■ Catheterization shows increased PAP and PAWP. ■ Confirmation by increased oxygen saturation of the right ventricle and pulmonary artery.	■ Surgical correction, IABP, nitroglycerin, nitroprusside, low-dose inotropic agents, or pacemaker
Pericarditis or Dressler's syndrome	■ Auscultation reveals a friction rub. ■ Chest pain is relieved by sitting up.	■ Aspirin

(continued)

COMPLICATIONS OF MYOCARDIAL INFARCTION *(continued)*

Complication	Diagnosis	Treatment
Ventricular aneurysm	▪ Chest X-ray may show cardiomegaly. ▪ ECG may show arrhythmias and persistent ST-segment elevation. ▪ Left ventriculography shows altered or paradoxical left ventricular motion.	▪ Cardioversion, defibrillation, antiarrhythmics, vasodilators, anticoagulants, cardiac glycosides, and diuretics (If conservative treatment fails, surgical resection is necessary.)
Thromboembolism	▪ Severe dyspnea and chest pain or neurologic changes. ▪ Nuclear scan shows ventilation-perfusion mismatch. ▪ Angiography shows arterial blockage.	▪ Oxygen and heparin

the myocardium; and ventricular aneurysm. Up to several months after infarction, Dressler's syndrome may develop (pericarditis, pericardial friction rub, chest pain, fever, leukocytosis and, possibly, pleurisy or pneumonitis).

Diagnosis

CONFIRMING DIAGNOSIS
Persistent chest pain, elevated ST segment on electrocardiogram (ECG), and elevated total creatine kinase (CK) and CK-MB levels over a 72-hour period usually confirm MI. Troponin T or troponin I is also used in the diagnosis because both are specific to cardiac necrosis, and levels rise 6 to 8 hours after onset of ischemia.

Auscultation may reveal diminished heart sounds, gallops and, in papillary dysfunction, the apical systolic murmur of mitral insufficiency over the mitral valve area.

When clinical features are equivocal, assume that the patient had an MI until tests rule it out. Diagnostic laboratory results include:
▪ serial 12-lead ECG — ECG abnormalities may be absent or inconclusive during the first few hours after an MI. When present, characteristic abnormalities include serial ST-segment depression in non–Q-wave (subendocardial) MI and ST-segment elevation in Q-wave (transmural) MI.
▪ serial serum enzyme levels — CK levels are elevated, specifically, the CK-MB isoenzyme.
▪ echocardiography — may show ventricular wall motion abnormalities in patients with a Q-wave (transmural) MI.
▪ nuclear ventriculography scans (multiple gated acquisition or radionuclide ventriculography) — using I.V. radioactive substance, can identify acutely damaged muscle by picking up radioactive nucleotide, which appears as a "hot spot" on the film; useful in localizing a recent MI.

Treatment

The goals of treatment are to relieve chest pain, stabilize heart rhythm, reduce cardiac workload, revascularize the coronary artery, and preserve myocardial tissue. Arrhythmias, the predominant problem during the first 48 hours after the infarction, may require antiarrhythmics, possibly a pacemaker and, rarely, cardioversion. Arrhythmias are best detected using a 12-lead ECG.

To preserve myocardial tissue in ST elevation MI, fibrinolytic therapy should be started I.V. within 30 minutes of arrival in the emergency department, if not contraindicated. Fibrinolytic therapy includes a choice of streptokinase, alteplase, urokinase, tenecteplase, or reteplase. (See *Comparing thrombolytics,* pages 1104 and 1105.)

Primary percutaneous transluminal coronary angioplasty is a Class I recommendation as an alternative to thrombolytic therapy only if performed in a timely manner by physicians skilled in the procedure and supported by experienced personnel in high-volume centers.

Other treatments consist of:
- lidocaine, vasopressin, or amiodarone for ventricular arrhythmias, or other drugs, such as procainamide, quinidine, or disopyramide
- antiplatelet therapy with glycoprotein IIb-IIIa inhibitors, such as ticlopidine and clopidogrel for non-ST-elevation MI
- atropine I.V. or a temporary pacemaker for heart block or bradycardia
- nitroglycerin (sublingual, topical, transdermal, or I.V.); calcium channel blockers, such as nifedipine, verapamil, or diltiazem (sublingual, oral, or I.V.); or isosorbide dinitrate (sublingual, oral, or I.V.) to relieve pain by redistributing blood to ischemic areas of the myocardium, increasing cardiac output, and reducing myocardial workload
- heparin I.V. (usually follows thrombolytic therapy)
- morphine I.V. for pain and sedation
- bed rest with bedside commode to decrease cardiac workload
- oxygen administration at a modest flow rate for 2 to 3 hours (a lower concentration is necessary if the patient has chronic obstructive pulmonary disease)
- angiotensin-converting enzyme inhibitors for patients with large anterior wall MIs and for those with an MI and a left ventricular ejection fraction less than 40%
- drugs to increase myocardial contractility or blood pressure
- beta-adrenergic blockers, such as propranolol or atenolol, after acute MI to help prevent reinfarction by reducing the heart's workload
- aspirin to inhibit platelet aggregation (should be initiated immediately and continued for years)
- pulmonary artery catheterization to detect left- or right-sided heart failure and to monitor the patient's response to treatment.

Special considerations

Care for patients who have suffered an MI is directed toward detecting complications, preventing further myocardial damage, and promoting comfort, rest, and emotional well-being. Most MI patients receive treatment in the intensive care unit (ICU), where they're under constant observation for complications.

- On admission to the ICU, monitor and record the patient's ECG, blood pressure, temperature, and heart and breath sounds.
- Assess and record the severity and duration of pain, and administer analgesics. Avoid I.M. injections; absorption from the muscle is unpredictable and bleeding is likely if the patient is receiving thrombolytic therapy.
- Check the patient's blood pressure after giving nitroglycerin, especially the first dose.
- Frequently monitor the ECG to detect rate changes or arrhythmias. Place rhythm strips in the patient's chart periodically for evaluation.
- During episodes of chest pain, obtain 12-lead ECG (before and after nitroglycerin therapy as well), blood pressure, and pulmonary artery catheter measurements and monitor them for changes.
- Watch for signs and symptoms of fluid retention (crackles, cough, tachypnea, and edema), which may indicate impending heart failure. Carefully monitor daily weight, intake and output, respirations, serum enzyme levels, and blood pressure. Auscultate for adventitious breath sounds periodically (patients on bed rest frequently have atelectatic crackles, which disappear after coughing), for S_3 or S_4 gallops, and for new-onset heart murmurs.
- Organize patient care and activities to maximize periods of uninterrupted rest.
- Initiate a cardiac rehabilitation program. This usually includes education regarding heart disease, exercise, and emotional support for the patient and his family.

COMPARING THROMBOLYTICS

If your patient has suffered a myocardial infarction (MI), you must intervene promptly to minimize cardiac damage and avert death. If appropriate, prepare the patient for thrombolytic therapy as ordered. Thrombolytic drugs enhance the body's natural ability to dispose of blood clots. To lyse (dissolve) fibrin, the essential component of a clot, tissue activators convert plasminogen to plasmin. A nonspecific protease, plasmin degrades fibrin, fibrinogen, and procoagulant factors (such as factors V, VII, and XII).

Candidates for thrombolytic therapy include patients with acute ST-segment elevation and chest pain that has lasted no more than 6 hours. Timely use of thrombolytic agents can restore myocardial perfusion and prevent further injury. When effective, thrombolytic agents relieve chest pain, restore the ST segment to baseline, and induce reperfusion arrhythmias within 30 to 45 minutes.

Contraindications to thrombolytic therapy include surgery within the past 2 months, active bleeding, a history of stroke, intracranial neoplasm, arteriovenous malformation, aneurysm, or uncontrolled hypertension.

Here's how selected thrombolytics open occluded coronary arteries in patients with an acute MI.

Alteplase

This naturally occurring enzyme has been cloned and produced as a drug, alteplase (tissue plasminogen activator). Binding to plasminogen, it catalyzes the conversion of plasminogen to plasmin in the presence of fibrin. Because of its strong affinity for fibrin, alteplase concentrates at the clot site, resulting in a minimal decrease in the fibrinogen level.

This thrombolytic has a half-life of 5 minutes, so maintaining coronary artery patency depends on continued anticoagulation with heparin. Alteplase doesn't induce antigenic responses; doses may be repeated at any time.

Reteplase

Reteplase, recombinant plasminogen activator, has a half-life of 13 to 16 minutes. Its longer half-life allows it to be administered as a bolus. Two boluses are required.

Anistreplase

Anistreplase is a partially synthetic thrombolytic drug that's composed of a complex of streptokinase bound to human plasminogen.

This complex binds to fibrin and promotes plasminogen conversion to plasmin. But the dose needed to lyse coronary artery clots can cause systemic clot lysis, characterized by fibrinogen depletion. This results in bleeding complications.

Anistreplase has the longest half-life (90 minutes). Because it's partially composed of streptokinase, a foreign protein, anistreplase is antigenic and may cause an allergic reaction. The per-dose cost is less than that for alteplase.

■ Ask the dietary department to provide a clear liquid diet until nausea subsides. A low-cholesterol, low-sodium, low-fat, high-fiber diet may be prescribed.

■ Provide a stool softener to prevent straining during defecation, which causes vagal stimulation and may slow the heart rate. Allow use of a bedside commode and provide as much privacy as possible.

■ Assist with range-of-motion exercises. If the patient is completely immobilized by a severe MI, turn him often. Antiembolism stockings help prevent venostasis and thrombophlebitis.

■ Provide emotional support and help reduce stress and anxiety; administer tranquilizers as needed. Explain procedures and answer questions. Explaining the ICU

This drug's main advantage is ease of administration: only a single bolus is required.

Streptokinase

Streptokinase, a thrombolytic, is a bacterial protein that binds to circulating plasminogen and catalyzes plasmin formation. Its low specificity for fibrin induces a systemic lytic state and increases the risk of bleeding.

The half-life is approximately 20 minutes. Like anistreplase, streptokinase is antigenic.

Tenecteplase

Tenecteplase is a modified form of human tissue plasminogen activator that binds to fibrin and converts plasminogen to plasmin. It's given as a single bolus dose.

Urokinase

Naturally produced by the human kidney, urokinase promotes thrombolysis by directly activating the conversion of plasminogen to plasmin.

With a serum half-life of 10 to 20 minutes, urokinase is rapidly cleared by the kidneys and liver. Unlike anistreplase and streptokinase, it doesn't induce an antigenic response. Urokinase isn't given through a peripheral I.V. line to treat an acute MI, but patients who undergo cardiac catheterization may receive it directly in a coronary artery.

environment and routine can ease anxiety. Involve the patient's family in his care as much as possible.

To prepare the patient for discharge:
■ Thoroughly explain dosages and therapy to promote compliance with the prescribed medication regimen and other treatment measures. Warn about drug adverse effects and advise the patient to watch for and report signs of toxicity (anorexia, nausea, vomiting, and yellow vision, for example, if the patient is receiving digoxin).
■ Review dietary restrictions with the patient. If he must follow a low-sodium or low-fat and low-cholesterol diet, provide a list of foods that he should avoid. Ask the dietitian to speak to the patient and his family.
■ Counsel the patient to resume sexual activity progressively.
■ Advise the patient to report typical or atypical chest pain. Postinfarction syndrome may develop, producing chest pain that must be differentiated from recurrent MI, pulmonary infarct, or heart failure.
■ If the patient has a Holter monitor in place, explain its purpose and use.
■ Stress the need to stop smoking.
■ Encourage participation in a cardiac rehabilitation program.
■ Review follow-up procedures, such as office visits and treadmill testing, with the patient.

Heart failure

Heart failure is a syndrome characterized by myocardial dysfunction that leads to impaired pump performance (diminished cardiac output) or to frank heart failure and abnormal circulatory congestion. Congestion of systemic venous circulation may result in peripheral edema or hepatomegaly; congestion of pulmonary circulation may cause pulmonary edema, an acute life-threatening emergency. Pump failure usually occurs in a damaged left ventricle (left-sided heart failure) but may occur in the right ventricle (right-sided heart failure) either as a primary disorder or secondary to left-sided heart failure. Sometimes, left- and right-sided heart failure develop simultaneously. (See *What happens in heart failure,* pages 1106 and 1107.)

Although heart failure may be acute (as a direct result of myocardial infarction [MI]), it's generally a chronic disorder associated with sodium and water retention by the kidneys. Advances in diagnostic and therapeutic techniques have greatly improved the outlook for patients with heart

PATHOPHYSIOLOGY
WHAT HAPPENS IN HEART FAILURE

Heart failure occurs when cardiac output is inadequate to meet the body's needs. The pathophysiology of heart failure is shown in the flow chart below.

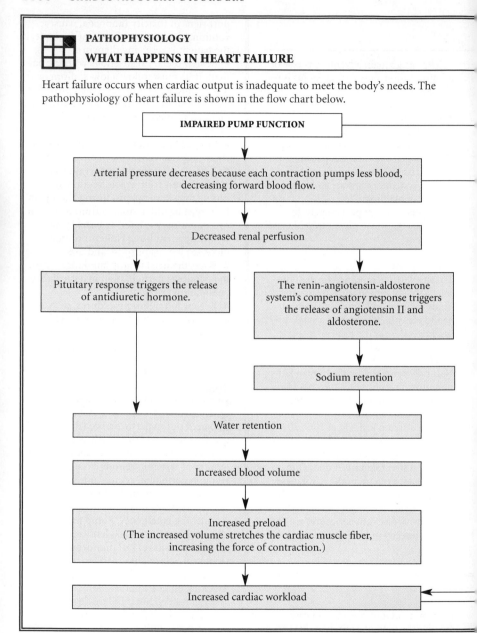

failure, but the prognosis still depends on the underlying cause and its response to treatment.

Causes and incidence

Heart failure may result from a primary abnormality of the heart muscle such as an infarction, inadequate myocardial perfusion due to coronary artery disease, or cardiomyopathy. Other causes include:

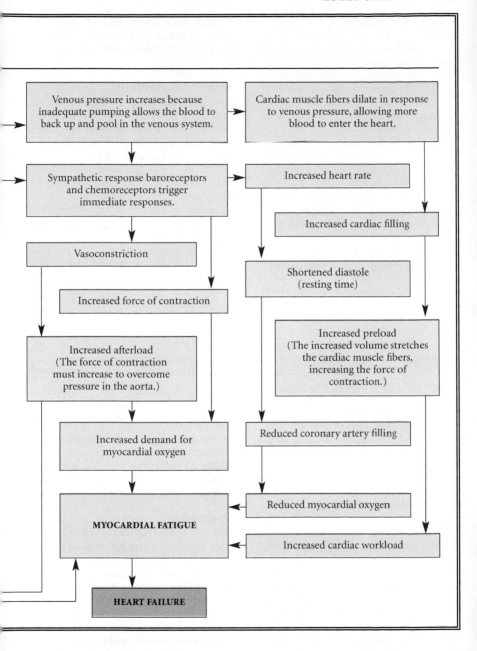

■ diastolic dysfunction, preserved ejection fraction, impairment of ventricular filling by diminished relaxation or reduced compliance seen with hypertrophic cardiomyopathy, myocardial hypertrophy, and pericardial restriction

■ mechanical disturbances in ventricular filling during diastole when there's too little blood for the ventricle to pump, as in mitral stenosis secondary to rheumatic heart disease or constrictive pericarditis and atrial fibrillation

■ systolic hemodynamic disturbances, such as excessive cardiac workload due to volume overloading or pressure overload that limit the heart's pumping ability. These disturbances can result from mitral or aortic insufficiency, which causes volume overloading, and aortic stenosis or systemic hypertension, which result in increased resistance to ventricular emptying.

Reduced cardiac output triggers compensatory mechanisms, such as ventricular dilation, hypertrophy, increased sympathetic activity, and activation of the renin-angiotensin-aldosterone system. These mechanisms improve cardiac output at the expense of increased ventricular work. In cardiac dilation, an increase in end-diastolic ventricular volume (preload) causes increased stroke work and stroke volume during contraction, stretching cardiac muscle fibers beyond optimum limits and producing pulmonary congestion and pulmonary hypertension, which in turn lead to right-sided heart failure.

In ventricular hypertrophy, an increase in muscle mass or diameter of the left ventricle allows the heart to pump against increased resistance (impedance) to the outflow of blood. An increase in ventricular diastolic pressure necessary to fill the enlarged ventricle may compromise diastolic coronary blood flow, limiting the oxygen supply to the ventricle and causing ischemia and impaired muscle contractility.

Increased sympathetic activity occurs as a response to decreased cardiac output and blood pressure by enhancing peripheral vascular resistance, contractility, heart rate, and venous return. Signs of increased sympathetic activity, such as cool extremities and clamminess, may indicate impending heart failure. Increased sympathetic activity also restricts blood flow to the kidneys, which respond by reducing the glomerular filtration rate and increasing tubular reabsorption of salt and water, in turn expanding the circulating blood volume. This renal mechanism, if unchecked, can aggravate congestion and produce overt edema.

Chronic heart failure may worsen as a result of respiratory tract infections, pulmonary embolism, stress, increased sodium or water intake, or failure to adhere to the prescribed treatment regimen.

Heart failure affects approximately 2 of every 100 people between ages 27 and 74. It becomes more common with advancing age.

Signs and symptoms

Left-sided heart failure primarily produces pulmonary signs and symptoms; right-sided heart failure, primarily systemic signs and symptoms. However, heart failure often affects both sides of the heart.

Clinical signs of left-sided heart failure include dyspnea, orthopnea, crackles, possibly wheezing, hypoxia, respiratory acidosis, cough, cyanosis or pallor, palpitations, arrhythmias, elevated blood pressure, and pulsus alternans.

Clinical signs of right-sided heart failure include dependent peripheral edema, hepatomegaly, splenomegaly, jugular vein distention, ascites, slow weight gain, arrhythmias, positive hepatojugular reflex, abdominal distention, nausea, vomiting, anorexia, weakness, fatigue, dizziness, and syncope.

Complications typically may include pulmonary edema (See *Pulmonary edema: How to intervene,* pages 1110 and 1111.) venostasis, with predisposition to thromboembolism (associated primarily with prolonged bed rest); cerebral insufficiency; and renal insufficiency, with severe electrolyte imbalance.

 ALERT *Excessive fluid can accumulate in the pericardium, requiring removal through pericardiocentesis.*

Diagnosis

■ Electrocardiography may reflect heart strain or enlargement, ischemia, or old MI. It may also reveal atrial enlargement, tachycardia, and extrasystoles.
■ Chest X-ray shows increased pulmonary vascular markings, interstitial edema, or pleural effusion and cardiomegaly.
■ Pulmonary artery monitoring typically demonstrates elevated pulmonary artery and pulmonary artery wedge pressures, left ventricular end-diastolic pressure in left-sided heart failure, and elevated right atrial pressure or central venous pressure in right-sided heart failure.

■ Echocardiogram may demonstrate wall motion abnormalities and chamber dilation.

Other tests that may also demonstrate enlargement of the heart or decreased functioning include chest computed tomography scan, cardiac magnetic resonance imaging, or nuclear scans, such as multiple-gated acquisition scanning and radionuclide ventriculography.

Treatment
The goal of therapy is to improve pump function by reversing the compensatory mechanisms producing the clinical effects, underlying disorders, and precipitating factors. Heart failure can be quickly controlled by treatment consisting of:

■ angiotensin-converting enzyme inhibitors to decrease peripheral vascular resistance

■ antiembolism stockings to prevent venostasis and thromboembolus formation

■ bed rest for acute heart failure

■ carvedilol, a nonselective beta-adrenergic blocker with alpha-receptor blockade to reduce mortality and improve quality of life

■ digoxin or dopamine to strengthen myocardial contractility

■ diuresis to reduce total blood volume and circulatory congestion

■ inotropic agents, such as dobutamine and milrinone, given I.V. to improve the heart's ability to pump

■ nesiritide, a recombinant form of endogenous human B-type natriuretic peptide, to reduce sodium through its diuretic action

■ vasodilators to increase cardiac output by reducing the impedance to ventricular outflow (afterload).

Excess fluid can be removed through dialysis if necessary. Circulatory assistance can be provided by implanted devices, such as the intra-aortic balloon pump and the left ventricular assist device, but they're only temporary solutions.

Left ventricular remodeling surgery may also be performed. This surgical technique involves cutting a wedge about the size of a small slice of pie out of the left ventricle of an enlarged heart. The remainder of the heart is sewn together. The result is a smaller organ that's able to pump blood more efficiently. This procedure offers promising results, especially for those whose only alternative may be a heart transplant.

Special considerations
During the acute phase of heart failure:

■ Place the patient in Fowler's position and give him supplemental oxygen to help him breathe more easily.

■ Weigh the patient daily and check for peripheral edema. Carefully monitor I.V. intake and urine output, vital signs, and mental status. Auscultate the heart for abnormal sounds (S_3 gallop) and the lungs for crackles or rhonchi. Report changes at once.

■ Frequently monitor blood urea nitrogen, creatinine, and serum potassium, sodium, chloride, and magnesium levels.

■ Make sure the patient has continuous cardiac monitoring during acute and advanced stages to identify and treat arrhythmias promptly.

■ To prevent deep vein thrombosis due to vascular congestion, assist the patient with range-of-motion exercises. Enforce bed rest and apply antiembolism stockings. Check regularly for calf pain and tenderness.

■ Allow adequate rest periods.
To prepare the patient for discharge:

■ Advise the patient to avoid foods high in sodium, such as canned or commercially prepared foods and dairy products, to curb fluid overload.

■ Encourage participation in an outpatient cardiac rehabilitation program.

■ Explain to the patient that the potassium he loses through diuretic therapy may need to be replaced by taking a prescribed potassium supplement and eating high-potassium foods, such as bananas and apricots.

■ Stress the need for regular checkups.

■ Stress the importance of taking digoxin exactly as prescribed. Tell the patient to watch for and immediately report signs of toxicity, such as anorexia, vomiting, and yellow vision.

■ Tell the patient to notify the physician promptly if his pulse is unusually irregular or measures less than 60 beats/minute; if he experiences dizziness, blurred vision,

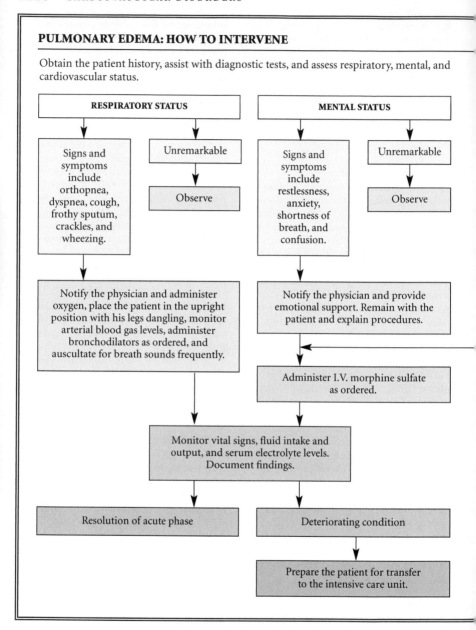

PULMONARY EDEMA: HOW TO INTERVENE

Obtain the patient history, assist with diagnostic tests, and assess respiratory, mental, and cardiovascular status.

RESPIRATORY STATUS

Signs and symptoms include orthopnea, dyspnea, cough, frothy sputum, crackles, and wheezing.

Unremarkable

Observe

Notify the physician and administer oxygen, place the patient in the upright position with his legs dangling, monitor arterial blood gas levels, administer bronchodilators as ordered, and auscultate for breath sounds frequently.

MENTAL STATUS

Signs and symptoms include restlessness, anxiety, shortness of breath, and confusion.

Unremarkable

Observe

Notify the physician and provide emotional support. Remain with the patient and explain procedures.

Administer I.V. morphine sulfate as ordered.

Monitor vital signs, fluid intake and output, and serum electrolyte levels. Document findings.

Resolution of acute phase

Deteriorating condition

Prepare the patient for transfer to the intensive care unit.

shortness of breath, a persistent dry cough, palpitations, increased fatigue, paroxysmal nocturnal dyspnea, swollen ankles, or decreased urine output; or if he notices rapid weight gain (3 to 5 lb [1.5 to 2.5 kg] in 1 week).

Dilated cardiomyopathy

Dilated cardiomyopathy results from extensively damaged myocardial muscle fibers. This disorder interferes with myocardial metabolism and grossly dilates all four chambers of the heart, giving the

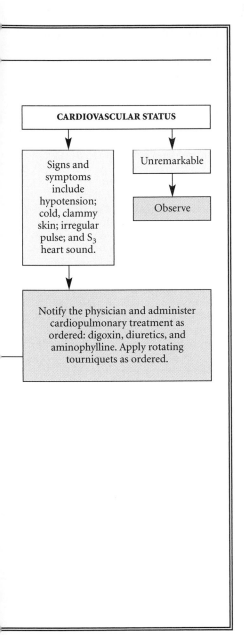

CARDIOVASCULAR STATUS

Signs and symptoms include hypotension; cold, clammy skin; irregular pulse; and S₃ heart sound.

Unremarkable

Observe

Notify the physician and administer cardiopulmonary treatment as ordered: digoxin, diuretics, and aminophylline. Apply rotating tourniquets as ordered.

Causes and incidence

The cause of most cardiomyopathies is unknown. Occasionally, dilated cardiomyopathy results from myocardial destruction by toxic, infectious, or metabolic agents, such as certain viruses, endocrine and electrolyte disorders, and nutritional deficiencies. Other causes include muscle disorders (myasthenia gravis, progressive muscular dystrophy, and myotonic dystrophy), infiltrative disorders (hemochromatosis and amyloidosis), and sarcoidosis.

Cardiomyopathy may also be a complication of alcoholism. In such cases, it may improve with abstinence from alcohol but recurs when the patient resumes drinking. How viruses induce cardiomyopathy is unclear, but researchers suspect a link between viral myocarditis and subsequent dilated cardiomyopathy, especially after infection with poliovirus, coxsackievirus B, influenza virus, or human immunodeficiency virus.

Metabolic cardiomyopathies are related to endocrine and electrolyte disorders and nutritional deficiencies. Thus, dilated cardiomyopathy may develop in patients with hyperthyroidism, pheochromocytoma, beriberi (thiamine deficiency), or kwashiorkor (protein deficiency). Cardiomyopathy may also result from rheumatic fever, especially among children with myocarditis.

Antepartal or postpartal cardiomyopathy may develop during the last trimester or within months after delivery. Its cause is unknown, but it occurs most frequently in multiparous women older than age 30, particularly those with malnutrition or preeclampsia. In these patients, cardiomegaly and heart failure may reverse with treatment, allowing a subsequent normal pregnancy. If cardiomegaly persists despite treatment, the prognosis is poor.

Dilated cardiomyopathy occurs in 2 of every 100 people and affects all ages and sexes. It's most common in adult men.

Signs and symptoms

In dilated cardiomyopathy, the heart ejects blood less efficiently than normal. Consequently, a large volume of blood remains in the left ventricle after systole, causing signs of heart failure — both left-sided (short-

heart a globular appearance and shape. In this disorder, hypertrophy may be present. Dilated cardiomyopathy leads to intractable heart failure, arrhythmias, and emboli. Because this disease isn't usually diagnosed until it's in the advanced stages, the patient's prognosis is generally poor.

ness of breath, orthopnea, dyspnea on exertion, paroxysmal nocturnal dyspnea, fatigue, and an irritating dry cough at night) and right-sided (edema, liver engorgement, and jugular vein distention). Dilated cardiomyopathy also produces peripheral cyanosis and sinus tachycardia or atrial fibrillation at rest in some patients secondary to low cardiac output. Auscultation reveals diffuse apical impulses, pansystolic murmur (mitral and tricuspid insufficiency secondary to cardiomegaly and weak papillary muscles), and S_3 and S_4 gallop rhythms.

Diagnosis
No single test confirms dilated cardiomyopathy. Diagnosis requires elimination of other possible causes of heart failure and arrhythmias.

■ Electrocardiography (ECG) and angiography rule out ischemic heart disease; ECG may also show biventricular hypertrophy, sinus tachycardia, atrial enlargement and, in 20% of patients, atrial fibrillation and bundle-branch block.

■ Chest X-ray shows cardiomegaly — usually affecting all heart chambers — and may demonstrate pulmonary congestion, pleural or pericardial effusion, or pulmonary venous hypertension.

■ Chest computed tomography scan or echocardiography identifies left ventricular thrombi, global hypokinesia, and degree of left ventricular dilation.

■ Nuclear heart scans, such as multiple-gated acquisition scanning and ventriculography, show heart enlargement, lung congestion, heart failure, and decreased movement or functioning of the heart.

Treatment
Therapeutic goals include correcting the underlying causes and improving the heart's pumping ability with digoxin, diuretics, oxygen, and a sodium-restricted diet. Other options may involve bed rest and steroids. Vasodilators reduce preload and afterload, thereby decreasing congestion and increasing cardiac output. Acute heart failure requires vasodilation with nitroprusside or nitroglycerin I.V. Long-term treatment may include prazosin, hydralazine, isosorbide dinitrate, angiotensin-converting enzyme inhibitors, and anticoagulants.

When these treatments fail, therapy may require a heart transplant for carefully selected patients. Cardiomyoplasty, which wraps the latissimus dorsi muscle around the ventricles, assists the ventricle to effectively pump blood. A cardiomyostimulator delivers bursts of electrical impulses during systole to contract the muscle.

Special considerations
In the patient with acute failure:

■ Monitor for signs of progressive failure (increasing crackles and dyspnea and increased jugular vein distention) and compromised renal perfusion (oliguria, elevated blood urea nitrogen and creatinine levels, and electrolyte imbalances). Weigh the patient daily.

■ If the patient is receiving vasodilators, check blood pressure and heart rate. If he becomes hypotensive, stop the infusion and place him in a supine position, with legs elevated to increase venous return and to ensure cerebral blood flow.

■ If the patient is receiving diuretics, monitor for signs of resolving congestion (decreased crackles and dyspnea) or too vigorous diuresis. Check serum potassium level for hypokalemia, especially if therapy includes digoxin.

■ Therapeutic restrictions and an uncertain prognosis usually cause profound anxiety and depression, so offer support and let the patient express his feelings. Be flexible with visiting hours.

■ Before discharge, teach the patient about his illness and its treatment. Emphasize the need to avoid alcohol, smoking, to restrict sodium intake, to watch for weight gain (a weight gain of 3 lb [1.4 kg] over 1 to 2 days indicates fluid accumulation), and to take digoxin as prescribed, and watch for its adverse effects (anorexia, nausea, vomiting, and yellow vision).

■ Encourage family members to learn cardiopulmonary resuscitation.

Hypertrophic cardiomyopathy

This primary disease of cardiac muscle, also called *idiopathic hypertrophic subaortic stenosis,* is characterized by disproportionate, asymmetrical thickening of the interventricular septum, particularly in the left ventricle's free wall. In hypertrophic cardiomyopathy, cardiac output may be low, normal, or high, depending on whether stenosis is obstructive or nonobstructive. If cardiac output is normal or high, the disorder may go undetected for years; but low cardiac output may lead to potentially fatal heart failure. The disease course varies; some patients progressively deteriorate; others remain stable for years.

Causes and incidence

Despite being designated as idiopathic, in almost all cases, hypertrophic cardiomyopathy may be inherited as a non–sex-linked autosomal dominant trait. Most patients have obstructive disease, resulting from effects of ventricular septal hypertrophy and the movement of the anterior mitral valve leaflet into the outflow tract during systole. Eventually, left ventricular dysfunction, from rigidity and decreased compliance, causes pump failure.

This disorder affects 2 to 5 of every 1,000 people.

Signs and symptoms

Clinical features of the disorder may not appear until it's well advanced, when atrial dilation and, possibly, atrial fibrillation abruptly reduce blood flow to the left ventricle. Reduced inflow and subsequent low output may produce angina pectoris, arrhythmias, dyspnea, orthopnea, syncope, heart failure, and death. Auscultation reveals a medium-pitched systolic ejection murmur along the left sternal border and at the apex; palpation reveals a peripheral pulse with a characteristic double impulse (pulsus biferiens) and, with atrial fibrillation, an irregular pulse.

Diagnosis

Diagnosis depends on typical clinical findings and these test results:

- Echocardiography (most useful) shows increased thickness of the intra-ventricular septum and abnormal motion of the anterior mitral leaflet during systole, occluding left ventricular outflow in obstructive disease.
- Cardiac catheterization reveals elevated left ventricular end-diastolic pressure and, possibly, mitral insufficiency.
- Electrocardiography usually shows left ventricular hypertrophy, T-wave inversion, left anterior hemiblock, Q waves in precordial and inferior leads, ventricular arrhythmias and, possibly, atrial fibrillation.
- Auscultation confirms an early systolic murmur.

Treatment

The goals of treatment are to relax the ventricle and to relieve outflow tract obstruction. Agents such as propranolol, a beta-adrenergic blocker, slow heart rate and increase ventricular filling by relaxing the obstructing muscle, thereby reducing angina, syncope, dyspnea, and arrhythmias. However, propranolol may aggravate symptoms of cardiac decompensation. Atrial fibrillation necessitates cardioversion to treat the arrhythmia and, because of the high risk of systemic embolism, anticoagulant therapy until fibrillation subsides. Because vasodilators such as nitroglycerin reduce venous return by permitting pooling of blood in the periphery, decreasing ventricular volume and chamber size, and may cause further obstruction, they're contraindicated in patients with hypertrophic cardiomyopathy. Also contraindicated are sympathetic stimulators such as isoproterenol, which enhance cardiac contractility and myocardial demands for oxygen, intensifying the obstruction. Although quinidine is used to suppress ventricular arrhythmia, disopyramide is preferred because of its negative inotropic properties. Patients with potentially lethal arrhythmias may need an implantable-cardioverter defibrillator to prevent sudden death.

If drug therapy fails, surgery is indicated. Ventricular myotomy (resection of the hypertrophied septum) or ventricular myectomy (removal of the hypertrophied septum) alone or combined with mitral valve replacement may ease outflow tract obstruction and relieve symptoms. However, ventricular myotomy may cause complications, such as complete heart block and ventricular septal defect.

Special considerations

■ Because syncope or sudden death may follow well-tolerated exercise, warn such patients against strenuous physical activity such as running.

■ Administer medications as prescribed. *Caution:* Avoid nitroglycerin, digoxin, and diuretics because they can worsen obstruction. Warn the patient not to stop taking propranolol abruptly, because doing so may increase myocardial demands. To determine the patient's tolerance for an increased dosage of propranolol, take his pulse to check for bradycardia. Also take his blood pressure while he's supine and standing (a drop in blood pressure [more than 10 mm Hg] when standing may indicate orthostatic hypotension).

■ Before dental work or surgery, tell the patient to discuss prophylaxis for subacute infective endocarditis with his health care provider.

■ Provide psychological support. If the patient is hospitalized for a long time, be flexible with visiting hours and encourage occasional weekends away from the hospital, if possible. Refer the patient for psychosocial counseling to help him and his family accept his restricted lifestyle and poor prognosis.

■ If the patient is a child, have his parents arrange for him to continue his studies in the health care facility.

■ Because sudden cardiac arrest is possible, urge the patient's family to learn cardiopulmonary resuscitation.

Restrictive cardiomyopathy

Restrictive cardiomyopathy, a disorder of the myocardial musculature, is characterized by restricted ventricular filling (the result of left ventricular hypertrophy) and endocardial fibrosis and thickening. If severe, it's irreversible. The average survival after diagnosis is 9 years.

Causes and incidence

An extremely rare disorder, primary restrictive cardiomyopathy is of unknown etiology. However, restrictive cardiomyopathy syndrome, a manifestation of amyloidosis, results from infiltration of amyloid into the intracellular spaces in the myocardium, endocardium, and subendocardium.

In both forms of restrictive cardiomyopathy, the myocardium becomes rigid, with poor distention during diastole, inhibiting complete ventricular filling, and fails to contract completely during systole, resulting in low cardiac output.

Restrictive cardiomyopathy is rare. It's most common in children and young adults. Natives of Africa, South America, and India are at increased risk.

Signs and symptoms

Because it lowers cardiac output and leads to heart failure, restrictive cardiomyopathy produces fatigue, dyspnea, orthopnea, chest pain, generalized edema, liver engorgement, peripheral cyanosis, pallor, S_3 or S_4 gallop rhythms, and systolic murmurs of mitral and tricuspid insufficiency.

Diagnosis

■ In advanced stages of this disease, chest X-ray shows massive cardiomegaly, affecting all four chambers of the heart; pericardial effusion; and pulmonary congestion.

■ Echocardiography, computed tomography scan, or magnetic resonance imaging rules out constrictive pericarditis as the cause of restricted filling by detecting increased left ventricular muscle mass and differences in end-diastolic pressures between the ventricles.

■ Electrocardiography may show low-voltage complexes, hypertrophy, atrioventricular conduction defects, or arrhythmias.

■ Arterial pulsation reveals blunt carotid upstroke with small volume.

■ Cardiac catheterization shows increased left ventricular end-diastolic pressure and rules out constrictive pericarditis as the cause of restricted filling.

Restrictive cardiomyopathy may be difficult to differentiate from constrictive pericarditis. A biopsy of heart muscle may be used to confirm the diagnosis. A cardiac catheterization procedure can also help differentiate the type of cardiomyopathy through simultaneous left- and right-heart catheterization. In some cases, surgical exploration and biopsies are the only means to distinguish the type of cardiomyopathy or to differentiate it from pericarditis.

Treatment

Although no therapy currently exists for restricted ventricular filling, cardiac glycosides, diuretics, and a restricted sodium diet are beneficial by easing the symptoms of heart failure.

Oral vasodilators—such as isosorbide dinitrate, prazosin, and hydralazine—may control intractable heart failure. Anticoagulant therapy may be necessary to prevent thrombophlebitis in the patient on prolonged bed rest. Steroids or chemotherapy may help with the underlying disease process. A heart transplant may be considered in those with poor myocardial functioning.

Special considerations

■ In the acute phase, monitor heart rate and rhythm, blood pressure, urine output, and pulmonary artery pressure readings to help guide treatment.

■ Give psychological support. Provide appropriate diversionary activities for the patient restricted to prolonged bed rest. Because a poor prognosis may cause profound anxiety and depression, be especially supportive and understanding, and encourage the patient to express his fears. Refer him for psychosocial counseling, as necessary, for assistance in coping with his restricted lifestyle. Be flexible with visiting hours whenever possible.

■ Before discharge, teach the patient to watch for and report signs of digoxin toxicity (anorexia, nausea, vomiting, and yellow vision); to record and report weight gain; and, if sodium restriction is ordered, to avoid canned foods, pickles, smoked meats, and use of table salt.

CARDIAC COMPLICATIONS

Hypovolemic shock

In hypovolemic shock, reduced intravascular blood volume causes circulatory dysfunction and inadequate tissue perfusion. Without sufficient blood or fluid replacement, hypovolemic shock syndrome may lead to irreversible cerebral and renal damage, cardiac arrest and, ultimately, death. Hypovolemic shock requires early recognition of signs and symptoms and prompt, aggressive treatment to improve the prognosis. (See *What happens in hypovolemic shock,* page 1116.)

Causes

Hypovolemic shock usually results from acute blood loss—about one-fifth of total volume. Such massive blood loss may result from GI bleeding, internal hemorrhage (hemothorax and hemoperitoneum), external hemorrhage (accidental or surgical trauma), or from any condition that reduces circulating intravascular plasma volume or other body fluids such as in severe burns. Other underlying causes of hypovolemic shock include intestinal obstruction, peritonitis, acute pancreatitis, ascites and dehydration from excessive perspiration, severe diarrhea or protracted vomiting, diabetes insipidus, diuresis, or inadequate fluid intake.

Signs and symptoms

Hypovolemic shock produces a syndrome of hypotension, with narrowing pulse pressure; decreased sensorium; tachycardia; rapid, shallow respirations; reduced urine output (less than 25 ml/hour); and cold, pale, clammy skin. Metabolic acidosis with an accumulation of lactic acid develops as a result of tissue anoxia, as cellular metabolism shifts from aerobic to anaerobic pathways. Disseminated intravascular coagulation (DIC) is a possible complication of hypovolemic shock.

PATHOPHYSIOLOGY
WHAT HAPPENS IN HYPOVOLEMIC SHOCK

In hypovolemic shock, vascular fluid volume loss causes extreme tissue hypoperfusion. Internal fluid losses can result from hemorrhage or third space fluid shifting. External fluid loss can result from severe bleeding or from severe diarrhea, diuresis, or vomiting. Inadequate vascular volume leads to decreased venous return and cardiac output. The resulting drop in arterial blood pressure activates the body's compensatory mechanisms in an attempt to increase vascular volume. If compensation is unsuccessful, decompensation and death may occur.

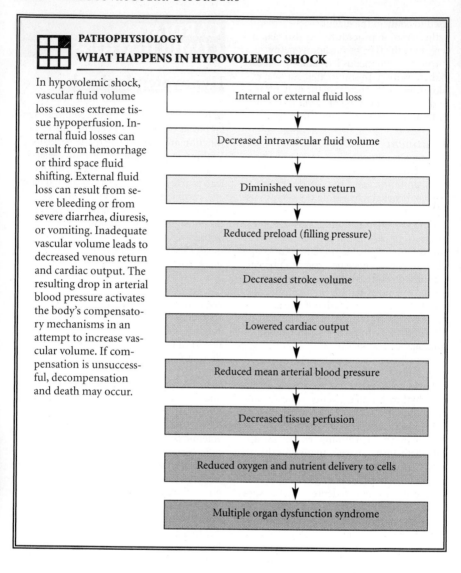

Internal or external fluid loss

↓

Decreased intravascular fluid volume

↓

Diminished venous return

↓

Reduced preload (filling pressure)

↓

Decreased stroke volume

↓

Lowered cardiac output

↓

Reduced mean arterial blood pressure

↓

Decreased tissue perfusion

↓

Reduced oxygen and nutrient delivery to cells

↓

Multiple organ dysfunction syndrome

Diagnosis

No single symptom or diagnostic test establishes the diagnosis or severity of shock. Characteristic laboratory findings include:
- elevated potassium, serum lactate, and blood urea nitrogen levels
- increased urine specific gravity (more than 1.020) and urine osmolality
- decreased blood pH and partial pressure of arterial oxygen and increased partial pressure of arterial carbon dioxide.

In addition, gastroscopy, aspiration of gastric contents through a nasogastric tube, computed tomography scan, and X-rays identify internal bleeding sites; coagulation studies may detect coagulopathy from DIC. Echocardiography or right-heart catheterization can help differentiate between hypovolemic and cardiogenic shock.

USING A PNEUMATIC ANTISHOCK GARMENT

A pneumatic antishock garment counteracts bleeding and hypovolemia by slowing or stopping arterial bleeding; by forcing any available blood from the lower body to the heart, brain, and other vital organs; and by preventing return of the available circulating blood volume to the lower extremities.

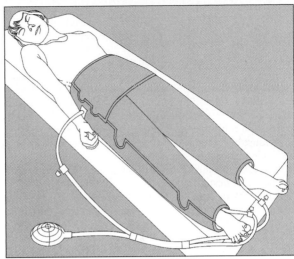

Do's

■ While the patient is wearing a pneumatic antishock garment, monitor blood pressure, apical and radial pulse rates, and respirations; check extremities for pedal pulses, color, warmth, and numbness; and make sure the garment isn't too constricting.

■ Remove the garment only when a physician is present, fluids are available for transfusion, and anesthesia and surgical teams are available. The compartments are deflated slowly and only one section at a time while the patient is monitored closely.

■ To clean, wash with warm soap and water, air-dry, and store.

Don'ts

■ Don't apply the garment if positions or wounds show or suggest major intrathoracic or intracranial vascular injury or if the patient has open extremity bleeding, pulmonary edema, or trauma above the application site. It may be used during pregnancy; however, the abdominal compartment should *not* be inflated.

■ When cleaning, don't autoclave or use solvents.

Treatment

Emergency treatment measures must include prompt and adequate blood and fluid replacement to restore intravascular volume and raise blood pressure. Saline solution or lactated Ringer's solution, then possibly plasma proteins (albumin) or other plasma expanders, may produce adequate volume expansion until whole blood can be matched. A rapid solution infusion system can provide these crystalloids or colloids at high flow rates. Application of a pneumatic antishock garment may be helpful. (See *Using a pneumatic antishock garment.*) Dopamine, dobutamine, epinephrine, and norepinephrine can help increase blood pressure and cardiac output after fluid resuscitation measures are done. Treatment may also include oxygen administration, identification of bleeding site, control of bleeding by direct measures (such as application of pressure and elevation of an extremity) and, possibly, surgery.

Special considerations

Management of hypovolemic shock necessitates prompt, aggressive supportive measures and careful assessment and monitoring of vital signs. Follow these priorities:

■ Check for a patent airway and adequate circulation. If blood pressure and heart rate are absent, start cardiopulmonary resuscitation.

■ Record blood pressure, pulse rate, peripheral pulses, respiratory rate, and other vital signs every 15 minutes and the electrocardiograph continuously. Systolic blood pressure lower than 80 mm Hg usually results in inadequate coronary artery blood flow, cardiac ischemia, arrhythmias, and further complications of low cardiac output. When blood pressure drops below 80 mm Hg, increase the oxygen flow rate and notify the physician immediately. A progressive drop in blood pressure, accompanied by a thready pulse, generally signals inadequate cardiac output from reduced intravascular volume. Notify the physician and increase the infusion rate.

■ Start I.V. lines with normal saline or lactated Ringer's solution, using a large-bore catheter (14G), which allows easier administration of later blood transfusions. (*Caution:* Don't start I.V. lines in the legs of a patient in shock who has suffered abdominal trauma, because infused fluid may escape through the ruptured vessel into the abdomen.)

■ An indwelling urinary catheter may be inserted to measure hourly urine output. If output is less than 30 ml/hour in adults, increase the fluid infusion rate, but watch for signs of fluid overload such as an increase in pulmonary artery wedge pressure (PAWP). Notify the physician if urine output doesn't improve. An osmotic diuretic such as mannitol may be ordered to increase renal blood flow and urine output. Determine how much fluid to give by checking blood pressure, urine output, central venous pressure (CVP), or PAWP. (To increase accuracy, CVP should be measured at the level of the right atrium, using the same reference point on the chest each time.)

■ Draw an arterial blood sample to measure blood gas levels. Administer oxygen by face mask or airway to ensure adequate oxygenation of tissues. Adjust the oxygen flow rate to a higher or lower level, as blood gas measurements indicate.

■ Draw venous blood for complete blood count and electrolyte, type and crossmatch, and coagulation studies.

■ During therapy, assess skin color and temperature, and note changes. Cold, clammy skin may be a sign of continuing peripheral vascular constriction, indicating progressive shock.

■ Watch for signs of impending coagulopathy (petechiae, bruising, and bleeding or oozing from gums or venipuncture sites).

■ Explain procedures and their purpose. Throughout these emergency measures, provide emotional support to the patient and his family.

Cardiogenic shock

Sometimes called *pump failure,* cardiogenic shock is a condition of diminished cardiac output that severely impairs tissue perfusion. It reflects severe left-sided heart failure and occurs as a serious complication in 5% to 10% of all patients hospitalized with acute myocardial infarction (MI). Historically, mortality for cardiogenic shock had been 80% to 90%, but recent studies indicate that the rate has dropped to 56% to 67% due to the advent of thrombolytics, improved interventional procedures, and better therapies. Mortality is expected to decline even further.

Causes and incidence

Cardiogenic shock can result from any condition that causes significant left ventricular dysfunction with reduced cardiac output, such as MI (most common), myocardial ischemia, papillary muscle dysfunction, or end-stage cardiomyopathy. Regardless of the underlying cause, left ventricular dysfunction sets into motion a series of compensatory mechanisms that attempt to increase cardiac output and, in turn, maintain vital organ function. (See *What happens in cardiogenic shock.*) As cardiac output falls in left ventricular dysfunction, aortic and carotid baroreceptors initiate sympathetic nervous responses, which in-

PATHOPHYSIOLOGY
WHAT HAPPENS IN CARDIOGENIC SHOCK

When the myocardium can't contract sufficiently to maintain adequate cardiac output, stroke volume decreases and the heart can't eject an adequate volume of blood with each contraction. The blood backs up behind the weakened left ventricle, increasing preload and causing pulmonary congestion. In addition, to compensate for the drop in stroke volume, the heart rate increases in an attempt to maintain cardiac output. As a result of the diminished stroke volume, coronary artery perfusion and collateral blood flow decrease. All of these mechanisms increase the heart's workload and enhance left-sided heart failure. The result is myocardial hypoxia, further decreased cardiac output, and a triggering of compensatory mechanisms to prevent decompensation and death.

```
                        Initial insult
                             │
                             ▼
                  Decreased myocardial
                      contractility
                             │
                             ▼
                    Decreased stroke
                        volume
              ┌──────────────┴──────────────┐
              ▼                              ▼
      Decreased left                 Increased heart rate
    ventricular emptying                     │
              │                              ▼
              ▼                       Decreased coronary
      Left ventricular               artery perfusion and
    dilation and backup of            collateral blood flow
          blood                              │
              │                              ▼
              ▼                       Myocardial hypoxia
      Increased preload                      │
              │                              ▼
              ▼                       Decreased cardiac
    Pulmonary congestion                   output
                                             │
                                             ▼
                                        Compensation
                                             │
                                             ▼
                                    Decompensation and
                                          death
```

crease heart rate, left ventricular filling pressure, and peripheral resistance to flow, to enhance venous return to the heart. These compensatory responses initially stabilize the patient but later cause deterioration with rising oxygen demands of the already compromised myocardium. These events comprise a vicious circle of low cardiac output, sympathetic compensation, myocardial ischemia, and even lower cardiac output.

Incidence of cardiogenic shock is higher in men than in women because of their higher incidence of coronary artery disease. However, among people with MI, women have a higher incidence of cardiogenic shock than men.

Signs and symptoms

Cardiogenic shock produces signs of poor tissue perfusion: cold, pale, clammy skin; a decrease in systolic blood pressure to 30 mm Hg below baseline, or a sustained reading below 80 mm Hg not attributable to medication; tachycardia; rapid, shallow respirations; oliguria (less than 20 ml/hour); restlessness; mental confusion and obtundation; narrowing pulse pressure; and cyanosis. Although many of these clinical features also occur in heart failure and other shock syndromes, they're usually more profound in cardiogenic shock.

Diagnosis

Auscultation may detect gallop rhythm, faint heart sounds and, possibly, if the shock results from rupture of the ventricular septum or papillary muscles, a holosystolic murmur.

- Pulmonary artery pressure (PAP) monitoring may show increased PAP, and increased pulmonary artery wedge pressure (PAWP), reflecting a rise in left ventricular end-diastolic pressure (preload) and increased resistance to left ventricular emptying (afterload) due to ineffective pumping and increased peripheral vascular resistance. Thermodilution technique measures decreased cardiac output.
- Invasive arterial pressure monitoring may indicate hypotension due to impaired ventricular ejection.
- Arterial blood gas (ABG) analysis may show metabolic acidosis and hypoxia.
- Electrocardiography may show possible evidence of acute MI, ischemia, or ventricular aneurysm.
- Echocardiography can determine left ventricular function and reveal valvular abnormalities.
- Enzyme levels may show elevated creatine kinase, lactate dehydrogenase, aspartate aminotransferase, and alanine aminotransferase, which point MI or ischemia and suggest heart failure or shock. Troponin I, troponin T, and isoenzyme values may confirm acute MI.

Additional tests determine other conditions that can lead to pump dysfunction and failure, such as cardiac arrhythmias, cardiac tamponade, papillary muscle infarct or rupture, ventricular septal rupture, pulmonary emboli, venous pooling (associated with vasodilators and continuous intermittent positive-pressure breathing), and hypovolemia.

Treatment

The aim of treatment is to enhance cardiovascular status by increasing cardiac output, improving myocardial perfusion, and decreasing cardiac workload with combinations of various cardiovascular drugs and mechanical-assist techniques. Myocardial reperfusion can be accomplished by percutaneous transluminal coronary angioplasty, stents, thrombolytic therapy, or bypass grafting. Drug therapy may include dopamine I.V., a vasopressor that increases cardiac output, blood pressure, and renal blood flow; amrinone or dobutamine I.V., inotropic agents that increases myocardial contractility; norepinephrine, when a more potent vasoconstrictor is necessary; and nitroprusside I.V., a vasodilator that may be used with a vasopressor to further improve cardiac output by decreasing peripheral vascular resistance (afterload) and reducing left ventricular end-diastolic pressure (preload). However, the patient's blood pressure must be adequate to support nitroprusside therapy and must be monitored closely.

The intra-aortic balloon pump (IABP) is a mechanical-assist device that attempts to improve coronary artery perfusion and decrease cardiac workload. (See *Intra-aortic balloon pump*.) The inflatable balloon pump is percutaneously or surgically inserted through the femoral artery into the descending thoracic aorta. The balloon inflates during diastole to increase coronary artery perfusion pressure and deflates before systole (before the aortic valve opens) to reduce resistance to ejection (afterload) and reduce cardiac workload. Improved ventricular ejection, which significantly improves cardiac output, and a subsequent vasodilation in the peripheral vasculature lead to lower preload volume.

When drug therapy and IABP insertion fail, treatment may require the use of a ventricular assist device. This device (which may be either temporary or permanent) diverts systemic blood flow from a diseased ventricle into a centrifugal pump.

INTRA-AORTIC BALLOON PUMP

An effective method of reducing myocardial oxygen consumption, the intra-aortic balloon pump (IABP) approximates the heart's action in response to an electrocardiograph signal. It inflates during ventricular diastole, displacing blood proximally and increasing coronary artery perfusion. It deflates before systole, decreasing aortic pressure and resistance to ventricular flow. The end result is decreased ventricular workload.

The patient remains supine during IABP therapy, and the extremity must remain extended to prevent catheter kinking.

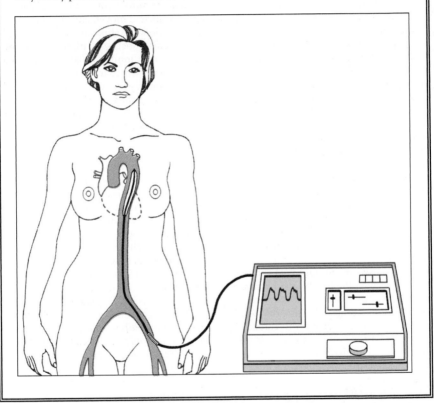

It assists the heart's pumping action rather than replaces it.

Special considerations
■ At the first sign of cardiogenic shock, check the patient's blood pressure and heart rate. If the patient is hypotensive or is having difficulty breathing, ensure a patent I.V. line and a patent airway, and provide oxygen to promote tissue oxygenation. Notify the physician immediately.

■ Monitor ABG values to measure oxygenation and detect acidosis from poor tissue perfusion. Increase oxygen delivery as indicated. Check complete blood count and electrolytes levels.

■ After diagnosis, monitor cardiac rhythm continuously and assess skin color, temperature, and other vital signs often. Watch for a drop in systolic blood pressure to less than 80 mm Hg (usually compromising cardiac output further). Report hypotension immediately.

■ An indwelling urinary catheter may be inserted to measure urine output. Notify the physician if output drops below 30 ml/hour.

■ Using a pulmonary artery catheter, closely monitor PAP, PAWP and, if equipment is available, cardiac output. A high PAWP indicates heart failure and should be reported.

■ When a patient is on the IABP, reposition him often and perform passive range-of-motion exercises to prevent skin breakdown. However, don't flex the patient's "ballooned" leg at the hip because this may displace or fracture the catheter. Assess pedal pulses and skin temperature and color to make sure circulation to the leg is adequate. Check the dressing on the insertion site frequently for bleeding and change it according to facility protocol. Also, check the site for hematoma or signs of infection, and culture any drainage.

■ After the patient becomes hemodynamically stable, the frequency of balloon inflation is gradually reduced to wean him from the IABP. During weaning, carefully watch for monitor changes, chest pain, and other signs of recurring cardiac ischemia and shock.

■ Provide psychological support and reassurance because the patient and his family may be anxious about the intensive care unit, IABP, and other tubes and devices. To ease emotional stress, plan your care to allow frequent rest periods, and provide as much privacy as possible.

Ventricular aneurysm

A ventricular aneurysm is an outpouching, almost always of the left ventricle, that produces ventricular wall dysfunction in about 20% of patients after myocardial infarction (MI). Ventricular aneurysm may develop within weeks after MI. Untreated ventricular aneurysm can lead to arrhythmias, systemic embolization, or heart failure, and may cause sudden death. Resection improves the prognosis in patients with heart failure or refractory patients who have developed ventricular arrhythmias.

Causes

When MI destroys a large muscular section of the left ventricle, necrosis reduces the ventricular wall to a thin sheath of fibrous tissue. Under intracardiac pressure, this thin layer stretches and forms a separate noncontractile sac (aneurysm). Abnormal muscular wall movement accompanies ventricular aneurysm and includes akinesia (lack of movement), dyskinesia (paradoxical movement), asynergia (decreased and inadequate movement), and asynchrony (uncoordinated movement). During systolic ejection, the abnormal muscular wall movements associated with the aneurysm cause the remaining normally functioning myocardial fibers to increase the force of contraction in order to maintain stroke volume and cardiac output. At the same time, a portion of the stroke volume is lost to passive distention of the noncontractile sac.

Signs and symptoms

Ventricular aneurysm may cause arrhythmias — such as premature ventricular contractions or ventricular tachycardia — palpitations, signs of cardiac dysfunction (weakness on exertion, fatigue, and angina) and, occasionally, a visible or palpable systolic precordial bulge. This condition may also lead to left ventricular dysfunction, with chronic heart failure (dyspnea, fatigue, edema, crackles, gallop rhythm, and jugular vein distention); pulmonary edema; systemic embolization; and, with left-sided heart failure, pulsus alternans. Ventricular aneurysms enlarge but seldom rupture.

Diagnosis

Persistent ventricular arrhythmias, onset of heart failure, or systemic embolization in a patient with left-sided heart failure and a history of MI strongly suggests ventricular aneurysm. Indicative tests include the following:

■ Left ventriculography reveals left ventricular enlargement, with an area of akinesia or dyskinesia (during cineangiography) and diminished cardiac function.

■ Electrocardiography may show persistent ST-T wave elevations after infarction.

- Chest X-ray may demonstrate an abnormal bulge distorting the heart's contour if the aneurysm is large; the X-ray may be normal if the aneurysm is small.
- Noninvasive nuclear cardiology scan may indicate the site of infarction and suggest the area of aneurysm.
- Echocardiography shows abnormal motion in the left ventricular wall.

Treatment
Depending on the aneurysm's size and the complications, treatment may necessitate only routine medical examination to follow the patient's condition or aggressive measures for intractable ventricular arrhythmias, heart failure, and emboli.

Emergency treatment of ventricular arrhythmia includes antiarrhythmics I.V. or cardioversion. Preventive treatment continues with oral antiarrhythmics, such as procainamide, quinidine, or disopyramide.

Emergency treatment for heart failure with pulmonary edema includes oxygen, cardiac glycosides I.V., furosemide I.V., morphine I.V. and, when necessary, nitroprusside I.V. and intubation. Maintenance therapy may include nitrates, prazosin, and oral hydralazine. Systemic embolization requires anticoagulation therapy or embolectomy. Refractory ventricular tachycardia, heart failure, recurrent arterial embolization, and persistent angina with coronary artery occlusion may necessitate surgery, of which the most effective procedure is aneurysmectomy with myocardial revascularization.

Special considerations
- If ventricular tachycardia occurs, administer a prescribed antiarrhythmic such as lidocaine. Monitor blood pressure and heart rate. If cardiac arrest develops, initiate cardiopulmonary resuscitation (CPR) and call for assistance, resuscitative equipment, and medication.
- In a patient with heart failure, closely monitor vital signs, heart sounds, intake and output, fluid and electrolyte balances, and blood urea nitrogen and creatinine levels. Because of the threat of systemic embolization, frequently check peripheral pulses and the color and temperature of extremities. Be alert for sudden changes in

sensorium that indicate cerebral embolization and for any signs that suggest renal failure or progressive MI.
- If arrhythmias necessitate cardioversion, use a sufficient amount of conducting jelly to prevent chest burns. If the patient is conscious, give diazepam or methohexital I.V., as ordered, before cardioversion. Explain that cardioversion is a lifesaving method using brief electroshock to the heart. If the patient is receiving antiarrhythmics, check appropriate laboratory tests. For instance, if the patient takes procainamide, check antinuclear antibodies because this drug may induce symptoms that mimic lupus erythematosus.

If the patient is scheduled to undergo resection:
- Before surgery, explain expected postoperative care in the intensive care unit (including use of such things as endotracheal tube, ventilator, hemodynamic monitoring, chest tubes, and drainage bottle).
- After surgery, monitor vital signs, intake and output, heart sounds, and pulmonary artery catheter. Watch for signs of infection, such as fever and drainage.

To prepare the patient for discharge:
- Teach him how to check for pulse irregularity and rate changes. Encourage him to follow his prescribed medication regimen—even during the night—and to watch for adverse effects.
- Because arrhythmias can cause sudden death, refer the family to a community-based CPR training program.
- Provide psychological support for the patient and his family.

Cardiac tamponade

In cardiac tamponade, a rapid, unchecked rise in intrapericardial pressure impairs diastolic filling of the heart. The rise in pressure usually results from blood or fluid accumulation in the pericardial sac. If fluid accumulates rapidly, this condition requires emergency lifesaving measures to prevent death. A slow accumulation and rise in pressure, as in pericardial effusion associated with malignant tumors, may not produce immediate symptoms, because the fibrous wall of the pericardial sac can gradually stretch to accommodate as much as 1 to 2 L of fluid.

Causes and incidence

Increased intrapericardial pressure and cardiac tamponade may be idiopathic (Dressler's syndrome) or may result from:

- effusion (in cancer, bacterial infections, tuberculosis and, rarely, acute rheumatic fever)
- hemorrhage from trauma (such as gunshot or stab wounds of the chest and perforation by catheter during cardiac or central venous catheterization or postcardiac surgery)
- hemorrhage from nontraumatic causes (such as rupture of the heart or great vessels or anticoagulant therapy in a patient with pericarditis)
- acute myocardial infarction (MI)
- end stage lung cancer
- heart tumors
- radiation therapy
- hypothyroidism
- systemic lupus erythematosus
- uremia.

Cardiac tamponade occurs in 2 of every 10,000 people.

Signs and symptoms

Cardiac tamponade classically produces increased venous pressure with jugular vein distention, reduced arterial blood pressure, muffled heart sounds on auscultation, and pulsus paradoxus (an abnormal inspiratory drop in systemic blood pressure greater than 15 mm Hg). These classic symptoms represent failure of physiologic compensatory mechanisms to override the effects of rapidly rising pericardial pressure, which limits diastolic filling of the ventricles and reduces stroke volume to a critically low level. Generally, ventricular end-systolic volume may drop because of inadequate preload. The increasing pericardial pressure is transmitted equally across the heart cavities, producing a matching rise in intracardiac pressure, especially atrial and end-diastolic ventricular pressures. Cardiac tamponade may also cause dyspnea, diaphoresis, pallor or cyanosis, anxiety, tachycardia, narrow pulse pressure, restlessness, and hepatomegaly, but the lung fields will

be clear. The patient typically sits upright and leans forward.

Diagnosis

- Chest X-ray shows slightly widened mediastinum and cardiomegaly.
- Electrocardiography (ECG) is rarely diagnostic of tamponade but is useful in ruling out other cardiac disorders. It may reveal changes produced by acute pericarditis.
- Pulmonary artery catheterization detects increased right atrial pressure, right ventricular diastolic pressure, and central venous pressure (CVP).
- Echocardiography, computed tomography scan, or magnetic resonance imaging shows pericardial effusion with signs of right ventricular and atrial compression.

Treatment

The goal of treatment is to relieve intrapericardial pressure and cardiac compression by removing accumulated blood or fluid. Pericardiocentesis (needle aspiration of the pericardial cavity) or surgical creation of an opening (pericardiectomy or pericardial window) dramatically improves systemic arterial pressure and cardiac output with aspiration of as little as 25 ml of fluid. Such treatment necessitates continuous hemodynamic and ECG monitoring in the intensive care unit. Trial volume loading with temporary I.V. normal saline solution with albumin, and perhaps an inotropic drug, such as isoproterenol or dopamine, is necessary in the hypotensive patient to maintain cardiac output. Although these drugs normally improve myocardial function, they may further compromise an ischemic myocardium after MI.

Depending on the cause of tamponade, additional treatment may include:

- in traumatic injury — blood transfusion or a thoracotomy to drain reaccumulating fluid or to repair bleeding sites
- in heparin-induced tamponade — the heparin antagonist protamine sulfate
- in warfarin-induced tamponade — vitamin K.

Resection of a portion or all of the pericardium to allow full communication with the pleura may be needed if repeated pericardiocentesis fails to prevent recurrence.

Special considerations

If the patient needs pericardiocentesis:

■ Explain the procedure to him. Keep a pericardial aspiration needle attached to a 50-ml syringe by a three-way stopcock, an ECG machine, and an emergency cart with a defibrillator at the bedside. Make sure the equipment is turned on and ready for immediate use. Position him at a 45- to 60-degree angle. Connect the precordial ECG lead to the hub of the aspiration needle with an alligator clamp and connecting wire, and assist with fluid aspiration. When the needle touches the myocardium, you'll see an ST-segment elevation or premature ventricular contractions.

■ Monitor blood pressure and CVP during and after pericardiocentesis. Infuse I.V. solutions, as prescribed, to maintain blood pressure. Watch for a decrease in CVP and a concomitant rise in blood pressure, which indicate relief of cardiac compression.

■ Watch for complications of pericardiocentesis, such as ventricular fibrillation, vasovagal response, or coronary artery or cardiac chamber puncture. Closely monitor ECG changes, blood pressure, pulse rate, level of consciousness, and urine output.

If the patient needs thoracotomy:

■ Explain the procedure to him. Tell him what to expect postoperatively (chest tubes, drainage bottles, and oxygen administration). Teach him how to turn, deep breathe, and cough.

■ Give antibiotics, protamine sulfate, or vitamin K, as ordered.

■ Postoperatively, monitor critical parameters, such as vital signs and arterial blood gas values, and assess heart and breath sounds. Give pain medication as ordered. Maintain the chest drainage system and be alert for complications, such as hemorrhage and arrhythmias.

Cardiac arrhythmias

In cardiac arrhythmias (sometimes called *cardiac dysrhythmias),* abnormal electrical conduction or automaticity changes heart rate and rhythm. (See *Normal cardiac conduction,* page 1126.) Arrhythmias vary in severity, from those that are mild, asymptomatic, and require no treatment (such as sinus arrhythmia, in which heart rate increases and decreases with respiration) to catastrophic ventricular fibrillation, which necessitates immediate resuscitation. Arrhythmias are generally classified according to their origin (ventricular or supraventricular). Their effect on cardiac output and blood pressure, partially influenced by the origin site, determines their clinical significance. (See *Types of cardiac arrhythmias,* pages 1127 to 1134.)

Causes

Arrhythmias may be congenital or they may result from one of several factors, including myocardial ischemia, myocardial infarction, or organic heart disease. Drug ingestion (cocaine, amphetamines, caffeine, beta-blockers, psychotropics, sympathomimetics), drug toxicity, or degeneration of the conductive tissue necessary to maintain normal heart rhythm (sick sinus syndrome) can sometimes precipitate arrhythmias. People with imbalances of blood chemistries or those with a history of cardiac conditions (coronary artery disease or heart valve disorders) are at higher risk for developing arrhythmias.

Signs and symptoms

Signs and symptoms of cardiac arrhythmias include palpitations, fainting, lightheadedness, dizziness, chest pain, shortness of breath, changes in pulse patterns, paleness, and the temporary absence of breathing. However, the patient with a cardiac arrhythmia may be asymptomatic until the development of sudden cardiac arrest.

Diagnosis

Diagnosis is made by tests that reveal the arrhythmia, such as 12-lead electrocardiography. Ambulatory cardiac monitoring (Holter monitoring), echocardiography, electrophysiology studies, and coronary angiography may also confirm or rule out suspected causes of arrhythmias and help determine treatment.

NORMAL CARDIAC CONDUCTION

Each electrical impulse travels from the sinoatrial node (1) through the intra-atrial tracts (2), producing atrial contraction. The impulse slows momentarily as it passes through the atrioventricular junction (3) to the bundle of His (4). Then, it descends the left and right bundle branches (5) and reaches the Purkinje fibers (6), stimulating ventricular contraction.

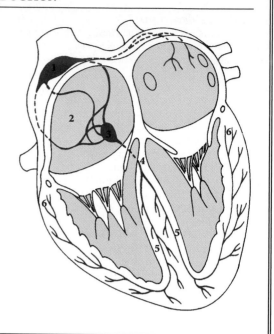

Special considerations

■ Assess an unmonitored patient for rhythm disturbances.

■ If the patient's pulse is abnormally rapid, slow, or irregular, watch for signs of hypoperfusion, such as altered level of consciousness (LOC), hypotension, and diminished urine output.

■ Document arrhythmias in a monitored patient, and assess for possible causes and effects.

■ When life-threatening arrhythmias develop, rapidly assess LOC, respirations, and pulse rate.

■ Initiate cardiopulmonary resuscitation if indicated.

■ Evaluate the patient for altered cardiac output resulting from arrhythmias.

■ Administer medications as ordered and prepare to assist with medical procedures, if indicated (for example, cardioversion).

■ Monitor for predisposing factors — such as fluid and electrolyte imbalance — and signs of drug toxicity, especially with digoxin. If you suspect drug toxicity, report such signs to the physician immediately and withhold the next dose.

■ To prevent arrhythmias in a postoperative cardiac patient, provide adequate oxygen and reduce the heart's workload while carefully maintaining metabolic, neurologic, respiratory, and hemodynamic status.

■ Consider sedation for transcutaneous pacing if appropriate.

■ To avoid temporary pacemaker malfunction, install a fresh battery before each insertion. Carefully secure the external catheter wires and the pacemaker box. Assess the threshold daily. Watch closely for premature contractions, a sign of myocardial irritation.

■ To avert permanent pacemaker malfunction, restrict the patient's activity after insertion as ordered. Monitor the pulse rate regularly and watch for signs of decreased cardiac output.

■ If the patient has a permanent pacemaker, warn him about environmental hazards, as indicated by the pacemaker manufactur-
(Text continues on page 1134.)

TYPES OF CARDIAC ARRHYTHMIAS

This chart reviews many common cardiac arrhythmias and outlines their features, causes, and treatments. Use a normal electrocardiogram strip, if available, to compare normal cardiac rhythm configurations with the rhythm strips below. Characteristics of normal rhythm include:

- ventricular and atrial rates of 60 to 100 beats/minute
- regular and uniform QRS complexes and P waves
- PR interval of 0.12 to 0.2 second
- QRS duration < 0.12 second
- identical atrial and ventricular rates, with constant PR interval.

Arrhythmia and features	Causes	Treatment
Sinus arrhythmia 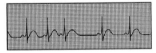 ■ Irregular atrial and ventricular rhythms ■ Normal P wave preceding each QRS complex	■ A normal variation of normal sinus rhythm in athletes, children, and elderly people ■ Also seen in digoxin toxicity and inferior wall myocardial infarction (MI)	■ Atropine if rate decreases below 40 beats/minute and patient is symptomatic (for example, has hypotension)
Sinus tachycardia 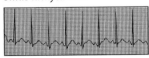 ■ Atrial and ventricular rhythms regular ■ Rate > 100 beats/minute; rarely, > 160 beats/minute ■ Normal P wave preceding each QRS complex	■ Normal physiologic response to fever, exercise, anxiety, pain, dehydration; may also accompany shock, left-sided heart failure, cardiac tamponade, hyperthyroidism, anemia, hypovolemia, pulmonary embolism, anterior wall MI ■ May also occur with atropine, epinephrine, isoproterenol, quinidine, caffeine, alcohol, and nicotine use	■ Correction of underlying cause ■ Beta-adrenergic blockers or calcium channel blockers for symptomatic patients
Sinus bradycardia 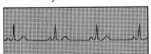 ■ Regular atrial and ventricular rhythms ■ Rate < 60 beats/minute ■ Normal P wave preceding each QRS complex	■ Normal in well-conditioned heart, as in an athlete ■ Increased intracranial pressure; increased vagal tone due to straining during defecation, vomiting, intubation, mechanical ventilation; sick sinus syndrome; hypothyroidism; inferior wall MI ■ May also occur with anticholinesterase, beta blocker, digoxin, and morphine use	■ For low cardiac output, dizziness, weakness, altered level of consciousness, or low blood pressure: follow advanced cardiac life support (ACLS) protocol for administration of atropine ■ Temporary pacemaker; may need to be evaluated for permanent pacemaker at a later time

(continued)

TYPES OF CARDIAC ARRHYTHMIAS *(continued)*

Arrhythmia and features	Causes	Treatment
Sinoatrial (SA) arrest or block (sinus arrest) 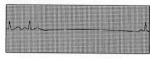 ■ Atrial and ventricular rhythms normal except for missing complex ■ Normal P wave preceding each QRS complex ■ Pause not equal to a multiple of the previous sinus rhythm	■ Acute infection ■ Coronary artery disease, degenerative heart disease, acute inferior wall MI ■ Vagal stimulation, Valsalva's maneuver, carotid sinus massage ■ Digoxin, quinidine, or salicylate toxicity ■ Pesticide poisoning ■ Pharyngeal irritation caused by endotracheal (ET) intubation ■ Sick sinus syndrome	■ Treat symptoms with atropine I.V. ■ Temporary pacemaker; consider permanent pacemaker for repeated episodes
Wandering atrial pacemaker 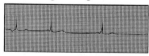 ■ Atrial and ventricular rhythms vary slightly ■ Irregular PR interval ■ P waves irregular with changing configuration, indicating that they aren't all from SA node or single atrial focus; may appear after the QRS complex ■ QRS complexes uniform in shape but irregular in rhythm	■ Rheumatic carditis due to inflammation involving the SA node ■ Digoxin toxicity ■ Sick sinus syndrome	■ No treatment if patient is asymptomatic ■ Treatment of underlying cause if patient is symptomatic
Premature atrial contraction (PAC) 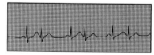 ■ Premature, abnormal-looking P waves that differ in configuration from normal P waves ■ QRS complexes after P waves, except in very early or blocked PACs ■ P wave often buried in the preceding T wave or identified in the preceding T wave	■ Coronary or valvular heart disease, atrial ischemia, coronary atherosclerosis, heart failure, acute respiratory failure, chronic obstructive pulmonary disease (COPD), electrolyte imbalance, and hypoxia ■ Digoxin toxicity; use of aminophylline, adrenergics, or caffeine ■ Anxiety	■ Usually no treatment is needed ■ Treatment of underlying cause if patient is symptomatic

TYPES OF CARDIAC ARRHYTHMIAS *(continued)*

Arrhythmia and features	Causes	Treatment

Paroxysmal supraventricular tachycardia

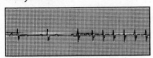

- Atrial and ventricular rhythms regular
- Heart rate > 160 beats/minute; rarely exceeds 250 beats/minute
- P waves regular but aberrant; difficult to differentiate from preceding T wave
- P wave preceding each QRS complex
- Sudden onset and termination of arrhythmia
- When a normal P wave is present, it's called *paroxysmal atrial tachycardia;* when a normal P wave isn't present, it's called *paroxysmal junctional tachycardia.*

Causes

- Intrinsic abnormality of atrioventricular (AV) conduction system
- Physical or psychological stress, hypoxia, hypokalemia, cardiomyopathy, congenital heart disease, MI, valvular disease, Wolff-Parkinson-White syndrome, cor pulmonale, hyperthyroidism, systemic hypertension
- Digoxin toxicity; use of caffeine, marijuana, or central nervous system stimulants

Treatment

- If patient is unstable, prepare for immediate cardioversion
- If patient is stable, vagal stimulation, Valsalva's maneuver, carotid sinus massage
- Adenosine by rapid I.V. bolus injection to rapidly convert arrhythmia
- If patient has a normal ejection fraction, consider calcium channel blockers, beta-adrenergic blockers, or amiodarone
- If patient has an ejection fraction less than 40%, consider amiodarone

Atrial flutter

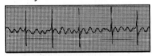

- Atrial rhythm regular; rate, 250 to 400 beats/minute
- Ventricular rate variable, depending on degree of AV block (usually 60 to 100 beats/minute)
- Sawtooth P wave configuration possible (F waves)
- QRS complexes uniform in shape but often irregular in rate

Causes

- Heart failure, tricuspid or mitral valve disease, pulmonary embolism, cor pulmonale, inferior wall MI, carditis
- Digoxin toxicity

Treatment

- If patient is unstable with a ventricular rate > 150 beats/minute, prepare for immediate cardioversion
- If patient is stable, drug therapy may include calcium channel blockers, beta-adrenergic blockers, or antiarrhythmics
- Anticoagulation therapy may be necessary

(continued)

TYPES OF CARDIAC ARRHYTHMIAS *(continued)*

Arrhythmia and features	Causes	Treatment
Atrial fibrillation 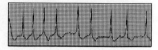 ▪ Atrial rhythm grossly irregular; rate > 400 beats/minute ▪ Ventricular rhythm grossly irregular ▪ QRS complexes of uniform configuration and duration ▪ PR interval indiscernible ▪ No P waves, or P waves that appear as erratic, irregular, baseline fibrillatory waves	▪ Heart failure, COPD, thyrotoxicosis, constrictive pericarditis, ischemic heart disease, sepsis, pulmonary embolus, rheumatic heart disease, hypertension, mitral stenosis, atrial irritation, complication of coronary bypass or valve replacement surgery	▪ If patient is unstable with a ventricular rate > 150 beats/minute, prepare for immediate cardioversion ▪ If patient is stable, drug therapy may include calcium channel blockers, beta-adrenergic blockers, digoxin, procainamide, quinidine, ibutilide, or amiodarone ▪ Consider anticoagulation to prevent emboli ▪ Dual chamber atrial pacing, implantable atrial pacemaker, or surgical maze procedure may also be used
Junctional rhythm 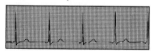 ▪ Atrial and ventricular rhythms regular ▪ Atrial rate 40 to 60 beats/minute ▪ Ventricular rate usually 40 to 60 beats/minute (60 to 100 beats/minute is accelerated junctional rhythm) ▪ P waves preceding, hidden within (absent), or after QRS complex; usually inverted if visible ▪ PR interval (when present) < 0.12 second ▪ QRS complex configuration and duration normal, except in aberrant conduction	▪ Inferior wall MI or ischemia, hypoxia, vagal stimulation, sick sinus syndrome ▪ Acute rheumatic fever ▪ Valve surgery ▪ Digoxin toxicity	▪ Correction of underlying cause ▪ Atropine for symptomatic slow rate ▪ Pacemaker insertion if patient is refractory to drugs ▪ Discontinuation of digoxin if appropriate

TYPES OF CARDIAC ARRHYTHMIAS *(continued)*

Arrhythmia and features	Causes	Treatment

Premature junctional contractions

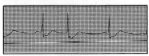

- MI or ischemia
- Digoxin toxicity and excessive caffeine or amphetamine use

- Correction of underlying cause
- Discontinuation of digoxin if appropriate

- Atrial and ventricular rhythms irregular
- P waves inverted; may precede, be hidden within, or follow QRS complex
- PR interval < 0.12 second if P wave precedes QRS complex
- QRS complex configuration and duration normal

Junctional tachycardia

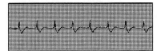

- Atrial rate > 100 beats/minute; however, P wave may be absent, hidden in QRS complex, or preceding T wave
- Ventricular rate > 100 beats/minute
- P wave inverted
- QRS complex configuration and duration normal
- Onset of rhythm often sudden, occurring in bursts

- Myocarditis, cardiomyopathy, inferior wall MI or ischemia, acute rheumatic fever, complication of valve replacement surgery
- Digoxin toxicity

- Cardioversion if ventricular rate is > 150 or if patient is symptomatic
- Amiodarone, beta-adrenergic blockers, or calcium channel blockers if patient is stable
- Discontinuation of digoxin if appropriate

First-degree AV block

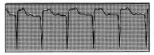

- Atrial and ventricular rhythms regular
- PR interval > 0.20 second
- P wave preceding each QRS complex
- QRS complex normal

- Inferior wall MI or ischemia or infarction, hypothyroidism, hypokalemia, hyperkalemia
- Digoxin toxicity; use of quinidine, procainamide, beta-adrenergic blockers, calcium channel blockers, or amiodarone

- Correction of underlying cause
- Possibly atropine if PR interval exceeds 0.26 second or symptomatic bradycardia develops
- Cautious use of digoxin, calcium channel blockers, and beta-adrenergic blockers

(continued)

TYPES OF CARDIAC ARRHYTHMIAS *(continued)*

Arrhythmia and features	Causes	Treatment

Second-degree AV block
Mobitz I (Wenckebach)

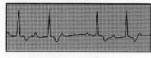

- Atrial rhythm regular
- Ventricular rhythm irregular
- Atrial rate exceeds ventricular rate
- PR interval progressively, but only slightly, longer with each cycle until QRS complex disappears (dropped beat); PR interval shorter after dropped beat

- Inferior wall MI, cardiac surgery, acute rheumatic fever, and vagal stimulation
- Digoxin toxicity; use of propranolol, quinidine, or procainamide

- Treatment of underlying cause
- Atropine or temporary pacemaker for symptomatic bradycardia
- Discontinuation of digoxin if appropriate

Second-degree AV block
Mobitz II

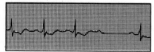

- Atrial rhythm regular
- Ventricular rhythm regular or irregular, with varying degree of block
- P-P interval constant
- QRS complexes periodically absent

- Severe coronary artery disease, anterior wall MI, acute myocarditis
- Digoxin toxicity

- Atropine, epinephrine, and dopamine for symptomatic bradycardia
- Temporary or permanent pacemaker for symptomatic bradycardia
- Discontinuation of digoxin if appropriate

Third-degree AV block
(complete heart block)

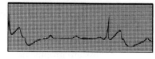

- Atrial rhythm regular
- Ventricular rhythm regular and rate slower than atrial rate
- No relation between P waves and QRS complexes
- No constant PR interval
- QRS interval normal (nodal pacemaker) or wide and bizarre (ventricular pacemaker)

- Inferior or anterior wall MI, congenital abnormality, rheumatic fever, hypoxia, postoperative complication of mitral valve replacement, Lev's disease (fibrosis and calcification that spreads from cardiac structures to the conductive tissue), Lenegre's disease (conductive tissue fibrosis)
- Digoxin toxicity

- Atropine, epinephrine, and dopamine for symptomatic bradycardia
- Temporary or permanent pacemaker for symptomatic bradycardia

TYPES OF CARDIAC ARRHYTHMIAS *(continued)*

Arrhythmia and features	Causes	Treatment

Premature ventricular contraction (PVC)

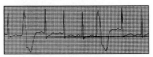

- Atrial rhythm regular
- Ventricular rhythm irregular
- QRS complex premature, usually followed by a complete compensatory pause
- QRS complex wide and distorted, usually > 0.14 second
- Premature QRS complexes occurring singly, in pairs, or in threes; alternating with normal beats; focus from one or more sites
- Ominous when clustered, multifocal, with R wave on T pattern

- Heart failure; old or acute myocardial ischemia, infarction, or contusion; myocardial irritation by ventricular catheter such as a pacemaker; hypercapnia; hypokalemia, hypocalcemia
- Drug toxicity (cardiac glycosides, aminophylline, tricyclic antidepressants, beta-adrenergics [bisoproterenol or dopamine])
- Caffeine, tobacco, or alcohol use
- Psychological stress, anxiety, pain, exercise

- If warranted, procainamide, lidocaine, or amiodarone I.V.
- Treatment of underlying cause
- Discontinuation of drug causing toxicity
- Potassium chloride I.V. if PVC induced by hypokalemia
- Magnesium sulfate I.V. if PVC induced by hypomagnesemia

Ventricular tachycardia (VT)

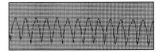

- Ventricular rate 140 to 220 beats/minute, regular or irregular
- QRS complexes wide, bizarre, and independent of P waves
- P waves not discernible
- May start and stop suddenly

- Myocardial ischemia, infarction, or aneurysm; coronary artery disease; rheumatic heart disease; mitral valve prolapse; heart failure; cardiomyopathy; ventricular catheters; hypokalemia; hypercalcemia; pulmonary embolism
- Digoxin, procainamide, epinephrine, or quinidine toxicity
- Anxiety

- Pulseless: Initiate cardiopulmonary resuscitation (CPR); follow ACLS protocol for defibrillation, ET intubation, and administration of epinephrine or vasopressin, followed by amiodarone or lidocaine; if ineffective, magnesium sulfate or procainamide
- With pulse: If hemodynamically stable monomorphic VT, follow ACLS protocol for administration of procainamide, sotalol, amiodarone, or lidocaine; if drugs are ineffective, initiate synchronized cardioversion
- If polymorphic VT, follow ACLS protocol for administration of beta-adrenergic blockers, lidocaine, amiodarone, procainamide, or sotalol; if drugs are ineffective, initiate cardioversion,

(continued)

TYPES OF CARDIAC ARRHYTHMIAS *(continued)*

Arrhythmia and features	Causes	Treatment
Ventricular fibrillation 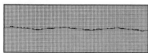 ■ Ventricular rhythm and rate rapid and chaotic ■ QRS complexes wide and irregular; no visible P waves	■ Myocardial ischemia or infarction, R-on-T phenomenon, untreated ventricular tachycardia, hypokalemia, hyperkalemia, hypercalcemia, alkalosis, electric shock, hypothermia ■ Digoxin, epinephrine, or quinidine toxicity	■ Pulseless: Initiate CPR; follow ACLS protocol for defibrillation, ET intubation, and administration of epinephrine or vasopressin, lidocaine, or amiodarone; if ineffective, magnesium sulfate or procainamide
Asystole ■ No atrial or ventricular rate or rhythm ■ No discernible P waves, QRS complexes, or T waves	■ Myocardial ischemia or infarction, aortic valve disease, heart failure, hypoxemia, hypokalemia, severe acidosis, electric shock, ventricular arrhythmias, AV block, pulmonary embolism, heart rupture, cardiac tamponade, hyperkalemia, electromechanical dissociation ■ Cocaine overdose	■ Continue CPR; follow ACLS protocol for ET intubation, transcutaneous pacing, administration of epinephrine, and atropine

er. Although hazards may not present a problem, in doubtful situations, 24-hour Holter monitoring may be helpful. Tell the patient to report light-headedness or syncope and stress the importance of regular checkups.
■ Compare the patient's cardiac status (pulse, blood pressure, and cardiac output) with the cardiac rhythm before and after treatments.

VASCULAR DISORDERS

Thoracic aortic aneurysm

Thoracic aortic aneurysm is an abnormal widening of the ascending, transverse, or descending part of the aorta. Aneurysm of the ascending aorta is the most common type and has the highest mortality. Aneurysms may be *dissecting,* a hemorrhagic separation in the aortic wall, usually within the medial layer; *saccular,* an outpouching of the arterial wall, with a narrow neck; or *fusiform,* a spindle-shaped enlargement encompassing the entire aortic circumference. (See *Types of aortic aneurysms.*) Some aneurysms progress to serious and, eventually, lethal complications, such as rupture of an untreated thoracic dissecting aneurysm into the pericardium, with resulting tamponade.

Causes and incidence
Thoracic aortic aneurysms commonly result from atherosclerosis, which weakens the aortic wall and gradually distends the lumen. An intimal tear in the ascending aorta initiates dissecting aneurysm in about 60% of the patients. Regardless of causation, these aneurysms affect 6 out of every 100,000 people.

TYPES OF AORTIC ANEURYSMS

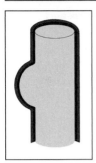 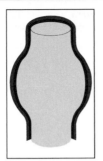 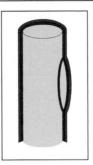 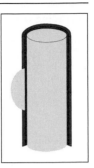

Saccular
Unilateral pouch-like bulge with a narrow neck

Fusiform
A spindle-shaped bulge encompassing the vessel's entire diameter

Dissecting
A hemorrhagic separation of the medial layer of the vessel wall, which creates a false lumen

False aneurysm
A pulsating hematoma resulting from trauma and often mistaken for an abdominal aneurysm

 ELDER TIP *Ascending aortic aneurysms, the most common type, are usually seen in hypertensive men younger than age 60. Descending aortic aneurysms, usually found just below the origin of the subclavian artery, are most common in elderly men who are hypertensive.*

Descending aortic aneurysms are also seen in younger patients with a history of traumatic chest injury; less often in those with infection. Transverse aortic aneurysms are the least common type.

Other causes include:
■ fungal infection (mycotic aneurysms) of the aortic arch and descending segments
■ congenital disorders, such as coarctation of the aorta and Marfan syndrome
■ trauma, usually of the descending thoracic aorta, from an accident that shears the aorta transversely (acceleration-deceleration injuries)
■ syphilis, usually of the ascending aorta (uncommon because of antibiotics)
■ hypertension (in dissecting aneurysm).

Signs and symptoms
The most common symptom of thoracic aortic aneurysm is pain. With ascending aneurysm, the pain is described as severe, boring, and ripping and extends to the neck, shoulders, lower back, or abdomen but seldom radiates to the jaw and arms. Pain is more severe on the right side.

Other signs of ascending aneurysm may include bradycardia, aortic insufficiency, pericardial friction rub caused by a hemopericardium, unequal intensities of the right carotid and left radial pulses, and a difference in blood pressure between the right and left arms. These signs are absent in descending aneurysm. If dissection involves the carotids, an abrupt onset of neurologic deficits may occur.

With descending aneurysm, pain usually starts suddenly between the shoulder blades and may radiate to the chest; it's described as sharp and tearing. Transverse aneurysm causes a sudden, sharp, tearing pain radiating to the shoulders. It may also cause hoarseness, dyspnea, dysphagia, and a dry cough because of compression of surrounding structures in this area. (See *Clinical characteristics of thoracic dissection*, page 1136.)

Diagnosis
Diagnosis relies on patient history, clinical features, and appropriate tests. In an

CLINICAL CHARACTERISTICS OF THORACIC DISSECTION

Ascending aorta	Descending aorta	Transverse aorta
Character of pain		
Severe, boring, ripping, extending to neck, shoulders, lower back, or abdomen (rarely to jaw and arms); more severe on right side	Sudden onset, sharp, tearing, usually between the shoulder blades; may radiate to the chest; most diagnostic feature	Sudden onset, sharp, boring, tearing, radiates to shoulders
Other symptoms and effects		
If dissection involves carotids, abrupt onset of neurologic deficit (usually intermittent); bradycardia, aortic insufficiency, and hemopericardium detected by pericardial friction rub; unequal intensity of right and left carotid pulses and radial pulses; difference in blood pressure, especially systolic, between right and left arms	Aortic insufficiency without murmur, hemopericardium, or pleural friction rub; carotid and radial pulses and blood pressure in both arms tend to stay equal	Hoarseness, dyspnea, pain, dysphagia, and dry cough resulting from compression of surrounding structures
Diagnostic features		
Chest X-ray		
Best diagnostic tool; shows widening of mediastinum, enlargement of ascending aorta	Shows widening of mediastinum, descending aorta larger than ascending	Shows widening of mediastinum, descending aorta larger than ascending, widened transverse arch
Aortography		
Shows false lumen; narrowing of lumen of aorta in ascending section	Shows false lumen; narrowing of lumen of aorta in descending section	Shows false lumen, narrowing of lumen of aorta in transverse arch
Treatment		
This is a medical emergency requiring immediate, aggressive treatment to reduce blood pressure (usually with nitroprusside or trimethaphan). Surgical repair is also required.	Surgical repair is required but less urgent than for the ascending dissection. Nitroprusside and propranolol may be used to control hypertension if bradycardia and heart failure are absent.	Immediate surgical repair (mortality as high as 50%) and control of hypertension are required.

asymptomatic patient, diagnosis often occurs accidentally when chest X-rays show widening of the aorta. Other tests help confirm aneurysm:

■ Aortography, the most definitive test, shows the lumen of the aneurysm, its size and location, and the false lumen in dissecting aneurysm.

■ Electrocardiography (ECG) helps distinguish thoracic aneurysm from myocardial infarction.

■ Echocardiography may help identify dissecting aneurysm of the aortic root.

■ Hemoglobin levels may be normal or low, due to blood loss from a leaking aneurysm.

■ Computed tomography scan can confirm and locate the aneurysm and may be used to monitor its progression.

■ Magnetic resonance imaging may aid diagnosis.

■ Transesophageal echocardiography is used to diagnose and size an aneurysm in either the ascending or the descending aorta.

Treatment

Dissecting aortic aneurysm is an emergency that requires prompt surgery and stabilizing measures: antihypertensives such as nitroprusside; negative inotropic agents that decrease contractility force such as propranolol; oxygen for respiratory distress; opioids for pain; I.V. fluids and, possibly, whole blood transfusions.

Surgery consists of resecting the aneurysm, restoring normal blood flow through a Dacron or Teflon graft replacement and, with aortic valve insufficiency, replacing the aortic valve. Groin catheter placement may be used for aortic stenting. This procedure, which may be used for aneurysms of the descending aorta, eliminates the need for a chest incision.

Postoperative measures include careful monitoring and continuous assessment in the intensive care unit, antibiotics, endotracheal (ET) and chest tubes, ECG monitoring, and pulmonary artery catheterization.

Long-term management includes treatment of underlying conditions, such as heart disease and diabetes.

Special considerations

■ Monitor blood pressure, pulmonary artery wedge pressure (PAWP), and central venous pressure (CVP). Assess pain, breathing, and carotid, radial, and femoral pulses.

■ Make sure laboratory tests include complete blood count, differential, electrolyte levels, type and crossmatching for whole blood, arterial blood gas studies, and urinalysis.

■ Insert an indwelling urinary catheter. Administer dextrose 5% in water or lactated Ringer's solution, and antibiotics, as ordered. Carefully monitor nitroprusside I.V.; use a separate I.V. line for infusion. Adjust the dose by slowly increasing the infusion rate. Meanwhile, check blood pressure every 5 minutes until it stabilizes. With suspected bleeding from aneurysm, give whole blood transfusion.

■ Explain diagnostic tests. If surgery is scheduled, explain the procedure and expected postoperative care (I.V. lines, ET and drainage tubes, cardiac monitoring, and ventilation).

After repair of thoracic aneurysm:

■ Assess level of consciousness. Monitor vital signs; pulmonary artery pressure, PAWP, and CVP; pulse rate; urine output; and pain.

■ Check respiratory function. Carefully observe and record type and amount of chest-tube drainage, and frequently assess heart and breath sounds.

■ Monitor I.V. therapy.

■ Give medications as appropriate.

■ Watch for signs of infection, especially fever, and excessive wound drainage.

■ Assist with range-of-motion exercises of legs to prevent thromboembolic phenomenon due to venostasis during prolonged bed rest.

■ After stabilization of vital signs and respiration, encourage and assist the patient in turning, coughing, and deep breathing. If necessary, provide intermittent positive-pressure breathing to promote lung expansion. Help the patient walk as soon as he's able.

■ Before discharge, ensure compliance with antihypertensive therapy by explaining the need for such drugs and the expected adverse effects. Teach the patient how to monitor his blood pressure. Refer him to community agencies for continued support and assistance, as needed.

■ Throughout hospitalization, offer the patient and his family psychological support. Answer all of their questions honestly and provide reassurance.

Abdominal aneurysm

Abdominal aneurysm, an abnormal dilation in the arterial wall, generally occurs in the aorta between the renal arteries and iliac branches. Rupture — in which the aneurysm breaks open, resulting in profuse bleeding — is a common complication that occurs in larger aneurysms. Dissection occurs when the artery's lining tears, and blood leaks into the walls.

Causes and incidence
Abdominal aortic aneurysms result from arteriosclerosis, hypertension, congenital weakening, cystic medial necrosis, trauma, syphilis, and other infections. In children, this disorder can result from blunt abdominal injury or Marfan syndrome. These aneurysms develop slowly. First, a focal weakness in the muscular layer of the aorta (tunica media), due to degenerative changes, allows the inner layer (tunica intima) and outer layer (tunica adventitia) to stretch outward. Blood pressure within the aorta progressively weakens the vessel walls and enlarges the aneurysm.

This disorder is four times more common in men than in women and is most prevalent in whites ages 40 to 70. Less than 50% of people with a ruptured abdominal aortic aneurysm survive.

Signs and symptoms
Although abdominal aneurysms usually don't produce symptoms, most are evident (unless the patient is obese) as a pulsating mass in the periumbilical area, accompanied by a systolic bruit over the aorta. Some tenderness may be present on deep palpation. A large aneurysm may produce symptoms that mimic renal calculi, lumbar disk disease, and duodenal compression. Abdominal aneurysms rarely cause diminished peripheral pulses or claudication, unless embolization occurs.

Lumbar pain that radiates to the flank and groin from pressure on lumbar nerves may signify enlargement and imminent rupture. If the aneurysm ruptures into the peritoneal cavity, it causes severe, persistent abdominal and back pain, mimicking renal or ureteral colic. Signs of hemorrhage — such as weakness, sweating, tachycardia, and hypotension — may be subtle because rupture into the retroperitoneal space produces a tamponade effect that prevents continued hemorrhage. Patients with such rupture may remain stable for hours before shock and death occur, although 20% die immediately.

Diagnosis
Because abdominal aneurysms seldom produce symptoms, they're commonly detected accidentally as the result of an X-ray or a routine physical examination.

CONFIRMING DIAGNOSIS
Several tests can confirm a suspected abdominal aneurysm. Serial ultrasound (sonography) *can accurately determine the aneurysm's size, shape, and location. Anteroposterior and lateral X-rays of the abdomen can detect aortic calcification, which outlines the mass, at least 75% of the time. Aortography shows the condition of vessels proximal and distal to the aneurysm and the aneurysm's extent but may underestimate aneurysm diameter because it visualizes only the flow channel and not the surrounding clot. Computed tomography scan is used to diagnose and size the aneurysm. Magnetic resonance imaging can be used as an alternative to aortography.*

Treatment
Usually, abdominal aneurysm requires resection of the aneurysm and replacement of the damaged aortic section with a Dacron graft. (See *Abdominal aneurysms: Before and after surgery.* Also see *Endovascular grafting for repair of an abdominal aortic aneurysm,* page 1140.) If the aneurysm is small and asymptomatic, surgery may be delayed and the aneurysm may be followed and allowed to expand to a certain size because of possible surgical complications; however, small aneurysms may

ABDOMINAL ANEURYSMS: BEFORE AND AFTER SURGERY

During surgery, a prosthetic graft replaces or encloses the weakened area.

Before surgery

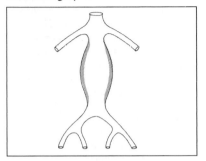

Aneurysm below renal arteries and above bifurcation

After surgery

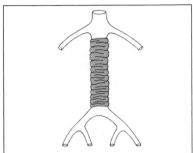

The prosthesis extends distal to the renal arteries to above the aortic bifurcation.

Before surgery

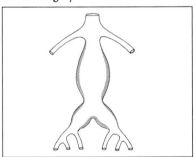

Aneurysm below renal arteries involving the iliac branches

After surgery

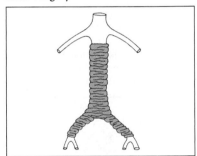

The prosthesis extends to the common femoral arteries.

Before surgery

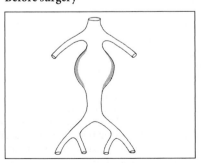

Small aneurysm in a patient with poor distal runoff (poor risk)

After surgery

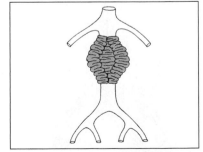

The external prosthesis encircles the aneurysm and is held in place with sutures.

ENDOVASCULAR GRAFTING FOR REPAIR OF AN ABDOMINAL AORTIC ANEURYSM

Endovascular grafting is a minimally invasive procedure for the repair of an abdominal aortic aneurysm. This procedure reinforces the walls of the aorta to prevent rupture and prevent expansion of the aneurysm.

Endovascular grafting is performed with fluoroscopic guidance: Using a guide wire, a delivery catheter with an attached compressed graft is inserted through a small incision into the femoral or iliac artery. The delivery catheter is advanced into the aorta, where it's positioned across the aneurysm. A balloon on the catheter expands the graft and affixes it to the vessel wall.

The procedure generally takes 2 to 3 hours to perform. Patients are instructed to walk the first day after surgery and are generally discharged from the facility in 1 to 3 days.

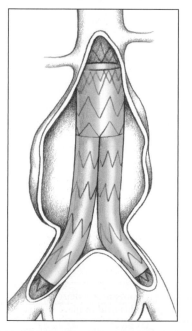

also rupture. Because of this risk, surgical repair or replacement is recommended for symptomatic patients or for patients with aneurysms greater than 5 cm in diameter.

Stenting is also a treatment option. It can be performed without an abdominal incision by introducing the catheters through arteries in the groin. However, not all patients with abdominal aortic aneurysms are candidates for this treatment.

Regular physical examination and ultrasound checks are necessary to detect enlargement, which may forewarn rupture. Large aneurysms or those that produce symptoms pose a significant risk of rupture and necessitate immediate repair. In patients with poor distal runoff, external grafting may be done.

Risk factor modification is fundamental in the medical management of abdominal aneurysm, including control of hypocholesterolemia and hypertension. Beta-adrenergic blockers are commonly prescribed to reduce the risk of aneurysm expansion and rupture.

Special considerations
Abdominal aneurysm requires meticulous preoperative and postoperative care, psychological support, and comprehensive patient teaching. Following diagnosis, if rupture isn't imminent, elective surgery allows time for additional preoperative tests to evaluate the patient's clinical status.

■ Monitor vital signs, and type and cross-match blood.

■ Use only gentle abdominal palpation.

■ As ordered, obtain renal function tests (blood urea nitrogen, creatinine, and electrolyte levels), blood samples (complete blood count with differential), electrocardiogram and cardiac evaluation, baseline pulmonary function tests, and arterial blood gas (ABG) analysis.

■ Be alert for signs of rupture, which may be immediately fatal. Watch closely for signs of acute blood loss (decreasing blood pressure; increasing pulse and respiratory rate; cool, clammy skin; restlessness; and decreased sensorium).

■ If rupture does occur, the first priority is to get the patient to surgery immediately. A pneumatic antishock garment may be used while transporting him to surgery. Surgery allows direct compression of the aorta to control hemorrhage. Large amounts of blood may be needed during the resuscitative period to replace blood loss. In such a patient, renal failure caused by ischemia is a major postoperative complication, possibly requiring hemodialysis.

■ Before elective surgery, weigh the patient, insert an indwelling urinary catheter and an I.V. line, and assist with insertion of an arterial line and pulmonary artery catheter to monitor fluid and hemodynamic balance. Give prophylactic antibiotics as ordered.

■ Explain the surgical procedure and the expected postoperative care in the intensive care unit (ICU) for patients undergoing complex abdominal surgery (I.V. lines, endotracheal [ET] and nasogastric [NG] intubation, and mechanical ventilation).

■ After surgery, in the ICU, closely monitor vital signs, intake and hourly output, neurologic status (level of consciousness, pupil size, and sensation in arms and legs), and ABG values. Assess the depth, rate, and character of respirations and breath sounds at least every hour.

■ Watch for signs of bleeding (increased pulse and respiratory rates and hypotension) and back pain, which may indicate the graft is tearing. Check abdominal dressings for excessive bleeding or drainage. Be alert for temperature elevations and other signs of infection. After NG intubation for intestinal decompression, irrigate the tube frequently to ensure patency. Record the amount and type of drainage.

■ Suction the ET tube often. If the patient can breathe unassisted and has good breath sounds and adequate ABG values, tidal volume, and vital capacity 24 hours after surgery, he will be extubated and will require oxygen by mask.

■ Weigh the patient daily to evaluate fluid balance.

■ Help the patient walk as soon as he's able (generally the second day after surgery).

■ Provide psychological support for the patient and his family. Help ease their fears about the ICU, the threat of impending rupture, and surgery by providing appropriate explanations and answering all questions.

Femoral and popliteal aneurysms

Femoral and popliteal aneurysms (sometimes called *peripheral arterial aneurysms*) are the end result of progressive atherosclerotic changes occurring in the walls (medial layer) of these major peripheral arteries. These aneurysmal formations may be *fusiform* (spindle-shaped) or *saccular* (pouchlike); the fusiform type is three times more common. They may be singular or multiple segmental lesions, often affecting both legs, and may accompany other arterial aneurysms located in the abdominal aorta or iliac arteries. (See *Arteries of the leg,* page 1142.)

This condition occurs most frequently in men older than age 50. The clinical course is usually progressive, eventually ending in thrombosis, embolization, and gangrene. Elective surgery before complications arise greatly improves the prognosis.

Causes

Femoral and popliteal aneurysms are usually secondary to atherosclerosis. Rarely, they result from congenital weakness in the arterial wall. They may also result from trauma (blunt or penetrating), bacterial infection, or peripheral vascular reconstructive surgery (which causes "suture line" aneurysms, or false aneurysms, in which a blood clot forms a second lumen).

Signs and symptoms

Popliteal aneurysms may cause pain in the popliteal space when they're large enough to compress the medial popliteal nerve and edema and venous distention if the vein is compressed. Femoral and popliteal aneurysms can produce symptoms of severe ischemia in the leg or foot due to acute thrombosis within the aneurysmal sac, embolization of mural thrombus fragments and, rarely, rupture. Symptoms of acute aneurysmal thrombosis include severe pain, loss of pulse and color, coldness in the affected leg or foot, and gangrene. Distal petechial hemorrhages may develop from aneurysmal emboli.

ARTERIES OF THE LEG

FRONT VIEW

BACK VIEW

Abdominal aorta

Common iliac artery

Internal iliac artery

External iliac artery

Deep femoral artery

Superficial femoral artery

Popliteal artery

Anterior tibial artery

Dorsalis pedis

Deep femoral artery

Superficial femoral artery

Popliteal artery

Posterior tibial artery

Medial plantar artery

Lateral plantar artery

Diagnosis

Diagnosis is usually confirmed by bilateral palpation that reveals a pulsating mass above or below the inguinal ligament in femoral aneurysm. When thrombosis has occurred, palpation detects a firm, nonpulsating mass. Arteriography or ultrasound may be indicated in doubtful situations. Arteriography may also detect associated aneurysms, especially those in the abdominal aorta and the iliac arteries. Ultrasound may be helpful in determining the size of the popliteal or femoral artery.

Treatment

Femoral and popliteal aneurysms require surgical bypass and reconstruction of the artery, usually with an autogenous saphenous vein graft replacement. Arterial occlusion that causes severe ischemia and gangrene may require leg amputation.

Special considerations

Before corrective surgery:
- Assess and record circulatory status, noting the location and quality of peripheral pulses in the affected arm or leg.
- Administer prophylactic antibiotics or anticoagulants, as ordered.
- Discuss expected postoperative procedures and review the explanation of the surgery.

After arterial surgery:
- Monitor carefully for early signs of thrombosis or graft occlusion (loss of pulse, decreased skin temperature and sensation, and severe pain) and infection (fever).
- Palpate distal pulses at least every hour for the first 24 hours and then as frequently as ordered. Correlate these findings with preoperative circulatory assessment. Mark the sites on the patient's skin where pulses are palpable to facilitate repeated checks.
- Help the patient walk soon after surgery to prevent venostasis and possible thrombus formation.

To prepare the patient for discharge:
- Tell the patient to immediately report any recurrence of symptoms because the saphenous vein graft replacement can fail or another aneurysm may develop.
- Explain to the patient with popliteal artery resection that swelling may persist for some time. If antiembolism stockings are ordered, make sure they fit properly and teach the patient how to apply them. Warn against wearing constrictive apparel.
- If the patient is receiving anticoagulants, suggest measures to prevent bleeding such as using an electric razor. Tell him to report any signs of bleeding immediately (bleeding gums, tarry stools, and easy bruising). Explain the importance of follow-up blood studies to monitor anticoagulant therapy. Warn him to avoid trauma, tobacco, and aspirin.

Thrombophlebitis

An acute condition characterized by inflammation and thrombus formation, thrombophlebitis may occur in deep (intermuscular or intramuscular) or superficial (subcutaneous) veins. Deep vein thrombosis (DVT) or thrombophlebitis affects small veins, such as the soleal venous sinuses, or large veins, such as the vena cava and the femoral, iliac, and subclavian veins, causing venous insufficiency. (See *Chronic venous insufficiency,* page 1144.) This disorder is typically progressive, leading to pulmonary embolism, a potentially lethal complication. Superficial thrombophlebitis is usually self-limiting and seldom leads to pulmonary embolism. Thrombophlebitis often begins with localized inflammation alone (phlebitis), but such inflammation rapidly provokes thrombus formation. Rarely, venous thrombosis develops without associated inflammation of the vein (phlebothrombosis).

Causes and incidence

A thrombus occurs when an alteration in the epithelial lining causes platelet aggregation and consequent fibrin entrapment of red and white blood cells and additional platelets. Thrombus formation is more rapid in areas where blood flow is slower, due to greater contact between platelet and thrombin accumulation. The rapidly expanding thrombus initiates a chemical inflammatory process in the vessel epithelium, which leads to fibrosis. The enlarging clot may occlude the vessel lumen partially

CHRONIC VENOUS INSUFFICIENCY

Chronic venous insufficiency results from the valvular destruction of deep vein thrombophlebitis, usually in the iliac and femoral veins, and occasionally the saphenous veins. It's often accompanied by incompetence of the communicating veins at the ankle, causing increased venous pressure and fluid migration into the interstitial tissue. Clinical effects include chronic swelling of the affected leg from edema, leading to tissue fibrosis, and induration; skin discoloration from extravasation of blood in subcutaneous tissue; and stasis ulcers around the ankle.

Treatment of small ulcers includes bed rest, elevation of the legs, warm soaks, and antimicrobial therapy for infection. Treatment to counteract increased venous pressure, the result of reflux from the deep venous system to surface veins, may include compression dressings, such as a sponge rubber pressure dressing or a zinc gelatin boot (Unna's boot). This therapy begins after massive swelling subsides with leg elevation and bed rest.

Large stasis ulcers unresponsive to conservative treatment may require excision and skin grafting. Patient care includes daily inspection to assess healing. Other care measures are the same as for varicose veins.

or totally, or it may detach and embolize to lodge elsewhere in the systemic circulation.

DVT may be idiopathic, but it usually results from endothelial damage, accelerated blood clotting, and reduced blood flow. Predisposing factors are prolonged bed rest, trauma, surgery, childbirth, and use of hormonal contraceptives such as estrogens. It occurs in about 80 of every 100,000 people; 1 of every 20 persons is affected at some point during his lifetime. Males are at slightly greater risk than females. People older than age 40 are also at increased risk.

Causes of superficial thrombophlebitis include trauma, infection, I.V. drug abuse, and chemical irritation due to extensive use of the I.V. route for medications and diagnostic tests.

Signs and symptoms

In both types of thrombophlebitis, clinical features vary with the site and length of the affected vein. Although DVT may occur asymptomatically, it may also produce severe pain, fever, chills, malaise and, possibly, swelling and cyanosis of the affected arm or leg. Superficial thrombophlebitis produces visible and palpable signs, such as heat, pain, swelling, rubor, tenderness, and induration along the length of the affected vein. Varicose veins may also be present. (See *Varicose veins.*) Extensive vein involvement may cause lymphadenitis.

Diagnosis

Some patients may display signs of inflammation and, possibly, a positive Homans' sign (pain on dorsiflexion of the foot) during physical examination; others are asymptomatic. Essential laboratory tests include:

- Duplex Doppler ultrasonography and impedance plethysmography make it possible to noninvasively examine the major veins (but not calf veins).
- Plethysmography shows decreased circulation distal to the affected area; this test is more sensitive than ultrasound in detecting DVT.

 CONFIRMING DIAGNOSIS
Phlebography, which shows filling defects and diverted blood flow, usually confirms the diagnosis.

Diagnosis must also rule out arterial occlusive disease, lymphangitis, cellulitis, and myositis.

Diagnosis of superficial thrombophlebitis is based on physical examination (redness and warmth over the affected area, palpable vein, and pain during palpation or compression).

Treatment

The goals of treatment are to control thrombus development, prevent complica-

VARICOSE VEINS

Varicose veins are dilated, tortuous veins, usually affecting the subcutaneous leg veins — the saphenous veins and their branches. They can result from congenital weakness of the valves or venous wall, diseases of the venous system such as deep vein thrombophlebitis, conditions that produce prolonged venostasis such as pregnancy, or occupations that necessitate standing for an extended period.

Varicose veins may be asymptomatic or produce mild to severe leg symptoms, including a feeling of heaviness; cramps at night; diffuse, dull aching after prolonged standing or walking; aching during menses; fatigability; palpable nodules and, with deep-vein incompetency, orthostatic edema and stasis pigmentation of the calves and ankles.

Treatment

In mild to moderate varicose veins, antiembolism stockings or elastic bandages counteract pedal and ankle swelling by supporting the veins and improving circulation. An exercise program such as walking promotes muscular contraction and forces blood through the veins, thereby minimizing venous pooling. Severe varicose veins may necessitate stripping and ligation or, as an alternative to surgery, injection of a sclerosing agent into small affected vein segments.

To promote comfort and minimize worsening of varicosities:
■ Discourage the patient from wearing constrictive clothing.
■ Advise the patient to elevate his legs above heart level whenever possible and to avoid prolonged standing or sitting.

After stripping and ligation or after injection of a sclerosing agent:
■ To relieve pain, administer analgesics as ordered.
■ Frequently check circulation in toes (color and temperature) and observe elastic bandages for bleeding. When ordered, rewrap bandages at least once a shift, wrapping from toe to thigh, with the leg elevated.
■ Watch for signs of complications, such as sensory loss in the leg (which could indicate saphenous nerve damage), calf pain (thrombophlebitis), and fever (infection).

---

tions, relieve pain, and prevent recurrence of the disorder. Symptomatic measures include bed rest, with elevation of the affected arm or leg; warm, moist soaks to the affected area; and analgesics. After the acute episode of DVT subsides, the patient may resume activity while wearing antiembolism stockings that were applied before he got out of bed.

Treatment also includes anticoagulants (initially, heparin; later, warfarin) to prolong clotting time. Low-molecular-weight (LMW) heparin has been shown to be effective in treating DVT. Although LMW heparin is more expensive, it doesn't require monitoring for its anticoagulant effect. Full anticoagulant doses must be discontinued during any operative period because of the risk of hemorrhage. After some types of surgery, especially major abdominal or pelvic operations, prophylactic doses of anticoagulants may reduce the risk of DVT and pulmonary embolism. For lysis of acute, extensive DVT, treatment should include streptokinase. Rarely, DVT may cause complete venous occlusion, which necessitates venous interruption through simple ligation to vein plication, or clipping. Embolectomy and insertion of a vena caval umbrella or filter may also be done.

Therapy for severe superficial thrombophlebitis may include an anti-inflammatory drug such as indomethacin, antiembolism stockings, warm soaks, and elevation of the leg.

Special considerations

Patient teaching, identification of high-risk patients, and measures to prevent venostasis can prevent DVT; close monitoring of anticoagulant therapy can prevent serious complications such as internal hemorrhage.

■ Enforce bed rest as ordered, and elevate the patient's affected arm or leg. If you plan to use pillows for elevating the leg, place them so they support the entire length of the affected extremity to prevent possible compression of the popliteal space.

■ Apply warm soaks to increase circulation to the affected area and to relieve pain and inflammation. Give analgesics to relieve pain, as ordered.

■ Measure and record the affected arm or leg's circumference daily and compare this measurement to the other arm or leg. To ensure accuracy and consistency of serial measurements, mark the skin over the area and measure at the same spot daily.

■ Administer heparin I.V., as ordered, with an infusion monitor or pump to control the flow rate if necessary.

■ Measure partial thromboplastin time regularly for the patient on heparin therapy; prothrombin time and international normalized ratio (INR) for the patient on warfarin (therapeutic anticoagulation values are 1½ to 2 times control values for prothrombin time and an INR of 2 to 3). Watch for signs and symptoms of bleeding, such as dark, tarry stools; coffee-ground vomitus; and ecchymoses. Encourage the patient to use an electric razor and to avoid medications that contain aspirin.

■ Be alert for signs of pulmonary emboli (crackles, dyspnea, hemoptysis, sudden changes in mental status, restlessness, and hypotension).

To prepare the patient with thrombophlebitis for discharge:

■ Emphasize the importance of follow-up blood studies to monitor anticoagulant therapy.

■ If the patient is being discharged on heparin therapy, teach him or his family how to give subcutaneous injections. If he requires further assistance, arrange for a home health nurse.

■ Tell the patient to avoid prolonged sitting or standing to help prevent recurrence.

■ Teach the patient how to properly apply and use antiembolism stockings. Tell him to report any complications such as cold, blue toes.

■ To prevent thrombophlebitis in high-risk patients, perform range-of-motion exercises while the patient is on bed rest, use intermittent pneumatic calf massage during lengthy surgical or diagnostic procedures, apply antiembolism stockings postoperatively, and encourage early ambulation.

Raynaud's disease

Raynaud's disease is one of several primary arteriospastic disorders characterized by episodic vasospasm in the small peripheral arteries and arterioles, precipitated by exposure to cold or stress. This condition occurs bilaterally and usually affects the hands or, less often, the feet. Raynaud's disease is most prevalent in females, particularly those between puberty and age 40. It's a benign condition, requiring no specific treatment and causing no serious sequelae.

Raynaud's phenomenon, however, a condition commonly associated with several connective tissue disorders—such as scleroderma, systemic lupus erythematosus (SLE), or polymyositis—has a progressive course, leading to ischemia, gangrene, and amputation. Distinguishing between the two disorders is difficult because some patients who experience mild symptoms of Raynaud's disease for several years may later develop overt connective tissue disease—especially scleroderma.

Causes and incidence

Although the cause is unknown, several theories account for the reduced digital blood flow: intrinsic vascular wall hyperactivity to cold, increased vasomotor tone due to sympathetic stimulation, and antigen-antibody immune response (the most likely theory because abnormal immunologic test results accompany Raynaud's phenomenon). Risk factors include associated diseases (Buerger's disease, atherosclerosis, rheumatoid arthritis, scleroderma, and SLE) and smoking. This disorder affects females more often than males.

Signs and symptoms

After exposure to cold or stress, the skin on the fingers typically blanches and then becomes cyanotic before changing to red and before changing from cold to normal temperature. Numbness and tingling may also occur. These symptoms are relieved by warmth. In long-standing disease, trophic changes, such as sclerodactyly, ulcerations, or chronic paronychia, may result. Although it's extremely uncommon, minimal cutaneous gangrene necessitates amputation of one or more phalanges.

Diagnosis

Clinical criteria that establish Raynaud's disease include skin color changes induced by cold or stress; bilateral involvement; absence of gangrene or, if present, minimal cutaneous gangrene; normal arterial pulses; and patient history of clinical symptoms of longer than 2 years' duration. Diagnosis must also rule out secondary disease processes, such as chronic arterial occlusive or connective tissue disease.

Treatment

Initially, treatment consists of avoidance of cold, mechanical, or chemical injury; cessation of smoking; and reassurance that symptoms are benign. Because adverse drug effects, especially from vasodilators, may be more bothersome than the disease itself, drug therapy is reserved for unusually severe symptoms. Such therapy may include phenoxybenzamine or reserpine; low doses of nifedipine have been shown to be effective. Sympathectomy may be helpful when conservative modalities fail to prevent ischemic ulcers and becomes necessary in less than 25% of patients.

Special considerations

■ Warn the patient against exposure to the cold. Tell him to wear mittens or gloves in cold weather or when handling cold items or defrosting the freezer.

■ Advise the patient to avoid stressful situations and to stop smoking.

■ Instruct the patient to inspect the skin frequently and to seek immediate care for signs of skin breakdown or infection.

■ Teach the patient about drugs, their use, and their adverse effects.

■ Provide psychological support and reassurance to allay the patient's fear of amputation and disfigurement.

Buerger's disease

Buerger's disease (sometimes called *thromboangiitis obliterans*) — an inflammatory, nonatheromatous occlusive condition — causes segmental lesions and subsequent thrombus formation in the small and medium arteries (and sometimes the veins), resulting in decreased blood flow to the feet and legs. This disorder may produce ulceration and, eventually, gangrene.

Causes and incidence

Buerger's disease is caused by vasculitis, an inflammation of blood vessels, primarily of the hands and feet. The vessels become constricted or totally blocked, reducing blood flow to the tissues and resulting in pain and, eventually, damage.

This disorder occurs in 6 of every 10,000 people. Incidence is highest among males ages 20 to 40 who have a history of smoking or chewing tobacco. It may be associated with a history of Raynaud's disease and may occur in people with autoimmune disease.

Signs and symptoms

Buerger's disease typically produces intermittent claudication of the instep, which is aggravated by exercise and relieved by rest. During exposure to low temperature, the feet initially become cold, cyanotic, and numb; later, they redden, become hot, and tingle. Occasionally, Buerger's disease also affects the hands, possibly resulting in painful fingertip ulcerations. Associated signs and symptoms may include impaired peripheral pulses, migratory superficial thrombophlebitis and, in later stages, ulceration, muscle atrophy, and gangrene.

Diagnosis

Patient history and physical examination strongly suggest Buerger's disease. Supportive diagnostic tests include:

■ Doppler ultrasonography to show diminished circulation in the peripheral vessels

■ plethysmography to help detect decreased circulation in the peripheral vessels

■ angiography or arteriography to locate lesions and rule out atherosclerosis.

Treatment

The primary goals of treatment are to relieve symptoms and prevent complications. Such therapy may include an exercise program that uses gravity to fill and drain the blood vessels or, in severe disease, a lumbar sympathectomy to increase blood supply to the skin. Aspirin and vasodilators may also be used. Amputation may be necessary for nonhealing ulcers, intractable pain, or gangrene.

Special considerations

■ Strongly urge the patient to stop smoking to enhance the treatment's effectiveness. Symptoms may disappear if he stops his tobacco use. If necessary, refer him to a self-help group to stop smoking.

■ Warn the patient to avoid precipitating factors, such as emotional stress, exposure to extreme temperatures, and trauma.

■ Teach the patient proper foot care, especially the importance of wearing well-fitting shoes and cotton or wool socks. Show him how to inspect his feet daily for cuts, abrasions, and signs of skin breakdown, such as redness and soreness. Remind him to seek medical attention at once after any trauma.

■ If the patient has ulcers and gangrene, enforce bed rest and use a padded footboard or bed cradle to prevent pressure from bed linens. Protect the feet with soft padding. Wash them gently with a mild soap and tepid water, rinse thoroughly, and pat dry with a soft towel.

■ Provide emotional support. If necessary, refer the patient for psychological counseling to help him cope with restrictions imposed by this chronic disease. If he has undergone amputation, assess rehabilitative needs, especially regarding changes in body image. Refer him to physical therapists, occupational therapists, and social service agencies, as needed.

Arterial occlusive disease

Arterial occlusive disease is the obstruction or narrowing of the lumen of the aorta and its major branches, causing an interruption of blood flow, usually to the legs and feet. This disorder may affect the carotid, vertebral, innominate, subclavian, mesenteric, and celiac arteries. (See *Types of arterial occlusive disease.*) Occlusions may be acute or chronic and commonly cause severe ischemia, skin ulceration, and gangrene.

The prognosis depends on the occlusion's location, the development of collateral circulation to counteract reduced blood flow and, in acute disease, the time elapsed between occlusion and its removal.

Causes and incidence

Arterial occlusive disease is a common complication of atherosclerosis. The occlusive mechanism may be endogenous, due to emboli formation or thrombosis, or exogenous, due to trauma or fracture. Predisposing factors include smoking; aging; such conditions as hypertension, hyperlipidemia, and diabetes; and a family history of vascular disorders, myocardial infarction, or stroke.

Arterial occlusive disease has no racial predilection. Men older than 50 are at increased risk for intermittent claudication, a common sign of arterial occlusive disease.

Diagnosis

Diagnosis of arterial occlusive disease is usually indicated by patient history and physical examination.

Pertinent supportive diagnostic tests include the following:

■ Arteriography demonstrates the type (thrombus or embolus), location, and degree of obstruction and the collateral circulation. It's particularly useful in chronic disease or for evaluating candidates for reconstructive surgery.

■ Doppler ultrasonography and plethysmography are noninvasive tests that show

TYPES OF ARTERIAL OCCLUSIVE DISEASE

Site of occlusion	Signs and symptoms
Carotid arterial system ■ Internal carotids ■ External carotids	■ Absent or decreased pulsation with an auscultatory bruit over the affected vessels ■ Neurologic dysfunction: transient ischemic attacks (TIAs) due to reduced cerebral circulation producing unilateral sensory or motor dysfunction (transient monocular blindness, and hemiparesis), possible aphasia or dysarthria, confusion, decreased mentation, and headache (These are recurrent features that usually last 5 to 10 minutes but may persist up to 24 hours and may herald a stroke.)
Vertebrobasilar system ■ Vertebral arteries ■ Basilar arteries	■ Neurologic dysfunction: TIAs of the brain stem and cerebellum producing binocular vision disturbances, vertigo, dysarthria, and "drop attacks" (falling down without loss of consciousness); less common than carotid TIA
Innominate ■ Brachiocephalic artery	■ Indications of ischemia (claudication) of the right arm ■ Neurologic dysfunction: signs and symptoms of vertebrobasilar occlusion ■ Possible bruit over the right side of the neck
Subclavian artery	■ Clinical effects of vertebrobasilar occlusion and exercise-induced arm claudication ■ Subclavian steal syndrome (characterized by the backflow of blood from the brain through the vertebral artery on the same side as the occlusion, into the subclavian artery distal to the occlusion) ■ Possibly gangrene (usually limited to the digits)
Mesenteric artery ■ Superior (most commonly affected) ■ Celiac axis ■ Inferior	■ Bowel ischemia, infarct necrosis, and gangrene ■ Diarrhea ■ Leukocytosis ■ Nausea and vomiting ■ Shock due to massive intraluminal fluid and plasma loss ■ Sudden, acute abdominal pain
Aortic bifurcation (saddle block occlusion, a medical emergency associated with cardiac embolization)	■ Sensory and motor deficits (muscle weakness, numbness, paresthesias, and paralysis) in both legs ■ Signs of ischemia (sudden pain and cold, pale legs with decreased or absent peripheral pulses) in both legs
Iliac artery (Leriche's syndrome)	■ Absent or reduced femoral or distal pulses ■ Impotence ■ Intermittent claudication of the lower back, buttocks, and thighs, relieved by rest ■ Possible bruit over femoral arteries
Femoral and popliteal artery (associated with aneurysm formation)	■ Gangrene ■ Intermittent claudication of the calves on exertion ■ Ischemic pain in feet ■ Leg pallor and coolness; blanching of the feet on elevation ■ No palpable pulses in the ankles and feet ■ Pretrophic pain (heralds necrosis and ulceration)

decreased blood flow distal to the occlusion in acute disease.

■ Ophthalmodynamometry helps determine the degree of obstruction in the internal carotid artery by comparing ophthalmic artery pressure to brachial artery pressure on the affected side. More than a 20% difference between pressures suggests insufficiency.

■ EEG and computed tomography scan may be necessary to rule out brain lesions.

Treatment

Treatment depends on the obstruction's cause, location, and size. For mild chronic disease, supportive measures include elimination of smoking, hypertension control, and walking exercise. For carotid artery occlusion, antiplatelet therapy may begin with ticlopidine or clopidogrel and aspirin. For intermittent claudication of chronic occlusive disease, pentoxifylline and cilostazol may improve blood flow through the capillaries, particularly for patients who are poor candidates for surgery.

Acute arterial occlusive disease usually requires surgery to restore circulation to the affected area, for example:

■ Atherectomy — Excision of plaque using a drill or slicing mechanism.

■ Balloon angioplasty — Compression of the obstruction using balloon inflation.

■ Bypass graft — Blood flow is diverted through an anastomosed autogenous or Dacron graft past the thrombosed segment.

■ Combined therapy — Concomitant use of any of the above treatments.

■ Embolectomy — A balloon-tipped Fogarty catheter is used to remove thrombotic material from the artery. Embolectomy is used mainly for mesenteric, femoral, or popliteal artery occlusion.

■ Laser angioplasty — Use of excision and hot tip lasers to vaporize the obstruction.

■ Lumbar sympathectomy — An adjunct to surgery, depending on the sympathetic nervous system's condition.

■ Patch grafting — This procedure involves removal of the thrombosed arterial segment and replacement with an autogenous vein or Dacron graft.

■ Stents — Insertion of a mesh of wires that stretch and mold to the arterial wall to prevent reocclusion. This new adjunct follows laser angioplasty or atherectomy.

■ Thromboendarterectomy — Opening of the occluded artery and direct removal of the obstructing thrombus and the medial layer of the arterial wall; usually performed after angiography and commonly used with autogenous vein or Dacron bypass surgery (femoral-popliteal or aortofemoral).

■ Thrombolytic therapy — Lysis of any clot around or in the plaque by urokinase, streptokinase, or alteplase.

Amputation becomes necessary with failure of arterial reconstructive surgery or with the development of gangrene, persistent infection, or intractable pain.

Other therapy includes heparin to prevent emboli (for embolic occlusion) and bowel resection after restoration of blood flow (for mesenteric artery occlusion).

Special considerations

■ Provide comprehensive patient teaching, including proper foot care. Explain diagnostic tests and procedures. Advise the patient to stop smoking and to follow the prescribed medical regimen.

Preoperatively, during an acute episode:

■ Assess the patient's circulatory status by checking for the most distal pulses and by inspecting his skin color and temperature.

■ Provide pain relief as needed.

■ Administer heparin by continuous I.V. drip as ordered. Use an infusion monitor or pump to ensure the proper flow rate.

■ Wrap the patient's affected foot in soft cotton batting and reposition it frequently to prevent pressure on any one area. Strictly avoid elevating or applying heat to the affected leg.

■ Watch for signs of fluid and electrolyte imbalance, and monitor intake and output for signs of renal failure (urine output less than 30 ml/hour).

■ If the patient has carotid, innominate, vertebral, or subclavian artery occlusion, monitor him for signs of stroke, such as numbness in an arm or leg and intermittent blindness.

Postoperatively:

■ Monitor the patient's vital signs. Continuously assess his circulatory function by inspecting skin color and temperature and by checking for distal pulses. In charting, compare earlier assessments and observations. Watch closely for signs of hemorrhage (tachycardia and hypotension) and check dressings for excessive bleeding.

■ In carotid, innominate, vertebral, or subclavian artery occlusion, assess neurologic status frequently for changes in level of consciousness or muscle strength and pupil size.

■ In mesenteric artery occlusion, connect the nasogastric tube to low intermittent suction. Monitor intake and output (low urine output may indicate damage to renal arteries during surgery). Check bowel sounds for return of peristalsis. Increasing abdominal distention and tenderness may indicate extension of bowel ischemia with resulting gangrene, necessitating further excision, or it may indicate peritonitis.

■ In saddle block occlusion, check distal pulses for adequate circulation. Watch for signs of renal failure and mesenteric artery occlusion (severe abdominal pain), and for cardiac arrhythmias, which may precipitate embolus formation.

■ In iliac artery occlusion, monitor urine output for signs of renal failure from decreased perfusion to the kidneys as a result of surgery. Provide meticulous catheter care.

■ In both femoral and popliteal artery occlusions, assist with early ambulation, but discourage prolonged sitting.

■ After amputation, check the patient's stump carefully for drainage and record its color and amount, and the time. Elevate the stump as ordered, and administer adequate analgesic medication. Because phantom limb pain is common, explain this phenomenon to the patient.

■ When preparing the patient for discharge, instruct him to watch for signs of recurrence (pain, pallor, numbness, paralysis, and absence of pulse) that can result from graft occlusion or occlusion at another site. Warn him against wearing constrictive clothing.

Selected references

American Heart Association. "Introduction to the International Guidelines 2000 for CPR and ECC: A Consensus on Science," *Circulation* 102(Suppl. I):II-III, August 2000.

Cardiovascular Care Made Incredibly Easy. Philadelphia: Lippincott Williams & Wilkins, 2004.

Fuster, V., et al. *Atherothrombosis and Coronary Artery Disease,* 2nd ed. Philadelphia: Lippincott Williams & Wilkins, 2005.

Griffin, B.P., and Topol, E.J., eds. *Manual of Cardiovascular Medicine,* 2nd ed. Philadelphia: Lippincott Williams & Wilkins, 2004.

Heger, J.W., et al. *Cardiology,* 5th ed. Philadelphia: Lippincott Williams & Wilkins, 2004.

Just the Facts: ECG Interpretation. Philadelphia: Lippincott Williams & Wilkins, 2005.

Klabunde, R.E. *Cardiovascular Physiology Concepts.* Philadelphia: Lippincott Williams & Wilkins, 2005.

Mastering ACLS. Springhouse, Pa.: Springhouse Corp., 2002.

Sharis, P.J., and Cannon, C.P. *Evidence-Based Cardiology,* 2nd ed. Philadelphia: Lippincott Williams & Wilkins, 2004.

Khonsari, S. and Sintek, C. *Cardiac Surgery: Safeguards and Pitfalls in Operative Technique,* 3rd ed. Philadelphia: Lippincott Williams & Wilkins, 2003.

Woods, S.L., et al., eds. *Cardiac Nursing.* Philadelphia: Lippincott Williams & Wilkins, 2005.

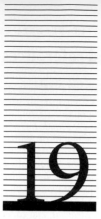

19

Eye disorders

Introduction *1153*

Eyelid and lacrimal ducts *1157*
Blepharitis *1157*
Exophthalmos *1158*
Ptosis *1159*
Orbital cellulitis *1160*
Dacryocystitis *1161*
Chalazion *1162*
Stye *1163*

Conjunctival disorders *1164*
Inclusion conjunctivitis *1164*
Conjunctivitis *1164*
Trachoma *1166*

Corneal disorders *1168*
Keratitis *1168*
Corneal abrasion *1169*
Corneal ulcers *1170*

**Uveal tract, retinal, and lens
   disorders** *1172*
Uveitis *1172*
Retinal detachment *1173*
Vascular retinopathies *1175*
Age-related macular degeneration *1178*
Cataract *1179*
Retinitis pigmentosa *1180*

Miscellaneous disorders *1181*
Optic atrophy *1181*
Extraocular motor nerve palsies *1182*
Glaucoma *1183*

Selected references *1186*

Introduction

Vision, the most complex sense, has recently been the focus of some of the greatest medical and surgical innovations. Disorders that affect the eye generally lead to vision loss or impairment; routine ophthalmic examinations and early treatment can help prevent it.

Review of anatomy

The visual system consists mainly of the bony orbit, which houses the eye; the contents of the orbit, including the eyeball, optic nerves, extraocular muscles, cranial nerves, blood vessels, orbital fat, and lacrimal system; and the eyelid, which covers the eye, moistens it, and protects it from injury.

The orbit (also called the *socket*) encloses the eye in a protective recess in the skull. Its seven bones — frontal, sphenoid, zygomatic, maxillary, palatine, ethmoid, and lacrimal — form a cone. The apex of this cone points toward the brain, and the cone's base forms the orbital rim. The periorbita covers the bones of the orbit.

Extraocular muscles hold the eyes in place and control their movement as described below:
- *superior rectus:* elevates the eye upward; adducts and rotates the eye inward
- *inferior rectus:* depresses the eye downward; adducts and rotates the eye outward
- *lateral rectus:* abducts or turns the eye outward (laterally)
- *medial rectus:* adducts or turns the eye inward (medially)
- *superior oblique:* rotates the eye inward; abducts and depresses the eye
- *inferior oblique:* rotates the eye outward; abducts and elevates the eye.

The actions of these muscles are mutually antagonistic: As one contracts, its opposing muscle relaxes.

 ELDER TIP *Eye structure and activity change with age. The eyes set deeper in their sockets or have laid down more fat, and the eyelids lose their elasticity and become saggy and wrinkled.*

Ocular layers

The eye has three structural layers: the sclera and cornea, the uveal tract, and the retina. (See *Cross section of the eye,* page 1154.)

The sclera is the dense, white, fibrous outer protective coat of the eye. It meets the cornea at the limbus (corneoscleral junction) anteriorly, and the dural sheath of the optic nerve posteriorly. The lamina cribrosa is a sievelike structure composed of a few strands of scleral tissue through which the optic nerve bundles pass. The sclera is covered by the episclera, a thin layer of fine elastic tissue.

 ELDER TIP *In older adults, lens changes occur typically with formation of a cataract. The vitreous body liquefies and pulls away from the retina, generating floating vitreous debris and peripheral vitreous detachments.*

The cornea is the transparent, avascular, curved layer of the eye that's continuous with the sclera. The cornea consists of five layers: the epithelium, which contains sensory nerves; Bowman's membrane, the basement membrane for the epithelial cells; the stroma, or supporting tissue (90% of the corneal structure); Descemet's membrane, containing many elastic fibers; and the endothelium, a single layer of cells that acts as a pump to maintain proper dehydration or detumescence of the cornea. Aqueous humor bathes the posterior surface of the cornea, maintaining intraocular pressure (IOP) by volume and rate of outflow. The anterior cornea is kept moist by the tear film. The cornea's sole function is to refract light rays.

ELDER TIP *Corneal sensitivity to touch decreases with age, and corneal curvature probably changes slightly also. It's believed that atrophy of the dilator muscle fibers and increased rigidity of the blood vessels of the iris reduce pupil size, decreasing the amount of light that reaches the retina. Consequently, higher levels of illumination may be needed to improve uncorrected visual acuity in the older adult.*

The middle layer of the eye, the uveal tract, is pigmented and vascular. It consists of the iris and the ciliary body in the anterior portion, and the choroid in the posterior portion. In the center of the iris is the

CROSS SECTION OF THE EYE

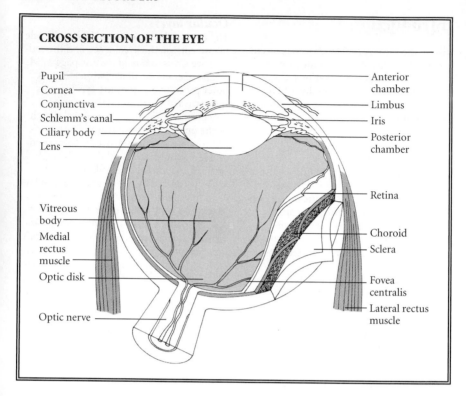

Pupil
Cornea
Conjunctiva
Schlemm's canal
Ciliary body
Lens

Anterior chamber
Limbus
Iris
Posterior chamber

Vitreous body
Medial rectus muscle
Optic disk
Optic nerve

Retina
Choroid
Sclera
Fovea centralis
Lateral rectus muscle

pupil. The sphincter and dilator muscles control the amount of light that enters the eye through the pupil, and the pupil itself allows aqueous humor to flow from the posterior chamber into the anterior chamber.

The angle formed by the anterior iris and the posterior corneal structures contains many minute collecting channels of the trabecular meshwork. Aqueous humor drains through these channels into an encircling venous system called the canal of Schlemm.

The ciliary body, which extends from the root of the iris to the ora serrata, produces aqueous humor and controls lens accommodation through its action on the zonular fibers. The choroid, the largest part of the uveal tract, is made up of blood vessels bound externally by the suprachoroid and internally by Bruch's membrane.

The retina is the neural coat of the eye. It receives visual images and transmits them to the brain for interpretation. It extends from the ora serrata to the optic nerve; the

retinal pigment epithelium (RPE) adheres lightly to the choroid. Located next to the RPE are rods and cones. Although both rods and cones are light receptors, they respond to light differently. Rods, scattered throughout the retina, respond to low levels of light and detect moving objects; cones, located in the fovea centralis, function best in brighter light and perceive finer details.

Three types of cones contain different visual pigments and react to specific light wavelengths: one type reacts to red light, one to green, and one to blue-violet. The eye mixes these colors into various shades; the cones can detect 150 shades.

ELDER TIP *Many elderly patients experience a loss of ability to discriminate blue-greens, and white objects appear yellowish; these patients may also have difficulty discriminating among pastels, violets, and yellow-greens.*

The lens and accommodation

The lens of the eye is biconvex, avascular, and transparent; the lens capsule is a semipermeable membrane that can admit water and electrolytes. The lens changes shape (accommodation) for near and far vision. For near vision, the ciliary body contracts and relaxes the zonules, the lens becomes spherical, the pupil constricts, and the eyes converge; for far vision, the ciliary body relaxes, the zonules tighten, the lens becomes flatter, the eyes straighten, and the pupils dilate. The lens refines the refraction necessary to focus a clear image on the retina.

The vitreous body, which is 99% water and a small amount of insoluble protein, constitutes two-thirds of the eye's volume. This transparent, gelatinous body gives the eye its shape and contributes to the refraction of light rays. The vitreous is firmly attached to the ora serrata of the ciliary body (anteriorly) and to the optic disk (posteriorly). The vitreous face contacts the lens; the vitreous gel rests against the retina.

Lacrimal apparatus and eyelids

The lacrimal apparatus consists of the lacrimal glands, upper and lower canaliculi, lacrimal sac, and nasolacrimal duct. The main gland, located in a shallow fossa beneath the superior temporal orbital rim, secretes reflex tears, which keep the cornea and conjunctiva moist. These tears flow through 12 to 14 excretory ducts and contain lysozyme, an enzyme that protects the conjunctiva from bacterial invasion. Multiple sebaceous glands in the eyelids produce an oily secretion that prevents tears from evaporating. With every blink, the eyelids direct the flow to the inner canthus, where the tears pool and then drain through a tiny opening called the punctum. The tears then pass through the canaliculi and lacrimal sac and down the nasolacrimal duct, which opens into the nasal cavity.

The eyelids (palpebrae) consist of tarsal plates that are composed of dense connective tissue. The orbital septum — the fascia behind the orbicularis oculi muscle — acts as a barrier between the lids and the orbit. The levator palpebrae muscle elevates the upper lid. The eyelids contain three types of glands:

- glands of Zeis — modified sebaceous glands connected to the follicles of the eyelashes
- meibomian glands — are sebaceous glands in the tarsal plates that secrete an oily substance as a tear film component (About 25 of these glands are found in the upper lid and about 20 in the lower lid.)
- Moll's glands — ordinary sweat glands.

The conjunctiva is the thin mucous membrane that lines the eyelids (palpebral conjunctiva), folds over at the fornix, and covers the surface of the eyeball (bulbar conjunctiva). The conjunctiva produces mucin, another component of the tear film. The ophthalmic, lacrimal, and multiple anastomoses of facial arteries supply blood to the lids. The space between the open lids is the palpebral fissure; the juncture of the upper and lower lids is the canthus. The junction near the nose is called the nasal, medial, or inner canthus; the junction on the temporal side, the lateral or external canthus.

ELDER TIP *Age-related vision changes are usually first noticed during the fifth decade of life and may include the inability to focus, narrowing of the visual field, reduced peripheral vision, and loss of iris elasticity producing decreased response to light and dark. In addition, as people age, production of any of the three tear film components may decrease, causing dry eyes.*

Depth perception

In normal binocular vision, a perceived image is projected onto the two foveae. Impulses then travel along the optic pathways to the occipital cortex, which perceives a single image. However, the cortex receives two images — each from a slightly different angle — giving the images perspective and providing depth perception.

Vision testing

Several tests assess visual acuity and identify visual defects:

- Ishihara's test determines color blindness by using a series of plates composed of a colored background, with a letter, number, or pattern of a contrasting color located in the center of each plate. The patient with deficient color perception can't perceive the differences in color or, consequently, the designs formed by the color contrasts.

- The Snellen chart or other eye charts evaluate visual acuity. Such charts use progressively smaller letters or symbols to determine central vision on a numerical scale. A person with normal acuity should be able to read the letters or recognize the symbols on the 20/20 line of the eye chart at a distance of 20 feet.

Subjective testing

Several tests accomplish subjective testing of the eyes:

- B-mode ultrasonography delineates retinal tumors, detachments, and vitreous hemorrhages — even in the presence of opacities of the cornea and lens. A handheld B-scanner has simplified ultrasonic examination of the eye, making it possible to perform such studies in the ophthalmologist's office.
- The convergence test locates the breaking point of fusion (before double vision occurs). For this test, the examiner holds a small object in front of the patient's nose and slowly brings it closer to the patient. The point at which the eyes "break" is termed the near point of convergence and is measured in prism diopters.
- The cover-uncover test assesses eye muscle misalignment or tendency toward misalignment. In this test, the patient stares at a small, fixed object — first from a distance of 20′ (6.1 m) and then from 1′ (0.3 m). The examiner covers the patient's eyes one at a time, noting any movement of the uncovered eye, the direction of any deviation, and the rate at which the eyes recover normal binocular vision when latent heterophoria is present.
- Duction test checks eye movement in all directions of gaze. While one eye is covered, the other eye follows a moving light. This test detects weakness of rotation due to muscle paralysis or structural dysfunction.
- Fluorescein angiography evaluates the blood vessels in the choroid and retina after I.V. injection of fluorescein dye; images of the dye-enhanced vasculature are recorded by rapid-sequence photographs of the fundus.

- Goldmann's applanation, Tonopen tonometry, and Schiøtz tonometry all measure IOP. After instilling a local anesthetic in the patient's eye, the examiner places the Schiøtz tonometer lightly on the corneal surface and measures the indentation of the cornea produced by a given weight. The Schiøtz tonometer has been largely replaced by an electronic Tonopen tonometer for bedside use. Applanation tonometry gauges the force required to flatten a small area of central cornea, and is the most accurate method of measuring IOP. For this test, a patient must be seated at a slit lamp and the cornea stained with fluorescein dye before the prism of the applanation tonometer touches the cornea and the examiner adjusts the controls until the two lines form an "S."
- Gonioscopy allows for direct visualization of the anterior chamber angle.
- The Maddox rod test assesses muscle dysfunction; it's especially useful in disclosing and measuring heterophoria (the tendency of the eyes to deviate). It can reveal horizontal, vertical and, especially, torsional deviations.
- Ophthalmodynamometry measures the relative central retinal artery pressures and indirectly assesses carotid artery flow on each side. This test has been largely supplanted by the color Doppler imaging test, which can assess blood flow velocities in ophthalmic vessels.
- Ophthalmoscopy — direct ophthalmoscopy or binocular indirect ophthalmoscopy allows examination of the interior of the eye after the pupil has been dilated with a mydriatic.
- Refraction tests may be performed with or without cycloplegics. In cycloplegic refraction, eyedrops weaken the accommodative power of the ciliary muscle. Lenses placed in front of the eye direct light rays onto the retina, thus focusing the image so that it can be transmitted along the visual pathway. A retinoscope may be used in the same way by directing a beam of light through the pupil onto the retina; the light's shadow is neutralized by placing the appropriate lens in front of the eye.
- Slit-lamp biomicroscopic examination allows a well-illuminated examination of

the eyelids and the anterior segment of the eyeball.

■ Visual field tests assess the function of the retina, the optic nerve, and the optic pathways when both central and peripheral visual fields are examined.

EYELID AND LACRIMAL DUCTS

Blepharitis

A common inflammation, blepharitis produces a red-rimmed appearance of the margins of the eyelids. It's frequently chronic and bilateral and can affect both upper and lower lids. Seborrheic blepharitis is characterized by formation of waxy scales and symptoms of burning and foreign-body sensation. Staphylococcal (ulcerative) blepharitis is characterized by formation of dry scales along the inflamed lid margins, which also have ulcerated areas and may be associated with keratoconjunctivitis sicca (KCS), a dry-eye syndrome. Both types may coexist. Blepharitis tends to recur and become chronic. It can be controlled if treatment begins before onset of ocular involvement.

Causes and incidence

Seborrheic blepharitis may be seen in conjunction with seborrhea of the scalp, eyebrows, and ears. It's common in elderly people and in people with red hair. Staphylococcal blepharitis is associated with *Staphylococcus aureus* infection and is more common in females than in males. Allergies and eyelash infestations with lice are less-common causes of blepharitis. Blepharitis may also be associated with repeated styes and chalazion.

Signs and symptoms

Clinical features of blepharitis include itching, burning, foreign-body sensation, and sticky, crusted eyelids on waking. This constant irritation results in unconscious rubbing of the eyes (causing reddened rims) or continual blinking. Other signs include

waxy scales in seborrheic blepharitis; and flaky scales on lashes, loss of lashes, and ulcerated areas on lid margins in ulcerative blepharitis. In association with KCS, dry eyes may also be a problem.

Diagnosis

Diagnosis depends on patient history and characteristic symptoms. In staphylococcal blepharitis, culture of ulcerated lid margin shows *S. aureus*.

Treatment

The goals of therapy are to control the disease and its underlying causes, maintain vision, and avoid secondary complications. Treatment depends on the type of blepharitis:

■ blepharitis resulting from pediculosis—removal of nits (with forceps) or application of ophthalmic physostigmine or other ointment as an insecticide (this may cause pupil constriction and, possibly, headache, conjunctival irritation, and blurred vision from the film of ointment on the cornea).

■ seborrheic blepharitis—daily lid hygiene (using a mild shampoo on a damp applicator stick or a washcloth) and hot compresses to remove scales from the lid margins; also, frequent shampooing of the scalp and eyebrows.

■ staphylococcal blepharitis—warm compresses and an antibiotic, such as tetracycline or erythromycin eye ointment, may be used. For some patients, systemic antibiotics are indicated. Patients with severe staphylococcal blepharitis may require antibiotic sensitivity studies.

Special considerations

■ Instruct the patient to gently remove scales from the lid margins daily, with an applicator stick or a clean washcloth.

■ Teach the patient the following method for applying warm compresses: First, run warm water into a clean bowl. Then, immerse a clean cloth in the water and wring it out. Place the warm cloth against the closed eyelid (be careful not to burn the skin). Hold the compress in place until it cools. Continue this procedure for 15 minutes.

- Antibiotic ophthalmic ointment should be applied after 15-minute application of warm compresses.
- Treatment for seborrheic blepharitis also requires attention to the face and scalp.

Exophthalmos

Exophthalmos (also called *proptosis*) is the unilateral or bilateral bulging or protrusion of the eyeballs or their apparent forward displacement (with lid retraction). The prognosis depends on the underlying cause.

Causes

Exophthalmos commonly results from hyperthyroidism, particularly ophthalmic Graves' disease in which the eyeballs are displaced forward and the lids retract. Unilateral exophthalmos may also result from trauma (such as fracture of the ethmoid bone, which allows air from the sinus to enter the orbital tissue, displacing soft tissue and the eyeball). Exophthalmos may also stem from hemorrhage, varicosities, thrombosis, and edema, all of which similarly displace one or both eyeballs.

Other systemic and ocular causes include:
- infection — orbital cellulitis, panophthalmitis, and infection of the lacrimal gland or orbital tissues
- parasitic cysts — in surrounding tissue
- pseudoexophthalmos paralysis of extraocular muscles — relaxation of eyeball retractors, congenital macrophthalmia, and high myopia
- tumors and neoplastic diseases — in children, rhabdomyosarcomas, leukemia, gliomas of the optic nerve, dermoid cysts, teratomas, metastatic neuroblastomas, and lymphoma; in adults, lacrimal gland tumors, mucoceles, cavernous hemangioma, meningiomas, metastatic carcinomas, and lymphoma.

Signs and symptoms

The obvious effect is a bulging eyeball, commonly with diplopia, if extraocular muscle edema causes misalignment. (See *Recognizing exophthalmos.*) A rim of the sclera may be visible below the upper lid as lid retraction occurs, and the patient may blink infrequently. Other symptoms depend on the cause: pain may accompany traumatic exophthalmos; a tumor may produce conjunctival hyperemia or chemosis; retraction of the upper lid predisposes to exposure keratitis. If exophthalmos is associated with cavernous sinus thrombosis, the patient may exhibit paresis of the muscles supplied by cranial nerves III, IV, and VI; limited ocular movement; and a septic-type (high) fever.

Diagnosis

Exophthalmos is usually obvious on physical examination; exophthalmometer readings confirm diagnosis by showing the degree of anterior projection and asymmetry between the eyes (normal bar readings range from 12 to 20 mm). The following diagnostic measures identify the cause:
- Computed tomography scan or magnetic resonance imaging detects swollen extraocular muscles or lesions within the orbit.
- Culture of discharge determines the infecting organism; sensitivity testing indicates appropriate antibiotic therapy.
- Biopsy of orbital tissue may be necessary if initial treatment fails.

Treatment

Eye trauma may require cold compresses for the first 24 hours, followed by warm compresses, and prophylactic antibiotic therapy. After edema subsides, surgery may be necessary in a small percentage of cases. Eye infection requires treatment with broad-spectrum antibiotics during the 24 hours preceding positive identification of the organism, followed by specific antibiotics. A patient with exophthalmos resulting from an orbital tumor may initially benefit from antibiotic or corticosteroid therapy. Eventually, surgical exploration of the orbit and excision of the tumor, enucleation, or exenteration may be necessary. Radiation and chemotherapy may be used when primary orbital tumors can't be fully excised as encapsulated lesions, such as in rhabdomyosarcoma lesions.

Treatment for Graves' disease may include antithyroid drug therapy or partial or total thyroidectomy to control hyperthy-

RECOGNIZING EXOPHTHALMOS

This photo shows the characteristic forward protrusion of the eyes from the orbit associated with exophthalmos.

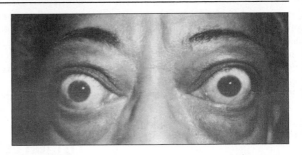

roidism; initial high doses of systemic corticosteroids, such as prednisone, for optic neuropathy and, if lid retraction is severe, protective lubricants.

Surgery may include orbital decompression (removal of the superior and lateral orbital walls) if vision is threatened, followed by lid (blepharoplasty) and muscle surgery.

Special considerations
- Administer medication as ordered.
- Record the patient's response to therapy.
- Apply cold and warm compresses, as ordered, for fracture or other trauma.
- Provide postoperative care.
- Explain tests and procedures and give emotional support.
- Protect the exposed cornea with lubricants to prevent corneal drying.

Ptosis

Ptosis (drooping of the upper eyelid) may be congenital or acquired, unilateral or bilateral, and constant or intermittent. Severe ptosis usually responds well to treatment; slight ptosis may require no treatment at all.

Causes and incidence
Congenital ptosis is transmitted as an autosomal dominant trait or results from a congenital anomaly in which the levator muscles of the eyelids fail to develop. This condition is usually unilateral.

Acquired ptosis may result from any of the following:
- advanced age (involutional ptosis, the most common form, usually seen in older patients following cataract surgery)
- mechanical factors that make the eyelid heavy, such as swelling caused by a foreign body on the palpebral surface of the eyelid or by edema, inflammation produced by a tumor or pseudotumor, or an extra fatty fold
- myogenic factors, such as muscular dystrophy or myasthenia gravis (in which the defect appears to be in humoral transmission at the myoneural junction)
- neurogenic (paralytic) factors from interference in innervation of the eyelid by the oculomotor nerve (cranial nerve III), most commonly due to trauma, diabetes, or carotid aneurysm
- nutritional factors, such as thiamine deficiency in chronic alcoholism, hyperemesis gravidarum, and other malnutrition-producing states.

Risk factors for ptosis include aging, diabetes, stroke, Horner's syndrome, myasthenia gravis, and cancer that affects nerve or muscle response.

Signs and symptoms
An infant with congenital ptosis has a smooth, flat upper eyelid, without the eyelid fold normally caused by the pull of the levator muscle; associated weakness of the superior rectus muscle isn't uncommon.

The child with unilateral ptosis that covers the pupil can develop an amblyopic eye from disuse or lack of eye stimulation. In bilateral ptosis, the child may elevate his brow in an attempt to compensate, wrinkling his forehead in an effort to raise the upper lid. Also, the child may tilt his head backward to see.

In myasthenia gravis, ptosis results from fatigue and characteristically appears in the evening, but is relieved by rest.

Ptosis due to oculomotor nerve damage produces a fixed, dilated pupil; divergent strabismus; and slight depression of the eyeball.

Diagnosis

A physical examination reveals upper lid retraction, and examination with the Hertel exophthalmometer reveals the degree of proptosis. Diagnosis also includes these tests to determine the underlying cause:

- digital subtraction angiography or magnetic resonance imaging—aneurysm
- glucose tolerance test—diabetes
- ophthalmologic examination—foreign bodies
- patient history—chronic alcoholism
- Tensilon test—myasthenia gravis (in acquired ptosis with no history of trauma).

Treatment

Slight ptosis that doesn't produce deformity or loss of vision requires no treatment. Severe ptosis that interferes with vision or is cosmetically undesirable usually necessitates resection of the weak levator muscles. Surgery to correct congenital ptosis is usually performed at age 3 or 4, but it may be done earlier if ptosis is unilateral because the completely occluded pupil may cause an amblyopic eye. If surgery is undesirable, special glasses with an attached suspended crutch on the frames may elevate the eyelid.

Effective treatment for ptosis also requires treatment for the underlying cause. For example, in patients with myasthenia gravis, neostigmine or steroids may be prescribed to increase the effect of acetylcholine and aid transmission of nerve impulses to muscles.

Special considerations

- Report any bleeding immediately. After surgery to correct ptosis, watch for blood on the pressure patch. (Some surgical procedures may not require a patch.) Apply ointment to the sutures as prescribed.
- Emphasize to the patient and his family the need to prevent accidental trauma to the surgical site until healing is complete (6 weeks). Suture line damage can precipitate recurrence of ptosis.

Orbital cellulitis

Orbital cellulitis is an acute infection of the orbital tissues and eyelids that doesn't involve the eyeball. With treatment, the prognosis is good; if untreated, the infection may spread to the cavernous sinus or the meninges, where it can be life-threatening.

Causes and incidence

Orbital cellulitis may result from bacterial, fungal, or parasitic infection. It can develop from direct inoculation, via the bloodstream, or spread from adjacent structures. Periorbital tissues may be inoculated as a result of surgery, foreign body trauma, and even animal or insect bites. The most common pathogens in children are *Haemophilus influenzae*, *Streptococcus pneumoniae*, and *Staphylococcus aureus*. In young children, it's spread from adjacent sinuses (especially the ethmoid air cells) and accounts for the majority of postseptal cellulitis cases. Immunosuppressed patients are also susceptible.

Signs and symptoms

Orbital cellulitis generally produces unilateral eyelid edema, hyperemia of the orbital tissues, reddened eyelids, and matted lashes. Although the eyeball is initially unaffected, proptosis develops later (because of edematous tissues within the bony confines of the orbit). Other indications include extreme orbital pain, impaired eye movement, chemosis, and purulent discharge from indurated areas. The severity of associated systemic symptoms (chills, fever, and malaise) varies according to the cause.

Complications include posterior extension, causing cavernous sinus thrombosis, panophthalmitis, meningitis, or brain abscess and, rarely, atrophy and subsequent loss of vision secondary to optic neuritis.

Diagnosis

Typical clinical features establish diagnosis. Computed tomography scan or magnetic resonance imaging of the sinuses and orbit tissues will determine if the cause of the cellulitis is preseptal or if deeper structures are involved, or if a tumor is the cause of swelling. Usually the patient will also be febrile with this type of infection. Wound culture and sensitivity testing determine the causative organism and specific antibiotic therapy. Other tests include white blood cell count, and ophthalmologic examination.

Treatment

Prompt treatment is necessary to prevent complications. Primary treatment consists of antibiotic therapy. Systemic antibiotics (I.V. or oral) and eyedrops or ointment will be ordered. Supportive therapy consists of fluids; warm, moist compresses; and bed rest. The patient should be monitored closely. If during the initial 48 to 72 hours of treatment no improvement is seen, adjustment of antibiotics guided by drug sensitivity should be considered. If an orbital abscess is present, surgical incision and drainage may be necessary.

Special considerations

■ Monitor vital signs at least every 4 hours, and maintain fluid and electrolyte balance.
■ Have the patient instill antibiotic eyedrops frequently during the day and apply ointment at night.
■ Apply compresses every 3 to 4 hours to localize inflammation and relieve discomfort. Teach the patient to apply these compresses. Give pain medication, as ordered, after assessing pain level.
■ Before discharge, stress the importance of completing prescribed antibiotic therapy. To prevent orbital cellulitis, tell the patient to maintain good general hygiene and to carefully clean abrasions and cuts that occur near the orbit.

Dacryocystitis

Dacryocystitis is an infection of the lacrimal sac. In infants, dacryocystitis results from congenital atresia of the nasolacrimal duct; in adults, it results from an obstruction (dacryostenosis) of the nasolacrimal duct (most common in women older than 40). It can be acute or chronic.

Causes and incidence

Atresia of the nasolacrimal ducts results from failure of canalization or, in the first few months of life, from blockage when the membrane that separates the lower part of the nasolacrimal duct and the inferior nasal meatus fails to open spontaneously before tear secretion. Bony obstruction of the duct may also occur.

In acute dacryocystitis, *Staphylococcus aureus* and, occasionally, beta-hemolytic streptococci are the cause. In chronic dacryocystitis, *Streptococcus pneumoniae* or, sometimes, a fungus — such as *Actinomyces* or *Candida albicans* — is the causative organism. Primary lumps and secondary tumors from sinuses, nose, and orbits have also been reported as causes.

Signs and symptoms

Dacryocystitis is extremely painful for the patient. The hallmark of both the acute and chronic forms of dacryocystitis is constant tearing. Other symptoms of dacryocystitis include inflammation and tenderness over the nasolacrimal sac; pressure over this area may fail to produce purulent discharge from the punctum.

Diagnosis

Clinical features and a physical examination suggest dacryocystitis. Culture of the discharged material demonstrates *Staphylococcus aureus* and, occasionally, beta-hemolytic streptococci in acute dacryocystitis, and *Streptococcus pneumoniae* or *C. albicans* in the chronic form. The white blood cell count may be elevated in the acute form; in the chronic form, it's gener-

RECOGNIZING CHALAZION

A chalazion is a nontender granulomatous inflammation of a meibomian gland on the upper or lower eyelid.

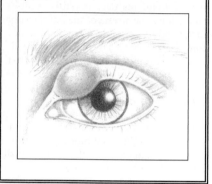

ally normal. An X-ray after injection of a radiopaque medium (dacryocystography) locates the atresia in infants.

Treatment

Treatment for acute dacryocystitis consists of warm compresses, topical and systemic antibiotic therapy and, occasionally, incision and drainage. Chronic dacryocystitis may eventually require dacryocystorhinostomy. Laser-assisted endoscopic dacryocystorhinostomy and balloon dilatation or probing of the nasolacrimal system may also be used.

Therapy for nasolacrimal duct obstruction in an infant consists of careful massage of the area over the lacrimal sac four times a day for 6 to 9 months. If this fails to open the duct, dilation of the punctum and probing of the duct are necessary.

Special considerations

■ Check the patient history for possible allergy to antibiotics before administration. Emphasize the importance of precise compliance with the prescribed antibiotic regimen.
■ Tell the adult patient what to expect after surgery: He'll have ice compresses over the surgical site and will have bruising and swelling.

■ Monitor blood loss by counting dressings used to collect the blood.
■ Apply ice compresses postoperatively. A small adhesive bandage may be placed over the suture line to protect it from damage.

Chalazion

A chalazion is a chronic granulomatous inflammation of a meibomian gland or gland of Zeis in the upper or lower eyelid. (There are approximately 100 of these glands located near the eyelashes.) This common eye disorder is characterized by localized swelling within the tarsal plate, or it may break through the conjunctival or skin side. Mild irritation and blurred vision usually develop slowly over several weeks. (See *Recognizing chalazion*.) A chalazion may become large enough to press on the eyeball, causing astigmatism. A large chalazion seldom subsides spontaneously. It's generally benign and chronic, and can occur at any age. In some patients, it's apt to recur.

Causes

Obstruction of the meibomian (sebaceous) gland duct causes a chalazion.

Signs and symptoms

A chalazion occurs as a painless, hard lump that usually points *toward* the conjunctival side of the eyelid. Eversion of the lid reveals a red or red-yellow elevated area on the conjunctival surface. Otherwise, it's seen as an indurated bump under the skin of the upper eyelid.

Diagnosis

Diagnosis requires visual examination and palpation of the eyelid, revealing a small bump or nodule. Persistently recurrent chalazions, especially in an adult, necessitate biopsy to rule out meibomian cancer.

Treatment

Initial treatment consists of application of warm compresses for 10 to 15 minutes at least four times a day to open the lumen of the gland, soften the hardened oils blocking the duct, and promote drainage and healing. If such therapy fails, or if the chalazion presses on the eyeball or causes a severe cosmetic problem, steroid injection or incision and curettage under local anesthetic may be necessary. After such surgery, a pressure eye patch applied for 4 to 6 hours controls bleeding and swelling. After removal of the patch, treatment again consists of warm compresses. Antibiotic eyedrops are occasionally prescribed before and after cyst removal, but otherwise are of little value.

Special considerations

■ Instruct the patient how to properly apply warm compresses: Tell him to take special care to avoid burning the skin, to always use a clean cloth, and to discard used compresses. Also tell him to start applying warm compresses at the first sign of lid irritation to increase the blood supply and keep the lumen open.

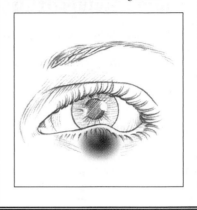

RECOGNIZING A STYE

A stye is a localized red, swollen, and tender abscess of the lid glands.

Stye

A localized, purulent staphylococcal infection, a stye (or hordeolum) can occur externally (in the lumen of the smaller glands of Zeis or in Moll's glands) or internally (in the larger meibomian gland). A stye can occur at any age. Generally, styes are self-limiting and respond well to hot, moist compresses. More than one may occur at the same time. If untreated, a stye can eventually lead to cellulitis of the eyelid. Styes can also develop into a chalazion if gland ducts are fully blocked.

Causes

Skin bacteria that enter eyelash hair follicles and cause inflammation can result in stye formation. Risk factors include blepharitis, diabetes and other chronic debilitating illnesses, and seborrhea.

Signs and symptoms

Typically, a stye produces redness, swelling, and pain. An abscess frequently forms at the lid margin, with an eyelash pointing outward from its center. (See *Recognizing a stye.*)

Diagnosis

Visual examination generally confirms this infection. Culture of purulent material from the abscess usually reveals a staphylococcal organism.

Treatment

Treatment consists of warm compresses applied for 10 to 15 minutes, four times a day for 3 to 4 days, to facilitate drainage of the abscess, to relieve pain and inflammation, and to promote suppuration. Drug therapy includes a topical sulfonamide or antibiotic eyedrops or ointment and, occasionally, a systemic antibiotic for secondary eyelid cellulitis. If conservative treatment fails, incision and drainage may be necessary.

Special considerations

■ Instruct the patient to use a clean cloth for each application of warm compresses and to dispose of it or launder it separately.
■ Warn against squeezing the stye; this spreads the infection and may cause cellulitis.
■ Teach the patient or his family members the proper technique for instilling eyedrops or ointments into the cul-de-sac of the lower eyelid.

CONJUNCTIVAL DISORDERS

Inclusion conjunctivitis

Inclusion conjunctivitis (also called *inclusion blennorrhea*) is an acute ocular inflammation resulting from infection by *Chlamydia trachomatis*. Although inclusion conjunctivitis occasionally becomes chronic, the prognosis is usually good.

Causes and incidence
C. trachomatis is an obligate intracellular organism of the lymphogranuloma venereum serotype group. Serotypes D through K are sexually transmitted, and secondary eye involvement in adults occurs in about 1 in 300 genital cases. Because contaminated cervical secretions infect the eyes of the neonate during birth, inclusion conjunctivitis is an important cause of ophthalmia neonatorum. Ocular chlamydial disease occurs most frequently in adults between ages 18 and 30.

Signs and symptoms
Inclusion conjunctivitis develops 5 to 12 days after contamination (it takes longer to develop than gonococcal ophthalmia). In a neonate, reddened eyelids and tearing with moderate mucoid discharge are presenting symptoms. In neonates, pseudomembranes may form, which can lead to conjunctival scarring. In adults, follicles appear inside the lower eyelids; such follicles don't form in infants because the lymphoid tissue isn't yet well developed. Children and adults also develop preauricular lymphadenopathy, and children may develop otitis media as a complication. Inclusion conjunctivitis may persist for weeks or months, possibly with superficial corneal involvement.

Diagnosis
Clinical features and a history of sexual contact with an infected individual suggest inclusion conjunctivitis.

 CONFIRMING DIAGNOSIS
Examination of Giemsa-stained conjunctival scraping reveals cytoplasmic inclusion bodies in conjunctival epithelial cells, and is effective in detecting chlamydial infection in infants. The direct fluorescent monoclonal antibody and enzyme-linked immunosorbent assay are most effective in adults.

Treatment
Because infection isn't limited to the eye in neonates, infants, or adults, systemic antimicrobial treatment is necessary. In infants, effective therapy is achieved with erythromycin. Adults may be given tetracycline, doxycycline, or erythromycin.

Prophylactic tetracycline or erythromycin ointment is applied once, 1 hour after delivery. However, this treatment hasn't been found to be significantly more effective than Credé's method (1% silver nitrate).

Special considerations
■ Keep the patient's eyes as clean as possible, using sterile technique. Clean the eyes from the inner to the outer canthus. Apply warm soaks as needed. Record the amount and color of drainage.
■ Remind the patient not to rub his eyes, which can irritate them.
■ If the patient's eyes are sensitive to light, keep the room dark or suggest that he wear dark glasses.

To prevent further spread of inclusion conjunctivitis:
■ Wash hands thoroughly before and after administering eye medications.
■ Suggest genital examination of the mother of an infected neonate or of any adult with inclusion conjunctivitis.
■ Obtain a history of recent sexual contacts, so they can be examined for chlamydial infection.

Conjunctivitis

Conjunctivitis is characterized by hyperemia of the conjunctiva due to infection, allergy, or chemical reactions. (See *Recognizing conjunctivitis.*) This disorder usually occurs as benign, self-limiting pinkeye; it may also be chronic, possibly indicating degenerative changes or damage from repeated acute attacks.

Causes and incidence

The most common causative organisms include:

- bacterial — *Staphylococcus aureus, Streptococcus pneumoniae, Neisseria gonorrhoeae, Neisseria meningitidis*
- chlamydial — *Chlamydia trachomatis* (inclusion conjunctivitis)
- viral — adenovirus types 3, 7, and 8; herpes simplex virus, type 1.

Other causes include allergic reactions to pollen, grass, topical medications, air pollutants, smoke, or unknown seasonal allergens (vernal conjunctivitis); environmental (wind, dust, and smoke) and occupational irritants (acids and alkalies); and a hypersensitivity to contact lenses or solutions.

Vernal conjunctivitis (so-called because symptoms tend to be worse in the spring) is a severe form of immunoglobulin E-mediated mast cell hypersensitivity reaction. This form of conjunctivitis is bilateral. It usually begins at age 3 to 5 years and persists for about 10 years. It's sometimes associated with other signs of allergy commonly related to pollens, asthma, and allergic rhinitis.

Epidemic keratoconjunctivitis is an acute, highly contagious viral conjunctivitis caused by adenovirus types 8 and 19. It's commonly complicated by visual loss due to corneal subepithelial infiltrates. Health care providers must be careful to wash their hands and sterilize equipment to prevent the spread of this disease.

In the Western hemisphere, conjunctivitis is probably the most common eye disorder.

Signs and symptoms

Conjunctivitis commonly produces hyperemia of the conjunctiva, sometimes accompanied by discharge, tearing and, with corneal involvement, pain and photophobia. It generally doesn't affect vision. Conjunctivitis usually begins in one eye and rapidly spreads to the other by contamination of towels, washcloths, or the patient's own hand.

Acute bacterial conjunctivitis (pinkeye) usually lasts only 2 weeks. The patient typically complains of itching, burning, and the sensation of a foreign body in his eye. The eyelids show a crust of sticky, mucopu-

---

RECOGNIZING CONJUNCTIVITIS

Itching is the hallmark of allergy. Giant papillae resembling cobblestones may be seen on the palpebral conjunctiva, as shown here.

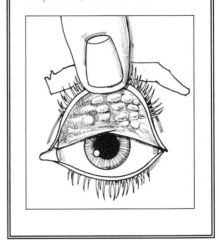

---

rulent discharge. If the disorder is due to *N. gonorrhoeae,* however, the patient exhibits a profuse, purulent discharge.

Viral conjunctivitis produces copious tearing with minimal exudate, and enlargement of the preauricular lymph node. Some viruses follow a chronic course and produce severe disabling disease; others last 2 to 3 weeks and are self-limiting.

Diagnosis

Physical examination reveals peripheral injection of the bulbar conjunctival vessels. In children, possible systemic symptoms include sore throat or fever, if the conjunctivitis is suspected of being of adenoviral origin.

Lymphocytes are predominant in stained smears of conjunctival scrapings if conjunctivitis is caused by a virus. Polymorphonuclear cells (neutrophils) predominate if conjunctivitis is due to bacteria; eosinophils, if it's allergy-related. Culture and sensitivity tests identify the causative bacterial organism and indicate appropriate antibiotic therapy.

Treatment

Treatment for conjunctivitis varies with the cause. Bacterial conjunctivitis requires topical application of the appropriate broad-spectrum antibiotic. Although viral conjunctivitis resists treatment, a sulfonamide or broad-spectrum antibiotic eyedrops may prevent a secondary infection. Patients may be contagious for several weeks after onset. The most important aspect of treatment is preventing transmission. Herpes simplex infection generally responds to treatment with trifluridine drops or vidarabine ointment or oral acyclovir, but the infection may persist for 2 to 3 weeks. Treatment for vernal (allergic) conjunctivitis includes administration of corticosteroid drops followed by cromolyn sodium, cold compresses to relieve itching and, occasionally, oral antihistamines.

Instillation of a one-time dose of erythromycin or 1% silver nitrate solution (Credé's procedure) into the eyes of neonates prevents gonococcal conjunctivitis.

Special considerations

■ Teach proper hand-washing technique because bacterial and viral conjunctivitis are highly contagious. Stress the risk of spreading infection to family members by sharing washcloths, towels, and pillows. Warn against rubbing the infected eye, which can spread the infection to the other eye and to other people.
■ Caution the patient who wears contact lenses to stop wearing the lenses while his eyes are infected.
■ Apply compresses and therapeutic ointment or drops, as ordered. Don't irrigate the eye, as this will spread the infection. Have the patient wash his hands before he uses the medication. Tell him to use clean washcloths or towels frequently so he doesn't infect his other eye.
■ Teach the patient to instill eyedrops and ointments correctly — without touching the bottle tip to his eye or lashes.
■ Remind the patient that the ointment will blur his vision.
■ Stress the importance of safety glasses for the patient who works near chemical irritants.
■ Notify public health authorities if cultures show *N. gonorrhoeae*.

Trachoma

The most common cause of preventable blindness in underdeveloped areas of the world, trachoma is a chronic form of keratoconjunctivitis. This infection is usually confined to the eye but may have a systemic component. Although trachoma itself is self-limiting, it causes permanent damage to the cornea and conjunctiva by scarring the lids, and it results in secondary infections that can lead to blindness. (See *What happens in trachoma.*) Early diagnosis and treatment (before trachoma results in scar formation) ensure recovery but without immunity to reinfection.

Causes and incidence

Trachoma results from infection by *Chlamydia trachomatis*, a gram-negative obligate-intracellular bacterium. These organisms are transmitted from eye to eye by flies and gnats and through hand-to-eye contact in endemic areas.

Trachoma is spread by close contact between family members or among schoolchildren. It's prevalent in Africa, Latin America, and Asia, particularly in children. In the United States, it's prevalent among Native Americans of the Southwest. Other predisposing factors include poverty and poor hygiene due to lack of water. Patients in hot, dusty climates are at greater risk.

Signs and symptoms

Trachoma begins with a mild infection resembling bacterial conjunctivitis (visible conjunctival follicles, red and edematous eyelids, pain, photophobia, tearing, and exudation).

After about 1 month, if the infection is untreated, conjunctival follicles enlarge into inflamed papillae that later become yellow or gray. At this stage, small blood vessels invade the cornea under the upper lid.

Eventually, severe scarring and contraction of the eyelids cause entropion; the eyelids turn inward and the lashes rub against the cornea, producing corneal scarring and visual distortion. In late stages, severe conjunctival scarring may obstruct the lacrimal ducts and cause dry eyes.

PATHOPHYSIOLOGY
WHAT HAPPENS IN TRACHOMA

Trachoma results from infection with *Chlamydia trachomatis* and in its early stages resembles bacterial conjunctivitis. If untreated, this chronic infection can spread to the cornea and lead to scarring and, eventually, to blindness.

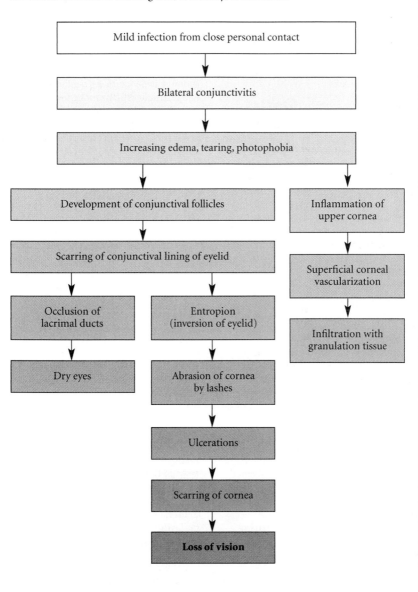

Diagnosis

Follicular conjunctivitis with corneal infiltration, and upper lid or conjunctival scarring suggest trachoma, especially in endemic areas, when these symptoms persist longer than 3 weeks.

 CONFIRMING DIAGNOSIS *Microscopic examination of a Giemsa-stained conjunctival scraping confirms the diagnosis by showing cytoplasmic inclusion bodies, some polymorphonuclear reaction, plasma cells, large macrophages containing phagocytosed debris, and follicle cells.*

Treatment

Primary treatment for trachoma consists of topical or systemic antibiotic therapy with erythromycin (and its derivatives), doxycycline, or sulfonamides. Severe entropion requires surgical correction.

 ALERT *Tetracycline is contraindicated in pregnant females, because it may adversely affect the fetus, and in children younger than age 7, in whom it may permanently discolor teeth.*

Because trachoma is contagious and reinfection is common, some physicians suggest treating entire villages with high incidence rates with antibiotic therapy.

Special considerations

Patient teaching is essential:

■ Emphasize the importance of hand washing and making the best use of available water supplies to maintain good personal hygiene. To prevent trachoma, warn the patient not to allow flies or gnats to settle around his eyes.

■ Because no definitive preventive measure exists (vaccines offer temporary and partial protection, at best), stress the need for strict compliance with the prescribed drug therapy.

■ If ordered, teach the patient or his family how to instill eyedrops correctly.

■ Stress the importance of not sharing contaminated items, such as towels, handkerchiefs, and eye makeup.

CORNEAL DISORDERS
Keratitis

An inflammation of the cornea, keratitis may result from bacterial, fungal, or viral infection. If untreated, the infection can lead to blindness.

Causes

The most common cause of keratitis is infection by herpes simplex virus, type 1 (known as *dendritic corneal ulcer* because of a characteristic branched lesion of the cornea resembling the veins of a leaf). Bacterial corneal ulcers frequently occur as a result of an infected corneal abrasion or a contaminated contact lens. Fungal keratitis is more frequently encountered in tropical climates. Poor lid closure can result in exposure keratitis. Chemicals accidentally splashed into the eye and exposure to ultraviolet light (sunlamps, sunlight, or welding arcs) also can produce keratitis. Vaccinial keratitis may result when the patient has red eye or periocular vesicles coinciding with a history of recent vaccine exposure (such as smallpox vaccination or close contact with a vaccine recipient).

Signs and symptoms

Keratitis is usually unilateral. The patient presents with decreased vision, discomfort ranging from mild irritation to acute pain, tearing, and photophobia. On gross examination with a penlight, the corneal light reflex may appear distorted. When keratitis results from exposure, it usually affects the lower portion of the cornea.

Diagnosis

 CONFIRMING DIAGNOSIS *Visual acuity may be decreased if the lesion is central. Slit-lamp examination confirms keratitis. Staining the eye with a sterile fluorescein strip enables the examiner to discern the extent and depth of the corneal lesion.*

Patient history may reveal a recent infection of the upper respiratory tract accompanied by cold sores, or eye irritation with the wearing of contact lenses. Culture may identify the virus.

Treatment

Treatment for acute keratitis due to herpes simplex virus consists of trifluridine eyedrops, vidarabine ointment, or oral acyclovir. A broad-spectrum antibiotic may prevent secondary bacterial infection. Dendritic keratitis may become chronic with recurrent episodes. Bacterial corneal ulcers require intense topical eyedrop instillation every half hour for the first 48 hours with 2 broad-spectrum antibiotics. Long-term topical therapy may be necessary. (Corticosteroid therapy is contraindicated in dendritic keratitis or any other viral or fungal disease of the cornea.) Fungal keratitis is treated with natamycin.

Exposure keratitis is treated with ointment at night and frequent instillation of artificial tears during the day. A plastic bubble shield may prevent tear evaporation. Vision may be restored by penetrating keratoplasty (corneal transplant) in blindness resulting from corneal scarring.

Special considerations

■ Protect the exposed corneas of unconscious patients by cleaning the eyes daily, applying moisturizing ointment, or covering the eyes with an eye shield.

■ Be aware that the patient with a red eye may have keratitis. Check for a history of contact lens wear, cold sores, or recent foreign-body sensation. Refer the patient for slit-lamp examination as soon as possible for intense treatment.

Corneal abrasion

A corneal abrasion is a scratch on the surface epithelium of the cornea. An abrasion, or foreign body in the eye, is the most common eye injury. With treatment, the prognosis is usually good.

Causes and incidence

A corneal abrasion usually results from a foreign body, such as a cinder or a piece of dust, dirt, or grit that becomes embedded under the eyelid. Even if the foreign body is washed out by tears, it may still injure the cornea. Small pieces of metal that get in the eyes of workers who don't wear protective glasses quickly form a rust ring on the cornea and cause corneal abrasion. Such abrasions also commonly occur in the eyes of people who fall asleep wearing hard contact lenses or whose lenses aren't fitted properly.

A corneal scratch produced by a fingernail, a piece of paper, or other organic substance may cause a persistent lesion. The epithelium doesn't always heal properly, and a recurrent corneal erosion may develop, with delayed effects more severe than the original injury.

In the United States, corneal abrasions are a common ophthalmologic cause of emergency department visits. Incidence is highest among younger, physically active individuals; corneal abrasions are rare in elderly people.

Signs and symptoms

A corneal abrasion typically produces redness, increased tearing, discomfort with blinking, a sensation of "something in the eye" and, because the cornea is richly endowed with nerve endings from the trigeminal nerve (cranial nerve V), pain disproportionate to the size of the injury. It may also affect visual acuity, depending on the size and location of the injury.

Diagnosis

History of eye trauma or prolonged wearing of contact lenses and typical symptoms suggest corneal abrasion.

CONFIRMING DIAGNOSIS
Staining the cornea with fluorescein stain confirms the diagnosis: The injured area appears green when examined with a flashlight. Slit-lamp examination discloses depth and allows measurement of the abrasion.

Examining the eye with a flashlight may reveal a foreign body on the cornea; the eyelid must be everted to check for a foreign body embedded under the lid.

Before beginning treatment, a test to determine visual acuity provides a medical baseline and a legal safeguard.

Treatment

Topical anesthetic eyedrops are instilled in the affected eye before removal of a superficial foreign body, using a foreign body spud. A rust ring on the cornea must be removed with an ophthalmic burr. When only partial removal is possible, reepithelialization lifts the ring again to the surface and allows complete removal the following day.

Treatment also includes instillation of broad-spectrum antibiotic eyedrops in the affected eye every 3 to 4 hours. Application of a pressure patch prevents further corneal irritation when the patient blinks. If the patient wears contact lenses, it may be advisable for him to abstain from wearing the lenses until the corneal abrasion heals.

Special considerations

- Assist with examination of the eye. Check visual acuity before beginning treatment.
- If a foreign body is visible, carefully irrigate with normal saline solution.
- Tell the patient with an eye patch to leave it in place for 6 to 12 hours. Warn that a patch alters depth perception, so advise caution in daily activities, such as climbing stairs or stepping off a curb.
- Reassure the patient that the corneal epithelium usually heals in 24 to 48 hours.
- Stress the importance of instilling antibiotic eyedrops, as ordered, because an untreated corneal abrasion, if infected, can lead to a corneal ulcer and permanent vision loss. Teach the patient the proper way to instill eye medications.
- Emphasize the importance of safety glasses to protect workers' eyes from flying fragments. Also review instructions for wearing and caring for contact lenses, to prevent further trauma.

Corneal ulcers

A major cause of blindness worldwide, ulcers produce corneal scarring or perforation. They occur in the central or marginal areas of the cornea, vary in shape and size, and may be singular or multiple. Marginal ulcers are the most common form. Prompt treatment (within hours of onset) can prevent visual impairment.

Causes

Corneal ulcers generally result from protozoan, bacterial, viral, or fungal infections.

Common bacterial sources include *Staphylococcus aureus, Pseudomonas aeruginosa, Streptococcus viridans, Streptococcus (Diplococcus) pneumoniae,* and *Moraxella liquefaciens;* viral sources comprise herpes simplex type 1, variola, vaccinia, and varicella-zoster viruses; and common fungal sources are *Candida, Fusarium,* and *Cephalosporium.*

Other causes include trauma, exposure, reactions to bacterial infections, toxins, trichiasis, entropion, allergens, and wearing of contact lenses. (See *What happens in corneal ulceration.*) Tuberculoprotein causes a classic phlyctenular keratoconjunctivitis, vitamin A deficiency results in xerophthalmia, and fifth cranial nerve lesions lead to neurotropic ulcers.

Signs and symptoms

Typically, corneal ulceration begins with pain (aggravated by blinking) and photophobia, followed by increased tearing. Eventually, central corneal ulceration produces pronounced visual blurring. The eye may appear injected. If a bacterial ulcer is present, purulent discharge is possible.

Diagnosis

A history of trauma or use of contact lenses and flashlight examination that reveals irregular corneal surface suggest corneal ulcer. Exudate may be present on the cornea, and a hypopyon (accumulation of white cells in the anterior chamber) may appear as a white crescent moon that moves when the head is tilted.

CONFIRMING DIAGNOSIS
Fluorescein dye, instilled in the conjunctival sac, stains the outline of the ulcer and confirms the diagnosis.

Culture and sensitivity testing of corneal scrapings may identify the causative bacteria or fungus, and may indicate appropriate antibiotic or antifungal therapy.

Treatment

Prompt treatment is essential for all forms of corneal ulcer to prevent complications and permanent visual impairment. Treatment usually consists of systemic and topical broad-spectrum antibiotics until culture results identify the causative organism. The goals of treatment are to eliminate the

PATHOPHYSIOLOGY
WHAT HAPPENS IN CORNEAL ULCERATION

Corneal ulcers can be caused by infection (protozoan, bacterial, viral, or fungal), trauma, exposure, toxins, contact lenses, or allergens. Scarring or perforation can cause changes in the eye structure and can lead to partial or total vision loss.

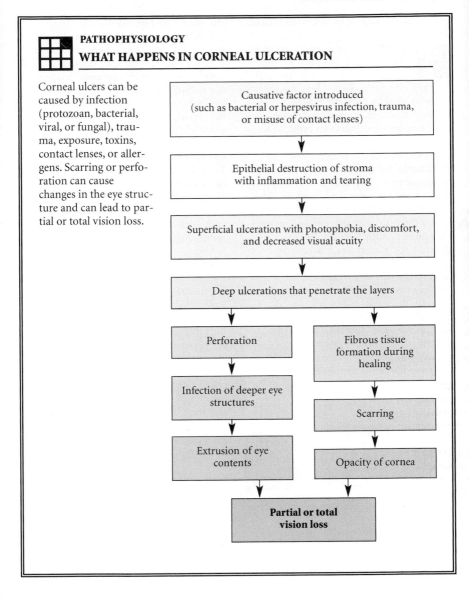

Causative factor introduced
(such as bacterial or herpesvirus infection, trauma, or misuse of contact lenses)

↓

Epithelial destruction of stroma
with inflammation and tearing

↓

Superficial ulceration with photophobia, discomfort, and decreased visual acuity

↓

Deep ulcerations that penetrate the layers

↓ ↓

Perforation

↓

Infection of deeper eye structures

↓

Extrusion of eye contents

Fibrous tissue formation during healing

↓

Scarring

↓

Opacity of cornea

↓ ↓

Partial or total vision loss

---

underlying cause of the ulcer and to relieve pain:

- Fungi — topical instillation of natamycin for *Fusarium, Cephalosporium,* and *Candida.*
- Herpes simplex type 1 virus — topical application of trifluridine drops or vidarabine ointment. Corneal ulcers resulting from a viral infection often recur, requiring further treatment with trifluridine.

- Hypovitaminosis A — correction of dietary deficiency or GI malabsorption of vitamin A.
- Infection by *P. aeruginosa* — polymyxin B and gentamicin, administered topically and by subconjunctival injection, or carbenicillin and tobramycin I.V. Because this type of corneal ulcer spreads so rapidly, it can cause corneal perforation and loss of the eye within 48 hours. Immediate treat-

ment and isolation of hospitalized patients are required.

> ⊙ **ALERT** *Treatment for a corneal ulcer due to bacterial infection should never include an eye patch because patching creates the dark, warm, moist environment ideal for bacterial growth.*

- Neurotropic ulcers or exposure keratitis — frequent instillation of artificial tears or lubricating ointments and use of a plastic bubble eye shield.
- Varicella-zoster virus — topical sulfonamide ointment applied three to four times daily to prevent secondary infection. These lesions are unilateral, following the pathway of the fifth cranial nerve, and are typically quite painful. Give analgesics as ordered. Associated anterior uveitis requires cycloplegic eyedrops. Watch for signs of secondary glaucoma (transient vision loss and halos around lights).

Special considerations

- Keep the room darkened and orient the patient as necessary.
- Teach the patient how to properly clean and wear his contact lenses to prevent a recurrence.

UVEAL TRACT, RETINAL, AND LENS DISORDERS

Uveitis

Uveitis is inflammation of the uveal tract. It occurs as anterior uveitis, which affects the iris (iritis) or both the iris and the ciliary body (iridocyclitis); as posterior uveitis, which affects the choroid (choroiditis) or both the choroid and the retina (chorioretinitis); or as panuveitis, which affects the entire uveal tract. Although clinical distinction isn't always possible, anterior uveitis occurs in two forms — granulomatous and nongranulomatous.

Granulomatous uveitis was once thought to be caused by tuberculosis bacilli; nongranulomatous uveitis, by streptococci. Although this isn't true, the terms are

still used. (See *Granulomatous and nongranulomatous uveitis.*) Untreated anterior uveitis may result in elevated intraocular pressure (IOP), leading to vision loss. With immediate treatment, anterior uveitis usually subsides after a few days to several weeks; however, recurrence can occur. Posterior uveitis may lead to vision loss if the macula is involved.

Causes and incidence

Typically, uveitis is idiopathic. However, it can result from allergy, bacteria, viruses, fungi, chemicals, trauma, or surgery; or it may be associated with systemic diseases, such as rheumatoid arthritis, ankylosing spondylitis, and toxoplasmosis.

Uveitis occurs in 15 of every 100,000 people.

Signs and symptoms

Anterior uveitis produces moderate to severe unilateral eye pain; severe ciliary injection; photophobia; tearing; a small, nonreactive pupil; and blurred vision (due to the increased number of cells in the aqueous humor). It sometimes produces deposits called keratic precipitates on the back of the cornea, which may be seen in the anterior chamber. The iris may adhere to the lens, causing posterior synechiae and pupillary distortion; pain and photophobia may occur. Onset may be acute or insidious.

Posterior uveitis begins insidiously, with complaints of slightly decreased or blurred vision or floating spots. Posterior uveitis may be acute or chronic, and it may affect one or both eyes. Retinal damage caused by lesions from toxoplasmosis and retinal detachments may occur. Refer the patient to an ophthalmologist for dilated fundus examination and treatment for local systemic diseases.

Diagnosis

> ⟨ℚ⟩ **CONFIRMING DIAGNOSIS** *In anterior and posterior uveitis, a slit-lamp examination shows a "flare and cell" pattern, which looks like particles dancing in a sunbeam. With a special lens, slit-lamp and ophthalmoscopic examination can also identify active inflammatory fundus lesions involving the retina and choroid, al-*

GRANULOMATOUS AND NONGRANULOMATOUS UVEITIS

Various factors that differentiate granulomatous and nongranulomatous uveitis are listed below.

Factor	Granulomatous	Nongranulomatous
Location	▪ Usually, posterior part of uveal tract	▪ Anterior part of the iris and ciliary body
Onset	▪ Insidious	▪ Acute
Pain	▪ None or slight	▪ Marked
Photophobia	▪ Slight	▪ Marked
Course	▪ Chronic	▪ Acute
Prognosis	▪ Fair to poor	▪ Good
Recurrence	▪ Occasional	▪ Common
Blurred vision	▪ Marked	▪ Moderate

though a hazy vitreous may obscure the view.

In posterior uveitis, serologic tests may be used to rule out toxoplasmosis.

Treatment

Uveitis requires vigorous and prompt management, which includes treatment for any known underlying cause — corticosteroids with antibiotic therapy for infectious diseases and suppression therapy for autoimmune diseases — and application of a topical cycloplegic, such as 1% atropine sulfate, and of topical corticosteroids applied three to four times daily. For severe uveitis, therapy includes oral systemic corticosteroids.

ALERT *Long-term steroid therapy can cause a rise in IOP or cataracts. Carefully monitor IOP during acute inflammation. If IOP rises, therapy should include an antiglaucoma medication, such as brimonidine (Alphagan), an alpha$_2$-adrenergic agonist, or dorzolamide (Trusopt), a sulfonamide.*

Occasionally, posterior uveitis requires systemic immunosuppression with azathioprine or cyclosporine.

Special considerations

- Encourage rest during the acute phase.
- Teach the patient the proper method of instilling eyedrops.
- Suggest the use of dark glasses to ease the discomfort of photophobia.
- Instruct the patient to watch for and report adverse effects of systemic corticosteroid therapy (for example, edema or muscle weakness).
- Stress the importance of follow-up care for IOP checks while the patient is taking steroids. Tell the patient to seek treatment immediately at the first sign of iritis.

Retinal detachment

Retinal detachment occurs when the outer retinal pigment epithelium splits from the neural retina, creating subretinal space. This space then fills with fluid, called *subretinal fluid*. Retinal detachment usually involves only one eye, but may later involve the other eye. Surgical reattachment is usually successful. However, the prognosis for good vision depends on which area of the retina has been affected.

Causes and incidence

Any retinal tear or hole allows the liquid vitreous to seep between the retinal layers, separating the retina from its choroidal blood supply. Predisposing factors include myopia, intraocular surgery, and trauma. In adults, retinal detachment usually results from degenerative changes of aging, which cause a spontaneous retinal hole. Perhaps the influence of trauma explains why retinal detachment is twice as common in males. Retinal detachment may also result from seepage of fluid into the subretinal space (because of inflammation, tumors, or systemic diseases) or from traction that's placed on the retina by vitreous bands or membranes (due to proliferative diabetic retinopathy, posterior uveitis, or a traumatic intraocular foreign body).

Retinal detachment is rare in children, but occasionally can develop as a result of retinopathy of prematurity, tumors (retinoblastomas), trauma, or myopia (which tends to run in families).

In the United States, approximately 10,000 people per year are affected by retinal detachments.

Signs and symptoms

Initially, the patient may complain of floating spots and recurrent flashes of light (photopsia). However, as detachment progresses, gradual, painless vision loss may be described as a veil, curtain, or cobweb that eliminates a portion of the visual field.

Diagnosis

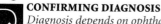 **CONFIRMING DIAGNOSIS** *Diagnosis depends on ophthalmoscopy after full pupil dilation. Examination shows the usually transparent retina as gray and opaque; in severe detachment, it reveals folds in the retina and ballooning out of the area. Indirect ophthalmoscopy is used to search for retinal tears. Ultrasound is performed if the lens is opaque.*

Treatment

Treatment depends on the location and severity of the detachment. It may include restriction of eye movements and complete bed rest until surgical reattachment is done. A hole in the peripheral retina can be treated with cryothermy; in the posterior portion, with laser therapy. Retinal detachment usually requires a scleral buckling procedure or a vitrectomy to reattach the retina. Basic salt solution is used to replace the retina while the vitreous is removed.

Certain types of uncomplicated retinal detachment may be treated by pneumatic retinopexy, in which an expansile gas is initially injected into the vitreous cavity and the patient's head is positioned to facilitate retina reattachment. This procedure can be performed under local anesthesia.

Special considerations

- Provide emotional support because the patient may be understandably distraught about his loss of vision.
- During transportation, position the patient's head so that the detached portion of the retina will fall back with the aid of gravity.
- To prepare for surgery, wash the patient's face with no-tears shampoo. Give antibiotics and cycloplegic-mydriatic eyedrops.
- Postoperatively, position the patient facedown on his right or left side and with the head of the bed raised. Discourage straining at stool, bending down, hard coughing, sneezing, or vomiting, which can raise intraocular pressure. Antiemetics may be indicated.
- Protect the patient's eye with a shield or glasses.
- To reduce edema and discomfort, apply ice packs as ordered. Administer pain medication, as ordered, for eye pain.
- After removing the eye shield, gently clean the eye with cycloplegic eyedrops and administer steroid-antibiotic eyedrops, as ordered. Use cold compresses to decrease swelling and pain.
- Administer analgesics as needed, and report persistent pain. Teach the patient how to properly instill eyedrops, and emphasize compliance and follow-up care. Suggest dark glasses to compensate for light sensitivity caused by cycloplegia.

ANATOMY OF VASCULAR RETINOPATHY

Vascular changes that occur with retinopathy, as seen by an ophthalmoscope, are depicted below.

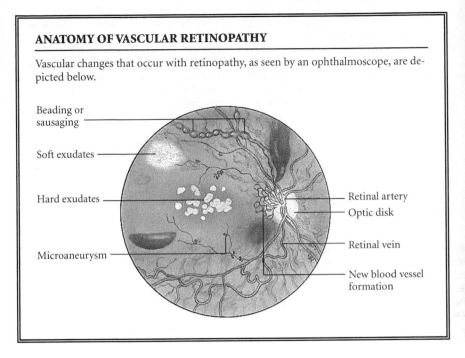

Beading or sausaging

Soft exudates

Hard exudates

Microaneurysm

Retinal artery

Optic disk

Retinal vein

New blood vessel formation

Vascular retinopathies

Vascular retinopathies are noninflammatory retinal disorders that result from interference with the blood supply to the eyes. The five distinct types of vascular retinopathy are central retinal artery occlusion, central retinal vein occlusion, diabetic retinopathy, hypertensive retinopathy, and sickle cell retinopathy.

Causes and incidence

When one of the arteries maintaining blood circulation in the retina becomes obstructed, the diminished blood flow causes visual deficits. (See *Anatomy of vascular retinopathy.*)

Central retinal artery occlusion may be idiopathic or may result from embolism, atherosclerosis, infection, or conditions that retard blood flow, such as temporal arteritis, carotid occlusion, and heart failure. This occlusion is rare, occurs unilaterally, and usually affects elderly patients. However, if it occurs in a younger person, the obstruction may have originated in the heart (such as embolization from plaque materi-

al from valve vegetations) and should be investigated accordingly.

Causes of central retinal vein occlusion include atherosclerosis, hypertension, optic disk edema, hypercoagulable states (polycythemia, leukemia, or sickle cell disease), glaucoma, retrobulbar compression (such as an orbital tumor), and drugs such as hormonal contraceptives. This form of vascular retinopathy is most prevalent in elderly patients and is characterized by impaired venous outflow.

Diabetic retinopathy results from juvenile or adult diabetes. Microcirculatory changes occur more rapidly when diabetes is poorly controlled. About 90% of patients with juvenile diabetes develop retinopathy within 20 years of onset of diabetes. In adults with diabetes, incidence increases with the duration of diabetes; 80% of patients who have had diabetes for 20 to 25 years develop retinopathy. This condition is a leading cause of acquired adult blindness.

Hypertensive retinopathy results from prolonged hypertensive disease, producing retinal vasospasm, and consequent damage and arteriolar narrowing.

Sickle cell retinopathy results from impaired ability of the sickled cell to pass through microvasculature, producing vaso-occlusion. This leads to microaneurysms, chorioretinal infarction, and retinal detachment.

Signs and symptoms

Central retinal artery occlusion produces sudden, painless, unilateral loss of vision (partial or complete). It may follow amaurosis fugax or transient episodes of unilateral loss of vision lasting from a few seconds to minutes, probably due to vasospasm. This condition typically causes permanent blindness. However, some patients experience spontaneous resolution within hours and regain partial vision.

Central retinal vein occlusion causes reduced visual acuity, allowing perception of only hand movement and light. This condition is painless, except when it results in secondary neovascular glaucoma (uncontrolled proliferation of weak blood vessels). The prognosis is poor—some patients with this condition develop secondary glaucoma within 3 to 4 months after occlusion.

Nonproliferative diabetic retinopathy produces changes in the lining of the retinal blood vessels that cause the vessels to leak plasma or fatty substances, which decrease or block blood flow (nonperfusion) within the retina. This disorder may also produce microaneurysms and small hemorrhages. Nonproliferative retinopathy causes no symptoms in some patients; in others, leakage of fluid into the macular region causes significant loss of central visual acuity (necessary for reading and driving) and diminished night vision.

Proliferative diabetic retinopathy produces fragile new blood vessels on the disk (neovascularization) and elsewhere in the fundus. These vessels can grow into the vitreous and then rupture, causing vitreous hemorrhage with corresponding sudden vision loss. Scar tissue that may form along the new blood vessels can pull on the retina, causing it to tear or even detach.

Symptoms of hypertensive retinopathy include blurred vision, often accompanied by headache. Ophthalmoscopic examination may reveal diffuse binocular narrowing, venular tortuosity, silver wire reflexes, macular stars, and swelling of the head of the optic nerve (disk edema). Severe, prolonged disease eventually produces blindness; mild, prolonged disease, visual defects.

Symptoms of sickle cell retinopathy include peripheral arteriolar occlusions, peripheral arteriovenous anastomoses, sea fan neurovascular fronds, vitreous hemorrhage as tractional forces and vitreous collapse tear fragile neovascular membranes and, with advanced disease, severe vitreous traction and retinal detachment.

Diagnosis

Check visual acuity and then vital signs, including blood pressure. Diagnosis is made on fundal examination with an ophthalmoscope. Determine if female patients are pregnant; hypertensive retinopathy may be an early sign of preeclampsia. (See *Diagnostic tests for vascular retinopathies.*)

Treatment

No treatment has been shown to control central retinal artery occlusion. However, an attempt is made to release the occlusion into the peripheral circulation. To reduce intraocular pressure, therapy includes acetazolamide I.V., eyeball massage, thrombolysis by intra-arterial injection or I.V., high concentrations of inhaled oxygen, and anterior chamber paracentesis (to try to move the arterial obstruction into the peripheral field).

Therapy for central retinal vein occlusion may include aspirin, which acts as a mild anticoagulant. Patients with central retinal vein occlusion have reported improved vision after direct injection of tissue plasminogen activator into the retinal venous system. Laser photocoagulation can reduce the risk of neovascular glaucoma for some patients whose eyes have widespread capillary nonperfusion.

Treatment for nonproliferative diabetic retinopathy is prophylactic. Careful control of blood glucose levels may reduce the severity of the retinopathy or delay its onset. Patients with early symptoms of microaneurysms should have frequent eye exam-

DIAGNOSTIC TESTS FOR VASCULAR RETINOPATHIES

Central retinal artery occlusion
- Ophthalmoscopy (direct or indirect): shows blockage of retinal arterioles during a transient attack.
- Retinal examination: within 2 hours of onset, shows clumps or segmentation in the artery; later, milky white retina around the disk due to swelling and necrosis of ganglion cells caused by reduced blood supply; also shows a cherry-red spot in the macula that subsides after several weeks.
- Color Doppler tests: evaluate carotid occlusion with no need for arteriography.
- Physical examination: reveals the underlying cause of vascular retinopathy, for example, diabetes or hypertension.

Central retinal vein occlusion
- Ophthalmoscopy (direct or indirect): shows flame-shaped hemorrhages, retinal vein engorgement, white patches among hemorrhages, and edema around the disk.
- Color Doppler tests: confirm or rule out occlusion of blood vessels.
- Physical examination: reveals the underlying cause.

Diabetic retinopathy
- Indirect ophthalmoscopic examination: shows retinal changes such as microaneurysms (earliest change), retinal hemorrhages and edema, venous dilation and beading, lipid exudates, fibrous bands in the vitreous, and growth of new blood vessels. Infarcts of the nerve fiber layer are observed.
- Fluorescein angiography: shows leakage of fluorescein from weak-walled vessels and "lights up" microaneurysms, differentiating them from true hemorrhages.
- History: of diabetes.

Hypertensive retinopathy
- Ophthalmoscopy (direct or indirect): in early stages, shows hard, shiny deposits; flame-shaped hemorrhages; silver wire appearance of narrowed arterioles; and nicking of veins where arteries cross them (atrioventricular nicking). In late stages, shows cotton wool patches, lipid exudates, retinal edema, papilledema due to ischemia and capillary insufficiency, hemorrhages, and microaneurysms in both eyes.
- Physical examination: reveals elevated blood pressure.
- History: of decreased vision, headache, and nausea.
- History: of hypertension, usually acute or malignant.

inations (three to four times per year); children with diabetes should have an annual eye examination.

Treatment for proliferative diabetic retinopathy or severe macular edema is laser photocoagulation, which cauterizes the leaking blood vessels. Laser treatment may be focal (aimed at new blood vessels) or panretinal (placing burns throughout the peripheral retina). Despite treatment, neovascularization continues to proliferate, and vitreous hemorrhage, with or without retinal detachment, may follow. If the blood isn't absorbed in 6 weeks to 3 months, vitrectomy may restore partial vision.

Treatment for hypertensive retinopathy includes control of blood pressure with appropriate drugs, diet, and exercise. Treating the systemic hypertension should improve the condition of the eyes. If left untreated, hypertensive retinopathy results in severe vision loss.

The treatment goal of sickle cell retinopathy is to reduce the risk of, or prevent or eliminate, retinal neovascularization. Patients with symptoms should be followed twice a year with ocular examinations and dilated retinal evaluation. Proliferative disease should be treated with fluorescein angiography and panretinal photocoagulation. Cryotherapy hasn't been proven to be effective and has a high complication rate.

Special considerations
■ Be sure to monitor a patient's blood pressure if he complains of occipital headache and blurred vision.

 ALERT *Arrange for immediate ophthalmologic evaluation when a patient complains of sudden, unilateral loss of vision. Blindness may be permanent if treatment is delayed.*
■ Encourage a diabetic patient to comply with the prescribed regimen.
■ For a patient with hypertensive retinopathy, stress the importance of complying with antihypertensive therapy.

Age-related macular degeneration

Macular degeneration is the atrophy or degeneration of the macular region of the retina. Two types of age-related macular degeneration occur. The dry or atrophic form is characterized by atrophic pigment epithelial changes and is most often associated with a slow, progressive, and mild vision loss. The wet, exudative form causes progressive visual distortion leading to vision loss. It's characterized by subretinal neovascularization that causes leakage, hemorrhage, and fibrovascular scar formation, which produce significant loss of central vision.

Causes and incidence
Age-related macular degeneration results from underlying pathologic changes that occur primarily at the level of the retinal pigment epithelium, Bruch's membrane, and the choriocapillaris in the macular region. Drusen (bumps), which are common in elderly people, appear as yellow deposits beneath the pigment epithelium and may be prominent in the macula. No predisposing conditions have been identified; however, some forms of the disorder are hereditary.

Macular degeneration is the most common cause of legal blindness in adults, accounting for about 12% of blindness cases in the United States and for about 17% of new blindness cases. It's also one of the causes of severe irreversible loss of central vision in elderly people — by age 75, almost 15% of people have this condition. Whites have the highest incidence. Other risk factors are family history and cigarette smoking.

Signs and symptoms
The patient notices a change in central vision. Initially, straight lines (for example, of buildings) become distorted; later, a blank area appears in the center of a printed page (central scotoma).

Diagnosis
■ Indirect ophthalmoscopy — fundus examination through a dilated pupil may reveal gross macular changes.
■ I.V. fluorescein angiography — sequential photographs may show leaking vessels as fluorescein dye flows into the tissues from the subretinal neovascular net.
■ Amsler's grid — used to monitor visual field loss.

Treatment
Laser photocoagulation reduces the incidence of severe vision loss in the patient with subretinal neovascularization, turning serous age-related macular degeneration to the dry form.

Photodynamic therapy, which can be performed in a physician's office, is an option for the patient with wet macular degeneration. In this procedure, verteporfin (a light-sensitive medication) is injected into a vein in the patient's arm and allowed to circulate to the eyes. The physician then shines a laser into the eyes, and the verteporfin produces a chemical reaction that destroys abnormal blood vessels. If the vessels regrow, the procedure can be repeated.

Special considerations
■ Inform the patient with bilateral central vision loss of the visual rehabilitation services available to him.
■ Special devices, such as low-vision optical aids, are available to improve the quali-

ty of life in the patient with good peripheral vision.

Cataract

The most common cause of correctable vision loss, a cataract is a gradually developing opacity of the lens or lens capsule of the eye. Cataracts commonly occur bilaterally, with each progressing independently. Exceptions are traumatic cataracts, which are usually unilateral, and congenital cataracts, which may remain stationary. The prognosis is generally good; surgery improves vision in 95% of affected people.

Causes and incidence
Cataracts have various causes:
- Senile cataracts develop in elderly patients, probably because of degenerative changes in the chemical state of lens proteins.
- Congenital cataracts occur in neonates as genetic defects or as a sequela of maternal rubella during the first trimester. They acquire them through autosomal dominant inheritance, which will occur even if only one parent passes it along. Fifty percent of children in such families are affected.
- Traumatic cataracts develop after a foreign body injures the lens with sufficient force to allow aqueous or vitreous humor to enter the lens capsule. Trauma may also dislocate the lens.
- Complicated cataracts develop as secondary effects in patients with uveitis, glaucoma, or retinitis pigmentosa, or in the course of a systemic disease, such as diabetes, hypoparathyroidism, or atopic dermatitis. They can also result from exposure to ionizing radiation or infrared rays.
- Toxic cataracts result from drug or chemical toxicity with prednisone, ergot alkaloids, dinitrophenol, naphthalene, phenothiazines, or pilocarpine or from extended exposure to ultraviolet rays.

Cataracts occur as part of the aging process and are most prevalent in people older than age 70.

Signs and symptoms
Characteristically, a patient with a cataract experiences painless, gradual blurring and loss of vision. As the cataract progresses, the normally black pupil appears hazy, and when a mature cataract develops, the white lens may be seen through the pupil. Some patients complain of blinding glare from headlights when they drive at night; others complain of poor reading vision, and of an unpleasant glare and poor vision in bright sunlight. Patients with central opacities report better vision in dim light than in bright light because the cataract is nuclear and, as the pupils dilate, patients can see around the lens opacity.

Diagnosis
On examination, visual acuity is decreased, and the lens opacity remains unnoticeable until the cataract is advanced.

 CONFIRMING DIAGNOSIS
Ophthalmoscopy or slit-lamp examination confirms the diagnosis by revealing a dark area in the normally homogeneous red reflex.

Treatment
Treatment consists of surgical extraction of the cataractous lens opacity and intraoperative correction of visual deficits. The current trend is to perform the surgery as a same-day procedure. Surgical procedures include the following:
- Extracapsular cataract extraction (ECCE) removes the anterior lens capsule and cortex, leaving the posterior capsule intact. With this procedure, a posterior chamber intraocular lens (IOL) is implanted where the patient's own lens used to be. (A posterior chamber IOL is currently the most common type used in the United States.) This procedure is appropriate for use in patients of all ages.
- Phacoemulsification uses ultrasonic vibrations to fragment and then emulsify the lens, which is then aspirated through a small incision.
- Intracapsular cataract extraction removes the entire lens within the intact capsule. This procedure is seldom performed today. ECCE with phacoemulsification has replaced it as the most commonly performed procedure.
- Discission and aspiration can still be used for children with soft cataracts, but

this procedure has largely been replaced by phacoemulsification.

Infection is the most serious complication of intraocular surgery. Wound dehiscence can occur but is seldom a complication because of the small incision and minute sutures that are used. Hyphema, pupillary block glaucoma, and retinal detachment still occasionally occur.

The patient with an IOL implant may experience improved vision shortly after surgery if there's no corneal or retinal pathology. Most IOLs correct for distance vision, but new IOLs are multifocal. However, the majority of patients will need either corrective reading glasses or a corrective contact lens, which will be fitted sometime between 4 and 6 weeks after surgery.

Where no IOL has been implanted, the patient may be given temporary aphakic cataract glasses; in about 4 to 8 weeks, he'll be refracted for his own glasses.

Some patients who have an extracapsular cataract extraction develop a secondary membrane in the posterior lens capsule (which has been left intact), which causes decreased visual acuity. This membrane can be removed by the Nd:YAG laser, which cuts an area out of the center of the membrane, thereby restoring vision. Laser therapy isn't used to remove a cataract.

Posterior capsular opacification occurs in approximately 15% to 20% of all patients within 2 years after cataract surgery.

Special considerations

After surgery to extract a cataract:
- Because the patient will be discharged after he recovers from anesthesia, remind him to return for a checkup the next day, and warn him to avoid activities that increase intraocular pressure such as straining.
- Urge the patient to protect the eye from accidental injury at night by wearing a plastic or metal shield with perforations; a shield or glasses should be worn for protection during the day.
- Before discharge, teach the patient to administer antibiotic ointment or drops to prevent infection and steroids to reduce inflammation; combination steroid-antibiotic eyedrops can also be used.
- Advise the patient to watch for the development of complications, such as a sharp pain in the eye uncontrolled by analgesics as a result of hyphema, or clouding in the anterior chamber (which may herald an infection), and to report them immediately.
- Caution the patient about activity restrictions, and advise him that it will take several weeks for him to receive his corrective reading glasses or lenses.

Retinitis pigmentosa

Retinitis pigmentosa is a group of hereditary disorders whose common feature is a gradual deterioration of the light-sensitive cells of the retina. Postmortem examination of the eyes reveals pigment cells that have clumped together as a result of the pigment epithelium budding off and settling within the layers of the retina. Retinitis pigmentosa often accompanies other hereditary disorders in several distinct syndromes — including Usher's syndrome, in which sight and hearing are both affected; and Laurence-Moon-Biedl syndrome (most common), which is typified by visual destruction from retinitis pigmentosa, with obesity, mental retardation, polydactyly, hypogenitalism, and spastic paraplegia.

Causes and incidence

Retinitis pigmentosa can be classified according to its inheritance pattern: autosomal dominant, autosomal recessive, and X-linked. Typically, in all forms of retinitis pigmentosa, the retinal rods slowly deteriorate. Clumps of pigment resembling bone corpuscles aggregate in the peripheral region of the retina and later involve the macular and peripheral areas. Visual symptoms usually appear between ages 10 and 30, though some children may become blind within the first year of life.

Retinitis pigmentosa affects 1 of every 4,000 people in the United States.

Signs and symptoms

Generally, night blindness occurs while the patient is in his teens. As the disease progresses, his visual field gradually constricts,

causing tunnel or "gun-barrel" vision.
Many people retain this tunnel of useful vision until quite late in life. The speed of vision loss varies considerably from person to person. However, blindness follows invasion of the macular region.

Diagnosis
A detailed family history may imply predisposition to retinitis pigmentosa. In the patient whose history suggests this condition, the following tests help confirm diagnosis.
■ Electroretinography shows a slower than normal or absent retinal response time.
■ Fluorescein angiography visualizes white dots (areas of dyspigmentation) in the epithelium.
■ Ophthalmoscopy may initially show normal fundi but later shows black pigmentary disturbance and white dots (dyspigmentation) in the epithelium.
■ Visual field testing (using a tangent screen) detects ring scotomata.

Treatment
No cure exists for retinitis pigmentosa. However, vitamin A and E supplementation may slow degeneration. Researchers are working on a procedure in which fetal retinal tissue is transplanted into people with retinitis pigmentosa, but its potential efficacy is unknown.

Special considerations
■ Teach the patient and his family about retinitis pigmentosa.
■ Encourage the patient to use sunglasses to protect the retina from ultraviolet light and to help preserve vision.
■ Explain that the disorder is hereditary, and suggest genetic counseling for adults who risk transmitting it to their children.
■ Encourage annual eye examinations to monitor the progress of the disease.
■ Warn the patient that he might not be able to drive a car safely at night.
■ Refer the patient to a social service agency or to the National Retinitis Pigmentosa Foundation for information and for counseling to prepare him for eventual blindness.
■ Because the prospect of blindness is frightening, your emotional support and guidance are indispensable.

MISCELLANEOUS DISORDERS

Optic atrophy

Optic atrophy, or degeneration of the optic nerve, can develop spontaneously (primary) or can follow inflammation or edema of the nerve head (secondary). Some forms of this condition may subside without treatment, but degeneration of the optic nerve is irreversible.

Causes
Optic atrophy usually results from central nervous system disorders (such as chiasmal tumors, syphilis, ischemic optic neuropathy, drugs, retinal vascular disease, or degenerative disease) or from end-stage glaucoma. Other causes include retinitis pigmentosa; chronic papilledema and papillitis; glaucoma; trauma; central retinal artery or vein occlusion that interrupts the blood supply to the optic nerve, causing degeneration of ganglion cells; ingestion of toxins, such as methanol and quinine; and deficiencies of vitamin B_{12}, amino acids, and zinc.
    There are several rare forms of hereditary optic atrophy that can affect children and young adults.

Signs and symptoms
Optic atrophy causes abrupt or gradual painless loss of visual field or visual acuity, with subtle changes in color vision.

Diagnosis
CONFIRMING DIAGNOSIS *Visual acuity testing reveals poor vision. An afferent pupillary defect is noted when pupils are examined. Fundus examination through a dilated pupil with an ophthalmoscope shows pallor of the nerve head from loss of microvascular circulation in the disk and deposit of fibrous or glial tissue. Visual field testing reveals a scotoma and, possibly, major visual field impairment.*

Treatment
Optic atrophy is irreversible, so treatment aims to correct the underlying cause and

prevent further vision loss. Steroids may be given to decrease inflammation and swelling, if the cause is found to be ischemic neuropathy. If a space-occupying lesion is the cause, neurosurgery may be required. In multiple sclerosis, optic neuritis often subsides spontaneously but may recur and improve repeatedly.

Special considerations
- Provide symptomatic care during diagnostic procedures and treatment. Assist the patient who's visually compromised to perform daily activities.
- Explain procedures, to minimize anxiety. Offer emotional support to help the patient deal with loss of vision.

Extraocular motor nerve palsies

Extraocular motor nerve palsies are dysfunctions of the third, fourth, and sixth cranial nerves. The oculomotor (third cranial) nerve innervates the inferior, medial, and superior rectus muscles; the inferior oblique extraocular muscles; the pupilloconstrictor muscles; and the levator palpebrae muscles. The trochlear (fourth cranial) nerve innervates the superior oblique muscles. The abducens (sixth cranial) nerve innervates the lateral rectus muscles. The superior oblique muscles control downward rotation, intorsion, and abduction of the eye. Complete dysfunction of the third cranial nerve is called total oculomotor ophthalmoplegia and may be associated with trauma, diabetes, or an intracranial aneurysm.

Causes and incidence
The most common extraocular motor nerve palsy affects the superior oblique muscle as a result of trauma. Other causes of these disorders vary, depending on the cranial nerve involved:
- Third nerve (oculomotor) palsy (acute ophthalmoplegia) may be congenital or acquired. Causes include oculomotor involvement resulting from intracranial tumors or aneurysms; diabetic neuropathy; and trauma.

- Sixth nerve (abducens) palsy commonly has an unknown etiology. Strokes are a common cause. Brain stem lesions, elevated intracranial pressure, inflamed petrous pyramid due to otitis media, cavernous sinus, orbital involvement with tumor and inflammation, or thyroid eye disease may be responsible for sixth nerve palsy.

There are approximately 4,500 cases of acquired extraocular motor nerve palsies in the United States. The incidence of congenital extraocular nerve palsies is unknown.

Signs and symptoms
The most characteristic clinical effect of extraocular motor nerve palsies is diplopia of recent onset, which varies in different visual fields, depending on the muscles affected.

Typically, the patient with third nerve palsy exhibits ptosis, exotropia (eye looks outward), pupil dilation, and unresponsiveness to light; the eye is unable to move and can't accommodate.

The patient with fourth nerve palsy displays diplopia and an inability to rotate the eye downward or upward. The head is tilted to the side opposite the involved area in superior oblique palsy.

Sixth nerve palsy causes one eye to turn; the eye can't abduct beyond the midline. To compensate for diplopia, the patient turns his head to the unaffected side and can develop torticollis.

Diagnosis
Diagnosis necessitates an orthoptic examination to isolate the involved muscle, a complete neuro-ophthalmologic examination, and a thorough patient history. Differential diagnosis of third, fourth, or sixth nerve palsy depends on the specific motor defect exhibited by the patient.

For all extraocular motor nerve palsies, a computed tomography scan or magnetic resonance imaging rules out tumors and may help detect the cause of the palsy, such as the cause of increased intracranial pressure. The patient is also evaluated for an aneurysm or diabetes. If sixth nerve palsy results from infection, culture and sensitivity tests identify the causative organism, and specific antibiotic therapy can be determined.

Treatment

Identification of the underlying cause is essential because treatment for extraocular motor nerve palsies varies accordingly. Neurosurgery is necessary if the cause is a brain tumor or an aneurysm. For infection, massive I.V. doses of antibiotics may be appropriate.

Special considerations

■ If the palsy results from thyroid eye disease, the patient must have normal thyroid levels before eye muscle surgery is attempted.

Glaucoma

Glaucoma is a group of disorders characterized by an abnormally high intraocular pressure (IOP), which can damage the optic nerve. If untreated, it can lead to gradual peripheral vision loss and, ultimately, blindness. (See *Blindness*.) Glaucoma occurs in several forms: chronic open-angle (primary), acute angle-closure, congenital (inherited as an autosomal recessive trait), and secondary to other causes. The prognosis for maintaining vision is good with early treatment.

Causes and incidence

Chronic open-angle glaucoma results from overproduction of aqueous humor or obstruction to its outflow through the trabecular meshwork or the canal of Schlemm. (See *Normal flow of aqueous humor,* page 1184.) This form of glaucoma, which is estimated to be present in 1% to 2% of people older than age 40, is frequently familial in origin and affects 90% of all patients with glaucoma. Diabetes and systemic hypertension have also been associated with this form of glaucoma.

Acute angle-closure (narrow-angle) glaucoma results from obstruction to the outflow of aqueous humor due to anatomically narrow angles between the anterior iris and the posterior corneal surface, shallow anterior chambers, a thickened iris that

> **BLINDNESS**
>
> Blindness affects 28 million people worldwide. In the United States, blindness is legally defined as optimal visual acuity of 20/200 or less in the better eye after best correction, or a visual field of 20 degrees or less in the better eye.
>
> According to the World Health Organization, the most common causes of preventable blindness worldwide are trachoma, cataracts, onchocerciasis (microfilarial infection transmitted by a blackfly and other species of *Simulium*), and xerophthalmia (dryness of conjunctiva and cornea from vitamin A deficiency).
>
> In the United States, the most common causes of acquired blindness are glaucoma, age-related macular degeneration, and diabetic retinopathy. However, the incidence of blindness from glaucoma is decreasing owing to early detection and treatment. Rarer causes of acquired blindness include herpes simplex keratitis, cataracts, and retinal detachment.

causes angle closure on pupil dilation, or a bulging iris that presses on the trabeculae, closing the angle (peripheral anterior synechiae).

Blacks are four times more likely to have this disorder than whites, and people with a family history of open-angle glaucoma are twice as likely to develop it than people without a family history of this disorder. The use of systemic anticholinergic medications, such as atropine or eye dilation drops, in a person who's already at high-risk for acute glaucoma increases the risk. Other risk factors include farsightedness and age-related changes that create an increase in intraocular pressure.

Congenital glaucoma occurs when there is an abnormal fluid drainage angle of the eye. It may be caused by congenital infec-

NORMAL FLOW OF AQUEOUS HUMOR

Aqueous humor, a plasmalike fluid produced by the ciliary epithelium of the ciliary body, flows from the posterior chamber to the anterior chamber through the pupil. Here it flows peripherally and filters through the trabecular meshwork to the canal of Schlemm, through which the fluid ultimately enters venous circulation.

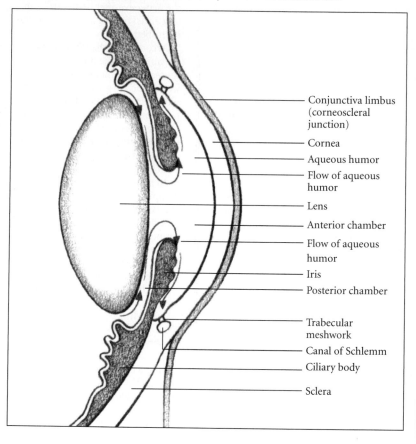

Conjunctiva limbus (corneoscleral junction)

Cornea

Aqueous humor

Flow of aqueous humor

Lens

Anterior chamber

Flow of aqueous humor

Iris

Posterior chamber

Trabecular meshwork

Canal of Schlemm

Ciliary body

Sclera

tions such as TORCH virus (*t*oxoplasmosis, *o*ther [varicella, mumps, parvovirus, human immunodeficiency virus], *r*ubella, *c*ytomegalovirus, and *h*erpes), Sturge-Weber syndrome, or retinopathy of prematurity.

Secondary glaucoma can result from uveitis, trauma, or drugs (such as steroids). Neovascularization in the angle can result from vein occlusion or diabetes.

Signs and symptoms

Chronic open-angle glaucoma is usually bilateral, with insidious onset and a slowly progressive course. Symptoms appear late in the disease and include mild aching in the eyes, loss of peripheral vision, seeing halos around lights, and reduced visual acuity (especially at night) that isn't correctable with glasses.

Acute angle-closure glaucoma typically has a rapid onset, constituting an ophthalmic emergency. Symptoms include acute pain in a unilaterally inflamed eye, with pressure over the eye, moderate pupil dilation that's nonreactive to light, a cloudy cornea, blurring and decreased visual acuity, photophobia, and seeing halos around lights. Increased IOP may induce nausea and vomiting, which may cause glaucoma to be misinterpreted as GI distress. Unless treated promptly, this acute form of glaucoma produces blindness in 3 to 5 days.

Diagnosis

 CONFIRMING DIAGNOSIS *Loss of peripheral vision and disk changes confirm that glaucoma is present.*
Diagnosis is made by:
- *testing IOP*
- *measuring the visual field and noting changes, such as an enlarged blind spot and loss of peripheral vision field*
- *observing changes in the cup/disk ratio of the optic nerve head.*

Relevant diagnostic tests include:
- Tonometry (using an applanation tonopen or air puff tonometer) — This test measures the IOP and provides a baseline for reference. Normal IOP ranges from 8 to 21 mm Hg. However, patients who fall within this normal range can develop signs and symptoms of glaucoma, and patients who have abnormally high pressure may have no clinical effects. Fingertip tension is another way to measure IOP. On gentle palpation of closed eyelids, one eye feels harder than the other in acute angle-closure glaucoma.
- Slit-lamp examination — The slit lamp facilitates examination of the anterior structures of the eye: the cornea, iris, and lens.
- Gonioscopy — By determining the angle of the anterior chamber of the eye, this test enables differentiation between chronic open-angle glaucoma and acute angle-closure glaucoma. The angle is normal in chronic open-angle glaucoma. However, in older patients, partial closure of the angle may occur, so that two forms of glaucoma may co-exist.

OPTIC DISK CHANGES

Ophthalmoscopy and slit-lamp examination show cupping of the optic disk, characteristic of chronic glaucoma.

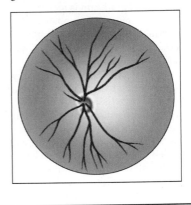

- Ophthalmoscopy — This test enables the examiner to look at the fundus to establish if there are any cup/disk ratio changes. (See *Optic disk changes.*) These changes appear later in chronic glaucoma if the disease isn't brought under control.
- Fundus photography — Pictures of the optic nerve head are made to track changes.
- Perimetry or visual field tests — These reveal the extent of damage to the optic neurons, signaled by an enlarged blind spot and loss of peripheral vision.

Treatment

For chronic open-angle glaucoma, treatment initially decreases IOP through the use of an alpha antagonist, brimonidine tartrate (Alphagan), and then beta blockers, such as timolol (contraindicated for asthmatics or patients with bradycardia) or betaxolol (Betoptic) to reduce aqueous humor production. A topical anhydrase inhibitor is used in preference to a systemic anhydrase inhibitor such as acetazolamide. A tubo-plast or tube shunt or valve may also be used. Miotic eyedrops such as pilocarpine facilitate the outflow of aqueous humor.

Patients who are unresponsive to drug therapy may be candidates for argon laser trabeculoplasty (ALT) or a surgical filtering procedure called trabeculectomy, which creates an opening for aqueous outflow. In ALT, an argon laser beam is focused on the trabecular meshwork of an open angle. This produces a thermal burn that changes the surface of the meshwork and increases the outflow of aqueous humor. In trabeculectomy, a flap of sclera is dissected free to expose the trabecular meshwork. Then this discrete tissue block is removed and a peripheral iridectomy is performed. This produces an opening for aqueous outflow under the conjunctiva, creating a filtering bleb. In chronic refractory glaucoma, a tubo-plast or tube shunt or valve is used to keep IOP within normal limits.

Acute angle-closure glaucoma is an ocular emergency requiring immediate treatment to lower the high IOP. Preoperative drug therapy lowers IOP with I.V. acetazolamide, pilocarpine (constricts the pupil, forcing the iris away from the trabeculae, allowing fluid to escape), timolol, and a topical steroid to quiet the inflammatory response, along with I.V. mannitol (20%) or oral glycerin (50%) to force fluid from the eye by making the blood hypertonic. Latanoprost is a topical medication that helps drain the aqueous outflow from the eye and lower the IOP. Oral medication or topical drops may be prescribed separately or in combination. Severe pain may necessitate administration of opioid analgesics. If pressure doesn't decrease with drug therapy, laser iridotomy or surgical peripheral iridectomy must be performed promptly to save the patient's vision. Iridectomy relieves pressure by excising part of the iris to reestablish aqueous humor outflow. A prophylactic iridectomy is performed a few days later on the other eye to prevent an acute episode of glaucoma in the normal eye.

Special considerations

■ Stress the importance of meticulous compliance with prescribed drug therapy to prevent an increase in IOP, resulting in disk changes and loss of vision.

■ For the patient with acute angle-closure glaucoma, give medications as ordered, and prepare him physically and psychologically for laser iridotomy or surgery.

■ Postoperative care after peripheral iridectomy includes cycloplegic eyedrops to relax the ciliary muscle and to decrease inflammation, thus preventing adhesions.

ALERT *Cycloplegics must be used only in the affected eye. The use of these drops in the normal eye may precipitate an attack of acute angle-closure glaucoma in this eye, threatening the patient's residual vision.*

■ Encourage ambulation immediately after surgery.

■ Following surgical filtering, postoperative care includes dilation and topical steroids to rest the pupil.

■ Stress the importance of glaucoma screening for early detection and prevention. All people older than age 35, especially those with family histories of glaucoma, should have an annual tonometric examination.

Selected references

Bartlett, J.D., et al. *Opthalmic Drug Facts 2004,* 5th ed. St. Louis: Facts and Comparisons, 2004.

Beers, M.H., et al., eds. *The Merck Manual of Diagnosis and Therapy,* 17th ed. Whitehouse Station, N.J.: Merck Research Laboratories, 1999.

Chono, J., et al. "Smallpox Vaccination and Adverse Reactions: Guidance for Clinicians." *Morbidity and Mortality Weekly Report* 52(RRO4):1-28, February 2003.

Foster, C.S., et al. *Smolin and Thoft's The Cornea: Scientific Foundations and Practice,* 4th ed. Philadelphia: Lippincott Williams & Wilkins, 2005.

Gupta, D. *Glaucoma Diagnosis and Management.* Philadelphia: Lippincott Williams & Wilkins, 2004.

Miller, N.R., and Newman, N.J. *Walsh and Hoyt's Clinical Neuro-Opthalmology,* 6th ed. Philadelphia: Lippincott Williams & Wilkins, 2005.

Ostler, H.B., et al. *Diseases of the Eye and Skin: A Color Atlas.* Philadelphia: Lippincott Williams & Wilkins, 2004.

Rootman, J. *Diseases of the Orbit: A Multidisciplinary Approach,* 2nd ed. Philadelphia: Lippincott Williams & Wilkins, 2003.

Tierney, L.M., et al. *Current Medical Diagnosis and Treatment 2004,* 43rd ed. New York: McGraw-Hill Book Co., 2004.

Wills Eye Hospital. *The Wills Eye Manual: Office and Emergency Diagnosis and Treatment of Eye Disease,* 4th ed. Philadelphia: Lippincott Williams & Wilkins, 2004.

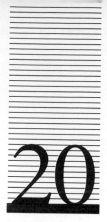

20

Ear, nose, and throat disorders

Introduction *1189*

External ear *1191*
Otitis externa *1191*
Benign tumors of the ear canal *1194*

Middle ear *1195*
Otitis media *1195*
Mastoiditis *1199*
Otosclerosis *1200*
Infectious myringitis *1201*

Inner ear *1202*
Ménière's disease *1202*
Labyrinthitis *1203*
Hearing loss *1204*
Motion sickness *1206*

Nose *1207*
Epistaxis *1207*
Septal perforation and deviation *1209*
Sinusitis *1211*
Nasal polyps *1213*
Nasal papillomas *1214*
Adenoid hyperplasia *1215*
Velopharyngeal insufficiency *1216*

Throat *1217*
Pharyngitis *1217*
Tonsillitis *1218*
Throat abscesses *1219*
Vocal cord paralysis *1221*
Vocal cord nodules and polyps *1222*
Laryngitis *1224*
Juvenile angiofibroma *1225*

Selected references *1226*

Introduction

Ear, nose, and throat disorders rarely prove fatal (except for those resulting from neoplasms, epiglottitis, and neck trauma), but they may cause serious social, cosmetic, and communication problems. Untreated hearing loss or deafness can drastically impair ability to interact with society. Ear disorders also have the ability to impair equilibrium. Nasal disorders can cause changes in facial features and interfere with breathing and tasting. Diseases arising in the throat may threaten airway patency and interfere with speech. In addition, these disorders can cause considerable discomfort and pain for the patient and require thorough assessment and prompt treatment.

The ear

Hearing begins when sound waves reach the tympanic membrane, which then vibrates the ossicles, incus, malleus, and stapes in the middle ear cavity. The stapes transmits these vibrations to the perilymphatic fluid in the inner ear by vibrating against the oval window. The vibrations then pass across the cochlea's fluid receptor cells in the basilar membrane, stimulating movement of the hair cells of the organ of Corti. The axons of the cochlear nerve terminate around the bases of those hair cells. Sound waves, which initiate impulses, travel over the auditory nerve (made up of the cochlear nerve and the vestibular nerve) to the temporal lobe of the brain.

The inner ear structures also maintain the body's equilibrium and balance through the fluid in the semicircular canals. This fluid is set in motion by body movement and stimulates nerve cells that line the canals. These cells, in turn, transmit impulses to the cerebellum of the brain by way of the vestibular branch of the eighth cranial nerve (the acoustic nerve).

Although the ear can respond to sounds that vibrate at frequencies from 20 to 20,000 hertz (Hz), the range of normal speech is from 250 to 4,000 Hz, with 70% falling between 500 and 2,000 Hz. The ratio between sound intensities, the decibel (dB) is the unit for expressing the relative intensity (loudness) of sounds. A faint

whisper registers 10 to 15 dB; average conversation, 50 to 60 dB; a shout, 85 to 90 dB. Hearing damage may follow exposure to sounds louder than 90 dB.

Assessment

After obtaining a thorough patient history of ear disease, inspect the auricle and surrounding tissue for deformities, lumps, and skin lesions. (See *Structures of the external ear.*) Ask the patient if he has ear pain. If you see inflammation, check for tenderness by moving the auricle and pressing on the tragus and the mastoid process. Check the ear canal for excessive cerumen, discharge, or foreign bodies.

Ask the patient if he has had episodes of vertigo or blurred vision. To test for vertigo, have the patient stand on one foot and close his eyes, or have him walk a straight line with his eyes closed. Ask him if he always falls to the same side and if the room seems to be spinning.

STRUCTURES OF THE EXTERNAL EAR

The structures of the external ear are depicted below.

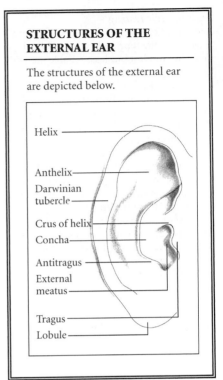

Helix

Anthelix

Darwinian tubercle

Crus of helix

Concha

Antitragus

External meatus

Tragus

Lobule

Audiometric testing

Audiometric testing evaluates hearing and determines the type and extent of hearing loss. The simplest but least reliable method for judging hearing acuity consists of covering one of the patient's ears, standing 18" to 24" (46 to 61 cm) from the uncovered ear, and whispering a short phrase or series of numbers. (Block the patient's vision to prevent lip reading.) Then ask the patient to repeat the phrase or series of numbers. To test hearing at both high and low frequencies, repeat the test in a normal speaking voice. (As an alternative, you can hold a ticking watch to the patient's ear.)

If you identify a hearing loss, further testing is necessary to determine if the loss is conductive or sensorineural. A conductive loss can result from faulty bone conduction (inability of the eighth cranial nerve to respond to sound waves traveling through the skull) or faulty air conduction (impaired transmission of sound through ear structures to the auditory nerve and, ultimately, the temporal lobe of the brain).

Sensorineural hearing loss results from damage to the cochlear or vestibulocochlear nerve, which can result from aging and prolonged exposure to high-frequency or loud noises.

The following tests assess bone and air conduction:

■ Impedance audiometry detects middle ear pathology, precisely determining the degree of tympanic membrane and middle ear mobility. One end of the impedance audiometer, a probe with three small tubes, is inserted into the external canal; the other end is attached to an oscillator. One tube delivers a low tone of variable intensity, the second contains a microphone, and the third, an air pump. A mobile tympanic membrane reflects minimal sound waves and produces a low-voltage curve on the graph. A tympanic membrane with decreased mobility reflects maximal sound waves and produces a high-voltage curve.

■ Pure tone audiometry uses an audiometer to produce a series of pure tones of calibrated decibels (dB) of loudness at different frequencies (125 to 8,000 Hz). These test tones are conveyed to the patient's ears through headphones or a bone conduction (sound) vibrator. Speech threshold represents the loudness at which a person with normal hearing can perceive the tone. Both air conduction and bone conduction are measured for each ear, and the results are plotted on a graph. If hearing is normal, the line is plotted at 0 dB. In adults, normal hearing may range from 0 to 25 dB.

■ Rinne test: The base of a lightly vibrating tuning fork is placed on the mastoid process (bone conduction). Then the fork is moved to the front of the meatus, where the patient should continue to hear the vibrations (air conduction). The patient must determine which sounds are louder. In a positive Rinne test, air conduction is greater than bone conduction, which may suggest sensorineural hearing loss. In a negative Rinne test, bone conduction is greater than air conduction, which may suggest a conductive loss.

■ Speech audiometry uses the same technique as pure tone audiometry, but with speech, instead of pure tones, transmitted through the headset. (A person with normal hearing can hear and repeat 88% to 100% of transmitted words.)

■ Tympanometry, using the impedance audiometer, measures tympanic membrane compliance with air pressure variations in the external canal and determines the degree of negative pressure in the middle ear.

■ Weber's test (used for testing unilateral hearing loss): The handle of a lightly vibrating tuning fork is placed on the midline of the forehead. Normally, the patient should hear sounds equally in both ears. With conductive hearing loss, sound lateralizes (localizes) to the ear with the poorest hearing. With sensorineural loss, sound lateralizes to the better functioning ear.

The nose

As air travels between the septum and the turbinates, it touches sensory hairs (cilia) in the mucosal surface, which then add, retain, or remove moisture and particles in the air to ensure delivery of humid, bacteria-free air to the pharynx and lungs. In addition, when air touches the mucosal cilia, the resultant stimulation of the first cranial nerve sends nerve impulses to the olfactory area of the frontal cortex, providing the sense of smell.

Assessment

Check the external nose for redness, edema, masses, or poor alignment. Marked septal cartilage depression may indicate saddle deformity due to septal destruction from trauma or congenital syphilis; extreme lateral deviation may result from injury. Red nostrils may indicate frequent nose blowing caused by allergies or infectious rhinitis. Dilated, engorged blood vessels may suggest alcoholism or constant exposure to the elements. A bulbous, discolored nose may be a sign of rosacea.

With a nasal speculum and adequate lighting, check nasal mucosa for pallor and edema or redness and inflammation, dried mucous plugs, furuncles, and polyps. Also, look for abnormal appearance of the capillaries and a deviated or perforated septum. Check for nasal discharge (assess color, consistency, and odor) and blood. Profuse, thin, watery discharge may indicate allergy or cold; excessive, thin, purulent discharge may indicate cold or chronic sinus infection.

Check for sinus inflammation by applying pressure to the nostrils, orbital rims, and cheeks. Pain after pressure applied above the upper orbital rims indicates frontal sinus irritation; pain after pressure applied to the cheeks, maxillary sinus irritation.

The throat

Parts of the throat include the pharynx, epiglottis, and larynx. The pharynx is the passageway for food to the esophagus and air to the larynx. The epiglottis (the lid of the larynx) diverts material away from the glottis during swallowing. The larynx produces sounds by vibrating expired air through the vocal cords. Changes in vocal cord length and air pressure affect pitch and voice intensity. The larynx also stimulates the vital cough reflex when a foreign body touches its sensitive mucosa.

Assessment

Using a bright light and a tongue blade, inspect the patient's mouth and throat. Look for inflammation or white patches, and any irregularities on the tongue or throat. Make sure the patient's airway isn't compromised and also assess vital signs. Watch for and immediately report signs of respiratory distress (dyspnea, tachycardia, tachypnea, inspiratory stridor, restlessness, and nasal flaring) and changes in voice or in skin color, such as circumoral or nail bed cyanosis. Assess symmetry of the tongue as well as function of the soft palate. The main diagnostic test used in throat assessment is a culture to identify the infective organism.

EXTERNAL EAR

Otitis externa

Otitis externa, inflammation of the skin of the external ear canal and auricle, may be acute or chronic. Also known as *external otitis* and *swimmer's ear,* it's most common in the summer. With treatment, acute otitis externa usually subsides within 7 days — although it may become chronic — and tends to recur.

Causes and incidence

Otitis externa usually results from bacteria, such as *Pseudomonas, Proteus vulgaris, Staphylococcus aureus,* and streptococci and, sometimes, from fungi, such as *Aspergillus niger* and *Candida albicans* (fungal otitis externa is most common in tropical regions). Occasionally, chronic otitis externa results from dermatologic conditions, such as seborrhea or psoriasis. Allergic reactions stemming from nickel or chromium earrings, chemicals in hair spray, cosmetics, hearing aids, and medications (such as sulfonamide and neomycin, which is commonly used to treat otitis externa) can also cause otitis externa.

Predisposing factors include:

■ swimming in contaminated water; cerumen creates a culture medium for the waterborne organism.

■ cleaning the ear canal with a cotton swab, bobby pin, finger, or other foreign object; this irritates the ear canal and, possibly, introduces the infecting microorganism.

- exposure to dust or hair care products (such as hair spray or other irritants), which causes the patient to scratch his ear, excoriating the auricle and canal.
- regular use of earphones, earplugs, or earmuffs, which trap moisture in the ear canal, creating a culture medium for infection (especially if earplugs don't fit properly).
- chronic drainage from a perforated tympanic membrane.
- perfumes or self-administered eardrops.

Signs and symptoms

Acute otitis externa characteristically produces moderate to severe pain that's exacerbated by manipulating the auricle or tragus, clenching the teeth, opening the mouth, or chewing. Its other clinical effects may include fever, foul-smelling discharge, crusting in the external ear, regional cellulitis, partial hearing loss, and itching. It's usually difficult to view the tympanic membrane because of pain in the external canal. Hearing acuity is normal unless complete occlusion has occurred.

Fungal otitis externa may be asymptomatic, although *A. niger* produces a black or gray, blotting, paperlike growth in the ear canal. In chronic otitis externa, pruritus replaces pain, and scratching may lead to scaling and skin thickening. Aural discharge may also occur.

Diagnosis

CONFIRMING DIAGNOSIS
Physical examination confirms otitis externa. In acute otitis externa, otoscopy reveals a swollen external ear canal (sometimes to the point of complete closure), periauricular lymphadenopathy (tender nodes anterior to the tragus, posterior to the ear, or in the upper neck) and, occasionally, regional cellulitis.

In fungal otitis externa, removal of the growth reveals thick red epithelium. Microscopic examination or culture and sensitivity tests can identify the causative organism and determine antibiotic treatment. Pain on palpation of the tragus or auricle distinguishes acute otitis externa

from acute otitis media. (See *Differentiating acute otitis externa from acute otitis media*.)

In chronic otitis externa, physical examination reveals thick red epithelium in the ear canal. Severe chronic otitis externa may reflect underlying diabetes mellitus, hypothyroidism, or nephritis. Microscopic examination or culture and sensitivity tests can identify the causative organism and help in the determination of antibiotic treatment.

Treatment

To relieve the pain of acute otitis externa, treatment includes heat therapy to the periauricular region (heat lamp; hot, damp compresses; or a heating pad), aspirin or acetaminophen, and codeine. Instillation of antibiotic eardrops (with or without hydrocortisone) follows cleaning of the ear and removal of debris. However, a corticosteroid helps reduce the inflammatory response. If fever persists or regional cellulitis or tender postauricular adenopathy develops, a systemic antibiotic is necessary.

If the ear canal is too edematous for the instillation of eardrops, an ear wick may be used for the first few days.

Topical treatment is generally required for otitis externa, as systemic antibiotics alone aren't sufficient. Analgesics, such as acetaminophen or ibuprofen, may be required temporarily.

As with other forms of this disorder, fungal otitis externa necessitates careful cleaning of the ear. Application of a keratolytic or 2% salicylic acid in cream containing nystatin may help treat otitis externa resulting from candidal organisms. Instillation of slightly acidic eardrops creates an unfavorable environment in the ear canal for most fungi as well as *Pseudomonas*. No specific treatment exists for otitis externa caused by *A. niger,* except repeated cleaning of the ear canal with baby oil.

In chronic otitis externa, primary treatment consists of cleaning the ear and removing debris. Supplemental therapy includes instillation of antibiotic eardrops or application of antibiotic ointment or cream (neomycin, bacitracin, or polymyxin

DIFFERENTIATING ACUTE OTITIS EXTERNA FROM ACUTE OTITIS MEDIA

Use the assessment findings shown below to help differentiate acute otitis externa from acute otitis media.

ACUTE OTITIS EXTERNA (OCCURS PRIMARILY IN SUMMER)

Swollen ear canal (may result in impaired hearing)

Painful tragus movement

Affects external ear

Discharge

Red or normal tympanic membrane

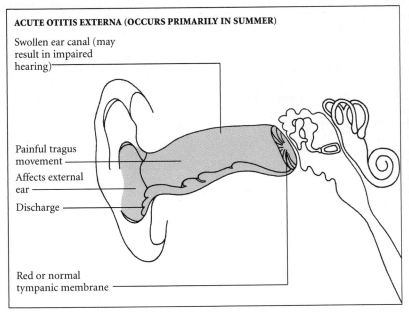

ACUTE OTITIS MEDIA (OCCURS PRIMARILY IN WINTER)

Affects middle ear

Painless tragus movement

Bulging or perforated tympanic membrane (results in impaired hearing)

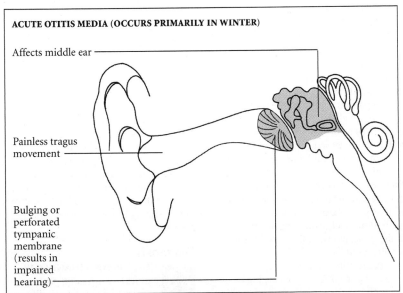

B, possibly combined with hydrocortisone). Another ointment contains phenol, salicylic acid, precipitated sulfur, and petroleum jelly and produces exfoliative and antipruritic effects.

For mild chronic otitis externa, treatment may include instillation of antibiotic eardrops once or twice weekly and wearing of specially fitted earplugs while the patient is showering, shampooing, or swimming.

Special considerations

If the patient has acute otitis externa:
- The patient shouldn't participate in any swimming activity.
- Have the patient return to the clinic in 1 week for evaluation of the tympanic membrane to make sure it's intact.
- Monitor vital signs, particularly temperature. Watch for and record the type and amount of aural drainage.
- Remove debris and gently clean the ear canal with mild Burow's solution (aluminum acetate). Place a wisp of cotton soaked with solution into the ear, and apply a saturated compress directly to the auricle. Afterward, dry the ear gently but thoroughly. (In severe otitis externa, such cleaning may be delayed until after initial treatment with antibiotic eardrops.)
- To instill eardrops in an adult, grasp the helix and pull upward and backward to straighten the canal. To instill eardrops in a child, pull the earlobe downward and backward. To ensure that the drops reach the epithelium, insert a wisp of cotton moistened with eardrops.
- Tell the patient to notify the physician if he develops an allergic reaction to the antibiotic drops or ointment, which may be indicated by increased swelling and discomfort of the area and worsening of other symptoms.

If the patient has chronic otitis externa, clean the ear thoroughly. Use wet soaks intermittently on oozing or infected skin. If the patient has a chronic fungal infection, clean the ear canal well, then apply an exfoliative ointment.

To prevent otitis externa:
- Suggest using lamb's wool earplugs coated with petroleum jelly, to keep water out of the ears when showering or shampooing.
- Tell the patient to wear earplugs or to keep his head above water when swimming and to instill two or three drops of 3% boric acid solution in 70% alcohol into his ear before and after swimming to toughen the skin of the external ear canal.
- Warn against cleaning the ears with cotton swabs or other objects.
- Urge prompt treatment for otitis media to prevent perforation of the tympanic membrane.
- If the patient is an elderly person or diabetic, evaluate him for malignant otitis externa.

 PEDIATRIC TIP *Children who have an intact tympanic membrane but are predisposed to otitis externa from swimming should instill two to three drops of a 1:1 solution of white vinegar and 70% ethyl alcohol into their ears before and after swimming.*

Benign tumors of the ear canal

Benign tumors may develop anywhere in the ear canal. Common types include keloids, osteomas, and sebaceous cysts; their causes vary. (See *Causes and characteristics of benign ear tumors.*) These tumors seldom become malignant; with proper treatment, the prognosis is excellent.

Signs and symptoms

A benign ear tumor is usually asymptomatic, unless it becomes infected, in which case pain, fever, or inflammation may result. (Pain is usually a sign of a malignant tumor.) If the tumor grows large enough to obstruct the ear canal by itself or through accumulated cerumen and debris, it may cause hearing loss and the sensation of pressure.

Diagnosis

CONFIRMING DIAGNOSIS
Clinical features and patient history suggest a benign tumor of the ear

CAUSES AND CHARACTERISTICS OF BENIGN EAR TUMORS

Tumor	Causes and incidence	Characteristics
Keloid	■ Surgery or trauma such as ear piercing ■ Most common in blacks	■ Hypertrophy and fibrosis of scar tissue ■ Commonly recurs
Osteoma	■ Idiopathic growth ■ Predisposing factor: swimming in cold water ■ Three times more common in males than in females ■ Seldom occurs before adolescence	■ Bony outgrowth from wall of external auditory meatus ■ Usually bilateral and multiple (exostoses) ■ May be circumscribed or diffuse, nondisplaceable, nontender
Sebaceous cyst	■ Obstruction of a sebaceous gland	■ Painless, circumscribed, round mass of variable size filled with oily, fatty, glandular secretions ■ May occur on external ear and outer third of external auditory canal

canal; *otoscopy confirms it. To rule out cancer, a biopsy may be necessary.*

Treatment

Generally, a benign tumor requires surgical excision if it obstructs the ear canal, is cosmetically undesirable, or becomes malignant.

Treatment for keloids may include surgery followed by repeated injections of long-acting steroids into the suture line. Excision must be complete, but even this may not prevent recurrence.

Surgical excision of an osteoma consists of elevating the skin from the surface of the bony growth and shaving the osteoma with a mechanical burr or drill.

Before surgery, a sebaceous cyst requires preliminary treatment with antibiotics, to reduce inflammation. To prevent recurrence, excision must be complete, including the sac or capsule of the cyst.

Special considerations

Because treatment for benign ear tumors generally doesn't require hospitalization, focus care on emotional support and providing appropriate patient education so that the patient follows his therapeutic plan properly when he's at home.

■ Thoroughly explain diagnostic procedures and treatment to the patient and his family. Reassure them and answer any questions they may have.

■ After surgery, instruct the patient in good aural hygiene. Until his ear is completely healed, advise him not to insert anything into his ear or allow water to get into it. Suggest that he cover his ears with a cap when showering.

■ Teach the patient how to recognize signs of infection, such as pain, fever, localized redness, and swelling. If he detects any of these signs, instruct him to report them immediately.

MIDDLE EAR

Otitis media

Otitis media, inflammation of the middle ear, may be suppurative or secretory, acute, persistent, unresponsive, or chronic. With prompt treatment, the prognosis for acute

SITE OF OTITIS MEDIA

The common site of otitis media is shown below.

Middle ear

Malleus

External ear canal

Tympanic membrane (eardrum)

Incus

Stapes

Eustachian tube

Semicircular canals

Cochlea

otitis media is excellent; however, prolonged accumulation of fluid within the middle ear cavity causes chronic otitis media and, possibly, perforation of the tympanic membrane. (See *Site of otitis media.*)

Chronic suppurative otitis media may lead to scarring, adhesions, and severe structural or functional ear damage. Chronic secretory otitis media, with its persistent inflammation and pressure, may cause conductive hearing loss.

Recurrent otitis media is defined as three near-acute otitis media episodes within 6 months or four episodes of acute otitis media within 1 year.

Otitis media with complications involves damage to middle ear structures (such as adhesions, retraction, pockets, cholesteatoma, and intratemporal and intracranial complications).

Causes and incidence

Otitis media results from disruption of eustachian tube patency. In the suppurative form, respiratory tract infection, allergic reaction, nasotracheal intubation, or positional changes allow nasopharyngeal flora to reflux through the eustachian tube and colonize the middle ear. Suppurative otitis media usually results from bacterial infection with pneumococcus, *Haemophilus influenzae* (the most common cause in children younger than age 6), *Moraxella catarrhalis,* beta-hemolytic streptococci, staphylococci (most common cause in children age 6 or older), or gram-negative bacteria. Predisposing factors include the normally wider, shorter, more horizontal eustachian tubes and increased lymphoid tissue in children, as well as anatomic anomalies. Chronic suppurative otitis media results from inadequate treatment for acute otitis episodes or from infection by resistant strains of bacteria or, rarely, tuberculosis.

Secretory otitis media results from obstruction of the eustachian tube. This causes a buildup of negative pressure in the middle ear that promotes transudation of sterile serous fluid from blood vessels in the membrane of the middle ear. Such effusion may be secondary to eustachian tube dysfunction from viral infection or allergy. It may also follow barotrauma (pressure injury caused by the inability to equalize pressures between the environment and the middle ear), as occurs during rapid aircraft descent in a person with an upper respiratory tract infection or during rapid underwater ascent in scuba diving (barotitis media).

Chronic secretory otitis media follows persistent eustachian tube dysfunction from mechanical obstruction (adenoidal tissue overgrowth or tumors), edema (allergic rhinitis or chronic sinus infection), or inadequate treatment for acute suppurative otitis media.

Acute otitis media is common in children; its incidence rises during the winter months, paralleling the seasonal rise in nonbacterial respiratory tract infections. Chronic secretory otitis media most commonly occurs in children with tympanostomy tubes or those with a perforated tympanic membrane.

Signs and symptoms

Clinical features of acute suppurative otitis media include severe, deep, throbbing pain (from pressure behind the tympanic membrane); signs of upper respiratory tract infection (sneezing or coughing); mild to very high fever; hearing loss (usually mild and conductive); tinnitus; dizziness; nausea; and vomiting. Other possible effects include bulging of the tympanic membrane, with concomitant erythema, and purulent drainage in the ear canal from tympanic membrane rupture. However, many patients are asymptomatic.

Acute secretory otitis media produces a severe conductive hearing loss — which varies from 15 to 35 dB, depending on the thickness and amount of fluid in the middle ear cavity — and, possibly, a sensation of fullness in the ear and popping, crackling, or clicking sounds on swallowing or with jaw movement. Accumulation of fluid may also cause the patient to hear an echo when he speaks and to experience a vague feeling of top-heaviness.

The cumulative effects of chronic otitis media include thickening and scarring of the tympanic membrane, decreased or absent tympanic membrane mobility, cholesteatoma (a cystlike mass in the middle ear) and, in chronic suppurative otitis media, a painless, purulent discharge. The extent of associated conductive hearing loss varies with the size and type of tympanic membrane perforation and ossicular destruction.

If the tympanic membrane has ruptured, the patient may state that the pain has suddenly stopped. Complications may include abscesses (brain, subperiosteal, and epidural), sigmoid sinus or jugular vein thrombosis, septicemia, meningitis, suppurative labyrinthitis, facial paralysis, and otitis externa.

 PEDIATRIC TIP *The following factors increase a child's risk of developing otitis media:*

■ *acute otitis media in the first year of life (recurrent otitis media)*
■ *day care*
■ *family history of middle ear disease*
■ *formula feeding*
■ *male gender*
■ *sibling history of otitis media*
■ *smoking in the household.*

Acute otitis media may not produce any symptoms in the first few months of life; irritability may be the only indication of earache.

Diagnosis

In acute suppurative otitis media, otoscopy reveals obscured or distorted bony landmarks of the tympanic membrane. Pneumatoscopy can show decreased tympanic membrane mobility, but this procedure is painful with an obviously bulging, erythematous tympanic membrane. The pain pattern is diagnostically significant: For example, in acute suppurative otitis media, pulling the auricle *doesn't* exacerbate the pain. A culture of the ear drainage identifies the causative organism.

In acute secretory otitis media, otoscopic examination reveals tympanic membrane retraction, which causes the bony landmarks to appear more prominent. Examination also detects clear or amber fluid behind the tympanic membrane. If hemorrhage into the middle ear has occurred, as in barotrauma, the tympanic membrane appears blue-black.

In chronic otitis media, patient history discloses recurrent or unresolved otitis media. Otoscopy shows thickening, sometimes scarring, and decreased mobility of the tympanic membrane; pneumatoscopy shows decreased or absent tympanic membrane movement. A history of recent air travel or scuba diving suggests barotitis media.

Tympanocentesis for microbiologic diagnosis is recommended for treatment failures and may be followed by myringotomy. Tympanometry, acoustic reflex measurement, or acoustic reflexometry may be needed to document the presence of fluid in the middle ear. White blood cell count is higher in bacterial otitis media than in sterile otitis media. Mastoid X-rays or computed tomography scan of the head or mastoids may show the spreading of the infection beyond the middle ear.

Treatment

In acute suppurative otitis media, antibiotic therapy includes amoxicillin. In areas with a high incidence of beta-lactamase-producing *H. influenzae* and in patients who aren't responding to ampicillin or amoxicillin, amoxicillin/clavulanate potassium may be used. For those who are allergic to penicillin derivatives, therapy may include cefaclor or co-trimoxazole. Severe, painful bulging of the tympanic membrane usually necessitates myringotomy. Broad-spectrum antibiotics can help prevent acute suppurative otitis media in high-risk patients. A single dose of ceftriaxone 50 mg/kg is effective against major pathogens but is expensive and is reserved for very sick infants. In the patient with recurring otitis media, antibiotics must be used with discretion to prevent development of resistant strains of bacteria.

In acute secretory otitis media, inflation of the eustachian tube using Valsalva's maneuver several times a day may be the only treatment required. Otherwise, nasopharyngeal decongestant therapy may be helpful. It should continue for at least 2 weeks and, sometimes, indefinitely, with periodic evaluation. If decongestant therapy fails, myringotomy and aspiration of middle ear fluid are necessary, followed by insertion of a polyethylene tube into the tympanic membrane, for immediate and prolonged equalization of pressure. The tube falls out spontaneously after 9 to 12 months. Concomitant treatment for the underlying cause (such as elimination of allergens, or adenoidectomy for hypertrophied adenoids) may also be helpful in correcting this disorder.

Treatment for chronic otitis media includes broad-spectrum antibiotics, such as amoxicillin/clavulanate potassium or cefuroxime, for exacerbations of acute otitis media; elimination of eustachian tube obstruction; treatment for otitis externa; myringoplasty and tympanoplasty to reconstruct middle ear structures when thickening and scarring are present and, possibly, mastoidectomy. Cholesteatoma requires excision.

Special considerations

■ Explain all diagnostic tests and procedures. After myringotomy, maintain drainage flow. Don't place cotton or plugs deeply into the ear canal; however, sterile cotton may be placed loosely in the external ear to absorb drainage. To prevent infection, change the cotton whenever it gets damp, and wash hands before and after giving ear care. Watch for and report headache, fever, severe pain, or disorientation.

■ After tympanoplasty, reinforce dressings, and observe for excessive bleeding from the ear canal. Administer analgesics as needed. Warn the patient against blowing his nose or getting the ear wet when bathing.

■ Encourage the patient to complete the prescribed course of antibiotic treatment.

If nasopharyngeal decongestants are ordered, teach correct instillation.

- Suggest application of heat to the ear to relieve pain.
- Advise the patient with acute secretory otitis media to watch for and immediately report pain and fever — signs of secondary infection.

To prevent otitis media:

- Teach the patient how to recognize upper respiratory tract infections, and encourage early treatment.
- Instruct the parents not to feed the infant in a supine position or put him to bed with a bottle. This prevents reflux of nasopharyngeal flora.
- To promote eustachian tube patency, instruct the patient to perform Valsalva's maneuver several times daily.
- Identify and treat allergies.

Mastoiditis

Mastoiditis is a bacterial infection and inflammation of the air cells of the mastoid antrum. Although the prognosis is good with early treatment, possible complications include meningitis, facial paralysis, brain abscess, and suppurative labyrinthitis.

Causes and incidence

Bacteria that cause mastoiditis include pneumococci, *Haemophilus influenzae, Moraxella catarrhalis,* beta-hemolytic streptococci, staphylococci, and gram-negative organisms. Mastoiditis is usually a complication of chronic otitis media; less frequently, it develops after acute otitis media. An accumulation of pus under pressure in the middle ear cavity results in necrosis of adjacent tissue and extension of the infection into the mastoid cells. Chronic systemic diseases or immunosuppression may also lead to mastoiditis. Anaerobic organisms play a role in chronic mastoiditis.

PEDIATRIC TIP *Acute otitis media increases a child's risk of developing mastoiditis. If mastoiditis does occur in infants younger than age 1, the swelling occurs superior to the ear and pushes the pinna downward instead of outward. I.V.*

antibiotic treatment choice includes ampicillin or cefuroxime. Before antibiotics, mastoiditis was one of the leading causes of death in children; now, it's uncommon and less dangerous.

Signs and symptoms

Primary clinical features include a dull ache and tenderness in the area of the mastoid process, low-grade fever, headache, and a thick, purulent discharge that gradually becomes more profuse, possibly leading to otitis externa. Postauricular erythema and edema may push the auricle out from the head; pressure within the edematous mastoid antrum may produce swelling and obstruction of the external ear canal, causing conductive hearing loss.

Diagnosis

X-rays or computed tomography scan of the mastoid area reveal hazy mastoid air cells; the bony walls between the cells appear decalcified. Audiometric testing may reveal a conductive hearing loss. Physical examination shows a dull, thickened, and edematous tympanic membrane, if the membrane isn't concealed by obstruction. During examination, the external ear canal is cleaned; persistent oozing into the canal indicates perforation of the tympanic membrane.

Treatment

Treatment for mastoiditis consists of intense parenteral antibiotic therapy. Reasonable initial antibiotic choices include ceftriaxone with nafcillin or clindamycin. If bone damage is minimal, myringotomy or tympanocentesis drains purulent fluid and provides a specimen of discharge for culture and sensitivity testing. Recurrent or persistent infection or signs of intracranial complications necessitate simple mastoidectomy. This procedure involves removal of the diseased bone and cleaning of the affected area, after which a drain is inserted.

A chronically inflamed mastoid requires radical mastoidectomy (excision of the posterior wall of the ear canal, remnants of the tympanic membrane, and the malleus and incus, although these bones are usually destroyed by infection before surgery). The stapes and facial nerve remain intact. Radical mastoidectomy, which is seldom necessary because of antibiotic therapy, doesn't drastically affect the patient's hearing because significant hearing loss precedes surgery. With either surgical procedure, the patient continues oral antibiotic therapy for several weeks after surgery and facility discharge. The prognosis is good if treatment is started early.

Indications for immediate surgical intervention include meningitis, brain abscess, cavernous sinus thrombosis, acute suppurative labyrinthitis, and facial palsy.

Special considerations
■ After simple mastoidectomy, give pain medication as needed. Check wound drainage and reinforce dressings (the surgeon usually changes the dressing daily and removes the drain in 72 hours). Check the patient's hearing, and watch for signs of complications, especially infection (either localized or extending to the brain); facial nerve paralysis, with unilateral facial drooping; bleeding; and vertigo, especially when the patient stands.
■ After radical mastoidectomy, the wound is packed with petroleum gauze or gauze treated with an antibiotic ointment. Give pain medication before the packing is removed, on the fourth or fifth postoperative day.
■ Because of stimulation to the inner ear during surgery, the patient may feel dizzy and nauseated for several days afterward. Keep the side rails up, and assist the patient with ambulation. Also, give antiemetics as needed.
■ Before discharge, teach the patient and his family how to change and care for the dressing. Urge compliance with the prescribed antibiotic treatment, and promote regular follow-up care.
■ If the patient is an elderly person or diabetic, evaluate him for malignant otitis externa.

Otosclerosis

The most common cause of chronic, progressive conductive hearing loss, otosclerosis is the slow formation of spongy bone in the otic capsule, particularly at the oval window. With surgery, the prognosis is good.

Causes and incidence
Otosclerosis appears to result from a genetic factor transmitted as an autosomal dominant trait; many patients report family histories of hearing loss (excluding presbycusis). Pregnancy may trigger onset of this condition.

Otosclerosis occurs in at least 10% of the U.S. population. It's three times more prevalent in females than in males, usually affecting people between ages 15 and 30. Whites are most susceptible.

Signs and symptoms
Spongy bone in the otic capsule immobilizes the footplate of the normally mobile stapes, disrupting the conduction of vibrations from the tympanic membrane to the cochlea. This causes progressive unilateral hearing loss, which may advance to bilateral deafness. Other symptoms include tinnitus and paracusis of Willis (hearing conversation better in a noisy environment than in a quiet one).

Diagnosis
Early diagnosis is based on a Rinne test that shows bone conduction lasting longer than air conduction (normally, the reverse is true). As otosclerosis progresses, bone conduction also deteriorates. Audiometric testing reveals hearing loss ranging from 60 dB in early stages to total loss. Weber's test detects sound lateralizing to the more affected ear. Physical examination reveals a normal tympanic membrane. Head computed tomography scan and X-ray help distinguish otosclerosis from other causes of hearing loss.

Treatment
Treatment consists of stapedectomy (removal of the stapes) and insertion of a prosthesis to restore partial or total hear-

ing. This procedure is performed on only one ear at a time, beginning with the ear that has suffered greater damage. Alternative surgery includes stapedotomy (creation of a small hole in the stapes' footplate), through which a wire and piston are inserted. Recent procedural innovations involve laser surgery. Postoperatively, treatment includes antibiotics to prevent infection. If surgery isn't possible, a hearing aid (air conduction aid with molded ear insert receiver) enables the patient to hear conversation in normal surroundings, although this therapy isn't as effective as stapedectomy.

Special considerations

- During the first 24 hours after surgery, keep the patient supine, with the affected ear facing upward (to maintain the position of the graft). Enforce bed rest with bathroom privileges for 48 hours. Because the patient may be dizzy, keep the side rails up, and assist him with ambulation. Assess for pain and vertigo, which may be relieved with repositioning or prescribed medication.
- Tell the patient that his hearing won't return until edema subsides and packing is removed.
- Before discharge, instruct the patient to avoid loud noises and sudden pressure changes (such as those that occur while diving or flying) until healing is complete (usually 6 months). Advise the patient not to blow his nose for at least 1 week to prevent contaminated air and bacteria from entering the eustachian tube.
- Stress the importance of protecting the ears against cold; avoiding any activities that provoke dizziness, such as straining, bending, or heavy lifting and, if possible, avoiding contact with anyone who has an upper respiratory tract infection. Teach the patient and his family how to change the external ear dressing (eye or gauze pad) and care for the incision. Emphasize the need to complete the prescribed antibiotic regimen and to return for scheduled follow-up care.

Infectious myringitis

Acute infectious myringitis is characterized by inflammation, hemorrhage, and effusion of fluid into the tissue at the end of the external ear canal and the tympanic membrane. This self-limiting disorder (resolving spontaneously within 3 days to 2 weeks) commonly follows acute otitis media or upper respiratory tract infection.

Chronic granular myringitis, a rare inflammation of the squamous layer of the tympanic membrane, causes gradual hearing loss. Without specific treatment, this condition can lead to stenosis of the ear canal, as granulation extends from the tympanic membrane to the external ear.

Causes and incidence

Acute infectious myringitis usually follows viral infection but may also result from infection with bacteria (pneumococcus, *Haemophilus influenzae*, beta-hemolytic streptococci, staphylococci) or any other organism that can cause acute otitis media. Myringitis is a rare sequela of atypical pneumonia caused by *Mycoplasma pneumoniae*. The cause of chronic granular myringitis is unknown.

Acute infectious myringitis frequently occurs epidemically in children.

Signs and symptoms

Acute infectious myringitis begins with severe ear pain, commonly accompanied by tenderness over the mastoid process. Small, reddened, inflamed blebs form in the canal, on the tympanic membrane and, with bacterial invasion, in the middle ear. Fever and hearing loss are rare unless fluid accumulates in the middle ear, or a large bleb totally obstructs the external auditory meatus. Spontaneous rupture of these blebs may cause bloody discharge. Chronic granular myringitis produces pruritus, purulent discharge, and gradual hearing loss.

Diagnosis

CONFIRMING DIAGNOSIS *Diagnosis of acute infectious myringitis is based on physical examination showing characteristic blebs and a typical patient history. Culture and sensitivity* *testing of exudate identifies secondary infection. In chronic granular myringitis, physical examination may reveal granulation extending from the tympanic membrane to the external ear.*

Treatment

Hospitalization usually isn't required for acute infectious myringitis. Treatment consists of measures to relieve pain: analgesics, such as aspirin or acetaminophen, and application of heat to the external ear are usually sufficient, but severe pain may necessitate use of codeine.

ALERT *Aspirin and combination aspirin products aren't recommended for people younger than age 19 during episodes of fever-causing illnesses because the use of aspirin has been linked to Reye's syndrome.*

Systemic or topical antibiotics prevent or treat secondary infection. Incision of blebs and evacuation of serum and blood may relieve pressure and help drain exudate but don't speed recovery.

Treatment for chronic granular myringitis consists of systemic antibiotics or local anti-inflammatory/antibiotic combination eardrops, and surgical excision and cautery. If stenosis is present, surgical reconstruction is necessary.

Special considerations

■ Stress the importance of completing the prescribed antibiotic therapy.
■ Teach the patient how to instill topical antibiotics (eardrops). When necessary, explain incision of blebs.
■ To help prevent acute infectious myringitis, advise early treatment for acute otitis media.

INNER EAR

Ménière's disease

Ménière's disease, a labyrinthine dysfunction also known as *endolymphatic hydrops,* produces severe vertigo, sensorineural hearing loss, and tinnitus. After multiple attacks over several years, this disorder

leads to residual tinnitus and hearing loss. Usually, only one ear is involved.

Causes and incidence

The exact cause of Ménière's disease is unknown. It may result from overproduction or decreased absorption of endolymph, which causes endolymphatic hydrops or endolymphatic hypertension, with consequent degeneration of the vestibular and cochlear hair cells. This condition may also stem from autonomic nervous system dysfunction that produces a temporary constriction of blood vessels supplying the inner ear. In some cases, Ménière's disease may be related to otitis media, syphilis, or head injury. Risk factors include recent viral illness, respiratory infection, stress, fatigue, use of prescription or nonprescription drugs (such as aspirin), and a history of allergies, smoking, and alcohol use. There also may be genetic risk factors: In some women, premenstrual edema may precipitate attacks of Ménière's disease.

In the United States, about 100,000 people per year develop Ménière's disease.

Signs and symptoms

Ménière's disease produces three characteristic effects: severe episodic vertigo, tinnitus, and sensorineural hearing loss. A feeling of fullness or blockage in the ear is also common. Violent paroxysmal attacks last from 10 minutes to several hours. During an acute attack, other symptoms include severe nausea, vomiting, sweating, giddiness, and nystagmus. Vertigo may cause loss of balance and falling to the affected side. Symptoms tend to wax and wane as the endolymphatic pressure rises and falls. To lessen these symptoms, the patient may assume a characteristic posture — lying on the side of the unaffected ear and looking in the direction of the affected ear.

Initially, the patient may be asymptomatic between attacks, except for residual tinnitus that worsens during an attack. Such attacks may occur several times a year, or remissions may last as long as several years. These attacks become less frequent as hearing loss progresses (usually unilaterally); they may cease when hearing loss is total. All symptoms are aggravated by motion.

Diagnosis

Presence of all three typical symptoms suggests Ménière's disease. Audiometric studies indicate a sensorineural hearing loss and loss of discrimination and recruitment. Selected studies such as electronystagmography, electrocochleography, computed tomography scan, magnetic resonance imaging, or X-rays of the internal meatus may be necessary for differential diagnosis.

Laboratory studies, including thyroid and lipid studies, may be performed to rule out other conditions such as *Treponema pallidum*.

Caloric testing may reveal loss or impairment of thermally induced nystagmus on the involved side. However, it's important not to overlook an acoustic tumor, which produces an identical clinical picture.

Treatment

Treatment with atropine may stop an attack in 20 to 30 minutes. Epinephrine or diphenhydramine may be necessary in a severe attack; dimenhydrinate, meclizine, diphenhydramine, or diazepam may be effective in a milder attack.

Long-term management includes use of a diuretic or vasodilator and restricted sodium intake (less than 2 g/day). A typical diuretic regime is hydrochlorothiazide 500 to 100 mg daily. Prophylactic antihistamines or mild sedatives (phenobarbital, diazepam) may also be helpful. If Ménière's disease persists after 2 years of treatment, produces incapacitating vertigo, or resists medical management, surgery may be necessary. Destruction of the affected labyrinth permanently relieves symptoms but results in irreversible hearing loss. Systemic streptomycin is reserved for the patient with bilateral disease for whom no other treatment can be considered. If a patient fails medical therapy and remains disabled by his vertigo, surgical decompression of the endolymphatic sac may bring relief.

Special considerations

If the patient is in the hospital during an attack of Ménière's disease:
- Advise him against reading and exposure to glaring lights, to reduce dizziness.
- Keep the side rails of the patient's bed up to prevent falls. Tell him not to get out of bed or walk without assistance.
- Instruct the patient to avoid sudden position changes and any tasks that vertigo makes hazardous because an attack can begin quite rapidly. Hazardous activities, such as driving and climbing, should be avoided until one week after symptoms disappear.
- Before surgery, if the patient is vomiting, record fluid intake and output and characteristics of vomitus. Administer antiemetics as needed, and give small amounts of fluid frequently.
- After surgery, record intake and output carefully. Tell the patient to expect dizziness and nausea for 1 or 2 days after surgery. Give prophylactic antibiotics and antiemetics, as ordered.

Labyrinthitis

Labyrinthitis, an inflammation of the labyrinth of the inner ear, frequently incapacitates the patient by producing severe vertigo that lasts for 3 to 5 days; symptoms gradually subside over a 3- to 6-week period. Viral labyrinthitis is commonly associated with upper respiratory tract infections.

Causes

Labyrinthitis is usually caused by viral infection. It may be a primary infection, the result of trauma, or a complication of influenza, otitis media, or meningitis. In chronic otitis media, cholesteatoma formation erodes the bone of the labyrinth, allowing bacteria to enter from the middle ear. Toxic drug ingestion is another possible cause of labyrinthitis and neuronitis.

Signs and symptoms

Because the inner ear controls both hearing and balance, this infection typically produces severe vertigo (with any movement of the head) and sensorineural hearing loss. Vertigo begins gradually but peaks within 48 hours, causing loss of balance and falling in the direction of the affected ear. Other associated signs and symptoms include spontaneous nystagmus, with jerking movements of the eyes toward the unaffected ear, and nausea, vomiting, and giddiness. With cholesteatoma, signs of middle ear disease may appear. With severe bacterial infection, purulent drainage, increased salivation, generalized malaise, and perspiration can occur. To minimize symptoms such as giddiness and nystagmus, the patient may assume a characteristic posture—lying on the side of the unaffected ear and looking in the direction of the affected ear.

Diagnosis

A typical clinical picture and a history of upper respiratory tract infection suggest labyrinthitis. Typical diagnostic measures include culture and sensitivity testing to identify the infecting organism, if purulent drainage is present, and audiometric testing. When an infectious etiology can't be found, additional testing must be done to rule out a brain lesion or Ménière's disease.

Differentiation from other causes of dizziness or vertigo may include head computed tomography (CT) scan or magnetic resonance imaging, audiology or audiometry testing, caloric stimulation tests, electronystagmography, EEG, and evoked auditory potential studies.

Treatment

Symptomatic treatment includes bed rest, with the head immobilized between pillows, and antibiotics to combat diffuse purulent labyrinthitis. Oral fluids can prevent dehydration caused by vomiting. For severe nausea and vomiting, I.V. fluids may be necessary. Medications that help reduce symptoms include antihistamines, anticholinergics, sedative-hypnotics, and antiemetics; benzodiazepines help control vertigo.

When conservative management fails, treatment necessitates surgical excision of the cholesteatoma and drainage of the infected areas of the middle and inner ear. Prevention is possible by early and vigor-ous treatment for predisposing conditions, such as otitis media and any local or systemic infection.

Special considerations

- Keep the side rails up to prevent falls. Tell the patient to keep still and rest during attacks and to avoid sudden position changes.
- If vomiting is severe, administer antiemetics as ordered. Record intake and output, and give I.V. fluids as ordered.
- During an attack, dim the lighting and tell the patient to avoid reading.
- Tell the patient that recovery may take as long as 6 weeks. During this time, he should limit activities that vertigo may make hazardous. Hazardous activities, such as driving and climbing, should be avoided until one week after symptoms disappear.
- If recovery doesn't occur within 4 to 6 weeks, a CT scan should be performed to rule out an intracranial lesion.

Hearing loss

Hearing loss results from a mechanical or nervous impediment to the transmission of sound waves. The major forms of hearing loss are classified as *conductive loss* (interrupted passage of sound from the external ear to the junction of the stapes and oval window), *sensorineural loss* (impaired cochlea or acoustic [eighth cranial] nerve dysfunction, causing failure of transmission of sound impulses within the inner ear or brain), or *mixed loss* (combined dysfunction of conduction and sensorineural transmission). Hearing loss may be partial or total and is calculated from this American Medical Association formula: Hearing is 1.5% impaired for every decibel that the pure tone average exceeds 25 dB.

Causes and incidence

Congenital hearing loss may be transmitted as a dominant, autosomal dominant, autosomal recessive, or sex-linked recessive trait. Hearing loss in neonates may also result from trauma, toxicity, or infection during pregnancy or delivery. Predisposing factors include a family history of hearing loss or known hereditary disorders (otosclerosis, for example), maternal exposure to rubella or syphilis during pregnancy, use of ototoxic drugs during pregnancy, prolonged fetal anoxia during delivery, and congenital abnormalities of the ears, nose, or throat. Premature or low-birth-weight neonates are most likely to have structural or functional hearing impairment; those with scrum bilirubin levels above 20 mg/dl also risk hearing impairment from the toxic effect of high serum bilirubin levels on the brain. In addition, trauma during delivery may cause intracranial hemorrhage and may damage the cochlea or the acoustic nerve.

Sudden deafness refers to sudden hearing loss in a person with no prior hearing impairment. This condition is considered a medical emergency because prompt treatment may restore full hearing. Its causes and predisposing factors may include:

- acute infections, especially mumps (most common cause of unilateral sensorineural hearing loss in children), and other bacterial and viral infections, such as rubella, rubeola, influenza, herpes zoster, and infectious mononucleosis; and mycoplasma infections
- blood dyscrasias (leukemia, hypercoagulation)
- head trauma or brain tumors
- metabolic disorders (diabetes mellitus, hypothyroidism, hyperlipoproteinemia)
- neurologic disorders (multiple sclerosis, neurosyphilis)
- ototoxic drugs (tobramycin, streptomycin, quinine, gentamicin, furosemide, ethacrynic acid)
- vascular disorders (hypertension, arteriosclerosis).

Noise-induced hearing loss, which may be transient or permanent, may follow prolonged exposure to loud noise (85 to 90 dB) or brief exposure to extremely loud noise (greater than 90 dB). Such hearing loss is common in workers subjected to constant industrial noise and in military personnel, hunters, and rock musicians.

Presbycusis, an otologic effect of aging, results from a loss of hair cells in the organ of Corti. This disorder causes progressive, symmetrical, bilateral sensorineural hearing loss, usually of high-frequency tones.

Minor decreases in hearing are common after age 20. Some deafness due to nerve damage occurs in one of every five people by age 55.

Signs and symptoms

Although congenital hearing loss may produce no obvious signs of hearing impairment at birth, a deficient response to auditory stimuli generally becomes apparent within 2 to 3 days. As the child grows older, hearing loss impairs speech development.

Sudden deafness may be conductive, sensorineural, or mixed, depending on etiology. Associated clinical features depend on the underlying cause.

Noise-induced hearing loss causes sensorineural damage, the extent of which depends on the duration and intensity of the noise. Initially, the patient loses perception of certain frequencies (around 4,000 Hz) but, with continued exposure, eventually loses perception of all frequencies.

Presbycusis usually produces tinnitus and the inability to understand the spoken word.

 PEDIATRIC TIP *The behavior of an infant who's deaf may appear normal and mislead the parents as well as the professional, especially if the infant has autosomal recessive deafness and is the first child of carrier parents.*

Diagnosis

CONFIRMING DIAGNOSIS *Patient, family, and occupational histories and a complete audiologic examination usually provide ample evidence of hearing loss and suggest possible causes or predisposing factors.*

The Weber, Rinne, and specialized audiologic tests differentiate between conductive and sensorineural hearing loss.

Treatment

After the underlying cause is identified, therapy for congenital hearing loss refractory to surgery consists of developing the patient's ability to communicate through sign language, speech reading, or other effective means. Measures to prevent congenital hearing loss include aggressively immunizing children against rubella to reduce the risk of maternal exposure during pregnancy; educating pregnant women about the dangers of exposure to drugs, chemicals, or infection; and careful monitoring during labor and delivery to prevent fetal anoxia.

Treatment for sudden deafness requires prompt identification of the underlying cause. Prevention necessitates educating patients and health care professionals about the many causes of sudden deafness and the ways to recognize and treat them.

Hyperbilirubinemia can be controlled by phototherapy and exchange transfusions. Children need the appropriate immunizations. Medications that may be ototoxic should be used judiciously in children and monitored closely. Reduction of exposure to loud noises generally prevents high-frequency hearing loss.

In people with noise-induced hearing loss, overnight rest usually restores normal hearing in those who have been exposed to noise levels greater than 90 dB for several hours; but not in those who have been exposed to such noise repeatedly. As hearing deteriorates, treatment must include speech and hearing rehabilitation, because hearing aids are seldom helpful. Prevention of noise-induced hearing loss requires public recognition of the dangers of noise exposure and insistence on the use, as mandated by law, of protective devices such as earplugs during occupational exposure to noise.

Amplifying sound, as with a hearing aid, helps some patients with presbycusis, but many patients have an intolerance to loud noise and wouldn't be helped by a hearing aid.

Special considerations

■ When speaking to a patient with hearing loss who can read lips, stand directly in front of him, with the light on your face, and speak slowly and distinctly. If possible, speak to him at eye level. Approach the patient within his visual range, and elicit his attention by raising your arm or waving; touching him may be unnecessarily startling.

■ Make other staff members and facility personnel aware of the patient's disability and his established method of communication. Carefully explain diagnostic tests and facility procedures in a way the patient understands.

■ Make sure the patient with a hearing loss is in an area where he can observe unit activities and people approaching because such a patient depends totally on visual clues.

■ When addressing an older patient, speak slowly and distinctly in a low tone; avoid shouting.

■ Provide emotional support and encouragement to the patient learning to use a hearing aid. Teach him how the aid works and how to maintain it.

■ Refer children with suspected hearing loss to an audiologist or otolaryngologist for further evaluation. Any child who fails a language screening examination should be referred to a speech pathologist for language evaluation. The child with a mild language delay may be involved with a home language-enrichment program.

■ To help prevent hearing loss, watch for signs of hearing impairment in the patient receiving ototoxic drugs. Emphasize the danger of excessive exposure to noise; stress the danger to pregnant women of exposure to drugs, chemicals, and infection (especially rubella); and encourage the use of protective devices in a noisy environment.

Motion sickness

Motion sickness is characterized by loss of equilibrium associated with nausea and vomiting that results from irregular or rhythmic movements or from the sensation of motion. Removal of the stimulus restores normal equilibrium. Motion sickness also can be induced when patterns of motion differ from what the patient has previously experienced.

Causes and incidence

Motion sickness may result from excessive stimulation of the labyrinthine receptors of the inner ear by certain motions, such as those experienced in a car, boat, plane, or swing. The disorder may also be caused by confusion in the cerebellum from conflicting sensory input—the visual stimulus (a moving horizon) conflicts with labyrinthine perception. Predisposing factors include tension or fear, offensive odors, or sights and sounds associated with a previous attack. Motion sickness from cars, elevators, trains, and swings is most common in children; from boats and airplanes in adults. People who suffer from one kind of motion sickness aren't necessarily susceptible to other types.

Signs and symptoms
Typically, motion sickness induces nausea, vomiting, headache, dizziness, fatigue, diaphoresis and, occasionally, difficulty in breathing, leading to a sensation of suffocation. These symptoms usually subside when the precipitating stimulus is removed, but they may persist for several hours or days.

Treatment
The best way to treat the disorder is to stop the motion that's causing it. If this isn't possible, the patient will benefit from lying down, closing his eyes, and trying to sleep. Antiemetics, such as dimenhydrinate, cyclizine, meclizine, and scopolamine (transdermal patch), may prevent or relieve motion sickness.

Special considerations
■ Tell the patient to avoid exposure to precipitating motion whenever possible. The traveler can minimize motion sickness by sitting where motion is least apparent (near the wing section in an aircraft, in the center of a boat, or in the front seat of an automobile). Instruct him to keep his head still and his eyes closed or focused on a distant and stationary object. An elevated car seat may help prevent motion sickness in a child by allowing him to see out the front window.
■ Instruct the patient to avoid eating or drinking for at least 4 hours before traveling and to take an antiemetic 30 to 60 minutes before traveling, or to apply a transdermal scopolamine patch at least 4 hours

before traveling. Tell the patient with prostate enlargement or glaucoma to consult a physician or pharmacist before taking antiemetics.

NOSE

Epistaxis

Epistaxis, commonly known as a *nosebleed*, may be a primary disorder or may occur secondary to another condition. Such bleeding in children generally originates in the anterior nasal septum and tends to be mild. In adults, such bleeding is most likely to originate in the posterior septum and can be severe. Epistaxis is twice as common in children as in adults.

Causes
Epistaxis usually follows trauma from external or internal causes: a blow to the nose, nose picking, or insertion of a foreign body; low humidity; or allergies, colds, or sinusitis. Less commonly, it follows polyps; acute or chronic infections such as sinusitis or rhinitis, which cause congestion and eventual bleeding of the capillary blood vessels; or inhalation of chemicals that irritate the nasal mucosa.

Predisposing factors include anticoagulant therapy, hypertension, long-term use of aspirin, high altitudes and dry climates, sclerotic vessel disease, Hodgkin's disease, hereditary hemorrhagic telangiectasia, neoplastic disorders (such as juvenile nasopharyngeal angiofibromas), scurvy, vitamin K deficiency, rheumatic fever, and blood dyscrasias (hemophilia, purpura, leukemia, and anemias).

Signs and symptoms
Blood oozing from the nostrils usually originates in the anterior nose and is bright red. Blood from the back of the throat originates in the posterior area and may be dark or bright red (commonly mistaken for hemoptysis due to expectoration). Epistaxis is generally unilateral, except when it's due to dyscrasia or severe trauma. In severe epistaxis, blood may seep behind

INSERTING AN ANTERIOR-POSTERIOR NASAL PACK

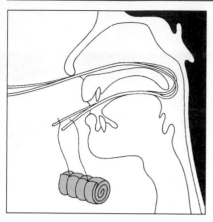

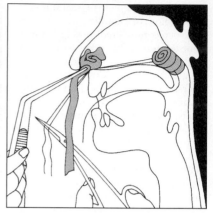

The first step in the insertion of an anterior-posterior nasal pack is the insertion of catheters into the nostrils. After the catheters are drawn through the mouth, a suture from the pack is tied to each (as shown above).

This positions the pack in place as the catheters are drawn back through the nostrils. While the sutures are held tightly, packing is inserted into the anterior nose (as shown above).

the nasal septum; it may also appear in the middle ear and in the corners of the eyes.

Associated clinical effects depend on the severity of bleeding. Moderate blood loss may produce light-headedness, dizziness, and slight respiratory difficulty; severe hemorrhage causes hypotension, rapid and bounding pulse, dyspnea, and pallor. Bleeding is considered severe if it persists longer than 10 minutes after pressure is applied and causes blood loss as great as 1 L/hour in adults. Exsanguination (bleeding to death) from epistaxis is rare.

Diagnosis

CONFIRMING DIAGNOSIS
Although simple observation confirms epistaxis, inspection with a bright light and a nasal speculum is necessary to locate the site of bleeding.

Relevant laboratory values include:
■ gradual reduction in hemoglobin levels and hematocrit (HCT; usually inaccurate immediately following epistaxis because of hemoconcentration)
■ decreased platelet count in the patient with blood dyscrasia
■ prothrombin time and partial thromboplastin time showing a coagulation time twice the control, because of a bleeding disorder or anticoagulant therapy.

Diagnosis must rule out underlying systemic causes of epistaxis, especially disseminated intravascular coagulation and rheumatic fever. Bruises or concomitant bleeding elsewhere probably indicates a hematologic disorder.

 PEDIATRIC TIP *Bleeding tests are indicated if any of the following are present:*
■ *family history of a bleeding disorder*
■ *medical history of easy bleeding*
■ *spontaneous bleeding at other sites*
■ *bleeding that won't clot with direct pressure by the physician*
■ *bleeding that lasts longer than 30 minutes*

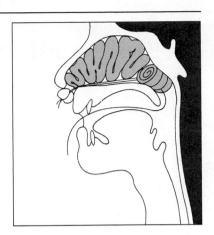

The sutures are then secured around a dental roll; the middle suture extends from the mouth (as shown above) and is taped to the cheek.

■ *onset before age 2 or a drop in HCT due to epistaxis.*

Treatment

Mild nosebleeds that occur spontaneously may be treated by gently squeezing the soft portion of the nose between the thumb and finger for 5 to 10 minutes while the patient leans forward slightly (to avoid swallowing the blood) and breathes through his mouth.

For anterior bleeding, treatment consists of application to the bleeding site of a cotton ball saturated with epinephrine, and external pressure, followed by cauterization with electrocautery or a silver nitrate stick. If these measures don't control the bleeding, petroleum gauze nasal packing may be needed.

For posterior bleeding, therapy includes gauze packing inserted through the nose, or postnasal packing inserted through the mouth, depending on the bleeding site. (Gauze packing generally remains in place

for 24 to 48 hours; postnasal packing, 3 to 5 days.) (See *Inserting an anterior-posterior nasal pack.*) An alternate method, the nasal balloon catheter, also controls bleeding effectively. Antibiotics may be appropriate if packing must remain in place for longer than 24 hours. If local measures fail to control bleeding, additional treatment may include supplemental vitamin K and, for severe bleeding, blood transfusions and surgical ligation or embolization of a bleeding artery.

Special considerations

To control epistaxis:
■ Elevate the patient's head 45 degrees.
■ Continuously compress the soft portion of the nares against the septum for 5 to 10 minutes. Apply an ice collar or cold, wet compresses to the nose. If bleeding continues after 10 minutes of pressure, notify the physician.
■ Administer oxygen as needed, and monitor saturation levels.
■ Monitor vital signs and skin color; record blood loss.
■ Tell the patient to breathe through his mouth and not to swallow blood, talk, or blow his nose.
■ Keep vasoconstrictors, such as phenylephrine, handy.
■ Reassure the patient and his family that epistaxis usually looks worse than it is.

To prevent recurrence of epistaxis:
■ Instruct the patient not to pick his nose or insert foreign objects into it, and to avoid bending or lifting. Emphasize the need for follow-up examinations and periodic blood studies after an episode of epistaxis. Advise prompt treatment for nasal infection or irritation.
■ Suggest humidifiers for people who live in dry climates or at high elevations, or whose homes are heated with circulating hot air.

Septal perforation and deviation

Perforated septum, a hole in the nasal septum between the two air passages, usually occurs in the anterior cartilaginous septum

SEPTAL PERFORATION

In the photograph at right, the nasal septum shows obvious perforation of the cartilage between the two air passages.

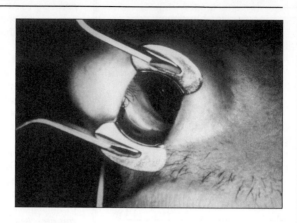

but may occur in the bony septum. Deviated septum, a shift from the midline, is common in most adults. This condition may be severe enough to obstruct the passage of air through the nostrils. With surgical correction, the prognosis for either perforated or deviated septum is good. (See *Septal perforation.*)

Causes and incidence
Generally, perforated septum is caused by traumatic irritation, most commonly resulting from excessive nose picking; less frequently, it results from repeated cauterization for epistaxis or from penetrating septal injury. It may also result from perichondritis, an infection that gradually erodes the perichondrial layer and cartilage, finally forming an ulcer that perforates the septum. Other causes of septal perforation include syphilis, tuberculosis, untreated septal hematoma, inhalation of irritating chemicals, cocaine snorting, chronic nasal infections, nasal carcinoma, granuloma, and chronic sinusitis.

Deviated septum commonly develops during normal growth, as the septum shifts from one side to the other. Consequently, few adults have perfectly straight septa. Nasal trauma resulting from a fall, a blow to the nose, or surgery further exaggerates

the deviation. Congenital deviated septum is rare.

Signs and symptoms
A small septal perforation is usually asymptomatic but may produce a whistle on inspiration. A large perforation causes rhinitis, epistaxis, nasal crusting, and watery discharge.

The patient with a deviated septum may develop a crooked nose, as the midline deflects to one side. The predominant symptom of severe deflection, however, is nasal obstruction. Other manifestations include a sensation of fullness in the face, shortness of breath, stertor (snoring or laborious breathing), nasal discharge, recurring epistaxis, infection, sinusitis, and headache.

Diagnosis
Although clinical features suggest septal perforation or deviation, confirmation requires inspection of the nasal mucosa with a bright light and a nasal speculum.

Treatment
Symptomatic treatment for perforated septum includes decongestants to reduce nasal congestion by local vasoconstriction, local application of lanolin or petroleum jelly to prevent ulceration and crusting, and antibiotics to combat infection. Surgery may

be necessary to graft part of the perichondrial layer over the perforation. Also, a plastic or Silastic "button" prosthesis may be used to close the perforation.

Symptomatic treatment for deviated septum usually includes analgesics to relieve headache, decongestants to minimize secretions and, as necessary, vasoconstrictors, nasal packing, or cautery to control hemorrhage. Manipulation of the nasal septum at birth can correct congenital deviated septum.

Corrective surgical procedures include:
- reconstruction of the nasal septum by submucous resection to reposition the nasal septal cartilage and relieve nasal obstruction.
- rhinoplasty to correct nasal structure deformity by intranasal incisions.
- septoplasty to relieve nasal obstruction and enhance cosmetic appearance.

Special considerations
- In the patient with perforated septum, use a cotton applicator to apply petroleum jelly to the nasal mucosa to minimize crusting and ulceration.
- Warn the patient with perforation or severe deviation against blowing his nose. To relieve nasal congestion, instill saline nosedrops and suggest use of a humidifier. Give decongestants as ordered.
- To treat epistaxis, have the patient sit upright, provide an emesis basin, and instruct the patient to expectorate any blood. Compress the outer portion of the nose against the septum for 10 to 15 minutes, and apply ice packs. If bleeding persists, notify the physician.
- If corrective surgery is scheduled, prepare the patient to expect postoperative facial edema, periorbital bruising, and nasal packing, which remains in place for 12 to 24 hours. The patient must breathe through his mouth. After surgery for deviated septum, the patient may also have a splint on his nose.
- To reduce or prevent edema and promote drainage, place the patient in semi-Fowler's position, and use a cool-mist vaporizer to liquefy secretions and facilitate normal breathing. To lessen facial edema and pain, place crushed ice in a rubber glove or a small ice bag, and apply the glove or ice bag intermittently over the eyes and nose for 24 hours.
- Because the patient is breathing through his mouth, provide frequent mouth care.
- Change the mustache dressing or drip pad as needed. Record the color, consistency, and amount of drainage. While nasal packing is in place, expect slight, bright red drainage, with clots. After packing is removed, watch for purulent discharge, an indication of infection.
- Watch for and report excessive swallowing, hematoma, or a falling or flapping septum (depressed, or soft and unstable septum). Intranasal examination is necessary to detect hematoma formation. Any of these complications requires surgical correction.
- Administer sedatives and analgesics as needed. Because of its anticoagulant properties, aspirin is contraindicated after surgery for septal deviation or perforation.
- Nose blowing may cause bruising and swelling even after nasal packing is removed. After surgery, the patient must limit physical activity for 2 or 3 days, and if he's a smoker, he must stop smoking for at least 2 days.
- Instruct the patient to sneeze with his mouth open and to avoid bending over at the waist. (Advise him to stoop to pick up fallen objects.)

Sinusitis

Sinusitis — inflammation of the paranasal sinuses — may be acute, subacute, chronic, allergic, or hyperplastic. Acute sinusitis usually results from the common cold and lingers in subacute form in only about 10% of patients. Chronic sinusitis follows persistent bacterial infection; allergic sinusitis accompanies allergic rhinitis; hyperplastic sinusitis is a combination of purulent acute sinusitis and allergic sinusitis or rhinitis. The prognosis is good for all types.

Causes and incidence
Sinusitis usually results from viral or bacterial infection. The bacteria responsible for acute sinusitis are usually pneumococci,

other streptococci, *Haemophilus influenzae*, and *Moraxella catarrhalis*. Staphylococci and gram-negative bacteria are more likely to cause sinusitis in chronic cases or in intensive care patients.

Predisposing factors include any condition that interferes with drainage and ventilation of the sinuses, such as chronic nasal edema, deviated septum, viscous mucus, nasal polyps, allergic rhinitis, nasal intubation, or debilitation due to chemotherapy, malnutrition, diabetes, blood dyscrasias, cystic fibrosis, human immunodeficiency virus or other immunodeficiency disorders, or chronic use of steroids. Bacterial invasion commonly occurs as a result of the conditions listed above or after a viral infection. It may also result from swimming in contaminated water.

Other risk factors for developing sinusitis include a history of asthma, overuse of nasal decongestants, presence of a foreign body in the nose, frequent swimming or diving, dental work, pregnancy, changes in altitude (flying or climbing), air pollution and smoke, gastroesophageal reflux disease, and having a deviated nasal septum, nasal bone spur, or polyp.

Each year, more than 30 million adults and children get sinusitis.

 PEDIATRIC TIP *The incidence of both acute and chronic sinusitis increases in later childhood. Sinusitis may be more prevalent in children who have had tonsils and adenoids removed.*

Signs and symptoms
The primary indication of acute sinusitis is nasal congestion, followed by a gradual buildup of pressure in the affected sinus. For 24 to 48 hours after onset, nasal discharge may be present and later may become purulent. Associated symptoms include malaise, sore throat, headache, and low-grade fever of 99° to 99.5° F [37.2° to 37.5° C]).

Characteristic pain depends on the affected sinus: maxillary sinusitis causes pain over the cheeks and upper teeth; ethmoid sinusitis, pain over the eyes; frontal sinusitis, pain over the eyebrows; and sphenoid sinusitis (rare), pain behind the eyes.

Purulent nasal drainage that continues for longer than 3 weeks after an acute infection subsides suggests *subacute sinusitis*. Other clinical features of the subacute form include nasal congestion, vague facial discomfort, fatigue, and a nonproductive cough.

The effects of *chronic sinusitis* are similar to those of acute sinusitis, but the chronic form causes continuous mucopurulent discharge.

The effects of *allergic sinusitis* are the same as those of allergic rhinitis. In both conditions, the prominent symptoms are sneezing, frontal headache, watery nasal discharge, and a stuffy, burning, itchy nose.

In *hyperplastic sinusitis*, bacterial growth on the diseased tissue causes pronounced tissue edema; thickening of the mucosal lining and the development of mucosal polyps combine to produce chronic stuffiness of the nose, in addition to headaches.

Diagnosis
The following measures are useful:
- Antral puncture promotes drainage of purulent material. It may also be used to provide a specimen for culture and sensitivity testing of the infecting organism, but it's seldom performed.
- Nasal examination reveals inflammation and pus.
- Sinus X-rays reveal cloudiness in the affected sinus, air and fluid, and any thickening of the mucosal lining.
- Transillumination is a simple diagnostic tool that involves shining a light into the patient's mouth with his lips closed around it. Infected sinuses look dark and normal sinuses transilluminate.
- Ultrasound, computed tomography scan, magnetic resonance imaging, and X-rays aid in diagnosing suspected complications.

Treatment
Local decongestants usually are tried before systemic decongestants; steam inhalation may also be helpful. Antibiotics are necessary to combat purulent or persistent infection. Amoxicillin and amoxicillin/clavulanate potassium are usually the antibiotics of choice. Other possible therapy

includes cefixime for responsive infections or if beta-lactamase-producing bacteria are present. Because sinusitis is a deep-seated infection, antibiotics should be given for 10 days to 2 weeks, with the exception of azithromycin, which is given for 5 days. Local applications of heat may help to relieve pain and congestion. In subacute sinusitis, antibiotics and decongestants may be helpful.

Treatment for allergic sinusitis must include treatment for allergic rhinitis—administration of antihistamines, identification of allergens by skin testing, and desensitization by immunotherapy. Severe allergic symptoms may require treatment with corticosteroids and epinephrine.

In both chronic sinusitis and hyperplastic sinusitis, using antihistamines, antibiotics, and a steroid nasal spray may relieve pain and congestion. If subacute infection persists, the sinuses may be irrigated. If irrigation fails to relieve symptoms, endoscopic sinus surgery may be required to obtain a histologic diagnosis, remove polyps, and provide adequate ventilation of the infected sinuses. Partial or total resection of the middle turbinate as well as more radical procedures, such as total sphenoethmoidectomy, may be performed.

Special considerations

■ Enforce bed rest, and encourage the patient to drink plenty of fluids to promote drainage. Don't elevate the head of the bed more than 30 degrees.

■ To relieve pain and promote drainage, apply warm compresses continuously, or four times daily for 2-hour intervals. Also, give analgesics and antihistamines as needed.

■ Watch for and report complications, such as vomiting, chills, fever, edema of the forehead or eyelids, blurred or double vision, and personality changes.

■ If surgery is necessary, tell the patient what to expect postoperatively: nasal packing will be in place for 12 to 24 hours following surgery; he'll have to breathe through his mouth and won't be able to blow his nose. After surgery, monitor for excessive drainage or bleeding and watch for complications.

■ To prevent edema and promote drainage, place the patient in semi-Fowler's position. To relieve edema and pain and to minimize bleeding, apply ice compresses or a rubber glove filled with ice chips over the nose, and iced saline gauze over the eyes. Continue these measures for 24 hours.

■ Frequently change the mustache dressing or drip pad, and record the consistency, amount, and color of drainage (expect scant, bright red, and clotty drainage).

■ Because the patient will be breathing through his mouth, provide meticulous mouth care.

■ Tell the patient that even after the packing is removed, nose blowing may cause bleeding and swelling. If the patient is a smoker, instruct him not to smoke for at least 2 or 3 days after surgery.

■ Tell the patient to finish the prescribed antibiotics, even if his symptoms disappear.

Nasal polyps

Benign and edematous growths, nasal polyps are usually multiple, mobile, and bilateral. Nasal polyps may become large and numerous enough to cause nasal distention and enlargement of the bony framework, possibly occluding the airway.

Causes and incidence

Nasal polyps are usually produced by the continuous pressure resulting from a chronic allergy that causes prolonged mucous membrane edema in the nose and sinuses. Other predisposing factors include chronic sinusitis, chronic rhinitis, and recurrent nasal infections.

Nasal polyps are more common in adults than in children and tend to recur. They're also commonly seen in patients with long-term allergic rhinitis. About 1 in 4 people with cystic fibrosis have nasal polyps.

Signs and symptoms

Nasal obstruction is the primary indication of nasal polyps. Such obstruction causes anosmia, a sensation of fullness in the face, nasal discharge, headache, and shortness of breath. Associated clinical features are usually the same as those of allergic rhinitis.

Diagnosis

Diagnosis of nasal polyps is aided by the following tests:

- Examination with a nasal speculum shows a dry, red surface, with clear or gray growths. Large growths may resemble tumors.
- X-rays of sinuses and nasal passages reveal soft tissue shadows over the affected areas.

Nasal polyps occurring in children require further testing to rule out cystic fibrosis and Peutz-Jeghers syndrome.

Treatment

Generally, treatment consists of corticosteroids (either by direct injection into the polyps or by local spray) to temporarily reduce the polyp. A short course of oral corticosteroids (such as prednisone) may be beneficial. Treatment for the underlying cause may include antihistamines to control allergy, and antibiotic therapy if infection is present. Local application of an astringent shrinks hypertrophied tissue. However, medical management alone is seldom effective.

Consequently, the treatment of choice is polypectomy, which is usually performed under a local anesthetic. The use of surgical lasers is becoming more popular. Continued recurrence may require surgical opening of the ethmoid, sphenoid, and maxillary sinuses and evacuation of diseased tissue.

Special considerations

- Administer antihistamines, as ordered, for the patient with allergies. Prepare the patient for scheduled surgery by telling him what to expect postoperatively, such as nasal packing for 1 to 2 days after surgery.

After surgery:

- Monitor for excessive bleeding or other drainage, and promote patient comfort.
- Elevate the head of the bed to facilitate breathing, reduce swelling, and promote adequate drainage. Change the mustache dressing or drip pad, as needed, and record the consistency, amount, and color of nasal drainage.

- Intermittently apply ice compresses over the nostrils to lessen swelling, prevent bleeding, and relieve pain.
- If nasal bleeding occurs — most likely after packing is removed — sit the patient upright, monitor his vital signs, and advise him not to swallow blood. Compress the outside of his nose against the septum for 10 to 15 minutes. If bleeding persists, nasal packing may be necessary.

To prevent nasal polyps, instruct patients with allergies to avoid exposure to allergens and to take antihistamines at the first sign of an allergic reaction. Also, advise them to avoid overuse of nose drops and sprays.

Nasal papillomas

A papilloma is a benign epithelial tissue overgrowth within the intranasal mucosa. Inverted papillomas grow into the underlying tissue, usually at the junction of the antrum and the maxillary sinus; they generally occur singly but sometimes are associated with squamous cell cancer. Exophytic papillomas, which also tend to occur singly, arise from epithelial tissue, commonly on the surface of the nasal septum.

Causes and incidence

A papilloma may arise as a benign precursor of a neoplasm or as a response to tissue injury or viral infection, but its cause is unknown. Both types of papillomas are most prevalent in males. Recurrence is common, even after surgical excision.

Signs and symptoms

Both inverted and exophytic papillomas typically produce symptoms related to unilateral nasal obstruction — congestion, postnasal drip, headache, shortness of breath, dyspnea and, rarely, severe respiratory distress, nasal drainage, and infection. Epistaxis is most likely to occur with exophytic papillomas. Occasionally hemorrhage may be the presenting symptom.

Diagnosis

On examination of the nasal mucosa, inverted papillomas usually appear large, bulky, highly vascular, and edematous; color varies from dark red to gray; and consistency, from firm to friable. Exophytic papillomas are usually raised, firm, and rubbery; pink to gray; and securely attached by a broad or pedunculated base to the mucous membrane.

 PEDIATRIC TIP *Juvenile angiofibroma is a benign vascular tumor that arises in the nasopharynx and occurs most commonly in adolescent males. Nasal obstruction and hemorrhage may occur as with nasal papillomas. Any adolescent male who continues to have recurrent episodes of epistaxis should be assessed for juvenile angiofibroma. Medical management involves surgical excision, with preoperative embolization to reduce bleeding.*

 CONFIRMING DIAGNOSIS *Tissue biopsy followed by histologic examination of excised tissue confirms the diagnosis.*

Treatment

The most effective treatment is wide surgical excision or diathermy, with careful inspection of adjacent tissues and sinuses to rule out extension. The use of surgical lasers is becoming more popular. Ibuprofen or acetaminophen and decongestants may relieve symptoms.

Special considerations

■ If bleeding occurs, have the patient sit upright, and instruct him to expectorate blood into an emesis basin. Compress both sides of his nose against the septum for 10 to 15 minutes, and apply ice compresses to the nose. If the bleeding doesn't stop, notify the physician.

■ Check for airway obstruction. Place your hand under the patient's nostrils to assess air exchange, and watch for signs of mild shortness of breath.

■ If surgery is scheduled, tell the patient what to expect postoperatively. Instruct him not to blow his nose. (Packing is usually removed 12 to 24 hours after surgery.)

■ Postoperatively, monitor vital signs and respiratory status. Use pulse oximetry to monitor oxygen saturation levels. As needed, administer analgesics and facilitate breathing with a cool-mist vaporizer. Provide mouth care.

■ Frequently change the mustache dressing or drip pad, to ensure proper absorption of drainage. Record the type and amount of drainage. While the nasal packing is in place, expect scant, usually bright red, clotted drainage. Remember that the amount of drainage typically increases for a few hours after the packing is removed.

■ Because papillomas tend to recur, tell the patient to seek medical attention at the first sign of nasal discomfort, discharge, or congestion that doesn't subside with conservative treatment.

■ Encourage regular follow-up visits to detect early signs of recurrence.

Adenoid hyperplasia

A fairly common childhood condition, adenoid hyperplasia (also known as *adenoid hypertrophy*) is enlargement of the lymphoid tissue of the nasopharynx. Normally, adenoidal tissue is small at birth (¾″ to 1¼″ [2 to 3 cm]), grows until the child reaches adolescence, and then begins to slowly atrophy. In adenoid hyperplasia, however, this tissue continues to grow. Enlarged adenoids commonly accompany tonsillitis.

Causes

The cause of adenoid hyperplasia is unknown, but contributing factors may include heredity, chronic infection, chronic nasal congestion, persistent allergy, insufficient aeration, and inefficient nasal breathing. Inflammation resulting from repeated infection increases the patient's risk of respiratory obstruction.

Signs and symptoms

Typically, adenoid hyperplasia produces symptoms of respiratory obstruction, especially mouth breathing, snoring at night, and frequent, prolonged nasal congestion. Persistent mouth breathing during the formative years produces voice alteration and distinctive changes in facial features — a slightly elongated face, open mouth, highly arched palate, shortened upper lip, and vacant expression.

Occasionally, the child is incapable of mouth breathing, snores loudly at night, and may eventually show effects of nocturnal respiratory insufficiency, such as intercostal retractions and nasal flaring; this may lead to pulmonary hypertension and cor pulmonale. Adenoid hyperplasia can also obstruct the eustachian tube and predispose to otitis media, which in turn can lead to fluctuating conductive hearing loss. Stasis of nasal secretions from adenoidal inflammation can lead to sinusitis.

Diagnosis

CONFIRMING DIAGNOSIS
Nasopharyngoscopy or rhinoscopy confirms adenoid hyperplasia by allowing visualization of abnormal tissue. Lateral pharyngeal X-rays show an obliterated nasopharyngeal air column.

Treatment

Adenoidectomy is the treatment of choice for adenoid hyperplasia and is commonly recommended for the patient with prolonged mouth breathing, nasal speech, adenoid facies, recurrent otitis media, constant nasopharyngitis, and nocturnal respiratory distress. This procedure usually eliminates recurrent nasal infections and ear complications and reverses any secondary hearing loss.

Special considerations

Care requires sympathetic preoperative care and diligent postoperative monitoring.

Before surgery:
■ Describe the facility routine, and arrange for the patient and his parents to tour relevant areas.
■ Explain adenoidectomy to the child, using illustrations if necessary, and detail the recovery process. Advise him that he'll probably need to be hospitalized. If facility protocol allows, encourage one parent to stay with the child and participate in his care.
After surgery:

■ Maintain a patent airway. Position the child on his side, with his head down, to prevent aspiration of draining secretions. Frequently check the throat for bleeding. Be alert for vomiting of old, partially digested blood (coffee-ground vomitus). Closely monitor vital signs, and report excessive bleeding, rise in pulse rate, drop in blood pressure, tachypnea, and restlessness.
■ If no bleeding occurs, offer cracked ice or water when the patient is fully awake.
■ Tell the parents that their child may temporarily have a nasal voice.

Velopharyngeal insufficiency

Velopharyngeal insufficiency results from failure of the velopharyngeal sphincter to close properly during speech, giving the voice a hypernasal quality and permitting nasal emission (air escape during pronunciation of consonants).

Causes and incidence

Velopharyngeal insufficiency can result from an inherited palate abnormality, or it can be acquired from tonsillectomy, adenoidectomy, or palatal paresis. It commonly occurs in people who undergo cleft palate surgery and those with submucous cleft palates. Middle ear disease and hearing loss frequently accompany this disorder.

Signs and symptoms

Generally, this condition causes unintelligible speech, marked by hypernasality, nasal emission, poor consonant definition, and a weak voice. The patient experiences dysphagia and, if velopharyngeal insufficiency is severe, he may regurgitate through the nose.

Diagnosis

Fiber-optic nasopharyngoscopy, which permits monitoring of velopharyngeal patency during speech, suggests this diagnosis. Ultrasound scanning, which shows air-tissue overlap, reflects the degree of velopharyngeal sphincter incompetence (an opening greater than 20 mm^2 results in unintelligible speech). Videofluoroscopy simultaneously records the movement of the velopharyngeal sphincter and the patient's speech.

Treatment
Treatment consists of corrective surgery, usually at age 6 or 7. The preferred surgical method is the pharyngeal flap procedure, which diverts a tissue flap from the pharynx to the soft palate. Children with velopharyngeal insufficiency shouldn't have adenoidectomy except in cases of life-threatening obstruction.

Other appropriate surgical procedures include:
- augmentation pharyngoplasty, which narrows the velopharyngeal opening by enlarging the pharyngeal wall with a retropharyngeal implant
- palatal push-back, which separates the hard and soft palates to allow insertion of an obturator, thus lengthening the soft palate
- pharyngoplasty, which rotates pharyngeal flaps to lengthen the soft palate and narrow the pharynx
- velopharyngeal sphincter reconstruction, which uses free muscle implantation to reconstruct the sphincter.

Surgery eliminates hypernasality and nasal emission, but speech abnormalities persist and usually necessitate speech therapy. Immediate postoperative therapy includes antibiotics and a clear, liquid diet for the first 3 days, followed by a soft diet for 2 weeks.

Special considerations
- After surgery for velopharyngeal insufficiency, maintain a patent airway (nasopharynx edema may obstruct the airway). Position the patient on his side, and suction the dependent side of his mouth, avoiding the pharynx.
- Control postoperative agitation, which may provoke pharyngeal bleeding, with sedation, as ordered.
- Administer high-humidity oxygen as ordered.
- Monitor vital signs frequently, and report any changes immediately. Observe for bleeding from the mouth or nose. Check intake and output, and watch for signs of dehydration.
- Advise the patient that preoperative and postoperative speech therapy require time and effort on his part, but with persistence and practice, his speech will improve. Before discharge, emphasize the importance of completing the prescribed antibiotic therapy.

THROAT

Pharyngitis

The most common throat disorder, pharyngitis is an acute or chronic inflammation of the pharynx. It frequently accompanies the common cold.

Causes and incidence
Pharyngitis is usually caused by a virus. The most common bacterial cause is group A beta-hemolytic streptococci. Other common causes include *Mycoplasma* and *Chlamydia*. In up to 30% of cases, no organism is identified.

Pharyngitis is widespread among adults who live or work in dusty or very dry environments, use their voices excessively, habitually use tobacco or alcohol, or suffer from chronic sinusitis, persistent coughs, or allergies.

Signs and symptoms
Pharyngitis produces a sore throat and slight difficulty in swallowing. Swallowing saliva is usually more painful than swallowing food. Pharyngitis may also cause the sensation of a lump in the throat as well as a constant, aggravating urge to swallow. Associated features may include mild fever, headache, muscle and joint pain, coryza, and rhinorrhea. Uncomplicated pharyngitis usually subsides in 3 to 10 days.

 PEDIATRIC TIP *More than 90% of cases of sore throat and fever in children are of viral origin. Associated symptoms usually include runny nose and nonproductive cough.*

Diagnosis

Physical examination of the pharynx reveals generalized redness and inflammation of the posterior wall, and red, edematous mucous membranes studded with white or yellow follicles. Exudate is usually confined to the lymphoid areas of the throat, sparing the tonsillar pillars. Bacterial pharyngitis usually produces a large amount of exudate.

A throat culture may be performed to identify bacterial organisms that may be the cause of the inflammation.

Treatment

Treatment for acute viral pharyngitis is usually symptomatic and consists mainly of rest, warm saline gargles, throat lozenges containing a mild anesthetic, plenty of fluids, and analgesics as needed. If the patient can't swallow fluids, I.V. hydration may be required.

Suspected bacterial pharyngitis requires rigorous treatment with penicillin or another broad-spectrum antibiotic because *Streptococcus* is the chief infecting organism. Antibiotic therapy should continue for 48 hours until culture results are back. If the culture (or a rapid strep test) is positive for group A beta-hemolytic streptococci, or if bacterial infection is suspected despite negative culture results, penicillin therapy should be continued for 10 days. This is to prevent the sequelae of acute rheumatic fever.

Chronic pharyngitis requires the same supportive measures as acute pharyngitis but with greater emphasis on eliminating the underlying cause, such as an allergen. Preventive measures include adequate humidification and avoiding excessive exposure to air conditioning. In addition, the patient should be urged to stop smoking.

Special considerations

■ Administer analgesics and warm saline gargles, as ordered and as appropriate.
■ Encourage the patient to drink plenty of fluids. Scrupulously monitor intake and output, and watch for signs of dehydration.
■ Provide meticulous mouth care to prevent dry lips and oral pyoderma, and maintain a restful environment.

■ Obtain throat cultures, and administer antibiotics as needed. If the patient has acute bacterial pharyngitis, emphasize the importance of completing the full course of antibiotic therapy.
■ Teach the patient with chronic pharyngitis how to minimize sources of throat irritation in the environment such as by using a bedside humidifier.
■ Refer the patient to a self-help group to stop smoking if appropriate.
■ Children attending school should receive at least 24 hours of therapy before being allowed to return to school.
■ If the patient has exhibited three or more documented bacterial infections within 6 months, consider daily penicillin prophylaxis during the winter months. Also, consider treatment of carriers who live in closed or semiclosed communities.

Tonsillitis

Tonsillitis — inflammation of the tonsils — can be acute or chronic. The uncomplicated acute form usually lasts 4 to 6 days. The presence of proven chronic tonsillitis justifies tonsillectomy, the only effective treatment. Tonsils tend to hypertrophy during childhood and atrophy after puberty.

Causes and incidence

Tonsillitis generally results from infection with group A beta-hemolytic streptococci but can result from other bacteria or viruses or from oral anaerobes. It commonly affects children between ages 5 and 10.

Signs and symptoms

Acute tonsillitis commonly begins with a mild to severe sore throat. A very young child, unable to describe a sore throat, may stop eating. Tonsillitis may also produce dysphagia, fever, swelling and tenderness of the lymph glands in the submandibular area, muscle and joint pain, chills, malaise, headache, and pain (frequently referred to the ears). Excess secretions may elicit the complaint of a constant urge to swallow; the back of the throat may feel constricted. Such discomfort usually subsides after 72 hours.

Chronic tonsillitis produces a recurrent sore throat and purulent drainage in the tonsillar crypts. Frequent attacks of acute tonsillitis may also occur. Complications include obstruction from tonsillar hypertrophy and peritonsillar abscess.

Diagnosis

Diagnostic confirmation requires a thorough throat examination that reveals:
- generalized inflammation of the pharyngeal wall
- swollen tonsils that project from between the pillars of the fauces and exude white or yellow follicles
- purulent drainage when pressure is applied to the tonsillar pillars
- possible edematous and inflamed uvula.

Culture may determine the infecting organism and indicate appropriate antibiotic therapy. Leukocytosis is also usually present. Differential diagnosis rules out infectious mononucleosis and diphtheria.

Treatment

Treatment for acute tonsillitis requires rest, adequate fluid intake, administration of ibuprofen or acetaminophen and, for bacterial infection, antibiotics. When the causative organism is group A beta-hemolytic streptococcus, penicillin is the drug of choice (another broad-spectrum antibiotic may be substituted). Most oral anaerobes also respond to penicillin. To prevent complications, antibiotic therapy should continue for 10 to 14 days.

Chronic tonsillitis or the development of complications (obstructions from tonsillar hypertrophy, peritonsillar abscess) may require a tonsillectomy, but only after the patient has been free from tonsillar or respiratory tract infections for 3 to 4 weeks.

Special considerations

- Despite dysphagia, urge the patient to drink plenty of fluids, especially if he has a fever. Offer a child ice cream and flavored drinks and ices. Suggest gargling with warm salt water to soothe the throat, unless it exacerbates pain. Make sure the patient and his parents understand the importance of completing the prescribed course of antibiotic therapy.
- Before tonsillectomy, explain to the adult patient that a local anesthetic prevents pain but allows a sensation of pressure during surgery. Warn the patient to expect considerable throat discomfort and some bleeding postoperatively. Watch for continuous swallowing, a sign of heavy bleeding.
- For the pediatric patient, keep your explanation simple and nonthreatening. Show him the operating and recovery areas, and briefly explain the facility routine. Most facilities allow one parent to stay with the child.
- Postoperatively, maintain a patent airway. To prevent aspiration, place the patient on his side. Monitor vital signs frequently, and check for bleeding. Immediately report excessive bleeding, increased pulse rate, or dropping blood pressure. After he's fully alert and the gag reflex has returned, allow him to drink water. Later, urge him to drink plenty of nonirritating fluids, to ambulate, and to take frequent deep breaths to prevent pulmonary complications. Give pain medication as needed.
- Before discharge, provide the patient or his parents with written instructions on home care. Tell them to expect a white scab to form in the throat between 5 and 10 days postoperatively, and to report bleeding, ear discomfort, or a fever that lasts longer than 3 days.

Throat abscesses

Throat abscesses may be peritonsillar (quinsy) or retropharyngeal. Peritonsillar abscesses form in the connective tissue space between the tonsil capsule and the constrictor muscle of the pharynx. Retropharyngeal abscesses, or abscesses of the potential space, form between the posterior pharyngeal wall and the prevertebral fascia. With treatment, the prognosis for both types of abscesses is good.

Causes and incidence

Peritonsillar abscess is a complication of acute tonsillitis, usually after streptococcal or staphylococcal infection. It occurs more commonly in adolescents and young adults than in children.

Acute retropharyngeal abscess results from infection in the retropharyngeal lymph glands, which may follow an upper respiratory tract bacterial infection. Most common pathogens are beta-hemolytic *Streptococcus* and *Staphylococcus aureus.* These lymph glands begin to atrophy after age 2. Acute retropharyngeal abscess most commonly affects infants and children younger than age 2.

Chronic retropharyngeal abscess may result from tuberculosis of the cervical spine (Pott's disease) and may occur at any age.

Signs and symptoms
Key symptoms of peritonsillar abscess include severe throat pain, occasional ear pain on the same side as the abscess, and tenderness of the submandibular gland. Dysphagia causes drooling. Trismus may occur as a result of the spread of edema and infection from the peritonsillar space to the pterygoid muscles. Other effects include fever, chills, malaise, rancid breath, nausea, muffled speech, dehydration, cervical adenopathy, and localized or systemic sepsis.

Clinical features of retropharyngeal abscess include pain, dysphagia, fever and, when the abscess is located in the upper pharynx, nasal obstruction; with a low-positioned abscess, dyspnea, progressive inspiratory stridor (from laryngeal obstruction), neck hyperextension and, in children, drooling and muffled crying occur. Other symptoms in children may include gurgling respirations, dyspnea and dysphagia, respiratory symptoms, and fever. A very large abscess may press on the larynx, causing edema, or may erode into major vessels, causing sudden death from asphyxia or aspiration.

Diagnosis
Diagnosis of peritonsillar abscess usually begins with a patient history of bacterial pharyngitis. Examination of the throat shows swelling of the soft palate on the abscessed side, with displacement of the uvula to the opposite side; red, edematous mucous membranes; and tonsil displacement toward the midline. Culture may reveal streptococcal or staphylococcal infection.

Diagnosis of retropharyngeal abscess is based on patient history of nasopharyngitis or pharyngitis and on physical examination revealing a soft, red bulging of the posterior pharyngeal wall. X-rays show the larynx pushed forward and a widened space between the posterior pharyngeal wall and vertebra. If neck pain or stiffness occurs, look for extension to the epidural space or the cervical vertebrae. Culture and sensitivity tests isolate the causative organism and reveal the appropriate antibiotic.

Treatment
For early-stage peritonsillar abscess, large doses of penicillin or another broad-spectrum antibiotic are necessary. If the patient is immunocompromised or has been repeatedly hospitalized, antibiotic therapy should include coverage for staphylococci and gram-negative organisms. For late-stage abscess, with cellulitis of the tonsillar space, primary treatment is usually incision and drainage under a local anesthetic, followed by antibiotic therapy for 7 to 10 days. Tonsillectomy, scheduled no sooner than 1 month after healing, prevents recurrence but is recommended only after several episodes.

In acute retropharyngeal abscess, the primary treatment is incision and drainage through the pharyngeal wall. It's considered a surgical emergency. In chronic retropharyngeal abscess, drainage is performed through an external incision behind the sternomastoid muscle. During incision and drainage, strong, continuous mouth suction is necessary to prevent aspiration of pus, and the head should be kept down. Postoperative drug therapy includes I.V. antibiotics (usually penicillin or clindamycin) and analgesics.

Special considerations
■ Be alert for signs of respiratory obstruction (inspiratory stridor, dyspnea, retractions and nasal flaring, increasing restlessness, and cyanosis). Keep emergency airway equipment nearby.
■ Explain the drainage procedure to the patient and his parents. Because the proce-

dure is usually done under local anesthesia, the patient may be apprehensive.
- Assist with incision and drainage. To allow easy expectoration and suction of pus and blood, place the patient in a semirecumbent or sitting position.

After incision and drainage:
- Give antibiotics, analgesics, and antipyretics, as ordered. Stress the importance of completing the full course of prescribed antibiotic therapy.
- Monitor vital signs, and report significant changes or bleeding. Assess pain, and treat accordingly.
- If the patient is unable to swallow, ensure adequate hydration with I.V. therapy. Monitor fluid intake and output, and watch for dehydration.
- Provide meticulous mouth care. Apply petroleum jelly to the patient's lips. Promote healing with warm saline gargles or throat irrigations for 24 to 36 hours after incision and drainage. Encourage adequate rest.

Vocal cord paralysis

Vocal cord paralysis results from disease of or injury to the superior or, most commonly, the recurrent laryngeal nerve. It may also be congenital.

Causes
Vocal cord paralysis commonly results from the accidental severing of the recurrent laryngeal nerve, or of one of its extralaryngeal branches, during thyroidectomy. Other causes include pressure from a thoracic aortic aneurysm or from an enlarged atrium (in patients with mitral stenosis), bronchial or esophageal carcinoma, hypertrophy of the thyroid gland, trauma (such as neck injuries) and intubation, and neuritis due to infections or metallic poisoning. Vocal cord paralysis can also result from hysteria and, rarely, lesions of the central nervous system.

Signs and symptoms
Unilateral paralysis, the most common form, may cause vocal weakness and hoarseness. Bilateral paralysis typically

produces vocal weakness and incapacitating airway obstruction if the cords become paralyzed in the adducted position.

 PEDIATRIC TIP *Children may present with hoarseness, aspiration, and stridor. If the paralysis is unilateral, it typically involves the left recurrent laryngeal nerve. In unilateral paralysis, airway intervention involving intubation and tracheostomy is rarely indicated; it's usually required if the paralysis is bilateral.*

Diagnosis
The patient history and characteristic features suggest vocal cord paralysis.

 CONFIRMING DIAGNOSIS *Visualization by indirect laryngoscopy shows one or both cords fixed in an adducted or partially abducted position and confirms the diagnosis.*

X-ray or computed tomography scan detect abnormalities in the mediastinum that may be responsible for the injury.

Treatment
Treatment for unilateral vocal cord paralysis consists of injection of Teflon into the paralyzed cord, under direct laryngoscopy. This procedure enlarges the cord and brings it closer to the other cord, which usually strengthens the voice and protects the airway from aspiration. Thyroplasty also serves to reposition the vocal cord, but in this procedure an implant is placed through a neck incision. The ansa cervicalis nerve transfer allows for reinnervation of the muscles of the vocal cord. Bilateral cord paralysis in an adducted position necessitates a tracheostomy.

Alternative treatments for adults include endoscopic arytenoidectomy to open the glottis, and lateral fixation of the arytenoid cartilage through an external neck incision. Excision or fixation of the arytenoid cartilage improves airway patency but produces residual voice impairment.

Treatment for hysterical aphonia may include psychotherapy and hypnosis.

Special considerations
If the patient chooses direct laryngoscopy and Teflon injection, explain these procedures thoroughly. Tell him these measures

will improve his voice but won't restore it to normal. Patients are sometimes placed on voice rest for 24 to 48 hours to reduce stress on the vocal cords, which would increase the edema and might lead to airway obstruction.

Many patients with bilateral cord paralysis prefer to keep a tracheostomy instead of having an arytenoidectomy; voice quality is generally better with a tracheostomy alone than after corrective surgery.

If the patient is scheduled to undergo a tracheostomy:

- Explain the procedure thoroughly, and offer reassurance. Because the procedure is performed under a local anesthetic, the patient may be apprehensive.
- Teach the patient how to suction, clean, and change the tracheostomy tube.
- Reassure the patient that he can still speak by covering the lumen of the tracheostomy tube with his finger or a tracheostomy plug.

If the patient elects to have an arytenoidectomy, explain the procedure thoroughly. Advise the patient that the tracheostomy will remain in place until the edema has subsided and the airway is patent.

Vocal cord nodules and polyps

Vocal cord nodules result from hypertrophy of fibrous tissue and form at the point where the cords come together forcibly. Vocal cord polyps are chronic, subepithelial, edematous masses. Both nodules and polyps have a good prognosis unless continued voice abuse causes recurrence, with subsequent scarring and permanent hoarseness.

Causes and incidence

Vocal cord nodules and polyps usually result from voice abuse, especially in the presence of infection. Consequently, they're most common in teachers, singers, and sports fans, and in energetic children (ages 8 to 12) who continually shout while playing. Polyps are common in adults who smoke, live in dry climates, or have allergies.

 PEDIATRIC TIP *In children, papillomas of the larynx (benign warty growths) are the most common laryngeal neoplasm. Suspected causes include human papillomavirus types 6, 11, and 16. The virus may be acquired during birth because many mothers have a history of condylomata acuminata at the time of delivery.*

Signs and symptoms

Nodules and polyps inhibit the approximation of vocal cords and produce painless hoarseness. The voice may also develop a breathy or husky quality.

Diagnosis

Persistent hoarseness suggests vocal cord nodules and polyps; visualization by indirect laryngoscopy confirms it. In the patient with vocal cord nodules, laryngoscopy initially shows small red nodes; later, white solid nodes on one or both cords. (See *Vocal cord nodules.*) In the patient with polyps, laryngoscopy reveals unilateral or, occasionally, bilateral, sessile or pedunculated polyps of varying size, anywhere on the vocal cords.

Treatment

Conservative management of small vocal cord nodules and polyps includes humidification, speech therapy (voice rest, training to reduce the intensity and duration of voice production), and treatment for any underlying allergies.

When conservative treatment fails to relieve hoarseness, nodules or polyps require removal under direct laryngoscopy. Microlaryngoscopy may be done for small lesions, to avoid injuring the vocal cord surface. If nodules or polyps are bilateral, excision may be performed in two stages: one cord is allowed to heal before excision of polyps on the other cord. Two-stage excision prevents laryngeal web, which occurs when epithelial tissue is removed from adjacent cord surfaces, and these surfaces grow together. For children, treatment consists of speech therapy. If possible, surgery should be delayed until the child is old enough to benefit from voice training, or

VOCAL CORD NODULES

The most common site of vocal cord nodules is the point of maximal vibration and impact (junction of the anterior one-third and the posterior two-thirds of the vocal cord).

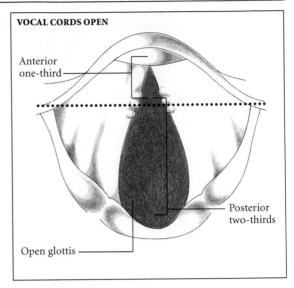

VOCAL CORDS OPEN

Anterior one-third

Posterior two-thirds

Open glottis

Vocal cord nodules affect the voice by inhibiting proper closure of the vocal cords during phonation.

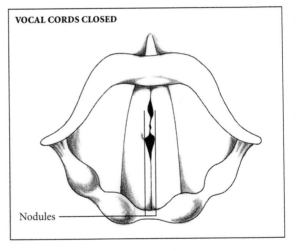

VOCAL CORDS CLOSED

Nodules

until he can understand the need to abstain from voice abuse.

Special considerations
■ Postoperatively, stress the importance of resting the voice for 10 to 14 days while the vocal cords heal. Provide an alternative means of communication—Magic Slate, pad and pencil, or alphabet board. Place a sign over the bed to remind visitors that the patient shouldn't talk. Mark the intercom so other facility personnel are aware that the patient can't answer. Minimize the

need to speak by trying to anticipate the patient's needs.
- If the patient is a smoker, encourage him to stop smoking entirely or, at the very least, to refrain from smoking during recovery from surgery.
- Use a vaporizer to increase humidity and decrease throat irritation.
- Make sure the patient receives speech therapy after healing if necessary, because continued voice abuse causes recurrence of growths.

Laryngitis

A common disorder, laryngitis is an acute or chronic inflammation of the vocal cords. Acute laryngitis may occur as an isolated infection or as part of a generalized bacterial or viral upper respiratory tract infection. Repeated attacks of acute laryngitis produce inflammatory changes associated with chronic laryngitis.

 ALERT *Several forms of laryngitis occur in children and can lead to significant or fatal respiratory obstruction, such as croup and epiglottiditis.*

Causes
Acute laryngitis usually results from infection (primarily viral) or excessive use of the voice, an occupational hazard in certain vocations (teaching, public speaking, or singing, for example). It may also result from leisure activities (such as cheering at a sports event), inhalation of smoke or fumes, or aspiration of caustic chemicals. Chronic laryngitis may be caused by chronic upper respiratory tract disorders (sinusitis, bronchitis, nasal polyps, or allergy), mouth breathing, smoking, constant exposure to dust or other irritants, and alcohol abuse.

Signs and symptoms
Acute laryngitis typically begins with hoarseness, ranging from mild to complete loss of voice. Associated clinical features include pain (especially when swallowing or speaking), a persistent dry cough, fever, laryngeal edema, and malaise. In chronic laryngitis, persistent hoarseness is usually the only symptom.

Diagnosis
CONFIRMING DIAGNOSIS
Indirect laryngoscopy confirms the diagnosis by revealing red, inflamed and, occasionally, hemorrhagic vocal cords, with rounded rather than sharp edges and exudate. Bilateral swelling may be present.

In severe cases or if toxicity is a concern, a culture of the exudate is obtained. Consider 24-hour pH probe testing in chronic laryngitis and gastroesophageal reflux disease (GERD). Also consider biopsy in chronic laryngitis in an adult with a history of smoking or alcohol abuse.

Treatment
Primary treatment consists of resting the voice. For viral infection, symptomatic care includes analgesics and throat lozenges for pain relief. Bacterial infection requires antibiotic therapy. Severe, acute laryngitis may necessitate hospitalization. When laryngeal edema results in airway obstruction, a tracheostomy may be necessary. In chronic laryngitis, effective treatment must eliminate the underlying cause. Antacids or histamine-2 blockers may be used if GERD is the cause. Steam inhalation may also prove beneficial as are smoking cessation, reducing alcohol intake, and job change or modification if warranted.

Special considerations
- Explain to the patient why he shouldn't talk, and place a sign over the bed to remind others of this restriction. Provide a Magic Slate or a pad and pencil for communication. Mark the intercom panel so other facility personnel are aware that the patient can't answer. Minimize the need to talk by trying to anticipate the patient's needs.
- For the patient with a bacterial infection, stress the importance of completing the full course of antibiotic therapy.
- Suggest that the patient maintain adequate humidification by using a vaporizer or humidifier during the winter, by avoiding air conditioning during the summer

(because it dehumidifies), by using medicated throat lozenges, and by not smoking.
■ Obtain a detailed patient history to help determine the cause of chronic laryngitis. Encourage the patient to modify predisposing habits, especially to stop smoking.
■ Provide the patient with assistance for smoking cessation as well as for modification of other predisposing habits or occupational hazards.

Juvenile angiofibroma

An uncommon disorder, juvenile angiofibroma is a highly vascular, nasopharyngeal tumor made up of masses of fibrous tissue that contain many thin-walled blood vessels. The prognosis is good with treatment.

Causes and incidence
A type of hemangioma, this tumor grows on one side of the posterior nares and may completely fill the nasopharynx, nose, paranasal sinuses and, possibly, the orbit. More commonly sessile than polypoid, juvenile angiofibroma is nonencapsulated; it invades surrounding tissue.

Juvenile angiofibroma is typically found in adolescent males and is extremely rare in females. It's associated with nasal obstruction and epistaxis.

Signs and symptoms
Juvenile angiofibroma produces unilateral or bilateral nasal obstruction and severe recurrent epistaxis, usually between ages 7 and 21. Recurrent epistaxis eventually causes secondary anemia. Associated effects include purulent rhinorrhea, facial deformity, and nasal speech. Serous otitis media and hearing loss may result from eustachian tube obstruction.

Diagnosis
A nasopharyngeal mirror or nasal speculum permits visualization of the tumor. X-rays show a bowing of the posterior wall of the maxillary sinus. Three-plane magnetic resonance imaging and computed tomography scans determine the extent of the tumors, which are seldom limited to the nasopharynx. Angiography determines the size and location of the tumor and shows the source of vascularization.

 ALERT *Tumor biopsy is contraindicated because of the risk of hemorrhage.*

Treatment
Surgical procedures range from avulsion to cryosurgical techniques. Surgical excision is preferred after embolization with Teflon or an absorbable gelatin sponge to decrease vascularization. Whichever surgical method is used, this tumor must be removed in its entirety and not in pieces.

Preoperative hormonal therapy may decrease the tumor's size and vascularity. Blood transfusions may be necessary during avulsion. Radiation therapy produces only a temporary regression in an angiofibroma but is the treatment of choice if the tumor has expanded into the cranium or orbit. Because the tumor is multilobular and locally invasive, it recurs in about 30% of patients during the first year after treatment, but rarely after 2 years.

Special considerations
■ Explain all diagnostic and surgical procedures. Provide emotional support; severe epistaxis frightens many people to the point of panic. Monitor hemoglobin levels and hematocrit for anemia.
■ After surgery, immediately report excessive bleeding. Make sure an adequate supply of typed and crossmatched blood is available for transfusion.
■ Monitor for any change in vital signs. Provide good oral hygiene, and use a bedside vaporizer to raise humidity.
■ During blood transfusion, watch for transfusion reactions, such as fever, pruritus, chills, or a rash. If any of these reactions occur, discontinue the blood transfusion and notify the physician immediately.
■ Teach the patient's family how to apply pressure over the affected area, and instruct them to seek immediate medical attention if bleeding occurs after discharge. Stress the importance of providing adequate humidification at home to keep the nasal mucosa moist.

Selected references

Bess, F.H., and Humes, L.E. *Audiology: The Fundamentals,* 3rd ed. Philadelphia: Lippincott Williams & Wilkins, 2003.

Layland, M. *The Washington Manual Otolaryngology Survival Guide.* Philadelphia: Lippincott Williams & Wilkins, 2004.

Lucente, F.E., et al. *Essentials of Otolaryngology,* 5th ed. Philadelphia: Lippincott Williams & Wilkins, 2004.

Woodson, G.E. *Ear, Nose, and Throat Disorders in Primary Care.* Philadelphia: W.B. Saunders Co., 2001.

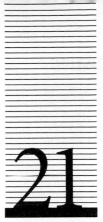

21

Skin disorders

Introduction *1228*

Bacterial infections *1232*
Impetigo *1232*
Folliculitis, furunculosis, and
  carbunculosis *1234*
Staphylococcal scalded skin
  syndrome *1236*

Fungal infections *1237*
Tinea versicolor *1237*
Dermatophytosis *1239*

Parasitic infestations *1241*
Scabies *1241*
Cutaneous larva migrans *1243*
Pediculosis *1244*

Follicular and glandular disorders *1246*
Acne vulgaris *1246*
Hirsutism *1248*
Alopecia *1250*
Rosacea *1251*

Pigmentation disorders *1252*
Vitiligo *1252*
Melasma *1255*
Photosensitivity reactions *1255*

Inflammatory reactions *1256*
Dermatitis *1256*

Miscellaneous disorders *1262*
Toxic epidermal necrolysis *1262*
Warts *1263*
Psoriasis *1265*
Lichen planus *1268*
Corns and calluses *1269*
Pityriasis rosea *1270*
Hyperhidrosis *1271*
Pressure ulcers *1273*

Selected references *1276*

Introduction

Skin is man's front-line protective barrier between internal structures and the external environment. It's tough, resilient, and virtually impermeable to aqueous solutions, bacteria, or toxic compounds. It also performs many vital functions. Skin protects against trauma, regulates body temperature, serves as an organ of excretion and sensation, and synthesizes vitamin D in the presence of ultraviolet light. Skin varies in thickness and other qualities from one part of the body to another, which often accounts for the distribution of skin diseases.

Skin has three primary layers: epidermis, dermis, and subcutaneous tissue. The epidermis (the outermost layer) produces keratin as its primary function. This layer is generally thin but is thicker in areas subject to constant pressure or friction, such as the soles and palms. The epidermis contains two sublayers: the stratum corneum, an outer horny layer of keratin that protects the body against harmful environmental substances and restricts water loss, and the cellular stratum, where keratin cells are synthesized. The basement membrane lies beneath the cellular stratum and serves to attach the epidermis to the dermis.

The cellular stratum, the deepest layer of the epidermis, consists of the basal layer, where mitosis takes place; the stratum spinosum, where cells begin to flatten, and fibrils — precursors of keratin — start to appear; and the stratum granulosum, made up of cells containing deeply staining granules of keratohyalin, which are generally thought to become the keratin that forms the stratum corneum. A skin cell moves from the basal layer of the cellular stratum to the stratum corneum in about 14 days. After another 14 days, normal wear and tear on the skin causes it to slough off. The epidermis also contains melanocytes, which produce the melanin that gives the skin its color, and Langerhans cells, which are involved in a variety of immunologic reactions.

The dermis, the second primary layer of the skin, consists of two fibrous proteins, fibroblasts, and an intervening ground substance. The proteins are collagen, which strengthens the skin to prevent it from tearing, and elastin to give it resilience. The ground substance, which makes the skin soft and compressible, contains primarily jellylike mucopolysaccharides. Two distinct layers constitute the dermis: the papillary dermis (top layer) and the reticular dermis (bottom layer).

Subcutaneous tissue, the third primary layer of the skin, consists mainly of fat (containing mostly triglycerides), which provides heat, insulation, shock absorption, and a reserve of calories. Both sensory and motor nerves (autonomic fibers) are found in the dermis and the subcutaneous tissue.

Nails, glands, and hair

Nails are epidermal cells converted to hard keratin. The bed on which the nail rests is highly vascular, making the nail appear pink; the whitish, crescent-shaped area extending beyond the proximal nail fold, called the *lunula* — most visible in the thumbnail — marks the end of the matrix, the site of mitosis and of nail growth.

Sebaceous glands, found everywhere on the body (but mostly on the face and scalp) except the palms and soles, serve as appendages of the dermis. These glands generally excrete sebum into hair follicles, but in some cases, they empty directly onto the skin surface. Sebum is an oily substance that helps keep the skin and hair from drying out and prevents water and heat loss. Sebaceous glands abound on the scalp, forehead, cheeks, chin, back, and genitalia, and may be stimulated by sex hormones — primarily testosterone.

The dermis and subcutaneous tissue contain eccrine and apocrine glands, and hair. Eccrine sweat glands open directly onto the skin and regulate body temperature. Innervated by sympathetic nerves, these sweat glands are distributed throughout the body, except for the lips, ears, and parts of the genitalia. They secrete a hypertonic solution made up mostly of water and sodium chloride; the prime stimulus for eccrine gland secretion is heat. Other stimuli include muscular exertion and emotional stress.

Apocrine sweat glands appear chiefly in the axillae and genitalia; they're responsible for producing body odor and are stimulated by emotional stress. The sweat produced is sterile but undergoes bacterial decomposition on the skin surface. These glands become functional after puberty. (Ceruminous glands, located in the external ear canal, appear to be modified sweat glands and secrete a waxy substance known as *cerumen*.)

Hair grows on most of the body, except for the palms, the soles, and parts of the genitalia. An individual hair consists of a shaft (a column of keratinized cells), a root (embedded in the dermis), the hair follicle (the root and its covering), and the hair papilla (a loop of capillaries at the base of the follicle). Mitosis at the base of the follicle causes the hair to grow; the papilla provides nourishment for mitosis. Small bundles of involuntary muscles known as *arrectores pilorum* cling to hair follicles. When these muscles contract, usually during moments of fear or shock, the hairs stand on end, and the person is said to have goose bumps or gooseflesh. Melanocytes in the matrix (inner core) of the hair bulb produce melanin, which passes into the innermost layers of the hair and is responsible for hair color. Dark hair contains mostly true melanin. Blond and red hair contains variants of melanin that have iron and more sulfur. Gray hair results from pigment loss due to a decline of tyrosinase, which is required for melanin synthesis. White hair occurs when air bubbles accumulate in the center of the hair shaft.

Vascular influence

The skin is served by a vast arteriovenous network, extending from subcutaneous tissue to the dermis. These blood vessels provide oxygen and nutrients to sensory nerves (which control touch, temperature, and pain), motor nerves (which control the activities of sweat glands, the arterioles, and smooth muscles of the skin), and skin appendages. Blood flow also influences skin coloring because the amount of oxygen carried to capillaries in the dermis can produce transient changes in color. For example, decreased oxygen supply can turn the skin pale or bluish; increased oxygen can turn it pink or ruddy.

Assessing skin disorders

Assessment begins with a thorough patient history to determine whether a skin disorder is an acute flare-up, a recurrent problem, or a chronic condition. Ask the patient how long he has had the disorder; how a typical flare-up or attack begins; whether or not it itches; and what medications— systemic or topical—have been used to treat it. Also, find out if any of his family members, friends, or contacts have the same disorder, and if he lives or works in an environment that could cause the condition. Also ask about hobbies.

When examining a patient with a skin disorder, be sure to look everywhere— mucous membranes, hair, scalp, axillae, groin, palms, soles, and nails. Note moisture, temperature, texture, thickness, mobility, edema, turgor, and any irregularities in skin color. Look for skin lesions; if you find a lesion, record its color, size, and location. (See *Primary skin lesions*, page 1230. Also see *Secondary changes in primary skin lesions*, page 1231.) Try to determine which is the primary lesion—the one that appeared first—which always starts in normal skin. The patient might be able to point it out.

If more than one lesion is in evidence, note the pattern of distribution. Lesions can be localized (isolated), regional, general, or universal (total), involving the entire skin, hair, and nails. Also, observe whether the lesions are unilateral or bilateral and symmetrical or asymmetrical; also note the arrangement of the lesions (clustered or linear configuration, for example).

Diagnostic aids

After simple observation, and examination of the affected area of the skin with a dermatoscope for morphologic detail, the following clinical diagnostic techniques may help to identify skin disorders:

■ Biopsy determines histology of cells, and may be diagnostic, confirmatory, or inconclusive, depending on the disease.

PRIMARY SKIN LESIONS

The most common primary skin lesions are illustrated below:

Macule
(flat, circumscribed, discolored area < 1 cm in diameter)

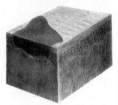

Patch — flat area of skin with change in color > 1 cm in diameter

Vesicle
(serous fluid-filled lesion)

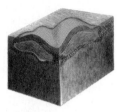

Bulla (> 1 cm) — larger circumscribed area containing free serous fluid

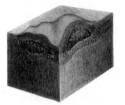

Pustule (size varies) — lesion containing purulent fluid

Papule
(solid, elevated mass usually < 1 cm in diameter)

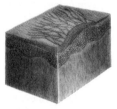

Plaque — forms by extensive confluence of papules > 1 cm in diameter

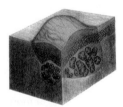

Nodule, tumor, or cyst palpable as a solid lesion in the dermis or subcutaneous tissue — if < 2 cm, it's called a *nodule;* > 2 cm, it's called a *tumor;* if filled with fluid or semi-solid material, it's called a *cyst.*

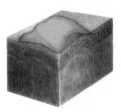

Wheal — circumscribed area of edema, usually transient

■ Diascopy, in which a lesion is covered with a microscopic slide or piece of clear plastic, helps determine whether dilated capillaries or extravasated blood is causing the redness of a lesion.

■ Gram's stains and exudate cultures help identify the organism responsible for an underlying infection.
■ Microscopic immunofluorescence identifies immunoglobulins and elastic tissue in

SECONDARY CHANGES IN PRIMARY SKIN LESIONS

Erosion
Circum-
scribed,
partial loss
of epidermis

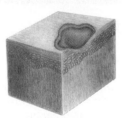

Scale
Loose frag-
ments of ker-
atin in stratum
corneum

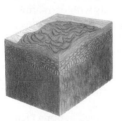

Ulcer
Irregularly
sized and
shaped excava-
tions penetrat-
ing into der-
mis

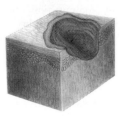

Lichenification
Thick and
roughened
skin, exaggerat-
ed skin lines

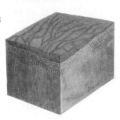

Fissure
Moist or dry
deep linear
cleavage that
extends into
dermis

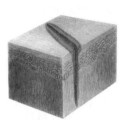

Atrophy
Thin skin with-
out normal
markings

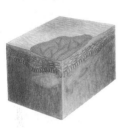

Excoriation
Abrasion or
scratch mark
(linear break
produced
manually)

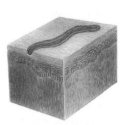

Scar
Permanent fi-
brous tissue at
site of healed
injury

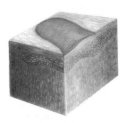

Crust
Variously col-
ored collec-
tions of dried
serum, cellular
debris, or
blood

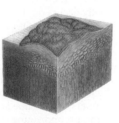

Keloid
Hypertrophied
scars

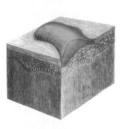

detecting skin manifestations of immunologically mediated disease.

■ Patch tests identify contact sensitivity (usually with dermatitis).

■ Potassium hydroxide preparations permit examination for mycelia in fungal infections.

■ Side-lighting shows minor elevations or depressions in lesions; it also helps determine the configuration and degree of eruption.

■ Subdued lighting highlights the difference between normal skin and circumscribed lesions that are hypopigmented or hyperpigmented.

■ Wood's light examination reveals yellow, green, or blue-green fluorescence when an area is infected with certain dermatophytes (fungi).

Special considerations

When assessing a skin disorder, keep in mind its distressing social and psychological implications. Unlike internal disorders, such as cardiac disease or diabetes mellitus, a skin condition is usually obvious and disfiguring. Understandably, the psychological implications are most acute when skin disorders affect the face — especially during adolescence, an emotionally turbulent time of life. However, such disorders can also create tremendous psychological problems for adults. A skin disease usually interferes with a person's ability to work because the condition affects the hands or because it distresses the patient to such an extent that he can't function.

For these reasons, be empathetic and accepting. Above all, don't be afraid to touch such a patient; most skin disorders aren't contagious. Touching the patient naturally and without hesitation helps show your acceptance of the dermatologic condition. Such acceptance is no less important than your patient teaching about the disease and your guidance and help with carrying out prescribed treatment.

BACTERIAL INFECTIONS

Impetigo

A contagious, superficial skin infection, impetigo occurs in nonbullous and bullous forms. This vesiculopustular eruptive disorder spreads most easily among infants, young children, and elderly people. Predisposing factors, such as poor hygiene, anemia, malnutrition, and a warm climate, favor outbreaks of this infection, most of which occur during the late summer and early fall. Impetigo can complicate chickenpox, eczema, or other skin conditions marked by open lesions.

Causes and incidence

Coagulase-positive *Staphylococcus aureus* and, less commonly, group A beta-hemolytic streptococci usually produce nonbullous impetigo; *S. aureus* (especially phage type 71) generally causes bullous impetigo.

In the United States, impetigo occurs most often in southern states. It often causes deeper dermal inflammation in blacks than in whites and may result in postinflammatory hypopigmentation or hyperpigmentation.

Signs and symptoms

Common nonbullous impetigo typically begins with a small red macule that turns into a vesicle or pustule. When the vesicle breaks, a thick yellow crust forms from the exudate. (See *Recognizing impetigo*.) Autoinoculation may cause satellite lesions. Although it can occur anywhere, impetigo usually occurs on the face, around the mouth and nose. Other features include pruritus, burning, and regional lymphadenopathy.

A rare but serious complication of streptococcal impetigo is glomerulonephritis, which is more likely to occur when many members of the same family have impetigo. Infants and young children may develop aural impetigo or otitis externa; the lesions usually clear without treatment in 2

RECOGNIZING IMPETIGO

In impetigo, when the vesicles break, crust forms from the exudate. This infection is especially contagious among young children.

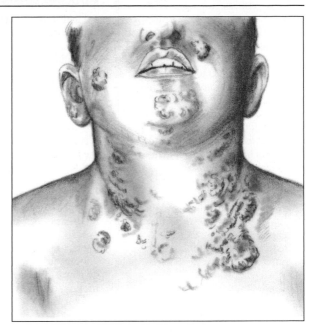

to 3 weeks, unless an underlying disorder such as eczema is present. Scarlet fever also may occur.

In bullous impetigo, a thin-walled vesicle opens, and a thin, clear crust forms from the exudate. The lesion consists of a central clearing, circumscribed by an outer rim — much like a ringworm lesion — and commonly appears on the face or other exposed areas. Both forms usually produce painless itching; they may appear simultaneously and be clinically indistinguishable.

Ecthyma is a skin infection that resembles impetigo but extends into the dermis and takes longer to resolve. These lesions are painful and more common on distal extremities. (See *Ecthyma,* page 1234.)

Diagnosis

Culture and sensitivity testing of fluid or denuded skin may indicate the most appropriate antibiotic, but therapy shouldn't be delayed for laboratory results, which can take 3 days. White blood cell count may be elevated in the presence of infection.

Treatment

Topical mupirocin is the treatment of choice if the lesions aren't too extensive. It's highly effective against group A beta-hemolytic streptococcus and *Staphylococcus aureus,* including methicillin-resistant *S. aureus.* Mupirocin also eliminates nasal carriers of these organisms. Extensive or nonresolving lesions require systemic antibiotics.

Therapy may also include removal of the exudate by washing the lesions two or three times a day with soap and water (or antibacterial soap) or, for stubborn crusts, warm soaks or compresses of normal saline or a diluted soap solution.

Special considerations

■ Urge the patient not to scratch, because this spreads impetigo. Advise parents to cut

ECTHYMA

Ecthyma is a superficial skin infection that usually causes scarring. It commonly occurs in persons with poor hygiene or living in crowded conditions and generally results from infection by *Staphylococcus aureus* or group A beta-hemolytic streptococci. Ecthyma differs from impetigo in that its characteristic ulcer results from deeper penetration of the skin by the infecting organism (involving the lower epidermis and dermis), and the overlying crust tends to be piled high (1 to 3 cm). These lesions are usually found on the legs after a scratch or bug bite. Autoinoculation can transmit ecthyma to other parts of the body, especially to sites that have been scratched open. Therapy is basically the same as for impetigo, but response may be slower. Parenteral antibiotics (usually a penicillinase-resistant penicillin) are also used.

their child's fingernails and cover his hands with socks or mittens to prevent scratching.

■ Give medications as ordered. Remember to check for medication allergy. Stress the need to continue prescribed medications for 7 to 10 days, even after lesions have healed.

■ Teach the patient or his family how to care for impetiginous lesions. To prevent further spread of this highly contagious infection, encourage frequent bathing using a bactericidal soap. Tell the patient not to share towels, washcloths, or bed linens with family members. Emphasize the importance of following proper hand-washing technique.

■ Check family members for impetigo. If this infection is present in a school-age child, notify his school.

Folliculitis, furunculosis, and carbunculosis

Folliculitis is a bacterial infection of the hair follicle that causes the formation of a pustule. The infection can be superficial (follicular impetigo or Bockhart's impetigo) or deep (sycosis barbae). Folliculitis may also lead to the development of furuncles (furunculosis), commonly known as *boils*, or *carbuncles* (carbunculosis), which involve multiple contiguous hair follicles. The prognosis depends on the severity of the infection and on the patient's physical condition and ability to resist infection.

Causes

The most common cause of folliculitis, furunculosis, or carbunculosis is coagulase-positive *Staphylococcus aureus*. Predisposing factors include an infected wound, poor hygiene, debilitation, diabetes, alcoholism, occlusive cosmetics, tight clothes, friction, chafing, exposure to chemicals, and treatment for skin lesions with tar or with occlusive therapy, using steroids. Furunculosis often follows folliculitis exacerbated by irritation, pressure, friction, or perspiration. Carbunculosis follows persistent *S. aureus* infection and furunculosis.

Signs and symptoms

Pustules of folliculitis usually appear in a hair follicle on the scalp, arms, and legs in children; on the face of bearded men (sycosis barbae); and on the eyelids (styes). Deep folliculitis may be painful.

Folliculitis may progress to the hard, painful nodules of furunculosis, which commonly develop on the neck, face, axillae, and buttocks. For several days these nodules enlarge, and then rupture, discharging pus and necrotic material. After the nodules rupture, pain subsides, but erythema and edema may persist for days or weeks.

Carbunculosis is marked by extremely painful, deep abscesses that drain through multiple openings onto the skin surface, usually around several hair follicles. Fever and malaise may accompany these lesions. (See *Follicular skin infections.*)

FOLLICULAR SKIN INFECTIONS

Degree of hair follicle involvement in bacterial skin infection ranges from superficial erythema and pustule of a single follicle to deep abscesses (carbuncles) involving several follicles.

| Superficial folliculitis (erythema and pustule in a single follicle) | Deep folliculitis (extensive follicular involvement) | Furuncle (red, tender nodule surrounding a follicle with one draining point) | Carbuncle (deep follicular abscesses of several follicles with several draining points) |

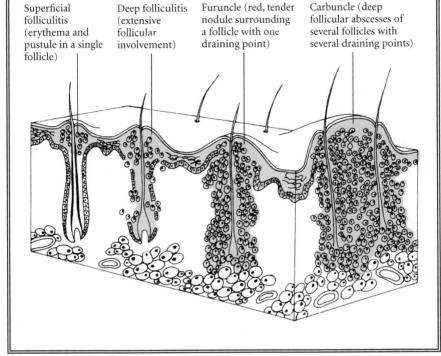

Diagnosis

CONFIRMING DIAGNOSIS *The obvious skin lesion confirms folliculitis, furunculosis, or carbunculosis. Wound culture shows S. aureus; sensitivity will help guide antibiotic therapy.*

In carbunculosis, patient history reveals preexistent furunculosis. A complete blood count may reveal an elevated white blood cell count (leukocytosis).

Treatment

Treatment for folliculitis consists of cleaning the infected area thoroughly with antibacterial soap and water or benzoyl peroxide; applying warm, wet compresses to promote vasodilation and drainage from the lesions; topical antibiotics such as

mupirocin ointment and, in extensive infection or if a furuncle or carbuncle has developed, systemic antibiotics. Use sensitivity results to guide therapy, but begin treatment before receiving results.

Furunculosis and carbunculosis may also require incision and drainage of ripe lesions if the lesions don't drain after the application of warm, wet compresses. They may also require topical antibiotics after drainage.

Special considerations

Care for patients with folliculitis, furunculosis, and carbunculosis is basically supportive and emphasizes teaching the patient scrupulous personal and family hygiene measures. Taking the necessary precautions to prevent spreading infection is also an important part of care.

■ Caution the patient never to squeeze a boil because this may cause it to rupture into the surrounding area.

■ To avoid spreading bacteria to family members, urge the patient not to share towels and washcloths. Tell him that these items should be laundered in hot water before being reused. The patient should change his clothes and bedsheets daily, and these also should be washed in hot water. Encourage the patient to change dressings frequently and to discard them promptly in paper bags.

■ Advise the patient with recurrent furunculosis to have a physical examination because an underlying disease, such as diabetes or human immunodeficiency virus, may be present.

In blacks, trauma resulting from such hairstyles as cornrowing (gathering the hair into tight braids or tufts) can cause folliculitis.

Staphylococcal scalded skin syndrome

Staphylococcal scalded skin syndrome (SSSS), also known as *Ritter's disease* or *Ritter-Lyell syndrome,* is marked by epidermal erythema, peeling, and necrosis that give the skin a scalded appearance. This severe skin disorder follows a consistent pattern of progression, and most patients recover fully. Mortality is 2% to 3%, with death usually resulting from complications of fluid and electrolyte loss, sepsis, and involvement of other body systems.

Causes and incidence

The causative organism in SSSS is group 2 *Staphylococcus aureus,* primarily phage type 71, which produces exotoxins that cause detachment of the epidermis. Predisposing factors may include impaired immunity and renal insufficiency — present to some extent in the normal neonate because of immature development of these systems.

SSSS is most prevalent in infants age 1 to 3 months but may develop in children. It's uncommon in adults.

Signs and symptoms

SSSS can usually be traced to a prodromal upper respiratory tract infection, possibly with concomitant purulent conjunctivitis. Cutaneous changes progress through three stages:

■ Erythema: Erythema, which may begin diffusely or as a scarlatiniform rash, usually becomes visible around the mouth and other orifices and may spread in widening circles over the entire body surface. The skin becomes tender; Nikolsky's sign (sloughing of the skin when friction is applied) may appear.

■ Exfoliation (24 to 48 hours later): In the more common, localized form of this disease, superficial erosions with a red, moist base and minimal crusting occur, generally around body orifices, and may spread to exposed areas of the skin. (See *Identifying staphylococcal scalded skin syndrome.*) In the more severe forms of this disease, large, flaccid bullae erupt and may spread to cover extensive areas of the body. These bullae eventually rupture, revealing sections of denuded skin; mucous membranes are spared.

■ Desquamation: In this final stage, affected areas dry up, and powdery scales form. Normal skin replaces these scales in 5 to 7 days.

Diagnosis

Diagnosis requires careful observation of the three-stage progression of this disease. Results of exfoliative cytology and biopsy aid in differential diagnosis, ruling out erythema multiforme and drug-induced toxic epidermal necrolysis, both of which are similar to SSSS.

CONFIRMING DIAGNOSIS
Isolation of group 2 S. aureus on cultures of skin lesions confirms the diagnosis. However, skin lesions sometimes appear sterile.

Treatment

Treatment includes systemic antibiotics, usually penicillinase-resistant penicillin.

IDENTIFYING STAPHYLOCOCCAL SCALDED SKIN SYNDROME

Staphylococcal scalded skin syndrome is a severe skin disorder that commonly affects infants and children. The illustration below shows the typical scalded skin appearance, with areas of denuded skin found in an infant.

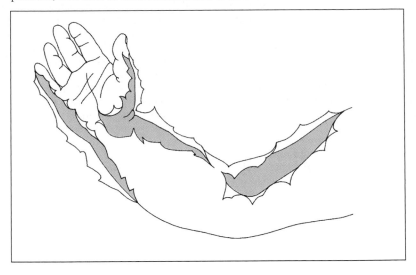

Severe cases require hospitalization and I.V. antibiotics. Oral antibiotics should be adequate for milder cases. Skin lubrication with a non–alcohol-based preparation is beneficial. Washing or bathing should be done sparingly. Replacement measures to maintain fluid and electrolyte balance are necessary.

 PEDIATRIC TIP *Admission is appropriate for neonates and young children with extensive sloughing.*

Special considerations
■ Carefully monitor intake and output to assess fluid and electrolyte balance. In severe cases, I.V. fluid replacement may be necessary.
■ Check vital signs. Be especially alert for a sudden rise in temperature, indicating sepsis, which requires prompt, aggressive treatment.
■ Maintain skin integrity. Use strict sterile technique to preclude secondary infection, especially during the exfoliative stage, be-

cause of open lesions. To prevent friction and sloughing of the skin, leave affected areas uncovered or loosely covered. Place cotton between severely affected fingers and toes to prevent webbing.
■ Gently débride exfoliated areas, especially those that have become necrotic.
■ Reassure the parents that complications are rare and residual scars are unlikely.

 PEDIATRIC TIP *Provide special care for the neonate, if required, including placement in a warming infant incubator to maintain body temperature and provide isolation.*

FUNGAL INFECTIONS

Tinea versicolor

A chronic, superficial, fungal infection, tinea versicolor (also known as *pityriasis versicolor*) may produce a multicolored rash, commonly on the upper trunk. Recurrence is common.

Causes and incidence

The agent that causes tinea versicolor is *Pityrosporum orbiculare*, also known as *P. ovale* and *Malassezia furfur*. Whether this condition is infectious or merely a proliferation of normal skin fungi is uncertain. Tinea versicolor is more common in hot climates — tropical countries or in those with high humidity — and associated with increased sweating. It usually affects adolescents and young men when sebaceous gland activity is at its highest.

Signs and symptoms

Tinea versicolor typically produces raised or macular, round or oval, slightly scaly lesions on the upper trunk, which may extend to the lower abdomen, neck, arms, groin, thigh, genitalia and, rarely, the face. These lesions are usually tawny but may range from hypopigmented (white) patches in dark-skinned patients to hyperpigmented (brown) patches in fair-skinned patients. Some areas don't tan when exposed to sunlight, causing the cosmetic defect for which most people seek medical help. Inflammation, burning, and itching are possible but usually absent.

Diagnosis

Visualization of blue-green fluorescent lesions during Wood's light examination strongly suggests tinea versicolor. However, if the patient has recently showered, this fluorescence may not show because the chemical that causes fluorescence is water-soluble.

CONFIRMING DIAGNOSIS
Microscopic examination of skin scrapings prepared in potassium hydroxide solution confirms the disorder by showing hyphae, clusters of yeast, and large numbers of variously sized spores (a combination referred to as "spaghetti and meatballs").

Treatment

The most economical and effective treatment is selenium sulfide lotion 2.5% applied once a day for seven days. It's left on the skin for 10 minutes, then rinsed off thoroughly. In persistent cases, therapy may require a single 12- or 24-hour application of this lotion, repeated once a week for 4 weeks. Either treatment may cause temporary redness and irritation.

Other treatments include the following: sodium thiosulfate 25% solution, applied twice daily to affected areas for 2 to 4 weeks; sulfur salicylic shampoo applied as a lotion at bedtime each night and washed off each morning for 2 weeks; zinc pyrithione shampoo 1% lathered into affected areas for 5 minutes before showering, and repeated every day for 2 weeks; or imidazole antifungal agents applied twice daily for 2 weeks.

Ketoconazole and other azole-based creams, such as topical ketoconazole, may be applied once or twice daily for 2 weeks. Oral ketoconazole or another oral azole-based medication, such as oral ketoconazole, may be used if the patient has extensive disease that fails to respond to other therapies.

Special considerations

■ Instruct the patient to apply selenium sulfide lotion as ordered. Tell him that this medication may cause temporary adverse effects.

■ Assure the patient that once his fungal infection is cured, discolored areas will gradually blend in after exposure to the sun or ultraviolet light.

■ Because recurrence of tinea versicolor is common, advise the patient to watch for new areas of discoloration.

■ Teach the patient proper hand-washing technique, and encourage good personal hygiene.

■ Stress the importance of not scratching or picking lesions to avoid the risk of skin breaks and secondary bacterial infections.

■ Provide written instructions for using prescribed medications. Tell the patient to contact the physician if adverse reactions occur.

Dermatophytosis

Dermatophytosis, commonly called *tinea*, may affect the scalp (tinea capitis), body (tinea corporis), nails (tinea unguium), hands (tinea manuum), feet (tinea pedis), groin (tinea cruris), and bearded skin (tinea barbae). With effective treatment, the cure rate is very high, although about 20% of infected people develop chronic conditions.

Causes and incidence

Tinea infections (except for tinea versicolor) result from dermatophytes (fungi) of the genera *Trichophyton, Microsporum,* and *Epidermophyton.* Transmission can occur through contact with infected lesions, household cats and dogs, and soiled or contaminated articles, such as shoes, towels, or shower stalls.

Tinea infections are prevalent in the United States. They're more common in males than in females.

Signs and symptoms

Lesions vary in appearance depending on the site of invasion (inside or outside the hair shaft), duration of infection, level of host resistance, and amount of inflammatory response. Tinea capitis ranges in appearance from broken-off hairs with little scaling to severe painful, inflammatory, pus-filled masses (kerions) covering the entire scalp. Partial hair loss occurs in all cases. The cardinal clue is broken-off hairs.

Tinea corporis produces flat lesions on the skin at any site except the scalp, bearded skin, hands, or feet. These lesions may be dry and scaly or moist and crusty; as they enlarge, their centers heal, causing the classic ring-shaped appearance. In tinea unguium (onychomycosis), infection typically starts at the tip of one or more toenails (fingernail infection is less common) and produces gradual thickening, discoloration, and crumbling of the nail, with accumulation of subungual debris. Eventually, the nail may be destroyed completely.

Tinea pedis, or *athlete's foot,* causes scaling and blisters between the toes. Severe infection may result in inflammation, with severe itching and pain on walking. A dry,

squamous inflammation may affect the entire sole. (See *Athlete's foot,* page 1240.) Tinea manuum produces scaling patches and hyperkeratosis on the palmar surface. It's usually unilateral and associated with tinea pedis. Tinea cruris (jock itch) produces red, raised, sharply defined, itchy or burning lesions in the groin that may extend to the buttocks, inner thighs, and the external genitalia. Warm weather, obesity, and tight clothing encourage fungus growth. Tinea barbae is an uncommon infection that affects the bearded facial area of men.

Diagnosis

CONFIRMING DIAGNOSIS
Microscopic examination of lesion scrapings prepared in potassium hydroxide solution will reveal branching fungal hyphae. Gently heating the slide helps separate epithelial cells and hyphae. Lowering the microscope condenser and dimming the light make hyphae easier to identify, as does adding a drop of ink to the potassium hydroxide.

Other diagnostic procedures include Wood's light examination (useful in only about 5% of cases of tinea capitis) and culture of the infecting organism, which is important for identifying hair and nail fungal infections.

Treatment

Tinea infections respond to a wide variety of medications. Typically, infections of the skin (hands, body, feet, and groin) require only topical therapy. Infections of the hair and nails, skin infections causing chronic thickening of the skin, and other unresolving infections require oral antifungal therapy.

Topical preparations are commonly azole-based, though other preparations are available. Oral therapy includes azole-based medications and terbinafine. Griseofulvin is falling out of favor because newer products are easier to use and have a shorter duration of therapy.

ALERT *Caution must be taken when using systemic antifungals: liver enzyme levels must be monitored before and throughout treatment if*

ATHLETE'S FOOT

Dermatophytosis of the feet (tinea pedis) is popularly called athlete's foot. This infection causes macerated, scaling lesions, which may spread from the interdigital spaces to the sole. Diagnosis must rule out other possible causes, such as eczema, psoriasis, contact dermatitis, and maceration by tight, ill-fitting shoes.

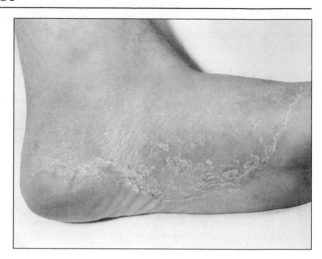

therapy is expected to extend more than 2 months, and chronic medications must be monitored because of the antifungal's potential effect on blood levels.

Treatment should continue from several days to 2 weeks after lesions have resolved. Topical agents with soothing and cooling effects may be used with systemic therapy for infections with severe itching and burning; they may be discontinued when the immediate discomfort resolves.

Special considerations

Management of tinea infections requires medication compliance, observation for sensitivity reactions, observation for secondary bacterial infections, and patient teaching. Specific care varies by site of infection:

■ For tinea barbae: Suggest that the patient let his beard grow (whiskers may be trimmed with scissors, not a razor). If the patient insists that he must shave, advise him to use an electric razor instead of a blade.

■ For tinea capitis: If the condition worsens, discontinue medications and notify the physician. Use good hand-washing technique, and teach the patient to do the same. Spores of tinea capitis are shed in the air around an infected patient or may spread on contaminated clothing and other personal articles. To prevent spread of infection to others, advise him to wash his towels, bedclothes, and combs frequently in hot water and to avoid sharing them. Suggest that family members be checked for tinea capitis.

■ For tinea corporis: Use abdominal pads between skin folds for the patient with excessive abdominal girth; change pads frequently. Check the patient daily for excoriated, newly denuded areas of skin. Apply wet Burow's compresses two or three times daily to decrease inflammation and help remove scales.

■ For tinea cruris: Instruct the patient to dry the affected area thoroughly after bathing and to evenly apply antifungal powder after applying the topical antifungal agent. Advise him to wear loose-fitting clothing, which should be changed frequently and washed in hot water.

- For tinea pedis: Encourage the patient to expose his feet to air whenever possible, and to wear sandals or leather shoes and clean, white cotton socks. Instruct the patient to wash his feet twice daily and, after drying them thoroughly, to apply antifungal cream followed by antifungal powder to absorb perspiration and prevent excoriation. Tell him to allow his shoes to dry out by alternating pairs every other daily. Also tell him to wear shower shoes when using public facilities.
- For tinea unguium: Keep nails short and straight. Gently remove debris under the nails with an emery board. Prepare the patient for prolonged therapy.

PARASITIC INFESTATIONS

Scabies

A common skin infection, scabies results from infestation with *Sarcoptes scabiei var. hominis* (itch mite), which provokes a sensitivity reaction. It's transmitted through skin or sexual contact.

Causes and incidence

Mites can live their entire life cycles in the skin of humans, causing chronic infection. (The adult mite can survive without a human host for only 2 or 3 days.) The female mite burrows into the skin to lay her eggs, from which larvae emerge to copulate and then reburrow under the skin. (See *Scabies: Cause and effect,* page 1242.)

Scabies occurs worldwide, primarily in environments marked by overcrowding and poor hygiene, and can be endemic.

Signs and symptoms

Typically, scabies causes itching, which intensifies at night. Characteristic lesions are usually excoriated and may appear as erythematous nodules. These threadlike lesions are approximately 1 cm long and generally occur between fingers, on flexor surfaces of the wrists, on elbows, in axillary folds, at the waistline, on nipples and but-

tocks in females, and on genitalia in males. In infants, the burrows (lesions) may appear on the head and neck.

Intense scratching can lead to severe excoriation and secondary bacterial infection. Itching may become generalized secondary to sensitization.

Diagnosis

CONFIRMING DIAGNOSIS *Visual examination of the contents of the scabietic burrow may reveal the itch mite. If not, a drop of mineral oil placed over the burrow, followed by superficial scraping and examination of expressed material under a low-power microscope, may reveal ova, or mite feces. However, excoriation or inflammation of the burrow often makes such identification difficult. If diagnostic tests offer no positive identification of the mite and if scabies is still suspected (for example, if family members and close contacts of the patient also report itching), skin clearing that occurs after a therapeutic trial of a pediculicide confirms the diagnosis.*

Treatment

Generally, treatment for scabies consists of application of a pediculicide — permethrin, lindane cream, or crotamiton — in a thin layer over the entire skin surface from the neck down. Lindane and permethrin are left on the skin for 8 to 12 hours. Crotamiton is applied nightly for 2 consecutive nights and washed off 24 hours after the second application. To make certain that all areas have been treated, this application should be repeated in approximately 1 week.

Lindane is an effective scabicide and when used properly may be applied safely to children, but shouldn't be used in children younger than age 2 or pregnant or nursing mothers because of potential neurologic toxicity. It also shouldn't be applied immediately after a shower. A 6% to 10% solution of sulfur in petrolatum may be used if patients object to using lindane, but they should be advised that sulfur is messy and odorous.

Persistent pruritus (due to mite sensitization or contact dermatitis) may develop from repeated use of pediculicides rather

SCABIES: CAUSE AND EFFECT

Infestation with *Sarcoptes scabiei* —the itch mite — causes scabies. This mite (shown enlarged below) has a hard shell and measures a microscopic 0.1 mm. The illustration above right shows the erythematous nodules with excoriation that appear in patients with scabies. These lesions are usually highly pruritic.

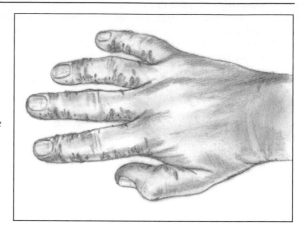

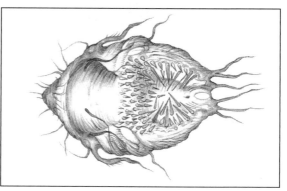

than from continued infection. An antipruritic emollient, topical steroid, or oral antihistamine can reduce itching; intralesional steroids may resolve erythematous nodules.

Special considerations

■ Instruct the patient to apply permethrin, crotamiton, or lindane cream or lotion from the neck down, covering his entire body. He must wait 15 minutes before dressing and avoid bathing for 8 to 12 hours or longer, depending on the treatment used. Contaminated clothing and linens must be washed in hot water or dry cleaned.

■ Tell the patient not to apply lindane cream if his skin is raw or inflamed. Advise him that if skin irritation or hypersensitivity reaction develops, he should notify the physician immediately, discontinue using the drug, and thoroughly wash it off his skin.

■ Suggest to the patient that his family members and other close personal be checked for possible symptoms.

■ If a hospitalized patient has scabies, prevent transmission to other patients: Practice good hand-washing technique or wear gloves when touching the patient; observe wound and skin precautions for 24 hours after treatment with a pediculicide; gas autoclave blood pressure cuffs before using them on other patients; isolate linens until the patient is noninfectious; and thoroughly disinfect the patient's room after discharge.

Cutaneous larva migrans

Cutaneous larva migrans, also known as *creeping eruption,* is a skin reaction to infestation by nematodes (hookworms or roundworms) that usually infect dogs and cats. Eruptions associated with cutaneous larva migrans clear completely with treatment.

Causes and incidence

Under favorable conditions — warmth, moisture, sandy soil — hookworm or roundworm ova present in feces of affected animals (such as dogs and cats) and hatch into larvae, which can then burrow into human skin on contact. After penetrating its host, the larva becomes trapped under the skin, unable to reach the intestines to complete its normal life cycle.

The parasite then begins to move, producing the peculiar, tunnel-like lesions that are alternately meandering and linear, reflecting the nematode's persistent and unsuccessful attempts to escape its host.

Signs and symptoms

A transient rash or, possibly, a small vesicle appears at the point of penetration, usually on an exposed area that has come in contact with the ground, such as the feet, legs, or buttocks. The incubation period is typically 1 to 6 days. The parasite may be active almost as soon as it enters the skin. Local pruritus begins within hours following penetration.

As the parasite migrates, it etches a noticeable thin, raised, red line on the skin, which may become vesicular and encrusted. Pruritus quickly develops, often with crusting and secondary infection following excoriation. Onset is usually characterized by slight itching that develops into intermittent stinging pain as the thin, red lines develop. The larva's apparently random path can cover from 1 mm to 1 cm a day. Penetration of more than one larva may involve a much larger area of the skin, marking it with many tracks.

Diagnosis

Characteristic migratory lesions strongly suggest cutaneous larva migrans. A thorough patient history usually reveals contact with warm, moist soil within the past several months.

Treatment

Topical application of thiabendazole, ivermectin, or albendazole is effective. The suspension is applied to lesions and the immediate surrounding areas four times daily for 1 week. Oral thiabendazole given in two divided doses for 3 to 5 days is effective. Oral ivermectin and albendazole are equally effective. Tell the patient that adverse effects of systemic thiabendazole include nausea, vomiting, abdominal pain, and dizziness.

Special considerations

Prevention requires patient teaching about the existence of these parasites, sanitation of beaches and sandboxes, and proper pet care.

■ Reassure the patient, especially if he's sensitive about his appearance, that larva migrans lesions usually clear 1 to 2 weeks after treatment. Stress the importance of adhering to the treatment regimen exactly as ordered.

■ Have the patient's nails cut short to prevent skin breaks and secondary bacterial infection from scratching. Apply cool, moist compresses to alleviate itching.

■ Be alert for possible adverse reactions associated with systemic treatment, including nausea, vomiting, abdominal pain, and dizziness.

■ Encourage the patient to verbalize feelings about the infestation, including embarrassment, fear of rejection by others, and body image disturbance.

TYPES OF LICE

Head louse
Pediculus humanus capitis (head louse) is similar in appearance to *Pediculus humanus corporis.*

Body louse
Pediculus humanus corporis (body louse) has a long abdomen and all its legs are approximately the same length.

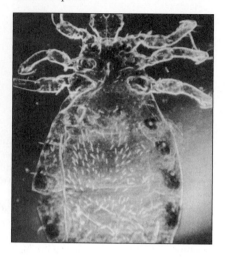

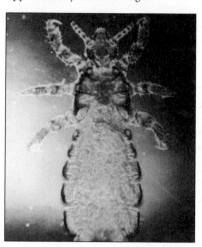

■ Instruct the patient and his family in good hand-washing technique, and stress the importance of preventing the spread of the infection among family members.

Pediculosis

Pediculosis is caused by parasitic forms of lice: *Pediculus humanus capitis* causes pediculosis capitis (head lice); *Pediculus humanus corporis* causes pediculosis corporis (body lice); and *Phthirus pubis* causes pediculosis pubis (crab lice). (See *Types of lice.*) These lice feed on human blood and lay their eggs (nits) on body hairs or clothing fibers. After the nits hatch, the lice must feed within 24 hours or die; they mature in about 2 to 3 weeks. When a louse bites, it injects a toxin into the skin that produces mild irritation and a purpuric spot. Repeated bites cause sensitization to the toxin, leading to more serious inflammation. Treatment can effectively eliminate lice.

Causes and incidence

P. humanus capitis (most common species) feeds on the scalp and, rarely, in the eyebrows, eyelashes, and beard. It's most commonly seen on the back of the head and neck and behind the ears. This form of pediculosis is caused by overcrowded conditions and poor personal hygiene, and commonly affects children, especially girls. It spreads through shared clothing, hats, combs, and hairbrushes.

P. humanus corporis lives in the seams of clothing, next to the skin, leaving only to feed on blood. Common causes include prolonged wearing of the same clothing (which might occur in cold climates), overcrowding, and poor personal hygiene. It spreads through shared clothing and bedsheets.

P. pubis is primarily found in pubic hairs, but this species may extend to the eyebrows, eyelashes, and axillary or body hair. Pediculosis pubis is transmitted through sexual intercourse or by contact

In severe cases, headache, fever, and malaise may accompany cutaneous symptoms.

Pediculosis pubis causes skin irritation from scratching, which is usually more obvious than the bites. Small gray-blue spots (maculae caeruleae) may appear on the thighs or upper body. Small red spots are often seen in the underclothing.

Diagnosis

Pediculosis is visible on physical examination:
- in pediculosis capitis: oval, grayish nits that can't be shaken loose like dandruff (the closer the nits are to the end of the hair shaft, the longer the infection has been present, because the ova are laid close to the scalp)
- in pediculosis corporis: characteristic skin lesions; nits found on clothing
- in pediculosis pubis: nits attached to pubic hairs, which feel coarse and grainy to the touch.

Treatment

Lindane, pyrethrin, permethrin, and malathion, in shampoo or lotion preparations, are all effective against lice. Shampoos should be applied to the infected skin or hair, lathered, then washed off in 5 minutes. Lotions should be applied over the entire affected area, then washed off after 10 minutes. Treatments should be repeated in 7 to 10 days.

Permethrin may be used for treating head lice. Saturate the hair and scalp and rinse after 10 minutes. Malathion lotion is also effective when applied to dry hair and washed out in 8 to 10 hours. After treatment, all nits (louse eggs) should be combed out of the hair with a metal nit comb. Nit removal may be aided by pre-rinsing with a pre-rinse solution containing formic acid, or dipping the comb in vinegar. Normal laundering of clothes and bedclothes in hot water after treatment is sufficient to remove adult lice as well as nits.

Special considerations

- Teach the patient how to use the creams, ointments, powders, and shampoos that eliminate lice. To prevent self-infestation,

---

Pubic louse
Phthirus pubis (pubic or "crab lice") is slightly translucent; its first set of legs is shorter than its second or third.

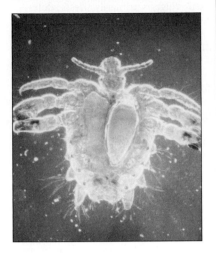

with clothes, bedsheets, or towels harboring lice.

Signs and symptoms

Clinical features of pediculosis capitis include itching; excoriation (with severe itching); matted, foul-smelling, lusterless hair (in severe cases); occipital and cervical lymphadenopathy (posterior cervical lymphadenopathy without obvious disease is characteristic); and a rash on the trunk, probably due to sensitization. Adult lice migrate from the scalp and deposit oval, gray-white nits on the proximal one-third of hair shafts.

Pediculosis corporis initially produces small, red papules (usually on the shoulders, trunk, or buttocks). Later, wheals (probably a sensitivity reaction) may develop. Untreated pediculosis corporis may lead to vertical excoriations and ultimately to dry, discolored, thickly encrusted, scaly skin, with bacterial infection and scarring.

avoid prolonged contact with the patient's hair, clothing, and bedsheets.

■ Ask the patient with pediculosis pubis for a history of recent sexual contacts, so that they can be examined and treated.

■ The patient should be tested for other sexually transmitted diseases, including human immunodeficiency virus.

To prevent the spread of pediculosis to other hospitalized persons, examine all high-risk patients on admission, especially elderly people who depend on others for care, those admitted from nursing homes, and people who live in crowded conditions.

FOLLICULAR AND GLANDULAR DISORDERS

Acne vulgaris

Acne vulgaris is an inflammatory disease of the sebaceous follicles. The prognosis is good with treatment.

Causes and incidence

The cause of acne is multifactorial, but theories regarding dietary influences appear to be groundless. Predisposing factors include heredity; hormonal contraceptives (many females experience an acne flare-up during their first few menstrual cycles after starting or discontinuing hormonal contraceptives); androgen stimulation; certain drugs, including corticosteroids, corticotropin, androgens, iodides, bromides, trimethadione, phenytoin, isoniazid, lithium, and halothane; cobalt irradiation; and hyperalimentation. Other possible factors are exposure to heavy oils, greases, or tars; trauma or rubbing from tight clothing; cosmetics; emotional stress; and unfavorable climate.

More is known about the pathogenesis of acne. (See *What happens in acne.*) Androgens stimulate sebaceous gland growth and production of sebum, which is secreted into dilated hair follicles that contain bacteria. The bacteria, usually *Propionibac-*terium acnes and *Staphylococcus epidermidis* (which are normal skin flora), secrete lipase. This enzyme interacts with sebum to produce free fatty acids, which provoke inflammation. Also, the hair follicles produce more keratin, which joins with the sebum to form a plug in the dilated follicle.

Acne vulgaris primarily affects adolescents (usually between ages 15 and 18), although lesions can appear as early as age 8. Although acne strikes boys more often and more severely than girls, it usually occurs in girls at an earlier age and tends to last longer, sometimes into adulthood.

Signs and symptoms

The acne plug may appear as a closed comedo, or whitehead (if it doesn't protrude from the follicle and is covered by the epidermis), or as an open comedo, or blackhead (if it does protrude and isn't covered by the epidermis). The black coloration is caused by the melanin or pigment of the follicle. Rupture or leakage of an enlarged plug into the dermis produces inflammation and characteristic acne pustules, papules or, in severe forms, acne cysts or abscesses. Chronic, recurring lesions produce acne scars.

Diagnosis

CONFIRMING DIAGNOSIS *The appearance of characteristic acne lesions, especially in an adolescent patient, confirms the presence of acne vulgaris.*

Treatment

Current therapy for acne includes topical and oral agents. Topical retinoic acid (tretinoin) is the treatment of choice for noninflammatory acne consisting of open and closed comedones. Benzoyl peroxide is antibacterial and is used primarily for inflammatory acne, including papules, pustules, and cysts. Topical antibiotics are effective for mild pustular and comedone acne. Tetracycline, erythromycin, clindamycin, meclocycline, and benzamycin are all available in topical forms. Systemic antibiotics, such as tetracycline, minocycline, clindamycin, erythromycin, ampicillin, cephalosporins, co-trimoxazole, and

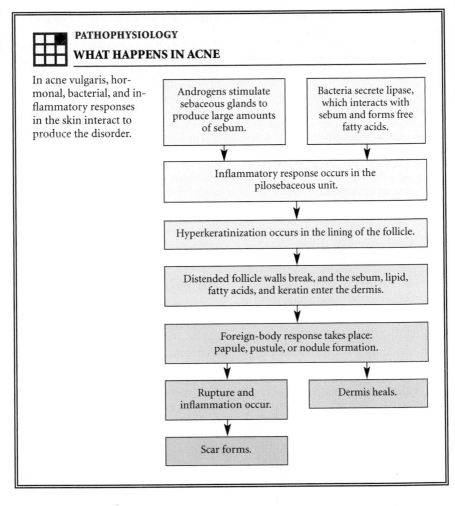

PATHOPHYSIOLOGY
WHAT HAPPENS IN ACNE

In acne vulgaris, hormonal, bacterial, and inflammatory responses in the skin interact to produce the disorder.

Androgens stimulate sebaceous glands to produce large amounts of sebum.

Bacteria secrete lipase, which interacts with sebum and forms free fatty acids.

Inflammatory response occurs in the pilosebaceous unit.

Hyperkeratinization occurs in the lining of the follicle.

Distended follicle walls break, and the sebum, lipid, fatty acids, and keratin enter the dermis.

Foreign-body response takes place: papule, pustule, or nodule formation.

Rupture and inflammation occur.

Dermis heals.

Scar forms.

systemic retinoids may help reduce the effects of acne.

Systemic therapy consists primarily of antibiotics, usually tetracycline (which also exhibits an anti-inflammatory effect), to decrease bacterial growth until the patient is in remission; then a lower dosage is used for long-term maintenance.

ALERT *Tetracycline is contraindicated during pregnancy because it discolors the teeth of the fetus. Erythromycin and ampicillin are alternatives for these patients. Exacerbation of pustules or abscesses during either type of antibiotic therapy requires a culture to identify a possible secondary bacterial infection.*

Oral isotretinoin combats acne by inhibiting sebaceous gland function and keratinization. However, because of its severe adverse effects, the 16- to 20-week course of isotretinoin is limited to those with severe papulopustular or cystic acne who don't respond to conventional therapy. Because this drug is known to cause birth defects, the manufacturer, with Food and Drug Administration approval, recommends the following precautions: pregnancy testing before dispensing; dispensing of only a 30-day supply; repeat pregnancy testing throughout the treatment period; effective contraception during treatment;

and informed consent of the patient or parents regarding the drug's adverse effects.

A serum triglyceride level should be measured before therapy with isotretinoin begins and at intervals throughout its course.

Females may benefit from the administration of estrogens to inhibit androgen activity. Improvement rarely occurs before 2 to 4 months, and exacerbations may follow its discontinuation. Unfortunately, the high estrogen doses that are required present a major risk of severe adverse effects.

Other treatments for acne vulgaris include intralesional or oral corticosteroids, vitamin A and zinc supplements, exposure to ultraviolet light (but never when a photosensitizing agent such as tretinoin is being used), cryotherapy, and surgery.

Special considerations

The main focus of care is teaching about the disorder as well as its treatment and prevention.

- Check the patient's drug history because certain medications such as hormonal contraceptives may cause an acne flare-up.
- Try to identify predisposing factors that may be eliminated or modified.
- Explain the causes of acne to the patient and his family. Make sure they understand that the prescribed treatment is more likely to improve acne than a strict diet and fanatical scrubbing with soap and water. Provide written instructions regarding treatment.
- Instruct the patient receiving tretinoin to apply it at least 30 minutes after washing his face and at least 1 hour before bedtime. Warn against using it around the eyes or lips. After treatments, the skin should look pink and dry. If it appears red or starts to peel, the preparation may have to be weakened or applied less often. Advise the patient to avoid exposure to sunlight or to use a sunscreening agent. If the prescribed regimen includes tretinoin and benzoyl peroxide, avoid skin irritation by using one preparation in the morning and the other at night.
- Instruct the patient to take tetracycline on an empty stomach and not to take it with antacids or milk because it interacts

with their metallic ions and is then poorly absorbed.

- Tell the patient who's taking isotretinoin to avoid vitamin A supplements, which can worsen any adverse effects. Also, teach how to deal with the dry skin and mucous membranes that usually occur during treatment. Tell the female patient about the severe risk of teratogenicity. Monitor liver function and lipid levels.
- Inform the patient that acne takes a long time to clear—even years for complete resolution. Encourage continued local skin care even after acne clears. Explain the adverse effects of all drugs.
- Pay special attention to the patient's perception of his physical appearance, and offer emotional support.

Hirsutism

A distressing disorder usually found in women and children, hirsutism is the excessive growth of body hair, typically in an adult male distribution pattern. This condition commonly occurs spontaneously but may also develop as a secondary disorder of various underlying diseases. It must always be distinguished from hypertrichosis. The prognosis varies with the cause and effectiveness of treatment.

Causes

Idiopathic hirsutism probably stems from a hereditary trait because the patient usually has a family history of the disorder. Causes of secondary hirsutism include endocrine abnormalities related to pituitary dysfunction (acromegaly or precocious puberty), adrenal dysfunction (Cushing's disease, congenital adrenal hyperplasia, or Cushing's syndrome), or ovarian lesions (such as polycystic ovary syndrome or ovarian neoplasm); prolactinoma; and iatrogenic factors (such as the use of minoxidil, androgenic steroids, testosterone, diazoxide, glucocorticoids, and hormonal contraceptives). Other kinds of hirsutism have been reported. (See *Hypertrichosis*.)

Signs and symptoms

Hirsutism typically produces enlarged hair follicles as well as enlargement and hyperpigmentation of the hairs themselves. Excessive facial hair growth is the complaint for which most patients seek medical help. Generally, hirsutism involves appearance of thick, pigmented hair in the beard area, upper back, shoulders, sternum, axillae, and pubic area. Frontotemporal scalp hair recession is often a coexisting condition. Patterns of hirsutism vary widely, depending on the patient's race and age. Elderly women commonly show increased hair growth on the chin and upper lip. In secondary hirsutism, signs of masculinization may appear — deepening of the voice, increased muscle mass, increased size of genitalia, menstrual irregularity, and decreased breast size.

Diagnosis

A family history of hirsutism, absence of menstrual abnormalities or signs of masculinization, and a normal pelvic examination strongly suggest idiopathic hirsutism. Tests for secondary hirsutism depend on associated symptoms that suggest an underlying disorder. About 90% of women with hirsutism have an elevated free testosterone level.

Treatment

At the patient's request, treatment for idiopathic hirsutism consists of eliminating excess hair by scissors, shaving, or depilatory creams, or removal of the entire hair shaft with tweezers or wax. However, removal with laser is the most effective method. Bleaching with hydrogen peroxide may also be satisfactory. Electrolysis can destroy hair bulbs permanently, but it works best when only a few hairs need to be removed. (A history of keloid formation contraindicates this procedure.) Hirsutism due to elevated androgen levels may require low-dose dexamethasone or prednisone, hormonal contraceptives, or androgen receptor–competitive inhibitors — such as spironolactone, cyproterone acetate, or cimetidine — however, these drugs vary in effectiveness.

HYPERTRICHOSIS

Hypertrichosis is a localized or generalized condition in males and females that's marked by excessive hair growth in areas that aren't androgen-sensitive. Localized hypertrichosis usually results from local trauma, chemical irritation, or hormonal stimulation; pigmented nevi (Becker's nevus, for example) may also contain hairs. Generalized hypertrichosis results from neurologic or psychiatric disorders, such as encephalitis, multiple sclerosis, concussion, anorexia nervosa, or schizophrenia; contributing factors include juvenile hypothyroidism, porphyria cutanea tarda, and the use of drugs such as phenytoin.

Hypertrichosis lanuginosa is a generalized proliferation of fine, lanugo-type hair (sometimes called *down* or *woolly hair*). Such hair may be present at birth but generally disappears shortly thereafter. This condition may become chronic, with persistent lanugo-type hair growing over the entire body, or may develop suddenly later in life; it is very rare and usually results from malignancy.

Treatment for secondary hirsutism varies, depending on the nature of the underlying disorder.

Special considerations

Care for patients with idiopathic hirsutism focuses on emotional support and patient teaching; care for patients with secondary hirsutism depends on the treatment for the underlying disease.

■ Provide emotional support by being sensitive to the patient's feelings about her appearance.
■ Watch for signs of contact dermatitis in patients being treated with depilatory creams, especially elderly people. Also,

watch for infection of hair follicles after hair removal with tweezers or wax.
- Suggest consulting a cosmetologist about makeup or bleaching agents.

Alopecia

Alopecia, or hair loss, usually occurs on the scalp but can also occur on bearded areas, eyebrows, and eyelashes. Hair loss elsewhere on the body is less common and less conspicuous. In the nonscarring form of this disorder (noncicatricial alopecia), the hair follicle can generally regrow hair. However, scarring alopecia involves tissue destruction, such as inflammation, scarring, and atrophy, and usually destroys the hair follicle, making hair loss irreversible.

Causes and incidence

The most common form of nonscarring alopecia is male-pattern alopecia, which appears to be related to androgen levels and to aging. Genetic predisposition commonly influences the time of onset, degree of baldness, speed with which it spreads, and pattern of hair loss. Women may experience diffuse thinning over the top of the scalp.

Other forms of nonscarring alopecia include:
- physiologic alopecia (usually temporary): sudden hair loss in infants, loss of straight hairline in adolescents, and diffuse hair loss after childbirth
- alopecia areata (idiopathic form): generally reversible and self-limiting; occurs most frequently in young and middle-age adults of both sexes (See *Alopecia areata.*)
- trichotillomania: compulsive pulling out of one's own hair; most common in children
- traction alopecia: localized areas of hair loss due to chronic use of tight braids (such as cornrows) or other hair styles. This condition may also result in scarring alopecia.

Predisposing factors of nonscarring alopecia also include radiation, many types of drug therapies and drug reactions, bacterial and fungal infections, psoriasis, seborrhea, and endocrine disorders, such as

thyroid, parathyroid, and pituitary dysfunctions.

Scarring alopecia causes irreversible hair loss. It may result from physical or chemical trauma and chronic tension on a hair shaft, as occurs in braiding. Diseases that produce alopecia include destructive skin tumors, granulomas, lupus erythematosus, scleroderma, follicular lichen planus, and severe fungal, bacterial, or viral infections, such as kerion, folliculitis, or herpes simplex.

Signs and symptoms

In male-pattern alopecia, hair loss is gradual and usually affects the thinner, shorter, and less pigmented hairs of the frontal and parietal portions of the scalp. In women, hair loss is generally more diffuse; completely bald areas are uncommon but may occur.

Alopecia areata affects small patches of the scalp but may also occur as alopecia totalis, which involves the entire scalp and eyebrows, or as alopecia universalis, which involves the entire body. Although mild erythema may occur initially, affected areas of scalp or skin appear normal. "Exclamation point" hairs (loose hairs with dark, rough, brushlike tips on narrow, less pigmented shafts) occur at the periphery of new patches. Regrowth hairs are thin and may be white or gray. They're usually replaced by normal hair.

In trichotillomania, patchy, incomplete areas of hair loss with many broken hairs appear on the scalp but may occur on other areas such as the eyebrows.

Diagnosis

CONFIRMING DIAGNOSIS
Physical examination is usually sufficient to confirm alopecia. In trichotillomania, an occlusive dressing can establish the diagnosis by allowing new hair to grow, revealing that the hair is being pulled out. Diagnosis must also identify any underlying disorder.

Treatment

Topical application of minoxidil, a peripheral vasodilator more typically used as an oral antihypertensive, has limited success

ALOPECIA AREATA

"Exclamation point" hairs often border new patches of alopecia areata. Not seen in any other type of alopecia, these hairs indicate the patch is expanding.

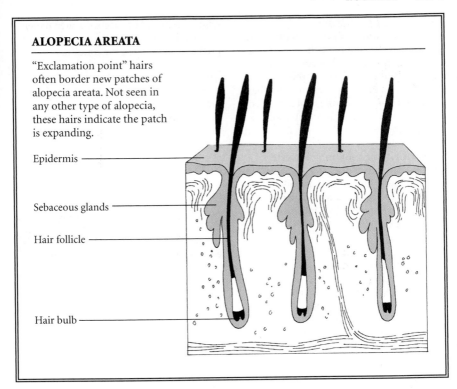

Epidermis

Sebaceous glands

Hair follicle

Hair bulb

in treating male-pattern alopecia. An alternative treatment is surgical redistribution of hair follicles by autografting. Oral finasteride has been shown to reverse androgenic loss, but it's approved only for use in men.

In alopecia areata, minoxidil is effective, although treatment is often unnecessary because spontaneous regrowth is common. Intralesional corticosteroid injections are beneficial for small patches and may produce regrowth in 4 to 6 weeks. Anthralin, topical high-potency corticosteroids, systemic corticosteroids, topical cyclosporine, oral inosiplex, and topical nitrogen mustard all have been used in treating alopecia areata. Hair loss that persists for more than a year has a poor prognosis for regrowth. In trichotillomania, an occlusive dressing encourages normal hair growth, simply by identifying the cause of hair loss; clomipramine may be effective for short-term treatment. Treatment for other types of alopecia varies according to the underlying cause.

Special considerations

■ Reassure a woman with female-pattern alopecia that it doesn't lead to total baldness. Suggest that she wear a wig.
■ If the patient has alopecia areata, explain the disorder and give reassurance that complete regrowth is possible.

Rosacea

A chronic skin eruption, rosacea produces flushing and dilation of the small blood vessels in the face, especially the nose and cheeks. Papules and pustules may also occur, but without the characteristic comedones of acne vulgaris. Ocular involvement may result in blepharitis, conjunctivitis, uveitis, or keratitis. Rosacea usually spreads slowly and rarely subsides spontaneously.

Causes and incidence

Although the cause of rosacea is unknown, stress, infection, vitamin deficiency, menopause, and endocrine abnormalities can aggravate this condition. Anything that produces flushing—for example, hot beverages, such as tea or coffee; tobacco; alcohol; spicy foods; physical activity; sunlight; and extreme heat or cold—can also aggravate rosacea.

Rosacea is most common in white women between ages 30 and 50. When it occurs in men, however, it's usually more severe and often associated with rhinophyma, which is characterized by dilated follicles and thickened, bulbous skin on the nose.

Signs and symptoms

Rosacea generally begins with periodic flushing across the central oval of the face, accompanied later by telangiectasia, papules, pustules, and nodules. Rhinophyma is commonly associated with severe untreated rosacea but may occur alone. Rhinophyma usually appears first on the lower half of the nose, and produces red, thickened skin and follicular enlargement. It's found almost exclusively in men older than age 40. Related ocular lesions are uncommon.

Diagnosis

CONFIRMING DIAGNOSIS *Typical vascular and acneiform lesions—without the comedones characteristically associated with acne vulgaris—and rhinophyma in severe cases confirm rosacea.*

Treatment

Treatment for the acneiform component of rosacea consists of oral tetracycline or erythromycin in gradually decreasing doses over 1 to 2 months as symptoms subside. Resistant cases can be treated with oral minocycline or doxycycline. Isotretinoin is also effective, but its use is limited to those with severe disease. Topical metronidazole gel helps the papules, pustules, and erythema. Sulfacet-R lotion, available in flesh tones, controls pustules and hides redness. It can be used alone or together with oral antibiotics. Other treatments include electrolysis to destroy large, dilated blood vessels and removal of excess tissue in patients with rhinophyma. Topical hydrocortisone preparations worsen the condition.

Special considerations

■ Instruct the patient to avoid spicy foods, hot beverages, alcohol, extended sun exposure, and other possible causes of flushing.
■ Assess the effect of rosacea on body image. Because it's always apparent on the face, support is essential.
■ Encourage the use of sunscreen.

PIGMENTATION DISORDERS

Vitiligo

Marked by stark-white skin patches that may cause a serious cosmetic problem, vitiligo results from the destruction and loss of pigment cells. It shows no racial preference, but the distinctive patches are most noticeable in blacks. Repigmentation therapy, which is widely used in treating vitiligo, may necessitate several summers of exposure to sunlight; the effects of this treatment may not be permanent.

Causes and incidence

Although the cause of vitiligo is unknown, inheritance seems to be a definite etiologic factor because about 30% of patients with vitiligo have family members with the same condition. Other theories implicate enzymatic self-destructing mechanisms, autoimmune mechanisms, and abnormal neurogenic stimuli.

Some link exists between vitiligo and many other disorders that it often accompanies—thyroid dysfunction, pernicious anemia, Addison's disease, aseptic meningitis, diabetes mellitus, photophobia, hearing defects, alopecia areata, uveitis, chronic mucocutaneous candidiasis, and halo nevi.

The most frequently reported precipitating factor is a stressful physical or psychological event—severe sunburn, surgery, pregnancy, loss of a job, bereavement, or some other source of distress. Chemical

RECOGNIZING VITILIGO

This illustration shows characteristic depigmented skin patches in vitiligo. These patches are usually bilaterally symmetrical, with distinct borders.

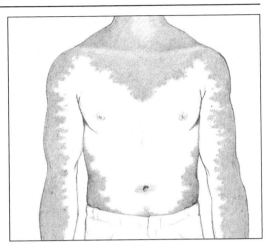

agents, such as phenols and catechols, may also cause this condition.

Vitiligo affects about 1% of the population in the United States, usually people between ages 10 and 30, with peak incidence around age 20. It affects men and women equally, but women are more likely to seek treatment.

Signs and symptoms

Vitiligo produces depigmented or stark-white patches on the skin; on fair-skinned whites, these are almost imperceptible. Lesions are usually bilaterally symmetrical with sharp borders, which occasionally are hyperpigmented. Lesions that are small initially can enlarge and even progress to total depigmentation (universal vitiligo).

These unique patches generally appear over bony prominences on the back of the hands; on the face, the axillae, genitalia, nipples, or umbilicus; around orifices (such as the eyes, mouth, and anus); within body folds; and at sites of trauma. The hair within these lesions may also turn white. Because hair follicles and certain parts of the eyes also contain pigment cells, vitiligo may be associated with premature gray hair

and ocular pigmentary changes. (See *Recognizing vitiligo*.)

Diagnosis

Diagnosis requires an accurate history of onset and of associated illnesses, a family history, and observation of characteristic lesions. Other skin disorders such as tinea versicolor must be ruled out.

 CONFIRMING DIAGNOSIS *In fair-skinned patients, Wood's light examination in a darkened room detects vitiliginous patches; depigmented skin reflects the light, and pigmented skin absorbs it. Biopsy will show normal skin except for the absence of melanocytes. If autoimmune or endocrine disturbances are suspected, laboratory studies (such as thyroid studies) are appropriate.*

Treatment

Repigmentation therapy combines systemic or topical psoralen compounds (trimethylpsoralen or 8-methoxypsoralen) with exposure to sunlight or artificial ultraviolet light, wavelength A (UVA). New pigment rises from hair follicles and appears on the skin as small freckles, which gradually enlarge and coalesce. Body parts containing few hair follicles (such as the fingertips) may resist this therapy.

Because psoralens and UVA affect the entire skin surface, systemic therapy enhances the contrast between normal skin, which turns darker than usual, and white, vitiliginous skin. Use of sunscreen on normal skin may minimize contrast while preventing sunburn.

Topical class I glucosteroid ointments may be used for single or small macules. Monitor patients on this therapy for skin atrophy or telangiectasia development.

Depigmentation therapy is suggested for patients with vitiligo affecting more than 50% of the body surface. A cream containing 20% monobenzone permanently destroys pigment cells in unaffected areas of the skin and produces a uniform skin tone. This medication is applied initially to a small area of normal skin once daily to test for unfavorable reactions such as contact dermatitis. In the absence of adverse effects, the patient begins applying the cream twice daily to those areas he wishes to depigment first. Eventually, the entire skin may be depigmented to achieve a uniform color. *Note:* Depigmentation is permanent and results in extreme photosensitivity. Patients may wish to take daily B-carotene to impart an off-white color to the chalk-white skin.

Commercial cosmetics may also help de-emphasize vitiliginous skin. Some patients prefer dyes because these remain on the skin for several days, although the results aren't always satisfactory. Although often impractical, complete avoidance of exposure to sunlight through the use of screening agents and protective clothing may minimize vitiliginous lesions in whites.

Special considerations

■ Instruct the patient to use psoralen medications three or four times weekly. (*Note:* Systemic psoralens should be taken 2 hours before exposure to sun; topical solutions should be applied 30 to 60 minutes before exposure.) Warn him to use a sunscreen (sun protection factor [SPF] 8 to 10) to protect both affected and normal skin during exposure and to wear sunglasses after taking the medication. If periorbital areas require exposure, tell the patient to keep his eyes closed during treatment.

■ Suggest that the patient receiving depigmentation therapy wear protective clothing and use a sunscreen (SPF 15). Explain the therapy thoroughly, and allow the patient plenty of time to decide whether to undergo this treatment. Make sure he understands that the results of depigmentation are permanent and that he must thereafter protect his skin from the adverse effects of sunlight.

■ Caution the patient about buying commercial cosmetics or dyes without trying them first because some may not be suitable.

 PEDIATRIC TIP *For the child with vitiligo, modify repigmentation therapy to avoid unnecessary restrictions. Tell parents to give the initial dose of psoralen medication at 1 p.m. and then let the child go out to play as usual. After this, medication should be given 30 minutes earlier each day of treatment, provided the child's skin doesn't turn more than slightly pink from exposure. If marked erythema develops, parents should discontinue treatment and notify the physician. Eventually, the child should be able to take the medication at 9:30 a.m. and play outdoors the rest of the day without adverse effects. Tell the parents the child should wear clothing that permits maximum exposure of vitiliginous areas to the sun.*

■ Remind patients undergoing repigmentation therapy that exposure to sunlight also darkens normal skin. After being exposed to UVA for the prescribed amount of time, the patient should apply a sunscreen if he plans to be exposed to sunlight also. If sunburn occurs, advise the patient to discontinue therapy temporarily and to apply open wet dressings (using thin sheeting) to affected areas for 15 to 20 minutes, four or five times daily or as necessary for comfort. After application of wet dressings, allow the skin to air dry. Suggest application of a soothing lubricating cream or lotion while the skin is still slightly moist.

■ Reinforce patient teaching with written instructions.

■ Be sensitive to the patient's emotional needs, but avoid promoting unrealistic hope for a total cure.

Melasma

A patchy, hypermelanotic skin disorder, melasma (also known as *chloasma* or *mask of pregnancy*) can pose a serious cosmetic problem. It may be chronic but is never life-threatening.

Causes and incidence

The cause of melasma is unknown, but onset is most common in young adults. Histologically, hyperpigmentation results from increased melanin production, although the number of melanocytes remains normal. Melasma may be related to the increased hormonal levels associated with pregnancy, menopause, ovarian cancer, and the use of hormonal contraceptives. Progestational agents, phenytoin, and mephenytoin may also contribute to this disorder. Exposure to sunlight stimulates melasma, but it may develop without any apparent predisposing factor. Patients with acquired immunodeficiency syndrome have an increased incidence of similar hyperpigmentation.

Melasma affects females more commonly than males. Although it tends to occur equally in all races, the light-brown color characteristic of melasma is most evident in dark-skinned whites.

Signs and symptoms

Typically, melasma produces large, brown, irregular patches, symmetrically distributed on the forehead, cheeks, and sides of the nose. Less commonly, these patches may occur on the neck, upper lip, temples and, occasionally, on the dorsa of the forearms.

Diagnosis

CONFIRMING DIAGNOSIS
Observation of characteristic dark patches on the face usually confirms melasma. The patient history may reveal predisposing factors. Wood's lamp examination accentuates the hyperpigmentation.

Treatment

Treatment consists primarily of application of bleaching agents containing 2% to 4% hydroquinone in combination with tretinoin or glycolic acid to inhibit melanin synthesis. This medication is applied twice daily for up to 8 weeks. Adjunctive measures include avoidance of exposure to sunlight, use of opaque sunscreens, and discontinuation of hormonal contraceptives.

Special considerations

■ Tell the patient that melasma associated with pregnancy usually clears within a few months after delivery and may not return with subsequent pregnancies.
■ Advise the patient to avoid exposure by using sunscreens and wearing protective clothing. Bleaching agents may help but may require repeated treatments to maintain the desired effect. Cosmetics may help mask deep pigmentation.
■ Reassure the patient that melasma is treatable. It may fade spontaneously with protection from sunlight, postpartum, and after discontinuing hormonal contraceptives. Serial photographs help show the patient that patches are improving.

Photosensitivity reactions

A photosensitivity reaction is a skin eruption that can be a toxic or allergic response to light alone or to light and chemicals. A phototoxic reaction is a dose-related primary response. A photoallergic reaction is an uncommon, acquired immune response that isn't dose-related — even slight exposure can cause a severe reaction.

Causes

Certain chemicals can cause a photosensitivity reaction, including dyes, coal tar, and furocoumarin compounds found in plants. The list of drugs that can cause photosensitivity reactions is extensive and includes many drugs within each of the following general categories: antibiotics (especially tetracycline), antidepressants, antihistamines, anticancer agents, antiparasitic agents, antipsychotic agents, diuretics, hypoglycemics, nonsteroidal anti-inflammatories, sunscreens, and miscellaneous agents, such as cardiac glycosides, hormonal contraceptives, and acne medications.

Berlock dermatitis, a specific photosensitivity reaction, results from the use of oil of bergamot—a common component of perfumes, colognes, and pomades.

Signs and symptoms

Immediately after exposure, a phototoxic reaction causes a burning sensation followed by erythema (sunburn-type reaction), edema, desquamation, and hyperpigmentation. Berlock dermatitis produces an acute reaction with erythematous vesicles that later become hyperpigmented.

Photoallergic reactions may take one of two forms. Developing 2 hours to 5 days after light exposure, polymorphous light eruption (PMLE) produces erythema, papules, vesicles, urticaria, and eczematous lesions on exposed areas; pruritus may persist for 1 to 2 weeks. Solar urticaria begins minutes after exposure and lasts about an hour; erythema and wheals follow itching and burning sensations.

Diagnosis

Characteristic skin eruptions in sun-exposed areas and a patient history of recent exposure to light or certain chemicals suggest a photosensitivity reaction. A phototopatch test for ultraviolet A and B (UVA and UVB) done while the patient is on the drug may aid diagnosis and identify the causative light wavelength. Other studies must rule out connective tissue disease, such as lupus erythematosus and porphyrias.

Treatment

For many patients, treatment involves a sunscreen, protective clothing, and minimal exposure to sunlight while the patient continues on the drug. For others, progressive exposure to sunlight can thicken the skin and produce a tan that interferes with photoallergens and prevents further eruptions.

Withdrawal of the causative agent and treatment with oral steroids usually provides relief. The patient should be advised not to use the causative agent again if it's known, even though this may limit the patient's treatment options.

Antimalarial drugs, beta-carotene, and PUVA (psoralen and UVA) may be used to treat PMLE. Treatment for solar urticaria may also require PUVA. Although hyperpigmentation usually fades in several months, hydroquinone preparations can hasten the process.

Special considerations

- To prevent reactions, advise the patient to avoid prolonged exposure to light.
- Tell the patient to inform his physician about sensitivity to any drugs.

INFLAMMATORY REACTIONS

Dermatitis

Inflammation of the skin, dermatitis occurs in several forms: atopic (discussed here), seborrheic, nummular, contact, chronic, localized neurodermatitis, exfoliative, and stasis. (See *Types of dermatitis*, pages 1258 to 1261.) Atopic dermatitis (atopic or infantile eczema, neurodermatitis constitutionalis, or Besnier's prurigo) is a chronic inflammatory response often associated with other atopic diseases, such as bronchial asthma and allergic rhinitis.

Causes and incidence

The cause of atopic dermatitis is unknown, but a genetic predisposition may be exacerbated by such factors as food allergies, infections, irritating chemicals, temperature and humidity, and emotions. Approximately 10% of childhood cases are due to allergy to certain foods, particularly eggs, peanuts, milk, fish, soy, and wheat. Atopic dermatitis tends to flare up in response to extremes in temperature and humidity.

Other causes of flare-ups are sweating and psychological stress.

An important secondary cause of atopic dermatitis is irritation, which seems to change the epidermal structure, allowing immunoglobulin (Ig) E activity to increase. Consequently, chronic skin irritation usually continues even after exposure to the allergen has ended or after the irritation has been systemically controlled.

Atopic dermatitis is most common in infants, usually developing between ages 1 month and 1 year, commonly in those with strong family histories of atopic disease. At least half of those cases clear by age 36 months. These children often acquire other atopic disorders as they grow older. Typically, this form of dermatitis flares and subsides repeatedly before finally resolving during adolescence. However, it can persist into adulthood. In adults, it's generally chronic or recurring.

Signs and symptoms

Atopic skin lesions generally begin as erythematous areas on excessively dry skin. In children, such lesions typically appear on the forehead, cheeks, and extensor surfaces of the arms and legs; in adults, at flexion points (antecubital fossa, popliteal area, and neck).

During flare-ups, pruritus and scratching cause edema, crusting, and scaling. Eventually, chronic atopic lesions lead to multiple areas of dry, scaly skin, with white dermatographia, blanching, and lichenification.

Common secondary conditions associated with atopic dermatitis include viral, fungal, or bacterial infections, and ocular disorders.

Because of intense pruritus, the upper eyelid is commonly hyperpigmented and swollen, and a double fold occurs under the lower lid (Morgan-Dennie folds, Morgan folds, Dennie pleats, or Mongolian lines). Atopic cataracts are unusual but may develop between ages 20 and 40.

Kaposi's varicelliform eruption, a potentially fatal, generalized viral infection, may develop if the patient with atopic dermatitis comes in contact with a person who's infected with herpes simplex.

Diagnosis

A family history of allergy and chronic inflammation suggests atopic dermatitis. Typical distribution of skin lesions rules out other inflammatory skin lesions, such as diaper rash (lesions are confined to the diapered area), seborrheic dermatitis (no pigmentation changes, or lichenification occurs in chronic lesions), and chronic contact dermatitis (lesions affect hands and forearms, sparing antecubital and popliteal areas). Serum IgE levels are usually elevated.

Treatment

Effective treatment for atopic lesions consists of eliminating allergens and avoiding irritants, extreme temperature and humidity changes, and other precipitating factors; local and systemic measures relieve itching and inflammation. Antihistamines relieve itching and induce more restful sleep. Topical application of a corticosteroid ointment, especially after bathing, often alleviates inflammation. Between steroid doses, application of a moisturizing cream can help retain moisture. Systemic corticosteroid therapy should be used only during extreme exacerbations. Topical tacrolimus and pimecrolimus (an immunosuppressant known as a *topical immunomodulator*) are new agents used in patients older than age 2 who are intolerant of or unresponsive to conventional therapy. Weak tar preparations and ultraviolet B light therapy are used to increase the thickness of the stratum corneum. Antibiotics are appropriate if a bacterial agent has been cultured.

Special considerations

■ Warn the patient that drowsiness is possible with the use of antihistamines to relieve daytime itching. If nocturnal itching interferes with sleep, suggest methods for inducing natural sleep, such as drinking a glass of warm milk, to prevent overuse of sedatives.

(*Text continues on page 1260.*)

TYPES OF DERMATITIS

Type	Causes	Signs and symptoms
Seborrheic dermatitis An acute or subacute skin disease that affects areas where sebaceous glands are most active—such as the scalp and face—and occasionally other areas, and is characterized by lesions covered with yellow or brownish gray scales.	■ Unknown; stress and neurologic conditions may be predisposing factors; may be related to the yeast *Pityrosporum ovale*	■ Eruptions in areas with many sebaceous glands (usually scalp, face, and trunk) and in skin folds ■ Itching, redness, and inflammation of affected areas; lesions may appear greasy; fissures may occur ■ Indistinct, occasionally yellowish, scaly patches from excess stratum corneum (dandruff may be mild seborrheic dermatitis) ■ Generally worse in winter
Nummular dermatitis (discoid eczema, nummular eczema) A chronic form of dermatitis characterized by inflammation of coin-shaped, vesicular, crusted scales and, possibly, pruritic lesions.	■ Possibly precipitated by stress, skin dryness, irritants, scratching, or bathing with hot water	■ Round, nummular (coin-shaped) lesions, usually on arms and legs, with distinct borders of crusts and scales ■ Possible oozing and severe itching ■ Summertime remissions common, with wintertime recurrence
Contact dermatitis Often sharply demarcated inflammation and irritation of the skin caused by contact with substances to which the skin is sensitive, such as perfumes, soaps, plants, or chemicals.	■ Mild irritants: chronic exposure to detergents or solvents ■ Strong irritants: damage on contact with acids or alkalis ■ Allergens: sensitization after repeated exposure	■ Mild irritants and allergens: erythema and small vesicles that ooze, scale, and itch ■ Strong irritants: blisters and ulcerations ■ Classic allergic response: clearly defined lesions, with straight lines following points of contact ■ Severe allergic reaction: marked edema of affected areas
Chronic dermatitis Characterized by inflammatory eruptions of the hands and feet.	■ Usually unknown but may result from progressive contact dermatitis ■ Secondary (possibly perpetuating) factors: trauma, infections, redistribution of normal flora, photosensitivity, and food sensitivity	■ Thick, lichenified, single or multiple lesions on any part of body (often on hands) ■ Inflammation and scaling ■ Recurrence following long remissions

Diagnosis	Treatment and intervention
■ Patient history and physical findings, especially distribution of lesions in sebaceous gland areas, confirm seborrheic dermatitis. ■ Diagnosis must rule out psoriasis.	■ Removal of scales with frequent washing and shampooing with selenium sulfide suspension (most effective), zinc pyrithione, or tar and salicylic acid shampoo ■ Application of fluorinated corticosteroids to nonhairy areas
■ Physical findings and patient history confirm nummular dermatitis; a middle-age or older patient may have a history of atopic dermatitis. ■ Diagnosis must rule out fungal infections, atopic or contact dermatitis, and psoriasis.	■ Elimination of known irritants ■ Measures to relieve dry skin: increased humidification, limited frequency of baths and use of bland soap and bath oils, and application of emollients ■ Application of wet dressings in acute phase ■ Topical corticosteroids (occlusive dressings or intralesional injections) for persistent lesions ■ Tar preparations and antihistamines to control itching ■ Antibiotics for secondary infection ■ Other interventions as for atopic dermatitis
■ Patient history, patch testing to identify allergens, and shape and distribution of lesions suggest contact dermatitis.	■ Elimination of known allergens and decreased exposure to irritants, wearing protective clothing such as gloves, and washing immediately after contact with irritants or allergens ■ Topical anti-inflammatory agents (including corticosteroids); systemic corticosteroids for edema, bullae, or very extensive outbreaks; antihistamines; and local applications of Burow's solution (for blisters) ■ Sensitization to topical medications may occur ■ Other interventions as for atopic dermatitis
■ No characteristic pattern or course; diagnosis relies on detailed patient history and physical findings.	■ Antibiotics for secondary infection ■ Avoidance of excessive washing and drying of hands and of accumulation of soaps and detergents under rings ■ Use of emollients with topical steroids ■ Other interventions as for contact dermatitis

(continued)

TYPES OF DERMATITIS (continued)

Type	Causes	Signs and symptoms
Localized neurodermatitis (lichen simplex chronicus, essential pruritus)		
Superficial inflammation of the skin characterized by itching and papular eruptions that appear on thickened, hyperpigmented skin.	▪ Chronic scratching or rubbing of primary lesion or insect bite, or other skin irritation	▪ Intense, sometimes continual scratching ▪ Thick, sharp-bordered, possibly dry, scaly lesions with raised papules ▪ Usually affects easily reached areas, such as ankles, lower legs, anogenital area, back of neck, and ears
Exfoliative dermatitis		
Severe, chronic skin inflammation characterized by redness and widespread erythema and scaling.	▪ Usually, preexisting skin lesions progress to exfoliative stage, such as in contact dermatitis, drug reaction, lymphoma, or leukemia	▪ Generalized dermatitis, with acute loss of stratum corneum, and erythema and scaling ▪ Sensation of tight skin ▪ Hair loss ▪ Possible fever, sensitivity to cold, shivering, gynecomastia, and lymphadenopathy
Stasis dermatitis		
A condition caused by impaired venous circulation and characterized by eczema of the legs with edema, hyperpigmentation, and persistent inflammation.	▪ Secondary to peripheral vascular diseases affecting legs, such as recurrent thrombophlebitis and resultant chronic venous insufficiency	▪ Varicosities and edema common, but obvious vascular insufficiency not always present ▪ Usually affects the lower leg, just above internal malleolus, or sites of trauma or irritation ▪ Early signs: dusky red deposits of hemosiderin in skin, with itching and dimpling of subcutaneous tissue; later signs: edema, redness, and scaling of large area of legs ▪ Possible fissures, crusts, and ulcers

▪ Complement medical treatment by helping the patient set up an individual schedule and plan for daily skin care. Instruct the patient to bathe in plain water, according to the severity of the lesions, and to bathe with a special nonfatty soap and tepid water (96° F [35.6° C]) but to avoid using any soap when lesions are acutely inflamed. Advise the patient to shampoo frequently and apply corticosteroid solution to the scalp afterward, to keep fingernails short to limit excoriation and secondary infections caused by scratching, and to lubricate his skin after a tub bath. Advise the patient to avoid using any perfume or makeup that causes burning or itching.
▪ To help clear lichenified skin, apply occlusive dressings (such as plastic film) intermittently. This treatment requires a physician's order, experience in dermato-

Diagnosis	Treatment and intervention
■ Physical findings confirm diagnosis.	■ Scratching must stop; then lesions will disappear in about 2 weeks ■ Fixed dressing or Unna's boot to cover affected area ■ Topical corticosteroids under occlusion or by intralesional injection ■ Antihistamines and open wet dressings ■ Emollients ■ Inform patient about underlying cause
■ Diagnosis requires identification of the underlying cause.	■ Severe cases: may require hospitalization with protective isolation and hygienic measures to prevent secondary bacterial infection ■ Open wet dressings, with colloidal baths ■ Bland lotions over topical corticosteroids ■ Maintenance of constant environmental temperature to prevent chilling or overheating ■ Careful monitoring of renal and cardiac status ■ Systemic antibiotics and steroids ■ Other interventions as for atopic dermatitis
■ Diagnosis requires positive history of venous insufficiency and physical findings such as varicosities.	■ Measures to prevent venous stasis: avoidance of prolonged sitting or standing, use of support stockings, weight reduction in obese patients, and increasing of activity ■ Corrective surgery for underlying cause ■ After ulcer develops, encourage rest periods, with legs elevated; open wet dressings; Unna's boot (zinc gelatin dressing provides continuous pressure to affected areas); and antibiotics for secondary infection after wound culture

logic treatment, and can't be used in all treatment modalities.

■ Inform the patient that irritants, such as detergents and wool, and emotional stress, exacerbate atopic dermatitis.

■ Be careful not to show any anxiety or revulsion when touching the lesions during treatment. Help the patient accept his altered body image, and encourage him to verbalize his feelings. Remember, coping with disfigurement is extremely difficult, especially for children and adolescents. Arrange for counseling, if necessary, to help the patient deal with this distressing condition more effectively.

MISCELLANEOUS DISORDERS

Toxic epidermal necrolysis

Toxic epidermal necrolysis (TEN) is a rare, severe skin disorder that causes epidermal erythema, superficial necrosis, and skin erosions. Mortality is high (30%), especially among debilitated and elderly patients. Reepithelialization is slow, and residual scarring is common. TEN primarily affects adults. Some experts consider TEN to be a maximal form of Stevens-Johnson syndrome (SJS), with SJS being a maximal variant of erythema multiforme major.

Causes and incidence

In 80% of cases, TEN is determined to result from a drug reaction — most commonly to sulfonamides, penicillins, barbiturates, hydantoins, procainamide, isoniazid, nonsteroidal anti-inflammatory drugs, or allopurinol. Numerous other drugs have also been implicated, although 5% of patients with TEN report no drug use. It may also result from chemical exposure, viral infection, mycoplasma pneumonia, or immunization.

TEN may reflect an immune response, or it may be related to overwhelming physiologic stress (coexisting sepsis, neoplastic diseases, and drug treatment).

The annual worldwide incidence of TENS is 1 to 3 cases for every 1 million people.

Signs and symptoms

Early symptoms include inflammation of the mucous membranes, a burning sensation in the conjunctivae, malaise, fever, and generalized skin tenderness. After such prodromal symptoms, TEN erupts in three phases:
- diffuse, erythematous rash
- vesiculation and blistering
- large-scale epidermal necrolysis and desquamation.

Large, flaccid bullae that rupture easily expose extensive areas of denuded skin, permitting both loss of tissue fluids and electrolytes and widespread systemic involvement. Systemic complications may include bronchopneumonia, pulmonary edema, GI and esophageal hemorrhage, shock, renal failure, sepsis, and disseminated intravascular coagulation; these conditions markedly increase the likelihood of mortality.

Diagnosis

CONFIRMING DIAGNOSIS *Early diagnosis is very important and is based on the patient's clinical status at the peak stage of the disease. Nikolsky's sign (skin sloughs off with slight friction) is present in erythematous areas. Culture and Gram stain of lesions determine whether infection is present. Supportive findings include leukocytosis, elevated levels of alanine aminotransferase and aspartate aminotransferase, albuminuria, and fluid and electrolyte imbalances.*

Exfoliative cytology and biopsy aid in ruling out erythema multiforme and exfoliative dermatitis.

Treatment

Treatment consists of transferring the patient to a burn center or an intensive care unit and providing I.V. fluid replacement to maintain fluid and electrolyte balance. Xenografts should be used to prevent pain and infection and to provide the framework for reepithelialization. High doses of I.V. immunoglobulins may halt progression if given early in the course of illness. Steroids may be appropriate initially, but should be discontinued as soon as healing occurs. Use of steroids may decrease survival rates only secondary to increased incidence of infections and other complications. Necrotic skin should be débrided. The patient also should stop using suspected drugs.

Special considerations

- Frequently assess hematocrit and hemoglobin, electrolyte, serum protein, and blood gas levels.
- Monitor vital signs, central venous pressure, and urine output. Watch for signs of renal failure (decreased urine output) and

bleeding. Report fever immediately, and obtain blood cultures and sensitivity tests promptly, as ordered, to detect and treat septic infection.
■ Prevent secondary infection with appropriate precautions. Use systemic antibiotics for specific identified infections only.
■ Maintain skin integrity as much as possible. The patient shouldn't wear clothing and should be covered loosely to prevent friction and sloughing of skin. A low air-loss or air-fluidized bed is helpful.
■ Administer analgesics as needed. Wounds will be virtually pain-free after the dermis is covered by the xenograft.
■ Provide eye care hourly to remove exudate. Because ocular lesions are common, the ophthalmologist should examine the patent's eyes daily.
■ Ensure that suspected drugs are never administered.
■ Encourage the patient to wear a medical alert bracelet.

Warts

Warts, also known as *verrucae,* are common, benign, viral infections of the skin and adjacent mucous membranes. The prognosis varies: Some warts disappear readily with treatment; others necessitate more vigorous and prolonged treatment. Some warts demonstrate spontaneous resolution.

Causes and incidence

Warts are caused by infection with the human papillomavirus, a group of ether-resistant, deoxyribonucleic acid-containing papovaviruses. Mode of transmission is probably through direct contact, but autoinoculation is possible.

Although their incidence is highest in children and young adults, warts may occur at any age.

Signs and symptoms

Clinical manifestations depend on the type of wart and its location:
■ common (verruca vulgaris): rough, elevated, rounded surface; appears most frequently on extremities, particularly hands

and fingers; most prevalent in children and young adults
■ condyloma acuminatum (moist wart or genital wart): usually small, pink to red, moist, and soft; may occur singly or in large cauliflower-like clusters on the penis, scrotum, vulva, cervix, vagina, and anus; can also occur on oral mucosa following oral-genital exposure; considered a sexually transmitted disease
■ digitate: fingerlike, horny projection arising from a pea-shaped base; occurs on scalp or near hairline
■ filiform: single, thin, threadlike projection; commonly occurs around the face and neck
■ flat (also known as *juvenile* or *verruca plana):* multiple groupings of up to several hundred slightly raised lesions with smooth, flat, or slightly rounded tops; common on the face, neck, chest, knees, dorsa of hands, wrists, and flexor surfaces of the forearms; usually occur in children but can affect adults; often linear distribution because of spread from scratching or shaving
■ periungual: rough, irregularly shaped, elevated surface; occurs around edges of fingernails and toenails; when severe, may extend under nail and lift it off nail bed, causing pain
■ plantar: slightly elevated or flat; occur singly or in large clusters (mosaic warts), primarily at pressure points of feet.

Diagnosis

CONFIRMING DIAGNOSIS *Visual examination usually confirms the diagnosis. Plantar warts can be differentiated from corns and calluses by certain distinguishing features. Plantar warts obliterate natural lines of the skin, may contain red or black capillary dots that are easily discernible if the surface of the wart is shaved down with a scalpel, and are painful on application of pressure. Both plantar warts and corns have a soft, pulpy core surrounded by a thick callous ring; plantar warts and calluses are flush with the skin surface.*

Anal warts require anoscopy or sigmoidoscopy to rule out internal involvement, which may necessitate surgery. Women with vulvar lesions require examination of

REMOVING WARTS BY ELECTROSURGERY

1. Injection of 1% to 2% lidocaine under and around the wart, avoiding the wart itself.

2. Electrodesiccation of the wart.

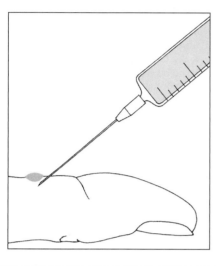

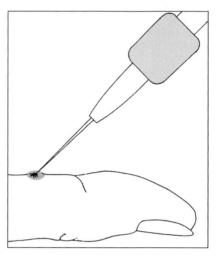

the vagina and cervix, including a Papanicolaou smear.

Treatment

Treatment for warts varies according to the location, size, number, pain level (present and projected), history of therapy, the patient's age, and compliance with treatment. Most persons eventually develop an immune response that causes warts to disappear spontaneously and require no treatment.

Treatment may include:

■ Electrodesiccation and curettage: High-frequency electric current destroys the wart and is followed by surgical removal of dead tissue at the base and application of an antibiotic ointment (such as polysporin), covered with a bandage, for 48 hours. This method is effective for common, filiform and, occasionally, plantar warts. (See *Removing warts by electrosurgery*.)

■ Cryotherapy: Liquid nitrogen kills the wart; the resulting dried blister is peeled off several days later. If initial treatment isn't

successful, it can be repeated at 2- to 4-week intervals. This method is useful either for periungual warts or for common warts on the face, extremities, penis, vagina, or anus.

■ Acid therapy (primary or adjunctive): The patient applies plaster patches impregnated with acid (such as 40% salicylic acid plasters) or acid drops (such as 5% to 16.7% salicylic acid in flexible collodion or trichloroacetic or dichloroacetic acids), every 12 to 24 hours for 2 to 4 weeks. This method isn't recommended for areas where perspiration is heavy, for those parts that are likely to get wet, or for exposed body parts where patches are cosmetically undesirable.

■ 25% podophyllin in compound with tincture of benzoin (for venereal warts): The podophyllin solution is applied on moist warts. The patient must lie still while it dries, leave it on for 4 hours, and then wash it off with soap and water. Treatment may be repeated every 3 to 4 days and, in some cases, must be left on a maximum of

3. Removal of the wart tissue with a curette and small, curved scissors.

4. Light desiccation of the area to control bleeding and prevent recurrence.

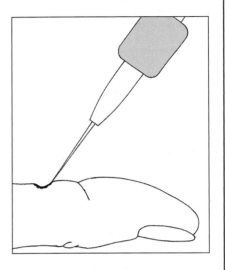

24 hours, depending on the patient's tolerance. Avoid using this drug on pregnant patients.

During acid or podophyllin therapy, the patient should protect the surrounding area with petroleum jelly or sodium bicarbonate (baking soda). A small amount of 25% to 50% trichloroacetic acid (for venereal warts) is applied to the wart. After the wart turns white, the acid is neutralized with baking soda or water.

■ Carbon dioxide laser therapy: This treatment has successfully treated genital warts.

The use of antiviral drugs is under investigation; suggestion and hypnosis are occasionally successful, especially with children. Patients can apply topical imiquimod cream to sites that aren't thickly keratinized. It's applied at bedtime three times per week. Imiquimod can be used alternately with a topical retinoid such as tazarotene, which may increase effectiveness.

Occlusion may be beneficial to persistent warts.

Special considerations
■ Conscientious adherence to prescribed therapy is essential. The patient's sexual partner may also require treatment. Encourage the patient to seek counseling if applicable.

Psoriasis

Psoriasis is a chronic, recurrent disease marked by epidermal proliferation. Its lesions, which appear as erythematous papules and plaques covered with silvery scales, vary widely in severity and distribution. Psoriasis is characterized by recurring partial remissions and exacerbations. Flare-ups are usually related to specific systemic and environmental factors but may be unpredictable; they can usually be controlled with therapy.

Causes and incidence
The tendency to develop psoriasis is genetically determined. Researchers have discov-

ered a significantly higher-than-normal incidence of certain human leukocyte antigens (HLAs) in families with psoriasis, suggesting a possible immune disorder. Onset of the disease is also influenced by environmental factors. Trauma can trigger the isomorphic effect or Koebner's phenomenon, in which lesions develop at sites of injury. Infections, especially those resulting from beta-hemolytic streptococci, may cause a flare of guttate (drop-shaped) lesions. Other contributing factors include pregnancy, endocrine changes, climate (cold weather tends to exacerbate psoriasis), and emotional stress.

Generally, a skin cell takes 14 days to move from the basal layer to the stratum corneum, where, after 14 days of normal wear and tear, it's sloughed off. The life cycle of a normal skin cell is 28 days, compared with only 4 days for a psoriatic skin cell. This markedly shortened cycle doesn't allow time for the cell to mature. Consequently, the stratum corneum becomes thick and flaky, producing the cardinal manifestations of psoriasis.

Psoriasis affects approximately 2% of the population in the United States, and incidence is higher in whites than other races. Although this disorder is most common in young adults, it may strike at any age, including infancy.

Signs and symptoms

The most common complaint of the patient with psoriasis is itching and, occasionally, pain from dry, cracked, encrusted lesions. Psoriatic lesions are erythematous and usually form well-defined plaques, sometimes covering large areas of the body. (See *Psoriatic plaques*.) Such lesions most commonly appear on the scalp, chest, elbows, knees, shins, back, and buttocks. The plaques consist of characteristic silver scales that either flake off easily or can thicken, covering the lesion. Removal of psoriatic scales frequently produces fine bleeding points (Auspitz sign). Occasionally, small guttate lesions appear, either alone or with plaques; these lesions are typically thin and erythematous, with few scales. Widespread shedding of scales is common in exfoliative or erythrodermic psoriasis and may also develop in chronic psoriasis.

Rarely, psoriasis becomes pustular, taking one of two forms. In localized pustular (Barber's) psoriasis, pustules appear on the palms and soles and remain sterile until opened. In generalized pustular (*von Zumbusch's*) psoriasis, which often occurs with fever, leukocytosis, and malaise, groups of pustules coalesce to form lakes of pus on red skin. These pustules also remain sterile until opened and commonly involve the tongue and oral mucosa.

In about 30% of patients, psoriasis spreads to the fingernails, producing small indentations and yellow or brown discoloration. In severe cases, the accumulation of thick, crumbly debris under the nail, causes it to separate from the nail bed.

Some patients with psoriasis develop arthritic symptoms (psoriatic arthritis), usually in one or more joints of the fingers or toes, or sometimes in the sacroiliac joints, which may progress to spondylitis. Such patients may complain of morning stiffness. Joint symptoms show no consistent linkage to the course of the cutaneous manifestations of psoriasis; they demonstrate remissions and exacerbations similar to those of rheumatoid arthritis.

Diagnosis

Diagnosis depends on patient history, appearance of the lesions and, if needed, the results of skin biopsy. Typically, serum uric acid level is elevated as a result of accelerated nucleic acid degradation, but indications of gout are absent. HLA-Cw6, B-13, and B-w57 may be present in early-onset psoriasis. Sudden onset of psoriasis may be associated with human immunodeficiency virus.

Treatment

Treatment depends on the type of psoriasis, the extent of the disease and the patient's response to it, and what effect the disease has on the patient's lifestyle. No permanent cure exists, and all methods of treatment are merely palliative. Ideally, all patients should see a dermatologist at least once.

Removal of psoriatic scales necessitates application of occlusive ointment bases, such as petroleum jelly, salicylic acid preparations, or preparations containing urea. Baker P & S liquid (phenol, sodium chloride, and liquid paraffin), applied to the scalp at bedtime, or liquid carbonis detergens in Nivea oil applied for 6 to 8 hours, is also effective. Shampoo or tar-based preparations are also used. These medications soften the scales, which can then be removed by scrubbing them carefully with a soft brush while bathing. Some preparations, such as tar-based preparations, can be used in whirlpools for extensively involved areas.

Methods to retard rapid cell production include exposure to ultraviolet light (UVB or natural sunlight) to the point of minimal erythema. Tar preparations or crude coal tar itself may be applied to affected areas about 15 minutes before exposure or may be left on overnight and wiped off the next morning. A thin layer of petroleum jelly may be applied before UVB exposure (the most common treatment for generalized psoriasis). Exposure time can increase gradually. Outpatient or day treatment with UVB prevents long hospitalizations and prolongs remission.

Steroid creams and ointments are useful to control psoriasis. A potent fluorinated steroid works well, except on the face and intertriginous areas. These creams require application twice daily, preferably after bathing to facilitate absorption, and overnight use of occlusive dressings, such as plastic wrap, plastic gloves or booties, or a vinyl exercise suit (under direct medical or nursing supervision). Small, stubborn plaques may require intralesional steroid injections. Anthralin, combined with a paste mixture, may be used for well-defined plaques but must not be applied to unaffected areas because it causes injury and stains normal skin. Apply petroleum jelly around the affected skin before applying anthralin. Commonly used concurrently with steroids, anthralin is applied at night and steroids during the day.

In a patient with severe chronic psoriasis, the Goeckerman regimen — which combines tar baths and UVB treatments —

PSORIATIC PLAQUES

In this patient with psoriasis, plaques consisting of silver scales cover a large area of the face.

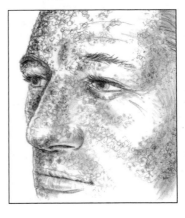

may help achieve the longest remission and clear the skin in 3 to 5 weeks. The Ingram technique is a variation of this treatment, using anthralin instead of tar. A therapy called PUVA combines administration of psoralens with exposure to high-intensity UVA. As a last resort, a cytotoxin, usually methotrexate or cyclosporine, an immunosuppressant, may help severe, refractory psoriasis.

Etretinate, a retinoid compound, is effective in treating extensive cases of psoriasis. However, because this drug is a strong teratogen, it's unsafe for use in women of childbearing age. It also has numerous adverse effects that many patients find intolerable. Tacarotene, a newer topical retinoid, combined with a medium-strength topical corticosteroid is also effective.

Low-dose antihistamines, oatmeal baths, emollients, and open wet dressings may help relieve pruritus. Aspirin and local heat help alleviate the pain of psoriatic arthritis; severe cases may require nonsteroidal anti-inflammatory drugs.

Therapy for psoriasis of the scalp consists of a tar shampoo followed by application of a steroid lotion; ketoconazole and anthralin may also be effective. No effective treatment exists for psoriasis of the nails.

Special considerations

Design your patient's care plan to include patient teaching and careful monitoring for adverse effects of therapy.

■ Make sure the patient understands his prescribed therapy; provide written instructions to avoid confusion. Teach correct application of prescribed ointments, creams, and lotions. A steroid cream, for example, should be applied in a thin film and rubbed gently into the skin until the cream disappears. All topical medications, especially those containing anthralin and tar, should be applied with a downward motion to avoid rubbing them into the follicles. Gloves must be worn because anthralin stains and injures the skin. After application, the patient may dust himself with powder to prevent anthralin from rubbing off on his clothes. Warn the patient never to put an occlusive dressing over anthralin. Suggest use of mineral oil, then soap and water, to remove anthralin. Caution the patient to avoid scrubbing his skin vigorously, to prevent Koebner's phenomenon. If a medication has been applied to the scales to soften them, suggest the patient use a soft brush to remove them.

■ Watch for adverse effects, especially allergic reactions to anthralin, atrophy and acne from steroids, and burning, itching, nausea, and squamous cell epitheliomas from PUVA. Initially, evaluate the patient on methotrexate weekly, then monthly for red blood cell, white blood cell, and platelet counts because cytotoxins may cause hepatic or bone marrow toxicity. Liver biopsy may be done to assess the effects of methotrexate.

■ Caution the patient receiving PUVA therapy to stay out of the sun on the day of treatment, and to protect his eyes with sunglasses that screen UVA for 24 hours after treatment. Tell him to wear goggles during exposure to this light.

■ Be aware that psoriasis can cause psychological problems. Assure the patient that psoriasis isn't contagious and, although exacerbations and remissions occur, they're controllable with treatment.

However, be sure he understands there's no cure. Also, because stressful situations tend to exacerbate psoriasis, help the patient learn to cope with these situations. Explain the relationship between psoriasis and arthritis, but point out that psoriasis causes no other systemic disturbances. Refer all patients to the National Psoriasis Foundation, which provides information and directs patients to local chapters.

Lichen planus

A benign but pruritic skin eruption, lichen planus is a relatively rare disorder that usually produces scaling, purple papules marked by white lines or spots. The features of these lesions are called the "4 Ps" — purple, polygonal, pruritic, and papule.

In most patients, lichen planus resolves spontaneously in 6 to 18 months. In a few, chronic lichen planus may persist for several years.

Causes and incidence

The cause of lichen planus is unknown. Eruptions similar to lichen planus have been induced by arsenic, bismuth, gold, quinidine, propranolol, and naproxen. Exposure to developers used in color photography may likewise cause an eruption that's indistinguishable from lichen planus.

Lichen planus is found in all geographic areas, with equal distribution among races. Eruptions of lesions with features characteristic of lichen planus occur most often in middle-age people and are uncommon in young and elderly people.

Signs and symptoms

Lichen planus may develop suddenly or insidiously. Initial lesions commonly appear on the arms or legs (generally on the wrist and medial sides of the thighs) and evolve into the generalized eruption of flat, glistening, purple papules marked with white lines or spots (Wickham's striae). These lesions may be linear from scratching or may coalesce into plaques. Lesions often affect the mucous membranes (especially the buccal mucosa), male genitalia and, less often, the nails. These lesions are painful, especially when ulcers develop. Mild to severe pruritus is common.

Diagnosis

 CONFIRMING DIAGNOSIS *Although characteristic skin lesions usually establish the diagnosis of lichen planus, confirmation may require a skin biopsy.*

Treatment

Treatment is essentially symptomatic. The goal of therapy is to relieve itching with topical fluorinated steroids and occlusive dressings, intralesional injections of steroids, oatmeal baths, and antihistamines. Erosive oral lesions should be treated with triamcinolone acetonide in Orabase twice daily. Generalized severely pruritic skin lesions may be treated with systemic corticosteroids. An initial dosage of oral prednisone may be prescribed; thereafter, the dosage is decreased by approximately one-third each week. If the patient experiences a recurrence of itching after the drug is discontinued, he'll be given a low dose every other morning. If a drug is suspected as the cause, it should be discontinued.

Special considerations

■ Administer medications as ordered, and inform the patient of possible adverse effects, especially drowsiness produced by antihistamines.
■ Provide emotional support and reassure the patient that lichen planus, although annoying, is usually a benign, self-limiting condition, although lesions may persist for months or years.

Corns and calluses

Usually located on areas of repeated trauma (especially the feet), corns and calluses are acquired skin conditions marked by hyperkeratosis of the stratum corneum. The prognosis is good with proper foot care.

Causes and incidence

A corn (also known as a *clavus*) is a hyperkeratotic area that usually results from external pressure, such as that from ill-fitting shoes or, less commonly, from internal pressure, such as that caused by a protruding underlying bone (due to arthritis for example). A callus is an area of thickened skin, generally found on the foot or hand, produced by external pressure or friction. Persons whose activities produce repeated trauma (for example, manual laborers or guitarists) commonly develop calluses.

The severity of a corn or callus depends on the degree and duration of trauma.

Signs and symptoms

Both corns and calluses cause pain through pressure placed on underlying tissue by localized thickened skin. Corns contain a central keratinous core, are smaller and more clearly defined than calluses, and are usually more painful. The pain they cause may be dull and constant or sharp when pressure is applied. "Soft" corns are caused by the pressure of a bony prominence. They appear as whitish thickenings and are commonly found between the toes, most often in the fourth interdigital web. "Hard" corns are sharply delineated and conical, and appear most frequently over the dorsolateral aspect of the fifth toe.

Calluses have indefinite borders and may be quite large. They usually produce dull pain on pressure, rather than constant pain. Although calluses commonly appear over plantar warts, they're distinguished from these warts by normal skin markings.

Diagnosis

Diagnosis depends on careful physical examination of the affected area and on patient history revealing chronic trauma.

Treatment

Surgical debridement may be performed to remove the nucleus of a corn, usually under a local anesthetic. In intermittent debridement, keratolytics — usually 40% salicylic acid plasters — are applied to affected areas. Injections of corticosteroids beneath the corn may be necessary to relieve pain. However, the simplest and best treatment

(See *Aids for relieving painful pressure.*)

AIDS FOR RELIEVING PAINFUL PRESSURE

Both metatarsal and corn pads can help relieve painful pressure. Commercial products available include, from left to right, foam toe cap, foam toe sleeve, soft corn shield, and hard corn (fifth toe) shield.

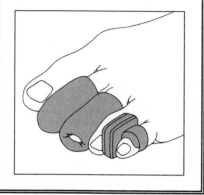

---

is essentially preventive — avoidance of trauma. Corns and calluses disappear after the source of trauma has been removed. Metatarsal pads may redistribute the weight-bearing areas of the foot; corn pads may prevent painful pressure. (See *Aids for relieving painful pressure.*)

Patients with persistent corns or calluses require referral to a podiatrist or dermatologist; those with corns or calluses caused by a bony malformation, as in arthritis, require orthopedic consultation.

Special considerations

■ Teach the patient how to apply salicylic acid plasters. Make sure the plaster is large enough to cover the affected area. Place the sticky side down on the foot, then cover the plaster with adhesive tape. Plasters are usually taken off after an overnight application but may be left in place for as long as 7 days. After removing the plaster, the patient should soak the area in water and abrade the soft, macerated skin with a towel or pumice stone. He should then reapply the plaster and repeat the entire procedure un-

til he has removed all the hyperkeratotic skin. Warn the patient against removing corns or calluses with a sharp instrument such as a razor blade.

■ Advise the patient to wear properly fitted shoes. Suggest the use of metatarsal or corn pads to relieve pressure. Refer to a podiatrist, dermatologist, or orthopedist, if necessary.

■ Assure the patient that good foot care can correct this condition.

Pityriasis rosea

An acute, self-limiting, inflammatory skin disease, pityriasis rosea usually produces a "herald" patch — which usually goes undetected — followed by a generalized eruption of papulosquamous lesions.

Causes and incidence

The cause of pityriasis rosea is unknown, but the brief course of the disease and the virtual absence of recurrence suggest a viral agent (herpes virus 7 is suspected) or an autoimmune disorder.

Although this noncontagious disorder may develop at any age, it's most apt to occur in adolescents and young adults. Incidence rises in the spring and fall.

Signs and symptoms

Pityriasis typically begins with an erythematous "herald" patch, which may appear anywhere on the body, although it occurs most commonly on the trunk. Although this slightly raised, oval lesion is about 2 to 6 cm in diameter, approximately 25% of patients don't notice it. A few days to several weeks later, yellow-tan or erythematous patches with scaly edges (about 0.5 to 1 cm in diameter) erupt on the trunk and extremities — and, rarely, on the face, hands, and feet in adolescents. Eruption continues for 7 to 10 days, and the patches persist for 2 to 6 weeks. Occasionally, these patches are macular, vesicular, or urticarial. A characteristic of this disease is the arrangement of lesions, which produces a pattern similar to that of a pine tree. Accompanying pruritus, if present, is usually mild but may be severe.

Diagnosis

Characteristic skin lesions support the diagnosis. Differential diagnosis must also rule out secondary syphilis (through serologic testing), dermatophytosis, and drug reaction.

Treatment

Treatment focuses on relief of pruritus, with emollients, oatmeal baths, antihistamines, topical steroids, and occasionally exposure to ultraviolet light or sunlight. Rarely, if inflammation is severe, systemic corticosteroids may be required.

Special considerations

■ Reassure the patient that pityriasis rosea isn't contagious, spontaneous remission usually occurs in 4 to 12 weeks, and lesions generally don't recur.

■ Urge the patient not to scratch. Advise him to avoid hot baths because they may intensify itching. Encourage the use of antipruritics.

Hyperhidrosis

Hyperhidrosis is the excessive secretion of sweat from the eccrine glands. It usually occurs in the axillae (typically after puberty) and on the palms and soles (often starting during infancy or childhood). Abnormal and excessive heat loss can occur, causing most patients to have body temperatures less than 98.6° F (37° C).

Causes and incidence

Genetic factors may contribute to the development of hyperhidrosis and, in susceptible individuals, emotional stress appears to be the most prominent cause, although most patients aren't anxious. Increased central nervous system (CNS) impulses may provoke excessive release of acetylcholine, producing a heightened sweat response. Exercise and a hot climate can cause profuse sweating in these patients. Certain drugs (such as antipyretics, emetics, meperidine, and anticholinesterases) and certain foods (such as tomato sauce, chocolate, coffee, and spicy foods) have been known to increase sweating.

In addition, hyperhidrosis commonly occurs as a clinical manifestation of an underlying disorder. Infections and chronic diseases, such as tuberculosis, malaria, or lymphoma, may cause excessive nighttime sweating. A person with diabetes commonly demonstrates hyperhidrosis during a hypoglycemic crisis. Other predisposing conditions include hyperthyroidism, pheochromocytomas; cardiovascular disorders, such as shock or heart failure; CNS disturbances (generally lesions of the hypothalamus); withdrawal from drugs or alcohol; menopause; and Graves' disease.

Hyperhidrosis occurs in up to 1% of the U.S. population.

Signs and symptoms

Axillary hyperhidrosis frequently produces such extreme sweating that patients often ruin their clothes in 1 day and develop contact dermatitis from clothing dyes; similarly, hyperhidrosis of the soles can easily damage a pair of shoes. Profuse sweating from both the soles and palms hinders the patient's ability to work and interact socially. Patients with this condition often report increased emotional strain.

Diagnosis

 CONFIRMING DIAGNOSIS
Clinical observations and patient history confirm hyperhidrosis.

Treatment

The treatment of choice is application of 20% aluminum chloride in absolute ethanol. (Most antiperspirants contain a 5% solution.) Formaldehyde may also be used but may lead to allergic contact sensitization. Glutaraldehyde produces less contact sensitivity than formaldehyde but stains the skin; it's used more often on the feet than on the hands, as a soak or applied directly several times a week and then weekly as needed.

Iontophoresis (low-level electric current applied locally to skin surfaces) reduces sweat secretion at the site. Repeated treatments will be necessary for sustained relief.

Therapy sometimes includes anticholinergics, except in patients with glaucoma or prostatic hypertrophy. Severe hyperhidrosis

PRESSURE POINTS: COMMON SITES OF PRESSURE ULCERS

Pressure ulcers may develop in any of these 16 pressure points. To prevent sores, reposition the patient frequently, and carefully check for any change in the patient's skin tone.

Shoulder blade

Ischial tuberosity

Sacrum

Posterior knee

Foot

Sacrum

Heel

---

unresponsive to conservative therapy may require local axillary removal of sweat glands or, as a last resort, a cervicothoracic or lumbar sympathectomy.

Special considerations

■ Provide support and reassurance because hyperhidrosis may be socially embarrassing.

■ Tell the patient to apply aluminum chloride in absolute ethanol nightly to dry axillae, soles, or palms. The area should be covered with plastic wrap for 6 to 8 hours, preferably overnight, then washed with soap and water. Tell him to repeat this procedure for several nights, until profuse daytime sweating subsides. Frequency of treatments can then be reduced.

■ Advise the patient with hyperhidrosis of the soles to wear leather sandals and white or colorfast cotton socks.

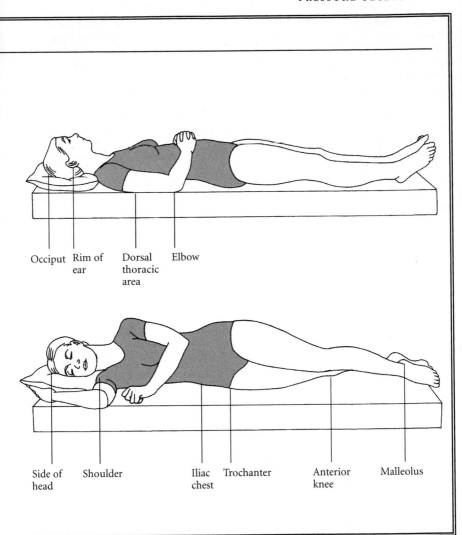

| Occiput | Rim of ear | Dorsal thoracic area | Elbow |

| Side of head | Shoulder | Iliac chest | Trochanter | Anterior knee | Malleolus |

Pressure ulcers

Pressure ulcers, commonly called *pressure sores* or *bedsores,* are localized areas of cellular necrosis that occur most often in the skin and subcutaneous tissue over bony prominences. These ulcers may be superficial, caused by local skin irritation with subsequent surface maceration, or deep, originating in underlying tissue. Deep lesions typically go undetected until they penetrate the skin; but, by then, they've usually caused subcutaneous damage.

Causes and incidence

Most pressure ulcers are caused by pressure, particularly over bony prominences, that interrupts normal circulatory function, leading to ischemia of the underlying structures of skin, fat, and muscles. (See *Pressure points: Common sites of pressure ulcers.*) The intensity and duration of such pressure govern the severity of the ulcer;

pressure exerted over an area for a moderate period (1 to 2 hours) produces tissue ischemia and increased capillary pressure, leading to edema and multiple small-vessel thromboses. An inflammatory reaction gives way to ulceration and necrosis of ischemic cells. In turn, necrotic tissue predisposes to bacterial invasion and subsequent infection.

The patient's position determines the pressure exerted on the tissues. For example, if the head of the bed is elevated, or the patient assumes a slumped position, gravity pulls his weight downward and forward. This shearing force causes deep ulcers due to ischemic changes in the muscles and subcutaneous tissues, and occurs most often over the sacrum and ischial tuberosities.

Predisposing conditions for pressure ulcers include altered mobility, inadequate nutrition (leading to weight loss, subsequent reduction of subcutaneous tissue and muscle bulk and, possibly, a poorly functioning immune system), and a breakdown in skin or subcutaneous tissue (as a result of edema, incontinence, fever, pathologic conditions, or obesity).

Pressure ulcers occur in 10% to 17% of all hospitalized patients and 20% to 40% of all nursing home patients. Patients living at home aren't free from risk, either: 20% of all pressure ulcers occur in the home. In the United States, there are approximately 2 million new cases of pressure ulcers diagnosed every year.

Signs and symptoms

Pressure ulcers commonly develop over bony prominences. Early features of superficial lesions are shiny, erythematous changes over the compressed area, caused by localized vasodilation when pressure is relieved. Superficial erythema progresses to small blisters or erosions and, ultimately, to necrosis and ulceration.

An inflamed area on the skin's surface may be the first sign of underlying damage when pressure is exerted between deep tissue and bone. Bacteria in a compressed site cause inflammation and, eventually, infection, which leads to further necrosis. A foul-smelling, purulent discharge may seep from a lesion that penetrates the skin from beneath. Infected, necrotic tissue prevents healthy granulation of scar tissue; a black eschar may develop around and over the lesion.

Diagnosis

Pressure ulcers are obvious on physical examination. Wound culture and sensitivity testing of the exudate in the ulcer identify infecting organisms and antibiotics that may be needed. If severe hypoproteinemia is suspected, total serum protein values and serum albumin studies may be appropriate.

Treatment

Successful treatment must relieve pressure on the affected area, keep the area clean and dry, and promote healing. (See *Special aids for preventing and treating pressure ulcers.*)

Special considerations

- During each shift, check the skin of bedridden patients for possible changes in color, turgor, temperature, and sensation. Examine an existing ulcer for any change in size or degree of damage. When using pressure relief aids or topical agents, explain their function to the patient.
- Prevent pressure ulcers by repositioning the bedridden patient at least every 2 hours around the clock. To minimize the effects of a shearing force, use a footboard and raise the head of the bed to an angle not exceeding 60 degrees. Also, use a draw or pull sheet to turn the patient or to pull him up. Keep the patient's knees slightly flexed for short periods. Perform passive range-of-motion exercises, or encourage the patient to do active exercises if possible.
- To prevent pressure ulcers in immobilized patients, use pressure relief aids on their beds.
- Provide meticulous skin care. Keep the skin clean and dry without the use of harsh soaps. Gently massaging the skin around the affected area — not on it — promotes healing. Thoroughly rub moisturizing lotions into the skin to prevent maceration of the skin surface. Change bed linens frequently for patients who are diaphoretic or

SPECIAL AIDS FOR PREVENTING AND TREATING PRESSURE ULCERS

Pressure relief aids

- *Gel flotation pads* disperse pressure over a greater skin surface area; convenient and adaptable for home and wheelchair use.
- *Alternating pressure mattress* contains tubelike sections, running lengthwise, that deflate and reinflate, changing areas of pressure. Use mattress with a single untucked sheet because layers of linen decrease its effectiveness.
- *Convoluted foam mattress* minimizes area of skin pressure with its alternating areas of depression and elevation: soft, elevated foam areas cushion skin; depressed areas relieve pressure. This mattress should be used with a single, loosely tucked sheet and is adaptable for home and wheelchair use. If the patient is incontinent, cover the mattress with the provided plastic sleeve.
- *Spanco mattress* has polyester fibers with silicon tubes to decrease pressure without limiting the patient's position. It has no weight limitation.
- *Sheepskin* is soft, dry, absorbent, and easy to clean. It should be in direct contact with the patient's skin. It's available in sizes to fit elbows and heels and is adaptable for home use.
- *Air-fluidized bed* supports the patient at a subcapillary pressure point and provides a warm, relaxing, therapeutic airflow. The bed is filled with beads that move when the air flows. It eliminates friction and maceration.
- *Low air-loss beds,* such as Flexicare and Accucare, slow the drying of any saline

soaks, and elderly patients often experience less disorientation than with high air-loss beds. The head of the bed can be elevated so there's less chance of aspiration, especially in patients who require tube feeding. Patients can get out of bed more easily and can be moved more easily on low air-loss surfaces.

Topical care

- Gentle soap
- Hydrogel dressings (Biolex wound gel, FlexiGel)
- Zinc oxide cream
- Absorbable gelatin sponge
- Collagen dressings (Kollagen-Medfil Pads)
- Composite dressings (Alldress, Stratasorb)
- Wound filter dressings (Catrix 10 ointment, IODOSORB gel)
- Topical antibiotics (*only* when infection is confirmed by culture and sensitivity tests)
- Silver sulfadiazine cream (antimicrobial agent) for necrotic areas
- Water vapor–permeable dressings
- Transparent film dressings

Skin-damaging agents to avoid

- Harsh alkaline soaps
- Alcohol-based products (can cause vasoconstriction)
- Tincture of benzoin (may cause painful erosions)
- Hexachlorophene (may irritate the central nervous system)
- Petroleum gauze

---

incontinent. Use a fecal incontinence bag for incontinent patients.

- Clean open lesions with a 3% solution of hydrogen peroxide or normal saline solution. Dressings, if needed, should be porous and lightly taped to healthy skin. Debridement of necrotic tissue may be

necessary to allow healing. One method is to apply open wet dressings and allow them to dry on the ulcer. Removal of the dressings mechanically débrides exudate and necrotic tissue. Other methods include surgical debridement with a fine scalpel blade and chemical debridement using proteolytic enzyme agents.

■ Encourage adequate intake of food and fluids to maintain body weight and promote healing. Consult with the dietary department to provide a diet that promotes granulation of new tissue. Encourage the debilitated patient to eat frequent, small meals that include protein- and calorie-rich supplements. Assist weakened patients with their meals.

Selected references

Barnhill, R.L. *Textbook of Dermatopathology,* 2nd ed. New York: McGraw Hill Book Co., 2004.

Burns, T., et al., eds. *Rook's Textbook of Dermatology,* 7th ed. Cambridge, Mass.: Blackwell Publishers, 2004.

Goodheart, H.P. *Goodheart's Photoguide of Common Skin Disorders: Diagnosis and Management,* 2nd ed. Philadelphia: Lippincott Williams & Wilkins, 2003.

Lee, B. *Manual of Wound Management and Healing.* New York: McGraw Hill Book Co., 2005.

Murphy, G.F., et al. *Lever's Histopathology of the Skin,* 9th ed. Philadelphia: Lippincott Williams & Wilkins, 2005.

Rakel, R.E., and Bope, E.T., eds. *Conn's Current Therapy 2004.* Philadelphia: W.B. Saunders Co., 2004.

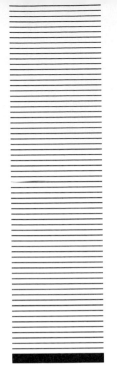

Appendices
Acknowledgments
Index

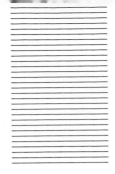

Cultural considerations in patient care

As a health care professional, you'll typically interact with a diverse, multicultural patient population regardless of the particular setting in which you work. Each culture has its own unique set of beliefs about health and illness, dietary practices, and other matters that you should take into consideration when providing care.

This appendix summarizes the beliefs and customs of six common cultures in the United States, including African Americans, Arab Americans, Chinese Americans, Iranian Americans, Japanese Americans, and Mexican Americans. Understanding these cultures will help you provide appropriate interventions without compromising your patients' cultural integrity.

Cultural group	Health and illness philosophy	Dietary practices	Other considerations
African Americans	■ May believe illness is related to supernatural causes, such as punishment from God or an evil spell ■ May believe illness is related to one of three areas: environmental hazards, divine punishment, and impaired social relationships ■ Believe health is a feeling of well-being ■ May seek advice and remedies from faith or folk healers	■ May have food restrictions based on religious beliefs, such as not eating pork if Muslim ■ May view cooked greens as good for health	■ Tend to be affectionate, as shown by touching and hugging friends and loved ones ■ If Muslim, may need to have head covered at all times ■ Respect elders, especially for their wisdom ■ Primary religions: Baptist, other Protestant denominations, Muslim

Cultural group	Health and illness philosophy	Dietary practices	Other considerations
Arab Americans	■ Believe health is a gift from God and that one should care for self by eating right and minimizing stressors ■ May believe illness is caused by the evil eye, bad luck, stress, or an imbalance between hot and cold or moist and dry ■ May believe whatever happens in life is destiny or God's will ■ If Muslim, after death, family may request body turned to face the holy city of Mecca ■ May assume passive role as patient ■ May use amulets to ward off evil eye during illness ■ Believe in complete rest and relieving self of all responsibilities during an illness ■ Tend to express pain vocally; may have low pain threshold	■ Don't mix milk and fish, sweet and sour, or hot and cold ■ Don't use ice in drinks; believe hot soup can help recovery ■ If Muslim, prohibited from drinking alcohol and eating pork ■ Favor coffee, bread, and fresh food cooked with spices	■ Respect elders and professionals ■ Traditional women may avoid eye contact with male strangers. ■ Use same-sex family members as interpreters ■ Burial, not cremation, preferred ■ Primary religions: Muslim, Christian (Greek Orthodox, Protestant)
Chinese Americans	■ Believe health is a balance of Yin and Yang and that illness stems from an imbalance of these elements; believe good health requires harmony between body, mind, and spirit ■ May use herbalists or acupuncturists before seeking medical help; ginseng root is a common home remedy ■ May use good luck objects, such as jade or rope tied around waist ■ Family expected to take care of patient, who assumes a passive role ■ Tend not to readily express pain; stoic by nature ■ May believe suffering before death atones for past sins and that suffering may occur in an afterlife if it didn't occur while alive	■ Staples are rice, noodles, and vegetables; tend to use chopsticks ■ Choose foods to help balance the Yin (cold) and Yang (hot) ■ Drink hot liquids, especially when sick ■ Lactose intolerance common	■ Health care providers should keep a comfortable distance when approaching patient ■ Elders shouldn't be addressed by first name (a sign of disrespect) ■ Lack of eye contact may be a sign of respect ■ Tend to be very modest; best to use same-sex clinicians ■ Primary religions: Buddhist, Catholic, Protestant
Iranian Americans	■ Believe illness stems from an imbalance of hot and cold foods; proper food combinations important in daily life ■ May use home or humoral cures before seeing a physician ■ Show great respect for health care providers ■ May seek alternative therapies and advice ■ Pain expressed with grimaces and moans	■ Choose foods based on humoral theory of balancing hot and cold ■ Prefer dairy products, rice, and wheat breads ■ May avoid pork and alcohol	■ Elders should be greeted first as sign of respect ■ Concept of shame may prevent full disclosure of an illness ■ Tend to be modest and reserved; best to use same-sex clinicians ■ Primary religion: Shiite Muslim

Cultural group	Health and illness philosophy	Dietary practices	Other considerations
Japanese Americans	■ Believe that health is a balance of oneself, society, and the universe ■ May believe illness is karma, resulting from behavior in present or past life ■ May believe certain food combinations cause illness ■ May use prayer beads if Buddhist ■ May use tea to treat stomach ailments and constipation ■ May not complain of symptoms until severe	■ Eat rice with most meals; may use chopsticks ■ Diet high in salt; low in sugar, fat, animal protein, and cholesterol ■ Favor tofu, fish, soy sauce, and green tea ■ Lactose intolerance common	■ Usually quiet and polite; may ask few questions about care, deferring to health care providers ■ Family is vital ■ Elderly may nod but not necessarily understand ■ Very modest; tend to avoid touching; best to use same-sex clinicians ■ Primary religions: Buddhist, Shinto, Christian
Mexican Americans	■ Believe that health is influenced by environment, fate, and God's will ■ May believe in Galen's theory that the four humors in the body — blood, phlegm, yellow bile, and black bile — must be kept in balance ■ May use herbal teas and soup to aid in recuperation ■ May self-medicate because prescription drug sales aren't controlled in Mexico ■ May express pain by nonverbal cues ■ Family may want to keep seriousness of illness from patient ■ May believe healing is a state of equilibrium in the universe where the forces of "hot," "cold," "wet," and "dry" must be balanced ■ May believe in *mal ojo*, the evil eye, which is believed to occur when a person with special powers voluntarily or involuntarily injures a child by looking at and admiring him while not also touching him	■ Beans and tortillas are staples ■ Eat lots of fresh fruits and vegetables	■ Women are especially modest ■ Use same-sex family members as interpreters ■ May be bilingual ■ Value physical presence; important to embrace, touch, and see relations face to face; togetherness important ■ Primary religion: Roman Catholic

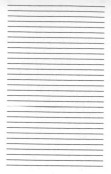

Rare diseases

Disease	Description
Addison-Schilder disease: adrenoleukodystrophy	Adrenal atrophy and diffuse degeneration of the brain in infancy or adolescence; characterized by loss of myelin and progressive loss of cerebral function, leading to spasticity, optic neuritis, blindness, and dementia
African trypanosomiasis: sleeping sickness	Febrile illness followed months or years later by progressive neurologic impairment and death; the Gambian form, found in west and central Africa, causes daytime drowsiness and nighttime insomnia and progresses to coma; the Rhodesian form, found in east Africa, is more virulent
Albers-Schönberg disease: osteopetrosis, marble bone disease	Rare heterogeneous bone disorder marked by disorganization of bone structure that causes dense sclerotic bones vulnerable to recurrent fractures; in severe cases, the bone marrow cavity may be obliterated; malignant variant begins in utero and progresses rapidly to cause marked anemia, hydrocephalus, cranial nerve involvement, hepatosplenomegaly, and fatal infection; benign variant causes milder anemia and fewer neurologic abnormalities
Alport's syndrome	Hereditary nephritis characterized by recurrent gross or microscopic hematuria; associated with deafness, albuminuria, and progressive azotemia
American trypanosomiasis: Chagas' disease	Febrile parasitic illness prevalent in Central and South America; cardiomyopathy may occur; megaesophagus and megacolon may develop many years later; can be severe in children
Arc-welders' disease: siderosis	Benign pneumoconiosis that can occur in iron ore miners, welders, metal grinders, and polishers from the inhalation and retention of iron
Armstrong's disease: lymphocytic choriomeningitis	Form of meningitis, usually occurring in adults ages 20 to 40 during fall and winter; usually asymptomatic or mild, although myocarditis and severe meningoencephalitis can occur; can spread to fetus with congenital infection, resulting in hydrocephalus
Ataxia telangiectasia: Louis-Bar's syndrome	Progressive, severe ataxia with telangiectasia of the face, earlobes, and conjunctivae; chronic recurrent sinopulmonary infections occur; ataxia usually occurs before age 2 but may not develop until as late as age 9; degree of immunodeficiency determines rate of deterioration

Cause	Treatment
Transmitted as X-linked recessive disorder	Symptomatic and supportive treatment; bone marrow transplant in boys; adrenal hormones; fatal in 1 to 10 years
Trypanosoma brucei rhodesiense and *T. brucei gambiense* transmitted by tsetse fly bite	Melarsoprol or pentamidine
Malignant variant transmitted as autosomal recessive trait, benign variant transmitted as autosomal dominant trait; increased bone mass secondary to defect in remodeling bone, resulting in thickened cortices; in the intermediate type, the disease is associated with renal tubular acidosis and cerebral calcification	Transfusion of nucleated marrow cells from a healthy, clinically normal donor (almost always a sibling); high doses of calcitriol have been used with some success in patients with lethal forms of the disease
Transmitted as X-linked autosomal trait	Supportive and symptomatic; antibiotic therapy for infection; antihypertensive therapy; protein-restricted diet; dialysis or renal transplant; avoidance of ototoxic drugs
Trypanosoma cruzi transmitted by insect; can also be transmitted through the transfusion of blood donated by a person who's infected	Nifurtimox or benznidazole in acute phase; supportive treatment in chronic phase
Inhalation and retention of iron after exposure to iron oxide fumes and dust	Supportive and symptomatic treatment; limiting or preventing exposure to iron dust or fumes with approved industrial respirators prevents progression of this disease
Infection caused by lymphocytic choriomeningitis virus (a member of the family *Arenaviridae*) that follows exposure to food or dust contaminated by an infected common house mouse	Supportive and symptomatic treatment; infection can be prevented by careful hand washing (although mode of transmission may be airborne); corticosteroids and ribavirin may be considered in some cases
Transmitted as autosomal recessive disorder; a genetic mutation found in the ATM gene	Supportive treatment with early, aggressive antibiotic therapy to prevent or control recurrent infections; immune globulin; fetal thymus transplant or histocompatible bone marrow transplant

Disease	Description
Barometer-maker's disease: chronic mercury poisoning	Soreness of gums, loosening of teeth, salivation, fetid breath, abdominal cramping and diarrhea, weakness, ataxia, intention tremors, irritability and depression, reproductive failures, birth defects (especially developmental neurologic damage), and death
Basal cell carcinoma of the eye	Common extraorbital cancer affecting the eyelid, conjunctivae, and cornea
Bauxite workers' disease: bauxite pneumoconiosis, Shaver's disease	Occupational disorder causing rapid and progressive pneumoconiosis and leading to empyema; may be accompanied by pneumothorax; puts patient at increased risk for blood and bladder cancers
Behr's disease: degeneration of the macula retinae	Familial spastic paraplegia with or without optic atrophy; hyperactive deep tendon reflexes and sensory disturbances in adolescents and adults
Berylliosis: Beryllium poisoning and beryllium disease	Systemic granulomatous disorder that's a form of pneumoconiosis with dominant pulmonary manifestations; two forms: acute nonspecific pneumonitis and chronic noncaseating granulomatous disease with interstitial fibrosis; death may result from respiratory failure and cor pulmonale
Blinding filarial disease: onchocerciasis, river blindness	Invasion of eye tissues by the filarial worm, which is enclosed in fibrous cysts or nodules; lesions also develop on the skin and, in severe infection, lead to chronic pruritus and disfiguring skin lesions
Bouillaud's syndrome: rheumatic endocarditis	Manifests as a heart murmur of either mitral or aortic insufficiency; pericarditis and heart failure are seen in severe cases
Breisky's disease: kraurosis vulvae	Vulval atrophy and dryness of skin and mucous membranes, causing shrinkage of the vaginal outlet; histopathologically identical to lichen sclerosis
Brill's disease: Brill-Zinsser disease, latent or recrudescent typhus	Relapse of typhus, which can occur years after the primary attack
Brown-Symmers disease	Acute serous encephalitis in children
Budd-Chiari syndrome	Hepatic vein obstruction that impairs blood flow out of the liver, producing massive ascites and hepatomegaly; may be acute or chronic

Cause	Treatment
Mercury poisoning resulting from chronic exposure to mercury or its vapors (possibly from batteries, thermometers, or dental amalgams) or to contaminated fish or fungicides used on seeds	Induce emesis or evacuate stomach, lavage with milk or sodium bicarbonate, and administer polythiol resins; penicillamine is the chelating agent of choice but dimercaprol is also effective; neurologic toxicity isn't considered reversible, although some practitioners recommend a trial dose of penicillamine
Unknown, but predisposing factors include exposure to sunlight, radiation, chemicals, and other carcinogens	Surgery; possibly radiation therapy
Inhalation of dust particles of alumina and silica (bauxite), the chief source of aluminum	Elimination of exposure to bauxite
Hereditary form of cerebellar ataxia	No confirmed treatment; vitamin B therapy is sometimes indicated
Inhalation or absorption of beryllium; severity depends on amount inhaled or absorbed	Beryllium ulcer requires excision or curettage; acute form requires prompt corticosteroid therapy, oxygen and, possibly, mechanical ventilation; chronic form is treated with corticosteroids
Onchocerca volvulus transmitted by the blackfly (*Simulium* and *Eusimulium*)	Microfilaricidal or macrofilaricidal agents, such as Ivermectin, Suramin, and diethylcarbamazine
Delayed sequel to pharyngeal infection by group B streptococci	Although no specific cure is available, a course of penicillin should still be given to eliminate group A streptococci; additionally, supportive therapy to reduce morbidity and mortality should be provided
Probable hypoestrogen	Surgery
Rickettsia prowazekii	Tetracycline, chloramphenicol, analgesics, antipyretics
Viral pathogens (rabies, measles, mumps, rubella, influenza)	Supportive care; control of intracranial pressure; correction of metabolic problems, disseminated intravascular coagulation, bleeding, renal failure, pulmonary emboli, and pneumonia; invariably fatal
Any condition or medication that obstructs blood flow from hepatic veins; acute form due to acute thrombosis of main hepatic vein or inferior vena cava; chronic due to fibrosis of intrahepatic veins	Surgery to shunt hepatic blood flow and remove obstruction; if congenital, transcardiac membranectomy or percutaneous stent placement for patients with inferior vena cava web; liver transplant may be recommended for patients with marked hepatocellular dysfunction

Disease	Description
Burkitt's tumor: Burkitt's lymphoma	Undifferentiated malignant lymphoma that usually begins as a large mass in the jaw (African Burkitt's) or as an abdominal mass (American Burkitt's)
Cat-scratch fever: cat-scratch disease	Subacute self-limiting disease characterized by a primary local lesion and regional lymphadenopathy; more common in children and young adults in contact with cats (90% of cases); disseminated form, bacillary angiomatosis, found in people who are immunocompromised, such as those infected with the human immunodeficiency virus
Central core disease: Shy-Magee syndrome	Rare muscle disease in which severe hypotonia causes weakness and arrests motor development in infancy; lack of oxidative enzymes in central core of each muscle fiber is diagnostic
Charcot-Marie-Tooth disease	Neuropathic (peroneal) muscular atrophy characterized by progressive weakness of the distal muscles of the arms and feet; most common form of the muscular dystrophies
Chédiak-Higashi syndrome	Characterized by morphological changes in granulocytes that impair the ability to respond to chemotaxis and to digest or kill invading organisms; associated with partial albinism
Chester's disease: cerebrotendinous xanthomatosis	Form of leukodystrophy indicated by excessive accumulation of lipids in the long bones; results in progressive cerebellar ataxia, dementia, mental retardation, spinal cord paresis, tendon xanthomas, and cataracts
Chiari-Frommel syndrome	Postpartum condition marked by uterine atrophy, persistent lactation, galactorrhea, prolonged amenorrhea, and low levels of urinary estrogen and gonadotropin
Choriocarcinoma	Rapidly metastasizing malignant tumor of placental tissue that typically causes profuse vaginal and intra-abdominal bleeding
Chromomycosis: chromoblastomycosis	Slowly spreading fungal infection of the skin and subcutaneous tissues; produces cauliflower-like lesions on the legs or arms and may spread to the brain, causing an abscess
Cockayne's syndrome	Hereditary syndrome consisting of dwarfism with retinal atrophy and deafness; associated with progeria, prognathism, mental retardation, photosensitivity, and accelerated atherosclerosis
Concato's disease	Progressive malignant polyserositis with large effusions into the pericardium, pleura, and peritoneum; associated with tuberculosis
Conradi-Hunermann syndrome: dysplasia epiphysealis punctata	Abnormal development of the secondary bone-forming center, marked by depressions or pinpoint structures

Cause	Treatment
Unknown, but Epstein-Barr virus suspected in some cases	Chemotherapy; radiation therapy; surgical resection in extensive local disease; in patients with a relapse, autologous bone marrow transplantation
Bartonella henoele; flea-borne transmission to kittens creates a feline reservoir for the disease	Symptomatic treatment; if patient is ill, can use ciprofloxacin, doxycycline, co-trimoxazole, erythromycin, cefoxitin, cefotaxime, mezlocillin, aminoglycosides, or antimycobacterials
Transmitted as autosomal dominant trait	Symptomatic and supportive treatment; genetic testing is available; recognition of this disease is important because patients with it have a well-established predisposition for malignant hyperthermia during anesthesia
Transmitted as autosomal dominant trait	Supportive treatment, including counseling, braces for foot drop, or orthopedic surgery to stabilize the foot and treat fractures
Transmitted as autosomal recessive trait; mutations found in CHS1 gene	Vigorous early treatment with antimicrobials and surgical drainage; large doses of vitamin C
Transmitted as autosomal recessive trait that causes disturbances of lipid metabolism	Chenodeoxycholic acid to arrest and reverse progression of disease
Possibly pituitary dysfunction or tumor	Treatment of underlying illness; bromocriptine to prevent osteoporosis
Possibly hydatidiform mole, abortion, fetal-maternal histoincompatibility, inherited factors, or infections; more common with complete molar pregnancy	Chemotherapy, suction to empty uterine contents, hysterectomy; serial chest X-rays; monitoring for progressively decreasing B-hCG levels
Phialophora verrucosa, Fonsecaea pedrosoi, F. compacta, and *Cladosporium carrioni;* found in warm climates, especially in South America; usually introduced through an injury, such as splinter or a thorn in the skin	Cryosurgery with liquid nitrogen; oral itraconazole (alone or with flucytosine); heat therapy; terbinafine has been shown to be effective, but posaconazole may be slightly superior
Transmitted as autosomal recessive trait	Effective treatment unknown; symptomatic treatment, establishment of protective environment
Mycobacterium tuberculosis	Thoracentesis; parenteral or oral antitubercular antibiotics, such as para-aminosalicylate and ethionamide
Transmitted as autosomal dominant and X-linked dominant trait	Supportive treatment ensuring adequate calcium intake

Disease	Description
Contact ulcers	Erosions on the laryngeal mucosa over the vocal cords, producing hoarseness, mild dysphagia, and gradual tissue necrosis
Copper deficiency anemia: hypocupremia	Nutritional deficiency that impairs hemoglobin synthesis and causes shortness of breath, pallor, fatigue, edema, poor wound healing, and anorexia; if prolonged, can cause poor mental development in infants and mental deterioration in adults
Crocq's disease: acrocyanosis, Cassirer syndrome	Symmetrical cyanosis of the hands and feet; distinguished from Raynaud's disease by persistent discoloration
Csillag's disease: lichen sclerosus et atrophicus	Acute inflammatory dermatitis, such as heat rash, prickly heat, miliaria rubra; chronic atrophic and lichenoid dermatitis
Cystinuria	Inborn error of amino acid transport in the kidneys and intestine that allows excessive urinary excretion of cystine and other dibasic amino acids; results in recurrent cystine renal calculi
Czerny's disease	Joint pain with swelling
Dengue: breakbone or dandy fever	Acute febrile disease with myalgia and arthralgia; endemic during the warmer months in the tropics and subtropics; rarely fatal unless it progresses to hemorrhagic shock syndrome
Dubois' disease: congenital syphilis	Vesicular bulbous eruptions resulting in a macerated appearance in the stillborn neonate if acquired in utero; may not manifest until age 2 years or, possibly, even later; associated with hepatosplenomegaly, osteochondritis, hemolytic anemia, thrombocytopenia, and cranial nerve palsies
Duhring's disease: dermatitis herpetiformis	Chronic inflammatory disease marked by erythematous, papular, vesicular, bulbous, or pustular lesions, with tendency toward grouping and associated with itching and burning; usually symmetrical, with eruptions in elbows, knees, sacrum, buttocks, and occiput
Dukes' disease: fourth disease, Filatov-Dukes disease	Marked by myalgia, headache, fever, pharyngitis, conjunctivitis, generalized adenopathy and desquamation following confluent raised erythema
Durand's disease: Durand-Nicholas-Favie disease	Venereal disease marked by involvement of the inguinal gland with an extruding lesion; found worldwide, but incidence higher in tropical and subtropical regions
Duroziez's disease: congenital mitral stenosis	Narrowing orifice of the mitral valve that obstructs blood flow, from atrium to ventricle
Eales disease: peripheral neovascular retinopathy	Condition marked by recurrent hemorrhages into the retina and vitreous; mainly affects males in the second and third decades of life; most cases spontaneous and unilateral; some cases associated with trauma or stress, but also occurs after awakening

Cause	Treatment
Vocal strain, laryngeal trauma, or emotional stress; prolonged alteration may lead to granulomas	Supportive treatment with absolute voice rest, adequate humidification, and aerosol therapy; granulomas tend to recur after surgical removal
Diseases associated with low protein levels; substantial protein loss; decreased GI absorption of copper; total parenteral nutrition without copper supplement; or Wilson's disease	Copper sulfate; supportive treatment of associated symptoms; treatment of underlying cause
Vasospastic disturbance of smaller arterioles of the skin; may be due to dysregulation of the nervous system; more prevalent in females than in males	Protection from exposure to cold, occasionally relieved by warmth
Keratin obstruction of sweat ducts	Symptomatic treatment, including cool environment, application of calamine lotion, and desquamation by ultraviolet rays
Transmitted as autosomal recessive trait	Supportive treatment, including increasing fluid intake, sodium bicarbonate administration, alkaline-ash diet, and penicillamine; surgical removal of calculi
Serous effusion in a joint space or cavity	Treatment of inflammation; aspiration of joint space
Group B arborviruses transmitted by the female *Aedes* mosquito	Symptomatic treatment; nonaspirin analgesics; I.V. fluid replacement; complete bed rest
Treponema pallidum, a spirochete obtained by venereal contact of the mother and transmitted from her to the fetus via the placenta	Penicillin G or, in allergic patients, either desensitize to penicillin or seek infectious disease consultation
Associated with intestinal sensitivity to dietary gluten (celiac sprue)	Sulfa-based antibiotics; strict gluten-free diet
Most likely a viral exanthema of the coxsackievirus or echovirus group	Symptomatic and supportive treatment
Chlamydia trachomatis (serologic type L_1-3)	Symptomatic and supportive treatment; antiviral agent specific to chlamydia
Congenital	Surgery, if possible; otherwise, supportive treatment
Etiology unknown	Treatment of underlying causes

Disease	Description
Economo's disease: lethargic encephalitis	Epidemic encephalitis marked by increasing languor, apathy, and drowsiness, progressing to lethargy; accompanied by ophthalmoplegia; usually occurs in winter
Elevator disease	Form of occupational pneumoconiosis affecting people who work in grain elevators
Engel-Recklinghausen disease: osteitis fibrosa cystica generalisata	Fibrous degeneration of bone, with the formation of cysts and fibrous nodules on affected bone; effective monitoring and control of hyperparathyroidism have made diseases even rarer
Eosinophilic endomyocardial disease: Löffler's endocarditis, Loeffler's endocarditis	Form of progressive endocarditis denoted by a highly increased number of eosinophilic granulocytes in the blood; fibrosis and thickening of the endocardium occur; cardiomegaly and heart failure may be present
Epstein-Barr virus: mononucleosis	Classic heterophil-positive infectious mononucleosis, occasionally complicated by neurologic diseases, such as encephalitis or transverse myelitis
Erysipeloid	Acute, self-limiting skin infection most common in butchers, farmers, cooks, fishermen, and others who handle infected material; may progress to infective endocarditis or affect other body systems if primary lesions aren't treated
Erythrasma	Superficial, bacterial skin infection that usually affects the skin folds, especially in the groin, axillae, and toe webs
Eulenberg's disease: paramyotonia congenita, Thomsen's disease	Slowly progressive disease of skeletal muscles; similar to muscular dystrophy; muscle stiffness in hands, legs, and eyelids is most prominent manifestation
Fabry's disease	Renal disorder that produces malfunctions of the proximal renal tubules, leading to hyperkalemia, hypernatremia, glycosuria, phosphaturia, aminoaciduria, uricosuria, bicarbonate wasting and retarded growth and development, and rickets
Fanconi's syndrome: de Toni-Fanconi syndrome	Disorder of fat storage related to a deficiency of enzyme alpha-galactosidase A; characterized by glycolipid accumulation in body tissues; results in clouding of the cornea, burning sensations of hands and feet, small raised purple blemishes on the skin, impaired arterial circulation, and renal and GI involvement
Fifth disease: erythema infectiosum	Contagious disease characterized by rose-colored eruptions diffused over the skin, usually starting on the cheeks; mainly affects children ages 4 to 10; infection in a patient who's pregnant can cause fetal hydrops and increase the risk of fetal death in the first half of pregnancy

Cause	Treatment
Pathogen not clearly identified, but may be arthropod-borne virus or sequela of influenza, rubella, varicella, or vaccinia	Symptomatic treatment, including appropriate antibiotics for secondary infection
Inhalation of dust particles, causing irritation and inflammation of respiratory tract	Avoidance of exposure to dust
Marked osteoclastic activity secondary to parathyroid hyperfunction, with calcium and phosphorus metabolic disturbances	Control of parathyroid hyperactivity; may require surgery if patient develops impaired renal function, bone demineralization, or significant hypertension
Unknown	Suppression of eosinophilia with prednisolone or hydroxyurea; digoxin; diuretics; medical and surgical therapy for cardiac complications should be used as indicated
Epstein-Barr virus	Symptomatic treatment; generally benign course
Erysipelothrix rhusiopathiae (insidiosa) transmitted by contact with infected animals	Penicillin or erythromycin in combination with rifampin if the patient has penicillin allergy; the patient with the systemic form may need valve replacement surgery or other surgery depending on the organ involved
Corynebacterium minutissimum	Topical antibiotics; treatment with oral erythromycin or tetracycline often produces quick resolution; antibacterial soap to prevent recurrence
Transmitted as autosomal dominant trait	Treatment with quinine sulfate, procainamide, tocainide, mexiletine, or phenytoin may help
Transmitted as X-linked recessive trait	Symptomatic treatment with low-dose phenytoin or carbamazepine for pain in hands and feet; metoclopramide or nutritional supplement for GI hyperactivity; enzyme replacement therapy
If diagnosed as a child, may be congenital; if diagnosed as an adult, considered acquired and may be secondary to Wilson's disease, cystinosis, galactosemia, or exposure to a toxins as in heavy metal poisoning	Symptomatic treatment with replacement therapy, vitamin D for rickets, and aluminum hydroxide for hyperphosphatemia; treatment of underlying cause for acquired form; dialysis as necessary
Human parvovirus B19, probably transmitted by respiratory tract	Symptomatic treatment; screening of donated blood, which might prevent transfusion-related transmission; transfusion if aplastic crisis; immune globulin I.V. if immunocompromised; intra-arterial blood transfusion if fetal hydrops present

Disease	Description
File-cutter's disease	Lead poisoning from inhalation of lead particles that arise during file cutting
Fish-skin disease: ichthyosis vulgaris	Condition of dry and scaly skin resembling fish skin; several forms, including vulgaris and lamellar
Flax-dresser's disease: byssinosis	Pulmonary disorder of flax-dressers or textile workers
Flecked retina syndrome	Group of retinal disorders, including fundus flavimaculatus, fundus albipunctatus, drusen, and congenital macular degeneration, all of which may be primary abnormalities of retinal pigment epithelium
Fleischner's disease	Inflammation of bone and cartilage affecting the middle phalanges of the hand
Friedländer's disease: endarteritis obliterans	Chronic, progressive thickening of the intima, leading to stenosis or obstruction of the lumen
Friedrich's disease: paramyoclonus multiplex, Friedrich's ataxia	Ataxic gait, cerebellar dysfunction, leg weakness, sensory disturbances in the limbs, and depressed tendon reflexes
Geotrichosis	Fungal infection affecting the mouth, throat, lungs, or intestines
Gerlier's disease: endemic paralytic vertigo, paralyzing vertigo	Nervous system disorder marked by pain, vertigo, paresis, and muscle contractions
Glioma of the optic nerve	Slow-growing tumor that causes progressive vision loss
Glossopharyngeal neuralgia	Disease of the ninth cranial (glossopharyngeal) nerve that produces paroxysms of pain in the ear, posterior pharynx, base of the tongue, or jaws; sometimes accompanied by syncope
Glucose-6-phosphate dehydrogenase (G6PD) deficiency	Deficiency of the red blood cell enzyme G6PD, which causes anemia; common in people of African or Mediterranean descent
Graefe's sign: ophthalmoplegia progressiva	Gradual paralysis of the eye, affecting first one eye muscle, then the other
Grinder's disease: pneumoconiosis	Permanent deposition of particles in the lungs
Habermann's disease	Sudden onset of a polymorphous skin eruption of macules, papules, and occasionally vesicles, with hemorrhage

Cause	Treatment
Inhalation of lead particles	Avoidance of exposure to lead; chelating agents should be used for moderate to high-level poisoning
Hereditary form is an autosomal dominant genetic disorder; acquired form seen in adulthood usually associated with internal disease such as malignancy	Alphahydroxy acids (lactic, glycolic, or pyruvic acids) to help hydrate the skin; removal of scales by keratolytics; propylene glycol; topical retinoids; treatment of underlying systemic condition for acquired form
Inhalation of dust from cotton or other vegetable fibers, such as flax or hemp	Avoidance of exposure to source; bronchodilators to manage symptoms (corticosteroids in severe cases)
Congenital	Supportive and symptomatic treatment
Unknown	Anti-inflammatory agents (including steroids in severe cases); analgesics
Trauma, pyogenic bacterial infection, infective thrombi, or syphilis	Endarterectomy
Central nervous system damage secondary to trauma or infection; may be hereditary	Treatment of underlying disease; no specific treatment for hereditary form
Geotrichum candidum	Gentian violet for oral, throat, or intestinal infections; oral potassium iodide for pulmonary infections
Disease of the internal ear from pressure of cerumen on the drum membrane	Symptomatic treatment, including scopolamine to combat nausea
Unknown	Surgical excision; radiation therapy
Unknown	Surgery; carbamazepine, phenytoin
Transmitted as an X-linked trait	Avoidance of known oxidant drugs, including primaquine, salicylates, sulfonamides, nitrofurans, phenacetin, naphthalene
Usually secondary to brain lesions or mitochondrial disorders	Treatment of underlying disease; corrective lenses
Inhalation of dust particles	Irreversible pulmonary disease; eliminating exposure to dust particles can prevent further irritation of tissues
Virus resembling smallpox	Supportive treatment, possibly isolation

Disease	Description
Hagner's disease	Obscure bone disease resembling acromegaly; associated with increased soft-tissue growth after puberty, increased metabolic rate, and increased sweating and sebaceous activity
Heavy chain disease	Neoplasms of the lymphoplasmacytes, in which abnormal proliferation occurs among cells that produce immunoglobulins, causing incomplete heavy chains and no light chains in their molecular structure
Heerfordt's syndrome: Uveoparotid fever	Variant of sarcoidosis manifested by parotid swelling and single or multiple palsies of cranial nerves
Hemangioma of the eye	In children, tumors not encapsulated, grow quickly in the first year, and then regress by about age 7; in adults, tumors encapsulated
Hemochromatosis: bronze diabetes, Recklinghausen-Applebaum disease	Disorder characterized by iron overload in parenchymal cells, leading to cirrhosis, diabetes, cardiomegaly with heart failure and arrhythmias, and increased skin pigmentation
Hemoglobin C-thalassemia disease	Simultaneous heterozygosity for hemoglobin C and thalassemia; characterized by mild hemolytic anemia and persistent splenomegaly
Henderson-Jones disease: osteochondromatosis	Presence of numerous benign cartilaginous tumors in the joint cavity or in the bursa of a tendon sheath
Hereditary spherocytosis	Anemia resulting in increased red blood cell membrane permeability and intracellular hypertonicity; characterized by slight jaundice, splenomegaly, and cholelithiasis
Heubner's disease	Syphilitic inflammation of tunica intima of cerebral arteries
Hoffa's disease	Proliferation of fatty tissue (solitary lipoma) in the knee joint
Hutchinson-Gifford disease: progeria	Premature old age marked by small stature, wrinkled skin, and gray hair, with attitude and appearance of old age in very young children
Hutinel's disease	Tuberculous pericarditis, with cirrhosis of the liver in children
Hydatid disease, alveolar	Infection characterized by invasion and destruction of tissue by cysts, which undergo endogenous budding and form an aggregate of innumerable small cysts that honeycomb the affected organ — usually the liver — and may metastasize
Hydatid disease, unilocal: echinococcus granulosus, hydatidosus	Infection causing marked formation of single or multiple unilocular cysts
Iceland disease: epidemic neuromyasthenia, benign myalgic encephalomyelitis	Marked by headaches, muscle pain, low-grade fever, lymphadenopathy, fatigue, and paresthesia; outbreaks occur in summer, usually in young women

Cause	Treatment
Growth hormone-secreting tumors that develop after puberty	Treatment of cardiovascular complications; surgery and irradiation (proton beam or heavy particle treatment and supravoltage) for large tumors
Possibly microorganisms and immune deficiency syndrome due to malnutrition or genetic predisposition	Supportive and palliative treatment with chemotherapy, radiation therapy, antibiotics, and steroids
Impaired regulation of thymus-derived lymphocytes (T cells) and bone-marrow–derived lymphocytes (B cells)	Adrenal corticosteroids to suppress inflammation and control symptoms
Unknown	Surgical excision for adults; no treatment for children
Erythropoietic disorders, hepatic disorders that increase iron absorption, autosomal recessive inheritance	Phlebotomy to remove excess iron; chelating agents such as deferoxamine
Hereditary and congenital	Supportive treatment, including transfusions for severe anemia and folate therapy
Irritation and trauma	Resection of tumor with curettage and bone grafts
Transmitted as autosomal dominant trait	Splenectomy; supplementation with folic acid
Treponema pallidum	Supportive treatment, including antibiotic therapy
Tissue trauma	Aspiration or surgery
Unknown	No known treatment
Mycobacterium tuberculosis	Tuberculostatic agents
Infection by *Echinococcus multilocularis* (larvae)	Symptomatic treatment and surgery; usually fatal; high-dose mebendazole may be used in patients with medical problems that preclude surgery, or in cases where surgery wouldn't be indicated
Infection by *Echinococcus granulosis* (larvae); hydatid tapeworm in dogs and cats	Surgery; drug therapy with an antihelmintic, such as albendazole or mebendazole
Probably infection but possibly psychosocial phenomenon	Symptomatic treatment

Disease	Description
Intestinal lymphangiectasia	Dilation and possible rupture of intestinal lymphatic vessels, resulting in hypoproteinemia and steatorrhea due to loss of fat and albumin into the intestinal lumen
Interstitial cystitis	Inflammation of the bladder wall occurring most often in women and marked by urinary frequency and urgency and abdominal, urethral, or vaginal pain; dyspareunia possibly also occurring; urine cultures and urinalysis are normal; cystoscopic examination revealing pinpoint hemorrhages on distended bladder wall
Isambert's disease: tuberculosis laryngitis	Acute miliary tuberculosis of the larynx and pharynx
Jaffee-Lichtenstein disease: cystic osteofibromatosis	Form of polyostotic fibrous dysplasia marked by an enlarged medullary cavity with a thin cortex, which is filled with fibrous tissue (fibroma)
Jaksch's syndrome: Anemia pseudoleukemia infantum, Jaksch's anemia, van Jaksch's syndrome	Syndrome of anisocytosis, peripheral red blood cell immaturity, leukocytosis, and hepatosplenomegaly that usually occurs in children younger than age 3
Jansen's disease: metaphyseal dysostosis	Skeletal abnormality with nearly normal epiphyses in which the metaphyseal tissues are replaced by masses of cartilage
Jensen's disease: retinochoroiditis juxtapapillaris	Inflammation of the retina and choroid marked by small inflammatory areas on the fundus close to the papilla
Juvenile angiofibroma: benign nasal tumor	Highly vascular, nasopharyngeal tumor that causes nasal obstruction and severe recurrent epistaxis; capable of eroding bone
Keratoconus	Degenerative eye disorder typified by thinning and anterior protrusion of the cornea, causing major changes in the refractive power of the eye and requiring frequent eyeglass changes
Keratosis pilaris: keratosis follicularis, Darier's disease	Skin condition marked by formation of horny plugs in the orifices of hair follicles; lesions appearing primarily on the lateral aspects of the upper arms, thighs, and buttocks; may also occur on face; more severe in the winter months
Kienböck's disease: lunatomalacia	Slowly progressive osteochondrosis of the semilunar (carpal lunate) bone from avascular necrosis
Köhler's bone disease: tarsal scaphoiditis, epiphysitis juvenilis	Osteochondrosis of the tarsal navicular bone in children, occurring at about age 5

Cause	Treatment
Congenital or may be acquired when obstruction, valvular heart disease, or constrictive pericarditis increases pressure on the lymphatics	No-fat diet; replacement of dietary sources of long-chain triglycerides with medium-chain triglycerides
Unknown	Symptomatic treatment (anti-inflammatory drugs, antispasmodics, antihistamines, and muscle relaxants)
Mycobacterium tuberculosis	Tuberculostatic agents
May be a lipoid granuloma	Symptomatic and supportive treatment; surgery
Malnutrition, chronic infection, malabsorption, hemoglobinopathies	Treatment of underlying causes
Unknown	Surgery
Unknown; probably an autoimmune process	Steroids may induce improvements
Unknown	Surgery
Possibly genetic inheritance and systemic and ocular associations; risk factors include eye rubbing, ocular allergies, and use of contact lenses	Hard contact lenses or glasses with high astigmatic correction; possibly, corneal graft or transplantation
Genetic follicular disease but may be transmitted as autosomal dominant trait	No specific therapy; keratolytic lotions to prevent cracking, drying, and skin breakdown possibly useful
Degenerative process precipitated by trauma	Anti-inflammatories and immobilization of wrist for several months (if ineffective, surgery)
Unknown but trauma suspected	Protection of foot from excessive use or trauma; if pain is severe, plaster cast may be required for 6 to 8 weeks; oral analgesics as needed; complete spontaneous recovery may occur

Disease	Description
Krabbe's disease: globoid cell leukodystrophy	Rapidly progressive cerebral demyelination with large globoid bodies in the white matter; associated with irritability, rigidity, tonic-clonic seizures, blindness, deafness, and progressive mental deterioration
Kugelberg-Welander syndrome: type III spinal muscular atrophy	Slowly progressive muscular atrophy resulting from lesions of the anterior horns of the spinal cord; usual onset in preschool or adolescent years
Kümmell's disease: posttraumatic spondylitis	Intercostal neuralgia with spinal pain and motor disturbances in the legs
Kuru	Chronic, progressive, and fatal neurologic disease found only in New Guinea
Larsen's disease: Sinding-Larsen and Johanssen syndrome, Larsen-Johansson disease, patellar chondropathy	Accessory center of ossification within the patella, associated with flat facies and short metacarpals
Leiner's disease: erythroderma desquamativum	Generalized exfoliative dermatitis and erythroderma, chiefly affecting breast-fed neonates; probably identical to severe seborrheic dermatitis
Leishmaniasis	Group of infectious disorders; cutaneous (skin lesions), mucocutaneous (mucosal ulcerations), and visceral forms (subacute, acute, and chronic)
Lenegre's disease	Acquired complete heart block
Leptospirosis	Infectious disease that causes meningitis, hepatitis, nephritis, or febrile disease; may be mild (anicteric) or severe (icteric or Weil's disease)
Lesch-Nyhan syndrome	Disorder of purine metabolism marked by behavioral problems that include cognitive dysfunction and aggressive and impulsive behaviors; also includes self-injurious behaviors, spasticity, hyperuricemia, and excessive uricaciduria
Letterer-Siwe disease: nonlipid reticuloendotheliosis; disseminated histiocytosis X	Hemorrhagic tendency with eczematoid skin eruptions, lymph node enlargement, hepatosplenomegaly, and progressive anemia; occurs mainly in infants

Cause	Treatment
Genetic deficiency of galactocerebrosiderase, an enzyme for myelin metabolism	Symptomatic treatment; bone marrow transplantation improves diagnosis, but death usually occurs before age 2
Transmitted as autosomal recessive or dominant trait	Supportive treatment with physical therapy; bracing or special appliances may help; normal life span probable
Compression fracture of the vertebrae	Treatment of fracture; extension of spine; pain relief
Caused by a prion, a naturally occurring protein considered the infectious agent and cause of spongiform encephalopathy; thought to be associated with cannibalism of the Fore culture in New	No effective treatment; invariably fatal
Unknown	Supportive treatment; surgery
Unknown, but inherited dysfunction or deficiency in the C5 component of complement has been implicated	Symptomatic treatment for fluid and heat loss; biotin appears useful
Intracellular parasites (*Leishmania*) transmitted by sandflies	Antiparasitics, including sodium antimony gluconate, amphotericin B, or such antiprotozoals as pentamidine; supportive treatment for lesions; transfusions for severe anemia
Primary sclerodegeneration of the conduction system	Artificial pacemaker; supportive treatment
Bacteria of genus *Leptospira* transmitted by contact with water, soil, food, or vegetation contaminated with urine from an infected lower mammal	Doxycycline or ampicillin
Defective enzyme transmitted by female carriers as X-linked recessive trait	Allopurinol to control urine and sedimentation; baclofen and benzodiazepines for spasticity; symptomatic and supportive treatment, such as behavioral modification and medications for behavior treatment; few patients live beyond age 40 and most die suddenly
Acute, disseminated form of histiocytosis X, an intense proliferation of reticulohistiocytic cells	Symptomatic and supportive treatment of anemia; local radiation is effective for osseous lesions; corticosteroids should be used to treat lung involvement

Disease	Description
Lewandowsky-Lutz disease: epidermodysplasia verruciformis	May manifest as flat-topped papules that vary in color from pink to brown, resembling verruca plana; have a tendency to become malignant; they increase in number and coalesce to form large plaques or scales on the knees, elbows, and trunk; often associated with mental retardation
Lichtheim's disease: Lichtheim's syndrome	Subacute degeneration of the spinal cord associated with pernicious anemia
Li-Fraumeni syndrome	Inherited syndrome predisposing patient to lung, breast, and soft-tissue cancers
Little's disease: cerebral palsy	Form of cerebral spastic paralysis and stiffness of the limbs associated with muscle weakness, seizures, bilateral athetosis, and mental deficiencies
Ludwig's angina	Infection of the sublingual and submandibular spaces characterized by brawny induration of the submaxillary region, edema of the sublingual floor of the mouth, and elevation of the tongue
Lung fluke disease: Paragonimus westermani, P. heterotrema	Parasitic hemoptysis, or oriental hemoptysis from pulmonary cysts
MacLean-Maxwell disease	Chronic condition of the calcaneus marked by enlargement of the posterior third and by sensitivity to pressure
Macroglobulinemia: Waldenström's macroglobulinemia	Malignant neoplastic disease of plasma and lymphoid cells that produces immunoglobulin M antibodies; may produce no symptoms or diverse signs and symptoms
Malibu disease: surfer's knots, surfer's knees	Hyperplastic, fibrosing granulomas occurring over bony prominences of the feet and legs of surfers
Malignant melanoma of the eye	Malignant tumor stemming from the melanocytes in the uvea, retina, or iris
Maple syrup urine disease	Enzyme defect in the metabolism of the branched chain amino acids, resulting in mental and physical retardation, reflex changes, feeding difficulties, characteristic odor of urine and perspiration, seizures, and death; four clinical phenotypes: classic, intermediate, intermittent, and thiamine-responsive
Marburg disease: Marburg virus disease; Marburg hemorrhagic fever	Severe viral disease characterized by fever, malaise, myalgia, headache, pharyngitis, vomiting, diarrhea, and rash, often accompanied by hepatic damage and renal failure, encephalitis, and multiorgan dysfunction
Medullary cystic disease: familial juvenile nephronophthisis	Congenital renal disorder marked by cyst formation, primarily in the medulla and the corticomedullary junction, with insidious onset of uremia that causes death between ages 4 and 14

Cause	Treatment
Autosomal recessive trait with impaired cell immunity; about 15 human papillomaviruses are implicated	No effective treatment
Vitamin B_{12} deficiency	Correction of vitamin B_{12} deficiency
Inherited family trait, deletion of tumor-suppression gene (chromosome 17)	Treatment specific to cancer
Congenital, resulting from birth trauma, fetal anoxia, or maternal illness during pregnancy	Preventive measures; symptomatic treatment
Causative bacteria include many gram-negative and anaerobic organisms, streptococci, and staphylococci	Significant airway obstruction may require tracheotomy; high doses of penicillin G given I.V., sometimes in combination with other drugs; incision and drainage to relieve pressure in affected tissues
Infestation by trematodes or flukes (Flukes may be classified as blood flukes, liver flukes, lung flukes, or intestinal flukes depending on location in the infected host)	Praziquantel is the drug of choice; symptomatic and supportive treatment of hemoptysis is usually necessary; surgery may be needed for complications
Trauma	Supportive shoes; surgery; avoidance of prolonged standing; high-impact exercises
Unknown but genetic predisposition suspected	Plasmapheresis for hyperviscosity; chemotherapy; interefron alpha; asymptomatic patients need no specific therapy
Common among surfers who paddle in a kneeling position	Supportive shoes; avoidance of prolonged standing
Unknown, but excessive exposure to sunlight is a risk factor	Laser or radiation therapy; chemotherapy; surgical excision; eye enucleation
Decarboxylation of the corresponding α-ketoacids by the branched-chain α-keto acid dehydrogenase components; transmitted as autosomal recessive trait	Supportive treatment; controlled intake of branched chain amino acids; peritoneal dialysis, hemodialysis, or both; one form is responsive to early initiation of thiamine
Zoonotic (animal-borne) ribonucleic acid virus of the filovirus family; initially discovered in exposure to African green monkeys	Symptomatic and supportive treatment; usually fatal
Transmitted as autosomal recessive or dominant trait	Symptomatic treatment: erythropoietin for anemia, recombinant growth hormone for growth retardation, peritoneal dialysis or hemodialysis; transplantation

Disease	Description
Megaloblastic anemia	Folic acid or vitamin B$_{12}$ deficiency that alters the nucleic acid production needed for erythrocyte maturation in bone marrow
Meyer-Betz disease: idiopathic or familial myoglobinuria	Myoglobinuria that may be precipitated by strenuous exertion or possibly by infection; marked by tenderness, swelling, and muscle weakness
Microdrepanocytic disease: sickle cell thalassemia	Anemia involving simultaneous heterozygosity for hemoglobin and thalassemia
Milroy's disease: congenital lymphedema	Chronic lymphatic obstruction causing lymphedema of the legs; sometimes associated with edema of the arms, trunk, and face
Minamata disease	Severe neurologic disorder characterized by peripheral and circumoral paresthesia, ataxia, mental disabilities, and loss of peripheral vision
Minor's disease: tremor familiaris	Hematomyelia (hemorrhage into the spinal cord) involving the central parts of the spinal cord; marked by sudden onset of flaccid paralysis, with sensory disturbances
Morton's neuroma: metatarsalgia, forefoot neuroma	Pain over the ball of the foot, especially left plantar surface distally
Mule-spinner's disease	Warts or ulcers, especially on the scrotum, that tend to become malignant; common among operators of spinning mules in cotton mills
Mushroom picker's disease: farmer's lung, bird breeder's lung, extrinsic allergic alveolitis	Allergic respiratory disease of persons working with moldy compost prepared for growing mushrooms; chronic form leads to pulmonary fibrosis
Mycetoma: maduromycosis, Madura foot, watering can foot	Chronic infection of the skin, subcutaneous tissues, and bone, usually affecting the foot; results in sinus tracts of the foot; deformity may occur
Myelosclerosis	Sclerosis of the spinal cord; obliteration of the normal marrow cavity by the formation of small spicules of bone
Nezelof syndrome	Primary immunodeficiency disease characterized by absent T-cell function and variable B-cell function, with fairly normal immunoglobulin levels and little or no specific antibody production; failure to thrive and increased susceptibility to infection typical; usually fatal as a result of sepsis

Cause	Treatment
Cobalamin (vitamin B$_{12}$) deficiency, secondary to pernicious anemia and folate deficiency, resulting from poor diet, sprue, pregnancy, or antifolate medication	Folic acid or vitamin B$_{12}$ supplementation
Unknown; familial tendencies possible	Bed rest; anti-inflammatory agents, steroids in extreme cases, analgesics for pain
Hereditary transmission	Management of anemia
Congenital and hereditary; transmitted as autosomal dominant trait	Microsurgery to rechannel lymph flow; supportive care; compression stockings
Alkyl mercury poisoning	Avoidance of causative agents; supportive and symptomatic treatment; chelation therapy with dimercaprol or 2,3-dimercaptosuccinic acid for acute cases; exchange transfusions; usually fatal
Usually seen with vascular malformation, blood dyscrasia, and in people on anticoagulants; possibly inheritable	Treatment of underlying disease; supportive treatment
Repeated injury	Supportive shoes; analgesics; perineural injections of long-acting corticosteroids with local anesthetics; arch support or orthotics; surgical excision if needed
Found in cotton textile workers who had frequent scrotal contact with mineral oils on a long-term basis while working on a machine called the *mule*	Chemotherapy; radiotherapy; bone marrow transplantation; surgery if needed
Airborne irritant, usually mold spores: *Micropolyspora faeni* or *Thermoactinomyces vulgaris*	Surgery; chemotherapy as indicated
Actinomycetes or fungi found in soil and plant material of tropical region	Supportive and symptomatic treatment; avoidance of exposure to allergen; glucocorticosteroids in chronic forms
Unknown	Antibiotics for actinomycetoma (streptomycin, co-trimoxazole, amikacin, rifampin, minocycline); itraconazole or ketoconazole for eumycetoma from fungi; surgery for affected tissue or amputation if bone is involved
May be transmitted as autosomal recessive trait	Symptomatic treatment (usually includes antibiotics for infection and monthly treatment with immune globulin or fresh frozen plasma infusions); bone marrow transplantation

Disease	Description
Niemann-Pick disease: sphingomyelin lipidosis	Lipid storage disorder resulting in abnormal accumulation of sphingomyelin in reticuloendothelial cells; most common in people of Ashkenazi Jewish ancestry; occurs in five different phenotypes, each with slightly different symptoms but characterized by pulmonary infiltrates, brownish skin, and sea blue histiocytes
Norrie's disease: atrophia bulborum hereditaria; retinal dysplasia	Bilateral blindness from absence of retinal ganglion cells; associated with cataracts, bilateral leukokoria, micro-ophthalmia, and mental retardation; represents inherited form of persistent hyperplastic primary vitreous
Nystagmus	Recurring, involuntary eyeball movement that may be jerking or pendular
Olivopontocerebellar atrophy	Progressively deteriorating neurologic disease marked by ataxia, dysarthria, and an action tremor that develops late in middle life; usually normal deep tendon reflexes; associated with occasional rigidity and other extrapyramidal signs
Opitz's disease	Thrombophlebitic splenomegaly
Osteitis pubis	Inflammation of the pubic symphysis and surrounding muscle insertions; painful condition characterized by bony resorption and spontaneous reossification; excruciating pain radiating along the adductor aspect of both thighs; pain intensified by movement, especially abduction
Otto's disease: arthrokatadysis, Otto pelvis	Osteoarthritic protrusion of the acetabulum into the pelvic cavity; onset during puberty or later with progressive and bilateral loss of hip joint movement without pain and deformity on hip flexion and abduction
Owren's disease: parahemophilia	Rare hemorrhagic tendency resulting from deficiency of coagulation factor V; death may occur
Paracoccidioidomycosis: South American blastomycosis	Fungal infection of the skin, lungs, mucous membranes, lymphatics, and viscera, seen primarily in the tropical forests of South America and Mexico
Paroxysmal nocturnal hemoglobinuria	Red cell breakdown with release of hemoglobin in the urine, resulting in dark-colored urine in the morning; symptoms include hemolytic anemia, thrombosis of large vessels, and a deficiency of hematopoiesis resulting in anemia (pancytopenia)
Pelizaeus-Merzbacher disease: sudanophilic leukodystrophy	Hyperplastic centrolobular sclerosis marked by nystagmus, ataxia, tremors, choreoathetotic movements, parkinsonian facies, and mental deterioration; begins early in life and occurs primarily in males

Cause	Treatment
Transmitted as autosomal recessive trait	Supportive and symptomatic treatment; possibly liver transplantation in an infant with type A
Transmitted as X-linked trait	No known treatment
May be congenital or acquired; jerking nystagmus results from excessive stimulation of the vestibular apparatus in the inner ear, lesions of the brain stem or cerebellum, drugs and alcohol toxicity, and congenital neurologic disorder; pendular nystagmus results from improper transmission of visual impulses to the brain in the presence of corneal opacification, high astigmatism, congenital cataract, or congenital anomalies of optic disk or bilateral macular lesions	Correction of the underlying cause if possible; eyeglasses for vision disturbances
Transmitted as autosomal dominant trait	No definitive therapy; death usually follows aspiration pneumonia secondary to loss of cough reflex
Thrombosis of the splenic vein	Symptomatic and supportive treatment, including anticoagulation
Cause unknown; repetitive microtrauma or shearing force to the pubic symphysis, which can happen while participating in sports involving running and kicking, may be a contributing factor	Symptomatic treatment; nonsteroidal anti-inflammatory drugs or cyclo-oxygenase-2 (COX-2) inhibitors, corticosteroids
Degenerative osteoarthritic changes, probably hereditary	Supportive treatment; surgery if night traction and rest are ineffective
Transmitted as autosomal recessive trait	Supportive treatment
Paracoccidioides brasiliensis	Ketoconazole, itraconazole, fluconazole; amphotericin B given I.V. for extremely ill patients
Unknown; possibly acquired clonal stem cell disorder	Symptomatic treatment with corticosteroids; androgen therapy; oral iron supplements and folic acid; transfusions; treatment of thrombotic complications
Familial transmission as an X-linked recessive trait, caused by mutations of the PLP gene located on the long arm of the X chromosome (Xq 22)	No specific treatment; supportive care, such as physical therapy, orthotics, and antispasticity agents; severely affected patients need airway protection and anticonvulsant therapy

Disease	Description
Pellegrini's disease: Pellegrini-Stieda disease, Köhler-Stieda-Pellegrini disease	Ossification of the superior portion of the medial collateral ligament of the knee with pain, swelling, tenderness, and limited motion; a calcified mass develops within weeks
Pemphigus	Chronic blistering disease that causes superficial and deep lesions; pemphigus vulgaris, most common form of this disease, can be fatal
Perrin-Ferraton disease: snapping hip; iliotibial band syndrome	Condition marked by slippage of the hip joint; sometimes occurs with an audible snap (due to slipping of a tendonous band over the greater trochanter)
Progressive multifocal leukoencephalopathy	Demyelination of the white substance of the brain, producing sensory aphasia, cortical blindness, deafness, weakness, spasticity of the limbs and, eventually, complete paralysis, dementia, and coma; primarily affects patients who are immunosuppressed
Pulseless disease: Takayasu arteritis	Progressive changes of the aorta and its branches resulting in decreased or absent radial pulse bilaterally with pain in arm and forearm; inflammation of carotid arteries cause vision problems, dizziness, or stroke; aneurysms and hypertension occur
Purtscher's disease: Purtscher's angiopathic retinopathy	Retinal hemorrhagic and vasoocclusive vasculopathy with edema, white retinal patches, and severe vision loss
Q fever	Rickettsial disease with acute and chronic stages, affecting respiratory as well as GI and cardiac systems
Rat-bite fever: sodoku	Gram-negative bacterial infection that occurs 1 to 3 weeks after contact with secretions (urine, oral, or conjunctival) or bite from an infected animal (rat, squirrel, weasel, gerbil), causing chills, fever, headache, muscle pain, maculopapular rash on extremities and painful joints
Refsum's disease: type IV hereditary sensorimotor neuropathy	Defect in metabolism of phytanic acid, marked by chronic polyneuritis, retinitis pigmentosa, and cerebellar signs (mild ataxia) with persistent elevation of protein levels in cerebrospinal fluid
Retinoblastoma	Most common intraocular cancer in children, arising from retinal gum cells; white pupil (leukokoria), poorly aligned eyes (strabismus), or a red and painful eye may be first indications
Rhabdomyosarcoma	Malignant tumors of muscle; areas affected include genitourinary tract, extremities, trunk, and retroperitoneum; in children, head and neck soft tissue sarcoma most common
Rhinosporidiosis	Fungal infection producing a chronic granulomatous infection that occurs as painless, vascularized, friable, and often large tumorlike lesions; most common in southern India and Sri Lanka
Richter's syndrome	Chronic lymphocytic leukemia that evolves into an aggressive lymphoma

Cause	Treatment
Trauma, such as a complication of athletic injuries	Surgical correction; supportive treatment
Autoimmune disorder; occasionally caused by reaction to such medications as penicillamine, captopril, carbidopa, and levodopa	Corticosteroids, immunosuppressants; antibiotics for secondary skin infections; plasmapheresis; dapsone for pemphigus foliaceus
Unknown	No effective treatment
Common human polyomavirus, JC virus	Symptomatic and supportive treatment
Unknown, but appears to be related to autoimmunity	Steroids, immunosuppressants, surgery, angioplasty; angiotensin-converting enzyme inhibitors for hypertension
Trauma — usually blunt thoracic or head trauma — and such nontraumatic diseases as pancreatitis, embolization, and vasculitis; amniotic fluid aneurysm also a cause	Supportive treatment; treatment of underlying condition
Inhalation of infected particles by *Coxiella burnetii*; considered category B agent for biologic warfare	Appropriate antibiotic therapy (doxycycline or chloramphenicol); possibly valve replacement
Streptobacillus moniliformis or *Spirillum minor*	Penicillin or tetracycline
Transmitted as autosomal recessive trait	Symptomatic and supportive treatment; therapeutic plasma exchange; transplantation of α-hydroxylase containing tissue
Transmitted as autosomal dominant trait (deletion of q14 band of chromosome 13)	Radiotherapy, chemotherapy-based multimodality therapy, or cryotherapy; enucleation
Unknown	Radiation therapy; surgical excision
Rhinosporidium seeberi; acquired by exposure to stagnant water	Electrocauterization or surgical excision, followed by dapsone
Clonal evolution of original leukemia	Chemotherapy for the lymphoma

Disease	Description
Rickettsialpox	Mild self-limiting zoonotic febrile illness characterized by a papulovesicular skin rash at the location of a tick bite
Robles' disease: onchocerciasis	Onchocerciasis of the fibroid nodules, lymph, subcutaneous connective tissue (severe dermatitis and depigmentation), and eyes (river blindness)
Schanz's syndrome: Albert's disease	Inflammation of the Achilles tendon; walking is difficult
Sever's disease	Epiphysitis of the calcaneus in children when the growth plate is injured
Silo filler's disease	Pulmonary inflammation often associated with acute pulmonary edema
Smith-Strang disease: methionine malabsorption syndrome, Oasthouse urine disease	Defective methionine absorption, resulting in white hair, mental retardation, seizures, attacks of hyperpnea, and characteristic urine odor
Soft-tissue sarcoma	Soft-tissue malignancy of muscle, fat, connective tissue, blood vessels, and synovium; composed of tightly packed cells similar to embryonic connective tissue
Sponge-diver's disease: sponge dermatitis, Skevas-Zerfus disease	Burning, itching, erythema, necrosis, and ulceration of skin; common in Mediterranean divers
Stargardt's disease	Degeneration of the macula lutea marked by rapid loss of central visual activity and abnormal appearance and pigmentation of the macular area; peripheral vision remains intact
Strabismus: squint, heterotropia, cross-eye	Eye malalignment due to the absence of normal, parallel, or coordinated eye movement
Swediaur's disease: Schwediauer's disease	Inflammation of the calcaneal bursa
Tangier disease	Deficiency of high-density-lipoproteins in the serum with storage of cholesterol esters in the tonsils causing orange-yellow tonsillar hyperplasia, and in the liver and spleen, causing hepatosplenomegaly
Toxocariasis: visceral larva migrans	Chronic, frequently mild syndrome common in children involving roundworm migration from the intestine to various organs and tissues (visceral larva migrans); characterized by hepatosplenomegaly, eosinophilia, cough, difficulty sleeping, abdominal pain, and behavioral problems; ocular larva migrans can also occur, resulting in decreased vision, red eye or leukokoria (white pupil), retinal detachment, and vision loss

Cause	Treatment
Rickettsia akari transmitted by bites of mites carried by infected rodents	Chloramphenicol, doxycycline, ciprofloxacin, levofloxacin; supportive care
Onchocerca volvulus transmitted by the black fly	Ivermectin or diethylcarbamazine, albendazole or mebendazole; corticosteroids or antihistamines to relieve allergic reactions from microfilariae
Trauma	Symptomatic treatment with anti-inflammatory agents, steroids, analgesics; rest
Inflammation secondary to trauma or irritation	Treatment of underlying cause; orthotics, arch supports, or heel cups; stretching exercises
Inhalation of oxides of nitrogen and other gases that collect in silos	Corticosteroids; supportive respiratory treatment; volume expanders; oxygen may be required; methylene blue if methemoglobin exceeds 30%; avoidance of exposure to silo gases
Transmitted as autosomal recessive trait	No effective treatment
Unknown	Surgical resection; radiation therapy; chemotherapy with doxorubicin or dacarbazine
Irritation by toxins of sea anemones of the *Sagartia* and *Actinia* genera	Symptomatic treatment; dilute acetic acid; administration of antihistamines for hives and itching; oral and topical steroids
Usually autosomal recessive inheritance, but some cases possibly autosomal dominant and related to the abca4 gene	Symptomatic and supportive treatment, including corrective lenses
May be inherited; nonhereditary risk factors include trauma and vision problems	Depends on type, but may include patching, prescriptive lenses, surgery, eye exercises
Irritation of bursa	Symptomatic treatment, including application of warm, moist heat and administration of anti-inflammatory agents and analgesics; also, injections of corticosteroids with local anesthetics
Transmitted as autosomal recessive metabolic disorder	Dependent on symptoms; may include heart surgery, removal of organs, or gene therapy
Ingestion of *Toxocara* larvae, usually from dirt or sand; risk factors include eating without handwashing and living with or raising dogs and cats	Thiabendazole or mebendazole; albendazole; diethylcarbamazine; ocular surgery

Disease	Description
Trench fever: Wolhynia fever, shin bone fever, His-Werner disease, quintan fever	Fever with bone pain of the tibia, neck, and back, worsening with attacks; conjunctivitis, rash, splenomegaly, and hepatomegaly may also occur
Trevor's disease: dysplasia epiphysealis hemimelica	Rare developmental disorder affecting epiphyses in which the lesions increase until skeletal maturity; painless swelling occurs on the side of the joint (usually the knee), limiting movement
Trichuriasis: whipworm disease	Nematode infection of the caecum and the anterior parts of the large intestine, producing various GI effects
Tropical sprue	GI disorder that causes atrophy of the small intestine, resulting in malabsorption, malnutrition, and folic acid deficiency; characterized by bulky, pale, frothy stools with increased fecal fat and macrocytic anemia; occurs mainly in Puerto Rico, Cuba, Haiti, Dominican Republic, and India
Typhus, endemic: murine, rat or flea typhus	Mild form of typhus causing systemic illness characterized by fever, headache, rash, and myalgia
Typhus, epidemic: European, classic, or louse-borne typhus	Acute systemic illness that may lead to death; signs and symptoms include severe headache, high fever, myalgia, chills, hypotension, delirium, and rash
Typhus, scrub: Japanese river or flood fever, tsutsugamushi fever	Acute systemic disease occurring almost exclusively in the western Pacific, Japan, and Southeast Asia
Tyrosinemia	*Hereditary form:* results in liver failure and renal tubular failure, hypoglycemia, rickets, darkening of the skin, and mild mental retardation; occasionally causes liver cancer *Transient form:* usually occurs in premature neonates; marked by elevation of blood tyrosine levels
Verneuil's disease: hidradenitis supporativa	Disorder of the terminal follicular epithelium in skin with apocrine glands; characterized by comedo-like follicular occlusions, inflammation, mucopurulent discharge, and scarring
Vibrio vulnificus septicemia	Overwhelming sepsis in a cirrhotic patient who has ingested oysters; typically affects men older than age 40 in coastal states between May and October
Volkmann's disease: Volksmann's deformity	Deformity of the hand, fingers, or wrist caused by injury to the muscles of the forearm
Von Hippel-Lindau disease: cerebroretinal angiomatosis	Phakomatosis characterized by angiomatosis of the retina, cerebellum, spinal cord and, less commonly, cysts of the pancreas, kidneys, and other viscera; onset usually in third decade and marked by symptoms of retinal or cerebral tumors
Wegner's disease: Bednar-Parrot disease, Parrot's pseudoparalysis	Pseudoparalysis from osteochondrotic separation of the epiphyses; onset most common in first weeks of life and seldom after 3 months

Cause	Treatment
Bartonella quintana transmitted by body lice	Doxycycline, ceftriaxone, tetracycline, analgesics, antipyretics; delousing with lindane or other pediculicides; valve surgery if endocarditis occurs
Unknown	No known treatment
Ingestion of food contaminated with *Trichuris*	Mebendazole or albendazole
Unknown	Tetracycline or oxytetracycline; folic acid and vitamin B_{12}
Rickettsia typhi transmitted by bites of infected fleas or lice or by inhalation of contaminated flea feces	Tetracycline, doxycycline, or chloramphenicol; analgesics; antipyretics
Rickettsia prowazekii transmitted by *Pediculus humanus trichiura*	Tetracycline, doxycycline, or chloramphenicol; analgesics; antipyretics; delousing with lindane or other pediculicide
Rickettsia tsutsugamushi transmitted by mite larvae	Chloramphenicol or tetracycline (Resistance to doxycycline and chloramphenicol has appeared in northern Thailand.)
Autosomal recessive trait resulting in excess of tyrosine in blood and urine; gene maps to band 15q23-q25 identify 30 distinct mutations	Tyrosine and phenylalanine restriction; nitisinone (a tyrosine degradation inhibitor); genetic counseling; liver transplantation is last resort
Unknown	Supportive treatment; antiseptics, warm compresses with sodium chloride or Burrow's solution; irradiation; surgery; tetracycline, doxycycline; clindamycin, erythromycin, retinoids, sulfonamides, corticosteroids; hormone therapy
Vibrio vulnificus	Tetracycline or chloramphenicol
Trauma	Surgery
Transmitted as autosomal dominant trait	Early surgical intervention
Congenital syphilis	Effective treatment of syphilis during pregnancy; after delivery, neonate is also treated for syphilis

Disease	Description
Werdnig-Hoffmann disease: spinal muscular atrophy	Progressive degeneration of anterior horn cells and bulbar motor nuclei in a fetus or neonate; type 1 is most severe, as neonates are born with weak thin muscles and breathing problems; type 2 has less severe symptoms during early infancy, but becomes progressively weaker until the infant's death; type 3 is the least severe form, with signs and symptoms appearing after age 2 (weakening becomes more profound as the patient ages, but survival may be into early adulthood)
Whipple's disease: intestinal lipodystrophy, lipophagia granulomatosis	GI malabsorption disorder characterized by chronic diarrhea and progressive wasting, with skin pigmentation and polyarthralgia
Wilms' tumor: congenital nephroblastoma, embryonal adenomyosarcoma	Malignant mixed tumors of the kidneys, primarily affecting children; major signs — abdominal mass, enlarged abdomen, hypertension, vomiting, and hematuria
Wolman's disease: infantile form of acid lipase deficiency	A lysosomal storage disorder; hepatosplenomegaly, steatorrhea, and adrenal calcification manifested in the first weeks of life; results from accumulation of large amounts of lipids (especially cholesteryl esters and glycerides) in the liver, spleen, lymph nodes, and other tissues
Yaws: frambesia tropica	Chronic relapsing infection characterized by highly contagious primary and secondary cutaneous lesions and noncontagious tertiary lesions, as well as systemic signs and symptoms; primarily occurs in Africa, Asia, South America, and Oceania—where overcrowding and poor sanitation prevail in warm, humid tropical regions
Yellow fever	Flavivirus infection that causes sudden illness accompanied by fever, slow pulse rate, and headache, nausea, and vomiting; endemic in tropical Africa and Central and South America
Zygomycosis: phycomycosis, mucormycosis	Fungal infection most often seen in patients who are immunocompromised; several forms, including rhinocerebral, GI, pulmonary, and disseminated mucormycosis

Cause	Treatment
Transmitted as autosomal recessive trait	Symptomatic and supportive treatment, including physiotherapy and bracing; airway clearance is a priority due to secretions
Tropheryma whippelii	Appropriate antibiotic therapy; supportive therapy with fluid and electrolyte replacement; iron, folate, vitamin D, and magnesium supplementation
Wilms' tumor recessive oncogen WT_1 at 11p15 locus	Nephrectomy; radiation therapy; chemotherapy
Transmitted as autosomal recessive trait; transmission caused by mutations of a specific gene located on chromosome 10	No specific therapy; usually fatal by age 6 months
Treponema pertenue	Penicillin G benzathine, tetracycline, or erythromycin; after single penicillin injection, early lesions become noninfectious in 24 hours; tissue damage occurring later in yaws is irreversible
Flavivirus transmitted by *Haemagogus* mosquitoes in South America and *Aedes africanus* in Africa; the mosquitoes bite monkeys, which act as hosts for the virus, then the mosquitos bite humans, transmitting the disease	Supportive treatment for fluid volume and maintenance of normothermia; yellow fever vaccine; prevention of gastric bleeding with histamine-2 antagonists
Zygomycetes	Treatment of the underlying condition; amphotericin B; surgical removal of necrotic tissue

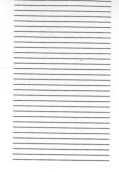

Community resources

Acquired immunodeficiency syndrome

National AIDS Hotline (Sponsored by the Centers of Disease Control and Prevention [CDC])
Phone: 800-342-AIDS; for Spanish speakers, 800-344-7432; for people who are hearing impaired, 800-243-7889
Web site: *www.ashastd.org/nah*

CDC National Prevention Information Network
P.O. Box 6003
Rockville, MD 20849-6003
Phone: 800-458-5231
Web site: *www.cdcnpin.org*

Association of Nurses in AIDS Care
3538 Ridgewood Rd.
Akron, Ohio 44333-3122
Phone: 800-260-6780
Web site: *www.anacnet.org*

Alcoholism

Al-Anon/Alateen Family Group Headquarters
1600 Corporate Landing Pkwy.
Virginia Beach, VA 23454-5617
Phone: 888-425-2666
Web site: *www.al-anon.alateen.org*

Alcoholics Anonymous
475 Riverside Dr., 11th Fl.
New York, NY 10115
Web site: *www.aa.org*

Arthritis

Arthritis Foundation
P.O. Box 7669
Atlanta, GA 30357-0669
Phone: 800-283-7800
Web site: *www.arthritis.org*

Asthma

Asthma and Allergy Foundation of America
1233 20th St., NW, Ste. 402
Washington, DC 20036
Phone: 800-7-ASTHMA
Web site: *www.aafa.org*

Birth defects

March of Dimes
1275 Mamaroneck Ave.
White Plains, NY 10605
Web site: *www.modimes.org*

Blindness

American Foundation for the Blind
11 Pennsylvania Plaza, Ste. 300
New York, NY 10001
Phone: 800-232-5463
Web site: *www.afb.org*

Cancer

American Cancer Society
1599 Clifton Rd., NE
Atlanta, GA 30329
Phone: 800-ACS-2345
Web site: *www.cancer.org*

Cerebral palsy
United Cerebral Palsy Association
1660 L St., NW, Ste. 700
Washington, DC 20036
Phone: 800-872-5827
Web site: *www.ucpa.org*

Diabetes
American Diabetes Association
1701 N. Beauregard St.
Alexandria, VA 22311
Phone: 800-DIABETES
Web site: *www.diabetes.org*

Juvenile Diabetes Research Foundation
International
120 Wall St.
New York, NY 10005-4001
Phone: 800-JDF-CURE
Web site: *www.jdf.org*

Eating disorders
Eating Disorders Awareness and
Prevention
603 Stewart St., Ste. 803
Seattle, WA 98101
Phone: 206-382-3587
Web site: *www.edap.org*

Epilepsy
Epilepsy Foundation
4351 Garden City Dr.
Landover, MD 20785-7223
Phone: 800-332-1000
Web site: *www.epilepsyfoundation.org*

Genetic disorders
Cleft Palate Foundation
1504 E. Franklin St., Ste. 102
Chapel Hill, NC 27514-2820
Phone: 919-933-9044
Web site: *www.cleftline.org*

Cystic Fibrosis Foundation
6931 Arlington Rd.
Bethesda, MD 20814
Phone: 800-FIGHT-CF
Web site: *www.cff.org*

National Down Syndrome Society
666 Broadway
New York, NY 10012
Phone: 800-221-4602
Web site: *www.ndss.org*

National Fragile X Foundation
P.O. Box 190488
San Francisco, CA 94119
Phone: 800-688-8765
Web site: *www.nfxf.org*

National Marfan Foundation
22 Manhasset Ave.
Port Washington, NY 11050
Phone: 800-8-MARFAN
Web site: *www.marfan.org*

National Tay-Sachs and Allied Diseases
Association
2001 Beacon St., Ste. 204
Brighton, MA 02135
Phone: 800-906-8723
Web site: *www.ntsad.org*

Osteogenesis Imperfecta Foundation
804 W. Diamond Ave., Ste. 210
Gaithersburg, MD 20878
Phone: 800-981-2663
Web site: *www.oif.org*

Hearing impairment
American Academy of Audiology
11730 Plaza America Dr., Ste. 300
Reston, VA 20190
Phone: 800-222-2336
Web site: *www.audiology.org*

American Speech-Language-Hearing
Association
10801 Rockville Pike
Rockville, MD 20852
Phone: 800-498-2071
Web site: *www.asha.org*

American Tinnitus Association
P.O. Box 5
Portland, OR 97207-0005
Phone: 800-634-8978
www.ata.org

Heart disease
American Heart Association
7272 Greenville Ave.
Dallas, TX 75231
Phone: 800-AHA-USA1
Web site: *www.americanheart.org*

Hemophilia
National Hemophilia Foundation
116 W. 32 St., 11th Fl.
New York, NY 10001
Phone: 800-42-HANDI
Web site: *www.hemophilia.org*

Huntington's disease
Huntington's Disease Society of America
158 W. 29 St., 7th Fl.
New York, NY 10001-5300
Phone: 800-345-4372
Web site: *www.hdsa.org*

Infectious diseases
Centers for Disease Control and
Prevention
1600 Clifton Rd.
Atlanta, GA 30333
Phone: 800-311-3435
Web site: *www.cdc.gov*

Lupus
Lupus Foundation of America
2000 L St., NW, Ste. 710
Washington, D.C. 20036
Phone: 202-349-1155
Web site: *www.lupus.org*

Lyme disease
Lyme Disease Foundation
P.O. Box 332
Tolland, CT 06084-0332
Phone: 860-870-0070
Web site: *www.lyme.org*

Mental retardation
Association for Retarded Citizens
1010 Wayne Ave., Ste. 650
Silver Spring, MD 20910
Phone: 301-565-3842
Web site: *www.thearc.org*

Multiple sclerosis
National Multiple Sclerosis Society
733 Third Ave.
New York, NY 10017
Phone: 800-FIGHT-MS
Web site: *www.nmss.org*

Muscular dystrophy
National Muscular Dystrophy Association
3300 E. Sunrise Dr.
Tucson, AZ 85718
Phone: 800-572-1717
Web site: *www.mdausa.org*

Myasthenia gravis
Myasthenia Gravis Foundation of America
1821 W. University Ave. West, Ste. S256
St. Paul, MN 55104
Phone: 800-541-5454
Web site: *www.myasthenia.org*

Neurofibromatosis
National Neurofibromatosis Foundation
95 Pine St., 16th Fl.
New York, NY 10005
Phone: 800-323-7938
Web site: *www.nf.org*

Osteoporosis
National Osteoporosis Foundation
1232 22nd St., NW
Washington, DC 20037-1292
Phone: 202-223-2226
Web site: *www.nof.org*

Parkinson's disease
National Parkinson Foundation
1501 NW 9th Ave., Bob Hope Rd.
Miami, FL 33136-1494
Phone: 800-327-4545
Web site: *www.parkinson.org*

Psoriasis
National Psoriasis Foundation
6600 SW 92nd Ave., Ste. 300
Portland, OR 97223-7195
Phone: 800-723-9166
Web site: *www.psoriasis.org*

Retinitis pigmentosa
Foundation Fighting Blindness
11435 Cronhill Dr.
Owings Mills, MD 21117-2220
Phone: 888-394-3937
Web site: *www.blindness.org*

Sickle cell anemia
Sickle Cell Disease Association of America
200 Corporate Pointe, Ste. 495
Culver City, CA 90230-8727
Phone: 800-421-8453
Web site: *www.sicklecelldisease.org*

Sjögren's syndrome
Sjögren's Syndrome Foundation
8120 Woodmont Ave.
Bethesda, MD 20814
Phone: 800-475-6473
Web site: *www.sjogrens.com*

Spina bifida
Spina Bifida Association of America
4590 MacArthur Blvd., NW, Ste. 250
Washington, DC 20007-4226
Phone: 800-621-3141
Web site: *www.sbaa.org*

Stroke
National Stroke Association
9707 E. Easter Lane
Englewood, CO 80112
Phone: 800-787-6537
Web site: *www.stroke.org*

Sudden infant death syndrome
SIDS Alliance
1314 Bedford Ave., Ste. 210
Baltimore, MD 21208
Phone: 800-221-7437
Web site: *www.sidsalliance.org*

Miscellaneous
American Red Cross
2025 E St., NW
Washington, DC 20006
Phone: 202-303-4498
Web site: *www.redcross.org*

Herpes Resource Center
P.O. Box 13827
Research Triangle Park, NC 27709
Phone: 919-361-8400
Web site: *www.ashastd.org/hrc*

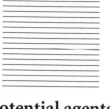

Potential agents of bioterrorism

Listed below are examples of biological agents that may be used as biological weapons and the major signs and symptoms for each.

POTENTIAL AGENTS	MAJOR ASSOCIATED SIGNS AND SYMPTOMS													
	Abdominal pain	Back pain	Blood pressure, decreased	Chest pain	Chills	Cough	Diarrhea, bloody	Diarrhea, watery	Diplopia	Dysarthria	Dysphagia	Dyspnea	Fever	Headache
Anthrax (cutaneous)													●	●
Anthrax (GI)	●						●						●	
Anthrax (inhalation)			●	●	●	●						●	●	
Botulism									●	●	●	●		
Cholera				●				●						
Plague (bubonic and septicemic)					●								●	
Plague (pneumonic)				●	●	●						●	●	●
Smallpox	●	●											●	●
Tularemia				●	●	●						●	●	●

Hematemesis	Hemoptysis	Lymphadenopathy	Malaise	Muscle spasms (muscle cramps)	Myalgias	Nausea	Oliguria	Papular rash (skin lesions)	Ptosis	Skin turgor, decreased	Stridor	Tachycardia	Tachypnea	Vomiting	Weakness
		●	●					●							
●					●									●	
											●				●
									●						●
				●			●			●		●		●	●
		●													
	●				●								●		
			●					●							
					●										

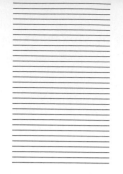

Acknowledgments

We thank the following people and companies for contributing the photographs that appear in the current and prior editions of *Professional Guide to Diseases*:

p. 139	John Murphy, Photographer
p. 712	Marc S. Lapayowker, MD, Temple University Hospital, Philadelphia
pp. 835, 840, 877, 1210	Consultant Magazine, Cliggott Publishing Co., Greenwich, Conn.
p. 915	Ron Hurst, Photographer, Little, Brown, & Co., Boston
pp. 997, 1004	Centers for Disease Control and Prevention, Atlanta
p. 1159	Joel I. Hamburger, MD, Northland Radioisotope Lab, Southfield, Mich.
p. 1240	Paul A. Cohen, Photographer
p. 1244, 1245	Reed and Carnrick, Kenilworth, N.J.

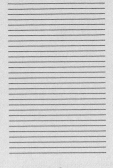

Index

A

ABCs, assessing, in trauma, 281-283
Abdominal aneurysm, 1138-1141
  repair of, 1139i, 1140i
Abdominal fat pad aspiration in amyloidosis, 903
Abdominal injuries, 299-301
  effects of, 299, 300i
  projectile pathway in, 299i
ABG analysis. *See* Arterial blood gas analysis.
ABO incompatibility, 988t
Abortion, 956-959
  in pregnancy-related cardiovascular disease, 970
Abortive poliomyelitis, 245. *See also* Poliomyelitis.
Abrasion, 332, 333t
Abruptio placentae, 967-969
  degrees of separation in, 967, 968i
Abscess
  amebic liver, 760
  anorectal, 738-739
  brain, 654-656
  intracranial, 654-656
  liver, 759-760
  lung, 548-549
  peritonsillar, 1219-1221
  retropharyngeal, 1219-1221
  of throat, 1219-1221
Absence seizures, 640-641
Acalculous cholecystitis, 767-769
Acceleration-deceleration cervical injuries, 292-293
Accommodation, 1155
Acetazolamide, 928
Acetylcholinesterase levels in neural tube defects, 40
Acetylcysteine as acetaminophen poisoning antidote, 755
Achilles tendon contracture, 610
Achilles tendon rupture, 302

Acid-base balance, regulation of, 773
Acid lipase deficiency, infantile form of, 1312-1313t
Acid phosphatase levels in prostatic cancer, 103
Acid therapy for warts, 1264, 1265
Acne vulgaris, 1246-1248
  pathophysiology of, 1247i
Acoustic neurinoma. *See* Schwannoma.
Acoustic neurofibromatosis, 8-10
  diagnostic criteria for, 9
Acquired adrenal virilism, 859
Acquired hypogammaglobulinemia, 390-391
Acquired immunodeficiency syndrome, 393-397
  common infections and neoplasms in, 394
  Kaposi's sarcoma and, 136-137
  tests for diagnosing and tracking, 396t
Acquired inflammatory heart disease, 1077-1086
Acrocyanosis, 1288-1289t
Acromegaly, 830-832
Actinic keratosis, 130, 131t
Actinomycosis, 185-186
Activated charcoal for poisoning, 325
Active retinochoroiditis, 268
Acute angle-closure glaucoma, 1184-1186
Acute coronary syndrome. *See* Myocardial infarction.
Acute coryza. *See* Common cold.
Acute dermal gangrene. *See* Necrotizing fasciitis.
Acute febrile respiratory illness, 227t. *See also* Adenovirus infection.
Acute follicular conjunctivitis, 227t. *See also* Adenovirus infection.
Acute glomerulonephritis, 786-787
Acute idiopathic polyneuritis. *See* Guillain-Barré syndrome.
Acute infarct imaging, 1063
Acute infective tubulointerstitial nephritis, 784-786
Acute intermittent porphyria, 905t

i refers to an illustration; t refers to a table.

Acute leukemia, 144-147
  forms of, 144
  predisposing factors to, 145
Acute pharyngoconjunctival fever, 227t. See
  also Adenovirus infection.
Acute poststreptococcal glomerulonephritis,
  786-787
Acute pyelonephritis, 784-786
Acute renal failure, 782-784
Acute respiratory disease, 227t. See also Aden-
  ovirus infection.
Acute respiratory distress syndrome, 521-524
  pathophysiology of, 522i
Acute respiratory failure in chronic obstructive
  pulmonary disease, 524-526. See also
  Chronic obstructive pulmonary disease.
Acute spasmodic laryngitis, 518
Acute sporadic encephalitis, 234. See also
  Herpes simplex.
Acute transverse myelitis, 659-660
Acute tubular necrosis, 787-789
  in transfusion reactions, 364
Acute tubulointerstitial nephritis, 787-789
Acyanotic defects, congenital, 1064-1072
Acyclovir
  for genital herpes, 1001
  for herpes zoster, 236
Adaptive Behavior Scale, 414
Addisonian crisis, 850, 851
  pituitary tumors and, 63
Addison's anemia, 1020-1023
Addison-Schilder disease, 1282-1283t
Addison's disease, 849-852
Adenoidectomy, 1216
Adenoid hyperplasia, 1215-1216
Adenoid hypertrophy, 1215-1216
Adenoviral pneumonia, 538-539t
Adenovirus infection, 226-227
  types of, 227t
ADHD. See Attention deficit hyperactivity
  disorder.
ADH. See Antidiuretic hormone.
Adolescent pregnancy, 970-972
Adrenal crisis, 850, 851
Adrenalectomy, 854, 856
Adrenal glands
  disorders of, 849-863
  hormones secreted by, 826-827
Adrenal hypofunction, 849-852
Adrenal insufficiency, 849-852
Adrenogenital syndrome, 858-861
  precocious puberty and, 945, 1013, 1014
Adrenoleukodystrophy, 1282-1283t
Adult group B streptococcal infections,
  170-171t
Adult respiratory distress syndrome. See Acute
  respiratory distress syndrome.

African Americans, cultural considerations
  for, 1279t
African trypanosomiasis, 1282-1283t
Afterload, 1059
Agammaglobulinemia, 390-391
Agglutination tests
  in amebiasis, 266
  in brucellosis, 203
  in cholera, 195
  in cytomegalovirus infection, 252
  in histoplasmosis, 218
  in mononucleosis, 249
  in salmonellosis, 189
  in shigellosis, 190
Agoraphobia, 459-461
  diagnostic criteria for, 460
Agranulocytosis, 1053-1055
AIDS. See Acquired immunodeficiency
  syndrome.
Airborne transmission, 154
  isolation precautions for, 157
Air-fluidized bed, 1275
Air-fluid lock syndrome, 721-722
Akathisia as antipsychotic adverse effect, 443
Akinesia in Parkinson's disease, 658
Akinetic seizure, 641
Alanine aminotransferase
  in abdominal injuries, 300
  in anorexia, 494
  in chest injuries, 296
  in kidney cancer, 94
  in liver cancer, 96
  in nonviral hepatitis, 755
  in toxic shock syndrome, 279
  in trichinosis, 269
  in viral hepatitis, 754
Albendazole
  for ascariasis, 272
  for enterobiasis, 274
  for hookworm disease, 271
  for taeniasis, 272
Albers-Schönberg disease, 1282-1283t
Albert's disease, 1308-1309t
Albinism, 20-21
Albumin levels
  in anorexia, 494
  in cystic fibrosis, 16
  in leprosy, 212
  nutritional status assessment and, 874
  in protein-calorie malnutrition, 889
Albumin transfusion for erythroblastosis
  fetalis, 990
Alcohol abuse, 432t. See also Alcohol-related
  disorder.
Alcoholic cirrhosis, 756
Alcoholics Anonymous, 428, 429

i refers to an illustration; t refers to a table.

Alcohol-related disorder, 426-431
  complications of, 427
Alcohol withdrawal, signs and symptoms
  of, 427-428, 429t, 431
Aldosterone
  function of, 773, 826
  hypersecretion of, 856-858
Alemtuzumab for chronic lymphocytic
  leukemia, 149
Alendronate for Paget's disease, 598
Alimentary tract. See Gastrointestinal tract.
Alkaline phosphatase levels
  in ankylosing spondylitis, 374
  in blastomycosis, 219
  in bone tumors, 124
  in breast cancer, 79
  in celiac disease, 715
  in gallbladder cancer, 102
  in Hodgkin's disease, 139
  in kidney cancer, 94
  in liver cancer, 96
  in nonviral hepatitis, 755
  normal values in, 776t
  in prostatic cancer, 104
  in renal infarction, 790
  in viral hepatitis, 754
Allergic angiitis, 385t
Allergic aspergillosis, 216, 217
Allergic disorders, 345-346, 350-364
Allergic purpura, 1040-1042
Allergic rhinitis, 354-356
Allergic transfusion reactions, 363-364
Allopurinol
  for chronic granulocytic leukemia, 148
  for chronic lymphocytic leukemia, 150
  for gout, 587
  for renal calculi, 793
Alopecia, 1250-1251, 1251i
Alpha-fetoprotein levels
  in liver cancer, 96
  in neural tube defects, 40
  in testicular cancer, 106
  as tumor marker, 50
Alport's syndrome, 1282-1283t
Alteplase, 1104
Alternating pressure mattress, 1275
Alzheimer's disease, 660-662
Amantadine for influenza, 228, 229
Amebiasis, 265-266
Amebic dysentery, 265-266
Amebic granuloma, 265-266
Amebic liver abscess, 760
Ameboma, 265-266
Amenorrhea, 951-952
  as anorexia complication, 493
  diagnosing, 953i
American trypanosomiasis, 1282-1283t

Amiloride for diabetes insipidus, 833
Amino acids, function of, 871t
Aminoglutethimide for Cushing's syndrome,
  854, 856
Aminophylline for anaphylaxis, 360
Ammonia intoxication in liver cancer, 97
Ammonia levels in hepatic encephalopathy, 764
Ammonium chloride
  for hypochloremia, 920
  for metabolic alkalosis, 927, 928
Amnesia
  in concussion, 285
  dissociative, 481-482
Amniocentesis
  in Down syndrome, 32
  genetic testing and, 7
  in neural tube defects, 40
  in Tay-Sachs disease, 17-18
Amniotic fluid analysis
  in erythroblastosis fetalis, 990
  in premature rupture of membranes, 977
Amphetamines
  abuse of, 435t
  for obesity, 888
Amputation
  for bone tumors, 124, 126
  for cold injuries, 315
  for snakebites, 327
  traumatic, 307-308
Amylase levels
  in abdominal injuries, 300
  in anorexia, 494
  in pancreatic cancer, 88
  in pancreatitis, 735
Amyloidosis, 902-903
Amyotrophic lateral sclerosis, 671-672
Anabolism, 870
Anaerobic cellulitis, 183
Anal fissure, 744
Analgesics for pain disorder, 476.
Anaphylactoid purpura, 1040-1041
Anaphylaxis, 359-361
Andersen's glycogen storage disease, 893t
Androgens
  for breast cancer, 80
  for endometriosis, 943
Anemia pseudoleukemia infantum, 1296-1297t
Anemia, 1020-1034
  aplastic, 1025-1028
  Blackfan-Diamond, 1025
  in chronic granulocytic leukemia, 147
  congenital hypoplastic, 1025
  Cooley's, 1030-1031
  copper deficiency, 1288-1289t
  erythroblastic, 1030-1031
  folic acid deficiency, 1024-1025
  hypoplastic, 1025-1028

Anemia *(continued)*
 iron deficiency, 1031-1034
 Jaksch's, 1296-1297t
 juvenile pernicious, 1020
 megaloblastic, 1302-1303t
 pernicious, 702, 1020-1023
 sickle cell, 21-25
 sideroblastic, 1028-1030, 1029i
 supportive management of patients
  with, 1034
Anencephaly, 39. *See also* Neural tube defects.
Angina
 forms of, 1097
 pain in, 1083, 1097
Angioedema, 361-362
Angiography
 in abdominal injuries, 300
 cerebral, 626
 in cerebral aneurysm, 633
 in cor pulmonale, 528
 in kidney cancer, 94
 in pancreatic cancer, 88
 in pituitary tumors, 63
 pulmonary, 511
 in pulmonary embolism, 544
 in pulmonary hypertension, 551
 in stroke, 644
Angiotensin-converting enzyme inhibitors for
  nephrotic syndrome, 797
Animal bites, first aid in, 251
Anion gap, 926
Anisocytosis, 1029
Anistreplase, 1104-1105
Ankylosing spondylitis, 373-375
Ann Arbor classification system for Hodgkin's
  disease, 140
Anorectal abscess, 738-739
Anorectal contracture, 741
Anorectal fistula, 738-739
Anorectal stenosis, 741
Anorectal stricture, 741
Anorexia nervosa, 492-495
 complications of, 493
 diagnostic criteria for, 494
 in protein-calorie malnutrition, 889
Anovulation, 948, 949
Antacids
 for gastritis, 702
 for hypocalcemia, 919
 for pancreatic cancer, 89
Anthracosilicosis, 567-569
Anthracosis, 567-569
Anthrax, 204
Antiandrogen therapy
 for breast cancer, 80
 for prostatic cancer, 104

Antianxiety drugs
 for generalized anxiety disorder, 463
 for panic disorder, 465
 for personality disorders, 488
 for phobias, 459-460
 for posttraumatic stress disorder, 469
Antibiotic therapy
 for acne, 1246-1247
 for actinomycosis, 185-186
 for acute pyelonephritis, 785
 for anthrax, 204
 for asthma, 353
 for brain abscess, 655
 for brucellosis, 203
 for campylobacteriosis, 205
 for cholera, 196
 for chronic granulomatous disease, 401
 for cor pulmonale, 529
 for encephalitis, 654
 for endocarditis, 1080-1081
 for epiglottiditis, 520
 for ehrlichiosis, 207
 for gonorrhea, 997
 for granulocytopenia, 1054-1055
 for *Haemophilus influenzae* infection, 198
 for legionnaires' disease, 531
 for listeriosis, 180
 for liver abscess, 760
 for lower urinary tract infection, 809
 for lung abscess, 549
 for Lyme disease, 208-209
 for mastitis, 983
 for meningitis, 648, 649
 for meningococcal infections, 177
 for near drowning, 319
 for necrotizing fasciitis, 174
 for nocardiosis, 186
 for ornithosis, 278
 for osteomyelitis, 592
 for otitis media, 1198
 for pancreatic cancer, 89
 for pancreatitis, 736
 for pelvic inflammatory disease, 950
 for peritonitis, 720
 for prostatitis, 819
 for *Pseudomonas* infections, 194
 for puerperal infection, 980
 for rheumatic fever, 1085
 for Rocky Mountain spotted fever, 258
 for salmonellosis, 189
 for septic arthritis, 583-584
 for septic shock, 197
 for shigellosis, 190-191
 for tetanus, 181
 for toxic shock syndrome, 279
 for tularemia, 206

i refers to an illustration; t refers to a table.

Antibiotic therapy (continued)
  for vancomycin-resistant enterococcus
    infection, 176
  for vesicoureteral reflux, 811
Antibody-dependent cytotoxicity, 346
Antibody tests
  in celiac disease, 715
  in female infertility, 949
  in giardiasis, 267
  in human immunodeficiency virus infection,
    395, 396t
  in juvenile rheumatoid arthritis, 372
  in latex allergy, 358
  in legionnaires' disease, 531
  in malaria, 263
  in rabies, 250
  in severe acute respiratory syndrome, 548
  in Sjögren's syndrome, 376
  in systemic lupus erythematosus, 378
Antibody titers
  in coccidioidomycosis, 220
  in cytomegalovirus infection, 252
  in herpangina, 243
  in infectious mononucleosis, 249
  in influenza, 228
  in Lassa fever, 253
  in legionnaires' disease, 531
  in mumps, 248
  in ornithosis, 278
  in parainfluenza, 226
  in plague, 202
  in poliomyelitis, 246
  in rabies, 250
  in respiratory syncytial virus infection, 224
  in Rocky Mountain spotted fever, 258
  in roseola infantum, 243
  in rubella, 238
  in rubeola, 240
  in smallpox, 241
  in trichinosis, 269
Anticholinergics
  for pancreatic cancer, 89
  for Parkinson's disease, 658
Anticholinesterase therapy
  for Alzheimer's disease, 661
  for myasthenia gravis, 670, 671
Anticoagulation therapy
  for cor pulmonale, 529
  for pregnancy-related cardiovascular
    disease, 969
  for pulmonary embolism, 545
  for renal infarction, 790
  for renal vein thrombosis, 795
Anticonvulsants
  for arteriovenous malformations, 637
  for bipolar disorders, 451
  for brain tumors, 61

Anticonvulsants (continued)
  for cerebral palsy, 628
  for epilepsy, 641
  for stroke, 645
Antidepressants
  for bipolar disorders, 454
  for major depression, 456, 459
  for migraine headache, 638
  for obsessive-compulsive disorder, 466
  for panic disorder, 465
Antidiabetic drug therapy
  for diabetes mellitus, 866-867
  pregnancy and, 974
Antidiuretic hormone. See also Vasopressin.
  deficiency of, 832-834
  excessive secretion of, 924-925
  function of, 773, 825-826
Anti-DNA test for systemic lupus erythemato-
    sus, 378
Antifungal therapy
  for aspergillosis, 217
  for blastomycosis, 219
  for candidiasis, 214
  for chronic granulomatous disease, 401-402
  for chronic mucocutaneous candidiasis, 398
  for coccidioidomycosis, 221
  for cryptococcosis, 215
  for dermatophytosis, 1239-1240
  for histoplasmosis, 218
  for sporotrichosis, 222
Antigenic variation, 228
Antigens, 341-342
Antigen tests
  in cryptococcosis, 215
  in histoplasmosis, 218
  in strongyloidiasis, 277
Antihistamines
  for allergic rhinitis, 356
  for atopic dermatitis, 357
  for dermatitis, 1257
  for transfusion reactions, 364
  for urticaria, 362
Antilymphocyte serum as immuno-
    suppressant, 349
Antimalarial drugs
  for malaria, 263, 264
  for rheumatoid arthritis, 366, 367t
Antimicrobial therapy. See also Antibiotic
    therapy.
  for leprosy, 212
  for plague, 202
  for pneumonia, 537, 539t
  for relapsing fever, 210
Antinuclear antibody tests
  in juvenile rheumatoid arthritis, 372
  in scleroderma, 383
  in systemic lupus erythematosus, 378

i refers to an illustration; t refers to a table.

Antipsychotic drugs
  adverse effects of, 443
  for delusional disorders, 447-448
  for schizophrenia, 441
Antipyretics
  for croup, 518
  for transfusion reaction, 364
  for tularemia, 206
Antiretroviral therapy for acquire immuno-
    deficiency syndrome, 395-396
Antisocial personality disorder, 485, 489
Antithymocyte globulin
  for aplastic anemias,1027
  as immunosuppressant, 349
Antithyroid drug therapy, 842-843
Antivenin therapy for snakebites, 327, 328
Antiviral therapy
  for herpes simples, 234
  for herpes zoster, 236
  for human immunodeficiency virus
      infection, 397
  for varicella, 232
Anxiety. *See* Generalized anxiety disorder.
Anxiety disorders, 459-471
Aortic aneurysm
  abdominal, 1138-1141
  thoracic, 1134-1138
  types of, 1135i
Aortic arch syndrome, 386t
Aortic insufficiency, 1087t, 1090
Aortic laceration or rupture, 296, 297
Aortic stenosis, 1087t, 1090
Aortic valve, 1058
Aortography
  in abdominal aneurysm, 1138
  in chest injuries, 296
  in thoracic dissection, 1136t
Aphthous stomatitis, 687, 689, 689i
Aplastic anemias, 1025-1028
Aplastic crisis in sickle cell anemia, 22-23
Apocrine glands, 1229
Appalachian Mountain disease, 217-218
Appendicitis, 718-719
Aqueous humor, 1154
  normal flow of, 1184i
Arab Americans, cultural considerations
      for, 1280t
Arc-welders' disease, 1282-1283t
ARDS. *See* Acute respiratory distress syndrome.
Argon laser trabeculoplasty, 1186
Ariboflavinosis, 877-879
Arm care, postoperative, 81
Arm fractures, 302-306
  classifying, 305
Armstrong's disease, 1282-1283t
Arnold-Chiari syndrome, 39, 631

Aromatase inhibitors for cancer, 54
Arousal disorder, 495-497
Arrhythmias, 1125-1134
  as myocardial infarction complication, 1101t
  types of, 1127-1134t
Arterial blood gas analysis, 510
  in abdominal injuries, 300
  in acute respiratory distress syndrome, 521
  in acute respiratory failure in chronic ob-
      structive pulmonary disease, 524, 525
  in asbestosis, 567
  in asphyxia, 318
  in asthma, 352
  in bronchiolitis obliterans, 542
  in chronic obstructive pulmonary disease,
      555t, 557t
  in cor pulmonale, 529
  in hemothorax, 549
  in infant respiratory distress syndrome, 515
  in metabolic acidosis, 926
  in metabolic alkalosis, 927
  in near drowning, 319
  in *Pneumocystis carinii* pneumonia, 260
  in pneumothorax, 536
  in pulmonary edema, 526
  in pulmonary embolism, 545
  in pulmonary fibrosis, 562
  in pulmonary hypertension, 550
  in respiratory acidosis, 533
  in respiratory alkalosis, 534
  in sarcoidosis, 546
  in septic shock, 197
Arterial occlusive disease, 1148-1151
  types of, 1149t
Arterial switch, 1076
Arteries, 1059, 1061
  of leg, 1142i
Arteriography. *See also* Cerebral arteriography.
  in bladder cancer, 98
  coronary, 1063
  in liver cancer, 97
  peripheral, 1064
Arteriovenous malformations, 635-637
Arthritis, types of, 584. *See also specific type.*
Arthrodesis, 366, 590
Arthrokatadysis, 1304-1305t
Arthro-ophthalmopathy, 13-14
Arthroplasty, 366, 369, 590
Arthroscopy, 574
Arytenoidectomy, 1221-1222
Asbestosis, 566-567
Ascariasis, 271-272
Ascites fluid aspiration in ovarian cancer, 118
Ascorbic acid. *See* Vitamin C.
Asherman's syndrome, 948
Asiatic cholera, 194-196

Aspartate aminotransferase
  in abdominal injuries, 300
  in anorexia, 494
  in chest injuries, 296
  in kidney cancer, 94
  in liver cancer, 96
  in Lyme disease, 208
  in nonviral hepatitis, 755
  in polymyositis, 388
  in toxic shock syndrome, 279
  in trichinosis, 269
  in viral hepatitis, 754
Aspergilloma, 216, 217
Aspergillosis, 216-217
  forms of, 216
Aspergillosis endophthalmitis, 216, 217
Asphyxia, 316, 318
Aspiration pneumonia, 538-539t
Aspirin
  for chronic granulocytic leukemia, 148
Aspirin
  for ankylosing spondylitis, 374
  for juvenile rheumatoid arthritis, 372
  for rheumatoid arthritis, 366, 367t
Asterixis, 764
Asthma, 350-354
  in chronic obstructive pulmonary disease,
    554-555t
  determining severity of, 351-352
  miner's, 567-569
Astrocytoma, 57t, 59, 61, 70. See also Brain tu-
    mors, malignant and Spinal neoplasms,
    malignant.
Asystole, 1134t
Ataxia telangiectasia, 1282-1283t
Ataxic cerebral palsy, 626, 627
Atelectasis, 531-533
Atherosclerosis, 1096
Athetoid cerebral palsy, 626, 627
Athlete's foot, 1239, 1240i, 1241
Atonic constipation, 732-733
Atopic dermatitis, 356-357
Atopic eczema. See Dermatitis.
Atria, 1058
Atrial balloon septostomy, 1076
Atrial fibrillation, 1130t
Atrial flutter, 1129t
Atrial septal defect, 1066-1068
Atrioventricular valves, 1058
Atrophia bulborum hereditaria, 1304-1305t
Atrophy, 1231i
Attention deficit hyperactivity disorder,
    422-424
  diagnostic criteria for, 423
Audiometric testing, 1190
Auditory brain stem–evoked response in
    Stickler's syndrome, 14

Auditory complications
  in Stickler's syndrome, 13
Auspitz sign, 1266
Autistic disorder, 418-422
  diagnostic criteria for, 421
Autografts, 310
Autoimmune disorders, 347, 350, 364-389
Autoimmune thrombocytopenia, 1046-1047
Autoimmune thyroiditis, 838
Autonomic nervous system, 617, 621
Autosomal dominant disorders, 8-14
  inheritance patterns in, 4-5, 5i
Autosomal recessive disorders, 14-25
  inheritance patterns in, 5, 5i
Autosplenectomy, 22
Aversion therapy, 468
  for alcohol-related disorder, 428
Avoidant personality disorder, 485, 489
Avulsion, 332, 333t
Azathioprine, 366
Azithromycin
  for chlamydial infections, 999
  for nonspecific genitourinary infections, 1007

B

Bacillary dysentery, 190-191
Bacteremia, 160-161t, 187, 188, 188t
Bacteria, 153
  tissue damage caused by, 154i
Bacterial contamination, transfusion reactions
    and, 363-364
Bacterial endocarditis. See Endocarditis.
Bacterial pneumonia, 538-539t
Balanitis
  penile cancer and, 107
  in Reiter's syndrome, 381
Balloon catheter dilation
  of prostate, 822
  for renovascular hypertension, 799
Balloon urethroplasty, 822
Bang's disease, 202-204
Barber's psoriasis, 1266
Barbiturate abuse, 433t
Barium studies, 684
  in amebiasis, 266
  in colorectal cancer, 93
  in corrosive esophagitis, 695
  in Crohn's disease, 711, 712i
  in diverticular disease, 717
  in esophageal cancer, 86
  in esophageal diverticulum, 698
  in fallopian tube cancer, 122
  in gastric cancer, 82
  in gastroesophageal reflux disease, 690-691
  in giardiasis, 267

Barium studies *(continued)*
  in hiatal hernia, 700
  in Hirschsprung's disease, 731
  in intestinal obstruction, 723
  in intussusception, 728
  in ovarian cancer, 118
  in peptic ulcers, 706
Barometer-maker's disease, 1284-1285t
Barrier precautions against infection, 155
Basal body temperature graph, 949
Basal cell carcinoma of the eye, 1284-1285t. *See also* Basal cell epithelioma.
Basal cell epithelioma, 129-130
  types of, 129
Basedow's disease. *See* Hyperthyroidism.
Basophil adenoma, 62
Basophils, 345, 1018, 1019i
Bauxite pneumoconiosis, 1284-1285t
Bauxite workers' disease, 1284-1285t
Beck Depression Inventory, 412
Becker's muscular dystrophy, 581-583
Bednar-Parrot disease, 1310-1311t
Bedsores. *See* Pressure ulcers.
Bee sting, 330-331t
Behavioral therapies, 468
Behçet's disease, 387t
Behr's disease, 1284-1285t
Bell's palsy, 676-678
  unilateral paralysis in, 677i
Bell's phenomenon, 677-678
Bence Jones protein, 127
Benign myalgic encephalomyelitis, 1294-1295t
Benign nasal tumor, 1296-1297t
Benign polycythemia, 1038-1039
Benign prostatic hyperplasia, 821-823
Benign prostatic hypertrophy, 821-823
Benign tumors, characteristics of, 47t
Benzodiazepines
  abuse of, 433t
  for generalized anxiety disorder, 463
Beriberi, 877, 878
Berlock dermatitis, 1256
Berylliosis, 1284-1285t
Beryllium disease, 1284-1285t
Beryllium poisoning, 1284-1285t
Besnier's prurigo. *See* Dermatitis.
Beta-adrenergic blockers
  for cardiac arrhythmias, 1127t, 1129t, 1130t, 1131t
  for chronic obstructive pulmonary disease, 555t
  for glaucoma, 1185
  for Marfan syndrome, 12
  for migraine headache, 638
  for panic disorder, 465
  for pheochromocytoma, 862
Beta$_2$-adrenergic agonists for asthma, 353

Bicarbonate levels
  in acute respiratory failure in chronic obstructive pulmonary disease, 525
  in hyperaldosteronism, 857
Bilateral massive epileptic myoclonus, 641
Bile, 684
Bile acid sequestrants, 900, 901
Bile duct cancer, 101-103
Bilharziasis. *See* Schistosomiasis.
Biliary cirrhosis, 756, 766, 767-769
Bilious typhoid, 209-210
Bilirubin levels
  in gallbladder cancer, 102
  in hyperbilirubinemia, 985
  in kidney cancer, 94
  in liver cancer, 96
  in nonviral hepatitis, 755
  in toxic shock syndrome, 279
  in transfusion reactions, 364
  in viral hepatitis, 754
Billroth II procedure, 83, 84-85
Binge-purge disorder. *See* Bulimia nervosa.
Biopsy
  in atopic dermatitis, 357
  in bone tumors, 124
  in brain tumors, 59
  in breast cancer, 80
  in bronchiolitis obliterans, 543
  in brucellosis, 203
  in cancer, 50. *See also specific cancer.*
  in cervical cancer, 109, 110
  in colorectal cancer, 92
  in cryptococcosis, 215
  in esophageal cancer, 86
  in giardiasis, 267
  in glycogen storage diseases, 893-894t, 894
  in Goodpasture's syndrome, 381
  in herpes simplex, 234
  in Hirschsprung's disease, 731
  in Hodgkin's disease, 139
  in Kaposi's sarcoma, 137
  in laryngeal cancer, 65
  in leprosy, 212
  in liver cancer, 96
  in lung cancer, 73
  in melanoma, 133
  in muscular dystrophy, 582
  in mycosis fungoides, 143
  in non-Hodgkin's lymphoma, 141
  in pancreatic cancer, 87
  in penile cancer, 108
  in polymyositis, 388
  in prostatic cancer, 103
  in pulmonary fibrosis, 561-562
  in Rocky Mountain spotted fever, 258
  in sarcoidosis, 546
  in scleroderma, 383

i refers to an illustration; t refers to a table.

Biopsy *(continued)*
  in severe combined immunodeficiency
    syndrome, 403
  in spinal neoplasms, 71
  in squamous cell carcinoma, 130
  in systemic lupus erythematosus, 379
  in testicular cancer, 106
  in trichinosis, 269
  in uterine cancer, 112
  in vaginal cancer, 116
  in viral hepatitis, 754
  in vulvar cancer, 121
Biotherapy
  as cancer therapy, 53
  for kidney cancer, 95
Bipolar disorders, 449-455
  depressive episodes in, 451, 454
  diagnostic criteria for, 452-453
  manic episodes in, 449-451, 454
  suicide risk in, 450, 451, 454
Bird breeder's lung, 1302-1303t
Black death. *See* Plague.
Blackfan-Diamond anemia, 1025
Black lung disease, 567-569
Blackwater fever as malaria complication, 263
Black widow spider bites, 330-331t
Bladder, 772
  congenital anomalies of, 814, 816-817i, 818
Bladder cancer, 98-101
  comparing staging systems for, 99t
Blalock-Taussig procedure, 1073, 1074
Blastomycosis, 218-220
Bleeding in hemophilia, 25
Bleeding time, 1022
  in anorexia, 494
  in platelet function disorders, 1048
  in snakebites, 326
  in Wiskott-Aldrich syndrome, 400
Blepharitis, 1157-1158
Blinding filarial disease, 1284-1285t
Blindness, 1183
Blood, 1015
  dysfunction of, 1017
  formation of, 1016
  function of, 1016
  tests for composition of, 1022
Blood alcohol level in alcohol-related
    disorder, 428
Blood culture
  in anthrax, 204
  in brucellosis, 203
  in candidiasis, 214
  in cryptococcosis, 215
  in endocarditis, 1080
  in *Haemophilus influenzae* infection, 198
  in lung abscess, 549
  in meningococcal infections, 177

Blood culture *(continued)*
  in methicillin-resistant staph infection, 166
  in pneumonia, 537
  in *Pseudomonas* infections, 194
  in Rocky Mountain spotted fever, 258
  in rubella, 238
  in septicemic plague, 202
  in septic shock, 197
  in tetanus, 181
  in toxic shock syndrome, 279
  in transfusion reactions, 364
  in tularemia, 206
Blood glucose levels
  classifying, 866
  in diabetes mellitus, 866
  in hypoglycemia, 896
  in metabolic syndrome, 907
  in osteomyelitis, 592
  in pancreatitis, 735
  stress and, 826
Blood pressure
  classifying, in hypertension, 1094t
  in pregnancy-induced hypertension, 962-963
Blood studies. *See also specific test.*
  in alcohol-related disorder, 428
  in anemias, 1021, 1026-1027, 1029, 1031,
    1032-1033
  in chronic lymphocytic leukemia, 149
  in chronic renal failure, 804
  in gas gangrene, 184
  in Hodgkin's disease, 139
  in mycosis fungoides, 143
  in polycythemias, 1036, 1039, 1040
  in Reye's syndrome, 664
  in systemic lupus erythematosus, 378
Blood transfusion reaction, 363-364
Blood typing, 1020
Blood urea nitrogen levels
  in alcohol-related disorder, 428
  in anorexia, 494
  in Goodpasture's syndrome, 381
  in hyperemesis gravidarum, 961
  in septic shock, 197
  in toxic shock syndrome, 279
  in vesicoureteral reflux, 811
B lymphocytes, 342-344, 354i
Bockhart's impetigo, 1234
Body dysmorphic disorder, 478-479
Body lice, 1244-1246, 1244i
Boils, 1234-1236
Bombesin, 687i
Bone cancer. *See* Bone tumors, primary
    malignant.
Bone culture
  in osteomyelitis, 592
  in sporotrichosis, 222
Bone disorders, 591-607

i refers to an illustration; t refers to a table.

Bone marrow aspiration and biopsy, 1022
in acute leukemia, 145
in anemias, 1021, 1027, 1029, 1029i, 1033
in chronic granulocytic leukemia, 148
in chronic lymphocytic leukemia, 149
in Gaucher's disease, 902
in multiple myeloma, 127
Bone marrow culture
in brucellosis, 203
Bone marrow studies, in radiation exposure,
322
Bone marrow transplantation, 1020, 1026-1027
for acute leukemia, 146
for chronic granulocytic leukemia, 148
for radiation exposure, 322
for severe combined immunodeficiency
syndrome, 403
Bone mineral density testing, 594
Bone pain
in bone tumors, 124
in multiple myeloma, 127
Bone resorption in hyperparathyroidism,
848, 848i
Bones, 571
brittle, 10-11, 303
structure of, 572i
Bone scan
in bone tumors, 124
in breast cancer, 79
in chronic granulomatous disease, 401
in Hodgkin's disease, 139
in Osgood-Schlatter disease, 597
in Paget's disease, 598
in prostatic cancer, 104
in spinal neoplasms, 71
Bone tumors, primary malignant, 123-127
types of, 125-126t
Borderline personality disorder, 485-486, 489
Botulinum toxin
for anal fissure, 744
for cerebral palsy, 628
for torticollis, 614
Botulinus antitoxin, 182, 183
Botulism, 182-183
Bouchard's nodes, 591i
Bougienage, 696
Bouillaud's syndrome, 1284-1285t
Bowel and bladder complications in spinal
neoplasms, 71
Bowen's disease, 130, 131t
Braces, 575
for epicondylitis, 609
for kyphosis, 601
for Legg-Calvé-Perthes disease, 595-596
for scoliosis, 606-607
Brain, 617-618
blood supply to, 618

Brain abscess, 654-656
Brain and spinal cord disorders, 642-668
Brain attack. *See* Stroke.
Brain scan, 626
in breast cancer, 79
in encephalitis, 654
in epilepsy, 641
in meningitis, 648
in stroke, 644
Brain stem, 618
Brain stimulator implantation, 659
Brain tumors, malignant, 56-62
comparing types of, 57-59t
Braxton Hicks contractions, 934
Breakbone fever, 1288-1289t
Breast cancer, 76-82
classifying, 76
doubling time in, 76
predisposing factors for, 76, 78-79
staging, 77-78
warning signs of, 79
Breast engorgement, 981-983
Breathing, 508-509, 509i
Breisky's disease, 1284-1285t
Breslow level method for measuring
melanomas, 133
Brill's disease, 1284-1285t
Brill-Zinsser disease, 1284-1285t
Brittle bones, 10-11, 303
Bromocriptine
for galactorrhea, 984
for pituitary tumors, 63
Bronchiectasis, 559-561
forms of, 559, 560i
Bronchodilators
for bronchiectasis, 560
for chronic obstructive pulmonary
disease, 557
for near drowning, 319
for silicosis, 566
Bronchoscopy, 510-511
in asphyxia, 318
in atelectasis, 532
in bronchiectasis, 560
in bronchiolitis obliterans, 543
in lung abscess, 549
in lung cancer, 73
in *Pneumocystis carinii* pneumonia, 260
in pneumonia, 537, 539t
Bronze diabetes, 1294-1295t
Brown recluse (violin) spider bites, 329-329t
Brown-Séquard's syndrome, 71
Brown-Symmers disease, 1284-1285t
Brucellosis, 202-204
Brudzinski's sign, 648i
Bruton's agammaglobulinemia, 389-390
Bryant's traction, 580, 581

Bubonic plague, 200, 201, 201t, 202. *See also*
  Plague.
Budd-Chiari syndrome, 758, 1284-1285t
Buerger's disease, 1147-1148
Bulbar paralytic poliomyelitis, 245. *See also*
  Poliomyelitis.
Bulbourethral glands, 994i
Bulimia nervosa, 490-492
  characteristic features in, 491
  diagnostic criteria for, 492
Bulla, 1230i
Bumetanide, 527
Bunionectomy, 600
Burkitt's lymphoma, 1286-1287t
Burkitt's tumor, 1286-1287t
Burns, 308-312
  classifying, 308
  estimating size of, 308-309
  fluid replacement for, 311
  gauging depth of, 308, 309i
  grafts for, 310
  types of, 308
Bursitis, 607-609
Buspirone, 463
Busulfan for chronic granulocytic
  leukemia, 148
Byssinosis, 1292-1293t

C

CA-125 as tumor marker, 50
Cabin fever, 209-210
Calcitonin, 598
Calcitonin assay in thyroid cancer, 69
Calcitriol
  for hyperparathyroidism, 849
  for hypocalcemia, 918
  for hypoparathyroidism, 846
Calcium channel blockers for migraine
  headache, 638
Calcium chloride for hypocalcemia, 918, 919
Calcium gluconate
  for DiGeorge syndrome, 393
  for hyperkalemia, 910
  for hypermagnesemia, 922
  for hypocalcemia, 918, 919
Calcium imbalance, 914-919
  clinical effects of, 914t
  diagnosing, 916-917i
Calcium levels
  in calcium imbalance, 918
  in leprosy, 212
  in non-Hodgkin's lymphoma, 141
Calcium pyrophosphate disease, 587
Calcium supplements
  for hyperparathyroidism, 849
  for hypoparathyroidism, 846

Calluses, 1269-1270
Campylobacteriosis, 205
Cancer. *See also specific type.*
  causes of, 48-49
  characteristics of, 47
  classifying, 47
  diagnosis of, 50
  hospice approach to, 55-56
  immune response and, 49-50
  maintaining nutrition and fluid balance
    in, 54
  major therapies for, 50-54, 52i
  metastasis of, 48-49i
  pain control and, 54-55
  prevalence and incidence of, 47
  psychological aspects of, 56
  staging and grading, 50
Candidal vaginitis, 939
Candidiasis, 213-215, 214t. *See also* Chronic
  mucocutaneous candidiasis.
  types of, 213
Candidosis. *See* Candidiasis.
Cannabinoid abuse, 432t
Capillaries, 1061
Capnography, 510
Carbamazepine
  for bipolar disorders, 451
  for epilepsy, 641
  for trigeminal neuralgia, 676
Carbohydrates
  function of, 871t
  metabolism of, 870
Carbon dioxide transport, 508-509
Carbon tetrachloride poisoning, 755
Carbuncles, 1234-1236
Carbunculosis, 1234-1236, 1235i
Carcinoembryonic antigen as tumor marker,
  50, 93
Cardiac amyloidosis, 903
Cardiac catheterization, 1063
  in congenital acyanotic defects, 1065, 1068,
    1069, 1071
  in congenital cyanotic defects, 1073,
    1075-1076
  in valvular heart disease, 1087-1090t
Cardiac cirrhosis, 756
Cardiac conduction, 1059, 1126i
Cardiac cycle, 1058-1059
Cardiac enzymes, 1063
Cardiac output, 1059
Cardiac rehabilitation programs, 1064
Cardiac tamponade, 1123-1125
Cardiogenic shock, 1118-1122
  as myocardial infarction complication, 1101t
  pathophysiology of, 1119i
Cardiomyoplasty, 1112
Cardiomyostimulator, 1112

i refers to an illustration; t refers to a table.

Cardiopulmonary resuscitation
  for asphyxia, 318
  for electric shock, 312
  for hypothermia, 315
  for near drowning, 319
Cardiovascular complications
  in anorexia, 493
  in Marfan syndrome, 12
  in respiratory acidosis, 533
  in velocardiofacial syndrome, 38
Cardiovascular disease in pregnancy, 969-970
Cardiovascular disorders, 1064-1151
  diagnostic tests for, 1062-1064, 1062i
  managing, 1064
Cardiovascular syphilis, 1003, 1004
Cardiovascular system, 1058
  assessment of, 1061-1062
  disorders of, 1064-1151
Carotid duplex in stroke, 644
Carpal tunnel, 611, 611i
Carpal tunnel syndrome, 611-612
Cassirer syndrome, 1288-1289t
Cast care, 305, 575, 578
Casts, 575
  for Achilles tendon contracture, 610
  for arm and leg fractures, 304
  for clubfoot, 577
  for dislocation, 306-307
  for Legg-Calvé-Perthes disease, 595, 596
Cast syndrome, 606
Catabolism, 870
Cataract, 1179-1180
Catatonic schizophrenia, 445. See also Schizo-
    phrenia.
Catecholamines levels in pheochromo-
    cytoma, 862
Catheter closure of atrial septal defect, 1068
Cat-scratch disease, 1286-1287t
Cat-scratch fever, 1286-1287t
Causalgia, 680-681
Ceftriaxone
  for chancroid, 1007
  for gonorrhea, 997
Celiac disease, 714-716
Celiac sprue, 714-716
Cell-mediated immune response, carcino-
    genesis and, 49
Cell-mediated immunity, 344
Central core disease, 1286-1287t
Central Mississippi Valley disease, 217-218
Central nervous system, 617
Central retinal artery occlusion, 1175,
    1176, 1177
Central retinal vein occlusion, 1175, 1176, 1177
Central venous pressure in septic shock, 197
Cerclage, 958, 975

Cerebellopontine angle tumor. See Schwan-
    noma.
Cerebellum, 618
Cerebral aneurysm, 631-635
  common sites of, 632i
  grading, 633
  surgical repair of, 634i
Cerebral arteriography, 626
  in arteriovenous malformation, 636
  in brain abscess, 655
  in cerebral aneurysm, 633
Cerebral contusion, 286-287
Cerebral palsy, 626-628, 1300-1301t
  causes of, 627
Cerebral radiation poisoning, 321
Cerebroretinal angiomatosis, 1310-1311t
Cerebrospinal fluid, 618
  circulation of, 629i
  in head trauma, 287, 288-289
Cerebrospinal fluid analysis
  in brain abscess, 655
  in cryptococcosis, 215
  in encephalitis, 654
  in Guillain-Barré syndrome, 667
  in herpes zoster, 236
  in listeriosis, 179, 180
  in meningitis, 648
  in meningococcal infections, 177
  in neurofibromatosis, 9
  in nocardiosis, 186
  in pituitary tumors, 63
  in poliomyelitis, 245, 246
  in Pseudomonas infections, 194
  in relapsing fever, 210
  in Reye's syndrome, 664
  in rubella, 238
  in spinal neoplasms, 71
  in tetanus, 181
  in trichinosis, 269-270
  in tuberculosis, 564
Cerebrotendinous xanthomatosis, 1286-1287t
Cerebrovascular accident. See Stroke.
Cerebrum, 618, 619i
Cervical cancer, 108-112
  staging, 110
Cervical intraepithelial neoplasia, 108-109
Cervicitis, 997-999, 1007-1008
Cervicofacial actinomycosis, 185
Cervix, 930, 931i
Cesarean birth, 978-979
Cesarean section, 978-979
Cestodiasis. See Taeniasis.
Chadwick's sign, 934
Chagas' disease, 1282-1283t
Chalazion, 1162-1163, 1162i
Chancroid, 1006-1007, 1006i
Charcot-Marie-Tooth disease, 1286-1287t

i refers to an illustration; t refers to a table.

Charcot's arthropathy, 588-589
Chédiak-Higashi syndrome, 20, 1286-1287t
Chemical burns, 308, 311. *See also* Burns.
Chemonucleolysis, 603, 604
Chemosurgery
  for basal cell epithelioma, 129-130
  for squamous cell carcinoma, 131
Chemotherapy
  for acute leukemia, 145-146
  adverse effects of, 51
  for bladder cancer, 100
  for bone tumors, 124
  for brain tumors, 61
  for breast cancer, 80
  as cancer treatment, 51-53
  for cervical cancer, 109
  for chronic granulocytic leukemia, 148
  for chronic lymphocytic leukemia, 149
  for colorectal cancer, 93
  for esophageal cancer, 86
  for fallopian tube cancer, 123
  for gastrointestinal cancers, 84
  for Hodgkin's disease, 140
  for Kaposi's sarcoma, 137
  for kidney cancer, 95
  for liver cancer, 97
  for lung cancer, 75, 76
  major agents used in, 51
  for melanoma, 136
  for multiple myeloma, 128
  for mycosis fungoides. 143
  for non-Hodgkin's lymphoma, 141-142
  for ovarian cancer, 119
  for pancreatic cancer, 89
  for penile cancer, 108
  for prostatic cancer, 104-105
  special considerations for, 51-53
  for testicular cancer, 106
  for thyroid cancer, 69
  for uterine cancer, 113
  for vaginal cancer, 116
  for vulvar cancer, 121
Chenodeoxycholic acid for cholelithiasis, 768
Chester's disease, 1286-1287t
Chest injuries, blunt, 294-297
  flail chest in, 295-296, 295i, 297
Chest physiotherapy, 514
  for asbestosis, 567
  for aspergillosis, 217
  for atelectasis, 532
  for bronchiectasis, 560-561
  for coal worker's pneumoconiosis, 568
  for common variable immunodeficiency, 391
  for cystic fibrosis, 16
  for lung abscess, 549
  for severe acute respiratory syndrome, 548
  for silicosis, 566

Chest physiotherapy *(continued)*
  for X-linked infantile hypogammaglobuline-
    mia, 390
Chest tube care, 552-553
Chest tube drainage, 513
  for empyema, 552
  for hemothorax, 549, 550
  for pleural effusion, 552
  for pneumothorax, 536
Chest wounds, penetrating, 298-299
Chest X-ray, 510. *See also* X-ray.
  in actinomycosis, 185
  in acute respiratory distress syndrome, 523
  in acute respiratory failure in chronic
    obstructive pulmonary disease, 525
  in asbestosis, 567
  in ascariasis, 272
  in aspergilloma, 217
  in asphyxia, 318
  in asthma, 352
  in atelectasis, 532
  in blastomycosis, 219
  in bronchiectasis, 559
  in bronchiolitis obliterans, 542
  in cardiovascular disorders, 1062
  in chest injuries, 296
  in chest wounds, 298
  in chronic obstructive pulmonary disease,
    555t, 557t
  in coal worker's pneumoconiosis, 568
  in coccidioidomycosis, 220
  in congenital acyanotic defects, 1065, 1067,
    1069, 1071
  in congenital cyanotic defects, 1073, 1075
  in cor pulmonale, 528
  in croup, 518
  in cryptococcosis, 215
  in cystic fibrosis, 16
  in fallopian tube cancer, 122
  in Goodpasture's syndrome, 381
  in *Hantavirus* pulmonary syndrome, 231
  in hemothorax, 549
  in Hodgkin's disease, 139
  in infant respiratory distress syndrome, 515
  in laryngeal cancer, 65
  in legionnaires' disease, 531
  in liver cancer, 96
  in lung abscess, 549
  in lung cancer, 73
  in nocardiosis, 186
  in ornithosis, 278
  in ovarian cancer, 118
  in pleural effusion, 552
  in *Pneumocystis carinii* pneumonia, 260
  in pneumonia, 537, 539t, 541t
  in pneumonic plague, 202
  in pneumothorax, 536

Chest X-ray *(continued)*
in poisoning, 323
in pulmonary edema, 526
in pulmonary embolism, 544
in pulmonary fibrosis, 562
in respiratory syncytial virus infection, 225
in sarcoidosis, 546
in scleroderma, 383
in severe acute respiratory syndrome, 547-548
in severe combined immunodeficiency disease, 402
in silicosis, 566
in snakebites, 326
in systemic lupus erythematosus, 379
in tracheoesophageal anomalies, 693-694
in tuberculosis, 564
in tularemia, 206
in urticaria, 362
in valvular heart disease, 1087-1090t
Chiari-Frommel syndrome, 1286-1287t
Chickenpox, 540-541t. *See also* Varicella.
Chinese Americans, cultural considerations for, 1280t
Chlamydiae, 153
Chlamydial infections, 997-999
Chloasma, 1255
Chloride imbalance, 919-921
Chloride levels
in chloride imbalance, 920
normal, 775t
in radiation exposure, 322
in renal disease, 775t
Chloroquine, 263
for amebiasis, 266
for malaria, 264
Cholangiocarcinoma, 96
Cholangiography, percutaneous transhepatic
in cholelithiasis, 767
in gallbladder cancer, 102
in gallbladder disease, 751
in hepatic disease, 750
Cholangiomas, 96
Cholangitis, 766, 767-769
Cholecystitis, 766, 767-769
Cholecystography
in cholelithiasis, 767
in gallbladder cancer, 102
in gallbladder disease, 751
in hepatic disease, 750
Cholecystojejunostomy, 89, 90-91
Choledochoduodenostomy, 89, 90-91
Choledochojejunostomy, 89, 90-91
Choledocholithiasis, 765, 767-769
sites of calculus formation in, 766i
Cholelithiasis, 765, 767-769
sites of calculus formation in, 766i

Cholera, 194-196
Cholesterol levels
in anorexia, 494
in hepatic disease, 748
in hyperlipoproteinemia, 899t
in leprosy, 212
Cholesterolosis, 766, 767-769
Cholestyramine, 900, 901
Chondrosarcoma, 124, 125t
Chordae tendineae, 1058
Chordoma, 124, 125t
Choriocarcinoma, 1286-1287t
Chorionic gonadotropin
in testicular cancer, 106
as tumor marker, 50
Chorionic villus sampling
genetic testing and, 7
in phenylketonuria, 19
in Tay-Sachs disease, 17-18
in velocardiofacial syndrome, 38
Choroiditis, 1172
Christmas disease, 25. *See also* Hemophilia.
Chromoblastomycosis, 1286-1287t
Chromomycosis, 1286-1287t
Chromophobe adenoma, 62
Chromosomal abnormalities, 6, 31-38
Chromosome analysis
in chronic granulocytic leukemia, 147
in Down syndrome, 32
in fragile X syndrome, 31
in Klinefelter's syndrome, 36
in neural tube defects, 40
in trisomy 13 syndrome, 35
in trisomy 18 syndrome, 34
in velocardiofacial syndrome, 38
Chromosomes, 2-3
Chronic bronchitis in chronic obstructive pulmonary disease, 554-555t
Chronic dermatitis, 1258-1259t
Chronic Epstein-Barr virus. *See* Chronic fatigue syndrome.
Chronic fatigue syndrome, 398-399
Centers for Disease Control and Prevention criteria for, 399
Chronic glomerulonephritis, 798-799
Chronic granular myringitis, 1201, 1202
Chronic granulocytic leukemia, 147-149
Chronic granulomatous disease, 401-402
Chronic lymphocytic leukemia, 149-150
Chronic mercury poisoning, 1284-1285t
Chronic motor or vocal tic disorder, 416, 418, 419
Chronic mucocutaneous candidiasis, 397-398. *See also* Candidiasis.
Chronic myelocytic leukemia, 147-149
Chronic myelogenous leukemia, 147-149

i refers to an illustration; t refers to a table.

Chronic obstructive lung disease. *See* Chronic obstructive pulmonary disease.
Chronic obstructive pulmonary disease, 553-558
  types of, 554-557t
Chronic open-angle glaucoma, 1184-1186
Chronic pancreatitis, 734
Chronic pyelonephritis, 785
Chronic renal failure, 802-805, 808
Chronic venous insufficiency, 1144
Churg-Strauss syndrome, 385t
Chvostek's sign, 846, 918i
Chymopapain, 603
Ciliary body, 1154, 1154i, 1155
Cimetidine for latex allergy, 358-359
Cinefluorography in tracheoesophageal anomalies, 694
Ciprofloxacin
  for chancroid, 1007
  for gonorrhea, 997
  for meningococcal infection prophylaxis, 177
Circulatory system, 1058
Circumcision, penile cancer and, 107
Cirrhosis, 756-757, 759
  liver cancer and, 96
Citric acid cycle, 870
Clam digger's itch, 276
Clark's staging system, 135i
Classic typhus, 1310-1311t
Clavus, 1269-1270
Cleft lip/palate, 42-44
  variations in, 42-43, 43i
Climacteric, 945
Clofazimine for leprosy, 212
Clofibrate for hyperlipoproteinemia, 900, 901
Clomiphene
  for abnormal premenopausal bleeding, 954
  for ovarian cysts, 941-942
Clonazepam
  for bipolar disorders, 451
  for epilepsy, 641
Clonidine for tic disorders, 418
Clonidine suppression test, 862
Closed reduction
  for dislocations, 306
  for fractures, 304
  for hip dysplasia, 580
Clostridium perfringens, growth cycle of, 183, 184i
Clozapine
  for delusional disorders, 448
  for schizophrenia, 441, 444
Clubfoot, 576-578
  types of orientation in, 576, 577i
Cluster headaches, 639t
Coagulation factor assays in hemophilia, 26
Coagulation factors, 1015, 1016t

Coagulation tests. *See also specific test.*
  in abdominal injuries, 300
  in disseminated intravascular coagulation, 1052
  in thrombocytopenia, 1045
  in von Willebrand's disease, 1049
Coal miner's disease, 567-569
Coal worker's pneumoconiosis, 567-569
Coarctation of the aorta, 1068-1070, 1070i
Cobalamin deficiency, 877-879
Cocaine abuse, 436t
Coccidioidal meningitis, 220
Coccidioidomycosis, 220-221
Cockayne's syndrome, 1286-1287t
Cognitive Capacity Screening Examination, 412
Cognitive complications in velocardiofacial syndrome, 38
Colchicine for gout, 586
Cold injuries, 313-316
  risk factors for, 314
Colectomy for colorectal cancer, 93-94
Collagen matrices for burns, 310
Colonic stasis, 732-733
Colonoscopy
  in colorectal cancer, 93
  in ulcerative colitis, 707
Colony-stimulating factors, 344
Colorado tick fever, 246-247
Colorectal cancer, 91-94
  staging, 92
Colostomy, caring for, 93-94
Colposcopy
  in cervical cancer, 109
  in vaginal cancer, 116
Common cold, 222-224
  pathophysiology of, 222, 223i
Common polypoid adenomas, 739, 740
Common variable immunodeficiency, 390-391
Communication barriers, 409-410
Compartment syndrome as fracture complication, 304
Complement deficiencies, 403-404
Complement fixation, 403
  in amebiasis, 266
  in Colorado tick fever, 247
  in histoplasmosis, 218
  in smallpox, 241
Complement system, 345
Complete abortion, 957
Complete blood count, 1022. *See also* Blood studies *and* White blood cell count.
  in acute leukemia, 145
  in ascariasis, 272
  in asthma, 352
  in chest wounds, 298
  in granulocytopenia, 1054
  in juvenile rheumatoid arthritis, 372

i refers to an illustration; t refers to a table.

Complete blood count *(continued)*
  in multiple myeloma, 127-128
  in non-Hodgkin's lymphoma, 141
  in open trauma wounds, 333t, 335t
  in rheumatoid arthritis, 366
  in systemic lupus erythematosus, 378
Complete heart block, 1132t
Complex regional pain syndrome, 680-681
Compression test, 612
Computed tomography scan, 413
  in abdominal injuries, 300
  in bladder cancer, 98
  in bone tumors, 124
  in breast cancer, 79
  in bronchiectasis, 559-560
  in chest injuries, 296
  in cholelithiasis, 767
  in chronic granulocytic leukemia, 148
  in chronic obstructive pulmonary
    disease, 557t
  in esophageal cancer, 86
  in head trauma, 285, 287, 288, 289
  in Hodgkin's disease, 139
  in Kaposi's sarcoma, 137
  in laryngeal cancer, 65
  in lung cancer, 73
  in necrotizing fasciitis, 174
  in neural tube defects, 40
  in neurofibromatosis, 9
  in osteomyelitis, 592
  in osteoporosis, 594
  in ovarian cancer, 118
  in pancreatic cancer, 88
  in pituitary tumors, 63
  in polycystic kidney disease, 781
  in pulmonary fibrosis, 562
  in renal calculi, 792
  in renal vein thrombosis, 794
  in schizophrenia, 439-440
  in spinal injuries, 294
  in spinal neoplasms, 71
  in stroke, 644
  in toxoplasmosis, 268
  in trisomy 13 syndrome, 35
  in vulvar cancer, 121
Concato's disease, 1286-1287t
Concussion, 285
Conduct disorder, 424-426
  diagnostic criteria for, 425
  risk factors for, 424
Conductive hearing loss, 1204
Condylomata acuminata, 1001-1002, 1263
Congenital acyanotic defects, 1064-1072
Congenital adrenal hyperplasia, 858
Congenital aganglionic megacolon, 730-732
Congenital bladder diverticulum, 817i
Congenital cyanotic defects, 1072-1077

Congenital hearing loss, 1204-1205, 1206
Congenital hypoplastic anemia, 1025
Congenital lymphedema, 1302-1303t
Congenital megacolon, 730-732
Congenital mitral stenosis, 1288-1289t
Congenital nephroblastoma, 1312-1313t
Congenital rubella syndrome, 237. *See also*
  Rubella.
Congenital syphilis, 1288-1289t
Congenital thymic hypoplasia, 392-393
Conjunctiva, 1154i, 1155
Conjunctival disorders, 1164-1168
Conjunctivitis, 1164-1166, 1165i
Conn's syndrome, 856-858
Conradi-Hunermann syndrome, 1286-1287t
Consumption coagulopathy. *See* Disseminated
  intravascular coagulation.
Contact dermatitis, 1258-1259t
Contact isolation precautions, 157
Contact transmission, 154
Contact ulcers, 1288-1289t
Continent ileostomy, 708
Continuous ambulatory peritoneal dialysis,
  804-805, 807i
Continuous arteriovenous hemodiafiltration,
  783
Continuous venovenous hemodiafiltration, 783
Convergence test, 1156
Conversion disorder, 473-475
  diagnostic criteria for, 474
Convoluted foam mattress, 1275
Cooley's anemia, 1030-1031
COPD. *See* Chronic obstructive pulmonary
  disease.
Coping mechanisms, 411
Copper deficiency anemia, 1288-1289t
Copper deposits in Wilson's disease, 762, 763
Coral snakebite, 325-329
Cori's glycogen storage disease, 893t
Cornea, 1153, 1154i
Corneal abrasion, 1169-1170
Corneal disorders, 1168-1172
Corneal ulcers, 1170-1172
  pathophysiology of, 1171i
Corns, 1269-1270
Coronary arteriography, 1063
Coronary artery disease, 1095-1100
Coronary artery spasm, 1096
Coronary brachytherapy, 1098
Cor pulmonale, 527-530
Corrosive esophagitis, 695-696
Corticospinal tract, 620
Corticosteroids
  adverse effects of, 543, 547
  for allergic rhinitis, 356
  for ankylosing spondylitis, 374
  for asthma, 353-354

Corticosteroids *(continued)*
  for atopic dermatitis, 357
  for Bell's palsy, 678
  for bronchiolitis obliterans, 543
  for brucellosis, 203
  for chronic obstructive pulmonary
    disease, 557
  for decompression sickness, 320
  for idiopathic thrombocytopenic
    purpura, 1047
  as immunosuppressants, 348-349
  for juvenile rheumatoid arthritis, 372
  for leprosy, 212
  for Marfan syndrome, 12
  for near drowning, 319
  for psoriatic arthritis, 373
  for sarcoidosis, 546
  for stroke, 645
  for systemic lupus erythematosus, 379
  for transfusion reactions, 364
  for urticaria, 362
Corticotropin, hypersecretion of, 852, 858
Corticotropin-secreting adenomas, 63
Corticotropin stimulation test, 851
Cortisol, 826
  in adrenal hypofunction, 851
  in Cushing's syndrome, 852, 854
Cortisone
  for adrenal hypofunction, 851
  for congenital adrenal hyperplasia, 860, 861
Coughing in respiratory conditions, 514
Cover-uncover test, 1156
Cowper's glands, 994i
Coxa plana, 595-596
Crab lice, 1244-1246, 1245i
Cranial nerve disorders, 674-680
Cranial nerve function, assessing, 623-624
Craniofacial complications in velocardiofacial
    syndrome, 37
Craniotomy
  aftercare for, 61, 64
  for skull fractures, 289
Creatine kinase
  in chest injuries, 296
  in muscular dystrophy, 582
  in myocardial infarction, 1102
  in polymyositis, 388
  in rhabdomyolysis, 615
  in toxic shock syndrome, 279
  in trichinosis, 269
Creatinine clearance
  in chronic renal failure, 804
  as measure of glomerular function, 772-773
Creatinine-height index, 874
Creatinine levels
  in anorexia, 494
  in Goodpasture's syndrome, 381

Creatinine levels *(continued)*
  in *Hantavirus* pulmonary syndrome, 231
  in septic shock, 197
  in toxic shock syndrome, 279
  in vesicoureteral reflux, 811
Credé's method, 813
Creeping eruption, 1243-1244
CREST syndrome, 382
Cretinism, 836-837
  iodine deficiency and, 886
Creutzfeldt-Jakob disease, 662-663
  variant of, 663
Crib death, 516-517
Crocq's disease, 1288-1289t
Crohn's disease, 711-712
  string sign in, 711, 712i
Cromolyn for allergic rhinitis, 356
Cross-eye, 1308-1309t
Crossmatching, 1020
Cross-McKusick-Breen syndrome, 20
Crotamiton for scabies, 1241, 1242
Croup, 518-520
  effect of, on upper airway, 519i
Crush wound, 332, 333t
Crust, 1231i
Cryohypophysectomy, 63
Cryoprecipitate for hemophilia, 26
Cryosurgery
  for basal cell epithelioma, 129
  for cervical cancer, 109, 110
Cryotherapy, 1264
Cryptococcosis, 215-216
Cryptogenic fibrosing alveolitis, 561-562
Cryptogenic organizing pneumonia, 542-543
Cryptomenorrhea, 951, 952
Cryptorchidism, 1010-1011
  testicular cancer and, 105
Csillag's disease, 1288-1289t
Culdocentesis, 960
Cultural considerations in patient care,
    1279-1281t
Cushingoid syndrome, symptoms of, 853i
Cushing's disease, 852, 854
Cushing's syndrome, 852-856
  diagnosing, 855i
  pituitary tumors and, 62, 63
  in thyroid cancer, 67
Cutaneous anthrax, 204
Cutaneous larva migrans, 1243-1244
Cyanotic defects, congenital, 1072-1077
Cyclophosphamide
  for Goodpasture's syndrome, 381
  for idiopathic bronchiolitis obliterans with
    organizing pneumonia, 543
  as immunosuppressant, 348
  for rheumatoid arthritis, 366
  for vasculitis, 387

i refers to an illustration; t refers to a table.

Cyclosporine as immunosuppressant, 349
Cyproheptadine for pituitary tumors, 63
Cystectomy for bladder cancer, 100
Cyst, 1230i
Cystic fibrosis, 14-17
  diagnostic criteria for, 16
  transmission risk for, 15t
Cystic osteofibromatosis, 1296-1297t
Cystinuria, 1288-1289t
Cystitis, 808-810
Cystometry, 777t
Cystoscopy, 777t
  in bladder cancer, 98, 100
  in kidney cancer, 94
  in vesicoureteral reflux, 811
Cystourethrography, 777t
  in abdominal injuries, 300
Cytokines, 344-345
Cytologic studies in esophageal cancer, 86
Cytomegalic inclusion disease, 251-253
Cytomegalovirus infection, 251-253
Cytomegalovirus mononucleosis, 252
Cytomegalovirus pneumonia, 540-541t
Cytotoxic drugs
  for ankylosing spondylitis, 374
  as cause of immunodeficiency, 348
  for juvenile rheumatoid arthritis, 372
Czerny's disease, 1288-1289t

D

Dacryocystitis, 1161-1162
Dandy fever, 1288-1289t
Darier's disease, 1296-1297t
Dark-field examination in syphilis, 1004, 1004i
Darling's disease, 217-218
D-dimer test, 1023
Deafness, sudden, 1205, 1206
Deamination, 871
Debridement
  for corns, 1269, 1270
  for necrotizing fasciitis, 174
  for snakebites, 327
Decompensation in pregnancy, 969
Decompression sickness, 319-320
Deep breathing in respiratory conditions, 514
Deep vein thrombosis, 1143-1146
Defibrillation
  in electric shock, 312
  paddles for, 313
Defibrination syndrome. See Disseminated
    intravascular coagulation.
Degenerative cardiovascular disorders,
    1091-1115
Delayed hypersensitivity, 347
Delirium as communication barrier, 409-410

Delusional disorders, 445-449
  diagnostic criteria for, 448
  themes of, 446
Delusions as communication barrier, 409
Demeclocycline for hyponatremia, 912
Dementia. See also Alzheimer's disease.
  as communication barrier, 410
  primary degenerative, 660-662
Dengue, 1288-1289t
Denis Browne splint, 577
Denver Developmental Screening test, 414-415
Deoxyribonucleic acid, 2i
  replication of, 3i
Deoxyribonucleic acid analysis
  in cystic fibrosis, 16
  in fragile X syndrome, 30
  in Huntington's disease, 657
Dependent personality disorder, 486, 489
Depersonalization disorder, 482-483
  diagnostic criteria for, 483
Depigmentation therapy, 1254
Depressant abuse, 432-434t
Depression
  in bipolar disorders, 451, 454
  diagnosing, 457
  major, 455-459
Depth perception, 1155
Dermatitis, 1256-1261
  types of, 1258-1261t
Dermatitis herpetiformis, 1288-1289t
Dermatomyositis, 388-389
Dermatophytosis, 1239-1241, 1240i
Dermis, 1228
Dermographism urticaria, 361
Desensitization. See Immunotherapy.
Desmopressin
  for diabetes insipidus, 833
  for hemophilia, 26, 27
  for von Willebrand disease, 1050
Desoxycorticosterone, 857, 861
Detached retina, 1173-1174
De Toni-Fanconi syndrome, 1290-1291t
Detoxification for substance abuse, 438
Developmental dysplasia of the hip, 578-581,
    579i
Deviated septum, 1209-1211
Dexamethasone
  for head trauma, 287, 289
  for meningitis, 648
  for spinal neoplasms, 71
Dexamethasone suppression test, 854
Diabetes insipidus, 832-834
  pituitary tumors and, 63
Diabetes mellitus, 864-868
  corticosteroid therapy and, 547
  foot care in, 867
  forms of, 864
  risk factors for, 865

i refers to an illustration; t refers to a table.

Diabetic retinopathy, 1175, 1176-1177
Dialysis, 776, 778, 808. *See also* Hemodialysis *and* Peritoneal dialysis.
Diaper rash. *See* Candidiasis.
Diaphragmatic rupture, 296
Diarrhea, 227t. *See also* Adenovirus infection.
Diascopy, 1230
Diastole, 1058-1059
Diazepam
  for epilepsy, 641
  for pancreatitis, 736
Diazoxide for hypoglycemia, 896
DIC. *See* Disseminated intravascular coagulation.
Dietary restrictions for phenylketonuria, 19
Diffuse interstitial fibrosis, 561-562
Diffuse systemic sclerosis, 382
DiGeorge syndrome, 37, 38, 392-393
Digestion, 684
Digestive hormones, primary source of, 686-687i
Digital rectal examination
  in colorectal cancer, 92
  in inactive colon, 733
  in prostatic cancer, 103
Digital subtraction angiography, 1063
  in neurologic disorders, 626
  in renovascular hypertension, 799
Digoxin, 529
Digoxin toxicity, signs of, 529
Dihydrotachysterol, 846
Dilatation and curettage
  for dysfunctional uterine bleeding, 955
  for hydatidiform mole, 964
  for postmenopausal bleeding, 956
Dilatation and evacuation for abortion, 958
Dilated cardiomyopathy, 1111-1113
Dilutional hyponatremia, 924-925
Diphenhydramine
  for anaphylaxis, 361
  for latex allergy, 358-359
  for transfusion reactions, 364
  for urticaria, 362
Diphtheria, 178-179
Diphtheria antitoxin, 178-179
Direct Coombs' test, 1022
Directly observed therapy, 564
Discoid eczema, 1258-1259t
Discoid lupus erythematosus, 377
Dislocations, 306-307, 306i
Disseminated aspergillosis, 216-217
Disseminated histiocytosis X, 1298-1299t
Disseminated intravascular coagulation, 1050-1053
  mechanisms of, 1051i
  in transfusion reactions, 364
Dissociative amnesia, 481-482
  diagnostic criteria for, 482
  types of, 481

Dissociative disorders, 479-490
Dissociative fugue, 480-481
  diagnostic criteria for, 481
Dissociative identity disorder, 479-480
  diagnostic criteria for, 480
Distal renal tubular acidosis, 801
Disulfiram, 428-429, 431
Diuretics
  for acute poststreptococcal glomerulo-nephritis, 787
  for coarctation of the aorta, 1069
  for heart failure, 1109
  for hyperaldosteronism, 858
  for hyperparathyroidism, 848
  for hypertension, 1094, 1095
  for hypervitaminosis D, 885
  for myocardial infarction, 1101t, 1102t
  for myocarditis, 1078
  for multiple myeloma, 128
  for near drowning, 319
  for pancreatic cancer, 89
  for patent ductus arteriosus, 1071
  for pernicious anemia, 1022-1023
  for pregnancy-related cardiovascular disease, 969
  for pulmonary edema, 527
  for renal calculi, 793
  for ventricular septal defect, 1065
Divarication traction, 580
Diverticular disease, 716-718
Diverticulitis, 716-718
Diverticulosis, 716-718
Donepezil for Alzheimer's disease, 661
Dopamine for anaphylaxis, 360
Dornase alfa for cystic fibrosis, 16
Down syndrome, 31-33
Doxycycline
  for gonorrhea, 997
  for nonspecific genitourinary infections, 1007
  for syphilis, 1004
Dressler's syndrome, 1124
  as myocardial infarction complication, 1101t
Droplet isolation precautions, 157
Drotrecogin alfa for septic shock, 197
Drug-induced hepatitis, 755-756
Dubois' disease, 1288-1289t
Duchenne's muscular dystrophy, 581-583
Duction test, 1156
Duhring's disease, 1288-1289t
Dukes cancer classification system, 92
Dukes' disease, 1288-1289t
Duodenal drainage, 751-752
Duodenal ulcers, 704, 705-706
Duplicated ureter, 815i
Durand-Nicholas-Favie disease, 1288-1289t
Durand's disease, 1288-1289t
Duroziez's disease, 1288-1289t
Dwarfism, 827-830

i refers to an illustration; t refers to a table.

Dyplasia epiphysealis punctata, 1286-1287t
Dysbetalipoproteinemia, 899t
Dysfunctional uterine bleeding, 954-955
Dysmenorrhea, 937-939
Dysmetabolic syndrome. *See* Metabolic
    syndrome.
Dyspareunia, 497-498
Dysphagia in esophageal cancer, 86
Dysplasia epiphysealis hemimelica, 1310-1311t
Dyspnea
    in asbestosis, 567
    in coal worker's pneumoconiosis, 568
    in silicosis, 565
Dysrhythmias. *See* Arrhythmias.
Dysthymic disorder, 456
Dystonia as antipsychotic adverse effect, 443

E

Eales disease, 1288-1289t
Ear
    anatomy of, 1189, 1189i
    assessment of, 1189
Ear disorders, 1191-1207
Eardrum, perforated, 292
Ear tumors, benign, 1194-1195, 1195t
Eastern equine encephalitis, 651
Eating Attitudes Test, 412
Eating disorders, 490-495
Ebola virus infection, 253-255
Eccrine glands, 1228
Echinococcus granulosus, 1294-1295t
Echocardiography, 1063
Echocardiography
    in atrial septal defect, 1067
    in cardiac tamponade, 1124
    in cardiogenic shock, 1120
    in chest injuries, 296
    in coarctation of the aorta, 1069
    in coronary artery disease, 1097
    in cor pulmonale, 528
    in heart failure, 1109
    in hypertrophic cardiomyopathy, 1113
    in hypovolemic shock, 1116
    in myocardial infarction, 1101t, 1102
    in patent ductus arteriosus, 1071
    in pulmonary edema, 526
    in restrictive cardiomyopathy, 1114
    in tetralogy of Fallot, 1073
    in thoracic aortic aneurysm, 1137
    in transposition of the great arteries, 1075
    in valvular heart disease, 1087-1090t
    in ventricular septal defect, 1065
    in ventricular aneurysm, 1123
Eclampsia, 962-964
Economo's disease, 1290-1291t
Ecthyma, 1233, 1234

Ectopic orifice of ureter, 815i
Ectopic pregnancy, 959-961
    implantation sites of, 960i
Edrophonium for myasthenia gravis, 670
Edwards' syndrome, 33-34
Ehrlichiosis, 206-207
Eisenmenger's syndrome, 1065-1066
Ejaculation, premature, 501-502
Electrical burns, 308, 311. *See also* Burns.
Electric shock, 312-313
Electrocardiography, 1062
    in acute respiratory failure in chronic
        obstructive pulmonary disease, 525
    in acute tubular necrosis, 788
    in anorexia, 494
    in calcium imbalance, 918
    in chest injuries, 296
    in chronic obstructive pulmonary disease,
        555t, 557t
    in congenital acyanotic defects, 1065, 1067,
        1069, 1071
    in congenital cyanotic defects, 1073, 1075
    in cor pulmonale, 529
    in cretinism, 837
    in electric shock, 312
    in near drowning, 319
    in polymyositis, 388
    positioning chest electrodes for, 1062i
    in pulmonary embolism, 544-545
    in pulmonary hypertension, 550-551
    in scleroderma, 383
    in septic shock, 197
    in snakebites, 326
    in stroke, 644
    in systemic lupus erythematosus, 379
    in valvular heart disease, 1087-1090t
Electroconvulsive therapy
    for bipolar disorders, 451
    for major depression, 456
Electrodesiccation and curettage
    for basal cell epithelioma, 129
    for squamous cell carcinoma, 131
    for warts, 1264, 1264-1265i
Electroencephalography, 413
    in Alzheimer's disease, 661
    in arteriovenous malformations, 636
    in autistic disorder, 419
    in Creutzfeldt-Jakob disease, 663
    in encephalitis, 654
    in epilepsy, 641
    in headache, 638
    in snakebites, 326
    in stroke, 644
Electrohydraulic shock wave lithotripsy, 768
Electrolyte levels
    in acute respiratory failure in chronic
        obstructive pulmonary disease, 525

i refers to an illustration; t refers to a table.

Electrolyte levels *(continued)*
in anorexia, 494
in bulimia, 491
in Crohn's disease, 711
in hyperemesis gravidarum, 961
in liver cancer, 97
in magnesium imbalance, 921-922
in near drowning, 319
in open trauma wounds, 335t
Electromyography, 626
in amyotrophic lateral sclerosis, 671
in botulism, 182
in muscular dystrophy, 582
in polymyositis, 388
Electronic fetal monitoring in pregnancy-
induced hypertension, 963
Electrophoresis
in multiple myeloma, 128
of serum proteins, 1023
in sickle cell anemia, 23
in systemic lupus erythematosus, 378
Electrophysiologic studies, 1064
Elevator disease, 1290-1291t
Embolectomy, 1150
Embolism as cause of stroke, 643
Embolization, 637
Embryo, 934
Embryonal adenomyosarcoma, 1312-1313t
Emergent category in triage, 281
Emetine for amebiasis, 266
Emphysema
in chronic obstructive pulmonary disease,
556-557t
types of, 558i
Empyema, 551-553
Encephalitis, 650-654
types of, 651-653
Encephalocele, 39, 40. *See also* Neural tube
defects.
Encephalopathy
hepatic, 764-765
in liver cancer, 97
portosystemic, 764-765
Endarterectomy for stroke, 644
Endarteritis obliterans, 1292-1293t
Endemic goiter, 839-840
Endemic paralytic vertigo, 1292-1293t
Endocarditis, 172-173t, 1079-1081
degenerative changes in, 1079, 1079i
Endocrine complications in pituitary
tumors, 62
Endocrine disorders, 827-868
Endocrine system
assessing dysfunctions of, 827
feedback mechanism of, 825, 825i
hormonal effects of, 825-827
hypothalamic control of, 824-825

Endogenous hypertriglyceridemia, 899t
Endolymphatic hydrops. *See* Ménière's disease.
Endometriosis, 942-943
stages of, 943
Endometritis, 980, 998
Endomyocardial biopsy, 1064
in myocarditis, 1078
Endoscopic retrograde cannulization of the
pancreas in bile duct cancer, 102
Endoscopic retrograde cholangiopancreatography, 685, 752
in gallbladder disorders, 767
in pancreatic cancer, 88
Endoscopy. *See also specific procedure.*
in bile duct cancer, 102
in corrosive esophagitis, 695
in esophageal cancer, 86
in gastric cancer, 83
in Kaposi's sarcoma, 137
Endotracheal intubation
for asphyxia, 318
for epiglottiditis, 520
for snakebites, 328
Endovascular grafting, 1140i
Engel-Recklinghausen disease, 1290-1291t
Entacapone for Parkinson's disease, 658
Enteric (oral-fecal) transmission, 154, 156
Enterobacteriaceae infections, 191-193
Enterobacterial infections, 191. *See also*
Enterobacteriaceae infections.
Enterobiasis, 273-274
Enterocolitis, 162-163t, 187, 188, 188t, 189
Enteroviruses, 245
Enuresis, functional, 417
Enzyme assay for phenylketonuria, 19
Enzyme deficiency, 402
Enzyme levels in renal infarction, 790
Enzyme-linked immunosorbent assay
in human immunodeficiency virus
infection, 395
in Lyme disease, 208
Eosinophil adenoma, 62
Eosinophilia myalgia syndrome, 382
Eosinophilic endomyocardial disease,
1290-1291t
Eosinophils, 345, 1018, 1019i
Ependymoma, 57t, 59, 61, 70. *See also* Brain
tumors, malignant *and* Spinal neo-
plasms, malignant.
Epicondylitis, 609-610
Epidemic cholera, 194-196
Epidemic keratoconjunctivitis, 227t, 1165. *See
also* Adenovirus infection.
Epidemic neuromyasthenia, 1294-1295t
Epidemic parotitis, 247-248
Epidermis, 1228
Epidermodysplasia verruciformis, 1300-1301t

i refers to an illustration; t refers to a table.

Epididymitis, 819-820, 999
Epididymo-orchitis, 248
Epidural hematoma, 286
Epiglottiditis, 520-521
Epilepsy, 640-642
  types of seizures in, 640-641
Epinephrine
  for anaphylaxis, 360, 361
  for arrhythmias, 1132t, 1134t
  for latex allergy, 359
  for transfusion reactions, 364
Epiphrenic diverticulum, 697, 698
Epiphysitis juvenilis, 1296-1297t
Epispadias, 817i
Epistaxis, 1207-1209
  inserting nasal pack for, 1208-1209i
Epstein-Barr virus, 1290-1291t
Erectile disorder, 499-501
Ergotamine, 638
Erosion, 1231i
Erotomanic delusions, 446
Erysipelas, 168-169t
Erysipeloid, 1290-1291t
Erythema in necrotizing fasciitis, 174
Erythema chronicum migrans, 207-208
Erythema infectiosum, 1290-1291t
Erythema marginatum, 1084
Erythema nodosum leprosum, 212. See also
  Leprosy.
Erythrasma, 1290-1291t
Erythremia. See Polycythemia vera.
Erythroblastic anemia, 1030-1031
Erythroblastosis fetalis, 987-991
Erythrocytes. See Red blood cells.
Erythrocyte sedimentation rate, 1023
  in ankylosing spondylitis, 374
  in blastomycosis, 219
  in bronchiolitis obliterans, 542
  in brucellosis, 203
  in chronic granulomatous disease, 401
  in coccidioidomycosis, 220
  in Crohn's disease, 711
  in gout, 586
  in juvenile rheumatoid arthritis, 372
  in leprosy, 212
  in Lyme disease, 208
  in osteomyelitis, 592
  in polymyositis, 388
  in psoriatic arthritis, 373
  in Reiter's syndrome, 382
  in relapsing fever, 210
  in rheumatoid arthritis, 366
  in scleroderma, 383
  in Sjögren's syndrome, 376
  in systemic lupus erythematosus, 378
Erythroderma desquamativum, 1298-1299t
Erythrohepatic porphyria, 905t

Erythromycin
  for chancroid, 1007
  for chlamydial infections, 999
  for gonorrhea, 997
  for inclusion conjunctivitis, 1164
  for rheumatic fever, 1085
  for rosacea, 1252
  for trachoma, 1168
Erythroplasia of Queyrat, 131t
  penile cancer and, 107
Erythropoiesis, 1017
Erythropoietic porphyria, 905t
Escherichia coli infections, 191-193
Esophageal atresia, 691-695, 692-693i
Esophageal cancer, 85-87
  staging, 86
Esophageal diverticula, 697-699
Esophageal stricture, 695-696
Esophageal varices, 758
Esophagogastrectomy, 86, 87
Esophagogastroduodenoscopy, 685
  in celiac disease, 715
  in esophageal cancer, 86
  in gastritis, 702
  in hiatal hernia, 700
  in Mallory-Weiss syndrome, 697
  in peptic ulcers, 706
Essential familial hypercholesterolemia, 899t
Essential pruritus, 1260-1261t
Essential thrombocytopenia, 1046-1047
Estrogen for breast cancer, 80
Estrogen replacement therapy, 947
Ethacrynic acid for hypercalcemia, 918
Ethambutol for tuberculosis, 564
Ethosuximide for epilepsy, 641
Etidronate for Paget's disease, 598
Etretinate for psoriasis, 1267
Eulenberg's disease, 1290-1291t
European blastomycosis, 215-216
European typhus, 1310-1311t
Evoked potentials, 624
Ewing's sarcoma, 124, 125t
Exanthema subitum. See Roseola infantum.
Exchange transfusion
  for erythroblastosis fetalis, 990, 991
  for hyperbilirubinemia, 985, 987
Excoriation, 1231i
Excretory urography, 777t
  in abdominal injuries, 300
  in acute pyelonephritis, 785
  in benign prostatic hyperplasia, 821
  in bladder cancer, 98
  in fallopian tube cancer, 122
  in hydronephrosis, 800
  in medullary sponge kidney, 779
  in multiple myeloma, 128
  in ovarian cancer, 118

i refers to an illustration; t refers to a table.

Excretory urography *(continued)*
  in polycystic kidney disease, 781
  in renal calculi, 792, 793
  in renal infarction, 790
  in renal vein thrombosis, 794
  in testicular cancer, 106
  in vesicoureteral reflux, 811
Exercise stress testing, 510, 1062-1063
Exfoliative dermatitis, 1260-1261t
Exhibitionism, 504
Exophthalmos, 842, 843, 844, 1158-1159, 1159i
Exstrophy of bladder, 816i
External otitis. *See* Otitis externa.
Extracapsular cataract extraction, 1179, 1180
Extracellular fluid, 872
Extracorporeal shock wave lithotripsy, 793
Extracorticospinal tract, 620
Extraocular motor nerve palsies, 1182-1183
Extraocular muscles, eye movement
       and, 1153, 1154i
Extrapyramidal system, 620
Extrinsic allergic alveolitis, 1302-1303t
Eye, anatomy and physiology of, 1153-1155,
       1154i
Eyelid disorders, 1157-1163
Eyelids, 1155

F

Fabry's disease, 1290-1291t
Facioscapulohumeral dystrophy, 581-583
Factitious disorders, 472
Factor concentrates for hemophilia, 26-27
Factor replacements products, 26
Falciparum malaria, 261, 263, 264. *See also*
       Malaria.
Fallopian tube cancer, 122-123
Fallopian tubes, 931, 931i
Familial broad-beta disease, 899t
Familial hyperbetalipoproteinemia, 899t
Familial juvenile nephronophthisis, 1300-1301t
Familial myoglobinuria, 1302-1303t
Famotidine for latex allergy, 359
Fanconi's syndrome, 1025, 1290-1291t
Farmer's lung, 1302-1303t
Fasciotomy for snakebites, 327
Fasting as obesity treatment, 887-888
Fasting blood glucose
  in anorexia, 494
  in diabetes mellitus, 866
  in pancreatic cancer, 89
Fasting hypoglycemia, 895, 896
Fat embolism as fracture complication, 303
Fat-induced hyperlipemia, 899t
Fats
  function of, 871t
  metabolism of, 870-871

Fat-soluble vitamins, functions of, 871t
Fatty liver, 760-762
  massive ascites in, 761i
Febrile nonhemolytic transfusion reactions,
       363-364
Fecal occult blood test
  in colorectal cancer, 93
  in gallbladder cancer, 102
  in pancreatic cancer, 89
Feedback system of endocrine system, 825, 825i
Female genitalia, 930-932, 931i
Female infertility, 947-949
Femoral aneurysm, 1141, 1143
Femoral hernia, 726i
Femoral thrombophlebitis, 980
Fenoprofen for rheumatoid arthritis, 366, 367t
Fen-phen, 888
Fetal cell transplantation, 658
Fetishism, 504
Fever in juvenile rheumatoid arthritis, 371
Fibrin degradation products, 1022
Fibrinogen levels, 1023
  in disseminated intravascular coagulation,
       1052
  in *Hantavirus* pulmonary syndrome, 230
  in malaria, 263
Fibrinolytic therapy, 1103, 1104-1105
Fibrin split products, 1022
Fibroids, 943-944
Fibromyomas, 943-944
Fibrosarcoma, 124, 126t
Fibrosis, hepatic, 756-757, 759
Fifth disease, 1290-1291t
Fight-or-flight response, 827
Filatov-Dukes disease, 1288-1289t
File-cutter's disease, 1292-1293t
Finasteride for benign prostatic hyper-
       plasia, 822
First-degree atrioventricular block, 1131t
Fish-skin disease, 1292-1293t
Fissure, 1231i
Fistulotomy, 739
Flaccid neurogenic bladder, 813
Flail chest, 295-296, 295i, 297
Flax-dresser's disease, 1292-1293t
Flea typhus, 1310-1311t
Flecked retina syndrome, 1292-1293t
Fleischner's disease, 1292-1293t
Flesh-eating bacteria. *See* Necrotizing fasciitis.
Flood fever, 1310-1311t
Flooding as behavioral therapy, 468
Fludrocortisone for congenital adrenal
       hyperplasia, 861
Fluid and electrolyte balance, 872-873
Fluid balance, maintaining, in cancer
       patient, 54

Fluid intake, restricted
  in hyponatremia, 912
  for syndrome of inappropriate antidiuretic
    hormone, 925
Fluid replacement therapy
  for burns, 310, 311
  for cholera, 196
  for decompression sickness, 320
  for heat syndrome, 316, 317t
  for hypovolemic shock, 1117, 1118
Fluorescein angiography, 1156
Fluorescence in situ hybridization for
  velocardiofacial syndrome, 38
Fluorescent antibody test
  in ehrlichiosis, 207
  in plague, 202
  in whooping cough, 200
Fluorescent treponemal antibody-absorption
  test, 1004
5-Fluorouracil for basal cell epithelioma, 129
Fluphenazine for delusional disorders, 448
Flu. See Influenza.
Focal glomerulosclerosis, 795-796
Focal polypoid hyperplasia, 739, 740
Folic acid
  foods high in, 1024t
  function of, 871t
Folic acid deficiency anemia, 1024-1025
Folic acid supplements
  for folic acid deficiency anemia, 1025
  recommendations for, 41
  for sickle cell anemia, 24
  for sideroblastic anemias, 1029
  for thalassemia, 1031
Follicular carcinoma, 67
Follicular cysts, 940, 941, 941i
Follicular disorders, 1246-1252
Follicular impetigo, 1234
Folliculitis, 1234-1236, 1235i
Food diary, allergic disorders and, 362
Food poisoning, 164-165t, 703-704. See also
  Botulism.
  Vibrio parahaemolyticus as cause of, 195
Footdrop, 610
Forefoot neuroma, 1302-1303t
Foscavir for genital herpes, 1001
Fourth disease, 1288-1289t
Fourth nerve (trochlear) palsy, 1182
Fowl-nest fever, 209-210
Fractured nose, 290-291
Fractures in osteogenesis imperfecta, 10-11
Fragile X syndrome, 29-31
  inheritance patterns in, 29-30
Frambesia tropica, 1312-1313t
Frederickson's hyperlipoproteinemia, 899t
Fresh frozen plasma for hemophilia, 26
Friedländer's disease, 1292-1293t

Friedrich's ataxia, 1292-1293t
Friedrich's disease, 1292-1293t
Frostbite, 313-316, 314i
Frotteurism, 504
Fructose intolerance, hereditary, 898
Fructose tolerance test, 898
Fulguration
  for bladder cancer, 98, 100
  for rectal polyps, 740
Functional Dementia Scale, 412
Functional encopresis, 417
Functional enuresis, 417
Functioning metastatic thyroid carcinoma, 841
Fungi, 153
Furosemide
  for hypercalcemia, 918
  for hypermagnesemia, 922
  for pulmonary edema, 527
  for rhabdomyolysis, 615
  for transfusion reactions, 364
Furunculosis, 1234-1236, 1235i

G

Gaisböck's syndrome, 1038-1039
Galactokinase-deficiency galactosemia, 890-892
Galactorrhea, 983-984
Galactosemia, 890-892
  diet for, 892
  metabolic pathway in, 890, 891i
Gallbladder, anatomy of, 750-751
Gallbladder cancer, 101-103
Gallbladder disorders, 765-769
  assessing for, 751
  diagnostic tests for, 751-752
Gallium scan in Pneumocystis carinii
    pneumonia, 260
Gallstone ileus, 766, 767-769
Gallstones. See Cholelithiasis.
Gardnerella vaginalis infection, 939
Gas gangrene, 183-185
  preventing, 185
Gastrectomy, 83, 84-85
Gastric analysis, 685
Gastric bypass surgery, 888, 908
Gastric cancer, 82-85
  sites of, 83i
  staging, 84
Gastric inhibitory peptide, 687i
Gastric lavage
  for asphyxia, 318
  for poisoning, 323, 325
Gastric resection, 83, 84-85
Gastric ulcers, 704, 705
Gastrin, 686i
Gastritis, 701-703

Gastroenteritis, 703-704
Gastroesophageal reflux disease, 689-691
  lower esophageal sphincter pressure and,
    689, 690i
Gastrografin swallow, 684
Gastrointestinal actinomycosis, 185
Gastrointestinal amyloidosis, 903
Gastrointestinal anthrax, 204
Gastrointestinal complications
  in alcohol-related disorder, 427
  in cystic fibrosis, 15
Gastrointestinal radiation exposure, 321
Gastrointestinal system, assessment of, 683-684
Gastrointestinal tract, 683
  anatomy and physiology of, 684
  histology of, 685
Gastrojejunostomy
  for gastric cancer, 83, 84-85
  for pancreatic cancer, 90
Gastroscopy in gastric cancer, 83
Gastrostomy for gastric cancer, 83, 84-85
Gastrostomy tube care, 87
Gaucher's disease, 901-902
Gel flotation pads, 1275
Gender identity disorders, 502
  diagnostic criteria for, 503
Generalized anxiety disorder, 461-463
  diagnostic criteria for, 462
Generalized salivary gland disease, 251-253
Generalized tonic-clonic seizure, 641
Genes, 2, 2i
Gene therapy for cystic fibrosis, 16
Genetic counseling, 7, 8
  for cleft lip/palate, 42
  for fragile X syndrome, 31
  for hemophilia. 27
  for Marfan syndrome, 12
  for phenylketonuria, 19-20
  for sickle cell anemia, 24-25
  for thalassemia, 1031
  for Wilson's disease, 763-764
Genetic disorders, 1-44
  chromosomal, 6
  detecting, 6-8
  multifactorial, 6
  patterns of transmission in, 4
  single-gene, 4
  types of, 3
Genetic testing, 6-8
Genital herpes, 234, 999-1001. See also Herpes
    simplex.
  cycle in, 1000i
Genitalia
  female, 930-932, 931i
  male, 994i
Genital warts, 1001-1002
Geotrichosis, 1292-1293t

GERD. See Gastroesophageal reflux disease.
Gerlier's disease, 1292-1293t
German measles. See Rubella.
Gestational diabetes, 865, 972-974
Gestational hypertension, 962-964
Giardia enteritis, 266-267
Giardiasis, 266-267
Gigantism, 830-832
Gilchrist's disease, 218-220
Gingivitis, 688t
Glasgow Coma Scale, 621-622, 622t
Glaucoma, 1183-1186, 1185i
Glioblastoma multiforme, 57t, 59, 61. See also
    Brain tumors, malignant.
Glioma of the optic nerve, 1292-1293t
Global Deterioration Scale, 412
Globoid cell leukodystrophy, 1298-1299t
Glomerulonephritis as lupus complication, 379
Glossitis, 688t
Glossopharyngeal neuralgia, 1292-1293t
Glucagon, 826
Gluconeogenesis, 870
Glucose-6-phosphate dehydrogenase
    deficiency, 1292-1293t
Glucose suppression test, 831
Gluten enteropathy, 714-716
Gluten-free diet, 715-716
Glycogenesis, 870
Glycogenolysis, 870
Glycogen storage diseases, 892-895
  rare forms of, 893-894t
Glycolysis, 870
GM_2 gangliosidosis, 17-18
Goeckerman regimen, 1267
Goldmann's applanation, 1156
Gold salts
  for juvenile rheumatoid arthritis, 372, 373
  for rheumatoid arthritis, 366, 368t
Gonadotropin-releasing hormone
    analogues, 944
Gonioscopy, 1156
Gonococcal ophthalmia neonatorum,
    995-996, 997
Gonococcal septicemia, 995
Gonorrhea, 995-997, 997i
  pathophysiology of, 996i
Goodpasture's syndrome, 380-381
Gout, 585-587
  tophaceous deposits in, 586, 586i
Gouty arthritis. See Gout.
Gower's sign, 581
Grading of tumor, 50
Graefe's sign, 1292-1293t
Graft-versus-host disease, 382
Grandiose delusions, 446
Grand mal seizure, 641
Granulocyte colony-stimulating factor, 1055

i refers to an illustration; t refers to a table.

Granulocyte-macrophage colony-stimulating factor, 1055
Granulocytes, 345
Granulocytopenia, 1053-1055
  in chronic lymphocytic leukemia, 149
Granuloma fungoides, 143-144
Granulomatosis, 385t
Granulomatous colitis. See Crohn's disease.
Granulosa-lutein cysts, 940, 941
Graves' disease. See Hyperthyroidism.
Grawitz's tumor. See Kidney cancer.
Grinder's disease, 1292-1293t
Grippe. See Influenza.
Ground itch, 270-271
Growth hormone
  deficiency, 828
  functions of, 826
  levels of, in hypopituitarism, 829
  oversecretion of, 830-832
Growth hormone–secreting adenomas, 63
Guillain-Barré syndrome, 666-668
  testing for thoracic sensation in, 667i
Gunther's disease, 904, 905t
Guthrie screening test, 19
Gynecologic disorders, 936-951
  diagnostic tests for, 935-936

H

Habermann's disease, 1292-1293t
Habitual abortion, 957, 958
Haemophilus influenzae infection, 198-199
Hagner's disease, 1294-1295t
Hair, 1229
Hair loss, 1250-1251, 1251i
Hallucinations as communication barrier, 409
Hallucinogen abuse, 434-435t
Hallux valgus, 599-600
Haloperidol
  for autistic disorder, 421
  for delusional disorders, 448
  for Huntington's disease, 657
  for tic disorders, 418
Hamman-Rich syndrome, 561-562
Hammer toe, 599
Hand care, postoperative, 81
Hansen's disease. See Leprosy.
Hantavirus pulmonary syndrome, 229-231
  screening criteria for, 230
Haptoglobin levels in transfusion reactions, 364
Hay fever, 354-356
Headache, 637-640
Head lice, 1244-1246, 1244i
Head-to-toe assessment in trauma, 283
Head trauma, 285-292
Health care–associated infections, 158

Hearing, mechanics of, 1189
Hearing loss, 1204-1206
  as communication barrier, 409
  forms of, 1204-1205
Heart, 1058
Heart attack. See Myocardial infarction.
Heart failure, 1105-1110
  as myocardial infarction complication, 1101t
  pathophysiology of, 1106-1107i
Heart rate, 1059
Heart sounds, 1059
Heat cramps, 316, 317t
Heat exhaustion, 316, 317t
Heatstroke, 316, 317t
Heat syndrome, 316
Heavy chain disease, 1294-1295t
Heberden's nodes, 591i
Heerfordt's syndrome, 1294-1295t
Hegar's sign, 934
Helicobacter pylori infection, 702
HELPP syndrome, 962
Hemangioma of the eye, 1294-1295t
Hematocrit, 874, 1022
  in abdominal injuries, 300
  in acute respiratory failure in chronic obstructive pulmonary disease, 525
  in chronic granulocytic leukemia, 148
  in cor pulmonale, 528, 529
  in Hantavirus pulmonary syndrome, 230
  in iron deficiency anemia, 1033
  in pancreatic cancer, 89
  in pernicious anemia, 1021
  in radiation exposure, 322
  in secondary polycythemia, 1040
  in snakebites, 326
  in spurious polycythemia, 1039
Hematologic complications in alcohol-related disorder, 427
Hematologic disorders, 1017, 1020-1056
Hematopoiesis, 1016
Hematopoietic growth factors for cancer, 53
Hematopoietic radiation exposure, 321
Hemin for porphyrias, 904
Hemipelvectomy, 124, 126
Hemochromatosis, 1294-1295t
Hemodialysis, 778, 806t. See also Dialysis.
  for acute renal failure, 783-784
  for chronic renal failure, 804-805
Hemoglobin C–thalassemia disease, 1294-1295t
Hemoglobin electrophoresis, 1022
Hemoglobin levels, 1022
  in abdominal injuries, 300
  in acute respiratory failure in chronic obstructive pulmonary disease, 525
  in anorexia, 494
  in chronic granulocytic leukemia, 148

Hemoglobin levels (continued)
in chronic lymphocytic leukemia, 149
in malaria, 263
in pancreatic cancer, 89
in radiation exposure, 322
in snakebites, 326
in transfusion reactions, 364
Hemolytic crisis in sickle cell anemia, 23
Hemolytic diseases of the neonate, 984-991
Hemolytic streptococcal gangrene. See
Necrotizing fasciitis.
Hemolytic transfusion reactions, 363-364
Hemophilia, 25-28
factor replacement products for, 26-27
inheritance patterns in, 25
parent education for, 28
Hemophilic arthrosis, 584
Hemorrhage as cause of stroke, 643
Hemorrhagic cystitis, 227t. See also Adenovirus
infection.
Hemorrhagic disorders, 1040-1053
Hemorrhoidectomy, 738
Hemorrhoids, 736-738
types of, 737i
Hemostasis
clotting mechanism and, 1018-1019
tests for production of, 1022-1023
Hemothorax, 296, 297, 549-550
Henderson-Jones disease, 1294-1295t
Henoch-Schönlein syndrome, 1040, 1041
Heparin
for pulmonary embolism, 545, 546
for renal vein thrombosis, 795
for stroke, 645
for thrombophlebitis, 1145
Hepatectomy, 97
Hepatic amyloidosis, 903
Hepatic carcinoma, 96-98
Hepatic coma, 764-765
Hepatic encephalopathy, 764-765
Hepatic failure, signs of, 895
Hepatic porphyria, 905-906t
Hepatic profile in viral hepatitis, 753-754
Hepatitis
nonviral, 755-756
viral, 752-755
Hepatoblastoma, 96
Hepatolenticular degeneration, 762-764
Hepatomas, 96
Hepatorenal glycogen storage disease, 892,
894-895
Hepatosplenomegaly in chronic granulocytic
leukemia, 147
Hereditary angioedema, 362
Hereditary coproporphyria, 906t
Hereditary fructose intolerance, 898

Hereditary hemorrhagic telangiectasia,
1042-1043
Hereditary polyposis, 739, 740
Hereditary spherocytosis, 1294-1295t
Heredity, analysis of, 1-3
Hermansky-Pudlak syndrome, 20
Hermaphrodism, 860
Hermaphroditism, 860
Herniated disk, 602-604
Herniated nucleus pulposus, 602-604
Hernioplasty, 727
Herniorrhaphy, 727
Herpangina, 243-244
Herpes simplex, 233-224
Herpes zoster, 234-236
skin lesions in, 235t
Herpetic keratoconjunctivitis, 234. See also
Herpes simplex.
Herpetic stomatitis, 233, 687, 689. See also
Herpes simplex.
Herpetic whitlow, 234. See also Herpes simplex.
Hers' glycogen storage disease, 893t
Heterotropia, 1308-1309t
Heubner's disease, 1294-1295t
Hexosaminidase deficiency, 17-18
Hiatal hernia, 699-701
types of, 699i
Hiatus hernia. See Hiatal hernia.
HIDA scan in gallbladder disorders, 767
Hidradenitis supporativa, 1310-1311t
High-bulk diet, 733
Highly active antiretroviral therapy for human
immunodeficiency virus infection, 395
Hip dysplasia, 578-581, 579i
Hirschsprung's disease, 730-732
Hirsutism, 1248-1250
Histology
in actinomycosis, 185
in amyloidosis, 903
in aspergillosis endophthalmitis, 217
in necrotizing fasciitis, 174
in Pneumocystis carinii pneumonia, 260
Histoplasmosis, 217-218
Histrionic personality disorder, 486, 489
His-Werner disease, 1310-1311t
Hives, 361-362
HIV infection. See Human immunodeficiency
virus infection.
Hoarseness in laryngeal cancer, 64, 65
Hodgkin's disease, 138-141
Reed-Sternberg cells and, 139i
staging, 140
Hoffa's disease, 1294-1295t
Homans' sign, 980
Homeostasis
assessing, 873
fluid and electrolyte balance and, 872

Homeostasis (*continued*)
  imbalance in, 908-928
  kidneys and, 772
  maintaining, 873-875
Hookworm disease, 270-271
Hordeolum, 1163, 1163i
Hormonal paraneoplastic syndromes, 73
Hormonal receptor assay, 79
Hormonal therapy. *See also* Hormone
    replacement therapy.
  as cancer treatment, 53-54
  for dysfunctional uterine bleeding, 955
  for dysmenorrhea, 938
  for hypogonadism, 1009
  for menopause, 947
  for ovarian cysts, 941
  for prostatic cancer, 104
  for uterine cancer, 113
Hormone levels
  in anorexia, 494
  in menopause, 946-947
Hormone replacement therapy. *See also*
    Hormonal therapy.
  for amenorrhea, 952
  for hypopituitarism, 829
  for osteoporosis, 594
Hospice care, 55-56
Host defense system, 341
Hoyne's sign, 245
Human chorionic gonadotropin
  in hydatidiform mole, 964
  in ovarian cysts, 941
  in spontaneous abortion, 957
Human immunodeficiency virus infection,
    393-397
  common infections and neoplasms in, 394
  tests for diagnosing and tracking, 396t
Human leukocyte antigen typing, 1020
Human leukocyte B27 antigen
  in ankylosing spondylitis, 374
  in juvenile rheumatoid arthritis, 372
  in Reiter's syndrome, 381, 382
Humoral immune response, carcinogenesis
    and, 49
Humoral immunity, 342. *See also* B lympho-
    cytes.
Hunchback, 600-602
Huntington's chorea, 656-657
Huntington's disease, 656-657
Hutchinson freckles. *See* Lentigo maligna.
Hutchinson-Gifford disease, 1294-1295t
Hutinel's disease, 1294-1295t
Hyaline membrane disease, 514-516
Hydatid disease, alveolar, 1294-1295t
Hydatid disease, unilocal, 1294-1295t
Hydatidiform mole, 964-965
Hydatidosus, 1294-1295t

Hydrocephalus, 628-631, 630i
Hydrochloric acid for metabolic alkalosis, 927
Hydrochlorothiazide in diabetes insipidus, 833
Hydrocortisone
  for adrenal hypofunction, 851
  for congenital adrenal hyperplasia, 860, 861
  for latex allergy, 359
Hydronephrosis, 800-801
Hydrophobia. *See* Rabies.
Hydrops fetalis, 987, 988-989, 990
Hydrops tubae profluens, 122
Hydrostatic reduction, 728-729
Hydroxychloroquine
  for juvenile rheumatoid arthritis, 372
  for rheumatoid arthritis, 366, 367t
  for systemic lupus erythematosus, 379
Hydroxyurea
  for chronic granulocytic leukemia, 148
  for sickle cell anemia, 24
Hydroxyzine for urticaria, 362
Hyperaldosteronism, 856-858
Hyperbaric oxygenation therapy
  for decompression sickness, 320
  for diabetic wounds, 867
  for gas gangrene, 184
  for necrotizing fasciitis, 174
Hyperbetalipoproteinemia, 899t
Hyperbilirubinemia, 984-987
  causes of, 985, 986
Hypercalcemia, 914-919, 914t, 916-917i
  in hyperparathyroidism, 847, 848
  in multiple myeloma, 128
Hypercarotenemia, 884-885
  in vitamin A replacement therapy, 876
Hyperchloremia, 919-921
Hyperemesis gravidarum, 961-962
Hypergonadotropic hypogonadism, 1008, 1009
Hyperhidrosis, 1271-1272
Hyperkalemia, 908-911, 909t
  in acute renal failure, 783
  in acute tubular necrosis, 788
Hyperlipoproteinemia, 898-901
  types of, 898, 899t
Hypermagnesemia, 921-923, 922t
Hypermenorrhea, 952, 954t, 955
Hypernatremia, 911-914, 912t
Hypernephroma. *See* Kidney cancer.
Hyperosmolar coma, 865, 867
Hyperosmolar hyperglycemic nonketotic
    syndrome, 865, 867
Hyperparathyroidism, 847-849
  bone resorption in, 848, 848i
Hyperphosphatemia, 923-924
Hyperpituitarism, 830-832
Hyperprolactinemia, 983-984
Hypersensitivity disorders, 345-347. *See also*
    Allergic disorders.

i refers to an illustration; t refers to a table.

Hypersensitivity reactions, classifying, 346-347t
Hypersensitivity vasculitis, 386t
Hypersplenism, 1055-1056
Hypertension, 1091-1095
  pregnancy-induced, 962-964
  stepped approach to treating, 1093-1095
Hypertensive crisis, 1095
  pathophysiology of, 1092-1093i
Hypertensive retinopathy, 1175-1176, 1177
Hyperthyroidism, 840-844
  forms of, 841
  thyroid cancer and, 69
Hypertrichosis, 1249
Hypertrophic cardiomyopathy, 1113-1114
Hypertrophic pulmonary osteoarthropathy, 73
Hypervitaminosis A, 884-885
  in vitamin A replacement therapy, 876
Hypervitaminosis D, 884-885
Hypocalcemia, 914-919, 914t
  DiGeorge syndrome and, 392
Hypochloremia, 919-921
Hypochondriasis, 476-478
  diagnostic criteria for, 477
Hypocupremia, 1288-1289t
Hypoglycemia, 895-898
  classifying, 895
  diagnosing, 897i
Hypogonadism, 1008-1009
Hypogonadotropic hypogonadism, 1008, 1009
Hypokalemia, 908-911, 909t
  in hyperaldosteronism, 857
Hypomagnesemia, 921-923, 922t
Hypomania, 451, 452-453
Hypomenorrhea, 952
Hyponatremia, 911-914, 912t, 913i
Hypoparathyroidism, 844-847
  DiGeorge syndrome and, 392
  pathophysiology of, 845i
Hypophosphatemia, 923-924
Hypophysectomy
  for Cushing's syndrome, 854
  for hyperpituitarism, 831, 832
  for multiple endocrine neoplasia, 864
Hypopituitarism, 827-830
  pituitary tumors and, 62-63
Hypoplastic anemias, 1025-1028
Hypospadias, 817i
Hypothalamic-pituitary-target organ axis, 825
Hypothalamus, 618, 824-825
Hypothermia, 313-316
  classifying severity of, 314
Hypothyroidism
  in adults, 834-836
  in children, 836-837
  iodine deficiency and, 886
  thyroid cancer and, 69

Hypovolemic shock, 1115-1118
  pathophysiology of, 1116i
Hypoxemia
  in acute respiratory distress syndrome, 521
  in acute respiratory failure in chronic
      obstructive pulmonary disease, 525
  in near drowning, 318
Hysterectomy
  for endometriosis, 943
  for pelvic inflammatory disease, 950
  for postmenopausal bleeding, 956
  for uterine leiomyomas, 944

I

Iatrogenic immunodeficiency, 348-349
Ibritumomab for non-Hodgkin's
    lymphoma, 142
Ibuprofen, 366, 367t
Iceland disease, 1294-1295t
Ichthyosis vulgaris, 1292-1293t
Idiopathic bronchiolitis obliterans with
    organizing pneumonia, 542-543
Idiopathic familial hyperlipoproteinemia, 899t
Idiopathic hypertrophic subaortic stenosis,
    1113-1114
Idiopathic interstitial pneumonitis, 561-562
Idiopathic myoglobinuria, 1302-1303t
Idiopathic pulmonary fibrosis, 561-562
Idiopathic steatorrhea, 714-716
Idiopathic thrombocytopenic purpura,
    1046-1047
IgA. See Immunoglobulin A.
Ileal conduit, caring for, 100-101
Ileoanal pull-through, 708
Iliotibial band syndrome, 1306-1307t
Imatinib for chronic granulocytic
    leukemia, 148
Immobility, coping with, 575-576
Immobilization
  for arm and leg fractures, 304
  for neck injury, 293
  for spinal injuries, 294
  for sprains, 302
Immune complex disease, 346-347
Immune disorders, 341-404
Immune globulin
  for common variable immunodeficiency, 391
  for X-linked infantile hypogammaglobuline-
      mia, 390
Immune response, 341
  carcinogenesis and, 49-50
  role of thymus in, 392
Immunization
  against infection, 156, 158
  for cholera, 195

Immunization (continued)
for influenza, 229
for measles, 238-239
for monkeypox, 242
for mumps, 248
for rabies, 251
for rubella, 238
schedule for, 159t
for smallpox, 241
for tetanus, 181
for whooping cough, 200
Immunodeficiency, 350, 389-404
with eczema and thrombocytopenia, 399-401
iatrogenic, 348-349
Immunodiffusion testing
in blastomycosis, 219
in coccidioidomycosis, 220
Immunoelectrophoresis
in common variable immunodeficiency, 391
in immunoglobulin A deficiency, 392
of serum proteins, 1023
in X-linked infantile hypogammaglobuline-mia, 390
Immunofluorescence
in cholera, 195
in complement deficiencies, 404
in Goodpasture's syndrome, 380
in infectious mononucleosis, 249
in legionnaires' disease, 531
in Lyme disease, 208
in shigellosis, 190
Immunoglobulin A
deficiency, 391-392
levels in ankylosing spondylitis, 374
Immunoglobulins , 342-344
in bronchiolitis obliterans, 542-543
in common variable immunodeficiency, 391
in immunoglobulin A deficiency, 392
in Lyme disease, 208
in severe combined immunodeficiency disease, 402-403
in Wiskott-Aldrich syndrome, 400
in X-linked infantile hypogammaglobuline-mia, 390
molecular structure of, 343i
Immunoglobulin E levels
in allergic rhinitis, 355
in atopic dermatitis, 357
Immunoglobulin M antibody capture enzyme-linked immunosorbent assay
in encephalitis, 650
in West Nile encephalitis, 256-257
Immunomodulators for atopic dermatitis, 357
Immunosuppressive therapy
for bronchiolitis obliterans, 543
for Goodpasture's syndrome, 381
for rheumatoid arthritis, 366, 368t

Immunosuppressive therapy (continued)
for sarcoidosis, 546-547
for scleroderma, 383
Immunosurveillance, 49
Immunotherapy. See also Biotherapy.
for allergic rhinitis, 356
for urticaria, 362
Impedance audiometry, 1190
Impedance plethysmography, 1064
Impetigo, 168-169t, 1232-1234, 1233i
Implosion therapy, 468
Impotence, 499-501
Inactive colon, 732-733
Incentive spirometry, 532
Incisional (ventral) hernia, 726i
Inclusion blennorrhea, 1164
Inclusion conjunctivitis, 1164
Incomplete abortion, 957
Indirect Coombs' test, 1022
Indomethacin
for ankylosing spondylitis, 374
for diabetes insipidus, 833
for rheumatoid arthritis, 366
Inevitable abortion, 957
Infant botulism, 182
Infantile eczema. See Dermatitis.
Infantile paralysis. See Poliomyelitis.
Infant respiratory distress syndrome, 514-516
Infarctive crisis in sickle cell anemia, 22
Infection, 152-279. See also specific infection.
assessment of, 158-160
Centers for Disease Control and Prevention isolation precautions for, 157
definition of, 152
factors that increase risk of, 152
health care–associated, 158
immunization against, 156, 158, 159t
kinds of, 153-154
preventing, 156, 158
sources of potential exposure to, 155
standard precautions for, 155-156
transmission of, 154, 156
variation in severity of, 152
Infectious arthritis, 583-585
Infectious parotitis, 247-248
Infectious polyneuritis. See Guillain-Barré syndrome.
Infective endocarditis. See Endocarditis.
Infertility
female, 947-949
male, 1012-1013
Inflammatory reactions, 1256-1261
Inflammatory response, 341
Influenza, 227-229, 540-541t
classifying viruses in, 228
immunization against, 229
Ingram technique, 1267

Inguinal hernia, 724-728
   common sites of, 726i
Inhalational anthrax, 204
Inheritance patterns
   autosomal dominant, 4-5, 5i
   autosomal recessive, 5, 5i
   in fragile X syndrome, 29-30
   in hemophilia, 25
   in sickle cell anemia, 21, 22i
   X-linked, 5-6, 5i
Insect bites and stings, 328-331t, 329
Insulin, 826
Insulinomas, 89
Insulin replacement
   for diabetes mellitus, 866
   for pancreatic cancer, 89
Insulin resistance syndrome. See Metabolic
   syndrome.
Intake and output assessment, 774
Interferons, 344
   for cancer, 53
   for chronic granulocytic leukemia, 148
   for Kaposi's sarcoma, 137
   for multiple myeloma, 128
Interleukins, 344
   for cancer, 53
Intermittent hydrarthrosis, 584
International Normalized Ratio, 1022
Intersexuality, 860
Interstitial cystitis, 1296-1297t
Intestinal enzymes, 684
Intestinal flu, 703-704
Intestinal lipodystrophy, 1312-1313t
Intestinal lymphangiectasia, 1296-1297t
Intestinal obstruction, 721-724
   symptom progression in, 724-725i
Intra-aortic balloon pump, 1120, 1121i, 1122
Intracapsular cataract extraction, 1179
Intracellular fluid, 872
Intracerebral hemorrhage, 286
Intracranial abscess, 654-656
Intracranial hemorrhage, 286
Intracranial pressure, increased, patho-
   physiology of, 60i, 625i
Intracranial pressure monitoring, 626
Intraocular lens implant, 1179, 1180
Intrauterine-intraperitoneal transfusion,
   990, 991
Intrinsic factor deficiency, 1020
Intrinsic renal failure, 782
Intussusception, 728-729
Invasive procedures, precautions for, 155
Iodine deficiency, 885-886
Iodine (^{131}I) therapy, 843
Iodoquinol for amebiasis, 266
Iontophoresis, 1271
Ipecac syrup for poisoning, 323, 325

Iranian Americans, cultural considerations
   for, 1280t
Iridectomy, 1186
Iridocyclitis, 1172
Iritis, 1172
Iron, absorption and storage of, 1032
Iron deficiency anemia, 1031-1034
Iron replacement therapy
   administering, 1035i
   for iron deficiency anemia, 1033
Irritable bowel syndrome, 713-714
Isambert's disease, 1296-1297t
Ishihara's test, 1155-1156
Islet cell tumors, 89
Isolation precautions, 157
Isoniazid for tuberculosis, 564
Isotretinoin
   for acne, 1247-1248
   for rosacea, 1252
Isoxsuprine for premature labor, 975
Ivermectin for strongyloidiasis, 277

J

Jaffee-Lichtenstein disease, 1296-1297t
Jaksch's anemia, 1296-1297t
Jaksch's syndrome, 1296-1297t
Janeway Type 3 dysgammaglobulinemia,
   391-392
Jansen's disease, 1296-1297t
Jantene procedure, 1076
Japanese Americans, cultural considerations
   for, 1281t
Japanese encephalitis, 652-653
Japanese river fever, 1310-1311t
Jarisch-Herxheimer reaction, 210
Jaundice, 985. See also Hyperbilirubinemia.
Jaw, dislocated or fractured, 291-292
Jealous delusions, 446
Jejunostomy, 83, 84-85
Jensen's disease, 1296-1297t
Jewett-Strong-Marshall staging system, 99t
Jock itch, 1239, 1240
Joint disorders, 583-591
Joints, 571-573
JSM staging system. See Jewett-Strong-Marshall
   staging system.
Junctional rhythm, 1130t
Junctional tachycardia, 1131t
Juvenile angiofibroma, 1215, 1225, 1296-1297t
Juvenile kyphosis, 600-602
Juvenile pernicious anemia, 1020
Juvenile polyps, 739, 740
Juvenile rheumatoid arthritis, 370-372

K

Kaplan therapy, 499
Kaposi's sarcoma, 136-138
   staging, 137
Kaposi's varicelliform eruption, 1257
Karyotype analysis, 7
Kawasaki disease, 386t
Kayser-Fleischer ring in Wilson's disease, 763i
Keloid, 1231i
Keratitis, 1168-1169
Keratoconus, 1296-1297t
Keratosis follicularis, 1296-1297t
Keratosis pilaris, 1296-1297t
Kernicterus, 984
Kernig's sign, 649i
Ketoacidosis, 865, 867
Ketoconazole
   for Cushing's syndrome, 854
   for tinea versicolor, 1238
17-Ketosteroid levels
   in abnormal premenopausal bleeding, 952
   in adrenogenital syndrome, 860
   in amenorrhea, 952
   in ovarian cysts, 941
   in precocious puberty, 945
Keyhole surgery, 1098
Kidney cancer, 94-96
   staging, 95
Kidneys
   anatomy of, 771, 771i
   blood supply to, 772
   homeostasis and, 772
   hormonal regulation of, 773
   innervation of, 772
Kidney stones. *See* Renal calculi.
Kidney transplantation, 778
Kidney-ureter-bladder radiography, 776
Kienböck's disease, 1296-1297t
Klebsiella pneumonia, 538-539t
Klinefelter's syndrome, 35-37
   fertilization in, 36i
Kock pouch, 708
Koebner's phenomenon, 1266
Kohler's bone disease, 1296-1297t
Kohler-Stieda-Pellegrini disease, 1306-1307t
Koplik's spots, 239-240
Krabbe's disease, 1298-1299t
Kraurosis vulvae, 1284-1285t
Kugelberg-Welander syndrome, 1298-1299t
Kümmell's disease, 1298-1299t
Kupffer cell sarcoma, 96
Kuru, 1298-1299t
Kwashiorkor, 888-890
Kyphosis, 600-602

L

Labor and delivery, 934-935
Labyrinthitis, 1203-1204
Laceration, 332, 334t
La Crosse encephalitis, 652
Lactate dehydrogenase
   in chest injuries, 296
   in liver cancer, 96
   in trichinosis, 269
Lactation, physiology of, 982i
Lactulose for hepatic encephalopathy, 765
Laënnec's cirrhosis, 756
Lambliasis, 266-267
Laminectomy
   for herniated disk, 603, 604
   for spinal neoplasms, 71
Landouzy-Dejerine dystrophy, 581-583
Landry-Guillain-Barré syndrome. *See* Guillain-Barré syndrome.
Language difficulties as communication
   barrier, 409
Laparoscopy, 935-936
Laparotomy
   for ectopic pregnancy, 960
   for ovarian cysts, 942
   for uterine leiomyomas, 944
Large-bowel obstruction, 721-724, 724-725i
Large intestine, function of, 684
Larsen-Johansson disease, 1298-1299t
Larsen's disease, 1298-1299t
Laryngeal cancer, 64-67
   classifying, 64
   staging, 66-67
Laryngeal tomography in laryngeal cancer, 65
Laryngectomy, aftercare for, 65-67
Laryngitis, 518, 1224-1225
Laryngography in laryngeal cancer, 65
Laryngoscopy in croup, 518
Laryngotracheobronchitis, 518
Lasegue test, 603
Laser angioplasty, 1097
Laser photocoagulation, 1178
Laser surgery
   for cervical cancer, 109, 110
   for laryngeal cancer, 65
Lassa fever, 253
Late benign syphilis, 1003, 1004
Late luteal phase dysphoric disorder, 936-937
Latent typhus, 1284-1285t
Latex, products that contain, 358
Latex allergy, 357-359
   people at risk for, 358
Laubenstein's staging system, 137
Laurence-Moon-Biedl syndrome, 1180
Laxatives for inactive colon, 733
Lazy colon, 732-733

i refers to an illustration; t refers to a table.

Lecithin/sphingomyelin ratio
  in gestational diabetes, 973
  in infant respiratory distress syndrome, 515
  in premature rupture of membranes, 977
Left ventricular papillary muscle rupture as
    myocardial infarction complication,
    1101t
Left ventricular remodeling surgery, 1109
Leg fractures, 302-306
  classifying, 305
Legg-Calvé-Perthes disease, 595-596
Legionnaires' disease, 530-531
  people at risk for, 530
Leiner's disease, 1298-1299t
Leishmaniasis, 1298-1299t
Lenegre's disease, 1298-1299t
Lens, 1154i, 1155
Lentigo maligna, 134
  melanoma and, 133
Leprosy, 210-213
  forms of, 211
Leptospirosis, 1298-1299t
Lesch-Nyhan syndrome, 1298-1299t
Lethargic encephalitis, 651, 1290-1291t
Letterer-Siwe disease, 1298-1299t
Leukapheresis for chronic granulocytic
    leukemia, 148
Leukemia. See specific type.
Leukemic reaction, 1018
Leukocyte alkaline phosphatase levels in
    chronic granulocytic leukemia, 147
Leukocytes. See White blood cells.
Leukocytosis
  in chronic granulocytic leukemia, 147
  in Haemophilus influenzae infection, 198
  in near drowning, 319
  in salmonellosis, 189
  in septic shock, 197
Leukopenia
  in chronic granulocytic leukemia, 147-148
  in Haemophilus influenzae infection, 198
  in salmonellosis, 189
Leukoplakia, 131t
  penile cancer and, 107
Leuprolide for prostatic cancer, 53-54
Level of consciousness, assessing, 621-622, 622t
Levodopa for Parkinson's disease, 658
Levothyroxine for hypothyroidism, 835,
    836, 837
Lewandowsky-Lutz disease, 1300-1301t
Lice, types of, 1244-1246, 1244-1245i
Lichenification, 1231i
Lichen planus, 1268-1269
Lichen sclerosus et atrophicus, 1288-1289t
Lichen simplex chronicus, 1260-1261t
Lichtheim's disease, 1300-1301t
Lichtheim's syndrome, 1300-1301t

Li-Fraumeni syndrome, 1300-1301t
Limb-girdle dystrophy, 581-583
Lindane
  for pediculosis, 1245
  for scabies, 1241, 1242
Lipase chain reaction, 996
Lipid nephrosis, 795
Lipogenesis, 870
Lipolysis, 870
Lipophagia granulomatosis, 1312-1313t
Lipoprotein levels in metabolic syndrome, 907
Listeriosis, 179-180
Lithium
  for bipolar disorders, 451, 454
  for hyponatremia, 912
Liver
  anatomy and physiology of, 747-748
  functions of, 748-749
Liver abscess, 759-760
Liver cancer, 96-98
Liver disorders, 752-765
  assessing for, 749-750
  diagnostic tests for, 750
Liver enzyme tests in cystic fibrosis, 16
Liver function studies, 750. See also specific tests.
  in alcohol-related disorder, 428
  in bile duct cancer, 102
  in breast cancer, 79
  in fatty liver, 761
  in gallbladder cancer, 102
  in infectious mononucleosis, 249
  in kidney cancer, 94
  in liver cancer, 96
  in ovarian cancer, 118
  in pancreatic cancer, 88-89
  in Reye's syndrome, 664
Liver scan, 750
  in chest injuries, 296
  in liver abscess, 760
  in liver cancer, 96
  in ovarian cancer, 118
Lobectomy
  for liver cancer, 97
  for lung cancer, 75-76
Lockjaw, 180-182
Loeffler's endocarditis, 1290-1291t
Löffler's endocarditis, 1290-1291t
Lou Gehrig disease, 671-672
Louis-Bar's syndrome, 1282-1283t
Louse-borne typhus, 1310-1311t
Low air-loss beds, 1275
Low-copper diet, 763
Lower urinary tract infection, 808-810
LSD abuse. See Lysergic acid diethylamide
    abuse.
Lucio's phenomenon, 212
Ludwig's angina, 1300-1301t

i refers to an illustration; t refers to a table.

Lugol's solution, 840
Lukes classification for non-Hodgkin's
    lymphoma, 142t
Lumbar puncture, 624, 626
    in acute leukemia, 145
    in brain tumors, 59
    in cerebral aneurysm, 633
    in herpes zoster, 236
    in meningitis, 648
    in multiple sclerosis, 672-673
    in neurofibromatosis, 9
    in nocardiosis, 186
    in spinal injuries, 294
    in spinal neoplasms, 71
Lumpectomy, 80
Lumpy jaw, 185
Lunatomalacia, 1296-1297t
Lung abscess, 548-549
Lung cancer, 72-76
    staging, 74
Lung fluke disease, 1300-1301t
Lung scan, 510
    in chest injuries, 296
    in Hodgkin's disease, 139
    in pulmonary embolism, 544
Lung volume reduction surgery, 558
Lupus erythematosus, 376-380
Lyme disease, 207-209
Lymphangiography
    in Hodgkin's disease, 139
    in ovarian cancer, 118
Lymphatic system, 1061
Lymphedema, exercises to prevent, 81
Lymphocytes, 1018, 1019i
Lymphocytic choriomeningitis, 647,
    1282-1283t
Lymphocytopenia, 1053-1055
Lymphocytosis in chronic lymphocytic
    leukemia, 149
Lymphogranuloma venereum, 998
Lymphopenia, 1053-1055
Lymphosarcomas. *See* Non-Hodgkin's
    lymphoma.
Lysergic acid diethylamide abuse, 434t

M

MacLean-Maxwell disease, 1300-1301t
Macroglobulinemia, 1300-1301t
Macrophages, 344
Macular degeneration, age-related, 1178-1179
Macula retinae degeneration, 1284-1285t
Macule, 1230i
Mad cow disease, 663
Maddox rod test, 1156
Madura foot, 1302-1303t

Maduromycosis, 1302-1303t
Magnesium imbalance, 921-923
    magnesium levels in, 921
    signs and symptoms of, 921-922, 922t
Magnesium sulfate
    for hypomagnesemia, 922
    for pregnancy-induced hypertension, 963
    for premature labor, 975, 976
Magnetic resonance imaging scan, 413-414
    in esophageal cancer, 86
    in head trauma, 285, 287, 288, 289
    in herniated disk, 603
    in kyphosis, 601
    in Legg-Calvé-Perthes disease, 595
    in necrotizing fasciitis, 174
    in neurofibromatosis, 9
    in osteomyelitis, 592
    in pancreatic cancer, 88
    in pituitary tumors, 63
    in polymyositis, 388
    in renal calculi, 792
    in schizophrenia, 439-440
    in spinal injuries, 294
    in spinal neoplasms, 71
    in stroke, 644
    in tendinitis, 608
    in toxoplasmosis, 268
    in trisomy 13 syndrome, 35
Major depression, 455-459
    diagnostic criteria for, 457
    suicide risk in, 455, 458
Major histocompatibility complex, 342
Malaria, 261-265
    pathophysiology of, 262i
    preventing, 264
Malathion lotion for pediculosis, 1245
Male genitalia
    anatomy of, 994i
    assessing, 993
Male infertility, 1012-1013
Male reproductive disorders, 1008-1014
Malibu disease, 1300-1301t
Malignant cutaneous reticulosis, 143-144
Malignant giant cell tumor, 124, 125t
Malignant hypertension, 1091
Malignant lymphomas. *See* Non-Hodgkin's
    lymphoma.
Malignant melanoma of the eye, 1300-1301t
Malignant neoplasms. *See* Cancer.
Malignant plasmacytoma, 127-129
Malignant tumors, characteristics of, 47t
Mallory-Weiss syndrome, 696-697
Malnutrition as anorexia complication, 493
Malta fever, 202-204
Mammography
    for breast cancer, 79
    in ovarian cancer, 118

Mannitol
  for cerebral contusion, 287
  for rhabdomyolysis, 615
  for transfusion reactions, 364
Manual traction, 574
Maple syrup urine disease, 1300-1301t
Marasmus, 888-890
Marble bone disease, 1282-1283t
Marburg disease, 1300-1301t
Marburg hemorrhagic fever, 1300-1301t
Marburg virus disease, 1300-1301t
Marfan syndrome, 11-13
Marie-Strümpel disease, 373-375
Marijuana abuse, 432t
Mask of pregnancy, 1255
Mast cells, 345
Mastectomy, 80
  postoperative care for, 80-81
Masters and Johnson therapy
  for arousal disorder, 497
  for premature ejaculation, 501
  for vaginismus, 499
Mastitis, 981-983
Mastoidectomy, 1199-1200
Mastoiditis, 1199-1200
Maternal drug use, effect of, on infant, 971i
McArdle's glycogen storage disease, 893t
Mean corpuscular hemoglobin, 1022
Mean corpuscular hemoglobin concentration, 1022
Mean corpuscular volume, 1022
Meares and Stamey technique, 818-819
Measles. See Rubeola.
Measles vaccine, administering, 239
Mebendazole
  for ascariasis, 272
  for enterobiasis, 274
  for hookworm disease, 271
  for trichinosis, 270
Mechanical ventilation, 513-514
  for acute respiratory distress syndrome, 523, 524
  for acute respiratory failure in chronic obstructive pulmonary disease, 525
  for asbestosis, 567
  for coal worker's pneumoconiosis, 569
  for cor pulmonale, 529
  for infant respiratory distress syndrome, 515, 516
  for respiratory acidosis, 534
  for silicosis, 566
Meckel's diverticulum, 717
Mediterranean disease, 1030-1031
Medroxyprogesterone
  for amenorrhea, 951
  for ovarian cysts, 942
  for precocious puberty, 945

Medullary carcinoma, 67
Medullary cystic disease, 1300-1301t
Medullary sponge kidney, 779
Medulloblastoma, 58t, 59. See also Brain tumors, malignant.
Megaloblastic anemia, 1302-1303t
Meiosis, 3i
Melanoma, malignant, 132-136
  Breslow level method for measuring, 133
  staging, 135i
  types of, 133
Melanotic freckles. See Lentigo maligna.
Melasma, 1255
Melioidosis, 193
Melphalan-prednisone combination for multiple myeloma, 128
Membranoproliferative glomerulonephritis, 796
Membranous glomerulonephritis, 795
Mendelian disorders. See Single-gene disorders.
Ménière's disease, 1202-1203
  risk factors for, 1202
Meningeal leukemia, 145, 146
Meningioma, 58t, 59, 61, 70-71. See also Brain tumors, malignant and Spinal neoplasms, malignant.
Meningitis, 172-173t, 646-650. See also Meningococcal infections.
  listeriosis and, 179, 180
Meningocele, 39, 40. See also Neural tube defects.
Meningococcal infections, 176-178
Meningococcemia, 176, 177
Meningomyelocele, 39, 40. See also Neural tube defects.
Menopause, 945-947
Menorrhagia, 952, 954t
Menstrual cycle, 932-933, 933i
Mental health. See also Psychiatric disorders.
  classifying disorders in, 407-408
  economic factors in, 407
  holistic care and, 408
  patient history and, 408, 410
  psychosocial assessment of, 408, 409-410
  social changes and, 407
Mental retardation, 414-416
  causes of, 415
  in Down syndrome, 32
  in fragile X syndrome, 29, 30
Mental status assessment, 410-412, 621
Meperidine
  for pancreatitis, 736
  for pregnancy-induced cardiovascular disease, 970
Metabolic acidosis, 925-927
Metabolic alkalosis, 927-928
Metabolic disorders, 890-908

Metabolic syndrome, 904, 906-908
  risk factors for, 906-907
Metabolism, 870. *See also specific type.*
Metaphyseal dysostosis, 1296-1297t
Metastasis, progression of, 48-49i
Metatarsalgia, 1302-1303t
Methicillin-resistant *Staphylococcus aureus*
  infection, 161, 164-167
  patients at risk for, 161, 164-165
Methionine malabsorption syndrome,
  1308-1309t
Methotrexate
  for psoriatic arthritis, 373
  for rheumatoid arthritis, 366, 368t
Metoclopramide for headache, 638
Metronidazole
  for amebiasis, 266
  for giardiasis, 267
  for nonspecific genitourinary infections, 1007
  for pseudomembranous enterocolitis, 713
  for trichomoniasis, 1005, 1006
Metrorrhagia, 952, 954t, 955
Metyrapone test, 851, 854
Mexican Americans, cultural considerations
  for, 1281t
Meyer-Betz disease, 1302-1303t
Microdiskectomy, 603, 604
Microdrepanocytic disease, 1302-1303t
Micrognathia in Stickler's syndrome, 13
Microvascular bypass, 644
Mifepristone for abortion, 958
Migraine headache, 637-640
  types of, 639t
Milroy's disease, 1302-1303t
Minamata disease, 1302-1303t
Miner's asthma, 567-569
Minimally invasive coronary artery bypass
  surgery, 1098
Mini-Mental Status Examination, 412
Minnesota Multiphasic Personality Inventory,
  412-413
Minor's disease, 1302-1303t
Minoxidil for hair loss, 1250-1251
Miscarriage, 956-959
Miscellaneous thyroiditis, 838
MI. *See* Myocardial infarction.
Missed abortion, 957
Missile injury, 332, 335t
Mitosis, 3i
Mitral insufficiency, 1086, 1088t
Mitral stenosis, 1086, 1088t
Mitral valve, 1058
Mitral valve prolapse syndrome, 1089t, 1090
Mixed hyperlipidemia, 899t
Mixed hypertriglyceridemia, 899t
Mobitz I, 1132t
Mobitz II, 1132t

Moles, types of, 134
Moniliasis. *See* Candidiasis.
Monkeypox, 241-242
Monoamine oxidase inhibitors for major
  depression, 456, 459
Monoclonal antibodies
  for cancer, 53
  for non-Hodgkin's lymphoma, 142
Monocytes, 1018, 1019i
Monocytosis in listeriosis, 179
Mononucleosis, infectious, 248-250,
  1290-1291t
Monospot test in infectious mono-
  nucleosis, 249
Mood disorders, 449-459
Morbilli. *See* Rubeola.
Morphine, 527
Morton's neuroma, 1302-1303t
Motion sickness, 1206-1207
Motor function, assessing, 622-623
Motor neuron disease, 671
Motor tics, 416
Mouth lesions in herpangina, 243, 244
Mucocutaneous lymph node syndrome, 386t
Mucormycosis, 1312-1313t
MUGA scanning. *See* Multiple-gated
  acquisition scanning.
Mule-spinner's disease, 1302-1303t
Multifactorial abnormalities, 6, 38-44
Multiple endocrine neoplasia, 863-864
Multiple-gated acquisition scanning, 1063
Multiple metabolic syndrome. *See* Metabolic
  syndrome.
Multiple myeloma, 127-129
Multiple neuritis, 678-680
Multiple personality disorder. *See* Dissociative
  identity disorder.
Multiple sclerosis, 672-674
  demyelination in, 672, 673i
Mumps, 247-248
Mumps meningitis, 248
Munchausen syndrome, 472
Mupirocin
  for folliculitis, 1235
  for impetigo, 1233
  for methicillin-resistant staph infection, 166
Murine typhus, 1310-1311t
Murray Valley encephalitis, 653
Muscle contraction, mechanism of, 573
Muscle relaxants for cerebral palsy, 628
Muscles, 573
Muscle-tendon ruptures, 302
Muscular dystrophy, 581-583
Musculoskeletal complications
  in Lyme disease, 208
  in polymyositis, 388
  in Reiter's syndrome, 381

i refers to an illustration; t refers to a table.

Musculoskeletal disorders, 571-615
  diagnostic tools for, 574
  patient care in, 574-575
Musculoskeletal system, assessing, 573-574
Mushroom picker's disease, 1302-1303t
Mustard procedure, 1076, 1076i, 1077
Myalgic encephalomyelitis. See Chronic fatigue
  syndrome.
Myasthenia gravis, 668-671
  impaired transmission in, 669i
Myasthenic crisis, 670
Mycetoma, 216, 217, 1302-1303t
Mycosis fungoides, 143-144
Myelitis, 659-660
Myelography, 574, 626
  in herniated disk, 603-604
  in neural tube defects, 40
  in neurofibromatosis, 9
  in spinal neoplasms, 71
Myelomatosis, 127-129
Myelomeningocele, 39, 40. See also Neural tube
  defects.
Myelosclerosis, 1302-1303t
Myelosuppressive therapy, 1036, 1038
Myocardial contusions, 296, 297
Myocardial imaging, 1063
Myocardial infarction, 1100-1105
  complications of, 1101-1102t
  pain in, 1083, 1100
  risk factors for, 1100
Myocarditis, 1077-1079
  diphtheria and, 179
Myoclonic seizure, 641
Myolysis, 944
Myomas, 943-944
Myositis, gas gangrene and, 183, 184
Myringitis, infectious, 1201-1202
Myxedema, signs of, 834, 835i
Myxedema coma, 835

N

Nails, 1228
Naltrexone, 428-429
Naproxen
  for headache, 638
  for rheumatoid arthritis, 367t
Narcissistic personality disorder, 486-487, 489
Narrow-angle glaucoma, 1184-1186
Nasal cultures in influenza, 228
Nasal papillomas, 1214-1215
Nasal polyps, 1213-1214
Nasogastric intubation, 685-686
Nasogastric lavage for hypothermia, 315
National Cancer Institute system, non-
      Hodgkin's lymphoma classification
      and, 142t

Near drowning, 318-319
Neck trauma, 292-293
Necrotizing enterocolitis, 709-711
Necrotizing fasciitis, 167, 172-175
  risk factors for contracting, 175
Necrotizing ulcerative gingivitis, 688t
Necrotizing vasculitis, 387t
Neonatal jaundice. See Hyperbilirubinemia.
Neonatal streptococcal infections, 170-171t
Neonate
  effect of maternal drug use on, 971i
  hemolytic diseases of, 984-991
  jaundice in, 984-987
Neoplasms, malignant. See Cancer.
Neostigmine for myasthenia gravis, 670
Nephrectomy, 94, 95-96
Nephrocarcinoma. See Kidney cancer.
Nephrogenic diabetes insipidus, 832-833
Nephrolithiasis. See Renal calculi.
Nephrons, 772
Nephrotic syndrome, 795-798
  pathophysiology of, 796i
Nephrotomography, 778t
  in kidney cancer, 94
Nephrotoxic injury, 787
Neural tube defects, 38-42
Neurilemoma. See Schwannoma.
Neurodermatitis, localized, 1260-1261t
Neurofibromatosis, 8-10
Neurogenic arthropathy, 588-589
Neurogenic bladder, 812-814
Neurohypophysis, 825-826, 832
Neuroleptic drugs. See Antipsychotic drugs.
Neuroleptic malignant syndrome, 443
Neurologic bladder dysfunction, 812-814
Neurologic complications
  in alcohol-related disorder, 427
  in leprosy, 211
  in Lyme disease, 208
  in pituitary tumors, 62
  in systemic lupus erythematosus, 378
Neurologic disorders, 617-681
Neurologic examination in head trauma, 285,
      287, 288
Neurologic function, assessing, 621
Neuromuscular complications
  in botulism, 182
  in tetanus, 180-181
Neuromuscular disorders, 668-674
Neuromuscular dysfunction of the lower
      urinary tract, 812-814
Neuron, 617, 617i
Neuropathic bladder, 812-814
Neurosyphilis, 1004
Neutropenia, 1053i
  in acute leukemia, 145
  in chronic granulocytic leukemia, 148

i refers to an illustration; t refers to a table.

Neutropenia (*continued*)
 in chronic lymphocytic leukemia, 149
Neutrophils, 345, 1018, 1019i
Nevi, types of, 134
Nezelof syndrome, 1302-1303t
Niacin
 function of, 871t
 for hyperlipoproteinemia, 900, 901
Niacinamide for niacin deficiency, 879
Niacin deficiency, 877-879
Niclosamide for taeniasis, 272
Nicotinic acid for hyperlipoproteinemia, 900
Niemann-Pick disease, 1304-1305t
Night blindness, 875, 876
Nikolsky's sign, 1262
Nitroblue tetrazolium test in chronic granulo-
  matous disease, 401
Nitrogen mustard for mycosis fungoides, 143
Nitroglycerin for coronary artery disease,
  1097, 1099
Nitroprusside
 for cor pulmonale, 529
 for pulmonary edema, 527
Nocardiosis, 186-187
Nodule, 1230i
Noise-induced hearing loss, 1205, 1206
Nongonococcal urethritis, 1007-1008
Non-Hodgkin's lymphoma, 141-143
 classifying, 142t
Nonlipid reticuloendotheliosis, 1298-1299t
Nonparalytic poliomyelitis, 245. *See also*
  Poliomyelitis.
Nonspecific genitourinary infections,
  1007-1008
Nonsteroidal anti-inflammatory drugs
 for ankylosing spondylitis, 374
 for bursitis, 608
 for carpal tunnel syndrome, 612
 for epicondylitis, 609
 for gout, 586
 for herniated disk, 603
 for juvenile rheumatoid arthritis, 372
 in myocarditis, 1078
 in peptic ulcers, 704, 706
 for pericarditis, 1082
 for psoriatic arthritis, 373
 for rheumatoid arthritis, 366, 367t
 for systemic lupus erythematosus, 379
 for tendinitis, 608
 for vasculitis, 387
Nonstress test, 963
Nontoxic goiter, 839-840
Nontropical sprue, 714-716
Nonurgent category in triage, 281
Nonviral hepatitis, 755-756
Norepinephrine for anaphylaxis, 360
Norrie's disease, 1304-1305t

North American blastomycosis, 218-220
Nose, 1190-1191
 assessment of, 1191
 fractured, 290-291
Nosebleed. *See* Epistaxis.
Nose disorders, 1207-1217
Nosocomial infections, 158
Nucleoside analogues for acquire immuno-
  deficiency syndrome, 395
Nummular dermatitis, 1258-1259t
Nummular eczema, 1258-1259t
Nutrition, maintaining, in cancer patient, 54
Nutritional cirrhosis, 756
Nutritional imbalance, 875-890
Nutritional status, assessing, 874
Nystagmus, 1304-1305t

O

Oasthouse urine disease, 1308-1309t
Obesity, 887-888
Obsessive-compulsive disorder, 465-468,
  487, 489
 diagnostic criteria for, 467
Ocular albinism, 20
Ocular complications
 in leprosy, 211, 212
 in Marfan syndrome, 12
 in Reiter's syndrome, 381-382
 in Sjögren's syndrome, 375
 in Stickler's syndrome, 13
Ocular toxoplasmosis, 268
Oculocutaneous albinism, 20
Ohio Valley disease, 217-218
Oil-retention enema for inactive colon, 733
Olanzapine, 443
 for personality disorders, 484
 for schizophrenia, 441
Oligodendroglioma, 58t, 59, 61. *See also* Brain
  tumors, malignant.
Oligomenorrhea, 952, 954t
Oligo-ovulation, 948
Olivopontocerebellar atrophy, 1304-1305t
Onchocerciasis, 1284-1285t, 1308-1309t
Onychomycosis, 1239, 1241. *See also*
  Candidiasis.
Oophoritis, 950-951
Open brain surgery, 637
Open reduction
 for dislocations,306
 for fractures, 304
 for hip dysplasia, 580
 for jaw fracture, 291
 for nose fracture, 290
Ophthalmodynamometry, 1156
 in arterial occlusive disease,1150

Ophthalmologic examination
  in neurofibromatosis, 9
  in pregnancy-induced hypertension, 963
  in Stickler's syndrome, 14
  in Tay-Sachs disease, 17
Ophthalmoplegia progressiva, 1292-1293t
Ophthalmoscopy, 1156
Opiate abuse, 434t
Opioids for pancreatic cancer, 89
Opitz's disease, 1304-1305t
Optic atrophy, 1181-1182
Optic disk, changes in, 1185i
Oral glucose tolerance test in diabetes
  mellitus, 866
Oral infections, 688t
Orbital cellulitis, 1160-1161
Orchiectomy, 106-107
Orchiopexy, 1010-1011
Orchitis, 819
Organic brain syndrome, 662
Orgasmic disorder, 495-497
Orlistat for metabolic syndrome, 907-908
Ornithosis, 277-278
Orthostatic hypotension as antipsychotic
  adverse effect, 443
Ortolani's sign, eliciting, 579
Oseltamivir for influenza, 228
Osgood-Schlatter disease, 596-597
Osler-Weber-Rendu syndrome, 1042-1043
Osmolality, 872-873
Osteitis deformans, 597-599
Osteitis fibrosa cystica generalisata, 1290-1291t
Osteitis pubis, 1304-1305t
Osteoarthritis, 589-591
  digital joint deformities in, 591i
  pathophysiology of, 590i
Osteochondromatosis, 1294-1295t
Osteochondrosis, 596-597
Osteogenesis imperfecta, 10-11
Osteogenic sarcoma, 124, 125t
Osteomalacia, 881-882
Osteomyelitis, 164-165t, 591-593
  common sites for, 592
Osteopetrosis, 1282-1283t
Osteoplasty, 590
Osteoporosis, 593-595
Osteotomy, 366, 368, 374, 590, 596
Ostium primum defect, 1066
Ostium secundum defect, 1066
Otitis externa, 1191-1194
  differentiating, from otitis media, 1193i
Otitis media, 172-173t, 1195-1199
  differentiating, from otitis externa, 1193i
  sites of, 1196i
Otosclerosis, 1200-1201
Otto pelvis, 1304-1305t
Otto's disease, 1304-1305t

Ovarian cancer, 117-120
  staging, 119
  types of, 117-118
Ovarian cysts, 940-942
Ovarian failure, infertility and, 948
Ovaries, 931-932, 931i
  hormones secreted by, 827
Owren's disease, 1304-1305t
Oxacillin, methicillin-resistant staph infection
  and, 166
Oxidative phosphorylation, 870
Oxygen therapy
  for acute respiratory distress syndrome, 523
  for acute respiratory failure in chronic
    obstructive pulmonary disease, 525
  for asbestosis, 567
  for asphyxia, 318
  for asthma, 353
  for bronchiolitis obliterans, 543
  for chronic obstructive pulmonary
    disease, 558
  for coal worker's pneumoconiosis, 569
  for cor pulmonale, 529
  for croup, 518
  for decompression sickness, 320
  for infant respiratory distress syndrome, 515
  for lung abscess, 549
  for pulmonary edema, 527
  for pulmonary fibrosis, 562
  for pulmonary hypertension, 551
  for silicosis, 566
  for transfusion reactions, 364
Oxygen transport, 508
Oxytocin
  for abortion, 958
  function of, 825
  for hydatidiform mole, 964
Oxyuriasis, 273-274

P

Packed cell volume, 1022
Paget's disease, 597-599
Pain
  cardiac, patterns of, 1083
  complex regional, 680-681
  in dysmenorrhea, 938
  in endometriosis, 942
  in herpes zoster, 235, 236
  in hyperlipoproteinemia, 900
  in necrotizing fasciitis, 174
  pelvic, 938
  in pericarditis, 1082, 1083
  in renal calculi, 792
  in spinal neoplasms, 71
  in thoracic aortic aneurysm, 1135, 1136t

i refers to an illustration; t refers to a table.

Pain control
  cancer patient and, 54-55
  for snakebites, 327
Pain disorder, 475-476
  diagnostic criteria for, 476
Painful crisis in sickle cell anemia, 22
Palatal push-back, 1217
Pallidotomy, 658-659
Pamidronate for Paget's disease, 598
Pancarditis, 1084
Pancreas
  anatomy of, 735i
  hormones secreted by, 826
Pancreatectomy
  for multiple endocrine neoplasia, 864
  for pancreatic cancer, 89, 90-91
Pancreatic cancer, 87-91
  staging, 90
  types of, 88t
Pancreatic disorders, 734-736, 863-868
Pancreatic enzymes, 684
  cystic fibrosis and, 14, 16
  for pancreatic cancer, 89
Pancreatitis, 734-736. See also Chronic
    pancreatitis.
Pancreatoduodenectomy, 89
Pancytopenia, 1025-1026
Panhypopituitarism, 827-830
Panic disorder, 463-465
  diagnostic criteria for, 464
Panuveitis, 1172
Papanicolaou test
  in cervical cancer, 109
  in fallopian tube cancer, 122
  in menopause, 946
  in ovarian cancer, 118
  in uterine cancer, 112
  in vaginal cancer, 116
  in vulvar cancer, 120
Papillary carcinoma, 67
Papule, 1230i
Paracoccidioidomycosis, 1304-1305t
Paradoxical breathing, flail chest and, 295i
Paraesophageal hernia, 699, 699i, 700
Paragonimus heterotrema, 1300-1301t
Paragonimus westermani, 1300-1301t
Parahemophilia, 1304-1305t
Parainfluenza, 225-226
Paralysis agitans, 657-659
Paralytic ileus, 722
Paralytic poliomyelitis, 245, 246. See also
    Poliomyelitis.
Paralyzing vertigo, 1292-1293t
Parametritis, 950-951, 980
Paramyoclonus multiplex, 1292-1293t
Paramyotonia congenita, 1290-1291t
Paranoid disorders. See Delusional disorders.

Paranoid personality disorder, 487, 489-490
Paranoid schizophrenia, 445, 448. See also
    Schizophrenia.
Paranoid thinking as communication
    barrier, 409
Paraphilias, 503-506
  diagnostic criteria for, 504-505
Parasitic infestations, 1241-1246
Parasympathetic nervous system, 621
Parathyroidectomy
  for hyperparathyroidism, 848, 849
  for multiple endocrine neoplasia, 864
Parathyroid glands
  disorders of, 844-849
  hormones secreted by, 826
Parathyroid hormone, 826
  deficiency of, 844-847
  oversecretion of, 847-849
Paratyphoid fever, 187, 188, 188t
Parkinsonism, 657-659
  drug-induced, as antipsychotic adverse
    effect, 443
Parkinson's disease, 657-659
Parkland formula for fluid replacement, 311
Parosteal osteogenic sarcoma, 124, 125t
Paroxysmal disorders, 637-642
Paroxysmal nocturnal hemoglobinuria,
    1304-1305t
Paroxysmal supraventricular tachycardia, 1129t
Parrot fever, 277-278
Parrot's pseudoparalysis, 1310-1311t
Partial thromboplastin time, 1022
  in *Hantavirus* pulmonary syndrome, 230
  in malaria, 263
  in septic shock, 197
  in snakebites, 326
Parturition, abnormalities of, 974-979
Patau's syndrome, 34-35
Patch, 1230i
Patch skin tests, 1232
Patellar chondropathy, 1298-1299t
Patent ductus arteriosus, 1070-1072
Pathologic jaundice, 984, 985
Patient-controlled analgesia, 55
Pediculosis, 1244-1246, 1244-1245i
Pedigree chart, 7
Pedophilia, 504-505
Pelizaeus-Merzbacher disease, 1304-1305t
Pellagra, 877, 877i, 878
Pellegrini's disease, 1306-1307t
Pellegrini-Stieda disease, 1306-1307t
Pelvic cellulitis, 980
Pelvic examination, 935
  in abnormal premenopausal bleeding, 954
  in abortion, 957
  in adolescent pregnancy, 972
  in amenorrhea, 951

i refers to an illustration; t refers to a table.

Pelvic examination (*continued*)
 in ectopic pregnancy, 960
 in endometriosis, 943
 to estimate gestational age, 934
 in placenta previa, 966
 in postmenopausal bleeding, 956
 in rape victim, 337
 in uterine leiomyomas, 944
 in vaginismus, 499
Pelvic exenteration, 113, 114
 for uterine cancer, 113
 for vaginal cancer, 116
Pelvic inflammatory disease, 950-951
Pelvic pain, causes of, 938
Pelvic thrombophlebitis, 980
Pemberton's sign, 839
Pemphigus, 1306-1307t
Penectomy, 108
Penicillamine
 for juvenile rheumatoid arthritis, 372
 for rheumatoid arthritis, 366
 for Wilson's disease, 763
Penicillin
 administration guidelines for, 359
 for peritonsillar abscess, 1220
 for pharyngitis, 1218
 for rheumatic fever, 1085
 for staphylococcal scalded skin
  syndrome, 1236
 for syphilis, 1004
 for tonsillitis, 1219
Penile cancer, 107-108
Penile horn, penile cancer and, 107
Peptic ulcers, 704-707
 development of, 705i
Percussion sounds, interpreting, 512-513t
Percutaneous transhepatic cholangiography,
  750, 751
 in gallbladder disorders, 767
Percutaneous transluminal coronary
  angioplasty, 1097, 1098-1099i
Percutaneous ultrasonic lithotripsy, 793
Percutaneous umbilical cord sampling, 990
Perforated septum, 1209-1211, 1210i
Pericardial friction rub, 1082
Pericardiectomy
 for cardiac tamponade, 1124
 for pericarditis, 1083
Pericardiocentesis, 1124, 1125
Pericarditis, 1081-1084
 as myocardial infarction complication, 1101t
 pain in, 1082, 1083
Pericardium, 1058
Periodontitis, 688t
Peripheral arteriography, 1064
Peripheral blood smear, 1022
Peripheral neovascular retinopathy, 1288-1289t

Peripheral nerve damage, 332
Peripheral nervous system, 617
Peripheral neuritis, 678-680
Peripheral neuropathy, 678-680
Peripheral stem cell rescue for multiple
  myeloma, 128
Peritoneal dialysis, 778, 806t. *See also* Dialysis.
 for acute renal failure, 783, 784
 for chronic renal failure, 804-805
Peritoneal lavage
 in abdominal injuries, 300
 for hypothermia, 315
Peritonitis, 719-721, 980
Peritonsillar abscess, 1219-1221
Permethrin
 for pediculosis,1245
 for scabies1241, 1242
Pernicious anemia, 702, 1020-1023
Perrin-Ferraton disease, 1306-1307t
Persecutory delusions, 446
Personality disorders, 483-490
 diagnostic criteria for, 485-488
Pertussis. *See* Whooping cough.
Pervasive developmental disorders, 420
Petit mal seizures, 640-641
pH
 in acute pyelonephritis, 785
 in acute renal failure, 782
 in chronic renal failure, 804
 in metabolic acidosis, 926
 in metabolic alkalosis, 927
 regulation of, 873
 in renal calculi, 793
Phacoemulsification, 1179
Phalen's wrist-flexion test, 612
Phantom breast syndrome, 81-82
Phantom limb syndrome, 126
Pharyngeal flap procedure, 1217
Pharyngitis, 1217-1218
Pharyngoplasty, 1217
Phencyclidine abuse, 435t
Phenobarbital for epilepsy, 641
Phenothiazine for Huntington's disease, 657
Phentermine for metabolic syndrome, 907
Phenylalanine levels in phenylketonuria, 18-19
Phenylketonuria, 18-20
Phenylpyruvic acid levels in phenylketonuria, 19
Phenytoin
 for arteriovenous malformations, 637
 for encephalitis, 654
 for epilepsy, 641, 642
 for trigeminal neuralgia, 676
Pheochromocytoma, 861-863
Phlebography, 1064
 in thrombophlebitis, 1144
Phlebotomy
 for polycythemia vera, 1036-1037

i refers to an illustration; t refers to a table.

Phlebotomy (continued)
  for secondary polycythemia, 1040
  for sideroblastic anemias, 1029
Phobias, 459-461
  diagnostic criteria for, 460-461
Phosphorus
  foods high in, 924t
  levels of, in phosphorus imbalance, 923
Phosphorus imbalance, 923-924
Photoallergic reaction, 1255-1256
Photodynamic therapy, 1178
  for bladder cancer, 100
  for esophageal cancer, 87
Photosensitivity reactions, 1255-1256
Phototherapy, 985, 986-987
Phototoxic reaction, 1255-1256
Phycomycosis, 1312-1313t
Physiologic jaundice, 984, 985
PID. See Pelvic inflammatory disease.
Pierre Robin syndrome. See Robin syndrome.
Pigmentation disorders, 1252-1256
Pigment cirrhosis, 756
Pilonidal disease, 741-742
Pimozide, 418, 448, 484
Pinkeye, 1164, 1165, 1166
Pinworm infection, 273-274
Piroxicam, 367t
Pituitary diabetes insipidus, 832-834
Pituitary gland
  disorders of, 827-844
  hormones secreted by, 824-825, 826
Pituitary hormones
  deficiency of, 827-830, 832-834
  oversecretion of, 830-832
Pituitary tumors, 62-64
  transsphenoidal surgery for, 63, 63i
Pit viper bites, 325-329
Pityriasis rosea, 1270-1271
Pityriasis versicolor, 1237-1238
PKU. See Phenylketonuria.
Placental abruption. See Abruptio placentae.
Placenta previa, 965-967
  types of, 965i
Plague, 200-202
  forms of, 200
  preventing, 202
Plantar wart, 1263
Plaque, 1230i
Plasma, 1015, 1018
Plasma cell myeloma, 127-129
Plasma cells, 1018
Plasma insulin immunoassay in pancreatic
    cancer, 89
Plasmapheresis, 1048, 1049
Platelet concentrate, 1048
Platelet count
  in anorexia, 494
  in chronic granulocytic leukemia, 148

Platelet count (continued)
  in ehrlichiosis, 207
  in Hantavirus pulmonary syndrome, 230
  in idiopathic thrombocytopenic purpura,
    1047
  in malaria, 263
  in meningococcal infections, 177
  in radiation exposure, 322
  in Rocky Mountain spotted fever, 258
  in septic shock, 197
  in snakebites, 326
  in systemic lupus erythematosus, 378
  in toxic shock syndrome, 279
  in Wiskott-Aldrich syndrome, 400
Platelet function disorders, 1047-1049
Platelet replacement therapy, 1048
Platelets, 1015, 1018
  decreased, causes of, 1046
Pleural biopsy, 511
Pleural effusion, 551-553
Pleural fluid analysis in pneumonia, 537
Pleural friction rub, 553
Pleurisy, 553
Pleuritis, 553
Plicamycin
  for hypercalcemia, 918
  for Paget's disease, 598
Pneumatic antishock garment, 1117i
Pneumatic retinopexy, 1174
Pneumococcal pneumonia, 170-171t
Pneumoconioses, 565-569, 1292-1293t
Pneumocystis carinii pneumonia, 259-261,
    538-539t
Pneumonectomy, 75-76
Pneumonia, 162-163t, 537-542
  classifying, 537
  types of, 538-541t
Pneumonic plague, 200, 201, 202. See also
    Plague.
Pneumothorax, 295, 297, 535-536. See also
    Tension pneumothorax.
  types of, 535
Podagra, 585
Podophyllum
  for genital warts, 1002
  for warts, 1264-1265
Poikilocytosis, 1029
Poisoning, 323-325
Poisonous plants, 324i
Poliomyelitis, 244-246
  vaccination against, 244
Polio. See Poliomyelitis.
Polyangiitis overlap syndrome, 385t
Polyarteritis nodosa, 385t
Polycystic kidney disease, 780-781, 780i
Polycystic ovarian disease, 941-942
Polycythemia rubra vera. See Polycythemia
    vera.

i refers to an illustration; t refers to a table.

Polycythemias, 1035-1040
Polycythemia vera, 1035-1038
  clinical features of, 1036, 1037t
Polymenorrhea, 952, 954t, 955
Polymerase chain reaction
  in fragile X syndrome, 30-31
  in severe acute respiratory syndrome, 548
Polymorphonuclear leukocytes, 345
Polymorphous light eruption, 1256
Polymyositis, 388-389
Polyneuritis, 678-680
Polysomnography, 510
Pompe's glycogen storage disease, 893t
Pontiac syndrome, 531
Popliteal aneurysm, 1141, 1143
Porphyria cutanea tarda, 906t
Porphyrias, 904
  types of, 905-906t
Portal cirrhosis, 756
Portal hypertension, 758
  circulation in, 759i
Portal vein manometry, 750
Portosystemic encephalopathy, 764-765
Positron emission tomography scan, 414
  in Alzheimer's disease, 661
  in esophageal cancer, 86
  in Hodgkin's disease, 139
  in Huntington's disease, 657
  in schizophrenia, 440
Postcholecystectomy syndrome, 767-769
Postcoital test, 949
Postconcussion syndrome, 285
Posthepatic cirrhosis, 756
Postherpetic neuralgia, 235, 236
Postmenopausal bleeding, 955-956
Postnecrotic cirrhosis, 756
Postpartum disorders, 979-984
Postpartum thyroiditis, 838
Postprandial hypoglycemia, 895
Postrenal failure, 782
Posttraumatic spondylitis, 1298-1299t
Posttraumatic stress disorder, 468-471
  diagnostic criteria for, 470
Postural drainage, 514
Postviral thrombocytopenia, 1046
Potassium chloride
  for hypochloremia, 920
  for hypokalemia, 910
Potassium hydroxide preparations for skin
    testing, 1232
  in dermatophytosis, 1239
  in tinea versicolor, 1238
Potassium imbalance, 908-911
  clinical effects of, 909t
Potassium iodide solution
  for iodine deficiency, 886
  for simple goiter, 840

Potassium levels
  in hyperaldosteronism, 857
  in potassium imbalance, 910
  in radiation exposure, 322
  in rhabdomyolysis, 615
Potassium phosphate for hypophosphatemia,
    923
Pouch ileostomy, 708
Powassan encephalitis, 652
Praziquantel
  for schistosomiasis, 276
  for taeniasis, 272
Precocious puberty
  in females, 944-945
  in males, 1013-1014
Prednisone
  as immunosuppressant, 348-349
  for latex allergy, 358
  for lichen planus, 1269
  for rheumatoid arthritis, 366
  for systemic lupus erythematosus, 379
  for vasculitis, 387
Preeclampsia, 962-964
Pregnancy
  adolescent, 970-972
  breast cancer and, 78
  cardiovascular disease in, 969-970
  cervical cancer and, 109
  diabetic complications during, 972-974
  disorders of, 956-974
  ectopic, 959-961
  fallopian tube cancer and, 122
  Hodgkin's disease and, 140-141
  listeriosis and, 179
  melanoma and, 133
  pheochromocytoma and, 862
  trimesters of, 934
Pregnancy-induced hypertension, 962-964
Pregnanetriol levels in adrenogenital
    syndrome, 860
Preload, 1059
Premature atrial contraction, 1128t
Premature ejaculation, 501-502
Premature junctional contractions, 1131t
Premature labor, 974-976
Premature rupture of membranes, 976-978
Premature ventricular contraction, 1133t
Premenopausal bleeding, abnormal, 952, 954
Premenstrual dysphoric disorder, 937
Premenstrual syndrome, 936-937
Prenatal syphilis, 1003
Prerenal failure, 782
Presbycusis, 1205, 1206
Pressure-relieving aids
  for corns, 1270, 1270i
  for pressure ulcers, 1275
Pressure sores. See Pressure ulcers.

Pressure ulcers, 1273-1276
  common sites of, 1272-1273i
  pressure-relief aids for, 1275
  preventing, in immobilized patient, 575
Preterm labor, 974-976
Preureteral vena cava, 815i
Primaquine, 263
  for malaria, 264
Primary degenerative dementia, 660-662
Primary polycythemia. *See* Polycythemia vera.
Proctitis, 745-746, 999
Proctoscopy
  in colorectal cancer, 93
  in hemorrhoids, 737
  in inactive colon, 733
  in shigellosis, 190
Proctosigmoidoscopy, 685
Progeria, 1294-1295t
Progesterone
  for breast cancer, 80
  function of, 931
  lactation and, 982i
  for menopause, 947
Progressive bulbar palsy, 671
Progressive massive fibrosis, 567-569
Progressive multifocal leukoencephalopathy,
      1306-1307t
Progressive muscular atrophy, 671
Progressive systemic sclerosis, 382-384
Prolactin-secreting adenomas, 63
Propranolol
  for hyperthyroidism, 843
  for hypertrophic cardiomyopathy, 1113
  for pheochromocytoma, 862
  for tetralogy of Fallot, 1073
  for thyroid cancer, 69
Proptosis. *See* Exophthalmos.
Prostatectomy, 104, 105
Prostate gland, 994i
Prostate-specific antigen, 50
  in prostatic cancer, 103
Prostatic cancer, 103-105
  staging, 104
Prostatism, 821
Prostatitis, 818-819, 999
Protease inhibitors for acquire immuno-
      deficiency syndrome, 396-397
Protein
  function of, 871t
  metabolism of, 871-872
Protein-calorie deficiency, 888-890
Protein-calorie malnutrition, 888-890
Protein deficiency, 888-890
Protein levels
  in anorexia, 494
  in non-Hodgkin's lymphoma, 141

Prothrombin time, 1022
  in kidney cancer, 94
  in malaria, 263
  in pancreatic cancer, 88
  in septic shock, 197
  in viral hepatitis, 754
Pro time, 1022. *See also* Prothrombin time.
Protoporphyria, 905t
Protozoa, 153
Proximal renal tubular acidosis, 801
Pruritus
  in enterobiasis, 274
  in mycosis fungoides, 144
Pruritus ani, 744-745
Pseudogout, 587
Pseudomembranous enterocolitis, 712-713
Pseudomonas infections, 193-194
  preventing, 194
Pseudopolycythemia, 1038-1039
Pseudoprecocious puberty
  in females, 944-945
  in males, 1013, 1014
Psittacosis, 277-278
Psoralen compounds, 1253-1254, 1256
Psoriasis, 1265-1268, 1267i
Psoriatic arthritis, 372-373, 1266
Psychiatric disorders, 407-506
  anxiety, 459-471
  delusional, 445-449
  dissociative, 479-490
  eating, 490-495
  of infancy, childhood, and adolescence,
      414-426
  mood, 449-459
  schizophrenic, 439-445
  sexual and gender identity, 495-506
  somatoform, 471-479
  substance-related, 426-439
Psychoactive drug abuse, 431, 436, 437-438. *See
      also* Substance abuse.
Psychological counseling for rape victim,
      338-339
Psychotic disorders, 439-449
Ptosis, 1159-1160
Pubic lice, 1244-1246, 1245i
Puerperal infection, 979-981
Pulmonary actinomycosis, 185
Pulmonary artery angiography, 511
Pulmonary artery catheterization
  in acute respiratory distress syndrome,
      521, 523
  in cardiogenic shock, 1120
  in cor pulmonale, 528
  in pulmonary edema, 526-527
  in pulmonary hypertension, 550, 551
  in septic shock, 197
Pulmonary circulation, 1058

i refers to an illustration; t refers to a table.

Pulmonary contusion, 296, 297
Pulmonary edema, 526-527
  in near drowning, 318
  treatment algorithm for, 1110-1111i
Pulmonary embolism, 543-546
  risk factors for, 544
Pulmonary function tests, 510
  in asbestosis, 567
  in asphyxia, 318
  in asthma, 352
  in bronchiectasis, 560
  in bronchiolitis obliterans, 542
  in chronic obstructive pulmonary disease,
    555t, 557t
  in coal worker's pneumoconiosis, 568
  in cor pulmonale, 529
  in cystic fibrosis, 16
  in pulmonary fibrosis, 562
  in pulmonary hypertension, 551
  in sarcoidosis, 546
  in scleroderma, 383
  in silicosis, 566
Pulmonary hypertension, 550-551
Pulmonic insufficiency, 1089t, 1090
Pulmonic stenosis, 1089t, 1090
Pulmonic valve, 1058
Pulseless disease, 1306-1307t
Pulse oximetry, 510
  in asthma, 352
Pulses, 1061
  amplitude scale for, 1061
  locating, 1060i
Pulsion diverticulum, 697-698
Pump failure. See Cardiogenic shock.
Puncture wound, 332, 335t
Pure tone audiometry, 1190
Purpura hemorrhagica, 1046-1047
Pursed-lip breathing, 514
Purtscher's angiopathic retinopathy,
    1306-1307t
Purtscher's disease, 1306-1307t
Pustule, 1230i
PUVA therapy, 1267, 1268
Pyelonephritis
  acute, 784-786
  chronic, 785
Pyloroplasty, 706
Pyramidal system, 620
Pyrantel for enterobiasis, 274
Pyrazinamide for tuberculosis, 564
Pyridoxine
  for sideroblastic anemias, 1029
  for Wilson's disease, 763
Pyridoxine deficiency, 877-879
Pyrimethamine, 263
  for malaria, 264

Q

Q fever, 1306-1307t
Quantified CD4+:CD8+ lymphocytes, 1023
Quick's test, 1022. *See also* Prothrombin time.
Quinine, 263
  for malaria, 264
Quinsy, 1219-1221
Quintan fever, 1310-1311t

R

Rabies, 250-251
  immunization against, 251
Radiation dermatitis, 322i
Radiation exposure, 320-322
  effects of, 320, 321t
Radiation therapy
  adverse effects of, 51, 52t
  for basal cell epithelioma, 129
  for brain tumors, 59-60
  for breast cancer, 80
  as cancer treatment, 50-51
  as cause of immunodeficiency, 349
  for cervical cancer, 109, 110-112
  for chronic lymphocytic leukemia, 149-150
  for colorectal cancer, 93
  external, preparing patient for, 53
  for fallopian tube cancer, 123
  for gastric cancer, 84
  for Hodgkin's disease, 140
  internal
    safe time for, 117i
    safety precautions for, 111i
  for Kaposi's sarcoma, 137
  for kidney cancer, 94-95
  for liver cancer, 97
  for lung cancer, 75, 76
  for melanoma, 136
  for multiple myeloma, 128
  for mycosis fungoides, 143
  for non-Hodgkin's lymphoma, 141
  for ovarian cancer, 119
  for penile cancer, 107, 108
  for pituitary tumors, 63
  for prostatic cancer, 104
  for squamous cell carcinoma, 131
  for testicular cancer, 106
  for uterine cancer, 113
  for vaginal cancer, 116
Radioactive iodine for radiation exposure, 322
Radioactive iodine uptake tests
  in hyperthyroidism, 842
  in hypothyroidism, 837
  in iodine deficiency, 886
  in simple goiter, 840

i refers to an illustration; t refers to a table.

Radioallergosorbent test in allergic rhinitis, 355-356
Radioimmunoprecipitation assay in human immunodeficiency virus infection, 395
Radioisotope scan in abdominal injuries, 300
Rape trauma syndrome, 335-339
  child as victim in, 336
  evidence collection in, 337-338
  legal considerations in, 338
Rapid plasma reagin test, 1004
Rappaport histologic classification for non-Hodgkin's lymphoma, 142t
Rash
  in cutaneous larva migrans, 1243
  in dermatomyositis, 388
  in juvenile rheumatoid arthritis, 371
  in monkeypox, 242
  in pediculosis, 1245
  in Rocky Mountain spotted fever, 258
  in roseola infantum, 242, 243
  in rubella, 237, 238
  in rubeola, 239-240
  in syphilis, 1003
  in systemic lupus erythematosus, 378, 378i
  in varicella, 232
Rashkind procedure, 1076
Rat-bite fever, 1306-1307t
Rat typhus, 1310-1311t
Raynaud's disease, 1146-1147
Raynaud's phenomenon, 1146
  scleroderma and, 383
Reactive hypoglycemia, 895, 896
Reactive polycythemia, 1039-1040
Recklinghausen-Applebaum disease, 1294-1295t
Recompression for decompression sickness, 320
Reconstructive breast surgery, 80
Recrudescent typhus, 1284-1285t
Rectal cancer. See Colorectal cancer.
Rectal polyps, 739-741
Rectal prolapse, 742-743
  types of, 743i
Red blood cells, 1015
  deficiency of, 1017, 1020-1034
  erythropoiesis and, 1017
  excess of, 1017, 1035-1040
  in sickle cell anemia, 21-22, 23i
  tests for function of, 1022
Reflex sympathetic dystrophy, 680-681
Reflux nephropathy, 810-811
Refraction tests, 1156
Refsum's disease, 1306-1307t
Regional enteritis. See Crohn's disease.
Reiter's syndrome, 381-382
Relapsing fever, 209-210
Relative polycythemia, 1038-1039

Remnant removal disease, 899t
Renal angiography, 778t
Renal biopsy, 778t
Renal calculi, 790-794
  effect of urine pH on formation of, 791i
  types of, 791-792, 792i
Renal cell carcinoma. See Kidney cancer.
Renal complications
  in multiple myeloma, 127
  in systemic lupus erythematosus, 378
Renal disease, 782-808
  assessment for, 774
  common symptoms of, 774t
  diagnostic tests for, 774, 776, 777-778t
  serum and urine values in, 775-776t
  treatment methods for, 776, 778
Renal failure
  acute, 782-784
  chronic, 802-805, 808
Renal infarction, 789-790
  sites of, 789i
Renal scan, 778t
Renal system, assessing, 773-774
Renal tubular acidosis, 801-802
Renal vein thrombosis, 794-795
Renin-angiotensin system, 773
Renovascular hypertension, 799-800
  in renal infarction, 790
Repigmentation therapy, 1253-1254
Reserpine for Huntington's disease, 657
Respiration, 508-509, 509i
Respiratory acidosis, 533-534
Respiratory alkalosis, 534-535
Respiratory center, 509-510
Respiratory complications
  cystic fibrosis and, 15
  in diphtheria, 178, 179
  in nocardiosis, 186
Respiratory disorders, 508-569
Respiratory syncytial virus infection, 224-225, 540-541t
Respiratory system
  assessment of, 511
  physical examination of, 511-512
Response prevention as behavioral therapy, 468
Restless leg syndrome, 803
Restrictive cardiomyopathy, 1114-1115
Reteplase, 1104
Reticular dysgenesis, 402
Reticular formation, 618
Reticulocyte count, 1022
Retina, 1154, 1154i
Retinal detachment, 1173, 1174
Retinal dysplasia, 1304-1305t
Retinitis pigmentosa, 1180-1181
Retinoblastoma, 1306-1307t
Retinochoroiditis juxtapapillaris, 1296-1297t

i refers to an illustration; t refers to a table.

Retinoic acid, 1246
Retrocaval ureter, 815i
Retrograde cystography in bladder cancer, 98
Retropharyngeal abscess, 1219-1221
Reverse transcriptase inhibitors for acquire
    immunodeficiency syndrome, 395
Rewarming guidelines, 315
Reye's syndrome, 663-666
    stages of treatment for, 665-666t
Rhabdomyolysis, 614-615
Rhabdomyosarcoma, 1306-1307t
Rheumatic endocarditis, 1284-1285t
Rheumatic fever, 1084-1086
Rheumatic heart disease, 1084-1086
Rheumatoid arthritis, 364-370
    drug therapy for, 367-368t
    joint deformities in, 365-366, 365i
Rheumatoid factor test
    in ankylosing spondylitis, 374
    in juvenile rheumatoid arthritis, 372
    in psoriatic arthritis, 373
    in rheumatoid arthritis, 366
    in scleroderma, 383
    in Sjögren's syndrome, 376
Rheumatoid spondylitis, 373-375
Rhinitis medicamentosa, 356
Rhinophyma, 1252
Rhinosporidiosis, 1306-1307t
Rh isoimmunization, 987
    pathophysiology of, 989i
    preventing, 990
Rh$_o$(D) immune globulin, 958
Rh system, 363
Rib fractures, 295-296, 297
Riboflavin
    deficiency of, 877-879
    function of, 871t
Richter's syndrome, 1306-1307t
Rickets, 881-882, 881i
Rickettsiae, 153
Rickettsialpox, 1308-1309t
Riedel's thyroiditis, 838
Rifampin
    for meningococcal infection prophylaxis, 177
    for tuberculosis, 564
Riluzole for amyotrophic lateral sclerosis, 672
Rimantadine for influenza, 228
Rinne test, 1190
Risedronate for Paget's disease, 598
Risperidone
    for autistic disorder, 421-422
    for personality disorders, 484
    for schizophrenia, 441
Risus sardonicus, 180-181
Ritodrine for premature labor, 975
Ritter-Lyell syndrome, 1236-1237, 1237i
Ritter's disease, 1236-1237, 1237i

Rituximab, 53
    for chronic lymphocytic leukemia, 149
    for non-Hodgkin's lymphoma, 142
Rivastigmine for Alzheimer's disease, 661
River blindness, 1284-1285t
Robin syndrome, 14, 43, 44
Robles' disease, 1308-1309t
Rocky Mountain spotted fever, 257-259
Rosacea, 1251-1252
Roscola infantum, 242 243
    incubation and duration of, 232t
Rotational atherectomy, 1097
Roundback, 600-602
Roundworm infection, 271-272
RU-486 for abortion, 958
Rubella, 236-238
    immunization against, 238
    incubation and duration of, 232t
Rubeola, 238-240, 540-541t
    immunization against, 239
    incubation and duration of, 232t
Ruptured disk, 602-604
Ruptures. *See* Inguinal hernia.

S

Salicylates for rheumatoid arthritis, 366, 367t
Salicylic acid plasters for warts, 1269, 1270
Saline infusion for hyponatremia, 912
Salmonellosis, 187-189
    preventing, 189
    types of, 188t
Salpingitis, 950-951, 998
Salpingo-oophorectomy
    for endometriosis, 943
    for ovarian cancer, 119, 120
    for pelvic inflammatory disease, 950
Salpingostomy, 960
Salt-losing congential adrenal hyperplasia, 858,
    859, 860-861
San Joaquin Valley fever, 220-221
Sarcoidosis, 546-547
Sarcomas of the bone. *See* Bone tumors,
    primary malignant.
SARS. *See* Severe acute respiratory syndrome.
Scabies, 1241-1243
    cause and effect of, 1241, 1242i
Scale, 1231i
Scar, 1231i
Scarlatina, 168-169t
Scarlet fever, 168-169t
Schanz's syndrome, 1308-1309t
Scheuermann's disease, 600-602
Schiller's test in uterine cancer, 112
Schilling test, 1021, 1023
Schiøtz tonometry, 1156
Schistosomal dermatitis, 276

Schistosomiasis, 274-276
  types of, 275t
Schizoid personality disorder, 488, 490
Schizophrenia, 439-445
  diagnostic criteria for, 442
  phases of, 440
Schizotypal personality disorder, 488, 490
Schönlein-Henoch purpura, 584
Schwannoma, 59t, 61, 70. *See also* Brain
    tumors, malignant *and* Spinal
    neoplasms, malignant.
Schwediauer's disease, 1308-1309t
Scintiphotography scan, 510
Sclera, 1153, 1154i
Scleroderma, 382-384
Scoliosis, 604-607
  measuring angle of curvature in, 605i
Scorpion sting, 330-331t
Screening for phenylketonuria, 19
Scrotum, 994i
Scurvy, 879-881, 880i
Seatworm infection, 273-274
Sebaceous glands, 1228
Seborrheic dermatitis, 1258-1259t
Secondary polycythemia, 1039-1040
Second-degree atrioventricular block, 1132t
Secretin, 686i
Secretory otitis media, 1196, 1197, 1198
Segmental breathing, 514
Seizure disorder. *See* Epilepsy.
Selective serotonin reuptake inhibitors
  for body dysmorphic disorder, 479
  for major depression, 456
  for personality disorders, 484, 488
Selegiline for Parkinson's disease, 658
Selenium sulfide lotion for tinea versicolor, 1238
Self-catheterization, intermittent, 813-814
Semans squeeze technique, 501
Semen analysis, 1012
Semilunar valves, 1058
Seminal vesicles, 994i
Senning procedure, 1076, 1077
Sensorineural hearing loss, 1204
Sensory deficits in spinal neoplasms, 71
Sensory function, assessing, 623
Septal deviation, 1209-1211
Septal perforation, 1209-1211, 1210i
Septic abortion, 957
Septic arthritis, 583-585
Septicemic plague, 200, 201, 202. *See also* Plague.
Septic shock, 196-198
Sequestration crisis in sickle cell anemia, 23, 24
Setting-sun sign, 630
Severe acute respiratory syndrome, 547-548
Severe combined immunodeficiency disease,
    402-403
Sever's disease, 1308-1309t

Sex hormone therapy for Marfan syndrome, 12
Sex reassignment, 502
Sex therapy
  for dyspareunia, 498
  for erectile disorder, 500
  for orgasmic disorder, 497
  types of, 995
Sexual assault. *See* Rape trauma syndrome.
Sexual history, obtaining, 993
Sexually transmitted diseases, 995-1008
Sexual masochism, 505
Sexual sadism, 505
Sézary syndrome, 143
Shaking palsy, 657-659
Shaver's disease, 1284-1285t
Sheehan's syndrome, 828
Sheepskin, 1275
Shigellosis, 190-191
Shin bone fever, 1310-1311t
Shingles. *See* Herpes zoster.
Shock lung. *See* Acute respiratory distress
    syndrome.
Shy-Magee syndrome, 1286-1287t
SIADH. *See* Syndrome of inappropriate
    antidiuretic hormone secretion.
Sibutramine for metabolic syndrome, 907, 908
Sickle cell anemia, 21-25
  autosplenectomy in, 22
  crises in, 22-23
  inheritance patterns in, 21, 22i
  red blood cells in, 21-22, 23i
Sickle cell retinopathy, 1176, 1177-1178
Sickle cell thalassemia, 1302-1303t
Sickle cell trait, 21
Sideroblastic anemias, 1028-1030, 1029i
Sideroblast test, 1022
Siderosis, 1282-1283t
SIDS. *See* Sudden infant death syndrome.
Sigmoidoscopy
  in amebiasis, 266
  in ameboma, 266
  in colorectal cancer, 93
  in pruritus ani, 746
  in shigellosis, 190
  in ulcerative colitis, 707
Sildenafil for erectile disorder, 500
Silent thyroiditis, 838, 841
Silicosis, 565-566
Silo filler's disease, 1308-1309t
Simple goiter, 839-840
Simple virilizing congenital adrenal hyper-
    plasia, 858-859, 860
Sims'-Huhner test, 949
Sinding-Larsen and Johanssen syndrome,
    1298-1299t
Single-gene disorders, 3, 4-6, 8-31
Sinoatrial arrest, 1128t

i refers to an illustration; t refers to a table.

Sinus arrest, 1128t
Sinus arrhythmia, 1127t
Sinus bradycardia, 1127t
Sinusitis, 1211-1213
  risk factors for, 1212
Sinus tachycardia, 1127t
Sinus venosus defect, 1066
Sipple's syndrome, 863-864
Sixth disease. See Roseola infantum.
Sixth nerve (abducens) palsy, 1182
Sjögren's syndrome, 375-376
Skeletal abnormalities
  in Marfan syndrome, 12
  in Stickler's syndrome, 13
Skeletal traction, 304, 574
Skevas-Zerfus disease, 1308-1309t
Skin
  anatomy of, 1228
  blood supply to, 1229
Skin disorders, 1232-1276
  assessing, 1229
  diagnostic aids for, 1229-1230, 1232
Skin grafts, 310
Skin infections, 164-165t
  bacterial, 1232-1237
  fungal, 1237-1241
Skin lesions
  in acne, 1246
  in allergic purpura, 1041, 1041i
  in angioedema, 362
  in atopic dermatitis, 357
  in carbunculosis, 1234, 1235i
  in chancroid, 1006, 1006i
  in cutaneous larva migrans, 1243
  in dermatitis, 1257
  in discoid lupus erythematosus, 377
  in folliculitis, 1234, 1235i
  in furunculosis, 1234, 1235i
  in genital herpes, 1000
  in herpes simplex, 233, 234
  in herpes zoster, 234-235, 235t
  in impetigo, 1232-1233, 1233i
  in leprosy, 211
  in lichen planus, 1268-1269
  in Lyme disease, 207-208
  in pediculosis, 1245
  in pityriasis rosea, 1270
  in porphyria, 904
  premalignant, 131t
  primary, 1230i
  in psoriasis, 1265, 1266
  in Reiter's syndrome, 382
  in rheumatic fever, 1084
  in scabies, 1241, 1242i
  secondary changes in, 1231i
  in smallpox, 241
  in syphilis, 1003

Skin lesions (continued)
  in systemic lupus erythematosus, 378
  in urticaria, 361-362
Skin tests
  in allergic rhinitis, 355
  in anthrax, 204
  in blastomycosis, 219
  in chronic obstructive pulmonary disease, 555t
  in coccidioidomycosis, 220
  for delayed hypersensitivity, 874
  in histoplasmosis, 218
  in plague, 201
  in trichinosis, 269
  in tuberculosis, 564
  in urticaria, 362
Skin traction, 304, 574
Skip lesions, 711
Skull fractures, 287-290
  classifying, 287
Skull X-ray, 624
  in hydrocephalus, 630
  in osteogenesis imperfecta, 11
  in pituitary tumors, 63
Sleeping sickness, 651, 1282-1283t
Sleep terrors, 417, 418
Sleepwalking, 417-418
Sliding hiatal hernia, 699, 699i, 700
Slings, 575
Slipped disk, 602-604
Slit-lamp examination, 1156-1157
  in Sjögren's syndrome, 376
  in Stickler's syndrome, 14
  in Wilson's disease, 763
Small-bowel obstruction, 721-724, 724-725i
Small-bowel series, 685
Small intestine, function of, 684
Smallpox, 240-241
  vaccination for, 240, 241, 242
Smith-Strang disease, 1308-1309t
Smoking
  as chronic obstructive pulmonary disease cause, 556
  counseling for, 76
  as lung cancer cause, 72-73
Snakebites, poisonous, 325-329, 326i
Snapping hip, 1306-1307t
Snellen chart, 1156
Social phobia, 459-461
  diagnostic criteria for, 460
Sodium bicarbonate
  for acute respiratory distress syndrome, 523
  for electric shock, 313
  for hyperchloremia, 920
  for hyperkalemia, 910
  for metabolic acidosis, 926
  for near drowning, 319
  for respiratory acidosis, 534

i refers to an illustration; t refers to a table.

Sodium imbalance, 911-914
  clinical effects of, 912t
  diagnosing, 913i
  sodium levels in, 912
Sodium polystyrene sulfonate, 910
Sodoku, 1306-1307t
Soft chancre, 1006-1007, 1006i
Soft-tissue sarcoma, 1308-1309t
Solar urticaria, 1256
Somatic delusions, 446
Somatic (voluntary) nervous system, 621
Somatization disorder, 471-473
  diagnostic criteria for, 473
Somatoform disorders, 471-479
Somatostatin, 687i
Somatrem for hypopituitarism, 829
South American blastomycosis, 1304-1305t
Southern tick–associated rash illness, 208
Spanco mattress, 1275
Spastic cerebral palsy, 626-627
Spastic colitis, 713-714
Spastic colon, 713-714
Speech audiometry, 1190
Speech therapy for laryngeal cancer, 65
Spermatic cords, 994i
Spermatogenesis, 1009i
Sphingomyelin lipidosis, 1304-1305t
Spica cast, caring for child in, 580
Spina bifida occulta, 39, 40. *See also* Neural
      tube defects.
Spinal cord, 618-621, 620i
Spinal cord tumors. *See* Spinal neoplasms,
      malignant.
Spinal fusion
  for herniated disk, 603, 604
  for kyphosis, 602
  for scoliosis, 606
Spinal injuries, 293-294
Spinal muscular atrophy, 1312-1313t
Spinal neoplasms, malignant, 70-72
Spinal nerves, 620-621
Spirochetes, 153
Spironolactone
  for hyperaldosteronism, 858
  for hypokalemia, 910
Spleen scan
  in chest injuries, 296
  in non-Hodgkin's lymphoma, 141
Splenectomy, 1056
  as cause of immunodeficiency, 349
  for chronic granulocytic leukemia, 148
  for hypersplenism, 1056
  for idiopathic thrombocytopenic purpura,
      1047
Splenomegalic polycythemia. *See* Polycythemia
      vera.
Splenomegaly, causes of, 1055

Splint, 575
  applying, 284
  for arm and leg fractures, 304
  for clubfoot, 577
  for dislocation, 306-307
  for hip dysplasia, 579-580
  for juvenile rheumatoid arthritis, 372
  for nose fracture, 290
Sponge dermatitis, 1308-1309t
Sponge-diver's disease, 1308-1309t
Spongioblastoma multiforme, 57t
Spontaneous abortion, 956-959
  types of, 957
Spontaneous pneumothorax, 535-536
Sporadic, goiter, 839-840
Sporotrichosis, 221-222, 222i
Sprains, 301-302
Spurious polycythemia, 1038-1039
Sputum analysis, 510
Sputum culture
  in allergic aspergillosis, 217
  in anthrax, 204
  in blastomycosis, 219
  in chronic obstructive pulmonary disease, 555t
  in cryptococcosis, 215
  in cystic fibrosis, 16
  in histoplasmosis, 218
  in lung abscess, 549
  in methicillin-resistant staph infection, 166
  in nocardiosis, 186
  in pneumonia, 537, 539t, 541t
  in pneumonic plague, 202
  in *Pseudomonas* infections, 194
  in sporotrichosis, 222
  in tuberculosis, 564
  in whooping cough, 199-200
Sputum cytology
  in allergic rhinitis, 355
  in lung cancer, 73
Squamous cell carcinoma, 130-132
  laryngeal cancer and, 64
  lung cancer and, 72
  staging, 132
Squint, 1308-1309t
SSKI. *See* Potassium iodide solution.
Stabilizing trauma patient, 283-284
Staining
  in actinomycosis, 185
  in candidiasis, 214
  in cervical cancer, 109
  in ehrlichiosis, 207
  in gas gangrene, 184
  in gonorrhea, 996
  in herpes zoster, 236
  in histoplasmosis, 218
  in lung abscess, 549
  in meningococcal infections, 177
  in necrotizing fasciitis, 174

Staining (*continued*)
in nocardiosis, 186
in pelvic inflammatory disease, 950
in plague, 201
in pneumonia, 537, 539t
in pneumonic plague, 202
in premature rupture of membranes, 977
in relapsing fever, 210
in septic arthritis, 583
in septicemic plague, 202
in uterine cancer, 112
in vaginal cancer, 116
in varicella, 232
in vulvar cancer, 121
Standard precautions, 155-156
Stapedectomy, 1200-1201
Staphylococcal infections, 160-161
comparison of, 160-165t
methicillin-resistant, 161, 164-167
Staphylococcal pneumonia, 538-539t
Staphylococcal scalded skin syndrome,
1236-1237, 1237i
Stargardt's disease, 1308-1309t
Stasis dermatitis, 1260-1261t
Status asthmaticus, 353, 354-355i
Status epilepticus, 641
Steatosis. *See* Fatty liver.
Stem cell transplantation for acute leukemia, 146
Stenosis of ureter, 816i
Stereotactic radiosurgery, 637
Stereotactic surgery, 59
Stickler's syndrome, 13-14
Still's disease, 370, 371. *See also* Juvenile
rheumatoid arthritis.
Stimulants
abuse of, 435-436t
for attention deficit hyperactivity disorder, 424
St. Louis encephalitis, 651-652
Stomatitis, 687, 689, 689i
Stool culture and examination
in abdominal injuries, 300
in ameboma, 266
in ascariasis, 272
in campylobacteriosis, 205
in cholera, 195
in cystic fibrosis, 16
in *Escherichia coli* infections, 192
in giardiasis, 267
in hookworm disease, 271
in poliomyelitis, 245
in schistosomiasis, 276
in shigellosis, 190
in strongyloidiasis, 277
in taeniasis, 272
in trichinosis, 269
in tularemia, 206
Stool softeners for stroke, 645

Stop-and-start technique, 501-502
Strabismus, 1308-1309t
Straight-leg–raising test, 603
Strains, 301-302
Strep throat, 168-169t
Streptococcal infections, 167
comparison of, 168-173t
Streptococcal pharyngitis, 168-169t
Streptococcal pneumonia, 538-539t
Streptococcal pyoderma, 168-169t
Streptokinase, 1105
Streptozocin for hypoglycemia, 896
Stress erythrocytosis, 1038-1039
Stress polycythemia, 1038-1039
Stress-related disorders in children, 417-418
Stress test, 963
Strictures of ureter, 816i
Stroke, 642-646
classifying, 644
Stroke-in-evolution, 644
Stroke volume, 1059
Strongyloidiasis, 276-277
Stump care, 126
Stuttering, 417
Stye, 1163, 1163i
Subacute granulomatous thyroiditis, 838
Subacute sclerosing panencephalitis, 240
Subacute thyroiditis, 841
Subcutaneous tissue, 1228
Subdural hematoma, 286
Subluxations, 306-307
Substance abuse, 431, 432-436t, 436-439
diagnostic criteria for, 430
Substance dependence, diagnostic criteria
for, 430
Substance intoxication, diagnostic criteria
for, 430
Substance P, 687i
Substance-related disorders, 426-439
Substance withdrawal, diagnostic criteria
for, 430
Subthalamotomy, 658-659
Sucrose hemolysis test, 1022
Sudanophilic leukodystrophy, 1304-1305t
Sudden infant death syndrome, 516-517
Suicide
prevention guidelines for, 458
risk of
in bipolar disorders, 450, 451, 454
in major depression, 455, 458
warning signs of, 412
Sulfasalazine
for ankylosing spondylitis, 374
for rheumatoid arthritis, 367t
Sulfonamide therapy for nocardiosis, 186, 187
Sulindac
for ankylosing spondylitis, 374
for rheumatoid arthritis, 367t

i refers to an illustration; t refers to a table.

Sulkowitch urine test, 918
Superficial thrombophlebitis, 1143-1146
Suppurative fasciitis. *See* Necrotizing fasciitis.
Suppurative otitis media, 1196-1198
Surfer's knees, 1300-1301t
Surfer's knots, 1300-1301t
Sweat gland dysfunction, cystic fibrosis and, 15
Sweat glands, 1228-1229
Swediaur's disease, 1308-1309t
Swimmer's ear. *See* Otitis externa.
Swimmer's itch, 276
Swiss-type agammaglobulinemia, 402
Sycosis barbae, 1234
Sydenham's chorea, 1084-1085
Sylvatic (wild rodent) plague, 201. *See also*
    Plague.
Sympathectomy for complex regional pain
    syndrome, 681
Sympathetic nervous system, 621
Syndrome of inappropriate antidiuretic
    hormone secretion, 826, 924-925
Syndrome X. *See* Metabolic syndrome.
Synergistic necrotizing cellulites. *See* Necrotiz-
    ing fasciitis.
Synovectomy, 366
Synovial fluid analysis
    in gout, 586
    in Reiter's syndrome, 382
    in rheumatoid arthritis, 366
    in septic arthritis, 583
Syphilis, 1002-1005, 1004i
    prenatal, 1003
Syphilitic chancres, 1003
Systemic circulation, 1058
Systemic lupus erythematosus, 376-380
    rash in, 378, 378i
    signs of, 377-378, 379
Systole, 1059

T

Tacarotene for psoriasis, 1267
Tacrine for Alzheimer's disease, 661
Taeniasis, 272-273
    types of, 273t
Takayasu's arteritis, 386t, 1306-1307t
Talipes. *See* Clubfoot.
Tamoxifen
    for breast cancer, 80
    for malignant neoplasms, 54
    for uterine cancer, 113
Tangier disease, 1308-1309t
Tapeworm disease. *See* Taeniasis.
Tardive dyskinesia as antipsychotic adverse
    effect, 443
Tarsal scaphoiditis, 1296-1297t
Tay-Sachs disease, 17-18

Teeth, reimplanting, 291
Teflon injection for throat disorder, 1221-1222
Temporal arteritis, 386t
Temporomandibular joint, displacement of,
    291-292
Tendinitis, 607-609
Tenecteplase, 1105
Tennis elbow, 609-610
Tensilon test, 670
Tension pneumothorax, 295-296, 297, 535-536
TENS. *See* Transcutaneous electrical nerve
    stimulation.
Tentorial herniation, 286
Terbutaline for premature labor, 975
Testes, 994i
    hormones secreted by, 827
    undescended, 1010-1011
Testicular cancer, 105-107
    staging, 106
Testicular torsion, 1011-1012, 1011i
Tetanus, 180-182
    immunization schedule for, 181
    prophylaxis for, 282t, 327
Tetany, 846, 847
Tetracycline
    for acne, 1247, 1248
    for amebiasis, 266
    for chlamydial infections, 999
    for rosacea, 1252
    for syphilis, 1004
Tetralogy of Fallot, 1072-1075
Thalamus, 618
Thalassemia, 1030-1031, 1030i
Thalidomide
    for leprosy, 212
    for multiple myeloma, 128
The "bends," 319-320
Theca-lutein cysts, 940-941
The "chokes," 320
Therapeutic abortion, 957, 958-959
    cardiac dysfunction and, 970
Therapeutic lifestyle change diet, 908t
Thermal burns, 308. *See also* Burns.
Thiabendazole
    for cutaneous larva migrans, 1243
    for strongyloidiasis, 277
Thiamine
    deficiency of, 876-879
    function of, 871t
Third-degree atrioventricular block, 1132t
Third nerve (oculomotor) palsy, 1182
Thomsen's disease, 1290-1291t
Thoracentesis, 511
    in empyema, 552
    for hemothorax, 549
    in lung cancer, 74
    in pleural effusion, 552
    for pleurisy, 553

i refers to an illustration; t refers to a table.

Thoracic aortic aneurysm, 1134-1138
  clinical characteristics of, 1136t
Thought disorders as communication
    barrier, 409
Thought stopping as behavioral therapy, 468
Thought switching as behavioral therapy, 468
Threadworm infection, 273-274, 276-277
Threatened abortion, 957
Throat, 1191
  assessment of, 1191
Throat abscesses, 1219-1221
Throat culture
  in croup, 518
  in diphtheria, 178
  in epiglottiditis, 520
  in influenza, 228
  in rubella, 238
Throat disorders, 1217-1225
Throat examination in epiglottiditis, 520
Thrombin time, 1022
Thromboangiitis obliterans, 1147-1148
Thrombocytes. *See* Platelets.
Thrombocytopenia, 1043-1046
  in acute leukemia, 145
  in chronic granulocytic leukemia, 147
  in chronic lymphocytic leukemia, 149, 150
  pathophysiology of, 1044-1045i
Thromboembolism as myocardial infarction
    complication, 1102t
Thromboendarterectomy
  for arterial occlusive disease, 1150
  for pulmonary embolism, 545
Thrombolytic therapy, 1103, 1104-1105
  for pulmonary embolism, 545
  for renal vein thrombosis, 795
Thrombophlebitis, 1143-1146
Thrombosis as cause of stroke, 643
Thrombus formation, 1143-1144
Thrombus-in-evolution, 644
Thrush, 213, 214t. *See also* Candidiasis.
Thymus, role of, in immune response, 392
Thyroid cancer, 67-70
  staging, 68
Thyroidectomy
  aftercare for, 69, 839
  for goiter, 840
  for hyperthyroidism, 843
  for Riedel's thyroiditis, 838
Thyroid gland
  disorders of, 834-844
  hormones secreted by, 826
Thyroid hormones
  function of, 826
  deficiency of, 834-837
  for thyroid cancer, 69
Thyroiditis, 837-839
Thyroid replacement therapy for hypothy-
    roidism, 835, 836, 837

Thyroid scan
  in hyperthyroidism, 842
  in hypothyroidism, 837
  in simple goiter, 840
  in thyroid cancer, 69
Thyroid-stimulating hormone levels
  in hyperthyroidism, 842
  in hypothyroidism, 835, 837
  in iodine deficiency, 886
  in simple goiter, 840
Thyroid-stimulating hormone–secreting
    pituitary tumor, 841
Thyroid storm, 840, 842, 843, 844
  pathophysiology of, 70i
Thyroplasty, 1221
Thyrotoxicosis. *See* Hyperthyroidism.
Thyrotoxicosis factitia, 841
Thyroxine levels
  in hyperthyroidism, 842
  in hypothyroidism, 835, 837
  in iodine deficiency, 886
  in simple goiter, 840
Tic disorders, 416, 418
  diagnostic criteria for, 419
Tic douloureux, 674-676
Tick bites, 328-329t
Tick-borne encephalitis, 653
Tick fever, 209-210
Ticlopidine for stroke, 645
Tics, classifying, 416
Tiludronate for Paget's disease, 598
Tinea infections, 1239-1231, 1240i
Tinea versicolor, 1237-1238
Tinel's sign, 612
Tissue culture and examination
  in amebiasis, 266
  in blastomycosis, 219
  in candidiasis, 214
  in disseminated aspergillosis, 217
  in herpes zoster, 236
  in histoplasmosis, 218
  in ornithosis, 278
  in toxoplasmosis, 268
Tissue plasminogen activator, 645
T lymphocytes, 344
TNM staging system, 50
Tocopherol. *See* Vitamin E.
Tolmetin for rheumatoid arthritis, 367t
Tonopen tonometry, 1156
Tonsillectomy, 1219
Tonsillitis, 1218-1219
Torticollis, 612-614, 613i
Torulosis, 215-216
Total oculomotor ophthalmoplegia, 1182
Total parenteral nutrition
  for cancer patient, 54
  for protein-calorie malnutrition, 889
Tourette syndrome, 416, 418, 419

i refers to an illustration; t refers to a table.

Tourniquet, guidelines for applying, 327
Toxic-acquired porphyria, 904, 905t
Toxic adenoma, 841
Toxic epidermal necrolysis, 1262-1263
Toxic hepatitis, 755-756
Toxic oil syndrome, 382
Toxicology screening, 412, 413
Toxicology tests
    in alcohol-related disorder, 428
    in asphyxia, 318
    in poisoning, 323
Toxic shock syndrome, 278-279
Toxocariasis, 1308-1309t
Toxoplasmosis, 267-269
Trabeculectomy, 1186
Tracheoesophageal anomalies, types of,
    692-693i
Tracheoesophageal fistula, 691-695, 692-693i
Tracheotomy for epiglottiditis, 520
Trachoma, 1166-1168
    pathophysiology of, 1167i
Trachoma inclusion conjunctivitis, 998
Traction, 574-575
    for arm and leg fractures, 304
    for dislocation, 306-307
    for hip dysplasia, 580, 581
    for spinal injuries, 294
Traction diverticulum, 697, 698
Transamination, 871
Transcutaneous electrical nerve stimulation for
    spinal neoplasms, 72
Transforming growth factor, 344-345
Transfusion reaction. *See specific type.*
Transfusion therapy
    for abortion, 958
    in acute tubular necrosis, 788
    for aplastic anemias, 1027
    blood components and, 1019-1029
    for chronic granulomatous disease, 401
    for complement deficiencies, 404
    in disseminated intravascular coagulation,
    1052
    for dysfunctional uterine bleeding, 955
    for hereditary hemorrhagic telangiectasia,
    1042, 1043
    for immunoglobulin A deficiency, 392
    for radiation exposure, 322
    for snakebites, 328
    for thalassemia, 1031
    for thrombocytopenia, 1045, 1046
    for von Willebrand's disease, 1049-1050
    for Wiskott-Aldrich syndrome, 400
Transient ischemic attack, 643
Transient tic disorder, 416, 418, 419
Transillumination
    in neural tube defects, 40
    in testicular cancer, 106

Transmission-based isolation precautions, 157
Transposition of the great arteries, 1075-1077
Transsphenoidal pituitary surgery, 63, 63i
Transurethral resection for bladder cancer,
    98, 100
Transvestic fetishism, 505
Trauma, 281-339
    assessing ABCs in, 281-283
    common mechanisms of, 281
    secondary assessment in, 283
    stabilizing patient in, 283-284
    tetanus prophylaxis in, 282t
    triage and, 281
Traumatic arthritis, 584
Traumatic pneumothorax, 535-536
Traveler's diarrhea, 703-704
Tremor familiaris, 1302-1303t
Trench fever, 1310-1311t
Trench mouth, 688t
Trendelenburg's sign, eliciting, 579
Tretinoin for acne, 1246
Trevor's disease, 1310-1311t
Triage in emergency care, 281
Trichinellosis, 269-270
Trichiniasis, 269-270
Trichinosis, 269-270
Trichomonal vaginitis, 939
Trichomoniasis, 1005-1006
Trichotillomania, 1250, 1251
Trichuriasis, 1310-1311t
Tricuspid insufficiency, 1089t, 1090
Tricuspid stenosis, 1090, 1090t
Tricuspid valve, 1058
Tricyclic antidepressants
    for body dysmorphic disorder, 479
    for generalized anxiety disorder, 463
    for major depression, 456, 459
Trigeminal nerve, function and distribution
    of, 675i
Trigeminal neuralgia, 674-676
Triiodothyronine levels
    in anorexia, 494
    in hyperthyroidism, 842
    in hypothyroidism, 835, 837
Trisomy 13 syndrome, 34-35
Trisomy 18 syndrome, 33-34
Trisomy 21, 31-33
Tropical sprue, 1310-1311t
Troponin levels, 1063-1064
    in myocardial infarction, 1102
Trousseau's sign, 846, 915i, 927
Truss, 727
Tsutsugamushi fever, 1310-1311t
Tuberculin skin tests, 564
Tuberculosis, 563-565
Tuberculosis laryngitis, 1296-1297t
Tularemia, 205-206

i refers to an illustration; t refers to a table.

Tumor necrosis factors, 344
Tumor, node, metastasis staging system, 50
Tumors, 1230i
  benign versus malignant, 47t
Turner's syndrome, 36
Tympanic membrane rupture, 292
Tympanometry, 1190
Type III spinal muscular atrophy, 1298-1299t
Type IV hereditary sensorimotor neuropathy,
    1306-1307t
Typhoid fever, 187, 188, 188t
Typhus
  endemic, 1310-1311t
  epidemic, 1310-1311t
  scrub, 1310-1311t
Tyrosinemia, 1310-1311t

U

Ulcer, 1231i
Ulcerative colitis, 707-709
Ultrafast computed tomography, 1064
Ultrasonography
  in abdominal injuries, 300
  in bladder cancer, 98
  in cholelithiasis, 767
  in fallopian tube cancer, 122
  in hip dysplasia, 579
  in neural tube defects, 40
  in osteogenesis imperfecta, 11
  in ovarian cancer, 118
  in pancreatic cancer, 87
  in pelvic inflammatory disease, 950
  in polycystic kidney disease, 781
  in pregnancy-induced hypertension, 963
  in pulmonary edema, 526
Umbilical hernia, 726i
Uncinariasis, 270-271
Undescended testes, 1010-1011
Undulant fever, 202-204
Unipolar disorder. See Major depression.
Upper gastrointestinal series, 685
  in volvulus, 730
Urea formation, 871
Uremic syndrome, 788
Ureter, 771-772, 77i
  congenital anomalies of, 814, 815-816i, 818
Ureterocele, 816i
Urethra, congenital anomalies of, 814, 817i, 818
Urethral syndrome, 998
Urethritis, 808-810, 997-999, 1007-1008
Urgent category in triage, 281
Uric acid levels
  in anorexia, 494
  in chronic granulocytic leukemia, 148
  in gout, 586
  in metabolic syndrome, 907

Uric acid levels (continued)
  in non-Hodgkin's lymphoma, 141
  in psoriatic arthritis, 373
Urinalysis
  in acute poststreptococcal glomerulo-
      nephritis, 786
  in acute pyelonephritis, 785
  in acute tubular necrosis, 788
  in anorexia, 494
  in bladder cancer, 98
  in chronic glomerulonephritis, 798
  in chronic renal failure, 804
  in diabetes insipidus, 833
  in epididymitis, 820
  in Goodpasture's syndrome, 381
  in lower urinary tract infection, 809
  in malaria, 263
  in medullary sponge kidney, 779
  in relapsing fever, 210
  in renal calculi, 793
  in renal infarction, 790
  in renal vein thrombosis, 794
  in rhabdomyolysis, 615
  in scleroderma, 383
  in snakebites, 326
  in systemic lupus erythematosus, 378
  in vesicoureteral reflux, 811
Urinary diversion, 776
  bladder cancer and, 100
  caring for, 100-101
Urine culture and examination
  in acute pyelonephritis, 785
  in cryptococcosis, 215
  in epididymitis, 820
  in methicillin-resistant staph infection, 166
  in multiple myeloma, 127
  in prostatitis, 818
  in Pseudomonas infections, 194
  in rubella, 238
  in schistosomiasis, 276
  in tuberculosis, 564
Urine osmolality in septic shock, 197
Urine output, maintaining, in electric shock,
    312-313
Urine specimen collection, 774, 776
Urobilinogen in gallbladder cancer, 102
Urodynamic studies in neurogenic bladder, 813
Urokinase, 1105
Urologic system, assessing, 773-774
Urticaria, 361-362
Usher's syndrome, 1180
Uterine artery embolization, 944
Uterine bleeding disorders, 951-956
Uterine cancer, 112-115
  staging, 113
Uterine leiomyomas, 943-944
Uterus, 930-931, 931i

i refers to an illustration; t refers to a table.

Uveal tract, 1153-1154, 1154i
Uveitis, 1172-1173, 1173t
Uveoparotid fever, 1294-1295t

V

Vagabond fever, 209-210
Vagina, 930, 931i
Vaginal cancer, 115-117
  staging, 116
Vaginismus, 498-499
Vaginitis, 939-940, 1007-1008
Vagotomy, 706
Valley fever, 220-221
Valproic acid
  for bipolar disorders, 451
  for epilepsy, 641
Valve disorders, 1086-1091
Valvular heart disease, 1086-1091
  types of, 1086, 1087-1090t, 1090
Vancomycin for methicillin-resistant staph
    infection, 167
Vancomycin-resistant enterococcus infection,
    175-176
  patients at risk for, 175
Vancomycin-resistant infections, 166
Van Jaksch's syndrome, 1296-1297t
Vaquez-Osler disease. See Polycythemia vera.
Varicella, 231-233, 540-541t
  immunization against, 233
  incubation and duration of, 232t
Varicose veins, 1145
Variegate porphyria, 906t
Variola, 240-241
Vascular disorders, 1134-1151
Vascular headaches, 637-640
Vascular retinopathies, 1175-1178
  anatomy of, 1175i
  diagnostic tests for, 1177
Vasculitis, 384-387
  types of, 385-387t
Vas deferens, 994i
Vasodilator therapy for pulmonary hyper-
    tension, 551
Vasoocclusive crisis in sickle cell anemia, 22
Vasopressin. See also Antidiuretic hormone.
  in diabetes insipidus, 832, 833
  for esophageal varices, 758
Vasopressors
  for pulmonary embolism, 545
  for septic shock, 197
Vector-borne transmission, 156
Veins, 1061
Velcade for multiple myeloma, 128
Velocardiofacial syndrome, 37-38
Velopharyngeal insufficiency, 1216-1217
Velopharyngeal sphincter reconstruction, 1217

Venereal Disease Research Laboratory slide
    test, 1004
Venereal warts, 1001-1002
Venezuelan equine encephalitis, 652
Ventilation, 508, 509i
Ventilation-perfusion scan, 510
Ventricles, 1058
Ventricular aneurysm, 1122-1123
  as myocardial infarction complication, 1102t
Ventricular assist device, 1120-1121
Ventricular fibrillation, 1134t
Ventricular myectomy, 1114
Ventricular myotomy, 1114
Ventricular septal defect, 1064-1066
Ventricular septal rupture as myocardial
    infarction complication, 1101t
Ventricular tachycardia, 1133t
Ventriculoatrial shunt, 630
Ventriculoperitoneal shunt, 630
Vernal conjunctivitis, 1165, 1166
Verneuil's disease, 1310-1311t
Verrucae. See Warts.
Vertebral epiphysitis, 600-602
Vertical banded gastroplasty, 888
Vesicle, 1230i
Vesicoureteral reflux, 810-812
Vibrio parahaemolyticus food poisoning, 195
Vibrio vulnificus septicemia, 1310-1311t
Villous adenomas, 739, 740
Vincent's angina, 688t
Vineland Social Maturity Scale, 415
Viral enteritis, 703-704
Viral hepatitis, 752-755
  forms of, 752-753
Viral pneumonia, 227t, 538-541t. See also
    Adenovirus infection.
Viruses, 153
Visceral larva migrans, 1308-1309t
Vision testing, 1155-1157
Visual field tests, 1157
Vitamin A
  deficiency of, 875-876
  function of, 871t, 884t
Vitamin B complex, recommended daily
    allowance of, 876
Vitamin B deficiencies, 876-879
Vitamin B$_{12}$ deficiency, 1020, 1021
Vitamin B$_{12}$ replacement therapy, 1022, 1023
Vitamin C
  deficiency of, 879-881, 880i
  function of, 871t
Vitamin D, 884t
  deficiency of, 881-882, 881i
  function of, 871t
Vitamin D supplements
  for hyperparathyroidism, 849
  for hypocalcemia, 918
  for hypoparathyroidism, 846

i refers to an illustration; t refers to a table.

Vitamin E
 deficiency of, 882-883
 function of, 871t
Vitamin K
 deficiency of, 883-884
 function of, 871t
Vitiligo, 1252-1255, 1253i
Vitreous body, 1154i, 1155
Vocal cord nodules, 1222-1224, 1223i
Vocal cord paralysis, 1221-1222
Vocal cord polyps, 1222-1224
Vocal tics, 416
Voiding cystourethrography in vesicoureteral
 reflux, 811
Volkmann's disease, 1310-1311t
Volksmann's deformity, 1310-1311t
Volvulus, 729-730
Von Economo's disease, 651
Von Gierke's glycogen storage disease, 892,
 894-895
Von Hippel-Lindau disease, 1310-1311t
Von Recklinghausen disease, 8-10
 diagnostic criteria for, 9
Von Willebrand's disease, 1049-1050
Von Zumbusch's psoriasis, 1266
Voyeurism, 505
Vulva, 930, 931i
Vulvar cancer, 120-122
 staging, 121
Vulvectomy, 121, 122
Vulvitis, 939-940
Vulvovaginitis, 939-940

W

Waldenström's macroglobulinemia, 1300-1301t
Wandering atrial pacemaker, 1128t
Warfarin
 for pulmonary embolism, 545
 for renal vein thrombosis, 795
 for stroke, 645
 for thrombophlebitis, 1145
Warts, 1263-1265
 removal of, 1264, 1264i
 types of, 1263
Wasp sting, 330-331t
Water deprivation test, 833
Watering can foot, 1302-1303t
Water regulation, hormonal control of, 773
Water-soluble vitamins, functions of, 871t
Weber's test, 1190
Wegener's granulomatosis, 385t
Wegner's disease, 1310-1311t
Weil-Felix reaction, 258
Wenckebach, 1132t
Werdnig-Hoffmann disease, 1312-1313t

Werlhof's disease, 1046-1047
Werner's syndrome, 863-864
Western equine encephalitis, 651
West Nile encephalitis, 255-257, 653
 transmission routes of virus that causes, 256i
Wheal, 1230i
Whiplash, 292-293
Whipple's disease, 1312-1313t
Whipple's operation, 89, 90-91
Whipworm disease, 1310-1311t
White blood cell count, 1023
 in abdominal injuries, 300
 in acute respiratory failure in chronic
  obstructive pulmonary disease, 525
 in anorexia, 494
 in appendicitis, 719
 in blastomycosis, 219
 in bronchiolitis obliterans, 542
 in brucellosis, 203
 in chronic granulocytic leukemia, 147-148
 in chronic granulomatous disease, 401
 in chronic lymphocytic leukemia, 149
 in coccidioidomycosis, 220
 in common cold, 224
 in Crohn's disease, 711
 in cryptococcosis, 215
 in ehrlichiosis, 207
 in epididymitis, 820
 in gout, 586
 in granulocytopenia, 1054
 in Hantavirus pulmonary syndrome, 230
 in Hodgkin's disease, 139
 in infectious mononucleosis, 249
 in lung abscess, 549
 in Lyme disease, 208
 in lymphocytopenia, 1054
 in malaria, 263
 in meningococcal infections, 177
 in nonviral hepatitis, 755
 in osteomyelitis, 592
 in plague, 202
 in pneumonia, 539t, 541t
 in poliomyelitis, 246
 in polymyositis, 388
 in rabies, 250-251
 in radiation exposure, 322
 in Reiter's syndrome, 382
 in relapsing fever, 210
 in Rocky Mountain spotted fever, 258
 in schistosomiasis, 276
 in septic arthritis, 583
 in snakebites, 326
 in tularemia, 206
 in viral hepatitis, 754
 in volvulus, 730
 in whooping cough, 200
White blood cell differential, 1023

i refers to an illustration; t refers to a table.

White blood cells, 1015
  deficiency of, 1018
  excess of, 1018
  function of, 1018
  testing function of, 1023
  types of, 1018, 1019i
Whooping cough, 199-200
  immunization against, 200
  stages of, 199
Widal's test, 189
Wilms' tumor, 1312-1313t
Wilson's disease, 762-764
Wiskott-Aldrich syndrome, 399-401
Wolhynia fever, 1310-1311t
Wolman's disease, 1312-1313t
Wood's light examination, 1232
  in tinea versicolor, 1238
  in vitiligo, 1253
Work practice precautions, 155-156
Wound botulism. *See* Botulism.
Wound culture
  in gas gangrene, 184
  in tetanus, 181
Wryneck, 612-614, 613i

X

Xanthoma tuberosum, 899t
Xerophthalmia, 875
Xeroradiography in laryngeal cancer, 65
X-linked agammaglobulinemia, 389-390
X-linked disorders, 25-31
  inheritance patterns in, 5-6, 5i
X-linked infantile hypogammaglobulinemia,
      389-390
X-rays
  in abdominal injuries, 300
  in acceleration-deceleration cervical
      injuries, 293
  in ameboma, 266
  in ankylosing spondylitis, 374
  in arm and leg fractures, 304
  in bone tumors, 124
  in common variable immunodeficiency, 391
  in cretinism, 837
  in dislocations and subluxations, 306
  in epiglottiditis, 520
  in esophageal cancer, 86
  in fallopian tube cancer, 122
  in gas gangrene, 184
  in gout, 586
  in head trauma, 290, 291
  in herniated disk, 603
  in hip dysplasia, 579
  in hyperparathyroidism, 848
  in intestinal obstruction, 723
  in juvenile rheumatoid arthritis, 372

X-rays (*continued*)
  in kyphosis, 601
  in Legg-Calvé-Perthes disease, 595
  in multiple myeloma, 128
  in necrotizing enterocolitis, 710
  in necrotizing fasciitis, 174
  in neural tube defects, 40
  in neurofibromatosis, 9
  in neurogenic arthropathy, 588
  in open trauma wounds, 333t, 335t
  in Osgood-Schlatter disease, 597
  in osteoarthritis, 589
  in osteogenesis imperfecta, 11
  in ovarian cancer, 118
  in Paget's disease, 598
  in peritonitis, 720
  in psoriatic arthritis, 373
  in radiation exposure, 322
  in Reiter's syndrome, 382
  in renal calculi, 792
  in rheumatoid arthritis, 366
  in scleroderma, 383
  in septic arthritis, 583
  in spinal injuries, 294
  in spinal neoplasms, 71
  in sprains, 302
  in tracheoesophageal anomalies, 694
  in vitamin D deficiency, 882
  in volvulus, 729

Y

Yaws, 1312-1313t
Yellow fever, 1312-1313t
Yellow jacket sting, 330-331t

Z

Zanamivir for influenza, 228
Zenker's diverticulum, 697-698
Zinc deficiency, 886-887
Z-track intramuscular technique, 1035i
Zygomycosis, 1312-1313t

i refers to an illustration; t refers to a table.